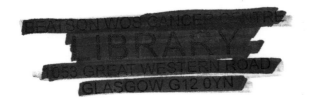
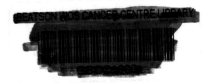

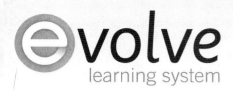

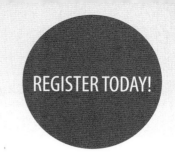

To access the free Evolve Resources, visit:

http://evolve.elsevier.com/ Washington+Leaver/principles

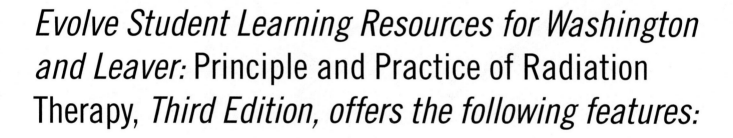

Evolve Student Learning Resources for Washington and Leaver: Principle and Practice of Radiation Therapy, *Third Edition, offers the following features:*

- **Answer Key to Review Questions**—This key provides answers to the review questions included at the end of each chapter.

- **Weblinks**—This exciting resource links you to websites that supplement the content of your textbook

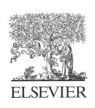

ELSEVIER

THIRD EDITION

PRINCIPLES and PRACTICE of
RADIATION
THERAPY

Charles M. Washington, MBA, RT(T), FASRT

Director, Clinical Services and Operations
Division of Radiation Oncology
The University of Texas MD Anderson Cancer Center
Houston, Texas

Dennis Leaver, MS, RT(R)(T), FASRT

Professor and Chairman
Department of Radiation Therapy
Southern Maine Community College
South Portland, Maine

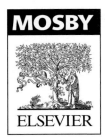

MOSBY

ELSEVIER

11830 Westline Industrial Drive
St. Louis, Missouri 63146

PRINCIPLES AND PRACTICE OF RADIATION THERAPY   ISBN: 978-0-323-05362-4

Library of Congress Cataloging-in-Publication Data

Principles and practice of radiation therapy / [edited by] Charles M. Washington, Dennis Leaver. — 3rd ed.
    p. ; cm.
  Includes bibliographical references and index.
  ISBN 978-0-323-05362-4 (hardcover : alk. paper) 1. Cancer—Radiotherapy. I. Washington, Charles M.
II. Leaver, Dennis T. III. Title: Radiation therapy.
  [DNLM: 1. Neoplasms—radiotherapy. 2. Radiation Oncology—methods. QZ 269 P9575 2010]
  RC271.R3P734 2010
  615.8'42--dc22

                                                                            2008050845

Acquisitions Editor: Jeanne Olson
Developmental Editor: Luke Held
Publishing Services Manager: Julie Eddy
Senior Project Manager: Laura Loveall
Designer: Paula Catalano

Printed in the United States

Last digit is the print number: 9   8   7   6   5   4   3   2   1

To those who have run and continue to run the race against cancer. We sincerely hope those who read this work will grow in the knowledge and understanding necessary to provide direction and compassion to their patients. Let us not grow tired in running our own race, but instead encourage those around us.

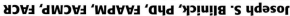

Contributors

Robert D. Adams, EdD, RT(R)(T), CMD
Assistant Professor
UNC Department of Radiation Oncology
University of North Carolina
Chapel Hill, North Carolina

Joy E. Anderson, MD
Assistant Professor of Radiation Oncology
University of Rochester
James P. Wilmont Cancer Center
Rochester, New York

Stacy L. Anderson, MS, RT(T), CMD
Associate Professor and Interim Chairperson
Medical Imaging and Radiation Sciences
University of Oklahoma Health Sciences Center
Oklahoma City, Oklahoma

Julius Armstrong, MBA, RT(T)
Program Chairman
Radiation Therapy Program
Bellevue Community College
Bellevue, Washington

Lisa Bartenhagen, MS, RT(R)(T)
Program Director, Radiation Therapist
Radiation Therapy Education, Radiation Oncology
University of Nebraska Medical Center, Nebraska Medical
Center
Omaha, Nebraska

Lana Havron Bass, BSRT(R)(T), CMD, FASRT
Medical Radiation Dosimetrist
Medical Physics and Dosimetry
Texas Oncology—Fort Worth
Fort Worth, Texas

E. Richard Bawiec, Jr., MS, DABR
Medical Physicist
Radiation Oncology
St. Edward Mercy Medical Center
Fort Smith, Arkansas

Susan B. Belinsky, EdD, RT(R)(T)
Associate Professor of Radiation Therapy, Director, Radiation
Therapy Program
School of Radiologic Sciences
Massachusetts College of Pharmacy and Health Sciences
Boston, Massachusetts

Joseph S. Blinick, PhD, FAAPM, FACMP, FACR
Chief Radiation Physicist
Maine Radiation Physics, Inc.
Portland, Maine

Leila Bussman-Yeakel, BS, RT(R)(T)
Director
Radiation Therapy
Mayo School of Health Science
Rochester, Minnesota

Shaun T. Caldwell, MS, RT(R)(T)
Assistant Professor
Program Director, Radiation Therapy
School of Health Sciences
MD Anderson Cancer Center
The University of Texas
Houston, Texas

Annette M. Coleman, MA, RT(T)
Product Manager
Radiation Oncology Charting and Imaging
IMPAC Medical Systems, Inc.
Cambridge, Massachusetts

Gay Dungey, MEd, BSc, DipTRad
Lecturer
Department of Radiation Therapy
University of Otago, Wellington

Stephanie Eatmon, EdD, RT(R)(T), FASRT
Associate Professor and Program Director
Health Science/Radiation Therapy
California State University
Long Beach, California

Correen Fraser, BS, RT(T), CMD
Certified Medical Dosimetrist
Radiation Oncology
Henry Ford Hospital
Detroit, Michigan

Michael T. Gillin, PhD
Professor, Deputy Chair, Chief of Clinical Services
Radiation Physics
MD Anderson Cancer Center
The University of Texas
Houston, Texas

Patricia J. Giordano, MS, RT(R)(T)
Assistant Professor/Program Director
Radiation Therapy
Gwynedd-Mercy College
Gwynedd Valley, Pennsylvania

Patton Griggs, BS
Physicist
Department of Radiation Oncology
Central Maine Medical Center
Lewiston, Maine

Sally Green, BS, RT(T)
Tenured Teaching Faculty
Radiation Therapy Program
Bellevue Community College
Bellevue, Washington

Ahmad Hammoud, BS, RT(T), CMD
Dosimetry Supervisor
Radiation Oncology
Karmanos Cancer Institute
Detroit, Michigan

Rosann Keller, MEd, RT(T)
Senior Lecturer
Radiation Therapy
Wayne State University
Detroit, Michigan

Adam F. Kempa, MEd, RT(T)
Program Director
Radiation Therapy Technology Wayne State University
Detroit, Michigan

Jane Koth, BS, RT(R)(T)
Clinical Education Coordinator
Radiation Therapy Technology
University of Nebraska Medical Center
Omaha, Nebraska

Deborah A. Kuban, MD
Professor of Radiation Therapy, Genitourinary Section Chief
MD Anderson Cancer Center
The University of Texas
Houston, Texas

Ronnie G. Lozano, MSRS, RT(T)
Chair and Associate Professor
Radiation Therapy
Texas State University
San Marcos, Texas

Shirlee E. Maihoff, MEd, RT(T)
Ret. Associate Professor/Program Director
Imaging & Therapeutic Science
University of Alabama at Birmingham
Birmingham, Alabama

Valerie Marable, BS, RT(T), CMD
Dosimetrist III
Department of Radiation Oncology
Providence Hospital
Southfield, Michigan

Mary Ann McKenney, RT(R)(T) (retired)
Radiation Oncology
Brigham and Women's Hospital
Boston, Massachusetts

Tammy Newell, BS, RT(T)
Radiation Therapist
Concord Hospital
Concord, New Hampshire

Sandy L. Piehl, MPA, RT(R)(T)
Radiation Therapy Program Director
Nursing and Health Professions
Indiana University Northwest
Gary, Indiana

Charlotte M. Prado, CMD
Medical Dosimetrist II
The Methodist Hospital
Houston, Texas

Karl L. Prado, PhD
Associate Professor
Department of Radiation Physics
MD Anderson Cancer Center
The University of Texas
Houston, Texas

Elizabeth G. Quate, MS
Manager, Imaging Physics/RSO
Maine Medical Center
Portland, ME

Narayan Sahoo, PhD
Associate Professor
Department of Radiation Physics
MD Anderson Cancer Center
The University of Texas
Houston, Texas

Judith M. Schneider, MS, RT(R)(T)
Clinical Assistant Professor/Clinical Coordinator
Health Professions Programs
Radiation Therapy Program
Indiana University School of Medicine
Indianapolis, Indiana

Donna Stinson, MPA, RT(R)(T)
Administration Director of Operations
Oncology Service Line
Bayhealth Medical Center
Milford, Delware

Megan L. Trad, MS, RS, RT(T)
Educational Coordinator/Instructor
School of Health Sciences
MD Anderson Cancer Center
The University of Texas
Houston, Texas

Nora Uricchio, MEd, RT(R)(T)
Director, Radiation Therapy Program
School of Allied Health
Hartford Hospital
Hartford, Connecticut

George M. Uschold, EdD, RT(T), FASRT
Associate Professor of Radiation Oncology
University of Rochester
James P. Wilmont Cancer Center
Rochester, New York

Amy C. Vonkadich, MEd, RT(T)
Program Director
Radiation Therapy
New Hampshire Technical Institute
Concord, New Hampshire

Paul E. Wallner, DO, FACR, FASTRO
Adjunct Professor
Department of Radiation Oncology
New York University School of Medicine
New York, New York

Bettye G. Wilson, MA Ed, RT(R)(CT), ARRT, RDMS, FASRT
Associate Professor
Clinical and Diagnostic Sciences
University of Alabama at Birmingham
School of Health Professions
Birmingham, Alabama

Jeffrey Young, MD
Maine Children's Cancer Program
Maine Medical Center
Portland, Maine

Hong Zhang, MD, PhD
Assistant Professor of Radiation Oncology
University of Rochester
James P. Wilmont Cancer Center
Rochester, New York

Cara Zeidman, RN, MSN
Chemotherapy Order Set Coordinator
Beth Israel Deaconess Medical Center
East Campus
Boston, Massachusetts

Tracy J. Bailey-Hauver, BSc (Hons), RT
Radiation Therapy
Howard University
Washington DC

Beverly Coker, MA, RT(R)(T)
Chairperson
Baptist College of Health Sciences
Memphis, Tennessee

Patricia A. Davis, BS, RT(R)
Clinical Instructor
University of Virginia Health System
Program of Radiography
Charlottesville, Virginia

Donna Kay Dunn, MS, RT(T)
Program Director
Indiana University School of Medicine
School of Allied Health Sciences
Radiation Therapy Program
Indianapolis, Indiana

Kathryn E. Frye-Oakley, MS(R)(T)
Assistant Professor
Weber State University
Ogden, Utah

Mark A. Graniero, BS, RTT
Orfit Industries America
Jericho, New York

Nancy Hawking, EdD, MEd, BSRT, RT(R)
Executive Director of Imaging Sciences
University of Arkansas
Fort Smith, Arkansas

Michelle Hutchings-Medina, MA, RT(T)
Radiation Oncology Sales Manager
IMPAC Medical Systems, Inc.
Sunnyvale, CA

Julie Kunkle, MSA, RT(R)(T)
Faculty
Baptist College of Health Sciences
Memphis, Tennessee

Geraldine M. Labonte, RT(T)(R)(M)
Therapist/Clinical Coordinator
Central Maine Medical Center,

Cynthia A. Rydholm Cancer Treatment Center
Lewiston, Maine

Kristi G. Moore, BSRT(R)(CT)
Educator, Radiology Technologist Instruction
University of Mississippi Medical Center
Jackson, Mississippi

Benjamin J. Morris, MSED, RT(R)(T)(CT)
Director, Skaggs Cancer Center
Skaggs Community Health Center
Springfield, Missouri

Selina McIntire Muccio, MEd, BA, RT(R)
Educational Course Developer, Diagnostic Radiology
University of Colorado at Denver & Health Sciences Center
Denver, Colorado

Karen M. Nelson, MS, RT(R)(T)
Program Manager of the Radiation Therapy Program
Hillsborough Community College
Tampa, Florida

Warren A. Parker, MA, ARRT(R)
Allied Health
St. Philip's College
San Antonio, Texas

Zachary D. Smith, MBA, RT(R)(T)
Director, Radiation Oncology
Baton Rouge General Pennington Cancer Center
Baton Rouge, Louisiana

Mattie J. Tabron, EdD, RT(R)(T), FASRT
Associate Professor and Chairman
Department of Radiation Therapy
Howard University
Washington, DC

Anne Marie Vann, MEd, RT(R)(T), CMD
Assistant Professor, Biomedical and Radiological Technologies
Medical College of Georgia
Augusta, Georgia

Tracy B. White, MS, RT(R)(T)
Radiation Therapy Program Director and Associate Professor
   of Radiologic Sciences
Arkansas State University
Jonesboro, Arkansas

Preface

Since the first edition of this text was published in 1996, the field of radiation therapy has experienced tremendous growth. Improvements in three-dimensional treatment planning, intensity-modulated radiation therapy, image-guided radiation therapy, particle therapies, brachytherapy, and patient immobilization have all allowed the radiation therapy team to enhance and improve clinical outcomes. More sophisticated electronic charting has allowed radiation therapists and medical dosimetrists to improve treatment-delivery documentation and quality-assurance practices. Although the face of radiation therapy has evolved through these advances, this textbook remains committed to its original purpose. It is still designed to contribute to a comprehensive understanding of cancer management, improve clinical techniques involved in delivering a prescribed dose of radiation therapy, and apply knowledge and complex concepts associated with radiation therapy treatment planning and delivery. As the methods of delivering a prescribed dose of radiation therapy have expanded and improved, so has the effort to localize the patient, deliver an accurate dose, and reproduce the daily treatment fields.

NEW TO THIS EDITION

Since the second edition, new chapters have been added and several chapters have been consolidated and additional information included. New chapters have been developed in the following:
- Special procedures, including image guided radiation therapy
- Intensity modulated radiation therapy
- CT simulation

Color inserts of important images have also been added to better demonstrate key aspects that are not easily conveyed in grayscale.

LEARNING AIDS

Pedagogical features, designed to enhance comprehension and critical thinking, are incorporated into each chapter. Elements retained from the second edition include the following:
- Chapter Outlines
- Key Terms lists
- Chapter Summaries that are bulleted for easier reference
- An updated Glossary that includes significant terms from all chapters
- Review Questions
- Questions to Ponder

Of particular note are the Review Questions and Questions to Ponder at the end of each chapter. Review Questions reinforce the cognitive information presented in the chapter, helping the reader incorporate the information into the basic understanding of radiation therapy concepts. The Questions to Ponder are open-ended, divergent questions intended to stimulate critical thinking and analytic judgment. Answers to the Review Questions are found on the companion website: http://evolve. elsevier.com/WashingtonLeaver/principles.

New features include the following:
- Chapter objectives that list the main topics in the chapter
- Spotlights throughout each chapter that highlight key information and/or direct readers to more information on important topics

In addition, each chapter offers a reference list, giving the reader additional information sources. In each edition, the focus of each chapter has been to present the comprehensive needs of the radiation therapy management team. In fact, dozens of experts in the field have contributed to this new edition, including radiation therapists, medical dosimetrists, physicists, radiation oncologists, nurses, and radiation therapy students.

ANCILLARIES

For Instructors

A robust instructor ancillary suite is available online on the companion website at http://evolve.elsevier.com/WashingtonLeaver/ principles, including the following:
- Instructor's Manual that contains content overviews of each chapter; learning competencies from the chapter objectives; teaching foci; materials to use for class; key terms lists from the chapters; lists of additional resources; critical thinking questions; as well as discussion topics, suggested class activities, and outside assignments
- Test Bank of approximately 1300 questions in .rtf and ExamView formats
- PowerPoint presentations for each chapter
- Image Collection of the figures from the book

For Students

The student site contains the Answer Key to the Review Questions from the text and links to websites pertinent to imaging sciences.

Charles M. Washington
Dennis Leaver

Acknowledgments

We are grateful to the contributors of the chapters and for the reviewers who offered helpful feedback and suggestions. We also offer special thanks to the editorial staff at Elsevier for their patience and valuable contributions during the preparation and production of this work.

Finally, it is our hope the expanded knowledge and progress in treatment planning, delivery, and patient care outlined in this work will ultimately enrich the patient's quality of life and reduce suffering from the effects of cancer.

Charles M. Washington
Dennis Leaver

Contents

Introduction to Radiation Therapy

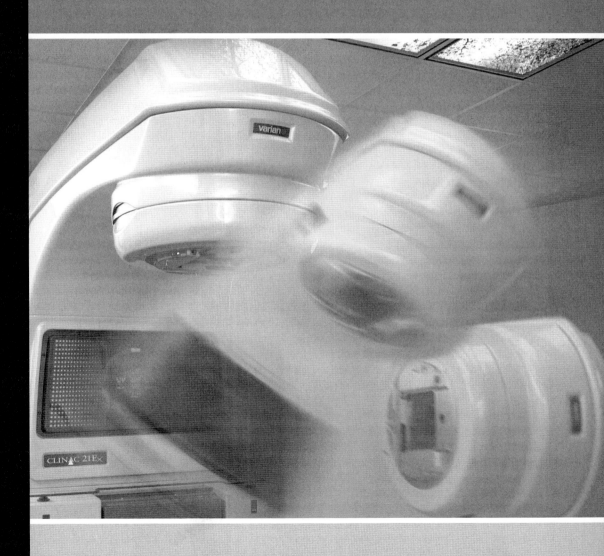

Cancer: An Overview

Stephanie Eatmon

Outline

Key Terms

Objectives

- Discuss how the changing theories of cancer affect treatment choices and outcome.
- Differentiate between benign and malignant tumors.
- Demonstrate a patient-focused solution to meet the needs of a patient in a given specific situation.
- Identify several local organizations that offer cancer patient resources.
- Explain what information physicians would need to know about a patient and his or her cancer to decide on an appropriate plan of treatment.

- Design a chart that details the strengths and weaknesses of the three major cancer treatments: radiation therapy, surgery, and chemotherapy.
- Discuss how each member of the radiation oncology team contributes to effective patient care and treatment.

Throughout recorded history, cancer has been a subject of investigation. Lacking current surgical techniques and diagnostic and laboratory equipment, early investigators relied on their senses to determine characteristics of the disease. Investigators were unable to thoroughly examine cells, so infections and other benign conditions were included in their category of cancer. Knowledge about these early observations, including examinations, diagnosis, and treatment, comes in part from Egyptian papyri dating back to 1600 BC.[6,9]

Initially, investigators believed that an excess of black bile caused cancer. This belief defined cancer as a systemic disease for which local treatment (such as surgery) only made the patient worse.[6,9] In light of this, cancer was considered to be fatal with little possibility of a cure. When investigators could not prove the existence of black bile, the theory of cancer as an initially localized disease emerged. With this theory came the possibility of treatment with a possible cure. However, because of the limited information available, few cures were accomplished.

In the fifth century BC, Hippocrates began the classification of tumors by observation. Later the discovery of the microscope enabled investigators to classify tumors on the basis of cellular characteristics.[9] Classification of tumors and their stages of growth will continue as technology advances.

The cause of this deadly disease remained a mystery, and, for many decades, people even thought that cancer was contagious. This theory brought isolation and shame to cancer victims. Although this belief has long since vanished, less than 30 years ago, patients expressed concern about spreading the disease to loved ones. Unfortunately, today many cancer patients still suffer discrimination in the workplace and when trying to obtain health insurance coverage.

With the ability to examine the genetic makeup of a cancer cell, scientists can determine many of the mutations that are responsible for a specific cancer initiation. This knowledge leads to earlier diagnosis in higher-risk individuals, improved screening examinations, and ultimately better treatment. In the future, it may be possible to develop designer drugs for individual cancers or provide drugs that will be effective in blocking specific cancer initiation in high-risk individuals.

BIOLOGIC PERSPECTIVE

Building on the work of early investigators and aided by technologic advances, researchers are able to diagnose many tumors in extremely early stages. In addition, scientists are able to examine the deoxyribonucleic acid (DNA) of cells obtained through biopsy to determine mechanisms causing uncontrolled growth. Although it is true that technology and knowledge about cancer has increased over the past decades, there is still much to be learned.

Theory of Cancer Initiation

Tumors are the result of abnormal cellular proliferation. This can occur because the process by which cellular differentiation takes place is abnormal or because a normally nondividing, mature cell begins to proliferate. **Cellular differentiation** occurs when a stem cell undergoes mitosis and divides into daughter cells. These cells continue to divide and differentiate until a mature cell with a specific function results. When this process is disrupted, the daughter cells may continue to divide with no resulting mature cell, thus causing abnormal cellular proliferation.

The cause of this cellular dysfunction has been the subject of research for many years. Researchers now know that "cancer is a disease of the genes."[5] Normal **somatic cells** (nonreproductive cells) contain genes that promote growth and genes that suppress growth, both of which are important to control the growth of a cell. In a tumor cell, this counterbalanced regulation is missing. Mutations occurring in genes that promote or suppress growth are implicated in the deregulation of cellular growth. Mutations in genes that promote growth force the proliferation of cells, whereas mutations to the genes that suppress growth allow unrestrained cellular growth. For many tumors, both mutations may be required for progression to full malignancy.[4,5,11-13]

The terms for the genes involved in the cancer process are *proto-oncogenes, oncogenes,* and *antioncogenes.* Proto-oncogenes are the normal genes that play a part in controlling normal growth and differentiation. These genes are the precursors of **oncogenes**, or cancer genes. The conversion of proto-oncogenes to oncogenes can occur through point mutations, translocations, and gene amplification, all of which are DNA mutations. Oncogenes are implicated in the abnormal proliferation of cells. Antioncogenes are also called *tumor-suppressor genes.* Inactivation of antioncogenes allows the malignant process to flourish.

 DNA point mutations, amplification, or translocations transform a proto-oncogene into an oncogene, resulting in unrestricted cellular growth.

What causes these mutations to occur? For somatic cells, exposure to carcinogens such as sunlight, radiation, and cigarette smoke is implicated. In some situations, such as the familial form of retinoblastoma, gene mutations are passed down through generations. Random mutations that occur during normal cellular replication can also lead to unregulated cellular growth.

Researchers have identified several gene mutations, including the gene implicated in the familial form of breast cancer. Using gene mapping and advanced technology, study in this area will continue. To understand the principles of cancer treatment, a review of the cell cycle and an overview of tumor growth are necessary.

Review of the Cell Cycle

Mammalian cells proliferate through the process of mitosis, or cellular division. The outcome of this process is two daughter cells that have identical chromosomes as the parent. The cell cycle consists of the period of time and the activities that take place between cell divisions. The cell cycle is broken up into five phases called G0, G1, S, G2, and M (Figure 1-1).

G0 is depicted outside of the cell cycle continuum because these cells are fully functioning but are not preparing for DNA replication. Most cells making up a tissue or organ are in the G0 phase. Given the proper stimulus, this reserve pool of cells can reenter the cell cycle and replicate.

G1, or the first growth phase, is characterized by rapid growth and active metabolism. The length of time that a cell remains in G1 is variable. Cells that are rapidly dividing spend little time in the first growth phase, whereas cells that are slow growing remain in G1 for a long period. The length of time spent in G1 varies from hours to years. During this time, the cell synthesizes the necessary ribonucleic acid (RNA) and proteins to carry out the function of the cell. Later in the first growth phase, the cell will commit to replication of DNA.

S phase, or synthesis, is the period in which DNA is replicated to ensure that the resulting daughter cells will have identical genetic material. G2, or the second growth phase, is the period in which the cell prepares for actual division. Enzymes and proteins are synthesized and the cell continues to grow and moves relatively quickly into the M, or mitotic, phase.

 Cells are most sensitive to radiation during G2 and M phases of the cell cycle.

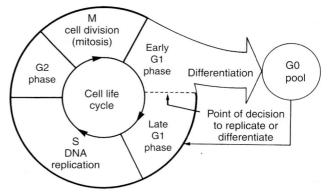

Figure 1-1. Cell generation cycle. (From Otto SE: *Oncology nursing*, ed 2, St. Louis, 1994, Mosby.)

Tumor Growth

When all cells are operating normally, there is a balance between cells that are dying and the replication of cells. Although tumor growth is a result of an imbalance between replication and cell death, the rate of growth is influenced by many factors. Malignant cells possess damaged genetic material, resulting in increased cell death. In addition, as the tumor grows larger, the blood and nutrient supply is inadequate, creating areas of **necrosis**, or dead tissue.

Initially, tumor growth is exponential, but as the tumor enlarges and outgrows the blood and nutrient supply, the rate of cell replication more closely equals the rate of cell death. This is demonstrated by the Gompertzian growth curve (Figure 1-2). Tumors that are clinically detectable are generally in the higher portion of the curve. Treatment reduces the number of cells, thus moving the tumor back down the curve where the growth rate is higher. Tumor cells that were previously in the G0 phase are prompted to reenter the cell cycle. Cells that are rapidly dividing are more sensitive to the effects of radiation and chemotherapy.[3]

 Cancer cells do not die after a programmed number of cell divisions as do normal cells. Hence, cancer cells have the ability to proliferate indefinitely.

Tumor Classification

Tumors are classified by their anatomic site, cell of origin, and biologic behavior. Tumors can originate from any cell; this accounts for the large variety of tumors. Well-differentiated tumors (those that closely resemble the cell of origin) can be easily classified according to their histology. Undifferentiated cells, however, do not resemble normal cells, so classification is more difficult. These tumors are called undifferentiated, or **anaplastic**.

Tumors are divided into two categories: benign or malignant (Table 1-1). **Benign** tumors are generally well differentiated and do not metastasize or invade surrounding normal tissue. Often, benign tumors are encapsulated and slow growing. Although most benign tumors do little harm to the host, some benign tumors of the brain (because of their location) are considered behaviorally malignant because of the adverse effect on the host. Benign tumors may be noted by the suffix *-oma*,

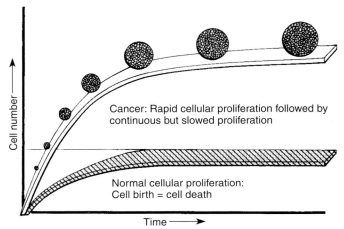

Figure 1-2. Gompertz' function as viewed by growth curve. (From Otto SE: *Oncology nursing*, ed 2, St. Louis, 1994, Mosby.)

Cell number

Cancer: Rapid cellular proliferation followed by continuous but slowed proliferation

Normal cellular proliferation: Cell birth = cell death

Time

Table 1-1 General Characteristics of Benign and Malignant Disease

Characteristics	Benign	Malignant
Local spread	Expanding, pushing	Infiltrative and invasive
Distant spread	Rare	Metastasize early or late by lymphatics, blood, or seeding
Differentiation	Well differentiated	Well differentiated to undifferentiated
Mitotic activity	Normal	Normal to increased mitotic rate
Morphology	Normal	Normal to pleomorphic
Effect on host	Little (depending on treatment and location of tumor)	Life threatening
Doubling time	Normal	Normal to accelerated

which is connected to the term indicating the cell of origin. For example, a *chondroma* is a benign tumor of the cartilage. Although this is a general rule, there are malignant tumors, such as melanoma, that end with the same suffix but are malignant.

Malignant tumors range from well differentiated to undifferentiated. They have the ability to **metastasize**, or spread to a site in the body distant from the primary site. Malignant tumors often invade and destroy normal surrounding tissue and, if left untreated, can cause the death of the host.

Tumors arising from mesenchymal cells are termed **sarcomas**. These cells include connective tissue such as cartilage and bone. An example is a chondrosarcoma or a sarcoma of the cartilage. Although blood and lymphatics are mesenchymal tissues, they are classified separately as leukemias and lymphomas.

Carcinomas are tumors that originate from the epithelium. These include all the tissues that cover a surface or line a cavity. For example, the aerodigestive tract is lined with squamous cell epithelium. Tumors originating from the lining are called *squamous cell carcinoma* of the primary site. An example is squamous cell carcinoma of the lung. Epithelial cells that are glandular are called **adenocarcinoma**. An example is the tissue lining the stomach. A tumor originating in the cells of this lining is called *adenocarcinoma of the stomach*. (Table 1-2 lists examples of nomenclature used in neoplastic classification.)

Table 1-2 Classifications of Neoplasms

Tissue of Origin	Benign	Malignant
Glandular epithelium	Adenoma	Adenocarcinoma
Squamous epithelium	Papilloma	Squamous cell carcinoma
Connective tissue smooth muscle	Leiomyoma	Leiomyosarcoma
Hematopoietic	—	Leukemia
Lymphoreticular	—	Lymphoma
Neural	Neuroma	Blastoma

Table 1-3	Histologies Associated with Common Anatomic Cancer Sites
Site	**Most Common Histology**
Oral cavity	Squamous cell carcinoma
Pharynx	Squamous cell carcinoma
Lung	Squamous cell carcinoma
Breast	Infiltrating ductal carcinoma
Colon and rectum	Adenocarcinoma
Anus	Squamous cell carcinoma
Cervix	Squamous cell carcinoma
Endometrium	Adenocarcinoma
Prostate	Adenocarcinoma
Brain	Astrocytoma

As in any classification system, some situations do not follow the rules. Examples include Hodgkin's disease, Wilms' tumor, and Ewing's sarcoma. This system of classification continues to change as more knowledge of the origin and behavior of tumors become available. (Table 1-3 lists histologies associated with common anatomic cancer sites.)

Cancer Outlook

The American Cancer Society[1] estimated that 1,437,180 new cases of cancer would be diagnosed in 2008. Of those patients, approximately 565,650 will die of their disease. It is estimated that 61% of individuals diagnosed with cancer will be cured. Skin cancer, excluding malignant melanoma, and most in situ cancers are not included in these numbers.[1]

Excluding carcinoma of the skin, the most common types of invasive cancers in the United States include prostate; lung; and colorectal in men and breast, lung, and colorectal in women.[1] These statistics are not static and change with environmental, lifestyle, technologic, and other influences in society. Lung cancer in the 1930s was much less prevalent than it was in the 1970s and 1980s. These differences can be explained by the increase in the number of cigarette smokers and improved diagnostic abilities. However, over the past 7 years, because of the improved educational programs and the decline of smoking in the United States, the incidence of lung cancer has dropped by approximately 17% in men and has not risen in women.[1] Invasive carcinoma of the cervix also decreased over the past 20 years as a result of the use of the Papanicolaou (Pap) smear. Currently, more carcinoma in situ, or preinvasive, cancers of the cervix are found than invasive tumors. These in situ carcinomas are not recorded in the American Cancer Society statistics.

Depending on the geographic location, the incidence of tumor sites also varies. For example, the incidence of stomach cancer is much greater in Japan than in the United States, and skin cancer is found more frequently in New Zealand than in Iceland. Diet and geographic environmental factors contribute to these tumor incidence differences.

PATIENT PERSPECTIVE

Although cancer is often a curable disease, the diagnosis is a life-changing event. In studying the various aspects of neoplasia, care providers can easily lose sight of the person behind the disease. The patient must be the focal point of all of the radiation therapist's actions. The highest level of quality care results from an in-depth knowledge of the disease process; psychosocial issues; patient care; and principles and practices of cancer management, including knowledge of radiation therapy as a treatment option. This knowledge provides the radiation therapist with the tools necessary for optimal treatment, care, and education of the cancer patient. Providing care that does not consider the whole person is unacceptable.

The Person Behind the Diagnosis

When providing treatment for a large number of people who develop cancer, care providers can easily forget that the patient has a life outside of treatment with concerns and worries continuing and adding to the emotional, social, psychological, physical, and financial burdens that come with his or her diagnosis. In addition, other medical concerns unrelated to cancer may complicate treatment and further burden the patient.

Factors such as age, culture, religion, support systems, education, and family background play important roles in medical treatment compliance, attitudes toward treatment, and responses to treatment. By knowing as much as possible about the patient and factors that influence the treatment outcome, the radiation therapist can provide quality patient care. For example, a female patient receiving treatment to the pelvic region may insist that male physicians or radiation therapists not be part of her treatment team. Although this would be an unusual situation and may present difficulties for the department, there may be some valid reasons for the patient's request such as a past history of sexual abuse or religious constraints. Once this information is obtained, the specific needs of this patient can be met, with the patient receiving quality care. Another example would be the patient who requests a treatment time not convenient for the department schedule. For a radiation therapist who has many patients to accommodate and a very tight schedule, this request may seem unreasonable. It may turn out that a working relative is providing daily transportation to the clinic and does not have a flexible work schedule. An appointment time that interferes with the relative's work schedule may lead to the loss of employment. In this example, there are three possible outcomes. First, the radiation therapist gives the patient an appointment time that fits the treatment schedule and lets the patient work out the transportation issues. Second, the radiation therapist gives the patient the requested appointment time and changes other patient appointments, or, third, the radiation therapist refers the patient and relative to community transportation resources and works with all parties to develop a plan for treatment. For reasons such as these, an in-depth knowledge of available patient resources is essential to ensure that all patients receive the care and help they need to deal with the disease and resulting life issues. The actual radiation treatment is only part of the radiation therapist's responsibility. A patient is not an organ with a cancer but a complete individual with a multitude of issues and needs that must be addressed. Because cancer affects the whole family, it is the responsibility of the radiation therapist to provide information and available resources to assist the patient and family in dealing with all the issues and challenges that a diagnosis of cancer brings. It is good to remember that sometimes it is the smallest act of compassion and connection with the patient and/or his or her family that will transform the radiation treatment experience from frightening and overwhelming to comforting and trusting.

Cancer Patient Resources

In each medical facility, there is generally a myriad of cancer support services. These services can include general education, cancer site–specific education, support groups, financial aid, transportation to and from treatment, and activity programs. Social work departments are available to assist with the financial, emotional, and logistic issues that arise, and community services through churches and other organizations are available to support individuals and their families. National organizations such as the American Cancer Society have established programs and information hotlines that are available to all patients. Caring for a cancer patient is often a 24-hour-a-day job, and it is essential that resources are available at all hours. Radiation therapists must become familiar with the services offered in their communities and nationally to better serve the patients and their family member caregivers. This is especially true for radiation therapists working at freestanding clinics not affiliated with a medical center. Unsupported caregivers often pay a heavy toll in terms of their own health and well-being. Educating patients and their families about available programs or services to address specific needs is an important component of quality care provided by the radiation therapist.

Two excellent national resources are:
- *American Cancer Society: http://www.cancer.org*
- *National Cancer Institute: http://cis.nci.nih.gov/*

ETIOLOGY AND EPIDEMIOLOGY

A tremendous amount of knowledge exists about factors that influence the development of cancer and the incidence at which it occurs. Etiology and epidemiology are the two areas of research that have contributed to the growing knowledge in these areas.

Etiology

Etiology is the study of the cause of disease. Although the cause of cancer is unknown, many carcinogenic agents and genetic factors have been identified. Experts use this information, as they have done with tobacco use, to establish prevention programs and identify high-risk individuals.

Etiology factors include cigarette smoke, human papillomavirus (HPV), alcohol, and sun exposure.

Etiologic and epidemiologic information is helpful in determining screening tests for early detection, producing patient education programs, and identifying target populations. An example is the set of guidelines of the American Cancer Society for screening mammograms to detect breast cancer in its early stages.

Epidemiology

Epidemiology is the study of disease incidence. National databases provide statistical information about patterns of cancer occurrence and death rates. With this information, researchers can determine the incidence of cancer occurrence in a population for factors such as age, gender, race, and geographic location. Researchers can also determine which specific type of cancer affects which specific group of people. An example is the higher incidence of prostate cancer in African-American males. Epidemiologic studies also help determine trends in disease such as the recent decrease of lung cancer in men and the decline of stomach cancer or the increase in malignant melanoma in the United States.

DETECTION AND DIAGNOSIS

Early detection and diagnosis are keys to the successful treatment of cancer. Generally, the earlier a tumor is discovered, the lower is the chance of metastasis or spread to other parts of the body. For some tumors such as carcinoma of the larynx, early symptoms cause the patient to seek medical care early in the course of the disease. As a result, the cure rate for early-stage glottic (or true vocal cord) tumors is extremely high. Cancer of the ovary, however, is associated with vague symptoms that could be the result of a number of medical problems. Therefore, a diagnosis is often made late in the course of the disease. Low cure rates for ovarian cancer reflect the results of late diagnosis.

Advances in medical diagnostic imaging allow physicians to see into the body and even visualize cellular activity. These increased capabilities have played a pivotal role in earlier detection and diagnosis of cancer.

Screening Examinations

To identify cancer in its earliest stages (before symptoms appear and while the chance of cure is greatest), screening tests are performed. Examples include the Pap smear for cervical cancer, fecal occult blood testing or colonoscopy for colorectal cancer, and mammograms for breast cancer. Unfortunately, for many cancers, screening examinations are not readily available because of the inaccessibility of the tumor or the high cost in relation to the information yield associated with the tests.

To be useful, screening examinations must be **sensitive** and **specific** for the tumors they identify. If an examination is sensitive, it can identify a tumor in its extremely early stages. For example, a Pap smear is sensitive because it can help detect carcinoma of the cervix before the disease becomes invasive. If a test is specific, it can identify a particular type of cancer. Carcinoembryonic antigen (CEA) may be elevated in a number of benign and malignant conditions. For this reason, the test is not specific, but it is the most sensitive test available for determining recurrences of colorectal cancer.

Screening tests may also yield **false-positive** or **false-negative** readings. A false-positive reading indicates disease when in reality none is present. A false-negative reading is the reverse; the test indicates no disease when in fact the disease is present.

For a screening test to be highly useful, it should be sensitive, specific, cost-effective, and accurate. The cost of the screening examination often limits its use to all but extremely high-risk populations.

In 2002, the National Cancer Institute began a national lung screening trial for high-risk individuals that compares standard chest radiography with spiral computed tomography (CT) as a screening tool. By February 2004, more than 50,000 individuals were enrolled in the study, and data are being collected.[7] The data will be analyzed over the next 8 years but already show that spiral CT is a more sensitive screening tool and allows much earlier diagnosis of cancer. Although this is very exciting, to be useful, the data will need to show that earlier diagnosis will decrease lung cancer mortality.

 A false-positive, sensitive but low-specificity screening examination results in the necessity for additional, often costly, diagnostic procedures to determine the diagnosis.

Workup Components

After a tumor is suspected, a workup, or series of diagnostic examinations, begins. The purposes of the workup are to determine the general health status of the patient and to collect as much information about the tumor as possible. To treat the patient effectively, the physician must know the type, location, and size of the tumor; the distance the tumor has invaded normal tissue; the presence or absence of spread to distant sites; the lymph node involvement if any; and amenability to specific treatment regimens. These questions are answered in the workup.

The workup depends on the type of cancer suspected and the symptoms experienced by the patient. The workup for a suspected lung tumor is different than that for a suspected prostate tumor. The same questions are answered, but because the two tumors are extremely different, the tests are based on the specific tumor characteristics. Additionally, the workup for an early stage tumor will be different from for later stage disease. The incidence of bone metastasis in a stage I breast cancer is extremely low, unlike stage IV disease. Therefore, the workup for stage I disease will not include a bone scan but would be ordered for stage IV disease.

 For patients who have lifestyle habits that include carcinogens such as cigarette smoking, alcohol, and chewing tobacco, the workup will include diagnostic procedures to rule out the possibility of second primary cancers.

With advancing technology, more information is available to the physician than ever before. As new technologies emerge and prove useful in the information-gathering process, treatment becomes more effective. Before CT or magnetic resonance imagining (MRI) became available, small tumor extension into normal lung tissues was not visible on chest radiographs. The physician had to make an educated guess about the extent of the tumor invasion and to treat the patient based on the suspected condition. As a result, treatment fields had to be larger to encompass all the suspected disease. Much of the guesswork is eliminated when using CT, so treatment volumes can include areas of known disease while limiting even more the areas of normal tissue, thereby producing a more effective treatment with fewer sequelae.

Today, with the added imaging tool of positron emission tomography (PET), physicians can identify very small foci of disease that may be active in other parts of the body undetectable to other forms of diagnostic imaging. PET has diagnostic value for tumors of the lung, head and neck, and breast, as well as for colorectal and esophageal tumors, lymphoma, and melanoma. The effectiveness of using PET for other tumor types is under investigation. Determining whether a suspicious posttreatment area is recurrent disease or expected tissue changes is another area in which PET excels.

Staging

Tumor staging is a means of defining the tumor size and extension at the time of diagnosis and is important for many reasons. Tumor staging provides a means of communication about tumors, helps in determining the best treatment, aids in predicting prognosis, and provides a means for continuing research. Staging systems have changed with advancing technologies and increased knowledge and will continue to progress as more information becomes known. For this reason, tumors that occur frequently have detailed staging classifications, whereas those that are rare have primitive or no working staging systems.

A common staging system adopted by the International Union Against Cancer (UICC) and the American Joint Committee on Cancer (AJCC) is the TNM system. The T category defines the size or extent of the primary tumor and is assigned numbers 1 through 4 or x. A T1 tumor is small and/or confined to a small area, whereas a T4 tumor is extremely large and/or extends into other tissues. The x indicates that there was an inability to obtain information necessary to make a determination. N designates the status of lymph nodes and the extent of lymph node involvement. A 0-through-4 or x designation exists depending on the extent of involvement, with N0 indicating that no positive nodes are present. N1 indicates positive nodes close to the site of the primary tumor, whereas N4 indicates positive nodes at more distant nodal sites. Nx indicates that the nodal status was not assessed. Not all cancers have the designation of N1 through N4. The natural history of a particular cancer and clinical treatment knowledge will affect the complexity of the staging system. M is the category that defines the presence and extent of metastasis. Again, the M category is generally categorized as 0, 1, or x depending on the extent of metastatic disease. The designation M0 indicates no evidence of metastatic disease was found, whereas M1 indicates disease distant from the primary tumor. Mx indicates that the presence or absence of metastasis was not assessed. Specific tumors with a detailed staging criteria may have an expanded M designation (Figure 1-3).

In the TNM staging are additional subcategories for commonly occurring tumors. Notations are often used to determine whether the staging was accomplished through clinical, surgical, or pathologic methods. Although the TNM system is widely used, numerous staging systems exist that more accurately detail important tumor characteristics for prognostic and treatment information. For example, the International Federation of Gynecology and Obstetrics (FIGO) system is more commonly used in the staging of gynecologic tumors.

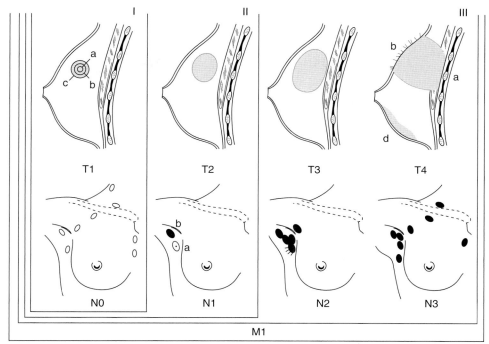

Figure 1-3. A diagrammatic depiction of the breast cancer staging system. (From Rubin P: *Clinical oncology*, ed 7, Philadelphia, 1993, WB Saunders.)

Surgical/Pathologic Staging

Surgical/pathologic staging offers the most accurate information about the tumor and the extent of disease spread. Although staging can be performed clinically, or without the use of invasive procedures, the status of the lymph nodes and micrometastatic spread would remain in question. During surgical staging, the physician has the opportunity to perform a biopsy of suspicious-looking tissue, obtain a sample of lymph nodes for microscopic examination, and observe the tumor and surrounding tissues and organs.

Ovarian disease may be staged surgically through the use of a laparotomy, or surgical exploration of the abdomen, because these tumors often spread by seeding into the abdomen. During the procedure, the primary tumor site is identified, tumor is removed, suspicious areas are biopsied, and fluid is introduced into the abdominal cavity to be removed and examined for cancer cells. The amount of tumor left behind following the surgery provides important treatment and prognostic information. The greater the amount of information obtained about the tumor, the more accurate the staging is likely to be, resulting in more effective treatment. Accurate staging is also able to limit aggressive treatment to only those patients who will benefit.

With the ability to look at a tumor's cellular DNA, even more information is becoming available to determine, even within a tumor type, which tumor is more sensitive to a particular treatment and which tumor has a greater chance of recurrence. As tumor cell DNA examination becomes standard practice, staging will change to include DNA characteristics, as well as clinical factors.

Grade

The **grade** of a tumor provides information about its aggressiveness and is based on the degree of differentiation. This is determined only by examining cells obtained through a biopsy under a microscope. For some tumors, such as high-grade astrocytoma, grade is the most important prognostic indicator. Grade is also more important than stage in bone and muscle tumors in determining treatment and prognosis.

 Grade can be determined only by examining tumor cells under a microscope.

The stage and grade offer an accurate picture of the tumor and its behavior. When physicians know the exact types of tumors with which they are dealing, treatment decisions can be made that effectively eradicate the tumors. (A detailed description of cancer detection and diagnosis is provided in Chapter 5.)

TREATMENT OPTIONS

Cancer treatment demands a multidisciplinary approach. Tumor boards were established so that cancer specialists can work together to review information about newly diagnosed tumors and devise effective treatment plans. Participants of a tumor board can include surgeons, radiation oncologists, medical oncologists, radiologists, pathologists, social workers, plastic surgeons, and other medical personnel. All of these individuals play key roles in developing a treatment plan that effectively treats the tumor while helping the patient maintain a high quality of life (Figure 1-4).

Surgery

As a local treatment modality, surgery plays a role in diagnosis, staging, primary treatment, **palliation**, and identification of treatment response. As a tool for diagnosis, surgery is used to perform a biopsy of a suspected mass to determine whether the

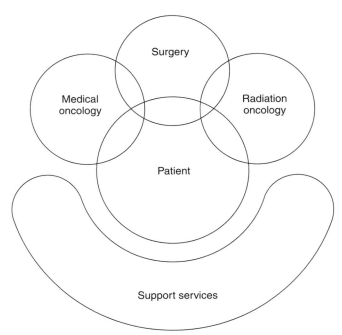

Figure 1-4. The cancer patient receives treatment and support from multiple sources during disease management.

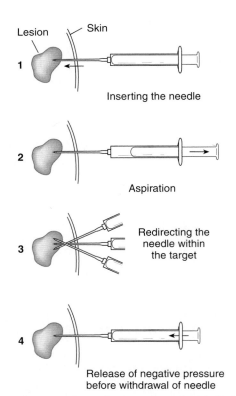

Figure 1-5. The steps in aspiration of a palpable lesion. Step 3 indicates the way that the needle should be redirected in the target, and step 4 emphasizes the importance of releasing the negative pressure before withdrawing the needle. (From Koss LG: Needle aspiration cytology of tumors at various body sites. In Silver CE et al, editors: *Current problems in surgery*, vol 22, Chicago, 1985, Year Book Medical Publishers.)

mass is malignant and, if so, the cellular origin. Many biopsy methods exist, and the characteristics of the suspected mass determine the use of a particular method.

To provide the most effective treatment, the histology and cellular characteristics must be identified. A few questions that a biopsy will answer are as follows: Is the tumor growing at the primary site or has it spread from another area in the body? Is the tumor slow growing or very aggressive? Is the tumor malignant? Once this information is known, an appropriate multidisciplinary treatment plan can be established.

Common **biopsy** methods include fine-needle aspiration, core needle, endoscopic, incisional, and excisional. The information obtained through a biopsy is essential for appropriate treatment management. A fine-needle aspiration biopsy would be used to determine the histology of a suspicious breast mass. During the biopsy, sample cells are collected in the needle from several areas of the suspected tumor (Figure 1-5). The cells are then transferred to a microscopic slide for further examination. This method of biopsy is relatively quick and easy, with minimal patient discomfort and healing time. The disadvantage is that the collected cells are examined without the benefit of their neighboring cells to provide a glimpse of the tumor architecture. There is also the chance that malignant cells will be seeded along the needle track as the needle is withdrawn from the tumor.

A large-gauge needle (14 or 16) is used to perform a core-needle biopsy. As the needle is inserted into the suspected tumor, a core of tissue is collected. The tissue obtained can be sectioned and examined under a microscope. Using this method, the tumor architecture is preserved, allowing identification of the tumor tissue of origin (Figure 1-6).

During endoscopic procedures, such as a bronchoscopy or colonoscopy, suspicious tissue can also be collected with the use of a flexible biopsy tool. The tool is passed through the scope, and tiny pincers are used to cut a small tissue sample. Tissue samples can then be frozen or imbedded in paraffin, sectioned, and examined under the microscope.

During an incisional biopsy, a sample of the tumor is removed with no attempt to remove the whole tumor. This method is often used with larger tumors or those that are locally advanced (Figure 1-7). In excisional biopsies, on the other hand, an attempt is made to remove the entire tumor and any possible local spread, as in the case of malignant melanoma. When a nevus, or mole, becomes suspicious by changing colors or growing larger, an excisional biopsy is performed. The nevi and normal surrounding tissue (to include a safe margin of underlying tissue) are removed **en bloc**, or as one piece.

Surgery plays a major role in the treatment of cancer. With advances in knowledge, equipment, and techniques, procedures that are performed are now less radical and are apt to be part of a multidisciplinary treatment plan. The success of surgical intervention is dependent on the medical condition; wishes of the patient; and size, extent, and the location of the tumor.

Not all patients are surgical candidates. Patients with preexisting medical conditions may have an unacceptable increase in surgical risk. For example, if the patient's pulmonary function is compromised, general anesthesia may be contraindicated and surgical procedures are impossible. In addition, as with any treatment modality, the patient may decide not to have surgery in favor of another type of treatment or no treatment at all.

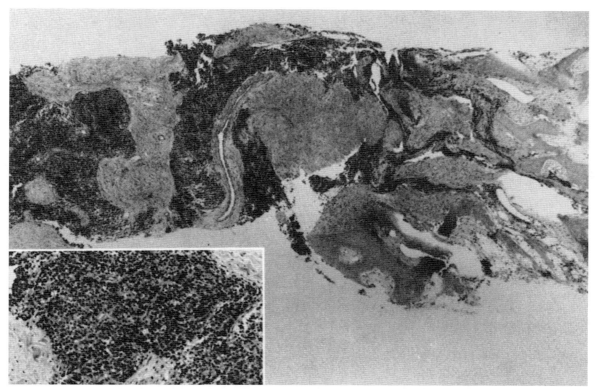

Figure 1-6. An example of the tissue core obtained by needle biopsy of a Ewing's sarcoma as seen microscopically. The insert demonstrates good preservation of cells. (From del Regato JA, Spjut HJ, Cox JD: *Ackerman and del Regato's cancer: diagnosis, treatment and prognosis,* ed 6, St. Louis, 1985, Mosby.)

 Risks associated with surgery include adverse reactions to anesthesia, infection, and potential loss of function.

Because surgery is a localized treatment, it is most successful with small tumors that have not spread to neighboring tissues or organs. During surgery, the physician attempts to remove the entire tumor and any microscopic spread, requiring the removal of normal tissue. As the size and/or extent of the tumor increases, more normal tissue must be removed, thus increasing the risk of the procedure. Surgical intervention may be the only treatment necessary if the tumor can be completely removed. If, however, the surgical margins are positive for cancer cells, the tumor has a high recurrence rate, or gross tumor was left, further treatment is necessary.

Before surgery, radiation therapy or chemotherapy may be given to increase the likelihood of a complete resection. The goals of radiation or chemotherapy in this case are to destroy microscopic and subclinical disease and shrink the tumor. Lower doses of radiation and/or chemotherapy are used to prevent complications during and following surgery.

The location of the tumor is an important factor in the success of surgical treatment. If a tumor is located in an area that is inaccessible or close to **critical structures** or **organs at risk** (vital organs or structures), surgery may not be possible. Damage to critical structures may be incompatible with life or may leave the patient in worse condition than before treatment. A cancer of the nasopharynx is located in an area in which

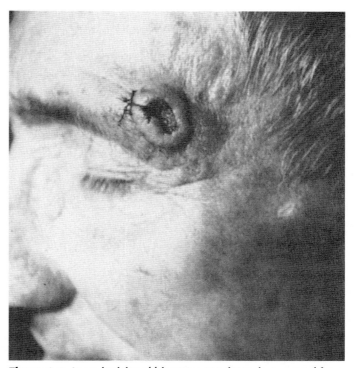

Figure 1-7. In an incisional biopsy, a specimen is removed from the edge of the tumor. (From del Regato JA, Spjut HJ, Cox JD: *Ackerman and del Regato's cancer: diagnosis, treatment and prognosis,* ed 6, St. Louis, 1985, Mosby.)

accessibility is difficult because the cancer is close to the base of the brain and the cranial nerves. For these reasons, patients with cancers of the nasopharynx are not good candidates for surgical intervention. With improved technology and procedures, however, location of the tumor continues to become less of a barrier to successful treatment.

Surgical palliation is used to relieve symptoms the patient may be experiencing as a result of the disease. Removing an obstruction of the bowel does not have a curative effect on the disease but provides the patient with symptom relief for an improved quality of life. Cutting nerves to reduce or eliminate pain caused by the tumor is another example of palliative surgery.

Radiation Therapy

Radiation therapy is a local treatment that can be used alone or with other treatment modalities. Benefits of radiation therapy include preservation of function and better cosmetic results. An early-stage laryngeal tumor can be effectively treated by surgery or radiation. Surgery may require removal of the vocal cords, thus leaving the patient without a voice. Radiation therapy, however, can obtain the same results while preserving the patient's voice. In the past, surgery for patients with prostate cancer commonly left the patient impotent with a high chance for incontinence. Radiation therapy can preserve function in a majority of sexually active males while providing an effective treatment.

Surgery and radiation therapy combined also obtain an optimal cosmetic result. In the past, breast cancer was usually treated with a radical mastectomy, leaving the patient disfigured. Currently, a common treatment for some types of breast cancer consists of a lumpectomy with axillary node dissection followed by radiation therapy, and this leaves the patient with minimal disfigurement and an equal chance of cure. Examination of the **sentinel node,** or the primary drainage lymph node, decreases the extent of an axillary node dissection. As a result, the patient experiences fewer range-of-motion deficits, and the risk of lymphedema is lowered.

Radiation therapy plays a major role in palliation, as in the case of bone metastasis. If the condition is left untreated, the patient may experience a great deal of pain and is at risk for pathologic bone fractures. Radiation therapy to these sites usually eliminates the pain and prevents fractures. If a tumor is pressing on nerves, radiation therapy is given to reduce the size of the tumor, thus eliminating pressure on the nerves and providing pain relief.

Radiation therapy is limited to a local area of treatment. Tumors that are diffuse throughout the body are not candidates for radiation therapy. Radiation therapy is further limited to areas in which a **tumoricidal** dose may be delivered without harming critical structures. Newer radiotherapy techniques of conformal therapy, intensity-modulated radiation therapy, stereotactic radiosurgery, and proton treatments take advantage of the advances in diagnostic medical imaging and are able to almost "paint the tumor" with radiation, which greatly spares the normal tissues. Patients treated with these techniques may experience fewer side effects than those treated using conventional radiation therapy techniques. All factors for a specific treatment plan must be examined to determine the most appropriate technique because one technique will not work for all types of treatments.

As with surgery, the patient's medical condition must be such that the patient can tolerate the treatment. If a patient is suffering from lung cancer and has little pulmonary function, radiation therapy may not be a suitable treatment option because it may further compromise the patient's ability to breathe. Numerous methods to deliver radiation exist. The two broad categories are external beam and brachytherapy.

Adverse long-term side effects of radiation are minimized by careful treatment planning and the use of appropriate fractionation schedules.

External Beam. Through the use of external beam x-rays, electrons, protons, or gamma rays can be delivered to the tumor. Linear accelerators are capable of producing x-rays within a specific energy range. Some treatment machines can produce multiple x-ray, or **photon**, energies in addition to a range of **electron** energies. Cyclotrons or similar equipment is needed for **proton** treatment. This treatment modality is housed in large cancer centers and will, with time, become more available. **Gamma rays** are produced by cobalt-60 machines; although they were the primary treatment machine 35 years ago, their numbers are limited today.

The difference between x-rays and gamma rays is the mechanism of production. X-rays are produced by the interaction of electrons striking a target, whereas gamma rays are produced through radioactive decay.

High-energy x-rays are used to treat tumors that are deeper in the body, whereas electrons are effective at delivering energy to superficial tumors. For tumors such as pancreatic cancer, electrons can be given at the time of surgery. Intraoperative radiotherapy is delivered directly to the tumor using a sterilized cone that is positioned during surgery. The cone is then attached to the accelerator, treatment is given, and the patient is returned to surgery for incision closure. This method allows a high dose to be delivered to the tumor while sparing the normal surrounding tissues. Not all tumors are amenable to this type of treatment because of their location, the extent of disease, or the patient's ability to withstand the rigors of surgery.

Treatment today is more precise and accurate than ever before. With the use of advanced treatment planning computers, sophisticated treatment equipment, and much better imaging technology, a high dose of radiation can be safely delivered to the tumor with minimal damage to surrounding normal tissue. Conformal therapy and intensity-modulated radiation therapy are two examples of recent advances. Very simply explained, these two techniques change the treatment field size and/or dose to vary with the shape of the tumor as the treatment machine is positioned or rotates around the body. These more current treatment techniques are covered in depth in Chapters 16 and 17.

Brachytherapy. Brachytherapy, or "short-distance therapy," uses radioactive materials such as cesium-137 (^{137}Cs), iridium-192 (^{192}Ir), palladium-103 (^{103}Pd), or iodine-125 (^{125}I). Through the use of brachytherapy, the radioactive sources can be placed next to or directly into the tumor. Because the energy of the radioactive sources is low, a high energy is delivered to the tumor, with the nearby normal tissues receiving very little dose. Brachytherapy is accomplished using a multitude of techniques.

During an interstitial implant, radioactive sources are placed directly into the tumor. The sources may remain in place permanently or they may be removed once the prescribed dose has been delivered. Treatment of prostate cancer is a good example for both of these methods. For a permanent implant, tiny seeds of ^{103}Pd or ^{125}I are placed in the prostate. These seeds remain in the prostate, with their radioactivity decreasing over time. Because of the low energy of the radioactive material, the patient poses no threat to his family and friends. Another patient with prostate cancer may be treated with a removable implant. At the time of surgery, needles are placed into the prostate through the perineum. Later, when the patient has left recovery and is in the appropriate hospital room, the radioactive sources are placed in the needles. The patient remains in the hospital with the sources in place until the prescribed dose has been delivered. Determination of the type of implant offered depends on the skill and preference of the radiation oncologist, the available resources, and the patient's wishes. Cancers of the head and neck and breast are amenable to interstitial implants.

High-dose afterloading equipment is available in many departments, eliminating the need for extended hospitalization. For example, during the lumpectomy for breast cancer, a special balloon is placed in the tumor bed. The balloon is attached to a catheter that extends outside of the patient's body. Later, when the patient has been discharged from the hospital, she will go for radiation therapy treatment. Treatment is delivered in a specially designed suite. Once all of the quality assurance tests have been completed to ensure a safe and accurate treatment, the catheter will be connected to the high-dose afterloading machine. The treatment begins when a radioactive source enters the catheter and travels into the balloon. The source will pause at predetermined spots, delivering the dose prescribed to the tumor bed.

Intracavitary implants are performed by placing the radioactive material in a body cavity, as in the case of treatment for cervical or endometrial cancers. Applicators are placed in the body cavity, often at the time of surgery, and later the radioactive sources are inserted and remain until the prescribed dose has been delivered. The prescribed dose can be delivered over several days as an inpatient procedure (low-dose brachytherapy) or, in one or more fractions, as an outpatient procedure (high-dose brachytherapy).

Interluminal brachytherapy is used when the radioactive material is placed within a body tube such as the esophagus or bronchial tree. The radioactive material is positioned in the lumen at the tumor site and removed once the prescribed dose is delivered. Another brachytherapy technique, intervascular brachytherapy, is used to prevent restenosis of blood vessels following angioplasty or stent placement.

 Brachytherapy provides a high dose to a small area, which spares normal surrounding tissue.

The tremendous arsenal of treatment delivery methods and the successful outcomes achieved make radiation therapy a major weapon in the fight against cancer. As the ability to detect and image a tumor improves, the precision of the treatment delivery methods will continue to advance. Treatments that are commonly used today were only dreams 20 years ago.

Chemotherapy

Unlike surgery and radiation therapy, chemotherapy is a **systemic treatment**. Using **cytotoxic** drugs and hormones, chemotherapy aims at killing cells of the primary tumor and those that may be circulating through the body. Chemotherapy may be administered as a primary treatment or as part of a multidisciplinary treatment plan. As with the other major cancer treatments, chemotherapy is most successful when the tumor burden is small. Most chemotherapy agents affect the cell during a specific phase of the cell cycle. Tumors that are rapidly dividing provide more opportunities for the cytotoxic effects to take place because more cells are in the cell cycle.

Administration of chemotherapeutic agents is accomplished through a variety of methods depending on the drugs prescribed. The route of administration depends on the drugs used, the type of cancer, and patient-related factors. Oral administration is the easiest method, but it requires full patient compliance in taking the drugs and in taking the drugs at the correct times. Injections can be self-administered by the patient or administered by the oncology nurse. Intraarterial administration requires an infusion pump connected to a catheter that has been placed in an artery near the tumor. Heparin, a blood thinner, is added to the cytotoxic agent to prevent clotting at the catheter site. Bladder cancer is often treated with an intracavitary administration whereby the chemotherapy drugs are instilled directly into the bladder. Cytotoxic drugs are introduced into the abdomen using an intraperitoneal administration through a catheter or implanted port. **Intrathecal** injection requires drugs to be instilled into the space containing cerebrospinal fluid. Although most chemotherapy drugs can be administered by the patient or a nurse, intrathecal administration is done only by a physician. One of the more common methods of drug installation is the intravenous (IV) route. Drugs may be administered using a syringe entering the vein directly or piggybacked with other fluids.

Chemotherapy agents are very toxic, and safety precautions must be taken during preparation and administration, such as the wearing of gloves, gowns, and face shields. Certain drugs have vesicant or blistering potential and if spilled on the skin or outside of the vein will cause ulceration, so extra precautions must be taken. For these reasons, patients coming to radiation therapy with IV lines for chemotherapy must be treated with extra care to preserve the patency of the IV line. Often these individuals have small, weak veins, so finding a site for the IV line is difficult at best. If a problem occurs with an IV line, the therapist should immediately call the nurse charged with the care of that patient to prevent total failure of the site. Precautions must also be taken when treating patients with portable infusion catheters (PIC lines) to prevent accidental dislodgment of the device.

 Chemotherapy administration methods depend on the types of drugs prescribed.

Chemotherapeutic Agents

Chemotherapeutic agents are classified by their action on the cell or their source and include alkylating agents, antimetabolites, antibiotics, hormonal agents, nitrosoureas, vinca alkaloids, and miscellaneous agents[3,8,10] (Table 1-4).

Alkylating agents were the first drugs identified to have anticancer activity. This class of drugs is related structurally to mustard gas; they are not cell cycle specific but rather work throughout the cycle. The mechanism of action is to bond with nucleic acids, thereby interfering with their action. Side effects include bone marrow depression, amenorrhea in women and azoospermia in men, and carcinogenesis. Administration of alkylating agents is associated with an increased risk of acute myelogenous leukemia and is related to the total drug dose. Examples of alkylating agents include nitrogen mustard, cyclophosphamide, and chlorambucil.

Antimetabolites act by interfering with the synthesis of new nucleic acids. They are cell cycle specific and are much more toxic to proliferating cells but are not associated with delayed bone marrow suppression or carcinogenesis. Side effects include gastrointestinal toxicity and acute bone marrow suppression. Examples of antimetabolites include methotrexate, often used with intrathecal administration, and 5-fluorouracil.

Antitumor antibiotics are derived from microbial fermentation. Antibiotics act on the DNA to disrupt DNA and RNA transcription. Although they are not cell cycle specific, the

Table 1-4	Chemotherapeutic Drug Classifications with Side Effects
Drugs	**Major Side Effects**
ALKYLATING AGENTS	
Carboplatin	Nausea and vomiting, bone marrow suppression, ototoxicity, neurotoxicity, and hyperuricemia
Chlorambucil	Myelosuppression and interstitial pneumonia-pulmonary fibrosis
Cisplatin	Neurotoxicity, myelosuppression, nephrotoxicity, nausea and vomiting, hypokalemia, and hypomagnesemia
Cyclophosphamide	Myelosuppression, anorexia, stomatitis, alopecia, gonadal suppression, nail hyperpigmentation, nausea and vomiting, diarrhea, and hemorrhagic cystitis
Dacarbazine	Nausea and vomiting, anorexia, vein irritation, alopecia, myelosuppression, facial flushing, and radiation recall
Melphalan	Hypersensitivity, nausea, myelosuppression, amenorrhea, pulmonary infiltrates, and sterility
Nitrogen mustard	Nausea and vomiting, fever, chills, anorexia, vesication, gonadal suppression, myelosuppression, hyperpigmentation, and alopecia
ANTIMETABOLITES	
Cytarabine	Myelosuppression, diarrhea, nausea and vomiting, alopecia, rash, fever, conjunctivitis, neurotoxicity, hepatotoxicity, pulmonary edema, and skin desquamation of the palms and soles of the feet
Methotrexate	Nausea and vomiting, oral ulcers
5-Fluorouracil (5-FU)	Oral and gastrointestinal ulcers, nausea and vomiting, diarrhea, alopecia, vein hyperpigmentation, and radiation recall
6-Mercaptopurine	Nausea and vomiting, anorexia, myelosuppression, diarrhea, hepatotoxicity, and hyperpigmentation
6-Thioguanine	Anorexia, stomatitis, rash, vein irritation, hepatotoxicity, myelosuppression, and nausea and vomiting
ANTITUMOR ANTIBIOTICS	
Bleomycin	Anaphylaxis, pneumonitis, pulmonary fibrosis, alopecia, stomatitis, anorexia, radiation recall, skin hyperpigmentation, fever, chills, and nausea and vomiting
Dactinomycin (actinomycin D)	Nausea and vomiting, stomatitis, vesication, alopecia, radiation recall, myelosuppression, and diarrhea
Doxorubicin	Myelosuppression, vesication, cardiotoxicity, stomatitis, alopecia, nausea and vomiting, radiation recall, and diarrhea
Mithramycin	Myelosuppression, hepatotoxicity, hyperpigmentation, nausea and vomiting, facial flushing, and nephrotoxicity
Mitomycin	Myelosuppression, vesication, nausea and vomiting, alopecia, pulmonary fibrosis, hepatotoxicity, stomatitis, and hyperuricemia
HORMONAL AGENTS	
Corticosteroids Dexamethasone Hydrocortisone Prednisone	Nausea, suppression of immune function, weight gain, hyperglycemia, increased appetite, cataracts, impaired wound healing, menstrual irregularity, and interruption in sleep and rest patterns
Antiandrogen Flutamide	Impotence and gynecomastia
Antiestrogen Tamoxifen Zoladex	Nausea and vomiting, hot flashes, fluid retention, changes in menstrual pattern, increase in bone pain, and hypercalcemia
Gonadotropin-releasing hormone Leuprolide	Impotence, decreased libido, increase in bone and tumor pain, genital atrophy, and gynecomastia

Table 1-4	**Chemotherapeutic Drug Classifications with Side Effects—cont'd**
Drugs	**Major Side Effects**
NITROSOUREAS	
Carmustine	Nausea and vomiting, vein irritation, myelosuppression, stomatitis, nephrotoxicity, and pulmonary fibrosis
Lomustine	Nausea and vomiting, stomatitis, anorexia, myelosuppression, pulmonary fibrosis, and nephrotoxicity
Streptozocin	Nausea and vomiting, fever, chills, nephrotoxicity, diarrhea, myelosuppression, and hypoglycemia
PLANT ALKALOID	
Etoposide	Nausea and vomiting, diarrhea, stomatitis, parotitis, anaphylaxis, hypotension, myelosuppression, radiation recall, hepatotoxicity, and alopecia
Taxol	Anaphylaxis, hypotension, nausea and vomiting, cardiotoxicity, myelosuppression, neurotoxicity, alopecia, stomatitis, and diarrhea
Vinblastine	Neurotoxicity, anorexia, myelosuppression, stomatitis, alopecia, gonadal suppression, peripheral neuropathy, and vesication
Vincristine	Neurotoxocity, constipation, myelosuppression, alopecia, vesication, peripheral neuropathy, and paralytic ileus
MISCELLANEOUS AGENTS	
Asparaginase	Anaphylaxis, nausea and vomiting, fever, chills, myelosuppression, hyperglycemia, abdominal pain, diarrhea, pancreatitis, and anorexia
Hydroxyurea	Nausea and vomiting, alopecia, myelosuppression, allergic reactions, radiation recall, rash, azotemia, and dysuria
Pentostatin	Nausea and vomiting, rash, myelosuppression, vein irritation, nephrotoxicity, and hyperuricemia
Procarbazine	Nausea and vomiting; stomatitis; peripheral neuropathy; and severe gastrointestinal and central nervous system effects if taken with foods containing tyramine, alcohol, or monoamine oxidase inhibitor
Topotecan	Diarrhea, nausea and vomiting, myelosuppression, anorexia, and influenza-like symptoms

effects of the antibiotics are more pronounced in the S or G2 phase. Examples of anticancer antibiotics include doxorubicin (Adriamycin), bleomycin, mitomycin C, and actinomycin D. Side effects include cardiac toxicity, skin ulceration with extravasation, pulmonary toxicities, bone marrow suppression, and increased effects of radiation therapy.

Hormonal agents act to eliminate or displace natural hormones. Steroid hormones are used to clinically manipulate cells by binding to specific intracellular receptors and interacting with DNA to change cellular function. The most common use is in the treatment of breast cancer when the tumor is positive for estrogen and progesterone receptors. Examples of hormonal agents include tamoxifen, flutamide, and megestrol acetate. Side effects include hot flashes, depression, loss of libido, and an increase in endometrial cancers.

Nitrosoureas are not cell cycle specific, but they are lipid soluble and able to cross the blood-brain barrier. Their action is similar to that of alkylating agents in that they interfere with DNA synthesis. Examples include carmustine (BCNU), lomustine (CCNU), and streptozocin. Side effects include delayed myelosuppression, gastrointestinal toxicity, and delayed nephrotoxicity.

Vinca alkaloids are derived from the periwinkle plant. By binding to a substance that is needed for mitosis and solute transport, the vinca alkaloids stop cell replication in metaphase. Neurotoxicity, severe ulceration of the skin (if extravasation occurs), and myelosuppression are the dose-limiting side effects. Examples include vincristine, vinblastine, and etoposide (VP-16).

Miscellaneous agents are a class of drugs that have varied action and are from a number of different sources. The platinum compounds such as cisplatin and carboplatin are included in this category, along with the taxanes such as paclitaxel and docetaxel. Cisplatin and carboplatin act similar to the alkylating agents with nephrotoxicity and myelosuppression as the dose-limiting side effects. The action of the taxanes is opposite of that of the vinca alkaloids and results in a disrupted mitosis, along with other cellular processes. Toxicities include neutropenia, cardiac toxicity, mucositis, alopecia, and neuropathy.

It is important for the radiation therapist to be familiar with the various chemotherapy drugs and how they interact with radiation therapy. The treatment for a breast cancer patient who has taken Adriamycin or bleomycin will be modified to take into account the synergistic effects of these drugs. Adriamycin is toxic to the heart and in combination with radiation therapy has a much greater toxic effect. The same is true for bleomycin and radiation therapy treatment to the lungs. Radiation therapy methods to minimize the toxic effects would include shielding or lowering the total dose.

 Some chemotherapy drugs can enhance the effects of radiation by increasing cellular sensitivity.

Chemotherapy Principles

Chemotherapy is used as a primary treatment and in combination with surgery and radiation therapy. Surgery is performed in an attempt to remove as much of the tumor as

Table 1-5	Concomitant Chemoradiotherapeutic Regimens	
Disease Site	**Chemotherapy**	**Radiation Therapy**
Anus	5-Fluorouracil (5-FU) 1000 mg/m^2 96-hr infusion in weeks 1 and 4; mitomycin C 10 mg first day of radiation therapy	4500 cGy in 4-5 weeks followed by perineal boost of 1500 cGy
Bladder	5-FU 1000 mg/m^2/day for 4 days in weeks 1 and 3; Cisplatin 25 mg/m^2/day in weeks 1 and 5	4000-6000 cGy in 5 weeks 4140 cGy in 4-5 weeks to whole pelvis plus 1000 cGy boost to bladder
Esophagus	5-FU 1000 mg/m^2 infusion plus mitomycin 10 mg/m^2 and/or cisplatin 75 mg/m^2 bolus	3000 cGy in 3 weeks to 6000 cGy in 6 weeks
Head and neck	5-FU 1000 mg/m^2 infusion plus mitomycin 10 mg/m^2 and/or cisplatin 60 mg/m^2 bolus	Hyperfractionated 125 cGy dose/twice daily; total dose of 6000-7200 cGy
Hodgkin's	Combination: nitrogen mustard, Oncovin, prednisone, procarbozine/Adriamycin, bleomycin, vinblastine, and dacarbazine	4000-4400 cGy over 4 weeks
Pancreas	Combination: 5-FU, mitomycin, and streptozocin infusion	4000-6000 cGy of split-course therapy
Rectal	Combination: 5-FU, lomustine, and mitomycin	4000-4700 cGy in 26 or 27 fractions
Non–small cell lung	Combination: cisplatin, carboplatin, etoposide, ifosfamide, and vincristine	Hyperfractionated 6000 cGy over 6 weeks

possible, decreasing the number of tumor cells. Chemotherapy drugs are then administered to eliminate the residual tumor cells at the primary site and those that are circulating throughout the body. In combination with radiation therapy, chemotherapeutic agents, such as doxorubicin, often act as **radiosensitizers** and increase the effects of treatment (Table 1-5). **Radioprotector** chemotherapeutic agents such as amifostine limit the effect of the radiation on the normal cells, decreasing treatment side effects.

Although single-agent chemotherapy is used occasionally, a combination of drugs is more often administered (Table 1-6). Each of the drugs selected for a particular treatment will have a known effect on the specific tumor treated. With **combination chemotherapy**, the physician can select drugs that act on the cell during different phases of the cell cycle, increasing the cell-killing potential. In addition, drugs with different known toxicities are used for maximum effectiveness, resulting in fewer side effects.

Table 1-6	Combination Chemotherapeutic Regimens	
Disease Site	**Drugs**	
Acute lymphocytic leukemia (induction)	Asparaginase, vincristine, prednisone, and daunorubicin	
Acute myelogenous leukemia (postinduction)	High-dose cytarabine, etoposide, and idarubicin	
Brain	PLV—Procarbazine, lomustine, and vincristine	
Breast	CAFVP—Cyclophosphamide, Adriamycin, 5-FU, vinblastine, and prednisone CMF—Cyclophosphamide, methotrexate, and 5-FU FUVAC—5-FU, vinblastine, Adriamycin, and cyclophosphamide	
Colorectal		
Adjuvant	5-FU and levamisole	
Metastatic	5-FU and leucovorin	
Hepatic metastases	Floxuridine and mitomycin (intraarterial)	
Ewing's sarcoma	CAV—Cyclophosphamide, Adriamycin, vincristine, and dactinomycin	
Hodgkin's	ABVD—Adriamycin, bleomycin, vinblastine, and dacarbazine MOPP—Nitrogen mustard, Oncovin, prednisone, and procarbazine	
Kaposi's sarcoma	ABV—Adriamycin, bleomycin, and vincristine	
Lung	ACE—Adriamycin, cyclophosphamide, and etoposide ICE—Ifosfamide, cylophosphamide, and etoposide CAV—Cyclophosphamide, Adriamycin, and vincristine CEP—Cyclophosphamide, etoposide, and cisplatin	
Lymphoma	CHOP-Bleo—Cylophosphamide, adriamycin, Oncovin, prednisome, and bleomycin PROMACE-CytaBOM—Prednisone, Oncovin, methotrexate, adriamycin, cyclophosphamide, etoposide, cytarabine, bleomycin, leucovorin, dexamethasone, and trimethoprim sulfa	
Myeloma	VAD—Vincristine, Adriamycin, and dexamethasone	
Testicular	VBP—Vinblastine, bleomycin, and cisplatin VPV-VP-16—Etoposide, cisplatin, and vinblastine	

Chemotherapeutic agents are being developed that target the specific cancer cell. Rather than acting on all cells, these drugs are aimed at the molecular differences that are found between the normal cells and the malignant cell.[2] These exciting agents have the potential of maximizing tumor cell kill while producing minimal long-term side effects.

Immunotherapy

Still in its infancy, immunotherapy carries great hope for the future. The goal of **immunotherapy** is to amplify the body's own disease-fighting system to destroy the cancer.

Cells at the forefront of the immune system are B, T, and natural killer cell lymphocytes. B cells produce the protein molecules or antibodies that circulate throughout the body, attacking and destroying foreign substances such as cancer. T cells, in response to contact with antigens found on the surface of a foreign substance, mature into killer cells that directly attack and destroy the foreign substance. Natural killer cells have the ability to spontaneously attack and destroy foreign substances.

Immunotherapy uses this knowledge to boost the naturally occurring defense mechanisms of the body. Monoclonal antibodies, for example, are produced to react to a specific antigen. The patient is given the monoclonal antibodies that seek out and destroy the specific antigen found on the surface of the tumor cells. Studies are also being conducted in which a cytotoxic agent is tagged to the antibody, so when the antibody attacks the antigen, additional cell kill occurs. Similarly, vaccines are available for specific tumors that boost the body's own immune response toward a specific tumor antigen.

Interferons are naturally occurring body proteins capable of killing or slowing the growth of cancer cells. Interferons administered to a patient can enhance the cytotoxic activity of the immune system and provide a means to make tumor cell antigens more easily identified by the immune system. Interleukin-2 is a growth factor that stimulates an increase in the number of lymphocytes, especially mature killer cells.

Although these three forms of immunotherapy are being used and researched, many other areas are currently under investigation.

PROGNOSIS

A **prognosis** is an estimation of the life expectancy of a cancer patient based on all the information obtained about the tumor and from clinical trials. A prognosis is, however, only an estimate. The duration of a person's life is a mystery, and thousands of cancer patients have outlived or underlived their estimated life expectancy.

Prognostic determination does not take into account the patient's mental attitude, which has an enormous impact on disease survivability.

Prognosis plays a role in the treatment plan. If a patient has a prognosis of 2 months, treatment is given in a manner such that the patient has the maximum time allowable to spend with family and friends. In this situation, a treatment lasting 7 weeks would likely be more intrusive than helpful. The goal of treatment is to eradicate the tumor or provide palliation while preserving quality of life for the patient. The prognosis provides the information to ensure that this goal is accomplished.

For patients and their families, this information provides a timeline to accomplish tasks or goals in preparation for impending death. This may include making a will, taking a long-awaited trip, and gathering family members from across the country. A patient's mental attitude plays an important role in the prognosis but is not a factor usually considered.

Factors specific to each tumor determine the prognosis. The **natural history** (the normal progression of a tumor without treatment) provides information about the tumor behavior. For example, some tumors grow slowly and cause the host few problems until late in the disease process, whereas other tumors grow rapidly and spread to distant sites at an early stage of tumor development. Generally, slow-growing tumors are associated with better prognoses than are tumors that have already metastasized at the time of presentation. Natural history information is also valuable in determining the most effective treatment for the patient, thus affecting the prognosis. For example, Hodgkin's disease has a systematic pattern of spread through the lymphatics. Therefore, radiation treatment of early-stage Hodgkin's disease may include the known area of involvement plus the next level of lymph nodes. With this information, the patient has a better chance for cure and a more favorable prognosis.

The method of treatment also determines the prognosis based on information obtained through clinical trials. As more effective treatment is delivered, the prognosis improves. As stated earlier, cancer demands a multidisciplinary approach to treatment. Finding the most effective combination of treatments has a profound effect on the prognosis.

Patterns of Spread

Growth characteristics and spread patterns of a tumor have important prognostic implications. Tumors that tend to remain localized are more easily treated and thus generally have a better prognosis than do those that are diffuse or spread to distant sites early in the development of the malignancy.

Tumors that are **exophytic**, or grow outward, have better prognoses than do those that invade and ulcerate underlying tissues because of the communication with blood vessels and lymphatics, which are the highways of cancer cell transport to distant sites. **Multicentric** tumors, or tumors that have more than one focus of disease, can be more difficult to treat because the volume of tissue required for treatment is larger to encompass the entire organ or region. In addition, detecting all the tumor foci that may be at different stages in the development process is difficult.

Tumor dissemination, or spread, can be accomplished through the blood, lymphatics, and seeding. Tumor cells invading blood or lymph vessels can be transported to distant sites in the body. The mechanisms responsible for these cells taking root and growing in one area and not another are not clear. However, many tumors have a propensity to spread to specific sites.

Prostate cancer commonly metastasizes to the bones. For this reason, a bone scan is included in the workup if evidence exists that metastasis has already occurred at the time of diagnosis. In addition, when the primary tumor is unknown and the

Table 1-7	Common Metastatic Sites of Primary Tumors
Primary Site	**Common Metastatic Sites**
Lung	Liver, adrenal glands, bone, and brain
Breast	Lungs, bone, and brain
Stomach	Liver
Anus	Liver and lungs
Bladder	Lungs, bone, and liver
Prostate	Bone, liver, and lungs
Uterine cervix	Lungs, bone, and liver

patient presents with metastatic disease, the sites of the metastasis give a clue about the primary tumor's location. Table 1-7 lists metastatic sites associated with common primary sites.

Tumor cells may also disseminate through seeding. Cells break off from the primary tumor and spread to new sites, where they grow. Ovarian cancer cells often spread to the abdominal cavity by this method, which is the reason that the staging laparotomy is an important diagnostic and staging tool. Cells from a medulloblastoma of the brain often seed into the spinal canal by means of the cerebrospinal fluid, thus necessitating the treatment of the spinal cord and brain.

Prognostic Factors

For each tumor, specific prognostic factors are based on the cellular and behavioral characteristics, tumor site, and patient-related factors. Determination of prognostic factors is made through clinical trials in which factors related to the disease and patient are statistically analyzed for a group of patients. With this method, factors that have the greatest influence on prognosis are determined.

Tumor-related factors that are often of prognostic significance include grade, stage, tumor size, status of lymph nodes, depth of invasion, and histology. Patient-related prognostic factors include age, gender, race, and medical condition. Each factor displays a different level of importance in specific tumors. For example, the main prognostic indicator for breast cancer is the status of the axillary lymph nodes, whereas for a soft tissue sarcoma, it is histologic grade.

CLINICAL TRIALS

Much of the progress made in the management of cancer is the result of carefully planned clinical trials. This type of research can be conducted at a single clinical site or in collaboration with many institutions. The advantage of collaboration is that a greater number of patients can participate in the study, thus increasing the significance of the results. Because cancer management is multidisciplinary, clinical trials are often a collaborative effort among disciplines. Research methodology for clinical trials can be accomplished through retrospective or prospective studies that examine randomized or nonrandomized samples of the population to be studied.

 Clinical trials provide research-based evidence about specific treatment effectiveness. It is through these trials that the most effective treatment with the fewest long-term side effects can be achieved.

Retrospective Studies

Studies that review information from a group of patients treated in the past are retrospective. The treatment has already been delivered, and the information is collected (often on a national basis) and analyzed. **Retrospective studies** have an advantage in that the information can be obtained rather quickly; the investigator does not have to wait years to see the results of a particular treatment. However, a number of drawbacks are apparent with retrospective studies and can lead to errors. Complete information about a treatment is not always easy to obtain and is often incomplete. Outside factors that may have influenced the treatment and results are not controlled and may not be accurately documented.

Prospective Studies

A clinical trial that is planned before treatment, with eligibility criteria for patient selection, is a **prospective study**. Investigators have the advantage of knowing the information that is essential to the study, thus leading to more complete and accurate documentation. In addition, better control of external factors that might influence the results of the study is possible. A disadvantage of prospective studies is the length of time needed to observe the results of a particular treatment. Depending on the length of the follow-up necessary to accurately assess the results, prospective trials can last 5 years or longer. The lung cancer screening study is an example of a prospective study.

Studies that examine the effectiveness of treatment are classified by the study objectives. **Phase I studies** are used to determine the maximum tolerance dose for a specific treatment. The end point can be either acute or long-term toxicity. **Phase II studies** are used to determine whether the Phase I treatment is significantly effective—given the acute and/or long-term side effects—to continue further study. **Phase III studies** are used to compare the experimental treatment with standard treatment using a randomized sample.

Randomized Studies

Clinical studies often include several methods of treatment to determine which method results in the best outcome. After meeting all eligibility requirements for the study, patients are randomly selected for one of the treatment arms. The purpose of randomization is to eliminate any unintentional "stacking of the deck" and increase the accuracy of results and conclusions. Although patients may have the same type, grade, stage, and extent of cancer, each person responds individually to the disease and treatment. Care providers cannot control these factors, but randomization helps minimize their effects on the end result. With randomization, each arm of the study has approximately equal numbers of individuals with varying reactions.

Survival Reporting

In the planning stages of a clinical trial, an end point must be established; otherwise, the study can continue indefinitely with no data analysis. Rates of survival at a set end point are one type of information used to determine the benefit of one treatment over another. Survival reporting, however, can be accomplished with many methods. With absolute survival reporting, patients alive at the end point and those who have died are counted.

Patients lost to follow-up are included, but the fact that patients may have died from other causes is not considered. Adjusted survival reporting includes patients who died from other causes and had **no evidence of disease (NED)** at the times of their deaths. Relative survival reporting involves the normal mortality rate of a similar group of people based on factors such as age, gender, and race.

In addition, survival reporting at the end point includes information about the status of the disease. At the end point the patient may be alive with NED, disease free, or alive with disease. Of equal importance is the information about treatment failures. Treatment failures are classified as local, locoregional, or distant and are based on tumor recurrences at the primary or nearby lymph node sites or metastatic disease. This information is valuable for ongoing clinical trials and for determining types of treatment techniques to prevent future failures.

THE RADIATION ONCOLOGY TEAM

The effectiveness of patient care and treatment is dependent on the teamwork of individuals in the entire radiation therapy department, the patient, and related medical professionals. From the receptionist to the physician, each individual has an important role in the goal of treating the person with cancer (Figure 1-8). The radiation oncologist has the overall responsibility for the patient's care and treatment. The patient is an important member of the team and works in collaboration by complying with treatment requirements and letting team members know the individual effects of treatment. The patient also brings into the treatment their family and support system that influence the treatment outcome. Community and national cancer support resources play a role in providing information and possible financial or emotional support following the cancer diagnosis. The support that is provided by these sources is important in the overall emotional and psychosocial wellness of the patient.

Each member of the radiation therapy team, under the direction of the oncologist, is essential in providing the most effective patient care and treatment. Team members work together collaboratively to share their expertise and contribute their abilities to the treatment process. Every day in every department, each of the radiation therapy team members has the opportunity to improve the quality of life for the cancer patient and his or her family. It may be answering a question, referring the patient to a support group, or giving a family member a hug. Each of these small actions has the potential to have a huge positive effect on the patient and his or her family.

When a patient enters the radiation therapy department, the first person he or she interacts with is the receptionist or secretary. Before the patient's arrival, this individual is involved in obtaining the patient's medical records and diagnostic images. The receptionist obtains insurance and the appropriate personal information and informs the other members of the radiation therapy team that the patient has arrived. The patient is taken to the consult/examination room to talk with the **radiation oncologist**. By the time the patient is in the examination room, the physician has become very familiar with the patient's medical history by talking with the patient's primary physician and reviewing all of the medical records. The physician reviews the medical findings with the patient and discusses treatment options that are available. The physician and patient will discuss the benefits of radiation therapy and the possible side effects. By the end of the consult and examination, the physician will have a treatment plan in mind and the patient will be sent on for treatment planning and/or simulation. A **medical dosimetrist** is responsible for designing the patient's treatment to accomplish the physician's prescription using the most effective techniques possible. A medical dosimetrist is often a radiation therapist who has had additional education but may also be an individual with a physics or medical physics background. The medical dosimetrist will work collaboratively with a **medical physicist**. The medical physicist is responsible for quality assurance of all radiotherapeutic equipment from acceptance testing and commissioning of new equipment to regularly scheduled calibration and testing of equipment already in the department. The medical physicist oversees all treatment planning and radiation safety programs and is involved with clinical physics procedures.

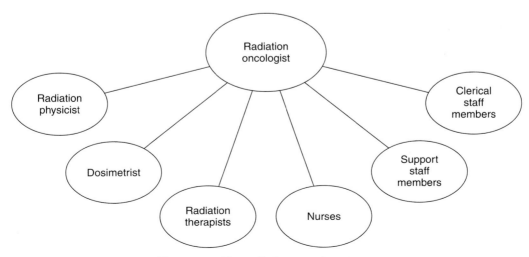

Figure 1-8. The radiation oncology team.

Before treatment, the patient will undergo a **simulation** or a procedure designed to delineate the treatment fields and construct any necessary immobilization or treatment devices. During a simulation, the **radiation therapist** is able to explain the simulation and treatment procedures and answer any questions the patient may have. Simulation provides an excellent time to assess the patient's medical condition and educational and support needs. Once the physician has approved of the treatment plan and simulation, the patient goes to the treatment machine. Depending on the purpose of treatment, the patient may be scheduled for 1 to 7 weeks of treatment. During treatment, the radiation oncologist generally sees the patient once a week to ensure that the treatment is progressing as expected. The radiation therapist sees the patient every day and is responsible for assessing the patient's reaction to treatment and the general medical condition. Radiation therapists and department nurses educate the patient about skin care, nutrition, and support services and provide appropriate referrals as necessary. Once the radiation therapy prescription has been completed, the patient will be scheduled for a follow-up appointment. The radiation oncologist may see the patient in follow-up for many years, or the primary physician may follow the patient.

Depending on the size of the department, the team may be very small or very large. In a small outpatient facility, the team may consist of a physician, radiation therapist, receptionist, and part-time physicist (see Figure 1-8). The role of the team members in this scenario is vastly different from that of the members in a large department with multiple physicians, treatment and simulation radiation therapists, medical dosimetrists, physicists, nurses, and clerical and support staff. Generally, as the department grows larger, the job description of the team members becomes more specific. In a large department, a radiation therapist's role may be limited to the actual treatment, and another radiation therapist is responsible for simulations. The role of the radiation therapist in dosimetry might be limited to treatment planning, calculations, and quality assurance procedures. In a large department, the role of the physician may also be limited to one area of expertise. For example, one physician might treat only those patients with head and neck tumors. In a small department, however, the radiation therapist's role will include treatment, simulation, treatment planning, patient care, and quality assurance. For the radiation therapist, there are opportunities for working in a number of different clinical sites, from free-standing clinics to university medical centers. Each center offers different opportunities and challenges for the radiation therapist who is willing to continue to learn and grow.

As an individual who is interested in joining the radiation therapy team, it is important to learn and understand as much as possible about all aspects of radiation therapy. It is not enough to "study for the exam," because the important examinations do not happen in the classroom but rather in the clinic, with real patients. Cancer patients deserve no less than the best that the radiation therapy team members have to offer.

SUMMARY

- Cancer has been studied for centuries and there is still much to be learned.

- Cancer occurs when normal cellular proliferation mechanisms break down.
- Cells that are rapidly dividing are more responsive to the effects of radiation and chemotherapy.
- Tumors are classified by their anatomic site, cell of origin, and biologic behavior.
- Benign tumors are generally well differentiated and do not harm the patient.
- Malignant tumors may be well differentiated to undifferentiated, may grow rapidly or very slowly, often metastasize, and invade surrounding tissues.
- Tumors are generally named for the tissue in which they arise.
- Remember that the patient has a life outside of the cancer diagnosis. His or her past, cultural mores, religious beliefs, and other factors will influence all aspects of the treatment trajectory.
- Patient support resources are available at local, regional, state, and national levels. Radiation therapists should be aware of these resources to better meet the needs of their patients.
- The stage of cancer defines the extent of the disease and is determined by the type of tumor.
- The grade of a tumor is determined following examination under a microscope and determines how aggressive a tumor will be.
- A multidiscipline approach to cancer treatment is essential. Working together, physicians from all disciplines develop treatment plans that best treat the cancer and preserve the quality of life for the patient.
- Clinical trials are important in gaining information regarding the effectiveness of treatment modalities and methods. This research furthers the knowledge base in the treatment of cancer.
- The radiation team encompasses those in the radiotherapy department and those associated with the patient and other health care providers. Communication and teamwork assist in providing the patient the best treatment and treatment experience possible.
- The radiation therapist has the ability to have a monumental and positive impact on each of the patients treated. This opportunity comes through accurate treatment, positive and engaging attitude, and genuine caring for patients.

Review Questions

1. How would a theory of cancer as an initially diffuse disease affect the treatment and outcome?
2. What are the characteristics of benign and malignant cells?
3. What would a primary tumor of the bone be called?
4. What would a tumor arising from cells lining the oral cavity be called?
5. What are the roles surgery plays in the overall management and treatment of cancer?
6. What is the role of radiation therapy in the treatment of cancer?
7. What is the role of chemotherapy in the treatment of cancer?
8. What is the difference between etiology and epidemiology?

9. What roles does the radiation therapist play in patient care and treatment?

The answers to the Review Questions can be found by logging on to our website at: *http://evolve.elsevier.com/Washington+Leaver/principles*

Questions to Ponder

1. What cancer patient resources are available in the hospital in which you work? What resources are available in your community?
2. Mr. Jones has a T2 tumor of the larynx, and Mrs. Smith has a T4 tumor of the larynx. What differences would you expect to see in the tumors and in the treatment plans for each of these patients?
3. What effects have etiology and epidemiology had on cigarette smoking?
4. How does a prognosis help or hinder a physician, care provider, or patient?
5. Analyze a clinical trial taking place in the hospital in which you work. What type of research is being done?
6. Discuss the process of carcinogenesis.
7. An 8-year-old child comes to your department for treatment. What factors need to be taken into account when scheduling an appointment?

REFERENCES

1. American Cancer Society: *Cancer facts and figures 2008* (website): http://www.cancer.org. Accessed October 2008.
2. Bunn PA: *New targeted therapies for lung cancer* (website): http://www.medscape.com in *Medscape-Hematology-Oncology eJournal.* Accessed August 20, 2002.
3. Cooper MR, Cooper MR: Systemic therapy. In Lenhard RE, Osteen RT, Gansler T, editors: *Clinical oncology,* Atlanta, 2001, The American Society.
4. Crowley LV: *An introduction to human disease: pathology and pathophysiology correlations,* ed 7, Boston, 2007, Jones & Bartlett.
5. Henshaw EC: The biology of cancer. In Rubin P, editor: *Clinical oncology: a multidisciplinary approach for physicians and students,* ed 7, Philadelphia, 1993, WB Saunders.
6. Kardinal CG, Strnad BN: Confrontation with cancer: historical and existential aspects. In Gross SC, Garb S, editors: *Cancer treatment and research in humanistic perspective,* New York, 1985, Springer Publishing.
7. National Cancer Institute National Lung Screening Trial: Questions and Answers (website): http://www.cancer.gov/news/center/NLSTQ. Accessed October 2008.
8. Raven RW: The development and practice of oncology. In Gross SC, Garb S, editors: *Cancer treatment and research in humanistic perspective,* New York, 1985, Springer Publishing.
9. Shagam JY: Principles of chemotherapy, *Radiat Therapist* 10:37-53, 2001.
10. Skeel RT: *Handbook of cancer chemotherapy,* ed 7, Philadelphia, 2007, Lippincott Williams & Wilkins.
11. Solomon E, Borrow J, Goddard AD: Chromosome aberrations and cancer, *Science* 254:1153-1159, 1991.
12. Weinberg RA: Tumor suppressor genes, *Science* 254:1138-1145, 1991.
13. Yunis JJ: The chromosomal basis of human neoplasia, *Science* 221:227-235, 1983.

BIBLIOGRAPHY

Aaronson SA: Growth factors and cancer, *Science* 254:1146-1152, 1991.

McCune CS, Chang AY: Basic concepts of tumor immunology and principles of immunotherapy. In Rubin P, editor: *Clinical oncology: a multidisciplinary approach for physicians and students,* ed 7, Philadelphia, 1993, WB Saunders.

Pajak T: Methodology of clinical trials. In Perez C, Brady L, editors: *Principles and practice of radiation oncology,* ed 2, Philadelphia, 1992, JB Lippincott.

Perez C, Brady L: Overview. In Perez C, Brady L, editors: *Principles and practice of radiation oncology,* ed 3, Philadelphia, 1998, JB Lippincott.

Ruben P, McDonald S, Keller J: Staging and classification of cancer: a unified approach. In Perez C, Brady L, editors: *Principles and practice of radiation oncology,* ed 4, Philadelphia, 2004, JB Lippincott.

Weiss DW: Immunological intervention in neoplasia. In Beers RF, Tilghman RC, Bassett EG, editors: *The role of immunological factors in viral and oncogenic processes. Seventh international symposium,* Baltimore, 1974, Johns Hopkins University Press.

The Ethics and Legal Considerations of Cancer Management

Bettye G. Wilson

Outline

Objectives

- List and define the terminology associated with the ethics and legal consideration of cancer management.
- Discuss the traditional ethical theories and models.
- Define *patient autonomy* and *informed consent*.
- Discuss advance directives.
- Differentiate between the types of living wills.
- Evaluate the patient care partnership to determine the scope of patient rights included therein.
- Explain how informed consent and patient autonomy are related.
- Recognize the role of the health care team in patient confidentiality.
- Apply HIPAA compliance standards in the clinical setting.
- Identify the stages of grief.
- Support dying patients and their families.
- Quote the legal doctrines applicable to patient care.
- Examine the role of risk management.
- Discuss medical records, their content, confidentiality of, and electronic record vulnerability.
- Determine the role of the Standards of Ethics and Practice Standards on the practice of radiation therapy.

Key Terms

Advance directives
Analytical model
Assault
Autonomy
Battery
Beneficence
Civil law
Code of Ethics
Collegial model
Confidentiality
Consequentialism
Contractual model
Covenant model
Deontology
Doctrine of foreseeability
Doctrine of personal liability
Doctrine of *res ipsa loquitur*
Doctrine of *respondeat superior*
Durable power of attorney for health care
Engineering model
Ethics
False imprisonment
Incident
Informed consent
Invasion of privacy
Justice
Laws
Legal concepts
Legal ethics
Libel
Living will
Medical record
Moral ethics
Negligence
Nonconsequentialism
Nonmaleficence
Practice standards
Priestly model
Risk management
Role fidelity
Scope of practice
Slander
Teleology
Tort law
Values
Veracity
Virtue ethics

A diagnosis of cancer is one of, if not the most, feared diagnoses any patient can receive. Although numerous advancements have been made in the treatment of these diseases, and there are many survivors, it is general knowledge that a cancer diagnosis is a life-altering event. Whether surgery, medical oncology, radiation oncology, or any combination of the three is used to treat the disease, patients often feel that they have little real control over the outcome. They are also acutely aware of the potential morbidity associated with treatment measures. One cancer patient may have summed up the experience of being diagnosed with cancer in a recent newspaper column she wrote about the event: "We cancer patients tend to recall our diagnosis day with the kind of clarity that comes with any catastrophic event. 'I'm sorry, but …,' the oncologist begins. Your heart races, or maybe it seems to stop. Your hands sweat. The noise of blood coursing through your veins deafens you to everything but the doctor's voice: 'You have cancer.' Just as most Americans can tell you where they were when JFK was shot or the twin towers fell, so can we recall, in often minute detail, that moment when our world stood still."[11]

A diagnosis of cancer changes a person's life in ways many can only imagine. Although the diagnosis does not mean that the disease is terminal, it is certainly bad news and a negative event. Dr. Elisabeth Kübler-Ross is perhaps the best known authority on the subject of dealing with those experiencing forms of grief. In her studies on people with terminal illnesses, she found that the emotional cycle experienced by those with terminal illnesses was not unique to them but is also found in those experiencing things they perceive as having a negative effect on their lives.[12] A diagnosis of cancer certainly fits the bill. The quest to beat the disease begins with personal courage and fortitude and with extensive involvement of dedicated health care professionals. Those who care for and treat cancer patients must understand their obligations as professionals. Not only must they care for and treat the patients, they must also deal with the emotions of the patients' families and other health care professionals. There are also legal issues that must be addressed and sometimes avoided, as will be discussed later in the chapter.

THE CASE FOR ETHICS IN RADIATION THERAPY

Every aspect of the world of health care is fast paced and ever changing, and radiation therapy is no exception. To provide quality patient care in this fast-paced dynamic world, all health care providers must keep abreast of the latest treatment developments and technological advancements. In addition, all must be well versed in the ethical and legal considerations of cancer management. Radiation therapists and radiation therapy students deal with patients who have specific needs related to their attempts to control catastrophic diseases that are taking over their lives and the lives of those close to them. Defining the roles and responsibilities of the radiation therapy student, the practicing radiation therapist, and other members of the radiation oncology team, as they care for their patients, is extremely important. In addition to developing the technical skills necessary to practice in the profession, members of the radiation oncology team must develop an understanding of the basic theories regarding ethics, patients' rights, and the scope of practice and code of ethics for radiation therapy. The medical-legal aspects of informed consent, record keeping, and confidentiality are also important.

Radiation therapists and medical imaging technologists are credentialed by the American Registry of Radiologic Technologists (ARRT). The ARRT uses the terms "Registered Technologists (RT) and Registered Radiologist Assistants (RRA)" to describe those certified under its umbrella. Upon certification, individuals may use the initials RT followed by the initial(s) designating their area(s) of certification. In radiation therapy, this would be RT(T) ARRT. The primary professional membership organization for those credentialed by the ARRT is the American Society of Radiologic Technologists (ASRT). The ASRT developed a code of ethics to guide radiation therapy students on elements of the field as they develop their knowledge and skills and to guide practicing radiation therapists in their professional conduct (Box 2-1). However, the Code of Ethics for Radiation Therapists does not list all principles and rules by which radiation therapists are governed. The ARRT developed a mission-based, more comprehensive document called the Standards of Ethics.[3] This document is published and enforced by the ARRT. The Standards of Ethics are applicable to individuals who are certified through the ARRT and are either currently registered or were previously. The Standards of Ethics also apply to applicants for ARRT examinations and certifications. The document is composed of a preamble and three parts or sections: Section A is the Code of Ethics, Section B contains the Rules of Ethics, and Section C describes the Administrative Procedures followed by the ARRT when an individual is accused of violating the Code as related to the established rules.

Box 2-1 **Code of Ethics for Radiation Therapists**

- The radiation therapist advances the principal objective of the profession to provide services to humanity with full respect for the dignity of mankind.
- The radiation therapist delivers patient care and service unrestricted by concerns of personal attributes or the nature of the disease or illness and nondiscriminatory with respect to race, color, creed, sex, age, disability, or national origin.
- The radiation therapist assesses situations; exercises care, discretion, and judgment; assumes responsibility for professional decisions; and acts in the best interest of the patient.
- The radiation therapist adheres to the tenets and domains of the scope of practice for radiation therapists.
- The radiation therapist actively engages in lifelong learning to maintain, improve, and enhance professional competence and knowledge.

The ARRT Code of Ethics contains 10 guiding principles (Box 2-2). As stated at the beginning of the code, "The Code of Ethics shall serve as a guide by which Registered Technologists and Candidates may evaluate their professional conduct as it relates to patients, health care consumers, employers, colleagues, and other members of the health care team."[6] This is quite a powerful and comprehensive statement. It is so inclusive that it seems be a guide as to how RTs and candidates should behave around everyone. Isn't everyone a potential consumer? Does this statement mean that professional behaviors extend into off-the-job activities? The answer to both of these questions is "yes." But it must be remembered that the Code of Ethics is aspirational, which simply means that the principles of the code are those to which the ARRT hopes RTs and candidates will aspire to or seek to achieve. On the other hand, mandatory rules do exist, in the second part or section of the Standards of Ethics. Appropriately, these rules are titled the Rules of Ethics. There are currently 22 Rules of Ethics (Box 2-3). These are true rules governing the professional behaviors of RTs, RRAs, and candidates for ARRT certification. The Rules of Ethics are not aspirational; they are enforceable. Those found in violation of the ARRT Rules of Ethics are subject to sanctions ranging from private reprimand to the most dreaded sanction of all—permanent revocation of certification. The rules not only cover activities in which an RT, an RRA, or a candidate might personally engage; they also cover activities of which individuals might be aware, although not personally involved in, but permit the activity to occur. A thorough examination and understanding of the ARRT Standards of Ethics must be an integral part of education in radiation therapy and imaging sciences. Students, especially those with questionable criminal activity in their background, unless the matter was adjudicated in juvenile court, should be encouraged to submit a preapplication for ARRT certification at least 6 months prior to graduation from their educational program. By doing so, their past criminal

The Code of Ethics is the first part of the Standards of Ethics. The Code of Ethics shall serve as a guide by which Registered Technologists and Candidates may evaluate their professional conduct as it relates to patients, health care consumers, employers, colleagues, and other members of the health care team. The Code of Ethics is intended to assist Registered Technologists and Candidates in maintaining a high level of ethical conduct and in providing for the protection, safety, and comfort of patients. The Code of Ethics is aspirational.

1. The radiologic technologist conducts herself or himself in a professional manner, responds to patient needs, and supports colleagues and associates in providing quality patient care.
2. The radiologic technologist acts to advance the principal objective of the profession to provide services to humanity with full respect for the dignity of mankind.
3. The radiologic technologist delivers patient care and service unrestricted by the concerns of personal attributes or the nature of the disease or illness, and without discrimination on the basis of sex, race, creed, religion, or socioeconomic status.
4. The radiologic technologist practices technology founded upon theoretical knowledge and concepts, uses equipment and accessories consistent with the purposes for which they were designed, and employs procedures and techniques appropriately.
5. The radiologic technologist assesses situations; exercises care, discretion, and judgment; assumes responsibility for professional decisions; and acts in the best interest of the patient.
6. The radiologic technologist acts as an agent through observation and communication to obtain pertinent information for the physician to aid in the diagnosis and treatment of the patient and recognizes that interpretation and diagnosis are outside of the scope of practice for the profession.
7. The radiologic technologist uses equipment and accessories, employs techniques and procedures, performs services in accordance with an accepted standard of practice, and demonstrates expertise in minimizing radiation exposure to the patient, self, and other members of the health care team.
8. The radiologic technologist practices ethical conduct appropriate to the profession and protects the patient's right to quality radiologic technology care.
9. The radiologic technologist respects confidences entrusted in the course of professional practice, respects the patient's right to privacy, and reveals confidential information only as required by the law or to protect the welfare of the individual or the community.
10. The radiologic technologist continually strives to improve knowledge and skills by participating in continuing education and professional activities, sharing knowledge with colleagues, and investigating new aspects of professional practice.

activity may be examined by the ARRT Ethics Staff and/or the ARRT Ethics Committee in the determination of whether the individual has violated the Rules of Ethics and whether he or she is eligible or ineligible for ARRT certification. The names of individuals sanctioned by the ARRT are published in the *Annual Report to Technologists* and may also be found on the ARRT website.

Any professional code of ethics serves two major functions: education and regulation. It educates persons in the profession who do not reflect on ethical implications of their actions unless something concrete is before them. It also educates other professionals and the general public regarding the ethical standards expected of a given profession.[24] Professional codes of conduct should accomplish several objectives: (1) describe the values held by the profession, (2) impose obligations on practitioners to accept the values and practices included within the code, and (3) hold professionals libel for adherence to those obligations with possible penalties for nonconformance.[26] It is an obligation of any profession to society to assist in the development of social attitudes and policies that govern not only the operation of the profession but also the expectations of the public.[6] Understanding ethical concepts and legal issues and developing interpersonal skills, through the study of the material in this chapter, should enable students and practicing radiation therapists to care for their patients humanely and compassionately while adhering to the professional code of ethics. After all, it is not just the cancer that is being cared for and treated—it is the patient.

ETHICAL ASPECTS OF CANCER MANAGEMENT
Definitions and Terminology

Webster's New Collegiate Dictionary[25] defines **ethics** as "(1) the discipline dealing with what is good and bad, moral duty, and obligation; (2) a set of moral principles or values; (3) a theory or system of moral values; and (4) the principles of conduct governing an individual or a group." Ethics for an individual derive from the person's values. There are four main sources of values: culture, experience, religion, and science.[26] Individuals gather an understanding of right and wrong from the cumulative experiences of life and develop patterns of approaching situations in which the complexities of right and wrong must be addressed.[27]

 Ethics are based on values.

In the study of ethics, a person must distinguish between **moral** and **legal ethics**. Morality has to do with conscience. It is a person's concept of right or wrong as it relates to conscience, God, a higher being, or a person's logical rationalization. *Morality* can be defined as fidelity to conscience. **Legal concepts** are defined as the sum of rules and regulations by which society is governed in any formal and legally binding manner. The law mandates certain acts and forbids other acts under penalties of criminal sanction. **Laws**, the foundation of which is ethics, are primarily concerned with the good of a society as a functioning unit.[7, 26]

 The foundation of law is ethics.

Box 2-3	Rules of Ethics

The Rules of Ethics form the second part of the Standards of Ethics. They are mandatory standards of minimally acceptable professional conduct for all present Registered Technologists, Registered Radiologist Assistants, and Candidates. Certification is a method of assuring the medical community and the public that an individual is qualified to practice within the profession. Because the public relies on certificates and registrations issued by the ARRT, it is essential that Registered Technologists and Candidates act consistently with these Rules of Ethics. These Rules of Ethics are intended to promote the protection, safety, and comfort of patients. The Rules of Ethics are enforceable. Registered Technologists, Registered Radiologist Assistants, and Candidates engaging on any of the following conduct or activities, or who permit the occurrence of the following conduct or activities with respect to them, have violated the Rules of Ethics and are subject to sanctions described hereunder.

1. Employing fraud or deceit in procuring or attempting to procure, maintain, renew, or obtain: reinstatement of certification or registration as issued by ARRT; employment in radiologic technology; or a state permit, license, or registration certificate to practice radiologic technology. This includes altering in any respect any document issued by the ARRT or any state or federal agency, or by indicating in writing certification or registration with the ARRT when that is not the case.

2. Subverting or attempting to subvert ARRT's examination process. Conduct that subverts or attempts to subvert ARRT's examination process includes, but is not limited to:
    (i) conduct that violates the security of ARRT examination materials, such as removing or attempting to remove examination materials from an examination room, or having unauthorized possession of any portion of or information concerning the future, current, or previously administered examination of ARRT; or disclosing what purports to be, or under all circumstances is likely to be understood by the recipient as, any portion of or "inside" information concerning any portion of a future, current, or previously administered examination of the ARRT;
    (ii) conduct that in any way compromises ordinary standards of test administration, such as communicating with another Candidate during administration of the examination, copying another Candidate's answers, permitting another Candidate to copy one's answers, or possessing unauthorized material; or
    (iii) impersonating a Candidate or permitting an impersonator to take the examination on one's own behalf.

3. Convictions, criminal proceedings, or military court-martials as described below:
    (i) Conviction of a crime including a felony, a gross misdemeanor, or a misdemeanor, with the sole exception of speeding and parking violations. All alcohol and/or drug related violations must be reported. Offenses that occurred while a juvenile and that are processed through the juvenile court system are not required to be reported to the ARRT.
    (ii) Criminal proceedings where finding a verdict of guilt is made or returned but the adjudication of guilt is either withheld, deferred, or not entered or the sentence is suspended or stayed; or a criminal proceeding where the individual enters a plea of guilty or nolo contendere (no contest).
    (iii) Military court-martials that involve substance abuse, any sex-related infractions, or patient-related infractions.

4. Failure to report to the ARRT that:
    (i) charges regarding the person's permit, license, or registration certificate to practice radiologic technology or any other medical or allied health profession are pending or have been resolved adversely to the individual in any state, territory, or country (including, but not limited to, imposed conditions, probation, suspension, or revocation); or
    (ii) that the individual has been refused a permit, license, or registration certificate to practice radiologic technology or any other medical or allied health profession by another state, territory, or country.

5. Failure or the inability to perform radiologic technology with reasonable skill and safety.

6. Engaging in unprofessional conduct, including, but not limited to:
    (i) a departure from or failure to conform to applicable federal, state, or local governmental rules regarding radiologic technology practice; or if no such rule exists, to the minimal standards of acceptable and prevailing radiologic technology practice;
    (ii) any radiologic technology practice that may create unnecessary danger to a patient's life, health, or safety; or
    (iii) any practice that is contrary to the ethical conduct appropriate to the profession that results in the termination from employment. Actual injury to a patient need not be established under this clause.

7. Delegating or accepting the delegation of a radiologic technology function or any other prescribed health care function when the delegation or acceptance could reasonably be expected to create an unnecessary danger to a patient's life, health, or safety. Actual injury to a patient need not be established under this clause.

8. Actual or potential inability to practice radiologic technology with reasonable skill and safety to patients by reason of illness; use of alcohol, drugs, chemicals, or any material; or as a result of any mental or physical condition.

9. Adjudication as mentally incompetent, mentally ill, a chemically dependent person, or a person dangerous to the public, by a court of competent jurisdiction.

10. Engaging in any unethical conduct, including, but not limited to, conduct likely to deceive, defraud, or harm the public; or demonstrating a willful or careless disregard for the health, welfare, or safety of a patient. Actual injury need not be established under this clause.

11. Engaging in conduct with a patient that is sexual or may reasonably be interpreted by the patient as sexual, or in any verbal behavior that is seductive or sexually demeaning to a patient; or engaging in sexual exploitation of a patient or former patient. This also applies to any unwanted sexual behavior, verbal or otherwise, that results in the termination of employment. This rule does not apply to pre-existing consensual relationships.

Continued

12. Revealing privileged communication from or relating to a former or current patient. Except when otherwise required or permitted by law.
13. Knowingly engaging or assisting a person to engage in, or otherwise participate in, abusive or fraudulent billing practices, including violations of federal Medicare and Medicaid laws or state medical assistance laws.
14. Improper management of patient records, including failure to maintain adequate patient records or to furnish a patient record or report required by law, or making, causing, or permitting anyone to make false, deceptive, or misleading entry in any patient record.
15. Knowingly aiding, assisting, advising, or allowing a person without a current and appropriate state permit, license, or registration certificate or a current certificate of registration with ARRT to engage in the practice of radiologic technology, in a jurisdiction which requires a person to have such a current and appropriate state permit, license, or registration certificate or a current and appropriate registration of certification with ARRT in order to practice radiologic technology in such jurisdiction.
16. Violating a rule adopted by any state board with competent jurisdiction, an order of such board, or state or federal law relating to the practice of radiologic technology, or any other medical or allied health professions, or a state or federal narcotics or controlled-substance law.
17. Knowingly providing false or misleading information that is directly related to the care of a former or current patient.
18. Practicing outside the scope of practice authorized by the individual's current state permit, license, or registration certificate, or the individual's current certificate of registration with ARRT.
19. Making a false statement or knowingly providing false information to ARRT or failing to cooperate with any investigation by ARRT or the Ethics Committee.
20. Engaging in false, fraudulent, deceptive, or misleading communications to any person regarding the individual's education, training, credentials, experience, or qualifications, or the status of the individual's state permit, license, or registration certificate in radiologic technology or certificate of registration with ARRT.
21. Knowing of a violation or probable violation of any Rule of Ethics by any Registered Technologist, Registered Radiologist Assistant, or Candidate and failing to promptly report in writing the same to the ARRT.
22. Failing to immediately report to his or her supervisor information concerning an error made in connection with imaging, treating, or caring for a patient. For purposes of this rule, errors include any departure from the standard of care that reasonably may be considered to be potentially harmful, unethical, or improper (commission). Errors also include behavior that is negligent or should have occurred in connection with a patient's care, but did not (omission). The duty to report under this rule exists whether or not the patient suffered any injury.

In dealing with ethical issues in cancer treatment, health care professionals should consider bioethics. *Miller-Keane Encyclopedia & Dictionary of Medicine, Nursing, & Allied Health, Sixth Edition*,[15] defines *bioethics* as the application of ethics to the bioethical sciences, medicine, nursing, and health care. It further states that the practical ethical questions raised in everyday health care are generally in the realm of bioethics. There are seven written principles associated with bioethics. Referred to as the *Principles of Biomedical Ethics,* the seven are inclusive of **autonomy**, **beneficence**, **confidentiality**, **justice**, **nonmaleficence**, **role fidelity**, and **veracity**.[4] It is generally desirable for those who practice in the health care setting to innately prescribe to the aforementioned principles. **Autonomy** emphasizes the right of patients to make decisions for themselves, free of interference by others. It also recognizes that patients are to be respected for their independence and freedom to control their own actions. Theoretically, each person should be recognized and respected for his or her social uniqueness and moral worth. In health care, this theory means that individuals should and must be respected for their abilities to make their own choices and develop their own plans for their lives.[6] **Beneficence** is defined as doing good, and calls on health care professionals to act in the best interest of patients, even when it might be inconvenient or sacrifices must be made. Palliative treatment may be considered a form of beneficence in radiation oncology because it helps relieve pain and suffering, thereby "doing good," but this can be viewed as a problem in some cases. When a patient has expressed no desire for prolongation of her or his life by any means, palliative treatment may not be viewed as a beneficent act. **Confidentiality** is the principle that relates to the knowledge that information revealed by a patient to a health care provider, or information that is learned in the course of a health care provider performing her or his duties, is private and should be held in confidence. To hold something in confidence basically means to keep it secret. A secret is information that a person has a right or an obligation to conceal. In health care, confidentiality is based on obligatory secrets, of which there are three types: natural, promised, and professional.[6] Natural secrets are those that involve information that is naturally harmful if it were to be revealed. Promised secrets are those that involve information that an individual has promised someone that they will not reveal. The professional secret is the type of secret that is of most importance in health care. Professional secrets are knowledge and information learned in the course of professional health care practice that if revealed would harm the patient, while also harming the profession and the society that depends on the profession for important care and services.[6] The obligation of health care providers to keep professional secrets is not only recognized within the frame of bioethics but also is seen as a patient right and is protected within the frame of law as well. In 1973, The American Hospital Association (AHA) constructed and adopted what became known as "A Patient's Bill of Rights." This document was further refined, revised, and copyrighted in 1992 and 1998. More recently, the document has again been revised and renamed as "The Patient Care Partnership." It is in the form of a patient brochure that is intended to provide patients with an explanation of what to expect during their stay in the hospital, and it explains their rights and responsibilities. The brochure is currently available in eight languages. The translation into multiple languages reflects the patient diversity within the health care population of the United States. The brochure contains the same tenets of "A Patient's Bill of Rights," with information included on the following patient rights and responsibilities:

- High-quality patient care
- A clean and safe environment
- Involvement in your care
- Protection of your privacy
- Help when you leave the hospital
- Help with your billing claim

As noted in the list of brochure topics above, protection of a patient's privacy is considered a patient right. The "Patient Care Partnership" is also related to other topics in ethics and will be discussed further in a later section of this chapter.

In 1996, the federal government became more involved in the regulation of health care with the passage of the Health Insurance Portability and Accountability Act (HIPAA), Public Law 104-191. Under this provision of health care law, overseen primarily by the U.S. Department of Health and Human Services (HHS), health care facilities, providers, and employees are mandated under penalty of law to publish rules to ensure (1) standardization of electronic patient administrative, financial, and health data; (2) creation of unique health identifiers for employees, health care providers, and health plans; and (3) security standards that protect the confidentiality and integrity of "individually identifiable health information," past, present, and future.[18]

All employees working in health care and students in health care educational programs are required to be trained in HIPAA regulatory requirements and compliance. At the heart of HIPAA regulations is confidentiality of health information. Confidentiality is the ethical principle that relates to all of the others.

> *Confidentiality is the ethical principle that binds all the seven bioethical principles.*

Justice is the ethical principle that relates to fairness and equal treatment for all. Essentially, the application of the bioethical principle of justice asks persons to ensure that fairness and equity are maintained among individuals.[22] Treating all patients as equals regardless of the nature of their illness, age, gender, sexual preference, socioeconomic status, religious preference, and the like is considered a form of justice. **Nonmaleficence** directs health care professionals to avoid harmful actions to patients. Professionals must avoid mishandling or mistreating patients in any manner that may be construed as harmful. Indeed, most health care professionals can recite the first part of the original Hippocratic Oath: "First, do no harm." **Role fidelity** is the principle that reminds health care professionals that they

must be faithful to their role in the health care environment. Health care professions have defined standards of practice, which will be discussed later in this chapter. The last of the seven principles of biomedical ethics is veracity. **Veracity** is truthfulness within the realm of health care practice. Under certain conditions, it is acceptable for confidentiality to be breached and veracity to be disregarded. These situations include, but are not exclusive to, civil cases, criminal cases, suspected child and elder abuse, and matters of public health and safety.[26] Even under the aforementioned conditions, health care professionals should safeguard as much patient information as they can by answering only the questions asked of them and disclosing only subpoenaed information.

Ethical Theories and Models

Ethics is the systematic study of morals (e.g., the rightness or wrongness of human conduct and character as known by natural reason), although many people believe that ethics simply means using common sense. A respectable value system and appropriate ethical behaviors are desirable traits for those serving in any health care profession. Ethical problem solving begins with an awareness of ethical issues in health care and is the sum of ethical knowledge, common sense, personal and professional values, practical wisdom, and learned skills.[23] Although an individual's personal system of decision making may be developed from values and experiences, it generally involves some understanding and application of basic principles common to formal ethical theories.[27]

Ethical theories may be divided into the following three broad groups:

1. teleology (consequentialism)
2. deontology (nonconsequentialism)
3. virtue ethics

Teleological ethical theories assert that the consequences of an act or action should be the major focus when deciding how to solve an ethical problem. Because of this, **teleology** is also called **consequentialism**. It has often been stated that teleologists believe that the ends justify the means. There are two forms of consequentialism: egoism and utilitarianism. In egoism, the best long-term interests of an individual are promoted. Egoists resolve that in evaluating an act or action for its moral value, the act or action must produce a greater ratio of good over bad for the individual, over the long term, than any of the possible alternatives. There are essentially two types of egoism: impersonal and personal. Impersonal egoists generally believe that everyone should choose to behave in a fashion that promotes her or his best long-term interest, whereas personal egoists pursue their own best long-term interests and perform in a manner that benefits only themselves. They usually make no attempt to advocate or control what others should do. Because the role of health care professionals is to serve others, the practice of egoism in any form is incompatible and undesirable. The ethical theory of utilitarianism holds that people should act to produce the greatest ratio of good to evil for everyone. Attributed to the work of Jeremy Bentham and his student John Mill, this theory is considered most applicable to ethical decision making in health care.[14] Bentham and Mill surmised that behaviors are right if they promote happiness and pleasure for everyone, and wrong to the extent that they do not produce pleasure, only pain. There are two categories or forms of utilitarianism: act and rule. Those practicing act utilitarianism believe that ethical behaviors should be geared toward performing acts that produce the greatest ratio of good to bad. The act itself, and its positive consequences, is their only genuine consideration. Rule utilitarianists believe that individuals should base their ethical choices on the consequences of a rule or rules under which an act or action falls, without primary consideration of the consequences. The so-called "rules" may be those derived from religious belief, such as the Ten Commandments; those offered by professional codes of conduct or ethics, such as the Code of Ethics for Radiation Therapists; those developed by professional organizations in the interest of their clients, such as the American Hospital Association's Patient Care Partnership; or what may be considered an arbitrary set of an individual's personal beliefs.[26] **Deontology**, or **nonconsequentialism**, uses formal rules of right and wrong for reasoning and problem solving. Developed by Immanuel Kant in its purest form, the ethical theory of deontology seeks to exclude the consideration of consequences when performing ethical acts or making ethical decisions. Kant surmised that morality is based on reason and that the principles derived from reason are universal and should be designated as universal truths. Because there was no definition or explanation of these truths, Kant created what he believed it should be: Kant's Categorical Imperative. The Categorical Imperative states that "… we should act in such a way as to will the maxim of our actions to become universal law." [10] A maxim is a statement of general truth, fundamental principle, or rule of conduct.[13] Although there are several maxims attributed to Kant, the one that is most relevant to the health care professions is: "We must always treat others as ends and not as means only."[10] Applying this maxim to health care professionals simply means that those adhering to this principle would never consider viewing their positions as just jobs for which they receive financial remuneration, but instead would consider each patient as an individual (autonomy) to whom a professional duty is owed (beneficience, confidentiality, justice, nonmaleficence, role fidelity, and veracity) and to which these principles of biomedical ethics should be applied. **Virtue ethics** is the use of practical wisdom for emotional and intellectual problem solving. Practical reasoning, consideration of consequences, rules established by society, and the effects that actions have on others play important parts in applying the theory of virtue ethics. This approach to problem solving serves the health care professional by integrating intellect, practical reasoning, and individual good.[23] Applying this theory to health care may be problematic, because instead of focusing on the acts or actions of individuals, this theory focuses on the individual performing the act or action.[8] Health care professionals work together as a team to provide patients with high-quality care. Promotion or consideration of self, like egoism, has no place in the health care professions.

Regardless of which values a person holds and to which ethical theory he or she prescribes, the person will face ethical problems that must be solved. Health care professionals, radiation therapists included, will face these types of problems almost daily. Many ethicists have described and identified numerous types of ethical problems. Four categories consistently traditionally emerged from the numerous types identified: ethical dilemmas, ethical dilemmas of justice, ethical distress, and locus of authority issues.[26] *Ethical dilemmas* arise when an individual is faced with an ethical situation to which there is more than one seemingly correct solution. The only problem is that all solutions cannot be applied, and choosing one precludes choosing the other(s). In ethical dilemmas, a choice must be made and implemented. Ethical problems associated with the distribution of benefits and burdens on a societal basis are called *ethical dilemmas of justice*. The most obvious manifestation of ethical dilemmas of justice in health care is that of allocation of scarce resources. *Ethical distress* occurs when there is a problem that has an obviously correct solution, but there are institutional constraints prohibiting its application. *Locus of authority* issues occur when there is a problem and there is a question as to whose authority the problem falls under. In other words: Whose job is it to clean up this mess or rectify this situation? No one wants to take the responsibility. In recent years, the past 15 to 20 or so, a new category of ethical problem has surfaced in health care—conflict of interest.[5] Conflicts of interest arise when an individual engages in an activity from which he or she could profit in several ways, such as when a conflict exists between a person's obligations to the public and his or her own self-interest. Consider the following example:

> Dr. Jones is a radiation oncologist at Intercollegial Medical Center. He also is part owner of a free-standing medical imaging center that has a PET-CT scanner. Dr. Jones refers all of his oncology patients to the free-standing center for frequent PET-CT scans. Could this possibly be a conflict of interest? It could be viewed as such, because by sending these patients to the free-standing center, Dr. Jones is increasing the income of the center, thereby increasing the profit margin of the owners, of which he is one. Joint venture and self-referrals are just two of the areas that have been identified as presenting the potential for conflicts of interest.[5] Physicians and other health care providers must be careful that their activities do not present conflicts of interest.

Models for ethical decision making involve different methods of interaction with the patient. The **engineering** or **analytical model** identifies the caregiver as a scientist dealing only in facts and does not consider the human aspect of the patient. The engineering model is a dehumanizing approach and is usually ineffective.[23] For example, with the engineering model the radiation therapist considers the patient only a lung or brain rather than an individual who has thoughts and feelings. This type of approach in the care of cancer patients is cold, unfeeling, and extremely inappropriate.

The **priestly model** provides the caregiver with a godlike, paternalist attitude that makes decisions *for* and not *with* the patient. This approach enhances the patient's feeling of loss of control by giving the caregiver not only medical expertise but also authority about moral issues.[23] An example of this model is the therapist or student forcing a patient to comply with planning or treatment procedures regardless of the patient's pain or discomfort because the physician ordered it or because the disease is known to respond to treatment. Patients must be allowed to make their own decisions regarding their treatment.

The **collegial model** presents a more cooperative method of pursuing health care for both provider and patient. It involves sharing, trust, and consideration of common goals. The collegial model gives more control to the patient while producing confidence and preserving dignity and respect.[23] For example, the therapist takes the extra time required to get acquainted with patients and listen to their needs. This knowledge enables the therapist to help patients cooperate with the demands of positioning for planning and treatment. Although the collegial model takes time, its application is crucial to the humane treatment of cancer patients.

The **contractual model** maintains a business relationship between the provider and patient. A contractual arrangement serves as the guideline for decision making and meeting obligations for services. With a contractual arrangement, information and responsibility are shared. This model requires compliance from the patient; however, the patient is in control of the decision making.[23] The contractual model is best represented by the process of informed consent. When provided with comprehensive and thorough information, competent patients will be able make decisions in an informed manner.

The **covenant model** recognizes areas of health care not always covered by a contract. A covenant relationship deals with an understanding between the patient and health care provider that is often based on traditional values and goals.[23] The covenant model is demonstrated by a patient trusting the caregiver to do what is right. This trust is often based on previous experience with health care, particularly cancer care procedures and treatment.

The role of the radiation therapist in regard to ethical decision making involves the application of professionalism, the selection of a personal theory of ethics, and the choice of a model for interaction with the patient. The difficulties encountered are the result of constant changes in health care, patient awareness, and evolving growth of radiation therapy in a highly technical and extremely impersonal world of health care.[23] Additional difficulties may arise when some health care professionals realize that they have never selected or examined which ethical theory that they subscribe to. To prescribe to an ethical theory, individuals must first examine their personal values. As mentioned earlier in this chapter, ethics are based on values and are derived from four main sources:

- Culture
- Experience
- Religion
- Science

Values are core beliefs concerning what is desirable and help assess the worth of intangibles.[26] They provide the foundation for decisions individuals make in their personal and professional lives.

It is not especially easy for people to examine and clarify their values. For that reason, several individuals have sought to develop a useful means of doing just that. One of those individuals was ethicist Louis Rath.[19] Rath, in the mid-1960s, developed what he termed *values clarification.* Rath formulated a values clarification exercise to assist individuals in discovering, analyzing, and prioritizing their personal values. The exercise contains questions that prompt individuals to make choices based on their particular feelings about specific topics and examine the feelings that were associated with their choices. By completing the exercise, Rath hoped that individuals would discover and be able to describe their values. He also sought to encourage these individuals to exhibit their discovered values daily. Discovering personal values will assist in the development of professional values. This will serve radiation therapists well as they provide quality patient care and treatment.

Patients should actively participate in their own care. Patients' awareness of their rights, their needs, and the availability of the many treatment options provides both opportunities and complications. As mentioned earlier, the AHA has published *The Patient Care Partnership: Understanding Expectations, Rights, and Responsibilities* (Box 2-4), and every medical institution has the responsibility to make this document available to its patients. Each patient's responsibility for the treatment process grows with the knowledge provided by patient education.[23]

PATIENT AUTONOMY AND INFORMED CONSENT

Cancer remains one of the most dreaded diseases and often evokes images of death, disfigurement, intolerable pain, and suffering. Approximately 35 years ago, the central ethical issue in caring for the cancer patient was whether to tell the patient that the diagnosis was cancer. Today, advancements in treatment, surgery, chemotherapy, and radiation therapy have resulted in longer periods of remission, improved survival, and even cures. This has generated more complex ethical issues.[22] More than half of all cancer patients ultimately need radiation therapy. The physician and patient must weigh the benefits of therapy against possible complications.[2]

The health care professional's ability to listen to patients sensitively, grasp the patient's truth, and honor that truth is indispensable, even across social, cultural, and age barriers. To be effective and supportive, physicians and caregivers must, in a sense, be masters of each patient's personal language. This ability to listen and communicate is an extremely important clinical skill that must be learned. There are at least three courses or areas within a radiation therapy program curriculum where these skills can be taught: patient care, ethics, and clinical education. Mastery of listening and communicating should be highly valued.[20]

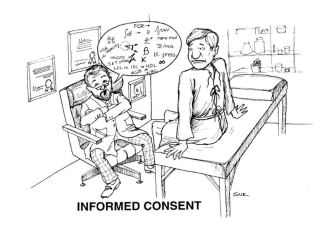

INFORMED CONSENT

Box 2-4	The Patient Care Partnership: Understanding Expectations, Rights and Responsibilities

When you need hospital care, your doctor and the nurses and other professionals at our hospital are committed to working with you and your family to meet your health care needs. Our dedicated doctors and staff serve the community in all its ethnic, religious and economic diversity. Our goal is for you and your family to have the same care and attention we would want for our families and ourselves.

The sections explain some of the basics about how you can expect to be treated during your hospital stay. They also cover what we will need from you to care for you better. If you have questions at any time, please ask them. Unasked or unanswered questions can add to the stress of being in the hospital. Your comfort and confidence in your care are very important to us.

WHAT TO EXPECT DURING YOUR HOSPITAL STAY

- **High quality hospital care.** Our first priority is to provide you the care you need, when you need it, with skill, compassion, and respect. Tell your caregivers if you have concerns about your care or if you have pain. You have the right to know the identity of doctors, nurses, and others involved in your care, as well as when they are students, residents, or other trainees.
- **A clean and safe environment.** Our hospital works hard to keep you safe. We use special policies and procedures to avoid mistakes in your care and keep you free from abuse or neglect. If anything unexpected and significant happens during your hospital stay, you will be told what happened and any resulting changes in your care will be discussed with you.
- **Involvement in your care.** You and your doctor often make decisions about your care before you go to the hospital. Other times, especially in emergencies, those decisions are made during your hospital stay. When decision-making takes place, it should include:
1. *Discussing your medical condition and information about medically appropriate treatment choices.* To make informed decisions with your doctor, you need to understand:
   1. The benefits and risks of each treatment.
   2. Whether your treatment is experimental or part of a research study.
   3. What you can reasonably expect from your treatment and any long-term effects it might have on your quality of life.
   4. What you and your family will need to do after you leave the hospital.
   5. The financial consequences of using uncovered services or out-of-network providers.
   Please tell your caregivers if you need more information about treatment choices.
2. *Discussing your treatment plan.* When you enter the hospital, you sign a general consent to treatment. In some cases, such as surgery or experimental treatment, you may be asked to confirm in writing that you understand what is planned and agree to it. This process protects your right to consent to or refuse a treatment. Your doctor will explain the medical consequences of refusing recommended treatment. It also protects your right to decide if you want to participate in a research study.
3. *Getting information from you.* Your caregivers need complete and correct information about your health and coverage so that they can make good decisions about your care. That includes:
   - Past illnesses, surgeries, or hospital stays.
   - Past allergic reactions.
   - Any medicines or dietary supplements (such as vitamins and herbs) that you are taking.
   - Any network or admission requirements under your health plan.
4. *Understanding your health care goals and values.* You may have health care goals and values or spiritual beliefs that are important to your well-being. They will be taken into account as much as possible throughout your hospital stay. Make sure your doctor, your family, and your care team, know your wishes.
5. *Understanding who should make decisions when you cannot.* If you have signed a health care power of attorney stating who should speak for you if you become unable to make health care decisions for yourself, or a "living will" or "advance directive" that states your wishes about end-of-life care, give copies to your doctor, your family and your care team. If you or your family need help making difficult decisions, counselors, chaplains and others are available to help.
- **Protection of your privacy.** We respect the confidentiality of your relationship with your doctor and other caregivers, and the sensitive information about your health and health care that are part of that relationship. State and federal laws and hospital operating policies protect the privacy of your medical information. You will receive a Notice of Privacy Practices that describes the ways that we use, disclose and safeguard patient information and that explains how you can obtain a copy of information from our records about your care.
- **Help preparing you and your family for when you leave the hospital.** Your doctor works with hospital staff and professionals in your community. You and your family also play an important role in your care. The success of your treatment often depends on your efforts to follow medication, diet and therapy plans. Your family may need to help care for you at home. You can expect us to help you identify sources of follow-up care and to let you know if our hospital has a financial interest in any referrals. As long as you agree that we can share information about your care with them, we will coordinate our activities with your caregivers outside the hospital. You can also expect to receive information and, where possible, training about the self-care you will need when you go home.
- **Help with your bill and filing insurance claims.** Our staff will file claims for you with health care insurers or other programs such as Medicare and Medicaid. They will also help your doctor with needed documentation. Hospital bills and insurance coverage are often confusing. If you have questions about your bill, contact our business office. If you need help understanding your insurance coverage or health plan, start with your insurance company or health benefits manager. If you do not have health coverage, we will try to help you and your family find financial help or make other arrangements. We need your help with collecting needed information and other requirements to obtain coverage or assistance.

While you are here, you will receive more detailed notices about some of the rights you have as a hospital patient and how to exercise them. We are always interested in improving. If you have questions, comments, or concerns, please contact _____.

Courtesy American Hospital Association, 2008.

Truth telling, which is required for informed consent, is an extremely curious principle. Many people have been taught from early childhood to tell the truth, but doing so is often extremely difficult and sometimes even seems wrong. Not long ago, lying to a patient about the cancer diagnosis was the norm. Caregivers believed that telling the truth would be destructive and that patients preferred ignorance of their conditions. Studies over the years, however, have conclusively documented that cancer patients want to know their diagnoses and do not suffer psychological injury as a result.[22]

As discussed earlier, the claim that each person is free to make life-directing decisions is known as the bioethical *principle of autonomy*. The concept of autonomy, understood in this sense, is crucial to ethics. Without some sense of autonomy, no sense of responsibility exists, and, without responsibility, ethics is not possible.[28] In conventional cancer therapy, patient autonomy is protected further by the practice of consent. The American Medical Association's principles of medical ethics imply the following about **informed consent:** a physician shall be dedicated to providing competent medical service with compassion and respect for human dignity; shall deal honestly with patients and colleagues; and shall make relevant information available to patients. Patients should be informed and educated about their conditions, should understand and approve their treatments, and should participate responsibly in their own care.[2] The basic element of informed consent is the patients' right to understand and participate in their own health care. Informed consent is a doctrine that has evolved sociologically and legally with the changing times. Every patient is entitled to receive information about a procedure or treatment before it is performed[17] (Box 2-5). Consent contains three important aspects: communication, ethics, and law.[26] The communication aspect of consent involves physicians or their agent telling the patient what he or she needs to know so that they may make a decision as to what course of action is best for him or her. The aspect of ethics in consent may involve conflict between the beneficent approach of the health care professional (doing good by providing the best level of care that they can) and patient autonomy (the patients right to make his or her own decisions), even those that many be considered bad ones, regarding his or her care. The law aspect is simply the fact that patients have legal rights that have been established through guidelines and the court system,

in the consent process. Although there are several types of consent, informed consent is the most critical. Informed consent must be secured in writing for all procedures, treatments, and research considered invasive and/or that pose significant risk(s).

   Informed consent MUST be secured in writing.

Informed consent is considered a procedure in which patients may agree to or refuse treatment based on information provided to them by their physician or designee(s). The patient must be fully informed concerning the nature of the procedure or treatment—the associated risks, including complications; side effects and potential mortality; desired outcome; and possible alternative procedures or treatments. To give consent a person must have the legal capacity to do so. The capacity is ensured if a person is a competent adult; the legal guardian or representative of an incompetent adult; an emancipated, married, or mature minor; the parent or legal guardian of a child; or an individual obligated by court order.[26]

Competency refers to the minimal mental, cognitive, or behavioral ability or trait required to assume responsibility. In general, the law recognizes only decisions or consents made by competent individuals. Persons older than the age of 18 are presumed to be competent; however, this may be disputed with evidence of mental illness or deficiency. If the individual's condition prevents the satisfaction of criteria for competency, the person may be deemed incompetent for the purpose of informed consent. Mental illness does not automatically render a person incompetent in all areas of functioning. Respect for autonomy demands that individuals, even if they are seriously mentally impaired, be allowed to make decisions of which they are capable. Minors are not generally considered legally competent and therefore require the consent of parents or designated guardians.[2] As noted earlier, there are exceptions to this. When a minor legally marries, he or she is considered an autonomous adult. The same applies to minors who petition the court and are granted emancipated or mature minor status. These minors generally do not live with their parents. In addition, minors serving in the uniformed services are also given autonomous adult status.[8]

A person's competency status may be altered if he or she is under the influence of certain medications, especially those used for pain control. The rule directing that a patient may not sign a document or give informed consent for a procedure after being medicated was established to protect the person going to surgery. Persons who have been premedicated for procedures are considered incompetent. However, persons experiencing intractable pain may be incapable of exercising autonomy until after they are medicated and pain free or experiencing pain control.[27]

The responsibility for obtaining informed consent from a patient clearly remains with the physician and cannot be delegated. However, it is known that many times other health care processionals secure informed consent for certain procedures. The legality of this can be challenged if the facility does not have appropriate written policies and procedures regarding the securing of informed consent by a nonphysician. The courts believe that a physician is in the best position to decide which

Box 2-5	Informed Consent

To give informed consent, the patient must be informed of the following[7]:
1. The nature of the procedure, treatment, or disease
2. The expectations of the recommended treatment and the likelihood of success
3. Reasonable alternatives available and the probable outcome in the absence of treatment
4. The particular known risks that are material to the informed decision about whether to accept or reject medical recommendations

information should be provided for a patient to make an informed choice. The scope of disclosure in any situation is a physician's responsibility. Some states, however, also have legislative standards or state statutes that articulate the information that the physician must tell a patient.[2]

 Informed consent MUST be secured by a physician, unless otherwise specified by facility policy and procedure or state law.

Often, a third person (a health care provider) is present during the informed consent session because patients are reluctant to question their physicians but will likely question the witness. The witness can then inform the physician about the patient's lack of understanding. The third-party signature is merely an attestation that the informed consent session took place and that the signature on the document is that of the patient.[2] The patient must be able to understand the information as presented, and no attempt must be made to influence the decision. In the United States today, obtaining true informed consent can present a real challenge due to language barriers (linguistic diversity). Medical interpreters and other services are seeing increased use as those seeking health care services in the United States continue to become more diverse. General agreement exists that informed consent is an active, shared decision-making process between the health care provider and patient. To give informed consent, patients must understand the information that is provided to them. Communication is key to the process and, when a patient and his or her health care providers cannot communicate due to language barriers, quality health care may be compromised. To deliver quality health care to everyone, all providers of health care must continuously seek better forms and more venues of communication.

Confidentiality

A struggle exists in medical practice between confidentiality and truthfulness. According to Garrett et al.,[6] truthfulness is summarized in two commands: "Do not lie" and "You must communicate with those who have a right to the truth." Truthfulness must not be the only consideration in discussing patients' rights and caregivers' obligations to patients. One of the major restrictions a health care profession imposes is strict confidence of medical and personal information about a patient. This information cannot be revealed without consent of the patient.

Breach of confidence is one of the major problems encountered in providing patient care and can result in legal problems. Information should not be discussed with other department personnel, except in the direct line of duty if it is requested from one ancillary department to another or with nursing service to meet specific medical needs. In the radiation therapy setting, staff members must be especially careful not to discuss patients in hallways or around the treatment area unless the discussion is directly related to the treatment. Unless a patient expressly and explicitly forbids such, health care professionals have the right to consult other health care providers in the effort to help the patient.[6] Staff members should never discuss information with their own families or friends, even in the most general terms, because doing so is a violation of confidentiality and HIPAA.

The patient's treatment chart should be kept in a secure area, inaccessible to anyone not involved in the treatment. Electronic patient records should only be accessed by those with a specific need to know the contents of the record, or by those required to document care within the record. Confidentiality issues must be stressed in every educational program at every opportunity.[7] Implementation of HIPAA regulations has provided more strict regulations regarding the confidentiality of patient information contained within standard or electronic form. All health care professionals and others who may be exposed to confidential information while working in the health care setting are required to receive HIPAA training. Noncompliance with HIPAA regulations is dealt with harshly. Violation of HIPAA policies can result in institutional sanctions and monetary fines, and individuals may be terminated for their violations. To help ensure HIPAA compliance, all health care employees and students undergo mandatory HIPAA training.

 ALL health care employees and students MUST receive mandatory HIPAA training.

There are some exceptions to confidentiality. These exceptions are generally grouped under four general headings: those commanded by state law, those arising from legal precedent, those resulting from a peculiar patient-provider relationship, and in cases of proportionate reason.[6] Exceptions may include particular types of wounds (e.g., gunshot and knife), certain communicable diseases (e.g., HIV, hepatitis, syphilis), acute poisonings (ingestion of caustic substances), automobile accidents, and abuse (especially child, elder, and spousal).[23] Subject to state law, confidentiality may also be overridden when the life or safety of the patient is endangered such as when knowledgeable intervention can prevent threatened suicide or self-injury. In addition, the moral obligation to prevent substantial and foreseeable harm to an innocent third party usually is greater than the moral obligation to protect confidentiality.[23]

Roles of Other Health Care Team Members

Patients and families dealing with cancer may be suddenly thrust into a new and potentially threatening world of blood tests, diagnostic procedures, therapeutic procedures, and specialists. A family physician or internist who is familiar with the patient's history and has established a trusting relationship with the patient can be a key member of the cancer-management team. This physician can help the patient and his or her family, make appropriate treatment decisions and can act as a liaison between the patient and others involved in the evaluation and treatment. If a patient does not have a physician to act as an advocate at the time of the cancer diagnosis, a physician should quickly be chosen to serve in this capacity throughout the course of the illness.[1]

In most situations, other health care professionals are available to help patients cope with the emotional effects of cancer. Nurses who spend much time at a patient's bedside can provide important information to the patient and physician. Social workers are invaluable in assessing the level of a family's psychological distress and their capacity to cope with the illness.[1] Community resources such as veteran patient programs (e.g., Reach to Recovery) that involve people who have coped with cancer in their own lives can provide valuable information and help reassure patients and their families. The local clergy may be able to provide spiritual guidance based on their knowledge of a particular patient's and family's needs.[1] Ultimately, most cancer patients will be treated by a radiation therapist. The therapists must not only treat the patient's body, they must also help provide emotional support, all within the scope of practice for the profession. The responsibilities and **scope of practice** of radiation therapists are included in Box 2-6.

DYING PATIENTS AND THEIR FAMILIES

Care for the dying patient and family has changed dramatically over the years with improvements in technology. The evolution of terminal care changed curing to caring, beginning with the publication of Dr. Elisabeth Kübler-Ross's book *On Death and Dying*.[21] Because radiation therapists and their students deal daily with terminally ill patients, they must explore questions concerning patients' rights, refusal of treatment, and quality of life and must understand the emotional state of cancer patients. A basic fear of dying is present in all humans. Patients fear the diagnosis, the treatment, the disease, and the death associated with it.[21] Dr. Kübler-Ross identified a Grief Cycle experienced by those with terminal illnesses and other catastrophic events that negatively affect their lives.[12] The Grief Cycle includes the following:

1. Shock	The initial reaction to hearing news of the bad event
2. Denial	Pretending that what is isn't
3. Anger	Outward demonstration of pent-up emotion and frustration
4. Bargaining	Trying to find a way out of the situation
5. Depression	Realization of the facts
5. Testing	Searching for realistic resolutions to the problem
6. Acceptance	Coping with situation and finding a way forward

Those in the Grief Cycle obviously experience highs and lows. It is a part of the radiation therapist's job to identify the cycles and to provide whatever type of emotional support necessary to get the patient through the cycles. A listening ear is often all patients require.

Although the final stage of a terminal illness is obvious, its beginning is less well defined. At some point during the treatment of patients who have metastatic cancer, the focus of management shifts from aggressive therapy to palliative care, from efforts to suppress tumor growth to attempts to control symptoms. Signals that the goals of treatment must be changed include the recognition of the tumor's progression, the failure of therapy to control the disease, the patient's deteriorating strength, and the patient's loss of interest in pursuing previously important objectives and pleasures. Rarely is this decision a difficult one; rather, it reflects the natural acceptance of the inevitability of patients' deaths on the part of families, caregivers, and patients themselves.[1] Indeed, Dr. Kübler-Ross identifies this acceptance as the last stage in the Grief Cycle.

Over the past decade, people in many countries have come to accept the notion that aggressive life support (i.e., prolonging life to the bitter end) is often not the right action to take. The ethic of allowing terminally ill patients to die with dignity has evolved. In recent years, the concept of the individual's right of self-determination has been central in the resuscitation issue. The medical and legal communities have recognized that self-determination is no more than an extension of the patient's right to informed consent. In the past, some physicians may have been placed in the extremely uncomfortable position of wanting to comply with a patient's wish to die in peace and dignity but fearing a malpractice suit by family members for failing to do all that should, could, or might have been done to prolong the life of the dying patient. The response to this dilemma, the **living will**, was created. The purpose of the living will is to allow the competent adult to provide direction to health care providers concerning his or her choice of treatment under certain conditions, should the individual no longer be competent by reason of illness or other infirmity, to make those decisions. The living will also provides patients' families with knowledge of what a person would or would not want done. The living will concept assumes that the individual executing the directive does the following:

1. Demonstrates competency at the time
2. Directs that no artificial or heroic measures be undertaken to preserve his or her life
3. Requests that medication be provided to relieve pain
4. Intends to relieve the hospital and physician of legal responsibility for complying with the directives in the living will
5. Has the signature witnessed by two disinterested individuals who are not related, are not mentioned in the last will, and have no claim on the estate[2]

In practice, actions to carry out a living will may involve withholding or discontinuing interventions such as ventilator support, chemotherapy, surgery, radiation therapy, and even assisted nutrition and hydration.[20] The decision to withhold curative therapy is based on the conclusion that the course of the patient's disease is irreversible and extraordinary measures to sustain life are not in the patient's best interest. To nullify the routinely mandatory order for cardiopulmonary resuscitation in the event of a cardiac arrest, many hospitals require the physician in charge of a terminally ill patient to issue a specific do-not-resuscitate (DNR) order. The Joint Commission requires that every hospital has a no-code (DNR) policy.[6] Plans for the patient's death, including issuance of the DNR order, should be made soon after the issue has been discussed with the patient and family. In most situations, patients and their families are relieved to know that every effort will be made to maintain the patient's comfort and that death will be peaceful.[1] The only problem with this is that often those treating the patient are not aware of the DNR order, and many times a patient may be resuscitated in the diagnostic imaging or radiation therapy department. To comply with a DNR, everyone involved in the patient's care must be made aware of its existence. All hospitals must have written policies and procedures describing the way that patients' rights are protected at their institutions. The living will is not the only document that can be used by individuals to guide the direction of their medical treatment should they become unable to do so.

Box 2-6	The Practice Standards for Medical Imaging and Radiation Therapy (Radiation Therapy Practice Standards)

The American Society of Radiologic Technologists (ASRT) initially developed and published what was known as the Scope of Practice for Medical Imaging and Radiation Therapy. Initially, the document covered the then current disciplines within medical imaging and radiation therapy. The name was changed to what is now known as the Practice Standards for Medical Imaging and Therapy (The Standards) and covers the initial disciplines, as well as those that were added since its inception, such as the Radiologist Assistant (RA). The newest version of the document was copyrighted in June of 2007. Each discipline has its own standards. It is imperative that every radiation therapy student and every practicing radiation therapist become familiar with the contents of this document in order to be knowledgeable regarding their standards of professional performance. The Standards is the defining document that guides therapists and students in their day-to-day responsibilities of caring for and treating their patients.

The structural elements of radiation therapy as a health profession in the contemporary health care delivery system in the United States include the following:
- A cognitive base
- A structured curriculum
- A professional credential
- A code of ethics
- Clinical practice autonomy
- Self-governance

The history of these elements combines in a complex structure that can be traced across historical time spans and contemporary functional boundaries. For example, in the history of radiography, radiation therapy was at one time an area of responsibility of the radiographer. This is no longer true today.

Curriculum of the discipline contains elements of physics, psychology, patient care, pathology, and others that cross horizontally through several medical specialties. The professional curriculum incorporates didactic and clinical elements and basic sciences that are reflective of contemporary practice in radiation therapy. The content and structural learning experiences facilitate attitudes and skills that prepare graduates to demonstrate a commitment to patient care and continued personal and professional development.

DESCRIPTION OF THE PROFESSION

Radiation therapy is the art and science of treatment delivery to individuals to restore, improve, and enhance performance; diminish or eradicate pathology; facilitate adaptation to the diagnosis of malignant disease; and promote and maintain health. Because the major focus of radiation therapy is the delivery of prescribed dosages of radiation to individuals from external beam and/or brachytherapy radiation sources or hyperthermia units, the radiation therapist's concern is with those factors that influence radiation dose delivery, individual well-being, and responsiveness to treatment, as well as those factors serving as barriers or impediments to treatment delivery.

The practice of radiation therapy is performed by competent radiation therapists who deliver care to the patient in the therapeutic setting and are responsible for the simulation, treatment planning, and administration of a prescribed course of radiation therapy and/or hyperthermia. Additional related settings where radiation therapists practice include education, management, industry, and research.

PROFESSIONAL CREDENTIAL

The initials RT(T) (ARRT) indicate a registered technologist in radiation therapy and certification as a radiation therapist by the American Registry of Radiologic Technologists.

PRACTICE STANDARDS

The practice standards define the practice and establish general criteria to determine compliance. Practice standards are authoritative statements established by the profession for judging the quality of practice, service, and education.

Professional practice constantly changes as a result of a number of factors including technological advances, market and economic forces, and statutory and regulatory mandates. Although a minimum standard of acceptable performance is appropriate and should be followed by all practitioners, it is inappropriate to assume that professional practice is the same in all regions of the United States. Community custom, state statute, or regulation may dictate practice parameters. *Wherever there is a conflict between these standards and state or local statutes and regulations, the state or local statutes and regulations supersede these standards.* Recognizing this, the profession has adopted standards that are general in nature.

A radiation therapist should, within the boundaries of all applicable legal requirements and restrictions, exercise individual thought, judgment, and discretion in the performance of the procedure.

FORMAT

The standards are divided into five sections: scope of practice, clinical performance, quality performance, professional performance, and advisory opinion.

Scope of Practice. The scope of practice delineates the parameters of the radiation therapy practice.

Clinical Performance Standards. The clinical performance standards define the activities of the practitioner in the care of patients and delivery of diagnostic and therapeutic procedures. This section incorporates patient assessment and management with procedural analysis, performance, and evaluation.

Quality Performance Standards. The quality performance standards define the activities of the practitioner in the technical areas of performance including equipment and material assessment, safety standards, and total quality management.

Professional Performance Standards. The professional performance standards define the activities of the practitioner in the areas of education, interpersonal relationships, self-assessment, and ethical behavior.

Advisory Opinion Statements. The advisory opinions are interpretations of the standards intended for clarification and guidance for specific practice issues.

Box 2-6	The Practice Standards for Medical Imaging and Radiation Therapy (Radiation Therapy Practice Standards)—cont'd

A profession's practice standards serve as a guide for appropriate practice. Standards provide role definition for practitioners that can be used by individual facilities to develop job descriptions and practice parameters. Those outside the therapeutic and radiation science community can use the standards as an overview of the role and responsibilities of the practitioner as defined by the profession.

Each section is divided into individual standards. The standards are numbered and followed by a term or set of terms that identify the standards, such as "assessment" or "analysis/determination." The next statement is the expected performance of the practitioner when performing the procedure or treatment. A rationale statement follows and explains why a practitioner should adhere to the particular standard of performance.

Criteria. Criteria are used in evaluating a practitioner's performance. Each set of criteria is divided into two parts: the general criteria and specific criteria. Both general and specific criteria should be used when evaluating performance.

General Criteria. General criteria are written in a style that applies to imaging and radiation therapy science practitioners. These criteria are the same in all sections of the standards and should be used for the appropriate area of practice.

Specific Criteria. Specific criteria meet the needs of the practitioners in the various areas of professional performance. While many areas of performance within imaging and radiation science are similar, others are not. The specific criteria are drafted with these differences in mind.

SCOPE OF PRACTICE

The curriculum base for a radiation therapist is that outlined in the ASRT Professional Curriculum for Radiation Therapy. Education program standards are those defined in the Essentials and Guidelines of an Accredited Educational Program for the Radiation Therapist. The scope of practice for radiation therapists includes:

1. Delivering radiation therapy treatments as prescribed by a radiation oncologist.
2. Performing simulation, treatment planning procedures, and dosimetric calculations.
3. Detecting and reporting significant changes in patients' conditions, and determining when to withhold treatment until the physician is consulted.
4. Monitoring doses to normal tissues within the irradiated volume to ensure tolerance levels are not exceeded.
5. Constructing/preparing immobilization, beam directional, and beam modification devices.
6. Performing quality assurance activities, detecting equipment malfunctions, and taking appropriate action.
7. Applying principles of radiation protection (as low as reasonably achievable, or ALARA) at all times.
8. Participating in brachytherapy procedures.
9. Practicing universal precautions in procedures.
10. Identifying and managing emergency situations.
11. Educating and monitoring students and other health care providers.
12. Educating patients, their families, and the public about radiation therapy.
13. Preparing and/or administering contrast media, and/or medications as prescribed by a licensed practitioner with the appropriate clinical and didactic education where state and/or institutional policy permits.
14. Performing venipuncture with the appropriate clinical and didactic education where state and/or institutional policy permits.
15. Administering medications at the physician's request according to policy.
16. Starting and maintaining intravenous (IV) access per orders when applicable.

RADIATION THERAPY CLINICAL PERFORMANCE STANDARDS
Standard One—Assessment
The practitioner collects pertinent data about the patient and the procedure.
Standard Two—Analysis/Determination
The practitioner analyzes the information obtained during the assessment phase and develops an action plan for completing the procedure
Standard Three—Patient Education
The practitioner provides information about the procedures and related health issues according to protocol.
Standard Four—Performance
The practitioner performs the action plan.
Standard Five—Evaluation
The practitioner determines whether the goals of the action plan have been achieved.
Standard Six—Implementation
The practitioner implements the revised action plan.
Standard Seven—Outcomes Measurement
The practitioner reviews and evaluates the outcome of the procedure.
Standard Eight—Documentation
The practitioner documents information about patient care, the procedure, and the final outcome.

RADIATION THERAPY QUALITY PERFORMANCE STANDARDS
Standard One—Assessment
The practitioner collects pertinent information regarding equipment, procedures, and the work environment.
Standard Two—Analysis/Determination
The practitioner analyzes information collected during the assessment phase to determine the need for changes to equipment, procedures, or the work environment.

Continued

Box 2-6	The Practice Standards for Medical Imaging and Radiation Therapy (Radiation Therapy Practice Standards)—cont'd

Standard Three—Education

The practitioner informs the patient, public, and other health care providers about procedures, equipment, and facilities.

Standard Four—Performance

The practitioner performs quality assurance activities.

Standard Five—Evaluation

The practitioner evaluates quality assurance results and establishes an appropriate action plan.

Standard Six—Implementation

The practitioner implements the quality assurance action plan for equipment, materials, and processes.

Standard Seven—Outcomes Measurement

The practitioner assesses the outcome of the quality management action plan for equipment, materials, and processes.

Standard Eight—Documentation

The practitioner documents quality assurance activities and results.

RADIATION THERAPY PROFESSIONAL PERFORMANCE STANDARDS

Standard One—Quality

The practitioner strives to provide optimal patient care.

Standard Two—Self-Assessment

The practitioner evaluates personal performance.

Standard Three—Education

The practitioner acquires and maintains current knowledge in clinical practice.

Standard Four—Collaboration and Collegiality

The practitioner promotes a positive, collaborative practice atmosphere with other members of the health care team.

Standard Five—Ethics

The practitioner adheres to the profession's accepted ethical standards.

Standard Six—Research and Innovation

The practitioner participates in the acquisition and dissemination of knowledge and the advancement of the profession.

ADVISORY OPINION STATEMENTS

Advisory opinions are interpretations of the standards intended for clarification and guidance for specific practice issues.

Reprinted and modified with permission of the American Society of Radiologic Technologists: *The Practice Standards for Medical Imaging and Radiation Therapy— Radiation Therapy Practice Standards,* Albuquerque, NM. © 2007, The American Society of Radiologic Technologists.

The **durable power of attorney for health care** is another such document. The durable power of attorney for health care is a legal document that allows an individual to designate anyone willing, 18 years of age or older, to be his or her surrogate and make decisions in matters of health care. The designee can be a family member, friend, or another trusted individual. The durable power can be used to accept or refuse treatment; however, the treatments that are desired or not desired must be specified in the document. Both the living will and the durable power of attorney for health care are considered **advance directives**. Both documents are useful in that they clearly describe the wishes of the patient when he or she was considered competent. These documents may also contain instructions for disposal of the body upon death, especially when an individual chooses to donate his or her body to medical science for research. This helps avoid treatment and other conflicts among families and surrogates.[6]

 Before treating a patient, always check the health care record for DNR orders and advance directives.

Hospice Care

During the Middle Ages, a hospice was a way station for travelers. Today a hospice represents an intermediate station for patients with terminal illnesses. The hospice movement began with programs to provide palliative and supportive care for terminally ill patients and their families. Hospice services include home, respite, and inpatient hospital care and support during bereavement. In addition to providing 24-hour care of the patient, the goal of hospice care is to help the dying patient live a full life and to offer hope, comfort, and a suitable setting for a peaceful, dignified death. The hospice team assists family members in caring for the patient by providing physical, emotional, psychological, and spiritual support. Several types of hospices are available, including free-standing facilities, institutionally based units, and community-based programs.[1]

Patients may enter the hospice on their own or may be referred by family members, physicians, hospital-affiliated continuing care coordinators and social workers, visiting nurses, friends, or clergy. Although admission criteria vary, they usually include the following: a terminal illness with an estimated life expectancy of 6 months or less; residence in a defined geographic area; access to a caregiver from immediate family members, relatives, friends, or neighbors; and the desire for the patient to remain at home during the last stage of the illness. On the initial assessment visit, a member of the hospice team obtains the patient's medical history and emotional and psychosocial histories of the patient and family and discusses nursing concerns. After the program begins, team members meet regularly to review the care plan for each patient and put into effect and supervise services for the patient and family.[1]

Most families prefer home care for dying relatives if they can rely on the supportive environment offered by a hospice. Institutionalization is perceived as impersonal and impractical, and acute care hospitals are not designed for the long-term care of terminal patients. A private home can be transformed to accommodate the level of care required, and nurses can instruct family members in physical care techniques, symptom management, nutrition, and medications. After the patient and family are made to feel confident and capable of managing the physical care, they can begin to address the emotional and spiritual issues surrounding death. During a patient's terminal illness, many problems arise, some of which test the hospice team's ingenuity and endurance. In general, however, simple remedies, common sense, good nursing care, preventive medicine, and the generous use of analgesia should be used to help reduce patient suffering.[1]

MEDICAL-LEGAL ASPECTS OF CANCER MANAGEMENT

Definitions and Terminology

Radiation therapists need to perform their duties with confidence even in today's litigious society. As consumers become more aware of the standards of care that they should receive and more cognizant about seeking legal compensation, health care professionals must become more knowledgeable about legal definitions concerning the standard of care.[17]

The type of law that governs noncriminal activities is known as **civil law**. One type of civil law is commonly called tort law. The word *tort* is an Old French word meaning "wrong."[8] In today's terms, a tort is considered a wrongful act committed against a person or a person's property, the one exception being breach of contract. **Tort law** is personal injury law. The act may be malicious and intentional or the result of negligence and disregard for the rights of others. Torts include conditions for which the law allows compensation to be paid to an individual damaged or injured by another. This type of law was created to preserve peace among individuals by providing a venue for assessing fault for wrongdoing (culpability), deter those who wrong others, and provide compensation for those injured.[26] Two types of torts exist: unintentional and intentional.[17] Unintentional torts are considered those acts that are not intentionally harmful, but still result in damage to property or injury to person. Examples of unintentional torts in the health care setting include failure of the health care provider to properly provide for the safety of a patient or failure to properly educate a patient, resulting in harm. Intentional torts are defined as willful acts committed against person or property. Health care providers incur duties incidental to their professional roles. The law does not consider the professional and patient to be on equal terms; greater legal burdens or duties are imposed on the health care provider.[2]

 Tort law is a type of civil law.

Several situations exist in which a tort action can be taken against the health care professional because of deliberate action. Intentional torts include assault, battery, false imprisonment, libel, slander, invasion of privacy, and intentional infliction of emotional distress.

Assault is defined as the threat of touching in an injurious way. If patients feel threatened and believe they will be touched in a harmful manner, justification may exist for a charge of assault. To avoid this, professionals must always explain what is going to happen and reassure the patient in any situation involving the threat of harm.[17] Radiation therapists must always seek permission to touch and treat a patient.

Battery consists of the actual act of harmful, unconsented, or unwarranted contact with an individual. Again, a clear explanation of what is to be done is essential. If the patient refuses to be touched, that wish must be respected. Battery implies that the touch is a willful act to harm or provoke, but even the most well-intentioned touch may fall into this category if the patient has expressly forbidden it. This should not prevent the therapist from placing a reassuring hand on the patient's shoulder, as long as the patient has not forbidden it and the therapist does not intend to harm or invade the patient's privacy. However, any procedure performed against a patient's will may be construed as battery.[17]

False imprisonment is the intentional confinement without authorization by a person who physically constricts another with force, threat of force, or confining clothing or structures. This becomes an issue if a patient wishes to leave and is not allowed to do so. Inappropriate use of physical restraints may also constitute false imprisonment. The confinement must be intentional and without legal justification. Freedom from unlawful restraint is a right protected by law. If the patient is improperly restrained, the law allows redress in the form of damages. Proof of all elements of false imprisonment must be established to support the claim that an illegal act was performed. False imprisonment requires proof that the alleged victim was really confined, that the confinement was intended by the perpetrator, and that consent was not obtained. If they are dangerous to themselves or others, patients may be restrained. An example of false imprisonment is a therapist using restraints on a patient without the patient's consent or without informing and obtaining consent from the family of a child.[17]

Libel is written defamation of character. Oral defamation is termed **slander**. These torts affect the reputation and good name of a person. The basic element of the tort of defamation is that the oral or written communication is made to a person other than the one defamed. The law recognizes certain relationships that require an individual to be allowed to speak without fear of being sued for defamation of character. For example, radiation oncology department supervisors who must evaluate employees or give references regarding an employee's work have a qualified privilege. Radiation therapists can protect themselves from this civil tort by using caution while conversing within the hearing of patients and their families.[17]

Invasion of privacy charges may result if confidentiality of information has not been maintained or the patient's body has been improperly and unnecessarily exposed or touched. Protection of the patient's modesty is vital during simulation, planning, and treatment procedures.[17] Health care providers must make sure that the patient is covered to the extent that treatment allows. Maintaining privacy is also extremely important in regard to video monitors in treatment areas. No one should ever be in the viewing area except authorized and necessary staff members.

Negligence refers to neglect or omission of reasonable care or caution. An unintentional injury to a patient may be negligence. The standard of reasonable care is based on the doctrine of the reasonably prudent person. This standard requires that a person perform as would any reasonable individual of ordinary prudence with comparable education and skill and under similar circumstances. In the relationship between a professional person and a patient, an implied contract exists to provide reasonable care. An act of negligence in the context of such a relationship is called *malpractice*. Negligence, as used in malpractice law, is not necessarily the same as carelessness. A person's conduct can be considered negligent in the legal sense even if the individual acts carefully. For example, if a therapist without prior education and training on a specific procedure attempts the procedure and does it carefully, the conduct can be deemed negligent if harm results to the patient.[17]

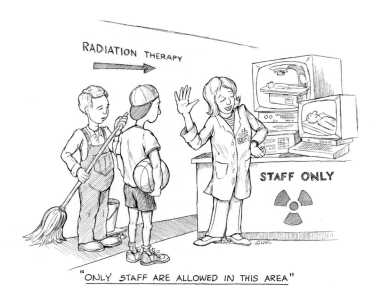

RADIATION THERAPY

STAFF ONLY

"ONLY STAFF ARE ALLOWED IN THIS AREA"

LEGAL DOCTRINES

Doctrine of Personal Liability

Radiation therapists should be concerned about the risk of being named as defendants in medical malpractice suits. Things can go wrong, and mistakes can be made. The legal responsibility of the radiation therapist is to give safe care to the patient.

The fundamental rule of law is that persons are liable for their own negligent conduct. This is known as the **doctrine of personal liability** and means that the law does not permit wrongdoers to avoid legal liability for their own actions even though someone else may also be sued and held legally liable for the wrongful conduct in question under another rule of law. Although they cannot be held liable for actions of hospitals or physicians, therapists can be held responsible and liable for their own negligent actions.[17]

Doctrine of *Respondeat Superior*

The **doctrine of *respondeat superior*** ("let the master answer") is a legal doctrine that holds that an employer is liable for negligent acts of employees that occur while they are carrying out orders or serving the interests of the employer. As early as 1698, courts declared that a master must respond to injuries and losses of persons caused by the master's servants. Nineteenth-century courts adopted the phrase *respondeat superior*, which is founded on the principle of social duty that all persons, whether by themselves or by their agents or servants, shall conduct their affairs in a manner not to injure others.[17] This principle is based on the concept that profit from others' work, and the duty to select and supervise employees, are joined in liability.[2]

Doctrine of *Res Ipsa Loquitur*

In a malpractice action for negligence, the plaintiff has the burden of proving that a standard of care exists for the treatment of the medical problem, the health care provider failed to abide by the standard, this failure was the direct cause of the patient's injury, and damage was incurred. The legal community describes the aforementioned as the steps in a medical malpractice lawsuit, such as duty, breach of duty, and causation and damages. If the alleged negligence involves matters outside general knowledge, an acceptable medical expert must establish these criteria. A long-accepted substitute for the medical expert has been the **doctrine of *res ipsa loquitur*,**[7] which means "the thing speaks for itself." Courts have decided to resolve the problem of expert unavailability in certain circumstances by applying *res ipsa loquitur,* which requires the defendant to explain the events and convince the court that no negligence was involved.[2] The Standards of Practice for Radiation Therapists may be used by either the defense or the prosecution to support or refute negligent behavior, as can expert witnesses. These standards are readily accessible to everyone via the ASRT website.

Doctrine of Foreseeability

The **doctrine of foreseeability** is a principle of law that holds an individual liable for all natural and proximate consequences of negligent acts to another individual to whom a duty is owed. The negligent acts could or should have been reasonably foreseen under the circumstances. A more simple definition is persons reasonably foreseeing that certain actions or inactions on their part could result in injury to others. In addition, the injury suffered must be related to the foreseeable injury. Routine radiation therapy equipment checks are important in overcoming this doctrine.[17]

RISK MANAGEMENT

Conceived little more that a decade ago, the concept of risk control, or **risk management**, was believed to be the key element in loss prevention from adverse medical incidents. Risk management links every quality-improvement program with measurable outcomes necessary to determine overall effectiveness. Effectiveness here means success in reducing patient injury. An acute care hospital or medical center has the duty to exercise such reasonable care in looking after and protecting the patient. The legal responsibility of any health care practitioner is safe care. Risk management, which is a matter of patient safety, is the process of avoiding or controlling the risk of financial loss to staff members and the hospital or medical center. Poor-quality care creates a risk of injury to patients and leads to increased financial liability. Risk management protects financial assets by managing insurance for potential liability by reducing liability through surveillance. The job of risk management is to identify actual and potential causes of accidents or incidents involving patients and employees and to implement programs to eliminate or reduce these occurrences.[17] The number one reason for medical liability (malpractice) claims in medical imaging and radiation therapy is patient falls.

Hospital liability and malpractice insurance, also known as *patient liability insurance,* is intended to cover all claims against the hospital that arise from the alleged negligence of physician staff members and employees. Many have discussed whether radiation therapists should carry malpractice insurance. In making that decision, persons must determine the extent of provisions for malpractice coverage in their institutions. According to the doctrine of *respondeat superior,* the employer is liable for employees' negligent acts during work. The authority and responsibility of a physician supervising and controlling the activities of the employee supersede those of the employer according to the doctrine of the borrowed servant. Regardless of the way these legal doctrines may be applied, the fundamental rule of law that every therapist should clearly know and understand is the doctrine of personal liability; persons are liable for their own negligent conduct, although most health care employees are covered under their employers' liability insurance. A wrongdoer may not be able to escape responsibility even though someone else may be sued and held legally responsible. In some situations, hospital insurers who have paid malpractice claims have successfully recovered damages from negligent employees by filing separate lawsuits against them.[17]

Hospital employees are instructed to report any patient injury to administration through the department manager. An incident report is routinely used to document unusual events in the hospital. An **incident** is defined as any happening that is not consistent with the routine operation of the hospital or the routine care of a particular patient. It may be an accident or a situation that could result in an accident.[23] Hospitals use incident reports in their accident-prevention programs to advise insurers of potential suits and prepare defenses against suits that might arise from documented incidents. Incident reports should be prepared according to the institution's published policies and procedures. An incident report is no place for opinion, accusation, or conjecture; it should contain only facts concerning the incident reported.[2] Incident reports should never be placed on the patient's written or electronic chart. There is usually written hospital and departmental procedure for completing and submitting incident reports. These reports ultimately end up in the office of risk management.

Incident reports should not be placed on patients' written or electronic health care record.

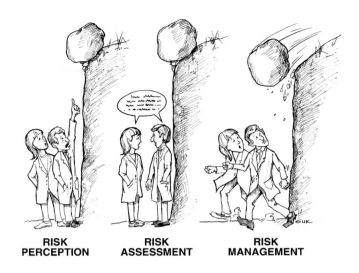

RISK PERCEPTION   **RISK ASSESSMENT**   **RISK MANAGEMENT**

MEDICAL RECORDS

The radiation oncology **medical record** is used to chronologically document the care and treatment rendered to the patient. All components of the patient's evaluation and cancer must be documented in the radiation oncology record. The format usually includes the following: a general information sheet listing the names of pertinent relatives, follow-up contacts, family physicians, and persons to notify in an emergency; an initial history and findings from the physical examination; reports of the pathology examinations, laboratory tests, diagnostic imaging procedures, and pertinent surgical procedures; photographs and anatomic drawings; medications currently used; correspondence with physicians and reimbursement organizations; treatment setup instructions; daily treatment logs; physics, treatment planning, and dosimetry data; progress notes during treatments; summaries of treatment; and reports of follow-up examinations. Patients' radiation oncology records must be maintained and secured in the department separate from hospital and clinic records to ensure ready access at any time.[9] Radiation oncology medical records are commonly maintained in both paper and electronic formats. Medical record entries should be made in clear and concise language that can be understood by all professional staff members attending the patient. Handwritten entries must be legible. An illegible record is worse than no record because it documents a failure by staff members to maintain a proper record and may severely weaken a hospital's or physician's defense in a negligence action. Entries into the paper record should be made in ink, and persons making entries should identify themselves clearly by placing their signatures after each entry. The hospital and physician should be able to determine who participates in each episode of patient care.[2] Entries should be made daily by the therapist operating the treatment machine. Any other therapist involved in the treatment of a patient, that day, should also check the entry for accuracy and initial the record.

Medical records are sometimes used by staff members to convey remarks inappropriate for a patient's chart. The following are examples of entries that should never be made:
- This is the third time therapist X has been negligent.
- Dr. A has mistreated this patient again.

- This patient is a chronic complainer and a nuisance.
- This patient smells, nursing staff should see that she gets a bath.

Such editorial comments are inevitably used against the physician and hospital in any negligence action filed by the patient. In addition, as the trend moves toward access by patients to their own medical records, patients are more likely to read and react with hostility to such comments.[2]

The general rule is to avoid the need for making corrections, but because humans are not perfect, corrections must be made from time to time. In the paper record, a staff member should simply draw a line through an incorrect entry because doing so allows others to identify what was initially written and corrected. The staff member should initial the correction, enter the time and date, and insert the correct information. Mistakes in the chart should not be erased, blacked out, or covered with a "white-out" product because doing so may create suspicion concerning the original entry.[2] Proper charting and documentation protocols should be taught in health care professional educational programs, as well as in the clinical setting. There are proper charting procedures.[27] The following lists contain information on charting information in the medical record in "always" and "never" categories.

Always

1. Write so that others can read what is written (legibly).
2. Use ink.
3. Use correct spelling and approved standard medical abbreviations.
4. Write accurate information: correct and precise.
5. Chart concisely.
6. Provide entries that are thorough.
7. Begin each new entry with the date and time (military notations) of the entry.
8. Chart information as it occurs.
9. Keep the information confidential.
10. Sign each entry with your name and title.

Never

1. Chart using a pencil.
2. Black-out, white-out, or erase entries.
3. Include unnecessary details.
4. Include critical comments about anyone, e.g., the patient, his or her family, or other health care professionals.
5. Leave blank spaces.
6. Use unapproved or improper abbreviations.
7. Record information for others.
8. Divulge patient information.
9. Use initials in place of your signature.

Charting and other documentation are written communication tools used to provide comprehensive health care data on an individual patient basis. Charting is the recording of patient information and observation regarding a specific patient in his or her long-term written or electronic record, such as the patient's chart. Documentation, on the other hand, is also the recording of any information relevant to patient care and treatment, but that information does not have to be entered into the patient chart.[26] There are forms used in a variety of health care

departments that are specific to the services offered by that department. These document are generally stored in the department only, for reference and use by that department only. What needs to be remembered most is that the patient's medical record is a legal document and as such is admissible in a court of law. It provides evidence concerning the care and treatment provided to the patient and the standards under which the care and treatment was administered.[16]

Radiation therapists under the direct supervision of the radiation oncologist and medical physicist carry out daily treatments. All treatment applications must be described in detail (orders) and signed by the responsible physician. Likewise, any changes in the planned treatment by the physician may require adjustment in immobilization, new calculations, and even a new treatment plan. Therefore, the therapist, physicist, and dosimetrist must be notified.[9]

SUMMARY

- The ethical and legal considerations in cancer management are numerous and varied. The development of professional ethical characteristics begins with the discovery of an individual's personal values.
- Ethics are based on values, and knowing one's own values serves to enhance a person's concept of right versus wrong. Professional ethics is an extension of personal ethics. Health care professionals innately prescribe to the Principles of Biomedical Ethics.
- Professional standards guide the practice of medical imaging and radiation therapy. The Standards of Ethics, including the Code of Ethics and the Rules of Ethics, along with the Practice Standards for Medical Imaging and Radiation Therapy, are the prevailing structured professional guides and rules under which medical imaging technologists, radiologist assistants, radiation therapists, and aspiring students perform their health care duties.
- In health care, failure to perform according to ethical and other professional standards subjects practitioners to penalties under the law.
- In addition to the development of technical knowledge and skills, the foundation of radiation oncology includes standards of conduct and ideals essential to meeting emotional and physical needs of patients.
- Radiation therapists must first view their profession as more than a job. Student therapists should not pursue a simple goal to just pass a series of examinations and eventually the registry or earn a degree. Student therapists should set goals that establish them as professionals.
- An ideal professional has superior technical knowledge and works in harmony and cooperation with peers, physicians, and other health care personnel. With the appropriate educational background and determination to excel, a person can practice professionalism and achieve technical excellence.
- By delivering excellent patient care within professional standards, quality patient care can be provided by a health care team that is focused on the needs of the patients, both emotionally and physically, while recognizing and respecting patient rights.

CASE I

Quality Care for All

As a student therapist, Susan observes many clinical situations. She is assigned to a treatment area that has an extremely high volume of patients. Susan observes that a staff member has treated a patient without an important treatment device in place. When she approaches the staff member about the situation, he mumbles something about the patient being palliative. Obviously, the treatment error must be corrected. How does Susan ethically and professionally handle this issue that her conscience dictates be addressed? Is this an ethical or a legal issue?

CASE II

You Really Need This Treatment

Sam is a staff radiation therapist in a large center. He has a patient on his treatment schedule who is uncooperative and verbally abusive to the staff members. It is time for the patient's treatment, but once in the treatment room he is refusing to cooperate by not getting into the position required and holding still. Sam knows the patient is uncomfortable and needs the treatment to relieve symptomatic disease. Should Sam restrain the patient and force him to have the treatment? What legal and ethical considerations are involved in Sam's final decision?

CASE III

To Tell or Not to Tell

Mrs. Smith is a 50-year-old woman with three adult children. She has been admitted to the hospital for tests to rule out cancer. While the tests are being processed, her husband and children meet with the doctor and ask him not to tell Mrs. Smith if the results are malignant. They tell him that she is afraid of cancer and that if she is given the diagnosis, she will become severely depressed and give up all desire to live. The physician is not comfortable with this request, but the family insists. The physician reluctantly agrees. What ethical and legal concepts are implicated in the family's request and physician's decision to comply with it?

CASE IV

Maintaining a Standard of Care

Currently employed in a small radiation oncology center, Sandra has the task of orienting a new employee to the department and the treatment machine to which she is assigned. The new radiation therapist, Jane, although older than Sandra, is newly graduated from an educational program and has recently taken the American Registry of Radiologic Technologists Examination for Radiation Therapy. She has not yet received her credentials but is certainly qualified to begin her position in the department. In the course of working with Jane, Sandra begins to realize that there are some physical limitations for Jane. She has freely shared that she has a degenerative problem with her hands and has some loss of strength. When Sandra begins to make some suggestions for modifying the handling of the custom blocks and other heavy treatment devices over the patient lying on the table, Jane becomes extremely defensive. Sandra is aware that the safety of her patients is at risk and she must take some action. Discuss what that action might be and whether this might be an ethical or a legal situation.

CASE V

Time Challenges in Treatment Delivery

A new patient is scheduled to start treatment on Jim's treatment machine on Monday. Everyone has warned him that the new patient is very angry and very difficult to schedule for procedures. He meets Mrs. Jones on Monday morning, greets her warmly, and does all that he can to put her at ease during the long process of starting her treatments. When the time comes for him to discuss her appointments, Mrs. Jones insists that she needs different appointment times daily. Jim carefully explains that they cannot accommodate quite that many changes in the schedule for the 7 weeks that she will be with them. Jim and Mrs. Jones reach an agreement that seems to satisfy them both. For the next several weeks Mrs. Jones arrives at a different time every day. Sometimes she calls to reschedule; sometimes she just comes in to the department. Jim and the other therapist he works with try very hard to accommodate their patient, but it is causing havoc with the rest of their schedule and inconveniencing most of their other patients. Jim approaches Mrs. Jones with the question of whether another appointment time would be better for her. Mrs. Jones quickly becomes verbally abusive, screaming that she wishes she had gone elsewhere for treatment. She shouts that she doesn't want to talk about this anymore and she is tired of being chastised every time she is 5 minutes late. Because this is the first time Jim or his partner has mentioned her tardiness, they are surprised at her reaction. Discuss how they should handle the situation. Consider whether they will be able to discuss this with Mrs. Jones or refer her to a supervisor, because she is so convinced that she has been harassed about her appointments since the beginning. What kind of legal or ethical issues does this case history contain?

CASE VI

A Call to Intervene

Jim is a radiation therapist at Mercy Hospital. He learns that his widowed, childless, 89-year-old neighbor, Mrs. Dysart, has been admitted to the hospital where he works. She has some type of heart ailment and is on oxygen and a heart monitor. Every day Jim goes to visit her. She asks him to read scripture to her and he does. Over a few days Mrs. Dysart tells Jim that she knows that her time on earth may be nearing the end. He tries to convince her that she has plenty of life left and to not give up. She confides in Jim that she does not want to be resuscitated should her heart stop beating. He asks whether she has an advance directive and she tells him no.

One evening after work Jim goes to visit Mrs. Dysart and she's not feeling well at all. She asks Jim to read to her again and he does so. In the midst of his reading, Mrs. Dysart starts to cough and clutch her chest. Jim stands up and goes to her, asking if she's OK. Suddenly, the heart monitor beeps a warning and Jim looks at the straight line it is showing. He then looks back at Mrs. Dysart, and she has passed out. What should Jim do? What would you do if you were Jim?

Review Questions

Multiple Choice

1. Which of the following does *not* govern ethics?
   a. professional codes
   b. popular science

c. Patient's Bill of Rights

d. technical practice

2. The foundation of law is:
   a. autonomy
   b. confidentiality
   c. justice
   d. ethics

3. Moral ethics are based on which of the following?
   a. right and wrong
   b. institutions
   c. legal rights
   d. codes

4. Which of the following is an ethical principle?
   a. justice
   b. individual freedom
   c. egoism
   d. confidentiality

5. Confidentiality, truth telling, and benevolence are which of the following?
   a. ethical principles
   b. legal rights
   c. ethical characteristics
   d. legal doctrines

6. A tort falls under which of the following?
   a. criminal law
   b. statutory law
   c. civil law
   d. common law

7. *Res ipsa loquitur* means which of the following?
   a. "Things speak for themselves."
   b. "The thing speaks for itself."
   c. "Do no harm."
   d. "No negligence was involved."

8. Which ethical theory group evaluates an activity by weighing good against bad?
   a. deontology
   b. teleology
   c. virtue ethics
   d. moral ethics

9. Which ethical model identifies the caregiver as a scientist dealing only with the facts and does *not* consider the human aspect of the patient?
   a. collegial
   b. convenent
   c. engineering
   d. priestly

10. Of the following, which model presents a more cooperative method of pursuing health care for patients and providers than the others?
    a. analytical
    b. engineering
    c. convenent
    d. collegial

11. Core beliefs concerning what is desirable and that help assess the worth of intangibles are called:
    a. prospects
    b. principles
    c. theories
    d. values

12. Informed consent must be secured:
    a. in writing
    b. verbally
    c. verbally and written
    d. upon admission

13. Consent to release a patient's health care records:
    a. must be secured from the patient orally
    b. must be secured from the patient in writing
    c. must be secured from the patient both orally and written
    d. is not required

14. Copies of incident reports should:
    a. be included in the patient's medical record
    b. sent to the floor on which the patient is housed
    c. given to the patient
    d. sent to the office of risk management

15. The acronym HIPAA stands for:
    a. Health Improvement Policy and Accountability Act
    b. Health Information Policy and Action Act
    c. Health Insurance Portability and Accountability Act
    d. Health Improvement Privacy and Action Act

The answers to the Review Questions can be found by logging on to our website at: *http://evolve.elsevier.com/Washington+Leaver/principles*

Questions to Ponder

1. What does deontology emphasize?

2. Discuss the difference between law and ethics, and describe a situation in which the two may be in conflict.

3. Discuss and compare the analytical and covenant models of ethical decision making. Discuss the way these models may be used in your profession and by whom.

4. What components are involved in ethical decision making for the radiation therapist?

5. Discuss the required elements that make up an informed consent.

6. Explain the purpose of the scope of practice as it pertains to your performance as a radiation therapist.

7. Compare and discuss the different settings available in hospice care.

8. Discuss the differences in assault and battery. What kind of action can be taken in response to either of these?

9. Analyze the difference between negligence and carelessness. Can careful behavior still result in a charge of negligence? Describe such an instance.

10. Explain the purpose of a medical record, and note the components of a complete radiation oncology record.

REFERENCES

1. American Cancer Society, Massachusetts Division: *Cancer manual,* ed 8, Boston, 1990, The American Cancer Society.

2. American College of Legal Medicine: *Legal medicine,* ed 5, St. Louis, 2001, Mosby.

3. American Registry of Radiologic Technologists: *The standards of ethics,* revised, St. Paul, 2004, The American Registry of Radiologic Technologists.

4. Beauchamp TL, Childers JF: *Principles of biomedical ethics,* ed 4, New York, 1994, Oxford University Press.

5. Edge RS, Groves JH: *Ethics of health care: a guide for clinical practice,* ed 2, New York, 1999, Delmar.

6. Garrett T, Baillie HW, Garrett R: *Healthcare ethics: principles and problems,* ed 4, Englewood Cliffs, NJ, 2001, Prentice Hall.

7. Gurley LT, Callaway WJ: *Introduction to radiologic technology,* ed 4, St. Louis, 1996, Mosby.

8. Hall JK: *Law and ethics for clinicians,* Amarillo, 2002, Jackhal Books.

9. Inter-Society Council for Radiation Oncology: *Radiation oncology in integrated cancer management, United States,* Philadelphia, 1991, The Inter-Society Council for Radiation Oncology.

10. Kant I: *Groundwork of the metaphysics of morals,* translated by JJ Patton, New York, 1964, Harper & Row.

11. Kemp K: My battle scars can help others, *The Birmingham News,* Sunday, September 2, 2007.

12. Kübler-Ross E: *On death and dying,* New York, 1969, Macmillan.

13. *Merriam-Webster's online dictionary* (website): http://mw1.merriam-webster.com/dictionary/maxim. Accessed June 2, 2007.

14. Mill JS: *On liberty: collected works of John Stuart Mill,* vol 18, Toronto, 1977, University of Toronto Press.

15. Miller BF, Keane CB: *Encyclopedia & dictionary of medicine, nursing, & allied health,* ed 6, Philadelphia, 1997, WB Saunders.

16. Norris J: *Mastering documentation,* Springhouse, PA, 1995, Springhouse Corporation.

17. Parelli RJ: *Medicolegal issues for radiographers,* ed 2, Dubuque, IA, 1994, Eastwind.

18. Phoenix Health Systems: *HIPAA advisory* (website): http://www.hipaadvisory.com/REGS/HIPAAprimer.htm. Accessed July 2, 2007.

19. Rath L, Simon S, Merrill H: *Values and teaching,* Columbus, OH, 1966, Charles E Merrill.

20. Roy DJ: Ethical issues in the treatment of cancer patients, *Bull World Health Organ* 67:341-346, 1989.

21. Slaby AE, Glicksman AS: *Adapting to life-threatening illness,* New York, 1985, Praeger.

22. Smith DH, McCarty K: In the care of cancer patients, *Primary Care Cancer* 19:821–833, 1992.

23. Towsley D, Cunningham E: *Biomedical ethics for radiographers,* Dubuque, IA, 1994, Eastwind.

24. Warner S: Code of ethics: professional and legal implications, *Radiol Technol* 52:485-494, 1981.

25. *Webster's new collegiate dictionary,* Springfield, MA, 1976, G & C Merriam.

26. Wilson B: *Ethics and basic law for medical imaging professionals,* Philadelphia, 1997, FA Davis.

27. Winter G, Glass E, Sakurai C: Ethical issues in oncology nursing practice: an overview of topics and strategies, *Oncol Nurs Forum* 20:21-34, 1993.

28. Wright R: *Human values in health care: the practice of ethics,* New York, 1987, McGraw-Hill.

Principles of Pathology

Patricia J. Giordano

Outline

Objectives

- Identify and describe the function of the cell and its various organelles.
- Define and discuss *homeostasis*.
- Define *inflammatory response*.
- Identify and discuss the most common cause of tissue damage.
- List the most common agents that cause tissue damage.
- Identify and discuss the characteristics of benign and malignant tumors.

- Compare and contrast carcinomas and sarcomas.
- Identify and discuss the four common viruses associated with neoplastic disease.
- List and discuss the three procedures most commonly used to diagnose cancer.
- Define and discuss *transcription* and *translation*.
- Discuss the function and relationship of DNA and RNA.
- Define *oncogene* and *tumor-suppressor gene*.

Key Terms

Cell cycle
Chromosomes
Cytoplasm
Endoplasmic reticulum
Extravasation
Genome
Golgi apparatus
Lysosomes
Mitochondria
Nuclear membrane
Nucleoli
Nucleotides
Nucleus
Oncogene
Organelles
Peroxisomes
Polypeptide
Proteins
Ribosome
Transcription
Translation
Tumor-suppressor gene
Vacuoles

Pathology is the branch of medicine devoted to the study and understanding of disease. More precisely, the discipline seeks to understand the effect of disease on the function of the human organism at all levels and relate functional alterations to changes perceived at the gross anatomic, cellular, and subcellular levels. This chapter considers briefly the history and evolution of the pathology of cancer,[1,3] discusses the cellular theory of disease, and examines the physiology of the neoplastic process. In addition, some of the practical aspects of establishing a pathologic diagnosis and using that information to classify and treat cancer are considered. Finally, this chapter provides an overview of subcellular molecular biology and its emerging effect on cancer.

Although disease theory and methods by which disease processes are studied have changed dramatically, humans have pursued these issues one way or another for well over 2000 years. As time passed, perceptions slowly changed. During the Middle Ages, semiscientific observations continued to be made and recorded, but evolution of the theory of disease was stagnant and treatment was based mostly on superstition or witchcraft. Prevailing theory and recorded observations were not considered at odds until the 16th and 17th centuries. After these contradictions were recognized and old ideas were challenged, the understanding of disease began to move rapidly forward, assisted by new technology that opened unimaginable frontiers.

The introduction of the microscope in the early 17th century made possible the observation of unicellular human anatomy, thus propelling pathology from its infancy into its childhood. This also made possible correlations between clinical manifestations of disease and gross anatomic findings and between gross pathology and microscopic observations. These correlations were further developed and refined during the 18th and 19th centuries as physicians began to comprehend the roles individual organs played in the expression of illness and began to introduce new theories of disease and to refine old ones. Practical application of these theories resulted in the development of the first scientifically sophisticated treatment of many diseases. A logarithmic growth took place in the 20th century in medical technology and understanding of disease processes.

Since 1970, another great advancement has been made to understand more completely the physiology of disease. This movement into an unfamiliar and even smaller microcosm has revealed the world of molecular biology, in which disease may be studied at a subcellular level not previously appreciated. This advancement, which has permitted study and observation of function at the molecular level, is at least as great as the development in the 17th century that refocused observations from the gross anatomic to the cellular level. The rate at which knowledge is expanding in molecular biology is so fast that only a regular review of the current scientific literature on the subject can provide up-to-date information. This chapter offers an overview of molecular biology and related enterprises to help the student or practitioner of radiation therapy understand vistas that lie ahead.

CELLS AND THE NATURE OF DISEASE

Every clinical disease has its inception with some kind of cellular injury or malfunction that ultimately is expressed at the molecular level of cellular function. To understand this chapter, the reader should be familiar with basic principles of elementary mammalian biology. A general understanding of the structure and function of the mammalian cell, including the several organelles (nucleus, endoplasmic reticulum, ribosomes, Golgi apparatus, mitochondria, lysosomes, peroxisomes, and vacuoles) and plasma membrane, is particularly important. Details of cellular form and function may be obtained from any modern textbook of general biology.

Cells differ greatly concerning functions they perform; however, they have certain characteristics in common. All cells share the ability to produce energy and maintain themselves in a state of normal function by elaborating a vast array of proteins and macromolecules that facilitate adaptation to physiologic or pathologic stress. As long as cells can maintain themselves in the range of normal function, they exist in a state of homeostasis. The homeostatic state represents a set of circumstances in which cellular processes associated with life proceed normally and in accordance with the function genetically assigned to that cell. In a typical cell, these functions include processes that provide nutrition, protection, communication, and sometimes, mobility and reproduction. All these processes are facilitated by the hundreds of macromolecules produced by each cell. Under prolonged or acute physiologic stress, this homeostasis may be maintained only with great difficulty. When a cell's adaptive mechanisms fail, changes in cellular structure become identifiable and a pathologic or disease state ensues.

Changes in cellular structure can usually be seen under the microscope and may be broadly divided into two categories: irreversible and reversible. *Irreversible* changes represent cellular death or changes that eventually prove lethal to the cell. Changes representing reversible injury are consistent with cell survival if the precipitating cause is corrected. Dead cells are recognized under the microscope because enzymes begin to destroy them. These enzymes may be derived from the dead cell

itself, or they may originate in other scavenging cells such as macrophages. Enzymatic action obliterates cellular detail. Irreversible changes signaling incipient cell death appear as a series of color alterations in typical cellular staining patterns and irregularities in the structure of the cell's nucleus. The nucleus under such circumstances may become fragmented, shriveled, or enzymatically destroyed. The changes of reversible cell damage may be subtler. They arise from internal loss of power caused by respiratory insufficiency. Cellular swelling is the hallmark of reversible damage and occurs as the damaged cellular membrane fails to properly regulate the concentration of sodium in the cell. As a consequence, water passes across the membrane to produce swelling. Swelling is followed by morphologic changes in the intracellular organelles and a decrease in the pH of the cell that can be identified by the application of special cellular stains. The radiation therapist must recognize that all these changes, whether reversible or irreversible, may occur in malignant and normal cells.

Inflammation

These changes in cellular form and function that represent a departure from homeostasis do not occur in a vacuum. They occur instead in the context of the aggregate physiology of the organism and therefore are subject to monitoring and response. In broad terms, the monitoring of and response to tissue damage is called the *inflammatory reaction*.[10,12] Its clinical features have been known since antiquity and have been described as rubor, calor, tumor, and dolor (i.e., redness, warmth, swelling, and pain). Although the clinical syndrome has not changed since Celsius described these cardinal features in the 1st century AD, much more is known about its purpose and physiology.

The inflammatory response is a complex, immunochemical reaction initiated by normal cells that have been injured or damaged. It has implications for the defense of the organism and repair of the injury or damage that initially provoked the reaction. The reaction may be intense or subdued depending on the magnitude and nature of the precipitating stimulus. If the reaction evolves completely over a few hours or days, it is acute. If it persists for longer periods, it is chronic. In either situation, the features of the reaction account for the well-known cardinal signs.

Inflammation begins as local vascular dilation that permits an increase in blood flow to the affected tissue. The increase in blood flow accounts not only for the redness and warmth that accompany inflammation but also for increases in intravascular pressure and permeability of the vascular membrane. These changes in pressure and permeability expedite the escape of fluid into the interstitial space to produce swelling. This interstitial fluid, which escapes through gaps between the endothelial cells lining small veins, is mostly water rich in proteins, polypeptides, and other low-molecular-weight substances called *inflammatory mediators* or *cytokines*. These latter substances, thought to be by-products of tissue injury, seem to play a role in nerve stimulation and pain production.

Many white blood cells (mostly neutrophils) and other phagocytes escape the vascular compartment with this fluid. These cells destroy bacteria and other microorganisms, neutralize toxins, and enzymatically destroy dead or dying tissue. When this phagocytic response accomplishes its physiologic objectives, it promotes the ingrowth of new capillaries and fibroblasts, which in turn facilitate tissue repair and a return to homeostasis. Tissue damage or injury initiates the cascade of events that constitute the inflammatory response. Without such an initiator, inflammation does not occur.

Many agents cause tissue damage leading to an inflammatory response. Among the most common agents are hypoxia, microbial infections, ionizing radiation, chemicals, allergic or immune reactions, and cancer.

The most common cause of tissue damage is hypoxia. Oxygen deprivation renders a living cell incapable of manufacturing energy. When insufficient energy is present to sustain the cell, intracellular organelles fail, the integrity of the cellular membrane is lost, and death results. Local hypoxia commonly results from vascular occlusive disease and trauma. Vascular occlusive disease is classically seen in acute myocardial infarction. Trauma is present, for example, in skin flap necrosis secondary to vascular damage at the time of a radical mastectomy. The radiation therapist sees generalized hypoxia as a result of cardiorespiratory compromise secondary to acute compression of the superior vena cava caused by lung cancer. If not promptly corrected, hypoxia of this magnitude results in death rather than localized tissue destruction and an ensuing inflammatory reaction. Similarly, other causes of generalized hypoxia such as carbon monoxide or cyanide poisoning, which prevent oxygen transport or use at the cellular level, do not involve inflammation.

Infections produced by bacteria and other microbes represent the most widely recognized cause of inflammation and commonly occur in patients undergoing radiation therapy. The many mechanisms of injury produced by microorganisms are complex and beyond the scope of this discussion; however, the bacterial cellulitis produced by minor injury to the edematous arm of a breast cancer patient who has undergone a radical mastectomy, an axillary lymph node dissection, and radiation therapy is often dramatic. Such an infection is commonly accompanied by all the cardinal signs of inflammation.

For the radiation therapist, the most obvious and frequently seen cause of tissue damage is ionizing radiation. Radiation is an agent of tissue damage used medically in a sophisticated fashion to achieve carefully delineated objectives. The primary objective is to lethally damage all cancer cells in a predefined volume of tissue, thus rendering the surviving normal tissue free of neoplastic disease. In pursuit of this objective, some damage is inevitably inflicted on normal tissues incorporated in the radiation portal. Such damage, whether to normal or neoplastic tissue, elicits an inflammatory response. In patients undergoing radiation therapy, this response may be intense and easily identified. More often, it is subtle or in deep tissues and not obvious.

Tissue Damage

Tissue damage produced by the use of chemicals or drugs is frequently encountered clinically. The list of agents responsible for such damage is long, and the mechanisms of injury are numerous. As with ionizing radiation, the judicious administration of certain chemotherapeutic agents may result in tissue destruction, thus having a tangible benefit for the patient. Chemical damage to superficial tissue may be observed after inadvertent extravasation of some chemotherapeutic agents. **Extravasation** is the accidental leakage of intravenous drugs into the tissue surrounding the venipuncture, either through a weak portion of the vein or because the needle has punctured the vein and the infusion goes directly into the surrounding tissue. These extravasations provoke an intense local inflammatory response. Moreover, the application of some dermatologic agents to the skin of patients undergoing radiation therapy may contribute to an easily seen inflammatory reaction in and beyond the radiation portal.

Immune reactions protect the host organism from biologic agents. These agents or antigens may be encountered in the external environment of the host or generated less frequently internally. Under normal circumstances, the intensity of the reaction confirms it to be a powerful mechanism of protection and tissue repair. Nevertheless, the reaction is often cytolytic and results in tissue damage. The normal immune reaction is subject to complex physiologic monitoring and control that promote the reaction's resolution when it is no longer a benefit to the host. Sometimes, however, when the reaction is caused by the presence of internally produced antigens, it can be a force that is destructive rather than beneficial to the organism.

A final, and perhaps less obvious, cause of tissue damage is neoplastic growth. One of the hallmarks of malignant tumors is local invasion and destruction of normal tissue. This destruction is accompanied by an inflammatory reaction that is usually of low intensity but microscopically identifiable. Occasionally, the classic signs of inflammation may be encountered in clinical malignancies. Inflammatory breast cancer typically exhibits, to a striking degree, the four cardinal signs of inflammation but is unaccompanied at the microscopic level by typical inflammatory cells, thus emphasizing once more the role of tissue damage rather than macrophages in provoking the inflammatory response.

The six important causes of cell damage (radiation, hypoxia, chemicals, microorganisms, immunologic reactions, and neoplasms) often share a final common pathway in the production of their damage. This pathway leads to the formation of free radicals, which are highly reactive molecular species that are usually intermediary products of oxygen metabolism. Free radicals, which may be produced directly by agents such as ionizing radiation or indirectly by enzymatic reactions in tissue, are destructive to nucleic acids and other vital cellular components.

THE PATHOLOGY OF NEOPLASMS
Neoplastic Diseases

Of the diseases that afflict mankind, cancer is of major importance. In the United States, it is the second leading cause of death. Furthermore, it is the primary disease with which radiation therapists deal. Accordingly, an understanding of the pathology of neoplastic disease is vital to therapists in the performance of their jobs and in their quests for professional maturity.

The term *cancer* applies to many different disease processes that seem to share some common characteristics. In fact, more than 100 types of cancer have been recognized and categorized.

The term *neoplasia* (meaning "new growth") applies to an abnormal process resulting in the formation of a neoplasm or tumor. In the neoplastic process, this new growth occurs beyond the limits of the normal growth pattern. The distinction between normal and neoplastic growth is usually, although not always, well defined and easily recognizable. Therefore, the process of neoplasia can be appreciated as one of disordered growth.

For the patient, the first and most important distinction between benign and malignant tumors involves the prognosis. Benign neoplasms seldom pose any threat to the host, even if left untreated. Several glaring inconsistencies notwithstanding, benign tumors usually carry descriptive names that end simply with *-oma*. These tumors tend to grow slowly and be composed of cells often appearing similar to the normal cells from which they arise. The size of benign tumors may persistently increase or inexplicably halt at a certain point. A benign tumor is usually surrounded by a distinct capsule of fibrous tissue that facilitates surgical removal if treatment is necessary. Although often large, these tumors do not invade surrounding tissue to produce direct destruction nor do they spread distantly to produce metastases.

However, characteristics of malignant tumors, which as a class are referred to as cancers, are much different. Cancers generally pose a serious, if not fatal, threat to the host. Therefore, they are seldom left untreated after discovery. Carcinomas arise in epithelial tissues and sarcomas arise in connective tissues. Cancers tend to grow rapidly, doubling in size over periods ranging from a few days to several months. They are composed of cells with microscopic characteristics decidedly different from normal cells that make up the tissue of origin. In fact, cancers may be so bizarre that they bear little, if any, resemblance to these normal cells. As cellular detail becomes more bizarre, the cell is said to be poorly differentiated compared with tumor cells more closely resembling the cells of origin, which are said to be well differentiated. Growth is incessant and proceeds with invasion and destruction of nearby tissues. The speed of growth correlates roughly with the differentiation of the cells (i.e., well-differentiated cancers tend to grow more slowly than poorly differentiated ones). A true limiting fibrous capsule of the type in benign tumors is lacking. Distant spread, or metastasis, of the cancer results from malignant cells gaining access to blood and lymphatic channels. Not all such cells survive to colonize distant tissues. The metastatic process is only partially understood but clearly more complex than the passive transport of cancer cells through nearby lymphatics or veins. Most cells gaining access to vascular channels never produce viable deposits of tumor cells in regional lymph nodes or more distant tissues. Instead, they are immunologically destroyed by internal surveillance mechanisms. Cancer cells arising in certain organs have a predilection for metastases to specific sites (i.e., cancers of the prostate and breast have a tendency to metastasize to bone). This specific metastatic potential is influenced by the biochemical interaction between proteins and polypeptides produced by both the tumor cells and the cells' populating sites of potential colonization. (See Table 3-1

Table 3-1	Characteristics of Benign and Malignant Tumors	
Characteristics	**Benign**	**Malignant**
Growth rate	Slow	Rapid
Mitoses	Few	Many
Nuclear chromatin	Normal	Increased
Differentiation	Good	Poor
Local growth	Expansive	Invasive
Encapsulation	Present	Absent
Destruction of tissue	Little	Much
Vessel invasion	None	Frequent
Metastases	None	Frequent
Effect on host	Often insignificant	Significant

From Damjanov I, Linder J: *Anderson's pathology,* ed 10, St. Louis, 1996, Mosby.

for a comparison of characteristics of benign and malignant tumors.)

Because benign tumors often require no treatment and have few radiation therapy implications, this chapter does not consider further their pathologic characteristics. Instead, subsequent attention is given to cancers, and their pathologic implications are considered from several points of view.

The term *cancer* in common use applies to the entire spectrum of malignant neoplastic processes. Cancers are broadly divided into carcinomas and sarcomas. The term *carcinoma* refers to a malignant tumor taking its origin from epithelial cells, which are widespread and generally considered to be cells that line surfaces. As such, epithelial cells cover most external surfaces, line most cavities, and form glands. From a functional standpoint, epithelial cells are protective, absorptive, or secretory. Because they are so widely distributed and metabolically active, epithelial cells give rise to a wide variety of tumor types that comprise most solid tumors encountered in clinical practice. Carcinomas tend to invade lymphatic channels more often than blood vessels; therefore, metastases are commonly found in lymph nodes. The designation of carcinoma by the pathologist may be modified by a preceding phrase or prefix further identifying the tissue of origin. For example, a cancer arising from cells lining the upper air and food passages may be designated a squamous cell carcinoma to identify further the nature of the epithelial surface from which the cancer arose. Similarly, a cancer with its origin internally in an organ such as the pancreas (for which surfaces are difficult to imagine) is designated an adenocarcinoma to indicate origin from the secretory epithelium that lines the individual pancreatic glands.

In contrast, the term *sarcoma* describes a neoplasm arising from cells other than those forming epithelial surfaces. From a practical point of view, these cells reside in connective tissue or the nervous system. Although such cells constitute the majority of the body by weight, they spawn relatively few malignant neoplasms. Sarcomas tend to metastasize via blood vessel invasion. This accounts for the frequent appearance of metastatic sarcoma in the lungs. Sarcomas may also carry a pathologic prefix more precisely designating the tissue of tumor origin.

For example, a malignant tumor arising in bone is termed an *osteosarcoma,* one arising in cartilage is termed a *chondrosarcoma,* and one originating from fat cells is termed a *liposarcoma* (see Table 3-2 for comprehensive nomenclature).

In describing carcinomas or sarcomas, the pathologist provides additional commentary about the nature of the neoplasm. This commentary is designed to provide guidance in the prognosis and treatment of the patient. In gross anatomic pathology, commentary is made about the size of the cancer and its apparent extent in tissues received from the surgeon. For example, a cancer of the kidney may be noted to have invaded the renal vein, a portion or all of which has been submitted to the pathologist along with the cancer. Comorbid changes in surrounding normal tissues such as abscess formations that might accompany perforated cancers of the colon are noted.

After examination under the microscope, cancer cells that exhibit no differentiation are called *anaplastic.* Similarly, the term *pleomorphic* describes the great variability in size and shape of these undifferentiated tumor cells. Nuclear abnormalities in cancer cells occur regularly. The nuclei of cancer cells may be assigned designations such as hyperchromatic, clumped, undergoing mitoses, and containing prominent nucleoli. These designations suggest circumstances that reflect malignant degeneration of cells.

Etiology

With so much descriptive terminology, it is perhaps surprising that so little is known about the causes of cancer. That unfortunate set of circumstances is, however, in rapid transition as a result of many advances in molecular biology. Nonetheless, the causes of cancer as presently understood are physiologically naive, incomplete, and more associative than precise. For example, some cancers are associated with exposure to certain chemicals such as those in tobacco smoke. Other cancers are associated with exposure to ionizing radiation in small-to-moderate doses. Still others are associated with viral infections. These associations are useful in describing possible risk factors in the environment, but they remain imprecise in elucidating molecular mechanics of carcinogenesis that allow useful therapeutic intervention.

Chemical carcinogenesis has been accepted as a clinical reality for many decades and was first suggested more than 200 years ago.[4,11] In the mid-18th century in England, Percivall Pott noted an association between scrotum cancer and the work done by chimney sweeps. In the early part of the 20th century, this association between cancer and products of hydrocarbon combustion was confirmed in Japan by Yamagiwa and Ichikawa, who were able to induce cancers in the skin of laboratory animals by the chronic application of coal tar.[13] Since that time, hundreds of chemicals that play roles in cancer induction have been identified and isolated.

Chemical carcinogenesis is not a simple process that proceeds in a linear fashion from point A to point B. Instead, it is a complex process in which interplay with other mechanisms of cancer induction is likely, if not probable. The rate and intensity of these processes vary from one tumor system to the next. Chemical carcinogens are mutagens (i.e., they can cause unusual changes in the deoxyribonucleic acid [DNA] of cells they attack).

Most chemical carcinogens are compounds containing atoms deficient in electrons and are therefore chemically active in the relatively electron-rich milieu that characterizes ribonucleic acid (RNA), DNA, and their products. Many of these chemicals occur naturally, but some are synthetic. Most of them require metabolic activation to assume their carcinogenic statures. Their action is thus somewhat indirect compared with a few compounds such as chemotherapeutic alkylating agents that can directly induce neoplasia. The number of chemical carcinogens is great. Some of the more important ones include polycyclic hydrocarbons produced by the combustion of fossil fuels and tobacco, alcohol, asbestos, nickel compounds, vinyl chloride, and nitrosamines and aflatoxins (both of which can be found in food).

Any of these chemical compounds may react with the DNA of a normal cell to produce a mutation. Having undergone such a mutation, a cell is not necessarily committed to neoplasia. Many mutations are not carcinogenic and, more important, are likely to be detected by cellular surveillance mechanisms that lead to their detection and repair. Some mutations, however, produce strategic damage sufficient to have potential neoplastic consequences. The chemical compound provoking such a mutation is called an *initiator;* the cell has undergone initiation. Initiation only conveys new potential to the cell; it does not produce an immediate cancer. In fact, the time between the initiating event and clinical appearance of the tumor may be many years or decades. The time between the two events is termed the *latent period.* During the latent period, initiated cells may appear normal under the microscope. At the same time, they may display subtle changes in their capacity to respond to mechanisms that usually regulate cell growth. Programmed cell death, or *apoptosis,* may not occur as it normally does, cellular differentiation may become irregular, and the action of another group of chemicals (called promoters) may influence cellular growth. Promoters are seldom carcinogens but have the effect of hastening and intensifying abnormal growth characteristics set in motion by the initiator. As a result, cell division accelerates beyond that normally seen under the influence of the initiator alone to produce a clone of cells displaying increased metabolic activity and early abnormal growth characteristics. In this clone, genetic evolution continues to produce occasional cells that behave more like those of a clinical malignancy. These cells in turn become ascendant and produce daughter cells with even more aggressive features. Whether or not they are augmented by the action of promoters, all these phenomena, which are set in motion by the initiator, culminate in the development of a clinical malignancy if given sufficient time.

The physiologist Francis Peyton Rous first demonstrated viral carcinogenesis in 1911.[10] He induced the growth of soft tissue sarcomas in a strain of normal chickens simply by injecting the chickens with a cell-free filtrate made from a tumor in another bird of the same strain. Unfortunately, the importance of this experiment was not immediately recognized because the entire sequence could not be reproduced in mammals. Moreover, because the particulate nature of viruses was not comprehensively understood at that time, Rous' experiment was relegated to the realm of curiosity. In a few years, Twort and d'Herelle[8] significantly advanced the scientific understanding of cell-free

Table 3-2	Nomenclature of Benign and Malignant Tumors	
Cell or Tissue of Origin	**Benign**	**Malignant**
TUMORS OF EPITHELIAL ORIGIN		
Squamous cells	Squamous cell papilloma	Squamous cell carcinoma
Basal cells	—	Basal cell carcinoma
Glandular or ductal epithelium	Adenoma	Adenocarcinoma
	Papillary adenoma	Papillary adenocarcinoma
	Cystadenoma	Cystadenocarcinoma
Transitional cells	Transitional cell papilloma	Transitional cell carcinoma
Bile duct	Bile duct adenoma	Bile duct carcinoma (cholangiocarcinoma)
Islets of Langerhans	Islet cell adenoma	Islet cell carcinoma
Liver cells	Liver cell adenoma	Hepatocellular carcinoma
Neuroectoderm	Nevus	Malignant melanoma
Placental epithelium	Hydatidiform mole	Choriocarcinoma
Renal epithelium	Renal tubular adenoma	Renal cell carcinoma (hypernephroma)
Respiratory tract	—	Bronchogenic carcinoma
SKIN ADNEXAL GLANDS		
Sweat glands	Syringoadenoma; sweat gland adenoma	Syringocarcinoma, sweat gland carcinoma
Sebaceous glands	Sebaceous gland adenoma	Sebaceous gland carcinoma
Germ cells (testis and ovary)	—	Seminoma (dysgerminoma)
		Embryonal carcinoma, yolk sac tumor
TUMORS OF MESENCHYMAL ORIGIN		
Hematopoietic/lymphoid tissues	—	Leukemias
		Lymphomas
		Hodgkin's disease
		Multiple myeloma
NEURAL AND RETINAL TISSUE		
Nerve sheath	Neurilemoma, neurofibroma	Malignant peripheral nerve sheath tumor
Nerve cells	Ganglioneuroma	Neuroblastoma
Retinal cells (cones)	—	Retinoblastoma
CONNECTIVE TISSUE		
Fibrous tissue	Fibroma	Fibrosarcoma
Fat	Lipoma	Liposarcoma
Bone	Osteoma	Osteogenic sarcoma
Cartilage	Chondroma	Chondrosarcoma
MUSCLE		
Smooth muscle	Leiomyoma	Leiomyosarcoma
Striated muscle	Rhabdomyoma	Rhabdomyosarcoma
ENDOTHELIAL AND RELATED TISSUES		
Blood vessels	Hemangioma	Angiosarcoma
		Kaposi's sarcoma
Lymph vessels	Lymphangioma	Lymphangiosarcoma
Synovia	—	Synoviosarcoma (synovioma)
Mesothelium	Benign mesothelioma	Malignant mesothelioma
Meninges	Meningioma	
Uncertain origin	—	Ewing's tumor
OTHER ORIGINS		
Renal anlage	—	Wilms' tumor
Trophoblast	Hydatidiform mole	Choriocarcinoma
Totipotential cells	Benign teratoma	Malignant teratoma

From Damjonov I, Linder J: *Anderson's pathology,* ed 10, St. Louis, 1996, Mosby.

filtrates by presenting data documenting the true nature of viruses as small packets of genetic material having the capacity to infect and sometimes destroy living cells. Twenty years later Shope and Bittner,[8] working independently, reported viral tumor induction in rabbits and mice, thus inviting more understanding of viral carcinogenesis in mammals.

In scientific laboratories today, many mammalian cell systems exist in which viral tumor induction can be demonstrated.[6] In humans, no specific cancers have been shown to be caused by a viral agent acting alone. However, scientists have discovered strong associations between several cancers and specific types of viruses.

As suggested by Twort and d'Herelle, viruses are simply small packets of genetic material enclosed in capsules. This genetic material may be DNA or RNA, but with either, the virus is an obligate parasite in need of a living cell to infect to reproduce itself. Some viruses can infect many kinds of cells in one or several species. For example, the rabies virus can infect rodents, dogs, and humans. Other viruses exhibit great specificity and can infect only certain cells in a single species. Regardless of the range of potential hosts, infection occurs after the genetic material in the virus gains access to the host cell. Inside the host cell, the viral **genome** assumes command of cellular function to replicate itself. In acute viral infections, this replication is rapid and not only produces hundreds of viral copies but also destroys the infected cell.

 Genome: *A genome is defined as the genetic complement found in the chromosomes of a given organism. (For more information, refer to Hall E:* Radiobiology for the Radiologist, *ed 6, Philadelphia, 2005, Lippincott Williams & Wilkins.)*

Genes of viral derivation that have become incorporated into chromosomes of the host cell and are concerned with the regulation of cell growth are called *viral oncogenes*. A few human cancers are associated with certain viral infections. The four common viruses widely distributed in nature and implicated in human neoplasia are the Epstein-Barr virus (EBV), the human papillomavirus (HPV), the hepatitis B virus (HBV), and the human T-cell leukemia type I virus (HTLV-I).

EBV causes acute infectious mononucleosis. This virus has a predilection for lymphocytes. In some of the lymphocytes, the genome of the virus may persist after the acute infection has resolved. Cell lines established from tumors in patients with Burkitt's lymphoma, immunoblastic lymphoma, and nasopharyngeal cancer often harbor this virus.

HPV is ubiquitous among higher vertebrates. Dozens of types have been recognized and recently classified. These viruses are associated with a variety of neoplasms ranging from simple warts to invasive cancer of the uterine cervix and probably play a role as initiator or promoter in a host of additional cancers arising from squamous cell epithelium.

HBV is endemic in Africa and Asia, continents in which chronic hepatitis is a major cause of mortality. In these same areas, the incidence of hepatocellular carcinoma among those infected with HBV is many times that of uninfected persons. The transitional cascade from HBV infection to the development of hepatocellular carcinoma is complex and remains to be completely elucidated. However, the epidemiologic evidence for an association between the two is overwhelming.

HTLV-I is endemic in Japan, Africa, and the West Indies and is an example of a retrovirus that plays a causal role in the development of human malignancy. Retroviruses are RNA viruses that uniquely carry their own enzyme systems. After invasion of a host cell, this enzyme (reverse transcriptase) allows retroviruses to transcribe their own RNA into DNA, which is then inserted into chromosomes of the host cell. This transcription is necessary because DNA (not RNA) is the functional material of genes.

Although each of these four viruses is associated with human cancer in a significant way, they all require the operation of cofactors to permit neoplastic expression. Complex pathologic interactions are required to defeat the function of normal cells programmed to prevent carcinogenesis.

Most cancers seem to arise spontaneously for reasons poorly understood (i.e., they are not induced by pure chemical nor pure viral mechanisms). Such cancers are considered to be caused by environmental factors. Of course, chemicals and viruses are constituents of the environment, so the classification is somewhat contrived. Nonetheless, among environmental factors that can cause cancer, few are better documented than radiant energy. Ionizing radiation has been known for decades to be carcinogenic.[4,7] The increased incidence of cancer in radiation workers and survivors of atomic bombing is legendary. Most of the radiation workers, whose exposure was chronic, received many small doses of radiation over long periods and subsequently developed cancers of hematologic origin (i.e., leukemias and lymphomas). In contrast, atomic bomb survivors received single large doses of whole-body radiation, which in addition to hematologic malignancies, induced solid tumors of the thyroid, breast, colon, and lung. All these cancers became manifest after latent periods ranging from a few years to several decades. These long, latent periods suggest that many cofactors are operative in radiation carcinogenesis.

Similar latent periods occur in cancers induced by ultraviolet radiation. Sunlight (the principal environmental source of ultraviolet radiation) has been implicated in the induction of all common cancers of the skin (i.e., basal cell carcinoma, squamous cell carcinoma, and malignant melanoma). These cancers arise only in skin lacking protective melanin pigment and therefore rarely occur in African Americans.

The mechanism by which radiant energy causes cancer is linked to its action as a mutagen. Energy absorbed by the cell's nucleus results in damage to the genetic material in the chromosomes, thus producing rearrangement or breakage in the strands of DNA. As in other situations that cause damage to DNA, intracellular mechanisms attempt to promote repair. When repair is incomplete in a cell surviving the radiation insult, the derangement of the genetic material may be perpetuated in much the same way that the incorporated genetic material of the virus is replicated by cells surviving viral infections. During the ensuing latent period, these altered cells are subject to the action

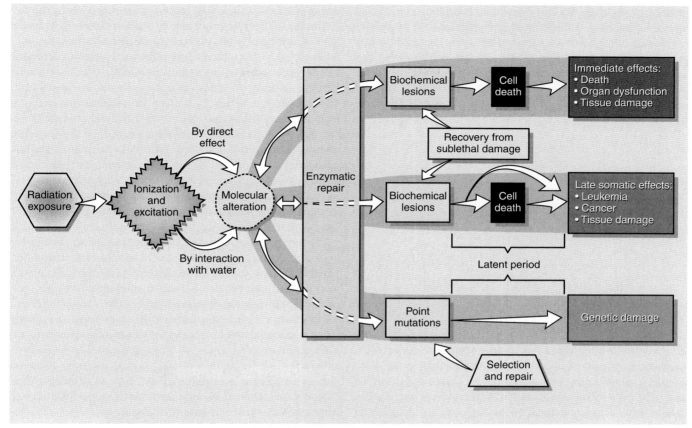

Figure 3-1. The sequence of events following radiation exposure of humans can lead to several radiation responses. At nearly every step, mechanisms for recovery and repair are available. (From Bushong SC: *Radiologic science for technologists*, ed 8, St. Louis, 2004, Mosby.)

of the entire spectrum of carcinogens and may eventually, under proper circumstances, exhibit neoplastic growth (Figure 3-1).

ESTABLISHING A PATHOLOGIC DIAGNOSIS

Little, if any, reason exists to treat cancer without first establishing a pathologic diagnosis. This entails the recovery of cells that the pathologist can identify as malignant.[3] The probable nature of an anatomic abnormality detected in the clinic on physical examination or identified on any of the several imaging studies commonly used in modern medicine can be predicted with considerable accuracy. However, verification of the clinical suspicion usually has significant therapeutic implications for the patient and physician and satisfies minimally the standards required medicolegally before a full-scale assault on cancer can be recommended or planned. More important, the clinical suspicion is sometimes incorrect, thus resulting in major modification of the proposed treatment program. For example, carcinoma of the lung is a disease that can be diagnosed with great regularity before any cells are recovered for examination. By careful consideration of all other available information (including age, symptoms, signs, smoking history, blood test results, and results of imaging studies such as radiographs and computed tomography scans), a malignancy of the lung can be diagnosed without much uncertainty. The conclusion might be made that little else

is required. However, several types of lung cancer exist, and the ability of the previously mentioned determinants to discriminate among them is considerably more limited than their ability to simply suggest the presence of a pulmonary malignancy. Each of the types of lung cancer has its own clinical and biologic characteristics, and these characteristics determine the best treatment and influence the outcome. Accordingly, recovering tumor cells for study to make appropriate recommendations to the patient becomes extremely important. The likely outcome of tissue recovery is only the documentation of a specific type of lung cancer, but the implications could be enormous for all concerned if the typical lung cancer turns out to be something else (i.e., a metastatic cancer or even a benign tumor). Pathologists are not always correct, but their tools for establishing a diagnosis of malignancy are the most powerful available in the medical armamentarium.

The acquisition of living cells to establish a diagnosis of malignancy is obviously a maneuver that is invasive or requires internal encroachment on the site harboring the tumor. This intrusion may be major or minor. The three procedures most commonly used to make a diagnosis of cancer (listed in ascending order of invasiveness) are (1) recovery of exfoliating cells, (2) fine-needle aspiration of malignant cells, and (3) open biopsy of the tumor. Attention to detail is necessary to obtain consistently good results from any of these procedures. The diagnosis depends on submitting to the pathologist representative portions of the tissue suspected of being cancerous. If inadequate samples are submitted, unfortunate inaccuracies in diagnosis are inevitable.

Exfoliative cytology is the study of single cells obtained from various surfaces or secretions shed by the tumor. The foremost example of exfoliative cytology is the Papanicolaou (Pap) smear, which is made for the early detection of cancer of the cervix and uterus. The usefulness of this technique has been proved over several decades.

Fine-needle aspiration is another recovery technique that results primarily in the acquisition of single cells. These cells are recovered through a fine needle inserted directly into the tumor. Because the needles are of small caliber, they can traverse most normal tissue without causing damage and therefore bring remote and relatively inaccessible tumors such as cancer of the pancreas into easy range.

Open biopsy (the most invasive of the three recovery procedures) is accomplished under direct vision. The tumor is surgically removed totally or partly.

Each of these procedures has its own set of variations, and some overlap of procedures is present from one to another. For example, a biopsy may be incisional with removal of only a piece of the tumor or excisional with removal of the entire tumor. Likewise, an incisional biopsy may be accomplished through a large-bore needle.

The tissue sample becomes the responsibility of pathologists who direct laboratory analysis of the specimen along several different pathways. Most important is the preparation of the sample for examination and study under the light microscope. This is usually accomplished by fixing the tissue or preserving its existing form and structure by immersing it in a solution such as formalin.

Specimens of solid tissue are fixed and then placed in hot liquid paraffin. After the paraffin cools and hardens, the tissue can be cut in extremely thin slices by a machine called a *microtome*. These slices are placed on glass slides, which are then immersed in an organic solvent, thus dissolving the paraffin. The resulting tissue sections may be treated with any of a vast number of stains to demonstrate specific features of cellular detail. Using the microscope, pathologists search for evidence of malignancy previously mentioned in this chapter.

Specimens of exfoliating cells or those obtained by fine-needle aspiration are smeared thinly on microscopic slides before being appropriately fixed and stained. In these preparations of single cells, attention is given not only to the size and shape of individual cells but also to the specific features of the nucleus and cytoplasm. Cells lacking uniformity of size, shape, and nuclear configuration may be suggestive of malignancy.

In tissue sections, departures from cellular and nuclear uniformity are also abnormal. In addition, the presence of a malignant tumor usually disturbs normal tissue architecture.

This disturbance is the result of malignant cells invading and destroying surrounding tissue. Some of this invasion may be into blood or lymph vessels, thereby suggesting the metastatic potential of the tumor. However, no single microscopic

abnormality is sufficient to establish the diagnosis of cancer in all instances. The job of pathologists often entails a highly complex and relatively subjective discrimination among a host of biologic variables, which together are predictive of the behavior of the process that is under study. Fortunately, pathologists have other tools to assist in this estimation. Among these tools is the flow cytometer, which is a piece of sophisticated electronic equipment that facilitates the extremely rapid passage of cells in suspension through a laser beam and past an array of detectors. These detectors analyze individual cells for predetermined characteristics such as size, DNA content, surface markers, cell-cycle position, and viability. In carefully selected test samples, abnormal DNA content, variation in cell size, and irregular cell-surface markers can furnish additional evidence of malignancy, identify incomplete responses to therapy, or document early tumor recurrence after treatment. As the molecular biology of the cancer cell is dissected and understood, additional techniques to assist the pathologist in determining the parameters of cell growth have been and continue to be developed. A detailed discussion of this new pathology is beyond the scope of this chapter. However, some of these innovative approaches are referenced in this chapter in the section on the biology of the cancer cell.

CLASSIFYING CANCER

The classification of neoplastic diseases is far from an exact science. Published systems of classification are intended as communication guidelines for those involved in cancer management rather than absolute frames of reference for the pathologist. Virtually all these systems contain many inconsistencies that lack rational explanation but over decades have become entrenched in medical jargon. Only time and experience will convey to the inquisitive radiation therapist an understanding of the full spectrum and meaning of these inconsistencies.

In describing the histopathology of various cancers, the pathologist not only assigns the tumor to a subset but also assigns to that particular tumor a grade and sometimes a stage. Tumor grade and stage are intended to serve as indices of outcome and are therefore of clinical importance.

Tumor grade is a specification that describes the apparent aggressiveness of the cancer as determined by cytologic and morphologic criteria. High-grade tumors are apt to be more aggressive than low-grade tumors. Now in common usage is a system that assigns a numeric value from 1 to 3. Tumors with low numeric designations are likely to be well differentiated, of lower metastatic potential, and easier to control. Conversely, grade 3, or high-grade, tumors appear poorly differentiated, may metastasize early, and may be extremely difficult to control.

Tumor stage is a description of the extent of the tumor at the time of diagnosis. Staging may be clinical, pathologic, or a combination of elements of both. Clinical stage is assigned on the basis of physical examination with or without the assistance of certain imaging studies, depending on the tumor. It is based on recognition of tumor size, invasiveness, and local or distant metastases. The clinical staging of a cancer may be verified and therefore converted to a pathologic stage by recovering appropriate tissue from one or more sites for study under the microscope. A more advanced stage of disease generally implies a worse prognosis. High-grade tumors are likely to be more advanced in stage at the time of diagnosis than low-grade tumors. Most of the time, however, the principal determinant of prognosis is the stage of disease rather than the grade.

Presently, two staging systems predominate. The first of these (the AJCC system) was developed by the American Joint Committee for Cancer Staging and End Results Reporting and represents the ongoing work of a consortium of specialty societies in American medicine. The other (the UICC system) is the work of an international agency known as the International Union Against Cancer. The two systems bear similarities and employ the basic elements of TNM staging introduced more than 50 years ago by Pierre Deniox. The TNM system specifies the extent or stage of a cancer by considering three categories: the primary tumor (T), the regional lymph nodes (N), and distant metastatic disease (M). In staging a particular tumor, the initial of each category is given a numerical subscript designating the extent of disease found in that anatomic compartment. For example, an early breast cancer of less than 2 cm in diameter that has spread neither locally nor distantly is assigned a stage of T1 N0 M0. These staging systems have many permutations and variations with unique meanings regarding tumors of specific sites.

BIOLOGY OF THE CANCER CELL

Considering the cancer cell to be an absolute biologic renegade wreaking havoc on one system after another is tempting. This temptation is resisted, however, by recalling that to exist as an entity at all, the cancer cell must participate in some of the same biologic processes sustaining the many normal cells around it.[5] Consequently, the biology of the cancer cell is best examined in the context of normal cellular function by noting deviations from normal function that cancer cells display.

Cells are diverse in size, shape, and function. Nevertheless, they have many common elements (Figure 3-2). All mammalian cells are surrounded by a cell or plasma membrane. All processes of life occur inside that membrane or on its surface and are accomplished by many specialized components called **organelles**. Within the plasma membrane is the **nucleus** of the cell containing the genetic material DNA that directs cellular metabolism. DNA is the material from which genes are made. Individual genes, which may number in the hundreds of thousands, are normally assigned specific positions or loci on protein structures called **chromosomes**. The cell nucleus also contains one or more **nucleoli**, which are organelles that facilitate **ribosome** assembly. A **nuclear membrane** encloses the nucleus. Between the nucleus and outer cell wall is a substance known as **cytoplasm**, which is a conglomerate of semiliquid material called *cytosol* and numerous extranuclear organelles. Woven throughout the cytoplasm is a filamentous membrane called the **endoplasmic reticulum**, which is continuous with the nuclear membrane and houses the ribosomes. Ribosomes are important organelles responsible for protein synthesis. Other important cytoplasmic organelles include the **Golgi apparatus**, **lysosomes**, **peroxisomes**, **vacuoles**, and **mitochondria**. The Golgi apparatus is important in the storage and management of intracellular chemical substances. Lysosomes play a role in intracellular digestion. Peroxisomes harbor specific enzyme systems, facilitating

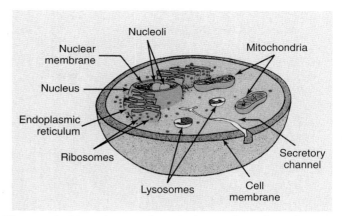

Figure 3-2. Note the membranes that enclose the cell proper and nucleus, respectively. A typical cell contains numerous organelles among which the endoplasmic reticulum, mitochondria, and lysosomes are prominent. The ribosomes, themselves important organelles, are represented by the many dots bordering the endoplasmic reticulum. (From Bushong SC: *Radiologic science for technologists*, ed 8, St. Louis, 2004, Mosby.)

certain metabolic processes, and vacuoles function in cytoplasmic storage. Mitochondria are the intracellular factories that produce adenosine triphosphate (ATP) from sugar and other organic fuels. ATP in turn is the source of energy that drives intracellular metabolism. Under ordinary circumstances, these components of the normal cell function together to maintain equilibrium, promote growth, and facilitate proliferation. All this occurs at one or more points during the cell cycle.

Classically, the **cell cycle** is the observable sequence of events pursued during the life span of a dividing cell.[2] The cycle is chronologically divided into four distinct phases: G1, S, G2, and M (Figure 3-3). G1 is the period before the duplication or synthesis of DNA in the nucleus. This phase is extremely variable in length and may be indistinguishable from G0, in which living cells are fully functional but simply not programmed for mitosis. The S phase is the period during which nuclear DNA is synthesized and chromosomes are duplicated. The G2 phase of the cell cycle commences after DNA synthesis is complete and continues until the cell begins to divide during the M phase. During G2, G1, and S, the cell is growing, producing proteins and organelles, and discharging its metabolic responsibilities. The shortest phase of the cell cycle is M, during which mitosis occurs. Whereas other phases may be measured in days or weeks, mitosis usually occurs in about 2 hours. With completion of mitosis, two identical daughter cells have been made. They in turn enter G1 to repeat the same sequence of events that led to their production.

 The radiation therapist should be cognizant that radiation is most effective on cells that are actively dividing (Law of Bergonié and Tribondeau). (Refer to Hall E: Radiobiology for the Radiologist, ed 6, Philadelphia, 2005, Lippincott Williams & Wilkins.)

During G1 the young daughter cell grows (i.e., increases in mass) and undergoes differentiation, or the expression of

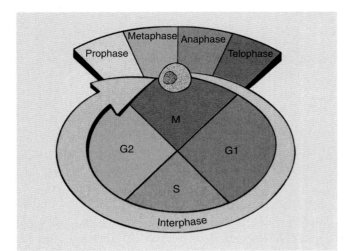

Figure 3-3. The cell's cycle progress through one cycle involves many phases. (From Bushong SC: *Radiologic science for technologists*, ed 8, St. Louis, 2004, Mosby.)

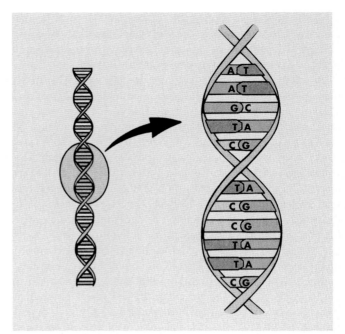

Figure 3-4. A schematic representation of the DNA double helix. *A*, Adenine; *C*, cytosine; *G*, guanine; *T*, thymine are paired nitrogenous bases. (From Bushong SC: *Radiologic science for technologists*, ed 8, St. Louis, 2004, Mosby.)

structural and functional specialization. The cell may prepare to proliferate or divide once more, but G1 is usually a point of restraint in cellular proliferation. Ordinarily, proliferation and differentiation are closely controlled by interrelated physiologic processes. They also tend to be reciprocal (i.e., the greater the differentiation, the less the proliferation). When these complex, cell cycle–related, intracellular mechanisms break down, reciprocity may be expressed in the uncontrolled proliferation of poorly differentiated cells.

Ultimately, these processes are controlled by molecular events predetermined by gene expression. Through the study and understanding of gene expression, molecular biology has evolved and dramatically expanded over the last two decades, and molecular biology has contributed greatly to the understanding of normal and malignant cells. (For a detailed discussion of gene form and function, refer to a standard college biology textbook.)

Genes that line chromosomes are composed of DNA, which is composed of a series of deoxyribonucleotides.[1,5] **Nucleotides** in general have three chemical components: a phosphate group, a molecule of sugar containing five carbon atoms, and a nitrogenous base. The five-carbon sugar may be deoxyribose or ribose, depending on whether the nucleic acid is DNA or RNA. Five nitrogenous bases—adenine, guanine, thymine, cytosine, and uracil—are in nucleotides. Adenine, guanine, thymine, and cytosine are in DNA. In RNA, uracil substitutes for thymine.

DNA is arranged in two complementary strands configured in the shape of a double helix (Figure 3-4). Nucleotides are present in a specific and unique sequence as far as nitrogenous bases are concerned. These bases connect the two strands of DNA and are complementary because chemical bonds that can form between the nitrogenous bases are exclusive. Adenine on one strand can combine only with thymine on the other. Similarly, guanine can combine only with cytosine. As a result, each strand bears in its structure the blueprint necessary to precisely reproduce the other strand. In the cell cycle, during synthesis, the strands are separated and each serves as a template to reproduce its complementary image; thus genetic replication is accomplished.

Proteins are the building blocks of life. They provide form and function for the organism and regulate growth and metabolism. Proteins are complex molecules composed of polypeptides. It is at the **polypeptide** level that the genetic expression has its impact, for it is the unique sequencing of the nucleotides along the length of a strand of DNA that determines the polypeptide configuration of all of the body proteins. Peptide information is encoded along the DNA strand in sequences called *codons.* Each codon is three nucleotides in length and represents a specific amino acid. Amino acids are the molecules from which peptides are made. RNA facilitates the transition from the code of DNA sequencing and codons to the structure of polypeptides and a protein molecule. In a process called **transcription**, enzymes in the cell nucleus facilitate the transfer of information from a strand of DNA to a strand of RNA. This particular type of RNA is called *messenger RNA* (mRNA). To become functional, this message-bearing strand of RNA undergoes splicing, during which the introns are excised. This excision results in a strand of RNA that contains only meaningful codons. After the splicing is complete, the mRNA leaves the nucleus for ribosomes in the cytoplasm.

 Transcription: *To learn more about the role of messenger RNA; mutations; and the role that UV light, chemicals, and other agents may play in causing mutations, go to www.ncc.gmu.edu/dna/transcri.htm.*

Ribosomes are the site of **translation** at which the message borne by the mRNA is apprehended by another type of RNA termed *transfer RNA* (tRNA) and is restated in the language of peptides. Transfer RNA is the form of RNA that transfers amino acids from the cytoplasm to the ribosome. In the sequence prescribed by the incoming mRNA, the tRNA supplies the ribosome with the specific amino acids to construct the required polypeptide. As the polypeptide grows in length, it begins to assume the three-dimensional configuration characteristic of the protein being constructed. After the required number of amino acids has been assembled and the three-dimensional folding and coiling has been completed, the resulting molecule may be a functional protein. In some situations the resulting protein undergoes enzymatic modification; in others, no such modification is required. In either situation, the result is a functional protein whose structure was determined by a unique sequence of nucleotides in the nucleus of the cell.

If the evident function of this newly made protein is to regulate cell growth by suppressing uncontrolled proliferation, such a protein is the product of a **tumor-suppressor gene**. Conversely, if the evident function is to accelerate cell growth, the responsible gene is termed an **oncogene** or perhaps its precursor, a proto-oncogene.[1,2] Tumor-suppressor genes and oncogenes are found in the normal genome. When both are properly located on the correct chromosome and accurately configured, cell growth and division proceed normally insofar as they are influenced by these proteins. If the genes become altered in location or configuration, the delicate balance between the proteins suppressing cell growth and those augmenting it may be destroyed.

DNA rearrangement occurs through mutations.[9] This rearrangement produces corresponding alterations in the resulting protein. In terms of neoplastic change, the genes most sensitive to mutation are oncogenes and tumor-suppressor genes. Oncogenes may be of viral derivation or part of the normal genome. In either situation, they have the potential to trigger malignant growth. Proto-oncogenes have similar potential but require some modification, usually by mutation, to function as oncogenes. Mutations may result in several types of genetic aberration, including gene amplification, chromosome translocation, gene transposition, and point mutations.

After mutation, gene amplification occurs when DNA replication becomes selective, thus resulting in overproduction and therefore overexpression of any gene. Amplification of an oncogene results in augmentation of cell growth. The *erb*B2 oncogene is often amplified in breast cancer, enhancing cell growth by elaboration of a protein that induces a favorable hormonal environment.

 Gene alterations: BRCA1 *and* BRCA2 *are gene alterations that are linked to hereditary breast and ovarian cancers. For more information, go to www.cancer.gov/cancertopics/ factsheet/risk/BRCA.*

Chromosome translocation results from mutations that cause chromosome breakage. The broken fragments may be juxtaposed from one chromosome to another and function abnormally. They may also facilitate oncogene expression. Translocations are frequently encountered in hematologic malignancies such as chronic myelogenous leukemia.

The pathology and pathophysiology of cancer are medical disciplines undergoing rapid expansion. Investigations of the molecular biologist have created a new understanding of the basic processes of life. With the discovery of each new gene and its protein product comes the potential to fit yet another piece into the biologic puzzle of cancer and its clinical management.

To keep abreast of these developments, the reader should monitor any of the several scientific publications devoted to providing understandable updates about cancer research.

SUMMARY

Having completed the sections of this chapter covering cells and the nature of disease, the pathology of neoplasia, establishment of a pathologic diagnosis, the classification of cancer, and the biology of the cancer cell, the reader should have a better understanding of pathology and how it affects cancer growth, cell patterns, and cancer cell classification.

- Cells differ greatly concerning functions they perform, but they have certain characteristics in common. All cells share the ability to produce energy and maintain themselves in a state of normal function called *homeostasis.*
- The inflammatory response is a complex, immunochemical reaction initiated by normal cells that have been injured or damaged. Its clinical features include redness, warmth, swelling, and pain.
- The six important causes of cell damage (radiation, hypoxia, chemicals, microorganisms, immunologic reactions, and neoplasms) often share a final common pathway in the production of their damage.
- The term *cancer* applies to many different disease processes that share some common characteristics. In fact, more than 100 types of cancer have been recognized and categorized. For the patient, the first and most important distinction between benign and malignant tumors involves the prognosis. Benign neoplasms seldom pose any threat to the host, even if left untreated.
- The term *carcinoma* refers to a malignant tumor taking its origin from epithelial cells, which are widespread and generally considered to be cells that line surfaces. In contrast, the term *sarcoma* describes a neoplasm arising from cells other than those forming epithelial surfaces. From a practical point of view, these cells reside in connective tissue or the nervous system.
- The three procedures most commonly used to make a diagnosis of cancer are (1) recovery of exfoliating cells, (2) fine-needle aspiration of malignant cells, and (3) open biopsy of the tumor.
- The cycle is chronologically divided into four distinct phases: G1, S, G2, and M.
- Through the study and understanding of DNA and gene expression, molecular biology has evolved and dramatically expanded over the last two decades, contributing greatly to the understanding of normal and malignant cells.

Review Questions

Multiple Choice

1. When cells maintain themselves in the range of normal function, they are said to be in a state of:
   a. homocarcinosis
   b. homeostasis
   c. hyperchromasia
   d. hypoesthesia

2. A tumor that tends to grow slowly is said to be:
   a. well differentiated
   b. moderately well differentiated
   c. moderately differentiated
   d. poorly differentiated
3. The most common cause of tissue damage is:
   a. microbial infection
   b. ionizing radiation
   c. allergic or immune reaction
   d. hypoxia
4. All of the following tumors arise from epithelial tissues except:
   a. leukemia
   b. cystadenocarcinoma
   c. choriocarcinoma
   d. transitional cell carcinoma
5. The chemical carcinogens that may be found in food are:
   1. asbestos
   2. polycyclic hydrocarbons
   3. alcohol
   4. nitrosamines
   5. aflatoxins
      a. 1 and 4
      b. 2 and 5
      c. 3 and 4
      d. 4 and 5
6. The organelle responsible for protein synthesis is (the):
   a. Golgi apparatus
   b. mitochondria
   c. ribosomes
   d. peroxisomes
7. The cell cycle phase, which is the period before the duplication or synthesis of DNA in the nucleus, is:
   a. G1
   b. S
   c. G2
   d. M
8. The process resulting in the transfer of genetic information from a molecule of DNA to a molecule of RNA is:
   a. translation
   b. transcription
   c. synthesis
   d. transfer
9. The process that results in the construction of a polypeptide in accordance with genetic information contained in a molecule of RNA is:
   a. translation
   b. transcription
   c. synthesis
   d. transfer
10. The gene that regulates the normal development and growth of cancerous tissues is a(n):
    a. proto-oncogene
    b. oncogene
    c. tumor-suppressor gene
11. The absence or inactivation of which gene leads to uncontrolled growth or neoplasm?
    a. proto-oncogene
    b. oncogene
    c. tumor-suppressor gene

The answers to the Review Questions can be found by logging on to our website at: *http://evolve.elsevier.com/Washington+Leaver/principles*

Questions to Ponder

1. What factors historically influenced the understanding of disease?
2. What is homeostasis?
3. Briefly discuss the metastatic process of malignant neoplasms.
4. Why is staging cancer important?
5. Describe the structure of DNA.
6. Discuss the cell cycle as it relates to radiation therapy.

REFERENCES

1. Baserga R: Principles of molecular cell biology of cancer: the cell cycle. In De Vita VT Jr, Hellman S, Rosenberg SA, editors: *Cancer: principles and practice of oncology,* ed 7, Philadelphia, 2004, JB Lippincott.
2. Bonfiglio TA, Terry R: The pathology of cancer. In Rubin P, editor: *Clinical oncology,* ed 8, Philadelphia, 2001, WB Saunders.
3. Campbell NA: *Biology,* ed 7, Riverside, CA, 2004, Benjamin/Cummings.
4. Hall EJ: Principles of carcinogenesis: physical. In De Vita VT Jr, Hellman S, Rosenberg SA, editors: *Cancer: principles and practice of oncology,* ed 7, Philadelphia, 2004. JB Lippincott.
5. Hill RP: The biology of cancer. In Rubin P, editor: *Clinical oncology,* ed 8, Philadelphia, 2001, WB Saunders.
6. Howley PM: Principles of carcinogenesis: viral. In De Vita VT Jr, Hellman S, Rosenberg SA, editors: *Cancer: principles and practice of oncology,* ed 7, Philadelphia, 2004, JB Lippincott.
7. Madri JA: Inflammation and healing. In Damjanov I, Linder J editors: *Anderson's pathology,* ed 10, St. Louis, 1995, Mosby.
8. Pennazio S: The origin of phage virology, *Rev Biol* 99(1): 103-29, 2006.
9. Perkins AS, Vande Woude GF: Principles of molecular cell biology of cancer: oncogenes. In De Vita VT Jr, Hellman S, Rosenberg SA, editors: *Cancer: principles and practice of oncology,* ed 7, Philadelphia, 2004, JB Lippincott.
10. Sheldon H: *Boyd's introduction to the study of disease,* ed 11, Philadelphia, 1992, Lea & Febiger.
11. Shields PG, Harris CC: Principles of carcinogenesis: chemical. In De Vita VT Jr, Hellman S, Rosenberg SA, editors: *Cancer: principles and practice of oncology,* ed 7, Philadelphia, 2004, JB Lippincott.
12. Vande Woude S, Vande Woude GF: Principles of molecular cell biology of cancer: introduction to methods in molecular biology. In De Vita VT Jr, Hellman S, Rosenberg SA, editors: *Cancer: principles and practice of oncology,* ed 7, Philadelphia, 2004, JB Lippincott.
13. Yamagiwa K, Ichikawa K: Experimental study of the pathogenesis of carcinoma, *CA Cancer J Clin* 27(3): 174-181, 1977.

BIBLIOGRAPHY

Anthony CP, Kolthoff NJ: *Textbook of anatomy and physiology,* ed 9, St. Louis, 1974, Mosby.
Boyd CM, Dalrymple GV: *Basic science principles of nuclear medicine,* St. Louis, 1974, Mosby.
del Regato JA, Spjut HJ, Cox JD: *Ackerman and del Regato's cancer: diagnosis, treatment, and prognosis,* ed 6, St. Louis, 1985, Mosby.
Kiemar V, Cotran RS, Robbins SL: *Basic pathology,* ed 5, Philadelphia, 1992, WB Saunders.

Overview of Radiobiology

Amy C. Vonkadich

Outline

Key Terms

Objectives

- Define *ionization* and list the rules of reactions to ionizing radiation.
- Define the term *radiobiology*.
- Compare and contrast direct ionization and indirect ionization.
- Define *LET*.
- Define *RBE*.
- Compare and contrast high-LET and low-LET radiation.
- List the types of DNA damage that may occur, including the consequences.
- List the gross structural changes to chromosomes.
- Diagram the cell cycle, labeling all phases.
- List the three categories of cellular response to radiation.
- Draw a cell survival curve for mammalian cells, and label the different components.

- State the three external factors that influence cellular response to radiation, and give examples of each.
- Explain the Law of Bergonié and Tribondeau.
- List each group of cell populations, and give an example of each.
- Compare and contrast the two components of tissues and organs.
- State the two phases of response to radiation.
- Compare and contrast the processes of repair and regeneration.
- List the three syndromes of total-body irradiation.
- Summarize the effects of radiation damage to the embryo and fetus.
- State the goal of radiation therapy.
- Define *tissue tolerance dose,* and list several factors that alter the tolerance of tissue to radiation.

INTERACTION OF RADIATION AND MATTER

Since the discovery of x-rays by Roentgen in 1895, scientists and clinicians have investigated the interaction of **ionizing* radiations** and various target materials, including biologic tissue. When discussing the interaction of radiation with matter, two terms must be described—ionization and excitation. In both ionization and excitation, the incoming radiation interacts with an atom. In ionization, the incoming radiation ejects an electron from the shell of the atom, thus causing the atom to be charged (ionized). In excitation, the electron in the outer shell of the atom is said to be excited (oscillating or vibrating) but is not ejected from the shell. *Radiation biology,* or *radiobiology,* has evolved since Roentgen's time and can be defined as the study of the sequence of events following the absorption of

---

*Ionization refers to the ejection of an electron from an atom, thus resulting in a charged particle or ion.

energy from ionizing radiations, the efforts of the organism to compensate, and the damage to the organism that may be produced.[64]

In evaluating the response of a living cell to ionizing radiation, the following must be considered[64]:

1. Radiation may or may not interact with a cell.
2. If an interaction occurs, damage may or may not be produced in the cell.
3. The initial energy deposition occurs extremely rapidly (much less than 1 second) and is nonselective or random in the cell, no specific areas of the cell are "chosen."
4. Visible tissue changes after irradiation are not usually distinguishable from those caused by other traumas. (The only exception to this may be cataracts, which are discussed later.)
5. Biologic changes that occur after irradiation do so after some time has elapsed. The duration of this latent period is inversely related to the dose administered and can range from minutes to years.

 For convenience, it is usual to classify ionizing radiations as electromagnetic or particulate.

Types of Interactions

When radiation initially interacts with a cell, the ionizations are direct or indirect.[27] When a beam of charged particles (alpha particles, protons, or electrons) is incident on living tissue, direct ionization (the result of the incident particle itself) of a critical target (**deoxyribonucleic acid [DNA]**) is highly probable because of the relatively densely ionizing nature of most particulate radiations. Direct effects predominate when neutrons compose the primary beam because the secondary particles produced (protons, alpha particles, or heavy nuclear fragments) from the neutron's interaction with the nucleus of the atom may cause damage directly to the DNA or other important macromolecules (large molecules) in the cell.

The other form of ionization is indirect because of the effects of specific secondary particles on the target. This mechanism predominates when the incident beam is composed of x-rays, gamma rays, or neutrons. These indirectly ionizing radiations give rise to fast (high energy), charged secondary particles that can then directly or indirectly cause ionizations in the critical target. Indirect effect occurs predominantly when x-rays or gamma rays compose the primary beam, thus producing fast electrons as the secondary particles that interact with the most abundant cellular medium, water (H_2O). Indirect effects involve a series of reactions known as **radiolysis** (splitting) of water. The initial event in radiolysis involves the ionization or ejection of an electron from a water molecule, thus producing a water ion (charged molecule):

$$H_2O \rightarrow H_2O^+ + 1e^-$$

The ejected electron (e^-), known as a *fast electron* because of its high energy, may now be absorbed by a second water molecule forming another water ion (H_2O^-):

$$e^- + H_2O \rightarrow H_2O^-$$

The pair of water ions produced are chemically unstable and tend to rapidly break down or dissociate into another ion

and a **free radical** (a highly reactive species with an unpaired valence [outer shell] electron):

$$H_2O^+ \rightarrow H^+ + OH^\bullet \text{ and } H_2O^- \rightarrow H^\bullet + OH^-$$

The free radical is symbolized by a dot (e.g., $H^\bullet$ or $OH^\bullet$).

The ion pair (H^+ and OH^-) may recombine, thus forming a normal water molecule with no net damage to the cell. The probability of recombination is high if the two ions are formed close to each other. If these ions persist in the cell, they can react with and damage important macromolecules.

Free radicals may also recombine like the previous ion pair, thus forming a normal water molecule:

$$H^\bullet + OH^\bullet \rightarrow H_2O$$

Free radicals may also combine with other nearby free radicals, thus forming a new molecule such as hydrogen peroxide that is toxic to the cell:

$$OH^\bullet + OH^\bullet \rightarrow H_2O_2 \text{ (hydrogen peroxide)}$$

Free radicals can participate in several other reactions involving normal cellular components, including DNA. Because the majority of the cell (80%) consists of water, the probability of damage by indirect effects is much greater than for direct effects with the use of indirectly ionizing radiations. Of the several reactions just presented for indirect effects, the predominant pathway that accounts for approximately two thirds of cellular damage involves the hydroxyl ($OH^\bullet$) radical. As discussed later, indirect effects predominate with sparsely ionizing or low **linear energy transfer (LET)** radiations and can be modified by physical, chemical, or biologic factors. It is important to keep in mind that due to the majority of the cell consisting of water, the probability of damage occurring through the indirect action is greater than the probability of damage through direct action.

 A free radical contains an unpaired electron in the outer shell; this makes it highly reactive.

Linear Energy Transfer and Relative Biologic Effectiveness

Depending on the composition of the incident beam of radiation, various secondary particles are produced in the cell. These secondary particles may directly or indirectly ionize the critical target. The physical properties of these secondary particles (mass and charge) give rise to a characteristic path of damage in the cell. Radiations can therefore be categorized by the rate at which energy is deposited by charged particles (incident or secondary) as they travel through matter. This is the LET of the radiation.[74] The LET is an average value calculated by dividing the energy deposited in kiloelectron volts (keV) by the distance traveled in micrometers (μm or 10^{-6} m). Sparsely ionizing radiations such as x-rays and gamma rays are therefore classified as low LET because the secondary electrons produced are small particles that deposit their energy over great distances in tissue. Typical LET values for sparsely ionizing radiations may range from 0.3 to 3.0 keV/μm.[63] Densely ionizing radiations, which include charged particles such as protons and alpha particles, are classified as high LET because these particles are much bulkier in terms of mass than electrons and therefore deposit their energy over much smaller distances in the cell (Figure 4-1). LET is therefore directly proportional to the square of the charge (Q) and inversely proportional to the square of the velocity (v). The previously described relationship is expressed in the following equation:

$$LET = Q^2/v^2$$

Typical LET values may range from 30 to 100 keV/μm or greater, depending on the particle energy. Generally, a large charged particle such as a proton or alpha particle does not penetrate nearly as far as a smaller charged particle (electron) and not quite as far as an uncharged particle of equal mass (neutron). Neutrons usually have intermediate LET values (usually within 5 to 20 keV/μm). As the neutron's energy increases, its penetration in tissue also increases; therefore, its LET decreases.

Knowing the LET of the radiation is important because the discovery was made early in the radiation therapy studies that different LET radiations produce different degrees of the same biologic response. In other words, equal doses of different LET radiations do not produce the same biologic response. This is called the **relative biologic effectiveness (RBE)** of the radiation.[27] The RBE relates the ability of radiations with different LETs delivered under the same conditions to produce the same biologic effect. The equation for determining the RBE of a test radiation is as follows:

$$RBE \text{ of test radiation} = \frac{\text{Dose from 250-keV x-ray}}{\text{Dose from test radiation to produce the same biologic effect}}$$

The test radiation referred to includes any type of radiation beam being used. The effectiveness of the beam is determined by a historical comparison with a 250-keV x-ray beam that was the primary radiation beam available in the early days of radiation therapy. For example, if 400 cGy of 250-keV x-rays and 200 cGy of neutrons both result in 50% cell kill, the RBE of the neutrons equals 2. This means that the neutrons are twice as effective as the x-rays. In general, as the LET of the radiation increases, so does its RBE. It is important to note that the biologic response, not the dose of radiation, is constant.

Radiation Effects on Deoxyribonucleic Acid

The key molecule in the nucleus of the cell for radiation damage is thought to be DNA. Damage to a key molecule may be lethal to a cell and has led to the development of a target theory for radiation damage. This theory states that when ionizing radiation interacts with or near a key molecule (DNA), the sensitive area is termed a *target*. An ionization event that occurs in the target is termed a *hit*. These terms are applied only under conditions in which radiation interacts with the target by direct effects. This theory does not account for damage to DNA that is the result of free radical–mediated pathways.

Regardless of whether DNA is damaged by direct or indirect effects caused by radiation, several types of damage can occur.[54] DNA is a large molecule with a well-known double-helix structure. The double helix consists of two strands, held together by hydrogen bonds between the bases. The "backbone" of each strand consists of alternating sugar and phosphate groups. Attached to this backbone are four bases, the sequence of which specifies the genetic code. Two of the bases are termed *pyrimidines*—these are thymine and cytosine. The remaining two bases are termed *purines*–these are adenine and guanine.[27] One form of damage involves the change in or loss of one or more of the four nitrogenous (nitrogen-containing) bases: adenine (A), thymine (T), cytosine (C), and guanine (G). A second form of damage may involve breakage of hydrogen bonds between the A-T and C-G base pairs, which function to keep the two DNA strands together. Bonds may also be broken between the components of the backbone of each DNA strand (i.e., between the deoxyribose sugar and phosphate groups connected to each base and known collectively as a *nucleotide*). This may lead to intrastrand or interstrand cross-linking of DNA.

The consequences of these types of DNA damage vary. Loss or change of a base results in a new base sequence, which can cause minor or major effects on protein synthesis. A change in base sequence not rectified by the cell is an example of a mutation (change in the genetic material). Agents such as ionizing radiation that cause mutations are mutagenic. Single-strand breaks in the DNA backbone (common after irradiation with low-LET radiations) may or may not be repaired. If they are not repaired, damage may occur. Single-strand breaks are more readily repaired than double-strand breaks, which are more apparent after exposure to high-LET radiations. The production of multiple-strand breaks compared with single-strand breaks correlates much more strongly with cell lethality. Radiation interaction with DNA does not always result in damage, and most of the damage can be and probably is repaired. Consequences of DNA damage in somatic (body) cells involve the irradiated organism or individual, whereas DNA damage in germ (reproductive) cells may also affect future generations.

Radiation Effects on Chromosomes

A review of the four phases of mitosis, which is a continuous process of organizing and arranging nuclear DNA during cell division, is helpful in understanding radiation effects on chromosomes. Figure 4-2 shows the major events of mitosis.

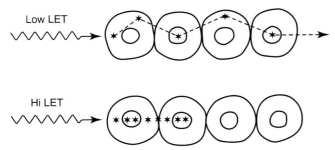

Figure 4-1. Comparative effects of low- and high-LET radiations on a population of cells. Low-LET radiation interacting with four cells emits an irregular path, whereas the straight path of high-LET radiation interacts with only two cells. High-LET radiation has produced two hits in the nuclei of two different cells, whereas low-LET radiation has produced only one hit in the same number of cells. (From Travis EL: *Primer of medical radiobiology,* ed 2, St. Louis, 1989, Mosby, with permission.)

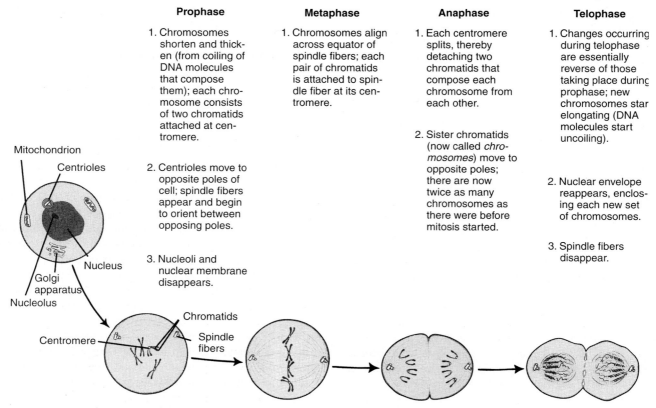

Figure 4-2. The major events of mitosis. (Modified from Thibodeau GA, Patton KT: *Anatomy and physiology,* ed 3, St. Louis, 1996, Mosby. Courtesy Joan M. Beck.)

Because DNA molecules form genes and thousands of genes compose a chromosome, studying genetic damage from ionizing radiation in terms of gross structural damage to chromosomes is often easiest.[19]

Early studies in this area often involved plant chromosomes because their small diploid number (number of chromosomes in each somatic cell) and large relative size facilitated study under the light microscope. The fact that radiation is an efficient breaker of chromosomes by indirect or direct pathways is now well documented. Gross structural changes in chromosomes are referred to as *aberrations, lesions,* or *anomalies.* A distinction also exists between chromosome and chromatid aberrations. A chromosome aberration occurs when radiation is administered to cells in the G1 phase or before the cell replicates its DNA in the S phase (cell duplication). A chromosome aberration may involve both daughter cells after mitosis, because if the break is not repaired, the cell replicates it during the S phase. A chromatid aberration results when radiation is administered to cells in the G2 phase or after they have completed DNA synthesis (cell duplication). This term applies to the arms (chromatids) of a replicated (duplicated) chromosome. In this situation, only one of the two daughter cells formed after cell division is affected if the damage is not repaired.

Structural changes induced in chromosomes by radiation include single breaks, multiple breaks, and a phenomenon known as *chromosome stickiness,* or *clumping.* Consequences of these structural changes may include healing with no damage and loss or rearrangement of genetic material.

A single radiation-induced break in any part of a chromosome results in two chromosome fragments. One fragment contains the centromere (the place the mitotic spindle attaches during mitosis), and the other (known as the *acentric fragment*) does not.[64] The rejoining of these fragments, termed *restitution,* has a high probability of occurring because of their proximity.[19] Approximately 95% of all single breaks heal by restitution with the result being no damage to the cell.

If irradiation occurs in G1 cells and restitution does not occur, both fragments are replicated during the S phase, thus resulting in four fragments (each with a broken end).[64] Two of these chromatids contain a centromere, whereas the other two do not. The two centromere-containing chromatids may now join, thus forming a dicentric fragment. The other two fragments may also join, thus forming an acentric fragment.

These structural aberrations become evident during the metaphase and anaphase stages of mitosis. Because the acentric fragment does not contain a centromere, the spindle fibers do not attach to it during the metaphase stage. Therefore, the genetic material it contains probably will not be transmitted to either daughter cell. The dicentric fragment, however, has two centromeres and will therefore be attached to the mitotic spindle at two sites instead of one. Therefore this fragment is pulled simultaneously toward both poles of the cell. The fragment between the two centromeres therefore becomes stretched, thus giving rise to a characteristic anaphase bridge, which eventually tears by the end of the anaphase stage, thus resulting in an unequal transmission of genetic information to each daughter cell (Figure 4-3).

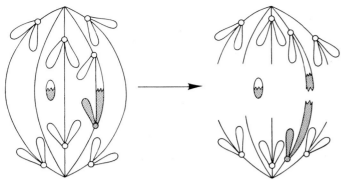

Figure 4-3. The fate of the dicentric and acentric fragments during anaphase, thus leading to anaphase bridge formation. The dicentric fragment attaches to the mitotic spindle at each centromere and is pulled toward both poles of the cell *(left)* and ultimately breaks again *(right)*. The acentric fragment does not attach to the spindle, thus resulting in loss of genetic material to the new daughter cells. (From Travis EL: *Primer of medical radiobiology,* ed 2, St. Louis, 1989, Mosby.)

A single break in one chromatid in two different chromosomes also produces four fragments. Two fragments contain a centromere and two do not.[64] Again, dicentric and acentric chromosomes may result by the joining of the broken fragments (Figure 4-4, A). In addition, the acentric fragment from one broken chromosome may join to a centromere-containing fragment of the other broken chromosome, thus forming a new normal-appearing chromosome. This rearrangement is known as *translocation* (Figure 4-4, B). Although translocation does not necessarily result in a loss of genetic information, the sequence

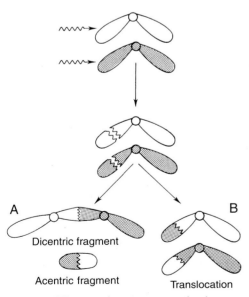

Figure 4-4. Two different chromosomes *(top)* may sustain a single break in one arm *(center)* and result in formation of dicentric and acentric fragments **(A)** or translocation of genetic material between the two **(B)**. In the latter process, two complete chromosomes are formed. However, the exchange of chromosome parts and therefore genetic information should be noted. (From Travis EL: *Primer of medical radiobiology,* ed 2, St. Louis, 1989, Mosby.)

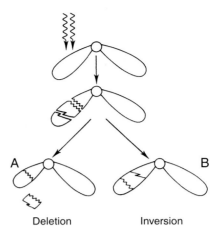

Deletion   Inversion

Figure 4-5. Two breaks occurring in the same arm of a chromosome *(top and middle)* may result in deletion of the fragment between the breaks **(A)** or inversion of the fragment, which is illustrated by the change in positions of the break lines **(B)**. (From Travis EL: *Primer of medical radiobiology,* ed 2, St. Louis, 1989, Mosby.)

of genes in the new translocated chromosome is different from the original sequence before radiation damage. The consequences of radiation-induced translocations can vary from no effects in somatic cells to malformed or nonviable offspring if these translocations occur in germ cells.

A double break in one arm (chromatid) of a chromosome results in three fragments, each with a broken end.[64] Of these three, one fragment contains the centromere and the other two are acentric. The major consequences of a double break are known as *deletions* and *inversions* (see Figure 4-3). A deletion of genetic material results when the fragment between the breaks is lost and the remaining two fragments join (Figure 4-5, A). The effect of a deletion varies depending on the amount and significance of the genetic information that was in the lost fragment. An inversion of genetic material results when the middle fragment with two broken ends turns around or inverts before rejoining the other two fragments (Figure 4-5, B). Although no loss of genetic material occurs after an inversion, the DNA base sequences, and therefore the gene sequence, are altered. This affects the types and amounts of critical proteins synthesized by the cell and can certainly affect the long-term viability of the cell.

Because of the random absorption of ionizing radiation in the cell, a single break can be induced in each chromatid of the same chromosome, thus again producing three fragments. The fragment with two broken ends contains the centromere and the other two fragments are acentric. This may result in the formation of a ring chromosome and an acentric chromosome[64] (Figure 4-6). The ring chromosome is replicated and transmitted to the daughter cells, whereas the acentric fragment and its genetic information are not passed on. If a replicated ring chromosome becomes tangled before the metaphase stage, unequal separation of each ring during the anaphase stage may result, therefore the daughter cells do not inherit equal amounts of genetic information.

Several factors influence the type and extent of chromosome damage induced by ionizing radiations. The number of single

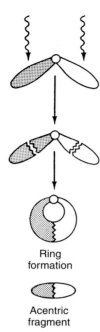

Figure 4-6. One possible consequence of breaks in both arms of a chromosome by radiation is that the broken arms join to form a ring. The remaining fragments join but are left without a centromere (acentric fragment). (From Travis EL: *Primer of medical radiobiology,* ed 2, St. Louis, 1989, Mosby.)

breaks produced is directly proportional to the total dose of radiation administered. The frequency of single breaks, or simple aberrations, also increases as the LET of the radiation decreases. Therefore, low-LET radiations such as x-rays and gamma rays produce a higher amount of simple versus complex (multiple break) aberrations.

Radiation Effects on Other Cell Components

Although nuclear DNA is the critical target for radiation-induced cell damage, other structures in the cell are also damaged by ionizing radiations and contribute to cell damage and death.[55] Among these cellular components is the plasma or cell membrane. Absorption of energy by the structural components of the plasma membrane (i.e., the phospholipid bilayer and proteins) can result in membrane damage and therefore changes in the permeability of the membrane with regard to the transport of substances in and out of the cell. Damage to the mitochondrial and lysosomal membranes in the cytoplasm can also result in drastic consequences to the cell. All cellular components (including vital proteins, enzymes, carbohydrates, and lipids) can undergo structural and functional changes after irradiation that can be deadly to the cell. Because the deposition of energy from secondary particles (electrons, protons, or alpha particles) is random in matter, any site in the cell can be at risk for damage from radiation exposure.

CELLULAR RESPONSE TO RADIATION

Since the mid-1950s, when Puck and Marcus[46] first irradiated human cervical carcinoma cells in a Petri dish, the response of human, animal, and plant cells to radiation has been intensely studied. The response of cells after irradiation can now be placed into one of three categories: division delay, interphase death, or reproductive failure.

 Puck and Marcus: *The line of cervical carcinoma cells that have been used since the 1950s are termed* HeLa *cells.*

Division Delay

Irradiated cells that involve a disruption in the mitotic index (MI), the ratio of the number of mitotic cells to the total number of cells in the irradiated population, is known as *division delay*. This results in cells in interphase at the time of irradiation to be delayed in the G2 phase. This is also known as *mitotic delay*.

The consequence of mitotic delay is a decrease in the MI for the population, which means that fewer cells than normal will enter mitosis and divide. Therefore, fewer new daughter cells will be produced. The magnitude of this response to radiation is dose dependent; the higher the radiation dose, the longer is the mitotic delay and therefore the greater is the decrease in MI. If the dose is less than 1000 cGy, most cell lines recover and eventually proceed through mitosis. This results in a higher-than-normal number of cells dividing and is termed *mitotic overshoot*.

Canti and Spear[12] first observed division delay in 1929 when they exposed chick fibroblasts in vitro to various doses of radiation. The mechanism behind division delay is thought to involve the inhibition or delay of DNA and/or protein synthesis after irradiation. Apparently, cells attempt to repair radiation damage before mitosis by stopping in the G2 phase to confirm that the DNA and proteins are intact. Any damage found is repaired during this phase of the cell cycle so that it does not disrupt cell division or possibly lead to cell death. Division delay occurs in both lethally and nonlethally damaged cells.

Interphase Death

If irradiation of the cell during the G1, S, or G2 phase results in death, this mode of response is termed an *interphase death*.[62] Interphase death is defined as the death of irradiated cells before these cells reach mitosis, also known as *nonmitotic* or *nondivision death*.[64] This form of cell response can occur in nondividing cells (such as adult nerve cells) and rapidly dividing cells. In general, radiosensitive cells (vegetative intermitotic [VIM] and differentiating intermitotic [DIM]) succumb to an interphase death at lower radiation doses than do radioresistant cells (reverting postmitotic [RPM] and fixed postmitotic [FPM]). The exception to this is the mature lymphocyte, which is sensitive to interphase death at a dose as low as 50 cGy. The mechanism of interphase death is not clear but may involve damage to one or more biochemical pathways involved in cell metabolism. In most cell types, interphase death is not the primary mode of response to irradiation.

Reproductive Failure

The third and most common end point for response of cells to radiation is **reproductive failure** (also known as *mitotic death*), which is defined as a decrease in the reproductive integrity or cells' ability to undergo a limited number of divisions after irradiation.[46]

This effect on the reproductive capacity of cells can be traced to the extent of chromosome damage induced by the radiation dose.

Apoptosis

Although unrelated to mitosis, because it is not an unsuccessful attempt by the cell to divide, another form of cell death that has been associated with the cellular response to radiation is apoptosis (programmed cell death). Cellular apoptosis appears to have gene (*p53* and *bcl-2*) involvement following exposure to radiation.[27] A characteristic apoptotic cell death involves nuclear fragmentation, cell lysis, and phagocytosis of the chromatin bodies by neighboring cells.[64]

Cell Survival Curves

The most common way of evaluating the cellular response to radiation was first introduced by Puck and Marcus[46] in 1956, when they irradiated human cervical cancer cells (known as *HeLa cells*) in vitro and plotted the results (number of colonies formed) on a semilogarithmic graph. Their results, termed a *survival curve,* was a plot of the radiation dose administered on the *x*-axis versus the surviving fraction (SF) of cells on the *y*-axis (Figure 4-7).

This survival curve is characteristic of the survival of cells exposed to low-LET radiations such as x-rays or gamma rays. A shoulder region or flattening of the curve occurs at doses below 150 cGy and indicates that cells must accumulate damage in multiple targets to be killed. Because this survival curve is graphed on a semilog plot, the linear portion of the curve (above a dose of 150 cGy) indicates that equal increases in dose causes equal decreases in the SF of cells but the absolute number of cells killed varies[64] (Table 4-1).

This exponential response of cells to radiation is due to the random probability of radiation interacting with critical targets in the cell. On irradiation of a cell population with *n* targets/cell (with *n* > 1), several results are observed:

Table 4-1	The Exponential Relationship Between a Radiation Dose and Surviving Fraction		
Original Cell Number	**Dose Delivered (Gy)**	**Fraction of Cells Killed**	**Number of Cells Killed**
1000,000	5	50	50,000
50,000	5	50	25,000
25,000	5	50	12,500
12,500	5	50	6,250
6,250	5	50	3,125

From Travis EL: *Primer of medical radiobiology,* ed 2, St. Louis, 1989, Mosby.

1. Some cells are lethally damaged (all targets are hit).
2. Some cells are sublethally damaged (a few targets are hit).
3. Some cells are not damaged (no targets are hit).

As the radiation dose increases, the probability of cellular targets being hit also increases.

Three important parameters that allow interpretation of survival curves are the **extrapolation number (*n*),** quasithreshold dose **(D$_q$)**, and **D$_o$** dose. A characteristic survival curve for cells exposed to x-rays is shown in Figure 4-8.[11]

The *n,* originally known as the *target number,* is determined by extrapolating the linear portion of the curve back until it intersects the *y*-axis. In Figure 4-8, the *n* equals 2, which theoretically means two critical targets are in the cell and must be inactivated. For mammalian cells exposed to x-rays, the *n* ranges from 2 to 10.

Another measure of cell response at low doses is the D$_q$. This parameter represents the dose at which survival becomes exponential. The D$_q$ is a measure of the width of the shoulder region of the survival curve and is determined by drawing a horizontal

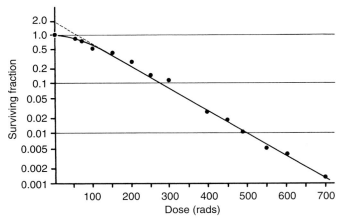

Figure 4-7. The first survival curve using HeLa cells by Puck and Marcus. Below 150 cGy the curve exhibits a shoulder region and becomes exponential (straight) at higher doses. (From Puck TT, Marcus TI: Action of x-rays on mammalian cells, *J Exp Med* 103:653, 1956.)

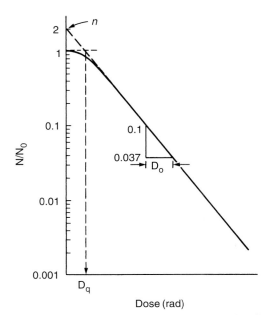

Figure 4-8. The multitarget, single-hit model of cell survival characteristic of low-LET radiations (x-rays and gamma rays). The parameters *n,* D$_o$, and D$_q$ should be noted. (From Bushong SC: *Radiologic science for technologists: physics, biology, and protection,* St. Louis, 2004, Mosby.)

line from an SF of 1 on the *y*-axis to the place it intersects the line extrapolated back from the linear portion of the curve for determination of *n*. The D_q is also a measure of the cell's ability to accumulate and repair sublethal damage.[7,21]

The third parameter, known as the D_o (or *D37*) *dose*, reduces the SF of cells by 63%. In other words, 37% of the cells survive. The D_o equals the reciprocal of the slope of the curve's linear portion and is a measure of the cells' radiosensitivity. Radiosensitive cells have a low D_o, whereas radioresistant cells have a high D_o. For mammalian cells, the D_o usually is between 100 and 220 cGy.[27]

Several equations describe the dose-response relationships expressed by survival curves.[11] The three survival-curve parameters are related by the equation $\log_e n = D_q/D_o$. The SF can be calculated as $SF = 1 - (1 - e^{-D/D_o})^n$. In this equation, *n* is the extrapolation number and *D* is the total dose.[11] This equation accurately predicts the response of complex cell types, including most mammalian cells in which the number of targets is presumed to be greater than one. (This is known as the *multitarget, single-hit model*.)

Factors Influencing Response

As proposed by Ancel and Vitemberger[3] in 1925, various external factors influence cellular response to radiation. This change in response is termed *conditional sensitivity*. Three groups of factors (physical, chemical, and biologic) can affect cellular radioresponse and therefore change the overall appearance of a cell line's survival curve and magnitude of the parameters *n*, D_q, and D_o.

Physical Factors. The response of cells to high-LET radiation differs from that seen after exposure to low-LET radiation.[9] The response of five mammalian cell lines to 300-kV x-rays and 15-MeV neutrons is shown in Figure 4-9. The shoulder region (D_q) is usually decreased or even absent after irradiation with high-LET radiations such as alpha particles and neutrons. In addition, survival curves tend to be steeper (the D_o is lower) after high-LET treatment. The effects of LET on biologic response are due to differences in the density of energy deposition in the cell. Because DNA is thought to be the critical target in cells, the most efficient radiation with the highest RBE induces two strand breaks in the DNA molecule, thus leading to a high probability of cell death. This optimal LET is thought to be approximately 160 keV/μm. Therefore, all radiations with LETs above or below the optimal level are less efficient (having a lower RBE) in terms of cell killing (Figure 4-10).

A second physical factor that influences cellular radioresponse is dose rate.[6] A dose-rate effect has been observed for reproductive failure, division delay, chromosome aberrations, and survival time after whole-body irradiation. Low dose rates are less efficient in producing damage than high dose rates. Survival curves generally shift to the right, thus becoming shallower (D_o increases), and the shoulder becomes indistinguishable at low dose rates (Figure 4-11). This change in the appearance of the survival curve is explained by the cells' ability to repair sublethal damage from radiation treatment during and after exposure when given at low enough dose rates.

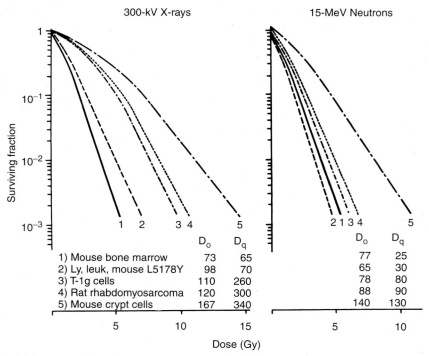

Figure 4-9. Survival curves for various types of mammalian cells irradiated with 33-kV x-rays or 15-MeV neutrons. The wide variability in the shoulder (D_q) and slope (D_o) seen in the x-ray survival curves is reduced after neutron irradiation. The D_o and D_q values shown are expressed in Gy. (From Broerse JJ, Barendsen GW: Current topics, *Radiat Res Q* 8:305-350, 1973.)

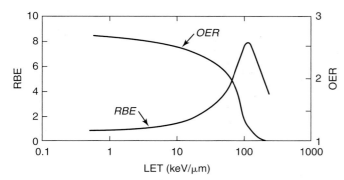

Figure 4-10. Demonstrates the relationship of OER and RBE as a function of LET. The data were obtained by using T1 kidney cells of human origin, irradiated with various naturally occurring alpha particles. (Redrawn from Barendsen GW: In Proceedings of the Conference on Particle Accelerators in Radiation Therapy. LA-5180-C. Washington, D.C., 1972, U.S. Atomic Energy Commission, Technical Information Center.)

This dose-rate effect is significant with low-LET radiations such as x-rays and gamma rays but is not observed with high-LET radiations.

Chemical Factors. Two major chemical factors influence cellular response to radiation. Certain chemicals that enhance response to radiation are known as **radiosensitizers**. Other chemicals, termed **radioprotectors**, have the opposite effect (i.e., they decrease the cellular response to radiation).

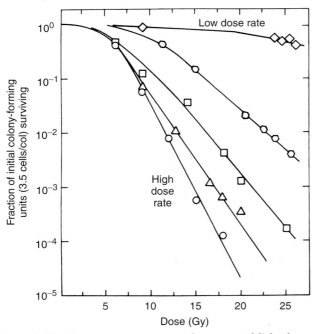

Figure 4-11. Dose-response curves for an established mammalian cell line irradiated with a wide range of dose rates from a high of 1.07 Gy/min to a low of 0.0036 Gy/min. Reducing the dose rate makes the survival curve more shallow and causes the shoulder to eventually disappear. (From Bedford JS, Mitchell JB: Dose-rate effects in synchronous mammalian cells in culture, *Radiat Res* 54:316-327, 1973.)

The most potent radiosensitizer to date is molecular oxygen. The oxygen effect has been observed in all organisms exposed to ionizing radiation.[73] Although the exact mechanism of the oxygen effect is unknown, the presence of oxygen may enhance the formation of free radicals and "fix" or make radiation damage permanent that would otherwise be reversible. This is also known as the oxygen fixation hypothesis. Oxygen must be present during the radiation exposure for sensitization to occur. The sensitizing effects of oxygen are most significant with low-LET radiations in which indirect effects caused by free radical formation predominate over direct effects.

Cell survival curves differ for oxic (normal oxygen level) versus hypoxic (reduced oxygen level) cell populations.[10] As the availability of oxygen decreases, cell response also decreases such that the survival curve shifts to the right because D_q and D_o increase. This effect is most pronounced with x-rays and gamma rays. The effects are less as the LET of the radiation increases (Figure 4-12). The magnitude of the oxygen effect is termed the **oxygen enhancement ratio (OER)**.[27] The OER compares the response of cells with radiation in the presence

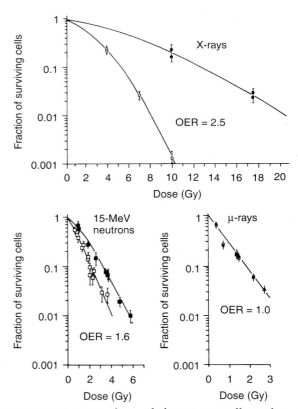

Figure 4-12. A comparison of the oxygen effect after x-ray, neutron, or alpha particle irradiation. The OER is highest after sparsely ionizing radiation (OER = 2.5), compared with densely ionizing radiations such as alpha particles (OER = 1.0). In the x-ray and neutron curves shown, the curve to the left represents the response of oxic cells and the curve to the right represents the hypoxic cell response. The oxic and hypoxic curves overlap when alpha particles are used. (From Broerse JJ, Barendsen GW, van Kersen GR: Survival of cultured human cells after irradiation with fast neutrons at different energies in hypoxic and oxygenated conditions, *Int J Radiat Biol* 13:559-572, 1967.)

and absence of oxygen. The equation for determining the OER for ionizing radiations is as follows:

$$OER = \frac{\text{Radiation dose under hypoxic/anoxic conditions}}{\text{Radiation dose under oxic conditions to}}$$
$$\text{produce the same biologic effect}$$

One common end point used for determination of the OER is the D_o. For example, if the $D_o = 300$ cGy under hypoxic conditions but is reduced to 100 cGy under oxic conditions, the OER for the radiation in the experiment is 300/100 = 3.0. For mammalian cells the OER for x-rays and gamma rays is generally 2.5 to 3.0. This means that hypoxic cells are 2.5 to 3.0 times more resistant than oxic cells to a dose of low-LET radiation. The oxygen effect is less significant with neutrons[25] (OER = 1.6) and may not be observable with high-LET radiations such as alpha particles (OER = 1.0). Figure 4-10 illustrates a strong correlation between the OER and RBE as a function of LET. This figure illustrates that the maximum RBE and the rapid decrease in OER occurs at an LET of approximately 100 keV/μm.

Whereas oxygenation conditions are easily modifiable with cells in vitro, measurements of oxygen levels (known as *oxygen tension* or Po_2) are more difficult to determine and modify in vivo. In vivo oxygen tensions of 20 to 30 μm Hg appear to render cells fully sensitive to low-LET radiations. The radiosensitivity of cells decreases as the Po_2 decreases, thus limiting the response of hypoxic cells in tumors treated with radiation.

Other compounds have also been tested as radiosensitizers. Most notable among these are halogenated pyrimidines and nitroimidazoles. Halogenated pyrimidines such as 5-bromo-deoxyuridine and 5-iododeoxyuridine are analogs of the DNA base thymidine.[29] These agents act as nonhypoxic cell sensitizers and are taken up by cycling cells during DNA synthesis (S phase). If enough of these compounds are substituted for thymidine, the DNA of the cell becomes more susceptible to radiation by a factor approaching 2. The rationale for the clinical use of these compounds is based on the shorter cycle times observed for tumor cells versus their normal cell counterparts. This should result in preferential uptake by tumors.

Nitroimidazoles such as misonidazole are oxygen-mimicking agents[1] (i.e., they behave chemically like oxygen in terms of indirect effects involving free radicals). In addition, nitroimidazoles may diffuse farther than oxygen from blood vessels, thereby reaching radioresistant hypoxic cells in a tumor. These agents are classified as *hypoxic cell sensitizers*. The idea behind their use is to selectively increase the radiosensitivity of hypoxic tumor cells. This desired selective sensitization of tumors has not been achieved in the clinic. Two major reasons for this are that (1) neither of these sensitizing agents exclusively localizes in malignant tissue and (2) both of these agents cause side effects at therapeutic doses. New and improved sensitizing agents that localize in malignant tissues without toxic side effects are under development in the United States and England.

In some clinical situations, attempts have been made to protect normal tissues instead of sensitizing tumors to a dose of radiation. The agents used are known as *radiation protectors,* or *dose-modifying compounds.*[43] The most important group of

protectors are sulfhydryls, agents that contain a free or potentially free sulfur (S) atom in their structure. Examples of sulfhydryls include cysteine, cysteamine, and WR-2721 (Amofostine). Sulfhydryls act as free radical scavengers that compete with oxygen for free radicals formed after the radiolysis of water. If the sulfhydryl binds to the free radical before the oxygen does, the free radical can decay back to a harmless chemical species instead of causing damage to vital structures in the cell. The ability of a radioprotector to diminish the effects of a dose of radiation is called the *dose reduction factor (DRF)*. The equation for determining the DRF is as follows[27]:

$$DRF = \frac{\text{Radiation dose with the radioprotector}}{\text{Radiation dose without the radioprotector}}$$
$$\text{to produce an equal biologic effect}$$

As with the oxygen effect, radioprotectors must be present during the irradiation. In practice, radioprotectors are administered at short time intervals (within 30 minutes) before radiation therapy. In general, this allows uptake by normal tissues so that they are protected without allowing enough time for significant tumor uptake. This therefore precludes protection of the tumor. If the radioprotector is effective, a DRF of 2.0 to 2.7 may be achieved, depending on the normal tissue that is involved. Similar to the oxygen effect, protection by sulfhydryls is much more significant against low-LET radiations that depend on free radical mechanisms, whereas little or no protection against high-LET radiations can be achieved. As with radiosensitizers, therapeutic doses of radioprotectors often cause side effects in patients. This has limited the widespread clinical use of radioprotectors.

 Examples of early radioprotectors were sodium cyanide, carbon monoxide, epinephrine, histamine, and serotonin because they all produced hypoxia in cells.

Biologic Factors. Cellular response is also affected by two important biologic factors: position in the cell cycle and ability to repair sublethal damage. Cellular radiosensitivity is dependent on the specific phase of the cell cycle containing the cells at the time of irradiation. (This is also referred to as *age response.*) In general, cells are most sensitive in the G2 and M phases, of intermediate sensitivity in the G1 phase, and most resistant in the S phase, especially during late S[57] (Figure 4-13). This variation in response of cells should not be discounted because the D_o for late S-phase cells may be as much as 2.5 times higher than for the same cells in the G2 and M phases. During irradiation of asynchronous cells with low doses, the majority of survivors are expected to be S-phase cells.

In addition to the variation in sensitivity caused by position in the cell cycle, Elkind and Sutton-Gilbert[21] showed in 1960 that cell survival increases if a dose of radiation is administered in fractions as a split dose instead of as a single dose (with the total dose remaining the same). Elkind and Sutton-Gilbert also showed that, depending on the time interval between each fraction, the survival curve parameters n, D_q, and D_o can remain the same as expected after a single-dose treatment. With low-LET radiations, Elkind and Sutton-Gilbert showed that the

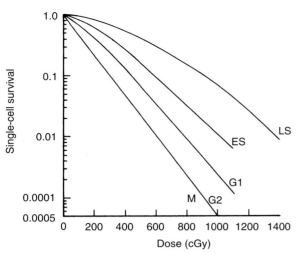

Figure 4-13. The effect of cell-cycle position on survival of a synchronous population of cells. The M and G2 phases are the most radiosensitive, whereas the early S period *(ES)* and late S period *(LS)* are the most resistant. (From Sinclair WK: Cyclic responses in mammalian cells in vitro, *Radiat Res* 33:620, 1968.)

shoulder on the survival curve repeated after each fraction. This indicated that cells were repairing sublethal damage from the first fraction before exposure to the second fraction.[21] This repair of sublethal damage after low-LET irradiation appears to be completed in most cell lines tested within several hours of each exposure depending on the dose/fraction. This repair of sublethal damage in normal tissues during fractionated radiation therapy in the clinic may account for the sparing of normal tissues relative to tumors. In addition, hypoxia reduces a cell's capacity to repair sublethal damage. This may partially account for the favorable tumor responses after fractionation compared with single-dose radiation therapy.

RADIOSENSITIVITY

Law of Bergonié and Tribondeau

In 1906, two scientists, Bergonié and Tribondeau,[8] performed experiments by using rodent testes to investigate reported clinical effects of radiation known at the time. Testes were chosen as the model for the experiments because they contain cells differing in function and mitotic activity. These cell types ranged from immature, mitotically active spermatogonia to mature, nondividing spermatozoa (sperm).

The results of the animal experiments indicated that immature, rapidly dividing cells were damaged at lower radiation doses than mature, nondividing cells. This result led to the formation of the **Law of Bergonié and Tribondeau**, which states that ionizing radiation is more effective against cells that (1) are actively mitotic, (2) are undifferentiated, and (3) have a long mitotic future. Bergonié and Tribondeau therefore defined radiosensitivity in terms of the mitotic activity and the level of differentiation. These two characteristics determined a normal cell's sensitivity to radiation. Therefore, cells dividing more often are more radiosensitive than cells dividing less often or not all.

The level of maturity or differentiation of a cell refers to its level of functional and/or structural specialization. According to Bergonié and Tribondeau, cells that are undifferentiated (i.e., immature cells whose primary function is to divide and replace more mature cells lost from the population) are extremely radiosensitive. These cells are also known as *stem* or *precursor cells.* In the testes, a spermatogonia is an example of a stem cell. A fully differentiated cell, known as an *end cell,* has a specialized structure or function, does not divide, and is radioresistant. Two examples of end cells are spermatozoa in the testes and erythrocytes in the circulating blood. In 1925, Ancel and Vitemberger[3] added to the findings of Bergonié and Tribondeau. Ancel and Vitemberger proposed that the environmental conditions of a cell before, during, or after radiation treatment could influence the extent and appearance of radiation damage. Current knowledge indicates that the expression of radiation damage generally occurs when the cell is stressed, usually during reproduction. The sensitivity of a cell to radiation can also be modified. This change in sensitivity is known as *conditional sensitivity.*

Cell Populations

In 1968, Rubin and Casarett[49] grouped mammalian cell populations into five basic categories based on radiation sensitivity (Table 4-2). The end point chosen was radiation-induced cell death. The most radiosensitive of these groups is known as *vegetative intermitotic (VIM) cells.* VIM cells are rapidly dividing, undifferentiated cells with short life spans. Examples include basal cells, crypt cells, erythroblasts, and type A spermatogonia.

The second most radiosensitive group is known as *differentiating intermitotic (DIM) cells.* These cells are also actively mitotic but a little more differentiated than VIM cells. In fact, VIM cells such as type A spermatogonia divide and mature into DIM cells such as type B spermatogonia.

The third group of cells, known as *multipotential connective tissue cells,* is intermediate in radiosensitivity. These cells (such as endothelial cells of blood vessels and fibroblasts of connective tissue) divide irregularly and are more differentiated than VIM and DIM cells.

The fourth group, *reverting postmitotic (RPM) cells,* normally do not divide but are capable of doing so. RPM cells typically live longer and are more differentiated than the three previously discussed groups. These cells, including liver cells, are relatively radioresistant. Another example of an RPM cell is the mature lymphocyte. This cell, however, is very radiosensitive despite its characteristics and is therefore an exception to the Law of Bergonié and Tribondeau.

The most radioresistant group of cells in the body are known as *fixed postmitotic (FPM) cells.* FPM cells are highly differentiated, do not divide, and may or may not be replaced when they die. Examples include certain nerve cells, muscle cells, erythrocytes, and spermatozoa.

Tissue and Organ Sensitivity

Because radiosensitivities of specific cells in the body are now known, that information can be used to determine radiosensitivities of organized tissues and organs. Structurally, tissues and

Table 4-2	Classification of Mammalian Cells According to Their Characteristics and Radiosensitivities		
Cell Type	**Characteristics**	**Examples**	**Radiosensitivity**
VIM	Divide regularly and rapidly, are undifferentiated, and do not differentiate between divisions	Type A spermatogonia, erythroblasts, crypt cells, and basal cells	Extremely high
DIM	Actively divide, are more differentiated than VIMs, and differentiate between divisions	Intermediate spermatogonia and myelocytes	High
Vessels/ connective tissue	Irregularly divide and are more differentiated than VIMs or DIMs	Endothelial cells and fibroblasts	Intermediate
RPM	Do not normally divide but retain capability of division and are variably differentiated	Parenchymal cells of liver and lymphocytes*	Low
FPM	Do not divide and are highly differentiated	Nerve cells, muscle cells, erythrocytes, and spermatozoa	Extremely low

From Travis EL: *Primer of medical radiobiology*, ed 2, St. Louis, 1989, Mosby.
*Lymphocytes, although classified as relatively radioresistant by their characteristics, are extremely radiosensitive.
DIM, Differentiating intermitotic; *FPM*, fixed postmitotic; *RPM*, reverting postmitotic; *VIM*, vegetative intermitotic.

organs are composed of two compartments: the parenchyma and stroma. The parenchymal compartment contains characteristic cells of that tissue or organ. VIM, DIM, RPM, and FPM cells are examples of parenchymal cells. The parenchyma is considered the functional unit of the cell. Regardless of the types of parenchymal cells in a tissue or organ, they also have a supporting stromal compartment.[61] The stroma consists of connective tissue and the vasculature and is generally considered intermediate in radiosensitivity, according to Rubin and Casarett.[49]

The radiosensitivity of a tissue or an organ is a function of the most sensitive cell it contains.[49] For example, the testes and bone marrow are considered radiosensitive because of the presence of VIM stem cells in their parenchymal compartments. In these two organs, parenchymal cells are damaged at lower radiation doses than stromal cells (fibroblasts and endothelial cells). Radiation-induced sterility in males can occur after high doses because of destruction of immature spermatogonia cells that were destined to become mature spermatozoa.[72] A decrease in circulating erythrocytes in the blood after irradiation is due to destruction of the more sensitive stem cell (erythroblast) in the bone marrow.[62]

Tissues and organs that contain only RPM or FPM parenchymal cells are therefore more radioresistant. Examples include the liver, muscle, brain, and spinal cord. In this situation, stromal cells are damaged at lower doses than parenchymal cells. Blood vessels in these organs become damaged, thus decreasing blood flow and therefore the supply of oxygen and nutrients to the parenchymal cells. Therefore, radiation-induced death of parenchymal cells in these organs is predominantly due to stromal damage. This form of indirect cell death is a significant mechanism of radiation damage in radioresistant tissues and organs.

SYSTEMIC RESPONSE TO RADIATION
Response and Healing

Response to ionizing radiation treatment refers to visible (detectable) structural and functional changes that a dose produces in a certain period. Response at all levels (whether in a cell, a tissue, an organ, a system, or the entire organism) is a function of the dose administered, the volume irradiated, and the time of observation after exposure. With the exception of cataracts of the ocular lens, radiation-induced changes are neither unique nor distinguishable from biologic effects caused by other forms of trauma.

Structural or morphologic response after irradiation is usually grouped into two phases: early or acute changes observed within 6 months of treatment and late or chronic changes occurring more than 6 months later.[64] The appearance of late changes is a consequence of early changes that were irreversible and progressive. The probability of late changes occurring depends on the dose administered, the volume irradiated, and the healing ability of the irradiated structure (organ).

Organ healing can occur after radiation exposure by the process of regeneration or repair.[64] *Regeneration* refers to the replacement of damaged cells by the same cell type. Regeneration results in partial or total reversal of early radiation changes and is likely to occur in organs containing actively dividing VIM and DIM parenchymal cells. Examples include the skin, small intestine, and bone marrow. Regeneration is the desired healing process and can restore an organ to its preirradiated state.

Irreversible early changes, however, heal by the process of repair. *Repair* refers to the replacement of damaged cells by a different cell type, thus resulting in scar formation or fibrosis. Healing by repair does not restore an organ to its preirradiated state. Repair can occur in any organ and is more likely after high doses (1000 cGy or higher) that destroy parenchymal cells, thus making regeneration impossible. Repair is the predominant healing process in radioresistant organs containing RPM and FPM parenchymal cells that do not divide or have lost the ability to do so.

Under conditions that produce massive and extensive damage to the organ, neither healing process may occur and tissue death or necrosis results. Therefore, the type of healing, if any, that occurs is a function of the dose received and volume of the organ receiving it.

The other important factor that must be considered is the time after the treatment. In general, radiosensitive organs (e.g., skin) respond faster and more severely than do radioresistant organs.[64] The reverse situation may hold true at a later time. For example, irradiation of skin and lung tissue with a dose of 2000 cGy induces severe early skin changes but minimal early lung changes (within 6 months). However, if the same tissues are examined 6 to 12 months after irradiation, minimal late changes are found in the skin but severe late changes are observed in the lung. This rate of response depends mostly on the cell cycle or generation times of the parenchymal cells in each organ. Because most cells die when attempting to divide after irradiation, cells with short cycle times show radiation damage sooner than cells with long cycle times. In comparing skin and lung parenchymal cells, cycle times are considerably shorter for parenchymal cells of the skin.

General Organ Changes

The most common early or acute changes after irradiation include inflammation, edema, and possible hemorrhaging in the exposed area. If doses are high enough, these early changes may progress to characteristic late or chronic changes, including fibrosis, atrophy, and ulceration. These late changes are not reversible and therefore are permanent. The most severe late response is tissue necrosis or death. The sensitivity of the most radiosensitive organ of a system determines the general response of that system in the body. The Radiation Therapy Oncology Group (RTOG)[16] has summarized the acute and chronic effects of radiation into various categories or grades based on the severity of the clinical response[65] (Tables 4-3 and 4-4).

TOTAL-BODY RESPONSE TO RADIATION

This section involves specific signs and symptoms induced by exposure of the entire body at one time to ionizing radiation. The total-body response to radiation is presented in terms of three radiation syndromes.[27] Characteristics of each syndrome are dependent on the dose received and exposure conditions. Three specific exposure conditions apply in dealing with radiation syndromes: (1) exposure must be acute (minutes); (2) total-body or nearly total-body exposure must occur; and (3) exposure must be from an external penetrating source rather than ingested, inhaled, or implanted radioactive sources.[64]

Radiation Syndromes in Humans

Although an abundance of animal data regarding the effects of total-body exposure to radiation exists, considerably less human data under the same conditions are available. However, human data are available from (1) industrial and laboratory accidents, (2) fallout from atomic bomb test sites, (3) therapeutic medical exposures, (4) individuals exposed at Hiroshima and Nagasaki, and (5) the nuclear reactor accident at Chernobyl in the Soviet Union. As with lower animals, humans suffer the three radiation syndromes if the same exposure conditions are met.[27] Table 4-5 contains a summary of the acute radiation syndromes in humans after whole-body irradiation.

Hematopoietic Syndrome. The hematopoietic syndrome in humans is induced by total-body doses of 100 to 1000 cGy.[27] The $LD_{50/60}$ for humans is estimated to be between 350 and 450 cGy but varies with age, health, and gender. Typically, females are more resistant than males, and the extremely young and old tend to be a little more sensitive than middle-aged persons. The prodromal stage or syndrome is observed within hours after exposure and is characterized by nausea and vomiting. The latent stage then occurs and lasts from a few days up to 3 weeks. Although the affected individual feels well at this time, bone marrow stem cells are dying. Peripheral blood cell counts decrease during the subsequent manifest illness stage at 3 to 5 weeks after exposure. Depression of all blood cell counts, termed *pancytopenia,* results in anemia (from a decreased number of erythrocytes), hemorrhaging (from a decreased number of platelets), and serious infection (from a decreased number of leukocytes).

The probability of survival decreases with an increasing dose. Most individuals receiving doses less than 300 cGy survive and eventually recover over the next 3 to 6 months. As the dose increases, the survival time decreases. After 300 to 500 cGy, death may occur in 4 to 6 weeks. After 500 to 1000 cGy, death is likely within 2 weeks.[64] No record exists of human survival when the total body dose exceeds 1000 cGy.[27] The primary causes of death from the hematopoietic syndrome are infection and hemorrhaging after destruction of the bone marrow.

Gastrointestinal Syndrome. If the total body dose is between 1000 and 10,000 cGy, the gastrointestinal syndrome is induced.[27] This syndrome may also be induced by a dose as low as 600 cGy and overlaps with the cerebrovascular syndrome at doses of 5000 cGy or more. The mean survival time for this syndrome is 3 to 10 days or up to 2 weeks with medical support and is largely independent of the actual dose received. The prodromal stage occurs within hours after exposure and is characterized by nausea, vomiting, diarrhea, and cramps. The latent stage then occurs 2 to 5 days after exposure. At 5 to 10 days after exposure, nausea, vomiting, diarrhea, and fever mark the manifest illness stage. Death occurs during the second week after exposure.

The gastrointestinal syndrome occurs as a result of damage to the gastrointestinal tract and bone marrow. As discussed previously, the small intestine is the most radiosensitive portion of the digestive system.[71] After exposure to doses in excess of 1000 cGy, severe depopulation of crypt cells leads to partial or complete denudation of the villi lining the lumen of the small intestine. Consequences of this damage include decreased absorption of materials across the intestinal wall, leakage of fluids into the lumen (resulting in dehydration), and overwhelming infection as bacteria gain access to the circulating blood. Significant changes in bone marrow also occur, highlighted by a severe decrease in circulating leukocytes. However, death occurs before the other peripheral blood cell counts significantly decrease. Despite attempts at regeneration of crypt cells in the small intestine, bone marrow damage likely leads to death as a result of the overwhelming infection, dehydration, and electrolyte imbalance.

Cerebrovascular Syndrome. The third and final radiation syndrome is the cerebrovascular syndrome. This syndrome, which was formerly known as the *central nervous system syndrome,* occurs exclusively after doses of 10,000 cGy or more but can overlap with the gastrointestinal syndrome because it can be induced by a dose as low as 5000 cGy.[27] Death after such high

Text continued on p. 74

Table 4-3	Radiation Therapy Oncology Group (RTOG) Acute Radiation Morbidity Scoring Criteria				
Organ/Tissue	**Grade 0**	**Grade 1**	**Grade 2**	**Grade 3**	**Grade 4**
Skin	No change over baseline	Follicular, faint or dull erythema; epilation; dry desquamation; decreased sweating	Tender or bright erythema; patchy, moist desquamation; moderate edema	Confluent, moist desquamation other than skin folds; pitting edema	Ulceration, hemorrhage, necrosis
Mucous membrane	No change over baseline	Injection/may experience mild pain not requiring analgesic	Patchy mucositis that may produce an inflammatory serosanguineous discharge; may experience moderate pain requiring analgesic	Confluent fibrinous mucositis; may include severe pain requiring narcotic	Ulceration, hemorrhage, necrosis
Eye	No change	Mild conjunctivitis with or without scleral injection; increased tearing	Moderate conjunctivitis with or without keratitis requiring steroids and/or antibiotics; dry eye requiring artificial tears; iritis with photophobia	Severe keratitis with corneal ulceration; objective decrease in visual acuity or in visual fields; acute glaucoma; panophthalmitis	Loss of vision (unilateral or bilateral)
Ear	No change over baseline	Mild external otitis with erythema; pruritus secondary to dry desquamation not requiring medication; audiogram unchanged from baseline	Moderate external otitis requiring topical medication; serious otitis media; hypoacusis on testing only	Severe external otitis with discharge or moist desquamation; symptomatic hypoacusis; tinnitus, not drug related	Deafness
Salivary gland	No change over baseline	Mild mouth dryness; slightly thickened saliva; may have slightly altered taste such as metallic taste; these changes not reflected in alteration in baseline feeding behavior, such as increased use of liquids with meals	Moderate to complete dryness; thick, sticky saliva; markedly altered taste	—	Acute salivary gland necrosis
Pharynx and esophagus	No change over baseline	Mild dysphagia or odynophagia; may require topical anesthetic or nonnarcotic analgesics; may require soft diet	Moderate dysphagia or odynophagia; may require narcotic analgesics; may require pureed or liquid diet	Severe dysphagia or odynophagia with dehydration or weight loss (>15% from pretreatment baseline) requiring NG feeding tube, IV fluids, or hyperalimentation	Complete obstruction, ulceration, perforation, fistula
Larynx	No change over baseline	Mild or intermittent hoarseness; cough not requiring antitussive; erythema of mucosa	Persistent hoarseness but able to vocalize; referred ear pain, sore throat, patchy fibrinous exudate, or mild arytenoid edema not requiring narcotic; cough requiring antitussive	Whispered speech; throat pain or referred ear pain requiring narcotic; confluent fibrinous exudate; marked arytenoid edema	Marked dyspnea, stridor, or hemoptysis with tracheostomy or intubation necessary

Table 4-3	Radiation Therapy Oncology Group (RTOG) Acute Radiation Morbidity Scoring Criteria—cont'd				
Organ/Tissue	**Grade 0**	**Grade 1**	**Grade 2**	**Grade 3**	**Grade 4**
Upper GI	No change	Anorexia with ≤5% weight loss from pretreatment baseline; nausea not requiring antiemetics; abdominal discomfort not requiring para-sympatholytic drugs or analgesics	Anorexia with ≤15% weight loss from pretreatment baseline; nausea and/or vomiting requiring antiemetics; abdominal pain requiring analgesics	Anorexia with >15% weight loss from pretreatment baseline or requiring NG tube or parenteral support; nausea and/or vomiting requiring tube or parenteral support; abdominal pain, severe despite medication; hematemesis or melena; abdominal distention (flat plate radiograph demonstrates distended bowel loops	Ileus, subacute or acute obstruction, perforation, GI bleeding requiring transfusion; abdominal pain requiring tube decompression or bowel diversion
Lower GI including pelvis	No change	Increased frequency or change in quality of bowel habits not requiring medication; rectal discomfort not requiring analgesics	Diarrhea requiring parasympatholytic drugs (e.g., Lomotil); mucous discharge not necessitating sanitary pads; rectal or abdominal pain requiring analgesics	Diarrhea requiring parenteral support; severe mucous or blood discharge necessitating sanitary bags; abdominal distention (flat plate radiograph demonstrates distended bowel loops)	Acute or subacute obstruction, fistula, or perforation; GI bleeding requiring transfusion; abdominal pain or tenesmus requiring tube decompression or bowel diversion
Lung	No change	Mild symptoms of dry cough or dyspnea on exertion	Persistent cough requiring narcotic, antitussive agents; dyspnea with minimal effort but not at rest	Severe cough unresponsive to narcotic antitussive agent or dyspnea at rest; clinical or radiologic evidence of acute pneumonitis; intermittent oxygen or steroids may be required	Severe respiratory insufficiency; continuous oxygen or assisted ventilation
Genitourinary	No change	Frequency of urination or nocturia twice pretreatment habit; dysuria, urgency not requiring medication	Frequency of urination or nocturia, which is less frequent than every hour; Dysuria, urgency, bladder spasm requiring local anesthetic (e.g., Pyridium)	Frequency with urgency and nocturia hourly or more frequently; dysuria, pelvic pain or bladder spasm requiring regular, frequent narcotic; gross hematuria with or without clot passage	Hematuria requiring transfusion; acute bladder obstruction not secondary to clot passage, ulceration, or necrosis
Heart	No change over baseline	Asymptomatic but objective evidence of ECG changes or pericardial abnormalities without evidence of other heart disease	Symptomatic with ECG changes and radiologic findings of congestive heart failure or pericardial disease; no specific treatment required	Congestive heart failure, angina pectoris, pericardial disease responding to therapy	Congestive heart failure, angina pectoris, pericardial disease, arrhythmias not responsive to nonsurgical measures
CNS	No change	Fully functional status (i.e., able to work) with minor neurologic findings, no medication needed	Neurologic findings present sufficient to require home care; nursing assistance may be required; medications including steroids; antiseizure agents may be required	Neurologic findings requiring hospitalization for initial management	Serious neurologic impairment that includes paralysis, coma, or seizures >3 per week despite medication; hospitalization required

Continued

Table 4-3	Radiation Therapy Oncology Group (RTOG) Acute Radiation Morbidity Scoring Criteria—cont'd				
Organ/Tissue	Grade 0	Grade 1	Grade 2	Grade 3	Grade 4
Hematologic WBC (×1000)	≥4.0	3.0-4.0	2.0-3.0	1.0-2.0	<1.0
Platetlets (×1000)	>100	75-100	50-75	25-50	<25 or spontaneous bleeding
Neutrophils	≥1.9	1.5-1.9	1.0-1.5	0.5-1.0	≤0.5 or sepsis
Hemoglobin (g %)	>11	11-9.5	9.5-7.5	7.5-5.0	—
Hematocrit (%)	≥32	28-32	≤28	Packed cell transfusion required	—

From Trotti A, Byhardt R, Stetz J, et al: Common toxicity criteria: version 2.0. An improved reference for grading the acute effects of cancer treatment: impact on radiotherapy, *Int J Radiat Oncol Biol Phys* 47:13-47, 2000.

CNS, Central nervous system; *ECG,* electrocardiogram; *GI,* gastrointestinal; *IV,* intravenous; *NG,* nasogastric.

Guidelines: The acute morbidity criteria are used to score and grade toxicity from radiation therapy. The criteria are relevant from day 1, the commencement of therapy, through day 90. Thereafter, the European Organization for Research and Treatment of Cancer (EORTC)/RTOG Criteria of Late Effects are to be used.

The evaluator must attempt to discriminate between disease- and treatment-related signs and symptoms.

An accurate baseline evaluation before commencement of therapy is necessary.

All toxicities grade 3, 4, or 5* must be verified by the principal investigator.

*Any toxicity that caused death is graded 5.

Table 4-4	Radiation Therapy Oncology Group/European Organization for Research and Treatment of Cancer Late Radiation Morbidity Scoring Schema					
Organ/Tissue	Grade 0	Grade 1	Grade 2	Grade 3	Grade 4	Grade 5
Skin	None	Slight atrophy; pigmentation change; some hair loss	Patch atrophy; moderate telangiectasia; total hair loss	Marked atrophy; gross telangiectasia	Ulceration	Death directly related to radiation late effect for all tissue types
Subcutaneous tissue	None	Slight induration (fibrosis) and loss of subcutaneous fat	Moderate fibrosis but asymptomatic; slight field contracture <10% linear reduction	Severe induration and loss of subcutaneous tissue; field contracture >10% linear measurement	Necrosis	
Mucous membrane	None	Slight atrophy and dryness	Moderate atrophy and telangiectasia; little mucus	Marked atrophy with complete dryness; severe telangiectasia	Ulceration	
Salivary glands	None	Slight dryness of mouth; good response on stimulation	Moderate dryness of mouth; poor response on stimulation	Complete dryness of mouth; no response on stimulation	Fibrosis	
Spinal cord	None	Mild Lhermitte's syndrome	Severe Lhermitte's syndrome	Objective neurologic findings at or below cord level treated	Mono- paraquadriplegia	
Brain	None	Mild headache; slight lethargy	Moderate headache; great lethargy	Severe headaches; severe CNS dysfunction (partial loss of power or dyskinesia)	Seizures or paralysis; coma	

Table 4-4			Radiation Therapy Oncology Group/European Organization for Research and Treatment of Cancer Late Radiation Morbidity Scoring Schema—cont'd			

Organ/Tissue	Grade 0	Grade 1	Grade 2	Grade 3	Grade 4	Grade 5
Eye	None	Asymptomatic cataract; minor corneal ulceration or keratitis	Symptomatic cataract; moderate corneal ulceration; minor retinopathy or glaucoma	Severe keratitis; severe retinopathy or detachment; severe glaucoma	Panophthalmitis; blindness	
Larynx	None	Hoarseness; slight arytenoid edema	Moderate arytenoid edema; chondritis	Severe edema; severe chondritis	Necrosis	
Lung	None	Asymptomatic or mild symptoms (dry cough); slight radiographic appearances	Moderate symptomatic fibrosis or pneumonitis (severe cough); low-grade fever; patchy radiographic appearances	Severe symptomatic fibrosis or pneumonitis; dense radiographic changes	Severe respiratory insufficiency; continuous O_2; assisted ventilation	
Heart	None	Asymptomatic or mild symptoms; transient T-wave inversion and ST changes; sinus tachycardia >110 beats/min (at rest)	Moderate angina on effort; mild pericarditis; normal heart size; persistent abnormal T wave and ST changes; low QRS	Severe angina; pericardial effusion; constrictive pericarditis; moderate heart failure; cardiac enlargement; ECG abnormalities	Tamponade; severe heart failure; severe constrictive pericarditis	
Esophagus	None	Mild fibrosis; slight difficulty in swallowing solids; no pain on swallowing	Unable to take solid food normally; swallowing semisolid food; dilation may be indicated	Severe fibrosis; able to swallow only liquids; may have pain on swallowing; dilation required	Necrosis; perforation; fistula	
Small and large intestine	None	Mild diarrhea; mild cramping; bowel movement 5 times daily; slight rectal discharge or bleeding	Moderate diarrhea and colic; bowel movement >5 times daily; excessive rectal mucus or intermittent bleeding	Obstruction or bleeding requiring surgery	Necrosis; perforation; fistula	
Liver	None	Mild lassitude; nausea; dyspepsia; slightly abnormal liver function	Moderate symptoms; some abnormal liver function tests; serum albumin normal	Disabling hepatitic insufficiency; liver function tests grossly abnormal; low albumin; edema or ascites	Necrosis; hepatic coma or encephalopathy	
Kidney	None	Transient albuminuria; no hypertension; mild impairment of renal function; urea 25-35 mg%; creatinine 1.5-2.0 mg%; creatinine clearance >75%	Persistent moderate albuminuria (2+); mild hypertension; no related anemia; moderate impairment of renal function; urea >36-60 mg%; creatinine clearance 50%-74%	Severe albuminuria; severe hypertension; persistent anemia <10 g%; severe renal failure; urea >60 mg%; creatinine >4.0 mg%; creatinine clearance <50%	Malignant hypertension; uremic coma; urea >100%	
Bladder	None	Slight epithelial atrophy; minor telangiectasia (microscopic hematuria)	Moderate frequency; generalized telangiectasia; intermittent macroscopic hematuria	Severe frequency and dysuria; severe generalized telangiectasia (often with petechiae); frequent hematuria; reduction in bladder capacity (<150 mL)	Necrosis; contracted bladder (capacity <100 mL); severe hemorrhagic cystitis	

Continued

Table 4-4	Radiation Therapy Oncology Group/European Organization for Research and Treatment of Cancer Late Radiation Morbidity Scoring Schema—cont'd					
Organ/Tissue	**Grade 0**	**Grade 1**	**Grade 2**	**Grade 3**	**Grade 4**	**Grade 5**
Bone	None	Asymptomatic; no growth retardation; reduced bone density	Moderate pain or tenderness; growth retardation; irregular bone sclerosis	Severe pain or tenderness; complete arrest of bone growth; dense bone sclerosis	Necrosis; spontaneous fracture	
Joint	None	Mild joint stiffness; slight limitation of movement	Moderate stiffness; intermittent or moderate joint pain; moderate limitation of movement	Severe joint stiffness; pain with severe limitation of movement	Necrosis; complete fixation	

From Trotti A, Byhardt R, Stetz J, et al: Common toxicity criteria: version 2.0. An improved reference for grading the acute effects of cancer treatment: impact on radiotherapy, *Int J Radiat Oncol Biol Phys* 47:13-47, 2000.
Cox JD, Stetz J, Pajak TF: Toxicity criteria of the Radiation Therapy Oncology Group (RTOG) and the European Organization for Research and Treatment of Cancer (EORTC), *Int J Radiat Oncol Biol Phys* 31:1341-1346, 1995.
CNS, Central nervous system; *ECG,* electrocardiogram.

total-body doses occurs in several days or less. The prodromal stage lasts only minutes to several hours (depending on the dose) and is characterized by nervousness, confusion, severe nausea and vomiting, loss of consciousness, and a burning sensation in the skin. The latent period (if distinguishable) lasts only several hours or less. Within 5 to 6 hours after exposure, the manifest illness stage begins and is characterized by watery diarrhea, convulsions, coma, and death.

The cause of death from the cerebrovascular syndrome is not completely known at this time. At autopsy, brain parenchymal cells appear almost completely normal despite the high dose. These parenchymal cells are extremely radioresistant FPM cells, according to Rubin and Casarett.[49] Autopsy findings show extensive blood vessel (stromal) damage in the brain, thus resulting in vasculitis, meningitis, and edema in the cranial vault. The resulting increase in intracranial pressure is probably the major cause of death. In addition, peripheral blood counts and the villi of the small intestine do not exhibit significant changes in these individuals when examined at autopsy. This is due to the exposed person not living long enough for these effects to become evident.

Response of the Embryo and Fetus

Radiation exposure can also damage the developing embryo and fetus in utero. Generally, in utero radiation damage is manifested as lethal effects, congenital abnormalities present at birth, or late effects observed years later. These effects can be produced by (1) irradiation of the sperm or ovum before fertilization, thus resulting in inherited effects, or (2) exposure of the fetus to radiation, thus resulting in congenital defects. This section deals only with congenital abnormalities resulting from radiation exposure.

Table 4-5	Summary of Acute Radiation Syndromes in Humans After Whole-Body Irradiation				
Syndrome	**Dose Range**	**Time of Death**	**Organ and System Damaged**	**Signs and Symptoms**	**Recovery Time**
Hematopoietic	100-1000 cGy*	3 weeks to 2 months	Bone marrow	Decreased number of stem cells in bone marrow, increased amount of fat in bone marrow, pancytopenia, anemia, hemorrhage, and infection	Dose dependent—3 weeks to 6 months; some individuals do not survive
Gastrointestinal	1000-5000 cGy†	3-10 days	Small intestine	Denudation of villi in small intestine, neutropenia, infection, bone marrow depression, electrolyte imbalance, and watery diarrhea	None
Cerebrovascular	>5000 cGy	<3 days	Brain	Vasculitis, edema, and meningitis	None

Modified from Travis EL: *Primer of medical radiobiology,* ed 2, St. Louis, 1989, Mosby.
*$LD_{50/60}$ for humans in this dose range (450 cGy).
†LD_{100} for humans in this dose range (1000 cGy).

Stages of Fetal Development. The husband-and-wife research team of Russell and Russell[51] divided fetal development into three stages: preimplantation, major organogenesis, and the fetal growth stage. Extensive mouse studies have established that the effect induced by radiation depends not only on the radiation dose, but also on the time of the exposure's occurrence during gestation.[50] In humans, the preimplantation stage occurs from conception (day 0) to 10 days after conception. During this time the fertilized ovum is actively dividing, thus forming a ball of highly undifferentiated cells.

The newly formed ball of cells, known as the *embryo,* then implants in the uterine wall and begins the major organogenesis stage (from day 10 to week 6). During this time, on specific gestational days, embryonic cells differentiate into the stem cells that eventually form each organ in the body. At the end of the sixth week, the embryo is known as a *fetus* and enters the fetal growth stage, in which it continues to grow until birth. The central nervous system in the fetus differs from that in the adult because the neuroblasts (stem cells) of the fetus are still mitotically active and not fully differentiated. Therefore, unlike that in the adult, the fetal central nervous system is responsive to radiation and can be damaged at relatively low doses.

Radiation Effects on Humans In Utero. Radiation effects on human embryos have been investigated with data sources that were described previously (atomic bomb survivors in Japan after World War II, fallout exposures, occupational exposures, and diagnostic or therapeutic exposures of pregnant women).[26,33] A definitive cause-and-effect relationship between radiation and a specific abnormality is difficult to prove in human beings. Two major reasons account for this: (1) the background incidence of spontaneous congenital abnormalities is approximately 6% and (2) radiation does not induce unique congenital abnormalities (excluding cataracts). Therefore, implicating a certain radiation exposure as the sole cause of a specific congenital abnormality is difficult. The results of animal studies have been extrapolated to humans to allow predictions with regard to effects that might occur in irradiated human embryos and fetuses (Figure 4-14). However, the assumption should not be made that in utero effects in mice will be observed under the same conditions in human beings. Viable comparisons may indicate that the mouse embryo is slightly more radioresistant than the human embryo. In addition, the mouse gestational period ends in 20 days versus 270 days or more in human beings. Therefore, although the same developmental stages occur for the most part in mice and humans, they certainly occur much more rapidly in mice.[64] This should be taken into account during comparisons of animal and human radiation effects in utero.

Unfortunately, human data exist for radiation effects from in utero exposure. A report in 1930 by Murphy and Goldstein[40] described congenital defects (microcephaly) attributed to radiation exposure in utero. In one study of children born to 11 women who were pregnant and received high doses from the bomb dropped in Hiroshima, 7 of the 11 children (64%) had microcephaly and were mentally retarded.[45] In another study of 30 children who were irradiated in utero at Nagasaki, 17 (57%) were affected (7 fetal deaths, 6 neonatal deaths, and 4 surviving

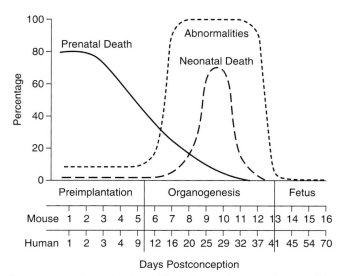

Figure 4-14. The induction of lethality and major abnormalities during in utero exposure on different gestational days in the mouse embryo using 2.0 Gy. Lower scale indicated Rugh's time estimates for the three stages in the human embryo. (From Travis EL: *Primer of medical radiobiology,* ed 2, Philadelphia, 1989, Mosby.)

children who were mentally retarded).[41] Table 4-6 illustrates the correlation between gestational stage and the probability of developing congenital malformations.

Dekaban[18] in 1968 studied children born to women irradiated with a therapeutic dose of 250 cGy during various stages of gestation. The results of this study indicated that exposure to the dose during the first 2 to 3 weeks of gestation produced a high frequency of prenatal death but few severe abnormalities in surviving children who were brought to term (similar to the mouse studies). Irradiation between 4 and 11 weeks correlated with severe central nervous system and skeletal abnormalities. The same dose (250 cGy) administered between the 11th and 16th week frequently resulted in mental retardation and microcephaly, whereas irradiation after the 20th week resulted in functional defects such as sterility.

Table 4-6	Summary of Radiation Effects on the Embryo and Fetus*		
Stage of Gestation	**Growth Retardation**	**Death**	**Microcephaly and Mental Retardation**
Preimplantation	None	Embryonic death and resorption	None
Organogenesis Fetal	Temporary Permanent	Neonatal death Approximately equal to the LD_{50} in adult	Very high risk High risk

*Summarized from Hall EJ, Giaccia AJ: *Radiobiology for the radiobiologist,* Philadelphia, 2005, Lippincott Williams & Wilkins.

The maximum permissible dose to the fetus during the entire gestational period from occupational exposure of the mother should not exceed 0.5 rem (5 mSv), with monthly exposure not exceeding 0.05 rem (0.5 mSv).

In summary, although difficult to prove conclusively, the embryo and fetus are considered to be the most radiosensitive forms of animals and humans. Radiation, if it must be administered during a known pregnancy, should be delayed as much as possible because the fetus is more radioresistant than the embryo. In 1993, the International Commission on Radiological Protection (ICRP) recommended the 28-day rule, which states that the safe period for exposure of the possibly pregnant uterus is 28 days after menstruation.[54] As mentioned previously, the most radiosensitive period for induction of abnormalities in humans is between days 23 and 37. These effects usually involve the central nervous system and most commonly include microcephaly, mental retardation, sensory organ damage, and stunted growth. Skeletal changes (bone) appear to be most prevalent when radiation is administered between weeks 3 and 20.

 In regard to fetal effects of radiation, the principal factors of importance are the dose and the stage of gestation at which it is delivered.

LATE EFFECTS OF RADIATION

The previous section dealt with the total-body response to high doses of radiation, which usually results in lethality. Of equal and possibly even more concern is the biologic response resulting from exposure to much lower doses of radiation. Because the latent period for an effect is inversely proportional to radiation dose, the biologic response to low doses is not observable for extended periods, ranging from years to generations.[27] These effects are therefore known as *late effects* and are termed *somatic effects* if body cells are involved or *genetic effects* if reproductive (germ) cells are involved.

 Latent period: *The time interval between irradiation and the appearance of a malignancy is known as the* latent period.

Somatic Effects (Carcinogenesis)

Historical Background. The most important late somatic effect induced by radiation is carcinogenesis.[14,66,68] Radiation is therefore classified as a *carcinogen,* or *cancer-causing agent.* In 1902 (only 7 years after Roentgen's discovery of the x-ray), the first reported case of radiation-induced carcinoma appeared in the literature. By 1910, at least 100 cases of skin cancer were reported in radiologists and radiation oncologists who were unaware of the potential hazards of this new modality.

Carcinogenesis is considered to be an all-or-nothing event. This means that any dose, no matter how low, has some potential of inducing cancer. Cancer induction is therefore a nonthreshold event with the probability of an effect increasing as the dose increases. Carcinogenesis is therefore an example of a stochastic effect, in which every dose carries some magnitude of risk.[27]

Sufficient human data exist to implicate radiation as a cancer-causing agent. Most of the early data involve occupational exposures by radiation scientists, clinicians, and therapists who were chronically exposed to various radiation sources before the risks of such exposures were known. Ionizing radiation has been implicated as a cause of skin cancer, leukemia, osteosarcoma, lung cancer, breast cancer, and thyroid cancer.

Leukemia. Radiation was first implicated as a cause of leukemia in 1911. That study involved 11 cases of leukemia in occupationally exposed individuals.[64] Atomic bomb survivors in Hiroshima and Nagasaki had higher incidences of leukemia than the nonexposed population.[27] Early radiologists in the United States who died between 1948 and 1961 had a much higher frequency of leukemia (300%) than the general population.[20,34] However, a similar study involving British radiologists showed no increased leukemia incidence in an early group (before 1921) compared with later groups who used some level of radiation safety.[13]

The latent period for leukemia induction by radiation is usually 4 to 7 years, with peak incidence approximately 7 to 10 years after exposure. This period is much shorter than that observed for radiation-induced solid tumors, which have latent periods ranging from 20 to 30 years or longer.[27]

Radiation induction of leukemia is somewhat specific in that only certain types of leukemia show an increased incidence in irradiated individuals. For example, only acute and chronic myeloid leukemia types are more prevalent in irradiated adults, whereas acute lymphocytic leukemia is more common in irradiated children.[15] Radiation exposure does not seem to affect the incidence of chronic lymphocytic leukemia. The available evidence suggests that leukemia induction is a nonthreshold (stochastic), linear response to radiation[62] (Figure 4-15). However, other cancers induced by radiation may follow a linear-quadratic rather than a linear relationship to radiation dose.[27]

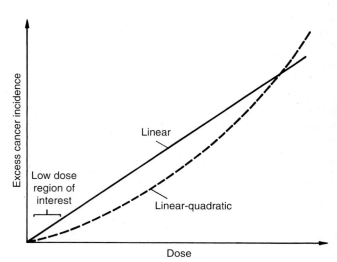

Figure 4-15. A schematic of the linear and linear-quadratic models used to extrapolate the incidence of cancer from high-dose data down to low doses. Both models fit high-dose data as well, but at low doses the estimated incidence depends on the model. (From Travis EL: *Primer of medical radiobiology,* ed 2, St. Louis, 1989, Mosby.)

Skin Carcinoma. The first reported case of radiation-induced skin cancer (which occurred on the hand of a radiologist) was in 1902.[42] Because early x-ray machines were crude, radiologists placed their hands in the beam path to check its efficiency. This led to early skin changes (erythema) that were used to gauge the output of the beam, but skin tumors were observed years later in many of these individuals. Patients treated with radiation for several benign conditions such as acne and ringworm of the scalp also showed an increased incidence of skin cancer years later.[2] As a result of modern radiation safety procedures, skin cancers in radiation workers are no longer observed.

 Skin cancer: *Squamous cell and basal cell carcinomas have been the most frequently observed skin cancers following radiation exposure.*

Osteosarcoma. The most striking example of radiation-induced osteosarcoma, or bone cancer, is given by the group of young female watch-dial painters who used radium to paint clock faces for a company in northern New Jersey from 1915 to 1930.[35] These workers regularly licked their brushes (which contained radium paint) to make the brush tip come to a point before painting the watch dials. This resulted in chronic ingestion of radium, which is a bone-seeking radioactive element.[24] Of the several hundred workers exposed this way, approximately 40 cases of osteosarcoma were observed years later. The dose response for bone cancer in this group followed a linear-quadratic relationship that was dependent on the activities of the two radium isotopes (^{226}Ra and ^{228}Ra) contained in the paint.[48]

Lung Carcinoma. More than 500 years ago, German pitchblende miners suffered from a condition known as *mountain sickness*, which was later determined to be lung cancer.[27] Inhaling chronic amounts of radon gas in the air of the mines, these miners exposed their lungs to high-LET alpha particles that were emitted as the radon decayed. Uranium miners in the United States who were studied from 1950 to 1967 also had an increased incidence of lung cancer, most likely for the same reasons.[52] Radon gas and its decay products are now known to be significant contributors (200 mrem/year) to annual background radiation levels and are the major risk factors for lung cancer in nonsmokers.

 Radon gas: *The naturally occurring deposits of radioactive materials in the rocks of the earth decay through a long series of steps until they reach a stable isotope of lead. One of these steps involves radon gas.*

Thyroid Carcinoma. Irradiation of enlarged thymuses in children before the 1930s over the dose range from 1200 to 6000 cGy was a popular treatment.[56,63] Unfortunately, a 100-fold increase in thyroid cancer was observed in these children. An increased incidence of thyroid cancer also occurred in individuals exposed as children from the bombs in Hiroshima and Nagasaki. Some of these individuals who developed thyroid cancer may have received doses as low as 100 cGy. Extensive follow-up is required to track the occurrence of these tumors because of their typical latent period of 10 to 20 years (which varies inversely with the dose that is received).

Breast Carcinoma. Three major groups of irradiated women with increased incidences of breast cancer seem to implicate radiation as the causative agent[27]: (1) irradiated female survivors in Hiroshima and Nagasaki, Japan; (2) Canadian women in a Nova Scotia sanitorium who had tuberculosis and were subjected to numerous fluoroscopic procedures; and (3) women treated for benign breast diseases such as postpartum mastitis. The best data that are available (with the Canadian study as the largest source) indicate that radiation induction of breast cancer most closely follows a linear dose-response relationship.[36]

Nonspecific Life-Shortening Effects

Research studies have shown that animals chronically exposed to low doses of radiation die younger than nonexposed animals.[47] Autopsy examinations (known as *necropsies* in animals) revealed a decreased number of parenchymal cells and blood vessels and an increased amount of connective tissue in organs. These changes resembled those seen in older animals and have been referred to as *radiation-induced aging*.[17] The effect on life span in these animals indicated a nonthreshold, linear relationship with radiation dose. However, more recent studies indicate that the life-shortening effect in these animals was probably due to cancer induction at moderate doses and organ atrophy, cell killing, and cell loss at high doses. Therefore, the life-shortening result can be explained by the occurrence of specific rather than nonspecific effects. Most of the human data available support the statement that specific causes of radiation-induced life shortening are identifiable, although some exceptions to this probably exist.

Genetic Effects

Somatic late effects can occur in an irradiated individual, and exposure of reproductive (germ) cells in that individual may affect future generations. As mentioned previously, ionizing radiation is a known mutagen (i.e., it can induce mutations in the genetic material [DNA/genes] found in the cell nucleus). Mutations (which are permanent, heritable [transmittable to subsequent generations], and generally detrimental) occur spontaneously in genes and DNA. The number of spontaneous mutations that occur in each generation of an organism is described as the *mutation frequency*, which can be increased by any mutagenic agent, including radiation.[30] If the mutation frequency in a generation is doubled by exposure to radiation, the radiation dose is then known as the *doubling dose*.[53] In humans, the doubling dose is estimated to range from 50 to 250 rem (0.5 to 2.5 Sv), with an average figure given as 100 rem (1.0 Sv).[27]

The classic study that demonstrated the mutagenic potential of radiation was performed by H. J. Müller[38] in 1927 and involved the use of the *Drosophila melanogaster*, or fruit fly. Müller irradiated male and female fruit flies under a number of conditions and observed the mutation frequencies in the next several generations. The fruit fly was used as the model for these experiments because it has a number of easily identifiable mutations such as those involving its wing shape and eye and body color. In addition, large populations of fruit flies can be maintained and bred relatively quickly and easily.

The results of Müller's fruit fly experiments (which have not been contradicted by subsequent studies with mice) include the following[38]:

1. Radiation does not produce new or unique mutations but increases the frequency of spontaneous mutations in each generation.
2. Mutation frequency is linearly related to radiation dose.
3. Radiation induction of mutations has no clear threshold; it is a stochastic effect like carcinogenesis.

In addition to Müller's experiments, subsequent animal studies have indicated that high dose rates can cause more genetic damage than low dose rates, males are more sensitive than females at low doses and low dose rates to genetic effects, and not all mutations show the same susceptibility to induction by radiation.[27] The estimated doubling dose for humans is based on extrapolations from the numerous animal experiments.

RADIATION THERAPY

Goal of Radiation Therapy

The goal of radiation therapy for cancer is to eradicate the tumor while not destroying normal tissues in the treatment field. This is easier said than done because radiation interaction in matter is a nonspecific, random process that does not distinguish between malignant and normal tissues. Biologic damage can be induced in tumor and normal tissues. Therefore, the tolerance of the normal tissue in the treatment field limits the dose that can be administered to the tumor. Several methods have been attempted to deal with this limiting factor during treatment so that more effective tumor treatments can be given. Several of these methods are discussed in this section.

General Tumor Characteristics

Parenchymal and Stromal Compartments. Like normal tissues, malignant tumors are composed of parenchymal and stromal compartments. A tumor parenchyma may contain up to four subpopulations or groups of cells.[64]

Cells belonging to group 1 are viable, actively mitotic (cycling) cells that are responsible for tumor growth. The percentage of group 1 cells in a tumor type usually varies from 30% to 50% and is termed the *growth fraction (GF)*.[37] The GF typically decreases as the size (volume) of the tumor increases.

Group 2 cells are typically viable but nondividing (not cycling). These cells, also known as *G0 cells*, have retained the ability to reenter the cell cycle and divide if properly stimulated.

Groups 3 and 4 are composed of nonviable cells. Group 3 cells appear structurally intact, whereas group 4 cells do not. Groups 3 and 4 cells therefore do not contribute to tumor growth.

The exact percentage of cells in each group varies with the size and type of tumor. In addition, each tumor contains a stromal compartment of blood vessels and connective tissue. In small, newly formed tumors the stroma may be entirely composed of normal host vessels, whereas large, older tumors contain a mix of normal and tumor vessels, or the supporting vasculature may be due to angiogenesis factors released by the tumor cells themselves. As discussed later, the tumor vasculature plays an important role in tumor growth and the oxygen effect.

Factors Affecting Tumor Growth. The rate at which tumors grow depends on three major factors: (1) the division rate of proliferating parenchymal cells, (2) the percentage of these cells in the tumor (GF), and (3) the degree of cell loss from the tumor.[58] The division rate of factor 1 cells in a tumor tends to be faster than the division rate for normal parenchymal cells from the same tissue.[32] For example, malignant skin cells cycle faster than normal skin cells. This might seem to imply that tumors have short doubling times (the time it takes to double in volume), but tumor doubling times in vivo are actually much longer than expected. The two major reasons for this are GF and cell loss. Although factor 1 cells have short cycle times versus normal cells of the same origin, only an average of 30% to 50% of all cells in the tumor are included in this category.[37] In addition, of the new cells produced by mitosis at the end of each cycle, up to 90% may be lost from the primary tumor itself. This cell-loss factor *(f)*, which is manifested by metastases, cell death, and exfoliation (shedding of cells as in gastrointestinal tumors), is thought to be the most significant in vivo factor with regard to tumor growth.[58] A high cell-loss factor slows the growth of the primary tumor, but if cells are lost by metastasis, new tumors form in other sites in the body and limit the curative potential of any treatment, including radiation therapy.

The Oxygen Effect. Tumor growth is characteristically unorganized compared with that of normal cells. During their early growth stages, tumors begin to outgrow their vascular supply. This results in differing levels of oxygen availability (known as *oxygen tension,* or PO_2) for the tumor cells depending on their proximity to functioning blood vessels. This was first observed clinically in 1955 by Thomlinson and Gray,[61] who examined human bronchial carcinoma specimens. Thomlinson and Gray observed that the amount of necrotic (dead) tissue in the tumor was related to the size of the tumor itself. A tumor with a radius of less than 100 µm did not contain necrotic areas. A tumor with a radius of greater than 160 µm showed a necrotic area surrounded by a viable rim of cells approximately 100 to 180 µm thick.

Thomlinson and Gray concluded that tumor cells located more than 200 µm from the nearest blood vessels (capillaries) are anoxic (no oxygen available) and unable to proliferate. These cells then die, thus forming the necrotic area. Tumor cells closest to blood vessels, however, are well oxygenated (known as *oxic* cells), are actively dividing, and compose the GF of the tumor. Between the oxic and anoxic cells are cells exposed to gradually decreasing oxygen tensions. These are known as *hypoxic cells.* Although hypoxic cells do not have normal levels of oxygen available to them, they are viable and capable of dividing. Data from animal tumors estimate that approximately 15% or more of the tumor-cell population may be hypoxic. This is known as the *hypoxic fraction* of the tumor.[67] Thomlinson and Gray's study estimated that the oxic, hypoxic, and anoxic populations in tumors were a result of the limited ability of oxygen to diffuse large distances in tissue. They estimated this diffusion distance of oxygen to be approximately 160 to 200 µm.[61] More recent studies indicate that a diffusion distance closer to 70 µm for oxygen may be more accurate.[27]

The vasculature network that forms in each growing tumor with factors such as division rate, GF, and cell loss ultimately gives rise to oxic, hypoxic, and anoxic cell populations in that tumor.

The radioresponse of a tumor depends (among other factors) on these cell populations. Anoxic cells do not contribute to the GF and therefore do not affect clinical outcome. Cells that are fully oxygenated (oxic) are highly radiosensitive to low-LET radiations (see the previous discussion on OER). The third group (viable hypoxic cells) is resistant to low-LET radiations by a factor of up to 2.5 to 3.0. The hypoxic fraction in each tumor is presumed to be responsible, at least in part, for tumor regrowth after radiation therapy. One of the reasons for the fractionation of a radiation dose is an attempt to increase the radioresponse of these hypoxic cells (see the discussion on reoxygenation).

Theory of Dose-Fractionation Techniques

Modern radiation therapy treatments are given in daily fractions over an extended period (up to 6 or 8 weeks) so that a high total dose is given to the tumor while ideally sparing normal tissues.[44] This technique, known as **fractionation**, originated in 1927 and replaced a single, high-dose radiation treatment. The type of tumor and tolerance of the normal tissue in the treatment field determine the total dose, size and number of fractions, and treatment duration.

A fractionated dose of radiation is less efficient biologically than a single dose. Therefore higher total doses are necessary during fractionation to produce the same damage compared with a single dose. For example, a single dose of 1000 cGy causes more damage than two fractions of 500 cGy separated by 24 hours, although the total delivered dose remains the same.

A typical fractionation scheme may involve a daily fraction size of 180 to 200 cGy given 5 times a week for 6 weeks for a total of 30 fractions. This results in a total treatment dose ranging from 5400 to 6000 cGy (54 to 60 Gy). Depending on the tumor to be treated, the actual total dose may be higher or lower than this. Hyperfractionated schedules for radiation include treatments BID (twice a day) and TID (three times a day). Hypofractionation involves the use of dose fractions substantially larger than the conventional level of around 2 Gy.[27]

The biologic effects on tissue from fractionated radiation therapy depend on the four Rs of radiation biology. These are repopulation, redistribution, repair, and reoxygenation.[70]

Repopulation. During protracted radiation therapy, surviving cells in the tumor and adjacent normal tissues may divide, thus repopulating these tissues partially or completely. Normal tissue repopulation is highly desirable and decreases the risk of late effects. Fractionated doses take advantage of normal tissue repopulation that occurs between fractions. This can result in the sparing of normal tissues in the treatment field.[70] In contrast, tumor repopulation is highly undesirable and contributes to tumor regrowth during or after treatment.

Redistribution. Irradiation of an asynchronous cell population (in which cells are distributed in all phases of the cell cycle) typically results in death to cells in the most sensitive phases (G2 and M), whereas more resistant cells (especially in late S) survive. This process, known as *partial synchronization*, results in a redistribution or reassortment of surviving cells after irradiation.[69] The ideal clinical situation for radiation treatment exists when tumor cells have moved into a sensitive phase and normal cells have moved into a resistant phase. Theoretically, the timing of each radiation fraction can be based on the progression of cells into a sensitive or resistant phase. However, because this cannot be determined clinically, the partial synchronization of cell populations by radiation and other modalities (e.g., hydroxyurea) that may occur has not yet been successfully exploited.

Repair of Sublethal Damage. Repair of sublethal damage has occurred within hours of radiation exposure in normal and tumor cells in vitro.[18] Fractionated radiation treatment takes advantage of repair processes in normal tissues that are active between radiation fractions. This partially accounts for the sparing effect on normal tissues that fractionation can achieve. Repair of sublethal damage is oxygen dependent (i.e., cells require a certain amount of oxygen to efficiently carry out repair mechanisms). Because a proportion of tumor cells are thought to be hypoxic, tumors in general are presumed to be incapable of repairing sublethal radiation damage as efficiently as normal tissues.[6] Although demonstrated in animal models, this differential repair between tumors and normal tissues may not be clinically significant in human tumors.

Reoxygenation. The fourth R of radiobiology, unlike the other three, is presumed to apply only to tumors. This phenomenon, termed *reoxygenation*, is the process by which hypoxic cells gain access to oxygen and become radiosensitive between radiation fractions.

As discussed previously, the OER for x-rays and gamma rays is 2.5 to 3.0 when delivered as a single dose. However, the OER decreases during fractionation of x-rays and gamma rays. This implies that a proportion of hypoxic cells reoxygenate and therefore become more sensitive to the next fraction. Although the exact mechanisms of reoxygenation are not clear, clinical trials of fractionated radiation therapy seem to indicate that tumor response is improved compared with that from single-dose treatment. During fractionation, the initial dose fraction should kill a significant proportion of well-oxygenated (oxic), radiosensitive cells near blood vessels in the tumor. The effects on hypoxic, radioresistant cells are considerably less from the same dose fraction. Therefore immediately after exposure the percentage of hypoxic tumor cells increases significantly and may even reach 100% for a short time. Within 24 hours, hypoxic cells somehow gain access to oxygen. Because cells nearest the blood vessels are likely killed by the radiation fraction, oxygen may diffuse beyond these dead cells and reach a percentage of the hypoxic cells. Studies on animal tumors have demonstrated that the hypoxic fraction reestablishes itself in the tumor, usually within 24 hours of treatment.[60] In other words, if a tumor had a hypoxic fraction of 15% before treatment, it eventually reestablishes this percentage after reoxygenation is complete. The standard time interval of 24 hours between radiation fractions in human tumors was extrapolated from animal experiments. This time interval coincides with the range of reoxygenation rates in animal tumors and presumably occurs in human tumors. Because healthy normal tissues do not usually have hypoxic cells, the process of reoxygenation does not apply to these tissues.

Methods of Improving Tumor Radioresponse. Reoxygenation does not rid the tumor of all hypoxic cells. If it did, fractionated treatments using low-LET radiations would be highly curative. Unfortunately, some tumors remain resistant to fractionated radiation therapy. This has given rise to a number of methods to overcome this persistent oxygen effect.

One early method involved the use of a chamber of hyperbaric (high-pressure) oxygen.[64] Patients were placed in sealed chambers containing pure oxygen at a pressure of 3 atmospheres. The rationale behind this was that the diffusion distance of oxygen would increase as a result of the high pressure used in the chamber so that it might reach the hypoxic areas in the tumor. However, this technique did not produce improved clinical results.

A related method involved the administration of perfluorochemicals (drugs that can carry oxygen) with 100% oxygen or carbogen (95% O_2/5% CO_2) breathing before and during radiation treatment.[64] The clinical results seemed to indicate improved response for several tumor types (most notably head and neck tumors), but the overall results were disappointing.

Radiosensitizers, radioprotectors, high-LET radiations, chemotherapy agents, and hyperthermia (heat) have all been used with varying degrees of success in terms of improved tumor response. However, each method is limited by biologic or technical constraints.[27]

Concept of Tolerance

Strandquist Isoeffect Curves. Although the preference of fractionated radiation treatments over high single doses is now established, the exact protocol for administration of fractionated doses continues to evolve. In 1944, Strandquist[59] made the first attempt to establish a relationship between radiation dose and treatment time. He developed plots of total dose (on a logarithmic scale) versus treatment duration (time in days on a linear scale) and called them isoeffect curves (Figure 4-16). These *isoeffect curves* related the treatment schedule in terms of total dose and time with the clinical outcome, including early effects, late effects, and tumor cure. The use of isoeffect curves led to treatment schedules for fractionated radiation therapy that gave a high probability of tumor control without exceeding the tolerance of normal tissue. Also during this time, the discovery was made that the tolerance of normal tissue is more dependent on the number and size of fractions than on the overall duration between the first and last fractions.

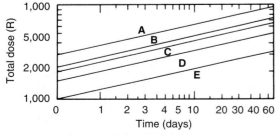

Figure 4-16. Isoeffect curves from Strandquist's data that relate various treatment schedules to the following clinical results: *A,* skin necrosis; *B,* cure of skin cancer; *C,* moist desquamation; *D,* dry desquamation; *E,* skin erythema. (From Strandquist M: Studien über die cumulative Wirkung der Röntgenstrahlen bei Fraktionierung, *Acta Radiol* 55[suppl]:1-300, 1944.)

Tolerance and Tolerance Dose. Because the radiation dose applied to the tumor mass is limited by the tolerance of the normal tissue in the treatment field, identifying doses that can be used on normal tissues and factors affecting these doses is important. Tolerance doses have therefore been established for normal tissues in terms of the total dose delivered by a standard fractionation schedule that causes a minimal (5%) or maximal (50%) complication rate within 5 years (**$TD_{5/5}$** or **$TD_{50/5}$**, respectively). These doses are commonly known as normal tissue tolerance doses (NTTDs). The $TD_{5/5}$ and $TD_{50/5}$ tolerance doses for various organs have been classified into mild to moderate and severe to fatal and are presented in Tables 4-7, 4-8, and 4-9, respectively.[31]

The NTTD is affected by two factors: the volume irradiated and fraction size. In terms of organ tolerance to radiation, the organ as a whole can tolerate higher radiation doses if the volume of the organ receiving that dose is small. As the volume of the organ affected by the treatment increases, the tolerance dose for the whole organ decreases. According to Rubin and Casarett,[49] for example, the $TD_{50/5}$ for the heart is 55 Gy if 60% of the heart is irradiated. If only 25% of the heart is irradiated, the $TD_{50/5}$ increases to approximately 80 Gy.

The other factor that affects the NTTD is the size of the daily radiation fraction used. In general, as the size of the daily fraction increases, cell killing increases, and the cell's ability to repair sublethal damage decreases, thus resulting in a decrease in the radiation tolerance of normal tissues.

Nominal Standard Dose. In an attempt to design treatment schedules that result in optimal tumor response with acceptable normal tissue damage, Ellis[22] in 1968 proposed the concept of nominal standard dose (NSD). Ellis derived the following equation from the isoeffect curves of Strandquist that took into account several parameters of fractionated radiation therapy:

$$D = NSD \times T^{0.11} \times N^{0.24}$$

In the equation, D is the total dose, NSD is the nominal standard dose, T is the overall treatment time in days between the first and last fractions, and N is the number of fractions.[22] Ellis[23] proposed the unit of rets (rad equivalent therapy) for NSD, and in many situations NSD1800 rets was considered the standard for comparison. The NSD equation allowed radiation oncologists to enter their treatment data, calculate the NSD for their centers, and compare this with other centers. The limitations of this concept, however, include the following: (1) the equation is based on connective tissue response and therefore is not useful for late-responding normal tissues and (2) the equation does not take into account the volume irradiated, which is critical to determining the tolerance of normal tissues. Although the NSD concept was popular in the 1970s, it is now useful for only an extremely limited number of clinical situations in radiation therapy.

PRESENT STATUS OF RADIATION THERAPY

The increasing popularity of intensity modulated radiation therapy (IMRT) has reduced radiation toxicity to surrounding tissues, altering the ratio of normal tissue dose to tumor dose. This has allowed the delivery of a higher dose without being

Table 4-7	Organs in Which Radiation Lesions Result in Mild to Moderate Morbidity

Organ	Injury	$TD_{5/5}$ (cGy)	$TD_{50/5}$ (cGy)	Whole or Partial Organ (Field Size/Length)
Articular cartilage	None	>50,000	>500,000	Joint surface
Bladder	Contracture	6000	8000	Whole
Breast (adult)	Atrophy	>5000	>10,000	Whole
Ear				
Middle	Serous otitis	5000	7000	Whole
Vestibular	Ménière's syndrome	6000	7000	Whole
Endocrine glands				
Thyroid	Reduced hormone production	4500	15,000	Whole
Adrenal	Reduced hormone production	>6000	—	Whole
Pituitary	Reduced hormone production	4500	20,000-30,000	Whole
Esophagus	Ulceration, stricture	6000	7500	75 cm²
Growing cartilage and bone (child)	Growth arrest	1000	3000	Whole
	Dwarfing	1000	3000	10 cm²
Mature cartilage and bone (adult)	Necrosis	6000	10,000	Whole
	Fracture, sclerosis	6000	10,000	10 cm²
Large arteries and veins	Sclerosis	>8000	>10,000	10 cm²
Lymph nodes and lymphatics	Atrophy, sclerosis	5000	>7000	Whole node
Muscle (child)	Atrophy	2000-3000	4000-5000	Whole
Muscle (adult)	Fibrosis	6000	8000	Whole
Oral cavity and pharynx	Ulceration	6000	8000	50 cm²
Ovary	Sterilization	200-300	635-1200	Whole
Peripheral nerves	Neuritis	6000	10,000	10 cm
Rectum	Ulcer, stricture	6000	8000	100 cm²
Salivary glands	Xerostomia	5000	7000	50 cm²
Skin	Acute and chronic dermatitis	5500	7000	100 cm²
Testis	Sterilization	100	200	Whole
Uterus	Stricture	7500	10000	5-10 cm

Modified from Rubin P, editor: *Clinical oncology: a multidisciplinary approach for physicians and students*, Philadelphia, 2001, WB Saunders.
$TD_{5/5}$, Tissue dose associated with a 5% injury rate within 5 years.
$TD_{50/5}$, Tissue dose associated with a 50% injury rate within 5 years.

Table 4-8	Organs in Which Radiation Lesions Result in Severe or Fatal Morbidity

Organ	Injury	$TD_{5/5}$ (in cGy)	$TD_{50/5}$ (in cGy)	Whole or Partial Organ (Field Size/Length)
Bone marrow	Aplasia, pancytopenia	250	450	Whole
		3000	4000	Segmental
Brain	Infarction, necrosis	5000-6000	6000-7000	Whole
Eye	Blindness			
Retina		5500	7000	Whole
Cornea		5000	>6000	Whole
Lens		500	1200	Whole or part
Fetus	Death	200	400	Whole
Heart	Pericarditis and pancarditis	4500	5500	60%
		7000	8000	25%
Intestine	Ulcer, perforation, and hemorrhage	4500	5500	400 cm²
		5000	6500	100 cm²
Kidney	Acute and chronic nephrosclerosis	1500	2000	Whole (strip)
		2000	2500	

Continued

Table 4-8	Organs in Which Radiation Lesions Results in Severe or Fatal Morbidity—cont'd			
Organ	**Injury**	**TD$_{5/5}$ (in cGy)**	**TD$_{50/5}$ (in cGy)**	**Whole or Partial Organ (Field Size/Length)**
Liver	Acute and chronic hepatitis	2500	4000	Whole
		1500	2000	Whole (strip)
Lung	Acute and chronic pneumonitis	3000	3500	100 cm^2
		1500	2500	Whole
Spinal cord	Infarction, necrosis	4500	5500	10 cm^2
Stomach	Perforation, ulcer, hemorrhage	4500	5500	100 cm^2
Uterus	Necrosis, perforation	>10,000	>20,000	Whole
Vagina	Ulcer, fistula	9000	>10,000	Whole

Modified from Rubin P, editor: *Clinical oncology: a multidisciplinary approach for physicians and students*, Philadelphia, 2001, WB Saunders.
TD$_{5/5}$, Tissue dose associated with a 5% injury rate within 5 years.
TD$_{50/5}$, Tissue dose associated with a 50% injury rate within 5 years.

regulated by the therapeutic ratio, as well as allowed higher and more effective radiation doses to be safely delivered to tumors with fewer side effects compared with conventional radiation therapy techniques. Taking advantage of IMRT relies critically on our knowledge of tumor and normal tissue dose-volume factors. A study by Hall and Wuu[27a,28,39] concluded that the lifetime risk of a radiation-induced carcinoma (secondary malignancy) following radiation therapy is approximately 1.75% for patients treated with IMRT.

A number of treatment techniques combine the use of radiation therapy with other modalities. This is now the method of choice for many human malignancies. Because of the limited

Table 4-9	Tolerance doses of Emami et al. (1991) predicted tolerance doses			
Organ	**Injury**	**TD$_{5/5}$ (cGy)**	**TD$_{50/5}$ (cGy)**	**Volume of Organ**
Bladder	Contracture	6500	8000	3/3
Brain	Necrosis	4500	6000	3/3
Colon	Obstruction/perforation	4500	5500	3/3
Ear	Acute serous otitis	3000	4000	3/3
Middle	Serous otitis	5500	6500	3/3
Vestibular	Ménière's syndrome	6000	7000	3/3
Endocrine glands (Thyroid)	Reduced hormone production	4500	8,000	3/3
Esophagus	Perforation, stricture	5500	6800	3/3
Heart	Pericarditis	4000	5000	3/3
Kidney	Nephritis	2300	2800	3/3
Larnyx	Necrosis	7000	8000	3/3
Cartilage	Edema	4500	8000	3/3
Liver	Liver failure	3000	4000	3/3
Lung	Pneumonitis	1750	2450	3/3
		3000	4000	2/3
		4500	6500	1/3
Optic chiasma	Blindness	4500	6500	3/3
Eye lens	Cataract	1000	1800	3/3
Optic nerve	Blindness	5000	6500	3/3
Retina	Blindness	4500	6500	3/3
Rectum	Ulcer, stricture	6000	8000	3/3
Salivary glands	Xerostomia	5000	7000	3/3
Skin	Necrosis/ulceration	5500	7000	100 cm^2
Small intestine	Obstruction/perforation	4000	5500	3/3
Spinal cord	Myelitis/necrosis	4500	—	20 cm
		5000	5000	10 cm/5 cm
Stomach	Ulceration/perforation	5000	6500	3/3

Modified from Emami B, et al: Tolerance of normal tissue to therapeutic radiation, *Int J Radiat Oncol Biol Phys* 21:109-122, 1991.
TD$_{5/5}$, Tissue dose associated with a 5% injury rate within 5 years.
TD$_{50/5}$, Tissue dose associated with a 50% injury rate within 5 years.

effect of low-LET radiations on hypoxic and S-phase tumor cells, the use of hyperthermia[4] and chemotherapeutic agents[27] in conjunction with radiation has increased with improved clinical results for a number of tumor types. In addition, the use of high-LET forms of radiation, such as protons, has certain benefits over conventional x-ray therapy.[5] The energy deposition of protons increases slowly with depth and reaches a sharp maximum near the end of the particles' range in a region called the *Bragg peak* (see Chapter 16). Clinical applications have attempted to use this Bragg peak region to maximize the delivery dose to the target organ while sparing the surrounding normal tissues. With the knowledge gained from clinical trials and preclinical experimentation, improvements in tumor responses and survival rates after radiation therapy continue to be realized.

SUMMARY

- In both ionization and excitation, the incoming radiation interacts with an atom. In ionization the incoming radiation ejects an electron from the shell of the atom, thus causing the atom to be charged (ionized). In excitation, the electron in the outer shell of the atom is said to be excited (oscillating or vibrating) but is not ejected from the shell.
- Radiation effects on tissue can be direct or indirect. When a beam of charged particles is incident on tissue, direct ionization of DNA is highly probable because of the relatively densely ionizing nature of most particulate radiations. Indirect effect occurs predominantly when x-rays or gamma rays compose the primary beam, thus producing fast electrons as the secondary particles that interact with water (H_2O). Indirect effects involve a series of reactions known as radiolysis (splitting) of water.
- A cell survival curve is a plot of the radiation dose administered on the *x*-axis versus the surviving fraction (SF) of cells on the *y*-axis. This survival curve is characteristic of the survival of cells exposed to low-LET radiations such as x-rays or gamma rays.
- The Law of Bergonié and Tribondeau states that ionizing radiation is more effective against cells that (1) are actively mitotic, (2) are undifferentiated, and (3) have a long mitotic future.
- The Radiation Therapy Oncology Group (RTOG) has summarized the acute and chronic effects of radiation into various categories or grades based on the severity of the clinical response (see Tables 4-3 and 4-4).
- There are three syndromes described in humans as a result to total-body irradiation: the hematopoietic syndrome in humans is induced by total-body doses of 100 to 1000 cGy. The gastrointestinal syndrome results if the total-body dose is between 1000 and 10,000 cGy. The cerebrovascular syndrome occurs exclusively above 10,000 cGy but can overlap with the gastrointestinal syndrome because it can be induced by a dose as low as 5000 cGy.
- Biologic response resulting from exposure to lower doses of radiation may not be observable for extended periods, ranging from years to generations. These effects are therefore known as late effects and are termed somatic effects if body cells are involved or genetic effects if reproductive cells are involved.
- The biologic effects on tissue from fractionated radiation therapy depend on the four Rs of radiation biology, which are repopulation, redistribution, repair, and reoxygenation.

Review Questions

1. The term that relates biologic response to the quality of radiation is:
   a. LET
   b. OER
   c. RBE
   d. TR
2. Generally, which is the most radiosensitive phase of the cell cycle?
   a. G1
   b. G2
   c. M
   d. S
3. Which of the following tissues is the most radiosensitive?
   a. muscle
   b. ocular lens
   c. liver
   d. bone and cartilage
4. Which of the following is *not* one of the four Rs of radiation therapy?
   a. reconfirmation
   b. reoxygenation
   c. redistribution
   d. repopulation
5. Strandquist's isoeffect curves are related to which of the following?
   a. oxygen enhancement
   b. translocation of DNA
   c. fractionation
   d. radiation syndromes
6. According to the Law of Bergonié and Tribondeau, ionizing radiation is more effective against cells that are:
   a. actively mitotic and differentiated and have a long mitotic future
   b. actively mitotic and differentiated and have a short mitotic future
   c. not actively mitotic and undifferentiated and have a long mitotic future
   d. actively mitotic and undifferentiated and have a long mitotic future
7. Which of the following particles do *not* contribute to the direct effect of radiation?
   a. protons
   b. positron
   c. alpha particles
   d. heavy nuclear fragments
8. Gross structural changes in chromosomes resulting from radiation damage are referred to as:
   a. chromosome stickiness or clumping
   b. aberrations, lesions, or anomalies
   c. deletions and inversions
   d. interphase death or replication failure

9. What is another term for the cellular response that results in the delay of division of cells in the cell cycle?
   a. mitotic delay
   b. interphase death
   c. reproductive failure
   d. apoptosis
10. Which are the most important parameters that allow interpretation of survival curves?
    I. extrapolation number *(n)*
    II. surviving fraction (SF)
    III. D_o (or D37)
    IV. quasi-threshold dose (D_q)
    V. oxygen enhancement ratio (OER)
    VI. linear energy transfer (LET)
    a. II, V, and VI
    b. II, III, and V
    c. I, III, and IV
    d. III, V, and VI

The answers to the Review Questions can be found by logging on to our website at: *http://evolve.elsevier.com/Washington+Leaver/ principles*

Questions to Ponder

1. Discuss the interactions of radiation and matter (specifically, the indirect and direct effects on the cellular level).
2. Describe the relationship between LET, RBE, and OER. Be able to graphically support your answer.
3. How does radiation sensitivity relate to the goals of radiation oncology in terms of tumor control and the sparing of normal tissue structures?
4. Relate the three graphic components of the cell survival curve (n, D_o, and D_q) to the administration of radiation treatments.
5. Describe the five classification of mammalian cells according to their radiosensitivities and characteristics, listing examples for each classification.
6. Briefly describe the three total-body responses to radiation. Remember to include the dose ranges at which each of these responses occur.

REFERENCES

1. Adams GE, et al: Electron-affinic sensitization. VII. A correlation between structures, one-electron reduction potentials, and the efficiencies of nitroimidazoles as hypoxic cell radiosensitizer, *Radiat Res* 67:9-20, 1976.
2. Albert RE, et al: Follow-up studies of patients treated by x-ray epilation for tinea capitis, *Arch Environ Health* 17:899-918, 1968.
3. Ancel P, Vitemberger P: Sur la radiosensibilitie cellulaire, *C R Soc Biol* 92:517, 1925.
4. Arcangeli G, et al: Tumor control and therapeutic gain with different schedules of combined radiotherapy and local external hyperthermia in human cancer, *Int J Radiat Oncol Biol Phys* 9:1125-1134, 1983.
5. Barendsen GW: *Proceedings of the Conference on Particle Accelerators in Radiation Therapy* (pp 120-125), LA-5180-C. Oak Ridge, Tenn, 1972, US Atomic Energy Commission, Technical Information Center.
6. Bedford JS, Mitchell JB: Dose-rate effects in synchronous mammalian cells in culture, *Radiat Res* 54:316-327, 1973.
7. Belli JA, et al: Radiation response of mammalian tumor cells. I. Repair of sublethal damage in vivo, *J Natl Cancer Inst* 38:673-682, 1967.
8. Bergonié J, Tribondeau L: De quelques resultats de la radiotherapie et essai de fixation d'une technique rationnelle, *C R Acad Sci (Paris)* 143:983, 1906.
9. Broerse JJ, Barendsen GW: Current topics, *Radiat Res Q* 8:305-350, 1973.
10. Broerse JJ, Barendsen GW, van Kersen GR: Survival of cultured human cells after irradiation with fast neutrons at different energies in hypoxic and oxygenated conditions, *Int J Radiat Biol* 13:559-572, 1967.
11. Bushong SC: *Radiologic science for technologists: physics, biology and protection,* ed 8, St. Louis, 2004, Mosby.
12. Canti RG, Spear FG: The effect of gamma irradiation on cell division in tissue culture in vitro, part II, *Proc R Soc Lond B Biol Sci* 105:93, 1929.
13. Court-Brown WM, Doll R: Expectation of life and mortality from cancer among British radiologists, *Br Med J* 2:181, 1958.
14. Court-Brown WM, Doll R: Mortality from cancer and other causes after radiotherapy from ankylosing spondylitis, *Br Med J* 2:1327, 1965.
15. Court-Brown WM, et al: The incidence of leukemia after the exposure to diagnostic radiation in utero, *Br Med J* 2:1599, 1960.
16. Cox JD, Stetz J, Pajak TF: Toxicity criteria of the Radiation Therapy Oncology Group (RTOG) and the European Organization for Research and Treatment of Cancer (EORTC), *Int J Radiat Oncol Biol Phys* 31:1341-1346, 1995.
17. Curtis HJ: *Radiation-induced aging in mice,* London, 1961, Butterworth.
18. Dekaban AS: Abnormalities in children exposed to x-irradiation during various stages of gestation: tentative timetable of radiation injury to the human fetus, *J Nucl Med* 9:471, 1968.
19. Dewey WC, Humphrey RM: Restitution of radiation-induced chromosomal damage in Chinese hamster cells related to the cell's life cycle, *Exp Cell Res* 35:262, 1964.
20. Dublin LI, Spiegelman M: Mortality of medical specialists, 1938-1942, *JAMA* 137:1519, 1948.
21. Elkind MM, Sutton-Gilbert H: Radiation response of mammalian cells grown in culture. I. Repair of x-ray damage in surviving Chinese hamster cells, *Radiat Res* 13:556, 1960.
22. Ellis F: Dose, time, and fractionation in radiotherapy. In Ebert M, Howard A, editors: *Current topics in radiation research,* Amsterdam, 1968, North Holland Publishing.
23. Ellis F: Nominal standard dose and the ret, *Br J Radiol* 44:101-108, 1971.
24. Evans RD, et al: Radiogenic tumors in the radium and mesothorium cases studied at MIT. In May CW, et al, editors: *Delayed effects of bone-seeking radionuclides,* Salt Lake City, 1969, University of Utah Press.
25. Field SB: The relative biological effectiveness of fast neutrons for mammalian tissues, *Radiology* 93:915-920, 1969.
26. Griem ML, et al: Analysis of the morbidity and mortality of children irradiated in fetal life, *Radiology* 88:347-349, 1967.
27. Hall EJ, Giaccia AJ: *Radiobiology for the radiologist,* ed 6, Philadelphia, 2005, Lippincott Williams & Wilkins.
27a. Hall EJ, Wuu CS: Radiation-induced second cancers: the impact of 3D-CRT and IMRT, *Int J Radiat Oncol Biol Phys* 56:83-88, 2003.
28. Khan F: *The physics of radiation therapy,* ed. 3, Philadelphia, 2003, Lippincott Williams & Wilkins.
29. Kinsella T, et al: The use of halogenated thymidine analog as clinical radiosensitizers: rationale, current status, and future prospects—nonhypoxic cell sensitizers, *Int J Radiat Oncol Biol Phys* 10:1399-1406, 1984.
30. Krall JF: Estimation of spontaneous and radiation-induced mutation rates in man, *Eugenics Q* 3:201, 1956.
31. Kramer S: Principles of radiation oncology and cancer radiotherapy. In Rubin P, editor: *Clinical oncology: a multidisciplinary approach for physicians and students,* Philadelphia, 1993, WB Saunders.
32. Lyskin AB, Mendelsohn ML: Comparison of cell cycle in induced carcinomas and their normal counterparts, *Cancer Res* 24:1131, 1964.
33. MacMahon B: Pre-natal x-ray exposure and childhood cancer, *J Natl Cancer Inst* 28:231, 1962.
34. March HC: Leukemia in radiologists in a 20-year period, *Am J Med Sci* 220:282, 1950.
35. Martland HS: Occurrence of malignancy in radioactive persons: general review of data gathered in study of radium dial painters, with special reference to occurrence of osteogenic sarcoma and interrelationship of certain blood diseases, *Am J Cancer* 15:2435, 1931.
36. McKenzie I: Breast cancer following multiple fluoroscopes, *Br J Cancer* 19:1, 1965.
37. Mendelsohn ML: The growth fraction: a new concept applied to tumors, *Science* 132:1496, 1960.

38. Müller HJ: On the relation between chromosome changes and gene mutations, *Brookhaven Symp Biol* 8:126, 1956.

39. Mundt A, Roeske J: *Intensity modulated radiation therapy: a clinical perspective*, London, 2005, BC Decker.

40. Murphy DP, Goldstein L: Micromelia in a child irradiated in utero, *Surg Gynecol Obstet* 50:79, 1930.

41. Otake M, Schull WJ: In utero exposure to A-bomb radiation and mental retardation: a reassessment, *Br J Radiol* 57:409-414, 1984.

42. Pack GT, Davis J: Radiation cancer of the skin, *Radiology* 84:436, 1965.

43. Patt HM, et al: Cysteine protection against x-irradiation, *Science* 110:213, 1949.

44. Peters LJ, Withers HR, Thames HD: Radiobiological considerations for multiple daily fractionation. In Kaercher KH, Kogelnik HD, Reinartz G, editors: *Progress in radio-oncology*, vol 2, New York, 1982, Raven Press.

45. Plummer C: Anomalies occurring in children exposed in utero to the atomic bomb at Hiroshima, *Pediatrics* 10:687, 1952.

46. Puck TT, Marcus TI: Action of x-rays on mammalian cells, *J Exp Med* 10:653, 1956.

47. Rotblat J, Lindop P: Long-term effects of a single whole body exposure of mice to ionizing radiation. II. Causes of death, *Proc R Soc Lond B Biol Sci* 154:350, 1961.

48. Rowland RE, Stehney AF, Lucas HF: Dose response relationships for radium-induced bone sarcomas, *Health Phys* 44:15-31, 1983.

49. Rubin P, Casarett GW: *Clinical radiation pathology*, vols 1 and 2, Philadelphia, 1968, WB Saunders.

50. Rugh R: X-ray-induced teratogenesis in the mouse and its possible significance to man, *Radiology* 99:433-443, 1971.

51. Russell LB, Russell WL: An analysis of the changing radiation response of the developing mouse embryo, *J Cell Physiol* 43(suppl 1):103-149, 1954.

52. Saccomanno G, et al: Lung cancer of uranium miners on the Colorado plateau, *Health Phys* 10:1195, 1964.

53. Schull WL, Otake M, Neal JV: Genetic effects of the atomic bomb: a reappraisal, *Science* 213:1220-1227, 1981.

54. Selman J: *The fundamentals of imaging physics and radiobiology*, ed 9, Springfield, 2000, Charles C Thomas.

55. Simic MG, Grossman L, Upton AC, editors: *Mechanisms of DNA damage and repair*, New York, 1986, Plenum Press.

56. Simpson CL, Hempelmann LH: The association of tumors and roentgen-ray treatment of the thorax in infancy, *Cancer* 10:42, 1957.

57. Sinclair WK: Cyclic x-ray responses in mammalian cells in vitro, *Radiat Res* 33:620-643, 1968.

58. Steel GG: Cell loss as a factor in the growth rate of human tumors, *Eur J Cancer* 3:381-387, 1967.

59. Strandquist M: Studien über die kumulative Wirkung der Roentgenstrahlen bei Fraktionierung, *Acta Radiol* 55(suppl):1-300, 1944.

60. Thomlinson RH: Effect of fractionated irradiation on the proportion of anoxic cells in an intact experimental tumor, *Br J Radiol* 39:158, 1966.

61. Thomlinson RH, Gray LH: The histological structure of some human lung cancers and the possible implications for radiotherapy, *Br J Cancer* 9:539, 1955.

62. Till JE, McCulloch EA: A direct measurement of the radiation sensitivity of normal mouse bone marrow cells, *Radiat Res* 14:213-222, 1961.

63. Toyooka ET, et al: Neoplasms in children treated with x-rays for thymic enlargement. II. Tumor incidence as a function of radiation factors, *J Natl Cancer Inst* 31:1357, 1963.

64. Travis EL: *Primer of medical radiobiology*, ed 2, St. Louis, 1989, Mosby.

65. Trotti A, et al: Common toxicity criteria: version 2.0. An improved reference for grading the acute effects of cancer treatment: impact on radiotherapy. *Int J Radiat Oncol Biol Phys* 47:13-47, 2000.

66. Upton AC: Radiation carcinogenesis. In Busch H, editor: *Methods in cancer research*, vol 4, New York, 1968, Academic Press.

67. Van Putten LM, Kahlman LF: Oxygenation status of transplantable tumor during fractionated radiotherapy, *J Natl Cancer Inst* 40:441-451, 1968.

68. Warren S: Radiation carcinogenesis, *Bull N Y Acad Med* 46:131-147, 1970.

69. Withers HR: Cell cycle redistribution as a factor of multi-fraction irradiation, *Radiology* 114:199-202, 1975.

70. Withers HR: The 4 R's of radiotherapy. In Lett JT, Adler H, editors: *Advances in radiation biology*, vol 5, San Francisco, 1975, Academic Press.

71. Withers HR, Elkind MM: Microcolony survival assay for cells of mouse intestinal mucosa exposed to radiation, *Int J Radiat Biol* 17:261-267, 1970.

72. Withers HR, et al: Radiation survival and regeneration characteristics of spermatogenic stem cells of mouse testis, *Radiat Res* 57:88-103, 1974.

73. Wright EA, Howard-Flanders P: The influence of oxygen on the radiosensitivity of mammalian tissues, *Acta Radiol (Stockholm)* 48:26, 1957.

74. Zirkle RE: Partial cell irradiation, *Adv Biol Med Phys* 5:103, 1957.

Detection and Diagnosis

Dennis Leaver

Outline

Key Terms

Objectives

- Discuss the three fundamental questions a physician would ask if someone were sick.
- Explain the value of the interview as a diagnostic tool.
- Describe the importance of the medical record.
- Compare and contrast the four aspects of the physical examination: inspection, palpation, percussion, and auscultation.
- Discuss the three levels of cancer screening.
- Explain the significance of sentinel node biopsy in the detection of breast cancer.
- Predict the possible consequences of a false-positive testing result in the use of the PSA marker for prostate cancer.

- Define *prevalence, incidence, sensitivity,* and *specificity*.
- Compare and contrast the benefits of digital mammography with screen-film mammography.
- Evaluate the various methods of screening for colorectal cancer.
- Discuss DNA testing for human papillomavirus and how it relates to cervical cancer.
- Describe how PET scanning differs from CT scanning in terms of anatomic structure and function.
- Compare MRI and CT as diagnostic tools.
- Describe the TNM system used for staging cancer, specifically the three components used to describe the extent of the disease.

INTRODUCTION TO DETECTION AND DIAGNOSIS

The 5-year relative survival rate for all cancers diagnosed between 1996 and 2003 is 66%, up from 50% in 1975 to 1977.[2] What will the survival rate be in 2022? The improvement in survival reflects the increased emphasis on detecting and diagnosing particular cancers at an earlier stage, the use of new treatment methods, and a better understanding of how some cancers behave. Survival rates will vary significantly by cancer type and stage at diagnosis, so careful observation of signs and symptoms may help diagnose a disease at an earlier stage. This ultimately should lead to better outcomes.

The detection and diagnosis of disease, especially cancer, have come to rely increasingly on two specialties: radiology and pathology. With recent advances in computer technology, diagnostic imaging and its application to the detection of disease provide increased effectiveness in managing diseases such as cancer. Medical imaging modalities include nuclear medicine studies, positron emission tomography (PET), mammography, computed tomography (CT), magnetic resonance imaging (MRI), ultrasound, and newer molecular imaging technologies. Some medical imaging modalities are able to show both anatomic detail and physiologic/functional detail. The physician is still needed to understand the application of these new imaging modalities and to establish a relationship with the patient.

The physician who wishes to help someone who is sick should try to answer these three fundamental questions, posed originally by Reinertsen and LeBlond.[6,21]
- "What's happening to me?"
- "What's going to happen to me?"
- "What can be done to improve what happens to me?"

The routine physical examination is an important tool in maintaining good health and detecting conditions or diseases early so that intervention is possible before the patient demonstrates signs or experiences more advanced symptoms. Early detection has proved important in cancer management. According to the American Cancer Society (ACS),[1] **prevention** and early detection are two of the most important and effective strategies of saving lives lost from cancer, diminishing suffering resulting from cancer, and eliminating cancer as a major health problem. Prevention includes measures that stop cancer from developing. Early detection includes examinations and tests intended to find the disease as early as possible, before it has spread. The earlier a cancer can be found, the more effectively it can be treated. This may result in fewer side effects. In fact, the relative survival rate for people with cancers for which the ACS has specific early detection recommendations (breast, colon, rectum, cervix, prostate, testes, and skin) is approximately 81%.[1] Early detection and effective **screening** (selecting appropriate tests, and studies to check for disease) programs translate into increased survival.

Broad cancer education may lead to less cancer incidence in our society. For example, limiting our exposure to harmful UV rays from the sun will reduce our risk of skin cancer. Smoking is the most preventable cause of death in our society. Certainly, our diet may play a role in preventing colon cancer. Find out more information by visiting the American Cancer Society at www.cancer.org.

The actual physical examination (whether routine or a result of the patient experiencing signs or symptoms) is a methodical process of detection that covers all the systems. A **sign** is "an objective finding as perceived by an examiner."[13] For example, the examining physician may notice signs such as a rash, feel a mass, or note the color of the patient's skin. A **symptom** is a "subjective indication of a disease or a change in condition as perceived by the patient."[13] For example, the patient may complain of pain, numbness, dysphagia, dyspnea, difficulty in sleeping, or lack of appetite. These are symptoms.

If a patient is experiencing symptoms, it is usually an indication that the condition or disease process is more advanced. If a set of signs or symptoms arises from a common cause, it is referred to as a **syndrome.** Many diseases share the same signs and symptoms. Grouping signs and symptoms into a syndrome with results of tests and medical procedures helps the physician eliminate some diseases and narrow the choices for a correct diagnosis.

A **diagnosis** is defined as the identification of a disease or condition. A diagnosis can be subjective or objective. A subjective diagnosis is based on several factors. The patient's complaints and medical history are considered subjective. The physician's preliminary diagnosis with no hard evidence for support is also considered subjective. An objective diagnosis is based on results of current medical procedures and tests (such as a tissue biopsy or laboratory data) and observations by the physician and other medical personnel.

The process for obtaining an objective diagnosis begins with the interview and physical examination to help assess the patient's current status and determine necessary steps (if any) to take. During a physical examination, the physician follows a methodical process that includes the acquisition of data or clues through the interview process, a review of past medical records, a physical examination, and a list of the patient's chief complaints.[8,21]

Each disease process has distinguishing features that may serve as "clues." The physician must search for clues that may correspond to a list of problems. The list is then used to generate hypotheses, which in turn may lead to a diagnosis. Clues are sought by taking a history, performing a physical examination, and ordering laboratory and medical imaging tests. The physician must then consider several hypotheses, which might explain the problems the patient is having in terms of diseases in another list called *differential diagnoses.* The clues or facts obtained during the interview, physical examination, and diagnostic testing are then used to support or refute each hypothetical disease in the differential diagnosis list in the hope of finally arriving at "the diagnosis."[21]

THE INTERVIEW AS A DIAGNOSTIC TOOL

The most powerful diagnostic tool of the physician is the initial interview. By this means, one learns the chronologic events and symptoms of the patient's illness. Diagnostic hypotheses are generated and tested as the patient's history unfolds, resulting in the formulation of the most likely diagnoses at the completion of the interview and testing.[14]

The physician must interview the patient to acquire accurate information. If the patient is too ill or handicapped to provide the information, the physician uses other sources such as family, friends, prior medical records, and other health care providers.

In the interview process, the physician asks questions and the patient provides answers. The physician determines the patient's chief complaints and current status and obtains the patient's medical and psychosocial history. The interview is also used to establish the physician-patient relationship and demonstrate to the patient a caring, empathetic attitude.[8,33] In a study of 103 cancer patients by Sapir et al.,[33] patients overwhelmingly expected their oncologists to be patient and skilled in diagnostic procedures (98%); tactful, considerate, and therapeutically skilled (90% to 95%); and skilled in the management of pain and the psychosocial consequences of cancer (75% to 85%). When there is bad news to be communicated, 92% of patients indicated that they would want disclosure, whereas 6% indicated that they would want the news withheld from them but passed onto a family member.[33] Evidence from studies like this reinforces the importance of the physician-patient relationship.

Allowing enough time for an interview is important. If the interview is rushed, the patient may believe that the physician is not empathetic. Not allowing enough time may limit the amount of information the physician is able to acquire. Interviewing requires active listening, which calls for minimal, if any, distractions. Telephone calls, interruptions by staff members, and loud noises can interfere with good communication.

The initial interview may be a long process in the radiation oncology setting, because the physician must not only assess the patient but also provide information regarding the goals, benefits, and risks involved in a course of radiation therapy. Radiation therapists; nurses; and midlevel practitioners, such as physician assistants or advanced practice nurses, may also interview the patient during the treatment process in an effort to obtain information about the patient's concerns, questions, and treatment-related side effects. The therapist must select words that are clear and mean the same thing to the patient. The meaning of words is relative. A radiation therapist may ask, "What medications are you taking?" The response may be "None," although the patient is taking aspirin for pain and an antacid for indigestion. In the patient's mind, these are not medications because they were not prescribed.

The objective of the interview is to obtain as much accurate information as possible. Avoiding technical jargon can mean the difference between a successful interview and one that fails to help the patient. During the interview, the patient's ability to communicate, level of understanding, and facial expressions should be assessed. One must also consider the reliability of the patient's responses. This requires skill in patient communication and observation, a technique that develops more over time and involves the use of verbal and nonverbal communication.

Verbal communication involves the manner, quality, and intonation of speech. Forms of nonverbal communication include facial expressions, posture, personal appearance, and manner of movement. Radiation therapists may be at a distinct advantage in assessing verbal and nonverbal communication from the patient because of daily interaction with the patient. Patients young and old will see their radiation therapist on average five to six times more often than their physician, assuming that the physician sees the patient during the initial consultation and weekly thereafter. This increased exposure to the therapist allows a sense of mutual confidence and trust to develop. In many situations, the patient may divulge more information to the therapist, especially concerning treatment-related side effects, pain management, and other issues important to the patient.

Observing nonverbal communication while the patient is talking can help determine the real meaning of the patient's words. The patient may say one thing but really mean another. For example, the radiation therapist asks the patient, "Are you having any pain?" The patient says, "No." However, the patient's appearance, posture, and facial expressions contradict the verbal response. The patient sits slouched over, grimaces during movement, and moves slowly with great deliberation. These are all nonverbal signs of pain. These signs may be related to a medical problem other than pain or a psychological problem, or they may simply have no significance. A slouched posture may indicate pain, low self-esteem, depression, or some other unexplained phenomenon. A grimace may be a psychological response to the question or physician, a sign of indigestion, or a facial tic. Slow, deliberate movement may mean unfamiliarity with the surroundings, discomfort, or distraction. Observing this type of nonverbal communication requires probing further to rule out pain.

Table 5-1	Examples of Facilitating Verbal Responses	
Type of Response	**Examples**
Minimal	"I see." "I understand."
Reflecting feelings	"I see you are very angry." "It is very scary."
Clarifications	"How bad did it hurt?" "This bothers you only at night?"

Some of the verbal responses that can facilitate the interview are minimal responses, reflecting feelings, and seeking clarification (Table 5-1). Responses that may hinder the interview are the use of social clichés, imposition of the interviewer's own values, and devaluing or minimizing the patient's feelings or responses (Table 5-2). In addition, the interviewer should present himself or herself as unhurried, interested, and sympathetic in an effort to obtain the patient's confidence and rapport.[21]

THE MEDICAL RECORD AND MEDICAL HISTORY

The medical record documents the patient's past medical experience. The format of the medical record may differ from institution to institution and according to whether the person was an inpatient or outpatient seen in the clinic or emergency department. It may be a paper or electronic chart or a combination of both forms.

The hospital medical record is a legal public document in that it is available to the medical staff; to medical departments of the hospital, clinic, and insurance companies; or by subpoena to a court of law.[31] Patients do not own their medical records, but they may review them on request and have copies released to other physicians. The medical record contains the medical history, results of laboratory tests and medical procedures, progress notes, copies of consent forms, correspondence, and even images produced in the radiation therapy department.

The format for taking a medical history may vary from physician to physician but should be done in a logical manner.

Table 5-2	Examples of Hindering Verbal Responses	
Type of Response	**Examples**
Social clichés	"You will feel better soon." "Don't worry, everything will be all right."
Imposing values	"You should not be having sex outside of marriage." "Someone your age should be more responsible."
Devaluing the patient's feelings or responses	"I wish I had a nickel for every time I heard this." "This is just part of the aging process."

Table 5-3	Information Gathered During the Medical History Interview
Type of Data	**Information Obtained**
Demographic data	Age, race, gender, marital status, and current occupation
Chief complaints	Symptoms, current illness, and current condition
Medical history	Childhood illnesses, allergies, immunizations, injuries, prior hospitalizations, psychological problems, and medications
Family history	Illnesses, causes of death, genetic disorders, and mental disorders
Personal history	Occupation, lifestyle, and sexual activity and preferences

Table 5-3 contains a summary of the type of information obtained that is important. This information may also become part of a separate radiation therapy paper or electronic chart.

The Need for Demographic Data

Demographic data provide an overview of the patient, including information on the patient's age, gender, race, and possibly national origin. The reason for obtaining demographic data is that certain disease conditions are found to be more prevalent for groups according to age, gender, race, and national origin.

For example, although cancer occurs at any age, the incidence is higher among older persons, especially those over the age of 65.[2] However, certain types of cancer occur more frequently in other age groups. The classic presentation of Wilms' tumor (a cancer of the kidney) is that of a healthy child in whom abdominal swelling is discovered by the child's mother, pediatrician, or family practitioner during a routine physical examination.[5,29]

Some types of cancer occur more frequently by gender. For example, men are affected more often than women by lung cancer, whereas the incidences of thyroid cancer are higher in women[29] (Table 5-4).

The incidence of cancer among races and nationalities varies. For example, the incidence of esophageal cancer is extremely high in the Bantu of Africa, China, Russia, Japan, Scotland, and the Caspian region of Iran.[29] In the United States, prostate cancer incidence rates are significantly higher in African-American men than in Caucasian men.[4]

The Importance of the Medical History

The medical history provides a snapshot of the patient's prior medical problems and treatments. The determination of prior medical problems may establish risk factors for acquiring diseases in the future. For example, a patient who has a long history of indigestion and gastric reflux caused by a hiatal hernia may be at risk for ulcers or carcinoma of the esophagus.[29,32] Gastric reflux is the backward flow of contents of the stomach into the esophagus. A hiatal hernia is a congenital or acquired condition that is the result of movement of the stomach through the esophageal hiatus of the diaphragm into the thorax.

Certain symptoms, illnesses, or conditions may indicate the possibility of a predisposing factor, **premalignant** condition (physiologic characteristics or predisposing factors that may lead to malignancy), **paraneoplastic syndrome** (a collection of symptoms that result from substances or hormones produced by the tumor, and they occur remotely from the tumor), or other risk factors.

Certain types of cancer appear to repeat in families. More than one sibling may develop leukemia. If the mother has breast cancer, the daughter is at a greater risk of developing the disease due to inherited genetic **mutations**, which are changes to the base pair sequence of either DNA or RNA and are passed down to descendants (*BRCA1* and *BRCA2*).[2,29,35] The risk of colon cancer increases with age and may be associated with certain inherited genetic mutations or a family history of colon cancer.[2]

The personal history encompasses the patient's lifestyle (past and present). The physician asks questions regarding dietary, exercise, alcohol, cigarette, and drug habits. The physician must also determine the patient's sexual activity, frequency, and preferences. Determining the patient's past occupations is important. For example, the patient may have been employed in an occupation that carried the risk of exposure to asbestos, disease, certain chemicals, or other carcinogens.

THE PHYSICAL EXAMINATION

The physical examination, medical history, and test results help the physician detect variations in the normal state of the patient. The physical examination is an extremely organized, detailed exploration of the patient's anatomic regions. Performing a physical examination requires all the physician's senses and skills.

The following paragraphs list some examples of aspects of the physical examination and information the physician may be seeking. The information in this section is extremely general and far from comprehensive regarding all aspects of the physical examination. Inspection, palpation, percussion, and auscultation are the four classic techniques of the physical examination.

Inspection

Inspection is the use of sight to observe. A distinction must be made between seeing and observing. Something may be seen but not observed. For example, a person may see a group of people, but on further observation of the group the person begins to make distinctions. The person may be able to say that 10 people were in the group and may then observe differences in gender, race, age, appearance, and behavior.

The physician observes the color of the patient's skin, which may indicate signs of a disease condition. Many diseases and conditions affect skin coloration. The skin may be dark, pale, gray, flushed, jaundiced, or cyanotic. Dark skin may be natural or caused by irritation of another medical condition. Pale skin may be natural or caused by anemia. Flushed or reddened skin may be caused by hormones, a reaction to external beam radiation therapy, infection, or burns. Jaundice, a yellow coloration of the skin, may be caused by obstruction of the bile ducts. Cyanosis, a blue coloration of the skin, may be caused by a lack of oxygen in the blood.

Table 5-4	Leading Sites of New Cancer Cases and Deaths—2008 Estimates*			
Estimated New Cases*		**Estimated Deaths**		
Male	**Female**	**Male**	**Female**
Prostate 186,320 (25%)	Breast 182,460 (26%)	Lung and bronchus 90,810 (31%)	Lung and bronchus 71,030 (26%)
Lung and bronchus 114,690 (14%)	Lung and bronchus 100,330 (14%)	Prostate 28,660 (10%)	Breast 40,480 (15%)
Colon and rectum 77,250 (10%)	Colon and rectum 71,560 (10%)	Colon and rectum 24,260 (8%)	Colon and rectum 25,700 (9%)
Urinary bladder 51,230 (7%)	Uterine corpus 40,100 (6%)	Pancreas 17,500 (6%)	Pancreas 16,790 (6%)
Non-Hodgkin's lymphoma 35,450 (5%)	Non-Hodgkin's lymphoma 30,670 (4%)	Liver and intrahepatic bile duct 12,570 (4%)	Ovary 15,520 (6%)
Melanoma of the skin 34,950 (5%)	Thyroid 28,410 (4%)	Leukemia 12,460 (4%)	Non-Hodkin's lymphoma 9,370 (3%)
Kidney and renal pelvis 33,130 (4%)	Melanoma of the skin 26,030 (4%)	Esophagus 11,250 (4%)	Leukemia 9,250 (3%)
Oral cavity and pharynx 25,310 (3%)	Ovary 21,650 (3%)	Urinary bladder 9,950 (3%)	Uterine corpus 7,470 (3%)
Leukemia 25,180 (3%)	Kidney and renal pelvis 21,260 (3%)	Non-Hodgkin's lymphoma 9,790 (3%)	Liver and intrahepatic bile duct 5,840 (2%)
Pancreas 18,770 (3%)	Leukemia 19,090 (3%)	Kidney and renal pelvis 8,100 (3%)	Brain and other nervous system 5,650 (2%)
All sites 745,180 (100%)	All sites 692,000 (100%)	All sites 294,120 (100%)	All sites 271,530 (100%)

From American Cancer Society, Inc., Surveillance Research, 2008.

*Excludes basal and squamous cell skin cancers and in situ carcinoma except urinary bladder.

Percentages may not total 100% due to rounding.

The physician looks for scarring or lesions such as warts, moles, ulcerations, tumors, and asymmetry on the surface of the skin. Scarring is an indication of prior medical procedures or injury. The presence of lesions or changes in warts and moles may be benign, a sign of malignant transformation, or cancer. Asymmetry may be an indication of edema, thrombosis, hematoma, injury, or an underlying tumor. Edema is a swelling of the tissue caused by the accumulation of excessive amounts of fluid. Thrombosis is the abnormal accumulation of blood factors in a blood vessel that causes a clot. A hematoma is the abnormal accumulation of blood in tissue from a blood vessel that has ruptured. An inspection may use the sense of smell to help in making a diagnosis. For example, the smell of the patient's breath, wound, urine, or sputum may indicate infection, ketoacidosis, or some other condition.

Olfactory (smell) inspection can be a valuable tool in the assessment process. Each time a patient is assessed, it provides an opportunity to train the four senses: sight, touch, hearing, and smell. Consider the following examples [21]:

- *Breath: Odors on the breath from acetone, alcohol, and other substances may lead to further questions and diagnosis.*
- *Sputum: Foul-smelling sputum suggests bronchiectasis (an abnormal stretching and enlarging of the respiratory passages caused by mucus blocking the airway, which may lead to infection and inflammation) or lung abscess.*

- *Vomitus: The gastric contents may emit odors of alcohol, phenol or other poisons, or the foul smell of fermenting food. A fecal smell from the vomitus may indicate an intestinal blockage.*
- *Feces: Particularly foul-smelling stools are common in pancreatic insufficiency.*
- *Urine: An ammonia odor in the urine may result from fermentation within the bladder.*
- *Pus: A nauseating sweet odor, like the smell of rotting apples, is evidence that pus is coming from a region of gas gangrene.*

Palpation

Palpation is the use of touch to acquire information about the patient. The physician palpates the patient by using the tips of the fingers. Light palpation is used for a superficial examination. Heavy pressure may be necessary for deep-seated structures. Through palpation, the physician tries to distinguish between hard and soft, rough and smooth, and warm and dry. Vibrations in the chest or abdomen can be felt through palpation. Palpation of an artery can help determine the pulse. Palpation is also used to determine whether pain is present. For example, the patient may not experience pain from an inflammatory process until pressure is applied or applied and released quickly. Areas where superficial lymph node groups exist, such as the neck, axilla, and groin, are important to palpate to determine whether there is any **lymphadenopathy** (swelling of any lymph nodes). The use of touch in these areas can help determine how many lymph nodes, if there are any, are palpable and whether they are mobile or fixed to underlying structures.

Percussion

Percussion is different from palpation in that percussion is the act of striking or tapping the patient gently. The purpose of percussion is to determine pain in underlying tissue or cause vibrations. Making a fist and pounding it gently over the kidney area does not normally produce pain. However, if the patient has an underlying kidney infection, percussion may produce pain.

Placing the examiner's third finger of one hand flat on the surface of the patient over the lung or abdomen produces another form of percussion. With the third finger of the other hand, the examiner gently raps the dorsal surface of the third finger that is resting on the patient. Depending on the location of the percussion, different sounds are produced. For example, if percussion is done over the lung (which is an air-filled cavity), the vibrations have a different sound from that of the abdominal cavity. Percussion over a normal lung produces a resonant sound, whereas percussion over the abdomen produces a distinctively duller sound. For the radiation therapist, percussion is helpful in determining the place the abdomen ends and the lung begins.

Auscultation

Auscultation is the act of listening to sounds within the body. With a stethoscope, the physician or nurse performs auscultation by listening to the lungs, heart, arteries, stomach, and bowel sounds. Sounds in the lungs vary depending on the presence or absence of air, fluid, and disease, producing distinct sounds to the trained ear. A pumping heart produces sounds that can be altered by changes or abnormalities of its structure and function.

Vital Signs

Vital signs are almost always taken during the physical examination. Vital signs include temperature, pulse, respirations, and blood pressure of the patient. These measurements of basic body functions can vary from patient to patient depending on the time of day and physical activity, condition, and age of the patient. Taking **baseline,** or initial, values at various times to establish the patient's norm is important.

Temperatures are taken orally, rectally, in the ear, on the skin, or in the axilla. Oral temperatures should not be taken on unreliable patients. This includes patients who are irrational, comatose, or prone to convulsions, as well as young children. Patients in these categories should have rectal or ear temperatures taken. The rectal temperature is considered the most accurate. Devices most commonly used for taking temperatures are glass and electronic thermometers. Electronic thermometers give much quicker readings than glass thermometers. The electronic ear thermometer can be used on adults and children. Temperatures are measured in Fahrenheit (F) or Celsius (C), and some values are given in ranges. Textbooks may list slightly different values for normal and abnormal temperatures (Table 5-5).

Factors observed during the taking of a pulse are rate, rhythm, size, and tension. Rate indicates the number of beats per second. Rhythm is the pattern of beats. Size has to do with the size of the pulse wave and volume of blood felt during the

Table 5-5	Normal Adult Values for Vital Signs	
Vital Signs	**Values**
Temperature	
Oral	96.8° to 98.6° F (36° to 37° C)
Rectal	99.6° F
Axillary	97.6° F
Pulse	60 to 90 beats/min
Respirations	10 to 20 breaths/min
Blood pressure	110 to 140 mm Hg / 60 to 80 mm Hg
Pain	Subjective scales may be used to indicate the intensity of pain

ventricular contraction of the heart. Tension refers to the compressibility of the artery (e.g., soft or hard)[9] (see Table 5-5).

Factors that are observed during the evaluation of respiration are rate, depth, rhythm, and character. Rate is the number of breaths that are taken in a minute. Depth refers to shallow or deep breathing. The deeper the breath, the greater is the amount of air that is inhaled. **Rhythm** refers to the regularity of breathing (slow, normal, or rapid). Character refers to the type of breathing from normal to labored[9] (see Table 5-5).

When blood pressure is taken, the systolic and diastolic pressures are noted. Systolic blood pressure represents the pressure in the blood vessels during the contraction of the heart and is the first sound heard through the stethoscope when taking a blood pressure. Diastolic pressure represents the pressure in the blood vessels during the relaxation phase of the heart after the contraction. The diastolic pressure is the last sound heard through the stethoscope when taking a blood pressure[9] (see Table 5-5).

Recognizing pain as a major, yet largely avoidable, public health problem, The Joint Commission (JC), formerly the Joint Commission on Accreditation of Healthcare Organizations (JCAHO), has developed standards that create new expectations for the assessment and management of pain in accredited hospitals and other health care settings. According to JC, pain is considered the "fifth" vital sign. Pain intensity ratings should be recorded along with temperature, pulse, respiration, and blood pressure. This should bring much needed attention to the undertreatment of pain.[19] JC provides accreditation for more than three fourths of the hospitals and medical centers in the United States. Standards have been developed for pain assessment and management. The standards received final JC approval in July 1999 and were first scored for compliance in 2001. Details of the standards involving pain assessment and management can be reviewed on their website (http://www.jointcommission.org/).

SCREENING

Cancer prevention that takes place in the United States is grouped into two important levels. The first level of cancer prevention is devoted to helping people maintain good health through education that encourages changes in lifestyle. Immunizations to prevent cancer, if they existed, would be encouraged.

The second level of cancer prevention is concerned with the early detection of conditions and disease. Early detection makes intervening and perhaps improving the outcome for the patient possible.

Cancer screening is part of the second level of health promotion.[41] Screening is the cornerstone of the diagnosis and management of the patient. It is done for large, asymptomatic populations at risk to detect deviations from the norm or signs of disease. Specific screening is performed for patients who are symptomatic, undergoing treatment, or being followed up. The determination to perform mass screening is based on the results obtained, cost-effectiveness, and risk to the patient. Areas of screening performed today are aimed at identifying cancer at its earliest stage, which translates into increased cure rates for most cancers.

Until the early 1960s, the only routine screening that was available for asymptomatic patients included a chest x-ray film, an electrocardiogram (ECG), a complete blood count (CBC), a blood chemistry test, a urinalysis, and a stool examination for occult blood. With the development of multichannel automated analyzers, many laboratory tests could be obtained for the same cost as that of the few tests that had been performed previously. Later studies questioned the value of performing such a large number of tests.[11,12] Many of the tests that were performed did not improve the outcome in asymptomatic outpatients.[14] For example, there has been an ongoing debate over the effectiveness of CT screening for lung cancer. This type of screening mechanism is costly and has resulted in a high number of false-positives. Has CT screening significantly reduced the number of deaths from lung cancer? The National Cancer Institute is currently performing a randomized clinical trial to study the effects of CT screening in detecting lung cancer.

Most screening studies can be grouped into two major categories: laboratory studies and medical imaging. Hundreds of laboratory tests and medical imaging procedures exist today. Discretion must be exercised in selecting appropriate tests to be done, and studies are not performed unless logical reasons exist for doing so.

The ACS believes that early detection examinations and tests can save lives and reduce suffering from cancers of the breast, colorectal, prostate, cervix, endometrial, testes, oral cavity, and skin. Some of these cancers can be found by self-examination, physical examination, and laboratory tests (such as mammography, the Papanicolaou [Pap] smear, and the prostate-specific antigen [PSA] blood test).[1] Cancer screening can be effective if a disease has a high incidence or prevalence in a population and the test has the ability to produce results having the appropriate **sensitivity** (defined as the ability of a test to give a true-positive result) and **specificity** (defined as the ability of the test to obtain a true-negative result). *Incidence* is defined as the number of new cases of a disease over a period, and *prevalence* is defined as the total number of cases of a disease at a certain time. Screening may be set up to determine the incidence of new cancer cases over a period. Screening for the prevalence of cancer determines the number of cases at a certain time.[18]

In the United States, one of eight women develops breast cancer, and one in eight men develops prostate cancer.[2]

Therefore, a significant portion of the population benefits from mass medical screening. If the disease is caught early enough, morbidity and mortality rates may be reduced. Mass screening for breast cancer in China is not effective because the at-risk population is low. However, the reverse is true for cancer of the esophagus; the number of persons at risk for cancer of the esophagus is extremely high in certain regions of China. Because the population at risk for cancer of the esophagus is much lower in the United States, mass screening for esophageal cancer would not be beneficial in terms of outcome and cost-effectiveness.

Areas where mass screening tools have received more attention in recent years include breast, lung, prostate, colon, cervix, gastric, and others. Mass screening is based on the specific results obtained, cost-effectiveness, and risk to the patient. Because areas of screening performed today are aimed at identifying cancer at its earliest stage, high-incidence cancers such as breast, lung, and prostate have received more attention.

Breast

For women 50 years and older, the ACS recommends an annual mammogram, which can demonstrate lesions before they can be palpated. There are few controlled studies evaluating the effectiveness of screening by self-breast examination (SBE) alone.[29] However, research has clearly demonstrated that screening mammography can improve survival rates.[25,29,32] High-quality mammography is the most effective technology available for the detection of breast cancer. There are several imaging technologies and other techniques under investigation to help improve the detection and diagnosis of breast cancer, some of which are used to assist with traditional mammography methods, including the following: ultrasound, digital mammography, MRI, PET, and image-guided breast biopsy.

In addition, as a type of secondary screening tool, surgeons are judging the usefulness of sentinel lymph node biopsy (SNB) as a means of assessing axillary node status once the primary has been detected.[16,25,34] The procedure, which has become more widely accepted in recent years, involves identifying and removing the sentinel lymph node(s) at the time of surgery and should be performed at a facility that has experience with the technique.[16,20]

The **sentinel lymph node** procedure focuses on finding lymph nodes that are the first to receive draining fluid from breast tumors and, therefore, the first to collect cancer cells. A blue dye or radioactive substance is injected near the tumor site and is then absorbed locally through the lymph system, traveling to the sentinel node(s). The node is then more easily identified by the surgeon so that it can be removed and examined for cancer cells (Figure 5-1). If there are no cancer cells present, an axillary lymph node dissection may not be necessary.[16,20] One recent study indicated no difference using the blue dye or combination of blue dye and radioactive substance.[40] Both procedures predicted the axillary lymph node status in early breast cancer with comparable success rates, accuracy, and false-negative rates. The combined technique facilitated quicker identification of sentinel lymph node; however, the dye technique alone can be used successfully in centers without nuclear medicine facilities.[40]

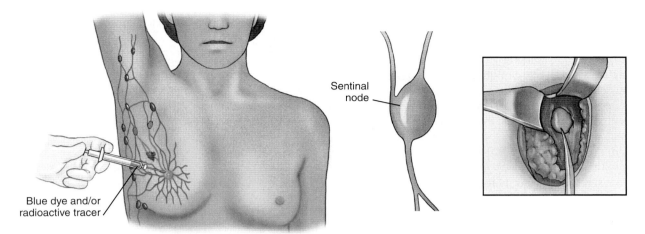

Sentinal node

Blue dye and/or radioactive tracer

Figure 5-1. The sentinel lymph node procedure focuses on finding lymph nodes that are the first to receive draining fluid from breast tumors. A blue dye or radioactive tracer is injected near the tumor site and is then absorbed locally, traveling to the sentinel node(s).

Lung

Screening for lung cancer has been used for decades without demonstrating overall survival benefit. However, improvements in the biologic understanding of lung tumors, the advent of multislice spiral CT scanning, and advances in the treatment of lung cancer have led many investigators to evaluate the use of CT in screening for lung cancer.[18,24,28,38,42] Several studies have shown a benefit using CT for screening lung cancer. One Japanese study reviewed the results of a 3-year study, using low-dose spiral CT for annual lung cancer screening. The CT screening program detected suspicious nodules in 3.5% to 5.1% of those scanned (3878 to 5483 total patients). Eighty-eight percent (55 of 60) of the lung cancers identified on screening and later surgically confirmed were American Joint Committee for Cancer Staging and End Results Reporting (AJCC) stage IA tumors.[38] Despite the small number of confirmed cancers overall, the use of low-dose spiral CT is able to detect cancers of the lung at a very early stage, when the cancer is more treatable.[4,38] More research is still needed to determine the most cost-effective method of early detection.

Prostate

Screening for prostate cancer, which is one of the leading causes of death in American men older than 50, remains controversial. The two most common methods used to screen for prostate cancer are digital rectal examination (DRE) and PSA blood test. Consensus is lacking on whom to screen, when to screen, and what to do if cancer is discovered.[39] Refinements to the sensitivity and specificity are needed to improve the effectiveness of the screening tools. PSA misses a significant number of prostate cancers and provides false-positive results in a large percentage of other cases.[35,39]

It is suggested that more than just the PSA value should be considered when screening for the presence of prostate cancer. Several studies have identified additional data, such as age, PSA level at the initial and repeat screening, prostate volume, number of positive DRE and TRUS (transurethral ultrasound) findings,

and number of previous negative biopsies.[31,39] The ACS's guidelines for testing for early prostate cancer detection were last updated in 2001 and recommend that PSA testing and DRE should be offered annually beginning at age 50 to men who have a life expectancy of at least 10 years and that a decision should be made between the physician and patient about the potential benefits, limitations, and harms associated with testing.[35] Potential harm can result from any diagnostic test if the specificity (probability of a negative test among patients without disease) is low. For example, a PSA performed on an asymptomatic 67-year-old patient returns a **false-positive** result, meaning the diagnostic test indicates there is disease, when in fact there is none.

The value of mass screening is determined by the number of the population at risk, cost of the studies, risks involved in the studies, and improvements in the morbidity and mortality rates.

 A sharp increase in prostate cancer incidence rates started in 1988 after the introduction of screening for prostate-specific antigen (PSA). This was not because more men actually developed prostate cancer, but because the new test found more cases at an earlier stage. Incidence leveled off after a few years and has recently started to decline. This is a pattern typically observed after the introduction of a new early detection test. Most importantly, death rates began to decline in recent years, possibly due to earlier detection.[1]

Sensitivity, Specificity, and Predictive Values

Other measures for determining the value of a study are the sensitivity, specificity, and predictive values. *Sensitivity* is defined as the ability of a test to give a true positive result when the disease is present. In other words, a person who tests positive for cancer from a high-sensitivity test probably has cancer. *Specificity* is defined as the ability of the test to obtain a true-negative result. When the results of a high-specificity test are negative, that person probably does not have cancer.[17]

The ideal situation is for a test to yield a high sensitivity and high specificity. However, that is almost impossible. Because of the morbidity and mortality rates of cancer, the ability to detect cancer early in all individuals tested is important. High sensitivity is selected when the disease prevalence is low. A positive finding of cancer from a high-sensitivity test can be confirmed by subjecting the patient to a second test of high specificity. High specificity is selected when the disease prevalence is high. Determining the sensitivity and specificity of the test can affect its *predictive value*. The predictive value of a positive test increases with an increase in the sensitivity and specificity of the test. Sensitivity and specificity are the most widely used statistics used to describe a diagnostic test. Unfortunately, they are not always helpful to clinicians trying to determine the probability of disease. Reviewing the definitions of prevalence, sensitivity, and specificity may be helpful:

- **Prevalence**—probability of disease in the entire population at any point in time
- **Incidence**—probability that a patient without disease develops the disease during an interval (approximately 1 in 225, or 1.4 million cancers, were predicted for 2008)
- **Sensitivity**—probability of a positive test among patients with disease
- **Specificity**—probability of a negative test among patients without disease

Common Sources of Errors

The sources of errors in medical studies are many. Any medical examination always has a margin of error in the results. The possibility of errors exists in the ordering of a study. Request forms must be filled out completely and correctly and may include the patient's demographic data, symptoms, or diagnosis if available and the purpose of the test.

Coordination of the patient's activities is important. Special consideration must be given to patients who are handicapped, disabled, diabetic, or infirm. Extra time may be necessary to accommodate these patients in scheduling a battery of activities before the study, preparing the patient, and performing the procedure. Care must be taken in the ordering of the study and test, coordination of activities, and preparation of the patient[11] (Table 5-6). For example, if a patient on the treatment schedule is receiving both radiation therapy and chemotherapy every fifth day, it may be helpful to the patient to attempt to schedule both appointments as close as possible on those days chemotherapy is scheduled, unless there are expected adverse side effects from combining both treatments too closely together.

The tests require coordination so that they do not interfere with each other. For example, a glucose tolerance test takes place over 2 hours, at which time blood must be drawn. If the patient is not available when the blood is to be drawn, the results of the test are invalid. Some tests must be done before others because they may interfere with the next test. Improper coordination may result in the patient having to go through an uncomfortable preparation for the test again. In addition, many of the tests are invasive, can be uncomfortable, and carry certain risks. Repeated radiographic procedures result in unnecessary exposure of the patient to ionizing radiation.[11]

Table 5-6	Actions that May Alter Test Results
Person Responsible	**Actions**
Caregiver	Incomplete or inaccurately filled-out requisitions
	Incomplete or inaccurate coordination of activities
	Incomplete or inaccurate patient instruction
	Incorrectly performed procedure
	Incorrect labeling of specimens
Patient	Incorrect interpretation of instructions
	Lack of cooperation
	Inability to follow instructions or noncompliance

THE AMERICAN CANCER SOCIETY'S RECOMMENDATIONS FOR DETECTING CANCER

The ACS strongly recommends mass screenings for breast, colorectal, prostate, cervical, and endometrial cancers. At present, no organization recommends testing for early lung cancer detection in asymptomatic individuals at risk for lung cancer. However, the growth of spiral CT to test for lung cancer detection in former and current smokers led the ACS to update its 2001 narrative on lung cancer testing emphasizing the importance of decisions among individuals at risk seeking testing.[35,36] Helping and educating people to stop smoking has the greatest effect on mortality statistics for lung cancer. Table 5-7 provides an excellent overview of recommendations for screening and detection by site and symptoms. In this next section, ACS guidelines for the early detection of cancer are discussed, specifically for breast, colorectal, prostate, and cervical cancers.[35]

Breast

Specific guidelines for the early detection of breast cancer in women (Table 5-8) emphasize a variety of procedures that begin after age 20 and consist of a combination of clinical breast examination, education to raise awareness of breast symptoms, and mammography beginning at age 40. New areas of research for breast screening have been advocated by many authors in an attempt to improve outcomes with the 185,000 breast cancers diagnosed each year, especially in the area of digital mammography.[22,25,30,35]

The first results of the Digital Mammographic Imaging Screening Trial (DMIST) were published in 2005. The goal of the research was to determine in a large prospective study whether digital technology improved diagnostic accuracy over screen-film mammography. The study was conducted at 33 sites in the United States and Canada and included 49,528 asymptomatic women. Women who agreed to be in the study were screened for breast cancer with both digital and screen-film mammography, and the examinations were interpreted independently by two radiologists. Previous studies comparing digital mammography with screen-film mammography have not found digital mammography to be significantly more accurate than

Table 5-7	American Cancer Society Screening Guidelines for the Early Detection of Cancer in Asymptomatic People

Site	Recommendation
Breast	• Yearly mammograms are recommended starting at age 40. The age at which screening should be stopped should be individualized by considering the potential risks and benefits of screening in the context of overall health status and longevity. • Clinical breast examination should be part of a periodic health examination approximately every 3 years for women in their 20s and 30s and every year for women 40 and older. • Women should know how their breasts normally feel and report any breast change promptly to their health care providers. Breast self-examination is an option for women starting in their 20s. • Screening MRI is recommended for women with an approximately 20%-25% or greater lifetime risk of breast cancer, including women with a strong family history of breast or ovarian cancer and women who were treated for Hodgkin's disease.
Colon and rectum	Beginning at age 50, men and women should begin screening with *one* of the examination schedules below: • A fecal occult blood test (FOBT) or fecal immunochemical test (FIT) every year • A flexible sigmoidoscopy (FSIG) every 5 years • Annual FOBT or FIT and FSIG every 5 years* • A double-contrast barium enema every 5 years • Colonoscopy every 10 years
Prostate	The PSA test and the digital rectal examination should be offered annually, beginning at age 50, to men who have a life expectancy of at least 10 years. Men at high risk (African-American men and men with a strong family history of one or more first-degree relatives diagnosed with prostate cancer at an early age) should begin testing at age 45. For both men at average risk and high risk, information should be provided about what is known and what is uncertain about the benefits and limitations of early detection and treatment of prostate cancer so that they can make an informed decision about testing.
Uterus	**Cervix:** Screening should begin approximately 3 years after a woman begins having vaginal intercourse, but no later than 21 years of age. Screening should be done every year with regular Pap tests or every 2 years using liquid-based tests. At or after age 30, women who have had 3 normal test results in a row may get screened every 2 to 3 years. Alternatively, cervical cancer screening with HPV DNA testing and conventional or liquid-based cytology could be performed every 3 years. However, doctors may suggest a woman get screened more often if she has certain risk factors, such as HIV infection or a weak immune system. Women aged 70 and older who have had 3 or more consecutive normal Pap tests in the last 10 years may choose to stop cervical cancer screening. Screening after total hysterectomy (with removal of the cervix) is not necessary unless the surgery was done as a treatment for cervical cancer. **Endometrium:** The American Cancer Society recommends that at the time of menopause all women should be informed about the risks and symptoms of endometrial cancer and strongly encouraged to report any unexpected bleeding or spotting to their physicians. Annual screening for endometrial cancer with endometrial biopsy beginning at age 35 should be offered to women with or at risk for hereditary nonpolyposis colon cancer (HNPCC).
Cancer-related checkup	For individuals undergoing periodic health examinations, a cancer-related checkup should include health counseling and, depending on a person's age and gender, might include examinations for cancers of the thyroid, oral cavity, skin, lymph nodes, testes, and ovaries, as well as for some nonmalignant diseases.

From *Cancer facts and figures,* Atlanta 2008, American Cancer Society, Inc.

DNA, Deoxyribonucleic acid; *HIV,* human immunodeficiency virus; *HPV,* human papillomavirus; *MRI,* magnetic resonance imaging; *PSA,* prostate-specific antigen.

* Combined testing is preferred over either annual FOBT or FIT, or FSIG every 5 years, alone. People who are at moderate or high risk for colorectal cancer should talk with a doctor about a different testing schedule.

American Cancer Society guidelines for early cancer detection are assessed annually in order to identify whether there is new scientific evidence sufficient to warrant a reevaluation of current recommendations. If evidence is sufficiently compelling to consider a change or clarification in a current guideline or the development of a new guideline, a formal procedure is initiated. Guidelines are formally evaluated every 5 years regardless of whether new evidence suggests a change in the existing recommendations. There are 9 steps in this procedure, and these "guidelines for guideline development" were formally established to provide a specific methodology for science and expert judgment to form the underpinnings of specific statements and recommendations from the Society. These procedures constitute a deliberate process to ensure that all Society recommendations have the same methodological and evidence-based process at their core. This process also employs a system for rating strength and consistency of evidence that is similar to that employed by the Agency for Health Care Research and Quality (AHCRQ) and the US Preventive Services Task Force (USPSTF).

screen-film mammography in the detection of breast cancer. The same was true in the 2005 DMIST study. However, there was some suggestion that digital mammography offered advantages over screen-film mammography by reducing the proportion of women recalled for further evaluation for positive findings.[22,30] This advantage is thought to be due to the ability of digital technology to manipulate the contrast in the image, allowing the physician to lighten or darken a portion of the image, as well as magnify areas of concern. Pisano et al.[30] did conclude that three subgroups of women may benefit from the accuracy of digital mammography over screen-film type mammography, primarily due to the ability to manipulate imaging factors such as contrast and density. The three subgroups are as follows:

• Women under the age of 50 years
• Premenopausal or perimenopausal women
• Women with heterogeneously dense or extremely dense breasts on mammography examination

Table 5-8	Methods for Breast Cancer Detection and Diagnosis[35]	
Method	**Description**	
Ultrasound	Ultrasound, also called sonography, is an imaging technique in which high-frequency sound waves are bounced off tissues and internal organs. Their echoes produce a picture called a sonogram. Ultrasound imaging of the breast is usually used to distinguish between solid tumors and fluid-filled cysts. Ultrasound can also be used to evaluate lumps that are hard to see on a mammogram. Sometimes, ultrasound is used as part of other diagnostic procedures, such as fine needle aspiration (also called needle biopsy). Fine-needle aspiration is the removal of tissue or fluid with a needle for examination under a microscope to check for signs of disease.	
Digital mammography	Digital mammography is a technique for recording x-ray images in computer code instead of on x-ray film, as with conventional mammography. The images are displayed on a computer monitor and can be enhanced (lightened or darkened) before they are printed on film. Images can also be manipulated by the radiologist to magnify or zoom in on an area needing more careful inspection. Digital mammography may have some advantages over conventional mammography, because the images can be stored and retrieved electronically, which makes long-distance consultations with other mammography specialists more convenient.	
Computer-aided detection	Computer-aided detection (CAD) involves the use of computers to bring suspicious areas on a mammogram to the radiologist's attention. It is used after the radiologist has done the initial review of the mammogram. Some devices scan the mammogram with a laser beam and convert it into a digital signal that is processed by a computer. The image is then displayed on a video monitor, with suspicious areas highlighted for the radiologist to review. The radiologist can compare the digital image with the conventional mammogram to see whether any of the highlighted areas were missed on the initial review and require further evaluation.	
MRI	In magnetic resonance imaging (MRI), a magnet linked to a computer creates detailed pictures of areas inside the body without the use of radiation. Each MRI produces hundreds of images of the breast from side-to-side, top-to-bottom, and front-to-back. The images are then interpreted by a radiologist.	
	During MRI of the breast, the patient lies on her stomach on the scanning table. The breast hangs into a depression in the table, which contains coils that detect the magnetic signal. The table is moved into a tube-like machine that contains the magnet. After an initial series of images has been taken, the patient may be given a contrast agent intravenously. The contrast agent is sometimes used to improve the visibility of a tumor. Additional images are then taken. The entire imaging session takes about 1 hour.	
	Breast MRI is not used for routine breast cancer screening, but clinical trials are being performed to determine whether MRI is valuable for screening certain women, such as young women at high risk for breast cancer. MRI cannot always accurately distinguish between cancer and benign (noncancerous) breast conditions. Like ultrasound, MRI cannot detect microcalcifications.	
	MRI is used primarily to evaluate breast implants for leaks or ruptures and to assess abnormal areas that are seen on a mammogram or are felt after breast surgery or radiation therapy. It can be used after breast cancer is diagnosed to determine the extent of the tumor in the breast. MRI is also sometimes useful in imaging dense breast tissue, which is often found in younger women, and in viewing breast abnormalities that can be felt but are not visible with conventional mammography or ultrasound.	

Breast cancer is the most common cancer among American women, except for skin cancers. The chance of developing invasive breast cancer at some time in a woman's life is approximately 1 in 8 (12%). Women living in North America have the highest rate of breast cancer in the world. At this time there are approximately 2.5 million breast cancer survivors in the United States.[1]

Colorectal

One barrier contributing to the low rate of colorectal screening is inadequate physician knowledge. In a recent study by Gennarelli et al.[12] regarding the ACS screening guidelines for average-risk and high-risk patients, knowledge about these guidelines was very low but did increase directly with the level of training of the physician providing care in a low-income minority community. Medical students obtained a mean score on the screening guidelines questionnaire of 32%, residents scored

higher at 49%, and attending internal medicine physicians received a 56%, calculated on the number of correct responses. Further educational efforts should be offered to these health professionals to increase the utilization of colorectal screening tools.

The ACS recommends that average-risk adults begin colorectal cancer screening at age 50 years, with one of the following options: (1) annual fecal occult blood test (FOBT) or fecal immunochemical test (FIT); (2) flexible sigmoidoscopy every 5 years; (3) annual FOBT or FIT, plus flexible sigmoidoscopy every 5 years; (4) double-contrast barium enema (DCBE) every 5 years; or (5) colonoscopy every 10 years.[35] Options for the patient may be based on the availability of the test and, to some degree, personal preference. Colonoscopy, which includes a somewhat uncomfortable bowel preparation, examines the entire colon from beginning to end, whereas the sigmoidoscopy examines the lower end of the colon with a flexible endoscope. These two procedures may also have the ability to further examine and/or take a biopsy sample of an area of concern. FOBT done at home or at the physician's office, perhaps following a DRE, has low sensitivity. This means a negative result with this type of diagnostic test may also provide false reassurance to the patient.[7,26,35]

Prostate

The ACS recommends that the PSA test or PSA test and DRE be done annually beginning at age 50 years for men who have a life expectancy of at least 10 years. In addition, they recommend that a discussion take place about the potential benefits, limitations, and harms associated with testing (false-positives). In men for whom DRE is an obstacle to testing, PSA alone is an acceptable alternative. In 2004, the proportion of men aged 50 years and older who reported having had a PSA test during the past year was 54%, and the prevalence of men who reported having a DRE was 50.5%.[35]

Cervical

The ACS guidelines for cervical cancer screening reflect the current understanding of the underlying epidemiology, in particular the causal role of human papillomavirus (HPV). The ACS recommends varying surveillance strategies based on a woman's age, her screening history, and the screening and diagnostic technologies she chooses and that screening should begin approximately 3 years after the onset of vaginal intercourse but no later than age 21 years. Annual screening with conventional cervical cytology smears, or biennial screening using liquid-based cytology, is recommended until age 30 years.[35] DNA testing for HPV is also available.

Women who chose to undergo HPV DNA testing should receive counseling and education about HPV and HPV testing. The following information should be discussed[35]:

- A positive HPV test result does not reflect the presence of a sexually transmitted disease, but rather a sexually acquired infection.
- Many who have had sexual intercourse have been exposed to HPV, and the infection is very common.
- HPV infection usually is not detectable or harmful. Most important, testing positive for HPV does not indicate the presence of cancer, nor will most women who test positive for an HPV infection develop advanced cervical cancer.

Research has been ongoing to develop and test a vaccine that would prevent infection with the most common high-risk subtypes of HPV, specifically HPV 16 and HPV 18, two subtypes believed to account for 70% of cervical cancer. Early results of the efficacy of the vaccine are very promising.[35]

LABORATORY STUDIES

Hundreds of laboratory studies are available today. Some studies are used to analyze the composition of the blood and bone marrow and rule out blood disorders. Blood studies are concerned with blood cells, whereas blood chemistry tests examine chemicals in the blood. Microbiologic studies are helpful in detecting specific organisms that may be causing an infection. Urine studies are done to analyze the composition and concentration of the urine. These are helpful in detecting diseases and disorders of the kidney and urinary system and endocrine or metabolic disorders. Fecal studies are done to examine the waste products of digestion and metabolic disorders. These studies are useful in detecting gastrointestinal diseases and disorders such as bleeding, obstruction, obstructive jaundice, and parasitic disease. Studies are also done to investigate the immune system. Immunologic studies examine the antigen-antibody reactions. Serologic tests are done to diagnose problems such as neoplastic disease, infectious disease, and allergic reactions. Baseline values should always be obtained to observe any deviation. Table 5-9 contains normal ranges for a CBC. The values may vary from institution to institution depending on the methods used.

MEDICAL IMAGING

The physiology and anatomy of the body can be imaged in many ways, and the procedures used can be extremely simple or complex. Every procedure provides some element of risk to the patient. For example, noninvasive procedures provide very little risk to the patient. Whereas an invasive procedure such as a biopsy provides some risk, the exact amount of acceptable risk depends on many factors. The physician and patient should discuss the risks and benefits of any diagnostic imaging procedure.

Electrical Impulses

Some medical imaging techniques use electrical impulses of the body to determine the ability of the heart, brain, and muscles to function. The ECG demonstrates the electrical conductivity of the heart muscle. This aids in the detection and diagnosis of heart disease. During the examination, wave patterns representing the electrical pulse are drawn on special paper. The physician studies the wave patterns to check for any deviations. The electroencephalogram (EEG) records brain-wave activity. The EEG helps detect and diagnose seizure disorders, brainstem disorders, brain lesions, and states of consciousness. An electromyogram (EMG) measures the

Table 5-9	Normal Ranges for Complete Blood Count	
Blood Component	**Range**
White blood cells	3,900 to 10,800/mm³
Red blood cells	3.90 to 5.40 million/mm³
Hemoglobin	12.0 to 16.0 g/dL
Hematocrit	37.0% to 47.0%
Differential white blood cells	
Neutrophils	42.0% to 72.0%
Lymphocytes	17.0% to 45.0%
Monocytes	3.0% to 10.0%
Eosinophils	0.0% to 12.0%
Basophils	0.0% to 2.0%
Platelets	150,000 to 425,000/mm³

electrical conductivity of the muscle, thus aiding in the detection and diagnosis of neuromuscular problems.

Nuclear Medicine Imaging

Nuclear medicine imaging introduces a special radionuclide (radioactive substance) into the patient. A radionuclide, or radiopharmaceutical, is an isotope that undergoes radioactive decay. In doing so, it gives off radiation, often in the form of gamma rays. It is an unstable element that attempts to reach stability by emitting several types of ionizing radiation. The radionuclide may be injected, swallowed, or inhaled, depending on the diagnostic procedure. After its introduction into the patient, the radionuclide follows a specific metabolic pathway in the body. Several minutes to several hours later, an imaging device is placed outside the patient's body, and the resultant radiation from the radionuclide is measured and imaged.

The three most common imaging devices are the gamma camera, rectilinear scanner, and PET scanner. The large circular gamma camera does not move and views the whole area of interest at one time. The rectilinear scanner starts at the top or bottom of the area of interest and then scans from side to side until the entire area of interest has been imaged. This method may be used to detect metastatic cancer in the bone. PET imaging has proved especially useful in oncology in recent years and is used more commonly as a diagnostic tool. This modality makes possible the viewing of the organ's function and blood flow in addition to the image of its anatomy.[5] Because PET images are more related to the organ's physiology, PET offers substantial advantages over other imaging modalities, such as CT and MRI, and often can distinguish between benign and malignant lesions when CT and MRI cannot.[15]

The PET scanner works by creating computerized images of chemical changes that take place in tissue. The patient is given an injection of a combination of a sugar (glucose) and a small amount of radioactive material. The radioactive sugar can help locate a tumor, because cancer cells take up or absorb sugar faster than other tissues in the body, and glucose is the essential building block for cell metabolism.[27]

After receiving the radioactive drug, the patient lies still for approximately 45 minutes while the drug circulates throughout the body. If a tumor is present, the radioactive sugar will accumulate in the tumor. Then, the patient lies on a table, which gradually moves through the PET scanner six or seven times during a 45-minute period, where the scanner detects the radiation and translates this information into the images that are interpreted by a radiologist.[27] Some investigators are reviewing the benefits of combining a PET scanner with the diagnostic abilities of a CT scanner in an effort to maximize the benefits of both imaging devices.

Routine Radiographic Studies

Routine radiographic studies consist of contrast and noncontrast types. The use of contrast media such as barium and iodine concentrated helps in the visualization of anatomy that is radiolucent. If the anatomic structure is radiolucent, the x-rays are not completely absorbed by the structure and therefore cannot be demonstrated on a radiograph. For example, gas and fecal material in the colon may be visualized without contrast. However, to visualize the structure, position, filling, and movement of the colon, a barium-based contrast agent is necessary. For the esophagus to be visible, the patient must drink barium. Bone has a relatively high density and can be demonstrated on a radiograph without the aid of contrast media.

Routine noncontrast studies consist of chest x-ray studiess; mammograms; radiographs of the abdomen that include the kidneys, ureters, and bladder (KUB); and radiographs of the skull, spine, and other bones. Contrast studies include, but are not limited to, the kidneys, upper and lower gastrointestinal tract, and blood vessels. Contrast examinations are also used in CT and MRI studies.

Computed Tomography

CT, which was first introduced in Great Britain in the early 1970s, was initially developed to study the brain in cross section. Since then, other applications have become useful, and today CT of the head, chest, abdomen, and pelvis is routine. The CT scanner digitizes a complex x-ray image and stores it in a computer. Scanners that can produce a three-dimensional image are available and are used for reconstructive surgery and radiation therapy treatment planning.

CT imaging has several advantages over routine radiography procedures. By rotating an x-ray tube 360 degrees around the patient, data are gathered that can be reconstructed digitally in more than one plane, allowing the physician to see structures in a three-dimensional display. This eliminates the problem of overlying structures commonly seen on radiographs and gives significantly more data to evaluate for diagnostic purposes. In addition, density data are more easily distinguished between air, soft tissue, and bone. In other words, one can see a greater degree of contrast of gray shades between various structures. CT scanning is also less expensive than MRI scanning.

Magnetic Resonance Imaging

MRI is a method of creating diagnostic images of the body by using a combination of radiofrequency waves and a strong magnetic field. Unlike nuclear medicine and radiology, MRI does not use ionizing radiation to produce an image. A major difference between the CT scanner and the MRI scanner is the ability of MRI scanners to obtain anatomic images in the sagittal plane. MRI units also have the ability to demonstrate soft tissue to a much greater degree than CT units. However, CT units can demonstrate bone better than MRI units.[10]

MRI has become increasingly popular clinically because it is a noninvasive procedure that has, to date, no harmful late side effects. In addition, the image quality is better in specific anatomic areas, such as the brain and spinal cord. The diagnostic scanning tool has several disadvantages compared with CT scanning: it is expensive to use; it cannot be used in patients with metallic devices, such as pacemakers; and it cannot be used with patients who are claustrophobic (however, new MRI systems with a more open design are available). MRI technology offers image reconstruction in multiple planes, including transverse, sagittal, and coronal.

Diagnostic Ultrasound

Diagnostic ultrasound is one of the least expensive imaging techniques. It is also quick and simple and usually causes only minimal patient discomfort. Ultrasound also differs from radiography in that its images are produced with high-frequency sound waves instead of ionizing radiation. Ultrasound, also called *sonography,* is an imaging technique in which high-frequency sound waves are bounced off tissues and internal organs, producing an image called a *sonogram.* During an ultrasound examination, the clinician spreads a thin coating of lubricating jelly over the area to be imaged. This improves the conduction of the sound waves. A handheld device called a transducer directs the sound waves through the skin toward specific tissues or organ. As the sound waves are reflected back from the tissues, the patterns formed by the waves create a two-dimensional image on a computer.[27] Ultrasound has been used for breast cancer screening and prostate localization and volume calculations.

In breast cancer screening, ultrasound may be used as part of other diagnostic procedures, such as mammography or fine-needle biopsy. Ultrasound is not used for routine breast cancer screening because it does not consistently detect certain early signs of cancer such as microcalcifications of calcium in the breast that cannot be felt but can be seen on a conventional mammogram. Sometimes, a cluster of microcalcifications may indicate that cancer is present.[27]

Ultrasound has been used extensively in gynecologic and prenatal imaging. Fetal weight, growth, and anatomy can be studied without exposure to ionizing radiation. The ability of ultrasound to demonstrate soft tissue structures is helpful in demonstrating gallstones, kidney stones, and tumors.

CANCER DIAGNOSIS

Histologic evidence is vital in making a diagnosis of cancer. Tissue for diagnosis is obtained through scraping, needle aspiration, needle biopsy, incisional biopsy, and excisional biopsy.

Exfoliative cells can be found in all parts of the body. These are cells that have been scraped off deliberately or sloughed off naturally. They are found in the urine, sputum, feces, and mucus.

Exfoliative cytologic studies are extremely helpful in identifying neoplastic disease, especially in the management of cervix and lung cancer. The only problem with cytologic studies is that individual cells are being viewed and the determination of cells as invasive or noninvasive is not possible.

Other methods of obtaining tissue are needle, incisional, and excisional biopsies. Needle biopsies and incisional biopsies can be done on an outpatient basis by using local anesthesia. Only small amounts of tissue can be obtained by needle and incisional biopsies. An **incisional biopsy** (see Figure 1-5) involves the removal of only a portion of the tumor for diagnosis. With all biopsy specimens, the sample is then viewed under a microscope by a pathologist. The tissue sample may be stained with chemicals to highlight specific parts of the cell's cytoplasm and nucleus or to amplify specific regions of DNA.

An **excisional biopsy** involves the removal of the entire tumor for diagnosis. This procedure provides for a more definitive diagnosis, because the margins of the tumor are examined by the pathologist to see whether the cancer has spread beyond the area biopsied. If the margins are "clear" or "negative," that means that no disease was found at the edges of the biopsy specimen. A "positive margin" means that disease was found at the edge of the specimen and that the tumor has directly invaded beyond the area biopsied. Additional investigation or treatment may be necessary.[23]

When cancer is detected, determining the presence of metastatic disease is necessary. The use of a tumor marker may help detect widespread disease. A **tumor marker** is a substance manufactured and released by the tumor. Tumor markers refer to a molecule that can be detected in serum, plasma, or other body fluid. Tumor markers are useful in detecting the presence of specific types of tissue, such as prostatic tissue in the case of PSA, in detecting metastatic disease, and in determining the effect of the treatment.

STAGING SYSTEMS

After a histologic diagnosis of cancer has been made, the cancer must be staged. **Staging** helps determine the anatomic extent of the disease. Treatment decisions are based on the histologic diagnosis and extent of the disease. The natural growth for most cancers if untreated is that they extend beyond their original site by direct extension and then to the lymphatic and circulatory systems. They ultimately metastasize to distant sites. Staging systems are based on this concept.[3]

Recommendations regarding staging of cancer by individual researchers, specialties, committees, and other groups have not been uniform. The major groups who have been involved in staging and are working together to establish common terminology are the International Union Against Cancer (UICC), the International Federation of Gynecology and Obstetrics (FIGO), and the AJCC.[3]

The AJCC's general definitions of the TNM system are shown in Table 5-10 (subdivisions are not included). Another part of

Table 5-10	TNM Clinical Classification
TNM Classification	**Description**
PRIMARY TUMOR (T)	
Tx	Primary tumor not assessable
T0	No evidence of primary tumor
Tis	Carcinoma in situ
T1, T2, T3, T4	Increasing size and/or local extent of the primary tumor
REGIONAL LYMPH NODES (N)	
Nx	Regional lymph nodes not assessable
N0	No regional lymph node metastasis
N1, N2, N3	Increasing involvement of regional lymph nodes
DISTANT METASTASIS (M)	
Mx	Presence of distant metastasis not assessable
M0	No distant metastasis
M1	Distant metastasis

From American Joint Committee on Cancer: *AJCC cancer staging manual,* ed 6, Chicago, 2002, American Joint Commission on Cancer.

Box 5-1	Histopathologic Grade (G)
Gx	Grade not assessable
G1	Well differentiated
G2	Moderately differentiated
G3	Poorly differentiated
G4	Undifferentiated

the staging system is the histologic type and histologic grade. *Histologic type* refers to cell type, and *histologic grade* refers to the differentiation of the cell. For example, the histologic type may be squamous cell carcinoma, and the histologic grade indicates the closeness of the cells' resemblance to a normal squamous cell. Box 5-1 lists the histopathologic grades.

Another aspect of the staging system is the use of stage 0 through stage IV. Stage 0 usually indicates carcinoma in situ. Stages I and II indicate the smallness of the tumor and/or involvement of early local and regional nodes with no distant **metastases** (defined as the spread of cancer beyond the primary site). Stage III indicates that the tumor is more extensive locally and may have regional node involvement. Stage IV indicates locally advanced tumors with invasion beyond the regional nodes to other areas. The categorizations of stage 0 through IV are often grouped with the TNM system of staging. For example, stage 0, Tis N0 M0, indicates an extremely localized early disease, whereas stage II, T2 N0 M0, indicates a more advanced disease. Stage IV, any T any N M1, indicates an extremely late advanced disease.

Using the TNM staging system for a specific type of cancer, the AJCC has grouped various combinations of the TNM designations to indicate a specific stage of the cancer. For example, using the AJCC staging system for breast cancer would yield the following TNM designations, grouped into four distinct stages (Note there are several combinations for most stage designation, especially for Stage IIA, IIB, and IIIA.):

Stage I	*T1 N0 M0*
Stage IIA	*T0 N1 M0, or T1 N1 M0, or T2 N0 M0*
Stage IIB	*T2 N1 M0, or T3 N0 M0*
Stage IIIA	*T0 N2 M0, or T1 N2 M0, or T2 N2 M0, or T3 N1 M0, or T3 N2 M0*
Stage IIIB	*T4, Any N M0, or Any T N3 M0*
Stage IV	*Any T, Any N M1*

There are several reasons for the precise clinical description and accurate classification (staging) of cancers, specifically:

- To aid the physician and radiation therapy team in the planning of the treatment.
- To provide some indication of prognosis. It may be one of many factors in determining prognosis.
- To assist in the evaluation of the results of treatment. It helps in comparing groups of cases, especially as it relates to various therapeutic procedures.
- To assist in the exchange of information from one treatment center to another.

SUMMARY

- Medicine is the accumulation of knowledge that has been developed through discovery, systematic scientific study, and research. These processes help detect, diagnose, treat, and manage disease.
- According to the ACS, prevention and early detection are effective strategies for saving lives lost from cancer, diminishing suffering, and eliminating cancer as a major health problem.
- Vital signs are almost always taken during the physical examination. They include temperature, pulse, respirations, blood pressure, and a pain assessment of the patient.
- Prevention includes measures that stop cancer from developing.
- Early detection includes examinations and tests intended to find the disease as early as possible. Screening examinations include mammography, the Papanicolaou (Pap) smear, and the prostate-specific antigen blood test.
- The sentinel lymph node procedure focuses on finding lymph nodes that are the first to receive draining fluid from breast tumors and, therefore, the first to collect cancer cells.
- After a diagnosis of cancer is made and the extent of the disease has been determined, appropriate treatment can be initiated. The TNM staging system is applied to the disease process in an effort to direct treatment options and predict outcomes from treatment.

Review Questions

Multiple Choice

1. Cancer screening can be effective if a disease has a high incidence or prevalence in a population and the test has the ability to produce results having the appropriate _____ and specificity.
   a. incidence
   b. sensitivity
   c. range
   d. cost factor

2. What are the factors that must be observed when taking the pulse?
   I. rate
   II. rhythm
   III. character
      a. I and II
      b. I and III
      c. II and III
      d. I, II, and III

3. Which of the following is *not* a screening procedure recommended by the American Cancer Society for the early detection of cancer?
   a. mammography for breast cancer
   b. Papanicolaou (Pap) smear
   c. prostate-specific antigen (PSA) blood test
   d. CT scanning for brain cancer

4. Which of the following statements is *false?*
   a. Ultrasonography uses high-frequency sound waves.
   b. CT scans have a higher resolution than radiographs.
   c. MRI scans use ionizing radiation.
   d. Most invasive procedures provide some risk to the patient.
5. What is the normal adult range for blood pressure?
   a. 110 to 140/60 to 80 mm Hg
   b. 130 to 160/90 to 99 mm Hg
   c. 90 to 100/60 to 80 mm Hg
   d. 115 to 150/60 to 90 mm Hg
6. Exfoliative cytology is a means of collecting tissue through:
   a. needle biopsy
   b. scraping cells
   c. incisional biopsy
   d. excisional biopsy
7. Factors that help facilitate the interview include all of the following *except:*
   a. the interviewer's ability to put the patient at ease
   b. the asking of clear and concise questions
   c. the use technical jargon
   d. the use of terminology having the same meaning to the patient and interviewer
8. Sensitivity, as it relates to screening examinations, is defined as:
   a. the ability of a test to give a true-positive result
   b. the ability of the test to obtain a true-negative result
   c. the number of new cases of a disease over a period
   d. the effectiveness of the therapist in assisting the patient toward understanding the test results
9. Mass screening is based on the all of the following *except:*
   a. specific results obtained
   b. cost-effectiveness
   c. risk to the patient
   d. geographic location
10. Which of the following are part of the medical record?
    I. results of laboratory tests
    II. medical history
    III. simulation and treatment-related images
    a. I and II
    b. I and III
    c. II and III
    d. I, II, and III

The answers to the Review Questions can be found by logging on to our website at: *http://evolve.elsevier.com/Washington+Leaver/ principles*

Questions to Ponder

1. Why do you think that the detection and diagnosis of disease, especially cancer, have come to rely more and more on two specialties—radiology and pathology?
2. Compare and contrast the elements of an interview in helping to make a diagnosis.
3. What is a sentinel node biopsy procedure, and why is it performed?

4. Predict the benefits of mass screening for at least three specific types of cancer.
5. Identify measures used to determine the value of a study.
6. Apply the general aspects of the TNM staging system in assisting with the treatment decision.
7. Compare the screening recommendations for the following cancer sites: breast, prostate, cervix, and colon.
8. Discuss at least three diagnostic imaging procedures used in the workup of a typical patient with breast cancer. Do the same for prostate cancer and colon cancer.

REFERENCES

1. American Cancer Society (website): http://www.cancer.org/. Accessed September 11, 2007.
2. American Cancer Society: *Cancer facts and figures,* Atlanta, 2008, American Cancer Society.
3. American Joint Commission on Cancer: *AJCC cancer staging manual,* ed 6, Chicago, 2002, American Joint Commission on Cancer.
4. Bellomi M, et al: Screening for lung cancer, *Cancer Imaging* 6:S9-S12, 2006.
5. Chao KSC, Perez CA, Brady LW: *Radiation oncology management decisions,* Philadelphia, 2001, Lippincott Williams & Wilkins.
6. Cohen JJ: Remembering the real questions, *Ann Intern Med* 128:563-566, 1998.
7. Collins JF, et al: Accuracy of screening for fecal occult blood on a single stool sample obtained by digital rectal examination: a comparison with recommended sampling practice, *Ann Intern Med* 142:81-85, 2005.
8. Detmar SB, et al: How are you feeling? Patients' and oncologists' preferences for discussing health-related quality-of-life issues, *J Clin Oncol* 18:3295-301, 2000.
9. Du Gas BW: *Introduction to patient care: a comprehensive approach to nursing,* ed 4, Philadelphia, 1983, WB Saunders.
10. Eisenberg RL: *Radiology: an illustrated history,* St. Louis, 1992, Mosby.
11. Fischbach F: *A manual of laboratory diagnostic tests,* ed 3, Philadelphia, 1988, JB Lippincott.
12. Gennarelli M, et al: Barriers to colorectal cancer screening: inadequate knowledge by physicians, *Mt Sinai J Med,* 72:36-44, 2005.
13. Glanze WD, editor: *Mosby's medical and nursing dictionary,* ed 2, St. Louis, 1986, Mosby.
14. Goldman L, Ausiello D, editors: *Cecil textbook of medicine,* ed 22, Philadelphia, 2004, WB Saunders.
15. Griffeth LK: Use of PET/CT scanning in cancer patients: technical and practical considerations, *BUMC Proc* 18:321-330, 2005.
16. Hartman LC, Loprinzi CL: *Mayo Clinic guide to women's cancer,* Rochester, MN, 2005, Mayo Foundation for Medical Education for Research.
17. Henry JB: *Clinical diagnosis and management by laboratory methods,* ed 18, Philadelphia, 1991, WB Saunders.
18. Hirsch FR, et al: Early detection of lung cancer: clinical perspectives of recent advances in biology and radiology, *Clin Cancer Res* 7:5-22, 2001.
19. Leaver DT: Cancer pain management in radiation oncology, *Radiat Therapist* 9:131-156, 2000.
20. Leaver DT: Women, cancer and fertility, *Radiat Therapist* 15:131-156, 2006.
21. LeBlond RF, DeGowin RL, Brown DD: *DeGowin's diagnostic examination,* ed 8, New York, 2004, McGraw-Hill.
22. Lewin JM, et al: Clinical comparison of full-field digital mammography and screen-film mammography for detection of breast cancer, *AJR Am J Roentgenol* 179:671-677, 2002.
23. Lewis SM, et al: *Medical-surgical nursing,* ed 6, St. Louis, 2007, Mosby.
24. Locklear D: New CT scanner drives lung study, *Advance Rad Sci Prof* March 5, 2001.
25. Moss S, et al: Effect of mammographic screening from age 40 years on breast cancer mortality at 10 years' follow-up: a randomised controlled trial, *Lancet* 368:2053-2060, 2006.

26. Nadel MR, et al: A national survey of primary care physicians' methods for screening for fecal occult blood, *Ann Intern Med* 142:86-94, 2005.

27. National Cancer Institute (website): http://www.cancer.gov/. Accessed September 11, 2007.

28. Patz EF, Goodman PC, Bepler G: Screening for lung cancer, *N Engl J Med* 343:1627-1633, 2000.

29. Perez C, Brady L, Halperin E, Schmidt-Ullrich R, editors: *Principles and practice of radiation oncology,* ed 4, Philadelphia, 2004, Lippincott Williams & Wilkins.

30. Pisano ED, et al: Diagnostic performance of digital versus film mammography for breast-cancer screening, *N Engl J Med* 353:1773-1783, 2005.

31. Roobol MJ, Schroder FH, Kranse R: A comparison of first and repeat (four years later) prostate cancer screening in a randomized cohort of a symptomatic men aged 55-75 years using a biopsy indication of 3.0 ng/ml (results of ERSPC, Rotterdam), *Prostate* 66:604-612, 2006.

32. Rubin P: *Clinical oncology: a multidisciplinary approach for physicians and students,* ed 8, Philadelphia, 2001, WB Saunders.

33. Sapir R, et al: Cancer patient expectations of and communication with oncologist and oncology nurses: the experience of an integrated oncology and palliative care service, *Support Care Cancer* 8:458-463, 2000.

34. Singletary SE: Systemic treatment after sentinel lymph node biopsy in breast cancer: who, what, and why? *J Am Coll Surg* 192:220-230, 2001.

35. Smith RA, Cokkinides V, Harmon JE: American Cancer Society guidelines for the early detection of cancer, *CA Cancer J Clin* 56:11-25, 2006.

36. Smith RA, et al: American Cancer Society guidelines for the early detection of cancer: update of early detection guidelines for prostate, colorectal, and endometrial cancers, *CA Cancer J Clin* 51:38-75, 2001.

37. Sochurek H: *Medicine's new vision,* Easton, PA, 1988, Mack Publishing.

38. Sone S, et al: Results of three-year screening programme for lung cancer using mobile low-dose spiral computed tomography scanner, *Br J Cancer* 84:25-32, 2001.

39. Toi NA, et al: Making sense of prostate specific antigen: improving its predictive value in patients undergoing prostate biopsy, *J Urol* 175: 489-494, 2006.

40. Varghese P, et al: Methylene blue dye versus combined dye-radioactive tracer technique for sentinel lymph node localisation in early breast cancer, *Eur J Surg Oncol* 33:147-152, 2007.

41. Varricchio CG, Hinds PS, editors: *A cancer source book for nurses,* ed 8, Atlanta, 2004, The American Cancer Society.

42. Wagner H, Ruckdeschel JC: Screening, early detection, and early intervention strategies for lung cancer, *Cancer Control* 2:493-502, 1995.

Medical Imaging

Dennis Leaver, Alan C. Miller[†]

Outline

Key Terms

Objectives

- List and describe the components and the operation of a radiographic, fluoroscopic, and computed tomography simulator.
- Describe the components of a typical x-ray tube and how x-rays are produced.
- Compare and contrast x-ray interactions in the diagnostic range with matter.
- Apply techniques to enhance image details and image distortion.
- Solve problems associated with magnification.
- Compare various imaging techniques, including conventional films, photostimulable plates, and flat

panel detectors, available for portal localization and verification in radiation oncology.
- Describe the concepts associated with digital image processing.
- Discuss the possible causes and health implications of darkroom chemical sensitivity.
- Explain the basic principles of image formation for each of the following modalities: computed tomography, magnetic resonance imaging, ultrasound, and nuclear medicine.

M edical imaging plays a critical role in the diagnosis and treatment of many cancer patients. In radiation therapy it provides a way to view the interior of the human body. The x-rays used in this process can penetrate matter and create an image on film or other digital receptors. This information helps members of the cancer management team achieve an important goal in radiation oncology: to maximize the radiation dose to the diseased tissue (cancer cells) and minimize the dose to the surrounding normal tissue.

Medical imaging has transformed in recent years due in part to advances in digital imaging technology. Advances in microprocessor speeds and computer memory that handle large amounts of data have increased almost exponentially each year. This is one of the reasons that digital imaging is possible for diagnostic medical procedures and radiation therapy imaging. Just as the sales of digital cameras continue to outpace the traditional 35-mm camera, medical imaging is experiencing a similar type of transformation.

With a digital camera, the image of a 5-year-old granddaughter can now be acquired in a matter of moments, with no processing at the photo lab; uploaded to the computer; and then sent via e-mail

[†]Deceased.

to grandma, who might live miles away. Digital images, obtained with a digital camera, cell phone, or a variety of medical devices, have reached a comparable quality in terms of clarity and resolution. A similar method of acquiring and sharing medical images has been slowly transforming medical imaging. Medical images can now be acquired in a matter of moments, with no chemical processing, and digitized and shared throughout the radiation therapy department.

A digital radiation therapy portal image taken on the treatment machine is of similar or slightly better quality than images acquired using traditional methods of film and cassettes. A computerized digital image of a patient in his or her radiation therapy treatment position can be captured in a matter of moments, uploaded to a computer to check or enhance the image quality, and then sent to a physician in another part of the hospital for viewing. This process is faster and more efficient than conventional methods of obtaining and viewing medical images. The ability to archive the digital image and transmit these images from one work station within the hospital to another is vastly better than the traditional methods of sharing and storing conventional simulation and portal images. [15]

Medical imaging modalities such as computed tomography (CT), magnetic resonance imaging (MRI), positron emission tomography (PET), and ultrasound use a variety of digital imaging concepts. Radiation therapy imaging is moving in the same direction, using devices that are smaller and more robust to produce higher-quality images.

In this chapter, several concepts are introduced, including the history of x-rays; their production; the design of the tube from which they are produced; their interaction with matter; the art of creating high-quality medical images (both conventional and digital); and the basic principles of image formation for CT, MRI, ultrasound, and nuclear medicine.

Types of Medical Imaging

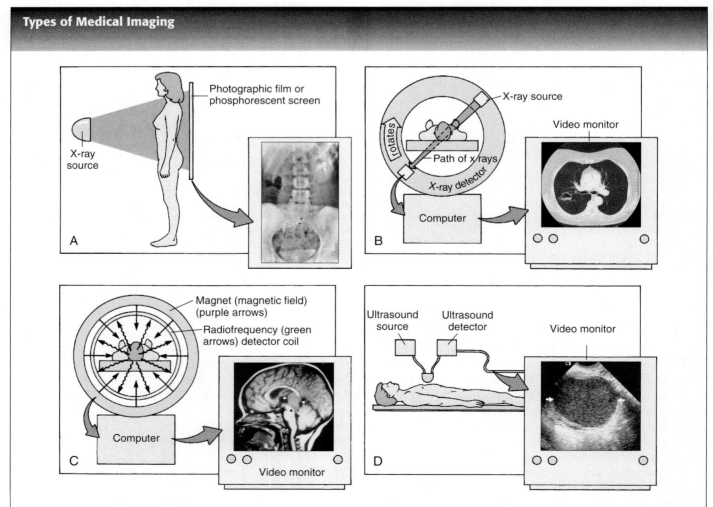

A, Radiography, or x-ray photography. **B,** Computed tomography (CT). **C,** Magnetic resonance imaging (MRI). **D,** Ultrasonography. (Modified from Thibodeau GA, Patton KT: *Anatomy & physiology,* ed 6, St. Louis, 2007, Mosby. Imaging scans from Eisenberg RL, Johnson NM: *Comprehensive radiographic anatomy,* ed 4, St. Louis, 2007, Mosby.)

HISTORIC OVERVIEW

Over 100 years ago in November 1895, a little-known German physicist tinkered in his laboratory at the University of Würzburg, Germany, with a fancy piece of glassware known as a *Hittorf-Crookes tube*. In communicating to his friend Theodor Boveri in early December 1895, Wilhelm Conrad Roentgen said, "I have discovered something interesting, but I do not know if my observations are correct."[15] After energizing his tube in the darkened laboratory, Roentgen noticed a strange green light emanating from a nearby piece of cardboard coated with phosphorescent material. This was hardly momentous because phosphorescence was a well-known event. However, when he passed a heavy piece of paper between the end of the tube and the cardboard coated with barium platinocyanide, the glow persisted. At that moment the scientist realized his newly found rays could pass through matter. He appropriately named them x-rays.

The essential elements of x-ray production have not changed in the intervening 100 years. However, x-rays have changed regarding their application in medicine. Modern x-ray tubes (Figure 6-1) still require a source of electrons (the cathode), a current capable of liberating them from their tungsten filament home, a target toward which they can be directed (the anode), and the extremely high voltage necessary to persuade this reluctant electron cloud to flow at the velocity required to produce x-rays.

RADIOGRAPHIC IMAGING CONCEPTS

Radiographic imaging rapidly expanded its role in diagnosing disease over the last half of the 20th century. More recently, digital imaging has begun to replace conventional methods of obtaining a medical image. The age of the computer and its advances in processing speed and memory storage capabilities have allowed the acquisition, storage, and mobility of digital imaging to expand rapidly. X-rays have a variety of diagnostic and therapeutic purposes, and, because of that, many modalities such as diagnostic radiology, nuclear medicine, mammography, cardiovascular imaging, and CT scanning exist to aid the physician in the precise diagnosis of disease. In addition, MRI and ultrasound, whose image is not based on x-rays' interaction with matter, greatly contribute to the diagnosis of disease.

Several types of x-rays are used therapeutically in radiation oncology and its treatment of malignant disease. In the 40- to 300-kVp range, x-rays are used for two purposes. The first purpose is the treatment of skin cancers and other superficial tumors (most other tumors are treated with gamma rays and much higher-energy x-rays above 1 million volts). The second purpose is the planning of a patient's treatment on the simulator. Two processes are used. With conventional simulation, x-ray fluoroscopy, radiographs, and a field-defining system are used to obtain important patient anatomic information. Second, during CT simulation, structural information related to the patient's anatomy are obtained using CT images. That digital information gathered during CT simulation is then directly linked to a computerized treatment planning system.

Conventional simulation provides geometries similar to those found on treatment machines. This is done with x-ray equipment in the 50- to 120-kVp range. Diagnostic-quality images displayed on a radiograph or television monitor allow part of the cancer management team to evaluate the geometry of

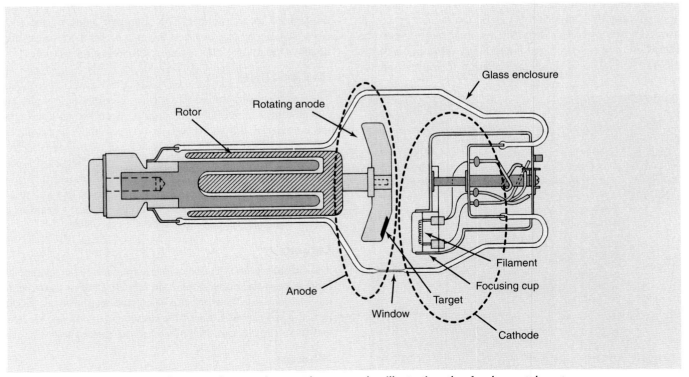

Figure 6-1. Diagram of a rotating-anode x-ray tube illustrating the fundamental parts. (From Bushong S: *Radiologic science for technologists: physics, biology, and protection,* ed 8, St. Louis, 2004, Mosby.)

| Box 6-1 | ACR Standards for Radiation Oncology Equipment |

"Radiation oncology, together with surgical, and medical oncology, are the three primary disciplines involved in cancer treatment. Radiation oncology with either curative or palliative intent is used to treat up to sixty percent (60%) of all cancer patients. The use of radiation therapy requires detailed attention to personnel, equipment, patient and personnel safety, and continuing staff education." The American College of Radiology (ACR) states, under the equipment section, that "high-energy and electron beams, a computer-based treatment planning system, simulation, dosimetry with direct participation of a qualified medical physicist, brachytherapy and ability to fabricate treatment aids must be available to patients in all facilities, either on site or through arrangements with another center. Regular maintenance and repair of equipment is mandatory and is also recommended as part of the ACR Standards for Radiation Oncology.[1] Radiation oncology equipment should include:

1. Megavoltage radiation therapy equipment for external beam therapy, e.g., a linear accelerator or cobalt-60 teletherapy unit.

If the cobalt-60 unit is the only megavoltage unit, it must have a treatment distance of 80 cm or more.
2. Electron beam or x-ray equipment for the treatment of skin lesions or superficial lesions.
3. Simulator capable of duplicating the setups of any megavoltage unit and producing radiographs or DRRs of the fields to be treated. Fluoroscopic capability is highly recommended.
4. Appropriate brachytherapy equipment for intracavitary and interstitial treatment (or arrangements for referral to appropriate facilities).
5. Computer dosimetry equipment capable of providing external beam isodose curves as well as brachytherapy isodose curves and 3-D radiation treatment planning.
6. Physics calibration devices for all equipment.
7. Beam-shaping devices.
8. Immobilization devices.

From the American College of Radiology: *ACR standards for radiation oncology*, Reston, VA, 2002, ACR Publications Department. Amended in 2006. The Standards of the American College of Radiology (ACR) are not rules, but guidelines that attempt to define principles of practice that should generally produce high-quality patient care.[1]

the actual treatment. One of the radiation therapy department's essential functions is to ensure that all definitive (curative) and many palliative treatments are planned with meticulous detail to optimize the treatment's outcome[1] (Box 6-1). The radiographic imaging capabilities of the conventional simulator allow the outlining of the tumor and a small volume of surrounding tissue to be documented and stored on a radiograph (Figure 6-2).

The major components of an imaging system on a conventional radiation therapy simulator are an x-ray tube and a fluoroscope. Although these two components can be found hard at work in most diagnostic radiology departments, their purpose is somewhat different in radiation oncology. X-ray tubes in diagnostic radiology settings and those on radiation therapy simulators are essentially the same devices. Both can produce the same mysterious rays that Roentgen found interesting in 1895.

CT simulation operates much differently from the conventional simulation method of recording an image using fluoroscopy and/or film. CT uses digital imaging techniques that require a computer with sufficient amounts of microprocessor speed and computer memory that can handle large quantities of data. A collimated x-ray beam is directed at the patient, and the attenuated beam is measured by detectors whose response is transmitted to a computer. The computer analyzes the signal from the detector, reconstructs the image, and then stores and/or displays the image. This is referred to as *digital imaging*.

X-RAY TUBE

The electrical production of x-rays is possible only under special conditions, including a source of electrons, an appropriate target material, a high voltage, and a vacuum.[5] The production of x-rays occurs inside the tube because of high-speed electrons colliding with a metal object called the *anode*. The components of the tube, the cathode and anode, are enclosed in a glass envelope and protective housing. A similar type of x-ray tube is used in both conventional and CT simulation. Let's examine the components of a typical x-ray tube.

Cathode

The **cathode** is one of the electrodes found in the x-ray tube and represents the negative side of the tube. It consists of two parts: the filament and focusing cup. As a first step in x-ray production, the primary function of the cathode is to produce electrons and focus the electron stream toward the metal anode.

Filament

The **filament** is a small coil of wire made of thoriated tungsten, which has an extremely high melting point (3380° C) (Figure 6-3). The coil of wire is a smaller version of that inside a light bulb

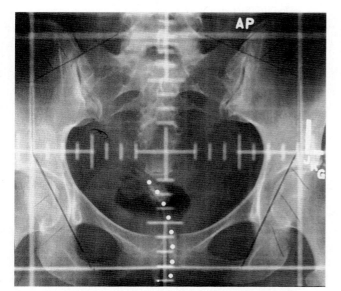

Figure 6-2. A conventional simulation radiograph used for treatment planning purposes. Note the field-defining wires outlining the tumor and a small volume of normal tissue.

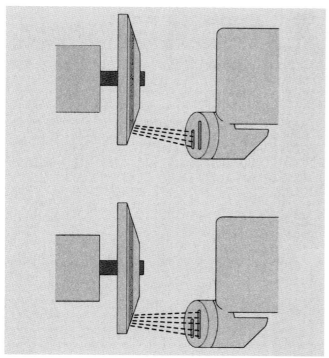

Figure 6-3. In a dual-focus x-ray tube, focal spot size is controlled by heating one of the two filaments. Note the size of the spot where the electron stream strikes the anode. (From Bushong S: *Radiologic science for technologists: physics, biology, and protection*, ed 8, St. Louis, 2004, Mosby.)

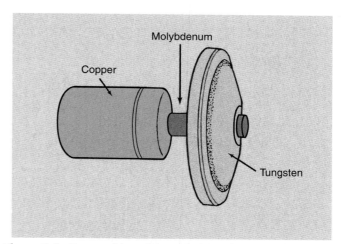

Figure 6-4. Composition of a rotating anode. (From Bushong S: *Radiologic science for technologists: physics, biology, and protection*, ed 8, St. Louis, 2004, Mosby.)

or toaster. A current, which heats the filament, is passed through the small coil of wire where electrons boil off and are emitted from the filament.

Most modern x-ray tubes have dual filaments, thus permitting the selection of a large or small source of electrons. The length and width of the filament control the ability of the x-ray tube to produce fine imaging detail. Most modern x-ray machines are equipped with a rotating anode tube having 0.6-mm (small) and 1.0-mm (large) focal spots. Other x-ray machines having focal spots as small as 0.1 mm and as large as 2.0 mm are also commercially available.[8] Using a small focal spot allows the radiation therapist to radiographically display fine detail. This is especially important in imaging the field-defining wires used to localize the treatment area during the conventional simulation process.

Focusing Cup. The selection of a small or large focal spot is associated with the small and large filaments, which are embedded in a small oval depression in the cathode assembly called a **focusing cup.** The negative charge of the focusing cup helps direct electrons toward the anode in a straighter, less-divergent path.

Anode

The **anode** is the positive side of the x-ray tube. It receives electrons from the cathode as a target, dissipates the great amount of heat as a result of x-ray production, and serves as the path for the flow of high voltage. Aspects of the anode assembly include the composition of the anode, the target, and the line-focus principle.

Composition. The anode is a circular disk composed of many different metals, each designed to contribute to the effectiveness of x-ray production (Figure 6-4). The rotating tungsten disk serves as the target and can range up to 13 cm in diameter. Rhenium-alloyed tungsten serves as the target focal-track material because of its ability as a thermal conductor and the source of x-ray photons. The rotor, which allows most anodes to reach 3400 revolutions per minute, is an excellent device to help dispel the great amounts of heat created.

Target. Electrons from the cathode strike the portion of the anode called the *target,* or *focal spot.* This is the point at which x-ray photons are produced and begin to fan out in a divergent path. Divergence of the x-rays from their focal spot is similar to the sun's divergent rays seen on a partly sunny day. As the rays get closer to the earth, they fan out more from their source, which is 93 million miles away. This is similar to how x-rays disperse as they move farther from their source.

Line-Focus Principle. The **focal spot** is the section of the target at which radiation is produced. With the use of a small focal spot, more detail is seen on the conventional simulation radiograph. Simultaneously, however, more heat is created by bombarding a smaller area of the target. To overcome the disadvantage of creating more heat and still maintain radiographic detail, the target is angled as shown in Figure 6-5. In this way, a larger geometric area can be heated while a small focal spot is maintained. Figure 6-5 displays the line-focus principle. The actual focal-spot size of the target is larger than the effective focal-spot size. Most x-ray tubes have a target angle from 7 to 20 degrees.[8,22]

Glass Envelope

The cathode and anode are in a vacuum in the x-ray tube. The removal of air from the glass envelope or x-ray tube permits the uninterrupted flow of electrons from the cathode to the anode. The efficiency of the tube is increased because no air molecules are floating around inside the x-ray tube to collide with the accelerated electrons. The tube may measure from 20 to 30 cm in length and be as large as 15 cm in diameter at the central portion.

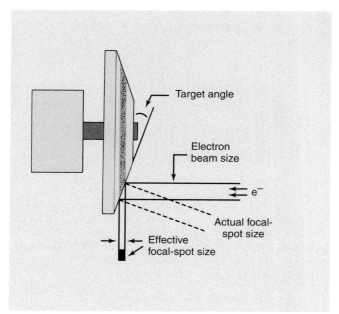

Figure 6-5. By angling the target of the rotating anode (thus taking advantage of the line-focus principle), a larger geometric area can be heated while a small focal spot is maintained. (From Bushong S: *Radiologic science for technologists: physics, biology, and protection*, ed 8, St. Louis, 2004, Mosby.)

Protective Housing

To control unwanted radiation leakage and electrical shock, the x-ray tube is mounted inside the protective housing. Lead lining in the protective housing helps prevent radiation leakage during an exposure. A special oil fills the space between the protective housing and glass envelope to insulate the high-voltage potential and provide additional cooling capacity.

Recommendations for Extending Tube Life

Proper care and use by the radiation therapist can extend the life of the x-ray tube, the cost of which may range from approximately $10,000 up to $120,000, depending on the type of x-ray tube and how heat capacity of the tube.[27] Several practical steps may extend the life of the x-ray tube (Box 6-2). The manufacturer's warm-up procedure should be followed to prevent excessive heat load on a cold anode; otherwise, serious damage can occur. Many systems have a digital display (measured in percent) of the heat capacity created on the tube after an exposure. This is a helpful tool in monitoring the **heat units** created, which is the capacity of the anode and tube housing to store thermal energy. The rotor switch should not be held before an exposure. Most x-ray systems do not permit an exposure until the rotor has reached its full revolutions per minute. When the rotor switch is depressed, thermionic emission of the electrons from the filament occurs and continues until an exposure is made. Any delay in exposure causes unnecessary wear on the filament and decreases the tube life. The use of low mA (filament current) values during an x-ray exposure decreases filament evaporation, thus extending tube life. Finally, making multiple exposures near the tube limit should be avoided; otherwise, unnecessary heat stress on the anode may occur and cause serious damage.

1. Follow the manufacturer's warm-up procedure to prevent heat damage to the anode.
2. Monitor the heat units created during repeated exposures.
3. Avoid holding the rotor switch before an exposure. Double-press switches should be completely depressed in one motion, and dual switches should have the exposure switch pressed first, and then the rotor switch.*
4. Use low mA (filament current) values whenever possible.
5. Avoid multiple exposures near the tube limit.

*From Carlton RR, McKenna-Adler A: *Principles of radiographic imaging*, ed 4, Albany, NY, 2005, Thompson Delmar Learning.

With x-ray production, large amounts of electrical energy are transferred to the x-ray tube. Only a small fraction (typically less than 1%) of the energy used in the x-ray tube is converted into x-rays; a large percentage appears in the form of heat. Excessive heat produced in the x-ray tube can cause damage. Most manufacturers place limits on the x-ray tube, once a certain number of heat units (HU) have been reached. Heat units on a conventional or CT simulator are a result of exposure factors such as:

$$Heat\ units\ (HU) = kVp \times mAs$$

X-RAY PRODUCTION

The essentials of x-ray generation are remarkably simple. They willingly follow the orderly progression of rules in the physical sciences. X-rays are just one of the many forms of electromagnetic energy organized according to wavelength on the electromagnetic spectrum (Figure 6-6). Initially, x-rays may appear to have little in common with their spectral cousins: radio waves and microwaves, visible light, cosmic radiation, and a host of other energy forms. However, all these radiant energies share certain properties. They all travel at the speed of light (3×10^{10} cm per second); they all take the form of a wave, each with its own characteristic undulating pattern expressed as wavelength (the distance between the crests in the wave) and frequency (the number of complete wave cycles per second); and they all consist of photons, which are minute bundles of pure energy having no mass and no electrical charge. The concept of something made up of nothing may be difficult to appreciate because humans tend to think in terms of objects or things, even at the atomic level. However, photons (or quanta) exist and constantly roam around us at the speed of light.

Understanding the unique relationship that exists between photon wavelength and frequency is essential to understanding the dramatically different behaviors observed in various forms of electromagnetic radiation. For example, microwave television signals can transmit sound and image information across great distances, but they cannot readily pass through matter without being deflected. In contrast, x-rays are capable of penetrating matter and altering its atomic structure through a process called *ionization* (the ejection of orbital electrons).

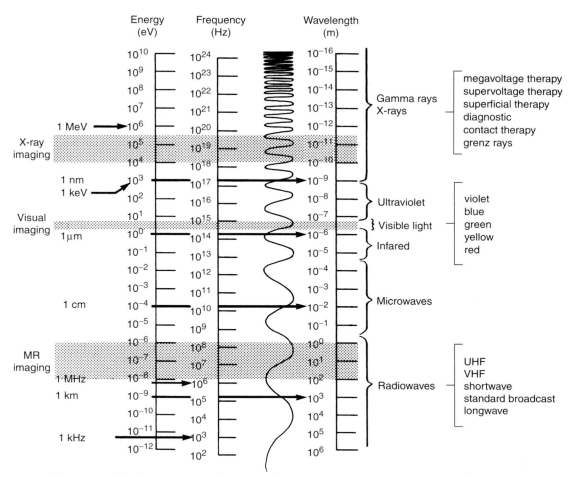

Figure 6-6. The electromagnetic spectrum demonstrates specific values of energy, frequency, and wavelength for some regions of the spectrum. (From Bushong S: *Radiologic science for technologists: physics, biology, and protection*, ed 8, St. Louis, 2004, Mosby.)

Because the velocity of all radiant energy forms is constant, the differing properties of radiant energy can be attributed only to variations in their wavelength and frequency.

X-ray radiations and gamma radiations are located at the high end of the spectrum and possess extremely short wavelengths. The relationship between wavelength and frequency is an inverse proportion (i.e., as wavelength decreases, frequency increases). In 1900, the German physicist Max Planck showed through his quantum theory that frequency and energy are directly proportional. Despite their constant velocities, different forms of electromagnetic radiation may have widely varying energies (from the low end of the spectrum [radio waves] to the high end [x-ray radiations, gamma radiations, and cosmic radiations]). As the wavelength decreases and frequency increases, so does the associated quantum energy.

X-rays are the classic form of artificially produced electromagnetic radiation. Unlike most spectral radiant energies, no spontaneous equivalent for x-rays exists in nature. They are purely a human-produced phenomenon. As described earlier in this chapter, producing x-rays is simple and requires only a source of electrons, a target at which to direct the electron stream, a high-vacuum glass tube, and a source of electricity of sufficient voltage.

Thermionic Emission

In an oversimplification, x-rays are produced when a stream of electrons liberated from the cathode is directed across the tube vacuum at extremely high speeds to interact with the anode. These cathode electrons are freed from the tungsten filament atoms in a process called **thermionic emission,** which refers to heat and the release of ions.

The process of liberating electrons through the application of heat is similar to that seen in an ordinary light bulb. An electrical current (mA) is applied to the filament, which, because of its resistance, begins to glow. As the current (which is the amount of electrical charge flowing over time) increases, the filament reaches the white-hot state necessary for outer-shell electrons to leave their orbits. This is known as *incandescence,* and the resulting electrons are called *thermions.* Thermionic emission begins when the filament circuit is energized.

Potential Difference

The electron cloud or space charge produced from the filament hovers in the vicinity of the cathode indefinitely unless something is done to encourage it to move. The motivating force comes the moment the exposure switch is depressed. High voltage, typically on the order of 70,000 to 120,000 V

(70 to 120 kVp), is applied to create a high potential difference between the negative cathode and positive anodes. kVp is the voltage that determines the kinetic energy of the electrons accelerated in the x-ray tube. According to the basic laws of electrodynamics, this causes the negatively charged electrons to be strongly repelled from the cathode and drawn at extreme speeds toward the attracting force of the positively charged anode. In modern three-phase radiographic equipment, the velocity of this electron stream can approach the speed of light.

Target Interaction

X-rays are produced when the kinetic energy of the moving electron stream is given up as it enters the nuclear field of the target anode. As noted earlier in the discussion of x-ray tube design, the anode (or target) is composed of materials selected for their high atomic number and high melting point. The former factor largely determines the energy efficiency of x-ray production resulting from interactions that take place in the tube. The latter minimizes the potential for damage from the intense heat that those interactions produce. More than 99% of the electrical energy applied to the tube is converted to heat, and only a tiny fraction (approximately 0.6% at diagnostic energy levels) becomes x-rays.

The principal interaction in x-ray production results in the output of **bremsstrahlung** (German for "breaking") radiation (Figure 6-7). Bremsstrahlung accounts for approximately 75% to 80% of the tube's output and is produced by the sudden deceleration of the high-speed electron as it is deflected around the nucleus of the tungsten atom. The therapist should remember that electrons have mass and moving electrons possess kinetic energy. When any moving object is abruptly slowed, the surplus energy must be given off. The greater the angle of deflection around the nucleus, the more pronounced the degree of deceleration and the more energy released. A somewhat remote analogy may be found in an automobile rounding a bend in the road. As the automobile slows, some energy is converted to heat through friction with the brakes and tires. This same vehicle suddenly negotiating a sharp curve may have to slow almost to a stop, thereby giving off most or all its kinetic energy. In the target atoms of the anode, the kinetic energy of the decelerating electron is given off as a bundle of pure energy, or an x-ray photon.

A second, lesser interaction also contributes to the production of x-rays. **Characteristic radiation** is created by the direct interaction of cathode electrons with inner-shell electrons of the target material. Some electrons may collide with tungsten orbital electrons that have sufficient energy to overcome their binding energy and eject them from orbit. This process is called *ionization* (Figure 6-8). When an inner-shell electron is ejected from orbit, other electrons (generally from adjacent shells) move in to fill the hole left. The energy of x-rays produced in this manner is dependent on the binding energy of the target atom's electrons. As the atomic number of an element increases, so does the energy level of each shell. This is the rationale for using materials of high atomic number (such as tungsten) in the targets of x-ray tubes. Binding energy drops with each successive electron orbit away from the nucleus. Outer-shell, or valence, electrons have an extremely low binding energy and are easily ejected from orbit. Therefore ionization events in the O or P shell of the tungsten atom do not produce characteristic x-ray photons of sufficient energy to be useful. Tungsten K-shell electrons, however, have a binding energy of 69.5 keV. When a K-shell electron is ejected from orbit and replaced with a tungsten L-shell electron, a surplus energy of 57.4 keV is released in the form of a characteristic x-ray photon.[4] Energies of this magnitude are well within the useful range for diagnostic x-rays. Table 6-1 summarizes the production of x-rays, which is mostly due to bremsstrahlung radiation.

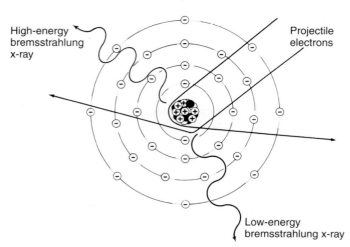

Figure 6-7. The bremsstrahlung interaction. (From Bushong S: *Radiologic science for technologists: physics, biology, and protection*, ed 4, St. Louis, 2004, Mosby.)

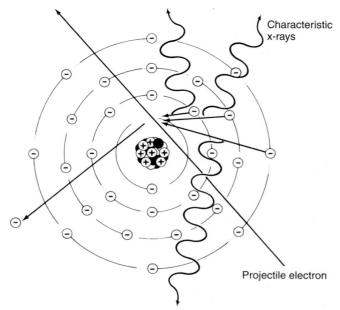

Figure 6-8. The characteristic interaction. (From Bushong S: *Radiologic science for technologists: physics, biology, and protection*, ed 8, St. Louis, 2004, Mosby.)

Table 6-1	Summary of X-Ray Production
Material	**Process**
Glass envelope	Establishes a vacuum
Anode	High-density target material
Cathode	Source of electrons
mA	Tube current
kVp	Tube voltage
X-ray tube	Electrons are accelerated in a vacuum toward the target; as the electrons are stopped suddenly, 75% to 80% of the target interaction is bremsstrahlung radiation, released in the form of x-rays

Physical Relationships in X-Ray Production

A basic premise of physics is that matter can be neither created nor destroyed; it can only change its state. Thanks to the efforts of Albert Einstein, matter's conversion to energy is now known. Einstein, the undeniable father of modern nuclear physics, proved mathematically the theoretical relationship between the kinetic energy of moving matter and the production of light quanta (photons). In his historic theory of relativity, Einstein demonstrated that matter accelerated to a sufficient velocity can become pure energy.

On a more practical level (applied to the production of x-rays), the velocity of the cathode stream is determined by the energy supplied in volts; as the voltage increases, so does the energy available for conversion into x-ray photons. As may be expected, high-energy photons pass through matter more readily than low-energy photons. The ability of the photon stream to pass through matter such as human body tissues is critical to the production of a useful image. This ability is generally called *penetration*. A radiation beam of high energy penetrates structures with greater ease than a weak, low-voltage beam. Although this may appear obvious, the theory behind it is of great importance in diagnostic radiography and radiation therapy.

As the potential difference (voltage) is increased across the x-ray tube vacuum, the velocity of the cathode electron stream is increased. The greater the speed of the moving matter, the greater the resultant energy of the photon stream produced by target interactions. As noted earlier, when mass is slowed or stopped, its energy must be given up in some form. In this situation, mass is converted to heat and photons. Increasing voltage (kVp) increases photon energy.

This energy is commonly termed *beam quality*. A beam of radiation produced by using high kVp is a high-quality beam (i.e., it contains a large percentage of highly penetrating, extremely energetic photons). However, quality addresses only half of the x-ray beam equation. The number of photons in the beam must be considered, and the way quality and quantity may interrelate in radiographic image production must be examined.

From an extremely early age, children are taught a simple mathematic premise: if five oranges are given to a friend, the friend will have five oranges (quantity). Explaining that three of the oranges are nice and juicy (high quality) and the other two are dry and useless (low quality) is more difficult. Such is the relationship between x-ray tube current and x-ray production. The relationship is purely a question of the number of photons in the stream.

Thankfully, the relationship between the number of cathode electrons released during thermionic emission and the production of x-ray photons is simple; they occur in direct proportion. As the operator of the radiation therapy conventional simulation equipment increases tube current, a predictable increase in the number of electrons released occurs. The relationship between current (expressed in mAs) and the quantity of electrons liberated is a direct proportion. The relationship has no bearing on beam energy, penetrating ability, or any other variable necessarily useful. For example, it may be simply a question of producing 10-to-the-billionth-power photons for a certain mAs. If the mAs is doubled, 20-to-the-billionth power photons are produced. The fact that many of these photons will not have sufficient energy to contribute to any useful radiographic image is irrelevant, but an important correlation exists among energy, quantity, and image production.

X-RAY INTERACTIONS WITH MATTER
Overview

The ability of an x-ray beam to produce a latent radiographic image on an image receptor depends on certain key properties characteristic of extremely short-wavelength, high-frequency forms of radiant energy.[4,9,25] X-rays travel in straight lines and diverge from a point of origin. (This is critical in understanding the geometrical principles discussed in the previous section.) X-rays are capable of causing certain substances to fluoresce, ionizing materials through which they pass, and causing chemical and biologic changes in tissue. These properties are the basis of x-ray interactions with matter.

As it passes through matter, the x-ray beam undergoes a gradual reduction in the number of photons or exposure rate. This process is termed *absorption* or, more correctly, **attenuation.** Photons in the original or primary beam may also be scattered (i.e., they may change direction as they collide with atoms in their path). In the human body, the rate of beam attenuation and degree of scattering is determined by tissue thickness, density, and effective atomic number. The net effect is a wide variation in the quantity of photons actually reaching the film. The nature of the tissues through which the beam must pass controls which photons strike and where they strike.

The human body is not a homogeneous structure. It consists of varying quantities of air, fat, water, muscle, and bone, each with its own absorption properties. A CT scan of the abdomen (Figure 6-9) provides an ideal demonstration of these differential absorption characteristics. Denser structures and those of higher-average atomic numbers appear as lighter areas on the image because of their higher rates of attenuation. Air (as a result of its extremely low density) and fat (as a result of its relatively low atomic number) appear as dark areas, whereas bone (which is dense and has a high atomic number [z]) appears as a light shadow on the film. This range in differential absorption makes the viewing of anatomic detail possible. From a practical standpoint, the goal of the radiation therapist in the conventional simulator is to select technical factors (appropriate kVp and mAs) that maximize the rate of differential

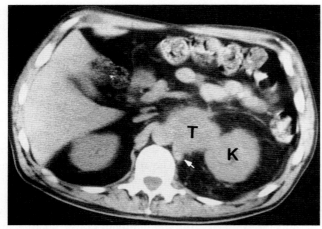

Figure 6-9. A transverse CT image demonstrates an adrenal carcinoma. Large soft tissue tumor (*T* and *arrow*) invades the medial aspect of the left kidney (*K*). (From Eisenberg RL, Johnson NM: *Comprehensive radiographic pathology*, ed 4, St. Louis, 2007, Mosby.)

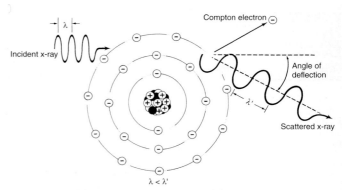

Figure 6-10. The Compton effect is produced when an x-ray photon interacts with an outer-shell orbital electron. The photon must possess sufficient energy to eject it from orbit and alter its own path. (From Bushong S: *Radiologic science for technologists: physics, biology, and protection*, ed 8, St. Louis, 2004, Mosby.)

absorption and increase the visibility of detail in the image. A CT simulation image may be electronically manipulated by using computer software to display varying degrees of black, gray, and white. Darker structures will still represent an area with a low atomic number and light shadows on the scan will represent tissue that is dense and has a high atomic number.

Interactions in the Diagnostic Range

For an appreciation of the importance of differential absorption, some understanding of x-ray photons at the subatomic level is important. In the diagnostic energy range, three interactions occur. Photons may be absorbed photoelectrically or undergo coherent (unmodified) or **Compton scattering** during an interaction. In general, a scattered photon is a bad photon. It rarely contributes to a useful image on the film, and therapists go to great lengths to minimize its detrimental effect.

Unfortunately, the predominant interaction in the diagnostic energy range is the Compton effect (Figure 6-10). Compton scattering is produced when an x-ray photon interacts with an outer-shell orbital electron with sufficient energy to eject the photon from orbit and alter its own path. The classic analogy is seen in the game of billiards, in which the cue ball collides with another ball and both fly off in different directions. In Compton scattering, the freed electron likely travels only an extremely short distance before attaching to another atom. At high kVp settings, the scattered photon may have enough energy remaining to interact with another atom (thus producing more scatter) or even exit the body part completely. If the photon reaches the film, it strikes it at random, thus producing unwanted density because the photon's path no longer corresponds accurately to the portion of anatomy through which it passed. In any situation, the scattered photon is a bad photon and detrimental to image quality.

Unmodified scattering (Figure 6-11) is of relatively little importance to diagnostic imaging. This scattering occurs at low energy levels (generally less than 10 keV), and the resultant scattered photons do not have sufficient energy remaining to

be emitted from the part. Coherent scattering (also called *Thomson* or *unmodified scattering*) results in a change in the incident photon's direction but no change in energy. In this interaction, not enough energy exists to eject an electron from its orbit.

As noted earlier, the only interaction with the capacity to produce a useful image on the film is **photoelectric effect**. This interaction, sometimes described as *true absorption*, occurs when the incident photon penetrates deep into the atom and ejects an inner-shell electron from orbit (Figure 6-12). Orbital electrons close to the nucleus have higher binding energies, and all the photon's energy is required to remove them from orbit. Because a photon is nothing more than a bundle of pure energy, it ceases to exist or is absorbed in the process if all its energy is given up. The energy is transferred to the electron, now termed a *photoelectron,* with a kinetic energy equal to the original energy of the incident photon. This photoelectron has sufficient energy to undergo a variety of other interactions that are beyond

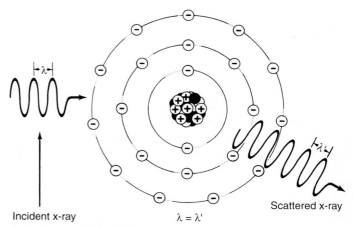

Figure 6-11. Unmodified scattering is an interaction between extremely low energy (generally less than 10 keV) and is of little importance in radiation therapy. (From Bushong S: *Radiologic science for technologists: physics, biology, and protection*, ed 8, St. Louis, 2004, Mosby.)

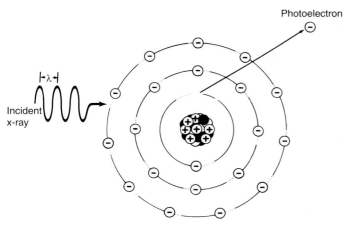

Photoelectron

Incident x-ray

Figure 6-12. The photoelectric effect, sometimes described as true absorption, occurs when the incident photon penetrates deep into the atom and ejects an inner-shell electron from orbit. (From Bushong S: *Radiologic science for technologists: physics, biology, and protection*, ed 8, St. Louis, 2004, Mosby.)

the scope of this chapter. It should be noted that the photoelectric effect is very dependent on the atomic number (z) of an atom. The more protons in the nucleus of an atom, the more probable an incident photon will be absorbed through the photoelectric effect. It is proportional to the atomic number of the material (z) on the order of z^3.

An atom is ionized when it loses or gains an electron. Ionization is an unstable atomic state, and the ionized atom seeks to stabilize itself by filling the hole left in its inner electron shell. This effort sets off a chain reaction that can lead to as many as six different ionizing events, each with its own subsequent release of pure energy (a new photon). In practice, most of these events possess insufficient energy to be of any radiographic significance. However, atoms of high atomic number with K-shell binding energies (K-energies) of 20 or 30 keV can easily produce secondary or characteristic photons energetic enough to reach the film or undergo additional ionizing events.

The human body is composed primarily of carbon, hydrogen, and oxygen atoms, and none of these materials has sufficiently high K-energies to produce secondary photons of any magnitude. For this reason, most photoelectric interactions in tissue result simply in absorption with no appreciable secondary effect. This is desirable because to clearly define anatomic structures of differing densities and atomic number on an image, their relative variation in absorption rates, however slight, must be used to the fullest imaging advantage.

Normal human anatomy provides a predictable variation in tissue densities. For example, kidneys can be seen in a radiograph of the abdomen not because of their density difference compared with the greater surrounding tissue but because they are outlined by a thin band of fat called the *adipose capsule*. Contrast materials such as iodine, barium, and other agents of high atomic number may be used to enhance the visibility of structures with similar composition that would otherwise remain unseen. Advanced imaging modalities such as CT scanning and MRI have done much to overcome this limitation in conventional diagnostic radiography.

 Attenuation of the radiation beam is the reduction of the number of photons remaining in the beam after passing through a given thickness of material. The amount of attenuation is the result of the thickness of the absorber (for example, the patient's body) and type of material irradiated (fat, bone, soft tissue, or air).

Imaging Pathology

Any diseased state in the body can dramatically alter the body's absorption characteristics. In many situations, the changes that accompany pathology can actually improve the image. This phenomenon is of obvious value in diagnostic radiography and can also prove useful in radiation therapy treatment planning. After all, localizing disease that is not visible with the use of x-rays is difficult.

Tissue changes that occur in pathology are often characterized as *additive* or *destructive* (Figure 6-13). Additive pathologies are those with increased tissue density and therefore appear as light regions on the radiograph or CT image. (The opposite is true with the reverse image on the television monitor during conventional simulation fluoroscopy, in which densities such as bone and tumor appear darker.) Most nonmalignant disease entities are additive. They include edema, Paget's disease, atelectasis, abscesses, pleural effusions, and several other common illnesses. Hilar masses commonly associated with lung tumors are universally additive, and any large, fluid-filled mass also appears as an additive pathology. Necrotic areas in a tumor are generally destructive in appearance (typical of a high-grade brain tumor called an *astrocytoma*), but the band of actively mitotic, highly vascularized malignant tissue that surrounds this dead mass is often seen as additive in density.

Unfortunately, definite rules for malignant disease imaging do not exist, because several tumors can cause increased tissue density. Certain cancers follow predictable patterns that can reliably guide the radiation oncologist and radiation therapist in their efforts to localize the lesion. Most patients with multiple myeloma or any osteolytic metastatic disease have a destructive pathologic disease. Metastases from breast and prostate cancer can sometimes be seen as pathologically additive or destructive in the radiographic image when they are present in bone (Figure 6-14). Certain sarcomas and other soft tissue tumors commonly differentiate poorly from surrounding tissues and are best localized by palpation and visual observation, although they can be seen radiographically through the use of low-kVp techniques.

The individual nature of healthy and diseased body tissues makes generalizations on levels of absorption difficult and possibly unwise. Far more important is the radiation therapist's understanding that dense structures absorb more photons photoelectrically and produce more Compton scattering. Conversely, tissues that are thin, less dense, and aged result in dramatically decreased attenuation and thus produce a disproportionately darker image.

FUNDAMENTALS OF IMAGING

The function of voltage (kVp) and current (mAs) in medical imaging involves the way more energetic photons (controlled by kVp) affect image receptors and the reason greater or lesser

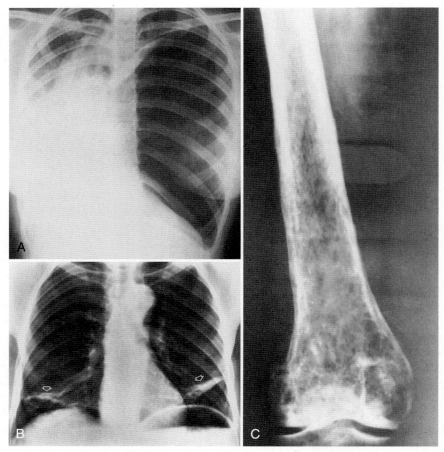

Figure 6-13. A, This pleural effusion in the left hemithorax is an example of an additive pathology. **B,** This illustration demonstrates atelectasis in the lower portion of both lungs (another example of an additive pathology [an opacity on the radiograph]). **C,** A Ewing's sarcoma has destroyed part of the distal femur. (From Eisenberg RL, Johnson NM: *Comprehensive radiographic pathology,* ed 4, St. Louis, 2007, Mosby.)

quantities of photons (controlled by mAs) make the image darker or lighter.[12,13] The explanation of these subjects focuses on the two most important concepts in radiographic imaging: density and contrast.

Density

Density is defined as the degree of darkening on the image. This is not to be confused with *tissue density,* which refers to the compactness of molecules in the atomic structure of different body parts. Image density is a relatively simple concept to grasp because it is easy to visualize. An image of high density is dark, and an image of low density is light. The rules governing density are equally straightforward. When more photons reach the image receptor, density increases; when fewer photons reach the image receptor, density decreases.

Many authors suggest that the principal factor governing image density is mAs (i.e., mAs equals the tube current in milliamperes multiplied by the time of exposure). Although mAs largely determines the quantity of photons in the primary beam, giving mAs an enormous amount of credit in the regulation of density is inaccurate because numerous other factors may have equal or greater effect. For example, source-to-image receptor

distance (SID), kVp, and grid ratio are important factors in conventional radiographic imaging. However, mAs has a clear and predictable role in image density. When all other factors remain the same, the relationship between mAs and density is a direct proportion (i.e., as mAs is doubled, so is the resulting density on the image). This makes mAs an extremely useful tool in the control of density and one that therapists find easy to use on the conventional simulator. By virtue of its convenience, this tool is also subject to abuse because as mAs is doubled to increase density so is the dose of radiation exposure to the patient.

In addition, kVp may be used to change image density. A far smaller increase in kVp is needed to significantly affect the image receptor than is required by using mAs. When all other factors remain the same, a kVp increase of only 15% doubles the radiographic density. To put this in perspective, a scenario in which the therapist is involved in a prostate localization procedure on the conventional simulator may be considered. In the anteroposterior (AP) projection, the therapist selects an mAs of 50 at 74 kVp. The resulting radiograph has insufficient density (too light) and must be repeated. The therapist may then use 100 mAs and 74 kVp or 50 mAs and 85 kVp to make the correction; either combination produces the same new

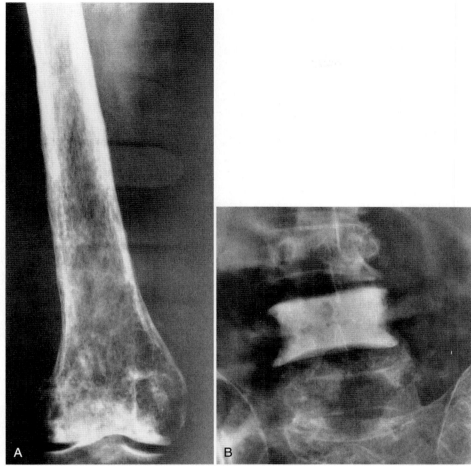

Figure 6-14. A, Diffuse punched-out osteolytic lesions caused from multiple myeloma are scattered throughout this view of the femur. **B,** Diffuse sclerosis of L4 vertebral body from metastatic carcinoma of the prostate. (From Eisenberg RL, Johnson NM: *Comprehensive radiographic pathology*, ed 4, St. Louis, 2007, Mosby.)

radiographic density. One choice may be preferable to the other, and several variables yet to be discussed determine the more desirable combination.

Distance

Another major extrinsic factor influencing density is *distance*, which refers to the gap between the focal spot (target) of the x-ray tube and the recording medium. The terminology used to describe this gap varies with the equipment in use and its application. Target-to-image receptor distance (TID), focal-film distance (FFD), and SID refer to the same idea.

Distance can have a profound effect on image density (Figure 6-15), and, although distance is a critical factor in diagnostic radiography when the radiographer may have to negotiate a variety of distance changes, it is less important to the radiation therapist who generally works with one or two fixed distances on the conventional simulator. Still, some discussion on the effect of distance is important, not only for its relationship to image density but also because of its vital influence on occupational exposure. The relationship between distance and density follows the **inverse square law,** which states that the intensity of the beam of radiation is inversely proportional to the square of the distance. Put more simply, when distance is doubled, the quantity of radiation reaching the image receptor (or occupationally exposed personnel) is reduced to one fourth. From a practical standpoint, a radiograph with a satisfactory image density using 100 mAs at 80 cm TID requires 400 mAs to produce the same density at 160 cm.

The inverse square law works because of the property of x-rays stating that they travel in straight lines and diverge from a point of origin. As distance is doubled, a quantity of radiation is spread over an area four times as great, thereby reducing the intensity of the beam in an area to one fourth its original value.

Contrast

Perhaps no element of medical imaging is more important or more misunderstood than contrast. **Contrast** is the element of imaging that provides visual evidence of the all-important differential absorption rates of various body tissues. Image contrast has been described as the tonal range of densities from black to white or the number of shades of gray in the image. Neither of these definitions (nor any of the others that have appeared in

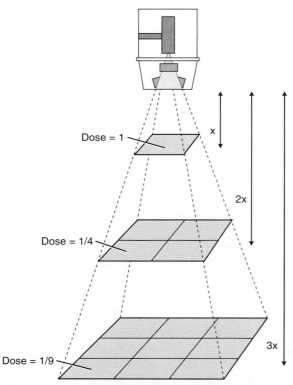

Figure 6-15. The inverse square law means as distance (D) is doubled, a quantity of radiation is spread over an area four times as great, thereby reducing the intensity of the beam in any area to one fourth its original value.

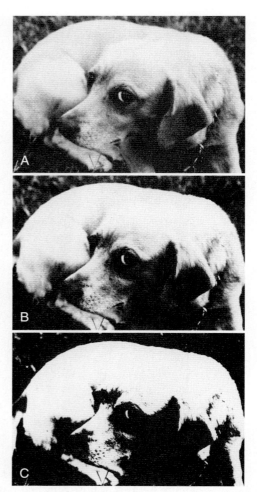

Figure 6-16. The dog pictured has been photographed to demonstrate differences in contrast. **A**, Low contrast. **B**, Moderate contrast. **C**, High contrast. (From Bushong S: *Radiologic science for technologists: physics, biology, and protection,* ed 8, St. Louis, 2004, Mosby.)

print over the years) provides an adequate description of the significance of contrast in defining information on the film.

When most homes had black-and-white television sets, describing the effect of contrast on a visible image was easier. With these old sets, contrast could be arbitrarily increased or decreased by the twist of a knob. Today, a similar demonstration can be conducted through black and white digital images. The amount of contrast can be adjusted using a variety of computer tools.

The dramatic variation in the three photographs in Figure 6-16 is clear. Figure 6-16 illustrates the difference between high and low contrast. The same ability to precisely define or destroy visible information exists in the medical imaging field and is the responsibility of the radiation therapist's correct application of technique.

Optimal contrast results when technical factors (primarily kVp) are selected that maximize the rate of differential absorption between body parts of varying tissue density and effective atomic number. Optimal kVp ranges exist for all body parts. The most important factor in determining optimal kVp is part thickness, but numerous other elements such as grid ratio and field size may also influence the selection (Table 6-2).

RECORDING MEDIA

One of the primary purposes of diagnostic-quality x-rays used in radiation oncology (as opposed to extremely high-energy x-rays used in the treatment of cancer) is to transfer information from a hard copy, electronically or digitally, to a member of the radiation oncology team. Today, the most common method of

Table 6-2	Factors Influencing Contrast and Density		
Factor	**Change**	**Result**
Kilovoltage peak	Increase kVp	Decrease contrast; Increase density
Part thickness	Increase thickness	Decrease contrast; Decrease density
Field size	Increase field size	Decrease contrast; Increase density (scatter)
Tissue density	Increase density	Decrease contrast; Decrease density
OID	Increase OID	Increase contrast; Decrease density

Note that the change in contrast results when a single factor is modified alone and without compensation of other factors. Multiple concurrent changes produce varying effects.

OID, Object-to-image receptor distance.

receiving and storing this information is through digital image processing. X-ray film is still used in many situations.

The construction and characteristics of x-ray film and photographic film are similar in that both are sensitive to light and radiation. However, x-ray film has a spectral response different from that of photographic film. In addition to conventional recording media (processing film), modern imaging technology has developed many other radiographic image receptors such as fluoroscopic screens, image intensifiers, photostimulable phosphor plates, scintillation and piezoelectric crystals, and flat panel detectors.[5,24,31] More recently, effort has been invested in developing and perfecting a digital imaging technology using newer imaging concepts.[22] With the use of CT simulation, fluoroscopy and film are replaced with digital imaging and digital reconstructed radiographs (DRRs), a type of computer image similar in appearance to a conventional radiograph but displayed on a video monitor or stored on x-ray film.[21] In digital imaging, radiation detectors whose electrical output is proportional to the radiation intensity are used to convert an output signal to a digital form that the computer can display as an image[4] (Figure 6-17).

Film

Conventional recording media (film, screens, and cassettes) used in capturing an x-ray image are discussed in this section. X-ray film has three major components: base, emulsion, and protective coating. The base is a rigid, transparent plastic coated with the emulsion (Figure 6-18). An x-ray film base must be flexible enough to maintain its size and shape during processing (immersion in a chemical solution) and handling yet strong enough to withstand repeated viewing on a radiographic illuminator. To help reduce eyestrain during viewing of the

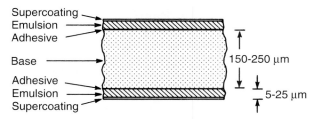

Figure 6-18. A cross-sectional view of x-ray film. The base is a rigid, transparent plastic coated with the emulsion. (From Bushong S: *Radiologic science for technologists: physics, biology, and protection*, ed 8, St. Louis, 2004, Mosby.)

radiographic image, a blue dye is added to the film during manufacturing. Before the film base is coated with the emulsion that contains the photosensitive crystals, a thin adhesive layer is applied to the base.

The emulsion is composed of gelatin and photosensitive silver halide crystals (Figure 6-19). The photosensitive crystals are suspended in the gelatin in much the same way as fruit is suspended in Jell-O during the preparation of a gelatin mold. The emulsion is spread onto the x-ray film in an extremely thin, even coating. The silver halide crystals must be evenly distributed over the surface of the film so that one area of the film is not more photosensitive than another. The gelatin also allows the water and other chemicals to reach the silver halide crystals during the film processing.

Approximately 95% of the photosensitive crystals are composed of silver bromide; the remainder consists of silver iodide. These crystals are the light-sensitive portion of the emulsion that allows it to interact with x-ray and light photons. These interactions are responsible primarily for the formation of the radiographic image on the film. To protect the image, a durable coating is applied to the emulsion to reduce the chance of damage from scratches, abrasions, and skin oils from handling.

Latent Image Formation. The remnant radiation (the amount of radiation leaving a patient after an x-ray exposure) that reaches the film's emulsion is responsible primarily for creating the latent image. The **latent image** is the image on the x-ray film that is not visible until the film is processed. The latent image exists on the film as an unseen change in the silver halide crystal's atomic structure. After processing, the invisible latent image becomes a manifest image, which contains a visible range of densities from black to white. The amount of radiation reaching the film after interaction with the patient greatly influences the degree of blackening on the film. This amount is proportional to the density and thickness of the anatomic part x-rayed. Denser and thicker parts of the body absorb more radiation and therefore allow less remnant radiation to reach the film. In many situations, the x-ray photons and light photons are responsible for interacting with the atomic structure of the silver halide crystals. The affected silver halide crystals indirectly make up the image. Although much is still unknown about critical mechanisms that control the formation of the latent image, the theory of sensitivity specks and their essential involvement in the image-formation process (proposed by Gurney and Mott in 1938) remains almost unchallenged.[5]

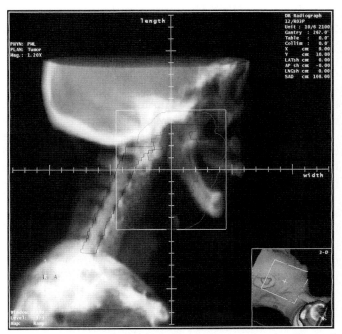

Figure 6-17. An example of a digital reconstructed radiograph (DRR) demonstrating the treatment area on a lateral neck field of a radiation therapy patient with a tumor in the tonsillar fossa.

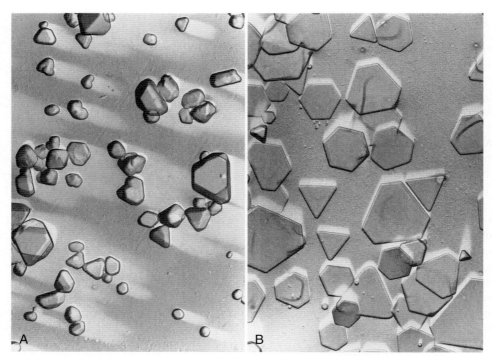

Figure 6-19. This is a photomicrograph of conventional silver halide crystals **(A)** and newer technology tabular grain silver halide crystals **(B)**, which result in the coverage of a larger surface area. (Courtesy Eastman Kodak Company.)

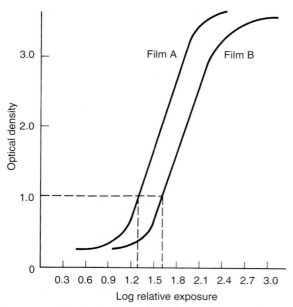

Figure 6-20. A characteristic curve shows the speed of a film. Film speed is the reciprocal of the exposure in roentgens needed to produce a density of 1.0. Notice that *film A* is faster than *film B*. (From Bushong S: *Radiologic science for technologists: physics, biology, and protection*, ed 8, St. Louis, 2004, Mosby.)

Film Characteristics. Important characteristics of x-ray film are speed, contrast, and latitude. **Sensitometry**, which is the measurement of the film's response to exposure and processing, provides a mechanism to analyze these characteristics within the normal exposure range of the film. Sensitometric evaluation of the film may also be part of a quality-assurance program designed to monitor the simulator's exposure system and performance of the processing unit.

The speed of two films can be compared through a graphic relationship called a *sensitometric, characteristic,* or *H & D curve* (Figure 6-20). Hurter and Driffield are two British photographers who in 1890 first described the relationship between exposure and density. This graph represents the measured density on a processed film compared with exposure. A special device called a **densitometer** measures the degree of blackening on the film. The readings from the densitometer, plotted on logarithmic graph paper, correlate to the characteristics of the film.

Another important characteristic of x-ray film is contrast, which is the ability of the film to record differences in density. Film emulsion manufactured to produce high contrast (mammography) or low contrast (a longer scale of grays) is designed to have its own unique response to exposure factors (kVp, mAs, distance). Low-contrast film provides more film latitude and is therefore more forgiving of errors in the selection of technical factors, whereas high-contrast film provides better image detail.[6,8]

Storage and Handling of Film. Several factors such as light, radiation, heat and humidity, shelf life, and proper handling influence the safe storage and handling of x-ray film. Most x-ray film must be stored and handled in the dark. A darkroom with an appropriate safelight (a special orange-red light that permits low-level illumination without fogging the film) is an essential component. A darkroom is needed not only for processing exposed simulation and port films but also for safely storing and handling the film. The unexposed film should be stored in a lightproof, lead-lined storage bin for added protection from light and radiation sources.

Intensifying Screens

Intensifying screens convert the invisible energy of an x-ray beam into visible light energy. Approximately 99% of the latent image on the x-ray film is formed because of this visible light created by intensifying screens. The process of using intensifying screens with film is especially important in diagnostic radiology, where imaging detail and limiting the dose to the patient is critical. Less exposure is required with film and screen systems than with direct-exposure film. These screens are commonly used in pairs to take full advantage of the double-coated emulsion on the film.

Intensifying screens are usually constructed of four distinct layers (Figure 6-21). A typical screen, designed to emit visible light when struck by x-rays, has a base, reflective layer, phosphor layer, and protective coating. The phosphor layer is key to the conversion power of the intensifying screen. This layer has the ability to absorb the energy of an incoming x-ray photon and emit light photons. The reflective layer increases the efficiency of the intensifying screen used in conventional imaging.

 In one form of digital imaging, a similar principle is used. Instead of the combination of intensifying screen and film used in conventional imaging, an x-ray image is captured on a phosphor imaging plate and the latent image is converted to an electrical signal, which is then processed by a computer.

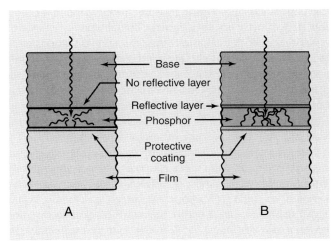

Figure 6-21. A, Intensifying screen without reflective layer. **B,** Intensifying screen with reflective layer. Screens without a reflective layer are not as efficient as those with a reflective layer because fewer light photons reach the film. (From Bushong S: *Radiologic science for technologists: physics, biology, and protection,* ed 8, St. Louis, 2004, Mosby.)

Screens Used in Radiation Therapy.

Three types of screens are used in radiation therapy: intensifying, lead, and copper screens. Intensifying screens, which are necessary in the production of diagnostic-quality radiographs, are used on the conventional simulator. In contrast, lead and copper screens are primarily used in portal imaging on the treatment unit.

Lead and copper screens are used primarily for port filming on high-energy radiation therapy equipment. They do not convert x-ray photons to light photons. The image quality of a portal image is considerably poor compared with that of a chest x-ray or a conventional simulator image. However, the image must be good enough to determine field boundaries of the treatment area in relationship to anatomic or bony landmarks. Taking regular portal images is good clinical practice and provides legal documentation of the patient's actual treatment area.

The thin metal screens can be used with screen-type or direct-exposure film. The lead and copper screens used in portal imaging can be mounted in a screen-type cassette with the intensifying screens removed or secured to a cardboard film holder. The screens can range in thickness from 0.1 to 0.5 mm for lead and up to 3 mm for copper.[23] The thin metal sheets act as an intensifying screen by ejecting electrons from the screen through photon interaction, thus providing an image on the film that represents the variation of beam intensity transmitted through the patient.[4] The ejected electrons from the screen do not have far to travel before reaching the film. High-energy photons used in portal imaging cause electrons produced farther in the patient to travel greater distances to the film emulsion. This adds to geometric blurring of the image. The copper screen absorbs some of these unwanted electrons and at the same time produces some of its own. Good screen-film contact is important to avoid poor image quality. Intensifying screens are used in the diagnostic photon range to produce conventional simulation images, whereas lead and copper screens are used in the megavoltage photon range to produce port films.

Cassettes

The **cassette** provides the light-tight conditions necessary for x-ray film and intensifying screens to work properly. The cassette, which opens like a book, is made of material with a low atomic number such as cardboard, plastic, and carbon fiber. Because of its low atomic number and strength, carbon fiber is also used as tabletop material for the conventional simulator and CT couches. The x-ray film is loaded between the front and back intensifying screens, which are mounted inside the sturdy cassette. Pressure pads, usually made of felt or a spongelike material, are mounted between each intensifying screen and the cassette cover. This design helps maintain good film-screen contact when the cassette is closed and loaded with film.

The back of the cassette is designed differently from the front of the cassette. Lead or other metal backing prevents unwanted scatter radiation from returning to the film or other image receptor after it has exited the cassette. This type of backscatter radiation can cause unnecessary fog and reduce image quality.

Photostimulable Plate

A **photostimulable plate** is a method using x-ray detectors that convert x-rays to a digital image. The flat plate contains a layer of phosphor material, which, when exposed to x-rays, stores the latent image as a distribution of electron charges. The number of trapped electrons is proportional to the amount of x-rays absorbed locally, constituting the latent image. Because of normal thermal motion, the electrons will slowly be liberated from the traps. The latent image should be readable up to 8 hours after the initial exposure, depending on the room temperature. The image plate is then inserted into a machine where a small helium-neon laser converts the stored electron energy to light energy. The emitted light energy is collected by a special photomultiplier tube and converted to an electrical signal, which is then digitized and stored on a computer.[28]

The photostimulable phosphor plate is also known as an *imaging plate, storage phosphor plate,* or *digital cassette.* The plate is reuseable. To prepare the plate for an x-ray exposure, the plate is exposed to high-intensity light to erase any previous image. The image plate is then placed in a cassette and may be used in the same manner as a film-screen exposure for both conventional simulation and portal imaging. Similar exposure techniques are used in each situation. For megavoltage images, the reuseable plate is placed inside the same cassette that is used to obtain portal imaging using film.[28]

Several advantages over the film-screen method of producing an image are seen with the phosphor imaging plate. With most exposures, a uniform density will be present on the plate despite overexposure and underexposure. This is one of the benefits of the system as compared with the conventional film-screen combination. If there is an underexposure, the digital system allows the addition of contrast, density, and brightness to modify the original image within a certain exposure latitude. Even if the original image was overexposed and too "dark," the digital image can be "lightened," by varying contrast and brightness using simple computer controls.

Flat Panel Detectors

Flat panel detectors (FPDs), using amorphous silicon and based on solid-state integrated circuit technology, have emerged as a significant improvement in image quality over conventional methods of film-screen combinations. The driving force behind this new technology is the portability of the digital image and improvement in image quality. Digital images can be transmitted over long distances, can be made available in multiple locations, and are easier to archive and integrate into the patient's electronic record. The FPDs used in radiation therapy are similar to those found in laptop computers, cell phones, personal digital assistants (PDAs), and camcorders. However, in radiation therapy the flat panel image receptor is of similar size to conventional film-screen receptors. As the technology improves with rapid advances in computer technology processing speed and the expanded use of thin-film transistor (TFT) technology, the application of FPD will continue to expand, especially in medical imaging. Today, FPDs are used in fluoroscopy in place of the traditional image intensifier, angiography, and with kV image-guided radiation therapy (IGRT).

Active-matrix liquid-crystal displays, which are commonly used in laptops, are the leading flat panel display technology. These displays use thin film transistor technology with amorphous silicon to convert the radiation beam exiting the patient

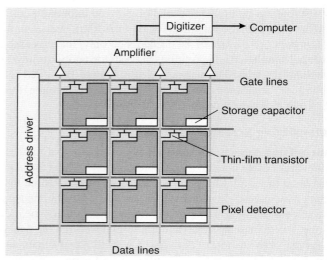

Figure 6-22. The active-matrix crystal display of pixels is read sequentially, one pixel at a time. (From Bushong SC, *Radiologic science for technologists: physics, biology, and protection*, ed 8, St. Louis, 2004, Mosby.)

to an electrical signal and finally to a digital image, which can be shared, stored, or manipulated to improve its image quality. The display (Figure 6-22) is composed of a grid (or matrix) of pixel detectors arranged in rows and columns called *address drives.* The greater the number of pixels in the matrix, the better the potential quality of the digital image. The latent image is stored in the TFT array and is read in sequence from one TFT to another through precise electronic control. These TFTs act as switches, which individually turn each pixel "on" (light) or "off" (dark), depending on the amount of radiation reaching the pixel.[4,31]

There are two approaches to converting the radiation beam exiting the patient to a digital image based on amorphous silicon TFT arrays—a direct and an indirect method. With the direct approach, the x-rays passing through the patient are converted directly to an electrical signal that generates the digital image. With the indirect digital imaging method, x-rays not absorbed by the patient interact with a layer of scintillation (a phosphor-based substance similar to that found in intensifying screens) material, which converts the x-ray photons to light. These light photons are then converted into electrons that in turn activate the TFTs and amorphous silicon generating electronic data used to create the digital image.

There are distinct advantages of flat panel detectors compared with other imaging methods, such as film-screen systems. Using film-screen methods, the x-rays exiting the patient are converted to light (phosphor intensifying screens), which deposit the latent image within the emulsion of the x-ray film. The final analog image is developed in a darkroom using various chemicals. Some information is lost or "blurred" due to the transfer of information between x-ray and light. Photostimulable plates capture an image using a phosphor plate, which is then scanned with a laser to convert the latent image into electrical signals used to generate a digital image. This image may easily become part of the patient's electronic record.

Table 6-3	Comparison of Digital and Analog Medical Imaging Methods	
Digital or Analog	**Detection Method**	**Conversion from X-Rays to Images**
Digital	Flat panel detector (direct)	X-rays → image
Digital	Flat panel detector (indirect)	X-rays → light → image
Digital	Image intensifier and TV camera	X-rays → light → image
Digital	Photostimulable plate	X-rays → latent image → light → image
Analog	Image intensifier	X-rays → light → latent image → image
Analog	Film and intensifying screen	X-rays → light → latent image → image

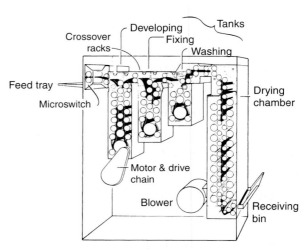

Figure 6-23. Diagram of a modern film processor demonstrating the major components. (From Bushong S: *Radiologic science for technologists: physics, biology, and protection*, ed 8, St. Louis, 2004, Mosby.)

With the direct approach of FPDs, the x-rays passing through the patient are converted directly to an electrical signal that generates the digital image. The direct approach FPD system possesses the most accurate conversion of x-ray data to a usable image, with little blurring and unwanted "noise" seen in the final image. Table 6-3 compares the analog and digital methods of converting x-rays to a usable image.

PROCESSING

Despite advances brought on by automation in the darkroom, some rudimentary understanding of film processing should remain a part of the future radiation therapist's curriculum. The standard textbook definition of radiographic film processing describes the procedure as the conversion of the latent image to a visible image.[4,5,29] The visible image must also be reasonably well preserved for storage.

Developer

The latent image is created when the remnant radiation reaching the intensifying screens of the cassette is converted to light. The light exposes the film in a pattern that precisely corresponds to the intensity of the remaining radiation beam after it passes through anatomy. Without delving too deeply into the chemistry involved, when the exposed film is placed in a developer solution, a reducing agent converts the light-sensitive silver halide crystals in the emulsion to black metallic silver. Unexposed crystals are chemically restrained from involvement in this process. However, if the film is exposed to white light at this time, the unfixed image is destroyed.

Fixer

The function of the fixer is to remove the unexposed silver halide from the film. (The silver washed off the film in this process is valuable, thus leading to the use of silver-recovery systems in most darkrooms.) The fixer also preserves the image by hardening the emulsion and neutralizing any developer remaining on the film. The film is then placed in a bath of running water to remove residual chemicals.

Automatic Processing

In approximately 90 seconds, the completely processed and preserved image emerges from the automatic processor, ready for viewing, analysis, and (ultimately) archival storage. The diagram of a modern film processor (Figure 6-23) is deceiving in its simplicity. Only a chain of rollers (the film-transport system) meandering through a row of three tanks is seen. However, this apparently simple processor took several major corporations nearly a generation to design and perfect.

Darkroom Chemical Sensitivity

The term "darkroom disease" was coined by radiographer Marjorie Gordon to refer to her illness caused by glutaraldehyde, sulfur dioxide, and solvent sensitivity. Generally, when individuals are processing films in the darkroom, they are exposed to higher levels of glutaraldehyde, acetic acid, formaldehyde, and sulfur dioxide. Although some may suggest that darkroom disease is on the decline with the introduction of digital imaging, it may be considered a form of multiple chemical sensitivity (MCS).[19]

MCS is generally acknowledged to be a condition in which individuals experience adverse reactions to low-level chemical exposure found in everyday substances. It involves two stages: initiation (causation) and triggering. Initiation is the initial sensitizing event caused by either massive exposure or multiple low-level exposures to the agent. Glutaraldehyde and sulfur dioxide exposure occurs in the darkroom, while simulation or portal images are being developed. Initiation is followed by triggering, which means that once sensitized, the immune system is somewhat compromised and that exposures to other agents, similar or dissimilar, cause symptoms.[19] Darkroom disease is rare but can be disabling in some.

Glutaraldehyde is used as a cold sterilant to disinfect and clean heat-sensitive equipment such as dialysis instruments; surgical instruments; suction bottles; bronchoscopes, endoscopes;

and ear, nose, and throat instruments. This chemical is also used as a tissue fixative in histology and pathology laboratories and as a hardening agent in the development of x-rays. Glutaraldehyde is a colorless, oily liquid with a pungent odor. Hospital workers use it most often in a diluted form mixed with water. The strength of glutaraldehyde and water solutions typically ranges from 1% to 50%, but other formulations are available.[26]

 The Occupational Safety and Health Administration (OSHA) publishes information regarding exposure to hazardous chemicals, respiratory standards, and general safety/health topics for health care facilities. Detailed information regarding occupational exposure to glutaraldehyde can be found at www.osha.gov or www.cdc.gov.

APPLICATIONS IN RADIATION ONCOLOGY

Producing quality images is not an easy task. Many components should be considered, such as geometric factors, control of unwanted scatter radiation, and problems associated with contrast and density of the image. An understanding of the many factors affecting the production of good-quality simulation radiographs and portal images is essential. In this section, a practical-application approach to these issues is explored.

Geometric Factors

Some principles in photography apply to radiography. Both areas require a certain intensity of light or x-ray energy and proper exposure time to create an image. A recorded image is possible in both situations because x-ray and visible-light photons travel in straight, divergent lines. This principle of divergence, in which photons move in straight but different directions from a common point (focal spot), contributes greatly to the magnification and distortion seen on simulation radiographs, image receptors, and port films. Two geometric factors are important in radiation oncology: magnification and distortion.

Magnification. All images on a radiograph, portal image, or LCD monitor appear larger than they are in reality. This condition is known as *magnification*. The images on the film represent objects in the path of the beam. These objects can be located closer to the common point source (e.g., objects near the multileaf collimator) or nearer to the film (anatomy in the patient). Figure 6-24 illustrates the principle of divergence, in which more tissue is exposed at the level of the lumbar vertebrae *(B)* than at the skin surface *(A)*. The degree of magnification depends on several factors, all of which have to do with the geometric arrangement of the x-ray target, the patient (object), and the medium on which the image is displayed.[2,30]

Magnification can be measured and expressed as a factor. Magnification is directly proportional to the distance of the object from the target or source and is dependent on the distance of the object from the film. The magnification factor is defined as follows:

Magnification factor = Image size/Object size

Example: If an object in the patient, such as the maximum width of a vertebral body, measures 5.3 cm and its image on the simulator film measures 7.5 cm, what is the magnification factor?

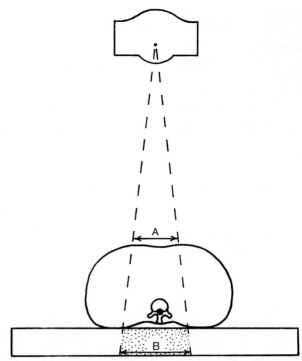

Figure 6-24. Divergence of an x-ray beam. More tissue is exposed as the beam exits the patient than at the anterior skin surface.

Answer:

Magnification factor = 7.5 cm/5.3 cm = 1.415

Another method of determining the magnification factor is using the geometric relationship between similar triangles. Two triangles are similar if the corresponding angles are equal and corresponding sides are proportional. Figure 6-24 illustrates a typical divergent x-ray beam used on the conventional simulator. In many radiation therapy imaging procedures, determining the size of an object (especially in a patient) is not possible. In these situations, the magnification factor can be calculated by using the ratio of target-to-image receptor distance (TID) and target-to-object distance (TOD):

Magnification factor = TID/TOD

Example: A radiograph taken at 140 cm TID during a conventional simulation procedure produces an image measuring 6.5 cm on the radiograph. The distance from the target (source) to the object is 100 cm. What is the magnification factor?

Answer:

Magnification factor = 140 cm/100 cm = 1.4

Magnification, expressed as a factor or ratio, is inherent in the production of all simulation images and portal images. This is due in part to limitations of the simulation and treatment equipment used in radiation oncology. A greater degree of magnification is tolerated in radiation oncology than in diagnostic radiology, in which loss of radiographic detail from magnification is more critical to image quality. The radiation therapist should posses an understanding of the practical applications of magnification and demonstrate the ability to measure its effects in the clinical setting.

Distortion. Distortion is a change in the size, shape, or appearance of the structures being examined. Magnification is a good example of size distortion. More magnification occurs with large TODs. Conversely, the greater the TID, the less is the magnification of the object on the image. For minimal distortion, the distance and angulation of the x-ray beam in relationship to the anatomic part (object) and image receptor must be given special attention.

Shape distortion is the misrepresentation of the actual shape of the structure being examined.[5] This occurs when the object plane or part examined is not parallel with the image plane. If these two planes are parallel, only size distortion occurs, and that distortion is directly proportional to the TOD and TID. Because of unequal magnification, shape distortion can be the result of the following two factors:

1. The angulation of the x-ray beam is in relationship to the part examined.
2. The object and image planes are not parallel in common anatomic projections such as AP, posteroanterior (PA), and lateral.

In radiation therapy treatment planning, angling the beam to avoid treating sensitive normal tissue structures is frequently necessary. When this occurs, a certain amount of shape distortion is observed on the image. No formula exists (as it does in magnification) to assess the amount of shape distortion. Instead, the assessment is based on the radiation therapist's understanding of normal radiographic anatomy in various situations. Figure 6-25, A, illustrates a common radiographic projection (AP), in which the object and image planes are closely parallel. Figure 6-25, B, illustrates shape distortion of a vertebral body when the simulator beam is angled 25 degrees. Greater shape distortion of an image is illustrated in Figure 6-25, C, in which the beam is angled 40 degrees from the vertical. The distortion that occurs in the thoracic vertebrae should be noted. In this situation, the objective in treatment planning may be to treat a lung mass while avoiding the spine (a sensitive critical structure).

Shape distortion can also occur when the object and image planes are not parallel. For example, in the pelvic region the obturator foramina are normally of equal size when imaged in the anterior or posterior projection. If the pelvic bones are rotated slightly, shape distortion can be detected in the image, especially in the shape of the obturator foramina openings. Figure 6-26 compares the amount of shape distortion as a result of unequal magnification when the object (the pelvis) and image planes are not parallel.

For reduction of the effects of distortion, the distances used for a specific procedure and angulation of the x-ray beam deserve particular attention. Otherwise, a misrepresentation of the size and shape of the anatomic part occurs. This misrepresentation, classified as size or shape distortion, can affect radiographic image quality. Other factors such as the selection of the focal-spot size can also contribute to distortion on the radiographic image.

Control of Scatter Radiation

During an exposure, some x-rays are absorbed photoelectrically, and others pass through the patient to reach the film. This is partially a result of the kilovoltage. If more photons pass through the patient, the radiographic image has a greater density. The opposite is true if fewer photons reach the film and more photons are absorbed in the body—radiographic density decreases. A considerable amount of the radiographic density on the film is due to scatter radiation, in which photons arrive at the film after bouncing off matter haphazardly. However, the density on the film from scatter photons does not directly correlate to the anatomic structures of interest. Instead, the unwanted scatter radiation decreases contrast and reduces image quality.

Reducing scatter or secondary radiation, which is created during a Compton interaction, is essential to improving image quality. Scatter photons are produced when an incoming primary photon interacts with an outer-shell electron and is forced to change direction. Sometimes that scattered photon never reaches the film or image receptor; other times, it does. When it reaches the film, scatter radiation reduces contrast by causing additional density on the film and fogging the image. The radiation therapist can create a better image by restricting the amount of scatter radiation reaching the film. Collimating the x-ray beam and using a grid reduces the effects of unwanted scatter radiation.

Less scatter radiation is produced by restricting the beam through careful collimation of the x-ray shutter blades. If fewer primary photons are emitted from the collimator head, fewer scatter photons are created. Collimating the primary x-ray beam is the first line of defense in controlling unwanted secondary radiation.[3,29] A grid absorbs scatter photons as a second line of defense. The grid, which acts like a filter by absorbing some photons, is placed between the film and patient. On some conventional simulator models, the grid is built into the cassette holder. Other models require the manual positioning of a grid in the cassette holder before exposure.

Several other factors influence image quality. The following three primary factors influence the amount of scatter radiation reaching the film: kilovoltage, irradiated material, and lead shutter size. If scatter radiation is to be controlled, understanding the influences of its production is important.

Kilovoltage. As x-ray energy increases, the penetrating ability of the beam increases. With extremely large patients, increasing the kVp considerably to penetrate the part being radiographed is sometimes necessary. When kVp increases, the amount of scatter radiation also increases and contrast decreases. More scatter radiation results with higher kVp because the percentage of x-rays undergoing Compton interactions also increases. For example, if the normal technical factors are not sufficient to penetrate an AP thorax, the radiation therapist can choose to increase kVp or mAs to compensate. An increase in mAs results in a higher radiation dose to the patient for that particular exposure, and a compensation in kVp increases the percentage of photons undergoing Compton interactions. Kilovoltage in the range of 60 to 90 kVp is appropriate for most examinations. Small increases in kVp of 10% to 15% or a larger increase in mAs may be all that is needed to sufficiently penetrate the anatomic part. In other situations, evidence of proper collimation on the radiograph and the use of a grid can help decrease the number of scatter photons.

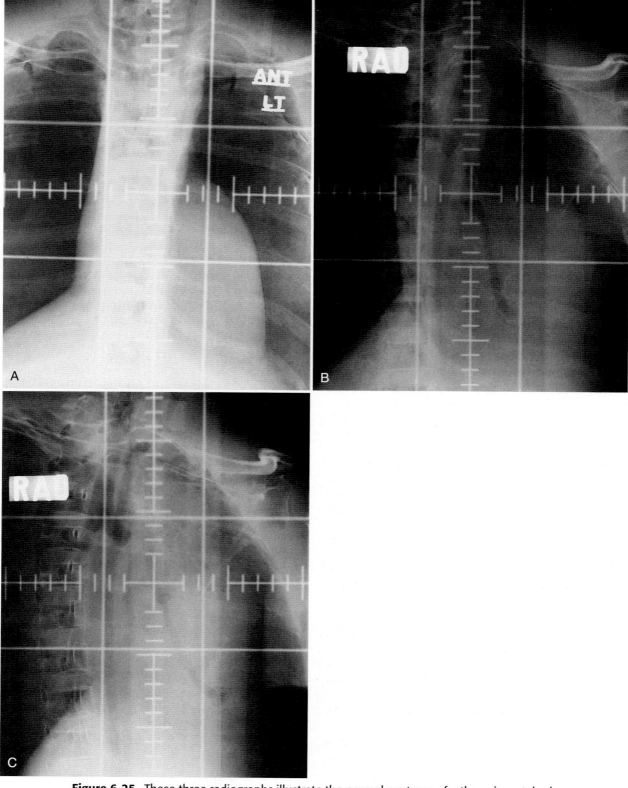

Figure 6-25. These three radiographs illustrate the normal anatomy of a thoracic vertebral body in the anteroposterior projection **(A)**, distorted anatomy with a 25-degree angulation of the beam **(B)**, and distorted anatomy with a 40-degree angulation of the beam **(C)**.

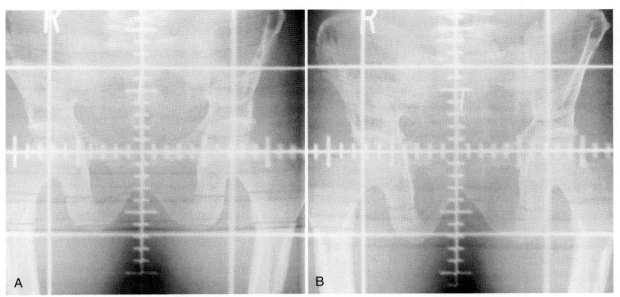

Figure 6-26. These two radiographs compare an anteroposterior projection of the pelvis **(A)** and shape distortion of the obturator foramina as a result of unequal magnification when the image and object plane are not parallel **(B)**. One obturator foramen appears smaller than the other because of rotation of the pelvis.

Irradiated Material. Large patients absorb and scatter more radiation than smaller patients. Not only does the amount of tissue irradiated influence the production of scatter but the density of the tissue irradiated also affects the quantity of scatter. As the volume of tissue irradiated and atomic number of the material irradiated increases, the amount of scatter increases.[16] The atomic number of the material irradiated affects the amount of scatter radiation produced because the x-ray photons have a greater chance of interacting with an electron in a material with a higher density. For example, more scatter occurs in the pelvis, which has more bone (higher atomic number), than in the thorax, which has more air (lower atomic number). The patient's thickness and the lead shutter field size greatly influence the volume of tissue irradiated. Larger patients and larger shutter openings produce more scatter.

Shutter Field Size. Unlike the patient's thickness, the lead shutter (diaphragm) field size and kilovoltage are under the control of the radiation therapist. As the lead shutter field size increases, the amount of scatter radiation increases because more radiation is available to interact with the patient. To improve image quality, radiographic evidence of collimation on the image or image intensifier (fluoroscopy) of the lead shutters is important. Restricting the beam through collimation reduces the quantity of primary photons available to produce scatter radiation. The restriction of the lead shutter opening to improve image quality is critical during fluoroscopy (Figure 6-27). When the beam size is not limited to the area under fluoroscopic examination, increased amounts of scatter reduce contrast and image quality, especially with large patient thicknesses.

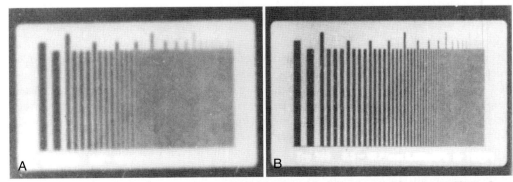

Figure 6-27. Small field sizes are particularly important in fluoroscopy. These spot films of a test pattern embedded in the middle of 20 cm of tissue-equivalent material were taken with full-field exposure and the x-ray beam restricted to the area of the pattern: full-field exposure **(A)** and beam restricted to the area of the pattern **(B)**. The radiograph in **B** is clearer because the smaller field size resulted in less scatter radiation. (From Bushong S: *Radiologic science for technologists: physics, biology, and protection*, ed 8, St. Louis, 2004, Mosby.)

IMAGE FORMATION FOR COMPUTED TOMOGRAPHY, MAGNETIC RESONANCE IMAGING, ULTRASOUND, AND NUCLEAR MEDICINE

In this section, an overview of the principles of medical imaging used in CT, MRI, ultrasound, and nuclear medicine are introduced. Many of the principles discussed here will be applied in other chapters, especially those in the practical application section. For example, some of the basic principles involved with ultrasound will be used to help students further understand the importance of localizing the prostate gland while learning about male genitourinary tumors in Chapter 37. In addition, the basic principles of imaging with computer technology and a description of each of the four important imaging modalities (CT, MRI, nuclear medicine, and ultrasound) as it relates to the administration of an applied dose of radiation and the treatment planning of that dose distribution in the body are discussed.

Imaging with Computer Technology

CT and MRI scans provide the most useful information for treatment planning purposes in radiation therapy. This information is invaluable for both simulation and treatment planning. Since the late 1970s, CT was used in the treatment planning process for radiation therapy patients. Sophisticated three-dimensional treatment planning is now a standard tool in all radiation therapy departments. CT-based treatment planning has since been supplemented with MRI and PET. By combining CT, MRI, and/or PET images in a way that overlays or electronically registers the information gathered from the same anatomic area, a better understanding of the structure and function of the tumor volume is possible. Combining CT, MRI, and/or PET images digitally is known as **image fusion**.

A CT scanner operates much differently from the conventional simulation method of recording an image with fluoroscopy or a radiograph. There is no image receptor such as a film or image intensifier. A collimated x-ray beam is directed at the patient, and the attenuated beam is measured by multiple rows of detectors whose response is transmitted to a computer. The computer analyzes the signal from the detector, reconstructs the image, and then stores and/or displays the image. This is referred to as *digital imaging*.

Digital Imaging. What does analog-to-digital conversion mean? Traditional direct reading devices are "analog," that is, they provide information in a nonnumeric format and are usually mechanical, electromechanical, or photographic. Examples include the arms on a clock, automobile odometer, conventional radiograph, and printed work. To provide a digital image, the analog image must undergo computerized conversion to a series of minute bits of information initially recorded as a series of binary numbers.

Converting a series of numbers to a viewable image is a long leap, one that would have been all but impossible 30 years ago. The numbers must be collected through some method of analog scan, stored, and then reconstructed to form **pixels** (picture elements). This provides the basic information necessary to make a two-dimensional image, the cornerstone of CT scanning technology. An even more complex system

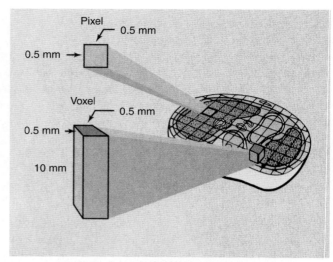

Figure 6-28. Each cell in a computed tomography (CT) scan is a two-dimensional representation (pixel) and a three-dimensional representation (voxel). (From Bushong S: *Radiologic science for technologists: physics, biology, and protection*, ed 8, St. Louis, 2004, Mosby.)

can create a three-dimensional image using **voxels** (volume elements) and is the basis for some CT imaging and most MRI. This permits the manipulation of images so that they may be viewed from all aspects. Figure 6-28 demonstrates that each cell in a CT scan is a two-dimensional representation (pixel) and a three-dimensional representation (voxel).

The relationship between the number of pixels or voxels is crucial to image quality. This is described as "resolution." The greater the number of pixels in the matrix, the higher is the resolution of the image. The downside is that high-resolution devices require either more time to reconstruct into an image or a more powerful computer.

Think of a "matrix" as a picture frame, exactly the same as a television or computer screen. Most televisions in the United States operate on 256 × 256 matrices. This is primitive and much too low for diagnostic imaging. A matrix of 512 × 512 pixels is common for fluoroscopy, but even that is unsatisfactory of high-resolution digital imaging. Generally, 1024 × 1024 is the minimum required, and, although higher matrices are available, the computing power required and reconstruction time make them impractical. The 1024 matrix is currently the size of choice for cardiac catheterization, CT, and other forms of digital imaging (Figure 6-29) and demonstrates increased resolution when using higher matrices used to reconstruct CT data and DRRs. Converting a series of numbers to a viewable image results in a viewable image, either viewed electronically or converted to a hard copy (paper or film). One critical advantage of DRRs is their ability to be moved and viewed electronically over the Internet or through e-mail.

Computed Tomography

Godfrey Hounsfield was a British physicist/engineer who shared the 1979 Nobel Peace Prize in physics with Alan Cormack, a Tufts University medical physicist, who had earlier developed the mathematics now used to reconstruct CT images.[12]

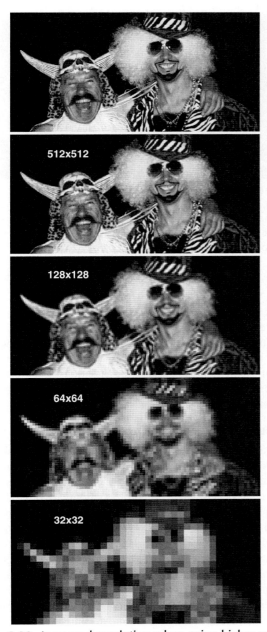

Figure 6-29. Increased resolution when using higher matrices used to reconstruct computed tomography (CT) data and digital reconstructed radiographs (DRRs). (From Bushong S: *Radiologic science for technologists: physics, biology, and protection*, ed 8, St. Louis, 2004, Mosby.)

Many scientists believe that William Oldendorf, a neuroscientist who developed a rudimentary CT scanner in the early 1960s, should have shared in the Noble Peace Prize for his efforts.[15] The use of CT scanners has provided a new window into viewing human anatomy. Today, this medical imaging tool has transformed the way we diagnose and treat disease.[17,20]

A conventional CT scanner consists of a rotating x-ray tube around the patient. Reconstruction yields a single image corresponding to an object's x-ray absorption along a straight but diverging line. As the x-ray tube rotates around the patient, a panel of detectors measures the amount of radiation exiting the patient. To acquire a complete volume, several acquisitions must be performed with a short table movement in between. Other more sophisticated and useful methods of CT scanning, such as spiral CT, cone-beam CT, and cardiac CT imaging, are available. As the CT scanner rotates around the patient, the transmission of x-rays through the patient are measured and recorded. The x-rays travel through different types of tissue, such as bone, soft tissue, and air-filled cavities, all with varying densities. Multiple measurements of x-ray transmission obtained from different angles of the x-ray source and detectors allow for the computation and representation of various tissue densities within the patient. Varying thicknesses detected by the transmission of the x-rays are also computed and represented as a cross-sectional image through the body.

A CT scan of the thorax (Figure 6-30) demonstrates three different windows for viewing. The data collected from the detectors, in terms of bone, soft tissue, and air, are the same in each image. It is the display of that information that has been manipulated by the computer to change the contrast and/or brightness of the image. By changing the contrast of the image through a process of electronic manipulation of the CT data, digital images can be processed to modify, enhance, or suppress some of their characteristics. This is especially useful in the thorax area, where it may be difficult to see lung detail and, at the same time examine anatomy around the heart and mediastinum. Other imaging modalities, such as MRI, may be performed in addition to CT, especially when the central nervous system or soft tissue detail is an area of interest.

Magnetic Resonance Imaging

Unlike x-rays and CT scans, which use radiation, MRI uses a large magnet and radiofrequency waves to produce an image. In 2003, Paul C. Lauterbur and Sir Peter Mansfield were awarded the Nobel Peace Prize in Medicine for their discoveries concerning MRI.[10]

An introduction to some of the basic principles of physics may be helpful in understanding the complexities of MRI technology. The human body is made up of many elements, such as carbon, hydrogen, oxygen, and others—all with specific and unique characteristics. In many cases, electrons orbit around a central nucleus of protons and neutrons. Because of this, both protons and neutrons behave like tiny magnets, as they spin about their own axis within the nucleus. Hence, these nuclei have what physicists call a "residual magnetic moment." Only those nuclei with an odd number of protons and neutrons behave as a small atomic magnet. Ordinary hydrogen with only one proton, and hence a net positive charge, has the strongest magnetic moment. Other nuclei with an odd number of nucleons (protons + neutrons) exhibit a smaller magnetic moment. Because the human body is composed mostly of H_2O (between 60% and 80%), there are an abundant number of hydrogen atoms expressing a magnetic moment. When the nuclei of hydrogen atoms or other atoms with weaker magnetic moments are placed in an intense magnetic field, they tend to align themselves either with or against the applied magnetic field, as is the case with the large and powerful magnets used in MRI.[10,15]

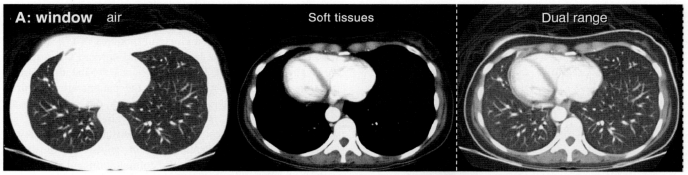

Figure 6-30. A CT scan of the thorax demonstrating three different windows for viewing. The data collected from the detectors, in terms of bone, soft tissue, and air, are the same in each image. It is the display of that information that has been manipulated by the computer to change the contrast of the image. (From Bidaut LM, Humm JL, Mageras GS, et al: Imaging in radiation oncology. In Leibel SA, Phillip TL, editors: *Textbook of radiation oncology*, ed 2, Philadelphia, 2004, Saunders.)

Pulses of radiofrequency (RF) energy are applied to the patient within the MRI scanner, and then the return signal from the patient is collected by a signal coil, measured, and reconstructed into an image. The RF energy returning from the patient is based on three characteristics: (1) the intensity of the signal (representative of the spin density related to the concentration of rotating nuclei within the patient); (2) the time constant T1, known as the *longitudinal relaxation time;* and (3) the time constant T2, known as the *transverse relaxation time.* These three characteristics form the basic parameters used to produce a magnetic resonance image. A variety of methods, known as *pulse sequences*, have been developed to apply the RF energy to a patient and to collect and measure the RF signal radiated from the patient. Pulse sequences yield images with valuable spatial and contrast information about atomic structure and function in the patient.[10,14] Figure 6-31 demonstrates a T2-weighted transverse MRI scan of the female pelvis.

MRI has the ability to display detailed anatomic information (in the sagittal, coronal, and transverse planes), such as the presence and extent of tumors, the shape of normal structures adjacent to the tumor volume, and the distinction between recurrent tumor and necrosis.[15] Its application has grown rapidly in recent years, especially with the ability to capture the MRI information and apply it to the radiation therapy treatment planning process either alone or fused with other imaging modalities such as CT or PET.

Positron Emission Tomography

PET is a form of imaging in which the physiology, metabolism, and biochemistry, rather than the anatomic structure, are displayed in the image. Physiology describes how a tissue, an organ, or a system may function. Anatomy is related to the structure of a specific tissue, system, or organ. CT imaging is an excellent example that displays anatomic structure and does so in detail.[15] The lack of detail in PET imaging is very noticeable compared with that of CT or MRI. PET imaging has significantly altered the diagnostic workup of cancer patients. The introduction of functional data into the radiation therapy treatment planning process is currently the focus of significant commercial, technical, and scientific development.[18]

PET takes advantage of the body's natural process of metabolism and labels some of the molecular building blocks of life; for example, the amount and rate of amino acids, molecular oxygen, or glucose used by the tissue or organ. This is done by labeling a radioactive nuclide, usually tagged to a specific gamma-emitting radioactive pharmaceutical selected for its tendency to concentrate in a specific tissue of interest in the patient. An analog of glucose, fluorine-18 fluorodeoxyglucose (FDG) is currently the most common agent used in PET imaging. Gamma rays emitted by FDG escape from the body and are measured by an external detector positioned very close to the patient. Malignant cells utilize more glucose to meet their energy needs. The measurement process yields a "physiologic map" of the accumulation, distribution, and excretion of the radioactive material in the organ or tissue of interest. Several types of radioactive tracers have been developed for imaging with PET, but most clinical oncology PET studies use FDG. The use of FDG to image glucose metabolism takes advantage of the observation

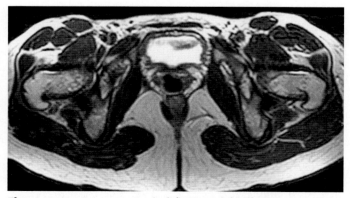

Figure 6-31. A transverse (axial) T2-weighted MRI scan of the female pelvis taken just inferior to the symphysis pubis. Note the normal anatomy of the bladder, vagina, and rectum. (From Kelley LL, Petersen CM: *Sectional anatomy for imaging professionals*, St. Louis, 2007, Mosby.)

Table 6-4	Normal Whole-Body FDG Distribution[7]	
Sites with Intense Activity	**Sites with Variable Activity**	
Brain	Salivary glands	
Liver (moderate)	Thyroid	
Kidneys (especially the collecting system)	Heart and vascular structures	
	Thymus (in children)	
Bladder	Spleen	
	Esophageal ampulla	
	Stomach	
	Bowel (especially the colon)	
	Endometrium (during menses)	
	Bone marrow	
	Muscles	
	Testicles	

FDG, Fluorine-18 fluorodeoxyglucose.

that malignant cells have higher rates of aerobic glycolysis than does normal tissue. Malignant cells need more glucose to meet their energy needs.[11,29]

PET images may be displayed in the transverse, sagittal, or coronal planes. Functional differences seen on the image may represent normal or abnormal pathology as areas of increased density. A thorough knowledge of normal anatomy and normal FDG distribution in the body is necessary before any evaluation of pathologic accumulations can be attempted. Table 6-4 lists organs and body structures where FDG normally accumulates. Figure 6-32 demonstrates normal distribution of FDG in

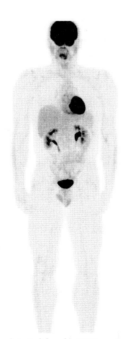

Figure 6-32. Normal total-body PET scan using FDG. Intense activity accumulates in the brain, salivary glands, left ventricular myocardium (variable), kidneys, and bladder. Moderate activity in this normal scan appears in the liver, spleen, and testicles. (From Christian PE, Waterstram-Rich KM: *Nuclear medicine and PET/CT*, ed 6, St. Louis, 2007, Mosby.)

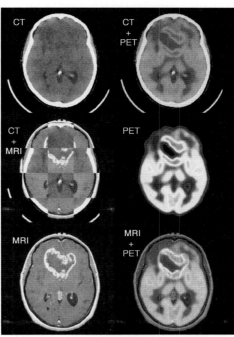

Figure 6-33. Registered or fused images of a brain tumor. Multiplanar reconstruction (side-by-side, checkerboard, and colorwash modes) of computed tomography (CT), magnetic resonance imaging (MRI), and positron emission tomography (PET) of the same patient after spatial registration. (See Color Plate 1.) (From Leibel SA, Phillips TL: *Textbook of radiation oncology*, ed 2, Philadelphia, 2004, Saunders.)

a total-body PET scan. Its application has grown rapidly in recent years, especially with the ability to capture the PET information and apply it to the radiation therapy treatment planning process either alone or fused with other imaging modalities such as CT or MRI (Figure 6-33).

Fusion of PET and CT images acquired separately has, in some cases, demonstrated problems with accurate tumor localization. The development of a dedicated CT/PET scanner has overcome many of the problems involved in fusing CT and PET images. In addition, combined CT/PET imaging has provided additional information in one study in reducing or expanding the tumor volume in 56% of patients. Using a dedicated CT/PET scanner that performs both imaging sequences during one examination provides both detailed structural information from the CT scan and functional information from the PET scan.[11]

Ultrasound

Ultrasound, also known as *sonography,* is a useful medical imaging tool for delineating surface contours and localizing internal structures such as the prostate gland. In this imaging technique, a transducer is used to generate a mechanical disturbance (pressure wave) that moves through the tissue. As the sound wave moves through the body, it encounters a variety of interfaces between tissue that reflect and **refract** (change the direction of) the ultrasound energy. The amount of energy reflected back to the transducer depends on the physical density of the tissue and the speed of the ultrasound through the tissue.

A piezoelectrical crystal within the transducer is used to create the ultrasound waves. The wave is initiated by applying a momentary electrical shock to the piezoelectrical crystal, which sets the crystal into a vibration mode. Ultrasound energy reflected from an interface between tissues returns as a pressure wave of reduced amplitude to the transducer, where a small electrical signal is generated, captured, and processed.[13]

The application of ultrasound is particularly useful in delineating tissues that differ only slightly. For example, ultrasonography is used to localize the prostate gland or prostate bed in the lower pelvis before external beam radiation treatment is administered before. It is also used to distinguish the difference between solid and cystic lesions in the breast following mammography. This works well, because the sound waves travel well through fluid-filled cavities and cysts.

Because the prostate gland moves relative to bony anatomy between the time of initial image acquisition for treatment planning and treatment delivery, real-time imaging, such as ultrasound, is commonly used to accurately localize the target at the time of treatment delivery. Freehand ultrasound imaging is used to acquire data at any anatomic orientation by either sliding or arcing the probe across the region of interest. One acquires many arbitrary two-dimensional images until enough images have been collected to fill a three-dimensional matrix covering the volume of interest. This information is then used through an in-room coordinate system each day to determine the absolute position of the prostate volume within the patient. Daily adjustments may be made relative to the linear accelerator isocenter.

Pressure variations applied in the suprapubic area during prostate localization procedures and the interuser (from one therapist to another) variation of the contour alignment process may affect the accuracy of prostate localization.

Medical imaging is a complex process. The application of knowledge and understanding concerning the production of x-rays, CT, MRI, and ultrasound and the creation of high-quality images is fundamental for the precision and accuracy necessary to deliver a prescribed dose of radiation therapy. Even as conventional recording media are replaced with a technology without film, the role of the radiation therapist in the art and science of medical imaging remains critical. Whether computer technology or conventional x-ray film is used, the goals of maximizing the radiation dose to the tumor and minimizing the dose to the surrounding normal tissue remain the same. The conventional simulator, CT simulator, and other diagnostic imaging equipment are essential tools in realizing this goal in radiation oncology. Correctly applying the principles and practice in medical imaging can lead to only improved patient outcomes.

SUMMARY

- X-rays have a variety of diagnostic and therapeutic purposes and, because of that, many modalities such as diagnostic radiology, nuclear medicine, mammography, cardiovascular imaging, and computed tomography (CT) scanning exist to aid the physician in the precise diagnosis of disease.
- X-rays are capable of causing certain substances to fluoresce, ionizing materials through which they pass,

and causing chemical and biologic changes in tissue. These properties are the basis of x-ray interactions with matter.

- In the production of x-rays, electrons are accelerated in a vacuum toward the target, and as the electrons are stopped suddenly, 75% to 80% of the target interaction is bremsstrahlung radiation, released in the form of x-rays.
- Target interactions include bremsstrahlung interactions, which occur with the nucleus, and characteristic radiation, which occurs mostly with inner-shell electrons of the target material.
- In the diagnostic energy range, three interactions occur. Photons may be absorbed photoelectrically or undergo coherent (unmodified) or Compton scattering during an interaction.
- The term "darkroom disease" was coined by radiographer Marjorie Gordon to refer to her illness caused by glutaraldehyde, sulfur dioxide, and solvent sensitivity. Generally, when individuals are processing films in the darkroom, they are exposed to higher-than-normal levels of glutaraldehyde, acetic acid, formaldehyde, and sulfur dioxide.
- Density is the overall blackening of the film or image receptor. Contrast is the tonal differences (scale of grays) between the blacks and whites on an image.
- Magnification can be measured and expressed as a factor. Magnification on a film is directly proportional to the distance of the object from the target or source and is dependent on the distance of the object from the film.
- CT and MRI scans provide the most useful information for treatment planning purposes in radiation therapy.
- Converting a series of numbers to a viewable image is the basis of digital imaging. The numbers are collected through some method of analog scan, stored, and then reconstructed to form pixels (picture elements). An even more complex system can create a three-dimensional image using voxels (volume elements) and is the basis for some CT imaging and most MRI imaging. This permits the manipulation of images so that they may be viewed from all aspects.
- Flat panel detectors, using amorphous silicon, are based on solid-state integrated circuit technology and thin-film transistor technology to produce useful digital images.
- Unlike x-rays and CT scans, which use radiation, MRI uses a large magnet and radiofrequency waves to produce an image.
- PET is a form of imaging in which the physiology, metabolism, and biochemistry, rather than the anatomic structure, are displayed in the image. Physiology describes how a tissue, organ, or system may function.
- Ultrasound, also known as *sonography,* is a useful medical imaging tool for delineating surface contours and localizing internal structures such as the prostate gland. In this imaging technique, a transducer is used to generate a mechanical disturbance (pressure wave) that moves through the tissue.

Review Questions

Multiple Choice

1. Which of the following additive or destructive conditions affect the radiographic image?
    I. hilar mass
    II. pneumonectomy
    III. edema
    IV. multiple myeloma
    V. atrophy
      a. I, II, and III
      b. II, III, and IV
      c. II, IV, and V
      d. I, II, III, IV, and V
2. A transducer with a piezoelectrical crystal best describes which of the following imaging modalities?
      a. MRI
      b. CT
      c. PET
      d. ultrasound (sonography)
3. Which of the following are considered x-ray interactions occurring with matter?
    I. bremsstrahlung x-rays
    II. Compton scattering
    III. photoelectrical absorption
    IV. rectification
      a. I and II
      b. II and III
      c. II, III, and IV
      d. I, III, and IV
4. An AP radiograph of the pelvis taken at 100 mAs and 67 kVp has too little density. Which of the following would increase the density of the image?
      a. 25 mAs
      b. 50 mAs
      c. 200 mAs
      d. 57 kVp
5. Which of the following *best* refers to the digital imaging process?
      a. analog image intensifier
      b. flat panel detector
      c. bremsstrahlung radiation effect
      d. characteristic radiation effect
6. If a radiograph taken at 120-cm TID produces an image measuring 3.5 cm on the radiograph through the use of a 90-cm TOD, what is the magnification factor?
      a. 0.75
      b. 1.33
      c. 2.63
      d. 4.66
7. Pulse radiofrequency techniques to help produce medical images *best* describes which of the following imaging modalities?
      a. MRI
      b. CT
      c. PET
      d. ultrasound

8. Amorphous silicon is commonly found in:
      a. intensifying screens
      b. photostimulable plates
      c. flat panel detectors
      d. x-ray target material
9. All of the following are methods of extending the life of an x-ray tube *except:*
      a. following manufacturer's warm-up procedure
      b. monitoring the heat units created during multiple exposures
      c. using high mA (filament current) values whenever possible
      d. avoiding multiple exposures near the tube limit
10. Bremsstrahlung interactions occur:
      a. at high energies within the patient
      b. at low energies within the patient
      c. within the x-ray target
      d. as electrons are "boiled off" the filament

The answers to the Review Questions can be found by logging on to our website at: *http://evolve.elsevier.com/Washington+Leaver/principles*

Questions to Ponder

1. Discuss the way that x-rays are used in radiation therapy. Are they different from those used in diagnostic radiology? Explain.
2. Discuss the conditions necessary for the production of x-rays.
3. Compare and contrast bremsstrahlung and characteristic target interactions.
4. Describe the two interactions in matter that have the most effect in the diagnostic imaging range.
5. Briefly explain the image production process involved in MRI, PET, and ultrasound.
6. Define the terms *pixel* and *voxel* and explain how they relate to digital imaging.

REFERENCES

1. American College of Radiology: *ACR standards for radiation oncology,* Reston, VA, 2002, American College of Radiology.
2. Bentel CG: *Radiation therapy planning,* New York, 1993, McGraw-Hill.
3. Bomford CK, et al: Treatment simulators, *Br J Radiol Suppl* 23:4-32, 1989.
4. Bushong SC: *Radiologic science for technologists: physics, biology, and protection,* ed 8, St. Louis, 2004, Mosby.
5. Carlton RR, McKenna-Adler A: *Principles of radiographic imaging,* ed 3, Albany, NY, 2001, Delmar.
6. Chow MF: The effect of a film's sensitivity to its speed, contrast, and latitude, *Can J Med Radiat Technol* 19:147-148, 1988.
7. Christian PE, Waterstram-Rich KM: *Nuclear medicine and PET/CT,* ed 6, St. Louis, 2007, Mosby.
8. Cullinan AM, Cullinan JE: *Producing quality radiographs,* ed 2, Philadelphia, 1993, JB Lippincott.
9. DeVos DC: *Basic principles of radiographic exposure,* Philadelphia, 1990, Lea & Febiger.
10. e-MRI (website): www.e-mri.org. Accessed August 6, 2007.
11. Francis IR, Brown RK, Avram AM: The clinical role of CT/PET in oncology: an update, *Cancer Imaging* 5:S68-S75, 2005.
12. Fuchs AW: Relationship of tissue thickness to kilovoltage, *Radiol Technol* 19:287, 1948.

13. Fuchs AW: The rationale of radiographic exposure, *Radiol Technol* 22:62, 1950.
14. Glasser O: *Dr WC Roentgen*, ed 2, Springfield, IL, 1972, Charles C Thomas.
15. Hendee WR, Ibbott GS, Hendee EG: *Diagnostic imaging and applications to radiation therapy*, ed 3, New York, 2005, John Wiley & Sons.
16. Hufton AP, et al: Low attenuation material for table tops, cassettes and grids: a review, *Radiography* 53:17, 1987.
17. Hunt M: Localization & field design using a CT simulator. In Coia L, editor: *A practical guide to CT simulation*, Madison, WI, 1995, Advanced Medical Publishing.
18. Jarritt PH, et al: The role of PET/CT scanning in radiotherapy planning, *Br J Radiol* 79:S27-S35, 2006.
19. Johnston JN, Killion JB: Hazards in the radiology department, *Radiol Technol* 76:134-144, 2005.
20. Kachelriess M: Clinical x-ray computed tomography. In Schlegel W, Bortfeld T, Grosu AL, editors: *New technologies in radiation oncology*. New York, 2006, Springer.
21. Karzmark CJ, Nunan CS, Tanabe E: *Medical electron accelerators*, Princeton, NJ, 1993, McGraw-Hill.
22. Khan FM: *The physics of radiation therapy*, ed 3, Baltimore, 2003, Lippincott Williams & Wilkins.
23. Kodera Y, Kunio D, Hwang-Ping C: Absolute speeds of screen-film systems and their absorbed-energy constants, *Radiology* 161:229-239, 1984.
24. Malott JC, Fodor J III: *The art and science of medical radiography*, ed 7, St. Louis, 1993, Mosby.
25. Nation Council on Radiation Protection and Measurements: *Medical x-ray, electron beam, and gamma-ray protection of energies up to 50 MeV (equipment design performance and use)*, NCRP Report No. 102, Bethesda, MD, 1989, The Council.
26. National Institute of Occupational Safety and Health (NIOSH): *Glutataldehyde occupational hazards in hospitals,* Washington, DC, 2001, DHHS (NIOSH) Publication No. 2001-115.
27. Oprax Medical International (website): www.opraxmedical.com/Parts/Tubes/CT/. Accessed July 8, 2007.
28. *Physics, techniques and procedures: photostimulable phosphor plate* (website): www.medcyclopaedia.com. Accessed November 20, 2007.
29. Selman J: *The fundamentals of imaging physics and radiobiology physics,* ed 9, Springfield, IL, 2000, Charles C Thomas.
30. Stears JG, et al: Radiologic exchange: resolution according to focal spot size, *Radiol Technol* 60:429-430, 1989.
31. *Thin film-transistor technology* (website): www.eecs.berkeley.edu/~tking/tft.html. Accessed November 24, 2007.

Treatment Delivery Equipment

Dennis Leaver

Outline

Objectives

- Discuss the historic development of radiation therapy treatment delivery equipment.
- Compare and contrast the clinical applications of kilovoltage equipment, including Grenz-ray therapy, contact therapy, superficial treatments, and orthovoltage therapy.
- Describe the four major components of the linear accelerator stand: the klystron, waveguide, circulator, and cooling system.
- Explain how x-rays are produced in the linear accelerator.
- Describe the major components located in the gantry of the linear accelerator, including the electron gun, accelerator structure (guide), and treatment head.
- Explain the concept of indexing as it relates to patient immobilization and positioning.
- Identify where multileaf collimators are located in the treatment head, and explain how they operate.
- Compare and contrast the use of older equipment such as the betatron, Van de Graaff generator, and cobalt unit.
- Discuss the characteristics of cobalt-60.
- Describe emergency procedures related to a cobalt-60 source that fails to retract.
- Discuss medical accelerator safety considerations.

Key Terms

HISTORIC OVERVIEW

The discovery of x-rays by Wilhelm Roentgen in 1895 and the subsequent therapeutic use of radiation have generated a variety of equipment. The features of each system mirrored the technology of the day while addressing the radiobiologic needs of the patient as closely as deemed necessary with the knowledge then available. In the relatively short period since the discovery of these mysterious rays, a great deal of specialized equipment has emerged. The application of this equipment has had most of its success in the treatment of malignant diseases.

This chapter discusses several aspects of related radiation therapy equipment, low-energy machines such as Grenz rays, contact therapy, superficial equipment, and orthovoltage machines. In addition, an overview of high-energy machines, including the Van de Graaff generator, betatron, and cobalt unit, is introduced. The operation of the modern linear accelerator is presented in detail.

EQUIPMENT DEVELOPMENT

Conventional low-energy equipment, which typically uses x-rays generated at voltages up to 300 kVp, has been used in radiation therapy since the turn of the 20th century. These kilovoltage units (low x-ray voltage radiation therapy treatment machines) include Grenz, contact, superficial, and orthovoltage machines. The use of this equipment dramatically decreased after 1950. This was due in part to the increased popularity of cobalt-60 units and subsequent development of the **linear accelerator** (a radiation therapy treatment machine that uses high-frequency electromagnetic waves to accelerate charged particles such as electrons to high energies via a linear tube). However, kilovoltage equipment is still part of many departments today, partly because of the low cost and simplicity of design compared with megavoltage units. The primary application of kilovoltage equipment is in the treatment of skin and superficial lesions.

The introduction of megavoltage therapy equipment, which generated x-ray beams of 1 MV or greater, was a natural progression from low-energy units. Although kilovoltage units were and are beneficial, they still have two principle limitations that are clinically essential: they could not reach deep-seated malignancies with an adequate dosage of radiation, and they did not spare skin and normal tissue. As a result, manufacturers began concentrating their efforts on addressing these and other shortcomings of low-energy equipment.

The early to middle part of the 20th century marked a period of tremendous development of equipment used to treat tumors (Figure 7-1). The physics community began experimenting with the acceleration of electrons, protons, neutrons, and heavy ions. An attempt was made in medicine to find a better way to deliver a curative dose of radiation therapy. In North America, the Van de Graaff (1937), betatron (1941), cobalt-60 (1951), and linear accelerator (1952) were introduced.[11]

Until the early to mid-1950s, most cancer patients undergoing radiation therapy were treated with low-energy equipment. Physicians did their best with the equipment available to them. Surgery was still the treatment of choice for most cancers.

CHARACTERISTICS OF KILOVOLTAGE X-RAY EQUIPMENT

Central-axis-depth dose and physical penumbra are related to beam quality. In treatment planning, the central-axis-depth dose distribution for a specific beam depends on the energy. The depth of an isodose curve increases with beam quality. For example, a 50% **isodose line** (a line representing various points of similar value in a beam along the central axis and elsewhere) for a 200-kVp beam reaches a deeper tumor than a 50% isodose curve of a 100-kVp orthovoltage beam. Orthovoltage beams demonstrate an increased scatter dose to the tissue outside the treatment region, thus exhibiting a marked disadvantage compared with megavoltage beams.[18] In other words, the absorbed dose in the medium outside the primary beam is greater for low-energy beams than for those of a higher energy.[13,14] Limited scatter outside the field for megavoltage beams occurs because of predominantly forward scattering of the beam.

CLINICAL APPLICATIONS OF KILOVOLTAGE EQUIPMENT

Grenz-Ray Therapy

In 1923, Gustav Bucky constructed an x-ray tube with a lithium borate window (Lindemann glass). The window permitted the transmission of long-wavelength x-rays, the physical properties of which Bucky later studied. Consequently, the rays became Bucky rays, or **Grenz rays** (low-energy x-rays having an energy of 10 to 15 kVp). This term comes from *Grenz,* a German word meaning "border." This was an accurate description because *Grenz* rays were thought at the time to lie within a gray zone between x-rays and ultraviolet radiation.

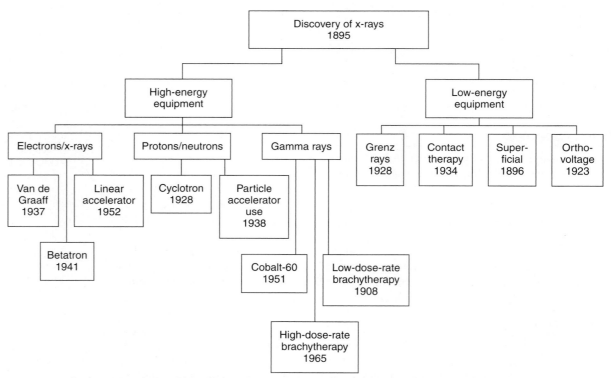

Figure 7-1. A timetable chart illustrates the development of high- and low-energy treatment equipment since the discovery of x-rays in 1895. Every effort has been made in researching the accuracy of the information in this chart. However, several sources and experts in the field sometimes disagree about the exact dates that equipment was introduced clinically. (For more information, refer to Bentel C: *Radiation therapy planning,* New York, 1993, McGraw-Hill; and Grigg EM: *The trail of the invisible light,* Springfield, IL, 1965, Charles C Thomas.)

The construction of a Grenz-ray tube and superficial tube is similar. In a Grenz-ray tube, the envelope is glass and the window is beryllium. Inherent filtration is approximately 0.1 mm aluminum (Al). Like the superficial and orthovoltage units, the quality of Grenz-ray measurements in terms of half-value layer (HVL) is expressed in millimeters of aluminum. Sometimes in dermatology, copper is the metal used to designate the HVL. The intensity of the radiation decreases when the kVp and mA decrease. This intensity also decreases when the distance is increased as a result of the inverse square law. Grenz rays are almost entirely absorbed in the first 2 μm of skin and have a useful depth-dose range of approximately 0.5 μm. The intensity falls off rapidly after this. Less than 2% is capable of reaching the sebaceous glands of the skin.

The application of Grenz rays characteristically is safe and painless for the patient and often yields visible results in 48 to 72 hours. The recommended fractionation involving approximately 200 roentgens (R) per session at weekly intervals totals 800 to 1000 R, followed by a 6-month period before additional treatment may occur. Grenz rays are especially effective for the treatment of inflammatory disorders, namely those involving Langerhans' cells. Grenz rays have also yielded positive results for Bowen's disease, patchy-stage mycosis fungoides, and herpes simplex.[5]

Contact Therapy

Clinical data on contact therapy are scarce. Figure 7-2 illustrates a handheld contact therapy unit. Historically, contact therapy

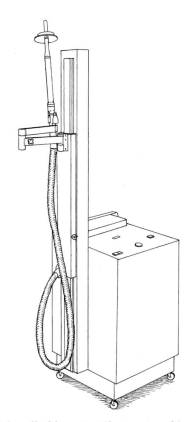

Figure 7-2. A handheld contact-therapy machine used to treat superficial skin lesions. The operators, one to monitor the patient and the other to hold the applicator, must wear protective shielding during the treatment application.

was primarily used to treat superficial skin lesions. The treatment machine derived its name because the treatment unit actually came in contact with the patient. Another use of contact therapy relates to endocavitary treatments for curative intent. This involves a limited group of patients with cancers of the low to middle third of the rectum (Figure 35-5). The rectal cancers treated are confined to the bowel wall in most situations. Papillon has established several criteria for treating rectal lesions by using low-energy x-rays.[22] These criteria are as follows: a maximum tumor size of 3 × 5 cm, a mobile lesion with no significant extension into the anal canal, and a well-differentiated to moderately well-differentiated exophytic tumor that is accessible by the treatment proctoscope (≤10 cm from anal verge). This treatment is especially desirable for the patient because it preserves the anal sphincter. (This may not be true with other methods.) On an outpatient basis, patients received four treatments of 3000 cGy each, separated by a 2-week interval. Papillon used a 50-kVp Philips contact unit. The source-skin distance (SSD) used was 4 cm with 0.50- to 1.0-mm aluminum filtration at a dose rate of 1000 cGy/min. A 3-cm applicator cone can deliver treatments directly to the rectal mucosa via the rectum. Overlapping fields existed if the size of the lesion exceeded the diameter of the applicator.[21] Chapter 35 provides additional details about the use of contact therapy in the treatment of rectal lesions.

Historically, Chaoul contact therapy was the treatment of choice for hemangiomas, especially in the dermatology department of the University Hospital in Munich, Germany. Fractionated doses of 300 to 500 R and total doses ranging from 1200 to 1500 R were delivered to patients in intervals of several days. Most patients showed visible improvement as evidenced by diminished lesion size and less elevation within 8 weeks of treatment. The Chaoul radiation technique was less hazardous than previously used orthovoltage techniques.[7] The popularity of this technique has decreased dramatically since 1975, because large studies have proved conclusively that spontaneous involution of strawberry angiomas (hemangioma simplex) occurs in 95% of cases after several years.[7]

Superficial Treatments

Superficial therapy relates to treatments with x-rays produced at potentials ranging from 50 to 150 kV. Usually, 1- to 6-μm-thick aluminum filters insert in a slot in the treatment head to harden the beam to the desired degree. The degree of hardening is measured in HVLs. Typical HVLs used in superficial treatments range from 1 to 8 mm of Al.[14] Superficial-treatment administration uses a cone or applicator. Cone sizes are generally 2 to 5 cm in diameter. Lead cutouts are tailored to fit the treatment area if needed. The cone lies directly on the skin or lead cutout and generally provides a SSD of 15 to 20 cm. Skin cancer and tumors no deeper than 0.5 cm are treated as a result of the rapid falloff of the radiation.

Three parameters are set at the console area for treatment delivery: kVp, mA (x-ray current measured in milliamperes), and treatment time. Superficial treatment and orthovoltage units are extremely reliable and free of electromechanical problems. This contributes to a lack of downtime, which is a problem more often with linear accelerators. The main difficulty encountered with the use of superficial units arises from having to lock down the unit after the cone is in position. Usually, the unit has a variety of handles or knobs (depending on the model) that require tightening while keeping the cone in place. This can be a challenge. Because no standard treatment table comes with the system, the patient can lie on a stretcher or sit in a chair for treatment, thus amplifying the difficulty of locking down all the knobs and positioning the patient and treatment equipment accurately.

Orthovoltage Therapy

Orthovoltage therapy describes treatment with x-rays produced at potentials ranging from 150 to 500 kV. Most orthovoltage equipment operates at 200 to 300 kV and 10 to 20 mA. Much like the superficial units, orthovoltage units use filters designed to achieve HVLs from 1 to 4 mm of copper (Cu).[3,14] Orthovoltage units can use external or del Regato cones to collimate the beam. In addition, a movable diaphragm consisting of lead plates can be used to adjust the field size. Conventionally, the SSD is 50 cm.

The types of tumors treated with orthovoltage units include skin, mouth, and cervical carcinoma (with the use of cones inserted into the patient). As with superficial treatments, the average treatment time can be seconds to several minutes depending on the filtered kV, prescribed dose, collimator, or cone size. The penetrating depth depends on the kV and filter. Usually, orthovoltage units experience limitation in the treatment of lesions deeper than 2 to 3 cm.

Orthovoltage units are still popular in many clinics and hospitals. They are reliable alternatives to the use of electrons in the treatment of many superficial skin lesions. Most skin lesions treated with orthovoltage units are squamous cell and basal cell cancers. Some clinicians prefer the orthovoltage unit for treating skin tumors because of beam characteristics, especially treatments requiring small fields.

In many departments in which kilovoltage equipment still exists, several treatment units may operate out of the same treatment room. Much of the equipment is older, compared with the design and appearance of modern megavoltage equipment. Historically, when orthovoltage was the highest energy available, treatments were limited by the skin's radiation tolerance. This limitation made the skin-sparing properties of cobalt teletherapy especially desirable and became the major reason for the modern trend to megavoltage beams.

 The 150- to 500-kV x-ray beam is usually better at treating superficial tumors such as skin cancer, because it limits the dose to normal tissue underneath. However, orthovoltage therapy is not as easy to find today in many radiation therapy centers because of the emphasis on the new methods of treating patients such as 3D-CRT, IMRT, and protons.

MEGAVOLTAGE EQUIPMENT

X-ray beams of 1 MV or greater can be classified as **megavoltage equipment**. Examples of clinical megavoltage machines are accelerators such as the linear accelerator (Figure 7-3), Van de Graaff generator, betatron, and cyclotron. Teletherapy units such as cobalt-60 are also classified as megavoltage treatment units.

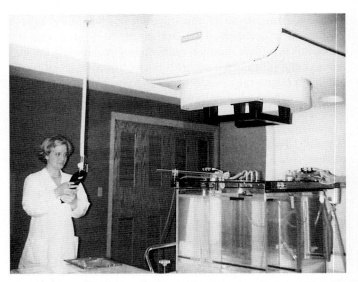

Figure 7-3. A linear accelerator, the Siemens Primus with rectangular water phantom used for measuring radiation beam characteristics.

Linear Accelerator

The term *linear accelerator* means that charged particles travel in straight lines as they gain energy from an alternating electromagnetic field. The linear accelerator (Figure 7-4) is distinguished from other types of particle accelerators such as the cyclotron, in which the particles travel in a spiral pattern, and the **betatron**, in which the particles travel in a circular pattern.[16]

In the linear accelerator, x-rays and electrons are generated and used to treat a variety of tumors.[4,16] The accelerator structure, which resembles a length of pipe, is the basic element of the linear accelerator. The **accelerator structure** allows

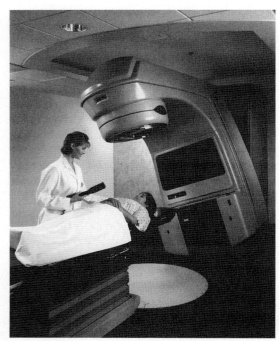

Figure 7-4. A linear accelerator, the 2300 CD. (Copyright ©2007, Varian Medical Systems, Inc. All rights reserved.)

electrons produced from a hot cathode to gain energy until they exit the far end of the hollow structure.[16] Understanding the proper use of this equipment is significant to the radiation therapist because it is one of the essential tools enabling the radiation therapist to deliver a prescribed dose of radiation.

Aspects of the linear accelerator that are discussed in this section include a history of the electron accelerator, its design features, and a description of the major components. An explanation of the key components in a linear accelerator provides a basic overview of its operation and will aid in the student's understanding of this complex piece of equipment. These components include the klystron, waveguide, circulator, water-cooling system, electron gun, accelerator structure, **bending magnet** (used in high-energy linear accelerators to bend the electron stream, sometimes at right angles so that it is pointed at the patient), flattening filter, scattering foil, and other accessories.

History. The first 100-cm source-axis-distance (SAD) "fully isocentric" linear accelerator was manufactured in the United States and installed in 1961 (Figure 7-5). With the linear accelerator, higher-energy beams can be generated with greater skin sparing, field edges are more sharply defined with less penumbra, and computer technology shapes the treatment beam and personnel receive less exposure to radiation leakage.

Development. The development of the linear accelerator has its roots in England and the United States. In these countries, many men and women have contributed significantly to the research and development of the linear accelerator. The magnetron and klystron proved invaluable in the development of and is an important component in the high-energy linear accelerator. The **klystron** is a form of radiowave amplifier that greatly multiplies the amount of introduced radiowaves. The **magnetron** and klystron are two special types of electron tubes that are used to provide microwave power to accelerate electrons. **Microwaves** are similar to ordinary radiowaves but have frequencies thousands of times higher. Microwave frequencies needed for linear accelerator operation are about 3 billion cycles per second (3000 MHz).[15] A major difference between the klystron and magnetron is that a klystron is a linear-beam

microwave amplifier requiring an external oscillator or radio-frequency (RF) source (driver), whereas the magnetron is an oscillator and amplifier. The introduction of the magnetron and klystron assisted in the transfer of energy needed to accelerate electrons, which in turn were converted to high-energy x-rays used in the medical application of the linear accelerator in the treatment of malignant disease.

Medical Application. In the late 1940s, the chief radiologist of Stanford's x-ray department, Dr. Henry Kaplan, became interested in the medical application of the linear accelerator. In addition, a working 1-MV linear accelerator was installed in 1948 at the Fermi Institute in Chicago. The mile-long waveguide, which ran under University Boulevard at the University of Chicago, provided photon and electron beams.[20] Work had also begun in England, but the Stanford University project proved most practical, partly because of the support of President Eisenhower in 1959 and subsequent funding by the U.S. Congress in 1961.

In 1948, the British Ministry of Health brought together the three main groups in England who were working on the linear accelerator project—the Medical Research Council (Dr. L.H. Gray), the Atomic Energy Research Establishment (D.W. Fry), and the Metropolitan Vickers Electric Company (later Associate Electrical Industries) (C.W. Miller). The resulting linear accelerator was installed at Hammersmith Hospital in London in June 1952. The first treatment was delivered on August 19, 1953, with an 8-MV photon beam. Another 4-MV linear accelerator was installed at Newcastle General Hospital (August 1953) and Christie Hospital in Manchester, England (October 1954). The first single gantry unit (Figure 7-6) could be rotated over an arc of 120 degrees by lowering part of the treatment room floor.[16]

The linear accelerator was introduced in England and the United States in the 1950s. In England a 2-MV magnetron and 3-m stationary accelerator were used to produce an output of 100 cGy/min with the 8-MV machine.[9,16] This was a major achievement, even by today's standards. In the United States, a linear accelerator was first clinically used at Stanford University Hospital in January 1956 to treat a child suffering from retinoblastoma. The patient was still disease free 32 years later.[10]

A joint venture between the British industrial work and the Stanford University group under the direction of C.S. Nunan produced the first ergonomic linear accelerator (a 6-MV, isocentric linear accelerator with the ability to rotate 360 degrees around a patient lying supine on the treatment couch).

The evolution of the linear accelerator is discussed in this section with reference to three types of linear accelerators: the early linear accelerators (1953 to 1961); second-generation, 360-degree rotational units (1962 to 1982); and new computer-driven, third-generation treatment machines.

Early Accelerators. The early linear accelerators were extremely large and bulky compared with today's design features. In 1952, the first linear accelerator was installed at Hammersmith Hospital in London and had an 8-MeV x-ray beam and limited gantry motion. Several other linear accelerators with improved design features were also installed in England in the early to mid-1950s. As mentioned previously, the Stanford University linear accelerator in the United States treated its first patient in 1956. Since then, several manufacturers have designed and built linear accelerators for clinical purposes.

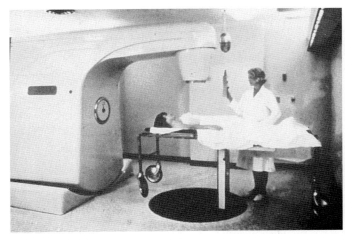

Figure 7-5. The first 100-cm SAD fully isocentric medical linear accelerator manufactured in the United States in 1961 by Varian Associates. (Courtesy Varian Medical Systems, Palo Alto, California.)

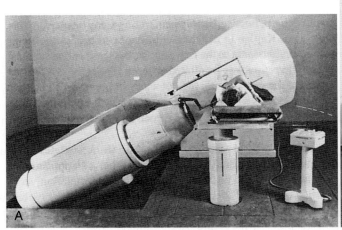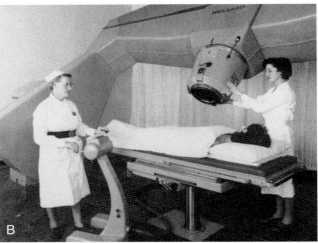

Figure 7-6. A, The first single gantry unit installed at Christie Hospital in Manchester, England, in October 1954. It could rotate over an arc of 120 degrees by lowering part of the treatment floor. **B**, The first clinical linear accelerator manufactured by Mullard (later purchased by Philips Medical Systems) in the United Kingdom, circa 1953. (A, Courtesy Christie Hospital, Manchester; B, courtesy Philips Medical Systems, Shelton, Connecticut.)

Second-Generation Accelerators. Second-generation linear accelerators can be referred to as the older 360-degree rotational units, which are less sophisticated than their modern offspring. These isocentric units, some of which are still operational today, allow treatment to a patient from any gantry angle. They offered an improvement in accuracy and dose delivery over the extremely early models, primarily because of their 360-degree rotational ability around an isocenter.

If two linear-accelerator models built between 1962 and 1982 were compared, many more similarities than differences would be observed, regardless of the manufacturer. Figure 7-7 illustrates two linear accelerators produced by different manufacturers. The similarities in design are related to their major features, such as gantry, treatment couch, and control console.

Second-generation linear accelerators are like some older cars on the road today. They may have more bumps, dents, and high mileage. They may work well at times but usually require a considerable amount of maintenance. An older car has the same basic components as a newer one, such as an engine, transmission, and operator's panel (with fewer knobs and buttons), to accomplish the task. A third-generation linear accelerator is like the newer car of today. The newer car is equipped with many of the basic components of the older, less-sophisticated automobile but has added features such as aerodynamic design, antilock brakes, and computer-integrated components.

Third-Generation Accelerators. In general, third-generation accelerators have improved accelerator-guide, magnet systems, and beam-modifying systems to provide wide ranges of beam energy, dose rate, field size, and operating modes with improved beam characteristics. These accelerators are highly reliable and have compact design features.[16] Today, linear accelerators account for more than 80% of all operational megavoltage treatment units in the world.[16,24]

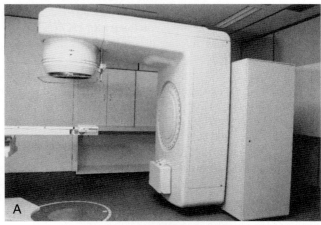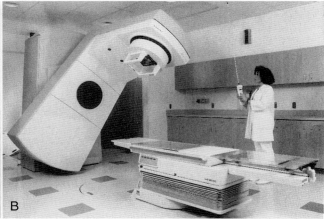

Figure 7-7. A, Philips 75/5 linear accelerator gantry and stand. **B**, Siemens Mevatron gantry, stand, and treatment couch. (A, Courtesy Philips Medical Systems, Shelton, Connecticut; B, courtesy Siemens Medical Systems, Concord, California.)

Third-generation, computer-driven linear accelerators are available with a wide variety of options, which may include dual photon energies, dynamic wedging, multileaf collimation, a choice of several electron energies, electronic portal verification systems, and image-guided apparatus. Because of the advances in three-dimensional treatment planning, some new linear accelerators provide additional features. Before some of these newer features are discussed, a basic understanding of components and design features of a linear accelerator are necessary.

Linear Accelerator Components

A typical linear accelerator (Figure 7-8) consists of a drive stand, gantry, treatment couch, and console electronic cabinet. Some linear accelerators may also have a modulator cabinet, which contains components that distribute and monitor primary electrical power and high-voltage pulses to the magnetron or klystron. Each of the components is critical to the total function and operation of the linear accelerator.

Design Features

In the treatment room, the major components of a linear accelerator can be divided into three specific areas: drive stand, gantry, and treatment couch (see Figure 7-8). A typical treatment room is designed with thick concrete walls for shielding purposes. In this space the gantry is mounted to the **stand**, which is secured to the floor. Most radiation therapy machines have three rotating parts: gantry, collimator, and couch.[1] The treatment unit is positioned in a way that permits 360-degree rotation of the gantry. A treatment couch is mounted on a rotational axis around the isocenter. This permits the positioning of a patient lying supine or prone on the treatment couch. One ceiling and two side lasers project small dots or lines onto predetermined marks (established during the simulation process) on the patient. Sometimes a fourth midsagittal laser is mounted opposite the drive stand, high on the wall in a way that directs a continuous line along the sagittal axis of the patient. This laser may be used to position the patient's midsagittal plane along the long axis of the treatment couch. One or more closed-circuit

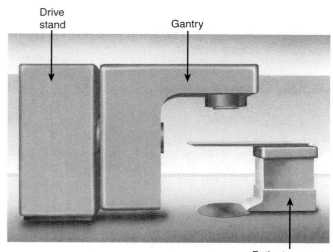

Figure 7-8. The major components of a linear accelerator include a drive stand, gantry, patient support assembly (treatment couch), control console (not shown), and modulator cabinet (also not shown). (Courtesy Robert Morton and Medical Physics Publishing Corp., Madison, Wisconsin.)

television cameras may be mounted on the wall of the treatment room to enable the radiation therapist to monitor the patient during treatment.

Drive Stand. The **gantry** rotates on a horizontal axis on bearings within the drive stand, which is firmly secured to the floor in the treatment room. The drive stand appears as a large, rectangular cabinet, at least as large as the gantry. As its name indicates, the drive stand is a stand containing the apparatus that drives the linear accelerator. The drive stand is usually open on both sides with swinging doors for easy access to gauges, valves, tanks, and buttons. Four major components are housed in the stand: the klystron, waveguide, circulator, and cooling system (Figure 7-9).

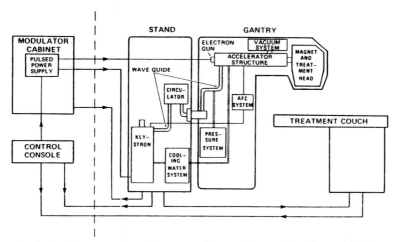

Figure 7-9. Block diagram of a linear accelerator illustrating the major components, including the stand, gantry, treatment couch, modulator cabinet, and control console. *AFC,* Automatic frequency control.(Courtesy Robert Morton and Medical Physics Publishing Corp., Madison, Wisconsin.)

The klystron provides the source of microwave power used to accelerate electrons.[16] This microwave power is directed into the circulator and out to the **waveguide**, much like a copper wire delivers electricity to an outlet in a home. However, the waveguide is usually a hollow, tubelike structure. A **circulator** is placed between the klystron and waveguide. It directs the RF energy into the waveguide and prevents any reflected microwaves from returning to the klystron, thus extending the life of the klystron. The circulator acts much like the valves found in human veins and the lymphatic system, which are designed to prevent the backflow of blood and lymphatic fluid.

The water-cooling system, which is actually a thermal-stability system, allows many components in the gantry and drive stand to operate at a constant temperature. Components cooled by circulating water include the accelerator structure, klystron, circulator, target, and other important assemblies and components. Often the water-cooling system is part of the hospital or medical center's water supply.

 If the engineering department within the hospital needed to shut down the water supply to the radiation therapy department temporarily to repair a valve in another part of the hospital, what would result? Discuss with other students in your class what impact a lack of water would have on the safe operation of a linear accelerator.

Gantry. The gantry is responsible primarily for directing the photon (x-ray) or electron beam at a patient's tumor. It can accomplish this through a single-rotational field or multiple-fixed fields positioned at the isocenter. For isocentric-type treatment, this point is usually positioned in the patient's tumor. The three translations of the **treatment couch** (left/right, up/down, and in/out) move the patient in relationship to the isocenter, thus allowing for precise patient positioning (Figure 7-10).

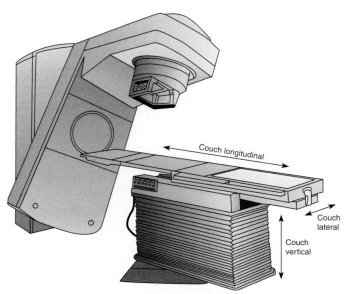

Figure 7-10. Three translations of the treatment couch are shown: in/out, up/down, and left/right. (Courtesy Siemens Medical Systems, Concord, California.)

The controls to the gantry motions are located on a control pendant(s) or the dedicated keyboard outside the room at the console area. Digital readings are also displayed. Gantry angle, collimator rotation, field size (defined by the X and Y collimators), and additional information are commonly displayed for easy reference at the throat of the gantry or on a separate monitor located in the treatment room.

The major components in the gantry are the electron gun, accelerator structure (guide), and treatment head (Figure 7-11).

Electron Gun. The **electron gun** is responsible for producing electrons and injecting them into the accelerator structure. Electron production in a diagnostic x-ray tube is similar to that in a linear accelerator. In the linear accelerator, the cathode is a spherically shaped structure made of a material with a high atomic number, such as tungsten. Tungsten is the element of choice because of the high temperatures required (between 800° and 1100° C). The anode, which carries a positive potential, is separated from the cathode to allow the focus electrode to direct the accelerated electrons through the beam hole in the anode.

Accelerator Guide. The accelerator guide, sometimes called the *accelerator structure,* can be mounted in the gantry horizontally, as illustrated in Figure 7-12 (high-energy machines), or vertically, as illustrated in Figure 7-13 (low-energy machines). Microwave power (produced in the klystron) is transported to the accelerator structure, in which corrugations are used to slow the waves (sometimes analogous to small jetties at a beach used to break up ocean waves). As a result, the crests of the microwave electrical field are made approximately synchronous with the flowing bunches of electrons.[16,27] After the flowing electrons leave the accelerator structure, they are directed toward the target (for photon production) or scattering foil (for electron production) located in the treatment head. In the gantry, x-rays are produced or a treatment beam of electrons is shaped.

 A vertically mounted accelerator structure provides a short distance to accelerate the electrons in a low-energy treatment machine, and a horizontally mounted accelerator structure provides a longer distance to accelerate electrons and equates to a higher-energy linear accelerator treatment machine.

Accelerator Structure. From basic radiologic physics, microwave means "extremely small wavelengths." Because the length of waves is inversely proportional to its energy, energy is high. The microwave frequency needed for the linear accelerator is in the range of 3 million cycles per second. Amplification that occurs in the accelerator structure is in the closed-ended, precision-crafted copper cavities (Figure 7-14). Here, the electrical power provides momentum to the low-level electron stream mixed with the microwaves. An alternating positive and negative electrical charge accelerates the electrons toward the treatment head. Medical linear accelerators accelerate by traveling or standing electromagnetic waves of frequencies in the microwave region. In the standing wave design, the microwave power is joined into the structure by side-coupling cavities, rather than through the beam aperture. This design tends to be more efficient than traveling wave design, but it can be more expensive.[25]

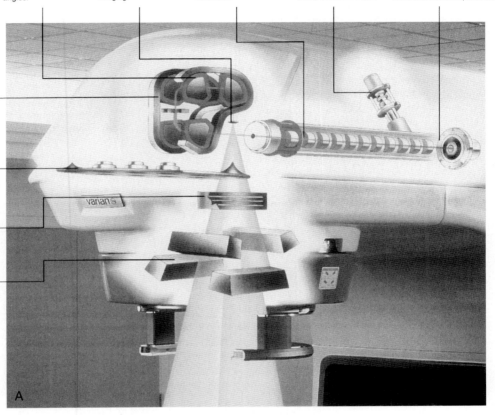

Steering System
Radial and transverse steering coils and a real-time feedback system ensure beam symmetry to within ±2% at all gantry angles.

Focal Spot Size
Even at maximum dose rate, the circular focal remains less than 3.0 mm, held constant by the achromatic bending magnet. Ensures optimal image quality for portal imaging.

Standing Wave Accelerator Guide
Maintains optimal bunching for different acceleration conditions, providing high dose rates, stable dosimetry, and low-stray radiation. Transport system minimizes power and electron source demands.

Energy Switch
Patented switch provides energies within the full therapeutic range, at consistently high, stable dose rates, even with low energy X-ray beams. Ensures optimal performance and spectral purity at both energies.

Gridded Electron Gun
Controls dose rate rapidly and accurately. Permits precise beam control for dynamic treatments because gun can be gated. Demountable, for cost-efffective replacement.

Achromatic Dual-Plane Bending Magnet
Unique design with ±3% energy slits ensures exact replication of the input beam for every treatment. Clinac 2300C/D design enhancements allow wider range of beam energies.

10-Port Carousel with Scattering Foils/Flattening Filters
Extra ports allow future specialized beams to be developed. New electron scattering foils provide homogeneous electron beams at therapeutic depths.

Ion Chamber
Two independently sealed chambers, impervious to temperature and pressure changes, monitor beam dosimetry to within 2% for long-term consistency and stability.

Asymmetric Jaws
Four independent collimators provide flexible beam definition of symmetric or asymmetric fields.

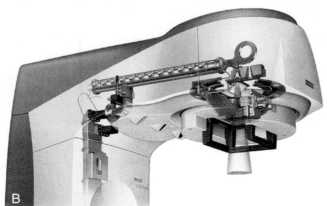

Figure 7-11. A, The major components of the gantry include the electron gun, accelerator guide, and treatment head, which includes components such as the bending magnet, beam-flattening filter, ion chamber, and upper-lower collimator jaws. **B**, Cross-sectional view of the accelerator structure, bending magnet, field light mirror, and multileaf collimator. (A, Courtesy Varian Medical Systems, Palo Alto, California; B, Courtesy of Siemens Medical Systems, Concord, California.)

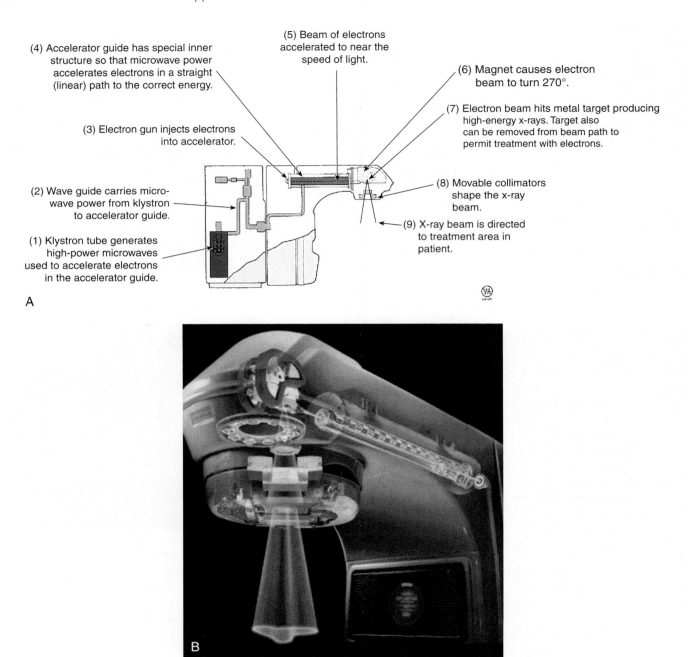

(4) Accelerator guide has special inner structure so that microwave power accelerates electrons in a straight (linear) path to the correct energy.

(5) Beam of electrons accelerated to near the speed of light.

(6) Magnet causes electron beam to turn 270°.

(3) Electron gun injects electrons into accelerator.

(7) Electron beam hits metal target producing high-energy x-rays. Target also can be removed from beam path to permit treatment with electrons.

(2) Wave guide carries micro-wave power from klystron to accelerator guide.

(8) Movable collimators shape the x-ray beam.

(1) Klystron tube generates high-power microwaves used to accelerate electrons in the accelerator guide.

(9) X-ray beam is directed to treatment area in patient.

A

B

Figure 7-12. A, This high-energy radiation therapy treatment machine illustrates the horizontally mounted accelerator structure and 270-degree bending magnet. **B,** The horizontally mounted accelerator structure and treatment head depict the path of the electron and x-ray beam. (Courtesy Varian Medical Systems.)

The length of the accelerator structure varies depending on the beam energy of the linear accelerator. The length may vary from 30 cm for a 4-MV unit to 1 m or more for high-energy units.[15,16] For high-energy linear accelerators, up to five cavities are sometimes used to accelerate the electron bunch enough to generate the desired microwave energy. The therapist should remember that as more cavities are used, higher energy is derived. After electrons leave the accelerator structure, they are directed toward the treatment head. The treatment head may contain various beam-shaping devices, radiation monitors, and possibly a bending magnet if a horizontal accelerator structure is used.

Treatment Head. Several components designed to shape and monitor the treatment beam are located in the treatment head (Figure 7-15). For photon therapy, these components may consist of a bending magnet; x-ray target; primary collimator; beam-flattening filter; ion chamber; secondary collimators; and one or more slots for wedges, blocks, and compensators.

The horizontal accelerator structure required for an 18-MV photon beam needs a bending magnet to direct the electrons vertically toward a supine patient for an anterior treatment (otherwise, the electrons would continue straight out, horizontally

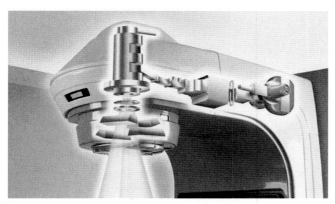

Figure 7-13. A low-energy linear accelerator demonstrates the vertically mounted, straight-through beam design, which eliminates the need for complex beam-bending magnet systems. (Courtesy Varian Medical Systems.)

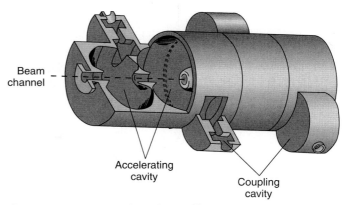

Figure 7-14. Cross section of a standing-wave accelerator structure used in high-energy treatment units. (Courtesy Siemens Corporation, Concord, California.)

through the treatment head of the gantry). A magnet system may bend the electron group through a net angle of approximately 90 to 270 degrees and onto the x-ray target (or scattering foil for electron production).[16] After emerging from the x-ray target, the x-rays produced are shaped by a primary collimator, which is designed to limit the maximum field size. A **beam-flattening filter** located on the carousel with the scattering foil (Figure 7-16) shapes the x-ray beam in its cross-sectional dimension. The beam flattening filter is a conical metal absorber that absorbs more photons from the central axis and fewer from

the periphery of the beam.[15] If the linear accelerator offers duel-energy photons, then two beam-flattening filters, one for each energy are used to provide more uniform treatment fields. Flattening filters have been constructed of tungsten, steel, lead, uranium, aluminum, or some combination of these metals depending on the x-ray energy.[23] The **scattering foil**, also positioned on the carousel, is used in the electron mode. When electrons are used for treatment instead of x-rays, the target is retracted and a scattering foil that matches the electron energy called for is moved in place to broaden the pencil-like electron

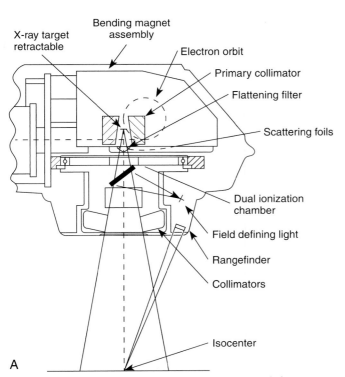

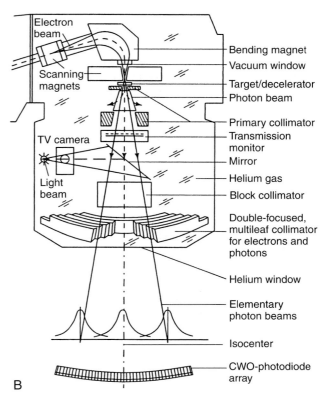

Figure 7-15. A, Cross section of the treatment head of a high-energy linear accelerator. **B,** Medical micotron. (A, Courtesy CJ Karzmark and Varian Associates, Palo Alto, California; B, courtesy A. Brahme and Scandinavian University Press, Stockholm.)

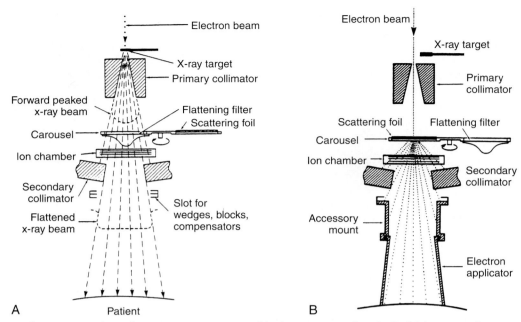

Figure 7-16. The subsystem components with the treatment head of a high-energy linear accelerator. **A**, Note the beam subsystem is in the x-ray mode, indicated by the position of the flattening filter. **B**, The subsystem in the electron mode is indicated by the position of the scattering foil. (Courtesy Robert Morton and Medical Physics Publishing Corp., Madison, Wisconsin.)

beam and produce a flat field across the treatment field. A different scattering foil is used for each electron energy. The scattering foil system usually consists of dual lead foils, where the first foil scatters most of the electrons with a minimum of bremsstrahlung x-rays. The second foil may be thicker in the central region to flatten the field. The small amount of bremsstrahlung contamination produced with an electron beam is usually less than 5% of the beam.[23]

An ion chamber monitors the beam for its symmetry in the right-left and inferior-superior direction. In most cases, the monitoring system consists of several transmission-type parallel plate ionization chambers. These chambers are used to monitor the integrated dose, the field symmetry, and the dose rate.[23] Secondary collimation is achieved through remote control to adjust the upper and lower collimator jaws, usually made of lead or depleted uranium. On newer units, secondary collimation may also be automatically set from the treatment console outside the room, using software to preset the patient's field size. Additional beam-shaping and modifying devices in addition to multileaf collimators (MLCs), such as a wedge, compensator, or custom shielding blocks, can be placed in slots just below the secondary collimators.

In addition, a field light is located in the treatment head. Light from a quartz-iodine bulb outlines the dimensions of the radiation field as it appears on the patient (Figure 7-17). This alignment of the radiation and light fields allows accurate positioning of the radiation field in relationship to skin marks or other reference points. When the secondary collimators are positioned to the desired width and length for the patient's setup, the reflected light field corresponds to the desired width

and length of the radiation field. MLCs or Cerrobend blocking may further define the light field to correspond to the desired treatment field shape.

Control Console. Monitoring and controlling of the linear accelerator occur at the control console. Located outside the treatment room, the control console may take the form of a digital display, push-button panel, and/or video display terminal (VDT) in which the machine status and patient-treatment information are incorporated into the computerized treatment unit. The ready state of the equipment allows the therapist to

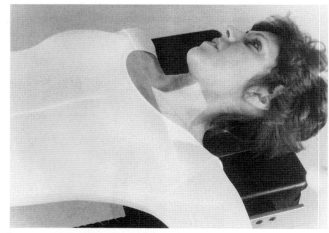

Figure 7-17. A light field, directed from a quartz-iodine bulb in the treatment head, corresponds to the radiation field in this anterior supraclavicular field. (Courtesy Varian Medical Systems.)

confirm the treatment parameters. All interlocks must be satisfied for the machine to allow the beam to be started. A lighted message on the VDT usually indicates that the machine is in the ready state. An indicator for the beam-on state remains on throughout the patient's treatment until the prescribed dose is delivered.

Monitoring the patient visually with a remote video monitor(s) and a sound system during treatment is essential. Both the visual and aural monitors must be functional to safely deliver a prescribed dose of radiation therapy. This is especially important for lengthy treatment sessions. Some treatment plans may take more than 20 minutes, depending on the number of beams used in the treatment plan.

Interlock displays can occur before or during a treatment. The **interlock system** is designed to protect the patient, staff members, and equipment from hazards. Patient-protection interlocks, including beam energy, beam symmetry, dose, and dose-rate monitoring, prevent radiation and mechanical hazards to the patient. For example, interlocks protect the patient against extremely high dose rates, especially if the treatment unit provides x-ray and electron beams. Because of the high electron-beam currents used for x-ray production, extremely high dose rates can result if the target or flattening filter does not intercept the beam. Machine interlocks protect the equipment from damage, which may include problems detected in the machine's high-voltage power supply, water-cooling system, or vacuum system.

Emergency off buttons, which can terminate irradiation and machine functions, are located on the control panel and at several other locations in the treatment room. These switches terminate all electrical power to the equipment and require a complete start-up procedure before the treatment machine can produce an electron or photon beam.

 As a radiation therapist, you witness the table begin to rise after the correct dose has been delivered for the first treatment field. You press the emergency "off" button located on the wall near the gantry, but nothing happens. What would you do next?

Besides displaying the operational mode of the treatment unit, the control console serves several other functions. It may provide a digital display for prescribed dose (monitor units), mechanical beam parameters such as collimator setting, MLC settings (on a separate monitor) or gantry angle, and possibly up to 50 other status messages.[16] Overall, the treatment control console provides a central location for controlling and operating the linear accelerator.

Treatment Couch. The treatment couch is the area on which patients are positioned to receive their radiation treatment. Several unique features of the treatment couch provide the tabletop with mobility. A standard feature allows the tabletop to move mechanically in a horizontal and lengthwise direction. This movement must be smooth and accurate with the patient in the treatment position, thus allowing for precise and exact positioning of the isocenter during treatment positioning. Many tabletops support up to 160 kg (350 lb) and range in width from 45 to 50 cm. If the couch width on the simulator is not similar to that of the treatment unit, reproducibility may become a problem, especially with large patients.

Some manufacturers offer the same **indexed carbon fiber couch** top for their simulator and treatment units. Indexing allows for increased accuracy in treatment setup reproducibility from simulation to treatment delivery and through multiple treatments over the course of daily radiation therapy delivery. The transfer of information, such as the exact location of immobilization devices, from simulation to the treatment machine is improved when devices are referenced or indexed to the treatment table. The patient and immobilization device are then "locked" into place on the treatment table using a system of numbered or lettered holes, or notches, along the lateral edge of the carbon fiber tabletop. In some models, moveable side rails allow all clinical setups, eliminating the need to reposition patients or to move the couch. The carbon fiber couch top facilitates higher image quality and improved dose distribution by reducing scatter radiation.[34] Indexing is essential for accurate treatment, especially where **intensity modulated radiation therapy (IMRT)** is used.

In addition, a set of local controls may be located on the treatment couch. These can mimic those of the conventional simulator unit as a pendant(s) (handheld control) suspended from the ceiling or attached to the base of the treatment couch. In some models, a portion of the local controls can be located on one or both sides of the treatment couch. In either situation, the controls should allow access to the mechanical movements and optical features of the treatment unit.

Although base support may differ, some treatment couches contain bellowlike curtain molding covering the motorized base that supports the horizontal tabletop. Other treatment couches may be mounted on a vertical column called a *ram*.

Modulator Cabinet. This important component of the linear accelerator is usually located in the treatment room and is the noisiest part of the ensemble. In some systems, the modulator cabinet contains three major components: the fan control, auxiliary power-distribution system, and primary power-distribution system. The fan-control switch automatically turns the fans off and on as the need arises for cooling the power distribution (auxiliary and primary) in the modulator cabinet. The auxiliary power-distribution panel contains the emergency off button that shuts off the power to the treatment unit.

Applied Technology

Computer-controlled accelerators include multimodality treatment units. Because of their increased flexibility in design and dose delivery, these accelerators are used by more radiation treatment centers. Dual-photon energies (ranging from a 4-MV low-energy x-ray beam to high-energy x-ray beams of 15 to 35 MV) provide the radiation oncologist with more options in treating a wide range of diseases. In addition, several electron energies ranging from 4 to 22 MeV are available to treat more superficial tumors. Table 7-1 categorizes linear accelerators based on energy. Multimodality treatment units offer several advantages. Because of their dual photon energies, they can provide backup for other treatment units that may experience downtime as a result of electrical, mechanical, or software problems. In addition, patients can be treated with multiple beam energies on the same treatment unit. In some centers with multiple treatment units, identical calibrations for each treatment

Table 7-1	Energy Range of Linear Accelerators
Energy Range	**Features**
Low	4 to 6 MV; x-rays
Medium	8 to 12 MV; x-rays and electrons
High	15 to 35 MV; x-rays, electrons, and special features

machine are completed to allow for additional flexibility in managing treatment delays.

State-of-the-Art Technologies. Numerous technologies are allowing radiation oncologists and radiation therapists to increase radiation doses to various tumor sites. These include conformal radiation therapy, dynamic wedging, independent jaws, MLCs, electronic portal imaging and **image-guided radiation therapy (IGRT)**.

Three-dimensional conformal radiation therapy (3D-CRT), in which the field shape and beam angle change as the gantry moves around the patient, requires sophisticated computer-controlled equipment. Conformal therapy has certain advantages over traditional forms of therapy (Figure 7-18). IMRT, which is a type of 3D-CRT, has provided a significant technologic advance in radiation therapy treatment planning. This method of delivering the prescribed dose of radiation therapy has proved beneficial in escalating the dose to the tumor volume and reducing the dose to normal tissue.[6,14,35] Traditionally, with the process of 3D-CRT, images from computed tomography (CT), magnetic resonance imaging (MRI), and positron emission tomography (PET) are transferred to treatment planning computers, where normal tissues and tumor volumes are defined. Treatment plans developed using 3D-CRT are done so with a "forward planning" process, where beam arrangements are tested by trial and error, until a satisfactory dose distribution is produced. This can be very time-consuming for complex cases. IMRT develops treatment plans using "inverse treatment planning."

With inverse treatment planning, the radiation oncologist selects dose parameters for normal tissues and the target volume and the computer "back calculates" the desired dose distribution and beam arrangements.[8,35] The IMRT targeting computer also adjusts the intensity of radiation beam across the field with the aid of MLC moving in and out of the beam portal under precise computer guidance.[18]

A **dynamic wedge** is used for computerized shaping of the treatment field (Figure 7-19). It has the ability, under computer control, to modify and shape the desired isodose distribution using the large field-defining collimator or jaw. The computer-controlled dynamic wedge can be used in place of a 15-, 30-, 45-, or 60-degree "hard" wedge. Dynamic wedges are designed in such a way that wedge-dose distributions using varying field sizes yield excellent wedged-isodose distributions compared with physical wedges.[17] This design relies strongly on computer software to vary the dose rate and mechanical motion of the collimator during treatment. When the beam is turned on, the dose rate and collimator setting are automatically set according to a pregenerated treatment plan. The field size changes to generate the desired wedge angle.

Dual asymmetric jaws provide a variety of options for treatment purposes. Traditionally, the upper and lower collimators, or *jaws,* moved symmetrically to define the width and length of a treatment field. However, for some treatments requiring abutting fields, independent motion of one or both sets of jaws may be desirable. A sharp, nondivergent field edge is obtained by closing one of the jaws to the beam's central axis, thereby shielding half the radiation field. This eliminates the need for heavy Cerrobend custom blocks. Use of the independent jaw motion necessitates accurate and precise treatment positioning to avoid treatment-field overlap. This technique may be useful in the treatment of the central nervous system, breast, sarcoma, and other sites requiring abutting fields. The dosimetry, treatment planning, and specifications of these asymmetrical fields are much more complex.[17,21]

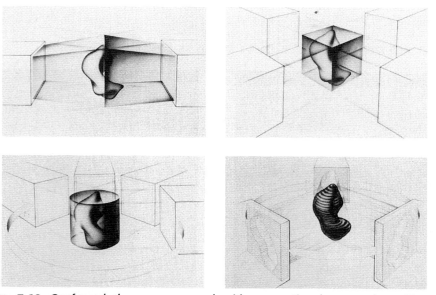

Figure 7-18. Conformal therapy compared with conventional approaches. (Courtesy Dr. Alan Lichter, University of Michigan, Ann Arbor, Michigan.)

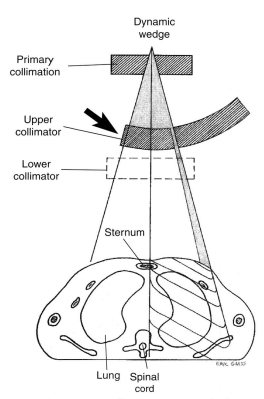

Figure 7-19. The upper collimator moves during treatment to create a dynamic wedge effect. (Courtesy Varian Medical Systems.)

Several **multileaf collimator (MLC)** systems exist that shield an area by using approximately 52 to 160 leaves. These heavy, metal collimator rods slide into place to form the desired field shape by projecting 0.5-cm to 2-cm beam widths per rod.[16] Figure 7-20 demonstrates a typical image created with an MLC. This beam-shaping technique is especially critical for full-field beam shaping using IMRT. Two concerns should be evaluated in using MLC beam shaping. Penumbra at the end of individual leaves may be increased depending on the angle of the leaf and its position within the treatment field (along the field edge or near the central portion of the treatment beam). Penumbra adds to a small amount of dose uncertainty along the edge of the shaped field. With multiple fields, as is common with 3D-CRT, the problem is minimized because the dose is spread out over multiple fields.[14] A second physics consideration is the interleaf transmission leakage. This may be on average of 2.5% and as high as 4% in some MLC configurations and should be considered when treating a large number of fields (especially using IMRT) requiring a higher number of monitor units to deliver the prescribed dose.[8,34,35]

 Some manufacturers provide multileaf collimators with 5-mm leaves in the central portion of the field and larger leaves on the perimeter of the field. This is helpful for conventional head and neck treatments, traditional conformal radiation therapy, and intricate IMRT techniques using small fields to deliver the dose.[34]

An **electronic portal imaging device (EPID)** is another method of improving treatment-field accuracy and verification. With older portal systems, cassettes are positioned in the slot under the treatment couch for anteroposterior (AP) films or placed in a cassette holder for posteroanterior (PA), lateral, and oblique field positions. With portal imaging technology, correct positioning of internal anatomic structures can be observed during the entire treatment process or checked by pretreatment imaging with the aid of computer software. Most electronic portal imaging systems are lightweight and come with a retracted arm along the gantry's axis (Figure 7-21). The arm is equipped with amorphous silicon (aSi) imaging technology, which provides a quick and accurate comparison of its images with reference images, without loss of patient data or duplicate entry. Images can be reviewed immediately online in the control room, or later with traditional offline review tools.[34] Despite the poor image quality common with regular port films (as a result of Compton and pair-production interactions), comparable quality images are possible using EPID. A new type of portal imaging process is available on some models, which provides superior radiographic detail and contrast compared with traditional EPID and is described in the section on IGRT.

The position of the image detector in relationship to the patient can affect image quality through magnification and scatter radiation. Bissonnette et al.[2] have shown that a magnification factor of 1.6 is optimal for television-based camera portal imaging systems. Swindell et al.[31] found that an object-image-receptor distance (OID) of 40 cm is sufficient to reduce the effects of scatter radiation on image quality. Attention to details such as scatter radiation and magnification is an important factor in improving an already somewhat poor image quality with traditional portal imaging.

Because it allows real-time monitoring of patients during treatment, portal imaging is also used to detect movement during treatment and to assess patient positional changes. In fact, in a study by Tinger et al.,[32] who examined systematic and random setup errors in patients treated with pelvic irradiation, EPID images were used to document field displacements. In this study using 547 images, there was no documented intra-treatment displacement in excess of 1 cm. However, intertreatment displacement exceeding 1 cm was documented in 23% of the patients in the AP, 16% in the superior-inferior, and 3% in the mediolateral direction. EPID are also used to detect patient movement, organ movement, and patient positioning in other areas such as the breast and abdomen.

Image-Guided Radiation Therapy. The newest imaging technology, IGRT, has the potential to improve the application of radiation therapy dose delivery. It may be used in a variety of forms, including EPID, an in-room CT scanner, KV cone-beam CT, MV cone-beam CT, ultrasound, and others. The rational for IGRT, is to image the patient just before treatment and compare the position of external setup marks and internal anatomy to the treatment plan. Shifts in patient position are made for each fraction just before treatment delivery. Recent studies have indicated that there is substantial interfractional and intrafractional variations in the shape, volume, and position of treatment targets and the normal surrounding tissue.[8] The cause of such variations may include respiratory motion, movement of the body or internal structures, weight loss, and radiation-induced changes such as tumor shrinkage. IGRT can track changes in patient positioning due to some of these variations.

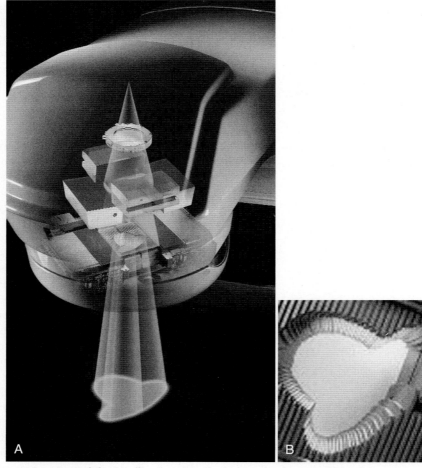

Figure 7-20. A, Multileaf collimator (MLC) shapes the beam within the treatment head under precise computer control. **B**, Leaf position is programmed to provide accurate beam shape and modify the beam intensity, especially during IMRT applications. (Courtesy Varian Medical Systems.)

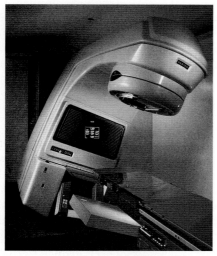

Figure 7-21. Fully retractable and collapsible gantry-mounted detector used in an electronic portal-imaging system. (Copyright ©2007, Varian Medical Systems, Inc. All rights reserved.)

Traditional EPID utilizing megavoltage (MV) x-ray beams are used to check patient position before or at the end of treatment. Disadvantages of the pretreatment MV imaging include high imaging dose (1 to 5 cGy) and poor image quality due to the high energy x-ray beams. All three major manufacturers—Elekta, Varian, and Seimens—are offering a type of kilovoltage x-ray imaging system that is installed at right angles to the treatment beam and may provide radiographic, fluoroscopic, and cone-beam CT modes to visualize patient anatomy.[14]

The use of on-board imagers (OBI), which use a source of kV x-rays and a flat panel image detector, represents a major breakthrough in radiation therapy portal imaging (Figure 7-22). The traditional MV x-ray beams used for EPIDs demonstrate poor image quality (poor contrast) and make bony anatomy difficult to see. The better-detailed kV image resembles conventional simulation images and diagnostic-quality x-ray images and provide more information related to soft tissue and bony anatomy comparison. Some centers used embedded fiducial markers to tract patient setup inaccuracies. The use of on-board imaging enables the tracking of these fiducial markers after the daily setup of the patient and before the delivery of treatment. With or without fiducial markers, this type of IGRT will allow daily checks of patient positioning prior to and/or during treatment for every patient scheduled on the treatment unit.[18]

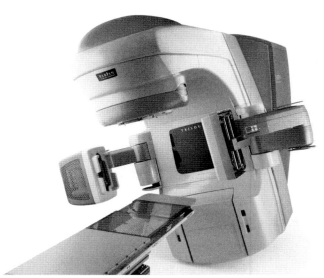

Figure 7-22. Varian's Trilogy system has a kV x-ray imaging system, which provides radiographic, fluoroscopic, and cone beam CT modes for tracking patient position. (Courtesy Varian Medical Systems.)

 Identification of radiographic anatomy is very important in comparing on-board images produced on the treatment machine with DRRs (produced at the time of simulation) or other images used as "masters" for comparison of the patient setup. Useful radiographic anatomy in the thorax includes the carina, which is located at the level of T4-5. Useful radiographic anatomy in the abdomen includes the iliac crest, which is located at the level of L4. (See Chapter 20 on Surface and Sectional Anatomy for additional information.)

Verification and Recording Devices. Computers are used to assist the radiation therapist in the verification of treatment parameters. If the average number of patients treated on a linear accelerator is assumed to be between 30 and 35 patients per day, and each patient may have an average of 20 separate parameters (e.g., gantry angle, treatment distance, field size), this equates to 600 to 700 parameters that must be matched each day. Verification systems not only allow incorrect setup parameters to be corrected before the machine is turned on but may also provide data in other areas, such as computer-assisted setup, recording of patient data, allowing for data transfer from the simulator or treatment planning computer, and assisting with quality control. See Chapter 27 on e-charting and image management for a more detailed discussion.

Medical Accelerator Safety Considerations

With the increased use of multimodality treatment units, potential hazards exist that usually are not present in single-modality treatment units.[26] Monitoring and controlling safe operating conditions for a computer-driven linear accelerator are more difficult than for the more conventional, electromechanical type.

Emergency Procedures. Emergency procedures, if implemented properly, can prevent a serious accident and possibly save a patient's life. Written emergency procedures should be located at or near the treatment-control console. (Some state regulatory agencies require this.) Radiation therapists should

be familiar with written procedures in the event of a patient emergency. Knowing the location of emergency stop buttons (inside and outside the treatment room) is critical in the event of a machine malfunction. Other emergencies involving the patient's medical condition may also require the therapist's attention.

Safety Considerations. Electrical, mechanical, and radiation-safety considerations must be more elaborate with multimodality treatment units because of the accelerator's increased flexibility. An example may better portray the need for more elaborate safety considerations.

The failure of some software can allow the delivery of large doses. For example, if a large electron-beam current intended for x-ray production is used for an electron treatment, an extremely large dose rate can result. If the scattering foil is in place or the beam scanning is operational, an estimated dose comparable with a typical 2-Gy dose fraction can be delivered to a patient in 0.03 second at 4000 Gy/min. This dose rate can create hazards for the patient. To address this type of problem, digital logic and microprocessors have been incorporated into the linear accelerator control and monitor functions.[26]

Potentially dangerous problems can result from **misadministration** of a prescribed radiation dose. A misadministration (incorrect application or delivery of a prescribed dose of radiation therapy) can be minor or major and may cause death or serious injury to the patient depending on the extent of the dose. The U.S. Food and Drug Administration defines an accident that can cause death or serious injury as a Class I hazard. If the risk of serious injury is low, because of human error or a linear accelerator malfunction, the accident is classified as a Class II hazard.[26]

The American Association of Physicists in Medicine (AAPM) Radiation Therapy Committee Task Group Number 35 has developed a list containing most of the causes of potentially life-threatening problems associated with electrical, mechanical, human, and software errors involving medical linear accelerators[26] (Table 7-2).

Table 7-2	**Medical Accelerator Hazards**	
Type	**Cause**	**Consequences**
Incorrect dose delivered	Electrical, software, and therapist	Serious injury, increased complications, genetic effects, second primary, and compromised tumor control
Dose delivered to the wrong area	Mechanical, software, patient motion, and therapist	Serious injury, increased complications, genetic effects, second primary, and compromised tumor control
Machine collision	Mechanical, software, patient motion, and therapist	Significant injury and death
Incorrect beam	Electrical, software, and therapist	Serious injury, increased complications, genetic effects, second primary, and compromised tumor control
General hazards	Electrical and mechanical	Significant injury and death

A comprehensive understanding of and familiarization with the design, characteristics, performance parameters, and control of the linear accelerator are essential for many of the members of the cancer-management team. In addition, the mechanical, electrical, software, and radiation-safety considerations are critical to applying the theory and operation of a linear accelerator to patients needing treatment.

Although the linear accelerator is the most widely accepted treatment machine in developed countries, it is worth discussing historic methods of delivering a tumoricidal dose, especially the megavoltage treatment machines, such as the betatron, Van de Graaff generator, and cobalt unit.

Betatron

The first betatron, developed by Kerst in 1941, produced x-rays of 2 MV.[19] Betatrons (megavoltage treatment units that can provide x-ray and electron therapy beams from less than 6 to more than 40 MeV) were initially used for radiation therapy in the early 1950s.[14,18] Besides medical uses, betatrons were applied to industrial radiography. Betatrons were used especially during World War II, when they provided the energy to x-ray thick castings and other metal sections of equipment used in wartime.

The operation of the betatron is based on the principle that an electron in a changing magnetic field experiences acceleration in a circular orbit.

One advantage of the betatron is the production of electrons for use with superficial tumors. In addition, x-rays can be used for hard-to-reach tumors at great depths. Betatrons capture and transport a smaller-than-average beam current compared with linear accelerators and are most often used for electron therapy. However, medical betatrons (Figure 7-23) can produce x-ray beams with energies more than 40 MV.[23]

The betatron generally used Lucite cones of various sizes, ranging from 15×15 cm to 8×8 cm at 100 SSD. Common tumors treated with the betatron included mostly gynecologic, bladder, and prostate carcinomas. The treatment times depended on the prescribed dose and diameter of the patient. They usually averaged 3 to 5 minutes and used a dose rate of

200 cGy/min. To compensate for the characteristically noisy machine, therapists applied cotton balls and ear mufflers for patients who wanted some noise reduction during treatments.

Van de Graaff Generator

Another historic medical accelerator, which has continued to diminish in popularity, is the Van de Graaff generator. In 1937, R.J. Van de Graaff, while working at the Massachusetts Institute of Technology, developed the first electrostatic linear accelerator. Accelerators may be circular or linear, and the linear type is electrostatic (such as the Van de Graaff) or electronic.[10]

The Van de Graaff is a constant potential electrostatic generator developed around the physical principle illustrated by the classic Faraday "ice bucket" experiment. The hemispheric high-voltage dome is analogous to the ice bucket (Figure 7-24). In the ice bucket experiment, electrons deposited inside the electrically conducted metal bucket (presumably used for carrying ice in earlier days) quickly move to the outside. The process can continue until a specified potential is attained or until there is a coronal breakdown of the air outside the bucket.[18]

These 2-MV units have a steel dome of about 3 feet in diameter and 5½ feet in height and are constructed nonisocentrically. Van de Graaff units use an external blocking tray to hold hand-placed blocks. Because no standard table is affixed to this unit, the patient lies on a stretcher underneath the machine or can even be placed in a chair if necessary. Blocking can be

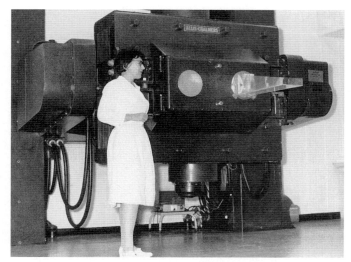

Figure 7-23. The Allis-Chalmers betatron. (Courtesy M.D. Anderson Cancer Center, Houston, Texas.)

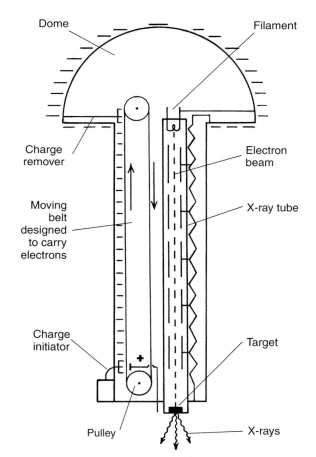

Figure 7-24. A schematic diagram of the Van de Graaff generator.

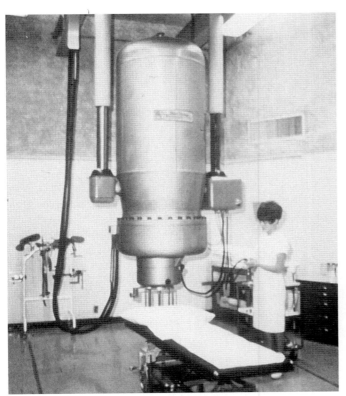

Figure 7-25. The Van de Graaff unit at the University Hospital in Oklahoma City, Oklahoma, was routinely used to treat seminoma, whole brain, and mantle fields. (Courtesy University Hospital, Oklahoma City, Oklahoma.)

dangerous because blocks frequently require stacking to approximate the treatment area. Van de Graaff units can operate at 200 cGy/min and provide a standard SSD of 100 cm, but they can also approximate much greater treatment distances. This was extremely useful in the treatment of extended fields needed to treat a variety of malignancies. The Van de Graaff unit (Figure 7-25) was routinely used to treat seminoma (a lengthy field in the abdomen and pelvis is used to treat this type of testicular cancer), whole brain, and mantle field (used to treat lymph nodes in the neck and thorax for Hodgkin's disease).

Arcing was frequent for radiation therapists warming up these units, which could sometimes require as long as 1 hour. When setting up a patient for treatment, the therapist used a front-pointer device to measure the distance to the patient. No optical distance indicator was available. However, the Van de Graaff unit could treat any tumor that other megavoltage equipment could treat. Its bulk made it cumbersome to use, and it was replaced by the isocentric linear accelerator, which is more popular today.

Cobalt Unit

Today, increasingly fewer cobalt-60 (^{60}Co) units are used for the treatment of cancer in the United States. In the 1980s, ^{60}Co units were the mainstay of most radiation oncology departments. The decrease began in the 1960s with the introduction of the linear accelerator, because linear accelerators provided better isodose distribution (greater dose to the tumor and less dose to normal tissue), faster dose rate, and more manageable radiation protection concerns. Despite the decline in popularity of ^{60}Co units

in the United States, they are the backbone of many radiation therapy departments in developing countries. This is probably due to the unit's cost, simpler design, and reliability.[30]

In the early 1950s, ^{60}Co units became popular because they could deliver a significant dose of radiation below the skin surface. Compared with earlier **teletherapy** (treatment at some distance) units such as radium and cesium treatment machines, ^{60}Co units were faster at delivering the dose and more cost-effective at producing and using the isotope. At the time, mining the ore necessary to produce a small amount of radium was extremely expensive. The ^{60}Co units were the first practical radiation therapy treatment units to provide a significant dose below the skin surface and simultaneously spare the skin the harsh effects of earlier methods. This allowed the radiation oncologist and radiation therapist to deliver larger doses of radiation to greater depths in tissue. When a greater percentage of dose occurs below the skin surface, the term **dose maximum (D_{max})** is used to describe the process. D_{max} is the depth of maximum buildup, in which 100% of the dose is deposited. For ^{60}Co, D_{max} occurs at 0.5 cm below the skin surface. This was a tremendous advantage over the other types of equipment (especially orthovoltage) used to treat cancer at the time.

To protect personnel, the ^{60}Co source must be shielded when the source is in the "off" position. Compared with linear accelerators and other electrically operated therapy equipment, these machines constantly emit radiation. A great deal of high-density material, such as lead or depleted uranium, surrounds the source in the head of the machine (Figure 7-26). To help the machine rotate smoothly and provide additional shielding, it must have a counterweight. In part, this is to balance the lead shielding in the head of the machine housing the radioactive ^{60}Co source. This counterweight, extending from the opposite end of the gantry in which the source is housed, is called a *beam stopper*. With the addition of a beam stopper, walls and ceilings in the treatment room did not require as much shielding. The beam stopper absorbed a significant amount of the radiation transmitted through the patient. Although it provided additional shielding and acted as a counterweight, the beam stopper had a number of drawbacks, including the difficulty associated with working around this cumbersome extension. The large beam stopper limited movement around the head of the gantry and could be a challenge at positioning a stretcher next to the treatment couch with the machine in the lateral position.

Application. Before the widespread distribution of linear accelerators, ^{60}Co units delivered radiation therapy treatments to all types of tumors. Because of its unique beam characteristics, the ^{60}Co unit was commonly used to treat cancers of the head and neck area, breast, spine, and extremities. In addition, areas just below the skin surface (where a deep penetration of the beam is not necessary) can be effectively treated with ^{60}Co.

Production. ^{60}Co is an artificially produced isotope. Like many other isotopes used in the diagnosis and treatment of disease, ^{60}Co becomes radioactive when its atomic number is altered. This may happen in a particle accelerator called a *cyclotron* or *nuclear reactor*. The production of ^{60}Co begins with the stable form of cobalt, which has an atomic mass number of 59. The atomic mass number is the sum of the number of protons and neutrons in the nucleus. After ^{59}Co is bombarded or irradiated

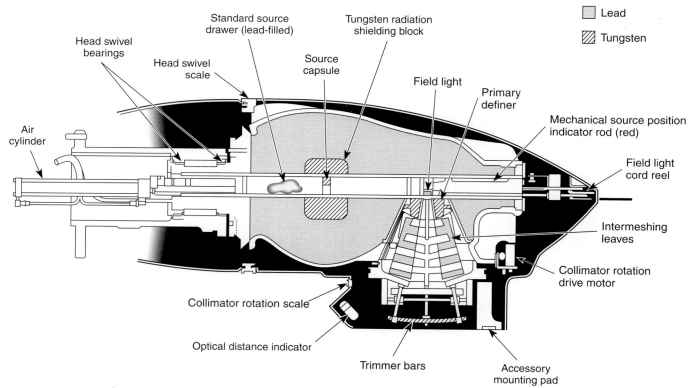

Lead

Tungsten

Head swivel
bearings

Head swivel
scale

Standard source
drawer (lead-filled)

Source
capsule

Tungsten radiation
shielding block

Field light

Primary
definer

Air
cylinder

Mechanical source position
indicator rod (red)

Field light
cord reel

Intermeshing
leaves

Collimator rotation
drive motor

Collimator rotation scale

Optical distance indicator

Trimmer bars

Accessory
mounting pad

Figure 7-26. A cross section of typical ^{60}Co components. (Courtesy Atomic Energy of Canada Limited, Medical Products, Kanata, Ontario, Canada.)

in a nuclear reactor with slow neutrons, the nucleus of ^{59}Co absorbs one neutron and becomes radioactive ^{60}Co. This can be expressed in the following formula:

$$^{59}Co + {}^{1}n \cong {}^{60}Co$$

As in any radioactive substance, ^{60}Co emits radiation in an effort to return to its more stable state.

^{60}Co activity may be expressed in curies (Ci), the historical unit of radioactivity, which equals 3.7×10^{10} becquerel (Bq). Bq, the standard international (SI) unit of radioactivity, equals 1 disintegration per second. Most sources have an activity of 750 to 9000 Ci and may be referred to as *kilocurie sources*.[28] In addition, the activity may be defined in rhm units (1 rhm unit represents 1 roentgen per hour at 1 m). The quality of the radiation produced by the source does not depend on the number of curies or rhms. With a 3000-Ci source, the equipment can be operated at an 80-cm distance and have a 10-cm depth dose of 56%.[12,14] Sources used in radiation therapy typically range from 3000 to 9000 Ci and have a specific activity of 75 to 200 Ci/g.

Specific activity is the number of transformations per second for each gram of radionuclide decaying at a fixed rate. Specific activity is the number of curies (Ci) per gram. The specific activity for a ^{60}Co source can be as high as 400 Ci/g, but for radiation therapy treatment, it is usually 200 Ci/g. A smaller source at the standard 80 SSD produces a beam of lower intensity requiring longer treatment time.

The radioactive ^{60}Co source and its shielding (in the form of a protective casing) are referred to as the *cobalt capsule*. The diameter of the capsule can range from 1 to 3 cm (Figure 7-27).

For radiation therapy purposes, 1.0 to 2.0 cm is preferred. The radioactive cobalt source contains disks, slugs, or pellets grouped in a cluster or solid cylinder, encased in a stainless steel capsule, and sealed by welding. The capsule is placed inside a second steel capsule that is also welded. The multiple layers of metal prevent leakage of the radioactive material and absorb the beta particles produced during the decay process.[14]

Characteristics. The radioactive ^{60}Co nucleus emits ionizing radiation in the form of high-energy gamma rays. ^{60}Co decays by first emitting a beta particle with an energy of 0.31 MeV that is absorbed in the source's steel capsule. After emitting the beta particle, the nucleus enters an excited state of nickel-60. The nickel-60 decays to a ground state by emitting two gamma rays per disintegration. Of the two gamma rays emitted, one has an energy of 1.17 MeV and the other is 1.33 MeV.[28] The beam can be considered polyenergetic or heterogeneous because more than one energy is decaying from the isotope. For practical purposes, the two energies are averaged to give an effective energy of 1.25 MeV.

Because ^{60}Co is a radioactive isotope, it has a half-life ($t_{1/2}$), the time necessary for a radioactive material to decay to half or 50% of its original activity. ^{60}Co decays to 50% of its activity after a $t_{1/2}$ of 5.26 years.[17] To compensate for the reduction in beam output each month, a correction factor of approximately 1% per month must be applied to the output. The correction factor increases the treatment time necessary to deliver the appropriate dose. To maintain adequate output for patient treatment and thus eliminate longer treatment times, the ^{60}Co source should be replaced at least every 5.3 years.

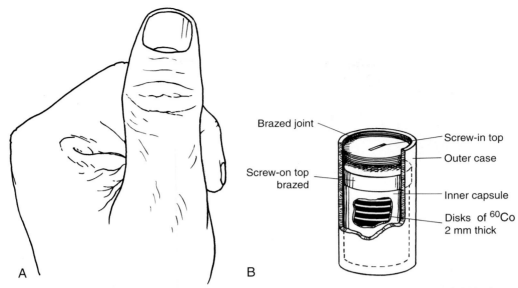

Figure 7-27. A, The radioactive ^{60}Co source or capsule can be compared in size with the end of a person's thumb. **B,** Double encapsulated teletherapy ^{60}Co source. (From Meredith WJ, Massey JB: *Fundamental physics of radiology,* St. Louis, 1977, Mosby.)

Electron equilibrium is another term used to describe D_{max}. As energy increases, so does the depth of electron equilibrium. For ^{60}Co, this point occurs at 0.5 cm below the skin surface. Table 7-3 describes the depth of D_{max} for a variety of beams.

Penumbra is the area at the edge of the radiation beam at which the dose rate changes rapidly as a function of distance from the beam axis.[8,14] Penumbra describes the edge of the field having full radiation intensity for the beam compared with the area at which the intensity falls to 0. Compared with the sharper field edge produced with linear accelerators, penumbra is a definite disadvantage in using ^{60}Co beams for radiation therapy treatments. Figure 7-28 demonstrates the difference between a ^{60}Co beam and a 6-MV linear accelerator beam. The sharp edge of the linear accelerator beam compared with the fuzzy edge (penumbra) of the cobalt beam should be noted.

The radioactive-source size contributes greatly to the degree of penumbra. The larger the source size, the larger is the penumbra. The following formula is used to determine the penumbra (P equals the penumbra size, S equals the source size, SSD equals the source-skin distance, and SDD equals the source-diaphragm [collimator] distance):

$$P = S(SSD - SDD)/SDD$$

Penumbra is the place where a lack of sharpness or fuzzy area occurs at the edge of the beam. The geometric blurring of the field edge occurs at the skin surface and greater depths in tissue. The geometric penumbra should be considered during the planning of the patient's treatment, especially where treatment fields will abut or match. An example can be made with the conventional simulator. During the planning process on the simulator, the field-defining wires outline the treatment volume. The wires outline the treatment area anatomically on a radiograph and visibly on the patient's skin. Different field sizes (slightly larger with the cobalt unit) are necessary to cover the same amount of tissue adequately on the cobalt machine as compared with a linear accelerator.

For radiation therapy beams using ^{60}Co, shielding blocks are most commonly made of Lipowitz metal. **Cerrobend** is a form of Lipowitz metal used for designing custom shielding blocks and consists of 50.0% bismuth, 26.7% lead, 13.3% tin, and 10.0% cadmium.[13] Cerrobend melts (70° C) at a much lower point than lead (327° C). Therefore, Cerrobend is easier and safer to use. However, cadmium (a toxic metal) can get into the bloodstream of individuals working with Lipowitz metal. Some manufacturers have a type of Lipowitz alloy without cadmium available for a slight increase in cost.

The Cerrobend used in custom block fabrication hardens quickly depending on the amount and degree of cooling applied to the alloy. Using the density ratio of Cerrobend to lead, a factor of 1.21 can be applied to the thickness of lead needed to attenuate 5% of the primary beam. For the most common megavoltage beams, a thickness of 7.5 cm of Cerrobend is used. This is equivalent to about 6 cm of lead.[14]

Table 7-3	Depth of Maximum Dose for Various Photon Energies	
Beam Energy	**D_{max} (cm below Skin Surface)**
Superficial	0.0
Orthovoltage	0.0
Cesium-137	0.1
Radium-226	0.1
Cobalt-60	0.5
4 MV	1.0
6 MV	1.5
10 MV	2.5
15 MV	3.0
20 MV	3.5
25 MV	5.0

From Stanton R, Stinson D: *Applied physics for radiation oncology,* Madison, WI, 1996, Medical Physics Publishing.

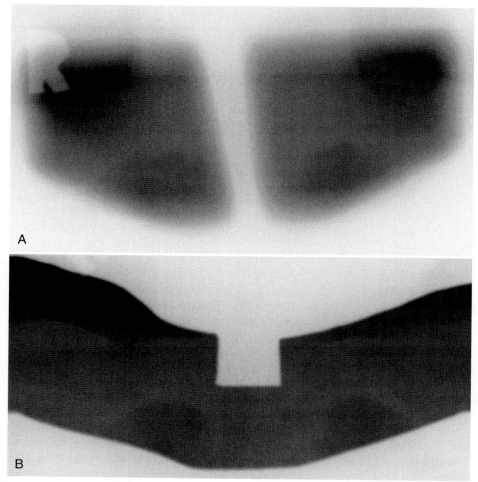

Figure 7-28. A, Port film taken with a ^{60}Co beam demonstrates the fuzzy field edges or penumbra. **B**, Port film taken with a 6-MV beam demonstrates the sharpness at the field edges or lack of penumbra.

Machine Design And Components.

Source Positioning. The most commonly used methods of delivering the source is the air-pressure (piston) method (Figure 7-29). The air-pressure method pushes a piston and thus the ^{60}Co source into the "on" position. A sliding drawer allows the source to be positioned over the collimator opening. In the "off" position, the source retracts back into the treatment head. In case of power failure, the air-driven piston automatically returns the source to the "off" position.

Travel Time. The time necessary to deliver the source from the "off," "on," or treatment position is defined as the travel time. To compensate for the travel time, a correction (shutter error) must be added to the calculation to deliver the prescribed dose. The shutter error allows for the total advancement and retraction of the source from the "off" position to the "on" position and back to the "off" position again. Depending on the manufacturer and method of source delivery, this may take place in about 0.2 second. If the travel time is neglected in the calculation used to deliver the prescribed dose, a small underdose may occur. Of course, the greater the number of fractions used to deliver the total dose, the greater the error in dose delivered.

Shielding. Because it constantly emits radiation, the ^{60}Co source must be shielded in a protective housing. The housing used for shielding and containing the device for positioning the source is referred to as the *source head*. The source head is a steel shell filled with lead or an alloy of lead, tungsten, and

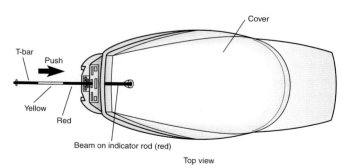

Figure 7-29. A ^{60}Co air-pressure (piston) drawer in the "on" position. (Courtesy Atomic Energy of Canada Limited, Medical Products, Kanata, Ontario, Canada.)

depleted uranium.[13] For adequate shielding, the housing may be up to 2 feet in diameter.[28] Radiation leakage around the source head should conform to Nuclear Regulatory Commission (NCR) guidelines.[33]

Machine Components. A multivaned or interleaf collimator is constructed as part of the source head to shape the size of the radiation beam. The collimator assists in reducing the penumbra associated with the source size. Trimmers or satellite collimators may be added to further sharpen the radiation-beam edge. Field size is defined by a light beam reflected from a light bulb to a small mirror. A tray holder is added below the collimators for field shaping by hand-placed lead or customized Cerrobend shielding blocks. Wedges made of lead, brass, or copper are placed in the path of the beam and shift or tilt the dose distribution from its normal shape. When needed, they are positioned in a separate slot in the block tray assembly.

Calibration and Leakage. A qualified radiation physicist must perform full calibration testing for radioactive ^{60}Co units annually. Full calibration may be done more frequently if (1) the source is replaced, (2) a 5% deviation is noticed during a spot check, and (3) a major repair requiring the removal or restoration of major components is done. A monthly output calibration should be done for a set of standard daily operating conditions. Measurements taken during a full calibration may include the following:

1. Radiation and light field coincidence
2. Timer accuracy
3. Exposure rate or dose rate to an accuracy of ±3% for various field sizes
4. Accuracy of distance-measuring devices used for treatment
5. Uniformity of the radiation field and its dependence of the orientation of the useful beam position around the head of the unit cannot exceed 2 mrem/hr at 1 m, with a maximum of 10 mrem/hr at 1 m at any measurable location. The maximum permissible leakage in the "on" position cannot exceed 0.1% of the useful beam at 1 m from the source. The 0.1% of the useful beam is the percentage of the actual output of the ^{60}Co source in cGy/min. For example, if the useful beam has an output of 197.3 cGy/min for the month of January, the maximum permissible leakage in the "on" position at 1 m from the source is 0.197 cGy/min.

A wipe test (or leak test) must be done twice a year on the sealed ^{60}Co source. If a source's seal is broken and leaking, it may have radiation contamination on the interleaf collimators. A wipe test is done, using long forceps, wiping the collimator edges with a filter paper, cloth pad, or cotton swab moistened with alcohol. A background radiation reading is done by using a survey meter calibrated with the same type of material as the one being tested. A reading is then taken of the wipe to determine its activity, with the acceptable level of activity less than 0.005 mCi. If the activity is higher, radiation contamination or leakage may have occurred and the unit must be removed from service until decontamination and repair can be completed.

Radiation Monitoring and Light System. Because it is a radioactive source that emits ionizing radiation, ^{60}Co requires not only a light system to show when the machine is "on" and "off" but also a monitoring system to detect radiation. The machine

"on" and "off" indicator lights must be on the console, at the head of the machine, and at the entrance to the treatment room. If the machine is "on," a red light must be lit. When the machine is "off," this light should show green. A radiation detector must be located in the treatment room. The detector is wired to a light outside the room near the console and door. The light must be blinking red if radiation is present and must be in view of the radiation therapist. Before entering the room, the therapist must be sure the "off" light is green and the blinking red light has stopped. Because a moment is necessary for the ^{60}Co source to retract into its "off" position, the green light comes on first, before the blinking red light stops. If the red light continues to blink for longer than a few seconds, the therapist must be ready to carry out an established emergency procedure. The source may not have retracted fully or properly.

Emergency Procedures. Emergency procedures must be established during the machine commissioning and before the unit is used for treatment. The emergency procedures must be posted at the machine console. These procedures must be developed by the radiation safety officer or radiation physicist and communicated to the radiation therapist and personnel responsible during a radiation emergency. No universal emergency procedure exists for a source that fails to return to the "off" position. Each department should develop and post emergency procedures. A sample procedure posted at the machine console is shown in Box 7-1.

Another procedure may include retracting the ^{60}Co source into the head source area with a T-bar. A T-bar is a steel rod

---

Box 7-1	Radiation Therapist Procedure for Cobalt-60 Emergency

A. If the console timer fails to terminate exposure, do the following:
1. PUSH EMERGENCY "OFF" BUTTON.
2. TURN CIRCUIT BREAKER OFF.
B. If the source drawer fails to close by shutting off electrical circuits, do the following:
1. OPEN TREATMENT ROOM DOOR.
   a. Use the hand crank if electrical power is off and if using a pneumatic door.
2. REMOVE PATIENT FROM ROOM.
   a. Verbally request that the patient get off the table and come to the treatment door.
   b. If the patient is unable to respond to a verbal command, enter the treatment room and quickly remove the patient. Do not stand in the path of the primary beam.
3. CLOSE TREATMENT ROOM DOOR.
   a. Use the hand crank if electrical power is off and if using a pneumatic door.
C. Notify the attending physician and radiation safety officer.
D. Secure the room against unauthorized entry by placing a DO NOT ENTER sign on the door, and secure or lock the door.

NOTE: This machine shall not be used unless the operating and emergency procedure manual is available in the control area. Operating personnel should familiarize themselves with this manual before operating this machine.

18 to 24 inches in length shaped like a T. The first 7 inches opposite the end of the T is painted red with the next 7 inches painted yellow (see Figure 7-29). In case of an emergency in which the source does not retract, the T-bar is placed in the source drawer at the top of the machine or source head. With the T end of the bar held in hand, forward pressure is applied to push the drawer backward into the off position. The ^{60}Co source can be considered relatively safe if no red paint is showing on the T-bar outside the machine or source-head cover. Before the ^{60}Co source is in the fully safe position, the yellow portion of the bar must be entirely inside the machine or source-head cover. Because of the complexity of this procedure, any radiation therapy personnel performing it may be exposed to a higher dose of radiation than under normal working conditions.

SUMMARY

- Ionizing radiation (in one form or another) has been used in the treatment of cancer almost from the time x-rays and radium were discovered.
- Historically, equipment evolved from low-energy, low-skin-sparing, unsophisticated systems (such as orthovoltage units) to today's computerized, megavoltage linear accelerators that can treat a variety of deep-seated tumors.
- In the treatment room, the major components of a linear accelerator can be divided into three specific areas: drive stand, gantry, and treatment couch.
- Four major components are housed in the stand: the klystron, waveguide, circulator, and cooling system.
- The major components in the gantry are the electron gun, accelerator structure (guide), and treatment head.
- The transfer of information, such as the exact location of immobilization devices, from simulation to the treatment machine is improved when devices are referenced or indexed to the treatment tabletop.
- Multileaf collimator systems are used to shield blocked area by using approximately 52 to 160 leaves. These heavy, metal collimator rods slide into place to form the desired field shape by projecting 0.5- to 2-cm beam widths per rod.
- New protocols are being formulated to reflect the enormous capabilities of radiation oncology equipment. The goal is to spare more normal tissue and deliver higher doses to the actual tumor volume. This will hopefully result in decreased morbidity and increased cure rates.
- Although the linear accelerator is the most widely accepted treatment machine in developed countries, older megavoltage treatment machines, such as the betatron, Van de Graaff generator, and cobalt unit are still used, especially in developing countries.
- The radioactive ^{60}Co nucleus emits ionizing radiation in the form of high-energy gamma rays, with a D_{max} of 0.5 cm. Of the two gamma rays emitted, one has an energy of 1.17 MeV and the other 1.33 MeV. For practical purposes, the two energies are averaged to give an effective energy of 1.25 MeV.

Review Questions

Multiple Choice

1. Which of the following does *not* relate to beam quality?
   a. penumbra
   b. kVp
   c. central-axis depth dose
   d. mA

2. Which of the following kilovoltage x-ray machines would be used to treat a skin cancer that was estimated to be nearly 2 cm in thickness?
   a. contact therapy
   b. superficial treatments
   c. orthovoltage therapy
   d. betatron

3. If an electron beam does *not* demonstrate consistency in dose across the treatment field, what might be at fault?
   a. scattering foil
   b. flattening filter
   c. wedge
   d. multileaf collimator

4. What is the average energy with which ^{60}Co emits gamma rays used for radiation therapy treatments?
   a. 1.17
   b. 1.25
   c. 1.33
   d. 2.50

5. Penumbra is related to which of the following?
   I. cobolt-60
   II. multileaf collimator
   III. klystron
   IV. magnetron
      a. I and II only
      b. II and III only
      c. III and IV only
      d. I, II, III, and IV

6. Which of the following would *not* be used for IGRT?
   a. EPID
   b. KV cone-beam CT
   c. ultrasound
   d. orthovoltage x-ray unit

7. When were linear accelerators first commercially available for clinical use?
   a. 1895
   b. 1930s
   c. 1950s
   d. 1980s

8. A beam-flattening filter is placed in the path of the beam when _____ are used for treatment purposes.
   a. protons
   b. electrons
   c. x-rays
   d. gamma rays

9. What does a klystron or magnetron produce?
   a. microwave power
   b. alternating current
   c. accelerated electrons and photons
   d. magnetic fields used to bend the beam

10. Trace the path of an electron in a linear accelerator by selecting the best route from the following.
    I. electron gun
    II. collimator
    III. accelerator guide
    IV. bending magnet
        a. I, II, III, IV
        b. I, III, IV, II
        c. II, I, IV, II
        d. III, I, II, IV

The answers to the Review Questions can be found by logging on to our website at: *http://evolve.elsevier.com/Washington+Leaver/ principles*

Questions to Ponder

1. Why do you think IGRT may be a better way to check the delivery of radiation therapy?
2. Discuss the application and use of the contact, superficial, and orthovoltage treatment units in radiation therapy.
3. Why must a monthly calculation correction be made for the ^{60}Co unit?
4. Discuss an emergency procedure for a source that fails to retract.
5. Discuss the integration of computerization and linear accelerator operation. What are the benefits and drawbacks?
6. Analyze the need, design, and operation of a linear accelerator cooling system.
7. What is ergonomy? Give some examples of other ergonomically designed tools in your department. What is the benefit of ergonomic designs?
8. Discuss the major components of the linear accelerator, including the klystron, waveguide, circulator, electron gun, accelerator guide, and bending magnet.
9. Describe the difference between a beam-flattening filter and a scattering foil.

REFERENCES

1. Bentel GC: *Patient positioning and immobilization in radiation oncology,* New York, 1999, McGraw-Hill.
2. Bissonnette JP, et al: Optimal radiographic magnification for portal imaging, *Med Phys* 21:1435-1445, 1994.
3. Bushong SC: *Radiologic science for technologists: physics, biology, and protection,* ed 8, St. Louis, 2004, Mosby.
4. Coia L, Moylan D: *Introduction to clinical radiation oncology,* Madison, WI, 1991, Medical Physics Publishing.
5. Edwards IK Jr, Edwards EK, Edwards SR: Grenz ray therapy, commentary, *Int J Dermatol* 29:17-18, 1990.
6. Elshaikh M, et al: Advanves in radiation oncology, *Annu Rev Med* 57:19-31, 2006.
7. Falco-Braun O, Schultze U: Contact radiotherapy of cutaneous hemangiomas, *Arch Dermatol Res* 253/254:237-246, 1975.
8. Fraass BA, Eisbruch A: Conformal therapy: treatment, planning, delivery, and clinical results. In Gunderson LL, Tepper JE, editors: *Clinical radiation oncology,* ed 2, Philadelphia, 2007, Churchill Livingstone.
9. Gington E: An informal history of the microwave electron accelerator for radiotherapy, *Proc Tenth Varian Users Meetings* 1(1):11-19, 1984.
10. Grigg FRN: *The trail of the invisible light: from x-olyahlen to radio (bio)logy,* Springfield, IL, 1965, Charles C Thomas.
11. Hansen WF: The changing role of the accelerator in radiation therapy, *IEEE Trans Nucl Sci* 30:1781-1783, 1983.
12. Jackson S: *Radiation oncology: a handbook for residents and the allied health professions,* St. Louis, 1985, Warren H Green.
13. Johns H, Cunningham J, Friedman M, editors: *Physics of radiology,* ed 4, Springfield, IL, 1983, Charles C Thomas.
14. Kahn FM: *Treatment planning in radiation oncology,* ed 2, Philadelphia, 2007, Lippincott Williams & Wilkins.
15. Karzmark CJ, Morton RJ: *A primer on theory and operation of linear accelerators in radiation therapy,* ed 2 Madison, WI, 1998, Medical Physics Publishing.
16. Karzmark CJ, Nunan CS, Tanabe E: *Medical electron accelerators,* New York, 1993, McGraw-Hill.
17. Klemp PFB, et al: Commissioning of a linear accelerator with independent jaws: computerized data collection and transfer to a planning computer, *Phys Med Biol* 33:865-871, 1988.
18. Klevehagen SC, Thaites DI: *Radiotherapy physics in practice,* Oxford, England, 1993, Oxford University Press.
19. Mallory MI: *Personal communication,* January 18, 1994.
20. Miller RA: *Personal communication,* January, 1995.
21. Palta JR, et al: Electron beam characteristics of a Philips SL 25, *Med Phys* 17:27-34, 1990.
22. Papillon J: *Rectal and anal cancers: conservative treatment by irradiation: an alternative to surgery,* Berlin, 1982, Springer-Verlag.
23. Perez CA, Brady LW: *Principles and practice of radiation oncology,* ed 4, Philadelphia, 2004, Lippincott Williams & Wilkins.
24. Podgorsak EB, Metcalfe P, Van Dyk J: Medical accelerators. In Van Dyk J, editor: *The modern technology of radiation oncology,* Madison, WI, 1999, Medical Physics Publishing.
25. Purdy JA: Principles of radiologic physics, dosimetry and treatment planning. In Perez CA, Brady LW, editors: *Principles and practice of radiation oncology,* ed 4, Philadelphia, 2004, Lippincott Williams &Wilkins.
26. Purdy JA, et al: Medical accelerator safety considerations: report of AAPM Radiation Therapy Committee Task Group No. 35, *Med Phys* 20:1261-1275, 1993.
27. Rajan G: *Advanced medical radiation dosimetry,* New Delhi, India, 1992, Pentice-Hall of India Private Limited.
28. Selman J: *Basis of physics of radiation therapy,* ed 2, Springfield, IL, 1976, Charles C Thomas.
29. Speight JL, Roach M 3rd: Advances in the treatment of localized prostate cancer: the role of anatomic and functional imaging in men managed with radiotherapy, *J Clin Oncol* 10:987-995, 2007.
30. Stanton R, Stinson D, editors: *Applied physics for radiation oncology,* Madison, WI, 1996, Medical Physics Publishing.
31. Swindell W, et al: The design of megavoltage projection imaging systems: some theoretical aspects, *Med Phys* 18:651-658, 1991.
32. Tinger A, et al: An analysis of intratreatment and intertreatment displacements in pelvic radiotherapy using electronic portal imaging, *Int J Radiat Oncol Biol Phys* 34:683-690, 1996.
33. United States Nuclear Regulation Commission: *Rules and regulations,* part 170, Washington, DC, 1994, The Author.
34. Varian Medical Systems (website): www.varian.com. Accessed January 10, 2008.
35. Xia P, Amols HI, Ling CC: Three dimensional conformal radiotherapy and intensity modulated radiotherapy. In Leibel SA, Phillips TL, editors: *Textbook of radiation oncology,* ed 2, Philadelphia, 2004, Saunders.

8 CHAPTER

Treatment Procedures

Annette M. Coleman

Outline

Radiation oncology record
Rationale for and documentation of treatment response
Electronic medical records
   Verify and record
   Quality assurance
Treatment session preparation
   Radiation prescription
   Treatment plan description and reference images
   Treatment record
   Verification images
The treatment room
The patient
   Identification
   Patient preparation and communication

Patient transfers
   Wheelchair transfers
   Stretcher transfers
Patient position, isocenter, and field placement
   Patient positioning
   Localization landmarks
   Positioning isocenter
   Verification imaging (setup)
Beam position and shape
   Multileaf collimators
   Blocks
   Verification imaging (portal)
Beam-modifying devices
   Bolus
   Compensators
   Wedges
   Transmission filters

Electron beam
   Collimation
   Internal shielding
   Bolus
   Electron beam shaping
Assessment and acceptance of treatment parameters
   Patient-monitoring systems
   Console
Treatment delivery
   Beam on and beam off
   Treatment interruptions
Common treatment techniques
   Multiple fields
   Adjacent fields
   Intensity-modulated radiation therapy
Treatment room maintenance
Summary

Key Terms

Beam modifiers
Beam's eye view
Collimation
Coplanar
Elapsed days
Feathering
Fiducial markers
Fractionation
Hinge angle
Immobilization devices
Interfraction
Interlocks
Intrafraction
Isocenter
Localization
Orthogonal
Positioning devices
Protraction
Stereoscopic
Treatment fields
Treatment number
Treatment record
Treatment technique
Triangulation
Verification imaging

Objectives

- Construct a plan of action for patient treatment setup and delivery.
- Describe the radiation therapist's role in the quality assurance program.
- Given a specific situation, select and describe the safest transfer method for the patient and the radiation therapist.
- Discriminate between the goals of setup and portal imaging.

- List and define beam-shaping and beam-modification devices.
- Compare treatment setup implications between photon and electron beams: (1) collimation, (2) bolus, and (3) adjacent fields.
- Describe multileaf collimators and their application as both beam-shaping and beam-modification devices in treatment delivery.
- List appropriate responses to treatment interruptions.

Radiation treatment delivery constitutes the core responsibility in the professional practice of the radiation therapist. Grounded in the planning, simulation, and administration of a prescribed course of radiation therapy, the practice of radiation therapy is an essential component of quality oncologic care. Conscientious attention to precision and reproducibility in simulation and treatment delivery and to the physiologic and psychological needs of patients highlights the radiation therapist's contribution to the cancer-management team. Radiation therapists deliver radiation therapy treatments, monitor and operate sophisticated radiation-producing equipment, and maintain detailed treatment records.

Quality care depends on the needs of the patient and the specialized knowledge and skills of the radiation therapist in the operation of equipment. The ability to reproduce treatment setups depends on abilities and limitations imposed by equipment, treatment beam geometry, and the patient. Proficiency in technical and patient care skills and a knowledge base in oncology, treatment planning, physics, radiation biology, and the legal consideration of practice are prerequisite to the formation of clinical judgment necessary for the execution of these responsibilities.

Well-developed organizational and communication skills enable successful coordination of individual patient treatments in the context of a varied patient load. The development of an action plan in

Box 8-1	Task Analysis of Treatment Procedures

1. Review the chart.
2. Prepare the room. Position immobilization devices on the treatment table and place treatment accessories within reach.
3. Greet and identify the patient.
4. Assist the patient onto the treatment table and into the prescribed position.
5. Locate surface landmarks.
6. Raise the couch, bringing the area to be treated to the beam area.
7. Refine the patient position relative to the isocenter using lasers, light field, and surface landmarks. Optionally perform setup verification procedures.
8. Rotate gantry and collimator to prescribed positions.
9. Position beam-shaping accessories and visually verify using the light field. Optionally perform portal verification procedures.
10. Position beam modifiers (wedge, compensator, and bolus).
11. Inform the patient that you are leaving and treatment will begin.
12. Monitor the patient.
13. Set appropriate machine controls and review correspondence with prescribed values in the record and verification system.
14. Initiate beam-on. Monitor patient and equipment function. When multiple fields are to be treated, do the following:
15. Validate parameters downloaded to accelerator and enable accelerator motion, or enter the room and check the patient, field position, and beam modifiers.
16. Repeat steps 8 through 14 for all fields until the completion of treatment.
17. Assist the patient from the couch and room.
18. Complete the treatment record.

the approach to treatment delivery assists the radiation therapist in ensuring thoroughness. A simple task analysis provides a method for organizing a plan of action (Box 8-1). Details and alternative pathways build on this foundation, addressing the complexities of individual treatment techniques, specialized equipment, and procedures.

RADIATION ONCOLOGY RECORD

Separate from the individual's hospital chart, a specialty chart is created and remains in the radiation oncology department. As the legal record of the patient's radiation treatment and associated medical care, its completeness, organization, and legibility are critical. Each page must clearly identify the patient by name and identification number. The radiation therapist recognizes the ethical and legal responsibility to maintain the patient's privacy and right to confidentiality of medical records. In general, access to information that is identifiable to an individual is restricted to caregivers to whom the patient has provided consent.

Rationale for and Documentation of Treatment Response

The rationale for radiation treatment includes a documented patient history including the results of diagnostic and staging procedures. Before receiving treatment, patients must receive an explanation of their status, treatment alternatives, and consequences associated with and without treatment to provide their informed consent to any procedures. This information must be presented in a manner that is understandable to the patient. As patient advocate, the radiation therapist verifies patient understanding of education delivered and ensures that informed consent has been attained and documented.

Patient response to treatment is monitored and recorded throughout and following completion of treatment. The physician, nurses, and radiation therapists document observations. Assessment records from weekly on-treatment visits with the radiation oncologist, records tracking the patient's weight and blood counts, and other indicators of treatment response are maintained. Radiation treatment responses often require medication, nutrition, or psychosocial intervention; all care activities are recorded in the chart. Other members of the treatment team such as nutritionists and social workers may also include their assessments and instructions in the radiation therapy chart.

Electronic Medical Records

Traditionally dependent on the handwritten or printed records of each member of the treatment team, computerized charting systems are rapidly integrating with the workflow of radiation oncology practices. These systems monitor and document experiences of the patient with the department. Information is stored in a centralized database from which it can be presented uniquely to each member of the treatment team, and access is limited only by the networking capabilities of the facility. The electronic medical record (EMR) in radiation oncology may be limited to clinical charting and radiation treatment details. A comprehensive EMR, however, includes all medical and administrative aspects of the patient's experience with the radiation treatment center: schedules, communications from referring physicians and external diagnostic facilities, and reimbursement information.

As with the written chart, electronic imaging records are also increasingly the norm. Digital diagnostic and planning images are transferable between computerized systems and complex imaging functions such as computed tomography (CT) and image registration and fusion have made their way to the megavoltage therapy room. Computed radiography using phosphor plates exposed in the same manner as film and electronic portal imaging devices (EPIDs) mounted opposite the head of the gantry, or a kilovolt x-ray source mounted to the gantry, convert x-ray information to digital information that can be displayed as an image on a computer screen. Electronic imaging systems rapidly produce static or real-time images of treatment volumes and computer manipulation of digital information enhances visualization, particularly beneficial to megavoltage imaging. These systems dramatically affect both treatment planning and delivery, providing the means to improve treatment accuracy.

With electronic charting, the medium but not the requirements of medical charting evolves. Traditional workflows come under scrutiny. Increasing access and quantity of information affect the responsibilities of team members, including the radiation therapist. Integral to the success of paperless and filmless radiation oncology departments, radiation therapists are actively participating in the examination and reengineering of patient care procedures. This evolution imposes new skill acquisition on practicing professionals and affects primary education requirements for those entering the profession.

Verify and Record

As accelerator capabilities and treatment plans increase in complexity, limitations of the paper record to track all treatment parameters are increasingly evident. The number of individual machine parameters alone is too large to be manually set, confirmed, and charted in the treatment history. The technical demands of modern treatment delivery require the integration of verification and record (V&R, R&V, or RV) systems.[5]

V&R systems provide validated parameters from the treatment plan for treatment machine setup and delivery. Machine settings are compared against those most recently prescribed for a particular field and prevent the initiation of the treatment beam if settings vary outside a specified tolerance range. Machine parameters typically monitored include monitor units, gantry position, collimator aperture and rotation settings, table position, arc versus fixed treatment, and use of beam modifiers. In addition, V&R systems can extend verification beyond the capabilities of the treatment machine, from patient identification to secondary equipment attached to, but not integrated with, the treatment machine itself. Treatment preferences may be definable, allowing selection of fields available for treatment and auto-setup of treatment parameters. Auto-sequencing of treatment fields presents the radiation therapist with the next set of treatment field parameters on completion of each field. For properly equipped accelerators, returning to the treatment room between fields is eliminated. Some accelerators are also capable of proceeding through an entire sequence of fields under the monitoring of the radiation therapist but without his or her intervention.

Providing significant functionality to aid in the accurate and efficient delivery of radiation therapy, V&R integration with the EMR changes the medium but not the requirements of treatment delivery charting. The patient's complete course of external beam radiation therapy is defined and recorded online for access at any time, but the accuracy of the record remains the responsibility of each professional contributing to its development. Data are confirmed at entry by the radiation therapist, always associated with a log-in and often with password-protected electronic signatures. Questioning and reviewing information at the time of data entry and on a regular schedule through the treatment course are just as critical as with manual records.

Quality Assurance

The treatment chart is a primary component of an institution's quality-assurance (QA) program. The QA program (see Chapter 19) consists of activities and documentation performed with the goal of optimizing patient care. The radiation therapist's primary role in the QA program is to ensure accuracy in the delivery of the radiation treatment plan as prescribed by a radiation oncologist. This requires reviewing patient records, monitoring the functioning of radiation-producing equipment, maintaining accuracy in the reproduction of treatment parameters, monitoring changes in patient status, and maintaining complete and accurate treatment records. The radiation

therapist communicates with the radiation oncology team through activities such as weekly chart reviews and through maintaining open lines of communication. Because their participation in QA activities is integral to the accomplishment of program goals, radiation therapists are represented on the departmental QA committee.[2,7]

Quality-management programs require that the treatment chart include information regarding the patient's history, including a diagnostic evaluation, rationale for treatment, detailed description of the treatment plan, and documentation of informed consent and the treatment delivered.[2,7] Normally, the radiation therapist does not begin treatment if any of this information is unavailable. Regular reviews of the entire chart are required of each member of the treatment team. Checklists of role responsibilities and schedules for review ensure completeness of chart reviews by the treatment team and are attached to every radiation therapy chart in written or electronic form. Examples of radiation therapist responsibilities to weekly chart reviews include monitoring verification of source-skin distance (SSD) and diode measurements and status of physics review, frequency of verification imaging and status of radiation oncologist review, accuracy of fractional and cumulative tracked dose, completion of physics chart checks, and verification of reimbursement charges submitted.

TREATMENT SESSION PREPARATION

Before initiating treatment, the radiation therapist reviews the treatment section of the chart for completeness and accuracy. The information necessary for the reproduction of the course of treatment by a qualified professional includes patient identification such as an identification photograph, a signed prescription, detailed patient- and equipment-positioning information, dosimetric plans, calculations, and the treatment history record.[7] The **treatment record** documents the delivery of treatments, recording fractional and cumulative doses, machine settings, verification imaging; and the ordering and implementation of prescribed changes.

Radiation Prescription

Radiation may be delivered only under the direct order of a radiation oncologist. Similar to drug and other therapies, radiation orders are written as prescriptions that must be signed by the radiation oncologist before the initiation of radiation treatment. No exceptions are allowed. The prescription must provide specific information to allow its interpretation by other qualified professionals, including the radiation therapist. The anatomic site and total radiation dose to be delivered with its **fractionation** (individual treatment dose) and **protraction** (time period over which the treatment will be given) schedule must be clearly stated. The prescription also identifies the **treatment technique** (number and orientation of treatment fields) to be applied. Information specifying beam energy, portal sizes and entry angles, and **beam modifiers** (devices that change the shape of the treatment field or distribution of radiation at depth) may be included in the prescription and with patient-positioning information.

As the dispenser of the radiation prescription, the radiation therapist accepts great responsibility. Radiation therapists must be knowledgeable of the effects of radiation on their patients, tumor-lethal doses, and limits of radiation tolerance for normal tissue. Prescriptions appearing to exceed these limits or deviate from standard practice should be reviewed with the physician before delivery. Care must be taken to eliminate any errors and to ensure delivery of safe treatment.

Changes in the treatment plan may be made any time during the course of treatment, and the radiation therapist is responsible for ensuring that changes are implemented as ordered. Therefore, the radiation therapist reviews the prescription immediately before the delivery of each treatment fraction. The physician's signature and date must accompany any changes in the prescription or treatment plan. With electronic charts, passwords protect the security of the physician's electronic signature. Common prescription changes include fractionation and total dose or the addition or deletion of a bolus or blocks. Changes affecting dose calculation require a review of the plan to ensure that corrections have been made before treatment delivery.

Treatment Plan Description and Reference Images

Treatment plans are composed of one or more **treatment fields** designed to maximize the dose delivered to the tumor while minimizing the dose to normal structures. Dose distributions and monitor-unit calculations prepared by the dosimetrist are to be reviewed and signed by at least two members of the treatment-planning team before being made available to the team at the treatment unit. Before treatment, the radiation therapist independently reviews the treatment plan for faithfulness of calculation factors with treatment parameters. Field sizes, beam modifiers, and treatment depths used in calculations must be consistent with those identified on the treatment setup instructions. Results may be further verified by direct dose measurements at the start of treatment using electronic diodes

or other dosimeters placed on the patient in the treatment field during treatment.

The treatment field, also called a *portal*, is the volume of tissue exposed to radiation from a single radiation beam. Each treatment field, or portal, is assigned an identifier and name indicating the prescription site and beam direction (Figure 8-1). A specific field identifier will be assigned only once to each patient, and new treatment fields progress sequentially as they are added to the patient record. Subscript letters, numbers, or prime marks (', ") may be used to denote changes in the field size, shape, or isocenter from the original field when the prescription volume and beam direction have not changed. The field description specifies field size, orientation of beam entry in patient coordinates, and beam modifiers to be used.

 Treatment field dimensions are stated width by length in centimeters.

A review of the treatment description is performed to ensure sufficient information is available for treatment plan reproduction before the initiation of the treatment. Where treatment definitions and records are duplicated between electronic and paper systems, consistency between the two records must be confirmed and monitored. Setup instructions, in addition to treatment field descriptions, include descriptive information with diagrams and/or photographs illustrating patient positioning and immobilization. Surface landmarks used to indicate the position of the isocenter and treatment target volumes must also be identified. If adjustments have been made to the original information, they must be clearly identified, signed, and dated by the radiation therapist.

 ICRU Reports 50 and 62 define treatment volumes to be used for prescribing and reporting radiation doses.

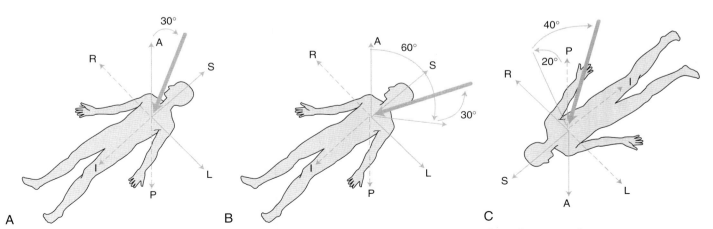

Figure 8-1. Three-dimensional beam nomenclature. Beams are named in reference to the patient coordinate system. **A**, The A30S beam is 30 degrees superior from the anterior axis. **B**, The A60L30S beam is 60 degrees left from the anterior axis and 30 degrees superior. **C**, The P20R40I beam is 20 degrees right from the posterior axis and 40 degrees inferior. (From Bourland D: Radiation Oncology Physics. In Gunderson LL, Tepper, JE, editors: *Clinical radiation oncology*, ed 2, Philadelphia, 2007, Churchill Livingstone.)

Treatment plans are further described with medical images. Reference images will be used to compare on-treatment images, verifying treatment position and documenting treatment delivery. Portal reference images display the **beam's eye view (BEV)** of the area to be irradiated and the treatment field shape and orientation as it passes through the patient. Setup reference images may be required in conjunction with portal reference images for verification of isocenter position where portal images are insufficient. Planar radiographs from simulation procedures or digital reconstructed radiographs (DRRs) from CT data by treatment planning or virtual simulation systems comprise traditional reference image sets. Radiographic landmarks such as bony references must be visible within and around the treatment area for comparison with exposures made on the treatment unit with the patient in treatment position.

The introduction of cone-beam CT and CT on rails systems to treatment rooms has greatly improved precision in the planning and delivery of radiation treatment. Rapid online imaging provides the radiation therapist with three-dimensional and soft tissue visualization. Computerized image registration calculates accurate setup corrections before positioning of treatment beams. With these systems, the planning CT scans themselves are necessary treatment reference images.

Treatment Record

Although the treatment plan and prescription direct the treatment, and the treatment record documents the course of its implementation, an inspection of the treatment record influences each subsequent treatment.

During treatment record review, the radiation therapist evaluates the completeness and accuracy of the treatment record to date and determines actions to be taken at the treatment session about to commence. Questions may include the following:

- "When was the last treatment?"
- "How far along is the patient in the course of treatment?"
- "Are verification images necessary?"
- "Have any changes to the prescription, treatment plan, or setup instructions been ordered?"

Radiation therapists monitor and record the dose delivered to the prescribed volume and critical structures or organs at risk near or in the treatment volume, and they respond to or initiate necessary changes in the treatment plan through consultation with the radiation oncologist. The radiation therapist must document and sign treatment plan changes in the treatment record when executed.

Records for individual treatments identify the date of treatment, **treatment number** (number of treatments delivered), and **elapsed days** (total time over which treatment is protracted). The fractional and total dose delivered must also be included. Notations are made regarding procedures completed on a particular treatment day, such as **verification imaging** (the documentation of treatment through radiographic or electronic imaging devices) and the addition or deletion of a block or other beam modifier. The radiation therapist records the radiation dose and parameters under which it was delivered at the completion of each treatment. All treatment record entries must be accompanied by the treating radiation therapist's signature or initials and the date. When multiple fractions are delivered on a day, the time of each delivery is also required.

Chart reviews include verification of previous entries. The most common written charting errors are those of addition or transposition and can often be seen in the dose record. Any corrections must leave the original entry legible. One line is drawn through the entry, followed by the correction, initials of the correcting individual, and the date. Because the chart is the primary document referenced in litigation processes, legible corrections and reasonable explanations are required. The use of correction fluid or other methods that hide original entries are viewed with suspicion and must be avoided. Charting corrections in electronic records must also be apparent in the treatment history. A process for voiding entries must retain an accurate representation of the original record while supporting documentation of what, by whom, and when corrections were made.

Attention to the dose delivered also provides the radiation therapist with expectations of the patient's physical reactions to the treatment. As the member of the treatment team who sees each patient with every treatment session, the radiation therapist has a significant responsibility in monitoring these reactions. The radiation therapist possesses a firm understanding of radiation reactions and intervention methods for their management. This understanding informs the decision to proceed or withhold treatment pending consultation with the radiation oncologist. The entire treatment team (including the oncologist and nursing staff members) monitors radiation reactions through review of blood counts or other lab tests; direct observation; and questioning of patients regarding their nutritional intake, skin reactions, and other associated symptoms.

Verification Images

The image file completes the treatment record. Setup and portal verification images perform a critical role in treatment execution and documentation, providing visual confirmation of reproduction of the planned treatment. Verification images are taken on the treatment unit with the patient in the treatment position and compared to reference images; clinical acceptance or change orders are generated from this assessment. Before treatment, the radiation therapist reviews the status of image review, implementing and documenting any treatment modification orders or calling unreviewed images to the attention of the radiation oncologist.

The quality of verification image communication between the radiation therapist and radiation oncologist is critical to treatment accuracy. The radiation therapist creates images demonstrating reproduction of the treatment **localization** (identification of hidden anatomy relative to observable or palpable surface landmarks), and the physician reviews, approving or directing changes. Radiation therapists' opportunity to exercise clinical judgment and skill when evaluating verification images may be limited by department policy. Increasingly, however, rapid production of images using electronic devices at the treatment unit is influencing the frequency of pretreatment (online) verification imaging and the involvement of the radiation therapist. Setup corrections are implemented before treatment and communicated to the radiation oncologist for offline review. Regardless of the autonomy of the radiation therapist's decision, within the United States, all images and change orders must be reviewed and signed by the physician.

Film imaging requires attention to equipment and technique. Radiographic film is selected for its relative exposure sensitivity and must be properly supported when positioned for use. Portal film reacts more slowly to radiation exposure than diagnostic film, allowing images to be created using the energies and dose rates used in therapeutic radiation exposures. Sensitivity of verification film (v-film) is even slower, allowing placement in the beam path through an entire exposure. Cassettes provide film stability for the film, may be hard or soft, and are usually lined with lead and/or copper to reduce film fog caused by backscatter. Films are positioned perpendicular to the central ray of the treatment beam, and source-film distance (SFD) is minimized or standardized depending on available equipment. Magnification markers, radiopaque indicators of known dimension, may be placed at the skin surface to determine magnification factors for an individual image. A graticule, however, is used more frequently.

 The graticule (bb tray or dot tray) is a calibrated device, a tray that fits into the collimator and provides radiographic representation of the central ray, aperture size, rotation, and magnification of the treatment aperture on the radiograph.

Radiopaque markers are aligned along the center width and length planes of the treatment aperture intersecting at the central ray. Photons are precisely blocked from exposing the radiograph at precisely positioned separations at a defined distance from the radiation source. Most commonly, unexposed marks include the central ray with additional markers calibrated to project at 1-cm increments along each axis at the source-axis distance (SAD) of the accelerator.

Time factors, poor image quality, and subjectivity in evaluation introduce limitations to precision using traditional film imaging techniques. Images created by megavoltage beams have poor contrast, making radiographic landmarks difficult to delineate. Films often are evaluated after treatment (offline), even on subsequent days, and offer no opportunity to correct for treatments already delivered. Even when films are taken immediately before treatment delivery (online), patient movement is possible while patients wait for the film processing and evaluation.

Electronic portal imaging offers many advantages to the practice of radiation therapy by allowing the radiation therapist and physician to verify isocenter position and treatment field alignment and to make adjustments much more quickly and accurately. Images are produced in seconds and displayed on a terminal at the treatment console (area located outside the treatment room), thus minimizing movement factors and the effect of frequent filming on the patient schedule.

Verification image interpretation is mostly a subjective process with room for variation in assessment between individuals. The traditional "side-by-side" evaluation of hanging film images produces qualitative results as the reviewer compares images of varying magnifications and static image quality. Electronic imaging introduces enhanced image quality and registration tools to reduce subjectivity and calculate corrections. Even with the introduction of these tools, the role of the radiation therapist and physician to accurately use them and to compare calculated results against their clinical assessment is critical.

Variation in patient position relative to the machine between treatments is expected and accommodated by planning normal tissue margins around the treatment target. These margins of normal tissue can be minimized by reducing treatment setup variation. Online image review most effectively minimizes the effect of daily setup variation, but the time factors may not outweigh this benefit for all treatment protocols. Setup variation is composed of systematic and random components. Systematic error is that which is consistently repeated and generally is the more significant source of treatment error. Where systematic variation for a patient setup is determined, changes can be made to setup instructions, applying precise offsets in couch position relative to the localization marks on the patient.

Systematic variation is the consistent component in daily setup variation, primarily resulting from translation of the planned treatment setup from the simulator to the treatment unit and patient positioning variables. Verification images taken before the first treatment generally assess systematic field shape errors that may be corrected against a single verification instance. Isocenter localization changes due to positioning factors between simulation and treatment, however, require imaging for several treatment sessions. Systematic variation is calculated by determining the average variation from several measurements. Consistent changes in the relative position of the isocenter to surface landmarks may then be corrected for during setup for subsequent treatment sessions. The remaining random variation includes inherent setup and organ motion variation that cannot be prospectively eliminated. The range of anticipated random error varies with anatomic site and must be accommodated in treatment planning. Random error is minimized by immobilization and increased use of online imaging techniques.

 Offline protocols determining systematic setup variation can identify setup adjustments producing more accurate results preimaging or pretreatment. The judicious combination of online and offline protocols with trend analysis can produce improved results for all patients.

THE TREATMENT ROOM

External-beam radiation therapy is accomplished through the use of sophisticated radiation-producing equipment such as linear accelerators. Newer technology is making alternative devices increasingly available, such as Tomotherapy, Cyberknife, and particle therapy units. All of these machines are engineered to facilitate the precise application of therapeutic radiation beams to well-defined treatment volumes, but the workhorse remains the linear accelerator.

Modern linear accelerators rotate around a fixed point. This point, **isocenter**, is the point of intersection of the three axes of rotation (gantry, collimator, and base of couch) of the treatment unit (see Chapter 7 for descriptions of isocentric treatment units). Isocentric mounting of treatment units facilitates the reproducibility of complex treatment plans. Accurate positioning of the treatment unit isocenter relative to the treatment plan isocenter allows redirection of the treatment beam to treat the target from multiple directions without moving the patient. These versatile units can accommodate extremely complex field arrangements.

The treatment room is also engineered around isocenter. A well-planned treatment room facilitates accessibility to treatment accessories and movement by the radiation therapists around this focal point. Shelves and storage cabinets form the perimeter; tables and counters do not obstruct access to and from the treatment unit. Treatment accessories are stored in consistent places and at heights that do not require radiation therapists to use step stools or ladders. An organized system for custom block storage facilitates quick retrieval. The radiation therapist accepts responsibility for the maintenance of the treatment room as part of the department's QA program.

Laser systems project points or lines of light from three or four sources along vertical and horizontal planes, intersecting at the treatment machine isocenter. Projecting from the walls and from the ceiling (or opposite the gantry), the lasers provide visual references to the location of isocenter, facilitating alignment of machine coordinates with external patient landmarks to align the accelerator's isocenter with its planned position within the patient. Red or green helium neon (HeNe) lasers are used. Green lasers project more sharply than red, with their shorter wavelength scattering less at the skin surface. HeNe lasers are not harmful to skin but do have the ability to damage vision. The laser source must not be looked directly into—this precaution applies to everyone entering the treatment room and must be communicated to patients.

A combination of standard and dim lighting is required in treatment rooms. Full, standard lighting provides safety for patients entering and exiting the room and assists radiation therapists in locating accessory equipment. Reducing the light in the treatment room improves the visualization of lasers and field light, thus assisting the patient positioning and treatment setup process. While treatment is in progress, full lights are on for visualization of the patient on the monitors.

Many room preparations are necessary before the arrival of the patient. The treatment setup dimensions, field size, gantry, collimator, and table positions are confirmed in the chart. The field size is typically set and the gantry positioned so that lasers are visible at isocenter and the field light crosshairs project in a vertical or lateral direction. The treatment table (couch) is raised or lowered appropriate to the patient's transportation method. Most treatment couches are designed with two window options to allow treatment fields to reach the patient without intercepting the couch. The primary window is open across the table and supported by bars on either side of the table, allowing treatment of most field arrangements. For oblique or rotational field arrangements that might pass through the side rails, an alternative configuration supports the center of the table with windows on either side. Mylar covers table windows, supporting the patient without attenuating the treatment beam. This support may be enhanced by carbon fiber wires beneath the Mylar.

The treatment table and positioning accessories must be cleaned with disinfectant cleaners after each use. Linens are replaced for each patient, covering the treatment table and keeping the treatment window clear. Universal precautions are practiced with all patients.

 Universal precautions are methods of infection control in which any human blood or body fluid is treated as if it were known to be infectious.

The radiation therapist is conscious that undiagnosed infections may be present in any individual and must handle all blood and body fluids as if they were infectious. Radiation therapists also remember the immunodeficient state of their patients and take responsibility for the prevention of disease transmission. The most important practice toward this goal is thorough hand washing after patient contact.

Positioning and **immobilization devices** such as sponges, casts, masks, and/or bite blocks matching those used at the simulation will be used to reproduce the planned treatment position and restrict movement. These are fitted to and positioned on the treatment table. Treatment accessories, including blocks, wedges, bolus, and compensators, are identified and brought out to a readily accessible location.

THE PATIENT

Identification

When room preparations are complete, the radiation therapist greets, confirms identification of the patient to be treated, and leads him or her to the treatment room. From first introductions, the radiation therapist initiates and is responsible for the rapport characterizing the radiation therapist–patient relationship. At least two methods of identification are used to confirm patient identity because many factors contribute to the possibility of misidentification. Patients may have the same or similar names, and illness or anxiety may hinder their ability to respond to their own name. As a result, the radiation therapist must be extremely cautious when identifying patients. The consequences of misidentification can range from discontent in the waiting room to misadministration of treatment.

The treatment chart includes an identification photograph for visual confirmation. The most important piece of identification for inpatients is their wrist bracelet, which is checked before the patient is moved into the treatment room. Outpatients typically carry identification cards to be checked and may be asked to state their own name. Bar-coding systems in conjunction with identification cards may be used with electronic charting and patient management systems to provide an independent confirmation of record selection.

Patient Preparation and Communication

As a professional caregiver, the radiation therapist seeks to establish with the patient a relationship that encourages confidence and cooperation. Patients entrust the radiation therapist with their care, typically over a period ranging from 2 to 8 weeks. Over this time, the radiation therapist is a resource for the patient and has the responsibility to develop a constructive patient-professional relationship, one that may provide the radiation therapist insight into the individual's experience and coping mechanisms. The radiation therapist has a great deal of control over the extent of this relationship and the patient's perception of quality of care. With this comes responsibility to anticipate questions and concerns associated with radiation treatments and to create an environment sensitive to the patient's needs.

The nature of their illness and anxiety surrounding the dangers of radiation make this no easy task. Observations of patient behavior may indicate needs for social support services or changes in the disease state. In the event of such changes, the physician must be notified. As a radiation oncology team member having the most frequent contact with the patient, the radiation therapist becomes the liaison, directing the patient to resources designed to meet his or her physical and psychosocial needs.

The radiation therapist demonstrates respect for the patient through clear communication of directions at a level understandable to the patient. Cultural sensitivity and linguistic competency are a high priority in health care today. Age, mental status, and native language must be considered in the effective presentation of instructions.[6] Understanding expectations during treatment empowers patients and fosters cooperation through feelings of mutual respect. Every effort must be extended to maximize patients' feelings of security. The patient is informed of the necessity of removal of restrictive clothing that may alter the position of skin marks and inhibit reproduction of the patient's position. If departmental practice requires the patient to undress before entering the treatment room, an explanation is given before the first treatment. The location of gowns or robes and a secure place for the patient's belongings are identified. Preparation for proximity to the gantry, machine motion, and sounds of treatment can reduce anxiety. At the outset, the patient is shown the audio and visual monitoring systems. Patients must be informed about safeguards to their privacy and reassured that although radiation therapists leave the room, contact will be maintained at all times.

Patients must be counseled from the start of treatment in the proper maintenance of skin marks, general skin care, and nutritional guidelines. Nursing personnel or radiation therapists may provide these services while being mindful of the limitations of their scope of practice. Appropriate decision making must be demonstrated in the practice of professional referrals. During the course of treatment, questioning skills may be used to discover the onset or severity of acute radiation reactions. Open-ended questions are formed to encourage dialogue, and brief answers by the patient may be followed with gently probing questions to develop a fuller picture of the patient's reactions to treatment. The radiation therapist is responsible for assessing the patient's verbal and observable responses (e.g., skin reactions, weight change, changes in demeanor) and evaluating whether treatment should continue or be withheld until the patient may be seen by the physician.

PATIENT TRANSFERS

Patients require varying assistance onto the treatment table. Most ambulatory patients require minimal assistance. Where extended-range treatment tables are in use, even the need for a step stool may be eliminated. Some patients may need only a supportive arm while walking, whereas others may arrive in a wheelchair or on a stretcher.

Mindful of the variety of auxiliary medical equipment the patient may be using, the therapist evaluates the transfer requirements. Although this equipment is most likely to be in extensive use by inpatients, outpatients may also be treated with oxygen or nutritional support and chemotherapy. Tubes and catheters must be recognized and carefully handled so as not to disrupt their placement or introduce infection.

In the planning of any transfer, the patient should be included when possible. Patients may be able to move themselves or have pain they wish the radiation therapist to consider. They may also have other suggestions to facilitate their safe transfer. In the initial planning of a patient transfer, the radiation therapist must assess his or her own need for assistance.

 Underestimating the need for assistance can result in injury to the patient and the caregiver.

For safe transfer of the patient to the treatment table, consider proper body mechanics of the patient and radiation therapist. General rules for lifting require the maintenance of a wide base of support with the feet apart and one foot placed slightly in front of the other. The weight to be moved is kept close to the lifter, who bends at the knees and hips rather than at the waist, while maintaining the normal curve at the lower back. Lifters should never twist or bend sideways while supporting weight.[4]

Wheelchair Transfers

For patients unable to stand unassisted, the radiation therapist prepares by positioning the wheelchair parallel to the table and locking its wheels. Foot rests are raised and the radiation therapist stands facing the patient. With the patient's feet together and radiation therapist's feet on either side, the radiation therapist leans forward and bends at the knees and hips, while maintaining the natural curve of the lower spine. The patient reaches around the radiation therapist's shoulders while the radiation therapist reaches under the patient's arms. The radiation therapist's arms are then locked around the patient's back. The patient is raised to his or her feet and pivoted 90 degrees so that the patient's back faces the table. Next, the patient is eased into a sitting position. With an arm behind the patient's shoulders and the other behind the knees, the radiation therapist turns and eases the patient into the supine position in one smooth motion.

If for any reason (e.g., paralysis, pain) the patient requires more assistance onto the table, the patient should be transported to the department with a stretcher. This is a safety consideration for the patient and caregivers.

Stretcher Transfers

Stretcher transfers should be completed with a minimum of two caregivers. The stretcher is placed alongside the treatment table with the side rails lowered and wheels locked. The table is positioned at the same level as the stretcher. If the patient can slide over, one radiation therapist may secure the stretcher while the other stands opposite the treatment table, providing assistance and ensuring that the patient does not fall.

Transfer of the immobile patient across the width of the treatment table and stretcher will force lifters to breach rules of good body mechanics. At some point the weight will be held away from the lifter's own center of gravity, and someone will push rather than pull the weight. The reach makes maintaining proper posture difficult. A draw sheet and slide board can assist the transfer of stretcher patients, reducing the risk of injury to the people performing the transfer. Slide board use is preferred when insufficient staff members are available for a safe lifting transfer. Slide boards are relatively thin sheets of plastic, large enough to support the patient but generally used only to bridge the space between the stretcher and treatment table so that the patient may be pulled rather than lifted from one to the other. Patients are positioned with their hands on their chest. The slide board is positioned by rolling the patient from the treatment table and placing the board under the draw sheet. After the patient is eased back onto the slide board, the board is pulled to the treatment table or the patient is slid across the bridge created over the gap between the stretcher and treatment table. The slide board must be removed if it is in the path of a treatment beam.

Slide boards should not be used if rolling places the patient at risk for injury. In this situation, the assistance of several trained individuals is necessary. The appropriate number of lifters depends on factors such as the size of the patient or special considerations such as pain. Lifters position themselves to maintain support of the patient's head, shoulders, hips, and feet during the entire lift. The draw sheet is pulled taut, edges are rolled and gripped firmly, and the team leader specifies a count so that everyone lifts at the same time. The patient is lifted just high enough to clear the treatment table and stretcher surfaces, moved over, and eased down. The radiation therapist ensures that the patient and any accessory equipment are secure before moving the stretcher away. Intravenous lines, catheters, oxygen, and other tubing are secured away from moving treatment machine parts.

PATIENT POSITION, ISOCENTER, AND FIELD PLACEMENT

Advances in imaging and treatment-planning computers encourage continued development in the precise planning of external-beam radiation treatments. With increasing confidence, the physician, dosimetrist, and radiation therapist focus beams to the target while minimizing the radiation delivered to surrounding normal tissues. V&R systems communicate with the treatment unit to verify and document the reproduction of treatment unit parameters for a specific plan. The clinical significance of these technical advances, however, will always be limited by the ability to translate them to the patient. Precision in the reproduction and immobilization of the treatment position, stability of surface landmarks, and exactitude in alignment of the patient with these references contribute greatly to variation in treatment delivery and thus represent the greatest obstacle to the application of advances in treatment planning. Management of these factors is a primary technical challenge for the radiation therapist.

Patient Positioning

Artificial devices (e.g., dentures, temporary prostheses) in the area of treatment should be removed before planning and treatment when possible. When prescribed, internal shielding is generally fitted to the patient and placed before positioning for treatment. For example, in the treatment of head and neck cancer with lateral ports, patients with metal fillings may benefit from the addition of internal shielding to reduce the dose on the buccal mucosa and tongue produced by increased electron scatter near the metal surface. A mouth guard made of wax and inlaid with a thin layer of tin can be prepared before the simulation and used throughout the treatment course to attenuate this scatter without significantly altering the dose distribution.

With the area to be treated over the appropriate window of the treatment couch, the patient is positioned straight and level. Positioning with the isocenter of the patient's treatment plan as close as possible to the center of the table provides the maximum clearance for techniques that require 360-degree gantry rotation around the patient.[6]

 Many opposing oblique or tangential fields may be accommodated without rotation of the treatment table by making lateral shifts of the patient (consequently isocenter) relative to the table surface.

For example, small angles off the vertical axis such as those used for lung boost fields may be accommodated by biasing the patient toward the side that the anterior field enters, or larger angles off the vertical axis (such as those used in breast tangents) may be accommodated by moving the patient closer to the treatment side.

The treatment description in the chart is used to reproduce a position consistent with that prescribed at the simulation (see Chapters 22 and 23). Configurations of positioning aids and immobilization devices must match those used at the simulation. External references rely on planar alignment; even slight variations of position can mean large discrepancies in the internal location that a surface landmark represents (Figure 8-2). Tools assisting position reproduction include descriptive statements such as supine versus prone, arm placement, and names and location of sponges or other positioning devices. Measurements indicating the relative position of anatomy (e.g., chin to suprasternal notch or slope of the sternum) may be used. Photographs taken at the simulation illustrate written descriptions. The precise reproduction of the treatment position is critical to the maintenance of the orientation of surface landmarks to internal targets.

Immobilization devices reproduce treatment position while restricting movement. The complexity of this task varies depending on the mobility of the anatomic site. Improvements in treatment planning and image evaluation methods are supporting increasingly narrow margins of normal tissue for setup variation, demanding increased immobilization for all treatment sites.

Comfort significantly affects the patient's ability to maintain the treatment position. Care is taken at the time of simulation to define a treatment position that the patient can tolerate for treatment. Considerations at the simulation include the general condition of the patient (e.g., age, disability, pain), location of normal structures, skin folds in the treatment fields, ability to treat all fields in one position, and reproducibility. The goal at treatment is to reproduce the planned position to ensure the coincidence of surface landmarks relative to the internal target. Even with the best planning, however, discomfort is not avoided for every patient. In these situations, the radiation therapist accommodates the patient's needs while maintaining the integrity of the planned position.

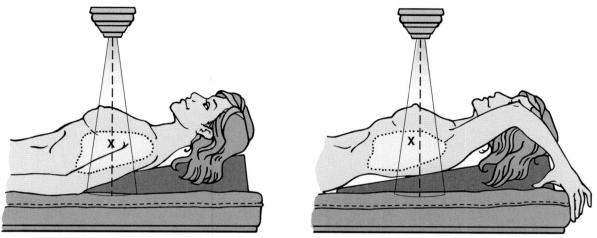

Figure 8-2. Change in patient position changes location of landmarks relative to point of interest.

Localization Landmarks

While patient dignity is maintained with drapes, external landmarks referenced in the treatment description are located. Localization landmarks include natural anatomy or artificial **fiducial markers** (fixed reference points against which other objects can be measured) positioned at a fixed relationship to unseen anatomy. Fiducials may be placed internally, at the skin surface, or fixed external to the patient. Landmarks may be maintained using a variety of permanent and nonpermanent methods.

The most common permanent references include visible and palpable anatomic landmarks (bones or other identifiable points that can be seen or felt and point to the location of hidden anatomy) or tiny permanent marks (tattoos) placed on the patient. Permanent marks are made using a small amount of dye introduced with a hypodermic needle just under the surface of the skin, within the dermis. Permanent marks allow patients to bathe normally during treatment without concerns of impacting their treatment. In addition to surface references, permanent implanted radiopaque markers such as gold seeds provide references for setup verification of the positioning of soft tissue structures, such as the prostate, that are mobile relative to surface or bony landmarks.

Permanent references have drawbacks to be considered, and judicial use is warranted. Implanting fiducials carries a risk of complications although the risk is low relative to the gains in treatment precision. The relative advantages of artificially produced surface marks such as tattoos, however, may be diminishing with current treatment methods. From the psychological perspective for the patient, cancer is increasingly a chronic condition and permanent marks are a reminder to the patient of a difficult period. Even the term *tattoo* has societal connotations and may be avoided when communicating the purpose of the procedure to the patient. From a quality-of-care perspective, although tattooing may provide some reference for follow-up assessment or subsequent treatment planning, these marks move relative to the treatment volume and do not provide precision in determination of exposed tissue. Alignment of any new treatment fields must be confirmed radiographically, further

weakening the long-term value of permanent visible marks.[1] Alternatively, semipermanent marks, or a combination of semipermanent with minimal permanent marks, may be used during treatment to mark triangulation coordinates, outline the field, or mark the field center and corners. Semipermanent marks must be maintained throughout the course of treatment and have the potential of removal or drift as they are reinforced. Permanent ink markers and paint pens easily mark skin and are difficult to remove; the variety of colors available can be useful for clarity against different skin tones. Clear patient-sensitive tape or markers with adhesives designed to resist removal while remaining gentle to sensitive skin may cover marks to aid in retention during bathing.

External fiducial markers may also be applied to certain forms of immobilization devices. Head frames that are screwed directly into the skull provide precise incremental references, which will not move relative to intracranial structures. Thermoplastic molds may also be designed with sufficient immobilization to ensure that marks will remain coincident with the treatment volume.

Positioning Isocenter

The isocenter of the treatment unit is defined in a static position. Because neither the isocenter nor its planned position in the patient can be directly visualized during treatment setup, coordinates distant to these points guide the setup process. Treatment volume alignment with the machine most often begins with a process of simple **triangulation**. Analogous to line of position navigation, the machine isocenter is located at the point of intersection of two lines with known coordinates, visible via the horizontal and vertical lasers. Similarly, the treatment isocenter is located relative to the three setup coordinates on the patient's surface or on the equipment fixed relative to his or her anatomy.

With the patient in the approximate treatment position and the localization landmarks identified, the treatment table is positioned to bring the patient close to the location for treatment. The room lights are dimmed and patient position is refined using lasers and the treatment-field light. Through the alignment of three fiducial landmarks on the patient relative to

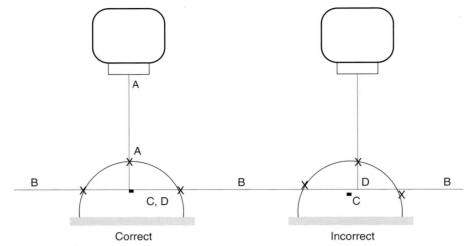

Figure 8-3. Three-point positioning: tattoos (x). *A,* Crosshairs. *B,* Lasers. *C,* Planned location of the isocenter. *D,* Actual location of isocenter.

three external references (lasers), the treatment position is reproduced.

With the patient in the precise treatment position, the isocenter is positioned relative to the localization landmarks. In some situations, the intersection of the planes identified by the three positioning points coincides with the treatment isocenter (Figure 8-3). For many clinical situations, however, this is not practical. Anatomic references are seldom so conveniently located, and many sites do not lend themselves to the reproducible placement of localization marks. Examples include mobile skin surfaces such as those of the breast, of the axilla, and of older or obese persons; sloping surfaces such as those treated with tangential fields; irregular surfaces; and areas covered by dressings. For these situations, a landmark and coordinate system may be used (Figure 8-4). The reproduction of isocenter placement is accomplished by aligning stable surface landmarks with lasers, defining a zero reference point. Table motions in the X, Y, and Z planes are made from that point. Z plane position may be determined from the table surface or the SSD from the gantry. Several methods may be used to determine SSD. An optical-distance indicator (ODI), or rangefinder, consists of a light that is projected onto the patient's skin and matched at the intersecting crosshairs that coincide with the central ray of the beam. Mechanical-distance indicators consist of incrementally marked rods or a measuring tape mounted to the collimator assembly extended to touch the patient's surface at the center of the treatment field. Couch movements direct the positioning of the isocenter, as demonstrated in Figure 8-4. Indexed couches with digital linear position readouts contribute valuable precision in making these adjustments.

Verification Imaging (Setup)

Verification of the position of isocenter is traditionally and most commonly accomplished by comparing a pair of planar images with corresponding reference images. **Stereoscopic** images are two images from different angles focused on the same point; **orthogonal** images are a special case of stereoscopic images with a 90-degree angle between them. These images may be a

subset of treatment portals or may be designed specifically for setup verification. A single planar image or pair of coplanar images with coincident (**coplanar**) central rays is insufficient to verify the position of a point in three-dimensional space. The position of isocenter on a planar image can be defined only in two dimensions along the central axis of the beam; its distance from the radiation source cannot be determined, and geometric distortion of the landmarks in each image as projected onto the uniform plane of the image skews perception further. An approximation of three-dimensional space (2D/2D or 2.5D) is made with the addition of a second image, rotated on isocenter from the first, identifying the position of isocenter as the

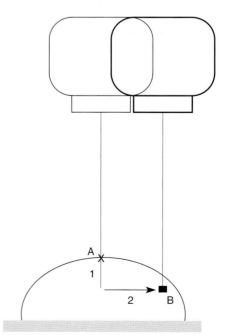

Figure 8-4. Landmark and coordinate method. *A,* Surface landmark (tattoo). *B,* Planned location of isocenter. *1,* Shift to depth; *2,* lateral shift.

intersection of the two central axes. Increasing the angle between the incident beams reduces the impact of geometric distortion across each planar image, improving the accuracy of results. Accuracy for planar image pairs is at its greatest with perpendicular, orthogonal, beam sets. Adding more projections also improves results, CT imaging producing the most accurate volumetric results.

Where setup verification is performed before treatment (online), setup variation is minimized. Image-guided radiation therapy (IGRT) techniques combine online verification with precise target localization to optimize corrections for **interfraction** changes in target position, changes occurring between treatment sessions. A variety of image- and non–image-based methods are used for precision in identifying the location of mobile soft tissues. EPIDs produce near real-time planar images on a computer screen for evaluation of treatment accuracy and can visualize implanted markers. Table position adjustments are applied as calculated from image findings and treatment proceeds.

Other IGRT techniques include ultrasound imaging, visualizing internal structures such as the bladder/prostate margin without the need to implant radiopaque markers. Cone-beam CT visualizes soft tissue with or without implanted markers and produces three-dimensional images for the most accurate positioning evaluation. Motion techniques in planar and CT imaging evaluate normal **intrafraction** (during treatment) motion, ensuring inclusion of the targeted treatment volume for the treatment to be delivered. Nonimaging radiofrequency tracking systems use implanted beacons to localize and track interfraction and intrafraction motion, allowing beam interruption should the tumor move outside of the path of the treatment beam.

BEAM POSITION AND SHAPE

The gantry and collimator are rotated to the positions defined in the treatment plan. Standard collimation systems using adjustable, divergent, and opposing jaws, often with the ability to be positioned asymmetrically around the central axis, allow the customizing of fields into a square or rectangle. Field (or jaw) size indicates the size and dimensions of the radiation field at the isocenter. Individuals and tumors, however, do not grow in squares and rectangles. Further field shaping is required for most treatments and may be accomplished using static multileaf collimation blocking, either custom or standard.

Multileaf Collimators

Linear accelerators equipped with multileaf collimator (MLC) (Figure 8-5) systems customize field shapes using "jaws" that have been sliced into a series of opposing leaves. Opposing banks of leaves form "leaf pairs." Each leaf is positioned independently, producing a variety of treatment field shapes. Space between leaves is a source of leakage radiation minimized by manufacturer engineering of an interlocking leaf design or by positioning the primary jaws outside of the field as backup jaws during treatment delivery. Leaf end shape supports production of a divergent field edge and will be rounded on systems that move leaves on a single plane. Leaf width is measured at the isocenter and has an impact on the smoothness of the contour of

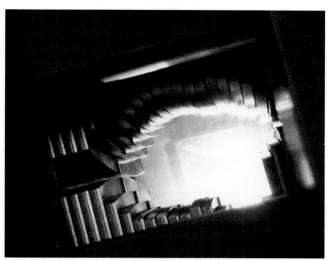

Figure 8-5. Multileaf collimator. (Courtesy of Elekta Systems.)

the exposed field edge. Micro-MLC units with leaf widths less than 5 mm provide greater refinement in field edge effects. These units are often removable offering flexibility for the treatment unit when the MLC is not needed. Number of leaf pairs, available leaf widths, specific characteristics, and control systems of MLCs vary between manufacturers, with some manufacturers offering several models. Because of the complexity of treatment procedures using MLCs, verification and record systems are usually in place. Control systems may be integrated with the accelerator console or may be separate, which has implications for selection of field parameters and MLC files as well as backup options should network access be interrupted.

By reducing the need for the positioning of heavy blocks, an MLC improves customization of treatment volumes and increases safety for patients and radiation therapists. MLCs controlled from the treatment console may be repositioned for each treatment field reducing individual treatment times and adding comfort for patients and efficiency in the department, all of which improves patient satisfaction.

Blocks

Individualization of treatment volumes may also be accomplished through the use of shielding blocks. Shielding blocks, used to shape photon or electron fields, take several forms. Materials range from spent uranium to lead and lead alloys used in the production of customized shielding blocks. Whereas a supply of standard lead blocks is among the necessary accessories in the treatment room, modern radiation therapy beam shaping requires the use of custom shielding or a static MLC. Blocks rest on or are screwed to plastic trays inserted into the accessory tray of the treatment-unit head. The required thickness of blocks varies based on the energy of the treatment beam and the attenuation coefficient of the block material. Full-shielding blocks are constructed to transmit less than 5% of the original beam.

A supply of standardized blocks occupy little space and accommodate emergency treatments until customized shielding or MLC plans can be created. Limitations include minimal

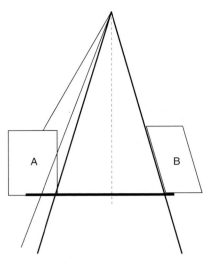

Figure 8-6. Blocks. *A*, Nondivergent (clinical). *B*, Divergent (custom).

variability in shape and size and perpendicular block sides increasing penumbra along the blocked field edges (see Figure 8-6, A). Standardized blocks are often placed on trays without a means of being secured to the tray, requiring attentiveness to removal before changing gantry position.

Lead alloys with low melting points are used in the construction of customized shielding blocks. Cutting systems mimic the geometric arrangement of the treatment beam, thus ensuring proper divergence and magnification at the treatment site. Cut block sides run parallel to the divergence of the treatment beam, reducing the penumbra caused by beam absorption through changing block thickness (Figure 8-6, B). Drawbacks of these systems include space requirements for fabrication and storage, hazards associated with lifting heavy equipment, and exposure to hazardous chemicals. The most common material used is Cerrobend (Lipowitz metal), an alloy with a low melting point and expansion characteristics.

 The interaction of the photon beam with materials produces scatter electrons that contaminate the photon beam and produce increased skin doses for patients. Low-energy electrons are absorbed in 15 cm of air; therefore, all beam-shaping and modification devices for photon beams must be secured a minimum of 20 cm from the surface of the patient.

 Cerrobend is composed of bismuth (50%), lead (26.7%), tin (13.3%), and cadmium (10%) and has a melting point of 165° F (74° C). Alternative alloys are available with similar characteristics with lower concentrations of toxic metals to further protect workers.

Verification Imaging (Portal)

Portal images are taken at the start of treatment and at regular intervals during its course to verify placement of isocenter and beam position, including beam shape. Frequency of portal imaging is based on department policy and professional judgment and varies among institutions. Partially based on historic studies showing a reduction in treatment errors associated with increased portal imaging—weekly portal imaging for radical cases—has become an accepted, although not universally implemented, standard.[2,3] Some clinical situations, such as unstable localization landmarks or the proximity of the treatment volume to critical structures, may require an increased frequency of portal or setup imaging. Finally, weekly portal filming cannot document variations in positioning of treatment fields. A review of daily portal images taken with an EPID has shown variations of greater than 1 cm in fields demonstrating excellent reproduction based on assessment of weekly films. Awareness of these limitations spurs the desire for increased frequency and precision in portal and setup imaging. The professional judgment of the radiation therapist is central in determining an appropriate imaging schedule with the radiation oncologist.

Portal images may be created using single- or double-exposure techniques. Single-exposure images may be used when sufficient landmarks for verification are located within the treatment area. The single-exposure image may be created using the same portal film/cassette combination as the double image, or, alternatively, verification film (v-film) may be positioned throughout the treatment exposure. The double-exposure technique yields a visualization of the treatment field and surrounding anatomy, thus increasing the landmarks available for interpretation but also increasing dose delivered to normal tissue. This technique is accomplished by producing a short exposure of the treatment area. A second exposure is taken after the removal of field-shaping and retracting collimator jaws.

BEAM-MODIFYING DEVICES

With assurance that the radiation is being directed to the prescribed volume, customization of dose delivery may require the addition of devices that modify the distribution of the radiation dose across the treatment field.

Bolus

In radiation therapy, *bolus* refers to materials whose interactions with the radiation beam mimic those of tissue. Bolus comes in many forms and has many applications. Common materials include paraffin wax, Vaseline gauze, wet gauze or towels, and water bags. Commercially available products developed specifically for use in radiation therapy are available in sheets of variable thicknesses (Figure 8-7) and powder forms that can be mixed with water and formed to meet specific needs. Flexibility in shaping is an advantage because bolus must conform to the treatment surface without air gaps.

Bolus of a thickness equal to the depth of maximum dose eliminates the skin-sparing effect of megavoltage photon beams. Bolus may be applied with this goal over entire treatment areas or simply over scars, superficial nodes, or other areas of concern. When bolus is applied in this fashion, the buildup of dose occurs within it, thus bringing the area of maximum dose deposition to the patient's surface.

Bolus may also be used to compensate for variations in surface contour or to eliminate air gaps in cavities. For example, surgical procedures leaving anatomic defects, such as those used for the removal of sinus or eye malignancies, produce

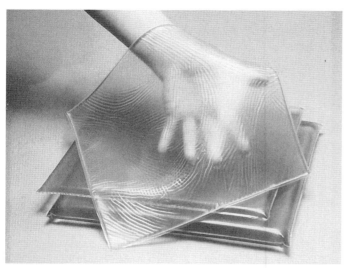

Figure 8-7. Bolus example: Superflab. (Courtesy Civco, Inc., Orange City, Iowa.)

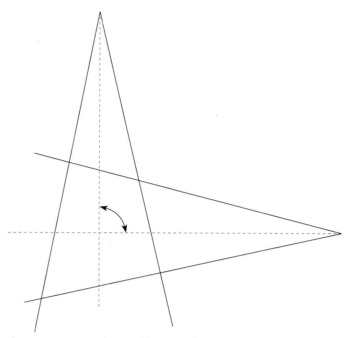

Figure 8-8. A 90-degree hinge angle.

significant irregularities. Filling the cavity with bolus material such as Vaseline gauze or a water-filled balloon significantly improves the dose distribution in the target volume. This application is useful only in situations in which the loss of skin sparing is acceptable or desired. When skin sparing is to be maintained, the creation of individualized compensators (a beam-modifier that changes radiation output relative to variations in attenuation over a changing patient contour) should be evaluated.

Compensators

The design of megavoltage treatment units produces a radiation beam delivering a relatively even dose across the plane perpendicular to the radiation beam. Patients, however, rarely provide a flat surface parallel with this ideal. Skewing of dose distribution caused by irregular surfaces can be compensated by using bolus material to produce a level treatment area; however, a loss of skin sparing accompanies this technique. To retain this important effect, compensating filters may be positioned in the head of the treatment unit, thus modifying the radiation beam to accommodate the contour of the patient. Compensating filters can be made from a variety of materials as long as the materials' equivalence to tissue absorption is known. Common materials include copper, brass, lead, and Lucite.

Tissue deficits in need of compensation are usually most significant over one dimension (width or length), and a set of standardized two-dimensional compensators meets the needs of many treatment situations. Custom compensators can easily be built for special situations. Strips of attenuating materials of known thicknesses are layered and mounted onto a tray.

Wedges

The primary goal of treatment planning is treating a target to an even (homogeneous) dose while minimizing the dose delivered to normal tissue. The orientation of multiple fields to one another during treatment may produce inhomogeneous dose distributions over the target volume. The isodose lines of a single treatment field on a flat surface are relatively parallel to the surface. When a second beam is positioned directly opposite this beam, the combined dose distribution is relatively even throughout the volume. However, as the **hinge angle** (measure of the angle between central rays of two intersecting treatment beams) (Figure 8-8) decreases, doses delivered to overlapping areas vary significantly, thus creating areas of high- and low-dose regions in the desired target volume.

Wedges appear similar to compensator filters; however, their application differs significantly. The wedge is designed to change the angle of the isodose curve relative to the beam axis at a specified depth within the patient. Wedges reduce the dose in areas of overlap between fields that have hinge angles less than 180 degrees. The thick end of the wedge, referred to as the *heel*, attenuates the greatest amount of radiation, thus drawing the isodose lines closer to the surface. Attenuation decreases along the wedge to the thin end, or *toe,* where the dose delivered to the patient will be relatively greater than the dose at the opposite side of the treatment field. When wedges are used, heels are typically positioned together.

Standard wedge systems use externally mounted wedges that the radiation therapist must position when required by the treatment plan. The manufacturer usually provides these wedges, which are customized for specific treatment units. Standard wedge sizes are 15, 30, 45, and 60 degrees.

Treatment units using internal wedging methods allow customizing of the wedge angle for each treatment plan. One system uses a 60-degree universal wedge placed in the beam path for a specified number of monitor units. The beam is interrupted to remove the wedge, and the remaining monitor units are delivered; the ratio of wedged-to-unwedged beam results in a custom wedge angle. Other systems use a virtual wedge system in which a dynamic, or moving, jaw starts at one side of the field and opens to a full field over the course of dose delivery. This effectively delivers a range of dose over the field.

The side of the field at which the jaw starts its movement allows the beam to pass to the patient for the longest time so that it correlates with the wedge toe.

Field sizes are limited with the use of compensators and wedges. Care must be taken to ensure that treatment fields do not extend beyond the heel or sides of either beam-modification device (flash or extension beyond the toe is acceptable).

Transmission Filters

Transmission filters are designed to allow the transmission of a predetermined percentage of the treatment beam to a portion of a treatment field and may be used throughout the course of the treatment. This allows the physician to treat structures that have varying radiosensitivity in proximity to one another at different dose rates from a single treatment field. For example, whole-abdomen radiation therapy induces significant gastrointestinal effects. By reducing the dose to the upper portion of the abdomen through the use of the transmission filter, patient tolerance is improved. The pelvis receives the dose at a higher rate, effectively completing the boost dose concurrently with the whole-abdomen treatment. When a transmission filter is used, fraction and total doses for each area must be written in the prescription and documented separately in the treatment record.

ELECTRON BEAM

Superficial treatment volumes may be addressed using electron beams. The physical characteristics of these beams provide rapid dose build-up, an area of uniform dose deposition, followed by rapid dose fall-off. The dose tends to bow or bulge laterally from the edge of the field. Setup procedures differ from penetrating beams with less reliance on isocenter. Gantry positions are defined to bring the beam surface as close to parallel with the treatment surface as possible, and collimation is brought closer to the treatment surface. Special considerations for electron beam treatments include beam collimation, shielding, and bolus requirements.

Collimation

The mass and charge of the electron give rise to increased interactions in air compared with those of the photon beam. This scattering of the electron beam necessitates the extension of **collimation** (field shaping) close to the treatment surface, improving radiation dose distribution by sharpening the dose gradient at the beam edges. Secondary collimation systems for electron therapy usually take the form of cones attached to the treatment-accessory tray of the gantry or trimmer bars adjustable to varying field sizes. Cones are limited to a few selected field sizes, generally squares. Trimmer bars attached to the collimator provide greater flexibility in field size, but the increased distance from the patient increases penumbra and lateral scattering of dose at depth. Cones or trimmer bars are usually secured on the treatment unit before the patient is positioned (Figure 8-9).

Internal Shielding

Sites such as the nares, auricle, eyelids, and lips are often treated with electron therapy. These structures are thin; underlying normal tissue such as the medial nasal membranes, skin behind

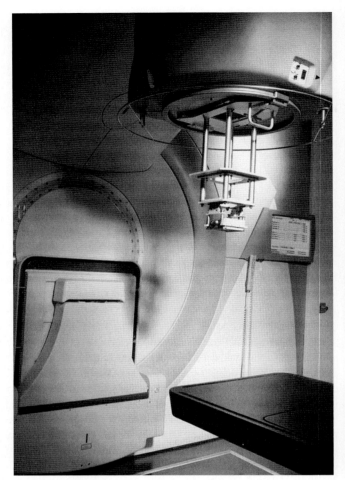

Figure 8-9. Electron cones. (Courtesy Elekta.)

the ear, optic lens, lacrimal ducts and glands, and gingiva must be protected from unnecessary radiation exposure. Shields may be produced to achieve this goal and placed between the tumor site and normal structures. The interaction of the electrons with the metal of these shields, however, produces low-energy scatter radiation that would increase the dose and reaction at the incident tissue surface. To absorb these low-energy photons, the shield must be covered with a low Z number material such as aluminum, tin, or paraffin wax. Because of the proximity of the beam collimation and the constraints of superficial beam alignment, these shields will typically be positioned before the treatment field itself is positioned.

Bolus

Although the materials used for bolus in electron therapy are the same as those used with photons, the applications differ. Three applications for bolus exist in electron therapy. First, as with photons, bolus may be used to eliminate skin sparing. However, because of the rapid buildup of dose with increasing electron energy, this is applicable only for low-energy electron beams. Second, the depth at which dose fall-off occurs can be customized by combining the choice of electron energy and using bolus to decrease the depth of penetration. Third, irregular surfaces and air cavities play havoc with the dose distribution of electron beams, and bolus may be used to fill in these irregularities. Bolus over an even contour will generally be positioned following beam alignment, whereas bolus to fill a cavity or irregular surface may require placement in advance.

Electron Beam Shaping

Field-shaping requirements for electron beam therapy differ significantly from photon requirements and may be referred to by several synonymous terms. Attenuated much more efficiently than photon beams, full shielding for electron beams requires lead thicknesses of only several millimeters (general rule: ½ energy in millimeters of lead). Electron shields, or field-defining apertures (FDAs), provide tertiary collimation and shape the electron treatment field. These may be cut and molded to the patient surface except in instances where the field area makes the weight of the cutout uncomfortable. Alternatively, field-defining apertures or "cutouts" can be designed to fit directly inside the electron cone. Planning of these field-shaping cutouts may be accomplished through simulation or clinical procedures. For clinical customization, the required field shape is drawn on a template positioned on the patient's surface with localization landmarks for later treatment reproduction. The template is then used to form a mold for creation of a Cerrobend cutout (Figure 8-10), which fits inside the base of the cone.

ASSESSMENT AND ACCEPTANCE OF TREATMENT PARAMETERS

The radiation therapist performs a final review of the treatment setup, verifying patient positioning, beam direction, and use of beam modifiers. If arc therapy is being applied, or if subsequent treatment fields will be positioned from outside the treatment room, the radiation therapist ensures free clearance for gantry motion throughout the treatment rotation. Once satisfied that the set parameters meet those prescribed by the treatment plan, the radiation therapist notifies the patient that he or she will exit the treatment room to administer the radiation. The radiation therapist reminds and reassures patients that they are being monitored at all times. An indication of the approximate

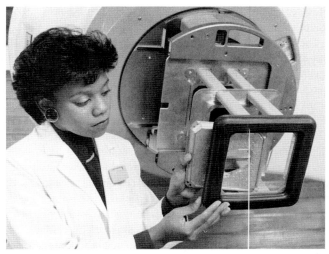

Figure 8-10. Electron cutouts. (Courtesy Varian Medical Systems.)

time that the beam will be on is reassuring. On confirmation that the patient is the only person in the treatment room, the radiation therapist exits and securely closes the door.

Patient-Monitoring Systems

To protect the radiation therapist from radiation exposure, the patient must be left alone at the treatment unit for the radiation delivery. In some situations (orthovoltage or other low-energy treatments), the radiation therapist may monitor treatment directly through leaded glass windows. This becomes impractical with megavoltage units, however, and indirect monitoring systems must be used. However, to maintain patient safety and accuracy of treatment, audio and visual contact is maintained at all times. At least two cameras are used to maintain visual contact with the patient. Generally, at least one camera will provide a long view of the whole patient, allowing observation of general distress or movement while another provides a closer view of the treatment field and observation of subtle patient movement.

A two-way communication system between the treatment room and console remains continuously audible to the operator. A switch allows the communication into the treatment room when necessary. A stop at the console area before the first treatment allows the radiation therapist to demonstrate monitoring systems to new patients, reassuring them that they are heard and seen during treatment delivery and that their privacy is being protected.

Console

Radiation delivery is controlled at the treatment console area located outside the treatment room. The configuration of the console varies widely among treatment units, from simple cobalt units with two timers and beam on-off lights to multiple computer-controlled screens displaying treatment unit and ancillary equipment parameters.

The console provides information to the radiation therapist regarding the status of the treatment unit. The use of beam modifiers may require verification of placement to release a safety interlock for treatment. **Interlocks** assist in meeting many safety parameters for treatment delivery, including the closing of doors, placement of proper beam modifiers (wedges, compensators, electron cones), and machine-operation requirements (water, vacuum, sulfur hexafluoride [SF6]). A lack of agreement with the requirements of any of these interlocks triggers a fault indicator on the console. Fault-light panels provide diagnostic information regarding proper functioning and the source of problems in the treatment unit.

Gauges and light panels provide further information regarding machine operation, including the dose rate during beam delivery. Although the maintenance of equipment is ultimately the responsibility of the radiation physicist, the monitoring of equipment functioning and reporting of problems to the physics or engineering department is a critical responsibility of the radiation therapist.[7] Any equipment malfunctions or setup errors affecting treatment delivery must be reported to the radiation oncologist, and corrective actions must be documented in writing. Malfunctions or errors resulting in misadministration must be reported following Nuclear Regulatory Commission (NRC) or state reporting requirements. Definitions of reportable events and misadministration may change over time so determination of a reportable event must be made by the radiation safety officer. Equipment malfunctions causing serious injury or death are reported through the U.S. Food and Drug Administration's Medical Device Reporting Act.

TREATMENT DELIVERY

Beam On and Beam Off

The radiation therapist sets the parameters for treatment delivery, or confirms settings downloaded from the V & R system, including the calculated primary and backup monitor unit (or timer) settings.

Initiation of the treatment beam requires turning a key, pressing a switch, or both. The console displays the dose rate and time or number of monitor units administered. Red "radiation on" lights in and outside the treatment room indicate the presence of radiation in the treatment room.

At beam on, ion chambers within the beam measure radiation output, displaying relative dose delivered in monitor units (MU). Primary, secondary, and backup systems function to interrupt the treatment beam after the prescribed dose has been delivered. Backup systems may be manually or automatically set depending on the sophistication of the treatment unit and function as safety interlocks, terminating the beam if the primary counter malfunctions. The accelerator is designed to deliver dose at specified rates; decreases in that rate may indicate problems. Backup systems include secondary ion chambers calibrated a percentage lower than the primary ion chamber and timers that interrupt the beam after a set period of time.

After radiation delivery to the first treatment port, the radiation therapist must assess the position of the patient and treatment unit for each subsequent field. Field size, table, gantry, and collimator angles are set, and treatment accessories are positioned. Capabilities of treatment units vary significantly. Some require radiation therapist reentry to the treatment room between every field for positioning of the machine and placement of treatment accessories. As computer control of field shaping through MLCs and beam modification through dynamic wedges, MLCs, and so forth become more widely available, the delivery of multiple treatment fields from the console becomes more prevalent. Bidirectional communication with external V&R systems is increasingly exploited by accelerators that accept online parameters for treatment field setup. With prescribed position values downloaded to the accelerator, the radiation therapist controls motion using motion-enabling functions at the accelerator console or on the pendant in the treatment room. Such auto-setup features reduce time for treatment and reduce potential for mispositioning of treatment variables but must be accompanied by diligence in observation of patient movement and proximity to moving equipment.

Treatment Interruptions

In the event of movement by the patient, improper machine motion, or failure of the unit to cease treatment at the prescribed dose, operator interruption of the treatment beam is necessary. Options for x-ray beam interruption include pressing the beam-off key, turning the operation key to the "off" position, or

opening the door to the treatment unit. If these actions fail to stop the beam, an emergency "off" switch must be used, thereby completely turning off the treatment unit. The use of the emergency "off" switch usually requires a warm-up period before reuse of the machine.

The beam may be resumed following an interruption or treatment may be terminated. The observations and decision-making of the treating radiation therapist determine the actions following beam interruption. Whenever possible, treatment will be resumed and completed. Resumption procedures are determined by the equipment and information system in place. Validation of settings, including monitor units, at interruption and resumption is the responsibility of the radiation therapist delivering treatment. When treatment termination is necessary, accurate recording of partial treatment is necessary. Subsequent treatments may require revision to produce final treatment intentions. Electronic and physical back-up monitor unit counters of the treatment unit are checked, and readouts are recorded in a manual system and compared with those transferred from the treatment unit to the V&R system. Any discrepancy must be recorded and reported to be followed by an investigation of the occurrence.

COMMON TREATMENT TECHNIQUES

The choice of field arrangement depends on the location of the tumor and nearby critical structures. As a member of the treatment planning team, the radiation therapist works with the radiation oncologist and dosimetrist to plan field arrangements within the capabilities of the treatment machine that cover target volumes while avoiding critical structures.

Multiple Fields

Most treatment plans require radiation delivery through more than one port to achieve sufficient dose homogeneity through the target volumes. Accuracy in multiple field irradiation is greatly enhanced with the use of isocentric treatment techniques. With the isocenter of the treatment unit precisely positioned in the target volumes, radiation beams can be aimed at the target from many directions without the patient being moved and accuracy compromised. The areas of overlap from these fields receive an increased dose relative to tissues receiving radiation from only one portal.

The most basic multiple-field technique is the parallel opposed portal (POP). POP fields are defined as those with a hinge angle of 180 degrees. These fields may enter the patient from any two directions relative to the patient and are often identified by those directions. Examples include right-and-left lateral (laterals or "lats"), anteroposterior and posteroanterior (AP/PA), and anterior oblique and posterior oblique (obliques). These are used for a great variety of treatment sites and usually require few treatment accessories other than blocks and compensators. Superficial volumes on curved surfaces such as the breast or ribs may require opposing fields, which flash off the surface of the patient. These fields are called *tangential fields, tangents,* or "*tangs.*" The hinge angle between tangential fields may vary slightly from 180 degrees, accommodating divergence of the beams and creating a coincident deep edge to the treated volume.

The four-field technique, sometimes referred to as a *four-field box* or *brick*, is commonly used in the treatment of deep-seated tumors of the pelvis or abdomen. These fields are arranged 90 degrees from one another and generally require no more than blocks for optimal dose distribution in the target volumes.

The wedge-pair technique changes the volume receiving radiation by decreasing the hinge angle between two treatment fields. The relative dose in the area formed between the narrowing hinge angle increases as the angle between the field pairs decreases (Figure 8-11). Overlapping isodose lines are parallel to the treatment surface, not parallel to one another, and combining them produces extremely high dose deposition in the shallow portion of the target relative to the dose deposited more deeply. By reducing the amount of radiation delivered to the shallow region, wedges distribute the dose more homogeneously throughout the target. Three-field techniques also often require the use of wedges to achieve the same dose-homogeneity goal.

Conformal therapy applies three-dimensional localization of the tumor volume. Using multiple fields, possibly in a noncoplanar arrangement, the volume is defined through the BEV and the field shaped to include the target with minimal normal tissue margins. Six or more fields may be used to increase dose to the target while producing sharp fall-off of dose to surrounding tissue. Immobilization devices are carefully designed, and treatment is delivered in the same manner as in other multiple-field techniques. With high-energy beams, dose distributions are comparable with arc therapy.

Arc therapy demonstrates the ultimate multiple-field technique. In standard arc therapy, radiation is delivered as the gantry moves through its arc of rotation, thus effectively delivering radiation through a continuous sequence of individual overlapping treatment portals. Verification of clearance of the patient; accessory medical equipment; the treatment table; and all stretchers, chairs, and stools must be completed before initiating the treatment beam. Visual monitors must be positioned so that the patient and motion of the gantry can be observed. The changing gantry angle must not obstruct monitoring of the treatment at any time.

Stereotactic radiosurgery (SRS) or fractionated stereotactic radiation therapy (SRT) uses sophisticated localization methods to reproduce the placement of the isocenter in the cranium with an accuracy of less than 1 mm. Linear accelerator–based SRS or SRT uses a series of non-coplanar arcs directed at the tumor by changing the treatment-table rotation between treatment arcs. The Gamma knife uses a series of fixed ^{60}Co sources to produce similar dose distributions. By distributing the dose delivered to normal tissue over greater areas, the area of high relative dose is increasingly focused on the target. In radiosurgery, a single large fraction of radiation dose can be delivered to the target without overdosing nearby normal tissue. With SRT, the radiobiologic benefits of fractionation is combined with advances in localization and definition of dose distribution.

Total-body irradiation (TBI) is accomplished through a variety of techniques. Patients must be positioned at an extended distance to produce a sufficiently large field size. On treatment units not specifically designed for this purpose, this usually means lying on the floor or standing or sitting against a treatment-room wall with the gantry rotated 90 degrees. To achieve dose homogeneity, patients must be treated with POP fields requiring repositioning halfway through the treatment. Several dedicated TBI treatment machines have been developed in centers with a high demand for this treatment. These machines simplify treatment by using fixed, extended-distance, double-headed treatment units to deliver radiation through both surfaces with the patient in a comfortable, constant position.

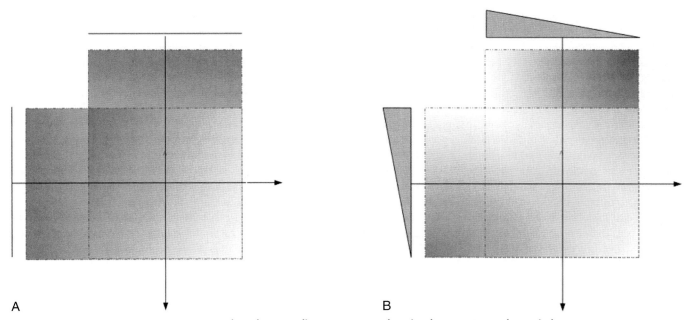

A   B

Figure 8-11. A, No wedge, dose gradient across overlapping beams. **B**, Wedge pair, homogeneity across overlapping region reduced.

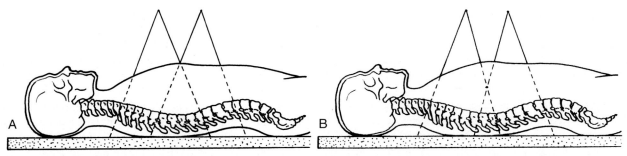

Figure 8-12. Matching adjacent treatment fields. **A**, Abutting a hot match. **B**, A calculated gap.

Adjacent Fields

The divergence of the photon beam poses geometrical problems during the alignment of adjacent treatment fields. Matching methods vary with clinical objectives. Methods include abutting fields at the surface and the use of gaps between fields with or without coplanar alignment of treatment-beam edges. **Feathering** (migration of the gap through the treatment course) may be used to blur dose inhomogeneities in a gapped area. The choice of gap technique and positioning of the gap depends on the location of tumor and critical structures.

Abutting field edges produces a "hot" match in which the diverging beams overlap immediately below the surface (Figure 8-12, A). This may be necessary in situations in which the tumor lies close to the skin surface near the position of the match. A primary example of this application is the treatment of head and neck cancer. The area of overlap must be carefully evaluated for the presence of critical structures and for the dose delivered to them with this technique. Care must be taken to avoid the overdose of critical structures.

When the area of low dose is acceptable at and near the surface, adjacent fields may be separated by a calculated gap (Figure 8-12, B) with treatment fields overlapping at a prescribed depth in the patient. The exact length of the gap must be calculated by knowing the length of each treatment field and depth at which the intersection of the fields is to be positioned (see Chapter 24 on dose calculations for more information).

Some clinical situations demand a precise alignment of the radiation beam at junctions. Areas of overdose and underdose arising from variations in the amount of overlap or space between fields may be unacceptable in these situations. Common examples include tangential breast techniques with matching supraclavicular fields and craniospinal irradiation (CSI). In each of these treatment techniques, positioning the planes of field edges coplanar to one another is useful. This may be accomplished through the use of blocks, independent jaws or gantry, collimator, and couch rotations. A nondivergent beam edge is achieved through the placement of an independent jaw at the isocenter or through the use of a block to the same point (Figure 8-13, A). These blocks may be called *half-beam blocks, central-axis blocks,* or *beam splitters.* Two fields with nondivergent beam edges may be abutted or separated by a standard gap. Limitations to the application of this method include techniques covering large target volumes, because jaw openings must be double the length of

the treatment area, and concerns regarding beam transmission through blocks.

For large field sizes such as those required for CSI, the flexibility of motion designed in the treatment unit is used. Rotation of the gantry, collimator, and table is coordinated to align treatment-field edges. With CSI as an example, the inferior field edges of the opposing cranial fields are made coplanar through the rotation of the couch toward the gantry while a rotation of the collimator aligns the same edge with the divergence of the posterior spine field (Figure 8-13, B and C). Although the abutting of these geometrically matched fields theoretically provides a perfect match without the inhomogeneity of other techniques, the risks of variations in setup must be recognized. Abutting may be desirable in clinical situations in which risks are low, but the presence of critical structures at the match may require the addition of a standard gap. The gap between geometrically aligned fields creates a low-dose area, or cold spot. This is reduced through the application of the feathering technique. The feathered gap moves through the course of treatment, thus varying the low-dose area and increasing the total dose that the area of the gap receives. Many methods are used with varied sequences, number of migrations, and gap sizes.[3]

Matching of electron fields poses different challenges than photon beams. The increased angle of scatter of electrons "bows" the isodose lines below the treatment surface. This bowing varies with energy and collimation. Junctions between multiple electron fields must be carefully modeled and planned, and feathering is routinely applied to spread out hot and cold spots.

Intensity-Modulated Radiation Therapy

The goal of radiation therapy treatment planning is to deliver an evenly distributed radiation dose to the target volume while minimizing the dose to surrounding normal tissue. Conventional and conformal treatment plans, including radiosurgery, accomplish this geometrically with the outline of each treatment field corresponding to the tumor volume. A relatively uniform dose is delivered to structures in the beam path. Normal tissue is protected by controlling beam direction and shape; areas in which treatment beams overlap receive an increased radiation dose relative to areas that receive radiation from only one field. (For a detailed discussion of radiation dose distribution, see Chapter 17.) Intensity-modulated radiation therapy (IMRT) alters this model by delivering nonuniform exposure across the BEV

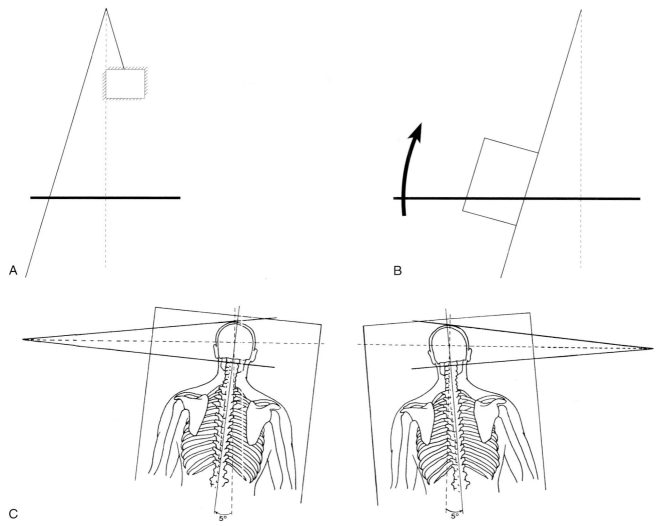

Figure 8-13. Geometric field matching. **A**, Half-beam block. **B**, Collimator rotation. **C**, Couch rotation.

using a variety of techniques and equipment. As radiation intensity is varied (*modulated*) across the exposed field, critical structures are protected. Areas of low dose in the target from one field are compensated by larger doses delivered through another gantry angle that does not intersect the protected structure. By producing several of these non-coplanar, intensity-modulated fields, high doses of radiation are delivered to targets that are irregularly shaped or close to critical structures. These nonuniform exposures create even dose distribution to target volumes with steep dose gradients to adjacent normal tissue. IMRT is an advanced form of three-dimensional conformal treatment planning that uses "inverse planning" techniques, where the clinical objectives are specified first and a computer program is used to automatically determine the optimal beam parameters needed for the desired dose distribution.

MLCs have revolutionized the delivery of radiation treatment. In addition to conventional field shaping, dynamic MLCs may be configured for motion through beam delivery. Alternatively, three-dimensional Cerrobend compensators may be generated to modulate the intensity of the beam at depth.

The plan for these compensators will be generated by a treatment planning system.

IMRT requires a committed program for delivery. The program is highly physics-intensive, requiring specially equipped accelerators and/or MLC units, inverse treatment planning, and sophisticated dose measurement and QA tools including V & R systems to manage large and complex treatment plans. For treatment delivery, immobilization and setup verification is emphasized. Variations in positioning and isocenter alignment have increased significance in delivery of dose to volumes with highly defined margins. For portal imaging, an outline of the irradiated area may be imaged to display a BEV of the "field" but does not offer the same information interpretable from traditional techniques.

Accelerators using MLCs to produce IMRT treatments may apply either of two methods. Segmental MLC (SMLC), or the *step and shoot* method, positions leaves in the first position, and the radiation therapist initiates the beam. As the first beamlet (a small photon-intensity element used to subdivide an IMRT beam for calculation purposes) is delivered, the beam turns off, the accelerator moves the leaves to the next position, turns the beam on and off, and so forth, proceeding through each leaf position until the treatment is delivered. The accelerator controls beam on/off throughout. An accelerator using dynamic MLC (DMLC) IMRT, sometimes called the *sliding window technique,* moves leaves through one beam on/off sequence. Operator intervention is similar in both accelerators, with the radiation therapist positioning the patient and the accelerator and initiating the beam once. Full-field IMRT using accelerators with appropriate MLC capabilities differs little in the setup and delivery of treatment from conventional treatment methods.

TREATMENT ROOM MAINTENANCE

Maintenance of the treatment room and its contents is the domain of the radiation therapist. In addition to monitoring the performance of the treatment unit, the radiation therapist must inspect treatment accessories for signs of wear or damage. Supplies of nonreusable or disposable items such as tape, laundry, and some bolus materials must be monitored.

Cleanliness and orderliness are essential to providing a safe treatment and work environment. Treatment accessories and positioning or immobilization devices coming in contact with patients must be cleaned and disinfected after each use. Sufficient shelf and cabinet space must be available to securely store equipment off the floor, and proper lighting levels must be maintained. Any unsafe conditions must be reported and corrected promptly.

SUMMARY

- The radiation therapist is an active participant in the treatment planning and delivery processes with a primary responsibility to the quality of care delivered to the patient. To meet the goals of treatment, whether palliative or curative, the radiation therapist remains vigilant in the accurate reproduction and administration of the treatment as prescribed by the physician.
- As the expert in treatment delivery, the radiation therapist is highly skilled in the use of megavoltage treatment units and accessories used to customize treatments for each patient. Through the delivery and documentation of treatment, monitoring of treatment-unit function, and inclusion on the departmental QA committee, radiation therapists actively participate in the ongoing goal of the radiation oncology team to continuously improve patient treatment and care.
- Safety and care in assessment of patient mobility, pain, or other factors affecting the patient's well-being are the responsibility of the radiation therapist. As the treatment team member interacting with the patient most frequently, the radiation therapist applies knowledge of the physical and emotional reactions to radiation treatment by addressing the needs and concerns of patients within the guidelines of their scope of practice. Patients are directed to the physician or other professionals as specific needs are discerned.
- Treatment room maintenance is critical to safe and efficient patient care and treatment delivery. The radiation therapist ensures accessibility and proper handling of treatment accessories, both standard and customized for an individual patient.
- Before the arrival of each patient to the treatment room, the radiation therapist carefully reviews the treatment record to determine the status of treatment already delivered and the prescribed plan to be administered during the imminent session. A plan of action is determined and prepared for, including collection and placement within easy reach of necessary positioning, beam-shaping and beam-modification devices for the individual patient; and determining the sequence of verification procedures and treatment field delivery to be performed.
- Responses to treatment interruptions are understood and appropriately applied with resumption protocols ranging from immediate to delayed to deferral of completion altogether.
- Technical advances in diagnostic imaging, treatment planning computers, and megavoltage treatment units have created great flexibility in the complexity of treatment plans that can be developed. Tumor volumes are identified and localized with greater confidence, and treatment beams are focused more narrowly. Normal tissue is increasingly spared from radiation exposure and damage. Reduction in setup error through the development and application of improvements in positioning, immobilization, and localization landmarks, then performing precise pretreatment setup verification, is attained through the diligence, knowledge, and precision of the radiation therapist.

Review Questions

Multiple Choice

1. The patient arrives in the radiation oncology department able to stand and walk several steps at a time. What is the *most* appropriate transportation and transfer method?
   a. walk with assistance
   b. wheelchair
   c. stretcher without slide board
   d. stretcher with slide board

2. Recommended setup landmarks include:
   I. tattoos
   II. palpable bony protrusions
   III. semipermanent ink marks
      a. I and II
      b. I and III
      c. II and III
      d. I, II, and III

3. Which of the following is added daily in the treatment record?
   I. treatment number
   II. cumulative dose
   III. elapsed days
      a. I and II
      b. I and III
      c. II and III
      d. I, II, and III

4. The period over which radiation is delivered is:
   a. fractionation
   b. exposure time
   c. protraction
   d. treatment time
5. Treatment beam shape and projection is verified through the process of:
   a. beam's eye view evaluation
   b. stereoscopic imaging
   c. cone-beam CT
   d. portal imaging
6. Wedge systems include all of the following *except:*
   a. global
   b. universal
   c. standard tray mounted
   d. virtual
7. Multileaf collimators may be used to accomplish which of the following?
   I. beam shape
   II. compensate for missing tissue
   III. vary dose delivered across the beam
     a. I and II
     b. I and III
     c. II and III
     d. I, II, and III
8. The feathering technique is used to accomplish which of the following?
   a. eliminate overlap
   b. increase dose to gapped region
   c. decrease dose to gapped region
   d. decrease dose in abutted fields
9. The angle between the central axes of two treatment beams is the:
   a. central angle
   b. gantry angle
   c. wedge angle
   d. hinge angle
10. Which of the following is *not* an application of bolus for electron treatments?
    a. eliminate skin sparing of high-energy electrons
    b. eliminate skin sparing of low-energy electrons

c. decrease depth of dose penetration
d. compensate for tissue deficits

The answers to the Review Questions can be found by logging on to our website at: *http://evolve.elsevier.com/Washington+Leaver/ principles*

Questions to Ponder

1. Differentiate between an immobilization device and a positioning aid.
2. Analyze information to be included in the radiation therapy treatment chart.
3. Discuss factors contributing to decisions regarding portal imaging frequency.
4. Discuss the role of the radiation therapist in continual improvement of the quality of patient care.
5. Practice converting closed- to open-ended questions.
6. Discuss systematic or random errors that verify and record systems might introduce to treatment delivery and the radiation therapist's role in reduction of these risks.

REFERENCES

1. David JE, Castle SKB, Mossi KM: Localization tattoos: an alternative method using flourescent inks, *Radiat Ther* 15:11-15, 2006.
2. Kutcher GJ, et al: Report of the AAPM Radiation Therapy Committee Task Group 40, *Med Phys* 21:581-618, 1994.
3. Marks JE, et al: The value of frequent treatment verification films in reducing localization error in the irradiation of complex fields, *Cancer* 37:2755, 1976.
4. Miller G, Hebert L: *Taking care of your back,* Bangor, ME, 1984, IMPACC.
5. Patton GA, Gaffney DK, Moeller JH: Facilitation of radiotherapeutic error by computerized record and verify systems, *Int J Radiat Oncol Biol Phys* 56:50-57, 2003.
6. Shams-Avari P: Linguistic and cultural competency, *Radiol Technol* 76:437-445, 2005.
7. Wizenberg MJ: *Quality assurance in radiation therapy: a manual for technologists,* Chicago, 1982, American College of Radiology.

CHAPTER 9

Radiation Therapy Education

Shaun T. Caldwell

Outline

Agencies that influence radiation therapy education
   American Society of Radiologic Technologists
   American Registry of Radiologic Technologists
Accreditation
   Regional or institutional accreditation

Programmatic accreditation
Consistency, Accuracy, Responsibility, and Excellence in Medical Imaging and Radiation Therapy (CARE)
Education in Radiation Oncology
Developing quality education programs and materials

Basic principles of design
Nine elements of good instruction
Summary

Objectives

- Define and identify *radiation therapy programmatic* and *institutional accreditation*.
- Discuss the importance of national minimum standards for education in radiation therapy.
- Describe best practices in radiation therapy education.

- Compare and contrast the foundation of knowledge for developing patient education materials, lectures, and other educational programs to better serve the communities of interest.

The education of the radiation therapist is the foundation of quality patient care, and it sets the direction for the profession. Over the years, the practice of radiation therapy technology has evolved from technologically simplistic to technologically sophisticated. With this sophistication, comes a greater complexity in patient setup and treatment. This shift to the highly complex treatment protocols has required the radiation therapy technologist to develop into a professional radiation therapist. Thus, the radiation therapist must demonstrate advanced technical competency, superior problem-solving skills, and appropriate patient care and education. The radiation therapist must also be prepared to educate colleagues, students, and his or her community. The purpose of this chapter is to define and identify appropriate radiation therapy programmatic and institutional accreditation; describe some of the best practices in radiation therapy education; and provide the student with a foundation of knowledge for developing patient education materials, lectures, and other educational programs in an effort to better serve the radiation oncology communities of interest.

AGENCIES THAT INFLUENCE RADIATION THERAPY EDUCATION

American Society of Radiologic Technologists

The primary agency responsible for developing the national curriculum in radiation therapy is the **American Society of Radiologic Technologists (ASRT)**. Established in 1920, as the American Society of Radiological Technicians, the organization's purpose was to bring technicians together to share thoughts and ideas related to the field.[3] From its initial 14 members in 1920, the ASRT has grown to a membership of more than 124,000 in 2007 of whom more than 12,000 are radiation therapists.[3,10] The ASRT's purpose has also grown to meet the demands of a growing profession as seen in their mission statement[4]:

> The mission of the American Society of Radiologic Technologists is to foster the professional growth of radiologic technologists by expanding knowledge through education, research and analysis; promoting exceptional leadership and service; and developing the radiologic technology community through shared ethics and values.

As the recognized professional organization, the ASRT appoints committees of qualified members representing all aspects of the profession to develop and update the Radiation Therapist's Practice Standards and Radiation Therapy Professional Curriculum. The Practice Standards define the context of the role a radiation therapist must work within. Under revision in 2007, the ASRT publishes the Introduction to Radiation Therapy Practice Standards on its website. These standards are divided into three primary categories: Clinical, Quality, and Professional Performance Standards. These categories are further subdivided into six or seven specific standards of Assessment, Analysis/Determination, Patient Education, Implementation, Evaluation, and Outcomes Measurement. Each standard identifies a minimum level of acceptable performance that should be followed by all radiation therapists. Box 9-1 provides a brief overview of these standards.

The Radiation Therapy Curriculum Committee is charged with the task of reviewing and updating the professional curriculum to ensure that the current principles and practices are defined for radiation therapy educators. The published curriculum includes outlines and objectives for the identified course content with a list of suggested resources, such as textbooks, media, and other educational products. The current Radiation Therapy Curriculum published in 2004 includes formal concepts in Mathematics, Computer Science, Written and Verbal Communication, General Physics, Research Methodology, Orientation to Radiation Therapy, Ethics and Law related to the practice, Medical Terminology, Radiation Therapy Patient Care, Radiation Protection, Pathology, Radiation Physics, Radiobiology, Medical Imaging and Processing, Principles and Practices of Radiation Therapy, Quality Management, Treatment Planning, Operational Issues in Radiation Therapy, Sectional Anatomy, and Clinical Practice.[7] The curriculum periodically undergos revisions to ensure that it reflects the needs of the practice. The most up-to-date curriculum is also published on the ASRT website (www.asrt.org).

American Registry of Radiologic Technologists

The world's largest credentialing body, the **American Registry of Radiologic Technologists (ARRT)**,[1] tests and certifies the radiation therapist for practice in the United States. The ARRT developed its first radiography certification examination in 1923 as a means to create a greater technical expertise and ethical

---

Box 9-1	Radiation Therapy Performance Standards

RADIATION THERAPY CLINICAL PERFORMANCE STANDARDS

Standard 1—Assessment
   The practitioner collects pertinent data about the patient and the procedure.
Standard 2—Analysis/Determination
   The practitioner analyzes the information obtained during the assessment phase and develops an action plan for completing the procedure.
Standard 3—Patient Education
   The practitioner provides information about the procedure to the patient, significant others, and health care providers.
Standard 4—Performance
   Quality patient services are provided through the safe and accurate implementation of a deliberate plan of action.
Standard 5—Evaluation
   The practitioner determines whether the goals of the action plan have been achieved.
Standard 6—Implementation
   The practitioner implements the revised action plan.
Standard 7—Outcomes Measurement
   The practitioner reviews and evaluates the outcome of the procedure.
Standard 8—Documentation
   The practitioner documents information about patient care, the procedure, and the final outcomes.

QUALITY PERFORMANCE STANDARDS

Standard 1—Assessment
   The practitioner collects pertinent information regarding equipment, procedures, and the work environment.
Standard 2—Analysis/Determination
   The practitioner analyzes information collected during the assessment phase and determines whether changes need to be made to equipment, procedures, or the work environment.

Standard 3—Education
   The practitioner informs the patient, public, and other health care providers about procedures, equipment, and facilities.
Standard 4—Performance
   The practitioner performs quality assurance activities or acquires information on equipment and materials.
Standard 5—Evaluation
   The practitioner evaluates quality assurance results and establishes an appropriate action plan.
Standard 6—Implementation
   The practitioner implements the quality assurance action plan.
Standard 7—Outcomes Measurement
   The practitioner assesses the outcome of the quality management action plan.

PROFESSIONAL PERFORMANCE STANDARDS

Standard 1—Quality
   The practitioner strives to provide optimal care to all patients.
Standard 2—Self-Assessment
   The practitioner evaluates personal performance.
Standard 3—Education
   The practitioner acquires and maintains current knowledge in clinical practice.
Standard 4—Collaboration and Collegiality
   The practitioner promotes a positive, collaborative practice atmosphere with the other members of the health care team.
Standard 5—Ethics
   The practitioner adheres to the profession's accepted Code of Ethics.
Standard 6—Research and Innovation
   The practitioner participates in acquisition, dissemination, and advancement of the professional knowledge base.

Derived from American Society of Radiologic Technologists: *The Practice Standards for Medical Imaging and Radiation Therapy*. https://www.asrt.org/content/ProfResources/PracticeIssues/standards.aspx.

standards in the profession. The organization has grown from 89 members in its first year to more than 265,000 in 2007.[1] The ARRT routinely conducts a practice analysis or job analysis of the radiation therapist. This analysis is a detailed inventory of commonly shared duties of radiation therapists nationwide. The data gathered identify the knowledge and skills required to practice as radiation therapists, educational and clinical requirements, and contents specifications specific to the radiation therapy certification examination. The **content specifications** are of particular interest to radiation therapy students because this document outlines the specific topics with corresponding number of questions that may appear on the ARRT certification examination. The up-to-date Content Specifications, Clinical Requirements, and Educational Requirements are published on the ARRT website (www.arrt.org). In addition, the ARRT currently publishes the eligibility requirements to sit for the examination in radiation therapy, which include (1) successful completion of a radiation therapy program that is accredited by a mechanism acceptable to the ARRT, (2) completion of specific competencies with an authorized educator's signature, and (3) declaration of ethical eligibility.[1] Upon successful completion of the certification examination, the radiation therapist must register annually with the organization and provide documentation of 24 hours of continuing education in the radiologic sciences every 2 years orphan to retain certification.

Only technologists who are currently registered may designate themselves as ARRT-registered technologists and use the initials "RT" after their name.[1] Although the educational pathways to certification in radiation therapy include hospital-based certificate, Associate of Applied Science degree, Associate of Science degree, and Bachelor of Science degree, the principles of delivering a sound education must be based on proven educational principles and meet the standards of education identified in the Professional Curriculum and the accrediting body's rules and government regulations. ARRT certifications awarded January 1, 2011, and thereafter will be time-limited to 10 years. Before the end of the 10-year period, the individual will be required to demonstrate continued qualifications to continue to hold the certification.

ARRT certifications that are awarded in advance of January 1, 2011, and that are kept currently registered, will not be subject to Continued Qualifications requirements.[2]

 Some states require continuing education for the therapist to maintain his or her state license. Guidelines regarding state licensure and state continuing education requirements are usually printed on the state's professional licensing website.

ACCREDITATION
Regional or Institutional Accreditation

One of the most important aspects in selecting an educational institution is the **accreditation** of the institution and its programs. Currently, the ARRT recognizes **regional accreditation** agencies of higher education and the Joint Review Committee on Education in Radiologic Technology as acceptable accreditation mechanisms to qualify an individual to sit for the radiation therapy certification examination.[11] Although both mechanisms are recognized, there are fundamental differences between them. The U.S. Department of Education recognizes six regional or institutional accreditation agencies that serve select regions of the United States: Middle States Association of Colleges and Schools, New England Association of Schools and Colleges, North Central Association of Colleges and Schools, Northwest Commission on Colleges and Universities, Western Association of Schools and Colleges, and Southern Association of Colleges and Schools (SACS). Figure 9-1 demonstrates the regional accreditor for each state. Although these six agencies are not identical in their philosophies, policies, or procedures, this chapter will focus on the information published by SACS to present a basic understanding of the institutional accreditation process. According to SACS, the purposes of institutional accreditation are to, "assure the college or university has a purpose in higher education, the financial resources, programs and services required to support and sustain that purpose. Institutional accreditation indicates that the college or university has developed clear educational objectives and degree offerings that support their mission."[11]

Institutional accreditation typically begins with determining the institution's integrity and commitment to quality enhancement. SACS states, "The Commission evaluates an institution and makes accreditation decisions based on the following: Compliance with the Principles of Accreditation, defined as integrity and commitment to quality enhancement, Compliance with the Core requirements, Compliance with the Comprehensive Standards and Compliance with additional Federal Requirements."[8] Compliance is determined by an offsite paper review and onsite review by peers from similar institutions. An outline of these items is listed in Box 9-2.

Programmatic Accreditation

The U.S. Department of Education recognizes only one agency as qualified to accredit programs in radiation therapy: the **Joint Review Committee on Education in Radiologic Technology (JRCERT)**. Unlike the regional accrediting bodies, JRCERT assesses the vitality of the institution and its mission and focuses on the quality of radiation therapy education delivered by the institution. The purpose of JRCERT is to promote excellence in education and to enhance quality and safety of patient care through the accreditation of educational programs.

Programmatic accreditation is the radiation therapy student's assurance that the program meets the minimum professional curriculum developed by ASRT. JRCERT has developed standards of accreditation similar to the institutional accreditation agencies. JRCERT states[11]:

> The Standards for an Accredited Educational Program in Radiologic Sciences are directed at the assessment of program and student outcomes. Using these STANDARDS, the goals of the accreditation process are to: protect the student and the public, stimulate programmatic improvement, provide protective measures for federal funding or financial aid, and promote academic excellence.

Programmatic accreditation is also a peer-review process. The peers chosen for offsite and onsite review of a program are selected from the radiation therapy community and formally educated in the accreditation process. Programs and institutions are required to publish their accreditation status with the

Regional acceditors

- Middle states
- New England
- North central
- Northwest
- Western
- Southern

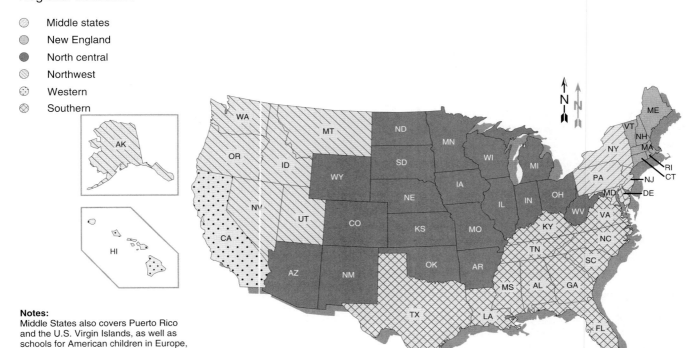

Notes:
Middle States also covers Puerto Rico and the U.S. Virgin Islands, as well as schools for American children in Europe, North Africa, and the Middle East. Western also covers Guam, American Samoa, Micronesia, Palau, and Northern Marianas Islands.

Figure 9-1. Representation of regional accreditors in the United States.

Box 9-2	The Principles of Accreditation: Foundation for Quality Enhancement

Southern Association of College and Schools
Commission on Colleges
Core Requirements
The Institution:
  Has degree-granting authority from the appropriate government agency
  Has a governing board and chief executive officer
  Has clearly defined and published mission statement
  Engages in ongoing, integrated, and intuition-wide research-based planning and evaluation processes that incorporate a systematic review of programs and services that results in continuing improvement and demonstrates that the institution is effectively accomplishing its mission
  Is in operation and has students enrolled in degree programs
  Offers one or more degree programs based on appropriate levels of credit hours
  Offers course content compatible with its mission
  Requires appropriate general education

  Provides instruction for required course work
  Has the appropriate number of faculty with acceptable credentials
  Has appropriate learning resources and services
  Provides student support services
  Has a sound financial base
  Has an acceptable Quality Enhancement Plan
  Evaluates student achievement
  Maintains a curriculum appropriate to its purpose and goals
  Makes calendars, grading, and refund policies available to students and the public
  Program length, that is appropriate to the degree offered
  Has adequate policies addressing written student complaints
  Has recruitment materials that are accurate
  Publishes the name of the primary accrediting agency with address and telephone number
  Is in compliance with Title IV of the 1998 Higher Education Amendments

Derived from Southern Association of Colleges and Schools. Available at www.sacscoc.org/pdf/PrinciplesOfAccreditation.pdf.

regional and programmatic organization, as well as provide the contact information of the accrediting agency. JRCERT's nine standards of accreditation are described in Box 9-3.

 Currently, New Jersey state regulations require that practicing radiation therapists graduate from a program accredited by JRCERT.

Consistency, Accuracy, Responsibility, and Excellence in Medical Imaging and Radiation Therapy (CARE)

In June 1997, the ASRT allocated $1 million to establish federally mandated minimum education and credentialing standards for all radiologic technologists, which includes radiation therapists. This new initiative was the catalyst for the development of the Alliance for Quality Medical Imaging and Radiation Therapy. Known as the Alliance, the organization consisting of 18 separate radiologic sciences associations drafted a bill to amend the 1981 Consumer Patient Radiation Health and Safety Act that was later named the Consumer Assurance of Radiologic Excellence bill.[4,6] According to ASRT:

> The **CARE bill** would require those who perform medical imaging and radiation therapy procedures to meet minimum federal education and credentialing standards in order to participate in federal health programs administered by the Department of Health and Human Services. These programs include Medicare and Medicaid. Under current law, education standards are voluntary and some states allow individuals to perform radiologic procedures without any formal education. Poor quality images can lead to misdiagnosis, additional testing, delays in treatment, and anxiety in patients, costing the U.S. health care system millions of dollars each year.

With the support of Senator Rick Lazio from New York, Senator Ted Kennedy from Massachusetts, and the grassroots efforts of the ASRT members, the U.S. Senate unanimously passed the bill during their 2007 session. Unfortunately, Congress adjourned before it could be heard in the House of Representatives and the bill died. The grassroots effort will continue until the bill is enacted into law.

EDUCATION IN RADIATION ONCOLOGY

Many radiation therapists are active participants in the formal clinical education setting of radiation therapy programs, are present at continuing education seminars, or publish new treatment techniques. A staff radiation therapist may be asked to provide formal or informal lectures on radiation therapy treatment techniques, procedures, or theories. Therefore, the educational responsibilities of the radiation therapist are complex and the importance of proper education techniques cannot be overemphasized.

Developing effective patient education materials plays an important role in radiation oncology and the patient's treatment. Providing the patient with well-planned and accurate educational information in the clinic helps ensure the desired treatment outcome. Formal patient education occurs not only in the patient consultation, simulation, and the first treatment but also throughout the patient's treatments and posttreatment follow-up.

Many assume patient education is the responsibility of the oncology nurse; however, the radiation therapist is the primary caregiver during the patient's daily treatments. Thus, radiation therapists must have the skills required for direct involvement in the design, development, and implementation of educational programs. These programs must meet the specific needs of the patient, general public, students studying radiologic sciences or other related fields of study, and health care professionals having direct contact with radiation oncology patients. The Radiation Therapy Clinical Practice Standards on Education[5] are detailed in Box 9-4 and show the radiation therapist's role and responsibilities in patient education.

Since the early 1990s, interactive education has technically evolved to enhance the learning experience through computer software programs that share ideas and techniques without regard to distance or time. Today, students and patients alike have a magnitude of resources at their fingertips. Accessing information about disease and treatment options has never been easier. Commercially available medical texts on CD-ROM and Internet resources have made the radiation therapist's role critical in helping the patient determine factual information from fiction.

Box 9-3	Standards for an Accredited Educational Program in Radiologic Sciences

STANDARD ONE—MISSION/GOALS, OUTCOMES, AND EFFECTIVENESS

The program, in support of its mission and goals, develops and implements a system of planning and evaluation to determine its effectiveness and uses the results for program improvement.

STANDARD TWO—PROGRAM INTEGRITY

The program demonstrates integrity in representations to communities of interest and the public, in pursuit of educational excellence, and in treatment of and respect for students, faculty, and staff.

STANDARD THREE—ORGANIZATION AND ADMINISTRATION

Organizational and administrative structures support quality and effectiveness of the educational process.

STANDARD FOUR—CURRICULUM AND ACADEMIC PRACTICES

The program's curriculum and academic practices promote the synthesis of theory, use of current technology, competent clinical practice, and professional values.

STANDARD FIVE—RESOURCES AND STUDENT SERVICES

The program's learning resources, learning environments, and student services are sufficient to support its mission and goals.

STANDARD SIX—HUMAN RESOURCES

The program has sufficient qualified faculty and staff with delineated responsibilities to support the program's mission and goals.

STANDARD SEVEN—STUDENTS

The program's and sponsoring institution's policies and procedures serve and protect the rights, health, and educational opportunities of all students.

STANDARD EIGHT—RADIATION SAFETY

Program policies and procedures are in compliance with federal and state radiation protection laws.

STANDARD NINE—FISCAL RESPONSIBILITY

The program and the sponsoring institution have adequate financial resources, demonstrate financial stability, and comply with obligations for Title IV federal funding, if applicable.

Adopted by the Joint Review Committee on Education in Radiologic Technology, January 1996, Revised 2001.

Box 9-4	Radiation Therapy Clinical Practice Standards on Education

CLINICAL PERFORMANCE STANDARDS

STANDARD THREE—PATIENT EDUCATION

The practitioner provides information about the procedure to the patient, significant others, and health care providers.

RATIONALE

Communication and education are necessary to establish a positive relationship with the patient, significant others, and health care providers.

GENERAL CRITERIA

The practitioner:

Verifies that the patient has consented to the procedure and fully understands its risks, benefits, alternatives, and follow-up. Verifies that written consent has been obtained when appropriate.

Provides accurate explanations and instructions at an appropriate time and at a level the patient can understand. Addresses and documents patient questions and concerns regarding the procedure when appropriate.

Refers questions about diagnosis, treatment, or prognosis to the patient's physician.

Provides appropriate information to any individual involved in the patient's care.

SPECIFIC CRITERIA

The practitioner:

Provides information regarding risks and benefits of radiation.

Instructs patient in the maintenance of treatment-field markings.

Provides information and instruction on proper skin care, diet, and self-care procedures.

Anticipates a patient's need for information and provides it throughout the treatment course.

QUALITY PERFORMANCE STANDARDS

STANDARD THREE—EDUCATION

The practitioner informs the patient, public, and other health care providers about procedures, equipment, and facilities.

RATIONALE

Open communication promotes safe practices.

GENERAL CRITERIA

The practitioner:

Elicits confidence and cooperation from the patient, the public, and other health care providers by providing timely communication and effective instruction.

Presents explanations and instructions at the learner's level of understanding and learning style.

SPECIFIC CRITERIA

The practitioner:

Informs the patient and significant others about appropriate and essential uses of radiation and corrects misconceptions.

Participates in instructing other health care providers about radiation protection procedures.

PROFESSIONAL PERFORMANCE STANDARDS

STANDARD THREE—EDUCATION

The practitioner acquires and maintains current knowledge in clinical practice.

RATIONALE

Advancements in medical sciences require enhancement of knowledge and skills through education.

GENERAL CRITERIA

The practitioner:

Demonstrates completion of the appropriate education related to clinical practice.

Maintains appropriate credentials and certification related to clinical practice.

Participates in educational activities to enhance knowledge, skills, and performance.

Shares knowledge and expertise with others.

SPECIFIC CRITERIA

The practitioner:

Demonstrates understanding of the functions and operations of equipment, accessories, treatment methods, and protocols.

Derived from American Society of Radiologic Technologists: *The Practice Standards for Medical Imaging and Radiation Therapy* (website): https://www.asrt.org/media/pdf/practicestds/GR06_OPI_Strds_RT_Adpd.pdf.

Life experiences, taken from day-to-day interactions, coupled with formal education provide the radiation therapist with a means of making a strong connection with the patient.

Developing Quality Education Programs and Materials

Historically, the oncology nurse has conducted formal patient education, and the radiation therapist reinforced knowledge and skills and presented new concepts while the patient was in clinic for his or her scheduled appointment. Today, the radiation therapist lectures to social groups, conducts radiation safety training to professionals providing direct patient care to brachytherapy patients, and lectures in university- and hospital-based radiologic sciences programs. In the past, commercially available videotapes and brochures have been given to the patient for reference. Although well meaning, these items typically are not patient specific and may not be the most effective method for teaching specific skills.

During the past decade, web-based learning has become a hot topic among medical centers for patient education and universities in offering formal curriculum. The opportunity to reach underserved populations in rural areas of the United States and throughout the world is one reason for the interest in web-based teaching. However, the computer may not always be the ideal delivery method for instructing patients on sensitive subjects or hands-on skills required for optimum healing or the application of radiation as a form of treatment.

Regardless of the mode of delivering the message, a radiation therapist must be efficient and effective in delivering his or her message and determining whether learning actually occurred. Specific steps, when followed correctly, will help ensure that the desired outcome from the delivered educational experience is successful. These steps are applicable to developing educational materials, public speaking engagements or seminars, academic courses for the radiation therapy student or associated health care professionals, and specific patient educational programs. Many institutions have written into the job descriptions and performance evaluation processes a requirement of the staff radiation therapist to actively engage in formal clinical and didactic education of radiation therapy students.

Basic Principles of Design

The **ADDIE model**, identified in Box 9-5, represents the Analysis, Design, Development, Implementation, and Evaluation of the curriculum. This model is a step-by-step order in which the radiation therapist can proceed in creating an educational tool for patients or students.

Analysis. A radiation therapist should understand the need for analysis in every educational event that he or she designs. Without substantiating a need for a patient education mechanism, course, or program, there is little benefit for its development. The saying, "Build it and they will come," is not based on fact. A formal needs assessment provides data to substantiate the necessity of the education to hospital or university administrators. Needs assessment should be performed during the analysis stage of the model and should answer some very important questions, such as the following:

- Does the patient or student lack the needed knowledge to complete the specific task?
- Are the patient's support system and the student's clinical or educational setting able to accommodate the additional skills or knowledge?
- Are there proper incentives, intrinsic or extrinsic, for learning?
- If the skill or knowledge is lacking, is there support for further education or training in this particular topic?
- Will the patients have religious, emotional, physical, developmental, or cultural issues that may hinder learning?
- Are there obvious questions that relate to the need for education in this area?

Box 9-5	The ADDIE Model of Instructional Design

- Analysis
  - Needs
  - Task
  - Audience
- Design
  - Objectives
  - Mode of delivery
- Development
  - Building the learning tool
- Implementation
  - Using the tool for the purpose for which it was designed
- Evaluation
  - Did the tool meet the desired outcomes?
  - Identifying needed refinements to the tool

The answers to these questions may come from data collected by surveying or interviewing former and current patients, students, front-line radiation therapists, supervisors, and education directors of medical institutions. Collected data also should define whether the education is truly needed and who needs it, while justifying the allocation of the institution's resources.

Additionally, information about the potential learner provides the radiation therapist with key information for making accurate decisions in the design step. Knowing specific information such as the learners' age range, ethnic background, gender, and education level will direct the therapist to develop a tool that is responsive in meeting the different learning styles and special needs of his or her students.

The educational product or course can benefit from a task analysis. This is the collection of the specific and detailed step-by-step documentation of accurately accomplishing the skill to be taught. It must be noted that the task analysis is only as accurate as the data collected from content experts who demonstrate the task or skill.[12]

Identify five vital functions of a task analysis, including inventorying tasks, describing tasks, selecting tasks, sequencing tasks and task components, and analyzing tasks and content level.

Inventorying tasks include the detailed documentation of the physical actions required to accurately complete the identified task. For example, a radiation therapist may inventory the task required to create custom blocks. The radiation therapist must observe a content expert, another radiation therapist or block room technician, as he or she creates the desired custom block. The therapist must identify each detailed step in the process. The required tasks must be assessed for their necessity in getting the desired outcome. Many times shortcuts or individual styles may introduce unnecessary steps into the project. These steps must be determined as beneficial to the learning outcome. Tasks must be sequenced in the proper order. Although it may not matter whether the holes on the block tray are predrilled, adjusting the target film-focus distance on the block cutter must be done before cutting the styrofoam with the heated wire to ensure the proper block size and divergence. Finally, analysis of the tasks and the knowledge and skills necessary for the accomplishment of each task must be done.

Design. The design step is the methodical blueprint of the course or product. The radiation therapist should document the details of the course or product. Descriptive narratives and storyboards provide effective tools in documenting the individual learning experiences within the product. This documentation becomes the primary means of communication during the development step. A radiation therapist actively involved in the design of specific patient education materials may want to invest in storyboarding computer software. However, simple hand drawings with detailed narratives can be effective.

Setting Objectives. The design step requires the creation of specific goals or objectives. Objectives must clearly state the purpose for learning as it relates to the completed analysis data. **Objectives** define the required behaviors needed to achieve the desired results and the knowledge, skills, and attitudes the students or patients must learn in the course or from the patient educational product. Objectives should address the cognitive, affective, and psychomotor domains of student learning as described in *Bloom's Taxonomy*.[14] In other words, the objectives should be written so that they address the student's knowledge, feelings or attitudes, and physical or hands-on skills required to accomplish mastery of the concept being taught. For example:

Upon completion of the training session, the student will:

1. Explain the importance of maintaining excellent oral hygiene during head and neck irradiation. (Cognitive)
2. Choose an appropriate oral hygiene regimen to follow during radiation therapy treatments. (Affective)
3. Properly demonstrate brushing, flossing, and oral rinsing as described in his or her oral hygiene regimen. (Psychomotor)

Rossett[15] suggested that objectives must answer many questions, including the following:

- Who can benefit from the course or product?
- What is required legally?
- What professional guidelines exist?
- Is the course voluntary or compulsory?
- Should levels of learning or rank be segregated in the course/product?
- How often should the learning experience be offered?
- What is the best timing for implementing the course or project?
- Under what conditions should the learning experience be provided?
- Who is best qualified to direct the learning?
- What items may be selected to enhance the learning environment (audiovisuals, computer-based training)?

The course or project design should be directed by the data obtained in the analysis step and follow the appropriate outlined objectives. The design should incorporate the appropriate facility and faculty along with educational materials used to optimally deliver the course effectively and efficiently. You may have noticed that a description of the final product has not been mentioned. Quality educational products and courses do not begin with a final picture in mind. The radiation therapist should not design the course around a specific mode of delivery such as a brochure or computer program. Remember that one form of a product may not meet all of your patient's needs. The product must be designed to meet the various learning styles, levels of comprehension, and physical and emotional conditions of the patient. In other words, the radiation therapist should let the information collected in the analysis step and the design steps dictate the development step.

Development. Development is the point at which the radiation therapist should take the design of the product and turn it into a tangible object. That is, the design is now formalized into the final product whether it be an instructional brochure, videotape, CD-ROM, or formal presentation. Professional multimedia developers, graphic artists, or other specialists may be recruited into the project at this point. However, once the project has been developed, it naturally evolves to the implementation step.

Implementation. The course or project is now ready to be used for the purpose for which it was designed. The therapist should deliver the course or product with the full intent of evaluating whether learning has actually occurred.

Implementation refers to all of the stages of the delivery of the education. Delivery is guided by the analysis and design phases of the model. This phase may include the delivery of the formal lecture, audio or video components, or electronic and written media. The design phase prescribes the appropriate delivery methods based on the analysis of the audience for which the education is intended. One must remember that delivering effective education may require multiple delivery methods to ensure that learning actually takes place.

Evaluation. Evaluating patient education products and educational courses is commonly overlooked. The information gained from evaluation is essential to the continued quality improvement. Although the evaluation step appears as the last step in the model, it is most effective when integrated throughout the entire design process. Evaluation is mandatory if the radiation therapist wants to substantiate the investment in the educational project. Proof that learning has occurred and the outcomes or goals of the project have been met is proved by the information gathered by the evaluation step. Kirkpatrick[13] defined a formula to ensure proper evaluation of educational and training programs by establishing four levels of evaluation, which provide summative and formative data collection procedures. These levels are as follows:

Level 1:   Reaction
Level 2:   Learning
Level 3:   Behavior
Level 4:   Results

Reaction refers to the participant's satisfaction with the educational offering, whether it is an informal training session, a single course, or an entire program. Learner feedback can easily be obtained using simple bubble-type sheets. The reaction evaluation serves to provide feedback from the student/patient's perception of the quality of the education delivered, the provided materials, and the delivery method.

Learning in an individual may be defined as increased knowledge or the proper use of a skill in conjunction with a change in attitude. The measurement of learning must be specifically designed for the target population. Standard examinations can measure knowledge, especially when using the practice of precourse and postcourse testing, providing an excellent method of measuring the amount of change in a learner's knowledge of a particular subject. The use of clinical or specific skills competencies provides an opportunity for the student/patient to demonstrate his or her understanding and ability to perform the specific skills contained in the program objectives. The radiation therapist can score these clinical competencies and can provide feedback regarding the program's effectiveness, while supplying suggestions for change.

Behavior refers to any noted and expected change that has been translated to the workplace. These changes are acquired during the educational program and then transfer to practice. Although Kirkpatrick[13] did not formally define this level, he alluded to its practice within his works.

Results, again not formally defined by Kirkpatrick, refer to the outcomes, particularly positive ones, that relate to education and practice. Operational efficiency, cost reduction, lower turnover, fewer grievances, and improved employee morale are representative of anticipated evaluative results.

Measuring learning and skills is not effective if a change in attitude toward performing the activity is not properly demonstrated; therefore, it may be necessary to obtain information regarding the student's attitude from other support individuals associated with the student. This support structure may include a patient's spouse, child, or supportive care provider. Clinical peers traditionally serve as mentors and evaluators within the radiation therapy student's clinical setting. Addressing the results of the evaluation is the essential step to evaluating the program's effectiveness as defined by its objectives.

Nine Elements of Good Instruction

Robert Gagné[9] identified the need for quality analysis, selection of appropriate media, and quality design of instructional events in the specific design of courses. This philosophy can be followed in creating formal courses for radiation therapy students, patients, or health care workers. When a course or patient educational event is being designed, during the analysis phase, it is important to recognize the prerequisite skills or knowledge needed in building the foundation of future learning. Throughout the course design process, Gagné offers the following nine suggestions[9]:

1. *Ascertain outcomes:* Identify the need for instruction. Correlate the needs and goals with the available resources and other imposed instructional constraints.
2. *Develop goals:* Implement identified goals into a framework of the curriculum.
3. *Course objectives are achieved through learning:* Human performance (intellectual skill, cognitive strategies, verbal information, attitudes, and motor skills) is considered in measuring outcomes.
4. *Goals and objectives:* Goals and objectives contribute to learning by allowing objectives to be systematically grouped in sections of similar types.
5. *Determine types of capabilities to be learned:* Identify learning conditions needed to create an optimal environment for learning and the appropriate sequence of instruction required.
6. *Instructional planning:* Design instructional units that are simple concepts that build upon themselves.
7. *Detailed planning of individuals' instructional events:* Focus is placed on arranging the external conditions that will best complement learning. Learner consideration is recognized and guides internal conditions of the instructional events or individual lessons.
8. *Assessment:* Development of procedures to identify what the students have learned. These procedures should be based on the objectives or, in other words, measurement and identification of what students have learned due to the instruction.
9. *System planning:* The course and individual design and the learning techniques should *complement* the program as a whole. Comprehensive instructional goals should be reflected within the course design and assessment.

Gagné[9] further suggests that a quality course should identify learning outcomes and the prerequisite skills or knowledge needed to accomplish each outcome; recognize the internal and external conditions and processes the learner needs to achieve the outcomes; specify the learning context and record the characteristics of the learners; select the media that will best support the learning environment; and develop methods to motivate the learner and obtain summative and formative data to objectively evaluate the effectiveness of instruction.

SUMMARY

- Formal radiation therapy programs have the option of institutional or programmatic accreditation. Many choose both to ensure the highest quality of education for the student.
- Technological sophistication has created a shift in radiation therapy education, creating a new environment of highly complex radiation treatments. Radiation therapists, now more than ever, must have an in-depth knowledge of treatment delivery and patient care. National minimum standards for educating radiation therapists are an important component in ensuring that this knowledge is properly instilled.
- Radiation therapists must also develop the skills necessary to deliver effective and efficient education to patients, the profession, and the community. The role of the radiation therapist continues to evolve, and the professional radiation therapist is taking on a larger role as a radiation oncology educator.

Review Questions

Multiple Choice

1. How many accreditation mechanisms does the U.S. Department of Education recognize for radiation therapy?
   a. 1
   b. 2
   c. 4
   d. 5
2. Which of the following is a sound educational design step that is *most often* overlooked in developing educational materials or programs?
   a. Analysis
   b. Implementation
   c. Design
   d. Evaluation
3. Which of the following are clinical performance standards for radiation therapists?
   I. collects pertinent data about the patient and procedure
   II. analyzes the information obtained during the assessment phase
   III. develops an action plan for completing the procedure
   a. I and II
   b. I and III
   c. II and III
   d. I, II, and III
4. Which organization is responsible for reviewing and updating the Radiation Therapy Curricula?
   a. ARRT
   b. ASRT
   c. JRCERT
   d. ADDIE

5. Once certified, how many continuing education credits must a radiation therapist earn to maintain his or her registry?
    a. 6 credits a year
    b. 12 credits a year
    c. 12 credits every 2 years
    d. 24 credits every 2 years
6. When looking at a formal evaluation process, which of the following refers to the participant's satisfaction with the educational offering, whether it is an informal training session, a single course, or an entire program?
    a. Results
    b. Behavior
    c. Reaction
    d. Learning
7. Which of the following represent the purpose of the Consistency, Accuracy, Responsibility, and Excellence in Medical Imaging and Radiation Therapy bill?
    I. require states to require a minimum education level for radiation therapists
    II. save the U.S. health care system and patient money
    III. prevent misdiagnosis and additional unnecessary testing
    a. I and II
    b. I and III
    c. II and III
    d. I, II, and III
8. The Performance Standards of a Radiation Therapist include which of the following: (Choose all that apply.)
    a. assessment of the patient's physical and emotional status
    b. education of patients and other professionals
    c. implementation of the treatment plan
    d. development of action plans to improve patient comfort and quality of care
9. An educational objective is defined as:
    a. the required behaviors needed to achieve the desired results as related to the knowledge, skills, and attitudes the student or patient will learn
    b. assessment of the patient's physical an emotional status
    c. development of an action plan to improve patient comfort and quality of care
    d. the national minimum standards for educating radiation therapists
10. The _____ outline(s) the specific topics with corresponding number of questions that may appear on the ARRT certification examination.
    a. outcomes
    b. content specifications
    c. radiation therapy curriculum
    d. JRCERT
    e. ASRT

The answers to the Review Questions can be found by logging on to our website at: *http://evolve.elsevier.com/Washington+Leaver/principles*

Questions to Ponder

1. Identify the accreditation agency for your educational program and determine the program's current accreditation status.

2. Compare and contrast institutional accreditation and regional accreditation.
3. Use the Nine Elements of Good Instruction to develop a formal presentation related to this chapter or a topic of special interest.
4. Discuss the importance of the radiation therapist's role in educating patients, students, and the public.
5. Jane, a seasoned radiation therapist, was assigned to prepare a community education program for radiation therapy treatment of the breast. She spent a great deal of time preparing a formal lecture with a quiz after to measure whether the audience learned something from her lecture. When she arrived to give her first lecture, she realized that approximately 50% of the audience were teenagers, and the other 50% were older women. After reviewing the quiz scores, she realized that half of the audience scored very well and the other half scored poorly. What stages of the ADDIE model did Jane skip?

REFERENCES

1. American Registry of Radiologic Technologists: *Certification eligibility requirements* (website): http://www.arrt.org. Accessed May 6, 2007.
2. American Registry of Radiologic Technologists: *CQ 2011, continued qualifications* (website): http://www.arrt.org. Accessed October 22, 2007.
3. American Society of Radiologic Technologists: *ASRT history* (website): https://asrt.org/content/abouthistory.aspx. Accessed May 6, 2007.
4. American Society of Radiologic Technologists: *ASRT vision, mission, care values, value propositions and strategic objective* (website): https://www.asrt.org/content/aboutasrt/MissionVisionValues.aspx. Accessed May 21, 2007.
5. American Society of Radiologic Technologists: *Introduction to the radiation therapy practice standards* (website): http://asrt.org. Accessed May 6, 2007.
6. American Society of Radiologic Technologists: *News release: Senators Enzi, Kennedy introduce 2007 CARE bill* (website): http://asrt.org/content/News/PressRoom/PR2007/radiologic070330.aspx. Accessed May 15, 2007.
7. American Society of Radiologic Technologists: *Radiation therapy professional education*, Albuquerque, NM, 2004, The Author (website): https://www.asrt.org/content/Educators/Curricula/RadiationTherapyRTT/therapy_curriculum.aspx. Accessed May 6, 2007.
8. Commission of Colleges Southern Association of Colleges and Schools: *The principles of accreditation: foundations for quality enhancement*, Decatur, GA, 2001, The Author.
9. Gagné RM: *Principles of instructional design*, New York, 1992, Holt, Rinehart and Winston.
10. Harris R: Personal communication, May 23, 2007.
11. Joint Review Committee on Education in Radiologic Technology: *Standards for an accredited educational program in radiologic sciences*, Chicago, 2002, The Author (website): http://www.jrcert.org. Accessed May 6, 2007.
12. Jonassen DH, Hannum WH: Analysis of task analysis procedures. In Anglin GJ, editor: *Instructional technology*, Englewood, CO, 1995, Libraries Unlimited.
13. Kirkpatrick DL: *Evaluating training programs*, San Francisco, 1994, Berrett-Koehler.
14. *Learning domains or Bloom's taxonomy* (website): http://www.nwlink.com/~Donclark/hrd/bloom.html. Accessed May 4, 2007.
15. Rossett A: Needs assessment. In, Anglin GJ, editor: *Instructional technology*, Englewood, CO, 1995, Libraries Unlimited.
16. Wolohan DD, Lung C: Senate passes CARE bill, but Congress adjourns, *ASRT Scanner* 39:6-9, 2007.

Infection Control in Radiation Oncology Facilities

Lana Havron Bass, Stacy L. Anderson

Outline

Definitions
Regulatory agencies and public oversight
Infection cycle and disease phases
Transmission routes
Defense mechanisms
  Nonspecific defense mechanisms
  Specific defense mechanisms
  Environmental factors contributing to nosocomial disease
Drug use and drug-resistant microorganisms
Health care facility epidemiology
Personnel and student health services and pertinent infectious diseases
  Hepatitis B virus
  Hepatitis C virus
  Other recommended vaccines for health care workers
  Tuberculosis

Health care worker removal from patient care
Varicella-zoster virus
Viral respiratory infections
Evolution of isolation practices
  Universal precautions
  Body substance isolation
  Comparison of universal precautions and body substance isolation
  Occupational Safety and Health Administration and bloodborne pathogens
Isolation chaos leads to a new isolation guideline
  Standard precautions
  Transmission-based precautions
Isolation fundamentals
  Hand hygiene
  Gloving
  Masks, respiratory protection, eye protection, and face shields

Gowns and protective apparel
Patient placement
Transport of infected patients
Patient care equipment and articles
Laundry
Routine cleaning of environment
Blood or body fluid spills
Student education
Handling exposure incidents related to HIV
Rights of the health care worker
Role of the central services department
Sterilization and disinfection techniques
  Heat
  Gas
  Radiation
  Chemical liquids
Sterility quality control measures
Summary

Key Terms

Antibodies
Antigen
Autoclaves
Carrier
Colonization
Convalescence
Droplet nuclei
Epidemiology
Fomite
Immune serum globulin
Incubation
Mantoux tuberculin skin test
Nosocomial
Pathogenicity
Recombinant deoxyribonucleic acid
Skin squames
Titers
Vector
Virulence

Objectives

- Define terms associated with epidemiology and infection control.
- Interpret and apply the processes of isolation techniques used in health care facilities.
- Discuss the evolution and necessity of standard precautions.
- Select protective equipment to be worn that is appropriate for a given medical procedure or situation.

- Use actions that will protect the patient, public, and yourself in regard to the transmission of disease.
- Identify processes used in the sterilization and disinfection of medical equipment and the medical environment.
- Describe laws and regulations that are in place to ensure a safe work environment for health care workers.

The concept of trying to control infectious disease in medical settings has a relatively long history and is associated with famous names such as Florence Nightingale and Joseph Lister. The focus remains the same today; that is, health care workers (HCWs) promote the surveillance, control, and prevention of infectious disease. This chapter emphasizes measures taken to protect the HCW, the patient, and the public. Regulatory agencies and legal aspects of infection control are also briefly discussed.

DEFINITIONS

In the hospital setting, the epidemiology department is responsible for infection control. The term *epidemiology* is historically related to the study of epidemics, such as the bubonic plague of the Middle Ages.[176] Today, **epidemiology** may be defined as the study of the distribution and determinants of diseases and injuries in human populations. To familiarize students with terminology pertinent to epidemiology, the following definitions need to be reviewed.

Infection involves the reproduction of microorganisms in the human body. *Disease* is the collective term used to describe related clinical signs and symptoms associated with an infectious agent or unknown etiology. A person who becomes infected typically develops specific clinical signs and symptoms that can be detected externally, and the body initiates an immune response internally. If a person develops an infection but has no clinically observable signs or symptoms, the infection is referred to as a *subclinical infection*. It is important to note that a subclinical infection does initiate an immune response within the body. Another type of infection, which does not provoke an immune response, is known as colonization. **Colonization** involves the reproduction of an infectious microorganism, but there is no interaction between the body and the microorganism that would result in a detectable immune response. The microorganism is simply present in or on the body and it is multiplying. A person who is colonized but not ill is known as a **carrier**. Carriers may be a source of infection on a short-term or even permanent basis.

The relevance of these sources of infection is that disease is disseminated not just by people who are obviously ill but also by those with subclinical infections and by those who are carriers. *Contamination* is defined as the presence of microorganisms on the body (commonly on hands) or on inanimate objects. It is the movement of people from one environment to another that spreads disease, either directly from the infected person or indirectly through the things that they come in contact with. By understanding the factors associated with the development of disease and its dissemination, control and prevention measures can be initiated.

Workers in the health care environment are especially interested in nosocomial infections. The term **nosocomial** was traditionally used to describe infections that developed in the hospital or to describe infections that were acquired in the hospital but did not develop until after discharge. Today, "hospital" is too restrictive and has been expanded to include ambulatory care settings and other health care settings. Nosocomial infections may be acquired not only by patients, but also by HCWs and visitors. Infections caught before a hospital admission but in which symptoms do not become apparent until after admission are not nosocomial; they are community related rather than hospital related. The primary goal of the epidemiology department is to decrease all preventable nosocomial infections. The hospital epidemiology team continuously monitors the number of infections that occur and investigates any abnormal occurrence or frequency to determine whether some action could have been taken to prevent the infection.

REGULATORY AGENCIES AND PUBLIC OVERSIGHT

The Centers for Disease Control and Prevention (CDC), a federal government agency located in Atlanta, Georgia, has been actively involved in helping hospital infection control personnel in investigating epidemics since the mid-1950s. Over time, this nationwide cooperative approach of hospitals and the CDC has lead to the formulation of very useful standards and guidelines, changes in federal and state laws, and many studies to monitor effectiveness of infection control measures.

The CDC has estimated that the nationwide nosocomial infection rate is 5.7%.[92] For larger hospitals with concentrated populations of gravely ill patients, the rate has been projected to be around 10%.[29] Investigators of the CDC Study of the Efficacy of Nosocomial Infection Control (SENIC) project, conducted from 1974 to 1983, estimated that nearly 2.1 million nosocomial infections occurred annually.[89] This figure of 2.1 million translates into a rate of 1 in every 20 patients and the eighth leading cause of death in the United States.[155]

A report from the Institute of Medicine (IOM) found that medical errors and hospital-acquired infections cost $17 to $29 billion in 1999.[103] The nation's largest advocacy group for senior citizens, the American Association of Retired Persons (AARP), spoke out about nosocomial infection in its January 2007 bulletin. The article, entitled "Dirty Hospitals," stated that 90,000 patients die annually from picking up something extra during their hospital stay.[83] The article also listed useful tips on ways to avoid getting infected that apply to all age groups.

Infections also erode hospital profits. Hospitals get paid per a diagnosis coding system. For a given procedure they are paid a preset amount based on a normal length of stay. If the patient has to stay days, weeks, or months longer to receive extended treatment caused by a nosocomial infection, then a hospital can actually lose money in treating a specific patient.

Since the landmark SENIC project, which focused on overall hospital infection rate, a move toward specific outcome objectives has been adopted as recommended by the Joint Commission on Accreditation of Healthcare Organizations (JCAHO) standards issued since the 1990s.[108] JCAHO is now known as The Joint Commission (TJC). This newer concept focuses on lowering the infection rate of something specific, for example, the number of infections in central venous catheters in patients receiving chemotherapy infusions.

SENIC established that hospitals with the lowest infection rates were the ones with the strongest surveillance, education, and prevention programs. Hospitals and outpatient centers are strongly encouraged to establish internal monitoring systems. The savings to be gained by patients, insurance companies, hospitals, and taxpayers are obvious. Reducing the number of nosocomial infections is a win-win situation for all parties involved.

As consumer advocate groups speak out across the country, more external monitoring is taking place. Many states have passed laws that require hospitals to disclose how often their patients get infections.[81] Public access will provide another incentive for an institution to work harder to lower its nosocomial rate. Regardless of the focus, what is important to remember is that 30% to 50% of nosocomial infections are preventable and are primarily caused by problems in patient care practices, such as handwashing.[90] Also emerging in the early 1990s from the voluntary public hospital experience of developing guidelines for infection control and surveillance associated with the SENIC project was a new, formal federal advisory CDC committee, the Hospital Infection Control Practices Advisory Committee (HICPAC).

Up to 50% of nosocomial infections are preventable.

When compared with hospital inpatients, most ambulatory care setting patients are not exposed to the shear number of invasive procedures or to the variety of medical devices that are known to pose significant infection risks. Time spent at an ambulatory care setting is usually limited and also serves as a factor in reducing the risk of acquiring a nosocomial infection. Nosocomial risk is low in ambulatory care settings overall, but special settings such as radiation oncology merit special attention because it may be important to identify those patients whose compromised immune status places them in a high-risk group.

Droplet spread of viral respiratory infections is especially dangerous to this high-risk group. These patients may benefit from reduced contact with other patients and visitors in the waiting room. It may even be prudent to consider permitting selected oncology patients to bypass the office waiting room entirely. Masks available at the front desk for anyone with sniffles, sneezing, or coughing is a practice now occurring in some centers.

INFECTION CYCLE AND DISEASE PHASES

Infectious disease cannot occur without the presence of an infectious agent, or *pathogen,* which is any of a wide range of small, primitive life forms. Pathogens may exist as bacteria; viruses; fungi; protozoa; algae; or lesser known agents such as chlamydiae, rickettsiae, and prions[76] (Figure 10-1). Of these, bacteria and viruses are most often the sources of nosocomial infections, with fungi next, and rarely protozoa or the other forms.[20] Several terms are associated with a disease and the infectious agent.

Pathogenicity describes the ability of an infectious agent to cause clinical disease. In other words, some agents readily cause clinical disease, whereas others may be present but not cause clinical disease. The term **virulence** describes the severity of a clinical disease and is typically expressed in terms of morbidity and mortality. *Dose* refers to the number of microorganisms; thus an *infective dose* is one in which enough microorganisms are present to elicit an infection. Microorganisms are also selective as to their host or the location at which they cause disease. The infectious agent may cause disease in animals but not in humans, vice versa, or in both. This selectivity is known as *host specificity.*

To remain viable, all microorganisms require a source and a reservoir; these may be the same or different. The *reservoir* is where the microorganism lives and reproduces. For example, the polio viral reservoir is human, never animal, whereas the rabies viral reservoir can be human or animal. The place from which the microorganism comes is known as the *source.* From the source it moves to the host; this transfer from the source to the host may be direct or indirect.

In the case of the common cold transmitted through a sneeze, the reservoir and source are the same. An example in which the reservoir and source are not the same is histoplasmosis, which is a fungal infection. In this situation a chicken can serve as the reservoir. The chicken's fecal droppings are deposited on soil and serve as the source. After drying, the wind carries the remains of the fecal droppings to a location where a human inhales them. Another example is hepatitis A virus (HAV); in this case the reservoir is often a cook who handles food. The food handled by the cook serves as the source of the infection.

A *host* is the person to whom the infectious agent is passed. Whether the host develops clinical disease depends on the body location at which the infectious agent is deposited and on the host's immune status and related defense mechanisms. If disease develops in the susceptible host, the host goes through three disease phases:

1. Incubation
2. Clinical disease
3. Convalescence

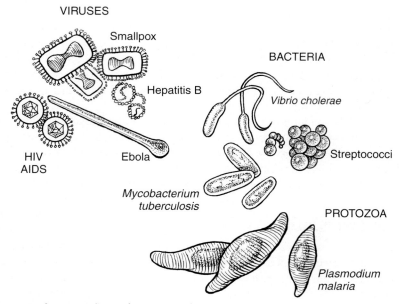

Figure 10-1. Microorganisms that cause disease come in a wide variety of shapes and sizes.

Incubation is the time interval between exposure and the appearance of the first symptom. The *clinical disease stage* is the time interval in which a person exhibits clinical signs and symptoms. **Convalescence** is the stage of recovery from the illness. Depending on the specific disease, a person may be infectious to others during any or a combination of the three disease phases.

In some diseases, such as hepatitis from hepatitis B virus (HBV), in which a chronic carrier state exists, a person who is apparently well can actually be disseminating disease. For disease to be passed to others, a *portal of exit* is necessary. Examples include the respiratory tract, gastrointestinal tract, blood, and skin.

After an exit portal is reached, transmission can take place. *Transmission* is defined as the movement of the infectious agent from the source to the host. To cause disease, the infectious agent must gain entrance to the body. The *entrance portal* can be through normal skin such as with *Leptospira* (one form is known as Fort Bragg fever due to the number of military personnel who developed it) or through broken skin such as with a needlestick in the transmission of HIV.[20] Agents also gain access through the respiratory system, gastrointestinal tract, urinary tract, or transplantation. Transmission of an infectious agent through these entry portals is also often associated with medications or equipment such as scopes or catheters. The complete cycle of infection is shown in Figure 10-2.

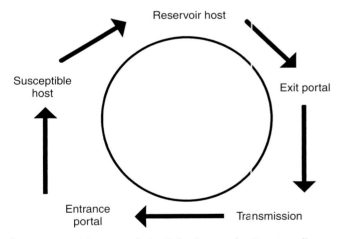

Figure 10-2. Diagram of the infection cycle. To stop disease, the cycle can be broken at any point.

TRANSMISSION ROUTES

Transmission routes vary from one disease to another. Five transmission routes are identified: *contact, droplet, common vehicle, airborne,* and *vectorborne*. Box 10-1 displays an outline of transmission routes. A specific disease may use one or more transmission modes.

Contact spread can be *direct* or *indirect*. Contact transmission is the most frequent and most important transmission route for the spread of nosocomial infections. In *direct contact* transmission, the susceptible host makes physical contact with the source of infection, either an infected or a colonized person.

Box 10-1	Transmission Routes

1. Contact
    Direct
    Indirect
2. Droplet (large)
3. Common vehicle (fomite)
4. Airborne
    Droplet nuclei
    Dust particles
    Skin squames
5. Vectorborne

Person-to-person spread can occur through simple touching such as helping a patient out of a wheelchair and onto the treatment couch. Mononucleosis transmitted through kissing and acquired immunodeficiency syndrome (AIDS) spread through sexual intercourse also are examples of direct contact transmission. *Indirect contact* transmission involves an intervening object that is contaminated from contact with an infectious agent and then comes into contact with another individual and results in a single infective episode. An example is a needlestick to an HCW after the needle has been used in a patient infected with human immunodeficiency virus (HIV).

Transmission by *droplet contact* involves the rapid transfer of the infectious agent through the air over short distances, such as in talking, coughing, or sneezing close to someone's face. The droplets consist of large, relatively heavy particles (larger than 5 μm) and thus are spread over short distances, typically 3 feet or less, and are deposited on the host's nasal mucosa, oral mucosa, and conjunctivae of the eye.[21] Rubella (also known as German measles or 3-day measles), colds, and influenza are commonly transmitted in this fashion. Suctioning of a patient with a head and neck cancer is another example of how large droplets can be created. Droplet contact involves large moist droplets, and because of their weight they do not linger in the air for long periods of time; thus, special air handling systems and ventilation are not required to prevent droplet transmission. Droplet contact transmission should not be confused with airborne transmission. Airborne transmission is an entirely different transmission route and will be discussed later in this chapter.

Another route of transmission is *common vehicle spread*. This type of transmission involves a contaminated inanimate vehicle, known as a **fomite**, for transmission of the infectious agent to multiple persons. The number of people infected distinguishes this type of transmission from indirect contact, which involves the spread of infection to only one person. In common vehicle spread, all the people are infected from a common fomite. Fomites include food, water, medications, and medical equipment and supplies. An example of historic significance is blood that was contaminated with HIV or HBV that was administered to several people before technology was developed to screen for the presence of these viruses.

Airborne transmission is spread that involves an infectious agent using the air as its means of dissemination and involves a long distance, which is typically described as 6 feet or greater, or even up to miles away. These airborne pathogens are either the remains of droplets (5 µm or smaller) that have evaporated **(droplet nuclei)** or the infectious agent is contained in dust particles, or sloughed **skin squames** (routinely shed superficial skin cells). These infectious microorganisms may also remain in the air for hours or even days and may become inhaled by or deposited on a susceptible host within the same room or even miles away.[20]

Special air handling and ventilation are required to prevent airborne transmission when droplet nuclei are involved. A susceptible host can catch rubeola (measles) and varicella viruses (chickenpox and shingles) just by being in the same room with an infected person. For these two infectious viral diseases, immune HCWs can safely care for infected patients; however, if susceptible HCWs must enter the room, they should wear respiratory protection. Tuberculosis (TB) is transmitted via droplet nuclei. TB has spread in hospitals because of air recirculation and low airflow rate.[88] All HCWs need to wear respiratory protection in the presence of a known or suspected infectious pulmonary TB patient.[145]

A lesser known example of airborne transmission is Legionnaire's disease, which causes death in 5% to 30% of cases. This acute bacterial disease is caused by *Legionella* and is associated with aerosol sources such as whirlpool spas, air conditioning units in large buildings, and other contained water sources used for drinking and bathing. The bacteria got its name in 1976 when many people attending an American Legion convention developed a deadly form of pneumonia-like illness.[30] Although the bacteria existed well before 1976, no one had detected it because no one was looking for it. Legionnaire's disease made the headlines again in 1994 when 1200 passengers were evacuated from a Royal Caribbean cruise ship. The pathogen was being carried throughout the ship through the air conditioning system.[123] In a 6-month period from November 2003 to May 2004, eight cases occurring after a cruise were reported to the CDC.[72] Each year, between 8000 and 18,000 cases are reported to the CDC. However, the actual number is believed to be much higher because many cases are not diagnosed and symptoms do not begin until 2 to 14 days after exposure. These factors, plus the dispersion of travelers to multiple states or countries, make it very difficult to recognize and then backtrack to its source.

Another airborne transmission route is that of skin squames. Our skin cells are always growing to replace aging cells that are located more superficially on our bodies and eventually sloughed off. If these sloughed skin cells are contaminated with a pathogen, they are capable of transmitting disease. In one study, skin squames were found to be the cause of several outbreaks of streptococcal wound infections and were eventually traced to hospital staff personnel.[20]

Dust particles containing the infectious agent are another means of airborne transmission. One example is *Histoplasma capsulatum,* the infectious fungal agent of the disease histoplasmosis. This fungal agent grows as a mold in soil containing bird droppings, such as in a chicken coop or pigeon roost. On a windy day, the dust containing the spores of this infectious fungal agent can be carried for miles to a susceptible host.[16]

In 2001, another airborne disease, anthrax, tragically made world headlines and took the life of a New York HCW and others. *Bacillus anthracis,* the infectious agent, is very resistant to adverse environmental conditions and disinfection and can remain viable in contaminated soil or on contaminated articles for many years.[16] Inhalation anthrax results from spore inhalation, and there is no evidence of transmission by person-to-person contact. A cell-free vaccine containing the protective antigen is available from the CDC.[16] Initially, the number of vaccines was very limited, but since then measures have been taken to mass-produce for future widespread distribution.

 Droplet contact and airborne transmission are differentiated from one another by particle size and by distance.

Vectorborne transmission involves a **vector** that transports an infectious agent to a host. An example of a vector is a fly that transports an infectious agent on its body or legs or an *Anopheles* mosquito that carries the malaria sporozoite, a protozoan parasite.[24] The malaria sporozoite enters the bloodstream of the human victim bitten by the mosquito. Other vectorborne disease examples include Lyme disease and Rocky Mountain spotted fever, which are carried by ticks containing the infectious agent. Because mosquitoes, flies, rats, and other vermin are not commonly found in U.S. health care facilities, vectorborne transmission is not nearly as common as it is in other parts of the world.

DEFENSE MECHANISMS
Nonspecific Defense Mechanisms

To establish an infection, the pathogen must successfully get by the host's defense mechanisms. The human body comes equipped with a wide variety of nonspecific defense mechanisms. For example, skin serves as a mechanical barrier and contains secretions that have antibacterial qualities. The upper respiratory system is full of cilia that facilitate the removal of pathogens. If the cilia are not successful, mucus aids in catching and removing pathogens. The respiratory system also protects against invasion through its secretions and defensive white cells that engulf and destroy pathogens. The gastrointestinal and urinary tracts are acidic and thus serve as a hostile environment to possible invaders. Even tears exhibit antibacterial activity and aid in the removal of pathogens.

Other nonspecific defense mechanisms include local inflammatory action and genetic, hormonal, and nutritional factors. Personal hygiene and behavioral habits influence the likelihood of developing disease. The age of a person also plays a role, with the extremely young and extremely old being most at risk. Alterations of any nonspecific defense mechanism through a skin break, surgery, chronic disease such as diabetes or immune deficiency disorders, or even medication to treat some diseases influence the host's susceptibility by lowering resistance to infectious disease processes.

Specific Defense Mechanisms

Immunity plays a critical role in reducing host susceptibility. Immunity exists in two forms: natural and artificial. Box 10-2 displays an outline of the different types of immunity.

1. Natural immunity: active disease
2. Artificial immunity
   - Active immunity: vaccine
   - Passive immunity
     i. Maternal antibodies
     ii. Antibody transferal to susceptible host

Natural immunity develops as a result of having acquired a specific disease. For example, children who have had rubella will never have it again. This is a fairly general rule for most acute viral infections, and such immunity usually persists for the lifetime of the host. Natural immunity can also develop after subclinical disease in which no readily apparent disease is observed. Unfortunately, all pathogens do not initiate lifelong immunity. Herpes simplex virus (cold sore) is a good example. After a herpes attack, the virus lies dormant until some event triggers another painful attack.

Artificial immunity can be further subdivided into active and passive immunity. Vaccines come in several forms: killed, toxoid, and attenuated live vaccines. *Active immunization* consists of vaccination with the altered pathogen or its products. The vaccine serves as the **antigen** (foreign substance) and thereby triggers the human body's immune system to create **antibodies**. Antibodies are specific; they work against only a specific antigen. The physiologic basis of this specificity resides in the unique sequences of amino acids that make a single antibody distinct from all other antibodies. T and B lymphocytes are the key white cells in the body's immune system.

The immune response requires careful study, and its complexity is beyond the scope of this chapter; however, it is well established that the B lymphocyte transforms itself into a plasma cell. Simply put, this cell is a highly active factory that synthesizes its own genetically unique type of antibody and sets it free into the body's fluids. The antibody then seeks the specific invading antigen. With some vaccines such as tetanus, a booster is necessary after a period of time because the number of antibodies **(titers)** drops to a level insufficient to provide adequate protection.

Historically, the earliest vaccine was developed to combat smallpox in 1796 by an English country doctor named Edward Jenner. Smallpox has since been eliminated from the world and exists only in such places as the CDC Level 4 research laboratories. For many decades before 1950, vaccines against diphtheria, tetanus, and pertussis formed the basic framework of U.S. public health. Later decades brought vaccines against poliomyelitis, measles, mumps, rubella, and chickenpox. Other vaccines are available for world travelers, research scientists, and military personnel. More recently, a vaccine against HBV was developed and must be offered by law to all at-risk HCWs. HBV vaccine has also been added to the list of recommended vaccines for newborns. Currently, immunologists have worked for more than two decades trying to develop an effective vaccine against HIV to curtail the worldwide AIDS pandemic.

To date, several experimental vaccines have been developed, although their effectiveness has yet to be determined.

Passive immunity, another form of artificial immunity, is defined as the transfer of protective antibodies from one host to a susceptible host. Examples include the administration of **immune serum globulin (ISG)** (e.g., a serum containing antibody) for the prophylaxis of measles, tetanus, and infectious HAV. The transfer of maternal antibodies to the fetus through the placenta is another form of passive immunity. Other substances available for passive immunization include antiserum against rabies administered after animal bites and antibiotics in known contacts of cases of TB, gonorrhea, and syphilis. Although it protects the individual from the disease in most cases or lessens disease severity, passive immunization does not protect against future infection nor does it prevent spread to others. Passive immunization typically has a short duration, usually several months at most, and thus active immunization is preferable whenever possible, such as in tetanus active vaccination.[20]

Environmental Factors Contributing to Nosocomial Disease

Environmental factors such as airflow, temperature, and humidity also influence links in the cycle of infection because they directly affect the pathogen and host. For example, measures directed at minimizing the risk of TB transmission within a hospital include the appropriate adjustment of airflow in designated rooms so that in any high-risk area, negative-pressure airflow occurs within the room. With the recent increase of classic TB, AIDS-related TB, and antibiotic-resistant strains of TB, the CDC has modified its guidelines. Hospitals are taking far greater protective measures to reduce the transmission of TB in the hospital environment.[43] Host susceptibility is also affected by environmental factors. For example, in winter months HCWs tend to stay indoors more often with doors and windows tightly closed. Centralized heating also tends to dry protective mucous membranes. This combination of reduced air circulation and dry membranes increases the risk of airborne diseases.

Many other environmental factors contribute to nosocomial disease. A person may enjoy the comfort and beauty of carpet in a radiation oncology department, but carpeting greatly increases the microbial level when compared with linoleum-like surfaces.[3,166] The presence of carpet has little, if any, affect on the amount of bacteria in the air of the carpeted area, so if no contact is made with the carpet, the risk of infection is usually negligible. However, carpets do present a greater infection risk to patients who use wheelchairs and pediatric patients who play or crawl on carpeted areas.[55]

Upholstered furniture should receive the same consideration as carpet. If it becomes soiled by body fluids, it should be discarded. Nonupholstered furniture should be routinely cleaned with an appropriate agent such as diluted bleach solution.[10] Fresh or dried flowers and potted plants may enhance the beauty of surroundings but harbor a multitude of microorganisms such as spores and bacteria. For this reason, flowers, potted plants, and fruit are often banned as a possible risk from high-risk areas such as bone marrow transplant wards and intensive care units.[112] Following this philosophy, flowers and fruit should be banned from any area in which immunosuppression is a concern.

Freshly laundered linen should be stored in a clean, closed closet or cabinet or a cart that remains covered. Linen is a nosocomial concern after it has been used. HCWs should use caution in handling used linen or paper by making sure it is not vigorously shaken and never handling it without gloves if it is contaminated with blood or other body fluids. Soiled linen should be placed in impervious Occupational Safety and Health Administration (OSHA)-approved bags. Bags should not be filled to capacity. A second bag is to be added if there is visible leakage. Fresh linen or paper should always be used for each patient.

 Used linen should never be vigorously shaken. Handle it with care and gloves if contaminated. Bag in room where used.

Other items routinely used in radiation therapy should also be considered as possible infection control hazards. For instance, custom-made bite blocks should be disinfected between each use on a single patient and then dried and stored in a clean, closed container.[160] If a custom-made device is deemed unnecessary, disposable one-use-only bite blocks are commercially available. Treatment tables and slide boards for transferring patients should be cleaned between each patient.

Tattooing or placing permanent ink dots to identify treatment portal or laser alignment is a routine patient care procedure that presents risk to the radiation therapist, as well as to the patient. The ink bottle must be treated as if it was a sterile container. Each patient must be tattooed with a fresh syringe and needle. After being used, the needle should never be reintroduced to the ink container. Likewise, drawing ink into a syringe and then changing needles between the tattooing of patients is a dangerous and unacceptable technique. The major infection hazard associated with traditional tattooing supplies is the nonsterile ink reservoir. A welcome advance over traditional methods is a tattooing device designed by a radiation therapist and marketed as SteriTatt. This device incorporates sterile, nontoxic ink that is contained in a sterile ink-dispensing pouch that looks somewhat like a mixture of an eyedropper and a syringe. This device is designed for single patient use and thus is an ideal tool for tattooing from an infection control point of view.[127]

 Sterile technique must be used in applying tattoos for patient alignment. Never recap a needle. The used needle should be discarded in a sharps container located in the room where used.

Ideally, bolus sheets should not be used on multiple patients. However, if bolus is to be reused, it must be wrapped in flexible plastic wrap to prevent the bolus material from being contaminated during use and then thoroughly disinfected before rewrapping for use on a subsequent patient. Another item often used on more than one patient is a pen or marker for drawing in a treatment port. If an item is contaminated by use on one patient, any harmful microorganisms can easily be spread to subsequent patients who need their treatment port markings reinforced. Some departments have solved this problem by issuing each patient a marker and placing it in a plastic, sealable bag that is kept with the patient's radiation treatment chart. The repeated use of marking pens and bolus would provide interesting data for epidemiologic studies.

 A pen used to apply marks on a patient's skin should never be used on multiple patients.

Thermoplastics were first used in a medical setting for splinting and casting of broken bones.[75] Later, their application as a way to prevent movement and improve position reproducibility was recognized in radiation therapy. The use of thermoplastic positioning devices for patient immobilization has steadily increased over the past two decades. A rigid sheet of thermoplastic material is placed in a hot water bath until it becomes pliable enough to mold over the patient's body surface. Once contact has been made with the patient's skin, the thermoplastic material should never be placed back in the water reservoir because cross contamination would occur. Although manufacturers may suggest that reforming is possible, to do so in the water reservoir is inappropriate. If reforming is necessary, it may be possible to use a separate disposable plastic container to hold the hot water for that specific patient. One rationale for concern is related to an opportunistic pathogen known as *Pseudomona.* Staphylococcal infections are also a worry.

 Never redip a thermoplastic material that has come into contact with a patient's skin. Always avoid cross contamination.

Pseudomonal infections have been well documented in contaminated water reservoirs such as hot tubs, swimming pools, and foot spas. These reservoirs typically maintain a water temperature range well below those used with thermoplastics and contribute to the frequency of *Pseudomonas* folliculitis. This skin condition appears within a half day to 2 days postexposure. The red, elevated lesions that make up the rash are sometimes pus filled and resolve quickly on their own in healthy people. Severe cases involving other body systems have occurred and even resulted in death and are usually found in immunocompromised people.[139,157]

When hot tub and spa safety measures are relaxed or ignored, *Pseudomonas* sets up residence and forms a protective slime layer to resist the effects of a subsequent chlorine application used to bring the water back up to a normal chlorine level.[177] Prophylactic measures include a constant flow of water or regular water replacement; maximum person capacity to accommodate chlorine ratios; draining the water; and applying superchlorination, brushing, and scrubbing. However, water tanks found in simulation do not have a constant water flow, are designed to be maintained at significantly higher temperatures than spas, do not have microorganism growth–retarding agents added to the water, and should never be subject to cross contamination.

A literature search did not yield any science-based studies of pseudomonal growth in simulation water tanks, but pseudomonal growth was found to be of interest to a TJC surveyor as noted in a communication on the Oncology Nursing Society website.[140] A temperature of 131° F for 1 hour is required to kill *Pseudomonas aeruginosa.*[167] Simulation water tanks are kept at temperatures in the range of 149° F to 165° F depending on the product used. This temperature range appears to be adequate to kill microorganisms of concern when carefully maintained.[141,182]

Until well-researched guidelines are available, possible prudent steps might include regularly scheduled draining, friction brushing and scrubbing, and chlorination followed with a thorough rinse of the water bath tank and its lid. A critical preventive step is not allowing the tank temperature to drop overnight or over weekends. Water tank temperatures should be continuously monitored and recorded, and the temperature-monitoring device should be periodically calibrated to ensure it is recording temperature correctly. It may even be possible to add something to the water to retard microorganism growth that would not interfere with the thermoplastic properties, but this has yet to be recommended. Further epidemiologic study and recommendations in cooperation with manufacturers are warranted at this time.

 Monitor the temperature of the thermoplastic water tank throughout the work day. Avoid temperature drops on weekends and holidays as well. Keep tanks clean.

The CDC is an excellent source for scientific literature relevant to infection control during construction, demolition, renovation, and repair of health care facilities.[10] To summarize, the best defense is a good offense. HCWs should take good care of their bodies to keep nonspecific defense mechanisms healthy, practice good personal hygiene and behavioral patterns, take advantage of active immunizations, and pay close attention to the work environment. Any strategy that workers can take to break a link in the cycle of infection helps protect not only themselves but also those for whom they care.

DRUG USE AND DRUG-RESISTANT MICROORGANISMS

Antibiotics have been in use for more than 60 years and have served as the main weapon in the medical world's arsenal against disease. Many of the once-terrifying killer diseases have become mere health inconveniences that, if diagnosed early enough, can be cured with pills or injections. Not too long ago, some people envisioned a future free of infectious disease. Then things began to change. Mutated germs and emerging diseases such as AIDS and a mysterious respiratory illness caused by the Hantavirus, once unheard of, began making the media headlines.[102] This led to many questions about the origins of these new and resurgent diseases and the reasons why antibiotics were not working as they once had. The answers to these questions required a review of the evolution of the use of antibiotics and other medications and a new understanding of the way that microorganisms function.

By changing their genetic makeup, microorganisms have found ways to resist the effects of medications. Many microorganisms have mutated and developed the ability to manufacture cell products that destroy the drugs that previously killed them.[99,123] (Figure 10-3). Mutations arise much faster in microorganisms than in humans because the time for a new generation to be created may be a matter of minutes compared with decades in humans. If mutations develop in their relatively short evolutionary processes that are beneficial in the struggle to survive against medications, the mutants are better suited to live

and reproduce. Others have picked up protective genes from other microorganisms[104,123] (see Figure 10-3).

People have also unwittingly helped in the development of drug-resistant microorganisms by not finishing prescribed medications and by demanding and receiving inappropriate antibiotics for illnesses. The tougher, remaining pathogens endure as the most fit to survive. Vaccines, like antibiotics, are challenged by mutating pathogens. This has been part of the problem in developing a successful vaccine for the continuously evolving HIV.

 Never stop a prescribed antibiotic early, even if you feel much better. Doing so helps create superinfections.

Because massive quantities of antibiotics and other drugs are used in medical settings, logic dictates that large proportions of these new mutating pathogens are responsible for nosocomial infections. This causes great concern because the patients who are the sickest are also the poorest equipped to fight these "superinfections." This is also alarming for HCWs and should serve as notice regarding the importance of the epidemiology department in helping protect workers and their patients. The CDC's Hospital Infection Control Practices Advisory Committee has also been addressing approaches to control resistant microorganisms in hospitals.[41,42] Through stringent adherence to infection control protocols, nosocomial infections can be reduced, thus lowering the overall cost of health care.

HEALTH CARE FACILITY EPIDEMIOLOGY

The Hospital Infections Branch of the CDC was established to help hospitals deal with nosocomial infections. Today's hospitals are required to establish an epidemiology division if they wish to be accredited by and meet TJC standards.[109] Even in non–TJC-accredited facilities, state health department or public health codes must be met for licensure, and requirements typically include some form of epidemiologic oversight.

State laws also govern the reporting of specific infectious diseases and the disposal of medical waste. In the past two decades, OSHA has focused its attention on health care facilities and the HCW more than ever before. In fact, OSHA mandated that employers of HCWs must offer the HBV vaccine.[133] Although current mandates do not specifically address students because they are not employees, common sense suggests that students are also at risk and should be vaccinated. Today's HCW can expect to undergo an employment physical, an epidemiologically related health and safety orientation, ongoing inservices on a regular basis, and routinely offered health services such as TB testing and checking of disease-related titers.

Even hospital reimbursement by third-party payers such as Medicare or Blue Cross/Blue Shield is affected by a health care facility's attention to the quality of care and quality assessment (QA). External reviewers such as the Health Care Financing Administration influence this reimbursement association. A staff radiation therapist, chief radiation therapist, or manager in a radiation oncology department can expect to participate at some level in the development or implementation of a QA or quality continuing improvement (QCI) program, with infection control being just one portion of the overall program.

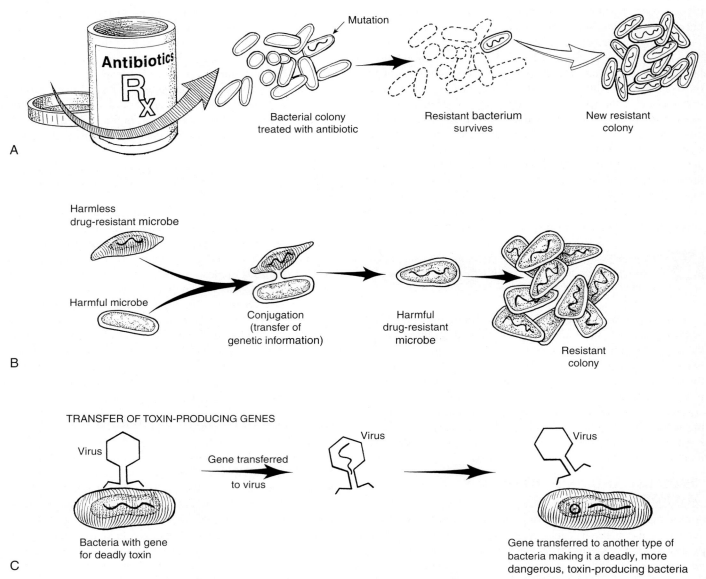

Figure 10-3. A, When antibiotics are used to treat a bacterial infection, most bacteria will die. However, mutated bacteria may survive and go on to produce more drug-resistant clones. **B,** The transfer of a drug-resistant gene from a harmless microbe to a harmful microbe through the conjugation process. **C,** A virus can carry a harmful trait to other types of bacteria, making them dangerous.

PERSONNEL AND STUDENT HEALTH SERVICES AND PERTINENT INFECTIOUS DISEASES

The employee health clinic and the epidemiology division of a health care facility have a vested interest in their HCWs because they are at risk of exposure to infectious disease in the work place and the community. If a HCW develops an infection, he or she poses a risk to patients, coworkers, friends, and family members. Because of the nature of their chosen profession, HCWs have frequent and prolonged direct contact with patients who harbor a multitude of infectious agents; thus HCWs are at great risk of exposure.

A health placement evaluation should be completed for hiring or for a new student before contact is made with patients.

Such an examination should determine that the potential HCW is able to perform the essential physical and mental functions of the position to ensure the safe and efficient performance of duties. The examination should also determine the worker's immunization status and medical history. A listing of recommended vaccines for HCWs is shown in Box 10-3. The following text highlights specific diseases against which HCWs and their patients must be protected.

Hepatitis B Virus

HBV infection is a major infectious occupational hazard of HCWs. Its transmission occurs through contact with blood and body fluids. HBV is a highly transmissible virus, and evidence has shown that this potentially deadly virus can live on surfaces

Box 10-3	Recommended Vaccines for Health Care Workers

HEPATITIS B (HB OR HBV)
- Recombinant vaccine; 3-dose series. Give at 0-, 1-, and 6-month intervals. Considered protected (positive) if HB surface antibody (anti-HB) is at least 10 mIU/mL at 1 to 2 months after dose no. 3.
- If anti-HB is less than 10 mIU/mL (negative), revaccinate and retest.
- If still negative after 6 doses (3 + 3), considered to be a nonresponder and at risk. If known or suspected clinical parenteral exposure, give HBIg prophylaxis.
- Is possible that nonresponder is actually infected (HBsAg positive) and should seek medical evaluation.

INFLUENZA (ANNUAL FLU SEASON)
- Preferred is the intramuscular trivalent (inactivated) influenza vaccine (TIV).
- Alternate is intranasal live, attenuated influenza vaccine (LAIV). Can use only if not pregnant and 49 years of age or younger.
- Give 1 dose of TIV or LAIV annually. Is modified annually for predicted flu type.

MMR (MEASLES, MUMPS, AND RUBELLA)
- Are all live-virus vaccines.
- If born in 1957 or later, considered immune only if: have had 2 doses of M and M vaccine (28 days apart) and 1 dose of R. Or have reliable physician diagnosed history. Or have serologic evidence of immunity.
- If born before 1957, probably had these diseases as a child. But still is recommended to get a dose of MMR vaccine (2 doses for a mumps outbreak). Or have reliable physician diagnosed history. Or have serologic evidence of immunity.

VARICELLA (CHICKENPOX)
- Varicella-zoster live-virus vaccine. Two doses (28 days apart). Or have reliable physician diagnosed history. Or have serologic evidence of immunity.

TETANUS/DIPHTHERIA/PERTUSSIS (PERTUSSIS IS WHOOPING COUGH)
- Tetanus (T) and diphtheria (d) are toxoid vaccines. Pertussis (P) is acellular vaccine (aproved by FDA in 2005).
- As child, probably received primary series (DTP, DTaP, DT, Td). Two intramuscular doses 4 weeks apart, then dose no. 3 given 6 to 12 months later.
- All HCWs need a Td booster every 10 years.
- As of February 2006, the ACIP has stated that all HCWs younger than 65 years with direct patient contact need to have a one-time dose of Tdap given intramuscularly. Radiation therapists are included in this initial target group. Vaccine is 92% effective. Is result of recent dramatic increase in number of pertussis cases and change in age distribution of pertussis.

Other vaccines are recommended for special groups of HCWs such as microbiologists and research scientists and include hepatitis A, BCG, meningococcal, typhoid, and vaccinia (smallpox).

Data from Centers for Disease Control and Prevention (CDC) website, March 2007 update. Also from CDC: *MMWR* 46(RR-18):1-42, 1997.
ACIP, Advisory Committee on Immunization Practices; *HBIg,* hepatitus B immune globulin; *HBsAg,* hepatitis B surface antigen.

at room temperature for 7 days.[18] In response to HCWs' concerns, the U.S. Department of Labor, OSHA, and the U.S. Department of Health and Human Services (DHHS) issued a Joint Advisory Notice in 1987 and began the rule-making process to regulate HBV exposure.[142] In 1987, the CDC recommended that HCWs be vaccinated. The final rule proposed by OSHA was printed in the *Federal Register* on December 6, 1991, and mandated that the HBV vaccine be made available to all at-risk HCWs.[133] Workers should understand that the HBV vaccine protects against only hepatitis B, not hepatitis C, hepatitis D, hepatitis E, and so on, for which no vaccine is available at this time.[126] Although all of these have similar names because they all cause liver inflammation, they are distinctly different viruses both genetically and clinically. As with any rule, an implementation deadline is set; thus mandatory implementation of HBV vaccination did not occur until July 6, 1992.[133]

In the mid-1980s, the CDC estimated that the total number of people infected with HBV annually in the United States was 280,000, with 8700 of those being HCWs. The annual CDC mortality rate for HCWs was approximately 200.[133] Morbidity associated with HBV includes chronic hepatitis, which is highly associated with hepatocellular (liver) cancer and other types of progressive liver damage or associated complications such as liver failure and liver cirrhosis, both of which can lead to death.[26] Due to voluntary vaccination since 1987, a very significant drop was seen by 1992; the number of infected HCWs had dropped

to 5020. Of this number, 6 people died with acute cases and 300 developed chronic hepatitis.[126] The latest available statistics show an estimated 51,000 total new infections in the United States for 2005.[164] With the HBV vaccine available by law to all at-risk HCWs, the morbidity and mortality rates will undoubtedly continue to drop significantly as they have in the general population.

A safe HBV vaccine derived from human plasma became available in the United States in 1982 and is effective in producing an HBV antibody in most healthy, susceptible people. In 1987, a **recombinant deoxyribonucleic acid (DNA)** vaccine became available.[133] Both vaccines are remarkably free of side effects, the most common being soreness at the injection site.[154] The HBV vaccine is of no use in HBV carriers or individuals who are immune to HBV.[174] Postvaccination testing should be performed 1 to 6 months after the three-part vaccination series to ascertain that immunity was conferred. Approximately 90% of healthy vaccinees develop protective antibodies after the series of three injections.[150] At this time, booster doses or periodic antibody status testing of vaccine is not recommended for HCWs with normal immune status who have demonstrated an antibody response following vaccination.[128] Postvaccination testing is recommended for persons whose medical care depends on concrete knowledge of their immune status. This includes an HCW who has a work-related incident connected to contact with blood.[27]

Hepatitis C Virus

Of increasing concern is the hepatitis C virus (HCV), which was identified in 1989.[2] As previously mentioned, no vaccine exists yet for HCV. Although the risks of transmission remain undefined, HCV appears to be transmitted not only through contact with blood and body fluids but also through household contact. Prevention tactics target risky sexual behavior, illegal intravenous and nasal drug use, body piercing, and tattooing.[128] Obviously, nosocomial and occupational exposures are of concern. Of particular importance is that HCV is associated with an extraordinarily high frequency of chronic infection leading to cirrhosis and primary hepatocellular carcinoma. The U.S. Food and Drug Administration (FDA) has recommended plasma screening for HCV since 1992.[2,175] The CDC has estimated that HCV is responsible for almost half of the annual liver transplants. While ongoing research for the development of a safe and effective vaccine continues, HCV has an exceptionally high mutation rate and elicits a weak immune response, both of which have made vaccine development an elusive challenge.

Other Recommended Vaccines for Health Care Workers

Other diseases for which immunizations are recommended for HCWs are influenza, measles, mumps, rubella, pertussis, tetanus, and diphtheria. In diseases for which no vaccine is available or for which the HCW has not received a vaccine or does not respond to a vaccine, prompt prophylaxis is advised. Diseases included in this group are HAV, HBV, HCV, meningococcal disease, and rabies.

Tuberculosis

At the turn of the century, TB was one of the leading causes of death. No effective vaccine exists for TB. The bacille Calmette-Guérin (BCG) vaccine, widely used outside the United States for several decades, confers varied and questionable degrees of protection, ranging from some degree of protection to no protection at all.[9,16]

The primary transmission route of TB is airborne droplet nuclei. The droplet nuclei are dispersed when people sneeze, cough, or talk. The risk of infection of an HCW depends on the number of droplet nuclei circulating in the air and the duration of time spent breathing the contaminated air. If exposed to TB, 5% to 10% of normal healthy individuals will actually develop the disease, half in the first 1 to 2 years after infection.[106] As a result of improved housing and nutrition, TB decreased in frequency until 1985, at which time the decline leveled off. Around 1985, TB made a dramatic reappearance.[87] To a large degree, its emergence was related to the AIDS epidemic, increased immigration, and inadequate precautions being taken at health care facilities. In a study conducted at Parkland Memorial Hospital in Dallas, Texas, and published in 1989, one patient admitted to the hospital's emergency department in April 1983 contributed to the development of active TB in six employees and one other patient, as well as positive conversion in at least 47 other employees.[88] Recirculation of air was deemed a major contributing factor in this specific transmission case. Based on the Parkland experience and CDC recommendations, many hospitals have redesigned airflow systems, and the employee health clinics of such hospitals now make TB surveillance among HCWs a high-level priority.[31,33-35]

Since the resurgence of TB during 1985 to 1992, the annual TB rate has steadily decreased. However, the proportion of TB cases among foreign-born persons has increased each year during 1993 to 2003 and has not changed much since.[43,57] Foreign-born persons lack access to medical services for a variety of reasons, which results in delays in diagnosis and treatment and in ongoing transmission of the disease.[32,60]

In 1994, the CDC published *Guidelines for Preventing the Transmission of Tuberculosis in Health-Care Facilities*.[43,57] There were many reasons for the new guidelines. In the mid-1980s to early 1990s, there was a resurgence of TB, including the documentation of several high-profile health care–associated outbreaks related to an increase in prevalence of TB and HIV coinfection. Individuals began to have lapse of disease. Surveillance studies indicated delays in diagnosis and treatment of persons with infectious TB and finally the emergence and transmission of multidrug-resistant (MDR) TB strains.

 No effective vaccine exists for TB. Multidrug-resistant TB is extremely dangerous and can be fatal.

The CDC later developed the *TB Respiratory Protection Program in Health Care Facilities—Administrator's Guide* (1999).[51,61] Because these guidelines recommended special particulate respirators (face masks) to protect the HCW, it fell under federal laws implemented to protect workers under the jurisdiction of OSHA. Jokes in the past about Darth Vader masks now had the ring of reality in the health care setting.

OSHA mandates that the minimum level of respiratory protection for TB will be a National Institute for Occupational Safety and Health (NIOSH)–certified N95 half-mask respirator.[38,51,184] NIOSH is the government agency that actually assesses, recommends, and tests respirators for OSHA. The N95 rating indicates that 95% of test particles will be stopped. OSHA also requires that HCWs who need to wear such masks be medically evaluated to wear them because of possible pulmonary- or cardiac-associated stresses on the user, receive training, and go through face-fitting procedures.[38,51,184] It is important to note that simple surgical masks are not respirators and are not certified as such. Also of importance is that men with beards are precluded from using some of the NIOSH-approved masks because an adequate seal cannot be maintained.[24,34,103] Masks labeled N, R, or P meet CDC guidelines, as do those that use high-efficiency particulate air (HEPA) filters, and may be obtained with or without exhalation valves. Four main mask designs are available as described in Box 10-4.

 OSHA-approved masks must be provided for contact with patients with active or suspected TB.

In 2005, the CDC, at the request of the Advisory Council for the Elimination of Tuberculosis (ACET), reviewed and updated the 1994 TB infection control document. The reassessment included the infection control guidelines for health care settings. The reasoning behind the update included the shifts in the epidemiology of TB, advances in the scientific understanding,

Box 10-4	Types of OSHA- and NIOSH-Approved Respirators for Protection Against Tuberculosis

DISPOSABLE PARTICULATE RESPIRATORS

Disposable, lightweight

Negative-pressure design

Half-mask or half-mask with face splatter shield

Can be used in sterile field area if there is no exhalation valve

REPLACEABLE PARTICULATE FILTER RESPIRATORS

Half-mask or half-mask with face splatter shield

Reusable, with single or dual filters that are replaced

Negative-pressure design

Has to be disinfected and inspected

Cannot be used in sterile field area

Communication may be difficult

Also comes in full facepiece design, which provides better seal and protection

POWERED AIR-PURIFYING RESPIRATORS (PAPRs)

Battery operated

Half or full facepiece designs

Has breathing tube and uses only HEPA filters

Usually more comfortable to wear and cooler

Easier to breathe

Cannot be used in sterile field area

Is not a true positive-pressure device, can be overbreathed when inhaling

Has to be disinfected and inspected

May be bulky and noisy

Communication may be difficult

Two types: tight fit and loose fit, which does accommodate facial hair (beard)

POSITIVE-PRESSURE SUPPLIED-AIR RESPIRATORS

Uses compressed air from a stationary source delivered through a hose

Much more protective

Should be used when the other types do not provide adequate protection

Minimal breathing effort

Should not be worn during sterile procedures

Must be disinfected and inspected

Modified from Centers for Disease Control and Prevention: *NIOSH TB respiratory protection program in health care facilities—administrator's guide* (DHHS Publication No. 99-143; pp vi-x, 1-37, 82-112), Cincinnati, 1999, National Institute for Occupational Safety and Health, HHS, Centers for Disease Control and Prevention.

HEPA, High-efficiency particulate air; *NIOSH*, National Institute for Occupational Safety and Health; *OSHA*, Occupational Safety and Health Administration.

and changes in health care practice over the past decade.[58] Box 10-5 indicates the changes in this report as compared with previous guidelines. The *Guidelines for Preventing the Transmission of* Mycobacterium tuberculosis *in Health-Care Settings, 2005* replaces all previous CDC guidelines for TB control in health settings.[32,38,57,58,143]

Risk classification should be used as part of the risk assessment to determine the need for a TB screening program for HCWs and the frequency of screening. There are three TB screening risk classifications: low risk, medium risk, and potential ongoing transmission.

The classification of low risk should be applied to settings in which persons with TB disease are not expected to be encountered; therefore, exposure to *Mycobacterium tuberculosis* is unlikely. The classification of medium risk should be applied to settings in which the risk assessment has determined that HCWs will or will possibly be exposed to persons with TB disease or to clinical specimens that might contain *M. tuberculosis.*

The classification of potential ongoing transmission should be temporarily applied to any setting if evidence suggests person-to-person transmission of *M. tuberculosis* has occurred in the setting during the preceding year. If uncertainty exists regarding whether to classify a setting as low risk or medium risk, the setting typically should be classified as medium risk.[146] Table 10-1 provides the guidelines for the TB screening procedures by classification of HCWs or the setting and includes the frequency of screening.[57]

Baseline testing for *M. tuberculosis* infection is recommended for all new HCWs (including students in health care education programs), regardless of the risk classification of the setting and can be conducted with the two-step tuberculin skin tests (TSTs) or blood assay for *M. tuberculosis* (BAMT).[52,168]

The TST consists of an intradermal **Mantoux tuberculin skin test** (purified protein derivative [PPD] of tuberculin). BAMT does not require two-step testing and is more specific than skin testing. BAMT that uses *M. tuberculosis*–specific antigens (i.e., QuantiFERON-QFTG) are not expected to result in false-positive results in persons vaccinated with Bacille Calmette-Guérin (BCG). Baseline test results should be documented, preferably within 10 days of HCWs of having patient contact (Table 10-2 provides indications).

 HCWs can be tested using a two-step skin test (TST) or a blood test (BAMT). A person with a positive test is at risk for developing active TB even years later; thus, treatment is highly encouraged before active TB develops.

To determine whether treatment for latent TB infection (LTBI) or a positive conversion is indicated, HCWs should be referred for medical and diagnostic evaluation according to the TST result criteria (see Table 10-2). In conjunction with a medical and diagnostic evaluation, HCWs with positive test results for *M. tuberculosis* should be considered for treatment of LTBI after TB disease has been excluded by further medical evaluation. HCWs cannot be compelled to take treatment for LTBI, but they should be encouraged to do so if they are eligible for treatment. Active TB is treated with an initial 2-month phase of four drugs such as isoniazid (INH), pyrazinamide (PZA), ethambutol (EMB), and rifampin (RIF) and at least a 4-month continuation phase of INH and RIF.[54,58]

All persons with a history of TB or positive TB test should be alerted that they are at risk of developing the disease in the future, even years later, and thus should promptly report any pulmonary symptoms. HCWs with active TB pose a risk to others and should be removed from work until adequate treatment is

Box 10-5	Changes Differentiating the 2005 Report of Guidelines for Preventing the Transmission of *Mycobacterium tuberculosis* in Health Care Settings from the 2004 Guidelines

- The risk assessment process includes the assessment of additional aspects of infection control.
- The term "tuberculin skin tests" (TSTs) is used instead of purified protein derivative (PPD).
- The whole-blood interferon gamma release assay (IGRA), QuantiFERON-TB Gold test (QFT-G) (Cellestis Limited, Carnegie, Victoria, Australia), is a Food and Drug Administration (FDA)–approved in vitro cytokine-based assay for cell-mediated immune reactivity to *M. tuberculosis* and might be used instead of TST in TB screening programs for HCWs. This IGRA is an example of a blood assay for *M. tuberculosis* (BAMT).
- The frequency of TB screening for HCWs has been decreased in various settings, and the criteria for determination of screening frequency have been changed.
- The scope of settings for which the guidelines apply has been broadened to include laboratories and additional outpatient and nontraditional facility–based settings.
- Criteria for serial testing for *M. tuberculosis* infection of HCWs are more clearly defined. In certain settings, this change will decrease the number of HCWs who need serial TB screening.
- These recommendations usually apply to an entire health care setting rather than areas within a setting.
- New terms, *airborne infection precautions (airborne precautions)* and *airborne infection isolation room (AII room),* are introduced.
- Recommendations for annual respirator training, initial respirator fit testing, and periodic respirator fit testing have been added.
- The evidence of the need for respirator fit testing is summarized.
- Information on ultraviolet germicidal irradiation (UVGI) and room-air recirculation units has been expanded.

Additional information regarding MDR (multidrug-resistant) TB and HIV infection has been included.
Adapted from *MMWR Recomm Rep* 54(RR-17):1-141, 2005.[57]

Table 10-1	Indications for Two-Step Tuberculin Skin Tests (TSTs)

Situation	Recommended Testing
No previous TST result	Two-step baseline TSTs
Previous negative TST result (documented or not) >12 months before new employment	Two-step baseline TSTs
Previous documented negative TST result 12 ≤ months before employment	Single TST needed for baseline testing; this test will be the second step
≥2 previous documented negative TSTs but most recent TST >12 months before new employment	Single TST; two-step testing is not necessary
Previous documented positive TST result	No TST
Previous undocumented positive TST result*	Two-step baseline TSTs
Previous BCG vaccination	Two-step baseline TSTs
Programs that use serial BAMT, including QFT† (or the previous version QFT)	See *MMWR Recomm Rep* 54(RR-17) supplement, "Use of QFT-G‡ for diagnosing *M. tuberculosis* infections in HCWs"

*For newly hired health care workers and other persons who will be tested on a routine basis (i.e., residents or staff of correctional or long-term care facilities), a previous TST is not a contraindication to a subsequent TST, unless the test was associated with severe ulceration or anaphylactic shock, which are substantially rare adverse events. If the previous positive TST result is not documented, administer TSTs or offer BAMT.
†QuantiFERON-TB test.
‡QuantiFERON-TB Gold test.
Adapted from *MMWR Recomm Rep* 54(RR-17):1-141, 2005.[57]

administered, cough has resolved, and sputum is free of bacilli in three consecutive smears.[138,154] In most infected HCWs or patients, respiratory secretions are no longer infectious 10 days after effective treatment.[154] Because of surveillance measures and changes in hospital practice, the number of TB cases has been on the decrease since 1992, and the number of MDR TB cases has been declining since 1998.[45,51,62]

Table 10-2	Interpretations of Tuberculin Skin Test and QuantiFERON–TB Results According to the Purpose of Testing for *M. tuberculosis* Infection in a Health Care Setting

Purpose of Testing	TST	QFT
1. Baseline	1. ≥10 mm is considered a positive result (either first or second step)	1. Positive (only one step)
2. Serial testing without known exposure	2. Increase of >10 mm is considered a positive result (TST conversion)	2. Change from negative to positive (QFT conversion)
3. Known exposure (close contact)	3. ≥10 mm is considered a positive result in persons who have a baseline TST result of 0 mm; an increase of ≥10 mm is considered a positive result in persons with a negative baseline TST result or previous follow-up screening TST result of ≥0 mm	3. Change to positive

QFT, QuantiFERON-TB, *TST,* tuberculin skin test. Adapted from *MMWR Recomm Rep* 54(RR-17):1-141, 2005.[57]

Health Care Worker Removal from Patient Care

With other diseases, infected HCWs should be removed from direct patient contact for variable time frames. These diseases include conjunctivitis, epidemic diarrhea, streptococcosis, HAV, herpes simplex of exposed skin areas such as the hands, measles, mumps, pertussis, rubella, rabies, *Staphylococcus aureus* skin lesions, and varicella zoster.

Varicella-Zoster Virus

Of these diseases, varicella-zoster virus (VZV) deserves special attention in a radiation oncology department. VZV is the pathogen that causes varicella zoster (chickenpox) and herpes zoster (shingles). VZV has an extremely high degree of communicability and is transmitted by the inhalation of small droplet nuclei or by direct contact with respiratory droplets or vesicle fluid.[91]

For children, chickenpox usually consists of a mild illness characterized by fever and a vesicular rash mainly on the body trunk. The rash may range from one or two vesicles to hundreds; thus, extremely light or subclinical infections may go undiagnosed. The skin lesions appear in groups at different times, so late and early lesions can be seen at the same time. In adults, chickenpox is typically more severe and the risk of complications is higher. Infection early in pregnancy is associated with neonatal complications and congenital malformations. In cancer patients, chickenpox can be life-threatening in children and adults as a result of an impaired immune system. If a nonimmune cancer patient is exposed, varicella-zoster immune globulin (VZIG) can be given to modify the disease.[33]

Shingles is a local manifestation of a recurrent, reactivated infection by the same virus. After a person has chickenpox, the VZV is thought to remain dormant in the cells of nerve root ganglia. Shingles usually is seen in middle age; however, children and even infants occasionally develop shingles. Painful rashes of blisters appear on the skin area supplied by the affected nerve. Clinically, especially in adults, pain and severe itching occur and often last for long periods after the lesions have crusted over and healed. A significant number of transplant or cancer patients, especially those with leukemia, lymphoma, or AIDS-related cancers, develop shingles as a result of immunosuppression.[26] In 2007, the FDA approved Zostavax, a vaccine for the herpes-zoster virus.[63]

Because VZV can be life-threatening to nonimmune cancer patients, HCWs, especially those in oncology or transplant departments, should have had documented varicella or should be able to show serologic evidence of immunity. Certainly only those workers who have a positive history should care for patients with VZV. If nonimmune HCWs are exposed to persons with chickenpox or shingles, these workers should be considered potentially infective during the incubation period. They should be should excluded from work beginning on the tenth day after exposure and should remain away from patient contact for the maximum incubation period of varicella, which is 21 days.[33]

In addition, infected workers should not return to work until all lesions have dried and crusted, which is usually 6 days from the onset of the rash.[33] VZIG can be used after exposure in nonimmune HCWs to lessen the severity of the disease if they develop it. If an HCW receives VZIG after exposure, the incubation period is prolonged; therefore he or she must be reassigned or furloughed for a longer time, typically 28 days after exposure.[33] In March 1995, the FDA approved a vaccine for chickenpox (trade name: Varivax) for use in the United States.[14]

VIRAL RESPIRATORY INFECTIONS

Viral respiratory infections are another major source of nosocomial infections. Although most people do not associate influenza specifically with the work environment, the issue should be addressed. Respiratory diseases, such as influenza, are associated with significant morbidity and mortality in older patients, patients with chronic underlying disease, and immunocompromised patients. In other words, patients of all ages seen in a radiation therapy department are at high risk for influenza and other respiratory viral infections. HCWs should not provide patient care if they have a fever, uncontrollable secretions, cough, or other communicable respiratory symptoms. Some institutions have created policies that allow managers to send an employee home to keep the remaining staff well. Likewise, outpatients who are coughing or who have other upper respiratory symptoms should be provided with a mask as a safety measure for the staff caring for them.

Respiratory viruses are spread through three major transmission modes: (1) direct contact via large droplets over a short distance; (2) airborne transmission, consisting of small droplet nuclei that can travel long distances; and (3) self-inoculation after contact with contaminated materials (this usually involves the hands transferring the virus to the mucous membranes of the eye or nose).

The common cold, croup, and viral pneumonia are all examples of infections caused by the influenza virus. Influenza is spread mainly by the airborne route via small particle aerosol, thus explaining explosive seasonal outbreaks of the flu. Two major types of influenza are recognized: type A and type B.[16] These two types of influenza are among the most communicable diseases of humans. Shedding of the influenza virus from an infected individual usually lasts 5 to 7 days after the onset of symptoms.[113] Because of the constantly changing nature of these viruses, new subtypes appear at irregular intervals. This translates to the need to develop different influenza vaccinations that will be effective against new mutated subtypes.

Prevention of winter influenza outbreaks consists of immunization programs initiated each year before the influenza season. Vaccination programs are typically aimed toward older persons, those with chronic disease states, those with respiratory diseases, and HCWs. Vaccine effectiveness ranges from 60% to 90%.[39] In persons not fully protected, the vaccine appears to reduce the severity of symptoms. Adequate serologic response typically takes place a couple of weeks after vaccination.

Unfortunately, HCWs often do not take advantage of free or low-cost vaccinations offered by employers. The workers are apparently reluctant to participate because of misinformation regarding the influenza vaccine's effectiveness and side effects. Famous quotes by the uninformed such as "The flu shot gave me the flu" and "Flu shots don't work" simply cannot be substantiated. On the other hand, substantial evidence supports the vaccine's effectiveness in preventing and decreasing morbidity.[39]

Flu shots never cause the flu. It is impossible because the vaccine is made from a killed virus. HCWs should get flu shots early in the flu season for greater protection.

The most commonly reported side effect is soreness at the injection site that lasts less than 24 hours. This temporary discomfort does not occur in all people and can be reduced or eliminated by premedication with ibuprophen or acetaminophen. Surely this is better than a week's sick leave; possible loss of income; and the health risk imposed on patients who are far more likely to develop serious complications, including death.

Perhaps with better educational programs, HCWs and the public will participate in greater numbers in annual flu prevention programs. In the event that an individual is not inoculated with the influenza vaccine, drugs such as amantadine and rimantadine are 70% to 90% effective in preventing influenza A to the same level of a vaccine or in decreasing the length of illness if administered within 24 to 48 hours after the onset of symptoms.[44] Amantadine and rimantadine are not effective against influenza B.[44,132]

EVOLUTION OF ISOLATION PRACTICES

Nosocomial infections have been a serious problem ever since sick patients were placed together in a hospital and a long time before the term *nosocomial* came about. Even in biblical times, the need to isolate or quarantine persons with leprosy was recognized. In the early part of the 20th century, HCWs wore special gowns, washed their hands with disinfecting agents, disinfected contaminated equipment, and practiced a wide variety of isolation or quarantine measures to contain contagious diseases such as TB. In 1970, the CDC published its first guidelines for nosocomial infections and isolation techniques.[31] These guidelines recommended the use of seven isolation categories based on the routes of disease transmission.

Because not all diseases in a given category required the same degree of precautions, this approach, although simple to understand and apply, resulted in overisolation for many patients. Over the next decade, it became evident that although this approach helped prevent the spread of classic contagious diseases, it neither addressed new drug-resistant pathogens or new syndromes nor focused on nosocomial infections in special care departments. Thus, in 1983 the CDC published new guidelines.[79] In this edition, many infections were moved or placed under new isolation categories. Three new categories were added: contact isolation, acid-fast bacilli (AFB) (another name for TB), and blood and body fluids. The protective isolation category was deleted. These significant changes encouraged the hospital's infection control committee to choose between category-specific and patient-specific isolation categories.

Universal Precautions

Then came AIDS. The onset of the HIV pandemic in the early 1980s drastically altered the way HCWs practiced overall infection control procedures. For the first time, emphasis was focused on applying blood and body fluid precautions to all persons. According to this new infection control approach now known as universal precautions (UP), all human blood and certain body fluids were to be treated as if they were known to be infectious for HIV, HBV, or other bloodborne pathogens.[34-37]

UP were intended to supplement rather than replace long-standing recommendations for the control of non-bloodborne pathogens. Although the old blood and body fluids isolation category was negated with the new concept, the earlier CDC category-specific or disease-specific isolation precautions remained intact. Later, in 1988, the CDC published an expanded UP guideline that addressed the prevention of needlesticks and the use of traditional gloves and gowns and placed new emphasis on masks, eye protection, and other protective equipment and procedures.[37]

Body Substance Isolation

Another system, known as *body substance isolation* (BSI), was proposed in 1987 at two hospitals, one in Seattle and the other in San Diego.[125] As its name implied, BSI concentrated on the isolation of all body fluids for all patients through protective equipment such as gloves. BSI also addressed the transmission of non–body fluid–associated pathogens such as those transmitted exclusively or in part by airborne transmission. In the BSI system, if a patient had an airborne infectious agent, a "stop" sign was placed on the door of the patient's room with further instructions to check with the nurse's station. The decision regarding the type of protective action to be taken was based on the specific patient, with the informed decision being made by the professional practitioners in charge of that patient. Decisions were guided by CDC isolation category-specific or disease-specific recommendations.

Comparison of Universal Precautions and Body Substance Isolation

Overall, many aspects of BSI were identical or extremely similar to the UP concept. BSI differed from UP in that the focus of UP was placed primarily on blood and body fluids implicated in the spread of bloodborne pathogens, whereas BSI focused on the isolation of all moist body substances in all patients. In other words, the term *universal* referred to all patients, not to all body fluids or all pathogens. UP did not apply to tears, sweat, saliva, feces, vomit, nasal secretions, or sputum unless visible blood was present.[34,35,37] On the other hand, BSI dealt with all body fluids. One major difference was the guideline for wearing gloves and washing hands. In the BSI system, hand washing was not required after removing gloves unless the glove's integrity had been broken and the hands were visibly soiled. This difference was interpreted by many as a disadvantage of using the BSI concept.

Occupational Safety and Health Administration and Bloodborne Pathogens

On December 6, 1991, OSHA published "29 CFR Part 1910.1030-Occupational Exposure to Bloodborne Pathogens, Final Rule" in the *Federal Register*.[42] For historic perspective, it is interesting to note that this OSHA mandate began in 1986 when various labor unions representing HCWs petitioned OSHA to adopt standards to protect them from what they perceived as dangerous work conditions. Although previous CDC recommendations on UP were not enforceable because they were simply recommendations, the newly published rules and regulations of the U.S. Department of Labor and OSHA were enforceable in terms of occupational exposure. OSHA chose to adopt the UP concept rather than the BSI concept. Major details of these OSHA requirements implemented on July 6, 1992, are addressed in the following text.[133] In late 1999, OSHA published another mandate on enforcement procedures that established policies and provided clarification to ensure that uniform inspection procedures are followed when an OSHA inspection occurs to review records related to bloodborne pathogens.[147]

At a minimum, UP must be followed precisely by all HCWs who are at risk of occupational exposure. Enforcement protects HCWs and those for whom they care. In addition, the medical facility can be faced with substantial fines and penalties for failure to comply with OSHA rules and regulations. OSHA requires that employers provide new HCWs with occupational exposure training at no cost and during working hours before the initial assignment to tasks in which occupational exposure can take place. Employers must also make the hepatitis B vaccine available at no cost to the HCW within 10 working days of the initial assignment. If an HCW declines the hepatitis B vaccine, he or she is required to sign a waiver. If an HCW changes his or her mind later, the employer must make the vaccine available at that time. Annual in-service training of an HCW is required within 1 year of previous training.[133]

The components of UP and their required application under a medical facility's exposure control plan include engineering controls, work practice controls, personal protective equipment, and housekeeping. Major highlights of OSHA's rules and regulations regarding bloodborne pathogens are shown in Box 10-6. The biohazard symbol is explained in Figure 10-4.

ISOLATION CHAOS LEADS TO A NEW ISOLATION GUIDELINE

The proponents of UP and BSI continued to debate their individual merits into the early 1990s. Some hospitals had incorporated parts or all of UP, some used parts or all of BSI, and others used various combinations. There was a lot of confusion about what precautions were needed for specific body fluids. Some hospitals stated that they practiced UP but in reality were using BSI or vice versa. Hand washing, precautions for airborne and droplet transmission, and implementation of TB transmission procedures were some of the important things lost through either omission or misinterpretation. In reviewing all the problems, it became readily apparent that a change was needed and that a quick fix to any of the existing approaches—UP, BSI, the CDC isolation guideline, or any other isolation system—would not be the answer.

HICPAC, established by the DHHS, issued a *Special Report: Guideline for Isolation Precautions in Hospitals* in January 1996.[101] This guideline consisted of two tiers of precautions. In the first and most important tier were precautions designed for the care of all hospital patients regardless of their diagnosis or presumed infection status; these were known as *standard precautions*.[101] The second tier, known as *transmission-based precautions*, consisted of precautions designed only for the care of specific patients.[101]

Standard Precautions

Standard precautions combined the major features of UP and BSI. As expected, standard precautions apply to (1) blood; (2) all body fluids, secretions, and excretions except sweat; (3) nonintact skin; and (4) mucous membranes. Standard precautions are designed to be the primary strategy to control nosocomial infection by reducing transmission risk from both known and unknown sources of infection. The major components of standard precautions are shown in Box 10-7.

Always practice standard precautions. Imagine that all patients have undiagnosed infections.

Transmission-Based Precautions

Transmission-based precautions are aimed at patients with a confirmed diagnosis or a suspected diagnosis of an epidemiologically important pathogen that warrants additional precautions beyond standard precautions. Box 10-8 lists some of the diseases that require transmission-based precautions. Airborne, droplet, and contact precautions are the three designated types of transmission-based precautions. Each of the three can be used alone or in combination for a disease that has more than one transmission route.

The revised guideline also lists specific clinical syndromes or conditions in both adult and pediatric patients that are associated with a high probability of harboring specific important pathogens. Examples of clinical syndromes and the appropriate transmission precaution approach needed are shown in Table 10-3. This empiric approach to admission and diagnosis is important because often a patient's definitive diagnosis cannot be made until a multitude of tests and procedures have been completed and may take several hours to several days. In the meanwhile, precautions can be taken to prevent the transmission of the disease if the suspected diagnosis ends up being the definitive diagnosis.

ISOLATION FUNDAMENTALS

Behind any effective isolation program are the basic practices and procedures used around the clock by all HCWs. If the following fundamental infection control measures are routinely observed, the risk of transmitting disease can be greatly diminished.

Hand Hygiene

One of the first official guidelines on hand hygiene for HCWs was a 1961 training film released by the U.S. Public Health Service.[66] During the 1980s, a renewed interest arose and the first national written guidelines were released.[22,80,171] Since then, many scientific studies, national guidelines, and even recent worldwide guidelines from the World Health Organization (WHO) have been published.[19,78,100,120-121,152] Over this almost 50-year history, the constant has been that hand hygiene remains the single most important way to prevent the spread of nosocomial infections in the health care setting. Hand hygiene consists of actions taken to reduce the transient flora that colonize the superficial layers of normal skin. The transient flora is acquired by HCWs during direct contact with patients or contact with contaminated environmental surfaces, which in turn are transferred to other patients or even the same patient through cross contamination if hand hygiene is inadequate or omitted.

1. Gloves that meet the FDA standard for medical gloves should be worn in any patient contact situation in which blood or other specified body fluid contact is possible. Other body fluids defined by OSHA are semen, cerebrospinal fluid, pericardial fluid, peritoneal fluid, pleural fluid, synovial fluid, amniotic fluid, saliva in dental procedures, vaginal secretions, any body fluid visibly contaminated with blood, and all body fluids in situations in which it is difficult or impossible to differentiate between body fluids. Other potentially hazardous materials include any unfixed tissue or organ from a human, cell or tissue cultures, and tissues from experimental animals infected with HIV or HBV. When touching any mucous membrane or broken skin surface, the person should wear gloves. The person should also wear gloves when handling any equipment or surface contaminated with blood or body fluid previously listed when performing any vascular or invasive procedure. Gloves should be changed after each patient and/or procedure.

2. Some people are allergic to regular gloves. If this is the case, the employer must provide hypoallergenic gloves, glove liners, powderless gloves, or other suitable alternatives.

3. Employers are required to provide readily accessible hand washing facilities. If this is not feasible, the employer is required to provide an appropriate antiseptic hand cleanser. If such a hand cleanser is used, employees should wash their hands with soap and running water as soon as possible.

4. Hands and any other skin surface should be washed thoroughly and immediately if accidentally contaminated with blood or any of the listed body fluids.

5. Extreme care should be taken when handling needles or any sharp instrument capable of causing injury. Contaminated needles or sharps should not be recapped, bent by hand, or removed from a syringe. Needles, sharps, and associated disposables should be placed in closable, leak-proof, puncture-resistant, specially labeled, or color-coded containers. If reusable needles must be used, recapping or needle removal must be done with a mechanical device that protects the hand or by using a one-handed technique. In general, it is always best to avoid using reusable sharps if possible. Reusable needles and sharps should likewise be placed in closable, leak-proof, puncture-resistant containers for transport to the sterilization department.

6. Masks and protective total eye shields or whole face shields must be worn to protect the mucous membranes of the eyes, nose, and mouth in any procedure in which spraying, spattering, or splashing with blood or other potentially infective materials could occur.

7. Personal protective equipment also includes gowns or, preferably, waterproof aprons that should be worn in any procedure in which spraying or splashing with blood or specified body fluid could occur. General work clothes are not considered protective. Surgical caps or hoods and shoe covers or boots must be worn in situations in which gross contamination can be reasonably foreseen.

8. Mouthpieces, resuscitation bags, or other ventilation devices should be available and used in any area in which the need for resuscitation is predictable. HCWs should not perform mouth-to-mouth resuscitation; instead, they should take a moment to get the appropriate equipment. (Note: There is no documentation of transmission following mouth-to-mouth resuscitation.)

9. Eating, drinking, smoking, applying cosmetics or lip balm, and handling contact lenses are prohibited in work areas having potential exposure hazards.

10. Contaminated laundry should be handled as little as possible with no shaking or other forms of agitation and bagged at the location at which it was used. The bag must be labeled or color coded sufficiently to permit identification of the bag's contents. The bag should be leak proof if the laundry is wet. Contaminated trash such as used bandages is to be handled with the same general precautions as laundry. The exceptions to labeling and color coding requirements are when the medical facility takes the BSI approach or considers all laundry and trash to be contaminated.

11. Potential infectious hazards must be communicated to employees through warning signs and labels. OSHA requires that the biohazard label be affixed to containers of regulated waste under specific conditions. The biohazard sign is displayed in Figure 10-4. The biohazard labels are fluorescent orange or orange red, with the lettering or symbols in contrasting color. Red bags or red containers are acceptable as substitutes for labels. If the medical facility practices BSI and it is understood that all specimens, used linen, and reusable equipment are treated as if potentially infectious, additional biohazard labeling or colored bags are not necessary.

12. OSHA mandates also address procedures that must be followed if an HCW is exposed.

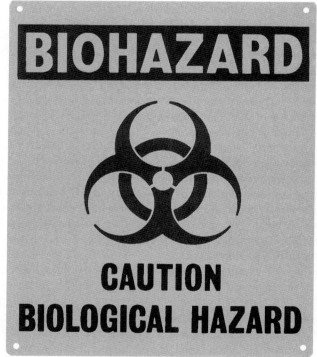

Figure 10-4. The biohazard symbol is used to remind HCWs to be cautious in areas in which the possibility of contamination exists. These reminders can be found anywhere infection control warrants them. The biohazard symbol is orange or orange red, except in special cases in which white, black, and red combinations are used.

Modified from the Department of Labor, Occupational Safety and Health Administration: Occupational exposure to bloodborne pathogens, final rule, 29 CFR Part 1910.1030, *Fed Reg* 56(235):64004, Washington, DC, 1991, The Department of Labor, Occupational Safety and Health Administration.
BSI, Body substance isolation; *FDA,* Food and Drug Administration; *HBV,* hepatitis B virus; *HIV,* human immunodeficiency virus; *OSHA,* Occupational Safety and Health Administration.

Box 10-7	Synopsis of Standard Precautions*

HAND WASHING

- Wash hands after touching blood, body fluids, secretions, or excretions (except sweat) whether gloves are worn or not.
- Wash hands immediately after gloves are removed, between patients, and when otherwise indicated to prevent the spread of microorganisms.
- Wash hands between tasks on the same patient to prevent cross contamination of different body sites.
- Use a plain (nonantimicrobial) soap for routine hand washing.
- Use an antimicrobial agent or a waterless antiseptic agent for special circumstances (such as when directed by the infection control department at your hospital to control outbreaks or hyperendemic infections).

GLOVES

- Clean, nonsterile gloves are adequate for most procedures.
- Wear gloves when touching blood, body fluids, secretions, excretions, and any contaminated items.
- Put on clean gloves just before touching mucous membranes or nonintact skin.
- Change gloves between tasks and procedures on the same patient after contact with material that may contain a high concentration of microorganisms.
- Remove gloves promptly and before touching noncontaminated items, equipment, and environmental surfaces and then immediately wash hands.

MASK, EYE PROTECTION, AND FACE SHIELD

- Wear these devices to protect mucous membranes of your eyes, nose, and mouth during procedures likely to generate splashes or sprays of blood, body fluids, secretions, or excretions.

GOWN

- A clean, nonsterile gown is adequate for most purposes.
- Wear a gown to protect your skin and to prevent soiling your clothing where splashes or sprays are likely.
- Select a gown that is appropriate for the amount of fluid likely to be encountered (cloth vs. plastic).
- Remove a soiled gown promptly.

PATIENT CARE EQUIPMENT

- Handle used equipment in a careful manner to prevent transfer of pathogens.
- Properly discard single-use items.
- Ensure that reusable equipment is not used again until it has been reprocessed.

ENVIRONMENTAL CONTROL

- This pertains to routine care, cleaning, and disinfection of environmental surfaces such as treatment couches, treatment equipment, and other frequently touched surfaces.

LINEN

- Handle, transport, and process used linen soiled with blood, body fluids, secretions, or excretions in a careful manner so as not to spread pathogens.

OCCUPATIONAL HEALTH AND BLOODBORNE PATHOGENS

- Take care to prevent injuries when using needles, scalpels, and other sharp or heavy instruments or devices.
- Never recap a used needle; do not manipulate a used needle using both hands or use any technique that involves directing the point of a needle toward any part of your body.
- Do use either a one-handed technique or a mechanical device designed for holding the needle sheath.
- Do not remove used needles from disposable syringes by hand and do not bend, break, or otherwise manipulate used needles by hand.
- Do place used needles, syringes, and other sharps into puncture-resistant containers, which should be located as close as possible to the area in which such items are used.
- Use mouthpieces, resuscitation bags, or other ventilation devices as an alternative to mouth-to-mouth resuscitation methods.

PATIENT PLACEMENT

- Place a patient who contaminates the environment or who does not (or cannot be expected to) assist in maintaining appropriate hygiene or environmental control in a private room or controlled environment.

*See Hospital Infection Control Practices Advisory Committee (HICPAC) guidelines for a complete listing of infections requiring precautions.

Most HCWs worldwide know that hand hygiene is mandatory in surgical settings, when blood is obviously present, or in other like "dirty" activities. However, transient pathogenic flora can be picked up by an HCW through lifting a patient, taking a pulse or blood pressure, touching a patient's hand or any skin surface, and touching a patient's gown or bed linen.[25,183] These so-called "clean" activities also contribute to the overall nosocomial rate and warrant hand hygiene measures after each episode.

Modern studies have focused on what product is best. Soap and water were the old standards and still play an active role, but now we also have medicated (antimicrobial) soap, alcohols, chlorhexidine, chloroxylenol, hexachlorophene, iodine and iodophors, quaternary ammonium compounds, triclosan, and other agents.[111] Other focal points include how the product is applied, what volume is needed, and how long the scrubbing

action should be performed. Skin irritation from hand hygiene products, especially soap and other detergents, can be addressed with the addition of emollients and humectants.[118,161] Whatever the final choice, antiseptic hygiene products used by HCWs are regulated by the FDA.[136]

Boxes 10-9, 10-10, and 10-11 outline recommendations currently endorsed by the CDC, HICPAC, Society for Healthcare Epidemiology of America (SHEA), Association for Professionals in Infection Control and Epidemiology (APIC), and Infectious Diseases Society of America (IDSA). These tables also meet recommendations in the 2005-2006 WHO draft on hand hygiene that was prepared by more than 100 international experts. In Boxes 10-9 and 10-10, emphasis is placed on work habits that are most likely to be encountered by a radiation therapist.[22] Surgical hand hygiene procedures have also changed substantially. The old days of 10-minute scrubs with a

Box 10-8	Diseases Requiring Transmission-Based Precautions

AIRBORNE PRECAUTIONS
- Measles
- Varicella (including disseminated zoster)*
- Tuberculosis

DROPLET PRECAUTIONS
- Diphtheria
- Pertussis
- Pneumonic plague
- Mumps
- Rubella
- Influenza
- Severe acute respiratory syndrome (SARS)
- Avian flu

CONTACT PRECAUTIONS
- Multidrug-resistant bacteria in gastrointestinal, respiratory, skin, or wound infections (of special interest to infection control experts at hospital, state, or national level)
- Enteric infections with a low infectious dose or prolonged environmental survival including *Escherichia coli* O157:H7, *Shigella,* and hepatitis A
- Skin infections that are highly contagious or that may occur on dry skin including herpes simplex virus, impetigo, scabies, zoster (disseminated or in the immunocompromised host)
- Viral hemorrhagic infections such as Ebola, Lassa, and Marburg

*Certain infections require more than one type of precaution. See Centers for Disease Control and Prevention (CDC) tuberculosis guidelines for details.
Adapted from CDC: Immunization of health-care workers, *MMWR* 46(RR-18): 1-42, 1997.

brush have been abandoned because the time and friction frequently lead to unacceptable skin damage and increased bacterial shedding.[98] Box 10-11 shows the highlights of current surgical hand antisepsis. As more studies and agents are analyzed, changes to these guidelines can be expected and are warranted.

Hand hygiene is the single most effective weapon for reducing nosocomial infection. Use hand agents and wash frequently.

In 1973, fingernails were shown to be the primary reservoir of microflora on the hands, even after intense washing.[86] The underside of the nail, the subungual region, has been shown to harbor the highest number of microorganisms.[84] Findings from more recent studies involving the use of fingernail polish and artificial nails have lead to hospital policies forbidding both. In 2000, Hedderwick et al.[93] conducted two separate studies. In study 1, HCWs wore artificial nails on one hand and native nails on the other for 15 days; nails on both hands were polished. Results showed that over the 15-day period, pathogens were increasingly likely to be isolated from artificial nails and in greater quantities. Study 2 was composed of HCWs who routinely wore polished acrylic nails and HCWs who did not. Once again, those with artificial nails were more likely to have a pathogen isolated than those with native nails (87% versus 43%). Today, most health care facilities with well-informed epidemiologic personnel have policies stating that nails must be neat and trimmed to a length typically around ¼ inch and that the wearing of artificial nails of any type is prohibited.

Fingernails should be natural, unpolished, short, and neat.

Also worth noting is that rings worn by HCWs have been studied to determine whether bacterial counts are higher in ring wearers than in those who do not wear rings. Several studies have shown that the area underneath the ring is more heavily populated by bacteria than on ringless fingers.[98,165] However, at this time it has not been firmly established whether the wearing of rings results in greater transmission of pathogens, and thus no recommendation has been made. Until further studies are performed, it would be prudent to wear fewer rings and to take special care to make sure that hand hygiene products reach the skin area under the ring.

Table 10-3	Clinical Syndrome or Condition Warranting Practical Precautions Until a Diagnosis is Confirmed*

Clinical Description	Suspected/Possible pathogen	Transmission Precautions
Skin or wound infection in which there is draining or an abscess that cannot be covered	*Staphylococcus aureus*	Contact
Diarrhea in an adult with a history of recent antibiotic use	*Clostridium difficile*	Contact
Rash or inflamed skin eruption generalized, cause unknown: maculopapular (reddish flat or raised bumps) with a head cold or inflammation of the nasal mucous membranes and fever	Rubeola (measles)	Airborne
Respiratory: cough, fever, upper lobe infiltrate in an HIV-negative or low risk for HIV patient	*Mycobacterium tuberculosis*	Airborne
Respiratory: sudden, reoccurring attacks or severe persistent cough during periods of pertussis activity	*Bordetella pertussis*	Droplet
Meningitis as characterized by loss of appetite, fever, intense headache, intolerance of light and sound, contracted pupils, delirium, retraction of the head, convulsions, and even coma	*Neisseria meningitidis*	Droplet

*Table examples are very limited. See Hospital Infection Control Practices Advisory Committee (HICPAC) guidelines for complete details.

Box 10-9	Actions and Indications for Hand Hygiene	
ACTION NEEDED	**INDICATION**
• Use alcohol-based hand rub (less skin irritation and more effective).	• Not visibly soiled • Simple routine touching of patient or patient environment • Before having direct contact with patient • Before inserting a urinary catheter or other invasive nonsurgical procedure • After contact with patient's intact skin (e.g., lifting or shaking hand) • When moving from contaminated body site to "clean" body site during same patient care • After contact with inanimate objects (including medical equipment) in the immediate vicinity of patient (e.g., bed rails, wheelchairs, treatment couch) • After removing gloves
Or alternately • Wash hands with water and soap (plain or antimicrobial).	• Visibly dirty or contaminated by blood or other body fluid/excretion, mucous membrane contact, nonintact skin, wound dressing • Before eating • After using restroom
• Antimicrobial-impregnated wipes/towelettes are not as effective as washing or alcohol hand rubs. • Nonalcohol-based hand rubs that smell good and are available in the stores/malls are not FDA approved unless so stated. • Alcohol-based hand rubs are flammable and should be stored only in approved areas.	

Adapted from WHO: *Advanced draft guidelines for hand hygiene in health care,* October 10, 2005, and Centers for Disease Control and Prevention: Guideline for hand hygiene in health-care settings, *MMWR* 51 (RR-16): 1-45, 2002.

With the development of blood-transmitted diseases, *Clostridium difficile*–associated diarrhea, MDR pathogens (e.g., vancomycin-resistant enterococci [VRE] and methicillin-resistant *Staphylococcus aureus* [MRSA]), legal actions by patients, and the cost of health care–associated infections, hand hygiene is in the health care and public spotlight. Patients and the public are very aware that HCWs are not always practicing hand hygiene as they should. Infection rates at specific hospitals and health care facilities are also becoming publicly available[81]; thus, it is very worthwhile at the institutional level to mount and maintain an active hand hygiene educational campaign. Institutions worldwide are revamping their HCW educational and safety strategies to promote adherence to hand hygiene protocols being implemented. Some facilities are actually monitoring employee compliance and counseling them for individual improvement in techniques; others are rewarding employees when goals are achieved, placing reminders and posters in the workplace, changing hygiene agents, and making agents more readily assessable through engineering controls/remodeling.[16,19,20,129] Facilities are also encouraged to provide hand lotions and creams to minimize hand irritation, which in turn discourages the practice of proper hand hygiene.[129] CDC guidelines also advocate that alcohol-based hand rubs be provided to HCWs who work in anticipated areas of high workload or high intensity.[22]

Gloving

There are several important reasons for the wearing of gloves. One is to provide the HCW a protective barrier and to keep his or her hands from becoming grossly contaminated. A second reason is to keep the patient safe from any microorganisms that may be present on the HCW's hands. A third reason is that when gloves are removed immediately after a patient contact and disposed of immediately, they cannot serve as a fomite and infect other patients. A massive increase in glove use has occurred since 1987 when OSHA mandated that gloves be made available and worn if blood or body fluids were present.[61]

The wearing of gloves does not guarantee safety, however, because they can have manufacturing defects too small to be seen and they can be easily torn or punctured by equipment. Hands can be easily and unknowingly contaminated upon glove removal. Because of these reasons, CDC guidelines state that hands should always be washed promptly after removing gloves. Both alcohol-based hand rubs and soap and water are ineffective against spore-forming bacteria. Recent widespread outbreaks of diarrhea caused by *C. difficile* throughout the United States have raised concerns, as does *B. anthracis* (anthrax).[107] *C. difficile* has been noted as the cause of death in some patients, and anthrax remains as a terrorist potential. When caring for patients infected with these pathogens, gloves are necessary.[61]

Gloves are usually made of latex, a natural rubber, or synthetic materials (e.g., vinyl, nitrile, and neoprene). With the increase of glove use, it was quickly realized that a significant and increasing number of HCWs were sensitive or even highly allergic to latex. Gloves must be available as powdered latex, powder-free latex, or synthetic to accommodate latex-sensitive HCWs.[143] The use of petroleum-based hand lotions or creams has been negatively associated with latex barrier protection and thus their use should be avoided.[80,110] Also of note is that the combination of some glove and hand hygiene products create an unpleasant, gritty feeling necessitating adjustment in product choices until a good combination has been achieved. Sharp or ragged nails should be avoided because they easily produce punctures or tears that are not visually detectable.

Gloves should always be removed before handling the hand pendant and couch controls, operating the accelerator console, answering the telephone, pushing the door close button, or touching any other treatment accessory. Two therapists typically make up the treatment team, so one can remove their gloves after a patient assist or lift and act as the "clean" therapist who

Box 10-10	Nonsurgical Hand Hygienic Technique and Characteristics
ALCOHOL-BASED HAND RUBS	**SOAP (DETERGENT) AND WATER WASHING**
• Current gold standard based on cost, effectiveness, and efficiency • Apply to palm, rub together to cover all surfaces of hands and fingers • Rub until completely dry • Use volume specified by manufacturer • Take less time to apply; come in pocket-size containers • Cause less skin irritation and dryness than water and soap	• Wet hands with water that is not hot (hot water is irritating to the skin) • Apply product covering all hand and finger surfaces • Rub hands together vigorously for at least 15 seconds (friction promotes removal of microorganisms) • Rinse well (more water usage removes more microorganisms) • Pat until completely dry with single-use, disposable towel (friction when drying irritates the skin) • Use paper towel to turn faucet off • Soap may be in bar, liquid, powdered, or leaflet form (if bar soap is used, a drainage rack should be in place) • Should be performed for every 10 to 15 alcohol-based hand rub applications • Should be followed with lotion/cream to decrease skin irritation

Modified from Centers for Disease Control and Prevention: *MMWR* 51 (RR-16): 1-45, 2002.

will be responsible for handling equipment. Alternately, both therapists can remove gloves as needed and put on another pair when indicated.

 Wear gloves when patient care dictates but not when handling accelerator controls or other objects. Apply hand hygiene after removing gloves.

Masks, Respiratory Protection, Eye Protection, and Face Shields

The use of masks is intended to prevent or decrease the risk of transmission of infectious agents through the air and applies to large droplet and small droplet nuclei. When a cloth or paper mask is worn to protect against infectious large particle droplets, it gradually becomes damp with exhalation respiratory moisture. Because transmission risk increases with the degree of wetness, damp masks should be replaced with dry ones as needed. A mask covering the mouth and nose is often combined with goggles or a face shield to protect the eyes. OSHA bloodborne pathogens final rule mandates the wearing of masks, eye protection, and face shields during activities likely to generate splashes or sprays.[133] Particulate respirators are needed to protect against pathogens that consist of small droplet nuclei.[85]

Gowns and Protective Apparel

Gowns are to be worn as a protective barrier over an HCW's uniform or street clothes. To protect clothing and underlying skin, one should anticipate the amount of fluid contamination and choose between ordinary cloth gowns and gowns that are impermeable to liquids. Leg coverings, boots, or shoe coverings are also needed when splashes or large quantities of liquids are present or anticipated. OSHA mandates that such apparel be made available to HCWs as needed and appropriate.[133]

Patient Placement

A vital component of any infection control plan is designating whether it is crucial for a patient to have a private room or not. When direct contact or indirect contact transmission pathogens are involved, a private room is needed when the source patient has poor hygiene practices, contaminates the environment, or cannot be expected to participate in infection control measures. If a private room is not available, then patients infected with the same pathogen can be housed together. A private room with special air handling and ventilation is important in airborne transmission diseases.

Transport of Infected Patients

Patients with epidemiologically significant microorganisms should leave their rooms only for essential procedures to

Box 10-11	Surgical Hand Antisepsis

• Remove rings, watches, and bracelets before starting scrub.
• Use nail cleaner under running water to clean under fingernails.
• Use either an antimicrobial soap or an alcohol-based hand rub with "persistent activity" (e.g., continues to work for a prolonged time period).
• Scrub all surfaces of hands, fingers, and forearms for time recommended by manufacturer (typically 2 to 6 minutes). Longer times (e.g., 10 minutes) are not necessary.
• If alcohol surgical hand rub is preferred, hands and forearms should be prewashed with a nonantimicrobial soap and dried completely before application of the alcohol agent.
• Hands, fingers, and forearms should be thoroughly dry before putting on sterile gloves.
• A brush to scrub with is not deemed necessary. Brushes and sponges may be used but are no longer required because they contribute to skin irritation.

Data from Centers for Disease Control and Prevention: *MMWR* 51 (RR-16): 1-45, 2002.

decrease the risk of transmission. For essential procedures, the patient should wear a mask, dressings, or whatever barrier is deemed necessary for the particular pathogen that he or she carries. The personnel in the hospital area performing the essential procedure should be notified in advance so that they can be prepared to receive the patient and the patient should receive instruction on how he or she can help prevent the spread of the pathogen to others.

Patient Care Equipment and Articles

Equipment and articles used for patient care require proper handling once contaminated. Many items are disposable, whereas others may be reused after reprocessing. The method of disposal or reprocessing is determined by the severity of the associated disease, the environmental stability of the pertinent pathogen, and the physical characteristics of the item. If a disposable item is sharp and could cause injury, it must be placed in a puncture-resistant container immediately after use to meet OSHA standards.[133] Other items may simply be bagged. Only one bag is needed if the bag is sturdy and the bag remains uncontaminated on the outside; if not, then two bags are used. Items that can be reprocessed are divided into three categories—critical, semicritical, and noncritical—and are covered in a later section of this chapter.

Laundry

Contaminated laundry presents a very low risk of disease transmission provided it is handled, transported, and laundered in a manner that prevents transfer of pathogens. OSHA also addresses how laundry is to be handled.[133] These federal standards state that used laundry is to be handled as little as possible with a minimum of agitation and bagged or placed in a container at the location where it is used. For a radiation therapy department, this translates to a container in every treatment room and every examination room. If laundry is contaminated and wet, gloves should be worn and the laundry must be placed in a bag, which prevents soak through or leakage. Contaminated laundry also has to be placed in labeled or color-coded bags unless the medical facility treats all laundry as if it was contaminated and all employees are aware of the practice.

Routine Cleaning of Environment

Equipment used on patients who have been placed on one or more of the transmission-based precautions should be cleaned in the same manner as patients on standard precautions unless the pathogen or the amount of environmental contamination is such that special procedures are necessary. In addition to routine cleaning, disinfectants may be required for specific pathogens that are capable of surviving in the inanimate environment for prolonged periods of time. Treatment tables and supporting rackets, prone pillows, breast boards, head and neck supports, and any other positioning device used on more than one specific patient should be cleaned after each patient contact.

Guidelines published by APIC list ethyl or isopropyl alcohol (70% to 90%), sodium hypochlorite (5.2% household bleach), diluted phenolic germicidal detergent solution, and diluted ionosphere germicidal detergent solution as appropriate products for low-level, noncritical items such as tabletops or blood pressure cuffs that come into contact with a patient's intact skin.[163] Method of cleaning and choice of cleaning products and disinfecting products should be determined based on recommendations of the infection care experts at the health care facility.

 Clean after treating each and every patient. Wipe down anything the patient makes contact with.

Blood or Body Fluid Spills

Blood or body fluid spills should be cleaned up immediately. OSHA does not specify a specific procedure or a single specific disinfectant. Either a disinfectant approved by the Environmental Protection Agency (EPA) for hospital use or a 1:10 fresh solution of household bleach (sodium hypochlorite) should be used, with 1 part bleach and 10 parts water.[133] Household bleach has a broad spectrum of antimicrobial activity and is inexpensive and fast acting; however, it is corrosive and is relatively unstable and therefore must be fresh to be effective. It is also inactivated by organic matter, which means that it becomes useless as it kills microorganisms; thus it does not provide a prolonged effect and must be available in an appropriate quantity for the size of the spill. Disinfectants labeled simply as germicides should not be used unless the germicide also happens to be a tuberculocide (meaning it is capable of killing the TB pathogen) to be in compliance with the OSHA compliance document.[144]

Student Education

Students should receive blood and body fluid instruction at the earliest stage of their professional education. Orientation to OSHA rules and regulations and medical facilities' overall infection control programs and hazardous materials programs should take place before active participation in the clinical component of education. In some educational programs, students rotate through multiple health care facilities. These programs must ensure that a student is thoroughly familiar with each facility's specific programs before any active participation occurs.

HANDLING EXPOSURE INCIDENTS RELATED TO HIV

The introduction in 1981 of the acronym AIDS and later the acronym HIV struck fear and anxiety in the community and in the health care setting. Since 1983, when the first case of occupational HIV infection was documented, HCWs have been flooded with information and literature about the risk that accompanies caring for HIV-positive patients.[4] Because these patients do not always have obvious characteristics of the disease, the only logical approach that an HCW can use for self-protection is to assume that all patients are HIV positive.

Since 1981, AIDS surveillance has been the cornerstone of national, state, and local efforts to monitor the scope and effect of the HIV epidemic. During 1998 and 1999, declines in AIDS rates began to level. This trend followed a period of sharp declines in reported cases after 1996, when highly effective antiretroviral therapies were introduced. At the end of 2005, an estimated 437,982 persons were living with AIDS. After a substantial decrease in the number of deaths among persons with

AIDS during the late 1990s, the rate of decrease declined through 2004. The number of deaths among persons with AIDS decreased 66% during 1995 to 2000. During 2001 to 2003, the number of reported deaths decreased an average of 5% annually; however, in 2004, the number of deaths increased 3% compared with the number reported in 2001. In 2005, reported deaths resumed a downward trend and decreased 17% compared with 2004 as illustrated in Figure 10-5.[59]

Preventing exposures to blood and body fluids is the primary means of preventing occupationally acquired HIV infection. Appropriate postexposure management is also an important element of workplace safety.[56] Because HCWs are human, accidents happen. When an exposure incident occurs, the first and most urgent question is, "What actions can be taken to decrease the risk of transmission?" In 1996, the first U.S. Public Health Service recommendations for the use of postexposure prophylaxis (PEP) after occupational exposure to HIV were published; these recommendations have been updated twice.[47,50,53] Since publication of the most recent guidelines in 2001, new antiretroviral agents have been approved by the FDA, and additional information has become available regarding the use and safety of HIV PEP. In August 2003, updated guidelines were recommended

for the management of occupational exposure to HIV specifically addressing PEP. Before any guidelines and recommendations are addressed, the definition of HCWs, exposure, and the risk of acquiring HIV should be reviewed.[56]

The definitions of *health care worker (HCW)* and *occupational exposures* have not changed from those used in 2001.[53] HCW refers to all paid and unpaid persons working in health care settings who have the potential for exposure to infectious materials (i.e., blood, tissue, specific body fluids, medical supplies, equipment, and environmental surfaces contaminated with these substances). An exposure that might place an HCW at risk for HIV infection is defined as a percutaneous injury (i.e., a needlestick or cut with a sharp object) or contact of mucous membrane or nonintact skin (i.e., exposed skin that is chapped, abraded, or afflicted with dermatitis) with blood, tissue, or other body fluids that are potentially infectious. In addition to blood and visibly bloody body fluids, semen and vaginal secretions also are considered potentially infectious.

The following fluids also are considered potentially infectious: cerebrospinal fluid, synovial fluid, pleural fluid, peritoneal fluid, pericardial fluid, and amniotic fluid. The risk for transmission of HIV infection from these fluids is unknown,

ACQUIRED IMMUNODEFICIENCY SYNDROME (AIDS). Incidence*—United States† and U.S. territories, 2005

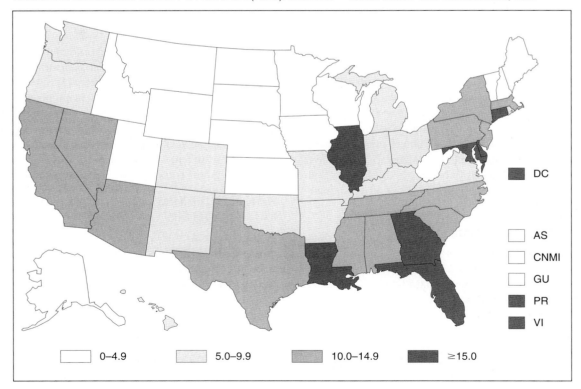

*Per 100,000 population.
†Includes 209 persons with unknown state of residence.

The highest AIDS rates were observed in the northeastern part of the country. High incidence (i.e., ≥15 cases per 100,000 population) also was reported in the southeastern states, the U.S. Virgin Islands, and Puerto Rico.

Figure 10-5. Acquired immunodeficiency syndrome incidence in the United States and U.S. territories, 2005. (Adapted from Centers for Disease Control and Prevention: Summary of notifiable diseases—United States, *MMWR* 54(53):2-92, 2005.[59])

and the potential risk to the HCW from occupational exposures has not been studied in health care settings.[65] Feces, nasal secretions, saliva, sputum, sweat, tears, urine and vomitus are not considered potentially infectious unless they are visibly bloody; the risk for transmission of HIV infection from these fluids and materials is low.[15,56] To date, no additional routes of transmission have been proved in occupational HIV exposure, and casual contact (such as a hand shake) that occurs with infected patients apparently poses no risk to the HCW.[12,13,115]

The risk of acquiring HBV has been statistically calculated to be 10 to 100 times greater than the risk of acquiring HIV. The risk of HBV after a needlestick involving blood from an HBV-positive patient has been estimated to be 5% to 43% compared with less than 0.3% (1 in 250) for HIV.[148] The risks for occupational transmission of HIV have been described; risks vary with the type and severity of exposure.[50,53] In studies of HCWs, the average risk for HIV transmission after a percutaneous exposure to HIV-infected blood has been estimated to be approximately 0.3% and after a mucous membrane exposure, approximately 0.09%.[53]

Percutaneous exposures account for 84% of occupationally acquired HIV cases, followed by mucocutaneous exposure (13%) and combined percutaneous and mucocutaneous exposure (3%).[40] Although episodes of HIV transmission after nonintact skin exposure have been documented, the average risk for transmission by this route is estimated to be less than the risk for mucous membrane exposures. The risk for transmission after exposure to fluids or tissues other than HIV-infected blood is probably considerably lower than for blood exposures.[56]

 Needlesticks account for 84% of job-related acquired HIV. There is no reason for a radiation therapist to ever recap a needle.

After an exposure, the type and severity of the exposure must be recorded because this information may eventually provide better epidemiologic data. For example, documenting the type of needle (e.g., hollow core, surgical), gauge of the needle, depth of penetration, volume of blood or body fluid, and source of fluid (e.g., semen, amniotic fluid) helps provide better analysis. Also important is whether the infective virus strain is known or suspected to be resistant to antiretroviral drugs.

Because the majority of occupational HIV exposures do not result in transmission of HIV, potential toxicity must be considered when prescribing PEP. Some hospitals have defined levels of HIV exposure to be used as guides in counseling the exposed HCW and in initiating prophylactic treatment (see typical exposure levels in Box 10-12).[11] A true occupational exposure requires that documented seroconversion take place. This means that the HCW tested negative for HIV shortly after an exposure and subsequently developed clinical and/or serologic evidence of HIV infection.

This documentation is necessary to sort out HCWs who may have unknowingly been positive for HIV at the time of exposure as a result of nonoccupational factors. In an analysis of 51 HCWs who experienced seroconversion, the average time was 65 days from exposure and 95% had seroconverted within 6 months.[23] In another report, HCWs tested negative at

Box 10-12	Situations for Which Expert Consultation* for HIV Postexposure Prophylaxis (PEP) is Advised

- Delayed (i.e., later than 24-36 hours) exposure report
  - Interval after which lack of benefit from PEP undefined
- Unknown source (i.e., needle in sharps disposal container or laundry)
  - Use of PEP to be decided on a case-by-case basis
  - Consider severity of exposure and epidemiologic likelihood of HIV exposure
  - Do not test needles or other sharp instruments for HIV
- Known or suspected pregnancy in the exposed person
  - Use of optimal PEP regimens not precluded
  - PEP not denied solely on basis of breastfeeding
- Resistance of the source virus to antiretroviral agents
  - Influence of drug resistance on transmission risk unknown
  - If source person's virus is known or suspected to be resistant to one or more of the drugs considered for PEP, selection of drugs to which the source person's virus is unlikely to be resistant recommended
  - Resistance testing of the source person's virus at the time of exposure not recommended
  - Initiation of PEP not to be delayed while awaiting any results of resistance testing
- Toxicity of the initial PEP regimen
  - Adverse symptoms (i.e., nausea and diarrhea) common with PEP
  - Symptoms often manageable without changing PEP regimen by prescribing antimotility or antiemetic agents
  - In other situations, modifying the dose interval (i.e., taking drugs after meals or administering a lower dose more frequently throughout the day, as recommended by the manufacturer) might help alleviate symptoms when they occur

*Either with local experts or by consulting the National Clinicians' Post-Exposure Prophylaxis Hotline (PEPline), telephone 888-448-4911.
Adapted from Centers for Disease Control and Prevention: Summary of notifiable diseases—United States, *MMWR* 54(53):2-92, 2005.[59]

6 months but went on to being seropositive by 12 months postexposure.[64]

Although no data are available demonstrating that first aid is effective in preventing the transmission of HIV, the use of first aid procedures is the only logical immediate management strategy. HCWs should be instructed to initiate decontamination procedures immediately if possible. Skin and injured wound sites that have been contaminated with blood or a body fluid should be washed with soap and water. Oral and nasal mucosal surfaces should be rinsed thoroughly with water. Eyes should be thoroughly rinsed with water, saline, or other suitable sterile solutions.

The application of an antiseptic is logical even though there is no evidence to show that antiseptic use decreases the risk of transmission. There also is no evidence that squeezing or making a wound bleed outwardly decreases risk. The use of a caustic substance such as bleach, injection of an antiseptic, or an application of a disinfectant at a wound site is discouraged.[49] A 1990 article reported a case in which an HCW poured undiluted bleach over a cut that involved blood from a patient with AIDS; despite this action the HCW still converted to HIV positive.[96]

When an exposure incident occurs, the employer must immediately make available to the HCW confidential medical evaluation and follow-up. If the incident involves a source individual, who is defined as any person, living or dead, whose blood or other potentially infectious body materials may be a source of exposure, the identification of the source individual will be made except when doing so is unfeasible or prohibited by law. If the source is known to be HIV positive, information from the medical records can be gathered and used to help plan the HCW's PEP for treatment. If the HIV status is unknown, the source's blood can be tested to determine whether the source is positive for HIV, but this can be done in some states only after consent is obtained.[82] Other states have passed legislation that allows HIV testing of the source after occupational exposure even if the source patient refuses to have the test performed.[94] Test results are to be made known to the HCW but the worker also must be advised on laws regarding the confidentiality of the source's identity, if known, and the infectious status.[133]

Rapid HIV testing of source patients can facilitate making timely decisions regarding use of HIV PEP after occupational exposures to sources of unknown HIV status. Early tests for HIV antibody may be negative; however, infection can usually be documented at an early stage by less widely available tests such as measuring p24 antigen, by HIV cultures, or by gene amplification studies.[82]

Immediately report any needlestick or body substance accidental exposure. Seek care quickly, because time is a factor. Know your rights.

The HCW should be evaluated to determine susceptibility to bloodborne pathogen infections. The blood of an exposed HCW should be tested if consent is obtained to establish an HIV baseline. If the source is determined to be negative and has not engaged in behaviors that are associated with a risk for HIV transmission, CDC guidelines state that baseline testing and follow-up is not needed. However, if the HCW is still concerned after counseling, serologic testing should be available. If the source has participated in risky behaviors and is currently testing negative, future testing of the HCW is warranted. The CDC recommends follow-up HIV antibody testing at 6 weeks, 3 months, and 6 months after exposure.[35] Delayed seroconversion, defined as the appearance of the HIV antibody at greater than 6 months, has been documented; thus some institutions test again at 12 months.

The rationale for testing after 6 months is that treatment may delay seroconversion. In addition, later testing often reassures the HCW.[82] Symptoms that are compatible with seroconversion include the following: an unexplained fever, lymphadenopathy, a rash, lymphopenia, and a sore throat. OSHA rules further state that if the worker consents to blood collection but not to an HIV test, the sample must be preserved for at least 90 days in case the HCW changes his or her mind.[133]

If it is determined that PEP is needed, it should be started in a matter of hours, not days. This urgency of treatment is based on animal studies and the reproductive cycle of the virus.

One study involving monkeys infected via a mucosal surface showed that the virus had migrated to regional lymph nodes within 24 to 28 hours and was present in circulating blood within 5 days.[49,169] This combined with the fact that HIV replication is rapid, approximately 2.5 days, and that 5000 viral particles are created in each replication demands that decision to treat must be implemented without delay.[49]

Antiretroviral agents from five classes of drugs are currently available to treat HIV infection.[137,185] These include the nucleoside reverse transcriptase inhibitors (NRTIs), nucleotide reverse transcriptase inhibitors (NtRTIs), nonnucleoside reverse transcriptase inhibitors (NNRTIs), protease inhibitors (PIs), and a single fusion inhibitor. The CDC guidelines include only antiretroviral agents approved by FDA for treatment of HIV infection. The recommendations in the most recent CDC report provide guidance for two or more drug PEP regimens on the basis of the level of risk for HIV transmission represented by the exposure as illustrated in Tables 10-4 and 10-5.[48,53,56,95]

Persons receiving PEP should complete a full 4-week regimen.[53] A substantial proportion of HCWs have been unable to complete a full 4-week course of HIV PEP as a result of toxicity and side effects.* Because all antiretroviral agents have been associated with side effects, the toxicity profile of these agents, including the frequency, severity, duration, and reversibility of side effects, is an important consideration in selection of an HIV PEP regimen. The symptom reported most frequently was nausea (26.5%), followed by malaise and fatigue (22.8%) (CDC, unpublished data, 2005). In addition, all approved antiretroviral agents might have potentially serious drug interactions when used with certain other drugs. This requires careful evaluation of concomitant medications, including over-the-counter medications and supplements (i.e., herbals), used by an exposed person before prescribing PEP and close monitoring for toxicity of anyone receiving these drugs.†

The management of exposed HCWs is extremely sensitive and complex. Workers should be treated on a priority basis in light of the extreme mental anguish associated with an HIV exposure. Psychological reactions include fear, anxiety, anger, depression, denial, sexual and sleep disturbances, suicide, and psychosis. Counseling must be available immediately and continuously for workers exposed to HIV. Some institutions have even set up 24-hour counseling hotlines for their exposed HCWs.[82]

Counseling of the HCW should also address lifestyle changes that should be made until seroconversion occurs or until enough time has passed (typically 6 months) for the worker to be deemed free of HIV infection. Lifestyle changes include no exchange of body fluids during sex; deferment of pregnancy; cessation of breastfeeding; no intimate kissing; no sharing of razors or toothbrushes; and no donation of blood, sperm, or organs. If the HCW is involved in an accident that results in bleeding, surfaces that are contaminated should be promptly disinfected.

In general, employees should be allowed to perform patient care duties except during times when their condition is infectious through non-bloodborne routes. For example, with

---

*References 122, 149, 156, 162, 173, and 179.
† References 4, 5, 56, 68-70, 73, 119, 124, 131, 151, 172 and 178.

Table 10-4	Recommended HIV Postexposure Prophylaxis (PEP) for Percutaneous Injuries				
	Infection Status of Source				
Exposure Type	**HIV-Positive, Class 1***	**HIV-Positive, Class 2***	**Source of Unknown HIV Status†**	**Unknown Source‡**	**HIV-Negative**
Less severe§	Recommended basic 2-drug PEP	Recommended expanded ≥3-drug PEP	Generally, no PEP warranted; however, consider basic 2-drug PEP¶ for source with HIV risk factors††	Generally, no PEP warranted; however, consider basic 2-drug PEP¶ in settings in which exposure to HIV-infected persons is likely	No PEP warranted
More severe**	Recommended expanded 3-drug PEP	Recommended expanded ≥3-drug PEP	Generally, no PEP warranted; however, consider basic 2-drug PEP¶ for source with HIV risk factors††	Generally, no PEP warranted; however, consider basic 2-drug PEP¶ in settings in which exposure to HIV-infected persons is likely	No PEP warranted

*HIV positive, class 1—asymptomatic HIV or known low viral load (i.e., <1500 ribonucleic acid copies/mL). HIV positive, class 2—symptomatic HIV infection, AIDS, acute seroconversion, or known high viral load. If drug resistance is a concern, obtain expert consultation. Initiation of PEP should not be delayed pending expert consultation and because expert consultation alone cannot substitute for face-to-face counseling, resources should be available to provide immediate evaluation and follow-up care for all exposures.
†For example, deceased source person with no samples available for HIV testing.
‡For example, a needle from a sharps disposal container.
§For example, a solid needle or superficial injury.
¶The recommendation "consider PEP" indicates that PEP is optional; a decision to initiate PEP should be based on a discussion between the exposed person and the treating clinician regarding the risks versus benefits of PEP.
††If PEP is offered and administered and the source is later determined to be HIV negative, PEP should be discontinued.
**For example, large-bore needle, deep puncture, visible blood on device, or needle used in patient's artery or vein.
Adapted from Centers for Disease Control and Prevention: Summary of notifiable diseases—United States, *MMWR* 54(53):2-92, 2005.[59]

infectious diarrhea, skin lesions, and pulmonary infections, work restrictions would be reasonable. In the case of a blood-borne infection status, such as HIV or HBV positive, employers are not allowed to discriminate against the employee. Employees are protected by section 504 of the Rehabilitation Act and the Americans with Disabilities Act, which prohibits discrimination against individuals with disabilities, including persons who are positive for HIV or HBV.[71] Employers must make every effort to maintain the employment of an individual as long as the individual is capable of performing the job and does not pose a reasonable threat of infection to others. At the same time, however, employees and students should take personal responsibility for their actions and not perform any procedure that could be dangerous to their coworkers or patients.[56]

RIGHTS OF THE HEALTH CARE WORKER

Today's HCW should never have to wonder what to do if an employer does not provide proper protection equipment, but if this occurs, HCWs have legal rights. OSHA helps provide job safety and health protection for employees by promoting safe and healthful working conditions throughout the nation. HCWs can lawfully refuse to work in truly unsafe conditions and have the right to insist on wearing protective equipment. However, HCWs cannot leave their job if they want their rights protected.[134]

HCWs must first inform their employer of the unsafe conditions. If an employer does not respond, the employee should contact OSHA to file a complaint and request that an inspection be conducted.[135] OSHA will withhold, on request, the name of the employee filing the complaint.[134] Before complaining, an HCW should be sure that the unsafe condition is indeed serious (i.e., the situation could have caused death or serious harm).

The opposite situation can also occur. On occasion, an HCW may have unreasonable fears and be overly cautious. Examples include the HCW who refuses to go anywhere near an AIDS patient or the worker who insists on wearing full-body protective gear when unnecessary. This type of reaction is usually caused by lack of proper education about the risk of transmission and proper protective actions that the HCW should take. The employer should let the HCW explain fears and perceptions and should then educate the HCW with the necessary information in understandable language. The HCW cannot be discharged or discriminated against in any way just because of a misperception or because of a complaint or a call to OSHA. HCWs who believe they have been discriminated against should file a complaint with their nearest OSHA office within 30 days of the alleged discriminatory act.[134] However, if after counseling and if the situation is deemed to be reasonably safe and proper equipment was provided, and the HCW still refuses to

Table 10-5	Recommended HIV Postexposure Prophylaxis (PEP) for Mucous Membrane Exposures and Nonintact Skin* Exposures

	Infection Status of Source				
Exposure Type	**HIV-Positive, Class 1[†]**	**HIV-Positive, Class 2[†]**	**Source of Unknown HIV Status[§]**	**Unknown Source[‖]**	**HIV-Negative**
Small volume**	Consider basic 2-drug PEP[††]	Recommend basic 2-drug PEP	Generally, no PEP warranted[§§]	Generally, no PEP warranted	No PEP warranted
Large volume[¶¶]	Recommend basic 2-drug PEP	Recommend expanded ≥3-drug PEP	Generally, no PEP warranted; however, consider basic 2-drug PEP[††] for source with HIV risk factors[§§]	Generally, no PEP warranted; however, consider basic 2-drug PEP[††] in settings in which exposure to HIV-infected persons is likely	No PEP warranted

*For skin exposures, follow-up is indicated only if evidence exists of compromised skin integrity (i.e., dermatitis, abrasion, or open wound).

[†]HIV positive, class 1—asymptomatic HIV or known low viral load (i.e., <1500 ribonucleic acid copies/mL). HIV positive, class 2—symptomatic HIV infection, AIDS, acute seroconversion, or known high viral load. If drug resistance is a concern, obtain expert consultation. Initiation of PEP should not be delayed pending expert consultation and because expert consultation alone cannot substitute for face-to-face counseling, resources should be available to provide immediate evaluation and follow-up care for all exposures.

[§]For example, deceased source person with no samples available for HIV testing.

[‖]For example, splash from inappropriately disposed blood.

[††]For example, a few drops.

[¶]The recommendation "consider PEP" indicates that PEP is optional; a decision to initiate PEP should be based on a discussion between the exposed person and the treating clinician regarding the risks versus benefits of PEP.

[§§]If PEP is offered and administered and the source is later determined to be HIV negative, PEP should be discontinued.

[¶¶]For example, a major blood splash.

Adapted from Centers for Disease Control and Prevention: Summary of notifiable diseases—United States, *MMWR* 54(53):2-92, 2005.[59]

provide care as in the AIDS patient example, the employer may have the right to dismiss the worker.

HCWs also have legal rights if they develop an occupationally acquired infection. Workers' Compensation laws, determined by each state, are in place to protect the employee. To be compensated in a case in which an HCW is disabled or killed, the injury must have occurred while practicing within his or her scope of practice. Bungee jumping off the 17th floor of the hospital during lunch hour, for example, would not be covered because it is outside the scope of practice of a radiation therapist. In most cases, HCWs do not have the right to file a negligence or criminal suit in addition to a Workers' Compensation claim unless they can prove that their employer intentionally disregarded an infection risk. The HCW must also be able to establish that the infection was actually acquired on the job, not in the community.

Another extremely important right HCWs have is complete confidentiality. To protect privacy, most health care facilities take special steps to avoid placing the HCW's "patient" chart where other employees have access to it. In addition, such a diagnosis would not be placed on computerized charting systems.

ROLE OF THE CENTRAL SERVICES DEPARTMENT

In the past, medical supplies and equipment that needed to be sterilized were often sterilized in an autoclave unit housed in the radiation oncology department. With the concerns of bloodborne pathogens and emerging diseases, health care centers have learned that it is far better to leave the reprocessing of medical supplies and equipment in the hands of experts. This area of expertise typically is housed in a department known as *central services,* or *central supply.* The central service department (CSD) is accountable for preparing, processing, sorting, and distributing medical supplies and equipment required in patient care. This central location not only is economical but also is subject to stringent levels of quality control according to TJC guidelines.[109]

A student or employee tour through a major hospital's CSD can be an extremely enlightening and educational experience. Contaminated equipment is first precleaned and decontaminated by trained, specially clothed workers. This clothing includes items such as waterproof aprons and face shields. Reprocessing may include disassembly and sending equipment through devices that remind a person of a commercial car wash complete with a presoak cycle, wash cycle, and dry cycle. Instruments are then prepared for sterilization by the most appropriate method. Ideally, each package sterilized is labeled with a control number in case any item needs to be recalled. The labeling process may also identify the sterilizing unit used, its load, the time and date an item was sterilized, the item's expiration date, and sometimes even the individual who packaged the item (Figure 10-6).

After a package has been disinfected or sterilized, it should be handled as little as possible and stored in a low-traffic, clean, dry, closed area. If an item comes into contact with something and becomes soiled, is dropped on the floor, is exposed to moisture, or is physically penetrated, it is deemed contaminated and

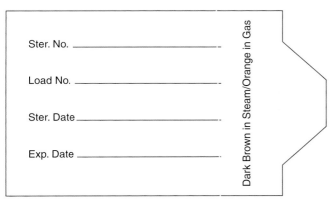

Ster. No. _____

Load No. _____

Ster. Date _____

Exp. Date _____

Dark Brown in Steam/Orange in Gas

Figure 10-6. Sterilization labels are used as part of the quality control program in a central services department. If an item must be recalled, it can be tracked by its control number.

should not be used. Sterile items should be stored away from the floor, ceiling, outside walls, vents, pipes, doors, and windows. The temperature should be 65° F to 72° F degrees with a relative humidity between 35% and 50%. Closed shelves are preferred over drawers because the risk of damaging a sterilized package is greater in opening and closing a drawer than opening the door to a cabinet. If a closed cabinet is not an option, open shelves are a feasible solution. Placing a plastic dust cover over the sterilized packages can decrease the chance of contamination.

Each health care facility determines the amount of time that a sterilized item can be stored. Important factors in determining shelf life include packaging material and an open or closed shelf design, both of which combined are more important than time alone. It is further assumed that after the opening of a sterilized package, sterile technique will be used and the date of expiration will be checked. Package dating assists in the rotation process, and the older items that have not yet expired should be used first. Commercially prepared items should be discarded upon reaching the expiration date provided by the manufacturer.

STERILIZATION AND DISINFECTION TECHNIQUES

Because a radiation therapist must routinely practice infection control techniques, an overview of sterilization and disinfection techniques is desirable and addressed in the following text. Every health care facility should have infection control policies and experts available for consultation. Simple questions regarding whether radiation oncology supplies should be single-use disposables or reprocessed can be answered by these experts. In addition, experts can advise the most economical route and the best method or product for each situation. Expertise is readily available from an institution's CSD and/or epidemiology department. Any policy developed within a radiation oncology department should be reviewed by these experts before the policy's implementation.

In general, medical supplies and equipment can be divided into risk categories based on an item's use. *Critical items* are products or instruments inserted into normally sterile areas of the body or into the bloodstream and must be sterile for use.

Items in this category include needles, surgical instruments, urinary catheters, and implants. *Semicritical items* are those that contact mucosal surfaces but do not ordinarily penetrate body mucosal surfaces. Nonintact skin is also included in this group. These include items such as endoscopes, thermometers, laryngoscopes, and anesthesia equipment. It is preferable to sterilize items in this category, but high-level disinfection may be used. *Noncritical items* do not ordinarily touch the patient or touch only the patient's intact skin; therefore, they do not need to be sterile. This category includes items such as tabletops, stethoscopes, and blood pressure cuffs.[163] The FDA requires that medical devices be sold with instructions stating whether the devices are single-use or reusable items and the way they must be processed if reusable.[17]

 Critical items, semicritical items, and noncritical items are labels used to classify risk of contamination for medical equipment utilization.

Sterilization is a process that destroys all microbial life forms, including resistant spores. Sterilization can be achieved through physical or chemical processes. There are no degrees of sterilization; an item is either sterile or it is not sterile. Processes used for sterilization include steam under pressure, dry heat, low-temperature sterilization (ethylene oxide gas or gas plasma), and specific liquid chemicals.

Disinfection is a process that reduces microbial life forms and can range from *high-level disinfection* to *intermediate-level disinfection* and even *low-level disinfection.*[97] Low-level disinfection is synonymous with sanitization. High-level disinfection eliminates all microbial life forms except situations in which there are high numbers of bacterial spores (such as anthrax terrorist attacks). Intermediate-level disinfection kills the TB bacterium, most viruses, and most fungi but not most bacterial spores. Low-level disinfection inactivates most bacteria, some viruses, and some fungi but is mostly ineffective against TB bacterium and bacterial spores. The major point to remember is that some microbial life forms cannot be eliminated by disinfection processes. In the health care setting, disinfection is typically achieved through the use of liquid chemicals or wet pasteurization (very hot water).

Antiseptics are different from disinfectants. The term *antiseptic* is reserved for antimicrobial substances applied to skin surfaces. Methods of sterilization and disinfection are addressed in the following text and differ with regard to the biocidal agent, biocidal action, contact between the biocidal agent and microorganism, and severity of treatment.[76] Regardless of whether sterilization or disinfection is appropriate for a given situation, neither process is likely to be successful if meticulous cleaning does not precede the process. Simple sorting, disassembly, soaking, scrubbing and brushing, rinsing and draining or drying is used prior to sterilization or disinfection processes. Foreign matter that remains after inadequate cleaning and processing generally renders an item unusable.

Heat

The use of heat, moist or dry, is the most reliable, available, and economical method of destroying microorganisms. Boiling water

(100° C, 212° F) is probably the oldest method used. Although boiling greatly decreases the number of microorganisms, it does not destroy all microorganisms, such as spores; thus boiling fits into the category of disinfectants rather than sterilants. In fact, temperatures lower than boiling (50° C to 70° C, 122° F to 158° F) are sufficient to kill most viruses, bacteria, and fungi.[97] HIV is destroyed by moist heat at 60° C (140° F) in 30 minutes, a temperature well below the requirement for boiling water.[67]

Hot water pasteurization is a process using water at a temperature of 145° F (63° C) for 30 minutes, but again it must be stressed that this is not considered to be a sterilization process.[163,181] Steam under pressure, however, is capable of destroying all life forms, provided that a proper combination of temperature and time is achieved. Older textbooks typically quoted a specific time, temperature, and pressure combination, and the student accepted this combination as an absolute. In reality, steam sterilization works as an inverse relationship and many combinations are equally effective; thus steam sterilization is analogous to the various time-dose relationships used in treating cancer. Simply put, the time required for sterilization decreases as the temperature increases.

With the special exception of an infectious life form known as a *prion* (proteinaceous infectious particle),which causes diseases such as Creutzfeldt-Jakob disease (CJD), no life forms survive if exposed to steam under pressure at 30 pounds per square inch (psi) at 121° C (250° F).[97] An exposure that lasts 15 to 20 minutes at this temperature is adequate for killing most life forms; however, the heat-resistant Creutzfeldt-Jakob agent requires 1 hour of exposure at a temperature of 132° C (270° F).[170]

The term *prion* (pronounced *pree-on*), which was introduced in 1982, is used to describe unique, infectious central nervous system (CNS) agents composed of protein but lacking identifiable nucleic acid.[180] Prions consist of long strands of protein that are normal components of brain and other tissues. They cause disease only when they go bad and start folding themselves into three-dimensional structures different from their normal structure.[180] CJD is a progressive, degenerative neurologic disorder and is believed to have a long incubation period. Once active symptoms begin, death follows in a matter of weeks to months. Symptoms present as rapidly progressing dementia, changing to coma then death, and there is no cure.

CJD has been associated with corneal transplants, dura mater graphs, pituitary growth hormone injections, and other neurosurgical procedures.[76] Extreme caution should be taken with brain tissue and CNS fluids because HCWs have died from an occupational exposure.[130] A better-known prion variant of CJD-related disease is bovine spongiform encephalopathy, commonly referred to as mad cow disease, which can be passed on to humans through contaminated beef products.[8] To summarize, sterilization combinations of pressure, temperature, and time are also influenced by the type of microorganism to be destroyed.

Steam sterilizers are commonly referred to as *steam autoclaves* and can be described as closed metal chambers. **Autoclaves** can be grouped into two general categories: gravity displacement and mechanically evacuated devices. The gravity displacement type requires a longer exposure time. Steam sterilization is the most commonly used method of sterilization used in health care

facilities because of its low cost, its absence of toxic residue, and the fact that it can be used to sterilize an extremely wide assortment of materials. A drying cycle follows exposure to the steam and is often the slowest portion of the autoclave cycle. Another device known as a *flash sterilizer*, or *flash autoclave*, can be used in an emergency situation. This device is operated at a higher temperature, and exposure time is only a few minutes. Flash autoclaving should not routinely be substituted for standard autoclaving procedures.

Cotton fabric and special steam-permeable plastics or paper can be used as packaging materials. Other criteria essential to the selection of appropriate packaging materials for any sterilization method include the resistance to puncture and tears, penetration by microorganisms, and absence of toxic or biologically harmful particles. Care must be exercised in packing items for steam sterilization to ensure that the steam can reach all surfaces and cavities of a specific item. For example, lids must be taken off containers and many items may require disassembly. Items in a package must be arranged loosely because overpacking may lead to nonsterilization.

Steam sterilization also has its limitations. Instruments with sharp points, such as needles, or cutting edges, such as scalpels, may be dulled. Oxidation and corrosion may also occur with certain metals. Powder and oil products should not be autoclaved because the steam has difficulty in penetrating such substances. Many products such as rubber and synthetic polymers are heat sensitive and could melt or deteriorate. Other products such as injectable solutions may lose their biologic usefulness when subjected to high heat levels.

Because of packing precautions, packaging material differences, product sensitivity to heat, and TJC quality control standards, comprehensive knowledge is required of anyone in charge of steam sterilization or any method of sterilization. For these reasons, sterilization is best done by experts, the employees of the CSD. Unfortunately, some centers operate units without expert advice and without biologic indicators (discussed at the end of this chapter) as a quality control measure.

Dry heat is also used for sterilization. Although its use has sharply declined since the introduction of single-use syringes and needles sterilized by other methods, dry heat is still useful for reusable needles, glass syringes, sharp cutting instruments and drills, powders and oily products, and metals that oxidize or corrode with exposure to moisture. The advantage of dry heat is its ability to penetrate solids, nonaqueous powders or oils, and closed containers. Its primary disadvantage when compared with steam is that higher temperatures and longer exposure times are required to achieve sterilization. A commonly quoted temperature is 160° C (320° F) with a time of 1 to 3 hours.[97]

As with steam sterilization, appropriate time and temperature combinations follow an inverse relationship. Similar to cooking in a home oven, aluminum foil or aluminum containers are commonly used for packaging. As with steam sterilization, items that are heat sensitive should be sterilized by other available techniques.

Incineration, another form of heat, is frequently applied to biohazardous waste materials generated in health care settings. Some incinerators are located on hospital grounds, but most are now located away from hospitals, residential areas, and high occupancy buildings. Because incinerators are typically located some distance away, designated vehicles are required to transport biohazardous waste to the incinerator site.

Gas

Gas sterilizers are available for medical products that cannot withstand high temperatures, such as endoscopes and plastic items. In recent times, the use of gas has become increasingly important in the health care setting and the commercial setting because of the use of a greater number of instruments and products that cannot tolerate high heat exposure. Gas is a more complex and expensive method than dry or wet heat. Ethylene oxide (usually written as ETOX or ETO) is the gas used in most gas sterilizers, and it sterilizes by alkylation, replacing a hydrogen atom that prevents the microorganism from metabolizing and/or reproducing.

In the past, ETOX was mixed with freon, but carbon dioxide (CO_2) is now used because of freon's harmful effect on the ozone layer. The operation of a gas sterilizer should be attempted only by qualified experts because the gases present fire and explosion hazards. In addition, the gas has a toxic effect on humans, is mutagenic, and is a suspected carcinogen, thus making it subject to strict OSHA regulations. Gas sterilizers are equipped with special detectors to alert personnel in the event of a gas leak.

Packages sterilized by gas are typically exposed for 4 to 12 hours at temperatures of 25° C to 60° C.[76,97] Other time and temperature combinations can be used because the process follows an inverse relationship. Packages are then aerated in special closed cabinets for 12 to 24 hours by heated, high air flows to dissipate any residual ETOX because of its tissue toxicity.[65] If special cabinet aeration is not available, the aeration process may take up to 7 days.[97] Gas should not be used to sterilize products that cannot withstand low heat.

To recap, gas is slower, more expensive, and has the possibility of toxic residue. Very few hospitals have an ethylene oxide sterilizer. Large medical institutions frequently cooperate and provide gas sterilization access to medium and small medical institutions to assist with cost. Gas sterilization is not applied to liquids or products packaged in gas impervious wrappers. Products can be wrapped in the same packaging materials used for steam sterilization.

Hydrogen peroxide gas plasma, a newer gas alternative, consists of gas in a highly charged vacuum state. Free radicals created interact with the microorganisms to destroy them. The entire process takes approximately 75 minutes, and there are no toxic emissions so no aeration is necessary. Very few units exist and there are associated technical problems.[1] They cannot be used with cellulose-based products such as paper and linen and may not be able to penetrate small lumens.

Radiation

Although not routinely used in the health care setting, ionizing radiation is widely applied at commercial industrial sites to medical products and equipment that cannot withstand heat. Gamma beams from cobalt-60 sources or linear accelerator photon and electron beams are used. Electrons are more limited in use because of their poorer penetration, and photon beams more than 10 MV are not used because they can induce significant radioactivity in the sterilized product through artificial nuclide production.[76]

Extremely high absorbed doses (kGy) are necessary because microorganisms are far more resistant to the effects of radiation than humans.[114]

The time required for sterilization depends on the unit's dose rate and the required absorbed dose. Packaging materials and the product contained within are sterilized. Caution must be employed in using radiation as a sterilant for medications because it may induce chemical changes by breaking chemical bonds and thus inactivate or modify some medications. An interesting student project is to check commercially prepared packages for a wide variety of single-use sterile (disposable) products to see how many were irradiated.

Radiation sterilization is used in the autosterilization of a strontium (^{90}Sr) applicator. After a strontium treatment for pterygium of the eye, the radioactive end of the applicator is wiped against a sterile alcohol pad to remove any biologic debris and then rinsed with sterile water. The surface radiation output emitted by a typical 50 mCi ^{90}Sr source is approximately 50 cGy per second, a rate high enough that it sterilizes itself with a dose of more than 4 million cGy in a 24-hour period.[105]

Nonionizing radiations such as ultraviolet (UV) and infrared light or microwave are also capable of killing microorganisms, but the wavelengths are too low to allow any significant penetration. UV sources are costly and require ongoing service and maintenance; thus they are not used for sterilization purposes except in a few extremely limited applications. Most viruses and bacteria are easily killed by UV when humidity is kept low. UV sources have been used in TB isolation areas, surgical suites, and burn units to keep microorganism concentrations down in the ambient air and general surface environment.

Chemical Liquids

Using chemicals for sterilization or disinfection is a relatively easy process. An item need only to be placed in a basin deep enough to completely submerge the item, with care taken to ensure that the chemical can reach all inner and outer surfaces and crevices. Caution should be exercised to ensure that the chemical does not damage the item to be processed or the basin containing the chemical itself. The most difficult part is selecting the best, most appropriate chemical. Therefore, a radiation therapist should contact a qualified CSD expert for input in choosing products and protocols for use.

Chemicals have an extremely wide range of antimicrobial action and are time sensitive. Very few can truly sterilize; the vast majority cannot, and those that can are known as *chemical sterilants*. The FDA has had the responsibility of overseeing the safety and effectiveness of any agent to be labeled and marketed as a liquid chemical sterilant or as a high-level disinfectant for critical and semicritical medical devices since 1993.[163] The EPA has assumed the main responsibility of overseeing and reviewing agents to be marketed as disinfectants for noncritical items. The FDA also regulates any agent registered and labeled as an antiseptic.[74]

The CDC cannot endorse specific products, but it can provide guidance in choosing products.[77] Other professional groups such as APIC also publish extremely useful guidelines.[159,163] Manufacturers are also responsible for furnishing recommendations on the reprocessing of items that they produce. Thus the chemical to be used on a specific item is based on expert guidelines, scientific literature, and manufacturer product information. Reliance on labels alone is insufficient and at times even misleading. Therefore caution should be used with wording such as "hospital strength disinfectant." "Hospital disinfectant" is preferred because this term indicates a higher level of disinfection.

Many chemical products may have other terminology on their labels that provides useful information about effectiveness. For example, a germicide is capable of killing microorganisms (germs) but does not specify what kind of germs. The term *bacteriostatic* is used to describe agents that inhibit the growth of bacteria but do not necessarily kill them. A bactericide is capable of killing nonsporulating bacteria, fungicides kill fungi and their spores, sporicides are agents that can kill bacterial spores, virucides make viruses noninfective, and tuberculocides kill TB bacteria and other acid-fast bacteria. Commonly used chemicals are addressed in the following text.

 Seek out experts on what chemical agents should be used in your treatment and simulation areas. Always follow written procedures.

Soap's usefulness as a disinfectant is limited because of its feeble antimicrobial action. The main merit of soap is that it aids in the removal of contamination buildup. Chlorine or chlorine compounds are widely used as disinfectants, and, although they are extremely effective against most microorganisms (including HIV and HBV), they are ineffective against spores and have an irritating odor. Alcohol, ethyl or isopropyl, is also ineffective against spores and some viruses. Iodine or iodine compounds may have sporicidal activity. In addition, some people are allergic to iodine and iodine compounds. Hexachlorophene is used for surgical hand disinfection but does not kill all microorganisms. Formaldehyde is effective against all microorganisms, but its vapors are extremely irritating. Alkaline glutaraldehyde (Cidex) can kill spores if they are exposed to it long enough, but it has a pungent odor and is time sensitive, which causes it to eventually lose effectiveness.

Some chemicals, when old and/or too diluted, even encourage rather than retard the growth of microorganisms. Some chemical disinfectants are extremely short acting, and others continue to retard the growth of microorganisms for variable lengths of time. Few special-use chemicals are effective as true sterilants. Because of the wide variability in the effectiveness of chemicals and their potential hazardous risks to HCWs, CSD experts should be contacted for advice on each situation to achieve the appropriate degree of asepsis.

Flexible scopes used in radiation oncology examination rooms deserve a special note of caution. Written procedures, documented training, test strips, and personal protective equipment need to be in place before cleaning a flexible endoscope. Meticulous care is required to ensure that an effective quality assurance process takes place, and a log is required that indicates the procedure, patient, date, serial number or other identifier of endoscope used, and the person performing the endoscopy.[163]

Another special note of caution is that liquid disinfectants and sterilants should not be used to clean brachytherapy devices

such as ovoids. These liquids are known to be capable of corroding the silver brazing that secures the ovoid to the ovoid handle.[117]

 Never accept responsibility for processing scopes or other medical equipment unless you have received proper, documented education for the task.

STERILITY QUALITY CONTROL MEASURES

Wide selections of chemical, mechanical, and biologic indicators are used externally and/or internally on packages subjected to a sterilization process. The purpose of the indicator is to alert an HCW that something went wrong during the sterilization process. External indicators are commonly used in heat, gas, and radiation sterilization processes and typically consist of an adhesive tape that darkens or changes color if exposed to a sterilization process (Figure 10-7). External indicators do not guarantee that sterility has been achieved; they indicate only that the package was exposed to the process. Internal indicators are strategically placed inside a package at a site that is least likely to be penetrated by steam or gas (Figure 10-8). Like external indicators, internal indicators do not guarantee that all microorganisms have been destroyed. Different types of external and internal indicators are commercially available for the different specific sterilization processes.

Biologic indicators are used to determine whether sterilization was achieved. A biologic indicator consists of a specially prepared strip coated with very hard to kill bacterial spores and is enclosed in a small container placed inside a test package. After the test package has gone through the sterilization process with other packages, a microbiologist or another qualified expert examines the biologic indicator to determine whether all the microorganisms were killed. If not, all packages are recalled by their processing number. Routine use of biologic indicators is required by external accrediting agencies such as TJC. These indicators are used daily in each sterilization unit cycle and after any repair on a particular unit. Biologic indicators, external and internal indicators, and close attention to proper time and temperature combinations are all needed to ensure that products and equipment are safe for patient use.

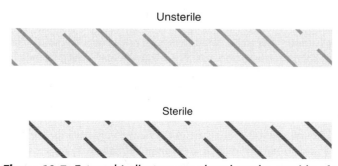

Figure 10-7. External Indicators are placed on the outside of a package to be sterilized. After exposure to the sterilization process, the tape darkens or changes color. An external indicator does not guarantee sterility; it indicates only that the package was exposed to the process. Different types of tape are used in different sterilization processes (e.g., gas, steam).

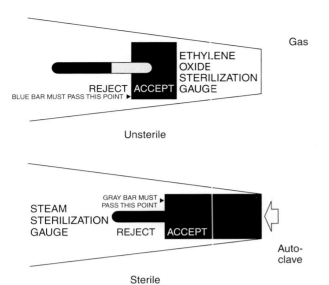

Gas

ETHYLENE OXIDE STERILIZATION GAUGE

BLUE BAR MUST PASS THIS POINT ▶ REJECT | ACCEPT

Unsterile

GRAY BAR MUST PASS THIS POINT ▶

STEAM STERILIZATION GAUGE REJECT | ACCEPT

Auto-clave

Sterile

Figure 10-8. Internal indicators are placed inside packages to be sterilized. They are placed in sites least likely to be reached by the sterilization process; internal indicators also do not guarantee sterility.

SUMMARY

- Epidemiology is a very important component to evaluate and study nosocomial infections.
- Nosocomial infections affect the patient, public, and health care worker physically and financially.
- Radiation therapists should accept the personal responsibility of making sure that their vaccines are complete and up to date annually to protect their patients and coworkers.
- The radiation therapist is responsible for ensuring that proper infection control measures are practiced in the treatment area environment.
- Standard precautions should be used in all patient care procedures.
- The single most important feature of avoiding disease transmission is continuous and meticulous hand hygiene.
- Radiation therapists should be well informed on sterilization and disinfection techniques that are used in their area and the equipment/supplies that they use.
- The radiation therapist should be capable of cleaning up blood and body fluid spills safely and efficiently.
- The radiation therapist should handle and transport laundry in a manner to minimize transmission of pathogens.
- The radiation therapist should be aware of his or her responsibility to report unsafe work conditions to his or her supervisor or outside agencies if needed.
- The radiation therapist should be well informed on what to do should he or she ever be involved in an accident such as a needlestick or blood spill.
- The radiation therapist should wear personnel protective apparel as appropriate to the situation by properly assessing the situation and anticipating what might be needed.
- The radiation therapist will provide a clean treatment couch and treatment accessories to each and every patient on a daily basis.

Review Questions

Multiple Choice

1. Which of the following is a government agency that legally oversees job safety and health protection of workers?
   a. CDC
   b. DEA
   c. JSHP
   d. OSHA
2. Which of the following viruses has been shown capable of living on environmentally friendly surfaces for as long as 7 days?
   a. human immunodeficiency
   b. hepatitis B
   c. influenza
   d. rubeola
3. The term used to describe the number of antibodies present in a blood sample is:
   a. antigen coefficient
   b. globulin factor
   c. immune serum level
   d. titers
4. An employer must provide particulate respirators to HCWs who must interact with a patient diagnosed with active:
   a. human immunodeficiency virus
   b. histoplasmosis
   c. hepatitis A
   d. tuberculosis
5. The concept known as universal precautions applies to:
   a. all body fluids
   b. all patients
   c. all blood and other certain body fluids in all patients
   d. all patients and all body fluids
6. If an HCW is stuck by a needle and consents to blood collection but not to an HIV test, the blood sample must be preserved by law for at least:
   a. 1 week
   b. 30 days
   c. 90 days
   d. 6 months
7. Alcohol-based hand rubs are indicated for all of the following clinical situations *except:*
   a. when the hands are visibly soiled
   b. preoperative cleaning of hands by surgical personnel
   c. before inserting urinary catheters, intravascular catheters, or other invasive devices
   d. after removing gloves
8. Which of the following statements regarding preoperative surgical hand antisepsis is *true?*
   a. Antimicrobial counts on hands are reduced as effectively with a 5-minute scrub as with a 10-minute scrub.
   b. A brush or sponge must be used when applying the antiseptic agent to adequately reduce bacterial counts on hands.
   c. Alcohol-based hand rubs for preoperative surgical scrub have been associated with increased surgical site infection rate.
   d. a and b are true.
   e. a and c are true.

Fill in the Blank

1. _____ is the name for the medical science field that studies the incidence, distribution, and determinants of disease.
2. An individual who is colonized but shows no immune response is known as a(n) _____.
3. Two nosocomial infectious diseases for which no vaccine is currently available are _____ and _____.
4. The three phases that a susceptible host goes through are _____, _____, and _____.
5. _____ is the gas that is routinely used for gas sterilization.

The answers to the Review Questions can be found by logging on to our website at: *http://evolve.elsevier.com/Washington+Leaver/principles*

Questions to Ponder

1. Discuss the differences between universal precautions and body substance isolation.
2. Using documented research, identify 10 infectious diseases that, if caught, result in lifelong immunity.
3. Compare and contrast the differences between killed, toxoid, and attenuated live vaccines.
4. Develop an infection control protocol for any clinical area task that must be addressed.
5. Compare labels on various liquid chemicals used for infection control in the medical setting and discuss what they can and cannot kill.
6. Compare the major differences between large droplet and droplet nuclei transmission.
7. Discuss what actions should be taken when an HCW develops hypersensitivity to latex.
8. Describe the use of sodium hypochlorite in a medical setting.
9. Discuss the significance of delayed seroconversion.

REFERENCES

1. Alfa M, et al: Comparison of ion plasma, vaporized hydrogen peroxide and 100% ethylene oxide sterilizers to the 12/88 ethylene oxide gas sterilizer, *Infect Control Hosp Epidemiol* 17:92-99, 1996.
2. Alter M: The detection, transmission and outcome of hepatitis C virus infection, *Infect Agents Dis* 2:155-156, 1993.
3. Anderson RL: Biological evaluation of carpeting, *Appl Microbiol* 18:180, 1969.
4. Andrade A, Flexner C: Progress in pharmacology and drug interactions from the 10th CROI, *Hopkins HIV Rep* 15(7):11, 2003.
5. Andrade A, Flexner CG: Genes, ethnicity, and efavirenz response: clinical pharmacology update from the 11th CROI, *Hopkins HIV Rep* 16:1-7, 2004.
6. Anonymous: Needlestick transmission of HTLV-III from a patient infected in Africa, *Lancet* 2:1376-1377, 1984.
7. Barnhart E, editor: *Physician's desk reference*, ed 49, Montvale, NJ, 1995, Medical Economics Data Production.
8. Bartholomew A: Mixed up over mad cow: how worried should you really be? Two experts sit down to hash it out, *Reader's Digest,* pp 104-109, August 2001.
9. Bartlett JG: *Pocketbook of infectious disease therapy,* Baltimore, 1991, Williams & Wilkins.
10. Bartley J, et al: APIC State-of-the-Art Report: The role of infection control during construction in health care facilities, *Am J Infect Control* 28:156, 2000.
11. Baylor University: *Human immunodeficiency virus (HIV) workplace guidelines,* Dallas, 1993, Department of Epidemiology, Baylor University Medical Center.
12. Beekmann SE, Henderson DK: HCWs and hepatitis: risk for infection and management of exposure, *Infect Dis Clin Pract* 1:424-428, 1992.
13. Beekmann SE, et al: Risky business: using necessarily imprecise casualty counts to estimate occupational risk of HIV-1 infection, *Infect Control Hosp Epidemiol* 11:371-379, 1990.
14. Beil L: FDA approves vaccine against chickenpox, 70 to 90% effectiveness expected, *Dallas Morning News*, p 1, March 18, 1995.
15. Bell DM: Occupational risk of human immunodeficiency virus infection in health-care workers: an overview, *Am J Med* 102(5B):9-15, 1997.
16. Benenson A, editor: *Control of communicable diseases in man,* ed 13, Washington DC, 1981, American Public Health Association.
17. Block S: Sterilization and preservation. In Favero MS, Bond WW, editors: *Chemical disinfection of medical and surgical materials,* ed 4, Philadelphia, 1991, Lea & Febiger.
18. Bond WW, et al: Inactivation of hepatitis B virus after drying and storage for one week, *Lancet* 1(8219):550-551, 1981 [letter].
19. Boyce JM: It is time for action: improving hand hygiene in hospitals, *Ann Intern Med* 130:153-155, 1999.
20. Brachman PS: Epidemiology of nosocomial infections. In Bennett JV, Brachman PS, editors: *Hospital infections,* ed 3, Boston, 1992, Little, Brown.
21. Brachman PS: Epidemiology of nosocomial infections. In Bennett JV, Brachman PS, editors: *Hospital infections,* ed 4, Philadelphia, 1998, Lippincott-Raven.
22. Bryan P, et al: Guidelines for hospital environmental control. Section 1. Antiseptics, handwashing and handwashing facilities. In Centers for Disease Control and Prevention (CDC), editor: *Centers for Disease Control Hospital Infection Program: Guidelines for prevention and control of nosocomial infections* (pp 6-10), Atlanta, 1981, CDC.
23. Busch MP, Satten GA: Time course of viremia and antibody seroconversion following human immunodeficiency virus exposure, *Am J Med* 102(suppl 5B):117-124, 1997.
24. Campbell CC: Malaria. In Hoeprich PD, Jordan MC, editors: *Infectious diseases,* ed 4, Philadelphia, 1989, JB Lippincott.
25. Casewell M, Phillips I: Hands as route of transmission for *Klebsiella* species, *Br Med J* 2:1315-17, 1977.
26. Cawson RA, et al: *Pathology: the mechanisms of disease,* ed 2, St Louis, 1989, Mosby.
27. Centers for Disease Control and Prevention: Viral hepatitis B vaccine: fact sheet (website): http://www.cdc.gov.ncidod/diseases/hepatitis/b/factvax.htm. Accessed August 15, 2007.
28. Centers for Disease Control and Prevention: Viral hepatitis: top 11 most frequently asked questions about viral hepatitis (website): http://www.cdc.gov/ncidod/diseases/hepatitis/common-faqs.htm. Accessed August 15, 2007.
29. Centers for Disease Control and Prevention: Feeding back surveillance data to prevent hospital-acquired infections (website). Retrieved July 11, 2007, from www.cdc.gov/ncidod/eid/vol7no2/gaynes.htm.
30. Centers for Disease Control and Prevention: Division of Bacterial and Mycotic Diseases: Legionellosis: Legionnaire's Disease (LD) and Pontiac Fever (website): http://www.cdc.gov/ncidod/dbmid/diseaseinfo/legionellosis-g.htm. Accessed July 11, 2007.
31. Centers for Disease Control and Prevention: Proceedings of the First International Conference on Nosocomial Infections, American Hospital Association, Atlanta, August 5-8, 1970.
32. Centers for Disease Control and Prevention: *Guidelines for prevention of TB transmission in hospitals,* Atlanta, 1982, US Department of Health and Human Services, Public Health Service.
33. Centers for Disease Control and Prevention: Recommendations of the Advisory Committee on Immunization Practices: varicella-zoster immune globulin for the prevention of chickenpox, *MMWR* 33:84-100, 1984.
34. Centers for Disease Control and Prevention: Recommendations for preventing transmission of infection in the human T-lymphotropic virus type III/lymphadenopathy-associated virus in the workplace, *MMWR* 34:681-695, 1985.

35. Centers for Disease Control and Prevention: Recommendations for prevention of HIV transmission in health care settings, *MMWR* 36(suppl 2S):1-19, 1987.

36. Centers for Disease Control and Prevention: Update: human immunodeficiency virus infections in health-care workers exposed to blood of infected patients, *MMWR* 36:285-289, 1987.

37. Centers for Disease Control and Prevention: Update: universal precautions for prevention of transmission of human immunodeficiency virus, hepatitis B virus, and other bloodborne pathogens in health care settings, *MMWR* 37:377-388, 1988.

38. Centers for Disease Control and Prevention: Guidelines for preventing the transmission of tuberculosis in healthcare settings, with special focus on HIV-related issues, *MMWR* 39(RR-17):1, 1990.

39. Centers for Disease Control and Prevention: Recommendations of the Immunization Practices Advisory Committee: prevention and control of influenza, *MMWR* 39(RR-7):1-15, 1990.

40. Centers for Disease Control and Prevention: Surveillance for occupationally acquired HIV infection—United States, 1981-1992, *MMWR* 41:823-825, 1992. Personal communication update with CDC National AIDS Clearinghouse, 1995.

41. Centers for Disease Control and Prevention: Hospital Infection Control Practices Advisory Committee: Agenda, *Fed Reg* 58:103, 1993.

42. Centers for Disease Control and Prevention: Hospital Infection Control Practices Advisory Committee: Meetings, *Fed Reg* 58:204, 1993.

43. Centers for Disease Control and Prevention: Guidelines for preventing the transmission of *Mycobacterium tuberculosis* in health-care facilities, *MMWR* 43(RR-13):69, 78-81, 1994.

44. Centers for Disease Control and Prevention: Prevention and control of influenza: part II. Antiviral agents—recommendations of the Advisory Committee on Immunization Practices (ACIP), *MMWR* 43(RR-15):1-10, 1994.

45. Centers for Disease Control and Prevention: Tuberculosis morbidity: United States, 1994, *MMWR* 44:387-389, 395, 1995.

46. Centers for Disease Control and Prevention: Hospital Infection Control Practices Advisory Committee: Guidelines for isolation precautions in hospitals, *Infect Cont Hosp Epidemiol* 17:53-80, 1996.

47. Centers for Disease Control and Prevention: Update: provisional Public Health Service recommendations for chemoprophylaxis after occupational exposure to HIV, *MMWR* 45:468-472, 1996.

48. Centers for Disease Control and Prevention: Guidelines for the use of antiretroviral agents in HIV-infected adults and adolescents, *MMWR* 46(RR-5):43-82, 1997.

49. Centers for Disease Control and Prevention: Public Health Service guidelines for the management of health-care workers exposed to HIV and recommendations for postexposure prophylaxis, *MMWR* 47(RR-7):1-28, 1998.

50. Centers for Disease Control and Prevention: Public Health Service guidelines for the management of health-care worker exposures to HIV and recommendations for postexposure prophylaxis, *MMWR* 47(RR-7):1-33, 1998.

51. Centers for Disease Control and Prevention: *NIOSH TB respiratory protection program in health care facilities—administrator's guide* (DHHS Publication No. 99-143), Cincinnati, 1999, National Institute for Occupational Safety and Health, HHS, CDC.

52. Centers for Disease Control and Prevention: American Thoracic Society: Targeted tuberculin testing and treatment of latent tuberculosis infection, *MMWR* 49(RR-6): 1–80, 2000.

53. Centers for Disease Control and Prevention: Updated US Public Health Service guidelines for the management of occupational exposures to HBV, HCV, and HIV and recommendations for postexposure prophylaxis, *MMWR* 50(RR-11):1-52, 2001.

54. Centers for Disease Control and Prevention: American Thoracic Society, Infectious Disease Society of America: Treatment of tuberculosis, *MMWR* 52(RR-11), 2003.

55. Centers for Disease and Control and Prevention: Guidelines for environmental infection control in health care facilities, recommendations of CDC and the Healthcare Infection Control Practices Advisory Committee (HICPAC), *MMWR* 52(RR-10), 2003.

56. Centers for Disease Control and Prevention: Updated US Public Health Service guidelines for the management of occupational exposures to HIV and recommendations for postexposure prophylaxis, *MMWR* 54(RR-9):1-17, 2005.

57. Centers for Disease Control and Prevention: Guidelines for preventing the transmission of *Mycobacterim tuberculosis* in health-care settings, *MMWR* 54(RR-17):1-141, 2005.

58. Centers for Disease Control and Prevention: Controlling tuberculosis in the United States: recommendations from the American Thoracic Society, CDC, and the Infectious Diseases Society of American, *MMWR* 54(RR-12):1-81, 2005.

59. Centers for Disease Control and Prevention: Summary of notifiable diseases—United States, *MMWR* 54(53):2-92, 2005.

60. Centers for Disease Control and Prevention: Trends in tuberculosis incidences—United States, 2006, *MMWR* 56(11):245-250, 2007.

61. Centers for Disease Control and Prevention: Guidelines for hand hygiene in health-care settings, *MMWR* 51(RR-16):29, 2002.

62. Chen SK, et al: Evaluation of single-use masks and respirators for protection of health care workers against mycobacterium aerosols, *Am J Infect Control* 22:65-74, 1994.

63. Cheney K: Skin so sad: shingles shot, *AARP* September-October:34, 2007.

64. Ciesielski CA, Metter RP: Duration of time between exposure and seroconversion in health-care workers with occupationally acquired infection with human immunodeficiency virus, *Am J Med* 102(suppl 5B):115-116, 1997.

65. Cooper JS: The role of radiation therapy in the management of patients who have AIDS. In Cox JD, editor: *Moss's radiation oncology: rationale, technique, results,* ed 7, St Louis, 1994, Mosby.

66. Coppage CM: *Hand washing in patient care* [motion picture], Washington, DC, 1961, US Public Health Service.

67. Cuthberton B, et al: Safety of albumin preparations manufactured from plasma not tested for HIV antibody, *Lancet* 2:41, 1987 [letter].

68. Dasgupta A, Okhuysen PC: Pharmacokinetic and other drug interactions in patients with AIDS, *Ther Drug Monit* 23:591-605, 2001.

69. de Maat MM, et al: Drug interactions between antiretroviral drugs and comedicated agents, *Clin Pharmacokinet* 42:223-282, 2003.

70. Edmunds-Obguokiri T: Understanding drug-drug interactions in the management of HIV disease, *HIV Clin* 14:1-4, 2002.

71. EEOC, Equal Employment Opportunity Commission: *A technical assistance manual on the employment provisions (title 1) of the Americans with Disabilities Act*, Washington, DC, 1992, Equal Employment Opportunity Commission.

72. Ewglinet C, et al: Cruise-ship-associated Legionnaire's disease, *JAMA* 294:November 2003-May 2004 (website): http://jama.ama-assn.org/cgi/content/full/294/24/3080. Accessed December 28, 2005.

73. Fichtenbaum CJ, Gerber JG: Interactions between antiretroviral drugs and drugs used for the therapy of the metabolic complications encountered during HIV infection, *Clin Pharmacokinet* 41:1195-1211, 2002.

74. Food and Drug Administration (FDA), Public Health Service (PHS), Environmental Protection Agency (EPA): Memorandum of understanding between the FDA, PHS, and the EPA, Washington, DC, June 4, 1993, FDA, PHS, EPA.

75. Fried DM, et al: Splinting using a new thermoplastic material, *J Am Phys Ther Assoc* 47(12):1123-1125, 1967.

76. Gardner JF, Peel MM: *Introduction to sterilization, disinfection and infection control,* ed 2, New York, 1991, Churchill Livingstone.

77. Garner JS, Favero MS: CDC guidelines for the prevention and control of nosocomial infections: guideline for handwashing and hospital environmental control, *Am J Infect Control* 14:110-129, 1986.

78. Garner JS: Hospital Infection Control Practices Advisory Committee: Guideline for isolation precautions in hospitals, *Infect Control Hosp Epidemiol* 17:53-80, 1996.

79. Garner JS, Simmons BP: CDC guidelines for isolation precautions in hospitals, *Infect Control* 4:245-325, 1983.

80. Garner JS, et al: CDC guideline for handwashing and hospital environmental control, *Infect Control* 7:231-243, 1986.

81. Garrett RT: Bill makes hospital reveal infections, *Dallas Morning News*, March 21, 2007.

82. Gerberding JL, Henderson DK: Management of occupational exposure to bloodborne pathogens: hepatitis B virus, hepatitis C virus and human immunodeficiency virus, *Clin Infect Dis* 14:1179-1185, 1992.

83. Greider K: Dirty hospitals, *AARP Bull* 48(1):12-14, 2007.

84. Gross A, Cutright DE, D'Alessandro SM: Effects of surgical scrub on microbial population under the fingernails, *Am J Surg* 138(3):463-467, 1979.

85. Guyton HG, Decker HM: Respiratory protection by five new contagion masks, *Appl Microbiol* 11:66-68, 1963.

86. Hahn JB: The source of the "resident" flora, *Hand* 5:247-252, 1973.

87. Haley CE: Drug resistant TB, Lecture at Baylor University Medical Center, Dallas, February 25, 1994.

88. Haley CE, et al: Tuberculosis epidemic among hospital personnel, *Infect Control Hosp Epidemiol* 10:204-210, 1989.

89. Haley RW: *Managing hospital infection control for cost*, Chicago, 1986, American Hospital Publishing.

90. Haley RW: The development of infection surveillance and control programs. In Bennett JV, Brachman PS, editors: *Hospital infections*, ed 3, Boston, 1992, Little, Brown.

91. Haley RW: The development of infection surveillance and control programs in hospital infection. In Bennett JV, Brachman PS, editors: *Hospital infections*, ed 4, Philadelphia, 1998, Lippincott-Raven.

92. Haley RW, et al: The efficacy of infection surveillance and control programs in preventing nosocomial infections in US hospitals, *Am J Epidemiol* 121:182-205, 1985.

93. Hedderwick SA, et al: Pathogenic organisms associated with artificial fingernails worn by healthcare workers, *Inf Control Hosp Epidemiol* 21:8:505-509, 2000.

94. Henderson DK: Zeroing in on the appropriate management of occupational exposure to HIV-1, *Infect Control Hosp Epidemiol* 11:175-177, 1990.

95. Henderson DK: Postexposure chemoprophylaxis for occupational exposure to human immunodeficiency virus type 1: current status and prospects for the future, *Am J Med* 91(suppl 3S):312-319, 1991.

96. Henderson DK, et al: The risk for occupational transmission of human immunodeficiency virus type 1 (HIV-1) associated with clinical procedures: a prospective evaluation, *Ann Intern Med* 113:740-746, 1990.

97. Hoeprich PD, Jordan MC: *Infectious diseases: a modern treatise on infectious processes*, ed 4, Philadelphia, 1989, JB Lippincott.

98. Hoffman PN, et al: Microorganisms isolated from skin under wedding rings worn by hospital staff, *Br Med J* 290:206-7, 1985.

99. Holmberg SD, et al: Health and economic impacts of antimicrobial resistance, *Rev Infect Dis* 9:1065, 1989.

100. Hospital Infection Control Practices Advisory Committee (HICPAC): Recommendations for preventing the spread of vancomycin resistance, *Infect Control Hosp Epidemiol* 16:105-113, 1995.

101. Hospital Infection Control Practices Advisory Committee: Guideline for isolation precautions in hospitals, *Infect Cont Hosp Epidemiol* 17:53-80, 1996.

102. Hughes JM: Hantavirus pulmonary syndrome: an emerging infectious disease, *Science* 262:850-851, 1993.

103. Institute of Medicine, editor: *To err is human*, Washington, DC, 1999, National Academy Press.

104. Jacoby GA, Archer GL: New mechanisms of bacterial resistance to antimicrobial agents, *N Engl J Med* 324:601, 1991.

105. James CD: Personal communication, 1995.

106. Jarvas WR: Nosocomial transmission of multidrug-resistant *Mycobacterium tuberculosis*, *Am J Infect Control* 23:146-151, 1995.

107. Johnson S, et al: Prospective controlled study of vinyl glove use to interrupt *Clostridium difficile* nosocomial transmission, *Am J Med* 88:137-140, 1990.

108. Joint Commission on Accreditation of Healthcare Organizations: Standards: infection control. In *Accreditation manual for hospitals*, Chicago, 1990, Joint Commission on Accreditation of Healthcare Organizations.

109. Joint Commission on Accreditation of Healthcare Organizations: *Accreditation manual for hospitals*, Chicago, 1995, Joint Commission on Accreditation of Healthcare Organizations.

110. Jones RD, et al: Moisturizing alcohol hand gels for surgical hand preparations, *AORN J* 71:584-599, 2000.

111. Kampf G, et al: Epidemiologic background of hand hygiene and evaluation of the most important agents for scrubs and rubs, *Clin Microbiol Rev* 17:863-893, 2004.

112. Kates SG, et al: Indigenous multiresistant bacteria from flowers in hospital and nonhospital environments, *Am J Infect Control* 19:156, 1991.

113. Kilbourne ED: The influenza virus and influenza. In Douglas RG Jr, editor: *Influenza in man*, New York, 1975, Academic.

114. Kollmorgen GM, Bedford JS: Cellular radiation biology. In Dalrymple GV, et al, editors: *Medical radiation biology*, Philadelphia, 1973, WB Saunders.

115. Koziol DE, Henderson DK: Risk analysis and occupational exposure to HIV and HBV, *Curr Opin Infect Dis* 6:506-510, 1993.

116. Kretzer EK, et al: Behavioral interventions to improve infection control practice, *Am J Infect Control* 26:2245-2253, 1998.

117. Kubiatowicz DO: Important safety information (business letter communication), St. Paul, MN, May 4, 1990, Medical Device Division, 3M Health Care.

118. Kutting B, et al: Effectiveness of skin protection creams as a preventive measure in occupational dermatitis: a critical update according to criteria of evidence based medicine, *Int Arch Occup Environ Health* 76:253-259, 2003.

119. Lange JMA, et al: Failure of zidovudine prophylaxis after accidental exposure to HIV-1, *N Engl J Med* 322:1375-1377, 1990.

120. Larson E: Guideline for use of topical antimicrobial agents, *Am J Infect Control* 23:251-269, 1995.

121. Larson EL, APIC Guidelines Committee: APIC guideline for handwashing and hand antisepsis in health care settings, *Am J Infect Control* 23:251-269, 1995.

122. Lee L, Henderson D: Tolerability of postexposure antiretroviral prophylaxis for occupational exposures to HIV, *Drug Safe* 24:587-597, 2001.

123. Lemonick MD: The killers all around, *Time*, pp 183-185, Sept 12, 1994.

124. Looke DFM, Grove DI: Failed prophylactic zidovudine after needlestick injury, *Lancet* 335:1280, 1990 [letter].

125. Lynch P, Jackson MM, Rogers JC: Rethinking the role of isolation precautions in the prevention of nosocomial infections, *Ann Intern Med* 107:243-246, 1987.

126. Mahy BWJ, Centers for Disease Control and Prevention: Overview of infectious diseases in the workplace. Lecture at Baylor University Medical Center, Dallas, February 25, 1994.

127. Matera JR: Sterile tattooing: improving quality of care, *Radiat Ther* 10:2:165-167, 2001.

128. Mayo Clinic Staff: Mayo Clinic: infectious disease: hepatitis C (website): http://www.mayoclinic.com/health/hepatitis-c/DS0097/DSECTION=9. Accessed August 13, 2007.

129. McCormick RD, et al: Double-blind, randomized trial of scheduled use of a novel barrier cream and an oil-containing lotion for protecting the hands of healthcare workers, *Am J Infect Control* 28:302-310, 2000.

130. Miller DC: Creutzfeldt-Jakob disease in histopathology technicians, *N Engl J Med* 318:853, 1988.

131. Moyle G, et al: Unexpected drug interactions and adverse events with antiretroviral drugs, *Lancet* 364:8-10, 2004.

132. Muldoon RL, Stanley ED, Jackson GG: Use and withdrawal of amantadine chemoprophylaxis during epidemic influenza A, *Am Rev Respir Dis* 133:487-491, 1976.

133. NARA, Department of Labor, Occupational Safety and Health Administration: Occupational exposure to bloodborne pathogens, Final rule, 29 CFR Part 1910.1030, *Fed Reg* 56(235):64004-64182, 1991.

134. NARA, Department of Labor, Occupational Safety and Health Administration: Title 29, code of federal regulations, part 1903.2, Washington DC, 1989, The Department of Labor, Occupational Safety and Health Administration.

135. NARA, Department of Labor, Occupational Safety and Health Administration: Title 29, code of federal regulations, part 1977.12, Washington DC, 1989, The Department of Labor, Occupational Safety and Health Administration.

136. NARA, Department of Labor, Occupational Safety and Health Administration: Proposed rules on TB transmission to and among HCWs, *Fed Reg* 59(219):58884-58935, 1994.

137. NIH: Panel on Clinical Practices for Treatment of HIV Infection: Guidelines for the use of antiretroviral agents in HIV-infected adults and adolescents (website): http://aidsinfo.nih.gov/guidelines/default_db2.asp?id=50. Accessed September 1, 2007.

138. Noble RC: Infectiousness of pulmonary tuberculosis after starting chemotherapy: review of the available data on an unresolved question, *Am J Infect Control* 9:6-10, 1981.

139. NZDS, New Zealand Dermatological Society Incorporated: Spa pool folliculitis (website): http://dermnetnz.org/acne/spapool-folliculitis.html. Accessed August 8, 2007.

140. Oncology Nursing Society: Where oncology nurses connect: radiation therapy: water bath related infection control issues (website): http://listserv.vc.ons.org/page/67034/:jsessionid=1dvu2jhs09un3?d_v=rm&d_mid+106477. Accessed January 9, 2007.

141. Orfit Industries (website): http://www.orfit.com/usa/radiotherapie/index.html. Accessed August 31, 2007.

142. OSHA, Department of Labor and the Department of Health and Human Services: Joint advisory notice: protection against occupational exposure to hepatitis B virus (HBV) and human immunodeficiency virus, *Fed Reg* 54:41818, October 30, 1987.

143. OSHA, Department of Labor, Occupational Safety and Health Administration: Occupational exposure to bloodborne pathogens, Final rule, 29 CFR Part 1910.1030, *Fed Reg* 64004-64182, 1991.

144. OSHA, Occupational Safety and Health Administration: *OSHA Instruction CPL 2-2.44C*, Washington DC, 1992, Office of Health Compliance Assistance.

145. OSHA, National Institute for Occupational Safety and Health, editor: TB study funding announcement, *Fed Reg* 148, 1993.

146. OSHA, Department of Labor, Occupational Safety and Health Administration: Proposed rules on TB transmission to and among HCWs, *Fed Reg* 58884-58935, 1994.

147. OSHA, US Department of Labor, OSHA: *Enforcement procedures for the occupational exposure to bloodborne pathogens*, OSHA Directive CPL 2-22.44D, Washington, DC, 1999, Occupational Safety and Health Administration.

148. Owens DK, Nease RF: Occupational exposure to human immunodeficiency virus and hepatitis B virus: a comparative analysis of risk, *Am J Med* 92:503-512, 1992.

149. Parkin JM, et al: Tolerability and side-effects of post-exposure prophylaxis for HIV infection, *Lancet* 355:722-723, 2000.

150. Patterson JV, Hierholzer WJ Jr: The hospital epidemiologist. In Bennett JV, Brachman PS, editors: *Hospital infections,* ed 3, Boston, 1992, Little, Brown.

151. Piscitelli SC, Gallicano KD: Interactions among drugs for HIV and opportunistic infections, *N Engl J Med* 334:984-996, 2001.

152. Pittet D, et al: Members of the Infection Control Program. Compliance with handwashing in a teaching hospital, *Ann Intern Med* 130:126-130, 1999.

153. Pittet D, et al: Effectiveness of a hospital-wide programme to improve compliance with hand hygiene, *Lancet* 356:1307-1312, 2000.

154. Polder JA, Tablan OC, Williams WW: Personnel health services. In Bennett JV, Brachman PS, editors: *Hospital infections,* ed 3, Boston, 1992, Little, Brown.

155. Price JH: Hospital's hidden danger, The Washington Times (website): www.hospitalinfection.org/press/022507/washington_times.htm. Accessed July 11, 2007.

156. Puro V: Post-exposure prophylaxis for HIV infection [letter], *Lancet* 355:1556-1557, 2000.

157. Qarah S, et al: *Pseudomonas aeruginosa infections,* December 12, 2005 (website): www.emedicine.com/med/topic1943.htm. Accessed August 1, 2007.

158. Rainey PM: HIV drug interactions: the good, the bad, and the other, *Ther Drug Monit* 24:26-31, 2002.

159. Rhame FS: The inanimate environment. In Bennett JV, Brachman PS, editors: *Hospital infections,* ed 3, Boston, 1992, Little, Brown.

160. Rhame FS: The inanimate environment. In Bennett JV, Brachman PS, editors: *Hospital infections,* ed 4, Philadelphia, 1998, Lippincott-Raven.

161. Rotter ML, et al: The influence of cosmetic additives on the acceptability of alcohol-based hand disinfectants, *J Hosp Infect* 18(suppl B):57-63, 1991.

162. Russi M, et al: Antiretroviral prophylaxis of health care workers at two urban medical centers, *J Occup Environ Med* 42:1092-1100, 2000.

163. Rutala WA: APIC guideline for selection and use of disinfectants, *Am J Infect Control* 24:313-342, 1996.

164. Saint Louis University: New investigational vaccine to prevent hepatitis C tested for first time in humans, November 17, 2003 (website): http://www.slu.edu/readstory/homepage/3472. Accessed August 13, 2007.

165. Salisbury DM, et al: The effect of rings on microbial load of health care worker's hands, *Am J Infect Control* 25:24-27, 1997.

166. Shaffer JG: Microbiology of hospital carpeting, *Health Lab Sci* 3:73, 1966.

167. Smith AL: *Principles of microbiology,* ed 7, St Louis, 1973, Mosby.

168. Snider DE Jr, Cauthen GM: Tuberculin skin testing of hospital employees: infection, "boosting," and two-step testing, *Am J Infect Control* 12:305-311, 1984.

169. Spira AI, et al: Cellular targets of infection and route of viral dissemination after an intravaginal inoculation of simian immunodeficiency virus into rhesus macaques, *J Exp Med* 183:215-225, 1996.

170. Steelman VM: Creutzfeldt-Jakob disease: recommendations for infection control, *Am J Infect Control* 22:312-318, 1994.

171. Steere AC, Mallison GF: Handwashing practices for the prevention of nosocomial infections, *Ann Intern Med* 83:683-690, 1975.

172. Struble KA, Pratt RD, Gitterman SR: Toxicity of antiretroviral agents, *Am J Med* 102(suppl 5B):65-67, 1997.

173. Swotinsky RB, et al: Occupational exposure to HIV: experience at a tertiary care center, *J Occup Environ Med* 40:1102-1109, 1998.

174. Szuness W, et al: Hepatitis B vaccine: demonstration of efficacy in a controlled clinical trial in a high risk population in the United States, *N Engl J Med* 303:833-841, 1980.

175. Taylor J: FDA Device Clearances: Hepatitis C test, laser-assisted lipolysis, percutaneous support catheter (website): http://www.medscape.com/viewarticle/559882. Accessed September 1, 2007.

176. Thomas CL, editor: *Taber's cyclopedic medical dictionary,* ed 1, Philadelphia, 1973, FA Davis.

177. Tubs R: *Pseudomonas* aka hot tub folliculitis (website): http://www.rhtubs.com/Pseudomonas.htm. Accessed August 1, 2007.

178. University of California at San Francisco Center for HIV Information. Database of antiretroviral drug interactions (website): http://hivinsite.ucsf.edu/InSite?page=ar-00-02. Accessed August 7, 2007.

179. Wang SA, Panlilio AL, Doi PA: Experience of health-care workers taking postexposure prophylaxis after occupational human immunodeficiency virus exposures: findings of the HIV Postexposure Prophylaxis Registry, *Infect Control Hosp Epidemiol* 21:780-785, 2000.

180. Washington P: Mad cow disease: engineered cattle avoid infection, *Star Telegram,* January 1, 2007. Reprint from Washington Post.

181. *Webster's New World Medical Dictionary,* Ames, IA, 2001, Wiley.

182. WFR/Aquaplast, WFR/Aquaplast Corporation (website): http://www.wfr-aquaplast.com/pages/protosheets.html. Accessed August 31, 2007.

183. WHO Guidelines on Hand Hygiene in Healthcare (Advanced Draft), *Part of the WHO Consultation on Hand Hygiene in Healthcare Global Patient Safety Challenge, 2005-2006: Clean Care is Safer Care,* Geneva, October 10, 2005, WHO World Alliance for Patient Safety Practice Guidelines.

184. Williams WW, Centers for Disease Control: CDC guidelines for infection control in hospital personnel, *Infect Control* 4(suppl):326-349, 1983.

185. Yeni PG, et al: Treatment for adult HIV infection: 2004 recommendations of the International AIDS Society-USA Panel, *JAMA* 292:251-265, 2004.

Patient Assessment

Shirlee E. Maihoff, Gay Dungey

Outline

Objectives

- Describe the attributes and responsibilities of an effective helper in a cancer health care setting.
- Demonstrate effective verbal and nonverbal communication in a range of contexts and age groups.
- Identify the determinants that make up the multidisciplinary approach to caring for the cancer patient.
- Discuss the importance of pain, psychosocial, nutritional, and cultural assessment with respect to

the cancer patient and identify how these are assessed and controlled in the health care setting.
- Discuss the importance of monitoring the patient while he or she is undergoing radiation therapy with respect to radiation dose and the expected timing of side effects.
- Discuss the relevance of culture to individual and group experience in society with particular reference to the cancer setting.

PATIENT ASSESSMENT DEFINED

The **assessment** of cancer patients and of systems in which they function provides the basis of effective cancer care.[34] The diagnosis of cancer can precipitate significant changes in the lives of the patient and family. These changes can be physiologic, psychological, and spiritual. To understand the effect of the cancer diagnosis on a patient, significant other, or family, the diagnosis must be considered a process rather than an event. That process is dynamic and continuous and changes over time.

Information obtained through a continuous, systematic assessment allows the health care provider to (1) determine the nature of a problem, (2) select an intervention for that problem, and (3) evaluate the effectiveness of the intervention. The assessment should be continued as long as interventions are needed and wanted by the patient to facilitate an optimal quality of life. Assessment can be accomplished most effectively through a multidisciplinary approach and requires the efforts of the entire oncology team, including surgical oncologists, medical oncologists, radiation oncologists, radiation therapists, oncology nurses, social workers, dietitians, and pastoral counselors.

Importance of Patient Assessment in Oncology

The assessment of cancer patients serves as the cornerstone for the structure of care. However, patient assessment is much more than obtaining a patient history. Patients come worried and often in pain. They feel extremely vulnerable and in need of help and understanding. Patients are often desperate to put their cancer problems behind them, receive treatment, and get on with their lives. They come hoping that health care providers will listen carefully and know the correct things to do to help them. Most patients want not only physical and psychological comfort but also another person to firmly stand alongside them with genuine empathy at this vulnerable time. They want someone to resonate with their distress. All this intense emotion is presented after initial contact with the patient. Most people use their coping skills, but few fully reveal the extent of their feelings. Most adults convey varying degrees of ability to remain in control in an environment that appears strange at best and terrifying at worst.

Establishing a Therapeutic Relationship

Health professionals must recognize that the patient feels at a distinct disadvantage and must respect, reassure, and support even those who convey an incredible sense of confidence and comfort. At an initial encounter with a patient, acceptance, interest, and genuineness are imperative to establishing a therapeutic and healing relationship, which is critical to the healing process. Verbal and nonverbal communication between the patient and therapist is the basis of an effective **therapeutic relationship.** Box 11-1 lists helpful behaviors in working with patients; Box 11-2 lists verbal and nonverbal behaviors that are not helpful.

To be effective in assessment, radiation therapists must use communication skills that involve hearing verbal messages, perceiving nonverbal messages, and responding verbally and nonverbally to both kinds of messages.

 The radiation therapist must be an effective listener to be able to successfully communicate with the patient via cognitive and affective avenues.

Various anthropologists believe that more than two thirds of any communication is transmitted nonverbally. Therefore, gestures, facial expressions, posture, personal appearance, and cultural characteristics must be interpreted to understand the patient. Nonverbal behavior provides clues to, but not conclusive proof of, underlying feelings. However, research has proved that nonverbal cues (Table 11-1) tend to be more reliable than verbal cues.

Simple phrases to respond to negative nonverbal cues include, "You seem to be upset" and "You appear to be unhappy." Box 11-3 provides an exercise for recognizing nonverbal cues.

Box 11-1	Helpful Behaviors

VERBAL
- Is nonjudgmental
- Uses understandable words
- Reflects and clarifies patient's statements
- Responds to real messages such as doubt and fear
- Summarizes or synthesizes the words of the patient
- Uses verbal reinforcers such as "I see" and "Yes"
- Gives information appropriately
- Uses humor at times to reduce tension
- Has moderately calm rate of speech
- Has moderate tone of voice

NONVERBAL
- Maintains good eye contact
- Touches appropriately
- Nods head occasionally
- Has animated facial expressions
- Smiles occasionally
- Uses occasional hand gestures

Box 11-2	Nonhelpful Behaviors

VERBAL
- Preaches
- Blames
- Placates
- Directs and demands
- Gives advice
- Has patronizing attitude
- Strays from topic
- Talks about self too much
- Overanalyzes or overinterprets
- Intellectualizes
- Uses words patient does not understand
- Probes and questions extensively, especially "why" questions
- Has unpleasant tone of voice

NONVERBAL
- Has poor eye contact
- Frowns
- Has expressionless face
- Has tight mouth
- Yawns
- Shakes pointed finger

Verbal messages are clearer than nonverbal messages. Verbal messages are composed of **cognitive** and **affective** content.

- *Cognitive* content is composed of the actual facts and words of the message. Affective content may be verbal or nonverbal and consists of feelings, attitudes, and behaviors. The difference in hearing only the obvious cognitive content of a verbal message and hearing the cognitive and underlying affective messages is the difference between being an ineffective or effective listener.
- *Affective* messages express feelings and emotions. These messages are much more difficult to communicate, hear, and perceive than cognitive messages.

Feelings can be grouped into four major categories: anger, sadness, fear, and happiness. One feeling commonly masks and covers up another. For example, anger may mask fear because fear is at the root of much anger. A cancer patient who appears

Table 11-1	Nonverbal Cues in a Communicative Relationship

Cue	Example
Eye contact*	Steady or shifty and avoiding
Eyes	Open, teary, closed, and excessively blinking
Body position	Relaxed, leaning (toward or away), and tense
Mouth	Loose, smiling, tight, and lip biting
Facial expression	Animated, pained, bland, and distant
Arms	Unfolded and folded
Body posture	Relaxed, slouching, and rigid
Voice	Slow, whispering, high-pitched, fast, and cracking
General appearance	Clean, neat, well-groomed, and sloppy

*Eye contact may vary in appropriateness based on cultural differences (e.g., Chinese persons do not consider eye contact appropriate with strangers, and Native Americans feel the eyes are the window to the soul).

Box 11-3	Exercise for Nonverbal Cues

What do the following gestures mean to you? When you have completed this exercise, compare your answers with those of your classmates. Do you have different perceptions?
1. A patient refuses to talk and avoids eye contact with you.
2. A patient looks directly into your eyes and stretches her hands out with the palms up.
3. The patient with whom you are talking holds one arm behind her back and clenches her hand tightly while using the other hand to make a fist at her side.
4. A patient walks into the examination room for a radiation therapy consultation with the doctor, sits erect, and clasps his folded arms across his chest before saying a word.
5. A patient sits in the waiting room, slouches in his chair, says nothing, and has tears streaming down his cheeks.

Reflective listening involves responding with empathy. *Empathy* is defined as identifying with the feelings, thoughts, or experiences of another person. To arrive at the way the other person feels, the health care provider may ask inwardly, "If I were in this person's position, how would I feel?" A critical part of empathy is sharing feelings about the person's verbal communication. For example, empathic responses include, "Yes, I understand that... I would feel angry, too," and "Yes, I'm glad that... It would make me feel good, too."

People rarely communicate in a direct manner concerning the thoughts and feelings that they are having. Reflective listening is a way for a person to listen and communicate effectively. The consequences of good reflective listening are as follows:

- The person becomes aware of small problems and prevents them from developing into major problems.
- The person is perceived by others as genuinely concerned, warm, understanding, and fair.
- The person has more knowledge about others, which helps in relating to them in a real way.

Reflective listening is not the only form of verbal response that radiation therapists can use. Reflective listening is essential to developing verbal responses appropriate for the issues involved. The following are 10 of the most commonly used and helpful verbal responses.

1. ***Minimal verbal response:*** *Minimal responses* are the verbal counterpart to the occasional head nodding. These are verbal clues such as "Yes," "Uh huh," and "I see" and indicate that the health care provider is listening to and understanding the patient.
2. ***Reflecting:*** *Reflecting* refers to health care providers communicating their understanding of the patient's concerns and perspectives. Health care workers can reflect the specific content or implied feelings of their nonverbal observations or communication they feel has been omitted or emphasized. The following are examples of reflecting: "You're feeling uncomfortable about finishing your treatments," "Sounds as

to be extremely angry may be afraid but not able to honestly show fear. Box 11-4 indicating cognitive and affective responses demonstrates the difference between the two levels of responding to patients.

Identifying underlying feelings in verbal messages is difficult at first and is related to a person's comfort level and proficiency in recognizing and expressing personal feelings. The health care professional must listen to patients' messages and identify their feelings rather than project personal feelings onto patients. This ability requires practice and awareness. Different people identify different underlying feelings for the same statement. Careful attention must be given to nonverbal and verbal cues when listening for the true feelings of patients.

 Affective communication involves feelings of anger, sadness, fear, and happiness. The radiation therapist needs to reflectively listen to the patient and to identify what the patient is feeling.

Box 11-4	Exercise for Cognitive and Affective Responses

1. Patient: My skin is getting really red. I think you're burning me up.
   Cognitive response: Are you putting that lotion on your skin?
   Affective response: I hear your discomfort. It sounds like you're uncomfortable with your skin change. These are normal and temporary, and we're watching it every day.
2. Patient: My throat is getting sore. How much more sore is it going to get? I don't want one of those feeding tubes.
   Cognitive response: Are you drinking acidic stuff, smoking, using your magic mouthwash?
   Affective response: Sounds like the idea of a feeding tube is really frightening. That's not what happens with sore throats. The worst scenario is if it gets too sore, you'll have a couple days off!
3. Patient: It's only the second day of treatment and I have diarrhea!
   Cognitive response: Well, what have you eaten?
   Affective response: It's really kind of early for any diarrhea. What else do you think might be causing the diarrhea? Let's see the doctor and ask what she thinks.
4. Patient: I'm still in so much pain! When does this radiation start to work?
   Cognitive response: Are you taking your pain medication?
   Affective response: I'm sorry you're hurting. Everybody is different and sometimes it takes longer to get pain relief.
5. Patient: I sure am having trouble going to sleep. Is that normal?
   Cognitive response: Well, how long is it taking you to go to sleep?
   Affective response: Tell me what kinds of things are going through your mind while you're going to sleep.
6. Patient: I have a question and it's probably stupid, but I'm going to ask it anyway.
   Cognitive response: No questions are stupid.
   Affective response: I always appreciate patients who ask questions. It helps me know the things that are important to you.

if you're really angry at this disease," and "You really resent being treated like you're sick."

3. ***Paraphrasing:*** A *paraphrase* is a verbal statement that is interchangeable with a patient's statement. The words may be synonyms of words the patient has used. Paraphrasing acknowledges to patients that they are really being heard. The following is an example:

Patient: "I had a really bad night last night."
Therapist: "Things didn't go well for you last night."

4. ***Probing:*** *Probing* is an open-ended statement used to obtain more information. It is most effective when using statements such as "I'm wondering about...," "Tell me more about that," and "Could you be saying...?" in a smooth and flowing style. These statements facilitate much more open conversation than asking "how," "what," "when," "where," or "who" questions.

5. ***Clarifying:*** *Clarifying* is used to obtain more information about vague, ambiguous, or conflicting statements. Examples include the following: "I'm confused about...," "I'm having trouble understanding...," "Is it that...?" and "Sounds to me like you're saying...."

6. ***Interpreting:*** *Interpreting* occurs when the therapist adds something to the patient's statement or tries to help the patient understand underlying feelings. Health care providers may share their interpretation, the meaning, or the facts, thus providing the patient with an opportunity to confirm, deny, or offer an alternative interpretation. The patient may respond by saying, "Yes, that's it" or "No, not that but...."

7. ***Checking out:*** *Checking out* occurs when therapists are genuinely confused about their perceptions of the patient's verbal or nonverbal behavior or have a hunch that should be examined. Examples are, "Does it seem as if...?" and "I have a hunch that this feeling is familiar to you; are you

saying...?" Therapists ask the patient to confirm or correct their perception or understanding of the patient's words.

8. ***Informing:*** *Informing* occurs when the therapist shares objective and factual information. An example is, "Your white blood cell count is extremely low, so it would be safer for you to avoid large crowds where the chances are higher of being exposed to bacteria and viruses."

9. ***Confronting:*** *Confronting* involves therapists making the patient aware that their observations are not consistent with the patient's words. This response must be done with respect for the patient and extreme tact so that a defensive response is not elicited. An example of this is, "You say you're angry and depressed, yet you're smiling."

10. ***Summarizing:*** By *summarizing* the therapist condenses and puts in order the information communicated. This is extremely helpful when a patient rambles and has difficulty conveying the sequence of events. An example is, "I hear you saying...."

Box 11-5 is designed to help the individual to learn to recognize and identify the types of major verbal responses just discussed. Box 11-6 is designed to help the individual to listen for feelings.

 By using the 10 verbal responses, empathetic communication can be accomplished.

THE MULTIDISCIPLINARY APPROACH TO THE ASSESSMENT OF CANCER PATIENTS

General Health Assessment

One method of health assessment is the self-report. In a self-report, individuals disclose their perception of what is being measured. Box 11-7 demonstrates a self-assessment tool that is

---

| **Box 11-5** | **Exercise for Recognizing and Identifying the Types of Major Verbal Responses** |

Read the following patient and therapist statements, and identify the therapist's response in each case as one of the 10 major verbal responses: minimal verbal response, paraphrasing, probing, reflecting, clarifying, checking out, interpreting, confronting, informing, or summarizing.*

1. Patient: I can't decide what to do. Nothing seems right.
   Caregiver: You're feeling pretty frustrated, and you want me to tell you what to do.
2. Patient: In our family the children don't do any of the work around the house.
   Caregiver: The children in your family don't do any housework.
3. Patient: My wife made me late for treatment today.
   Caregiver: Tell me more about that.
4. Patient: Do you think this is a good cancer center?
   Caregiver: The XYZ Association has ranked this cancer center number one in the state.
5. Patient: I guess that about covers it.
   Caregiver: Let's see if we can review what we've talked about today.... Does this seem right to you?

6. Patient: That's why I'm here. Dr. Jones said you were a good one to talk to.
   Caregiver: Let's see now. You want me to help you decide whether or not you should file for disability. Is that right?
7. Patient: Nobody in this world cares about anyone else.
   Caregiver: It's scary to feel that nobody at all cares about you.
8. Patient: Anyway, I'm unable to do it because it's too expensive. Besides, they won't help me anyway.
   Caregiver: Let me get this straight. You feel the tests will cost too much, and the results won't be worth the cost. Is that it?
9. Patient: I don't want to talk about it.
   Caregiver: You've told me that being open and honest about your illness is important to you, but you aren't willing to do that just now.
10. Patient: I have to go to the grocery store before picking up the children on the way home from my treatment.
    Caregiver: Oh, I see....

*See the Answer Key on the Evolve website for the answers to this exercise.

Box 11-6	Exercise for Listening for Feelings

For each of the following statements, write what you think the person is really feeling. Ask yourself, "What are the underlying feelings here?"*

1. The doctor told me to come over here and have all these tests. I'll sit over here and wait until you're ready for me.
2. Have you heard anything about the new social worker? I'm supposed to see her at 3 PM.
3. Coming for treatment just doesn't seem to be helping me.
4. Are you going to see me again this week, Doctor?
5. Only 2 more weeks and I'm finished with my treatments.

*Discuss your answers with a small group in your class. Then look at all the possible answers in the Answer Key on the Evolve website.

useful in decreasing documentation time by the oncology professional while eliciting comprehensive information.

An alternative assessment method is for the oncology practitioner to do an interview. This often is done by the oncology nurse or radiation oncologist, but a radiation therapist may also conduct the interview. The history includes the collection of data about the past and present health of each patient. A historical and physical evaluation should come from a referring physician, but a verification and current assessment should also be done.

Physical Assessment

Table 11-2 lists physical aspects a therapist is responsible to assess daily and interventions for treatment. Some assessments are relative to the area being treated with radiation therapy. Specific areas in the physical realm in which assessment of

Box 11-7	Functional Health Pattern Patient Self-Assessment*

HEALTH PERCEPTION AND HEALTH MANAGEMENT
- Who provides your health and dental care?
- How often do you see your doctor and dentist?
- List the medication(s) you take. How much? How often?
- How much alcohol do you drink in a week?
- Do you smoke cigarettes or cigars? If so, how much?
- What allergies do you have? What happens when you have an allergic reaction?
- What other medical problems do you have?

NUTRITIONAL METABOLIC PATTERN
- Are you on any special diet?
- What did you eat yesterday (over the past 24 hours)?
- How much fluid do you drink each day?
- List the vitamins you take each day.
- Have you noticed any changes in your appetite? If yes, describe.
- Have you noticed any changes in your weight? If yes, describe.
- What foods do you avoid?
- Who cooks your meals?
- Do you wear dentures or partial plates?
- How do you take care of your skin? (What creams, lotions, or powders are you using?)
- Do you take baths or showers? How often?

ELIMINATION PATTERN
- How often do you move your bowels?
- Do you have problems with diarrhea, constipation, or loss of control?
- What foods and medications do you use to regulate your bowels (laxatives, prunes, bran, and others)?
- How many times a day do you urinate?
- Have you had any changes such as loss of control, burning, frequency, or difficulty urinating?

ACTIVITY AND EXERCISE PATTERN
- Do you feel tired during the day? Is this new?
- What changes have you noticed in your energy level?
- What exercises do you do? How often?
- What do you do for relaxation and fun?
- Do you need help with ambulating, bathing, toileting, dressing, grooming, feeding, cooking, food shopping, housecleaning, or food preparation?

SLEEP AND REST PATTERN
- What time do you go to bed?
- What time do you get up?
- Do you have any problems sleeping?
- How do you feel when you wake up?
- Do you take any medications to help you sleep?

COGNITIVE AND PERCEPTUAL PATTERN
- Are you having problems hearing?
- Have you noticed any recent changes in your hearing?
- Do you use any hearing aids?
- Have you noticed any changes in your vision?
- How often do you have your eyes examined?
- Do you wear glasses or contact lenses?
- Are you experiencing any pain? If yes, where is the pain located? Describe it.
- What do you do to manage your pain?
- How does the pain affect your lifestyle?
- What is your occupation?

ROLES AND RELATIONSHIPS PATTERN
- What is your marital status?
- Do you have children and grandchildren?
- With whom do you live?
- What changes in your family roles or relationships have you noticed since your illness?
- How do you anticipate that the radiation treatment will affect your daily routine?
- What is the best time for your radiation treatment?

SELF-PERCEPTION AND CONCEPTUAL PATTERN
- How would you describe yourself?
- What are your strengths and weaknesses?

SEXUAL AND REPRODUCTIVE PATTERN
- Are you sexually active?
- Do you use any form of birth control?
- Have you had any changes in sexual relations?

COPING AND STRESS-MANAGEMENT PATTERN
- How do you handle major problems and stresses in your life?
- How are you coping with your life and diagnosis?
- What do you do to relax?
- What are your concerns regarding your treatment?

Box 11-7	Functional Health Pattern Patient Self-Assessment—cont'd

VALUE AND BELIEF PATTERN
- What is important in your life?
- Describe your spiritual needs.
- What part does religion play in your lifestyle?

LIFE AND LIFESTYLE PATTERNS
- Describe your usual day.
- What means of transportation do you have?

Modified from Hirshfield-Bartek J, Dow KH, Creaton E: Decreasing documentation time using a patient self-assessment tool, *Oncol Nurs Forum* 17:251-255, 1990. Courtesy Beth Israel Hospital, Boston, Massachusetts.
*In the actual form, space is provided for patients' responses.

the cancer patient is paramount include nutrition, pain, and biochemical balance (blood counts).

Nutritional Assessment

Nutritional assessment involves the multidisciplinary oncology team. Oncology nurses are in an ideal position for the initial assessment of cancer patients and referrals to the nutrition specialist, or dietitian. In addition, therapists' awareness and knowledge in this area enable them to monitor patients under treatment and make appropriate referrals when needed.

Maintaining a good nutritional status is one of the most difficult challenges in treating cancer patients. Nutritional assessment is the critical first step in developing a comprehensive approach to the nutritional management of individuals

Table 11-2	Components of Daily Physical Assessment—Specific and Nonspecific Effects	
Side Effects	**Dose**	**Interventions**
SPECIFIC EFFECTS		
Skin reactions	1600 cGy	Instruct the patient to do the following:
• Faint erythema	2000-3000 cGy	• Assess and monitor skin integrity and changes.
• Erythema	3000-4000 cGy	• Use a prescribed moisturizing lotion after showering, and avoid port marks.
• Dry desquamation	4000-6000 cGy	• Avoid creams that contain alcohol.
• Moist desquamation		• Avoid exposing the treated area to heat, cold, wind, soaps, deodorant, and razor shaving.
		If skin erythema occurs, do the following:
		• Use moisturizing lotion according to the physician's orders.
		• Protect skin from further irritation, and wear loose cotton clothes.
		If skin breakdown occurs, do the following:
		• If dry desquamation has occurred, continue to use moisturizing lotion.
		• If the skin is tender, use cortisone cream as directed.
		• For moist desquamation, use Burrow's compresses, silver sulfadiazine creams per the physician's prescriptions or moist healing techniques. (The physician may consider temporarily stopping further treatment.)
		• Try to aerate areas of skin breakdown, especially in skinfolds.
Epilation/alopecia (hair loss)	2000 cGy	Protect the scalp from heat, cold, and wind. Suggest an appropriate head covering.
		Do the following to minimize scalp irritation:
		• Avoid frequent shampooing.
		• Avoid using blow dryers, hairsprays, gels, or other hair preparations.
		• Apply moisturizing lotion to the scalp.
		Explore issues related to body image (e.g., getting a wig or hairpiece at the start of treatment).
Mouth changes	All occur between	Inspect the oral cavity.
• Stomatitis	2000 and 3000 cGy	Assess the presence of stomatitis, xerostomia, mucositis, and taste changes.
• Xerostomia		Instruct the patient about a soft, bland diet.
• Mucositis		
• Taste alterations		
Pharyngitis	2000-3000 cGy	Assess pain during swallowing (dysphagia).
Laryngitis	4000 cGy	Modify the diet to soft, nonspicy, and nonacidic foods.
Esophagitis	2000-3000 cGy	Use topical anesthetics and analgesics as prescribed (lidocaine mixed with Mylanta or Maalox [1:3]).
		Assess cough.
Nausea and vomiting	1000-2000 cGy	Anticipate nausea and vomiting in high-risk patients, and prevent nausea and vomiting by using antiemetics prophylactically before treatment and as needed continuously.
		Provide fluids to prevent dehydration.
		Refer or instruct the patient on a low-fat and low-sugar diet.
		Use nonpharmacologic measures such as relaxation and guided imagery.

Continued

Table 11-2	Components of Daily Physical Assessment—Specific and Nonspecific Effects—cont'd	
Side Effects	**Dose**	**Interventions**
Diarrhea/colic	2000-5000 cGy	Assess the bowel function.
Cystitis	3000-4000 cGy	• Instruct the patient on a low-residue diet for use as diarrhea occurs.
		• Use antispasmodic medications as prescribed.
		• Instruct the patient on perianal care.
		Assess the bladder function.
		• Monitor for urinary retention or hematuria.
		• Use antispasmodic medications as prescribed.
		• Monitor for bladder infections.
Pain	Associated with inflammatory reactions at varying doses	Assess the location and intensity. Instruct the patient on the importance of taking medications regularly.
NONSPECIFIC EFFECTS		
Skin pallor		Monitor low hemoglobin, white blood cell count, and platelet levels with weekly complete blood counts (CBCs).
Weight loss		Monitor once per week, and chart the results.
		Determine eating problems.
Fatigue		Assess the energy level.
		Determine periods of increased fatigue.
		Assist patients to pace activities and listen to their bodies.
		Ensure adequate nutritional intake.
Sleep		Assess normal sleep patterns and changes.
		Evaluate the cause of problems.

cGy, Centigray.

All doses are based on a 180 to 200-cGy daily fractionation schedule, and side effects will occur earlier if the patient is having or had chemotherapy.

with cancer. A complete list of components involved in nutritional assessment is outlined in Box 11-8.

If malnutrition is diagnosed, a plan of intervention is developed and implemented based on the information obtained in the nutritional assessment.

Weight loss is often the first physical change that alerts individuals with cancer to seek medical treatment. It is also frequently the first sign of malnutrition.

Specifically, the percent weight change is the most accurate measure of nutritional status. The percent weight change indicates

---

Box 11-8 Components of the Nutritional Assessment

MEDICAL HISTORY
- Duration and type of malignancy
- Frequency, type, and severity of complications (e.g., infections and draining lesions)
- Type and duration of therapy
- Specific chemotherapeutic agents used
- Radiation sites
- Antibiotics used
- Other drugs used
- Surgical procedures performed (site, type, and date)
- Side effects of therapy (diarrhea, anorexia, nausea, and vomiting)
- Concomitant medical conditions (diabetes, heart disease, liver failure, kidney failure, and infection)

PHYSICAL EXAMINATION
- General appearance
- Condition of hair
- Condition of skin
- Condition of teeth
- Condition of mouth, gums, and throat

- Edema
- Performance status
- Identification of nutritionally related problems (fistula, pain, stomatitis, xerostomia, infection, constipation diarrhea, nausea, vomiting, and obstruction)

DIETARY HISTORY
- 24-hour recall of foods eaten, including snacks
- Composition of food taken in 24 hours (calories and protein, caffeine, and liquor)
- Time of day meals and snacks are eaten
- Past or current diet modifications
- Self-feeding ability
- Special cancer diet
- Vitamins, minerals, or other supplements
- Modifications of diet or eating habits as a result of treatment or illness
- Foods withheld or given on the basis of personal or religious grounds (e.g., kosher, vegetarian)
- Food preferences
- Food allergies or intolerances

Box 11-8	Components of the Nutritional Assessment—cont'd

SOCIOECONOMIC HISTORY

- Number of persons living in the home (ages and relationships)
- Kitchen facilities
- Income
- Food purchased
- Food prepared
- Amount spent on food per month
- Outside provision of meals

ANTHROPOMETRIC DATA

- Height
- Weight
- Actual weight as percentage of ideal
- Weight change as percentage of usual
- Triceps skinfold measurement
- Actual triceps skinfold as percentage of standard
- Midarm circumference
- Midarm muscle circumference
- Actual midarm muscle circumference as percentage of standard

BIOCHEMICAL DATA

- Hematocrit
- Hemoglobin
- Serum albumin
- Serum transferrin
- Creatinine
- Creatinine height index
- Total lymphocyte count
- Delayed hypersensitivity response—skin testing
- Nitrogen balance
- Blood urea nitrogen
- Sodium, potassium, carbon dioxide, chloride
- Glucose

Modified from Groenwald SL, et al: *Nutritional disturbances: cancer nursing principles and practice,* ed 3, Boston, 1993, Jones & Bartlett.

the extent of tissue loss as a result of inadequate nutrition. For this reason, monitoring weight change weekly is imperative for patients who are undergoing radiation therapy. A calculation of a percent weight change is found in Table 11-3.

Nutritional Consequences of Cancer. Anorexia (loss of appetite resulting in weight loss) is a major contributor in the cause of cancer cachexia. **Cachexia** is a state of general ill health and malnutrition with early satiety; electrolyte and water imbalances; and progressive loss of body weight, fat, and muscle. Cachexia affects half to two thirds of patients with cancer.

Anorexia and taste alterations are two of the major causes of protein-calorie malnutrition in patients with cancer. The three forms of protein-calorie malnutrition are marasmus, kwashiorkor, and marasmus-kwashiorkor mix.

Marasmus, or calorie malnutrition, can be observed in patients who are slender or slightly underweight. It is characterized by weight loss of 7% to 10% and fat and muscle depletion. *Kwashiorkor,* or protein malnutrition, is seen in patients with an adequate intake of carbohydrates and fats but an inadequate intake of protein. Kwashiorkor in patients is often initially overlooked because they appear well nourished. This condition is characterized by retarded growth and development, muscle wasting, depigmentation of the hair and skin, edema, and depression of the cellular immune response. *Marasmus-kwashiorkor mix,* or protein and calorie malnutrition, is the most life-threatening form of malnutrition because it involves the depletion of fat and muscle stores and visceral protein stores. This condition is most commonly found in seriously ill, hospitalized patients who have had inadequate nutritional care throughout their illness. Marasmus-kwashiorkor mix is characterized by weight loss of 10% or greater in a 6-month period, decreased fat and muscle stores, depleted visceral protein stores, and depression of the cellular immune responses.

Pain Assessment

Pain, one of the most feared consequences of cancer, is a complex process that has biologic, social, and spiritual dimensions. All pain is real, regardless of its cause, and most pain is a combination of physiologic and psychogenic factors. This phenomenon is connected to the essence of human existence and often precipitates questions about the meaning of life itself. Pain holds a great deal of power with the cancer patient experiencing it.

Pain assessment has several purposes. First, it establishes a baseline for treatment and interventions. Second, it helps focus which interventions are best for the patient. Third, it enables the evaluation of chosen interventions. Pain assessment should be systematic, organized, and ongoing. In general, certain principles should be followed in evaluating the cancer patient who experiences pain (Box 11-9).

A multidimensional conceptualization of cancer pain as defined by Ahles et al.[1] aids in understanding the scope of cancer pain. They propose five dimensions to consider in assessing and managing the experience of cancer pain: (1) physiologic (organic cause of pain), (2) sensory (intensity, location, and quality), (3) affective (depression and anxiety), (4) cognitive

Table 11-3	Evaluation of Weight Change*	
Time	**Significant Weight Loss**	**Severe Weight Loss**
1 wk	1%-2%	>2%
1 mo	5%	>5%
3 mo	7.5%	>7.5%
6 mo	10%	>10%

From Blackburn GL, et al: Nutritional and metabolic assessment of the hospitalized patient, *J Parent Enteral Nutr* 1:17, 1977.
*Values charged are for percent weight change.

$$\text{Percent weight change} = \frac{\text{Usual weight} - \text{Actual weight}}{\text{Usual weight}} \times 100$$

- Believe the patient's complaint of pain.
- Take a careful history of the patient's pain complaint.
- Evaluate the patient's psychological state.
- Perform a careful medical and neurologic examination.
- Order and review appropriate diagnostic studies.
- Treat the pain to facilitate the appropriate workup.
- Reassess the patient's response to therapy.
- Individualize the diagnostic and therapeutic approaches.
- Discuss advance directives with the patient and family.

(the manner in which pain influences a person's thought processes and the way people view themselves or the meaning of pain), and (5) behavioral (pain-related behaviors such as medication intake and activity level).

McGuire[18] proposes a sixth dimension: sociocultural. This dimension involves the effects of cultural, social, and demographic factors that are related to the experience of pain.

Physiologic Dimension. Foley[10] described three types of pain (each with a different cause) observed in cancer patients: (1) pain associated with direct tumor involvement, (2) pain associated with cancer therapy, and (3) pain unrelated to the tumor or its treatment.

Two important characteristics of pain are related to the cause of pain: the duration and pattern of pain. *Duration* refers to whether pain is acute or chronic.

- *Acute* pain generally has a sudden onset with an identifiable cause lasting 3 to 6 months and responds to treatment with analgesic drug therapy and treatment of its precipitating cause.
- *Chronic* pain is the persistence of pain for more than 3 months with a less well-defined onset. Its cause may not be known.

The second characteristic related to the cause of pain (*the pattern of pain*) has three separate patterns: (1) brief, momentary, or transient; (2) rhythmic, periodic, or intermittent; and (3) continuous, steady, or constant. Melzack[20] first described these patterns in the McGill Pain Questionnaire (MPQ).

Sensory Dimension. The second dimension (sensory) as set forth by Ahles et al.[1] consists of pain location, intensity, and quality. The first component of establishing the location of pain is extremely important. One of the methods that can be used is to ask the patient to point with one finger to the site of the pain. Another method is to use a picture of the body and ask the patient to mark on the picture the location of the pain.

The second component is the intensity of the pain (i.e., the strength of its feeling). Intensity is the most commonly assessed aspect of pain. The goal is to translate the patient's description of intensity into numbers or words to provide an objective description. Visual analog scales (VASs) and categorical scales are commonly used to quantify the intensity of pain. A VAS rates 0 (no pain) to 10 (severe pain). A categorical scale also has a numerical system with 0 (no pain), 1 (mild), 2 (discomforting), 3 (distressing), 4 (horrible), and 5 (excruciating). Descriptions of the pain may be helpful in determining its origin and implementing effective measures for its control. For example, burning, hot pain may indicate the involvement of nerve tissue.

The third component of the sensory dimension is the quality of pain (i.e., the way it actually feels). In the MPQ, some of the most common terms used to describe the quality of pain are as follows: aching, hot-burning, sharp, tender, throbbing, cramping, stabbing, heavy, shooting and gnawing, splitting, tiring-exhausting, sickening, and fearful.

Affective Dimension. The third dimension (affective) as defined by Ahles et al.[1] consists of depression, anxiety, and other psychological factors or personality traits associated with pain. Anxiety and depression are critical factors that affect a patient's response to pain and ability to tolerate and cope with pain, because anxiety often increases pain. Assessing which measures can be taken to decrease the pain is essential.

Cognitive Dimension. The fourth dimension (cognitive) involves the way that pain influences thought processes or the way that people view themselves. A patient can be asked, "Are there any thoughts or images that may make your pain worse?" Some patients experience pain based on faulty logic. The following are examples of problem thinking by patients: "Nothing can be done to control the pain," "Pain is inevitable and should be tolerated," and "Doctors do not want to be bothered with complaints of pain." If undetected, these thoughts impair the assessment and management of pain.

Behavioral Dimension. The fifth dimension (behavioral) includes a variety of observable behaviors related to pain. The assessment of pain behavior can include verbal and nonverbal responses such as moans, grimaces, and complaints. Estimates of physical activity are also important aspects of pain behavior. Factors such as physical exercise, time spent in bed, and ability to do chores have been used to measure pain behavior. An excellent tool for this is the Karnofsky Performance Status[35] (Table 11-4).

Table 11-4	**Karnofsky Performance Status**
Score (%)	**Status**
100	Normal—no complaints and no evidence of disease
90	Ability to carry on normal activity—minor signs or symptoms of disease
80	Normal activity with effort—some signs or symptoms of disease
70	Self-care—inability to carry on normal activity or do active work
60	Occasional assistance required but ability to care for most needs
50	Considerable assistance and frequent medical care required
40	Disability—special care and assistance required
30	Severe disability—hospitalization indicated, although death not imminent
20	Extreme sickness—hospitalization and active supportive treatment neccessary
10	Moribund status—fatal processes progressing rapidly
0	Death

Modified from Yates JW, Chalmer B, McKegney FP: Evaluation of patients with advanced cancer using the Karnofsky Performance Status, *CA Cancer J Clin* 45:2220-2224, 1980.

The use of analgesics and other treatments should also be considered in the assessment of pain behavior. The type and amount of drug and the way the dose is scheduled are important. Patients are often afraid of narcotic pain medications and take them only after they are in pain. Therapists should encourage regular dosing and explain the importance of a stable blood-serum level, which is needed to interrupt the pain cycle. The duration of the effect of the drug and any mood change on administration should be noted.

Sociocultural Dimension. The last dimension (proposed by McGuire[18] and added to Ahles et al.'s five dimensions[1]) consists of a variety of ethnic, cultural, demographic, spiritual, and related factors that influence a person's perception of and response to pain. Cultural and religious practices have a strong influence on the pain experience. Overt actions are accepted in some cultures, whereas other cultures consider such actions weak. A general value held by many Americans is that a good patient does not complain when in pain; a complainer has lost self-control. Unfortunately, health care professionals sometimes directly reinforce these beliefs.

Age, gender, and race may provide different pain experiences. Research shows that females and older individuals have increased verbal expressions of pain.

In considering the six dimensions of cancer pain, a holistic and multidisciplinary approach to assessment and management is essential. As stated, many factors contribute to the pain experience.

The multidimensional concept of cancer pain necessitates the involvement of various health care disciplines in assessment and management. Input is needed from many health care providers, including oncologists, primary physicians, nurses, radiation therapists, social workers, pharmacists, psychologists, anesthesiologists, and occupational therapists.

Tools to assess pain must be simple, short, and relevant for the patient. Pain assessment tools can be classified according to the number of pain dimensions they assess. Multidimensional tools focus on two or more dimensions of the pain experience. Probably the most well-known and best example is the MPQ.[20]

The MPQ has the ability to assess in the sensory, cognitive, affective, and behavioral dimensions. Specifically, the MPQ elicits information about the location of pain; the intensity and periodicity of the pain; symptoms; effects on sleep, activity, and eating; and patterns of the analgesic used. Two long forms and a short form are used.

A similar multidimensional tool is the *Brief Pain Inventory (BPI)*.[5] The BPI was developed primarily for clinical use with patients in pain who were too ill to be subjected to long and exhausting assessment techniques. The BPI assesses the following dimensions: the history and site of pain; the intensity of pain at its worst, at its usual level, and at its present level; medications and treatments used to relieve the pain; the relief obtained; and the effect of pain on mood, interpersonal relations, walking, sleeping, working, and enjoyment of life. The BPI is a self-administered tool.

A third tool is the *Memorial Pain Assessment Card (MPAC)*.[9] The MPAC consists of three visual analog scales. It is a short, easy-to-administer tool that measures pain intensity, pain relief, and

mood by asking the patient to choose from a list of adjectives describing each. It can distinguish pain from psychological distress and can be used to study the subtle interaction of these factors.

A sample questionnaire for an initial pain assessment is shown in Figure 11-1.

Radiation therapists are vital in the ongoing assessment of a patient's pain. Therapists see patients every day and can evaluate the level of pain and the way the patient is responding. Being aware of personal beliefs and biases about pain, learning how to listen and communicate, and asking key questions are imperative skills for holistic health care providers.

Accurate assessment of pain is the first step toward understanding the experience as the patient perceives it. Good assessment promotes an essential therapeutic relationship between patient and caregiver. Assessment is the foundation in the process of finding an effective intervention for the devastating experience of pain for the cancer patient.

Pain assessment has six dimensions, and all are important to consider when treating the whole patient.

Blood Assessment

Hematologic changes in cancer patients are critical for ongoing assessments because hematopoietic tissue exhibits a rapid rate of cellular proliferation. Hematopoietic tissue is especially vulnerable to cancer treatments (chemotherapy and radiation therapy). A **myelosuppression,** a reduction in bone marrow function, often results. The changes that may occur can result in anemia, leukopenia, and thrombocytopenia.

Anemia is a decrease in the peripheral red blood cell count. Without sufficient red blood cells, the circulatory system's oxygen-carrying capacity is impaired. This is due to a decrease in the hemoglobin level in the red blood cell, which serves as the carrier of oxygen from the lungs to tissues. Patients usually experience pale skin, muscle weakness, and fatigue (probably the most pervasive symptom). Normal blood values are found in Table 11-5.

Leukopenia is a decrease in the white blood cell count, thus increasing the risk of infection for the cancer patient. Due to chemotherapy or the disease process itself, patients may already have compromised immune systems. Therefore, monitoring the white blood cell count during treatments is essential. (Refer to Table 11-5 for normal values.) As a consequence of the patients' inability to fight disease, they need to reduce their exposure risks. Patients should be told to have minimal contact with others, especially if someone is sick. Health care workers also need to keep a distance if sick and at work.

Thrombocytopenia is a reduction in the number of circulating platelets. This decrease may be caused by a failure of the bone marrow to produce megakaryocyte cells, the precursors of platelets. This can be a result of various factors, such as chemotherapy, radiation therapy, the disease, or stress. The most significant factor that determines the risk of bone marrow depression related to radiation therapy is the volume of productive bone marrow in the radiation field. Therefore with large fields, monitoring counts is extremely important. Normal values for platelets can be found in Table 11-5.

Date _____

Patient's Name _____   Age _____ Room _____

Diagnosis _____   Physician _____

Therapist /Nurse_____

Location The patient or therapist marks the drawing.

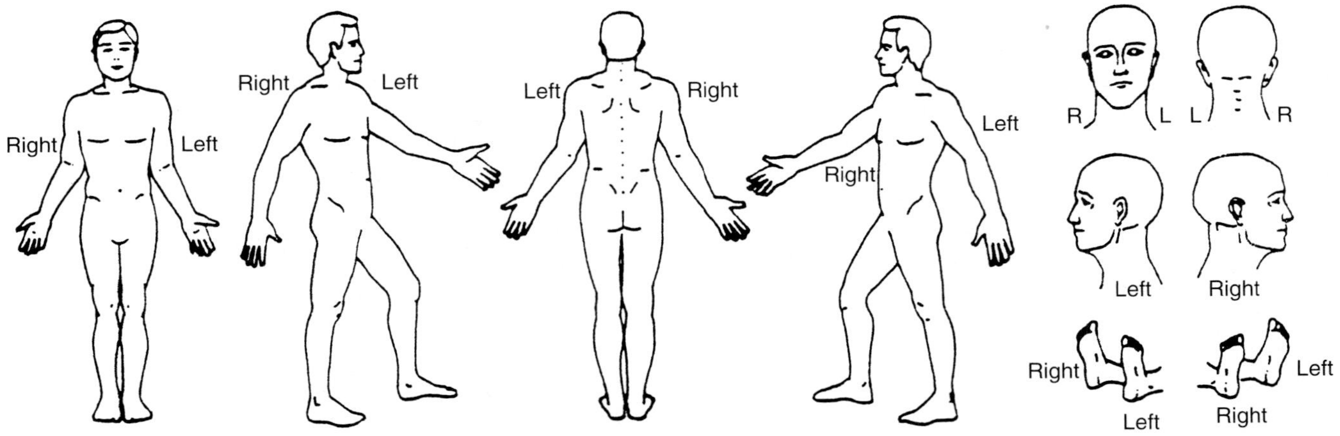

Intensity   The patient rates the pain.

Scale used: _____

Present level of pain: _____

Worst level of pain: _____

Best level of pain: _____

Acceptable level of pain: _____

Quality   Use the patient's own words (e.g., "prick," "ache," "burn," "throb," "pull," "sharp")

_____

Onset Duration, Variation, and Rhythms   _____

Manner of Expressing Pain _____

What Relieves the Pain? _____

What Causes or Increases the Pain? _____

Effects of Pain (Note the decreased function and decreased quality of life)

Accompanying symptoms (e.g., nausea): _____

Sleep: _____

Appetite: _____

Physical activity: _____

Relationship with others (e.g., irritability): _____

Emotions (e.g., angry, suicidal, crying): _____

Concentration: _____

Other: _____

Other Comments _____

Plan _____

Figure 11-1. Pain Assessment Questionnaire. (Modified from McCaffery M, Beebe A: *Pain: Clinical manual for nursing practice,* St. Louis, 1989, Mosby.)

Table 11-5	Normal Blood Values*	
Level		**Percentage/Range**
Hematocrit (Hct)		
Men		45 (38-54)
Women		40 (36-47)
Hemoglobin (Hgb)†		
Men		14-18 g/dL
Women		12-16 g/dL
Children		12-14 g/dL
Blood Counts	**Per Cubic Millimeter**	**Percentage**
Erythrocytes (RBCs)		
Men	5 (4.5-6) × 10	100
Women	4.5 (4.3-5.5) × 10	100
Reticulocytes	0-1	
Total leukocytes (WBCs)	5000-10,000	100
Polymorphonuclear leukocytes‡	2500-6000	40-60
Bands	0-500	0-5
Lymphocytes	1000-4000	20-40
Eosinophils	50-300	1-3
Basophils	0-100	0-1
Monocytes	200-800	4-8
Platelets	200,000-500,000 (severely low <20,000)	100

*Values may vary slightly according to the laboratory methods used.
†Severely low <7.5 g/dL.
‡Granulocytes, segmented neutrophils, and polymorphonuclear cells.
RBCs, Red blood cells; *WBCs,* white blood cells.

Psychosocial Assessment

Quality of Life. A growing attention to the quality of life of cancer patients reflects the changing attitude of society and health care personnel. The value of cancer treatments is judged not only on survival but also on the quality of that survival. The term **quality of life** has emerged in recent years to summarize the broad-based assessment of the combined effect of disease and treatment and the trade-off between the two.

Cancer and its treatment, perhaps more than any other medical condition, become a major determinant of a patient's quality of life. The suggestion has been made in the literature that the emotional repercussions of cancer far exceed those of any other disease, and the emotional suffering cancer generates may actually exceed the physical suffering it causes. Therefore, good quality-of-life information can make a major contribution in improving the management of cancer patients.

A more general definition of quality of life is a person's subjective sense of well-being derived from personal experience of life as a whole. The areas of life, or domains, most important to individuals resultantly have the most influence on their quality of life.

General agreement exists that the domains of quality of life for assessment should include physical, psychological, and social factors. In the physical domain, the quality of life is affected by loss of function, symptoms, and limited activity as a result of the disease process and physical effects of treatments. In the psychological domain, five major emotional themes have been identified: (1) fear and anxiety generated by the diagnosis and compounded by inadequate communication with caregivers, (2) loss of personal control associated with the need to be dependent on those administering treatment, (3) uncertainty about the outcome of treatments, (4) the physician's persistent enthusiasm for cure, and (5) the debilitating effect of standard cancer treatments. In addition, loss of self-esteem and feelings of anxiety, depression, resentment, anger, discouragement, helplessness, hopelessness, isolation, and rejection are common.

Assessment. Many measures are available to assess quality of life or health-related quality of life. This is, however, a double-edged sword. Those doing the assessing have choices and can choose tools based on specific characteristics of a particular disease site. However, this divides potential data and makes comparisons of studies and research much more difficult. The following are some of the assessment tools* available to examine quality of life.

Quality of Life Index. The Quality of Life Index (QLI)[25] focuses on the present (within the last week) quality of a person's life. It clusters 14 items in three groups: general physical condition, normal human quality, and general attitudes as they relate to general quality of life. The patient responds by placing an X on a linear slide. The QLI can be found in Figure 11-2.

Normal refers to the normal status before illness. The QLI is easy to use and practical. It has reliability and validity in its statistical components.

Functional Living Index—Cancer. The Functional Living Index—Cancer (FLIC)[29] is a 22-item scale on which patients indicate the effect of cancer on day-to-day living issues that assess the functional quality of life. It uses a 7-point Likert-type scale. This scale is often used in measuring attitudes and in the following ranges: strongly agree, agree, slightly agree, undecided, slightly disagree, disagree, and strongly disagree. This tool has been used extensively in oncology with predominantly positive results.

Functional Assessment of Cancer Therapy Scale. The Functional Assessment of Cancer Therapy (FACT) Scale[4] has 28 items and specifies subscales that reflect symptoms or problems associated with different diseases (head and neck, breast, bladder, colorectal, and lung cancers). The results yield information on the patient's well-being, social and family well-being, relationship with the physician, emotional well-being, and specific disease concerns. A form of this tool, called the *FACT–G,* can be found in Figure 11-3. This tool can also distinguish stages, metastatic from nonmetastatic diseases, and inpatients from outpatients.

Assessment tools can be used to determine the effect of cancer on the patient and result in additional interventions.

---

*These tools are several of the cancer-specific, health-related, quality-of-life measures and approaches that are yielding good results.

With respect to your general physical condition, please place an X on the line at the point that best shows what is happening to you at the present time (within the past week):

GENERAL PHYSICAL CONDITION

1. How much *pain* are you feeling?   None _____ Excruciating
2. How much *nausea* do you experience?   None _____ Constant nausea
3. How frequently do you *vomit?*   Not at all _____ Constant vomiting or retching
4. How much *strength* do you feel?   None _____ Normal for me
5. How much *appetite* do you have?   None _____ Normal for me

IMPORTANT HUMAN ACTIVITIES

6. Are you able to *work* at your usual tasks (e.g., housework, office work, and gardening)?   Not at all _____ Normal for me
7. Are you able to *eat?*   Not at all _____ Normal for me
8. Are you able to obtain *sexual* satisfaction?   Not at all _____ Normal for me
9. Are you able to *sleep* well?   Not at all _____ Normal for me

GENERAL QUALITY OF LIFE

10. How good is your quality of life (general QL)?   Extremely poor _____ Excellent
11. Are you having *fun* (e.g., hobbies, recreation, and social activities)?   Not at all _____ Normal for me
12. Is your life *satisfying?*   Not at all _____ Normal for me
13. Do you feel *useful?*   Not at all _____ Normal for me
14. Do you *worry about the cost* of medical care?   Not at all _____ A great deal

Figure 11-2. Quality of Life Index. (Modified from Padilla GV et al: Quality of Life index for patients with cancer, *Res Nurs Health* 6:117-126, 1983.)

Coping Strategies and Responses—The Patient. Over the past several decades, a great deal of interest has been focused on assessing an individual's psychosocial adjustments to illness. The areas that compose the realm of psychosocial issues are numerous.

The affective responses that occur most commonly among cancer patients are anxiety and depression. The discussion about tools for assessment focuses on these two major areas.

A working definition for *anxiety* is an individual responding to a perceived threat affectively at an emotional level with an increased level of arousal associated with vague, unpleasant, and uneasy feelings. The instrument used most often to measure anxiety in cancer patients is the State-Trait Anxiety Inventory (STAI).[31] The STAI is composed of two scales: the A-trait and A-state. On the A-state are 20 items with a 4-point scale with the following possible responses: not at all, somewhat, moderately so, and very much. Responses are summed to measure the way the patient feels at a particular moment. Scores demonstrate the level of transitory anxiety characterized by feelings of apprehension; tension; and autonomic nervous system–induced symptoms that are worry, nervousness, and apprehension. The A-trait inventory is designed to measure a general level of arousal and predict anxiety proneness. Construct validity and reliability are established for this tool.

Irwin et al.[14] conducted a study of 181 patients receiving external beam radiation and found that all patients (males and females) exhibited higher anxiety scores than nonpatient norms before treatment. In this sample, higher anxiety scores were reported among females over males before treatment began, 1 week after treatment was completed, and 2 months after the completion of therapy. In general, patients showed significantly higher anxiety during rather than after treatment.

Every patient brings a history of **coping strategies** to the cancer experience. Patients use whatever has worked for them in the past in managing their anxiety. Box 11-10 lists effective and noneffective coping strategies.

Depression is the second most common affective response in cancer patients. Depression is defined as the perceived loss of self-esteem resulting in a cluster of affective behavioral (change in appetite, sleep disturbances, lack of energy, withdrawal, and dependency) and cognitive (decreased ability to concentrate, indecisiveness, and suicidal ideas) responses. Depression plays a major role in the quality of life for cancer patients and their families. However, empirical and clinical reports indicate that depression is an underdiagnosed and probably undertreated response among persons with cancer.

Knowing the way to recognize depression is a critical skill for all oncology health care providers. Instances have been cited of patients with undiagnosed depression who returned home and committed suicide after receiving a radiation therapy treatment. The physicians, nurses, and therapists thought that the patient who was experiencing severe sequelae in the head and neck radiation treatments was just a "quiet person." The signs of depression were present, and no referral was made to a professional. The criteria for recognizing a depressed condition are the following (usually four of these are present nearly every day for at least 2 weeks):

1. Poor appetite or significant weight loss or increased appetite or significant weight gain

FACT-G (version 4)

Patient's Name _____ Age _____ Room _____

Diagnosis _____ Physician _____

Below is a list of statements that other people with your illness have said are important. By circling one (1) number per line, please indicate how true each statement has been for you during the past 7 days.

		Not at all	A little bit	Some-what	Quite a bit	Very much
PHYSICAL WELL-BEING						
GP1	I have a lack of energy	0	1	2	3	4
GP2	I have nausea	0	1	2	3	4
GP3	Because of my physical condition, I have trouble meeting the needs of my family	0	1	2	3	4
GP4	I have pain	0	1	2	3	4
GP5	I am bothered by side effects of treatment	0	1	2	3	4
GP6	I feel ill	0	1	2	3	4
GP7	I am forced to spend time in bed	0	1	2	3	4

		Not at all	A little bit	Some-what	Quite a bit	Very much
SOCIAL/FAMILY WELL-BEING						
GS1	I feel close to my friends	0	1	2	3	4
GS2	I get emotional support from my family	0	1	2	3	4
GS3	I get support from my friends	0	1	2	3	4
GS4	My family has accepted my illness	0	1	2	3	4
GS5	I am satisfied with family communication about my illness	0	1	2	3	4
GS6	I feel close to my partner (or the person who is my main support)	0	1	2	3	4
Q1	*Regardless of your current level of sexual activity, please answer the following question. If you prefer not to answer it, please check this box ☐ and go to the next section.*					
GS7	I am satisfied with my sex life	0	1	2	3	4

		Not at all	A little bit	Some-what	Quite a bit	Very much
EMOTIONAL WELL-BEING						
GE1	I feel sad	0	1	2	3	4
GE2	I am satisfied with how I am coping with my illness	0	1	2	3	4
GE3	I am losing hope in the fight against my illness	0	1	2	3	4
GE4	I feel nervous	0	1	2	3	4
GE5	I worry about dying	0	1	2	3	4
GE6	I worry that my condition will get worse	0	1	2	3	4

		Not at all	A little bit	Some-what	Quite a bit	Very much
FUNCTIONAL WELL-BEING						
GF1	I am able to work (include work at home)	0	1	2	3	4
GF2	My work (include work at home) is fulfilling	0	1	2	3	4
GF3	I am able to enjoy life	0	1	2	3	4
GF4	I have accepted my illness	0	1	2	3	4
GF5	I am sleeping well	0	1	2	3	4
GF6	I am enjoying the things I usually do for fun	0	1	2	3	4
GF7	I am content with the quality of my life right now	0	1	2	3	4

Figure 11-3. The FACT-G scale. (Courtesy Dr. David Cella. Copyright 1987, 1997.)

2. Insomnia or hypersomnia (e.g., difficulty with falling asleep, awakening 30 to 90 minutes before time to arise, awakening in the middle of the night with difficulty going back to sleep, increased time of sleep, frequent naps)

3. Psychomotor agitation or retardation (noticeable to others, not just subjective feelings)

4. Loss of interest or pleasure in usual activities or decrease in sexual drive

5. Loss of energy (fatigue)

Box 11-10 Effective and Noneffective Coping Strategies

EFFECTIVE STRATEGIES
- Information seeking
- Participation in religious activities
- Distraction
- Expression of emotions and feelings
- Positive thinking
- Conservation of energy
- Maintenance of independence
- Maintenance of control
- Goal setting

NONEFFECTIVE STRATEGIES
- Denial of emotions
- Minimization of symptoms
- Social isolation
- Passive acceptance
- Sleeping
- Substance abuse
- Avoidance of decision making
- Blame of others
- Excessive dependency

Modified from Miller JF: *Coping with chronic illness: overcoming powerlessness,* Philadelphia, 1983, FA Davis.

6. Feelings of worthlessness, self-reproach, or excessive or inappropriate guilt
7. Complaints or evidence of diminished ability to think or concentrate, such as slowed thinking or indecisiveness
8. Recurrent thoughts of death, suicidal ideation, wishes to be dead, or suicide attempt

The radiation therapist who sees and talks to the patient daily is in an excellent position to recognize signs of depression. Questions asked about a patient's eating or sleeping habits or energy level are essential. Therapists must listen and discern carefully the answers to these questions. The danger of routine is to ask how patients are doing and not hear what they are saying, whether through their words or nonverbal cues. Practicing and developing skills discussed in the first part of this chapter are critical for taking care of the whole patient.

Physiologic changes such as sleep disturbance, change in weight, appetite disturbance, and decreased energy are commonly experienced by cancer patients as a result of their disease or treatment. In addition, a level of depression is certainly appropriate because cancer represents to patients a potential loss of not only life but also body parts, image, function, roles, and relationships. The oncology team must assess whether the level of the depression is a change from previous functioning; the way this change occurs; and whether depression is persistent, occurs most of the day, occurs more days than not, and is present for at least a period of 2 weeks.

A variety of instruments are available to assess depression. These tools were designed for psychiatrically ill patients. Therefore, the data are limited somewhat with respect to oncology populations.

The first tool is the *Beck Depression Inventory (BDI).*[3] This is a 21-item self-report scale used to assess symptoms of depression. Each item is composed of a set of statements graduating in severity of symptoms and measured on a scale of 0 to 3 with the higher score representing a more severe symptom. Subjects choose the statement in the tool that best describes their present feelings. The responses are tallied, and a level of depression is assessed.

The second tool is the *Hamilton Rating Scale for Depression (HRS-D).*[11] It is a 17-item self-report scale used to assess cognitive, behavioral, and physiologic signs and symptoms of typical depression. The scores on each item are totaled to give a level of assessment of the depression.

Another tool is the *Psychosocial Adjustment to Illness Scale (PAIS).*[23] This tool is explicitly designed to assess a patient's psychosocial adjustment to medical illness in general. The PAIS is composed of 45 questions divided into the following six domains of psychosocial adjustment: health care orientation, vocational environment, domestic environment, sexual relationships, social environment, and psychological distress. Each of the domains is scored separately and summed. Morrow et al.'s study reveals that the PAIS indicates an acceptable degree of reliability and initial confidence of validity.[23]

Focusing on systematic and continuous assessment for signs and symptoms of psychosocial responses can improve the quality and quantity of survival for patients who have cancer.

 Anxiety and depression are very important and common affective responses to a diagnosis of cancer and should be assessed for by specialists.

Coping Strategies and Responses—The Family. The dynamics of a diagnosis of cancer reach beyond the patient and extend to the entire family. Responses will vary with respect to economic and psychosocial resources, across developmental stages of the family, and with differing demands of the illness.

Life for families of cancer patients becomes complex. Family members must often learn new roles; self-care skills; and ways of relating to and communicating with each other, friends, and the health care team. To support family members, an assessment of their functioning to reveal problem areas may be necessary.

Instruments for assessing the family include the *Family Functioning Index (FFI),*[27] the *Family APGAR* Questionnaire,[30] and the *Family Inventory of Resources for Management (FIRM).*[17] The FFI is a 15-item self-report instrument designed to assess the dynamics of family interaction in families that contain children. Questions are designed to assess marital satisfaction, frequency of disagreement, communication, problem solving, and feelings of closeness and happiness.

The Family APGAR Questionnaire[30] is a screening tool designed to assess the family from the view of the patient. The questionnaire consists of five questions on a 3-point scale. This tool does not assume institutional, structural, or cultural boundaries of a traditional family; therefore, it has a wide application to the many configurations of the modern family.

The *FIRM* is a 69-item self-report questionnaire designed to assess the ability of the family to deal with stressors. This self-report is a 4-point Likert scale evaluating four factors: family strengths (esteem and communication), mastery and health, extended family social support, and financial well-being.

---

*Adaptability, Partnership, Growth, Affection, and Resolve.

Rehabilitation. In cancer cases, the focus is most often on the disease rather than on its functional consequences. Cancer and its therapy can produce significant long-term and permanent functional losses, even in cases in which the goal is a cure. Each person with a disability needs opportunities for improving or at least maintaining functional ability, regardless of the cause of the disability. Often, little thought is given to aggressive rehabilitation of the cancer patient compared with patients having other conditions such as cardiac disease, a stroke, or a spinal cord injury. This occurs even though the 5-year survival rate for patients with cancer is currently approximately 50%. Rehabilitation in cancer is certainly relevant because the number of cancer survivors is growing.

Rehabilitation has been defined as the "dynamic process directed toward the goal of enabling persons to function at their maximum level within the limitations of their disease or disability in terms of their physical, mental, emotional, social and economic potential."[7]

In the early work by Mayer,[16] the concept was set forth that cancer rehabilitation should encompass the theme of quality of survival—not just a person's life span but also that individual's ability to live in the constraints of the disease. In their article, "Can life be the same after cancer treatment?" Veroness and Martino[33] stated that rehabilitation is the bridge leading the patient from diversity to normality. Mellette[19] expanded on the idea by suggesting that prevention, the initial avoidance of dysfunction, is the key word in discussing *rehabilitation*.

The National Cancer Rehabilitation Planning Conference, sponsored by the National Cancer Institute, identified four cancer-rehabilitation objectives[7]:
1. Psychological support after the diagnosis of cancer
2. Optimal physical functioning after the treatment of cancer
3. Early vocational counseling when indicated
4. Optimal social functioning as the ultimate goal of all cancer-control treatment

Probably one of the first major descriptions of a cancer-rehabilitation perspective is that of Dietz[6] in his book *Rehabilitation Oncology*. Dietz considers rehabilitation applicable to all patients who can learn and respond. He stressed "readaptation" as the synonym for rehabilitation because of widespread reluctance to view rehabilitation as relevant to the cancer patient. He further defined the term as accommodation or adjustment to personal needs for physical, psychological, financial, and vocational survival. Dietz defined the initial goals of rehabilitation as the elimination, reduction, or alleviation of disability, and he defined the ultimate goal as the reestablishment of patients as functional individuals in their environments. Rehabilitation should begin at the earliest possible time, and it should continue throughout the entire convalescence until maximal benefit can be achieved.

Romassas et al.[28] developed a method to be used for assessing the rehabilitation needs of oncology patients. They devised an oncology clinic patient checklist designed to include rehabilitation concepts in the patient-assessment process. The patients were asked information regarding the following areas: fatigue; pain; nutrition; speech and language; respiration; bowel and bladder management; transportation; mobility; self-care and home care; vocational and educational interests and activities; and emotional, family, and interpersonal relationships.

> **Box 11-11** **Ways to Develop Cultural Sensitivity**
>
> - Recognize that cultural diversity exists.
> - Demonstrate respect for persons as unique individuals with culture as one factor that contributes to their uniqueness.
> - Respect the unfamiliar.
> - Identify and examine your own cultural beliefs.
> - Recognize that some cultural groups have definitions of health and illness and practices attempting to promote health and cure illness. (These may differ significantly from the health caregiver's own definitions and practices.)
> - Be willing to modify health care delivery in keeping with the patient's cultural background.
> - Do not expect all members of one cultural group to behave in exactly the same way.
> - Appreciate that each person's cultural values are ingrained and therefore extremely difficult to change.

Modified from Stulc P: The family as bearer of culture. In Cookfair JN, editor: *Nursing process and practice in the community,* St. Louis, 1990, Mosby.

As in other assessments, the evaluation for rehabilitative purposes is a dynamic event. It should continue as new issues arise or past issues recur and is best accomplished by a multidisciplinary team meeting the specific needs of each patient.

Cultural Assessment

Cultural assessment refers to the systematic appraisal of the cultural beliefs, values, and practices of individuals and communities. Cultural beliefs and individual differences determine health behaviors in families and cultural groups. Many of the problems with health are the result of behavior and lifestyle.

Accepting and respecting patients for who they are is an important attribute of oncology caregivers. Being culturally sensitive is essential in caring for the whole patient. Box 11-11 lists ways to develop **cultural sensitivity**.

Cultural assessment has several key variables. Figure 11-4 demonstrates a model of cultural strata useful in examining these variables. In this model, values are the foundation of beliefs that includes attitudes and behaviors. Values, which are most difficult to assess, are established early in childhood through an unconscious process of socialization.

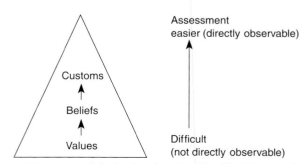

Figure 11-4. A model of cultural strata. (Modified from Bellack J, Edlund B, editors: *Nursing assessment and diagnosis*, Boston, 1992, Jones & Bartlett. Sudbury, MA. www.jbpub.com. Reprinted with permission.)

Beliefs that include knowledge, opinions, and faith about life are built on an individual's values. Based on their knowledge, opinions, and faith, people of different cultures view the origin, treatments, and responses to illness differently. Treatment of the whole cancer patient involves evaluating and understanding the patient's values and beliefs. This is especially important when these values and beliefs are different from or in direct conflict with those of the health care provider and may impair the care of the patient.

Customs that are the result of values and beliefs are the most observable and assessable. These customs include dietary habits, religious practices, communication patterns, family structure, and health practices.

An extremely simple and short assessment model is proposed by Kleinman et al.[15] They suggest the following questions:
- What do you think caused your problems?
- Why do you think your sickness started when it did?
- What does your sickness do to you? How does it work?
- How severe is your sickness? Will it have a long or short duration?
- What kind of treatment do you think you should receive?
- What are the most important results you hope to receive from this treatment?
- What are the chief problems your sickness has caused you?
- What do you fear most about your sickness?

A more thorough cultural assessment tool can be found in Box 11-12.

Cultural assessment enables the health care provider to develop a solid therapeutic relationship, which is a genuine collaborative effort between the patient and health care provider. This requires the person assessing to use good reflective listening skills and pay careful attention to all the cues. In addition, these cues need to be interpreted in the context of the patient's values, beliefs, and culture to be truly meaningful and helpful in treating and respecting the uniqueness of each cancer patient.

Spiritual Assessment

In a holistic approach to care for cancer patients, dimensions of the total person must be recognized and assessed. This includes the patient's spiritual concerns. In a presentation given at the White House Conference for Aging, Moberg[22] defined the *spiritual dimension* as pertaining to "man's inner resources especially his ultimate concern, the basic value around which all other values are focused, the central philosophy of life... which guides a person's conduct, the supernatural and nonmaterial dimensions of human nature." The spiritual dimension encompasses a person's need to find satisfactory answers to questions that revolve around the meaning of life, illness, and death.

To help explore this dimension, Stoll[32] developed guidelines for the spiritual assessment of patients. She suggested the

---

Box 11-12   Cultural Assessment Guide

HEALTH BELIEFS AND PRACTICES
- How does the client define health and illness?
- Are particular methods such as hygiene and self-care practices used to help maintain health?
- Are particular methods being used by the client for the treatment of illness?
- What are the attitudes toward preventive health measures such as immunizations?
- Do health topics exist to which the client may be particularly sensitive or that are considered taboo?
- What are the attitudes toward mental illness, pain, handicapping conditions, chronic disease, death, and dying?
- Is a person in the family responsible for various health-related decisions, such as places to go, persons to see, and advice to follow?

RELIGIOUS INFLUENCES AND SPECIAL RITUALS
- Does the client adhere to a particular religion?
- Does the client look to a significant person for guidance and support?
- Do any special religious practices or beliefs affect health care when the client is ill or dying?
- What events, rituals, and ceremonies (birth, baptism, puberty, marriage, and death) are considered important in the life cycle?

LANGUAGE AND COMMUNICATION
- What language is spoken in the home?
- How well does the client understand English (spoken or written)?
- Do special signs of demonstrating respect or disrespect exist?

- Is touch involved in communication?
- Are there culturally appropriate ways to enter and leave situations (including greetings, farewells, and convenient times to make a home visit)?

PARENTING STYLES AND THE ROLE OF FAMILY
- Who makes decisions in the family?
- What is the composition of the family? How many generations are considered a single family? Which relatives compose the family?
- When the marriage custom is practiced, what is the attitude about separation and divorce?
- What is the role of and attitude toward children in the family?
- When do children need to be disciplined or punished? How is this done? In what way is physical punishment used (if any)?
- Do parents demonstrate physical affection toward their children and each other?
- What major events are important to the family? How are these events celebrated?
- Do special beliefs and practices surround conception, pregnancy, childbirth, lactations, and child rearing?

DIETARY PRACTICES
- What does the family like to eat? Does everyone in the family have similar tastes in food?
- Who is responsible for food preparation?
- Are any foods forbidden by the culture? Are some foods a cultural requirement in observance of a rite or ceremony?
- How is food prepared and consumed?
- Do specific beliefs or preferences exist concerning food, such as those believed to cause or cure in illness?

From Stulc DM: The family as bearer of culture. In Cookfair JN, editor: *Nursing process and practice in the community*, St. Louis, 1990, Mosby.

importance of understanding four areas related to this search for meaning and spirituality in patients' lives: (1) patients' concepts of God or deity, (2) their source of hope and strength, (3) the significance of their religious practices, and (4) the relationship between their spiritual beliefs and state of health.

Stoll notes that spiritual topics are emotionally laden and should be handled in the assessment process accordingly. They should probably be introduced late in an interview, perhaps as a continuation of the psychosocial assessment. As with all questions asked patients, the basis for inquiry should be explained.

Spiritual support may bring comfort, peace, and, for some, the reason for suffering. To facilitate the essential spiritual aspects of caring, oncology health care providers should do the following:

1. Assist patients to experience their own spirituality.
2. Listen carefully to the patient's expression of belief.
3. If possible, provide an appropriate environment and quiet time for reflection and contemplation.
4. Assist the patient in finding resources for spiritual fulfillment.

The willingness to allow a patient or family to be themselves by being present and supporting them is an essential part of working in oncology. In the spiritual realm, presence implies an unconditional acceptance of persons. To be present with a cancer patient or the family is to listen or, in the broadest sense, to hear the communication clearly. Compassionate presence does not require many words. Sometimes it requires none.

Numerous tools are available for assessing spirituality. They include the Spiritual Well-Being Scale, the Religious Well-Being Scale,[26] the Existential Well-Being Scale,[8] Moberg's Indexes of Spiritual Well-Being,[22] and Hess' Spiritual Needs Survey.[13] Studies indicate a combination of these tools best yields the multifaceted nature of spirituality.

Hope. Hope is the key concept and an essential ingredient in the religious and spiritual aspects of care and a major component in the healing process. Spiritual persons inspire hope more by who they are than by their actions. Giving support with realistic hope is a powerful gift oncology caregivers can offer their patients. For some patients, hope is a major determinant between life and death.

A physician often becomes a symbol of hope. Through the physician's continued interest, the patient does not despair. The fear of being abandoned by this person of hope can clearly alter the patient's behavior. Patients may protect their relationships with their physicians by not questioning them, limiting their complaints to them, and treating them as they wish to perceive them — as miracle workers. When this occurs, the role of another member of the multidisciplinary team becomes paramount. Establishing a therapeutic relationship and applying good communication skills are essential in caring for this patient.

The literature and published research articles on hope number approximately 20. Of those articles, 10 involve patients with cancer. This suggests that cancer may have a greater effect on hope than other chronic illnesses. Key measurement instruments include the Nowotny Hope Scale,[24] Herth Hope Scale,[12] and Miller Hope Scale.[21]

The *Nowotny Hope Scale* is a 29-item scale designed to measure hope on six dimensions: confidence in outcomes, relationship to others, possibility of a future, spiritual beliefs, active involvement, and internal origin. This tool is a 4-point Likert-type scale that yields reliable and validated outcomes.

The *Herth Hope Scale* is a 32-item self-report scale to which patients respond, "does not apply to me" or "applies to me" to each item. A total hope score is attained by adding all the responses on each item. Reliability and validity estimates are determined. Herth's descriptive study investigated the relationship between hope and coping in 120 adult cancer patients receiving chemotherapy in a variety of care settings. A significant relationship was found between the level of hope and level of coping. In addition, patients with a strong religious faith had significantly higher mean scores on the Hearth Hope Scale than subjects with weak, unsure faith.

The *Miller Hope Scale* is a 40-item scale using a 5-point Likert format. The possible range of scores is 40 to 200, with a high score indicating high hope. Exemplary items include the statement, "I look forward to an enjoyable future." A low score item is, "I feel trapped, pinned down." The strength of this tool is strong reliability and validity.

Hope is a multidimensional construct that is more than goal attainment and has not been easily quantified. Hope is fundamental to meaning and transcendence for humans. For these reasons, including hope in holistic patient assessment is important.

 Awareness and respect for patient beliefs, values, and practices are essential in being an effective health care worker.

Special Cases in Assessment

Special attention must be given to meet the diverse needs of patients at different stages in life, because cancer is a group of diseases that affects individuals across the life span.

Children. To provide holistic care to a child with cancer, assessing the needs and concerns of the child's primary caregivers (usually the parents) is essential. Experiencing a life-threatening diagnosis for their child is an extremely stressful event for parents.

The assessment of children with cancer is a multidimensional task. Areas of functioning that should be considered are depression, withdrawal, anxiety, delinquency, achievement, family relations, and development.

The developmental level of children is directly related to the way they perceive, interpret, and respond to the diagnosis of cancer. A substantial amount of literature in nursing, medicine, psychiatry, psychology, and social work exists detailing the psychological effect of childhood cancer. The shock of diagnosis, discomfort and inconvenience of treatment, and burden of living with a life-threatening disease are sources of distress and disruption for the child with cancer, parents, siblings, and extended family members.

Those who provide health care to children with cancer have a key role in helping the child and family cope with situations. The study by Armstrong et al.[2] suggests that most children with cancer are normally adjusted. This is due in part to the caregivers' concern and help with coping.

Adolescents. Developmental theory suggests that adolescence is a crucial stage in the process of building self-esteem,

Box 11-13	Suggestions for Interviewing an Older Patient

- If feasible, gather preliminary data before the appointment. Request previous medical records, or have the patient or family complete a questionnaire at home or by telephone.
- Try to avoid making patients tell their story more than once.
- In the review of systems, ask about difficulty sleeping, incontinence, falling, depression, dizziness, and loss of energy.
- Pace the interview. An older patient may need extra time to formulate answers.
- If the patient has difficulty with open-ended questions, use yes-or-no or simple-choice questions.

- Encourage patients and their caregivers to bring a list of their main concerns and questions to help ensure that the issues important to them are discussed.
- Ask patients to bring with them all the medications they are taking (prescription and over-the-counter).
- Ask about the patient's functional status, such as eating, bathing, dressing, cooking, and shopping. Sudden changes in these areas are valuable diagnostic clues.
- Determine whether the patient is a caregiver. Many older women care for spouses, older parents, or grandchildren. Patients' willingness to report symptoms depends on whether they think they can afford to get sick.

Modified from Gastel B: *Working with your older patient: a clinician's handbook,* Bethesda, Md, 1994, National Institute on Aging, National Institutes of Health.

forming perceptions about body image, establishing autonomy, and developing social functions. The adolescent with cancer experiences a disruption of these vital processes. As a result, assessment for the adolescent must consider and address these unique areas. The adolescent with cancer may face a loss of self-esteem because of the unfamiliar patient role. This role can cause the adolescent to feel inferior and dependent, thus inhibiting the developmental task of establishing independence.

Relationships with others and self-perception can change as the adolescent goes through treatment and is hospitalized. The unpredictability and uncertainty of cancer can limit the adolescent's sense of control and autonomy. Changes in body image, disruption of activities, and prescribed therapies can have a profound effect on the adolescent's self-image. Rapid changes in physical appearance as a result of treatments, disfigurement caused by the disease or amputation, or reduction in weight can confuse and impair the adolescent's self-perception.

These are complex processes that must be assessed and incorporated into the plan of care for the adolescent. The health care team must promote growth and developmental maturity while recognizing the burden that cancer places on the adolescent in meeting developmental tasks.

Elderly. As individuals enter the later stages of life, the risk of developing cancer increases. Specific attention to the sociologic issues for older persons is crucial for appropriate assessment and treatment of cancer.

An important problem to assess in older persons is the amount of sensory and cognitive impairment that may be present. Assessing the ability of older patients to hear, see, or understand is paramount in their care. Recognizing any change from normal behaviors, usual routines, and social interactions is extremely important. Loss of physical health, limited economic resources, changes in family structure, and losses of social status greatly affect the quality of life for older persons. Obtaining a complete medical history that includes medications, the family health experience and history, the functional status, and current concerns is crucial to sound health care. Box 11-13 lists some suggestions for interviewing an older patient.

Ongoing communication is the key to assessing and working effectively with the older patient. The best way to promote ongoing communication is to communicate well from the start and to take time to establish a therapeutic and healing relationship.

 Special attention is imperative in caring for the young and the older patient.

SUMMARY

- Communication with the cancer patient can be achieved through verbal and nonverbal networks. The radiation therapist needs to be an effective listener to be able to successfully communicate with the patient via cognitive and affective means.
- Affective communication involves feelings of anger, sadness, fear, and happiness. The radiation therapist needs to reflectively listen to the patient and identify what the patient is feeling. By using the 10 verbal responses, the therapist will be able to communicate effectively with the patient and also be empathetic.
- Physical assessment of the patient on a daily bases by the radiation therapist is imperative to assess the onset of treatment-induced side effects. The therapist needs to be aware of all adjuvant treatments, such as chemotherapy, so that accurate patient assessment is made and the patient is referred to the doctor, dietitian, oncology nurse, or social worker for advice on caring for and treating any side effects.
- Pain assessment has six dimensions, and all are important to consider when treating the cancer patient as a whole being.
- Blood counts are affected by chemotherapy and radiation therapy and need to be monitored throughout a patient's treatment.
- Quality of life for the cancer patient needs careful assessment, and several tools can be used to determine the effect of cancer on the patient.
- Anxiety and depression are common affective responses and should be assessed by specialists.
- The family unit can also be disrupted by a cancer diagnosis, and some families need extra support to cope with the added dimension to family life. Assessment tools are available to help families determine whether they need help so that help can be established.

- As patients survive their cancer diagnoses, rehabilitation becomes a focus, and the aim is to encourage patients to function at their maximal level post-treatment.
- Awareness and respect for patient beliefs, values, and practices, even if they differ from the radiation therapist's values, are important aspects of being an effective health care worker. Cultural sensitivity can be achieved in various ways and involves aspects of spiritual assessment and hope.
- Cancer affects all age groups, and special needs must be met when dealing with all age groups, including children and the elderly.

CASE I

Paraganglioma Assessment

The patient is a 39-year-old white female with a history of paragangliomas: a resection was performed several years ago, and now a metastatic T8 was resected, presently a T2 lesion at C5-6.

Family History:

No known endocrine disorders, but mother and grandmother took diethylstilbestrol during pregnancy

Social History:

Smokes 10 cigarettes per day
Has 2 healthy daughters
Lives out of state and drives 4 hours for treatment
Has lost job and applied for disability/is waiting outcome
Sleeps in car when waiting for treatment due to no income/drives back after Tx

Physical Examination:

133 lb, pulse 74 beats/min, blood pressure (BP) 134/83 mm Hg, temp 98.4° F
Karnofsky status, Eastern Cooperative Oncology Group (ECOG) of 100
Still symptomatic pain with myelopathy impairing her walking and her strength

Treatment:

To T spine in 6/07 with 1500 cGy in 1 fx; to C spine 1600 cGy in 1 fx
Assess this patient's needs by applying the contents of this chapter.

CASE II

Multiple Metastasis Assessment

The patient is an 82-year-old white female with recurrent squamous cell carcinoma to the scalp with metastasis to the neck and supraclavicular fossa. A new chest wall nodule was noted.

History:

Patient has had 3 separate Mohs procedures to scalp
Radiation therapy followed with 6 MeV electrons, 6000 cGy total dose
Has had course of chemotherapy

Physical Examination:

110 lb, BP 128/68 mm Hg, temperature afebrile
Karnofsky Performance Scale status 80%, alert and oriented

Impression and Plan:

She has progressive disease that is growing rapidly.
Current plan is 5000 cGy intensity modulated radiation therapy (IMRT) to left neck
Assess this patient's needs by applying the contents of the chapter.

Review Questions

1. Define *patient assessment*.
2. Explain what is included in the cognitive content of a message. Give an example.
3. Explain what is involved in an empathic response.
4. State the 10 most common verbal responses in effective communication.
5. Explain the assessment responsibility of radiation therapists for daily treatment in the following areas—relate this to daily dose and fractionation and when the side effects might happen.
   - Skin reactions
   - Diarrhea
   - Alopecia
   - Fatigue
   - Cystitis
   - Pain
   - Sleep
   - Nausea
   - Skin pallor
   - Oral changes and vomiting
   - Weight loss
   - Pharyngitis and esophagitis
6. State the frequent first sign of malnutrition.
7. State two important characteristics related to the cause of pain.
8. Define leukopenia and explain its sign and symptoms.
9. State the major symptoms of depression.
10. List five ways to be culturally sensitive.

The answers to the Review Questions can be found by logging on to our website at: *http://evolve.elsevier.com/Washington+Leaver/principles*

Questions to Ponder

1. Why is doing an assessment in oncology important?
2. What is the basis of an effective therapeutic (communication) relationship?
3. Why is observing nonverbal communication so important?
4. What are the three purposes of pain assessment?
5. Why is rehabilitation of the cancer patient important?
6. What are four areas related to the search for meaning and spirituality in patients' lives?
7. Describe five helpful methods in interviewing an older patient.

REFERENCES

1. Ahles TA, Blanchard EB, Ruckdeschel JC: The multidimensional nature of cancer-related pain, *Pain* 17:277-288, 1983.
2. Armstrong GD, Wirt RD, Nesbit ME, Martinson IM: Multidimensional assessment of psychological problems in children with cancer, *Res Nurs Health* 5:205-211, 1982.

3. Beck AT, Beamesderfer A: Assessment of depression: the Depression Inventory. In Pichot P, Olivier-Martin R, editors: *Psychological measurements in psychopharmacology: modern problems in pharmacopsychiatry,* vol 7, New York, 1974, S. Karger.

4. Cella DF, Tulsky DS, Gray G, et al: The Functional Assessment of Cancer Therapy Scale: development and validation of the general measure, *J Clin Oncol* 11:570-579, 1993.

5. Daut RW, Cleeland CS, Flannery RC: Development of the Wisconsin Brief Pain Questionnaire to assess pain in cancer and other disease, *Pain* 17:197-210, 1983.

6. Dietz JH: *Rehabilitation oncology,* New York, 1981, John Wiley & Sons.

7. Dudas S, Carlson CE: Cancer rehabilitation, *Oncol Nurs Forum* 15:183-188, 1988.

8. Ellison CW: Spiritual well-being: conceptualization and measurement, *J Psychol Theol* 11:330-340, 1983.

9. Fishman B, Pasternak S, Wallenstein SL, et al: The Memorial Pain Assessment Card: a valid instrument for the evaluation of cancer pain, *Cancer* 60:1151-1158, 1987.

10. Foley KN: Pain syndromes in patients with cancer. In Bonica JJ, Ventafridda V, editors: *Advances in pain research and therapy,* vol 2, New York, 1979, Raven Press.

11. Hamilton M: A rating scale for depression, *J Neurol Neurosurg Psychiatry* 23:56-62, 1960.

12. Herth KA: The relationship between level of hope and level of coping response and other variables in patients with cancer, *Oncol Nurs Forum* 16:67-72, 1989.

13. Hess JS: Spiritual Needs Survey. In Fish S, Shelly JA, editors: *Spiritual care: the nurse's role,* Downers Grove, Ill, 1983, Intervarsity Press.

14. Irwin PH, et al: Sex differences in psychological distress during definitive radiation therapy for cancer, *J Psychosoc Oncol* 4:63-75, 1986.

15. Kleinman A, Eisenberg L, Good B: Culture, illness and care: clinical lessons from anthropologic and cross-cultural research, *Ann Intern Med* 88:251-258, 1978.

16. Mayer NH: Concepts in cancer rehabilitation, *Semin Oncol* 2:393-398, 1975.

17. McCubbin HI, Comew J: FIRM: Family Inventory of Resources for Management. In McCubbin HI, Thompson AI, editors: *Family assessment inventories for research and practice,* Madison, Wis, 1987, University of Wisconsin-Madison.

18. McGuire DB: Cancer-related pain: a multidimensional approach, *Dissert Abst Int* 48(3):Sec B:705, 1987.

19. Mellette SJ: Rehabilitation issues for cancer survivors: psychosocial challenges, *J Psychosoc Oncol* 7:93-109, 1989.

20. Melzack R: The McGill Pain Questionnaire: major properties and scoring methods, *Pain* 1:277-299, 1975.

21. Miller JF: Development of an instrument to measure hope, *Nurs Res* 37:6-9, 1988.

22. Moberg D: *Spiritual well-being: background and issues,* Washington DC, 1971, White House Conference on Aging.

23. Morrow GR, Chiarello RJ, Derogatis LR: A new scale for assessing patients' psychosocial adjustment to medical illness, *Psychol Med* 8:605-610, 1978.

24. Nowotny ML: Assessment of hope in patients with cancer: development of an instrument, *Oncol Nurs Forum* 16:57-61, 1989.

25. Padilla GV, Presant C, Grant MM, et al: Quality of Life Index for patients with cancer, *Res Nurs Health* 6:117-126, 1983.

26. Paloutzian R, Ellison CW: Spiritual well-being and quality of life. In Peplau LA, Perlman D, editors: *Loneliness: a sourcebook of current theory, research, and therapy,* New York, 1982, Wiley Interscience.

27. Pless IB, Satterwhite BB: A measure of family functioning and its application, *Soc Sci Med* 7:613-620, 1973.

28. Romassas ED, et al: A method for assessing the rehabilitation needs of oncology outpatients, *Oncol Nurs Forum* 10:17-21, 1983.

29. Schipper H, Clinch J, McMurray A, Levitt M: Measuring the quality of life of cancer patients: the Functional Living Index–Cancer: development and validation, *J Clin Oncol* 2:472-483, 1984.

30. Smilkstein F: The family APGAR: a proposal for a family function test and its use by physicians, *J Fam Pract* 6:1231-1239, 1978.

31. Spielberger C, Gorusch R, Lushene R: *Manual for the State-Trait Anxiety Inventory,* Palo Alto, Calif, 1970, Consulting Psychologists Press.

32. Stoll RI: Guidelines for spiritual assessment, *Am J Nurs* 79:1574-1577, 1979.

33. Veroness V, Martino G: Can life be the same after cancer treatment? *Tumori* 64:345-351, 1978.

34. Yasko JM: A model for the assessment of the client with cancer. In Yasko JM, editor: *Guidelines for cancer care symptom management,* Reston, Va, 1983, Reston Publishing.

35. Yates JW, Chalmer B, McKegney FP: Evaluation of patients with advanced cancer using the Karnofsky Performance Status, *CA Cancer J Clin* 45:2220-2224, 1980.

BIBLIOGRAPHY

The American Psychiatric Association: *Diagnostic and statistical manual of mental disorders (DSM IV–R),* ed 3, Washington, DC, 2000, The American Psychiatric Association.

Blackburn GL, et al: Nutritional and metabolic assessment of the hospitalized patient, *J Parenter Enteral Nutr* 1:17, 1977.

Gastel B: *Working with your older patient: a clinician's handbook,* Bethesda, Md, 1994, National Institute on Aging, National Institute on Health.

Gordon M: *Manual of nursing diagnosis,* New York, 1987, McGraw-Hill.

Groenwald SL, et al: *Nutritional disturbances: cancer nursing principles and practice,* ed 3, Boston, 1993, Jones & Bartlett.

Hirshfield-Bartek J, Dow KH, Creaton E: Decreasing documentation time using a patient self-assessment tool, *Oncol Nurs Forum* 17:251-255, 1990.

McCaffery M, Beebe A: *Pain: clinical manual for nursing practice,* St. Louis, 1989, Mosby.

Miller JF: *Coping with chronic illness: overcoming powerlessness,* Philadelphia, 1983, FA Davis.

Stulc DM: The family as bearer of culture. In Cookfair JN, editor: *Nursing process and practice in the community,* St. Louis, 1990, Mosby.

Trip-Reimer T: Cultural assessment. In Bellack J, Edlund B, editors: *Nursing assessment and diagnosis,* Boston, 1992, Jones & Bartlett.

CHAPTER 12

Pharmacology and Drug Administration

Sandy L. Piehl

Outline

Key Terms

Objectives

- Recognize common definitions and nomenclature associated with medications.
- Give an example of a trade name and a generic name of a medication typically used in radiation oncology.
- Identify the various classifications of drugs.
- Demonstrate how to look up a medication in a drug reference book.

- List the "Six Rights of Medication Administration."
- List the methods of drug administration.
- Prepare intravenous drugs for injection.
- Describe documentation procedures related to drug administration.
- Define abbreviations commonly used in drug administration.

The radiation therapist interacts closely with patients in radiation oncology and may be the first to notice adverse reactions or unusual symptoms as they appear. Competent patient care requires that the therapist have a general knowledge of pharmacology and specific details of each patient's medication history. With a basic understanding of medications and their common side effects, the therapist will be able to distinguish an expected side effect from an adverse reaction that requires medical intervention.

Although the administration of drugs is not primarily the role of the radiation therapist, it is a crucial part of overall patient care.[2] The therapist may administer medications specific to radiation therapy, such as contrast media, anesthetics, or intravenous (IV) fluids. To effectively care for the patient, the therapist must also be aware of all the drugs that a patient is taking and their purpose.

This chapter discusses general principles of medication administration. Its purpose is not to provide information about specific drugs but to identify the essential prerequisite knowledge the therapist must have to administer drugs safely to patients. Various aspects of assessment, preparation, and administration of medications are discussed. Finally, the legal aspects of medication administration are considered.

DRUG LEGISLATION

The Federal Food, Drug, and Cosmetic Act of 1938 and the Controlled Substance Act of 1971 govern the labeling, availability, and dispensation of all drugs in the United States.[12] Radiation therapists must remain current with information about the drugs in use in their profession. Safer and more effective drugs, such as nonionic contrast media, are continually being developed. Legislation requires extensive testing of all new drugs before they can be used on patients; however, the value and drawbacks of medications are proved through their actual daily use. The therapist administering these drugs plays an important role in providing feedback to the pharmacology community.

DRUG NOMENCLATURE

A **drug** is any substance that alters physiologic function, with the potential for affecting health. A **medication** is a drug administered for its therapeutic effects. All medications are drugs, but not all drugs are medications. **Pharmacology** is the science of drugs, including the sources, chemistry, and actions of drugs. The list of drugs available for medical use changes constantly as new formulas are developed. Each drug has at least four separate names—its chemical name (constituents of the chemical formula), **generic name** (coined by the original manufacturer), official name (usually the same as the generic name), and brand or trade name (the drug's name in official publications).[11,12,16] Several manufacturers may produce the same generic drug but call that drug by different brand names. Radiation therapists and all health professionals need to easily access this drug name information. The most commonly used resources are the *Physicians' Desk Reference (PDR)*, *United States Pharmacopoeia (USP)*, and specific drug packaging.

Chemical name: 4-[5-(4-methylphenyl)-3-(trifluoromethyl)-1H-pyrazol-1-yl]benzenesulfonamide
Generic name: Celecoxib
Brand name: Celebrex

PHARMACOLOGIC PRINCIPLES

The way in which drugs affect the body is called **pharmacodynamics**. Each drug has a unique molecular structure enabling it to interact with a specific enzyme or a corresponding cell type. The drug attaches itself to a target site in the body called the *receptor site* in the same way that two puzzle pieces interlock. The combined effect alters the behavior of the targeted cells or enzyme and causes physiologic changes in the patient.

The way that drugs travel through the body to their appropriate receptor sites is called **pharmacokinetics**. A drug must be administered so that the body can absorb it, distribute it to the necessary sites, metabolize it, and excrete the excess. Many individual factors cause these steps to vary within each patient; the effectiveness of and reaction to a drug may differ greatly from one patient to another.

Absorption

Every drug must be absorbed into the bloodstream to be effective. The dosage and speed of absorption depend on factors such as the route of entry, the pH of the recipient environment, the solubility of the formula, and the drug's interaction with body chemicals while in transit.[12,16]

Distribution

A drug travels through the circulatory system to its receptor site(s) and then connects with the molecular structure for which it was designed. The drug may need to bind with a certain protein or cross specific membranes to produce the desired response. Many drugs cross the placental villi and affect the fetus. Fewer drugs can cross the blood-brain barrier. Some medications may be stored in the tissues for later use.

Metabolism

"Metabolism, also referred to as biotransformation, is the process by which the body alters the chemical composition of a substance."[12] The liver detoxifies nearly all foreign substances entering the body, including drugs, and changes them into inactive, water-soluble compounds that can be excreted by the kidneys.[12] The breakdown of drugs into waste matter may also involve chemical processes and enzyme reactions in the blood and other organs such as the gallbladder, lungs, and intestines. If drugs accumulate or react synergistically with other substances in the body or the organs are damaged, metabolism and excretion of the drugs may be difficult.[16]

Excretion

The body excretes drugs and their by-products in a variety of ways. Most drugs leave the body through the kidneys. The lungs sometimes expel those drugs that break down into gases. The sweat glands, tear ducts, salivary glands, intestines, and mammary glands can also eliminate small quantities of drugs. The rate of excretion depends on the body's systems, the drug's half-life, and concentration in the tissues.

VARIABLES AFFECTING PATIENT RESPONSE

The caregiver must consider numerous factors that determine patient response to drugs. The following section discusses several of these factors, which also affect the optimal dose to be prescribed by the physician.

Patient-Related Variables

Age. Young children and older adults generally require smaller than average adult doses to achieve the same results, although for different reasons.

In children and infants, the organs are still developing. Children may be hypersensitive to medications, so administration of minimal doses and close monitoring of their responses is the usual process required to decrease the likelihood of an untoward event occurring. Determining dosages by using body weight is safer than using age, but this calculation remains imprecise because of the child's immature metabolism.[15] Administering the prescribed dose to children can be challenging, because they often have difficulty swallowing pills, spit out liquid preparations, reject suppositories, and fight injections.

Older adults may require smaller or, at times, larger doses. Age decreases the efficiency of their organs. Their circulation slows, enzymes are depleted, sensitivities develop, absorption becomes impaired, and the liver and kidneys can no longer detoxify efficiently.[11,12,15,16] In addition, elderly patients commonly take multiple medications that may interact negatively. Elderly patients should be monitored to ensure that the dosage of the medications they are taking is appropriate.

Weight and Physical Condition. Average doses are based on the median 150-lb, healthy adult. The dose must be adjusted for heavier or lighter patients, and body mass must be taken into account because obesity or excessive thinness affects circulation and organ efficiency. A damaged liver or kidneys, an electrolyte imbalance, poor circulation, nutritional deficiency, infection, and other physiologic disorders should be considered in the determination of the optimal dosage.[12]

Gender. Women have a lower average body weight than men and metabolize drugs differently. Women's hormone profiles and the amount and distribution of their body fat differ greatly from those of men and influence the dosage of medications needed. The difference in fluid balance between the genders is another important factor for figuring dosage. The added complication of pregnancy is critical because many drugs may affect the fetus.

Personal and Emotional Requirements. Patients react differently to drugs. Caffeine is a common example; some people can drink coffee all day and have no trouble sleeping, whereas others cannot tolerate caffeine. As a result, patients have unique needs and must be evaluated individually. For example, patients with negative attitudes or anxiety require higher levels of sedation than do calm patients with positive outlooks. Although some patients prefer to take minimum doses of medication, others see drugs as cure-alls.[15] Health care professionals must relate to patients as individuals and be alert to each patient's emotional response to the drugs administered.

Drug-Related Variables: Nontherapeutic Reactions

An important difference exists between unpleasant but expected side effects and adverse drug responses or complications. Side effects are expected reactions to medication; complications are *unexpected* reactions to medications that range from mild to severe.[12] In radiation therapy, the treatment, diagnostic contrast media used, and various medications taken before and after treatment can combine to produce toxicities and discomfort for the patient.

Allergic Reactions. Allergic reactions result from an immunologic reaction to a drug to which the patient has already been sensitized. In an allergic reaction, the drug acts as an antigen, and the body develops antibodies to that drug. The signs and symptoms of such a reaction may range from a light rash to life-threatening **anaphylactic shock**. Once an allergy develops, subsequent exposures to that drug cause increasingly severe symptoms. Penicillin is a common allergenic drug.

Tolerance. Tolerance occurs if the body adapts to a particular drug and requires ever-greater doses to achieve the desired effect. For example, the body develops a tolerance for narcotics extremely quickly. If overused, antibiotics become increasingly less effective by killing not only harmful bacteria but also the beneficial ones. Antibiotics may also leave the patient susceptible to further infection. Bacteria that survive antibiotic use can mutate within the patient into strains that are resistant to the antibiotic during subsequent use.[16] The patient may then need to switch to a different drug if the first one loses its effectiveness.

Cumulative Effect. A **cumulative effect** develops if the body is unable to detoxify and excrete a drug quickly enough or if too large a dose is taken.[15] Unless the dosage is adjusted, the drug accumulates in the tissues and can become toxic. In some cases the cumulative effect is desirable, such as with medications prescribed to prevent depression.

Idiosyncratic Effects. Idiosyncratic effects are the inexplicable and unpredictable symptoms caused by a genetic defect within the patient.[15] These symptoms are completely different from the expected symptoms and may even occur the first time a drug is given.

Dependence. Drug dependency can result from extensive exposure to a drug or a compulsion to continue taking a drug to feel good or to avoid feeling bad. Most persons who become drug dependent do so because of physiologic or psychological problems.

Drug Interactions. Drug interactions occurring between two or more drugs or a combination of food and drugs can create or produce positive or negative effects in patients. This interaction of drugs may result in synergism, which increases a drug's effects; interaction can also result in antagonism, which decreases a drug's effects. For example, alcohol and sedatives taken together produce a toxic reaction, whereas an antiemetic given with anesthesia can be therapeutic. Older adults commonly take many different medications, and the interactions of these drugs can cause a toxic shock situation. The person administering medications should *never* mix drugs without consulting a drug compatibility chart or checking with a pharmacist.

The therapist should also be familiar with the term **iatrogenic disease**. This disease results from long-term use of a drug that damages organs or causes other disorders over time.

In these nontherapeutic responses, the drugs used to treat disease may also cause disease. The therapist should remain aware of complications caused by drug administration.

PROFESSIONAL DRUG ASSESSMENT AND MANAGEMENT

Assessing the Patient's Medication History

The patient is the managing partner in the business of self-medication. Although the health care professional may educate and evaluate the patient regarding drug use, the patient is ultimately responsible for self-medication. If the patient is forgetful, confused, depressed, or taking several medications simultaneously or has inadequate diet and exercise habits, it may be difficult to differentiate between poor compliance and additional medical needs. For example, impaired liver or kidney function may indicate toxicity from drug overuse, lack of improvement from a prior disease, poor drug distribution because of sluggish circulation, an allergic reaction, damaged organs from alcohol or drug abuse, or a negative response from drug interaction. Assessment is further complicated because the person recording the medical history must rely on the patient's verbal description and inadequate recollection.

Despite these difficulties, the therapist must assess the patient's drug use during the patient evaluation by documenting every drug that the patient is taking (including alcohol) and looking especially for overuse and underuse of prescribed drugs.[3,5,11-12,16-17] Misuse of drugs can influence the outcome of radiologic diagnosis or treatment. An accurate medication history is essential to proper diagnosis and treatment (see Legal Aspects).

Applying the Six Rights of Medication Administration

The Six Rights of Medication Administration are as follows[5,7,11,12,15,16]:

1. To identify the *right* patient
2. To select the *right* medication
3. To give the *right* dose
4. To give the medication at the *right* time
5. To give the medication by the *right* route
6. To ensure *right* documentation

Each of these *rights* is discussed in greater detail later.

To properly identify the right patient, checking the name on the door or looking at the chart in the slot is not enough; the therapist should check the patient's identification bracelet *and* ask patient to give his or her name if possible. If the patient's name is called and the patient nods or smiles, this does not necessarily mean that the name has been called correctly. Other possibilities for such a response include: (1) the patient may have nodded or smiled in acknowledgment; (2) a patient may be too young to understand; or (3) he or she may not have a needed hearing aid in place, may not speak English as a primary language, or may be drowsy and misheard. Checking the patient's identification bracelet is *essential*.

The therapist does not bear the primary responsibility for choosing the correct dose; however, as with all caregivers, the therapist must continually watch for errors. Even if the physician or nurse (in the case of standing orders) has prescribed the drug, the therapist involved should *always* check the dosage.[11,12,15,16] As discussed earlier, extremely old or young patients have special dose requirements, as do people of different weights, genders, physical conditions, allergic statuses, and emotional conditions. The dose should *always* be double-checked.

Although a physician (not a therapist) must prescribe the medications, the therapist may confirm that the physician has ordered the proper drug for the patient and that the drug ordered is also the drug being administered. The patient may be the first to notice if a medication order seems different. A patient's concern can be a "red flag" for a therapist to check for a change in the medication or for an error. Every patient deserves to receive the correct medication every time. Therefore, the written order should always be checked against the patient's chart and the drug label.

Some drugs can be administered in more than one way; other drugs should be given only by a particular route. If a drug is administered incorrectly, the consequences may range from minor injury to death. In the radiologic sciences profession, a drug given by the wrong route can also skew a procedure's results. **Contrast media**, in particular, must be delivered to the proper location by the correct route to enhance the images that facilitate the diagnosis or treatment. Contrast media are any substances introduced into the body to make an organ, the surface of an organ, or materials within the lumen of an organ visible on imaging. The route of entry should *always* be double-checked.

Giving a drug at the wrong time can have serious consequences. Such consequences can include poor absorption, fluctuation of blood or serum levels, increased side effects, or less than optimal diagnostic capability in the case of contrast media. A drug that has been ordered before surgery or before a diagnostic procedure must be administered punctually because the procedure is scheduled for a particular time and depends on the drug's effect. Patients always deserve to receive medications *on time*.

Implementing Proper Emergency Procedures

If a drug emergency occurs, the therapist or another health care professional must follow proper emergency procedures. Each hospital and clinic has its own emergency codes and procedures. At the onset of an emergency, the therapist's first duty is to summon help by "calling a code." The therapist should know the location of emergency supplies within the area and the way to administer oxygen and perform cardiopulmonary resuscitation (CPR).

Recognizing symptoms and delivering the appropriate procedure are required skills for therapists.[2] If a reaction develops while a contrast medium is being administered, the therapist must stop the procedure immediately and call the oncologist. The patient must *never* be left alone.

Types of emergencies that the radiation therapist is most likely to encounter are as follows:

- *Asthma attack,* which produces tightness or pressure in the chest, mild to moderate shortness of breath, wheezing, and coughing.
- *Pulmonary edema,* which produces abnormal swelling of tissue in the lungs because of fluid buildup with symptoms of rapid, labored breathing; cough; and cyanosis.
- *Anaphylactic shock* produces symptoms such as nausea, vomiting, diarrhea, urticaria, shortness of breath, airway obstruction, and vascular shock.
- *Cardiac arrest* is when the heart stops beating suddenly and respiration and other body functions stop as a result.

The ability to handle medical emergencies improves with hands-on experience. All radiation therapists should seek extensive education in this area.

DRUG CATEGORIES RELEVANT TO RADIATION THERAPY

Oncology patients have specific symptoms or indications for certain types of drugs. In radiation therapy, for example, patients may require certain drugs (e.g., antidiarrheals and antiemetics) to relieve the symptoms of the therapy and other drugs (e.g., contrast media) to facilitate the pretherapy diagnosis and planning.

Pharmacologists classify drugs in the following ways: according to the effects of the drug on particular receptor sites or body systems, in terms of the symptoms that the drug relieves, or by chemical group.[1,5,17] These categories overlap; often a single drug can be used to treat multiple conditions, and several different drugs can be used to treat a single condition. The following categories of drugs contain common medications that are administered to oncology patients for conditions that may precede or relate to the radiation treatment.

Analgesics relieve pain. Narcotic analgesics (such as morphine, codeine, and meperidine [Demerol]) are given for moderate to severe pain and are derived from opium. These narcotic analgesics are not only addictive, but they can cause adverse side effects. Nonnarcotic analgesics, such as acetaminophen (Tylenol), propoxyphene (Darvon), and aspirin are not addictive but are also not strong enough to relieve severe pain.

Anesthetics suppress the sensation of feeling by acting on the central nervous system. General anesthetics, such as thiopental (Pentothal), depress the entire central nervous system, thereby rendering the patient unconscious allowing major surgery to be performed. Local anesthetics, such as procaine (Novocain), act only on the nerves in a small area. Lidocaine (Xylocaine), as a viscous solution, is used to treat inflamed mucous membranes in the mouth and pharynx.

Antianxiety drugs are mild tranquilizers that help calm anxious patients and relieve muscle spasms. Lorazepam (Ativan), diazepam (Valium), and chlordiazepoxide (Librium) are antianxiety drugs that may be used concurrently with radiation therapy treatments.

Antibiotics suppress the growth of bacteria. Examples include erythromycin, which is usually prescribed for respiratory tract infections, and penicillin and tetracycline, which are broad-spectrum antibiotics that are effective against a variety of bacterial infections.

Anticoagulants prevent blood from clotting too quickly in cases of thrombosis or if an IV line must be kept open. The most commonly used drugs in this category are warfarin (Coumadin), which is administered orally, and heparin, which is always administered by injection.

Anticonvulsants inhibit or control seizures. The most commonly used drugs in this category are clonazepam (Klonopin), which is used orally to prevent petit mal seizures, and phenytoin (Dilantin), which is administered orally or parenterally to treat grand mal seizures.

Antidepressants affect communication between cells in the brain. The drugs affect the neurotransmitters, which carry signals from one nerve cell to another and are involved in the control of mood and in other responses and functions, such as eating, sleep, pain, and thinking.

The most commonly used drugs categorized as antidepressants are fluoxetine (Prozac) and sertraline (Zoloft). Other antidepressants, such as amitriptyline (Elavil), act on the serotonin and norepinephrine. Antidepressants generally take a month or longer to work. In addition, they can be addictive, and they often react negatively with other drugs.

Antidiarrheal drugs control the gastrointestinal distress that often results from bacterial infections, the administration of other medications, or radiation therapy treatments. Two examples of antidiarrheal drugs are diphenoxylate (Lomotil) and loperamide (Imodium).

Antiemetics prevent nausea and vomiting and are most effective when given before symptoms develop. These are often used to alleviate side effects of radiation therapy and chemotherapy. Commonly used antiemetics include prochlorperazine (Compazine), promethazine (Phenergan), and ondansetron (Zofran).

Antifungals treat fungal infections, such as yeast or thrush. Ketoconazole (Nizoral) or nystatin may be given to patients with head and neck cancer who have oral thrush.

Antihistamines are usually used to treat allergies but can also be found in cold remedies and motion sickness tablets. Because many drugs trigger allergic reactions in susceptible patients, antihistamines are often administered to patients before surgery. Diphenhydramine (Benadryl), promethazine, and chlorpheniramine (Chlor-Trimeton) are common antihistamines.

Antihypertensives lower the blood pressure. Clonidine (Catapres), metoprolol (Lopressor), and reserpine (Serpasil) are all antihypertensives (hypertension can become a factor in many medical procedures).

Antiinflammatory drugs reduce inflammation. Although they do not work as quickly as corticosteroids, they may have fewer side effects. Commonly used antiinflammatory drugs include ibuprofen (Motrin), piroxicam (Feldene), and naproxen (Naprosyn).

Antineoplastic drugs are chemotherapeutic agents used by medical oncologists to treat cancer cells throughout the body. Chemotherapy, a treatment modality that uses antineoplastic drugs, can be extremely aggressive and cause adverse side effects because chemotherapy drugs affect the entire system.

Contrast media enhance the visibility of internal tissues for diagnostic imaging. Oncologists depend on these agents to pinpoint target areas for radiation therapy treatments.[1,5,9,17]

Corticosteroids reduce inflammation and are sometimes used to treat adrenal deficiency. Common examples of corticosteroids are dexamethasone (Decadron) and hydrocortisone (Solu-Cortef).

Diuretics remove fluid from the cells. They are used to treat edema and are often used with antihypertensives to lower blood pressure. Fluids and electrolytes must be watched closely for imbalance whenever diuretics are used. Commonly used diuretics include acetazolamide (Diamox), chlorothiazide (Diuril), and furosemide (Lasix).

Hormones are used to augment endocrine secretion. Estrogen (Premarin) is given to females; methyltestosterone is given to males. Sex hormones can also be used to treat neoplastic conditions in the opposite sex; that is, estrogens can be given to males and methyltestosterone can be given to females. Other hormone drugs include insulin, which is a hormone commonly used to treat diabetes, and levothyroxine (Synthroid), a hormone used to treat thyroid disorders.

Narcotics are federally controlled substances that relax the central nervous system and relieve pain. Some examples include codeine, meperidine, and morphine.

Radioactive isotopes that are used in nuclear medicine as diagnostic imaging agents include technetium-99m and iodine-131. Radioactive isotopes that are used in radiation therapy for therapeutic purposes include some of the following: palladium-103, iodine-125, iridium-192, and strontium-89.

Sedatives can calm anxious patients and relax the central nervous system, thereby inducing sleep or unconsciousness. Barbiturates, such as secobarbital (Seconal) and pentobarbital (Nembutal), can be addictive. Examples of nonbarbiturate sedatives include lorazepam, diphenhydramine, and midazolam (Versed). Chloral hydrate is the sedative most often used to sedate children.

Skin agents are used to keep the skin soft and supple while reducing the pain and itching caused by erythema. Some examples include hydrocortisone 1%, Aquaphor, and Eucerin.[6]

Tranquilizers relieve anxiety. Two examples are chlordiazepoxide and diazepam.

Vitamins and other supplements can act as drugs within the body and may have adverse effects if taken in excess or combined with other drugs.

CONTRAST MEDIA

Although some departments do not administer contrast agents, many do, and it often falls within the therapist's scope of practice. The next section focuses on contrast administration.

Contrast agents allow for the enhanced visibility of soft tissue and other areas with low natural contrast. Each diagnostic imaging examination has unique requirements, and every oncology department has its own protocols for the imaging procedures that are performed. The following are fundamental principles that every therapist must understand whenever dealing with radiographic contrast media.

Types of Contrast Agents

The two basic categories of contrast agents are negative (radiolucent) and positive (radiopaque).[1,5,17] Radiolucent agents have low atomic numbers and, as a result, are easily penetrated by x-rays. The spaces containing these compounds (usually in the form of gases) appear dark on radiographs. Air and carbon dioxide are the most common negative contrast media. Air alone can sometimes provide sufficient contrast for radiography of the larynx or other parts of the upper respiratory system.

Radiopaque agents have high atomic numbers and absorb x-ray photons, so the spaces filled with these agents appear opaque (white) on the film. For some procedures, negative and positive contrast media are given together to demonstrate certain internal structures. For example, diagnostic tests of the stomach and large intestine usually use barium sulfate combined with air or carbon dioxide as the contrast media.

Heavy Metal Salt

Barium sulfate, a heavy metal salt, is the most commonly used contrast agent for gastrointestinal tract examinations.[1,5,17] This contrast agent is delivered orally or rectally in an aqueous (water-based) suspension. Barium sulfate coats the lining of the alimentary organs, and because it is radiopaque, the contrast is extremely high. Hazards and inconveniences with the use of barium sulfate are that it requires additives to facilitate ingestion and prevent clumping and it must be concentrated to coat the organs. However, if it is too thick, barium sulfate will not flow easily and is difficult to swallow. Barium sulfate can irritate the colon and cause cramping. It can also stimulate the body to absorb too much fluid, thus leading to hypervolemia or pulmonary edema. Barium sulfate can cause constipation or peritonitis if used in patients with a perforation of the colon or vaginal rupture. If preexisting conditions contraindicate the use of barium sulfate, oncologists will prescribe water-soluble iodides instead.

Organic Iodides

As with barium sulfate, iodine atoms have been proved to be one of the best contrast elements for imaging. Iodine atoms attach to water-soluble carrier molecules or oil-based ethyl esters and dispatch to certain areas of the body. These atoms then displace water in the cells and absorb x-ray photons in those regions.

Most of the conventional, older compounds are highly toxic ionic iodine agents. These compounds are called ionic because their molecules split into two particles (i.e., one negatively charged particle and the other positively charged) whenever they come in contact with body fluids. This splitting results in twice as many iodine particles dissolving into solution in the plasma. The chemical structure of these particles pulls water from the cells, and, because so many of the offending particles exist, the fluid balance of the body may be severely affected. The **ionic contrast media** are said to have **high osmolality**, a high number of particles in solution.[1] A large amount of iodine provides greater contrast but also increases toxicity and viscosity. The most common ionic iodides used are meglumine iodine salts and various sodium iodine salts.

The charged ions discussed previously are irritants and can cause allergic reactions. Nonionic contrast media have been developed for this reason. **Nonionic contrast media** have **low osmolality**—the iodides remain intact instead of splitting—and therefore they agitate the cells less. No charged ions are introduced into the body. These agents are equally effective for imaging but cost much more than ionic agents, so some oncology departments reserve them for allergy-prone patients. Three common nonionic contrast agents are iopamidol, iodixanol, and iohexol.

Some contrast agents have characteristics of ionic and nonionic agents (called *ionic dimers*); they have low osmolality because the molecules are larger and do not have an osmotic (water-moving) effect, but they split and are therefore still ionic.[1,17] An example of this type of contrast agent is sodium meglumine ioxaglate.

Iodinated contrast media are generally viscous, especially at room temperature. This causes discomfort to the patient during injection, although the discomfort can be eased somewhat by preheating the solution to body temperature. Some iodinated contrast media are so viscous that they are best injected by a power injector.

The four aforementioned iodides are all aqueous. Iodinated contrast media can also be oil based. Oil-based agents do not dissolve in water and therefore stay in the body longer. They are unstable and decompose if exposed to light or heat. Although historically used for bronchography and myelography, oil-based contrast agents have limited use in modern departments.[8]

ABSORPTION AND DISTRIBUTION OF CONTRAST MEDIA

Each type of radiographic imaging requires specific contrast media and a sophisticated route of delivery. For example, when rapid systemic distribution is desired, an IV injection is used. Direct injection of contrast media allows optimal imaging of the organ or joint before the media are absorbed into the bloodstream and later excreted. If the intestinal tract is being imaged, ionic contrast media cause increased fluid in the intestines and increased intestinal contractions (peristalsis), thereby producing a better image.

For increased efficiency and decreased toxicity of contrast media the patient must comply with preparation instructions such as fasting and enemas. Compliance leads to diagnostic-quality images produced with the least possible contrast media. An accurate patient history helps determine the optimal dose, prevent unnecessary adverse reactions, and determine the correct route so that the distribution and metabolism of the contrast media illuminate the desired area. Table 12-1 shows some of the common procedures performed with contrast media.

Metabolic Elimination of Contrast Media

When large volumes of foreign materials must be introduced into the body to facilitate imaging, radiation therapy becomes invasive. Unlike drugs in the curative sense, contrast media are nontherapeutic toxic substances, and prompt elimination from the body limits toxic effects.

Excretion through the kidneys is the most common method of elimination; however, a catheter may be used to quickly drain large volumes of aqueous media found in the bladder.

Patient Reactions to Contrast Media

Water displaced by the osmotic action of iodine particles in the plasma is forced into cells or drawn to specific areas. The excess fluid can saturate and distend the blood vessels, inundate the vascular system and cause hypovolemia, or cause shock by withdrawing too much water from the vessels. The osmotic action of ionic molecules can also cause dramatic fluctuations in kidney function. Giving IV fluids can counteract these fluctuations in function.

Nonionic media or water-soluble ionic media are toxic to the kidneys. Patients with renal disease, diabetes, allergies, asthma, sickle cell anemia, thyroid disease, pregnancy, old age, hypertension, or coronary disease may suffer life-threatening reactions to contrast agents and should be carefully evaluated. Children and older adults are often unable to tolerate the dehydration caused by ionic contrast media.

Ionic iodine compounds can provoke allergic reactions ranging from **urticaria** (hives) to anaphylactic shock in susceptible patients. If a patient is going to react to contrast media, the reaction usually happens very quickly (i.e., within a few minutes of administration of the compound).

Classifications of the severity of adverse reactions* seen in contrast media administration are as follows:
- *Minor reactions* are those that usually require no treatment: nausea, retching, mild vomiting

- *Moderate reactions* are those that require some form of treatment, but there is no serious danger for the patient and response to treatment is usually rapid: fainting, chest or abdominal pain, headache, chills, severe vomiting, **dyspnea**, extensive urticaria, edema of the face and/or larynx
- *Severe reactions* are those for which there is a fear for the patient's life, and intensive treatment is required: **syncope**, convulsions, pulmonary edema, life-threatening cardiac arrhythmias, cardiac or respiratory arrest
- *Death*[10]

The therapist must be ready to take immediate remedial action if any of the previously mentioned symptoms begin to manifest.

ROUTES OF DRUG ADMINISTRATION

Radiation therapy patients may receive specific medications before or after the radiation treatments. Medications administered before radiation treatments are for sedation, cytoprotective, and diagnostic purposes; medications given after radiation treatments are palliative (i.e., for relief of distressing symptoms). Therapists must clearly understand the way to administer medications, whether their knowledge is firsthand or a supporting role.

Drugs may be administered via a variety of routes. General information regarding the numerous routes of administration and the effects of each can be found in clinical textbooks.* The following four administration routes are particularly important for radiation therapy and radiologic imaging:
- Oral
- Mucous membrane
- Topical
- Parenteral

The remainder of this chapter discusses these ways to administer drugs and related patient care issues.

Oral Administration

The oral route of administration is safe, simple, and convenient for both the patient and caregiver. Drugs taken by mouth absorb slowly into the bloodstream and are less potent but longer lasting than drugs given by injection.[1,5,7,11-12,15-17] The risk of infection is also less from oral administration than from any other route. Some patients are unable to take oral preparations because of vomiting or nausea, unconsciousness, intubation, required fasting before tests or surgery, difficulty swallowing, or refusal to cooperate. The latter two occurrences are especially common with children.

In radiation therapy, some types of contrast media used for pretreatment diagnosis *must* be administered orally, such as barium for esophageal or small bowel localization.[1,5,15] Palliative medications administered after the therapy are commonly given by mouth. Whenever oral medications are given, the caregiver should do the following:
1. Wash the hands.
2. Read the label and medication order before and after preparing the dose.

---

*Data from American Society of Radiologic Technologists.

*References 1, 3, 5, 7, 11-12, 15-17.

Table 12-1	Common Diagnostic Imaging Procedures that Use Contrast Media	
Procedure	**Route of Administration**	**Contrast Agent**
Cardiovascular	Intravascular	Diatrizoate meglumine 60% Diatrizoate sodium 50% Iopamidol 61.2% Iohexol
Arthrography	Direct injection	Diatrizoate meglumine 60% Sodium meglumine ioxaglate Air
Bronchography	Intratracheal catheter	Propyliodone oil
Cholangiography	IV	Iodipamide meglumine 10.3% Diatrizoate sodium 50%
Cholecystography	Oral	Ipodate sodium (500 mg) Iopanoic acid (500 mg)
Computed tomography	IV injection or infusion	Ioversol 68% Diatrizoate meglumine 60% Iohexol
Cystography	Urinary catheter	Iothalamate meglumine 17% Iothalamate sodium 17% Diatrizoate meglumine 17%
Discography	Direct injection	Diatrizoate meglumine 60% Diatrizoate sodium 60%
Esophagraphy	Oral	Barium sulfate 30%-50%
Hysterosalpingography	Cervical injection	Iothalamate meglumine 60%
Lymphography	Direct injection	Ethiodized oil
MRI	IV injection	Gadolinium and derivatives
Myelography	Intrathecal (lumbar puncture)	Iohexol
Pyelography	Instillation via catheter	Diatrizoate meglumine 20% Diatrizoate sodium 20% Methiodal sodium 20%
Sialography	Catheter	Iohexol
Splenoportography	Percutaneous injection Catheter	Diatrizoate meglumine 60% Diatrizoate sodium 50% Sodium meglumine ioxaglate
Upper and lower GI examination	Oral/rectal	Barium sulfate
Urography and nephrography	IV injection	Diatrizoate meglumine 60% Iodamide meglumine 24% Sodium meglumine ioxaglate Iohexol
Venography	IV injection	Ioxaglate meglumine Ioxaglate sodium Iohexol

GI, Gastrointestinal; *IV,* intravenous; *MRI,* magnetic resonance imaging.
Note: Some departments prefer to use nonionic contrast media on all of their patients in an effort to reduce patient reactions.

3. Identify the patient.
4. Check for allergies.
5. Assess the patient by checking and recording vital signs.
6. Prepare the medicine accurately without touching it directly.
7. Confirm the order with the physician.
8. Give water or other more palatable liquid, such as ice chips, orange juice, or a strong-tasting chaser, if indicated.
9. Elevate the patient's head if the patient is supine.
10. Observe and ensure that the medicine is swallowed and not aspirated.
11. Discard medication paraphernalia.
12. Rewash the hands.
13. Confirmation of medication administration is required. Record the medication administration in the patient's chart.

Some physicians encourage self-administration of drugs. However, the therapist should be aware that some depressed patients in particular might hide and store drugs for later suicide attempts.

Mucous Membrane Administration

Some drugs cannot be given orally because gastric secretions inactivate the medications or because the drugs have a bad taste or odor, damage teeth, or cause gastric distress. If a drug has one of these potential side effects, it can be given in a suppository form using alternate mucous membranes in the rectum or vagina.

Other methods of introducing drugs through the mucous membrane include the following:
- Inhalation in a medicated mist
- Direct application by swabbing
- Gargling
- Irrigating the target tissue by flushing with sterile or medicated fluid

Medications can also be dissolved under the tongue by sublingual administration. All these methods have a systemic effect, although some affect the system more rapidly than others. Regardless of the route used, the person administering the drug must never compromise sterility by touching the drug directly.

Topical Administration

Topical administration involves placement of the drug directly on the skin. This method is often needed after the skin is disturbed by radiation therapy.[6] Topical applications are also used for antiseptics preceding injections, ointments, lotions, and transdermal patches. Such patches can dispense scopolamine, estrogen, or nicotine slowly and at a constant level. If the caregiver is administering topical drugs, gloves should be worn to prevent absorption of the medication and introduction of infectious agents to the patient.

Parenteral Administration

Parenteral administration means that the medication bypasses the gastrointestinal tract. Taken literally, this includes the topical and some mucous membrane routes, but the word *parenteral* colloquially means "by injection."

A drug administered parenterally is absorbed rapidly and efficiently. None of the drug is destroyed by digestive enzymes, so the dose is usually smaller.[15-17] Medications are administered parenterally in the following situations:
- The drug would irritate the alimentary tract too much to be taken orally.
- A rapid effect is needed, such as during an emergency.
- Drugs need to be dispensed intravenously over time.
- The patient is unconscious or otherwise unable to take oral medications. For example, if the patient is fasting before surgery or tests, medication can be given by injection.

Parenteral administration carries with it the danger of infection from piercing the skin and an increased risk of unrecoverable error because of rapid absorption. Injections also cause genuine fear in some patients. Long-term parenteral therapy can also damage injection sites.

Parenteral administration is categorized by the depth of the injection and location of the injection site (Figure 12-1). The following are the four most common parenteral routes[17]:
- **Intradermal (ID)**—a shallow injection between the layers of the skin
- **Subcutaneous (SQ or SC)**—a 45- or 90-degree injection into the subcutaneous tissue just below the skin
- **Intramuscular (IM)**—a 90-degree injection into the muscle used for larger amounts or a quicker systemic effect

- **Intravenous (IV)**—an injection directly into the bloodstream that provides an immediate effect

The therapist may also become a member of a health care team that administers drugs by less common parenteral routes as well. Other routes pertaining to radiation oncology include the following:
- Intrathecal administration, in which medications are injected directly into the spinal canal, such as chemotherapeutic agents
- Intratracheal administration, in which medications are administered directly into the trachea
- Intracranial administration, in which medications are administered directly into the brain
- Catheterization, which includes urinary catheterization[6]

The physician or anesthesiologist performs the administration of drugs by these routes with the therapist acting as a support person.

IV ADMINISTRATION

Of the four parenteral routes, therapists most often use the IV route. IV injections, or **venipuncture**, are within the scope of practice for radiation therapists in most states.[2] This technique is best learned by hands-on experience.

When a patient requires ongoing IV therapy, a catheter is inserted into a peripheral vein where it can remain for a number of days. Every therapist should practice error-free preparation, use appropriate equipment and flawless venipuncture technique, and have a caring bedside manner. Even if all these requirements are met, venipuncture is still potentially hazardous. The advantage of having ongoing access is that the vein's integrity is broken only at the time of insertion. This catheter can be used for either intermittent medications, continuous infusions, or a combination of both. If continuous access is not required, the caregiver can disconnect the patient from the infusion using a heparin lock. The heparin lock has a self-seal for when it is not in use.

The therapist administering drugs through an IV route must never leave the patient alone during the procedure and must continuously monitor the patient.

Different methods of IV administration serve different purposes. The safest method is continuous infusion, in which the medication is mixed with a large volume of IV solution and given gradually over time. Second, a drug can be "piggybacked" (added) onto the main IV line by means of a special valve so that the medication can be administered intermittently at prescribed levels.[11,12,15-17] During drug administration, the volume of IV fluid administered is lowered. This process usually takes less than 1 hour, after which the volume is restored to the initial level.

A third method of IV injection is a bolus, or push, of a concentrated dose of medication injected by a syringe directly into the vein or through the IV port. This method requires diligent observation of the patient because the effect is rapid and can be irreversible.

Two major types of IV injections pertain to radiation therapists: drugs requiring dilution and drugs requiring delivery by IV bolus. Most contrast media, if not given orally, are injected by bolus. Drugs that are diluted or solutions for the maintenance of fluid levels are administered slowly by IV drip.

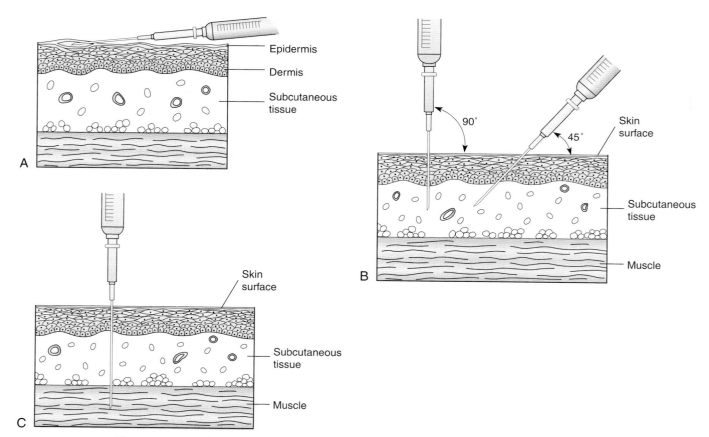

Figure 12-1. A, The syringe is positioned almost parallel to the skin with the bevel pointed upward for intradermal injections. The medication is deposited right under the skin, forming a small, raised area. **B,** The syringe is positioned at a 45- or 90-degree angle to the skin for subcutaneous injections. The medication is deposited in the subcutaneous tissue just below the skin. **C,** The syringe is positioned at a 90-degree angle for intramuscular injections. The medication is deposited in the muscular area just below the subcutaneous tissue.

Administering Bolus Injections

Certain medications, including contrast media, must be administered at full strength. If the patient has an IV line that is running a continuous infusion, the therapist must temporarily stop the infusion while the bolus is injected to avoid mixing the solutions. The IV line should remain in place because radiopaque materials are highly toxic and reactions can happen quickly. The IV line allows the patient to receive immediate remedial treatment should a negative reaction occur.

Bolus injection requires the same preliminaries discussed in regard to other routes of administration (i.e., checking the medication, identifying the patient, washing the hands). Proper preparation of the dose of contrast is required. IV contrast medication comes packaged in ampules or vials, each of which has its own specific requirements for use. An ampule contains a single dose of medicine; the tip is snapped off, and the drug is drawn into a syringe through a filter needle (Figure 12-2, A).

A vial has a rubber stopper, and the needle is inserted through that stopper to draw out the medicine (Figure 12-2, B) (usually multidose vials are not used because of possible contamination, but if the vial contains more than one dose, a new needle should be used and the stopper of the vial must be wiped with alcohol before every use). The vial should be dated and initialed at the time of use. It should be discarded within 24 hours of initial use.

If the medication is not directly delivered by a vein, an IV port (Figure 12-3, A and B) may be used. The injection port of the catheter should be wiped with alcohol or the heparin lock should be flushed with sterile saline, and then the drug may be slowly injected into the port. The correct rate for injecting the drug should be specified on the package or in the medication order. If the medication enters the vein too quickly, the body may go into speed shock, a severe, life-threatening reaction caused by the toxicity of the drug. Following injection, the port

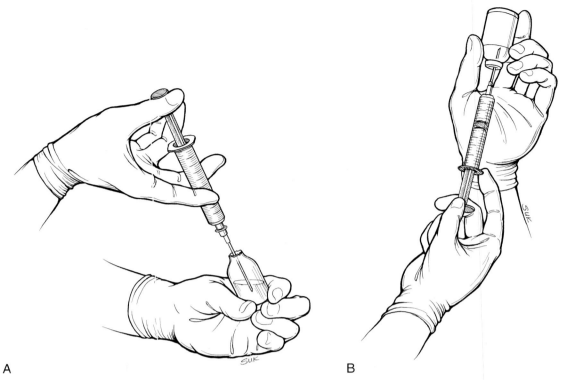

A   B

Figure 12-2. A, This drawing shows the way to remove the medication from an ampule. The medication is removed by pulling back on the plunger of the syringe. The therapist should be careful not to contaminate the needle when inserting and removing the needle from the ampule. **B,** This drawing shows the removal of medication from a vial. The rubber stopper must be cleaned with alcohol before the needle is inserted into the vial. The same amount of air must be injected into the vial as will be withdrawn to equalize the pressure in the vial.

should be again wiped with alcohol or the heparin lock should be flushed and refilled with heparin solution. Only then can the IV flow be restored.

Chemotherapy is often administered through a different type of vascular access port such as the Hickman, Groshong, Port-A-Cath, and PAS Port[15] (Figure 12-3, C).

IV Infusion and Venipuncture Equipment

Before the actual venipuncture or injection takes place, the health care professional must gather all the necessary equipment. Interruption of the procedure to find missing equipment is extremely unprofessional and erodes the patient's confidence in the caregiver. The IV equipment can be prepared with the tubing capped and ready to attach before the venipuncture is performed or after the IV port is in place. The timing of the preparation depends on institutional policy or the physician's orders.

In the case of an IV drip, required equipment includes IV tubing with a clamp on it, the vacoliter or plastic drip bag, a stand on which to hang the bag of solution, an IV filter, and a meter to measure the flow rate. The most common place for sterility to be compromised is in the two ends of the tubing; neither the end going into the sterile solution nor the end

connecting with the IV catheter should *ever* be touched, even with gloves.* If either end is inadvertently touched, it must be sterilized before use or discarded and replaced.

IV equipment varies according to the drug and dose. The equipment tray should include a tourniquet, antiseptic swabs, gloves, a syringe, a needle, cotton balls, the correct drug, and adhesive bandages. Any catheters, tubing, drip bottles, poles, and monitors required should also be in place before the procedure begins.

The type of medication and physical characteristics of the patient determine which instrument should be used for IV injection. For a one-time injection of 30 mL or less, a regular needle (i.e., 18 to 20 gauge, depending on the viscosity of the drug and size of the patient's veins) and a syringe should suffice. An infusion that takes place over a longer time requires a butterfly set, which is a special steel needle attached to two plastic "wings" taped to the skin. This butterfly set anchors the needle in the vein.

Whenever the infusion requires a large volume of fluid or must be administered over an extended period of time, a plastic catheter can be inserted into the vein. Because the tubing is flexible and soft, it allows the patient to move around and it

*References 1, 5, 7, 11, 13, 16-17.

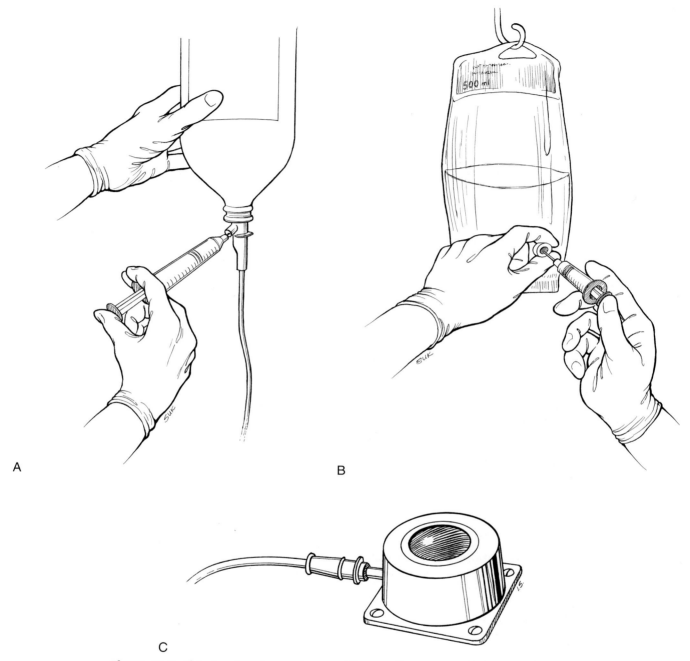

Figure 12-3. This drawing demonstrates adding medication to a bottle **(A)** or **(B)** bag of IV solution. **C**, Chemotherapy is often administered through a vascular access port.

is less irritating than a rigid, metal needle. Two kinds of venous catheters exist; one is a narrow tube inserted through a hollow needle, and the other has the needle through the tube. The through-the-needle catheter is generally longer and thinner and can be inserted deeper into the vein. This type of catheter is commonly used for antineoplastic drugs. After the catheter is in place and taped down, the needle is removed.

Dosage, Dose Calculation, and Dose Response

Medication charts list standard measurements (i.e., metric or apothecary), their abbreviations, and recommended doses for most common medicines. Table 12-2 lists common abbreviations used for prescribing medications.[5,12] Health care personnel must invariably calculate individual doses for their patients if the standard packaging differs from the amount ordered.

Table 12-2	Common Abbreviations Used for Prescribing Medications
Abbreviation	**Meaning**
a.c.	Before meals
bid	Twice a day
h	Hour
h.s.	At bedtime
IM	Intramuscular
IV	Intravenous
mL	Milliliter
p.c.	After meals
PO	By mouth
p.r.n.	As necessary
q	Every
q3h, q4h, and so on	Every 3 hours, every 4 hours, and so on
qh	Hourly
qid	Four times each day
qod	Every other day
stat	At once
SQ/SC	Subcutaneous
tid	Three times a day

To calculate the quantity ordered, the therapist or nurse must multiply or divide the dose required by the packaged amount (make sure the two are in the same unit of measurement). The math should *always* be double-checked by a second person.

Doses for children should be calculated according to the child's weight or body surface area. The latter is more accurate because it also takes into account the child's height and body density.[12,15]

Although the specifics of dose calculation are beyond the scope of this chapter, a good nursing text will explain the way to compute the correct dose.

Whenever drugs are administered intravenously, the dosages must be calculated according to the total volume of fluid the patient receives (except in the case of a bolus injection). This calculation must be carefully monitored because flow and absorption rates can fluctuate. Also, the drug must be given in the correct dilution, at the appropriate rate, and in the correct amount. Controlling the dosage in single injections or piggyback deliveries is easier than in long-term IV treatment.

Many factors can affect the delivery rate of an IV injection. The flow can be interrupted by a kink in the tubing, a clot in the needle or catheter, the needle tip pressing against the vein wall, or a problem at the site of entry. The drip rate may depend on the patient's absorption rate, which always varies greatly from one person to another. Sudden fluctuations in flow rates happen frequently because of mechanical problems with the equipment or because the patient dislodges the catheter. All these factors influence the accuracy of delivery whenever drugs are infused intravenously.

Initiation of IV Therapy

Patient Education. Before any IV drugs are administered, therapists should identify themselves to the patient, assess the

patient's condition, and explain the procedure. Assessment involves the following:
- Taking an allergy history (or reading the patient's chart if a history has already been taken)
- Taking the blood pressure for a baseline reading
- Determining whether the patient has had any medication that affects blood clotting
- Asking the patient (not the nurse) whether the patient has been fasting[1,7,9,12,16,17]

The physician is responsible for explaining the reason the procedure is needed; the therapist can ease any anxiety the patient may have by describing the process and answering questions. Iodinated contrast media can produce adverse reactions within minutes after being administered, so the therapist must ask the patient to report any symptoms that he or she may experience *before* administering the drug. It may help the patient to know some common sensations related to the medication and whether they are serious.

Site Selection for Venipuncture

The site chosen for venipuncture depends on the drug to be administered and the length of time that the IV line will be in place (Figure 12-4, A). The large antecubital vein in the arm is convenient for drawing blood or for injecting a single dose or viscous solution, but this vein is inappropriate for long-term IV therapy because it hinders the patient's mobility. The best choices for long-term infusion include sites above the anterior wrist (lower cephalic, accessory cephalic, and basilic veins) or veins on the posterior hand (basilic, metacarpal, and cephalic veins)[12] (Figure 12-4, B). If the patient is right-handed, putting the IV line into the left arm allows the patient to maintain use of the dominant arm.

Certain contraindications at a specific venipuncture site mean that a different site should be chosen. These contraindications include scar tissue or hematoma that necessitates injection above this site, infection or skin lesions that could introduce infection into the bloodstream, burns, collapsed veins, or veins too small for the chosen gauge of the needle. Special techniques apply if a patient has rolling veins, has **phlebitis**, is on dialysis, or is extremely obese. If the patient is taking blood thinners, extra compression is needed.

Venipuncture Technique

The venipuncture may be performed after the preliminaries, such as collection of supplies, patient identification, informing the patient of the procedure, and patient assessment, are completed. The procedure[13,17] is as follows:
1. Position the patient. The patient should be sitting or lying down, and the arm should be placed in a relaxed position. The arm may need to be anchored to an arm board if the patient is extremely active.
2. Determine the best site for the venipuncture.
3. Wash the hands and put on gloves. All **standard precautions** should be followed because of potential contact with body fluids. These precautions include wearing gloves, a mask, and protective eyewear; properly handling needles; and disposing of used equipment into containers for biohazardous material. Many institutions use safety needles, which eliminates recapping.

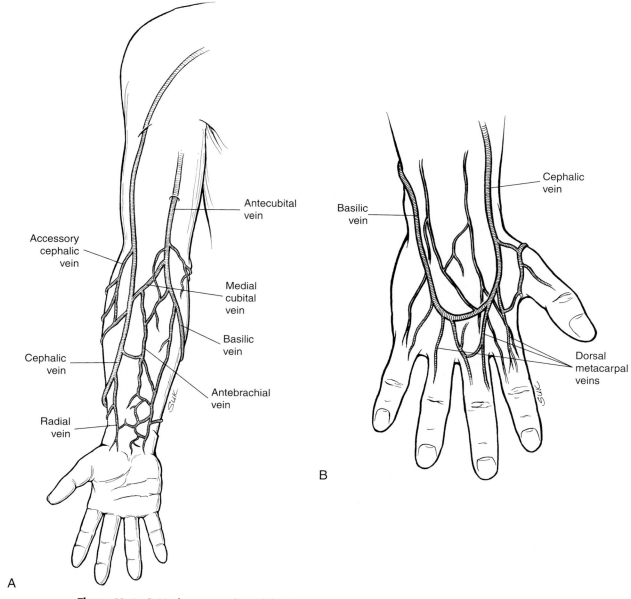

Figure 12-4. A, Venipuncture sites of the forearm. **B,** Venipuncture sites of the wrist and hand.

4. Apply the tourniquet tightly in a way that it can be removed with one hand. The tourniquet should be approximately 2 to 4 inches above the puncture site. Never leave a tourniquet on for more than 2 minutes.

5. It may be necessary to tap or stroke the vein or to have the patient make a fist to enhance distention of the vein (Figure 12-5).

6. Cleanse the skin with an antimicrobial solution (tincture of iodine 2%, 10% povidone-iodine, 70% isopropyl alcohol, or chlorhexidine) in small concentric circles outward to a radius of approximately 2 inches. Do not touch area again with a nonsterile object. If local anesthetic is being used, inject it intradermally at this time.

7. Verify that you have the proper medication.

8. Anchor the vein firmly above and below the puncture site with the thumb and index finger of your free hand. This will prevent the vein from "rolling."

9. Insert the needle parallel to the vein, bevel side up, at a 30-degree angle, and then flatten the needle to a 10- to 15-degree angle. If the angle is too shallow, the needle will skim between the skin and vein; if the angle is too deep, the needle will penetrate the posterior wall of the vein and cause bleeding into the tissues. When blood flows back into the syringe or hub of the cannula, the needle is in the vein. Allowing the blood to fill the hub before attaching tubing ensures that air bubbles are not trapped in the line.

10. Remove the needle from the catheter. Release the tourniquet and push the catheter deeper into the vein and up to the hub, if possible.

11. Attach IV tubing and place an antiseptic swab or patch over the puncture site, and fix the catheter in place with adhesive tape or, if injecting contrast media with a butterfly needle and syringe, proceed with the injection after securing the butterfly needle in place.

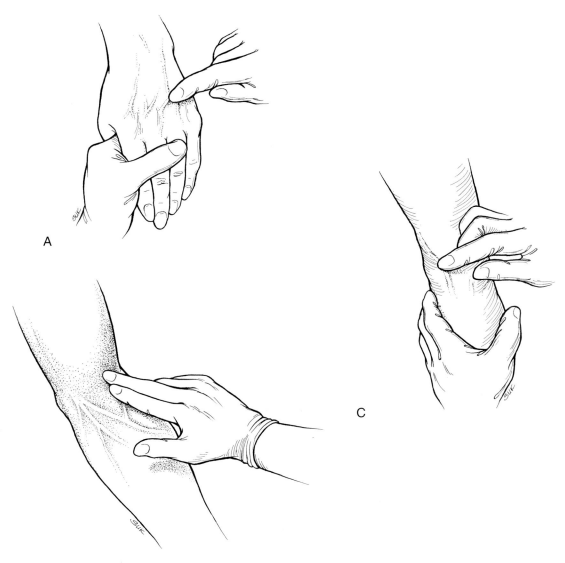

Figure 12-5. Techniques to distend veins include tapping the vein **(A)**, gently stroking the vein **(B)**, and having the patient make a fist **(C)**.

12. If the venipuncture is unsuccessful, withdraw the needle or catheter and immediately apply light pressure to the insertion site and remove the tourniquet.

Infusion of Medication

The procedure* for starting a drip infusion after venipuncture has been performed and an IV line is in place is as follows:
1. Wash the hands.
2. Double-check the patient's name. Assess the patient. Ask the patient about allergies to drugs.
3. Triple-check the physician's orders against the solution label.
4. Check the bag or vacoliter for an expiration date, signs of contamination (such as discoloration, cloudiness, or sediment), and cracks or leaks.

*References 1, 5, 7, 11, 13, 15, 16.

5. Put on gloves and follow all standard precautions according to institutional policy.
6. Remove the metal cap and rubber diaphragm from the bottle or bag without touching the rubber stopper.
7. Close the clamp on the tubing, attach the in-line filter, and insert the spike of the drip chamber into the rubber stopper without touching the sterile end.
8. Invert the fluid container and hang it on an IV pole 18 to 24 inches above the vein.
9. Remove the cap covering the lower end of the tubing, release the clamp, and allow the fluid to flow through the tube to get rid of air bubbles (if air is left in the tubing, it will be forced into the vein). Close the clamp. Attach the tubing to the IV line.
10. Monitor the flow until the desired rate is established.
11. Monitor the condition of the patient.

12. Discard used materials and gloves according to institutional policy.
13. Rewash hands.
14. Record the medication procedure in the patient's chart.

Hazards of IV Fluids

Perhaps the biggest challenge of administering drugs intravenously is to get the drug into the vein without introducing foreign microorganisms that can cause infection. No one should ever touch the fluid ports, needle, ends of tubing, or any other part of the equipment through which germs could pass into the bloodstream. Diligent observation of the venipuncture site allows the caregiver to recognize symptoms of sepsis at its earliest stage.

IV infusion carries unique hazards with it. Any swelling around the injection site accompanied by cool, pale skin and possibly hard patches or localized pain is a sign of **infiltration**.[17] This can occur if the catheter or IV needle has pulled out of the vein and the fluid has seeped into the adjacent subcutaneous tissue. Infiltration can also occur if the IV bottle is hung too high, the hydrostatic pressure is so great that the vein cannot absorb the fluid quickly enough, and the fluid saturates the surrounding tissue. If the therapist mistakenly misses the vein and injects contrast media into the tissues surrounding the vein, the result is a similar condition called **extravasation**, which is not only painful but can cause severe tissue damage.[11,12,15,16]

Other hazards of IV infusion include an allergic reaction to the drug, an air embolism caused by failure to eliminate air bubbles in the equipment, a metabolic or an electrolyte imbalance, edema caused by the dressing being too tight at the site or too much fluid, speed shock from too rapid a delivery, drug incompatibility, thrombus (blood clots), and phlebitis. Phlebitis can be prevented if the needle is a small enough gauge that the blood can flow around it. A "keep vein open" (KVO) drip keeps the blood from clotting at the site; likewise, the heparin in a heparin lock prevents the injection site and bloodstream from developing clots.

Sudden increases in fluid volume introduced by IV equipment can accidentally occur. If the patient is extremely frail or has a head trauma, a sudden overload can be fatal. Any time fluid is infused too quickly, the excess can collect in the lungs, thereby causing pulmonary edema. Rapid infusion can also result in an overdose of the medication. Too little fluid may result in dehydration or an insufficient dose of the required medication. These are only a few of the reasons that monitoring IV lines closely is crucial.

Discontinuation of IV Therapy

Because the potential for contamination is so high in IV therapy, the infusion set should be changed every 24 to 48 hours. If IV therapy must be continued for a longer period, changing to a new venipuncture site may be necessary, depending on the condition of the original site. Most of the drugs that therapists administer are infused over a short period of time, through a single site.

To remove the IV line, the therapist must gather the following supplies: sterile gauze pads, gloves, and tape. After the patient has been properly identified and informed of the procedure, these steps should be followed to discontinue IV therapy[1,12]:

1. Wash the hands.
2. Clamp off the IV tubing and remove the tape holding the catheter in place.
3. Put on gloves and follow standard precautions according to institutional policy.
4. Apply a folded gauze sponge over the insertion site and hold it down with your thumb. Grasp the needle or catheter and withdraw in one smooth motion.
5. Before taping the gauze, inspect the site.
6. Tape the gauze pad in place and elevate the patient's arm. Apply direct pressure for 1 to 2 minutes.
7. Dispose of the used IV materials properly.
8. Rewash the hands.
9. Record the appropriate information in the patient's chart.

LEGAL ASPECTS

In considering legal aspects, the scope of practice must be reviewed. The scope of practice for radiation therapists includes the delivery of radiation to treat disease. It also requires patient care, including providing comfort, dignity, education, monitoring, and documentation.[2] Increasingly, the practice of venipuncture and the administration of IV medications and contrast media are also included.

The therapist may not legally diagnose, interpret images, reveal test results to patients or family members, prescribe drugs, admit or discharge patients, or order tests. Those duties belong to the physician. The therapist, like every health care professional, is legally required to report incidents or errors and is allowed to act without liability in an emergency if no other care is available (the Good Samaritan laws).

The therapist is legally liable for administering competent treatments and accurately communicating with the patient. The two most common complaints leading to malpractice suits in radiology and oncology are false-negative or false-positive diagnoses of fractures or cancers and the misadministration of contrast media.[4] The oncologist does not bear these risks alone. The radiation therapist is part of the team and on the frontline of patient care.

Although radiation oncology team members cannot be held accountable for poor health results, they are liable if they act negligently or cause injury. Because the profession can be so hazardous, it is in everyone's best interest that efforts be taken to communicate *all* risks before any procedure or treatment takes place. Every precaution must be taken in the actual treatment of each patient.

Different states have different laws regulating the radiation therapist's scope of practice. You must adhere to state laws and institutional policies and procedures regarding venipuncture and the administration of medication.

Documentation of Administration

The medical record is a legal document and is evidence for the caregiver and patient in the event of confusion or litigation.[4,9] Therefore, it is in the therapist's best interest to make sure the information in the chart is thorough and accurate. For example, if the patient verbally informs the therapist of a sensitivity to iodine and the therapist fails to pass on the information or record it in the chart, the therapist could be held liable for adverse reactions. A previously documented sensitivity should be apparent in the patient's permanent record, and in this situation the therapist is responsible for noticing and making sure the physician is also aware of the sensitivity.[9]

The patient's chart or medical record is often the primary means of communication among the members of a health care team. Each patient is often treated by several different professionals, all of whom need to know the entire medical history to do their jobs effectively.

Accurate documentation protects the patient from errors in treatment; likewise, accurate documentation protects the caregivers from making procedural, ethical, or legal errors. Every medication, every treatment procedure, every diagnostic test, and even verbal communication should be documented in the patient's permanent medical record.

Although each medical institution is allowed to develop its own system of record keeping, certain standard contents are required by the various accrediting bodies in the medical profession; these include the following[14]:

1. Patient identification and demographic information.
2. Medical history, including family history, allergies, and previous illnesses.
3. Nature of the current complaint and a report of examinations and treatments.
4. Orders for and results of any tests or procedures.
5. Record of all medications, whether self-administered, prescribed, or professionally administered. The information should include but is not limited to time, route, dosage, site of administration, and caregiver's signature.
6. Physician's notes, instructions, and conclusions.
7. Informed consent form.

Documentation of any complications or adverse reactions to a medication is especially critical to the medical record of any patient.[1,4-5,9,12,15] A sensitivity to any medication must be prominently displayed in the patient's record. Remedial action taken to counteract the complication must also be recorded.

The therapist bears the responsibility for understanding the way to read the chart accurately and enter information in the record. A written error should not be erased or covered with correction fluid but should have a single line drawn through it and initialed (so that the original information is legible). The information should be rewritten, dated, and initialed.

Medical records are confidential and may not be released without the patient's consent. Orders of any kind *must* be signed by the attending health care professional.

Informed Consent

Radiation therapy and diagnostic imaging require informed consent from the patient. In addition to the general consent form the patient signs when entering a health care facility, each radiation therapy procedure requires a separate form in the patient's record.[17]

Especially in cases of radiation administration and ionic contrast media in which the potential risk is so high, a gray area exists about what constitutes "informed" consent. If a patient agrees in writing to receive ionic contrast media but suffers a reaction, the oncologist could be held liable if that oncologist failed to inform the patient that nonionic agents were available. The issue of cost (e.g., nonionic media costs considerably more than ionic media) should not determine how much the physician tells the patient. Open communication about risk and cost are part of the patient's legal rights.

Informed consent expectations and documentation vary by state and institution. Informed consent forms generally include the name of the authorized physician; a description of the procedure and associated medications; an assurance that the purpose, benefit, risk, and any alternative options have been imparted and understood; an area where patients can write in their words what the procedure entails; and a disclaimer, which does not always hold up in court, releasing the caregiver and facility from liability if complications develop or the treatment fails.

SUMMARY

The technique of venipuncture and assisting in the administration of IV drugs and contrast media are crucial skills required for the practice of radiation therapy. The descriptions in this chapter do not qualify a radiation therapist to perform those actions but are intended only as an overview. The therapist must study the principles of pharmacology and must have hands-on experience before performing these techniques on patients. The therapist who is knowledgeable in all pertinent aspects of drug administration contributes an invaluable service to the success of the radiation therapy team.

- Pharmacologic principles include absorption, distribution, metabolism, and excretion.
- Patient-related variables that affect response include age, weight, physical condition, gender, and personal and emotional requirements.
- Drug-related variables are allergic reaction, tolerance, cumulative effect, dependence, and drug interactions.
- The Six Rights of Medication Administration are to identify the right patient, select the right medication, give the right dose, give the right medication at the right time, give the medication by the right route, and document what you have done.
- Routes of drug administration are oral, mucous membrane, topical, and parenteral.
- Parenteral drug administration includes intradermal, subcutaneous, intramuscular, and intravenous.
- Patient assessment is imperative before the initiation of any intravenous therapy and should include an allergy history, baseline blood pressure reading, determination of whether the patient is taking any medication that could affect blood clotting, and if applicable, asking the patient whether he or she has been fasting.

Review Questions

Multiple Choice

1. Which of the following is *not* one of the rights of drug administration?
   a. right patient
   b. right route
   c. right time
   d. right syringe

2. Which of the following is *not* a patient-related variable affecting response to medications?
   a. weight
   b. physical condition
   c. tolerance
   d. emotional requirements
   e. age

3. The way in which drugs affect the body is called:
   a. pharmacokinetics
   b. metabolism
   c. pharmacodynamics
   d. drug effectiveness

4. Which of the following is *not* a parenteral route of administration for medications?
   a. subcutaneous
   b. instillation
   c. intravenous
   d. intramuscular

5. The type of drug given to cancer patients to relieve nausea and vomiting is a(n):
   a. antacid
   b. emetic
   c. cathartic
   d. antiemetic

6. The way a drug travels through the body to the appropriate receptor site is known as:
   a. pharmacodynamics
   b. excretion
   c. distribution
   d. pharmacokinetics

7. The abbreviation "qod" stands for:
   a. once daily
   b. once every other day
   c. daily
   d. none of the above

8. Which of the following is the correct category for the drug Imodium?
   a. analgesic
   b. antidiarrheal
   c. antianxiety
   d. anticoagulant

9. Which drug would be given to a patient who needs a blood thinner?
   a. Dilatin
   b. Decadron
   c. Heparin
   c. Zoloft

10. The escape of fluid from a vessel into the surrounding tissue, which can cause localized vasoconstriction, is termed:
    a. anaphylaxis
    b. extravasation
    c. edema
    d. hematoma

11. Which of the following is a parenternal route of administration?
    a. intravenous
    b. topical
    c. oral
    d. inhalation

The answers to the Review Questions can be found by logging on to our website at: *http://evolve.elsevier.com/Washington+Leaver/principles*

Questions to Ponder

1. You are charting a dose of medication administered in the oncology department. You recorded the wrong route of administration. You "white out" the error and rewrite the appropriate route to correct the record. Is this an acceptable method to correct the record? If not, what is the correct method?

2. Why is following standard precautions during drug administration important?

3. Discuss the importance of parenteral drug administration.

4. Compare the gender differences in the absorption of medications.

5. Analyze the differences between ionic and nonionic contrast media.

REFERENCES

1. Adler AM, Carlton RR, editors: *Introduction to radiologic sciences and patient care*, ed 2, Philadelphia, 2007, Saunders.
2. American Society of Radiologic Technologists: *Radiation therapy practice standard*, Albuquerque, 2007, The American Society of Radiologic Technologists.
3. Beebe RO, Funk DL: *Fundamentals of emergency care*, Albany, NY, 2001, Delmar.
4. Brice J: Imaging and the law: simple tactics minimize exposure to malpractice, *Diagn Imaging* 14(3):43-46, 1992.
5. Ehrlich RA, Daly JA, McCloskey ED: *Patient care in radiography with an introduction to medical imaging*, ed 6, St. Louis, 2004, Mosby.
6. Holleb A, Fink DJ, Murphy GP: *Clinical oncology: a multidisciplinary approach for physicians and students*, Atlanta, 1991, The American Cancer Society.
7. Kemp BB, Pillitteri A, Brown P: *Fundamentals of nursing: a framework for practice*, ed 2, Glenview, Ill, 1989, Scott, Foresman.
8. Kowalczyk N, Donnett KA: *Integrated patient care for the imaging professional*, St. Louis, 1996, Mosby.
9. Lucchese DR, Eikman EA: The medical-legal implications of contrast agent use, *Appl Radiol* 18(12):36-37, 1989.
10. Newman J, Hladik WB: *Pharmacology for the radiologic technologist, Part 3: adverse reactions to radiopaque contrast media*, Albuquerque, 1997, The American Society of Radiologic Technologists.
11. Perry AG, Potter PA: *Clinical nursing skills and techniques*, ed 5, St. Louis, 2006, Mosby.
12. Potter PA, Perry AG: *Fundamentals of nursing*, ed 6, St. Louis, 2005, Elsevier Mosby.
13. Roberts GH, Carson J: Venipuncture tips for radiologic technologists, *Radiol Technol* 65(2):107-115, 1993.
14. Schwartz HW: *Current concepts in radiology management*, Sudbury, Mass, 1992, American Healthcare Radiology Administrators.
15. Smith SF, Duell DJ: *Clinical nursing skills: nursing process model, basic to advanced skills*, ed 3, Norwalk, Conn, 1992, Appleton & Lange.
16. Taylor C, Lillis C, LeMone P: *Fundamentals of nursing: the art and science of nursing care*, ed 5, Philadelphia, 2005, JB Lippincott.
17. Torres LS: *Basic medical techniques and patient care in imaging technology*, ed 6, Philadelphia, 2003, Lippincott Williams & Wilkins.

Physics, Simulation, and Treatment Planning

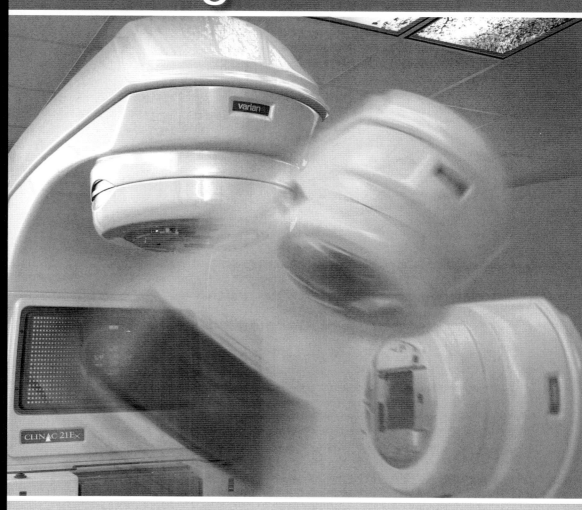

13

Applied Mathematics Review

Charles M. Washington, E. Richard Bawiec, Jr.

Outline

Review of mathematical
  concepts
    Algebraic equations with one
      unknown
    Ratios and proportions
    Inverse proportionality
    Direct proportionality

Trigonometric ratios and the
    right angle triangle
Linear interpolation
Working with exponents
Significant figures
Natural logarithms and the
    exponential function

Basic units
Measurements and experimental
    uncertainty
  Dimensional analysis
Practical examples of mathematics
    in radiation therapy
Summary

Objectives

* Explain why mathematics is involved in radiation therapy and explain its significance in conducting treatments.
* Compare and contrast the differences between direct proportionality and inverse proportionality.
* Describe the three most common trigonometric fractions associated with a right triangle and describe instances when they are used in treatment.
* Understand when to use linear interpolation in treatment.

* Explain how natural logarithms and exponential factors are inverses of each other.
* Compare and contrast the three categories of uncertainties in measurements.
* Explain two differences between accuracy and precision and how they are used in radiation therapy treatment.
* Describe why errors occur in radiation therapy.

Key Terms

Adjacent
Algebraic equation
Base
Cosine
Dimensional analysis
Direct proportionality
Exponent
Hypotenuse
Inverse proportionality
Linear interpolation
Logarithm
Opposite
Proportion
Ratio
Right triangle
Scientific notation
Significant figures
Sine
Tangent

The practice of radiation therapy requires the use of exact quantitative measurements for the accurate delivery of a therapeutic dose. Patient simulation, treatment planning, and quality assurance have a strong functional dependence on mathematics. Because of this fact, the radiation therapist and the medical dosimetrist must have a good working knowledge of basic, as well as advanced, mathematical skills to accurately perform their duties. This chapter serves as a review of the principles of the mathematical concepts pertinent to the delivery of ionizing radiation in cancer management. The emphasis is on practical application, not on teaching theoretical principles. This chapter reviews ratios and proportions, exponential functions, logarithms, basic units, uncertainty, and dimensional analysis. Appropriately, practical applications are emphasized. The initial sections are structured as a review and are not intended to "teach" math concepts. The reader is presumed to have a working knowledge of basic entry-level college algebra.

REVIEW OF MATHEMATICAL CONCEPTS

Algebraic Equations with One Unknown

In many situations, an **algebraic equation** is used to describe a physical phenomenon based on the interaction of several factors. For example, the dose to any point from a brachytherapy source requires knowledge of the source activity, source filtration, distance from the source to the point of calculation interest, and several other factors. The ability to solve an equation for the value of an unknown variable is important. The following "rules" of algebra are helpful in remembering how do to this:
* When an unknown is multiplied by some quantity, divide both sides of an equation by that quantity to isolate the unknown.
* When a quantity is added to an unknown, subtract that quantity from both sides of the equation to isolate the unknown. When the quantity is subtracted from the unknown, add it to both sides.
* When an equation appears in fractional form, that is, the unknown is divided by some quantity, cross multiply both sides by that quantity, then solve for the unknown.[3]

Algebraic manipulation is used commonly in radiation therapy, so the radiation therapist and medical dosimetrist should be comfortable solving these types of equations. An example of a typical algebraic manipulation scenario is shown in the practical examples at the end of this chapter.

Ratios and Proportions

A **ratio** is the comparison of two numbers, values, or terms. The ratio denotes a relationship between the two components. Often these relationships allow the radiation therapist to predict trends. The notation for writing a ratio of a value or term, *x*, to another value or term, *y*, is most often written as follows:

$$\frac{x}{y} \ or \ x{:}y$$

One important property of a ratio is that any ratio, x/y, remains unchanged if both terms undergo operations by the same number. For example, the ratio $32/80$ can be simplified to the ratio $2/5$ by dividing both the numerator and the denominator by 16, a common factor of both numbers.

If two ratios are equal, this is known as a **proportion**. A proportion can also be looked at as an equation relating two ratios. This principle can assist in solving for an unknown factor in a proportion. For example, examine the following proportion:

$$5{:}7 = n{:}49$$

This can be rewritten in a more recognizable form as follows:

$$\frac{5}{7} = \frac{n}{49}$$

By cross-multiplication, this proportion can be solved for *n*:

$$(49 \times 5) = 7n \ or \ 7n = (49 \times 5)$$
$$7n = 245$$
$$n = 35$$

In the clinical radiation therapy environment, inverse and direct proportions can occur in various ways. The concepts of inverse and direct proportionality are pertinent in the management of cancer with ionizing radiation, so a brief review of these concepts is beneficial.

Inverse Proportionality

Consider a hypothetical situation in which a number of aircraft must complete a trip of 1000 miles. Each aircraft travels at a different velocity. The time required for each plane to make the trip depends on that plane's velocity. Table 13-1 lists the times and velocities for each aircraft.

What simple relationship can we determine from these data? By examining the table, the following conclusions can be made:

- As velocity increases, time decreases.
- As velocity is doubled, time is halved.
- As velocity is quadrupled, time decreases by a factor of 4.

This example exhibits the concept of **inverse proportionality**. Velocity *(v)* is inversely proportional to time *(t)*. Mathematically, that is written as follows:

$$v \propto \frac{1}{t} \ or \ v = \frac{k}{t}$$

where *k* is a constant of proportionality. We can also relate two different aircrafts' velocities and times as an inverse proportion:

$$v_1 : v_2 = t_2 : t_1 \ or \ \frac{v_1}{v_2} = \frac{t_2}{t_1}$$

Example 2 in the practical examples section demonstrates inverse proportionality while solving for an unknown.

Inverse proportionality is commonly seen in radiation therapy. For example, depth and percentage depth dose are inversely related (as depth increases, percentage depth dose decreases) as are beam energy and penumbra width (as energy increases, the width of the beam's penumbra decreases). Another good example of inverse proportionality is the inverse square law, which states that the intensity of radiation from a point source varies inversely with the square of the distance from the source.

Direct Proportionality

The distance traveled by an aircraft moving at a constant velocity depends on the length of time that the aircraft is aloft. Suppose we consider an aircraft traveling at a constant velocity of 400 miles per hour. The time required for this aircraft to travel 100 miles is 0.25 hour; for 200 miles, the time is 0.5 hour; and so forth. Table 13-2 lists several distances and the time required by the aircraft to complete each distance.

Similar to the inverse proportionality example, conclusions can be reached from the data in this table, as follows:

- As time increases, distance increases.
- As time doubles, distance doubles.
- As time triples, distance triples.

Therefore, we say that distance *(D)* is directly proportional to time *(t)*. Mathematically, that is written as follows:

$$D \propto t \ or \ D = kt$$

Table 13-1	Aircraft Velocities and Times to Complete Trip	
Aircraft	Velocity (miles/hr)	Time (hr)
A	500	2.0
B	400	2.5
C	250	4.0
D	200	5.0
E	125	8.0

Table 13-2	Distance and Time Values for Aircraft	
Distance (miles)		Time (hr)
0		0.00
100		0.25
200		0.50
300		0.75
400		1.00

where k is the constant of proportionality. We can also relate two different distances and times as a direct proportion:

$$D_1 : D_2 = t_1 : t_2$$
$$or \frac{D_1}{D_2} = \frac{t_1}{t_2}$$

Example 3 in the practical examples section demonstrates direct proportionality while solving for an unknown.

Direct proportionality is also commonly seen in radiation therapy. For example, field size and percentage depth dose are directly proportional (as field size increases, percentage depth dose increases) as are beam energy and tissue air ratio (TAR) or tissue maximum ratio (TMR) (as energy increases, TAR and TMR increase). These relationships assume that all other related factors are constant.

Trigonometric Ratios and the Right Angle Triangle

Calculating angles, such as collimator and gantry angles, and depths and lengths that are related to these angles is common in setups during patient simulation and treatment. In many of these cases, a solution is derived by using the properties of a right triangle. A **right triangle** is a three-sided polygon on which one corner measures 90 degrees. The three most common functions associated with the right triangle are the **sine, cosine**, and **tangent**. Figure 13-1 diagrams these quantities. There are six quantities that describe a right triangle: the three angles (α, β, and the 90-degree angle) and the three lengths (line segments AB, AC, and BC). The sine, cosine, and tangent of an angle on a right triangle are defined mathematically (using the angle α, for example), as follows:

$$sin(\alpha) = \frac{\text{Opposite}}{\text{Hypotenuse}} = \frac{AC}{BC}$$
$$cos(\alpha) = \frac{\text{Adjacent}}{\text{Hypotenuse}} = \frac{AB}{BC}$$
$$tan(\alpha) = \frac{\text{Opposite}}{\text{Adjacent}} = \frac{AC}{AB}$$

In these equations, **opposite** refers to the length of the side of the right triangle that is opposite the specified angle, **hypotenuse** refers to the length of the longest side of the triangle, and **adjacent** refers to the length of the side of the right triangle that is close, or adjacent, to the specified angle.

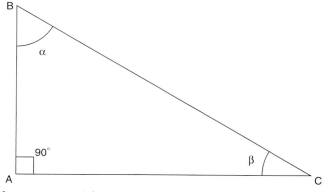

Figure 13-1. A right triangle.

To solve for any unknown quantity on a right triangle, only specific combinations of two of the five remaining quantities (excluding the 90-degree angle) must be known. One other characteristic of the right triangle is that the angles all add up to 180 degrees. Expressed mathematically, this is simply: $\alpha + \beta + 90 = 180$. Example 4 in the practical example section illustrates how one can determine unknown quantities in a right triangle.

Sine, cosine, and tangent are the primary trigonometric knowledge required of the radiation therapist and are used frequently for specific clinical functions such as matching the divergences of two abutting treatment fields or measuring the angle or thickness of a chest wall. Values of specific trigonometric functions can be determined either by looking them up in tables or by using a handheld scientific calculator. Because of the simplicity and common use of such calculators, this method for calculating the sine, cosine, or tangent of an angle is used here.[1]

Scientific calculators use the SIN, COS, and TAN keys. To obtain the specific trigonometric value desired, enter the known angle into the calculator in degrees and press the desired trigonometric function key. For example, to find the tangent of 30 degrees, type in the following:

| 3 | | 0 | | TAN | | = |

The calculator should display 0.57735. This means that the ratio of the opposite side of the 30-degree angle to the side adjacent to the 30 degrees is 0.57735. It is also possible to determine the measure of an angle by knowing the ratio between the two sides. If the ratio of the opposite side to the hypotenuse is 0.6, then the angle associated with this ratio can be calculated. Remember that the ratio opposite of the hypotenuse defines the sine of the angle. Therefore, sin α = 0.6. To calculate the angle, one simply needs the inverse sine of 0.6. This is obtained on most scientific calculators by pressing either the inverse sine $\boxed{\text{SIN}^{-1}}$ button or the $\boxed{\text{INV}}$ button followed by the sin $\boxed{\text{SIN}}$ button. For the example, the inverse sine of 0.6 is 36.87 degrees. Therefore, α = 36.87 degrees.

Success in understanding trigonometric functions and identities depends, to a large degree, on the clinical application. Trigonometric functions are the most difficult type of mathematical problems for many therapy practitioners. Practice through didactic work or experiencing these problems firsthand can aid the radiation therapist and medical dosimetrist in recognizing these problems and solving them when they occur.

Linear Interpolation

To determine many of the factors that are used often in the practice of radiation therapy, one must be able to find values from tables that contain these needed factors. Field-size dependence factors, TARs, TMRs, percentage-depth doses, and so forth are conveniently listed in easy-to-read tables. For example, a radiation therapist or medical dosimetrist can easily look up the TAR for a 10 × 10 cm field size at a 10-cm depth. However, the tables list the factors only in incremental values. What happens if the exact depth of calculation and/or field size is not listed in the table or lies between two table values? In this case, the radiation therapist or medical dosimetrist can use an approximate evaluation for the intermediate point. The process of calculating

unknown values from known values is called **linear interpolation**. Linear interpolation assumes the following[5]:
1. That two particular values are known
2. That the rate of change between the known values is constant
3. That an unknown data point must be found

The rate of change can be assumed as constant between the values typically used when finding the unknown value. To minimize any inherent rate of change and be more precise, it is important to use known values that are close together. In most tables used in radiation therapy dose calculations, algebraic ratios can be used to assist the radiation therapist and medical dosimetrist in finding the intermediate number. If a desired point is directly between two known points, a simple average of the two factors for the two respective points is all that is required to determine the new value. When the desired point is not directly between the two known points, the new value must be determined by simple ratios. The ratio of the difference between the unknown value and the upper and lower known values equals the ratio of the difference between the desired point and the upper and lower points in the table. In some cases, the number that we need may require a "double-interpolation" where the unknown value is between known values in two different directions. A TAR may be needed for a field size of 11×11 cm at a depth of 8.5 cm. In this case, values for the field size and depth needed are not listed in a TAR table and it is necessary to find values for one of the unknowns before the other can be calculated. Example 5 in the practical example section demonstrates how factors are interpolated from a table when the known values lie "above" and "below" the unknown value. Relationships are established between the known values, and these relationships must be maintained throughout the calculation to arrive at the correct factor.

Working with Exponents

An exponent, or "power," is a shorthand notation that represents the multiplication of a number by itself a given number of times. For example, $4^3 = 4 \times 4 \times 4 = 64$. In this case the superscript 3 represents the **exponent**, and the 4 represents the **base**. The 3 is also said to be the "power." One could verbally express 4^3 as "four raised to the third power." The following simple rules are important to remember when working with exponents:

1. $x^0 = 1$
2. $x^a \times x^b = x^{a+b}$
3. $(x^a)^b = x^{ab}$
4. $(xy)^a = x^a y^a$
5. $\left[\dfrac{x}{y}\right]^a = \dfrac{x^a}{y^b}$
6. $x^{-a} = \left[\dfrac{1}{x^a}\right]$ and $\left[\dfrac{1}{x^{-a}}\right] = x^a$

Scientific notation is a special use of exponents that uses base 10 notation. It is used to represent either very large or very small numbers.[2] Numbers written in scientific notation are written in the following form:

$$n.nnn \times 10^p$$

where *n.nnn* indicates the first four numerical values of the specified number. The power to which the base of 10 is raised (*p*) depends on the size of the specified number. For example, 2657.89 can be written in scientific notation as 2.65789×10^3; it can also be written as 26.5789×10^2. However, in the scientific community, placing only one number to the left of the decimal point is the preferred style. Example 6 in the practical example section illustrates the use of exponents.

Significant Figures

All measurements are approximations—no measuring device can give perfect measurements without some experimental uncertainty. In most radiation oncology physics measurements, this uncertainty is typically very small. The number of **significant figures** in a measurement or calculation is simply the number of figures that are known with some degree of reliability. The number 10.2 is said to have 3 significant figures. The number 10.20 is said to have 4 significant figures.

There are several rules for deciding the number of significant figures in a measured quantity:
1. All nonzero digits are significant: 1.234 g has 4 significant figures, 1.2 g has 2 significant figures.
2. Zeroes between nonzero digits are significant: 1002 kg has 4 significant figures, 3.07 mL has 3 significant figures.
3. Zeroes to the left of the first nonzero digits are not significant; such zeroes merely indicate the position of the decimal point: 0.001° C has only 1 significant figure, 0.012 g has 2 significant figures.
4. Zeroes to the right of a decimal point in a number are significant: 0.023 mL has 2 significant figures, 0.200 g has 3 significant figures.[6,7]
5. When a number ends in zeroes that are not to the right of a decimal point, the zeroes are not necessarily significant: 190 miles may be 2 or 3 significant figures, 5040 centigrays (cGy) may be 3 or 4 significant figures.

The last rule can be made clearer by the use of standard exponential, or scientific, notation. For example, depending on whether 3 or 4 significant figures is correct, we could write 5040 cGy as:

$$5.04 \times 10^3 \text{ cGy (3 significant figures)}$$
$$\text{or}$$
$$5.040 \times 10^3 \text{ cGy (4 significant figures)}$$

When combining measurements with different degrees of accuracy and precision (different number of significant figures), the accuracy of the final answer can be no greater than the least accurate measurement. This principle can be translated into the following rules:
- When measurements are added or subtracted, the answer can contain no more decimal places than the least accurate measurement.
- When measurements are multiplied or divided, the answer can contain no more significant figures than the least accurate measurement.[6,7]

Natural Logarithms and the Exponential Function

A **logarithm** operates as the reverse of exponential notation. While the example 4^3 is considered "four raised to the third power" in exponential notation and equals 64, the logarithm base 4 of 64 equals 3. In mathematical notation the logarithm is written as follows:

$$\log_b(N) = x$$

where b is the base, N is the desired product, and x is the power. In exponential notation, this is written as follows:

$$b^x = N$$

Certain physical processes have been discovered in nature that obey a special type of logarithmic, and thus exponential, behavior. A radioactive substance is said to decay exponentially.[1,3,4,8] This simply means that the physical process that occurs can be described by exponential notation. However, rather than the base being an integer, the base is a special number that was discovered by Euler, a mathematician. This special number is represented by the letter e and is called Euler's constant or the "base of the natural logarithms." Numerically, e is equal to 2.718272 …. Logarithms based on e are called "natural logarithms." Exponential function is the terminology used to describe e raised to a power and is written as follows:

$$e^x = N$$

A special notation is also given to the natural logarithm. The symbol ln is shorthand for "(natural) logarithm base e" and can be written as follows:

$$\ln(N) = x$$

These two equations can be combined to yield an important identity:

$$\ln(e^x) = x$$

In other words, the natural logarithm and the exponential functions are inverses of each other. The exponential function has a few important properties that can be beneficial to the radiation therapy practitioner:

- If the power (x) is greater than 0 (meaning the power is positive), then the value of e^x is greater than 1.
- If the power is less than 0 (meaning the power is negative), then the value of e^x is a number greater than 0 and less than 1.
- If the power is exactly 0, then the value of e^x is exactly equal to 1.
  To summarize:

$$e^x > 1 \text{ if } x > 0$$
$$0 < e^x < 1 \text{ if } x < 0$$
$$e^x = 1 \text{ if } x = 0$$

Example 7 in the practical example section demonstrates how to use the exponential function.

Basic Units

The system of basic units used most commonly in radiation therapy clinics is the metric or International System of Units (SI) system. This system is the world standard for scientific and technical work. The metric system is based on fundamental units of time, distance, mass, and electrical current and several derived units that are combinations of the four fundamental units.

In addition, prefixes may be added to the four fundamental units to represent large or small quantities of the fundamental units.[2-4,8]

The four fundamental units in the metric system are the second (time), the meter (distance), the kilogram (mass), and the ampere (electrical current). These units are defined internationally by standards kept at a laboratory near Paris, France. However, secondary standards are kept in national laboratories in most countries. In the United States, the National Institute of Standards and Technology (NIST) maintains the secondary standards.[2] Commonly used prefixes and their meanings are listed in Table 13-3.

Special units have been defined for the radiologic sciences. The Roentgen (r) is the unit of radiation exposure that represents a measure of the amount of ionization created by radiation in the air. A derived unit for exposure is the Coulomb/kilogram (C/kg). Thus, the relationship between these two quantities is 1 Roentgen = 2.58×10^{-4} C/kg.

The accepted unit of absorbed dose is the Gray (Gy). Absorbed dose describes the amount of radiation × energy absorbed by a medium. The Gray can be expressed in units as joule/kilogram (J/kg). An outdated unit that was replaced by the Gray is the rad. A rad is equal to 0.01 Gray or, restated, 100 rads equals 1 Gray. Therefore, 1 rad equals 1 cGy.[3]

The accepted unit of energy is the joule (J), which is equal to 1 kilogram-meter^2 per second^2 (1 kgm^2/s^2). A joule of energy is a rather large amount of energy, relative to the energies associated with radiation therapy. Therefore, another special "derived" unit is the electron volt (eV). The relationship between the electron volt and the joule is as follows:

$$1 \text{ eV} = 1.602 \times 10^{-19} \text{ J}$$

The kiloelectron volt (keV = 10^3 eV) and the megaelectron volt (MeV = 10 eV) are the most common energy units used in the radiation therapy clinic.[3]

Measurements and Experimental Uncertainty

During the course of a program in radiation therapy, a student eventually becomes familiar with certain quantities such as source-to-axis distance (SAD) and source-to-skin distance (SSD) measurements, as well as certain units such as absorbed dose (cGy), exposure (Roentgen), and activity (millicurie).[2-4,8] Different instruments can be used to measure these and various

Table 13-3	Numerical Prefixes Used with SI Units		
	Prefix	**Symbol**	**Multiplier**
	pico	p	10^{-12}
	nano	n	10^{-9}
	micro	μ	10^{-6}
	milli	m	10^{-3}
	centi	c	10^{-2}
	deci	d	10^{-1}
	kilo	k	10^{3}
	mega	M	10^{6}
	giga	G	10^{9}

SI, International System of Units.

other quantities. The process of taking a measurement is basically an attempt to determine a value or magnitude of known quantity.

For example, the quantity SSD is a physical measurement of distance. Suppose an SSD of 73.5 cm was measured from the source of radiation to the chest wall of a patient during the treatment simulation process. This indicates that the centimeter was used as a unit of length and that the distance to the skin surface was 73.5 times larger than this unit. Stated differently, a measurement is a comparison of the magnitude (how large or small) of a quantity with that of an accepted standard. In this measurement and in other measurements such as determining the temperature using a thermometer, the barometric pressure using a barometer, or the exposure rate using an exposure rate meter, an amount of uncertainty is inherent. Therefore, the measuring process requires that the person taking the measurement must have the knowledge that this uncertainty exists. Referring to the SSD measurement, the distance of 73.5 cm will contain error that is introduced not only by the measuring device but also by the fact that the patient will most probably be moving as a result of inhalation and exhalation. This inherent or built-in uncertainty in making a measurement is a characteristic of almost all of science. Uncertainties can be grouped into three categories: systematic errors, random errors, and blunders.

Systematic Errors. A systematic error is an error or uncertainty inherent within the measuring device. A systematic error always affects the measurement in the same way: the measurement will either be too large or too small, depending on the device. These errors are commonly obtained, for example, from one or more of the following: human biases such as vision inaccuracies; imperfect techniques that may occur, for example, during experimental setup; and unacceptable instrument calibrations. Stem leakage of an ionization chamber and the inaccuracy of reading an analog temperature meter on an annealing oven are examples of systematic errors.

Random Errors. Random errors, as the name implies, are a result of variations attributed to chance that are unavoidable. Random errors can either increase or decrease the result of a measurement. To correct for this type of error, a common practice is to take several measurements and average them. Random errors can also be reduced by making improvements in the measuring device and/or technique. An uncontrolled rapid change in temperature or barometric pressure, accidental movement of a patient during setup, and electronic noise are all examples of random errors.

Blunders. Blunders during measurement are those errors that occur as a result of human error in algebraic or arithmetic calculations or from improper use of a measuring device. Errors

such as these can be avoided by properly educating the individuals who will be making the measurements. They can also be avoided by comparing the measurements being made to previous measurements that are known to be correct or even comparing them with theoretical values. If large discrepancies exist between the correct values and the values that the individual is obtaining, then something must have been done incorrectly, and retracing the setup and procedure can be an easy way to remedy the error.

Accuracy and Precision of Measurements. Another facet of measurements that must be discussed is the importance of and the difference between the accuracy and precision of a measurement. When measurements are made, the individual must be concerned with how close the measurements are to the "true" value. Although the true value cannot be known exactly, theoretical calculations can define a value that is accepted as a true value. How close a measurement comes to this true value is referred to as *accuracy*. The precision of a measurement indicates how reproducible a particular measurement is or how consistent the measurement is.

Figure 13-2 illustrates the difference between accuracy and precision. The bull's-eye represents the "true value." The arrows represent measurements. In the first picture, the measurements are neither precise nor accurate. The arrows (measurements) did not hit the bull's-eye, nor did they land close to each other. In the second picture, the arrows were precise but inaccurate. They all hit close to the same location but were not close to the bull's-eye. In the third picture, the arrows were precise and accurate, because they were grouped together close to the bull's-eye.

As another example, consider the output measurement of a linear accelerator as performed by three therapists as part of the daily quality assurance program. After setting up the necessary apparatus and following the policy and procedure outline, the following data were gathered. Each therapist made four measurements with the ionization chamber to obtain an average value for the output and thereby eliminate random errors.

	Therapist A	Therapist B	Therapist C
	2.702	2.650	2.738
	2.701	2.660	2.578
	2.702	2.655	2.737
	2.702	2.651	2.579
Average	2.702	2.654	2.657

The accepted value for the output for that accelerator was 2.658. So a number of questions could be asked about the values obtained by the radiation therapists. Which therapist had the most accurate values? Which therapist had the most precise

Cobalt-60 is a live radioactive source that is still used today in the treatment of many malignancies. When working on these machines, the radiation therapist must remember that, because it is a live source, there is radioactive decay occurring all the time. In essence, the source is continually getting weaker. To make up for this, each month the treatment times must be increased to ensure that the same amount of dose is given throughout the patients' treatment. The decay rate is based on the knowledge that the half-life of a cobalt-60 source is 5.26 years; therefore the timer correction is –0.011 minute decay per month. The equation to determine the new timer setting is as follows:

$$\text{Timer setting} = \frac{\text{Prescribed dose per field}}{\text{Calibrated dose rate in cGy/min} \times \text{Depth factor} \times \text{Field size factors} \times \text{Beam attenuation}} + \text{Timer correction}$$

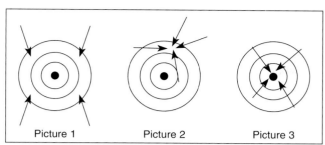

Figure 13-2. Representation of the contrast between accuracy and precision. *Picture 1* is neither accurate nor precise. *Picture 2* demonstrates precision but not accuracy. *Picture 3* illustrates both precision and accuracy.

values? Which therapist had the best overall results? The measurements made by Therapist A were more consistent and more precise because values do not differ by more than 0.001 from each other. However, the average results obtained by Therapists B and C were closer to the accepted value. Apparently, Therapists B and C were more accurate than Therapist A, although Therapist A was the most precise. By comparing the individual values that were obtained by Therapists B and C, one can see that Therapist C's values had a large range. Therefore, although Therapist C's average value was the closest to the accepted value, it was obtained through imprecise readings. Therefore, the values obtained by Therapist B are deemed the most acceptable because they were precise and accurate.

From this example, it is apparent that a measurement can be precise without being accurate and vice versa. Radiation therapy practitioners should be concerned not only with accuracy but also with precision. Discerning between the two is a function of analytic al judgment and critical thinking skills, both very important in the practice of radiation therapy.

Experimental Uncertainty. Because it is impossible to eliminate all systematic errors, random errors, and blunders, an absolutely accurate and precise measurement cannot be achieved. Although this seems disheartening to the scientist, there is a method that is accepted by the scientific community to handle this experimental uncertainty. It is common practice to measure the percent relative error in a measurement to discover the degree of accuracy. The percent relative error can be thought of as the percentage of error in a measurement relative to the accepted value. It is calculated by using the following equation:

$$\text{\% Relative error} = \left[\frac{\text{Experimental value} - \text{Accepted value}}{\text{Accepted value}} \right] \times 100$$

Look at the measurement result of Therapist A. The percent relative error in that result can be calculated as follows using the previous equation:

$$\text{\% Relative error} = \left[\frac{2.702 - 2.658}{2.658} \right] \times 100 = 1.65\%$$

The percent relative error in the result obtained by Therapist A was +1.65%. This means that the result was 1.65% higher than the accepted value. The percent relative errors in the results obtained by Therapists B and C can be calculated by the reader as −0.15% and −0.04%, respectively. Both of these values were low.

Dimensional Analysis

A technique that can be very useful in radiation therapy (as well as in many other branches of science) is dimensional analysis. **Dimensional analysis** is a process that involves the careful assessment of the units of measurement used in calculating a specific quantity. This technique involves canceling common units that appear in the numerator and denominator of an equation. When one or more quantities are manipulated to obtain a specified quantity, the units of the known quantities when combined must be equivalent to the unit of measurement of that specified quantity. For example, to obtain the specific quantity of velocity, one must divide distance by time. In other words, velocity is measured in meters per second, distance is measured in meters, and time is measured in seconds.[3]

When an equation is being used, it is important to ensure that all of the units when combined equate to the units desired. There are a few "rules of thumb" that can be used when analyzing the dimensions of an equation. First, any quantity divided by 1 is equal to the quantity itself. Next, any quantity divided by itself is equal to 1. In addition, the process of division is equivalent to multiplying the numerator by the inverse of the denominator.[2,3] Using these facts, one can cancel units in any equation until no cancellation possibility remains. The units that remain should be equivalent to the desired units. If this is not true, then an error must have occurred.

PRACTICAL EXAMPLES OF MATHEMATICS IN RADIATION THERAPY

Mathematical theories must be put into practice for the radiation therapist to really understand the concepts and what it means to radiation therapy practice. Several examples have been used throughout this chapter to help focus the content into useful information. This section of the chapter provides more in-depth analysis of practical application examples of mathematical principles as seen in radiation therapy.

Example 1—algebraic equations: For the value of an unknown to be determined, it is necessary to use the rules of algebra. For example, if a radiation therapist knows the total dose that a patient is to receive and the dose per fraction, then the number of treatments can be determined. Assume that the total dose is 5000 cGy and the daily dose is 200 cGy. The number of fractions can be determined from the following equation:

$$200 \text{ cGy/fraction} \times N(\text{fraction}) = 5000 \text{ cGy}$$

where *N* represents the number of fractions. To isolate the unknown *(N)*, the value of 200 can be divided out of both sides of the equation without disturbing the equality:

$$\frac{200 \text{ cGy/fraction}}{200 \text{ cGy/fraction}} \times N = \frac{5000 \text{ cGy}}{200 \text{ cGy/fraction}}$$

The first term in this equation is equal to 1, and any value multiplied by 1 equals that number. In addition, because the unit cGy appears in both the numerator and the denominator of the fraction on the right side of the equation, it can be canceled. The resulting equation is thus:

$$N = \frac{5000}{200} \times \frac{1}{1/\text{fraction}}$$

At this point, one other algebraic rule can be applied.

Any fraction that appears in the denominator of a fraction can be written as the reciprocal of that fraction. Therefore, our final answer becomes the following:

$$N = \frac{5000}{200} \text{ fraction} = 25 \text{ fraction}$$

So the radiation therapist knows that the patient has 25 fractions prescribed.

As already stated, values can be subtracted from both sides of an equation to find an answer. Suppose that a radiation therapist knows that the physician wants to deliver 200 cGy on a particular day and knows that on the previous day the patient received 250 cGy. Therefore the unknown can be determined from the following equation:

$$250 \text{ cGy} - X = 200 \text{ cGy}$$

Obviously, this is a simple problem, but it is used to illustrate a principle. From this point, one can subtract 250 cGy from both sides of the equation, as follows:

$$250 \text{ cGy} - X - 250 \text{ cGy} = 200 \text{ cGy} - 250 \text{ cGy}$$

Subtracting 250 from itself equals 0, and 0 added to any value simply equals that value. In addition, one can multiply both sides of an equation by the same value without disturbing the equality. Therefore, if both sides of the equation are multiplied by −1, the following results:

$$-X = 200 \text{ cGy} - 250 \text{ cGy} = -50 \text{ cGy}$$
$$(-1) \times -X = (-1) \times -50 \text{ cGy}$$
$$X = 50 \text{ cGy}$$

So the radiation therapist knows that the daily dose was reduced by 50 cGy.

Example 2—inverse proportionality: A radiation therapist just learned from a medical physicist that the therapy unit would be running at a dose rate of 400 cGy/min on a given day. The radiation therapist knows that the normal dose rate is 300 cGy/min and wonders how this new dose rate will affect the patient's treatment times. This example illustrates inverse proportionality. If a particular patient's treatments took 1.2 minutes with the normal dose rate of 300 cGy/min, then what would it be with the new dose rate? This can be solved by the following equation:

$$300 \text{ cGy/min} \times 1.2 \text{ min} = 360 \text{ cGy}$$
$$\frac{360 \text{ cGy}}{400 \text{ cGy/min}} = 0.9 \text{ minute}$$

Therefore, as the dose rate increases, treatment times decrease, which demonstrates the concept of inverse proportionality.

Example 3—direct proportionality: A radiation oncologist wants to increase the dose that a patient receives per fraction but does not want to change the total number of fractions. Assume that, originally, the physician had planned to give 200 cGy per fraction for 25 fractions, then decided that 230 cGy would achieve better results. Initially, the total dose would have been as follows:

$$200 \text{ cGy/fraction} \times 25 \text{ fractions} = 5000 \text{ cGy}$$

But because the dose per fraction was changed to 230 cGy, the total dose would also change:

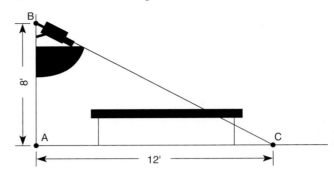

$$230 \text{ cGy/fraction} \times 25 \text{ fractions} = 5750 \text{ cGy}$$

Therefore, note that as the dose per fraction increases, the total dose increases. This is an example of direct proportionality.

Example 4—unknown quantities and the right triangle: A medical physicist wants to know at what angle a wall-mounted laser is directed at the floor. Assume that she also wants to know the distance from the laser to its intersection point on the floor. First, she measures the distance from the wall to the intersection point on the floor (segment AC measures 12 ft). Then she measures how far up the wall the laser is mounted (segment AB measures 8 ft).

From the trigonometric identities outlined in the text, the physicist knows that the tangent of the angle is equal to the length of the opposite side divided by the length of the adjacent side. That can be stated in mathematical form as follows:

$$\tan \beta = \frac{\text{Opposite}}{\text{Adjacent}}$$
$$\tan \beta = \frac{\text{Segment AC}}{\text{Segment AB}} = \frac{12 \text{ feet}}{8 \text{ feet}}$$
$$\tan \beta = 1.5$$
$$\tan \beta = \tan^{-1}(1.5)$$
$$\tan \beta = 56$$

Therefore, angle β is equal to 56 degrees. In addition, the physicist knows that the sine of β is equal to the length of the opposite side divided by the hypotenuse. This can be written as follows:

$$\sin \beta = \frac{\text{Opposite}}{\text{Hypotenuse}} = \frac{\text{Segment AC}}{\text{Segment BC}}$$

Because the length of segment BC is desired, the equation can be rewritten and solved for that length:

$$\text{Segment BC} = \frac{\text{Opposite}}{\sin \beta} = \frac{12 \text{ feet}}{\sin(56°)} = \frac{12}{0.829} = 14.5 \text{ feet}$$

Therefore, the distance from the laser's position on the beam wall to the point where the beam intersects the floor is 14.5 feet.

Example 5—linear interpolation: A medical dosimetrist wants to determine the output of a cobalt machine for two different field sizes for one specific date from the following output table. The field sizes are 12 × 12 cm and 19 × 19 cm. The desired date is March 30. Assume that this date is exactly halfway between March 15 and April 15.

Output (cGy/min) for Theratron 780 @ 80 cm in Air (SAD Treatment) 2009 (15th of Month)

Field size	Jan 15	Feb 15	Mar 15	Apr 15	May 15
5 × 5 cm	210.71	208.41	205.13	203.88	201.66
10 × 10 cm	218.58	216.19	213.83	211.50	209.19
12 × 12 cm	220.98	218.57	216.18	213.82	211.49
15 × 15 cm	224.48	222.03	219.60	217.21	214.83
20 × 20 cm	228.19	225.70	223.24	220.80	218.39

Because the 12 × 12 cm field size is listed on the table, the only step required to determine the output for that field size is to determine the intermediate value between the March 15 and April 15 outputs for that field size. The outputs for a 12 × 12 cm field size for March 15 and April 15 are 216.18 and 213.82 cGy/min, respectively. Therefore, the output for the 12 × 12 cm field size for March 30 is the simple average of the two outputs:

$$\frac{216.18 + 213.82}{2} = \frac{430.0}{2} = 215.00 \text{ cGy/min}$$

The first step in determining the desired output for the 19 × 19 cm field size is to determine the intermediate values of the output for March 30 for the field sizes nearest to 19 × 19 cm. These would be the 15 × 15 cm and 20 × 20 cm field sizes. The outputs for March 15 and April 15 for the 15 × 15 cm field size are 219.60 and 217.21 cGy/min, respectively, whereas the outputs for March 15 and April 15 for the 20 × 20 cm field size are 223.24 and 220.80 cGy/min, respectively. To determine the intermediate values for March 30 for each field size, the simple averages are calculated and can be shown to be 218.41 cGy/min for the 15 × 15 cm field size and 222.02 cGy/min for the 20 × 20 cm field size. The next step is to determine the ratio of how "far" the 19 × 19 cm field size is from either the smaller or the larger field size. For this example, we will choose the smaller field size. The 19 × 19 cm field size is 4 cm greater than the 15 × 15 cm field size. The difference between the 15 × 15 cm and 20 × 20 cm field sizes is 5 cm. Therefore the 19 × 19 cm field size is four fifths of the "distance" between the two known values, and thus the output for the 19 × 19 cm field size must also be four fifths of the "distance" between the two intermediate outputs that we just determined previously. It should be noted that the direction one would move on the table in going from a 15 × 15 cm² field size to a 20 × 20 cm² field size will be the same direction one would move on the table to determine the output, as well. Now, to calculate the desired output, one must know the distance between the two intermediate values and then multiply that distance by the field size distances ratio. This will give the desired output of 221.30 cGy/min:

$$222.02 \text{ cGy/min} - 218.41 \text{ cGy/min} = 3.61 \text{ cGy}$$
$$3.61 \text{ cGy/min} \times 4/5 = 2.89 \text{ cGy/min}$$
$$218.41 \text{ cGy/min} + 2.89 \text{ cGy/min} = 221.30 \text{ cGy/min}$$

Therefore, the output for March 30 for the 19 × 19 cm field size was 221.30 cGy/min.

Example 6—exponents: A brief example of the use of exponents is all that is demonstrated here. The primary use of exponents in the field of radiation therapy is in scientific notation.

If one must calculate the product of two numbers that are represented in scientific notation, some of the rules outlined in this chapter can be useful. For example, assume that a radiation physicist desires to determine the total amount of exposure produced by ionizing radiation in a specified mass of air. She knows that 1 Roentgen is equal to 2.58×10^{-4} Coulombs of charge liberated per kilogram of air present. She measured 3.23×10^{-2} Coulombs in 1 kilogram of air mass. Mathematically, this is written as follows:

$$\text{Exposure (x)} = \frac{3.23 \times 10^{-2} \text{ Coulombs}}{1 \text{ kg air}} \times \frac{1 \text{ Roentgen}}{2.58 \times 10^{-4} \text{ Coulombs/1 kg air}}$$
$$\text{Exposure (x)} = \frac{3.23 \times 10^{-2} \text{ Coulombs/1 kg air}}{2.58 \times 10^{-4} \text{ Coulombs/1 kg air}} \times 1 \text{ Roentgen}$$
$$\text{Exposure (x)} = 1.25 \times \frac{10^{-2}}{10^{-4}} \text{ Roentgen}$$

If a number with a negative exponent is in the denominator of a fraction, then that is the same as the same number with the equal positive exponent moved to the numerator of the equation:

$$\text{Exposure (x)} = 1.25 \times 10^{-2} \times 10^{4} \text{ Roentgen}$$
$$\text{Exposure (x)} = 1.25 \times 10^{(-2+4)} \text{ Roentgen}$$
$$\text{Exposure (x)} = 1.25 \times 10^{2} \text{ Roentgen} = 125 \text{ Roentgen}$$

Example 7—exponential functions: The decay of a radioactive substance behaves in an exponential manner. Therefore, if one wishes to calculate the amount of activity of a particular substance that remains after a specific amount of time, the following equation can be used:

$$A_t = A_0 \times e^{-\lambda t}$$

where A_t is the activity after time t, A_0 is the initial activity, and λ is the decay constant that is specific to the particular radioactive substance being used. As an example, assume that the activity of a sample of iridium-131 is known exactly 2 days after it was received from a manufacturer. Assume that we would like to know what the activity was when it arrived. The activity at the present is 5 Curies (Ci). Therefore, we know that $t = 2$ days and $A_t = 5$ Ci. In addition, the decay constant for iridium-131 is 8.6×10^{-2}/day. So plugging these values into the decay equation gives the following:

$$5 \text{ Ci} = A_0 \times e^{-(8.6 \times 10^{-2}/\text{day}) \times (2 \text{ days})}$$
$$5 \text{ Ci} = A_0 \times e^{-0.172}$$
$$A_0 = 5 \text{ Ci}/e^{-0.172} = \frac{5 \text{ Ci}}{0.842}$$
$$A_0 = 5.94 \text{ Ci}$$

Therefore, the activity on arrival 2 days earlier was 5.94 Ci. One can also determine the activity of the substance 2 days after the present date using the same equation. The reader can calculate this independently.

SUMMARY

- Although treatment planning and calculation checking are, for the most part, done by a member of the dosimetry or physics team, it is imperative that every member of the radiation therapy staff know how to perform the basic treatment calculations.
- With a basic knowledge of the calculations, a radiation therapist is able to determine whether a treatment dose looks correct for what is about to be treated; if something looks suspicious, the therapist can have another member of the treatment planning team verify the dose and possibly avoid a mistreatment.
- Emergent situations demand therapists to have a good working knowledge of treatment planning. These situations often occur outside of clinic hours or when radiation needs to be delivered very quickly, so it is up to the radiation therapists to calculate and administer the dose often without a treatment plan.

Review Questions

Multiple Choice

1. $(10^3)^5$ equals:
   a. 10^8
   b. 10^2
   c. 10^{15}
   d. 10^{-2}
2. Convert 910,000,000 to scientific notation.
   a. 9.1×10^8
   b. 9.01×10^7
   c. 91.0×10^8
   d. 9×10^7
3. If an instrument positioned 1 m from a point source is moved 50 cm closer to the source, the radiation intensity will be:
   a. increased by a factor of 4
   b. increased by a factor of 2
   c. decreased by a factor of 4
   d. decreased by a factor of 2
4. As the depth in tissue increases, the percentage depth dose values decreases. This is an example of:
   a. inverse proportionality
   b. direct proportionality
   c. interpolation
   d. none of the above
5. What is the ratio of 100 cGy to 500 cGy?
   a. 5:1
   b. 1:5

c. both a and b
d. neither a nor b
6. How many significant figures are there in 780,000,000?
   a. 2
   b. 3
   c. 6
   d. 9
7. How many significant figures are there in 0.0101?
   a. 2
   b. 3
   c. 4
   d. 5
8. Errors that occur as a result of human error in algebraic or arithmetic calculations or from improper use of a measuring device are:
   a. systematic errors
   b. random errors
   c. blunders
   d. precision
9. $\ln(e^x) = x$ is:
   a. true
   b. false
10. $\dfrac{10^x}{10^y} = 10^{x+y}$ is:
    a. true
    b. false

The answers to the Review Questions can be found by logging on to our website at: *http://evolve.elsevier.com/Washington+Leaver/principles*

REFERENCES

1. Bernier DR, Christian PE, Langan JK: *Nuclear medicine: technology and techniques,* ed 5, St. Louis, 2004, Mosby.
2. Bushong SC: *Radiologic science for technologists: physics, biology, and protection,* ed 8, St. Louis, 2004, Mosby.
3. Harris M: *Radiation therapy physics handbook,* Houston, 1992, The University of Texas M. D. Anderson Cancer Center.
4. Khan FM: *The physics of radiation therapy,* ed 3, Philadelphia, 2003, Lippincott Williams & Wilkins.
5. Linear interpolation (website): http://gpwiki.org/index.php/Linear_Interpolation. Accessed November 9, 2008.
6. Significant figures (website): http://www.chem.tamu.edu/class/fyp/mathrev/mr-sigfg.html. Accessed August 20, 2007.
7. Significant figures (website): http://academic.udayton.edu/VladimirBeninCHM/123_2002.htm. Accessed August 20, 2007.
8. Stanton R, Stinson D: *Applied physics for radiation oncology,* Madison, Wis, 1996, Medical Physics Publishing.

Introduction to Radiation Therapy Physics

Narayan Sahoo

Outline

Radiation quantities and units
Atomic physics
  Subatomic particles
  The model of atom
  Atomic energy levels
  Atomic nomenclature
  Nuclear forces
  Nuclear structure, stability, and
    isotopes
  Particle radiation
Electromagnetic radiation

Photons
  Physical characteristics of an
    electromagnetic wave
  Photon energy
Radioactivity
  The nuclear stability curve
  Types of radioactive decay
  Specification of radioactivity
  Exponential decay of
    radioactivity
  Radioactive equilibrium

Photon interactions
  The inverse square law
  Exponential attenuation
  X-ray beam quality
  Types of photon interactions
Other particle interactions
  Elastic and inelastic collisions
  Electron interactions
  Heavy charged particle interactions
  Neutron interactions
Summary

Key Terms

Atom
Atomic mass number
Atomic mass unit
Atomic number
Auger electron
Binding energy per
  nucleon
Bohr atom model
Bremsstrahlung
Characteristic radiation
Characteristic x-rays
Electrical charge
Electromagnetic radiation
Electron's binding
  energy
Excitation
Excited nuclear energy
  level
Frequency of the wave
Gamma rays (γ-rays)
Gravity
Ground state
Half-value layer
Heavy charged particle
Ionization
Mass equivalence
Neutron
Nuclear binding energy
Nuclear energy level
Nuclear force
Photon
Proton
Radioactivity
Rest mass
The strong force
The weak force
Wave-particle duality
Wavelength of the wave

Objectives

- Identify and describe the different sources of ionizing radiation.
- Convert units and measurements often needed in the field of radiation therapy.
- Identify types of forces responsible for interactions between particles.

- Define *binding energy, excitation,* and *ionization* and relate them to the field of radiation therapy.
- Differentiate and describe the different forms of radioactive decay.
- Identify and describe the different forms of photon interaction used in radiation therapy.

Radiation is the transmitted energy in the form of electromagnetic (EM) waves, charged and neutral particles from different sources, such as the sun and atoms. Radiation therapy involves the use of ionizing radiation that can ionize the medium it passes through, to deliver lethal dose to the target cells while keeping the normal tissue dose below its tolerance level as much as possible. This ionizing radiation can be from different sources such as x-rays; gamma rays; and electron, proton, or neutron beams, which are produced by accelerators and radioactive sources. The process of dose deposition in tissue involves complex interaction between the ionizing source and the molecules of the tissue. A good understanding of the source and nature of radiation, as well as the processes involved in the transport or interaction of the radiation in tissue, will help the radiation therapy practitioner in planning the radiation dose delivery to the target volume in the patient. The objective of this chapter is to describe some of the basic principles of radiation therapy physics.

RADIATION QUANTITIES AND UNITS

Four major quantities that are important in radiation physics are (1) radioactivity, (2) radiation exposure, (3) radiation absorbed dose, and (4) radiation dose equivalent. Every physical quantity is characterized by its magnitude and unit. Units are agreed-on standard quantities of measurements such as meters, seconds, and grams. From these fundamental units, the units of other quantities can be derived. There were two different systems of units before 1977, namely, the foot-pound-second (FPS) and the meter-kilogram-second (MKS) systems for length, mass, and time. In 1977, a new Système Internationale d'Unités (International System of Units, abbreviated as SI), was adopted to create a uniform worldwide standard.

According to SI units, the seven basic physical quantities are assigned the following units.
Length (l): meter (m)
Mass (m): kilogram (kg)
Time (t): second (s)
Electrical current (I): ampere (A)
Temperature (T): kelvin (K)
Amount of substance: mole (mol)
Luminous intensity: candela (cd)
All other physical quantities and their units can be derived from the above seven quantities and units. More information on SI units is available at http://physics.nist.gov/cuu/Units/index.html.

Example: Speed is the rate of change of position and is given by the ratio distance/time. Thus, it is quantified by l/t and its unit is m/s.

Practice: What will be the unit of momentum, which is mass multiplied by velocity?

The original units for each of the important radiation quantities of interest are given in Table 14-1 along with the new SI units and the conversion factors to change the original unit to the new one.

It is often necessary to convert between various systems and magnitudes of units.

Example: 1. How many minutes are in 2 hours 14 minutes?

$$2 \text{ hr} \times \frac{60 \text{ min}}{1 \text{ hr}} + 14 \text{ min} = 134 \text{ min}$$

2. How many meters are in 5.5 miles?

$$5.5 \text{ miles} \times \frac{5280 \text{ feet}}{1 \text{ mile}} \times \frac{12 \text{ inches}}{1 \text{ foot}} \times \frac{2.54 \text{ cm}}{1 \text{ inch}} \times \frac{1 \text{ meter}}{100 \text{ cm}} = 8851.4 \text{ m}$$

Throughout this chapter and this text you will find the opportunity to convert many types of units.

ATOMIC PHYSICS

Subatomic Particles

The smallest unit of an element that retains the properties of that element is called an **atom**. It is well known that an atom consists of electrons and a nucleus made of protons and neutrons.

The electrons, protons, and neutrons are called *subatomic particles.*[1-3] The electrons are considered to be elementary particles belonging to the class of particles called *leptons.* The neutrons and protons are composite particles and belong to the *hadron* group of particles. Hadrons are considered to be made up of constituent quarks bound together by gluons. Many types of subatomic particles have been discovered or postulated since the discovery of electrons in 1897 by J. J. Thomson.[2] The subatomic particles are classified into two groups—leptons and hadrons. There are four types of forces, which are responsible for the interaction between different particles:

1. **Gravity:** The force responsible for interaction between particles with nonzero mass and has infinite range.
2. **Electromagnetic (EM):** This force is responsible for interaction between electrically charged particles and particles with nonzero magnetic moments. It has infinite range. This force is responsible for the binding of the electrons and the nucleus to form the atoms, the binding of atoms to form molecules, and the binding of atoms and molecules to form liquids and solids. Production of light or EM radiation is a process associated with EM interactions.
3. **The strong force:** This is a short-ranged force that is responsible for interaction between neutron and proton and other particles belonging to the hadrons family.
4. **The weak force:** This is a short-ranged force that is responsible for interaction between elementary particles involving neutrinos or antineutrinos. This force is also responsible for radioactive decay of a neutron to a proton, an electron, and an antineutrino, called *beta decay.*

The strong force is the strongest among the four forces, followed by EM force, the weak force, and the weakest being gravity. The particles affected by the strong force are called *hadrons* and all others are grouped as *leptons.*

The subatomic particles important for radiation therapy are electrons, positrons, protons, neutrons, and photons. Rest mass and electrical charge are the properties of these particles with which we will be concerned. The **rest mass** refers to the mass (weight) of the particle when it is not moving. Einstein's theory of special relativity states that subatomic particles moving at high speeds will have increased mass. At this point, we will not need to concern ourselves with this theory, other than to know of it.

Table 14-1	Radiation Activity, Exposure, and Dose Units of Measurement		
Measured Property	**Old Unit**	**New SI Unit**	**Conversion Factor**
Radioactivity	Curie (Ci) = 3.73×10^{10} dps	becquerel (Bq) = 1 dps	1 Ci = 3.7×10^{10} Bq 1 Bq = 2.7×10^{-11} Ci
Radiation exposure	roentgen (R) = 2.58×10^{-4} C/kg	Coulomb/kg (C/kg)	1 R = 2.58×10^{-4} C/kg 1 C/kg = 3.88×10^{3} R
Radiation absorbed dose	rad = 100 erg/g	gray (Gy) = 1 J/kg	1 rad = 0.01 Gy 1 Gy = 100 rad
Radiation dose equivalent	rem = QF × rad	sievert (Sv) = QF × Gy	1 rem = 0.01 Sv Sv = 100 rem

From Christian PE, Waterstram-Rich KM, editors: *Nuclear medicine PET/CT: technology and techniques,* ed 6, St. Louis, 2007, Mosby.
dps, Disintegrations per second; *QF,* quality factor.

The mass of subatomic particles can be measured in terms of the standard metric system mass unit, the kilogram. For those more familiar with U.S. units of measure, 1 kg is equivalent to approximately 2.2 lb. Because of the very small masses of these particles, expressing them in kilograms would make these values very cumbersome to handle; therefore a quantity called the *atomic mass unit (amu)* was defined.

 *The **atomic mass unit** is defined such that the mass of an atom of carbon-12 is exactly 12.00 amu. As you may remember, the number of atoms in 12 grams of carbon-12 is equal to 6.022 × 10²³, which is Avogadro's number. Thus, mass of each carbon-12 atom = $12/(6.022 \times 10^{23})$ grams = $1.99 \times 10^{-23}/1000$ kg = 1.99×10^{-26} kg, which is equal to 12.00 amu. Thus,*

1 amu = $1.99 \times 10^{-26}/12$ kg = 1.66×10^{-27} kg

$$1 \text{ amu} = 1.66 \times 10^{-27} \text{ kg}$$

This relationship can be used to convert from one mass unit to another.[2]

Example: The mass of a proton is equal to 1.00727 amu. Express this mass in terms of kilograms.

$$(1.00727 \text{ amu}) \times \frac{1.66 \times 10^{-27} \text{ kg}}{(1 \text{ amu})} = 1.672 \times 10^{-27} \text{ kg}$$

The **electrical charge** is a fundamental property or character of subatomic particles. It determines the strength of their EM interaction just like the mass of particles determines the strength of their gravitational interaction. A particle can have positive, negative or zero charge. By definition or convention, the electron is assigned a negative charge and the proton has a positive charge. The electron and the proton have the same amount of electrical charge, 1.6×10^{-19} Coulombs (the Coulomb is the metric unit of electrical charge). The neutron, as the name implies, carries no electrical charge. Photons are quanta of EM energy of different frequencies and have zero rest mass and electrical charge. Two particles with an electrical charge of the same sign experience a repulsive EM force, whereas this force is attractive when the charges are of the opposite sign.

The radiation energy is transferred to any medium through its interaction with the atomic electrons and nucleus. A good understanding of the atomic structure will be helpful to understand the radiation interaction with matter.

The Model of Atom

Historically, J. J. Thomson proposed the first model of the atom, known as the *raisin bread* or *plum pudding model*. According to this model, the positive charges and negatively charged electrons are uniformly distributed in the spherical volume of the atom with a radius of a few angstroms. However, Geiger-Marsden's alpha particles scattering from a metal foil experiment proved this to be wrong by observing an unexpected large scattering probability at angles greater than 90 degrees, contrary to the prediction by Thomson's plum pudding model. It led Rutherford to propose a new model in 1911. According to the Rutherford model, the positive electrical charge (+Ze) in an atom is not uniformly distributed over the whole area of the atom but is localized in a small area with a diameter in the order of 10^{-14} m, called the *nucleus*. The negatively charged electrons are distributed in the remaining space of the spherical atomic volume with a diameter in the order of 10^{-10} m and are postulated to be rotating around the nucleus like the planets in the solar system. This model could explain very well the backscattering of the alpha particles from the metal foil as the result of Coulomb repulsion of the positively charged alpha particle from the localized positively charged nucleus. However, this model could not explain the stability of the atom. As the electrons are rotating around the nucleus, they will experience the centripetal acceleration, will continuously lose energy, and will eventually collapse to the nucleus. The Rutherford model also could not explain the discrete spectra of emitted radiation from atoms. In 1913, Neils Bohr attempted to explain the observed atomic spectra by combining the Rutherford atomic model with the newly postulated quantum theories of Einstein and Planck. This model, known as the *Bohr atom*, has since been replaced with complex quantum mechanical models of the atom; however, it is still an excellent way to derive a mental picture of the atom's structure. The Bohr atom seen in Figure 14-1 consists of a central core, called the *nucleus*, and the electrons in fixed orbits. The **Bohr atom model** is based on the following four assumptions or postulates.

1. Electrons surrounding the nucleus exist only in certain energy states or orbits.[1,4]
2. Electrons do not lose any energy when they reside in any of the allowed orbits.
3. When an electron moves from one orbit with higher energy to a lower-energy orbit, the atom emits radiation. The lost energy is seen as the atomic spectra.

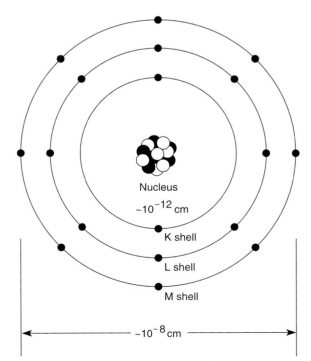

Figure 14-1. The Bohr atom model with central nucleus surrounded by the electron orbits. (From Christian PE, Waterstram-Rich KM, editors: *Nuclear medicine PET/CT: technology and techniques*, ed 6, St. Louis, 2007, Mosby.)

4. In any allowed orbit, the angular momentum (L) of the electron, which is the product of electron mass, its velocity, and the radius of its orbit, can have only quantized or fixed values and are given as an integer multiple of a fundamental constant, called *Planck's constant (h)*. The model was successful in predicting the energy levels of hydrogen and other hydrogen-like atoms and ions with single electrons, for example, singly ionized helium and doubly ionized lithium. The energy of the orbiting electron was derived to be as follows:

$$E_n = -13.6 \; eV(Z / n)^2$$

where Z is the number of protons in the nucleus and n is an integer known as the principal quantum number, which is related to the different available orbits for the electron to occupy. The ground state or the lowest energy state is n = 1; n > 1 corresponds to the excited states. Some energy has to be given to the atom for the electron to move from the ground state to different excited states. Similarly, when the electron moves from a higher n excited state to a lower n excited state or to the ground state with n = 1, some amount of energy has to be given up, leading to discrete observed spectra for these atoms and ions.

The Bohr atom model can also be used to predict qualitatively the binding energy of the electrons and the transition of electrons between the possible electron orbits or levels leading to the emission or absorption of photons for multielectron atoms and ions. For multielectron atoms, the electrons are assigned to different shells. The proton number Z in the equation is replaced by Z_{eff}, which is the effective proton number seen by the electrons in the outer shell to account for the screening of the net nuclear charge by electrons in the inner shells. The Bohr model, which was based on postulates without a solid physical foundation, has many limitations and could not explain many observed phenomena in atomic physics. It was replaced by the quantum mechanical model of atoms in which the electron in an atom or a molecule is described by its characteristic wave function and quantum numbers. The wave function or the atomic orbital gives a probabilistic description of the position of the electron around the nucleus under the influence of its attractive force and effect of the presence of other electrons. The wave function and the associated quantum numbers are obtained by solving the quantum mechanical many-body Schrödinger equation. The quantum numbers reflect the symmetry of the potential energy function of the electron and the restrictions imposed by the boundary conditions on the solution of the many-body equation. Presently, the electronic structure of any atom can be computed with a high level of accuracy due to the use of quantum mechanics and high-speed computers. The energy and spatial distribution of an electron in an atom depend on its four quantum numbers: principal quantum number *(n)*, azimuthal or orbital angular momentum quantum number *(l)*, magnetic quantum number *(m$_l$)*, and spin quantum number *(m$_s$)*. The three-dimensional nature of the orbital requires three quantum numbers n, l, and m to distinguish each orbital from the other, and m$_s$ is associated with the spinning nature of the electron. The principal quantum number determines the energy and size of the atomic orbital, has only nonzero positive integral values (n = 1, 2, ...),

and electrons with the same n are considered to belong to the same shell. Shells with n = 1, n = 2, n = 3, n = 4, n = 5, n = 6, and n = 7 are designated as K, L, M, N, O, P and Q shells. Energy of the shell increases with the increase in the value of n. The l quantum number determines the angular shape of the orbital and determines the angular momentum of the electron due to its orbital motion. The value of l depends on the n value of the orbital and can have integer values only between 0 and n − 1. For example, if n = 1, then l = 0. For n = 4, the allowed values of l are 0, 1, 2, and 3. The energy of the electron is also determined by the value of l of its orbital, and it increases with the increase of l. Electrons in an atom with the same value of l are considered to belong to the same subshell. The subshells are designated as s, p, d, and f for l = 0, 1, 2, and 3, respectively. The magnetic quantum number (m$_l$) is used to differentiate the orientation of the orbital in each subshell. It is used to describe the change in the energy of the electron under the influence of the external magnetic field. The energy of the electron without any external magnetic field in not affected by m$_l$. The allowed values of m$_l$ are integers between −l and +l. Thus, m$_l$ can have 2l + 1 values. For example, with l = 0, m$_l$ = 0, for l = 2, m$_l$ has five values: −2, −1, 0, 1, and 2. The number of allowed m$_l$ values determines the number of possible orbitals within a subshell. Every elementary particle-like electron has an intrinsic spin angular momentum. This can be thought of as a consequence of its own spinning motion similar to that of the earth around its own axis. This can have two values to describe either the clockwise or counterclockwise direction of electron spin. The two values are +1/2 or −1/2.

The electronic configuration or occupation of different allowed orbitals is governed by the principle that every electron would like to occupy an orbital that would lead to the lowest energy state of the atom called the *ground state*. Electrons also obey the Pauli exclusion principle, which states that no two electrons in an atom can have all of their four quantum numbers the same.

The orbital occupation of electrons in different atoms in the periodic table can be worked out with the aid of these principles and allowed values of different quantum numbers as discussed previously.

As seen in Figure 14-1, electron shells are numbered and are given letter names that represent, in increasing order, their distance from the nucleus.

The maximum number of electrons in any shell is determined by the formula 2n^2, where n is the shell number. As the atomic number increases, the number of electrons needed to keep the atom electrically neutral also increases. The rules by which the electrons fill the shells are as follows:
1. *No shell can contain more than its maximum number of electrons.*
2. *The outermost shell can contain no more than eight electrons.*

Example: Describe the electron shell configuration of an atom of stable nitrogen (Z = 7).

The first two electrons will fill the K shell. The five remaining electrons will fill five of the eight electron positions in the L shell.

Example: What is the electron configuration of an atom of electrically neutral cobalt (Z = 27)?

The K and L shells contain 10 electrons. The remaining 17 electrons would be spread between the M and N shells, even though the M shell can hold 18 electrons. This results from the second rule, which states that only 8 electrons can be in the outermost shell. Predicting the exact configuration of the electrons will involve using chemical principles, which we are not concerned with here. The important fact is that the electrons will be in four shells.

Practice: How many electronic shells are occupied in a neutral atom of oxygen with eight electrons?

 To learn more about structure of atoms, visit: http:// education.jlab.org/qa/atom_idx.html

Atomic Energy Levels

An **electron's binding energy** is the amount of energy required to remove that electron from the atom. The binding energy is different for each shell and depends on the makeup of the nucleus. The larger the number of positive charges in the nucleus, the greater the attraction of the electrons toward it, and thus the higher the binding energy. The electron binding energy has a negative value and is usually measured in kiloelectron volts (keV). It represents the amount of energy that must be added to the electron's total energy before the electron can begin to move away from the atom.

The electrons in the outermost shell of the atom are called *valence electrons* and are responsible for chemical reaction and bonding of the atom with other atoms. When some energy is imparted to the electrons of the atom, the electrons will move to higher-energy empty states, called *excited states,* and the atom will then reach an unstable state. This process is called **excitation**. Eventually, the excess energy will be given up as radiation by the electron to return to its ground state. The excitation of valence electrons will require less energy as compared with that for tightly bound core electrons. If sufficient energy is given to the atom, one or more electrons of the atom can overcome its (their) binding energy and can be completely removed from the atom. This process is called **ionization**. When a core electron is ionized, a vacancy in its shell is created. An electron from one of the higher-energy orbitals immediately fills this vacancy or hole. This transition is accompanied by emission of excess energy in the form of photons, known as **characteristic x-rays**. The energy of these photons is equal to the difference in the energy of the two orbitals involved in the transition. The excess energy can also knock out one of the outer electrons from the atom. Such an ejected electron is known as an **Auger electron** (pronounced "O-zhey").

 When atoms of any material are exposed to radiation, the electrons of the atom can get excited and ionized, leading to the energy transfer from the incident radiation to the medium.

Atomic Nomenclature

The atom consists of a nucleus and the orbiting electrons. The nucleus consists of protons and neutrons tightly bound together by a force known as the *strong nuclear force.* This force is strong enough at the extremely small distances found within the nucleus that it can hold together the positively charged protons that are trying to repel each other. Outside the nucleus, the strong nuclear force quickly becomes ineffective. The number of protons and neutrons within the nucleus defines the physical and chemical properties of the atom. Elements are substances made up entirely of atoms of a single kind. Some familiar substances that are elements include oxygen, carbon, helium, aluminum, and cobalt. All other substances are called *compounds* and are made up of various combinations of elements. As previously stated, each element contains a unique number of protons in its nucleus: carbon has six, oxygen has eight, and so forth. If a nucleus gains or loses protons, its elemental identity changes. For example, if a carbon atom gains a proton, it becomes a positive ion of nitrogen (which has seven protons). The number of protons in the nucleus is known as the **atomic number** of the atom. The number of protons and neutrons in the nucleus is termed the **atomic mass number**.

 The symbol used to identify an atom (X), its atomic number (Z), and atomic mass number (A) is as follows:

$$_Z^A X$$

The periodic table in Figure 14-2 is a listing of the elements and their symbols.

Nuclear Forces

The nucleus of the atom consists of protons and neutrons, which are together called *nucleons*. The protons are positively charged particles, and neutrons are neutral with no electrical charge. As you can imagine, the electrostatic force between the positively charged protons will repel each other. To hold a nucleus together, another force must be present. This force must be strong enough to overcome the electrostatic force that is attempting to break up the nucleus. This particular binding force is called the *nuclear force.* The **nuclear force** comes into play only over very short distances ($\cong 10^{-14}$ m). The nature of this force and others within the nucleus to hold the nucleus together is complex. This is not discussed in detail here, but the major force that holds the nucleus of an atom together is the nuclear force.

Nuclear Structure, Stability, and Isotopes

The arrangement of nucleons in the nucleus is described by the nuclear shell model. The nucleons occupy different shells in the nucleus with discrete energy levels like that in the atomic shell model. The total amount of energy that it takes to hold a nucleus together is called the **nuclear binding energy** and is measured in megaelectron volts (MeV). To compare the binding energy of one nucleus with another, one must calculate the binding energy per nucleon. The **binding energy per nucleon** is the binding energy divided by the atomic mass number. It should be noted that a peak at an atomic mass number of approximately 56 represents the most stable state of iron (Fe). A nucleus can have more energy than is required for stability; to illustrate this, one can think of a staircase. The **ground state** is the minimum amount of energy needed to keep the nucleons together. The bottom step represents the ground state of the nucleus. Higher and higher steps of the staircase represent higher and higher

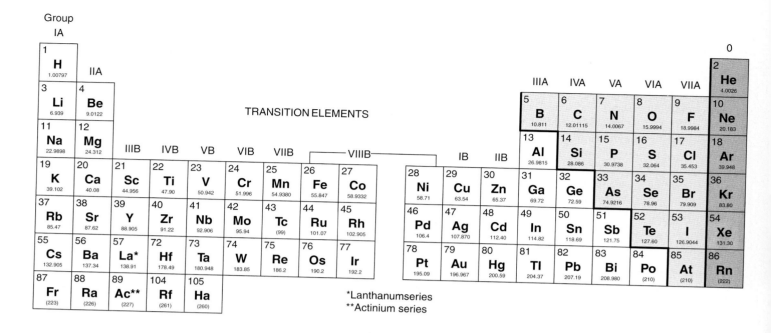

Figure 14-2. Periodic table of elements. (From Christian PE, Waterstram-Rich KM, editors: *Nuclear medicine PET/CT: technology and techniques*, ed 6, St. Louis, 2007, Mosby.)

energy states of the nucleus. As in a staircase, the steps have finite levels. The energy levels of a nucleus do not have transition zones between the steps, so the energy level of the nucleus must be one step or the other, not between. Each of the higher steps is called an **excited nuclear energy level**. As with an atom, if energy is imparted to the nucleus, some of the nucleons can move to higher-energy shells. Unstable nuclei or atoms are those that are not at their ground states. Similar to an atom, an excited nucleus tends to lose the excess energy and return to its ground state. This can be achieved in a number of ways, including radioactivity. **Radioactivity** is the emission of energy from the nucleus in the form of EM radiation or energetic particles.[4]

As can be imagined, any element can have different nuclear configurations. Atoms with the same atomic number but different atomic mass numbers are called *isotopes* of that atom.[2,4] Other nuclear configurations, related to the various combinations of atomic number and number of neutrons, are summarized in Table 14-2. An easy way to remember this table is to recall the next to last letter of the configuration—isoto**p**e, isoba**r**, isoto**n**e, and isom**e**r—which tells the value that remains constant (one must assume that **e** stands for everything). For example, when looking at isotopes, the Z, or atomic number, remains the same. Thus, the number of protons that define the element remains constant. In that case, the p (second from the end) becomes a quick reminder. The same is true for the others as well.

Particle Radiation

Radiation can be considered as both waves and particles. In 1925, de Broglie hypothesized the dual nature of matter. According to his principle, waves can behave like particles, and every particle can have a wavelike character. Thus, EM waves sometimes act as particles. These particles are termed as *photons*, and they have momentum like other particles. This is important to the definition of particle radiation, because it is the propagated energy that has a definite rest mass, a definite momentum (within limits), and a position at any time. This hypothesis is discussed in more detail later.

Table 14-2	Nuclear Configurations		
Name	**Z**	**A**	**N**
Isotope	Same	Different	Different
Isobar	Different	Same	Different
Isotone	Different	Same	Different
Isomer	Same	Same	Same

A, Atomic mass number; *N*, number of neutrons; *Z*, atomic number.

Radiation therapy uses radiation that can create ionization in the medium by removing electrons from the atomic shells of the target, which can then lead to breaking of chemical bonds and other damages leading to cell death. This radiation is classified as ionizing radiation *and all others are known as* nonionizing radiation. *Ionizing radiation is divided into two groups, namely directly ionizing radiation and indirectly ionizing radiation. The directly ionizing radiation, as the name indicates, produces the ionization itself; the group consists of charged particles such as electron, proton, and alpha particles and other heavy charged particles. The indirectly ionizing radiation group consists of neutral particles such as photons and neutrons, and the ionization by this group involves two steps. In the first step, their interactions with the electrons and nuclei of the target create charged particles such as electrons, positrons, protons, and other heavy ions in the medium. These released charged particles then create the actual ionization of the target atoms in the second step.*

ELECTROMAGNETIC RADIATION

Radiation is defined as energy that is emitted by an atom and travels through space. This energy can take the form of EM radiation or can be transferred to subatomic particles such as electrons and cause the particles to move away from the atom. This section covers the phenomenon of EM radiation.

Photons

A **photon** is any "packet" of energy traveling through space at the speed of light, 3×10^8 m/sec (in a vacuum). Although a photon can be envisioned as a particle, it has no mass of its own nor does it have an electrical charge. It has only its energy, which is a fixed quantity for that particular photon. Thus, high-energy photons can pass through miles of dense material unscathed, because they have no mass with which to "bump" into atoms and no electrical charges to attract or repel other particles that might interfere with their travels.

The nature of photons puzzled physicists until early in the 20th century, when a new branch of physics called *quantum mechanics* burst into prominence. This field of study was an attempt to explain atomic and nuclear phenomena on their own level rather than trying to make the physics of these extremely small and special bits of matter correspond to the physics of large objects such as automobiles or planets. One of the discoveries of the new science was that photons can be viewed in one of two ways, depending on the situation: either as massless particles, as described previously, or, alternatively, as waves, like the movements of a violin string or the human voice. Photons are a special case of a type of wave called an *electromagnetic wave,* which consists of an electrical field and a magnetic field traveling through space at right angles to each other[1] (Figure 14-3).

 *Photons exhibit the characteristics of a particle at times and the characteristics of a wave at other times. This phenomenon is known as **wave-particle duality**.*

Both of these manifestations of the photon and how they can be related to each other in a single equation are discussed in the following sections.

Physical Characteristics of an Electromagnetic Wave

An EM wave has three major distinguishing physical characteristics, which are closely interrelated. They are as follows:

1. The **frequency of the wave,** which is represented by the Greek letter ν (read as nu), is the number of times that the wave oscillates or cycles per second and is measured in units of cycles per second. Because the term "cycles" does not really have a unit, but is simply a number, the unit for frequency is 1/sec, called the *Hertz (Hz).*

2. The **wavelength of the wave** is the physical distance between peaks of the wave. Wavelength is represented by the Greek letter lambda (λ) and is measured in meters (m). Usually the waves that we will be working with have wavelengths of approximately one billionth of a meter, so to avoid having to constantly write very small numbers, we will express wavelengths in terms of the nanometer (nm), which is equal to 10^{-9} m. Another unit of wavelength seen frequently is the angstrom (Å), equal to 10^{-10} m, or 0.1 nm.

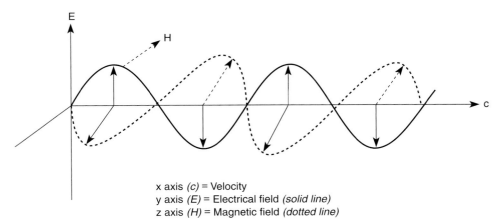

x axis *(c)* = Velocity
y axis *(E)* = Electrical field *(solid line)*
z axis *(H)* = Magnetic field *(dotted line)*

Figure 14-3. Electromagnetic wave component energy fields. (From Christian PE, Waterstram-Rich KM, editors: *Nuclear medicine PET/CT: technology and techniques,* ed 6, St. Louis, 2007, Mosby.)

3. The final important wave characteristic is the velocity of the wave as it travels through space. For our purposes, we will assume that all EM waves travel at the same speed, which is the speed of light in a vacuum, represented by the letter c and equal to 3×10^8 m/sec.

The relationship between these three quantities is as follows:

$$c = v\lambda$$

Note that if you rearrange the variables, there are two other forms of this equation:

$$v = \frac{c}{\lambda}$$

$$\lambda = \frac{c}{v}$$

Looking closely at these equations, you can see that the frequency v and wavelength λ of an EM wave are inversely related. As one gets larger, the other gets smaller. Table 14-3 lists some of the frequencies and wavelengths present in the range of known EM waves.

Example: Calculate the wavelength of an EM wave that has a frequency of 4.5×10^{14} Hz.

To calculate wavelength from frequency, we can use the equation $\lambda = \frac{c}{v}$:

$$\lambda = \frac{c}{v} = \frac{3 \times 10^8 \text{ m/s}}{4.5 \times 10^{14} \text{ Hz}} = 6.67 \times 10^{-7} \text{ m}$$

This answer could also be expressed in nanometers and angstroms:

$$(6.67 \times 10^{-7} \text{ m}) (1 \text{ nm}/10^{-9}\text{m}) = 667 \text{ nm, or } 6670 \text{ Å}$$

Example: An FM radio station broadcasts at a wavelength of 3.125 m. At what frequency will you find this station on your radio dial?

$$v = \frac{c}{\lambda} = \frac{3 \times 10^8 \text{ m/s}}{3.125 \text{ m}} = 96,000,000 \text{ Hz, or } 96 \times 10^6 \text{ Hz}$$

This station broadcasts at 96 megahertz (MHz).

Photon Energy

As stated previously, the energy of a photon is its major characteristic, especially from the viewpoint of radiation therapy physics. Fortunately, there are ways to calculate the energy of the wave when its other properties are known. The energy can, for example, be calculated when the frequency (v) of the wave is known, using the following equation:

$$E = hv$$

where E is the energy of the wave, and h is a constant called *Planck's constant*, which has the value 6.626×10^{-34} J • s; this is equivalent to 4.15×10^{-15} eV • s. Either value can be used, depending on whether you want the resultant energy in joules (J) or electron volts (eV).

A joule (J) is the metric system, or SI, unit of energy and is equivalent to 1 kg • m²/sec². This unit is typically used for applications involving "real-world" objects, such as billiard balls, cans of light beer, and space shuttles. However, the energies of EM waves are usually much smaller than the energies involved in these situations (with the possible exception of light beer), so another smaller unit is used. This unit is the eV and represents the amount of energy that one electron would pick up as it passed through an electrical field whose potential difference was 1 V. This unit will be the standard unit for photon energy in this text and is related to the joule as follows:

$$1 \text{ eV} = 1.6 \times 10^{-19} \text{ J, or } 1 \text{ J} = 6.25 \times 10^{18} \text{ eV}$$

Example: If an EM wave has a frequency of 1.8×10^{20} Hz, what are its wavelength and energy (in eV)?

$$\lambda = \frac{c}{v} = \frac{3 \times 10^8 \text{ m/s}}{1.8 \times 10^{20} \text{ Hz}} = 1.667 \times 10^{-12} \text{ m}$$

$$E = hv = (4.15 \times 10^{-15} \text{ eV • s}) (1.8 \times 10^{20} \text{ Hz})$$
$$= 747,000 \text{ eV} = 0.747 \text{ MeV}$$

Example: The photon emitted from the decay of the radioisotope ^{99m}Tc has an energy of approximately 142 keV. What are the frequency and wavelength of this photon?

Because we know that E = 142 keV = 142,000 eV, we can find v by the following:

$$v = \frac{E}{h} = \frac{142,000 \text{ eV}}{4.15 \times 10^{-15}\text{eV • s}} = 3.422 \times 10^{19} \text{ Hz}$$

Now λ can be found:

$$\lambda = \frac{c}{v} = \frac{3 \times 10^8 \text{ m/s}}{3.422 \times 10^{-19}\text{Hz}} = 8.77 \times 10^{-12} \text{ m}$$

 Another interesting fact about photons can be discovered using Einstein's theories of relativity, in which he postulated the famous equation for relating the mass of any object to the amount of energy that it can be converted into:

$$E = mc^2$$

where E is the energy, m is the mass of the object, and c is the speed of light. Note that, because c² has units of m²/sec², it is necessary to express the mass of the object in kilograms so that we obtain an answer in joules whenever using this equation.

This equation gave the first indication to the scientific world that matter and energy are really different aspects of the same thing and that one can be directly converted into the other.

Table 14-3	The Electromagnetic Spectrum	
Radiation	**Average λ (m)**	**Average v (Hz)**
Gamma rays	10^{-12}	10^{20}
Ultraviolet light	10^{-8}	10^{17}
Visible light	10^{-6}	10^{14}
Infrared light	10^{-5}	10^{13}
Microwaves	10^{-2}	10^{10}
Radio and television waves	10^{2}	10^{6}

From Christian PE, Waterstram-Rich KM, editors: *Nuclear medicine PET/CT: technology and techniques*, ed 6, St. Louis, 2007, Mosby.

This discovery has drastically changed the world in which we live by increasing our understanding of the universe and giving us the ability to harness the power of the stars in nuclear fusion reactions, which convert a small amount of matter directly into a huge amount of energy. Unfortunately, the only current use of this knowledge in any viable sense is the stockpile of "hydrogen bombs" present in our defense arsenals.

If you set this equation for E equal to the Planck equation and solve, you find that:

$$m = \frac{h\nu}{c^2}$$

With this equation, it is possible to calculate the **mass equivalence** of a photon. Although the photon has no actual mass, the equation allows one to treat the photon as if it actually had mass of its own—the more energy, the greater the mass equivalence. Thus, the previous equation neatly combines the particle and wave natures of the photon into a single, tidy equation.

Example: Calculate the mass equivalence of a photon of green light, with a nominal wavelength of 520 nm.

First, calculate the energy of this wave, letting $\nu = \frac{c}{\lambda}$:

$$E = \frac{hc}{\lambda} = \frac{(6.626 \times 10^{-34} \text{ J} \bullet \text{s})(3 \times 10^8 \text{ m/s})}{520 \times 10^{-15} \text{eV} \bullet \text{s}} = 3.823 \times 10^{-19} \text{ J}$$

Notice that to keep the units consistent, we have used the value for Planck's constant in joules. The SI unit of meters present in the photon wavelength will cancel out along with the seconds in others. Having found the energy, we can now calculate the mass equivalence by solving Einstein's equation for the mass:

$$m = \frac{E}{c^2} = \frac{(3.823 \times 10^{-19} \text{ J})}{(3 \times 10^8 \text{m/s})^2} = 4.248 \times 10^{-36} \text{ kg}$$

RADIOACTIVITY

Unstable atomic nuclei tend to seek their ground state, meaning that they tend to give off their excess energy until they reach a point at which the energy in the nucleus is just enough to maintain nuclear stability. The process by which they lose this energy is called radioactivity. Radioactivity may involve the emission of particles, EM radiation (photons), or a combination of the two. This section discusses the processes by which atoms rid themselves of this excess nuclear energy, and the mathematic methods used to describe them.

The Nuclear Stability Curve

The nuclear stability curve is shown in Figure 14-4. The vertical axis represents the atomic number (Z) of the atom, that is, the number of protons in the nucleus. The horizontal axis represents the number of neutrons (N) in the nucleus. The straight line represents the condition $N/Z = 1$, that is, atoms with the same number of neutrons and protons in the nucleus. The curved line shows the "line of stability"; atoms whose proton/neutron combinations place them on this line are stable and will not undergo radioactive decay, because they have no excess energy. The two lines are coincident at low values of Z, for example, Z less than 20, indicating that these atoms have identical numbers of protons and neutrons. As Z increases, however, the curve begins to

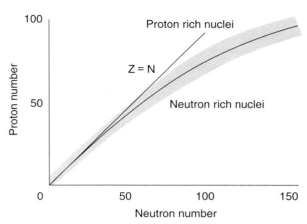

Figure 14-4. Nuclear stability curve. (From Christian PE, Waterstram-Rich KM, editors: *Nuclear medicine PET/CT: technology and techniques*, ed 6, St. Louis, 2007, Mosby.)

diverge from the "ideal" line, curving to the right. This indicates that, as the number of protons grows larger, more neutrons than protons are required to maintain stability, and the required neutron/proton ratio increases as Z increases. Atoms that do not meet this criterion appear at other positions on the graph, away from the stability curve; these represent unstable atoms. As these atoms lose energy, they will move closer to the stability curve, finally reaching a stable state.

 You may recall that the combinations called isotope, isobar, *and* isotone *refer to different arrangements of nuclear particles. Similarly, the terms* isotopic, isobaric, *and* isotonic *refer to types of transformations that change the atom to an isotope, isobar, or isotone of itself. For example, an isotopic transition is one in which the Z of the atom remains constant, but the atomic mass number (A) increases or decreases. Similarly, during an isobaric transition the A of the atom remains the same, and the Z and N change appropriately; during an isotonic transition, the N remains constant and Z (and therefore A) changes. By undergoing as many of these transitions as necessary, atoms can move from an unstable to a stable state.*

Types of Radioactive Decay

Alpha Decay. An alpha particle, symbolized by the Greek letter (α), consists of two neutrons and two protons bound together; this is equivalent to a helium atom (Z = 2) that has been stripped of its two electrons.[1-4] Large, unstable atoms that have a large amount of excess energy tend to undergo radioactive decay by the emission of α particles, which eliminates four nuclear particles and therefore a substantial amount (in nuclear terms) of excess energy. The equation for radioactive decay is as follows:

$$^A_Z X \rightarrow ^{A-4}_{Z-2} Y + ^4_2\alpha + Q$$

where Q represents the excess energy shed by the nucleus. This energy often appears in the form of photons, which, because of their nuclear origin, are called **gamma rays (γ-rays)**.

Examine this equation carefully. "Reading" it, it says that a nucleus X with a known A and Z decays to a new atom with atomic mass number A−4 and atomic number Z−2; the two missing protons and two missing neutrons appear as an α particle emitted from the nucleus. In addition, a certain amount of energy is given off, either in the form of kinetic energy (i.e., speed of the α particle) or as γ-rays or, more commonly, as a combination of the two. A key feature of this equation is that the numbers of protons, neutrons, and electrical charges on both sides of the arrow are equal. This is a critical feature of all radioactive decay equations: the two sides of the arrow must balance exactly in terms of number of particles, electrical charges, and energy. The most important thing to note, however, is that the original atom has now changed into a new element by the loss of two nuclear protons.

Example: An atom of uranium, U, undergoes α decay. What is the result?

$$^{238}_{92}\text{U} \rightarrow {}^{234}_{90}\text{Th} + {}^{4}_{2}\alpha + \gamma$$

The atom of uranium has been transformed into an atom of thorium.

Alpha decay occurs when the $^N/_Z$ ratio is too low, that is, when the atom falls "underneath" the stability curve on the $^N/_Z$ graph. By eliminating two neutrons and two protons, plus the associated energy, this transition increases the $^N/_Z$ ratio, attempting to correct for the too low $^N/_Z$ ratio that existed before the transition.

The energies of the α particles emitted by a given isotope are fixed and discrete. Even though an isotope may emit more than one α particle, each α particle will have one of a selection of fixed energies. This contrasts with beta (β) decay, described in the next two sections, in which essentially infinite numbers of particle energies are possible.

Beta-Minus Decay. Recall that a beta-minus (β−) particle is the same as an electron, the difference in name arising because of the difference in place of origin. An electron is found orbiting in the electron shells, whereas a β− particle is emitted as the result of a nuclear decay. To understand β− decay, think of a neutron as a "mixture" of a proton plus an electron:

$$n^0 \rightarrow p^+ + e^-$$

What essentially happens during a β− decay is that a neutron in the nucleus "decays" into a proton plus an electron, as shown. The proton remains in the nucleus, and the electron is ejected and leaves the atom; this ejected electron is called the *β⁻ particle.* The equation for β− decay is as follows:

$$^A_Z\text{X} \rightarrow {}^A_{Z+1}\text{Y} + {}^{0}_{-1}\beta + \upsilon_a$$

where the symbol υ_a stands for the emission of a tiny particle called the *antineutrino.* This particle carries away the energy that is left over when the β− does not carry away all of the atom's excess energy. You can see that when undergoing β− decay, the atom increases its Z by one, while maintaining the same A (having lost a neutron but gained a proton), making this an isobaric transition. Because of this property, the ratio $^N/_Z$ of this atom will decrease. Usually the daughter nucleus of a β− decay is itself radioactive and can undergo radioactive decay in many ways, typically by giving off its excess energy as γ-rays. In fact, there are very few isotopes that emit only β− particles; the majority are accompanied by γ-ray emission from the daughter nucleus.[1-4]

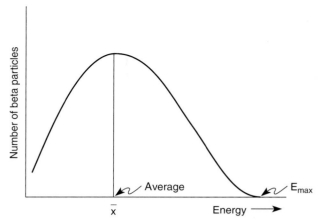

Figure 14-5. Beta particle energy spectrum. (From Christian PE, Waterstram-Rich KM, editors: *Nuclear medicine PET/CT: technology and techniques,* ed 6, St. Louis, 2007, Mosby.)

Example: Cobalt-60 decays by β− decay to an excited state of ⁶⁰Ni, which then decays by the emission of two high-energy γ-rays as follows:

$$^{60}_{27}\text{Co} \rightarrow {}^{60}_{28}\text{Ni} + {}^{0}_{-1}\beta + \nu \rightarrow {}^{60}_{28}\text{Ni} + 2\gamma$$

Beta-emitting isotopes do not give off β− particles of fixed energy as do alpha emitters. Instead, the emitted β− particles possess energies between 0 and a given maximum (E_{max}), creating what is called a *beta spectrum* (Figure 14-5). The average energy of the β− particle in the spectrum is approximately one third of E_{max}. The extra energy between E_{max} and the actual energy of the β− particle is carried away by the antineutrino (ν_a).

Beta-Plus Decay. There is a subatomic particle that has exactly the same characteristics as an electron, except that it possesses a positive electrical charge rather than a negative charge. This particle is called a *positron* and has the symbol β+. In addition, like a β−, it is ejected from an atomic nucleus; in this case, a nuclear proton decays into a neutron and a positron:

$$p^+ \rightarrow n^0 + \beta^+$$

So the equation for β+ decay is as follows:

$$^A_Z\text{X} \rightarrow {}^A_{Z-1}\text{Y} + {}^{0}_{+1}\beta + \nu$$

Because of the loss of a proton but the gain of a neutron, the atom retains the same A, but the Z of the atom decreases and the $^N/_Z$ ratio of the atom increases, making this an isobaric transition.[1]

Sodium-22 ($^{22}_{11}\text{Na}$) is a common radioactive isotope of natural sodium. It decays by β+ decay to a stable isotope of the gas neon, with the emission of a β+ particle and a γ-ray, as follows:

$$^{22}_{11}\text{Na} \rightarrow {}^{22}_{10}\text{Ne}^* + {}^{0}_{+1}\beta \rightarrow {}^{22}_{10}\text{Ne} + \gamma$$

As with β− decay, a spectrum of energies is emitted, with an average energy of one third E_{max}; the remainder of the energy is carried off by the neutrino (ν), as in β− decay.

Electron Capture. Although the Bohr model of the atom depicts the electrons as being in fixed orbits outside of the nucleus, according to theories of quantum mechanics it is possible that the electrons may, at some time, come very close to the nucleus. An electron that strays too close to the nucleus may be captured and combined with a proton, reversing the process for β⁻ decay:

$$p^+ + e^- \rightarrow n^0 + \nu$$

This process is known as *electron capture* and has the same result as β⁺ decay; in other words, the Z of the parent nucleus decreases by 1, and the $\frac{N}{Z}$ ratio of the atom increases.

Because of the proximity of the K shell to the nucleus, it is most likely that the captured electron will be taken from this shell, although it is possible to capture an electron from the L or M shell. When an electron is taken from one of the electron shells, it leaves a "hole" in the shell; this will place the atom in an unstable configuration in terms of energy, because an inner shell electron has lower energy than an outer shell electron. As a result, one of the electrons from an outer shell will "fall" toward the nucleus, moving from a higher energy state to a lower one, and this excess energy, no longer needed to maintain stability, will be given off in the form of an x-ray. This type of radiation is called **characteristic radiation** and is an important part of many radioactive decay schemes and radiation/matter interactions.

Isomeric Transition or Gamma Decay. An isomer is an atom with the identical Z and A of another atom but is currently in what is called a *metastable state*. This represents a daughter product of some other kind of decay that is itself in an excited state, but instead of instantly decaying by γ emission (see the example for β⁻ decay), it remains in this excited state for a given period of time and then decays. Such a nucleus is represented by a small "m" next to its atomic mass number, as in ^{99m}Tc. A nucleus that has no metastable state but decays instantly has an asterisk to the right of its chemical symbol (^{60}Ni*). Metastable isotopes, or isomers, usually decay by emitting the excess energy as a γ-ray.

^{99m}Tc is an isotope used daily in nuclear medicine procedures. It is a daughter product of ^{99}Mo, and the decay equation looks like this:

$$^{99}_{42}\text{Mo} \rightarrow {}^{99m}_{43}\text{Tc*} + {}^{0}_{-1}\beta + \nu \rightarrow {}^{99}_{43}\text{Tc} + \gamma$$

Specification of Radioactivity

To quantify the amount of radioactivity present in a given sample, in the early 20th century, the Curie was defined as the activity of 1 g of ^{226}Ra, the most well-known isotope in use at that time. Unfortunately, as measurement techniques improved, disputes arose as to exactly what the activity of 1 g of ^{226}Ra meant in terms of the number of radioactive atoms present. So eventually the unit of radioactivity, the Curie, was defined as follows:

$$1 \text{ Ci} = 3.7 \times 10^{10} \text{ dis/sec}$$

where *dis/sec* stands for nuclear disintegrations per second, that is, the number of atoms that undergo some kind of radioactive decay every second. Because disintegration is merely a quantity and does not have a unit, the Curie is numerically equal to 1/sec or sec⁻¹. In fact, the SI unit of radioactivity, the becquerel (Bq), is equal to 1 dis/sec. Because many disintegrations per second are present in even a small sample of radioactive material, the becquerel is a much smaller unit than the Curie. You can easily see that $1 \text{ Ci} = 3.7 \times 10^{10} \text{ Bq} = 37$ billion Bq.

For this reason, Ci still remains the popular unit of radioactivity, although we are supposed to use the SI units.

For various amounts of radioactive material, multiples of the Curie such as the millicurie (mCi, 10^{-3} Ci) and the microcurie (μCi, 10^{-6} Ci) are used. A typical nuclear medicine procedure uses amounts of radioactivity in the range of hundreds of millicuries, whereas a cobalt teletherapy machine uses a source of Co-60 of an activity in the range of 5000 to 6000 Ci.

Exponential Decay of Radioactivity

The amount of radioactivity present in a given sample is never a constant quantity but rather is being reduced continuously by the decay of the radioactive atoms in the sample.[2,4] This decay process follows a mathematical pattern known as *exponential behavior.* Any value that increases or decreases exponentially will double or halve its value within a certain amount of time; when that time interval passes again, the value will have further reduced by half or increased by two times. Although it is impossible to say exactly which atoms in a radioactive sample will decay at any given time, it is reasonably straightforward to determine what percentage of the atoms will remain after a given amount of time.

The equation of exponential decay of radioactivity is as follows:

$$A_t = A_0 e^{-\lambda t}$$

where A_t is the activity at time t; A_0 is the activity at time zero (when the activity was measured); and λ is a value known as the *exponential decay constant,* which is discussed in more detail later. The symbol e represents the base of the natural logarithms, which governs exponential behavior; it has the value e = 2.718282....

According to the rules of logarithms, e to any negative power will always be less than 1.000; e to a very small negative number power will be very close to 1.000, and many hand calculators will give the value of 1.000 in this case. However, the number should never be greater than 1.000; if this is the case, you have made a mathematical error, because radioactive decay will always result in a decrease in the amount of radioactivity present.

To make this point absolutely clear, we will use a little algebra to rearrange the previous equation:

$$\frac{A_t}{A_0} = e^{-\lambda t}$$

This says that the final amount of radioactivity divided by the initial amount is equal to the exponential side of the equation, which will always be between 0 and 1.

Another important principle in working with natural logarithms is that the inverse of the exponential function e is the natural logarithm *ln,* which makes

$$\ln(e^{\text{anything}}) = \text{Anything}$$

or in our case:

$$\ln(e^{-\lambda t}) = -\lambda t$$

Example: A radioactive sample is measured to contain 100 mCi of radioactivity. If the decay constant of this isotope is 0.115 hr⁻¹, how much activity will remain after 24 hours?

$$A_t = A_0 e^{-\lambda t} = (100 \text{ mCi}) e^{(-0.115)(24)} = 6.329 \text{ mCi}$$

Note the units on λ, which are time^{-1}. Because the units of t are in time and the units of λ are time^{-1}, these must cancel out, leaving the exponent of e with no units. To accomplish this, λ and t must be in the same unit of time, that is, minutes, hours, days, years, and so forth.

The λ is a constant for a given isotope, that is, all atoms of a given isotope will decay with the same λ, which will not change no matter what environmental conditions persist—you cannot change the λ of an isotope with heat, pressure, or any other known factors.

How can we use the exponential decay equation to derive the useful quantity, known as the *half-life* of an isotope? The half-life is the time required for the activity of any sample of a particular radioisotope to decay to half of its initial value. So the quantity we seek to solve for is t, the time, which we will give the special symbol t_h to represent half-life.

How do we solve the equation for half-life? We know that the activity after one half-life will be half of the initial activity, by definition. So, we can write the following:

$$\frac{A_t}{A_0} = 0.5$$

Knowing this, solve for t_h:

$$\frac{A_t}{A_0} = e^{-\lambda t}$$

$$0.5 = e^{-\lambda t_h}$$

$$\ln(0.5) = -\lambda^{t_h}$$

$$-0.693 = -\lambda^{t_h}$$

We now divide and cancel the minus signs to get the final solution:

$$t_h = \frac{0.693}{\lambda}$$

We can, if needed, rearrange this equation:

$$\lambda = \frac{0.693}{t_h}$$

You should go through this derivation several times and try it yourself, so that the method is clear. These equations are used frequently in calculations involving radioactive isotopes.

Example: A sample of an isotope with a half-life of 8.0 days is measured to have an activity of 25.0 mCi on Monday at noon. What would the activity be on Friday of that week, at noon?

Find λ using the previous equations with 4.0 days as the value for t:

$$\lambda = \frac{0.693}{t_h} = \frac{0.693}{8.0\ d} = 0.087\ d^{-1}$$

$$A_t = (25.0\ \text{mCi})e^{(-0.087\ d^{-1})(4.0\ d)} = 17.679\ \text{mCi}$$

The exponential decay equation is powerful, because it can be solved algebraically in a number of ways, depending on the results required. For example, if you take two activity readings from an isotope sample, you can call these A_0 and A_t, and the elapsed time between the two readings will be t. You can now find the decay constant and half-life of this isotope by rearranging the exponential decay equation into a new form:

$$\frac{A_t}{A_0} = e^{-\lambda t}$$

$$\ln \frac{A_t}{A_0} = e^{-\lambda t}$$

$$\ln \frac{A_t}{A_0} \times \frac{-1}{t} = \lambda$$

Note that we have made use of the relationship between ln and e, that is, that the natural log function and the exponential function are inverse functions—one will cancel the effect of the other. This allows us to find any unknown quantities that may exist in the exponent of the exponential function, such as λ or t. The previous equation can be used to find λ and therefore the half-life of the isotope.

Two readings of the activity of a radioactive sample are taken 40 hours apart. The first reading is 125.0 mCi; the second one is 1.232 mCi. Calculate the half-life of this isotope.

Find λ, then find t_h:

$$\ln \frac{A_t}{A_0} \times \frac{-1}{t} = \lambda$$

$$\ln \frac{1.232\ \text{mCi}}{125.0\ \text{mCi}} \times \frac{-1}{40.0\ \text{hr}} = \lambda$$

$$(-4.620)(-0.025) = 0.116\ \text{hr}^{-1} = \lambda$$

$$t_h = \frac{0.693}{0.116\ \text{hr}^{-1}} = 6.0\ \text{hr}$$

An isotope with a decay constant $\lambda = 0.043\ \text{hr}^{-1}$ is allowed to decay for 24 hours. The activity at the end of this period is measured as 17.8 mCi. What was the initial activity?

$$A_t = A_0 e^{-\lambda t}$$

$$17.8 = A_0 e^{(-0.043)(24)}$$

$$17.8 = A_0(0.356)$$

$$A_0 = 50\ \text{mCi}$$

A quantity called the *mean life* ($\bar{t}$) of the isotope is sometimes used in brachytherapy calculations involving short-lived isotopes (i.e., isotopes with short half-lives). The mean life $\bar{t}$ is related to the half-life and decay constant of the isotope as follows:

$$\bar{t} = 1.44 t_h = \frac{1}{\lambda}$$

Radioactive Equilibrium

It is common for some radioisotopes, especially high Z isotopes, to decay to daughter products that are themselves radioactive. An example of this process is ^{226}Ra, which is one of a number of isotopes along a "chain" of daughter products created when ^{238}U, found in nature, decays to ^{206}Pb over the course of millions of years. When parent and daughter isotopes exist in this manner, it is possible that a condition of equilibrium (i.e., balance) will be established in this system—the daughter and parent isotopes will begin to appear to decay with nearly the same half-lives and to have the same activities.

To illustrate this, consider the case of the decay of ^{226}Ra to ^{222}Rn via α decay:

$$^{226}_{88}\text{Ra} \rightarrow \, ^{222}_{86}\text{Rn} + \, ^{4}_{2}\alpha + Q$$

^{226}Ra has a half-life of more than 1600 years, whereas the half-life of the daughter ^{222}Rn is only approximately 3.8 days. A sample that starts out as pure radium begins to decay to radon, causing a buildup of radon. However, the radon decays with a shorter half-life and so will have a higher activity (number of disintegrations per second). Eventually the daughter product is so active that it essentially equals the activity of the parent. This condition is called *secular equilibrium* and can occur only when the half-life of the parent is much greater than the half-life of the daughter isotope, that is, when:

$$t_{hparent} \gg t_{hdaughter}$$

If the differences in parent and daughter half-life are not as dramatic but the parent is still longer lived than the daughter, the daughter activity will actually grow slightly larger than the parent activity and then appear to decay at the same rate (with the same half-life). This condition is called *transient equilibrium* and occurs when:

$$t_{hparent} > t_{hdaughter}$$

In the case $t_{hparent} < t_{hdaughter}$, no equilibrium can exist.

Radioactive equilibrium conditions can be exploited to provide a steady source of some radioisotopes used in nuclear medicine procedures. An excellent example of this is the use of "generators" that contain a source $^{99}_{42}$Mo, which decays by β^- decay to the metastable isotope $^{99}_{43}$Tc. The parent half-life of 67 hours is greater than the daughter half-life of 6 hours, so transient equilibrium is reached. Each week a fresh generator is delivered to the nuclear medicine department. At the beginning of each day, the technologist adds a solvent to the generator, which chemically separates the ^{99m}Tc from the ^{99}Mo, and the ^{99m}Tc is drawn off. ^{99m}Tc can then be used as a radioactive injection in a number of diagnostic studies. Of course, because the ^{99}Mo is decaying away, at the beginning of each day less ^{99m}Tc is available than the day before. So, at the end of the week, the generator is stored for further decay and then returned to the manufacturer when radiation levels reach acceptable levels.

 You can learn more about basic nuclear physics by visiting http://www.lbl.gov/abc/.

PHOTON INTERACTIONS

When a beam of radiation from any source strikes some material, a number of processes can occur that lead to transfer of energy from the radiation to the medium; this energy can then affect the medium in many ways. Biologic tissue, for example, may suffer damage to the nucleic acid structures (deoxyribonucleic acid [DNA]) and lose its ability to reproduce itself, thereby damaging the organism as a whole. Other materials may undergo physical or chemical changes as a result of the energy transfer, such as heating or disruption of crystal structures. This section discusses the ways in which photons (x-rays or γ-rays) interact with matter.

The Inverse Square Law

The intensity of flux of a radiation beam is defined as the number of photons in the beam per square centimeter. Note that this definition does not take into account the energy of the radiation in the beam, only the number of photons present in the beam at a given instant per square centimeter. So a beam can be called "low intensity" if it has just a few photons per square centimeter, even if the photons are very high energy; similarly, a "high-intensity" beam may consist entirely of a large number of very-low-energy photons. For practical purposes, the intensity of a radiation beam is usually measured in terms of the exposure rate (X, mR/hr) or dose rate (D, cGy/min) of the beam at that point, rather than the number of photons present.

Often in radiation therapy physics, we are interested in describing the intensity from a point source of radiation. A point source is a source that is so small (from the viewpoint of the observer) that it appears to have no area, and all photons coming from it appear to originate at the same point. In reality, most radiation sources have some finite area; however, if the distance from the source is large, it will appear to be a point. For example, a coin viewed from a distance of 3 m will appear to be a point. So, if the distance from the source to the point of interest is at least five times the physical size of the source, the source can be treated as a point source. This assumption greatly simplifies most radiation therapy calculations; because the distance from a radiation therapy source to the point of interest is rarely shorter than five times the source size, most sources can be considered point sources for our purposes. This is not always true in the case of internally implanted radioisotopes.

Given that we are working with a point source, the intensity of the radiation beam coming from this source can be determined first by assuming that the radiation is emitted isotropically from the source—that is, it is emitted evenly in all directions from the point source. If this is the case, the intensity of the beam at any distance from the source is calculated by dividing the number of photons coming from the source by the area of the sphere surrounding the source at that distance. If we let Δp represent the number of photons emitted by the point source in any instant, we can say that the intensity of the beam at distance d_1 from the point source is equal to the following:

$$I_1 = \text{Number of photons/Area of sphere} = \Delta p / 4\pi d_1^2$$

where $4\pi d_1^2$ is the area of the sphere of radius d_1.

How does the intensity change as we move closer to or farther away from our point source? If we assume that none of the photons are attenuated (taken out of the beam), then Δp will remain the same; only d, the distance from the point source, will change. If we call the new distance d_2, then the intensity at this point is equal to the following:

$$I_2 = \frac{\Delta p}{4\pi d_2^2}$$

So the change in intensity moving from distance d_1 to distance d_2 is the ratio of I_1 to I_2:

$$\frac{I_1}{I_2} = \left(\frac{\Delta p / 4\pi d_1^2}{\Delta p / 4\pi d_2^2} \right) = \left(\frac{d_2^2}{d_1^2} \right) = \left(\frac{d_2}{d_1} \right)^2$$

When we solve this equation for I_2, we get the following:

$$I_2 = I_1 \left(\frac{d_1}{d_2} \right)^2$$

This is one statement of the inverse square law, an important principle in radiation therapy physics.

 The basic idea of the inverse square law is that the intensity of a radiation beam in a nonabsorbing medium decreases or increases as the inverse of the square of the distance.[1]

A few examples should clarify the use of this principle.

Example: The intensity of a radiation beam is measured at 10.0 mR/hr at a distance of 10 cm. What will be the intensity of this beam at 20.0 cm?

Let $I_1 = 10$ mR/hr, $d_1 = 10.0$ cm, and $d_2 = 20.0$ cm. The intensity at d_2 will be as follows:

$$I_2 = (10.0 \text{ mR/hr}) \left(\frac{10.0 \text{ cm}}{20.0 \text{ cm}} \right)^2 = 2.5 \text{ mR/hr}$$

The intensity at twice the distance is one fourth of the original intensity.

If, in the preceding example, d_2 is equal to 5 cm (i.e., the new distance is closer to the source than the original), what will be the change in beam intensity?

With d_2 now equal to 5 cm, the solution becomes:

$$I_2 = (10.0 \text{ mR/hr}) \left(\frac{10.0 \text{ cm}}{5.0 \text{ cm}} \right)^2 = 40.0 \text{ mR/hr}$$

Because the distance change was in the opposite direction of the previous example, the intensity increased by four times.

The inverse square law, as indicated earlier, is an important factor in radiation therapy dose calculations.

Exponential Attenuation

The inverse square law is strictly correct only when certain conditions are met. For example, the size of radiation source must be small enough to be treated as a point source. In addition, we have assumed that none of the radiation emitted from the source is removed from the beam but rather continues outward from the source unmolested. When working with photons in air, this condition is met well enough that the inverse square law can be said to apply in most of these cases. For high-energy medical accelerators, the inverse square law applies to a limited degree when the photons are traveling in some material such as water or a patient. In most cases of photon interactions with material, however, the photons will indeed interact with the atoms of the material, giving up their energy and being removed from the beam. This process is called *attenuation*.

Earlier we saw that the decay of a radioactive source is an exponential function, described by the following equation:

$$A_t = A_0 e^{-\lambda t}$$

where λ is a constant for a given radioisotope and t is the time between measurements A_0 and A_t. This represents a statistical view of the problem; it is impossible to say exactly when each individual atom will decay, but large numbers of atoms can be described with high precision. The attenuation of radiation by a medium can also be described in this way. For this purpose, we define a quantity called the *linear attenuation coefficient* with the symbol μ. This describes the probability that each photon in the beam will interact with the medium and lose its energy, per centimeter of material that the photons pass through, and has units of cm^{-1}. It is not a constant like λ but instead depends greatly on the energy of the photon beam and the medium in which the interaction is taking place.

The extent of attenuation of a photon beam by a medium is then calculated by the following:

$$I_x = I_0 e^{-\mu x}$$

where I_0 is the intensity of the beam before striking the medium, I_x is the intensity after passing through the medium, μ is the linear attenuation coefficient for this beam energy and medium, and x is the thickness of the medium (in cm). Note that this equation is in exactly the same form as the equation for radioactive decay, indicating that the two processes are similar to each other in being statistical in nature, rather than exact.

Like the radioactive decay equation, the equation of attenuation can be used in many ways. Some examples are given subsequently.

Example: A beam of ^{60}Co photons is incident on a lead sheet 1.0 cm thick. If the initial dose rate of the cobalt beam (I_0) was 50 cGy/ min, what will the dose rate be after passing through the lead sheet if the value of μ for this beam in lead is 0.533 cm^{-1}?

$$I_x = I_0 e^{-\mu x}$$
$$I_x = (50) e^{(-0.533)(1.0)}$$
$$I_x = (50)(0.587)$$
$$I_x = 29.35 \text{ cGy/min}$$

Example: Using the data from the previous example, calculate the initial dose rate if the dose rate after passing through the lead sheet was measured to be 15.0 cGy/min.

From the previous example, $\mu = 0.533$ cm^{-1} and $x = 1.0$ cm:

$$I_x = I_0 e^{-\mu x}$$
$$15.0 = I_0 e^{(-0.533)(1.0)}$$
$$15.0 = I_0 (0.587)$$
$$I_0 = 25.55 \text{ cGy/min}$$

The μ values for materials and photon energies important in radiation therapy is provided in Table 14-4.

 The exponential radioactivity decay equation can be used to derive a special quantity, the half-life, *that describes the amount of time required for the isotope to decay to half of its original activity. In the same manner, we can define a quantity, called the **half-value layer (HVL)**, that is, the thickness of some added material required to reduce the beam intensity to half of its original value:*

$$HVL = \frac{0.693}{\mu}$$

Because μ depends on the energy of the beam and the material with which the radiation is interacting, HVL values must be defined by both energy and attenuating material. This procedure is fairly straightforward if the photon beam is monoenergetic, that is, if it consists of only a single-photon energy. Unfortunately, this is not the case with photon beams produced by most modern radiation therapy equipment, which produce polyenergetic beams

Table 14-4	Linear Attenuation Coefficients (μ)(cm⁻¹)				
Energy (MeV)	Water	Tissue	Aluminum	Copper	Lead
0.010	5.0660	5.360	71.1187	1964.0300	1507.4720
0.050	0.2245	0.2330	0.9803	22.9466	88.7330
0.100	0.1706	0.1760	0.4604	4.0759	62.0370
0.200	0.1370	0.1412	0.3306	1.4067	11.2612
0.500	0.0969	0.0998	0.2281	0.7500	1.8040
0.662	0.0857	0.0883	0.2013	0.6496	1.2314
0.800	0.0787	0.0810	0.1846	0.5914	0.9906
1.000	0.0707	0.0729	0.1660	0.5277	0.7963
1.250	0.0632	0.0651	0.1482	0.4704	0.6600
1.500	0.0575	0.0593	0.1352	0.4301	0.5873
2.000	0.0494	0.0510	0.1169	0.3763	0.5146
3.000	0.0397	0.0409	0.0955	0.3226	0.4737
4.000	0.0340	0.0350	0.0839	0.2975	0.4714
5.000	0.0303	0.0312	0.0767	0.2840	0.4805
8.000	0.0242	0.0249	0.0713	0.2715	0.5157
10.00	0.0222	0.0229	0.0626	0.2778	0.5544
20.00	0.0182	0.0186	0.0586	0.3055	0.6952
30.00	0.0171	0.0176	0.0594	0.3324	0.7952
50.00	0.0167	0.0172	0.0623	0.3692	0.9168
80.00	0.0169	0.0173	0.0656	0.4005	1.0122
100.0	0.0172	0.0177	0.0677	0.4184	1.0544

consisting of a wide spectrum of photon energies. Therefore, the HVL is usually simply measured for a given machine and beam energy and, in the case of low-energy x-ray units, is used to describe the characteristics of the treatment beam.

We know that exponential decay data plotted on a semilogarithmic graph paper yields a straight line. This technique can also be applied to exponential attenuation by plotting the percentage of radiation passing through a material as a function of the material thickness. By plotting data such as these, and drawing in the straight line formed by the data, the HVL of the beam can be determined experimentally. Once the graph is done, the thickness of material required to reduce the beam intensity to any fraction of its initial value can be found simply by reading the graph. If a large number of attenuation readings are taken, the curve may not actually display a single line but a series of line segments of decreasing slope. This effect results from the "hardening" of the beam, explained in the next section.

X-Ray Beam Quality

The HVL is an important quantity for photon beams and can be used as a description of "beam quality." Photon beams can be classified as "hard" or "soft" beams, depending on their HVL.[4] Although there are no strict rules for determining the hardness or softness of a radiation beam, a hard beam will have a higher HVL and higher penetrating ability than a soft beam.

This concept of beam hardness becomes more important when one considers the various factors involved. Softer beams have less penetrating ability and therefore will tend to deposit their energy in a medium fairly quickly. If the medium in question is actually a radiation therapy patient, this means that the skin dose to that patient will be increased. In some situations this is desirable; in many situations, however, it is not. Consider, for example, a conventional radiation therapy simulator

(or any diagnostic x-ray device). A soft beam will not penetrate adequately through the patient to the film but will instead leave a large amount of dose inside the patient without contributing any quality to the final film. In this setting, the technician should attempt to reduce the softness of the beam (and therefore the patient dose) without requiring a large increase in radiation exposure to take the film.

To understand one solution to these problems, consider a polyenergetic beam of radiation striking a medium such as lead. The beam consists of a large variety of x-ray energies—some low, some more energetic. As the beam passes through the lead, the softer x-rays (those with the lower energy) tend to be absorbed by the lead, whereas the harder x-rays, whose μ value is lower, are not as likely to be absorbed and may pass through the lead untouched. So if you examine the various energies in the beam before and after it passes through the lead, you can see that the beam exiting from the lead will have a higher average energy (i.e., fewer low-energy x-rays) and a larger HVL than the initial beam. By passing the beam through this lead attenuator, we have actually increased the overall HVL of the beam, although the intensity of the beam has probably been decreased. This effect is called *beam hardening* and is very important in the design and use of diagnostic and radiation therapy equipment.[2-4]

Low-energy x-ray units (diagnostic and superficial therapy) usually have a certain amount of "inherent filtration"; that is, there is some filtration material built into the machine. Usually this consists of the metal window where the radiation beam exits the inside chamber of the tube, where it is produced, together with a small amount of added filtration (usually aluminum) to harden the beam for use in patient diagnosis and treatment. High-energy x-ray units (linear accelerators and betatrons) have several devices in the treatment head that harden the beam, as well as change the distribution of the radiation within the field so that the dose across the patient is uniform. These devices assist in improving the uniformity of dose within the treatment volume while eliminating excessive dose in areas where tissue sparing is desirable.

Types of Photon Interactions

The exact mechanisms of the interactions of photons with the atoms of the irradiated medium are known to a large extent from the work performed in the late 19th and early 20th centuries by Thomson, Einstein, Compton, Rutherford, and many others. There are five photon interaction processes that occur in the energy range of concern in radiation therapy:

1. Thomson (coherent) scattering
2. Photoelectric scattering
3. Compton (incoherent) scattering
4. Pair production
5. Photodisintegration

Rayleigh (Coherent) Scattering. In Rayleigh scattering, the incident photon is of very low energy, not energetic enough to ionize the atom. The photon, coming into the region close to the atom, is absorbed, but because not enough energy is present to cause the release of any electrons, the atom re-emits a second photon of exactly the same energy as the incident photon but headed in a new direction. So, from the outside, it appears that the photon bounced off of the atom into another direction. In this case, no damage is done to the atom, so this interaction has no biologic effect. The interaction is called *coherent* because the wavelength and energy of the emitted photon are identical to those of the incident photon, a condition known in physics as *coherency.*

Photoelectric Scattering. The photoelectric effect was first described in detail by Einstein, who was awarded the Nobel Prize in Physics for the discovery—his other theories were believed to be too controversial and far-out for serious consideration (at the time). This interaction occurs exclusively at low photon energies (≤1 MeV) and is more relevant to diagnostic radiology than to radiation therapy.

In a photoelectric interaction (Figure 14-6), the incident photon interacts with an electron in the inner shells of the atom—usually the K or L shell—leading to transfer of all the energy of the photon to the electron. When the energy received by an electron in the shell is sufficient to overcome its binding energy, this electron is ejected from the atom with energy equal to the following:

$$E^{electron} = E^{photon} - E^{binding}$$

where $E^{electron}$ is the kinetic energy of the electron leaving the atom (related to its mass and speed), E^{photon} is the energy of the incident photon, and $E^{binding}$ is the binding energy of the involved electron shell. After ejection of the electron, there is a "hole" in the electron shell, which is then filled by outer shell electrons "falling" into it, losing energy in the process. The energy lost by these outer shell electrons usually appears as low-energy x-rays, called *characteristic radiation.*[1-4]

Whenever characteristic radiation is produced, there is a possibility that the characteristic x-ray photon may be absorbed by an orbital electron rather than leaving the atom. The electron, now having an excess of energy, will be ejected from the atom in place of the photon. An electron that leaves the atom in this manner is called an *Auger electron* and is capable of causing biologic damage on its own.

Compton (Incoherent) Scattering. Compton scattering is the most common photon interaction that occurs in the energy range used in radiation therapy.[4] In a Compton interaction, as shown in Figure 14-7, the incident photon interacts with an

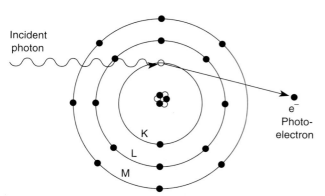

Figure 14-6. In the photoelectric effect, the incident photon is totally absorbed and transfers all of its energy to the resultant photoelectron. (From Christian PE, Waterstram-Rich KM, editors: *Nuclear medicine PET/CT: technology and techniques,* ed 6, St. Louis, 2007, Mosby.)

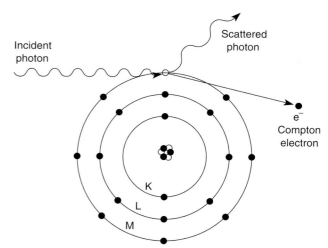

Figure 14-7. Compton scattering occurs in outer electron shells. The atom is left ionized. (From Christian PE, Waterstram-Rich KM, editors: *Nuclear medicine PET/CT: technology and techniques,* ed 6, St. Louis, 2007, Mosby.)

outer shell electron, that is, an electron very loosely bound to the atom (sometimes called a *free electron* because the binding energy of the electron is much less than the incident photon). This electron absorbs some of the photon's energy and is ejected from the outer shell, making an angle with the direction of the incident photon. The photon is scattered from its incident path and has different energy and wavelength than the incident photon. This interaction is also called *incoherent scattering.*

The ejected electron, also known as a *Compton electron,* and the scattered photon travel away from the atom at different angles, which can be calculated using several complex equations relating the angles and energies of the particles involved both before and after the interaction takes place. The equations for energy of the scattered photon (hv′) and the kinetic energy of the Compton electron (E_k) can be derived by using the physics principles of conservation of energy and momentum and are given subsequently.

$$hv' = hv \frac{1}{1 + \varepsilon(1 - \cos\theta)}, \quad E_k = hv \frac{\varepsilon(1 - \cos\theta)}{1 + \varepsilon(1 - \cos\theta)}$$

In the previous equation, hv is the energy of the incident photon; θ is the angle between the paths of the incident and scattered photons; and ε is equal to $hv/m_e c^2$, where m_e is the rest mass of the electron and $m_e c^2 = 0.511$ MeV.

The relation between the scattering angle (θ) of photon and scattering angle (ϕ) of the Compton electron with respect to the direction of the incident photon is given by the following equation:

$$\cot\phi = (1 + \varepsilon) \tan(\theta/2)$$

Although the mathematics of this process is complex, a few examples can show the effect of angle on the results of a Compton interaction:

1. *Direct hit on the target atom.* If the incident photon makes a direct hit on the atom, the Compton electron will go straight forward (in the same direction the incident photon was traveling) and carry away most of the energy, whereas the scattered photon will travel backward from the atom and

carry away a minimum of energy. This effect is called *backscatter*. At high photon energies (such as those from a typical therapy accelerator), the energy of the secondary photon approaches a maximum value of 0.255 MeV, and the number of photons that scatter directly back is very small.

2. *Grazing hit on the target atom.* A grazing hit on the atom by the incident photon will cause very little energy loss; most of the energy will be carried away by the scattered photon, which as a result will have nearly the same energy as the incident photon.

3. *90-degree scatter.* It is important for radiation protection purposes to look at what takes place when the scattered photon emerges at an angle 90 degrees to the incident photon. It turns out that the energy of this photon reaches a maximum value of 0.511 MeV and is essentially independent of the energy of the incident photon, even at very high photon energies.

Pair Production. Pair production interactions occur at high energies; in fact, they are physically impossible when the energy of the incident photon is less than 1.022 MeV.[1-4] In the pair production interaction (Figure 14-8), the incident photon passes close to the nucleus of the atom. When the photon interacts with the EM field of the nucleus, it is absorbed, and instantly the energy is re-emitted as an electron-positron pair (β^-, β^+), which is then ejected from the atom. If you use Einstein's equation $E = mc^2$, letting m equal the mass of an electron, you can calculate that the rest energy of an electron or positron (i.e., the energy needed to create one during an interaction) is equal to 0.511 MeV. Because two such particles are created, this explains why you must have at least two times that energy ($2m_ec^2$), or 1.022 MeV, for pair production interaction to occur. The leftover energy of the incident photon, after the 1.022 MeV has been used for creation of the electron-positron pair, is divided between the electron and positron. Electron-positron pair production can also occur under the influence of the EM field of the electrons in the target material and is called *triplet production.* The electron-positron pair and the electron with which the photon interacts share all the photon energy.

The triplet production has a threshold energy of $4m_ec^2$, or 2.044 MeV, and has a relatively small probability of occurrence as compared with other photon interactions in the target medium.

The electron created usually begins to interact with other atoms outside of the original atom, until it loses its excess energy and is absorbed. The positron, however, suffers a more interesting fate. When it has undergone several interactions and is moving somewhat more slowly than when it left the atom where the pair production interaction took place, it will collide with a free electron, creating an annihilation reaction. The positron is called an "antimatter" version of the electron, and when the two meet, both are destroyed, with the energy of the two being emitted as two photons of 0.511 MeV each, traveling at 180 degrees to each other (i.e., in opposite directions). These two photons will have further interactions with the atoms of the medium.

Photodisintegration. A photodisintegration reaction is one in which the photon strikes the nucleus of the target atom directly and is absorbed. The sudden absorption of this energy causes the nucleus to emit both neutrons and γ-rays in an attempt to maintain stability. This interaction occurs mainly in high Z materials and at usually higher energies (higher than 7 MeV), depending on the material. Thus it is a very unimportant interaction in tissue, where the Z_{eff} is approximately 7.42 (in other words, very low Z). However, it is extremely important when working with high-energy medical accelerators, those with photon or electron beam energies of 10 MeV or greater. Because of the high energies of these beams, combined with the massive amounts of high Z materials such as lead and tungsten in the beam production systems of these accelerators, a substantial neutron hazard to patients or personnel can occur. If you look at the inside of the treatment head of a high-energy linear accelerator, you will probably see some neutron shielding in the form of a borated plastic that slows down ("moderates") the neutrons so that they can be captured.

Effects of Combined Interactions. When a radiation beam interacts with a medium, no single type of photon interaction occurs; instead, the result is usually a combination of two or more of the previous interactions. The factor µ, discussed earlier, actually represents the combined effects of all of the possible interactions for a given energy and material:

$$\mu = \sigma_{coh} + \tau + \sigma_{inc} + \pi + \Pi$$

where σ_{coh} represents Thomson ("coherent") scattering; τ, photoelectric interactions; σ_{inc} the Compton ("incoherent") interactions; π, the pair production interactions; and Π, the photodisintegration and other high-energy reactions that we did not study here. Each of these symbols represents a probability that the photon, when it interacts with the medium, will undergo that type of reaction; µ describes the total probability of an interaction. Table 14-5 shows the relative importance of the three interactions of greatest concern in radiation therapy physics: the photoelectric, Compton, and pair production interactions.

As you can see from the table, at low energies, most photon interactions taking place are photoelectric (τ) interactions. However, as energy increases, the Compton (σ_{inc}) interaction quickly takes precedence and is itself slowly replaced by the pair production (π) and other interactions as the energy continues to increase.

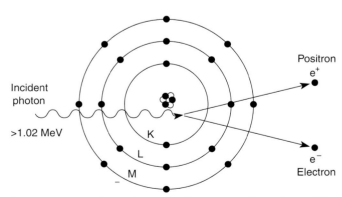

Figure 14-8. In the pair production interaction, the incident photon passes close to the nucleus of the atom and creates a positron-electron pair. The positron will undergo annihilation with another electron. (From Christian PE, Waterstram-Rich KM, editors: *Nuclear medicine PET/CT: technology and techniques,* ed 6, St. Louis, 2007, Mosby.)

Table 14-5	Relative Importance of Photon Interactions in Water (the Number of Each Type that Occurs per 100 Photons)		
Photon Energy (MeV)	τ	σ_{inc}	π
0.010	95	5	0
0.026	50	50	0
0.060	7	93	0
0.150	0	100	0
4.000	0	94	6
10.00	0	77	23
24.00	0	50	50
100.0	0	16	84

Most radiation therapy energies fall into the range of 1 to 5 MeV, where Compton predominates. You can also see this trend in Table 14-4, especially for lead; the values of μ start extremely high, drop to a minimum at energies around 4.0 MeV, then begin to climb again as the pair production interactions begin to produce more and more interactions as energy increases. You should keep this behavior of μ in mind when thinking about exponential attenuation problems.

The relative importance of different photon interactions with an attenuator depends on the energy of the photon, the atomic number (Z), and the electron density of the attenuating material.

The coherent scattering is important only for photons with energy less than 10 keV and high Z materials and has no significance in radiation therapy. The photoelectric interaction is known to dominate at low photon energies in keV ranges and in high Z materials. The Compton interaction plays the leading role for photon energies in the low MeV range, and the probability of this interaction is independent of Z but depends on the electrons per gram of the attenuating material. The pair production dominates for photon energies greater than 10 MeV in high Z material, with a threshold of 1.02 MeV. The photodisintegration usually occurs for a photon with energy in the MeV range and has a threshold energy that depends on the nuclei present in the material. The probability of this interaction is much smaller than that for pair production, but this interaction is the major source of neutron production in high-energy accelerators used for radiation therapy. As you can imagine, Compton interaction of photons plays an important role in imaging and radiation therapy and is responsible for the loss of contrast in diagnostic and megavoltage beam portal images. It is also the major process responsible for megavoltage therapeutic photon beam dose deposition in tissue.

OTHER PARTICLE INTERACTIONS

The interactions of nonphoton particulate radiation with matter differ considerably from those of photons because of the different nature of this particulate radiation. Although photons have no mass and no electrical charge, particles do have mass, and most

have some amount of electrical charge as well. As a result, interactions between particles and atoms tend to resemble "billiard ball" interactions, familiar to us on an everyday level. This section examines some of the interactions that take place in the cases of particle radiations used in radiation therapy, namely, electrons, protons, heavy charged particles, and neutrons. Among these, electron beam radiation therapy is widely used, proton beam therapy is gradually becoming popular, and heavy charged particle beam therapy and neutron beam therapies are available in a small number of radiation therapy centers in the world. The electrons, protons, and heavy charged particles such as carbon-12 are charged particles, and they interact with the orbital electrons and nuclei of the atoms in the material, which are also charged entities, through the Coulomb force. The collision or interaction of the particulate radiation with the atomic electrons of the material leads to excitation and ionization of the atoms. The interaction of charged particles with the nuclei can lead to their radiative energy loss through a process called *bremsstrahlung*. Heavy charged particles can also have a nuclear reaction with the nuclei of the material and can make them radioactive.

A neutron is electrically neutral with zero charge. The collision of neutrons with the nuclei of the atoms of the material produces protons or other heavy charged particles. These protons and heavy charged particles then deposit their energy in the material by different processes discussed previously. The neutron is thus an indirectly ionizing particle like a photon.

Elastic and Inelastic Collisions

The collisions of particle radiations can be likened to the collisions between large-scale objects such as billiard balls. Each ball can be described as possessing kinetic energy, that is, energy caused by its motion through space. When the balls collide, their directions and speeds will change depending on the conditions of the collision, and thus each ball may lose or gain kinetic energy; the total kinetic energy, however, may or may not remain the same before and after the collision. If no kinetic energy of the system is lost in the collision, the collision is elastic; if kinetic energy is lost from the system, the collision is inelastic.

Example: Two balls with kinetic energies equal to 10 J each collide. After the collision, one ball has a kinetic energy of 15 J, and the other has a kinetic energy of 5 J. Because the total kinetic energy in the system has not changed (20 J = 20 J), the collision was elastic.

If, in the same example, the kinetic energies of the two balls after the collision had been measured as 12 J and 6 J, this would have been an inelastic collision, because kinetic energy was lost during the collision (20 J > 18 J). The remaining 2 J of energy were converted into other forms of energy, such as vibrational energy or heat.

Note that, whether or not kinetic energy is conserved, the total energy of the system (which includes all other forms of energy such as heat) must remain the same. In the second example, the 2 J of kinetic energy lost to the billiard balls did not disappear but rather were converted into another form of energy. This concept is called the principle of conservation of energy and is one of the basic concepts of physics and chemistry.

The interactions between atoms and particle radiations can be classified in the same manner. If the total kinetic energies of the particle and atom are the same after the interaction, then an elastic collision has taken place; if not, the collision was inelastic. We next look at how these definitions apply in the cases of interactions of electrons, protons, heavy charged particles such as carbon-12 ion, and neutron radiations with a medium.

Electron Interactions

Electron-Electron Interactions. When electrons from a radiation source interact with the electrons in different shells of the atoms in the medium, they give up energy to those atomic electrons and are then deflected away from the atom in a new direction. Because they have given up energy to the atomic electron, the original electron is now moving at a slower speed (and therefore has less kinetic energy). The target electron in the atomic orbit may be "kicked up" to a shell farther from the nucleus (excitation) or may be ejected completely from the atom (ionization) if the energy gained from the incident electron is high enough for the process to occur. Remember that a "collision" between two particles does not necessarily mean that actual physical contact between the particles has occurred; a collision can also result if the EM fields of the two particles come close enough to interact with each other, a distance that may be several times larger than the physical size of these particles.

Recall from our study of the Compton interaction that outer shell electrons are considered as "free" electrons because their binding energies are very low compared with the energy of the incoming photons. If one of these free electrons is involved in the electron-electron interaction just described, the binding energy of the target electron is so small that it may be ignored; therefore the total kinetic energy of the incident and target electrons before and after the collision is taken to be same. In this case, the collision can be considered elastic. If, however, the interaction involved an electron in a shell close to the nucleus, the binding energy must be taken into account. In this case, because of the principle of conservation of energy already discussed, some of the kinetic energy of the original electron will be lost to overcome the binding energy of the target electron before the target electron can change shells or leave the atom, making this an inelastic collision because the final total kinetic energy of the particles is reduced from its initial value.

When the electron's energy is finally depleted by a series of collisions, an atom in its vicinity captures it.

Elastic Electron-Nuclei Collisions. In materials heavier than hydrogen (Z = 1), electrons with certain energies are more likely to undergo elastic scattering with the nuclei of atoms than with the atomic electrons. As with an electron-electron elastic collision (already described), the incident electrons lose a small amount of energy to the nucleus of the atom and bounce away with reduced energy. Because the nuclei are so much larger than electrons, the electron will retain a larger percentage of its energy than if it had collided with an electron and is more likely to bounce straight backward from the atom after the collision. This effect diminishes quickly as the energy of the incident electrons is increased, and, at energies in the range usually used in radiation therapy (4 to 25 MeV), the electrons interact mainly

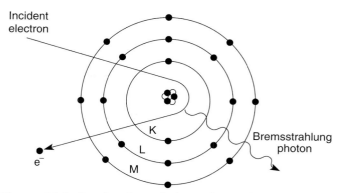

Figure 14-9. Deceleration of charged particle passing near nucleus results in release of energy in the form of bremsstrahlung radiation. (From Christian PE, Waterstram-Rich KM, editors: *Nuclear medicine PET/CT: technology and techniques*, ed 6, St. Louis, 2007, Mosby.)

by electron-electron scattering (discussed previously) or inelastic nuclear scattering (discussed later).

Inelastic Electron-Nuclei Collisions. High-energy electrons can pass close to the nucleus of a target atom, as seen in Figure 14-9, and be so strongly attracted by the charges in the nucleus that they will slow down, losing some of their kinetic energy; this energy will be emitted from the atom as a photon with energy (hv) equal to the energy lost by the electron when it slowed down.[1] This process is called **bremsstrahlung** (German for "braking radiation") and is the most important method of producing x-ray beams in therapy units.

The photon created in the bremsstrahlung process can be of any energy from 0 up to the energy of the incident electron and can emerge from the atom in any direction. Thus like β decay, bremsstrahlung produces not a single-energy x-ray but rather a spectrum of x-ray energies ranging from 0 to the energy of the incident electron beam. The average energy of the bremsstrahlung spectrum is approximately one third of the maximum possible energy (E_{max}).

When the electron beam is in the lower energy range (50 to 300 keV), the photons are emitted in a wide range of angles. As the electron beam energy increases, the photons tend to be emitted closer to the direction of the incident electron, a phenomenon known as *forward peaking* of the photon beam. This effect is very important in the design and use of high-energy photon machines such as linear accelerators and betatrons, because for the high-energy electron beams hitting the targets used in these machines, the bremsstrahlung photon beam is highly forward peaked.

Bremsstrahlung production is more likely in high Z materials such as lead or tungsten than in low Z materials such as water or tissue. For this reason, high Z materials can be bombarded with a beam of high-energy electrons to produce high-energy photon beams in radiation therapy machines. For low Z materials such as water or soft tissue, the bremsstrahlung production from electron beams is very small. The energy loss of electrons is mostly by ionization and excitation leading to energy deposition in the medium. The electrons lose approximately 2 MeV/cm in water or soft tissue.

X-rays are photons produced by the interaction of electrons with any material. The x-ray tubes and high-energy radiation therapy accelerators use a high-voltage power supply and the necessary technology to generate a narrow or focused high-energy electron beam, which then hits a high Z target to produce the x-ray beam for imaging and radiation therapy. The two atomic processes responsible for production of x-rays are (1) bremsstrahlung and (2) characteristic x-ray emission by atomic electrons. The physics of these processes were discussed earlier in this chapter. The x-ray energy spectra consist of the continuous bremsstrahlung photon energies between zero to the value of energy of the incident electron superimposed with the peaks at discrete energies of the characteristics radiation of the target. The efficiency of the x-ray production by this process is proportional to both the atomic number (Z) of the target and the strength of the applied high voltage. Usually, less than 1% of the kinetic energy of the electron is converted to x-rays or photons and the rest of it is converted to heat, thus requiring a good cooling system for the target to remove this heat. The direction of the x-ray beam emission depends on the energy of the incident electrons. In the keV energy range, most of the x-rays are emitted at a direction perpendicular to the path of the incident electron beam. In the MeV energy range, x-rays are emitted in the same direction as the incident electrons. Therefore, a reflectance target is used in diagnostic energy x-ray tubes, whereas a thick transmission-type target is used in therapy accelerators. The thick target not only stops the electrons but also hardens the beam by filtering out the low-energy components of the x-ray spectra. Suitable filters are also added to diagnostic and superficial kilovoltage therapy units to remove the unnecessary low-energy x-ray photons to harden the beam and reduce the skin dose to patients.

You can learn more about the physics of x-ray production by visiting http://www.colorado.edu/physics/2000/xray/making_xrays.html.

Heavy Charged Particle Interactions

Protons, alpha particles (helium nucleus with two protons and two neutrons), and heavier charged particles such as carbon-12 ions lose their energy by Coulomb interactions with atomic electrons and nuclei. In addition, they also undergo nuclear reactions with the nuclei. Like electrons, the heavy charged particles undergo multiple scattering due to elastic collisions with electrons and the nuclei without loss of energy. Because of their heavy mass, they undergo less multiple scattering compared with electrons. They deposit their energy in the medium mostly by ionization and excitation resulting from the inelastic collision with the atomic electrons. The inelastic collision of heavy charged particles with the nuclei of the medium creates nuclear fragments. These fragments usually deposit their energy locally. Unlike electrons, radiative bremsstrahlung energy loss is not significant for heavy charged particles. The rate of energy loss per unit path length is proportional to the square of the charge of the particle and inversely proportional to the square of the velocity of the particle. As the heavy charged particle slows down, the rate of energy loss increases leading to higher deposition of dose in the medium. Thus, these particles deposit the maximum dose when they are very close to being stopped in the medium or near the end of their range of travel, giving rise to a Bragg peak as shown in Figure 14-10. The dose beyond the Bragg peaks falls to zero very rapidly. This is one of the most desirable features of the dose distribution of heavy charged particles. These peaks can be broadened to any desirable width by combining the Bragg peaks of heavy charged particles with different energies with the help of range-modulating wheels or other

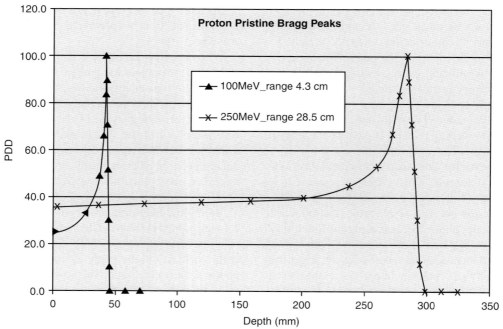

Figure 14-10. Depth-dose curve of a 250-MeV proton beam showing the Bragg peak. *PDD*, Percentage depth dose. (From N. Sahoo et al., private communication.)

energy-modulation schemes. The existence of Bragg peaks allows one to use these beams to deposit the maximum dose inside the target volume while reducing the dose beyond the target to a very small value.

Neutron Interactions

The neutron has zero electrical charge like the photon, but has a large mass relative to the electron. The neutron interacts with the nucleons of the atomic nucleus of the medium through the nuclear force. The neutrons cannot create any ionization by removing the atomic electrons themselves. However, when neutrons have a head-on collision with an atomic nucleus, it leads to generation of other charged particles such as protons and alpha particles. These secondary charged particles deposit their energy through inelastic collision with atomic electrons and the atomic nuclei. The transfer of energy from neutrons to the secondary particles is very high when they collide with the nuclei of a hydrogen atom, which is a proton with almost equal mass as a neutron. Thus, a neutron beam will deposit a higher dose to fatty tissue because of the high concentration of hydrogen atoms. A neutron loses very little energy when it collides with heavier nuclei. A nuclear reaction of a neutron with nuclei in the medium can lead to nuclear disintegration, giving rise to more neutrons, heavy charged particles, and γ-rays. As mentioned earlier, these secondary particles then deposit their energy in the medium. The dose distribution of the neutron beam is similar to that of γ-rays from a cobalt-60 source.

 You can learn about heavy particle therapy from: http://www-bd.fnal.gov/ntf/reference/hadrontreat.pdf

SUMMARY

To understand the discipline of radiation physics, one must be familiar with the developments, theories, and technologic advances that have taken place since Roentgen discovered the x-ray in 1895. From the Curies, who discovered radioactivity and determined the activity of 1 g of radium (^{226}Ra), to Bohr's attempt to explain the atom, to Einstein's work that earned him the Nobel Prize for photoelectric effect, the areas of atomic physics and nuclear physics has significantly contributed to the development and advances in diagnostic and therapeutic radiology. The knowledge of the interactions of radiation with subatomic particles is critical to understanding the scientific basis and intelligent use of radiation therapy. This chapter introduces the following concepts to provide the foundation for understanding the discipline of radiation physics.

- **The structure of the atom**: An atom consists of negatively charged electrons distributed in specific orbitals around a positively charged nucleus made of protons and neutrons. The laws of quantum mechanics determine the occupation of orbitals. The electrons play the vital role in determining structure and properties of materials important to radiation therapy physics. The protons and neutrons are bound together in the nucleus by a strong nuclear force. Atoms and nuclei are stable only when they are in their lowest energy ground state configurations. When they are in excited states, they tend to return to their respective ground states by emitting the excess energy as different kinds of radiation.

- **Radiation**: Radiation can be in the form of electromagnetic waves or particles. According to de Broglie's principle of wave particle duality, every particle has a wavelike character and vice versa. The characteristic wavelength (λ) of a particle is given by the equation $\lambda = h/p$, where h is Planck's constant and p is the momentum of the particle, which is equal to m × v, the product of the mass (m) of the particle with velocity (v). According to Einstein's mass-energy equivalence principle, any mass m has an equivalent energy E and vice versa, and they are related by the formula, $E = mc^2$. Some radiation can ionize the matter by removing the electrons from atomic shells of the target and are known as *ionizing radiation*. Ionizing radiation can be either directly ionizing like electrons, protons, and heavy charged particles, which are charged particles, or indirectly ionizing like photons and neutrons, which are neutral. Radiation therapy involves use of ionizing radiation only.

- **Photon**: The photon is the particle associated with an electromagnetic field and its energy is given by $E = h\nu$. The frequency ν of the photon is related to the wavelength of the electromagnetic wave by $\nu = c / \nu$.

- **Radioactivity**: Radioactivity is the process in which the unstable nuclei give up the excess energy in the form of radiation to move toward their stable ground state. Radioactive nuclei decay by emitting alpha particles (He-4 nucleus), beta particles (electrons or positrons), and gamma rays (photons), and these are known as alpha, beta, and gamma decay, respectively. Characteristic x-rays and Auger electrons are also produced from electronic shells of the atom during the radioactivity. Gamma rays are emitted from the nuclei, whereas x-rays are from electrons, and both consist of photons. Radioactivity can also be classified as isotopic, isotonic, isobaric, or isomeric transitions in which either the number of protons or neutrons or their sum or both remains unchanged, respectively, after the decay. All radioactivity is statistical in nature and follows an exponential decay law, with the activity (A) at any time (t) being determined from the initial activity A_0 from $A = A_0 e^{-\lambda t}$. The half-life of decay (t_h) = 0.693/λ, λ being the decay constant. The SI unit of activity is the becquerel (Bq) or disintegrations per second, but the Curie (Ci) is the old and widely used practical unit: $1 \text{ Ci} = 3.7 \times 10^{10}$ Bq.

- **Photon interactions**: When a beam of x-ray and gamma-ray photons strikes a target, some of the photons will (1) pass through the target without any interaction; (2) change the direction of motion without losing any energy by coherent Rayleigh scattering with electrons; (3) change direction and lose some energy by the incoherent Compton scattering with electrons; or (4) lose all their energy (a) by photoelectric effect or triplet production while interacting with the atomic electrons, or (b) by pair production or photodisintegration while interacting with the nuclei of the target. The probability of various photon interactions with the atomic electrons and nuclei of the target depends on the energy of the photon and atomic number Z of the target material. Among the interactions in which the photon loses some or all of its energy, the photoelectric effect is dominant at low photon energies in keV ranges, the Compton effect in the high keV to low MeV range, and the pair production in the high MeV range. The photonuclear interaction is responsible for neutron production in high-energy linear accelerators used in radiotherapy. The attenuation of a photon beam with an initial intensity of I_0 while passing through a target follows an exponential law, $I_x = I_0 e^{-\mu x}$. I_x is the intensity after the photon beam passes through a thickness of x cm in the medium, and μ is the linear attenuation constant of the medium. The quality of the photon beam or penetrating power of a photon beam can be specified by the beam's half-value layer (HVL), which is the thickness of the attenuator that reduces the beam intensity to half of its initial value. HVL is related to μ by the equation $HVL = 0.693/\mu$. Tenth value layer (TVL) is the thickness of the attenuator that reduces the beam intensity to 10% of its initial value and is related to μ by the equation $TVL = \ln(10)/\mu$.

- **Electron and heavy charged particle interaction**: Charged particles lose their energy while passing through the target medium predominantly through excitation and ionization of the atomic electrons. In addition interaction with the nuclei of the target atoms results in energy loss through emission of bremsstrahlung x-ray photons by electrons and production of nuclear fragments by heavy charged particles. The electrons also undergo multiple scattering without losing any significant amount of energy. Electrons lose approximately 2 MeV per cm of travel in water. Unlike photons, charged particles have finite ranges in the medium and their intensity falls to zero after this range. In addition, energy loss of heavier charged particles such as protons, alpha particles, and carbon-12 ions exhibit Bragg peaks at certain depths depending on their initial energy, making them attractive for conformal radiation therapy.

- **Neutron interaction**: Neutrons interact with the nuclei of the atoms in the target and lose their energy to the target nuclei by billiard ball–like collision processes. These collisions lead to production of charged particles such as protons, alpha particles, and gamma rays, which then deposit the energy by their interaction with the electrons and nuclei of the target medium. The dose distribution of neutrons in water is very similar to that of the photons from a cobalt-60 source.

- **Inverse square law**: According to the inverse square law, in a nonabsorbing medium such as air, the intensity of radiation from an effective point source at any distance d from the source is inversely proportional to the square of d. Thus, the intensity I_2 at a distance d_2 can be calculated from the intensity I_1 at a distance d_1 from the equation, $I_1/I_2 = d_2^2/d_1^2$.

Review Questions

Multiple Choice

1. How many seconds are there in 2.54 minutes?
   a. 174.0
   b. 114.0
   c. 152.4
   d. 92.4
   e. 254

2. Calculate the wavelength of an electromagnetic wave that has a frequency of 3.95×10^{14} Hz.
   a. 1.32×10^6 m
   b. 13.2×10^6 m
   c. 7.59×10^{-8} m
   d. 7.59×10^{-7} m
   e. 7.59×10^{-6} m

3. An FM radio station broadcasts at 102.0 MHz on your radio dial. What is the wavelength of the station's signal?
   a. 34.0 m
   b. 3.40 m
   c. 2.941 m
   d. 2.941×10^6 m
   e. 29.41 m

4. An electromagnetic wave has a frequency of 2.1×10^{21} Hz. What is the energy of the wave?
   a. 3.355×10^{54} eV
   b. 1.39×10^{12} eV
   c. 5.060×10^{35} eV
   d. 8.250 MeV
   e. 8.715 MeV

5. If an electromagnetic wave has an energy of 6 MeV, what would its wavelength be?
   a. 50 m
   b. 3.313×10^{-32} m
   c. 2.075×10^{-13} m
   d. 2.075×10^{-12} m
   e. 2.075×10^{-7} m

6. A sample of an isotope has a half-life of 74 days and is measured to have an activity of 8.675 Ci at noon on that day. What will the activity of the isotope be 94 days later at 6 PM?
   a. 4.338 Ci
   b. 3.588 Ci
   c. 3.596 Ci
   d. 5.034 Ci
   e. 2.37 Ci

7. The intensity of a radioactive beam is measured at a distance of 100 cm and found to be 250 mR/min. What will the intensity of this beam be at 105 cm?
   a. 226.8 mR/min
   b. 238.1 mR/min
   c. 205.7 mR/min
   d. 275.6 mR/min
   e. 262.5 mR/min

8. A 6-MeV photon beam is incident on a lead sheet 1.5 cm thick. If the initial dose rate of the beam is 300 cGy/min, what will the dose rate be after passing through the lead sheet if the linear attenuation coefficient for this beam in lead is 0.4911 cm⁻¹?
   a. 79.0 cGy/min
   b. 183.6 cGy/min
   c. 147.33 cGy/min
   d. 143.6 cGy/min
   e. 221.0 cGy/min

9. What is the HVL of the beam in question 8?
   a. 2.72 cm
   b. 4.07 cm
   c. 0.941 cm
   d. 1.386 cm
   e. 1.411 cm

10. In the problem given in question 8, what minimal thickness of lead is needed to reduce the dose rate to less than 9 cGy/min?
    a. 2 cm
    b. 10 cm
    c. 100 cm
    d. 7.0 cm
    e. 7.5 cm

The answers to the Review Questions can be found by logging on to our website at: *http://evolve.elsevier.com/Washington+Leaver/ principles*

Questions to Ponder

1. A portal radiograph (port film) is taken with a high-energy photon beam (MeV range). Why is the radiograph inferior in diagnostic quality when compared with a radiograph taken on a simulator (keV range)?

2. Explain the difference between the tenth value layer (TVL) of a material and its linear attenuation coefficient.

3. Explain the reason for using lead as a shielding material for x-ray rooms and/or vaults.

4. Explain the concept of the exponential decay constant and how it relates to half-life.

5. What feature of proton dose distribution makes it more attractive compared with electron and photon dose distribution.

REFERENCES

1. Christian PE, Waterstram-Rich KM, editors: *Nuclear medicine PET/CT: technology and techniques,* ed 6, St. Louis, 2007, Mosby.
2. Hendee WR, Ritenour R: *Medical imaging physics,* ed 3, St. Louis, 1992, Mosby.
3. Johns HE, Cunningham JR: *The physics of radiology,* ed 4, Springfield, Ill, 1983, Charles C Thomas.
4. Khan FM: *The physics of radiation therapy,* ed 2, Baltimore, 1992, Williams & Wilkins.

15 CHAPTER

Aspects of Brachytherapy

Charles M. Washington

Outline

Historic overview and perspective
Review of source strength
  specification
  Radioactive decay
Radioactive sources used in
  brachytherapy
  Radium
  Radium substitutes
The exposure rate from a
  radioactive source

High-dose-rate brachytherapy
Pulsed-dose-rate brachytherapy
Brachytherapy applicators and
  instruments
  External applicators or molds
  Interstitial applicators
  Intracavitary applicators
  Intravascular stent applications
Brachytherapy dosimetry and dose
  distribution

The Paterson-Parker
  (Manchester) system
The Quimby/Memorial
  dosimetry system
The Paris system
  Computer calculation methods
Radiation safety and quality
  assurance
Summary

Objectives

- Understand the importance of brachytherapy as an option for treatment.
- Be able to list advantages of brachytherapy versus external beam radiation therapy.
- Identify the different types of brachytherapy and what types of cancers are treated with each type.
- Recognize the most commonly used isotopes and their half-lives in brachytherapy.

- Describe how afterloading decreases exposure to staff and patients.
- Explain the disadvantages of using radium and the importance of radium substitutes.
- Compare and contrast high-dose brachytherapy versus low-dose brachytherapy.
- Describe the different types of intracavitary applicators.

HISTORIC OVERVIEW AND PERSPECTIVE

The discovery of x-rays by Roentgen in the late 19th century has proved, more than any other innovation, to have a dramatic effect on modern medicine. Shortly after the discovery of x-rays, Henri Becquerel and Pierre Curie began investigating the existence of similar rays produced by known fluorescent materials. Curie, in his experimentation, deliberately produced an ulcer on his arm and described in detail the various phases of a moist epidermitis and his recovery from it.[3] At that point he gave a small radium tube to a colleague and suggested he insert it into a tumor. Subsequently, several physicians began investigating the effects of these rays on malignant tumors, and the therapeutic use of ionizing radiation began.

The term **brachytherapy** refers to radiation therapy that involves placing radioactive material directly into or immediately adjacent to the tumor, rather than through external beams. *Brachy,* meaning "short," implies therapy at a short distance. Today, brachytherapy is a standard technique in the treatment of a large number of malignancies, including uterus and uterine cervix, lung, prostate, and breast. Brachytherapy use in cancer therapy is increasing and is paralleled by the increasing desire for organ preservation and acceptable cosmetic results.[7] In current oncology practice, there are many opportunities for medical dosimetrist and radiation therapist involvement in the practical application of brachytherapy. The scopes of practice for the medical dosimetrist and radiation therapist identify the need for critical thinking skills that involve the application of radiation through these means.

The major advantage of brachytherapy is that very high doses of radiation can be delivered locally to the tumor in a relatively short time, while very low doses are delivered in the surrounding tissue.[6,15] As the distance around the source of radiation increases, there is a dramatic reduction of dose absorbed in tissue. This adheres directly to the premise that in radiation therapy, homogeneous tumoricidal doses must be deposited in the tumor while sparing as much normal tissue as possible. Brachytherapy is commonly used to supplement the dose administered by external beam irradiation; this allows additional doses to be delivered to a well-defined volume of tumor tissue. Because the radiation administered in this way

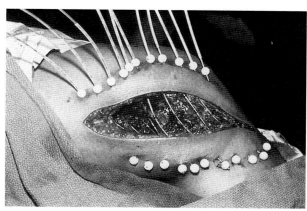

Figure 15-1. Example of interstitial catheters placed along a tumor bed of an extremity. Sources placed inside the catheters will deliver a high dose of radiation to the tumor bed and immediate surrounding area.

does not penetrate through overlying tissues to reach this volume, surrounding tissues are spared from increased doses of radiation.

Brachytherapy can be administered through several types of applications. **Interstitial brachytherapy** is characterized by the placement of radioactive sources directly into a tumor or tumor bed. Rigid needles or flexible tubes may be used in the actual placement of the sources (Figure 15-1). Interstitial brachytherapy is commonly used in the treatment of neck, breast, prostate, and skin tumors and soft tissue sarcomas.

 MammoSite is a brachytherapy procedure that is currently being used in patients with stage 1 or 2 breast cancer with limited or no nodal involvement. These patients must first have a lumpectomy and biopsy of regional lymph nodes to become a candidate. If chosen, they will undergo 10 treatments over 5 days, coming in twice a day. A balloon is placed into the cavity left by the lumpectomy. A catheter is placed in the balloon that allows for the introduction of the radioactive seed on a daily basis. After each treatment, the radioactive seeds are removed while the catheter and balloon remain in the patient. The patient is then free to go home and interact with family and friends. After the completion of the 5-day treatment, both the balloon and catheter are removed. The use of MammoSite brachytherapy for partial breast irradiation continues to increase.[12]

Intracavitary brachytherapy places radioactive sources within a body cavity for treatment. This type of brachytherapy has been the mainstay in treatment of cervical cancer for more than 50 years.[2] Closely associated with interstitial brachytherapy, **intraluminal brachytherapy** places sources of radiation within body tubes such as the esophagus, uterus, trachea, bronchus, and rectum. **Intravascular brachytherapy** is a rapidly emerging treatment modality with potential applications for peripheral vessel angioplasty, bypass graft anastomoses, and arteriovenous dialysis grafts in addition to its application for coronary vessels. The use of stents and radiation can reduce the rate of restenosis in the vessel. **Topical brachytherapy** places the radioactive sources on top of the area to be treated. Molds of the body part treated may be taken and prepared

to place the sources in definite arrangements to deliver the prescribed dose.

REVIEW OF SOURCE STRENGTH SPECIFICATION

Source strength specification plays three roles in brachytherapy. The first is to provide a commonly accepted standard means of describing quantities of emitted radiation. The second allows practitioners to form a basis for *computational dosimetry*, which is the calculation of dose with the aid of a computerized system. Third, source strength specification serves as a prescription parameter in brachytherapy.

The historic term used to describe activity in terms of number of disintegrations per unit time is the curie (Ci). The curie is 3.7×10^{10} disintegrations per second from 1 g of radium. The Système Internationale (SI) unit of activity is the becquerel (Bq). One becquerel equals one disintegration per second. Although the becquerel is the unit recommended for use, the curie is still commonly used in practice. Table 15-1 reviews the conversions commonly used.

Radioactive Decay

The key relationship in understanding radioactivity, which is a statistical process, is as follows:

$$\frac{\Delta N}{\Delta t} \propto N$$

where N is the number of atoms and t is the time. The change in the number of atoms per change in unit time is proportional to the number of atoms present. This proportion can be made into an equation by the addition of a constant, λ, called the **decay constant:**

$$\frac{\Delta N}{\Delta t} = -\lambda N$$

The negative sign is added because there are fewer atoms present after a given amount of time. The equation can be rearranged to solve for the gamma constant as follows:

$$\lambda = -\frac{\frac{\Delta N}{N}}{\Delta t}$$

Therefore, the decay constant can be expressed as the total number of atoms that decay per unit time. From this, the definition of activity and the formula for exponential decay are developed.

Table 15-1	Commonly Used Conversions Relating Curies to Becquerels	
Unit		**Definition**
1 curie (Ci)		3.7×10^{10} disintegration/sec
1 millicurie (mCi)		3.7×10^{7} disintegration/sec
1 microcurie (μCi)		3.7×10^{4} disintegration/sec
1 becquerel (Bq)		1 disintegration/sec
1 megabecquerel (MBq)		1×10^{6} disintegration/sec
1 mCi		37 MBq
1 gigabecquerel (GBq)		1×10^{9} disintegration/sec
1 Ci		37 GBq

Activity. Activity, A, is the rate of decay of a radioactive material or the change in the number of atoms in a certain amount of time and can be written as follows:

$$A = \frac{\Delta N}{\Delta t} = -\lambda N$$

The activity is directly proportional to the decay constant. So, as the decay constant increases, the activity increases.

The previous equation can also be rearranged and integrated to yield the exponential decay equation, as follows:

$$N = N_0 e^{-\lambda t}$$

A (activity) can be substituted for N (the number of atoms) to yield the following:

$$A = A_0 e^{-\lambda t}$$

This formula, as presented in Chapter 14, is commonly used to calculate activity of a radioisotope after some length of time has passed.

Half-life. The concept used to deal with the isotope disintegration is half-life. The **half-life** is the time period in which the activity decays to one half the original value. It is the essential value to use the decay formula for a particular isotope. Half-life ($t\frac{1}{2}$) is related to the decay constant by the following formula:

$$t\frac{1}{2} = \frac{0.693}{\lambda}$$

The relationship between activity and half-life is given by the formula:

$$A = \lambda N = \frac{0.693}{t\frac{1}{2}}$$

The relationship between half-life and activity is inversely proportional. In other words, as half-life increases, overall activity decreases.

Decay Formula. These mathematical expressions can be grouped together and allow the radiation therapist and medical dosimetrist to derive a formula that will relate radionuclide decay. This is called the *decay formula*, which is expressed by the following:

$$A = A_0 e^{-\left(\frac{0.693}{t\frac{1}{2}}\right)t}$$

where A_0 denotes the originally known activity, A is the current activity, $t\frac{1}{2}$ is the half-life, and t is the length of time passed since time of originally known activity. Table 15-2 lists isotopes commonly used in radiation therapy with their half-lives. The half-life will vary somewhat from different literature sources and from past to present, but these are fairly representative of what is in common use today. A good way to remember these concepts is to put them into practical use. It is important to make sure that the units used throughout the problem are consistent.

Example 1: Every year a new decayed value must be determined for clinical use of the cesium-137 tubes. The decay is always calculated from the original assayed value obtained when the source was received. One source was received on

Table 15-2	Commonly Used Isotopes
Isotope	**t½**
Radium-226	1622 years
Cobalt-60	5.27 years
Cesium-137	30.0 years
Iridium-192	73.83 days
Iodine-125	59.4 days
Palladium-103	16.99 days
Gold-198	2.7 days
Radon-222	3.82 days

February 18, 2003; that value was determined to be 69.5 mCi. What would be the activity for this source 365 days later?

$$A = A_0 \times e^{-\left(\frac{0.693}{t\frac{1}{2}}\right) \times t}$$

$$A = A_0 \times e^{-\left(\frac{0.693}{30\ yr}\right) \times 1\ yr}$$

$$A = 67.91\ mCi$$

Mean Life. Another concept related to half-life is mean life, which is complicated in explanation but useful and easy in calculation. **Mean life** is the average lifetime for the decay of radioactive atoms. It is the time period for a hypothetical source that decays at a constant rate equal to its initial activity to produce the same number of disintegrations as the exponentially decaying source that decays for an infinite period of time. It is primarily applicable to dose calculations in permanent implants, typically gold-198 and iodine-125. Theoretically, all of the dose is delivered over a very long time period because all the activity is not decayed away until the last unstable atom disintegrates. The treatment planning team needs a practical means of calculating a final dose. The relationship between mean life and half-life is as follows:

$$\text{Mean life} = t\frac{1}{2} \times 1.44$$

Example 2: 106 mCi of gold-198 is implanted into a pelvic mass. Determine the emitted radiation.

$$\text{Mean life of gold-198} = 1.44 \times (2.7\ \text{days}) = 3.89\ \text{days}$$

$$\text{Emitted radiation} = 106\ \text{mCi} \times 3.89\ \text{days} = 412.34\ \text{mCi-days}$$

Average Energy (E_{ave}). Another property of interest in isotope usage is the average energy of the emitted photons. This is derived from the decay schemes of each isotope. Any beta emission has already been eliminated by filtrating encapsulations, because radiation treatment is not accomplished with beta particles. Table 15-3 illustrates a list of the average energy for isotopes commonly used in brachytherapy.

RADIOACTIVE SOURCES USED IN BRACHYTHERAPY

Brachytherapy most commonly uses sealed radioactive sources within or adjacent to a tumor volume. A sealed source is one in which the radioactive material is encapsulated by welded ends.

Table 15-3	Average Energy of Isotopes Used in Brachytherapy	
Isotope		**E$_{ave}$ (MeV)**
Radium-226		0.830
Cobalt-60		1.253
Cesium-137		0.662
Iridium-192		0.380
Iodine-125		0.028
Palladium-103		0.021
Gold-198		0.412

Typically, the isotope is encased within metal casings that serve two main functions: (1) preventing escape of radioactivity and (2) absorption of beta particles. Figure 15-2 demonstrates a sealed source. The International Organization of Standardization (ISO) classifies sealed sources based on safety requirements. They also specify leak test methods, such as wipe tests, for sealed sources to be carried out at both the manufacturer and user levels.[20]

Most brachytherapy procedures were developed using radium-226, the first radioisotope to be isolated and identified. Other isotopes have come into use when nuclear reactor– produced isotopes became readily available. Most of the isotopes used in radiation therapy today have their dosimetry based on the original radium work and are referred to as **radium substitutes**. These substitutes offer several advantages over radium. Both radium and radium substitutes are described later in the chapter.

Radium

Radium ($^{226}_{88}$Ra) decays mainly by alpha emission and is part of a long decay chain that begins with natural uranium ($^{238}_{92}$U) and concludes in an isotope of stable lead ($^{206}_{82}$Pb). The half-life for radium is approximately 1622 years. As part of the process, radium decays to form radon, a heavy inert gas that further decays down to the stable lead atom. Radon gas has caused concern during home construction in the Midwest to the eastern seaboard.

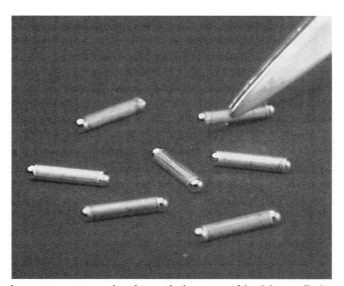

Figure 15-2. Example of a sealed source of ionizing radiation, iodine-125.

As ore deposits decay, the radioactive gas seeps up into the basements of the homes, causing serious health concerns.

Use of radium was very practical because it has a very high specific activity. **Specific activity** is defined as the activity per unit mass of a radioactive material (Ci/g). The specific activity dictates the total activity that a small source can have. Although some radionuclides might have some particular advantage for implantation, they may not be suitable because a small size and high activity may not be possible for that particular isotope. The disadvantage of radium concerns itself mainly with radiation hazards.[20] Radiation is produced by alpha emission and produces a daughter, radon-222 ($^{222}_{86}$Rn), which is a gas that can possibly leak from the encapsulated sources.

A typical radium source consists of a hollow needle or tube made of a metal such as platinum or stainless steel. Inside the tube, small capsules of radium salt are placed, giving the source a known activity. This activity, together with the thickness of the source capsule (known as the *filtration*), determines the dosimetric properties of the source and how it can be used in brachytherapy. Note that the area in which the radioactivity is packed is shorter that the total length of the source; the length of the area in which the radioactivity lies in the source is called the **active length** of the source and must be differentiated from the physical length, which is the total length of the source, end-to-end.[20]

The gamma (Γ) factor for radium-226 is 8.25 R • cm^2/mCi • hr, assuming a filtration of 0.5 mm of platinum. The filtration (shell thickness) of the radium source is very important, because the decay processes of radium-226 result in a large number of low-energy x-rays, which are easily filtered by any additional filtration. In other words, as you increase the filtration of the radium-226 source, the Γ factor will decrease as you eliminate more and more low-energy x-rays. If you have a radium-226 source with ±0.5 mm platinum filtration, the Γ factor from this source will change as follows: increase of 2% for each additional 0.1 mm of platinum added to 0.5 mm, and decrease of 2% for each 0.1 mm of platinum less than 0.5 mm.

Radium Sources. The amount of radioactivity in a radium source is expressed in milligrams of radium. In the definition of a curie, it was initially the amount of activity of 1 g of radium. Later, however, the definition of the curie was changed to exactly 3.7×10^{10} disintegrations/sec, whereas $^{226}_{88}$Ra decays with approximately 3.66×10^{10} disintegrations/sec. Despite this small discrepancy, in clinical situations it is assumed that 1 mg radium has an activity of 1 mCi.

When brachytherapy was becoming a popular treatment method, the manufacturers of radium sources decided on a standard for specifying the ways in which radium can be distributed inside a needle source. A full-strength source is defined as one that has 0.66 mg/cm of activity, and a half-strength source has 0.33 mg/cm of activity.

Example 3: A full-strength radium source has an active length of 3 cm. What is the activity of this source in milligrams?

$$A = (0.66 \text{ mg/cm}) (3.0 \text{ cm}) = 2.0 \text{ mg}$$

Sources that have the same concentration of radioactivity throughout their active length are called *uniform sources*. However, physicians soon found that it is convenient to have available some sources that had a nonuniform distribution of activity in them. Two other types of source were developed: the *Indian club source,* which is heavily loaded with activity at one end, and the *dumbbell source,* which has heavy loading at both ends, with lighter activity concentration in the middle. A nonuniform dose distribution allows for treatment plans to, in some cases, increase the dose to the tumor while keeping the dose to critical structures in the area minimal. These types of sources were all needles; that is, they were sharply pointed at one end and could be inserted directly into tumor tissue; the other end held an eyelet, to allow the source to be secured with sutures and easily removed (Figure 15-3).

The use of needle sources presents several problems from medical and radiation safety viewpoints. Because they are stiff, they must be inserted into areas of the body thick enough to accept them without bending them. The possibility of breakage is always present. In addition, the personnel loading the sources are continually exposed to radiation while performing the procedure, which is not in line with the recommended national policy of keeping medical radiation exposure to a minimum for both patients and staff. To avoid these problems, systems were developed to allow devices known as *applicators* to be inserted into the treatment area first, then loaded with radioactivity quickly and safely when the patient is back in his or her room (Figure 15-4). This technique, known as **afterloading,** led to the development of tube sources. These are small sources that are rounded on each end and contain larger amounts of activity than needle sources (up to 50 mg in a single source).

Some isotopes, such as radon-222 and gold-198, have very short half-lives and are implanted permanently rather than temporarily. Such sources are packaged in tiny versions of tube sources called *seeds,* which are usually approximately 3 to 5 mm long and the diameter of a pencil lead. These sources are implanted using a gunlike applicator that uses long needles to accurately position the seeds within the tumor during surgery. This type of therapy is often used in the case of prostate cancer, as well as other types of solid, localized tumors that can be reached surgically.

Radium Substitutes

The term **radium substitute** is used to indicate any isotope used for brachytherapy whose dosimetry is based on the original

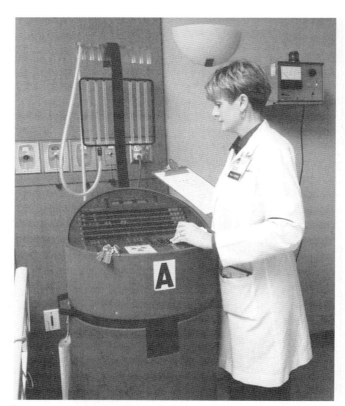

Figure 15-4. Afterloading unit.

radium work. These include, but are not confined to, the following: cesium-137, iridium-192, gold-198, and iodine-125. The activities of these isotopes are expressed in millicuries. However, when these isotopes were first introduced, an attempt to correlate the effect of these isotopes with that of radium was made, because all clinical experience up to that time involved the use of radium. A unit was defined, called *radium equivalence,* which is defined as follows:

$$\text{mg Ra eq} = (A_{isotope}, \text{mCi})\left(\frac{\Gamma_{isotope}}{\Gamma_{Ra}}\right)$$

where $A_{isotope}$ is the activity of the source in millicuries.

Example 4: What is the radium equivalence of a 25.0 mCi source of $^{137}_{55}\text{Cs}$?

$$\text{mg Ra eq} = (25.0 \text{ mCi})\left(\frac{3.28}{8.25}\right) = 9.939 \text{ mg Ra eq}$$

Cesium-137. Cesium-137 ($^{137}_{55}\text{Cs}$) is one of the most widely used of the radium substitutes and has largely replaced radium as the primary isotope for brachytherapy of the uterus and cervix. It has a primary photon energy of 662 keV, which is comparable with the average photon energy of radium (830 keV). This means that the cesium photon penetrates tissue in about the same manner as radium. In fact, when the depth dose along the transverse axes of the sources is calculated, the exposure in water to exposure in air ratio is the same for radium and cesium for depths up to 10 cm.[14] This makes the conversion from using radium to using cesium easier for radiation therapy practitioners.

Cesium has some positive advantages over radium. Although the average energy of radium is 830 keV, it emits a spectrum of

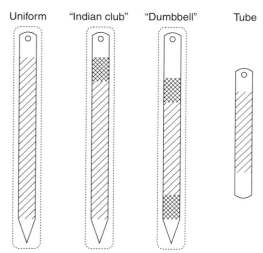

Figure 15-3. Typical radium sources. Note the depiction of the active length and physical length.

photon energies (0.047 to 2.45 MeV). Photon energies higher than 2 MeV result in a radiation safety hazard. The lower energy of cesium and the fact that it has no higher photon energy reduces the radiation safety hazard when this isotope is used. This same fact makes storing the isotope less of a problem than with radium. Cesium has a half-life of 30.0 years, so sources can be used for a long time; they decay by only approximately 2% per year. Because cesium is produced in nuclear reactor fuel as a natural by-product of nuclear fission, it can be chemically separated from spent nuclear fuel and is therefore widely available. Several manufacturers can provide cesium sources in a wide variety of needle or tube configurations. These facts, plus the wide use of cesium in educational institutions, make $^{137}_{55}$Cs very popular with hospital-based and privately owned radiation therapy practices.

Iridium-192. Iridium-192 ($^{192}_{77}$Ir) is supplied in the form of wires of iridium-platinum alloy or as small seeds of this alloy attached to a nylon ribbon with spacing of 1 cm between seeds. This radioisotope undergoes beta decay and has an average energy of 380 keV. The wire form combines flexibility with strength along with filtration characteristics that absorb the beta particles released. The half-life of 73.83 days is shorter than that of cesium, and it is used for temporary implants of easily reached tumor sites such as the breast and tongue.[20]

The usual technique for iridium wire implants is to insert into the tissue carrier needles that penetrate through the tumor area or, alternatively, flexible plastic catheters that can be looped though or around a tumor. Then the iridium wire or seed carrier is threaded into the catheter and left in place for a calculated amount of time. If needed, the wire or seed carrier can be cut to the proper length for insertion into the needles, an operation that requires great care to avoid spreading radioactivity around the work area or patient room. $^{192}_{77}$Ir is ordered in batches approximately every 2 months, and iridium whose activity is too low to use for treatment can be kept until it decays to a low activity level, then returned to the manufacturer. Because $^{192}_{77}$Ir is produced in a nuclear reactor, like cobalt, it can be reactivated for future use.

Cobalt-60. Cobalt-60 is a radionuclide that is not commonly used in today's brachytherapy applications. It undergoes a two-tiered beta decay after its neutron activation that produces 1.17- and 1.33-MeV gamma rays, averaging out to the commonly accepted 1.25 MeV. This radionuclide has a half-life of 5.27 years. Cobalt-60 has typically been used as an external beam radiation therapy source, but it has been used for ophthalmic applicators in some countries in needles and tubes. It has also seen some application in high-dose-rate applications. Although there is history of cobalt-60 use in brachytherapy applications, the isotope's main use in radiation therapy treatment delivery has been in external beam applications.

Gold-198. Gold ($^{198}_{79}$Au) is a popular replacement for $^{222}_{86}$Rn in permanent implants. It has a very short half-life of 2.7 days and a monoenergetic (only one energy produced) energy of 412 keV. It is normally supplied in the form of cylindrical grains or seeds encapsulated in platinum.[7,14] Like cesium, the lower photon energy makes radiation safety much less of a problem with gold than with radon, and more of the dose is absorbed locally. Because of the short half-life, gold seeds are shipped with very high activities, and by the time they are ready to be used they

have an activity of approximately 5 mCi/seed. Thus, gold gives the tissue a very high dose in a short time, a method called high-dose-rate therapy. The prostate can benefit from interstitial implants with permanent gold seeds because other isotopes would require surgical procedures for both insertion and removal of sources.[1]

Iodine-125. The use of iodine-125 ($^{125}_{53}$I) is becoming more common in interstitial seed implants.

In the past, enucleation (the surgical removal of the eye) was the main option in the treatment of ocular melanomas because, in general, melanomas are highly radioresistant. Enucleation not only is a very invasive surgery but also drastically changes a person's lifestyle. It has been discovered, however, that highly concentrated doses of radiation cause signs of regression in these tumors. Iodine-125 seeds are placed on cup-shaped plaque that sits directly on the eye. The seeds are able to deliver a dose of 8000 cGy over a 5- to 6-day period. The seeds put out approximately 50 to 100 cGy/hr, and iodine-125 is able to produce a more uniform exposure than the traditional source of cobalt-60.[18]

Iodine-125 is a radioisotope produced as a daughter product from the neutron activation of xenon-124 to xenon-125. The activated xenon-125 decays by electron capture to produce the daughter, iodine-125. This isotope decays by electron capture to produce useful 35.5-keV gamma rays. Because of the low energy of the isotope, whose half-life is 59.4 days, shielding requirements are minimal. The dose is deposited very close to the seeds, reducing the dose to structures next to the tumor. In addition, the dose from $^{125}_{53}$I is deposited over a longer period of time than a dose from $^{198}_{79}$Au, making iodine therapy a type of *low-dose-rate therapy,* which may cause a different biologic reaction than the same dose from gold.[16] Radiation therapy practitioner education in the use of iodine-125 is an important part of any brachytherapy program using this isotope.

Gold-198 and iodine-125 are used as replacements for radon ($^{222}_{86}$Rn) in seed sources.

$^{222}_{86}$Rn is a radioactive gas, making its use very dangerous. If a seed breaks, the radioactivity becomes airborne and can be inhaled, doing great damage to the sensitive tissues of the lung. Because of this very real problem, radon seeds are no longer used.

THE EXPOSURE RATE FROM A RADIOACTIVE SOURCE

Calculation of absorbed dose from radioactive sources can be done using any one of a number of methods, all of which are based on either calculation techniques or tables of measured data. A central component of the calculation techniques is the gamma factor (Γ factor), which can be defined as the exposure rate at 1 meter from a radioactive source of known activity. The units of the Γ factor are as follows:

$$\frac{\text{Roentgen} \cdot \text{cm}^2}{\text{mCi} \cdot \text{hr}}$$

The actual value of the Γ factor is different for each radioisotope; values for the radioisotopes most commonly used in radiation therapy are given in Table 15-4.

Table 15-4	Gamma Factors for Isotopes	
Isotope	**Γ Factor**	$\left(\dfrac{\text{Roentgen} \cdot \text{cm}^2}{\text{mCi} \cdot \text{hr}}\right)$
Radium-226	8.25	
Radon-222	8.25	
Cobalt-60	13.07	
Cesium-137	3.28	
Iridium-192	4.69	
Gold-198	2.327	

Although the units of the Γ factor may seem complex, they actually make the Γ factor a very useful and easily manipulated quantity. For example, to calculate the exposure rate (Roentgen/hr) at some distance from a radioactive source, the Γ factor can be used in the following equation:

$$\dot{X} = (\Gamma \text{ isotope})(A)(1/d)^2$$

where $\dot{X}$ is the exposure rate (recall that the dot over the X means "rate" in physics notation), d is the distance from the source to the point of calculation, and A is the activity of the source. Notice that if d is in centimeters and A is in millicuries, the units cancel neatly, leaving Roentgens/hr, which is the exposure rate. An example should clarify this process.

Example 5: Calculate the exposure rate at 10 cm from a cesium-137 source with an activity of 10 mCi.

Given that Γ of cesium = 3.26 R · cm²/mCi · hr, d = 10 cm, and A = 10 mCi:

$$\dot{X} = (3.26 \text{ R} \cdot \text{cm}^2/\text{mCi} \cdot \text{hr})(10 \text{ mCi})(1/10 \text{ cm})^2$$

$$\dot{X} = 0.326 \text{ R/hr} = 326.0 \text{ mR/hr}$$

By arranging the equation, you can find any of the four quantities included in the Γ factor if the other three are known. For example, if you know the total exposure, the distance from the source, and the activity of the source, the total time of exposure in hours could easily be calculated. Another typical use is to find the activity of a source by measuring the exposure rate at some distance and solving for the activity, as in Example 6.

Example 6: At 15 cm from an ^{192}Ir source, the exposure rate is 305 mR/hr (0.305 Roentgen/hr). What is the activity of this source?

With a value of 4.69 R · cm²/mCi · hr for Γ_{Ir}, solve for A:

$$0.305 \text{ R/hr} = (4.69 \text{ R} \cdot \text{cm}^2/\text{mCi} \cdot \text{hr})(A)(1/15 \text{ cm})^2$$

$$A = \frac{(0.305 \text{ R/hr})}{4.69 \text{ R} \cdot \text{cm}^2/\text{mCi} \cdot \text{hr})(1/15)^2}$$

$$A = 14.63 \text{ mCi}$$

An important limitation to the use of the Γ factor is that it is applicable only to a point source of radiation. A radioactive source can be considered a point source if the distance from the source to the calculation point is at least five times the length of the source. Therefore the size of the source will place a limitation on the distances at which the Γ factor can be applied.

HIGH-DOSE-RATE BRACHYTHERAPY

Brachytherapy is delivered either in a conventional low-dose-rate (LDR) regimen that lasts several days and requires a hospital stay or on an outpatient basis using high-dose-rate (HDR) brachytherapy equipment. Both techniques are practiced in hospital settings today, with an increasing use of HDR applications noted.

Although conventional LDR brachytherapy has a long history of use and success in head and neck, gynecologic, breast, and prostate cancers, HDR regimens are also used for management of these same diseases. HDR brachytherapy can be as effective as LDR brachytherapy and can have a very low risk of radiation injury. It is suggested that HDR treatment may be preferable to the LDR treatment because HDR brachytherapy can be given on a fractionated outpatient basis. The actual treatment delivery lasts approximately 5 to 10 minutes in contrast to a hospital stay that might take several days for LDR brachytherapy.[18]

In the HDR brachytherapy treatment, a device or holder is placed into the area to be treated. The device is connected to an HDR brachytherapy machine (Figure 15-5), and a single small, intense radiation source is loaded into it. A high dose of radiation is given over a short treatment time, with the actual time dependent on the intensity of the source. The radioactive source is withdrawn back into the brachytherapy machine after the treatment and is then disconnected from applicator in the tumor; the process can then be repeated for any other prescribed fractions. The use of HDR procedures can also be applied to intraoperative applications.[11,18]

The main cited advantages of HDR brachytherapy compared with LDR treatment is that HDR brachytherapy can be more convenient for the patient and treatment facility in terms of time and space requirements, making it less expensive with similar outcomes.[10,14,18]

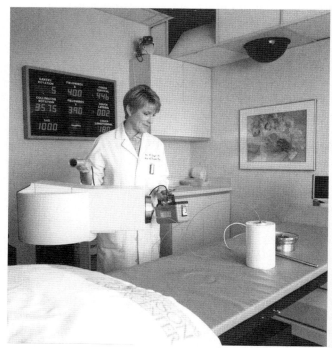

Figure 15-5. High-dose-rate (HDR) unit undergoing quality assurance (QA) tests.

PULSED-DOSE-RATE BRACHYTHERAPY

In recent years, brachytherapy has resurged in its popularity due to technical advances in computerization, and with it, the ability to even further increase the therapeutic advantage between tumor control and late effects. This application of brachytherapy takes advantage of computer-controlled remote afterloader technology. A single source that can be positioned at different dwell points along a catheter pathway for various times, known as *stepping*, is used to deliver a precise dose to the treatment volume. Although this is similar to the procedures used in HDR, this technique simulates a continuous LDR interstitial treatment lasting several days with a sequence of short HDR irradiations. The short applications over several hours, gives the technique the name, pulsed-dose-rate brachytherapy (PDR). [4]

PDR uses an irradiator and the principle of using one high-activity source that dwells under computer control through the catheters of an implant with dwell times set in various positions for a set amount of time. This occurs for short times, about 10 minutes each, every hour. The advantages of using this technique include:

- The patient is not irradiated for most of each hour.
- Fewer sources are needed.
- The computer control of the source facilitates optimal dose delivery.
- It is easy to correct for natural source decay.

Although the PDR treatment commonly takes longer than HDR, the protracted irradiation schedule, with a potentially wider therapeutic ratio than HDR, can reduce toxicity. [5,8] PDR offers flexible fractionation and a more straightforward technical approach; a single stepping source replaces multiple line sources, and advanced treatment planning (optimization, 3D treatment planning) is possible. [17] The use of PDR continues to increase and looks to eventually replace the continuous low-dose-rate applications that has been the foundation of traditional brachytherapy applications.

BRACHYTHERAPY APPLICATORS AND INSTRUMENTS

Just as there are various sources of radioisotopes that are used in radiation therapy, there are numerous methods of applying them in clinical practice. It has been apparent since the first uses of brachytherapy that applicator design is important in maintenance of source positioning and radiation safety. As stated earlier, there are several generalized methods of brachytherapy application: external or mold, interstitial, and intracavitary therapy. [14]

External Applicators or Molds

When a patient has a well-circumscribed surface lesion that requires a high localized dose, surface molds are commonly used. [3] External applicators usually are molded to fit snugly on the surface of the affected area, with areas specified for radio-isotope placement. These molds can be designed to incorporate shielding for adjacent sensitive structures so that they do not receive as high a dose as the lesion. These molds can be designed to fit any shape. Sometimes impressions are made of the body part so that a detailed anatomic template with custom isotope pathways can be designed.

Eye plaques are also a means of using radioisotopes with external application. Iodine-125 is used in the management of

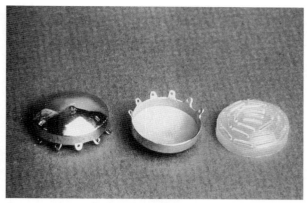

Figure 15-6. Typical plaque used in topical brachytherapy of the eye. The thin gold shielding is sufficient to block neighboring dose-limiting structures from the damaging effects of the low-energy isotope.

uveal melanoma of the eye. Brachytherapy is used in the management of this disease because of its ability to effectively treat tumors near the optic nerve and macula without causing loss of vision secondary to radiation-induced changes. The plaque carrier arranges the sources in appropriate positions so that adequate dose distributions are obtained (Figure 15-6). The efficacy of this treatment method is often compared with stereotactic and proton therapy procedures, conformal modalities that strive to also deposit high doses of radiation to the tumor while sparing normal and sensitive tissues and structures.

Areas commonly treated with external applicators include any areas on the skin, oral cavity, nasal cavity, hard palate, and orbital cavity, just to name a few. Ingenuity and creative thinking are typically used in creating applicators for treatment of these superficial lesions.

Interstitial Applicators

Interstitial brachytherapy places the radioactive sources directly into or adjacent to the tumor or tumor bed. There are both permanent and temporary applications of interstitial implants used in radiation therapy.

Permanent Implants. Permanent implantations are performed when the tumor to be treated is inaccessible, making the removal of the radioisotope impossible or impractical. Iodine-125, palladium-103, and gold-198 are ideally suited for permanent implants because of their short half-lives. The patient who receives these types of implants does not have to have a second surgical procedure to remove the isotopes. The tumor volumes to be treated commonly require placement of many sources, which requires a rapid and accurate means of application. To accomplish this, gun-type applicators with a long, hollow insertion needle is often used. Often computed tomography (CT) guided, the needle is pushed through the skin into the deep tumor, and the sources are inserted into the tumor. The needle is then withdrawn 5 to 10 mm, and the next source is inserted. This is repeated until the desired length and number of sources are applied. Permanent implants using iodine-125 and gold-198 are ideally suited for deep-seated lesions in the pelvis, abdomen, and lung. Figure 15-7 demonstrates images used in planning a gold-198 colorectal implant to address a recurrence.

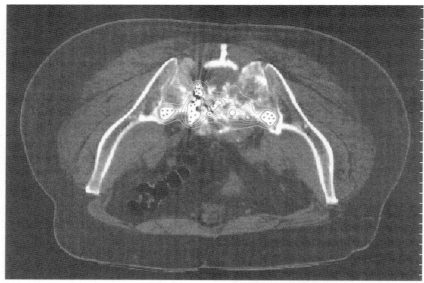

Figure 15-7. Gold-198 permanent seed implant. Note the small size and clustering of the source placement.

 According to a study released by the International Journal of Radiation Oncology, *more than 90% of men who were treated with permanent gold seed implants were still cancer free 8 years after the treatment. Radioactive seeds are placed in the prostate gland with the help of an ultrasound-guided technique and left in permanently. Patients reported being spared from side effects such as impotence and incontinence.*[19]

Temporary Implants. Temporary, removable implants are used in anatomic areas where there is no body cavity or orifice to accept radioactive sources.[3] The sources are placed directly into the tumor and tumor bed for a short period of time to deliver a high dose to the area. Radiation therapy boost fields often use this method of brachytherapy application.

Hollow stainless steel needles can be pushed through the tissues to accommodate catheters holding radioisotopes. Iridium-192 afterloading is used in most applications. The tubes are spaced 1 cm apart; several planes may be used, depending on the tumor size. Catheters are placed in the tubes before removal. When the stainless steel tubes are removed, the catheters are left in place, ready to accommodate dummy sources. Dummy sources are nonradioactive radiopaque seeds that can be seen on a radiographic image. The sources are aligned and spaced just as the radioactive seeds would be. This is done to enable visualization of source placement, to ensure that the implants are positioned correctly, and for treatment planning and dose calculation without unnecessary radiation exposure to the patient and personnel. This is the basic principle of remote afterloading. Table 15-5 outlines the advantages and disadvantages of remote afterloaders.

Once the placement is confirmed, the dummy sources can be replaced with the radioactive sources and left in place for the desired time. This technique is commonly used in, but not limited to, breast and chest wall irradiation.[3,13] Figure 15-8 demonstrates an iridium-192 breast implant radiograph. Anterior,

lateral, and posterior walls of the vagina are also treated with interstitial afterloading techniques (Figure 15-9).

To improve the accuracy of needle placement and to maintain position during treatment, stabilizers and guides can be used. These are popular in transperineal implants. In these applications, ultrasound and radiographic imaging can be used to confirm location and placement of sources. Figure 15-10 demonstrates a Syed-Neblett template radiograph. Cancers of the rectum, prostate, vagina, and urethra are commonly treated with this applicator.

Intracavitary Applicators

Insertion of radioactive sources into body cavities has been a viable component of radiation therapy for many years.[3,6] Several applicators have been designed and used, most for the treatment of gynecologic tumors. The designs used in the newer applicators allow for customized, intricate dose distributions maximizing the dose to the tumor and sparing the dose to adjacent, sensitive structures (such as the rectum and urinary bladder). Extensive knowledge of physics and anatomy are required to be effective in the dose delivery using this brachytherapy application.

Table 15-5	Advantages and Disadvantages of Remote Afterloading Systems	
Advantages		**Disadvantages**
Reduction or elimination of exposure to medical personnel		Remote afterloaders are expensive
Treatment techniques are more consistent		Increased maintenance costs
In HDR, allows outpatient treatment, thus lowering costs		In HDR, increased room shielding may be needed
In LDR, sources can be retracted in an emergency situation		

HDR, High-dose-rate; *LDR,* low-dose-rate.

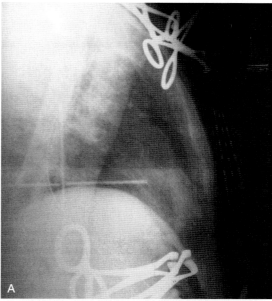

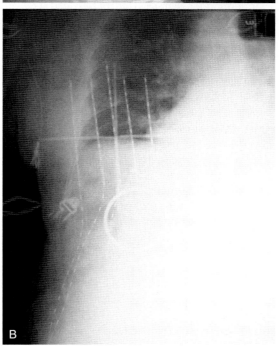

Figure 15-8. Iridium-192 breast implant. Note how the dummy sources can be seen and used for dose calculation. Magnification ring allows for accurate size perspective to be realized. **A**, Anterior. **B**, Lateral.

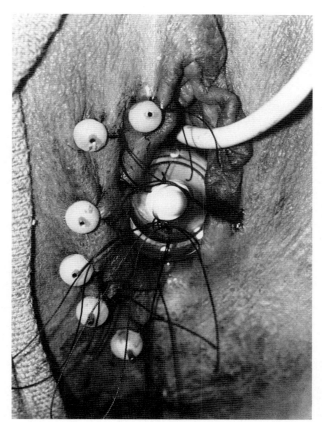

Figure 15-9. Delclos stainless steel needles for afterloading. Iridium implant of the lateral vaginal wall. Note Foley catheter and empty vaginal cylinder.

Tandem and Ovoids. Gynecologic malignancies are usually treated using standard apparatus; however, standardized applicators typically have room in their design for customized modifications. Gynecologic insertions are done with both LDR and HDR applications today.

A central tandem and a pair of lateral ovoids are commonly used in brachytherapy applications involving the cervix (Figure 15-11). The **tandem** is a long narrow tube that inserts into the opening of the cervix (cervical os) into the uterus. **Ovoids**, or

colpostats, are oval shaped and insert into the lateral fornices of the vagina. Both components are hollow and can accommodate several radioactive sources. The ovoids come in various sizes to accommodate the variances in anatomic structures (wide or narrow vaginas). These ovoids can have shielding that customizes the dose distributions in such a way that the dose to the urinary bladder and rectum is minimized. Tandems and ovoids are placed into the female anatomy and stabilized with packing. This packing (sterile gauze) not only stabilizes the apparatus during its 2- to 3-day placement in the vagina but also serves to displace the rectum and bladder from the sources. Remember that radioisotope emissions adhere to the inverse square law. The farther structures are from the sources, the less dose they will receive.

Location of the applicator is verified with radiographic images, and dose calculations can be performed (Figure 15-12). Once loaded with sources, the tandem and ovoids typically demonstrate a pear-shaped isodose distribution (Figure 15-13). Currently the standard treatment unit is the centigray (cGy) to a specific anatomic point or isodose line. The anatomic points used historically for cervical and uterine treatment are points A and B. Point A is located 2 cm superior and 2 cm lateral to the center of the cervical canal (at the cervical os) in the plane of the uterus. Point B was originally 3 cm lateral to point A but is currently noted as being 1 cm lateral to the medial aspect of the pelvic side wall (Figure 15-14). The dose at point B is typically

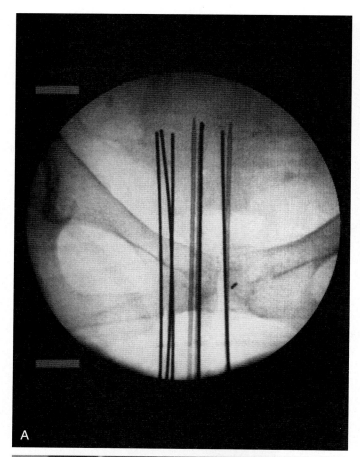

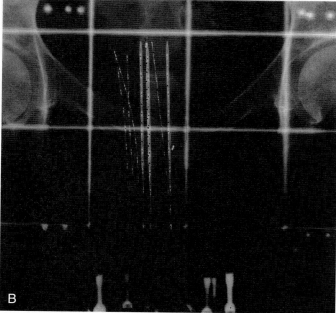

Figure 15-10. Radiograph of a Syed-Neblett template technique for a vaginal carcinoma. **A**, Radiograph of needle placement during surgery. **B**, Radiograph of stylets loaded with dummy iridium-192 sources.

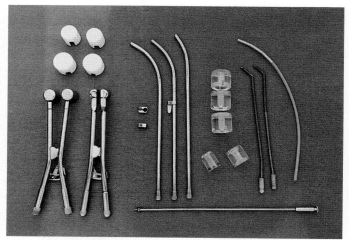

Figure 15-11. Fletcher Suit, Delclos Manual Afterloading System. From *left* to *right:* Small colpostats with additional caps for conversion to medium and large; microcolpostats; intrauterine "tandems"; Delclos and cylindrical colpostats (selected); colpostats carriers; tandem carrier. *Bottom:* (Horizontal) dead seed implanter and seeds. (From Fletcher GH: *Textbook of radiotherapy,* Baltimore, 1980, Williams & Wilkins.)

approximately one third that at point A. Although these points of dose specification have been used for years, their location is not standard in all patients. Anatomic differences can cause variances. Each case must be considered individually.

Vaginal Cylinders. There are a variety of customized applicators designed to give a high dose to vaginal lesions without giving excessive dose to the urinary bladder or rectum. The applicators are of different lengths, diameters, and shielding design. In other words, individual application of treatment is optimized. Several designs, such as the Delclos uterine-vaginal afterloading system, are designed for simultaneous treatment of the uterine cavity, cervix, and vaginal walls.[3] Vaginal cylinders can be used in conjunction with interstitial implants. The cylinder not only can place sources in proximity to diseased anatomy but it can also assist in the shielding of anatomy from radiation by both shielding material in the applicator and the application of the inverse square law.

A specialized type of intracavitary brachytherapy places sources within body tubes such as the esophagus, trachea, and biliary tract. Obstructive lesions can be addresses by placing radioactive sources onto or adjacent to the lesions. Pulsed HDR applications for these types of treatments using cesium-137 and iridium-192 have been performed successfully.

Intravascular Stent Applications

There are an increasing number of clinical trials evaluating the role of intravascular brachytherapy radiation following percutaneous transluminal coronary angioplasty (PTCA), an alternative to coronary artery bypass grafts (CABGs), to inhibit restenosis in coronary arteries. Although PTCA alone has benefits over CABG surgery, its effectiveness is limited by restenosis occurring in some patients after treatment. It is thought that the addition of radiation may reduce the rate of restenosis in patients receiving the stent therapy. This radiation dose may be delivered with either brachytherapy or external beam.

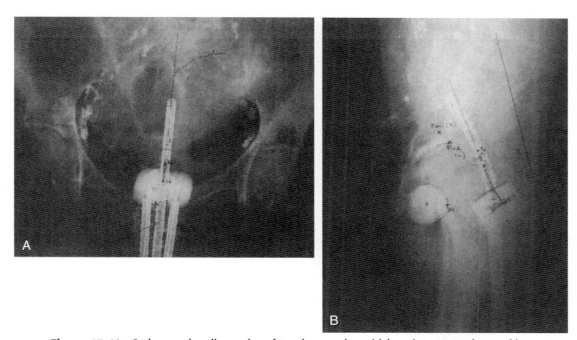

Figure 15-12. Orthogonal radiographs of tandem and ovoid location. Note the packing that serves to stabilize the placement of the applicators as well as "push" the urinary bladder and rectum out of the way. **A**, Anterior. **B**, Lateral. (From Cox JD: *Moss' radiation oncology*, ed 7, St. Louis, 1994, Mosby.)

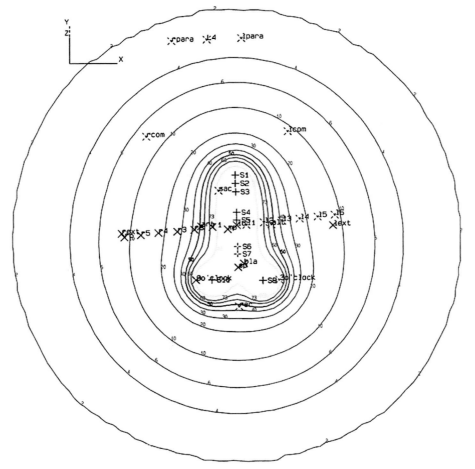

Figure 15-13. Pear-shaped isodose distribution obtained with the use of a tandem and ovoid applicator. Note that the fuller, inferior portion of the distribution can be attributed to the contribution of dose from the location of the ovoids.

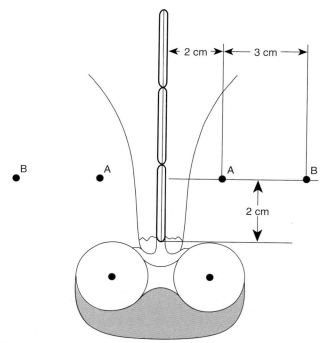

Figure 15-14. Diagram of points *A* and *B*.

However, because of cardiac motion, external beam may be better suited for irradiation of peripheral vessels than coronary vessels.[9]

Intravascular brachytherapy may be delivered with either catheter-based systems or radioactive stents. Catheter-based systems consist of a linear array of sources, such as ^{192}Ir, attached to a guide wire and inserted into the balloon catheter and pushed into place in the stented area. Other catheter-based systems under development include a number of beta sources, with phosphorus-32 (^{32}P), yttrium-90 (^{90}Y), and strontium-90/yttrium-90 (^{90}Sr/^{90}Y) receiving the most consideration at this time.[13]

BRACHYTHERAPY DOSIMETRY AND DOSE DISTRIBUTION

Dose distribution from radium-226 is the basis of all dose calculations in brachytherapy. As seen earlier, knowing the relationship of radium substitutes and radium allows the radiation therapy practitioner to deliver a dose to a patient accurately. A keen knowledge of anatomy and adherence to a few rules will provide the medical dosimetrist and radiation therapist to develop optimized treatment plans for patients. This section provides basic rules and generalized discussion of dosimetry and dose distribution for interstitial implants. Three systems are discussed: Paterson-Parker, Quimby, and Paris.

The Paterson-Parker (Manchester) System

Using the gamma factor of radium, it is possible to perform radium dosimetry calculations, assuming the point source approximations stated previously. However, for patient dosimetry a number of sources are typically used, and the accurate calculation of the dose distributions from these implants is a complex procedure. In addition, it requires that the radioactive sources be implanted in the patient before the calculations are done, so the physician, medical physicist, and medical dosimetrist

Table 15-6	Spacing Sources in a Paterson-Parker Planar Implant	
Area	**Activity in Periphery/Activity Over Area**
Area < 25 cm²	⅔
25 cm² < Area < 100 cm²	½
Area > 100 cm²	⅓

have no idea of how the patient is being treated until after the sources are already in place. In the 1930s, Ralston Paterson and H. M. Parker, at the Manchester Hospital in England, developed a series of guidelines and dosimetry methods known as the *Paterson-Parker* or *Manchester system* of radium dosimetry to remove these difficulties.

The Paterson-Parker system establishes a set of guidelines that, if followed, will provide a dose of ±10% within the implanted area. Implantation philosophy strives to deliver a uniform dose to a plane or volume. This system uses a nonuniform distribution of radioactive material to produce a uniform distribution of dose. The system assumes the use of linear sources to be implanted in tissue in planes or other geometric shapes and gives rules for placing the radium sources in each case. Then the system provides dose tables, which, if distribution rules have been followed, can be used to calculate the dose within the volume. Rules have been established for both planar and volume implants.[14]

Planar Implants. Planar arrangements of sources can be summarized in Table 15-6 for square and rectangular implants. In multiple plane implants, the planes should be 1 cm apart and parallel. If there is no crossing source at one or both ends, the area is reduced by 10% for each uncrossed end (Figure 15-15). If the plane is not square, the mg-hr is increased by the appropriate elongation factor for the ratio of long side to short side. Figure 15-16 depicts a single-plane implant.

For circular and near-circular areas, the activity should first be placed on the periphery, preferably using more than five

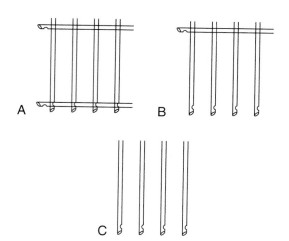

Figure 15-15. Planar implants. **A,** Both ends crossed. **B,** One crossed end (reduce treatment area calculation by 10%). **C,** No crossed ends (reduce treatment area in calculation by 20%).

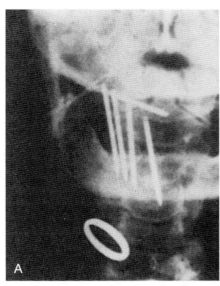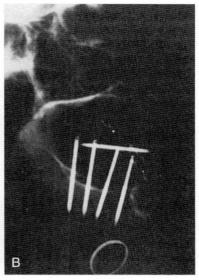

Figure 15-16. A, Image of a planar implant. **B,** Single-plane implant. (From Cox JD: *Moss' radiation oncology*, ed 7, St. Louis, 1994, Mosby.)

sources with spacing no greater than the treatment distance. Then more sources are arranged in an inner circle of half the diameter of the original area. Remaining sources go in the center. The distribution of activity is governed by the ratio of the diameter to the treatment distance. Parameters are outlined in Table 15-7.

Volume Implants. If the shape of the implanted volume resembles a three-dimensional shape more than a plane, it is called a *volume implant*. Shapes defined by the Paterson-Parker system include cylinders, ellipsoids (football-shaped volumes), spheres, and cubes, among others. This type of calculation is usually done for seed implants of the prostate and other implants in which the activity is evenly spread out inside an organ or structure. Similar to the planar implants, volume implants can have crossed ends. If there is no crossing source at one or both ends of the volume implant, the area used for calculations should be reduced by 7.5% for each uncrossed end. Figure 15-17 shows a multiplane implant.

The Quimby/Memorial Dosimetry System

The Quimby system is similar in concept to the Paterson-Parker system. It provides a set of tables used to calculate dose given a number of implant parameters such as area, volume, or total activity. However, in the Quimby system, the implant is assumed to be made up of a uniform distribution of activity within the implant,

giving a nonuniform distribution of dose. The Quimby system is used less frequently than the Paterson-Parker system but has been adapted into a system called the *Memorial system*, whose tables are based on computer calculations that take into account filtration at all angles, modern units of activity, and dose.

The Paris System

The Paris system was developed in the early 1920s and uses uniform distribution of the radiation sources, just as seen in the Quimby system.[3] The system is based on three principles:

1. The radioactive sources must be rectilinear and arranged so that their centers are in the same plane, which is perpendicular to the direction of the sources and is called the *central plane*. The dose is defined and calculated in this plane but not restricted to the plane.
2. The linear activity must be uniform along each source and the same for all sources.

Table 15-7	Circular Source Distribution in Paterson-Parker Circular Implant				
	Diameter/Distance (cm)				
Location	**1-3**	**3-6**	**6**	**7.5**	**10**
Outer circle (%)	100	95	80	75	70
Inner circle (%)	0	0	17	22	27
Center (%)	0	5	3	3	3

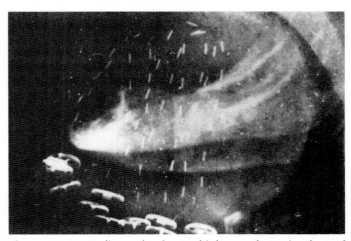

Figure 15-17. Radiograph of a multiplane volume implant of the tongue and floor of the mouth. (From Cox JD: *Moss' radiation oncology*, ed 7, St. Louis, 1994, Mosby.)

3. The radioactive sources must be spaced uniformly. This is the case even when more than one plane is used.

This system is intended for use with removable long line implants, such as ^{192}Ir wires. The system uses wider spacing for longer sources or larger treatment volumes, typically implanted in parallel lines.[14]

Computer Calculation Methods

In the 1970s, computers began to be used for calculating the dose distribution from a specific brachytherapy implant, using a method called the *Sievert integral*, which breaks a linear source into tiny components, calculates the dose at every point in the patient from every component, and adds these values to get the final result. Using computer methods, exact isodose distributions, such as those from external beam treatments, can be obtained for brachytherapy instead of relying on the somewhat general method of the Paterson-Parker tables. Today, most implant procedures have a computerized dose distribution produced, and this has become an important tool in adjusting each implant to the individual patent's needs. As with all computer calculations, however, it must be cautioned that the doses obtained should be checked periodically by hand, using the Paterson-Parker tables or another method; reliance on a computer can have serious consequences if the results are not verified in some way.

RADIATION SAFETY AND QUALITY ASSURANCE

The safe handling of radioactivity has been a matter of concern in hospitals for many years. Those small, seemingly harmless ribbons and tubes can cause a great hazard if not dealt with appropriately. The subject of practical radiation safety of brachytherapy merits a few generalized thoughts concerning this important aspect of therapeutic administration.

A good place to start would be a complete description of all brachytherapy sources in use on file. The uniformity of the source materials distribution should be checked by **autoradiograph**. An autoradiograph is a signature exposure of a radioactive source obtained by placing the source on an unexposed x-ray film for a period of time long enough to darken the film. The film may be scanned to check for dose uniformity.[1] The storage of the sources should facilitate source identification by type and strength. Appropriate documentation should be kept for source control from initial receipt through calibration, inventory, and disposal. Dose calculations should also be double-checked. A quality assurance program can be the difference between safe administration of radiation and a massive radiation disaster.

SUMMARY

- Brachytherapy is an art and a science that has evolved through the years into a specialized aspect of malignant disease management.
- The first brachytherapy procedure followed the discovery of radioactivity by only a few months.
- Today, brachytherapy is a standard technique in the treatment of a large number of malignancies through various means.
- Both naturally and artificially produced radioisotopes are used to deliver a high tumor dose while sparing normal

tissues, adhering to the very basic tenets of disease management with ionizing radiation.
- A resurgence in the use of brachytherapy dictates radiation therapy practitioners to be prepared to demonstrate a comprehensive knowledge of its uses because brachytherapy is an intricate part of cancer management today.
- Brachytherapy allows for patients to continue living their lives as they always have but yet not sacrifice the quality of their treatments.
- Brachytherapy has changed the preferred course of treatment for many early-stage cancers such as breast, cervical, and prostate, and with continued research the future is constantly looking brighter.

Review Questions

Multiple Choice

1. When using both tandem and ovoids in a gynecologic implant, the typical resultant dose distribution has the shape of a(n):
   a. oval
   b. rectangle
   c. butterfly
   d. pear
2. Afterloading techniques were developed primarily to reduce:
   a. the possibilities of loading errors
   b. the time required for an implant
   c. exposure to personnel
   d. exposure to nearby dose-limiting structures
3. Radium sources are leak tested as specified by regulatory agencies to check for:
   a. uranium-238
   b. radon-222
   c. radium-228
   d. lead-208
4. The key relationship for radioactivity states:
   a. The change in the number of atoms per change in unit time is proportional to the number of atoms present.
   b. The change in unit time per change in the number of atoms is proportional to the number of atoms present.
   c. The change in the number of atoms per change in unit time is equal to the number of disintegrations per second.
   d. The change per unit time per change in the number of atoms is proportional to the number of disintegrations per second.
5. The decay constant describes:
   a. the half-life of a particular radionuclide
   b. the number of ionizations produced in tissue per unit time
   c. the fraction of the number of atoms that decay per unit time
   d. none of the above
6. The average lifetime for the decay of radioactive atoms is the definition of:
   a. half-life
   b. decay constant
   c. specific activity
   d. mean life

7. The distance between the ends of radioactive material in a radioisotope tube is known as:
   a. permanent activity
   b. active length
   c. physical length
   d. filtration distance

8. A new batch of iridium-192 wire has arrived, and its calibration must be checked. The supplier states that the activity of the material was 0.351 mCi/seed 10 days earlier. What is the expected activity of the iridium-192 today?
   a. 0.002 mCi
   b. 9.970 mCi
   c. 0.320 mCi
   d. 0.007 mCi

9. Isotopes used in permanent implants are most common:
   a. iodine-125 and gold-198
   b. gold-198 and cesium-137
   c. cesium-137 and radium-226
   d. radium-226 and iodine-125

10. Packing in gynecologic implants serves which of the following purposes?
    I. spaces sources to even out dose distributions
    II. aids in pushing dose-sensitive structures farther from the sources
    III. provides stability of applicator placement
    a. I and II
    b. I and III
    c. II and III
    d. I, II, and III

The answers to the Review Questions can be found by logging on to our website at: *http://evolve.elsevier.com/Washington+Leaver/principles*

Questions to Ponder

1. Compare and contrast the dose distribution rules of the Paterson-Parker and Quimby systems.
2. Compare and contrast the use of radium and cesium as brachytherapy sources for treatment.
3. Describe the necessary criteria for a radioisotope to be used as a permanent implant.
4. How does the mean life differ from the half-life of an isotope?
5. Compare and contrast LDR and HDR brachytherapy applications and uses.

REFERENCES

1. Baltas D, Zamboglou N, Sakelliou L: *The physics of modern brachytherapy for oncology,* New York, 2007, Taylor & Francis.
2. Barillot I, Raynaud-Bougnoux A: The use of MRI in planning radiotherapy for gynaecological tumors, *Cancer Imaging* 6:100-106, 2006.
3. Bentel GC: *Radiation therapy planning,* ed 2, New York, 1996, Macmillan.
4. Brenner DJ: Radiation biology in brachytherapy, *J Surg Onc* 65:66-70, 1997.
5. Brenner DJ, Hall EJ: Conditions for the equivalence of continuous to pulsed low dose rate brachytherapy, *Int J Radiat Oncol Biol Phys* 20:181-190, 1991.
6. Devlin PM: *Brachytherapy applications and techniques,* Philadelphia, 2007, Lippincott Williams & Williams.
7. Fletcher DT et al: Valgus and varus deformity after wide-local excision, brachytherapy and external beam irradiation in two children with lower extremity synovial cell sarcomal, *BMC Cancer* 4: 57, 2004. Retrived July 24, 2008 from http://www.pubmedcentral.nih.gov/articlerender.fcgi?artid=518976.
8. Fowler J, Mount M: Pulsed brachytherapy: the conditions for no significant loss of therapeutic ratio compared with traditional low dose rate brachytherapy, *Int J Radiat Oncol Biol Phys* 23:661-669, 1992.
9. Grewe PH, et al: Human coronary morphology after beta radiation brachytherapy of in-stent restenosis, *Heart* 90: e32, 2004.
10. Grimm P, Sylvestor J: Advances in brachytherapy, *Urology* 6:37-48, 2004.
11. Harrison LB, Enker WE, Anderson LL: High-dose-rate intraoperative radiation therapy for colorectal cancer, *Oncology* 9: 679-683, 1995. Retrieved August 5, 2007, from Cancer Network at http://www.cancernetwork.com/display/article/10165/71118?pageNumber=1.
12. Harvard Health Medical School: MammoSite targeted radiation therapy (website): www.mammosite.com. Accessed August 21, 2007.
13. Hilaris BS, Nori D, Anderson LL: *Atlas of brachytherapy,* New York, 1992, Macmillan.
14. Khan FM: *The physics of radiation therapy,* ed 3, Philadelphia, 2003, Williams & Wilkins.
15. Kuerer HM, et al: Accelerated partial breast irradiation after conservative surgery for breast cancer, *Ann Surg* 239:338-351, 2004.
16. Larson DA, et al: Permanent iodine 125 brachytherapy in patients with progressive or recurrent glioblastoma multiforme, *Neuro Oncol* 6: 119-126, 2004.
17. Martin T, Kolotas C, Dannenberg T: New interstitial HDR brachytherapy technique for prostate cancer: CT based 3D planning after transrectal implantation, *Radiother Oncol* 52:257-260, 1999.
18. Robertson DM, et al: Radioactive iodine-125 as a therapeutic radiation source for management of intraocular tumors, *Trans Am Ophthalmol Soc* 79:294-306, 1981.
19. Science Daily: Prostate cancer patients see high survival rates with seed implants (website): http://www.sciencedaily.com/releases/2007/01/070131090556.htm. Accessed August 21, 2007.
20. Terk MD: Brachytherapy for prostate cancer, *Commun Oncol* 4:89-92, 2007.

BIBLIOGRAPHY

Ash D: Overviews of interstitial therapy, *Br J Radiol Suppl* 22:79-82, 1988.
Hall EF, Brenner DJ: The 1991 George Edelstyn Memorial Lecture: needles, wires and chips—advances in brachytherapy, *Clin Oncol* 4:249-256, 1992.
Hoefnagel CA: Radionuclide therapy revisited, *Eur J Nucl Med* 18:408-431, 1991.
Janjan NA, et al: Control of unresectable recurrent anorectal cancer with gold-198 seed implantation, *J Brachyther Int* 15:115-129, 1999.
Shiu MH, Hilaris BS: Brachytherapy and function-saving resection of soft tissue sarcoma arising in the limb, *Int J Radiat Oncol Biol Physics* 21: 1485-1492, 1991.
Trott NG: Radionuclides in brachytherapy: radium and after, *Br J Radiol Suppl* 21:1-54, 1987.

Special Procedures

Michael T. Gillin

Outline

Image-guided radiation therapy
Respiratory motion management

Stereotactic radiation therapy
Proton treatments

Summary

Objectives

- Provide a basic description of four different special procedures that address some of the limitations of conventional radiation therapy—image-guided radiation therapy, cranial and extracranial stereotactic radiation therapy, respiratory motion management, and proton therapy.
- State the options available for treatment unit imaging, both kilovoltage and megavoltage.
- Define *cone beam computed tomography (CBCT)*.
- Compare ultrasound imaging with kilovoltage imaging.

- List the advantages and disadvantages of fiducial guided treatment.
- Name the core elements of stereotactic guided treatments.
- Describe four-dimensional CT imaging.
- Present the basic concept of gated treatments.
- List the advantages and disadvantages of mechanical methods of motion management.
- State the potential advantages of proton therapy.

Key Terms

Cone beam CT (CBCT)
CT-on-rails
Electronic portal imaging devices (EPIDs)
Fiducial
Four-dimensional CT (4D CT)
Gated treatments
Image-guided radiation therapy (IGRT)
Image registration
Information flow
Kilovoltage (kV)
Megavoltage (MV)
Motion management
Passively modulated proton beams
Protons
Respiratory cycle
Stereotactic
Ultrasound
Volumetric imaging

R adiation oncology has evolved into a complex, integrated image-based treatment planning and treatment delivery enterprise. The time of the stand-alone treatment delivery system has passed. Now the modern treatment delivery unit is a network unto itself and a node with the wired world. The modern treatment delivery unit not only provides a therapeutic radiation beam but also controls its multileaf collimator, its megavoltage (MV) electronic portal imaging system, its kilovoltage (kV) imaging system, and its on/off gated treatment system. The modern accelerator communicates with the electronic medical record, as it downloads treatment parameters and reference images before treatment and uploads treatment delivered information and daily patient positioning images post-treatment. **Information flow** between multiple databases and primary information-generating systems has become an essential part of accurate treatment delivery in radiation oncology. Figure 16-1 is a schematic drawing of information flow in a radiation oncology practice. Figure 16-2 shows five different computer monitors and six different computer terminals, which are all part of a modern photon treatment delivery system.

Radiation is an effective treatment modality with potential morbidities. There are data that indicate, for specific patients, that higher doses will result in a higher rate of local control. To use radiation more effectively by reducing the side effects from the therapeutic doses delivered to the target and the surrounding tissue, the radiation treatment is becoming more focused; that is, targets are being planned using computed tomography (CT), magnetic resonance imaging (MRI), and positon emission tomography (PET) images, and patient positioning in the treatment position is being confirmed using a variety of imaging modalities in the treatment room. One goal in radiation oncology is to plan and deliver accurate and precise treatments. An accurate treatment is a treatment that deviates within acceptable limits from a standard. A precise treatment is a treatment that is in high agreement with the planned and other daily treatments. A precise treatment may miss the target completely. Thus, the goals of accurate and precise treatments are to plan and deliver treatments that are within acceptable limits and that are in high agreement with each other and with the plan (see Figure 13-2).

This chapter reviews developments in image-guided radiation therapy, stereotactic radiation therapy, the management of respiratory motion, and the basic principles of proton therapy. All of these developments are offered at an increasing number of institutions.

RADIATION ONCOLOGY INFORMATION FLOW

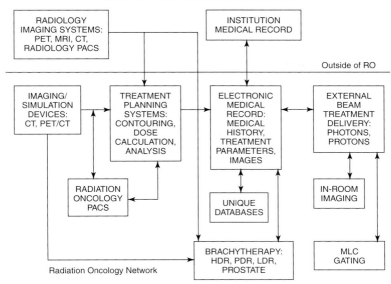

Figure 16-1. Typical information flow in radiation oncology. *CT,* Computed tomography; *HDR,* high-dose-rate; *LDR,* low-dose-rate; *MLC,* multileaf collimation; *MRI,* magnetic resonance imaging; *PACS,* Picture Archiving and Communication System; *PET,* positron emission tomography; *RO,* radiation oncology.

IMAGE-GUIDED RADIATION THERAPY

In the treatment room, **image-guided radiation therapy (IGRT)** has been available for decades. **Kilovoltage (KV)** x-ray units were mounted at an angle to the side of cobalt-60 units. The kV images produced by such devices provided the oncologist with more information (better resolution, higher-contrast images) upon which to make a decision regarding patient positioning with the patient in the treatment position. Figure 16-3 is an image of a kV x-ray tube mounted on the side of a Theratron 780-C cobalt unit.

Ultrasound imaging was commercially introduced approximately one decade ago for localization of the prostate, using a two-dimensional (2D) B-mode approach to image a thin slice of anatomy.[5,15,20] (Ultrasound imaging involves sending high-frequency sound waves into the body and recording the echo waves as the sound bounces back from various tissue interfaces.) Generally, the therapist positions the linear phased-array ultrasound transducer on the patient's anterior pelvic surface and views the ultrasound image on an in-room monitor. Figure 16-4 shows a therapist, whose face is blocked by the ultrasound monitor, holding the transducer in the pelvis of a male patient and acquiring either a sagittal or an axial image. In addition to the imaging system itself, these systems are designed to compare the position of the prostate and surrounding anatomy (bladder and rectum) with the patient on the treatment table with the position of these structures at the time of simulation. Because the treatment plan is based on the patient simulation images, the more the treatment delivery matches the plan, the better it is for the patient. To obtain better agreement between

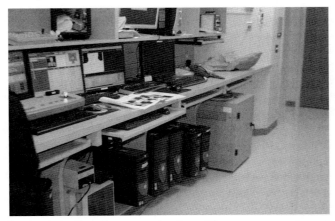

Figure 16-2. One linear accelerator with many computers. On the top shelf, there is one platform that contains programs written by the institution for specific image functions. On the bottom shelf, there are at least seven platforms, including one for the electronic medical record, one for respiratory monitoring, and several with specific imaging functions.

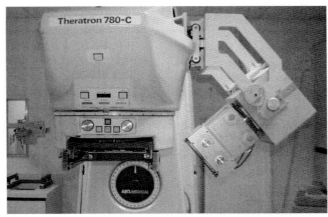

Figure 16-3. An x-ray tube and housing mounted on the side of a Theratron 780-C cobalt-60 unit.

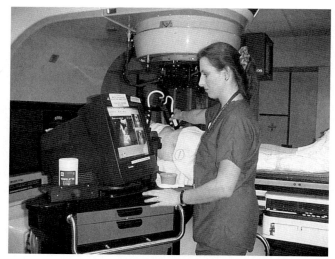

Figure 16-4. Therapist holding the ultrasound probe to locate the prostate with the patient in the treatment position.

the planned and delivered treatment, the ultrasound device must be registered **(image registration)** with the treatment delivery unit to know where in space its images of the prostate are, that is, to register the images with respect to the isocenter of the accelerator. Axial and sagittal ultrasound images are obtained and then overlaid with the contours of structures defined in the treatment planning process. Figure 16-5 displays an axial ultrasound image, together with contours of the bladder, prostate, and rectum, which were generated from the CT simulation images. The therapist can digitally move the ultrasound images to a position in which there is reasonable coincidence between the two data sets—the contours from the planning system and the ultrasound images appear to overlay each other. The treatment couch can then be shifted by these increments that have just been determined.

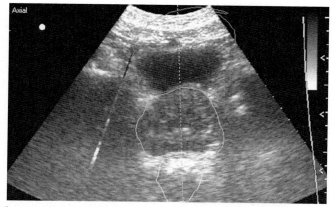

Figure 16-5. Axial ultrasound image with contours of the bladder, prostate, and rectum, which were generated in treatment planning. (See Color Plate 2.)

 The greater use of ultrasound and related new devices in the radiation treatment of prostate cancer has increased physicians' confidence that the patient's daily setup is truly replicating the patient's position during simulation. For example, the introduction of the bladder scanner, a handheld device that digitally reads how many milliliters of urine are in the bladder, allows the therapist to be confident that the patient is ready to be brought into the treatment room. If not, the patient can continue to drink while the therapist moves on to another patient, saving everyone time.

Such B-mode ultrasound systems have been widely accepted. They are available from several different manufacturers with several generations of such devices being available from a single vendor. There is general agreement that the added time required to image the patient, which can be several minutes, is justified by more precise patient setups.

Beam's eye view **megavoltage (MV)** planar imaging with a linear accelerator has been common for decades. The small focal spot size of the linear accelerator (linac) is capable of providing high-resolution images, but the soft tissue contrast was poor as a result of using x-rays produced by MV sources. Special films, which required a small number of monitor units (MUs), were developed for MV imaging. The films may have been placed in lead-lined cassettes or in paper cassettes. **Electronic portal imaging devices (EPIDs)** replaced films in many clinics within the last decade.[3] There are at least two different basic designs for EPIDs. One design obtains images using a scintillation screen and a television camera. The other design uses an amorphous silicon flat panel detector, which consists of an array of photodiodes that detect light from an x-ray–stimulated scintillator. Both approaches produce clinically useful MV images in a digital format. One great advantage of the digital format is that the images can be reviewed from multiple locations, as opposed to being available only on a piece of film, which must be carried to the review location.

The introduction of kV in-room planar x-ray systems as an integral part of a linear accelerator treatment delivery system developed slowly but now is well established commercially. Oncologists and supporting staff are generally more comfortable with reviewing kV images, because kV images provide better soft tissue contrast compared with MV images. Thus, in theory, kV images should provide an easier tool to ensure proper patient positioning on the treatment table. kV imaging systems have been implemented in several different ways.

One commercial planar image product, the Varian On-Board Imager, has the x-ray unit and image receptor system mounted using robotic arms on the accelerator gantry at 90 degrees from the MV x-ray beam with its EPID system. This is shown in Figure 16-6. Thus, kV and/or MV planar images can be taken with the patient in the treatment position. The gantry can be rotated, and two perpendicular kV images can be obtained. Reference images (e.g., digital reconstructed radiographs [DRRs]) can be downloaded from the treatment planning systems and used as the gold standard to compare against the kV images taken with the patient on the treatment table. Software tools are available to register the two different image sets

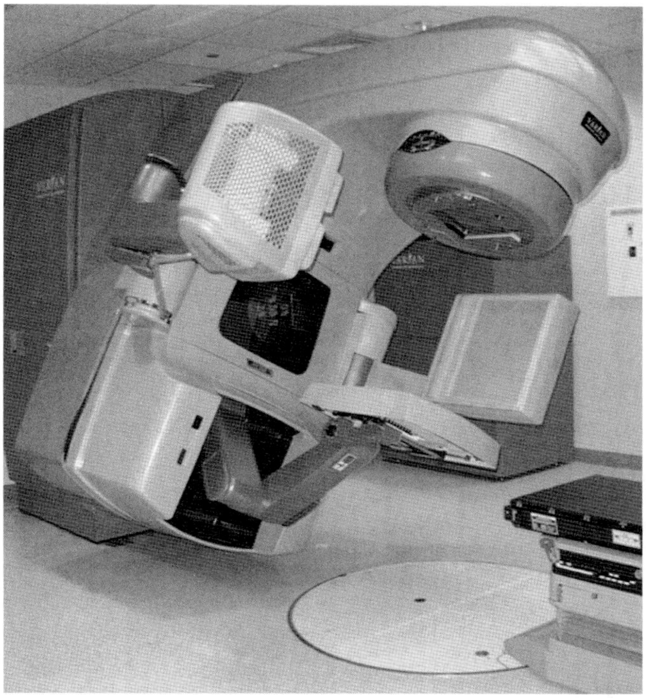

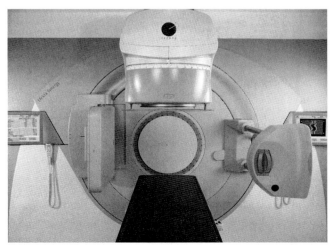

Figure 16-6. A Varian linear accelerator with the MV flat panel detector and a kV x-ray tube on the right of the accelerator C-arm and its kV flat panel detector on the left of the accelerator C-arm. The couch has been lowered for the purposes of this image.

and calculate the couch shifts to align the patient by superimposing the bony anatomy. At least one other accelerator vendor, Elekta, currently offers a similar kV product. This is shown in Figure 16-7.

Another commercial example of a planar image-guided x-ray system, the ExacTrac from BrainLAB, which is not attached to the accelerator, uses two floor-recessed x-ray units and two ceiling-mounted amorphous silicon flat panel detectors.

Images from this system can be analyzed and couch corrections calculated to position the patient before treatment. An infrared tracking system is used to track the patient during treatment.

In the treatment room, **volumetric imaging** (three-dimensional [3D] imaging as opposed to 2D imaging), using a CT unit, which is separate from the accelerator but that shares a registration system, has been available for more than 10 years. The first report by Uematsu et al.[23] was designed for frameless stereotactic radiation therapy. The treatment couch has two rotation axes—one for rotation about the accelerator isocenter and the other to rotate between the accelerator and the CT scanner. Figure 16-8 shows the treatment couch in the imaging position for within in the treatment room CT device. Another approach placed a CT simulator in the treatment room and used a sliding couch top to transport the patient between the CT scanner and the accelerator treatment table. There are at least two different commercial versions of the **CT-on-rails** approach, systems provided by GE and Siemens.[6,7,24] The accelerator treatment table is rotated 180 degrees and the CT unit moves on rails as the patient is imaged, while the couch is stationary. (This, of course, is just the opposite of the normal CT imaging technique, in which the CT unit is stationary and the couch moves the patient into the imaging position.) Such CT-on-rails systems, if used and maintained properly, can provide very accurate patient localizations with uncertainties less than 1 mm. The images obtained with the moving CT unit have almost the same quality as those obtained from a stationary CT unit, but the low-contrast resolution is worse compared with couch-moving CTs. Institutions have had to write their own software to calculate couch corrections for these systems, which represents a potential weakness of this approach. However, these systems can be used to deliver very precise treatments (e.g., metastasis to the vertebral body within 1 to 2 mm of the spinal cord).

There is one commercial product that combines CT imaging and treatment delivery using the same x-ray source, namely TomoTherapy, which is shown in Figure 16-9.[17] A continuous 360-degree ring gantry geometry, which is the CT scanner geometry,

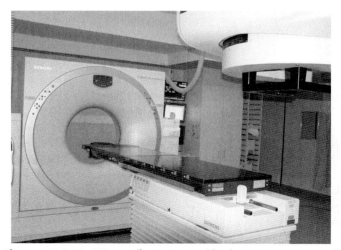

Figure 16-7. An Elekta accelerator with the kV imaging system perpendicular to the MV treatment and imaging system.

Figure 16-8. A CT-on-rails system with the treatment couch rotated to the imaging position. Note the treatment unit head is in the foreground.

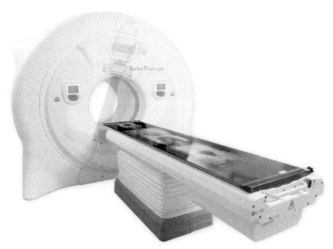

Figure 16-9. TomoTherapy Hi-Art imaging and treatment system, which uses the same MV source for computed tomography and for treatment. (Used with permission of TomoTherapy Incorporated.)

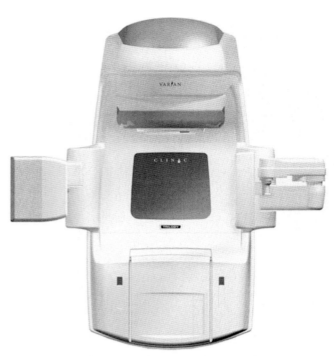

Figure 16-10. A linear accelerator with a kilovoltage source on the left and a flat panel detector on the right. The gantry rotates 360 degrees around the patient as a series of radiographs are taken. These radiographs are constructed into a three-dimensional computed tomography data set.

is used to support a straight-through 6-MV waveguide, which is used for both MV CT imaging and MV treatments. MV images have poor low-contrast resolution compared with kV images but are able to define the position of the patient on the treatment table. One benefit to MV images is that they avoid the metal artifacts that are present in kV images (e.g., from hip prostheses). Helical intensity-modulated radiation treatments are delivered after the patient is imaged. The treatment can be adjusted to match the position of the patient. This unit is designed to deliver only helical intensity-modulated radiation therapy (IMRT), as opposed to customized or rectangular fields, and the patient is moved through the imaging/treatment section in a manner similar to diagnostic CT imaging. This self-contained approach certainly conceptually is very appealing.

In the treatment room, volumetric imaging using an integrated accelerator with an x-ray system has recently become available using several different approaches. **Cone beam CT (CBCT)** differs from fan beam CT in that the CT detector is an area detector (a 2D extended digital array)[12] (Figure 16-10). At certain degree intervals during the rotation of the gantry, single projection images are acquired—for example, at every 1 degree. These different gantry angle images are slightly offset one from another and are the basis upon which a 3D volumetric data set is generated. The net result is a 3D reconstruction data set, which can project images in three orthogonal planes (axial, sagittal, and coronal). The rotation speed of the gantry remains at 1 revolution per minute, which is a standard specification for safety purposes. Thus, patient motion during this 1-minute revolution may cause a problem. In addition, x-rays, which are scattered in the patient, may degrade the resultant images, especially when imaging thick body parts such as the pelvis. However, the final product is a 3D CT data set with the patient in the treatment position.

This technology permits registration of two different 3D data sets. Registration is the process of aligning multiple data sets into a single coordinate system so that the spatial locations of corresponding points coincide. This is an important and

well-studied issue in medicine.[11] As a simple example of the rigid body registration of two images, consider an initial image of a penny on a table and a second image of the same penny on the same table that has been moved in the X and Y (lateral and longitudinal) directions. To register these two images, a calculation must be performed that determines the amount of displacement in the X and Y directions of the two images of the penny. This can be described as a geometric transformation. Rigid body registration is routinely performed with medical images (e.g., the PET image is registered with the CT image in a display of both data sets superimposed on each other). It is possible to register 2D image sets to address translational setup differences between the reference images and the daily image set. This is shown in Figure 16-11. Three-dimensional volumetric data sets can address both translational and rotational differences. In a radiation oncology application, the CT reference data set is taken at the time of simulation and is the basis of the treatment plan. The other 3D volumetric data set, which can be from CBCT or CT-on-rails, is taken with the patient on the treatment table before treatment.

The IGRT approaches, which have been described previously, rely on rigid body image registration, that is, registration of bony anatomy. Rigid body registration restricts the searched transformation to be a combination of translations in the X, Y, and Z directions and rotations, which are sufficient to describe the movement of solid objects. Many therapy treatment tables have rotation capabilities, which are limited to rotation about isocenter and do not provide for rotation about the long axis of the couch (pitch) or the short axis of the couch (roll). Rotation of

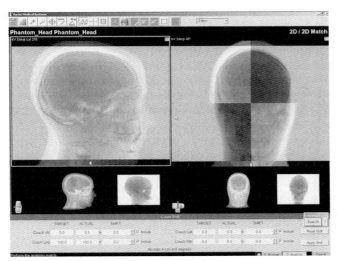

Figure 16-11. Two-dimensional reference images (anteroposterior and lateral) and daily images have been registered and fused. The couch shifts, which are designed to bring these two data sets into better alignment, is about to be calculated. (See Color Plate 3.)

the collimator may be able to address some of these limitations. There are some commercial therapy couches with 6 degrees of freedom, however.

Deformable image registration is a more difficult problem than rigid body registration. Consider an image of a dish of ice cream with candy embedded in the ice cream. Now consider a second image of this dish of ice cream and candy after this combination has melted and is almost liquid. Deformable registration is transformation that maps the current position of the candy in the deformed ice cream volume to the original position of the candy in the ice cream. One initial application of deformable image registration was the correlation of functional images in the brain, which have well-defined neuroanatomy, with images of a diseased brain. For model-based deformable registration, a surface in the 3D image data set is defined and then warped (bent and twisted) into alignment with features in the target image data set. There is also a pixel approach that maps on a pixel-by-pixel basis. Image warping is an active field of image processing in which an image is geometrically distorted to conform to a given specification. In most interactive warping systems, the user specifies the warp in a general way and then the software automatically interpolates this specification to produce the mapping. In radiation oncology, deformable image registration defines a transformation that deforms an image template, such as the daily CBCT image set, into alignment with the target image of interest, the 3D reference image set. It can be used to track radiation doses in the target and surrounding tissue during the 5 to 8 weeks of treatment, as the patient's anatomy changes. This permits the development of adaptive radiation therapy.[4]

In summary, today it is possible to image and analyze the patient's position on the treatment table and compare this in-room image set with the image set used for treatment planning. This should result in a more focused treatment, which avoids more normal tissue and limits toxicity. There will be changes in current practice as daily information on the patient is obtained and reviewed. As an example of the potential use of image-guided therapy, Barker et al.[2] reported on thrice-weekly CT scans of 15 patients with head and neck cancer. These patients demonstrated significant anatomic changes over the course of their treatment. The location of the center of the mass of the tumor changed during the course of treatment and the parotid glands shifted in the medial direction. The opportunity to adjust to these changes in the patient now awaits the development of clinical understanding of what to do to change the treatment plan and when to do it during the course of treatment.

RESPIRATORY MOTION MANAGEMENT

The systems described previously are designed to address interfraction motion (see Chapter 22), or the differences in the patient position between the treatment planning imaging study or the first day of treatment imaging study, the reference images, and the daily images. However, even if the patient position is in perfect agreement with the reference image data set, there remains the issue of intrafraction motion. Patients breathe and, as a consequence, the location of a number of organs changes. The organs whose location is affected by the breathing process may include the lungs, esophagus, liver, and pancreas. The breathing pattern of a patient can change significantly during treatment in reaction to the sequelae of the radiation treatment and medical oncology treatments. A healthy adult at rest breathes in and out, one **respiratory cycle**, approximately 12 to 16 times per minute or approximately 1 cycle every 4 seconds. Under normal circumstances, an adult inhales and exhales approximately 0.5 L of air in each respiratory cycle.

The management of respiratory motion has become an important topic in radiation oncology. The American Association of Physicists in Medicine published a report entitled, "The Management of Respiratory Motion in Radiation Oncology Report of AAPM Task Group 76."[13] A number of different approaches are available to address the uncertainties introduced by respiratory motion. The magnitude of respiratory motion, which is a 3D process, is very patient specific. Although generalizations may not be accurate, Ekberg et al.[9] found, for lesions in the lower lobe of the lung, respiratory motion up to 12 mm in the superoinferior direction and up to 5 mm in the anteroposterior and left and right lateral directions. Respiratory motion is not a significant issue for every patient. In a study of 22 patients, Stevens et al.[21] reported that 10 patients showed no tumor motion in the superoinferior direction. The range of superoinferior motion of the remaining 12 patients was from 3 to 22 mm.[21]

Gating has become very well known in the treatment of many types of cancers such as lung and esophagus and tumors in the abdomen. Physicians have now begun to use this same technology in the treatment of patients with breast cancer in monitoring not only the lung but the amount of cardiac tissue moving in and out of the treatment field as the patient breathes. With the implementation of respiratory gating in the treatment of breast cancer, physicians can still maintain adequate margins around breast tissue while also minimizing the dose to the heart.

A simple approach to managing motion is provided by abdominal compression. There is a commercial device that is designed to compress the abdomen and thus limit motion by limiting the amount of air that the patient can inhale. This forced shallow breathing technique was initially designed to manage motion for stereotactic lung and liver treatments. This device includes a rigid stereotactic body frame with an attached vacuum bag. A pressure plate is attached to the frame. The amount of abdominal compression is controlled by the position of the plate, which can be adjusted by a screw mechanism. There are published reports that describe the accuracy and reproducibility of this mechanical system.[18]

Given the emergence of the CT simulator as a common device within radiation oncology, CT is now widely used to study respiratory motion. There are at least three different CT approaches—slow CT scanning, two breath-hold CT studies with the patient at inhalation and at exhalation, and **four-dimensional CT (4D CT)**. The slow CT scanning technique involves operating the scanner at a low number of revolutions per second (1 revolution per second or greater) so that multiple respiration phases are recorded on the same axial image. The inhalation and exhalation breath-hold technique requires the patient to hold his or her breath in a reproducible manner as these two independent CT studies are performed. The data sets are then registered, and the target volume defined on one set is fused with the target volume on the second set. A typical 4D CT method uses an oversampled spiral CT with a pitch of 0.5, a scanner rotation time of 1.5 seconds, and an external respiratory signal. (*Pitch* is defined as the ratio of the table feed in millimeters per 360-degree rotation divided by the product of the number of detector rows multiplied by the slice collimator in millimeters. A pitch of 0.5 indicates that the same location in the body is in more than one axial image.) Each image obtained through a 4D CT study can be sorted into a bin that corresponds to the phase of the respiratory cycle at which the image was acquired. A complete set of such respiratory cycled images, the 4D CT data set, would display target motion during the breathing cycle. If 10 different image sets were acquired, then images would be available from peak inhale through mid-exhale to peak exhale to mid-inhale and back to peak inhale in 10 different complete image sets. One useful approach to track lung tumors is to use the maximum intensity projection (MIP), which is the maximum CT number found in a given voxel in the 4D CT data set, to visualize the volume encompassed by motion of the tumor. With a modern multislice CT scanner, a 4D CT scan can be obtained within 1 to 2 minutes. The consensus is that any approach that defines targets while considering motion is better than ignoring the effects of motion.

After treatment planning has been performed on a 4D CT study, the patient can be treated in such a manner as to account for respiratory motion. One simple approach is to define an internal target volume (ITV), which encompasses the maximum extent of the target through the breathing cycle. This is a conservative approach, which may include more normal tissue than is absolutely necessary. Another approach is **gated treatments**—that is, the radiation is turned on when the target is within the treatment volume and the radiation is turned off

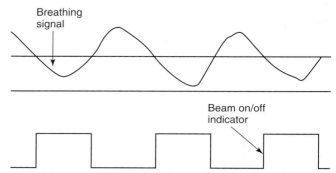

Figure 16-12. The *top trace* displays the breathing pattern of a patient. The *bottom trace* indicates when the accelerator is turned on and off. Note that the accelerator is on during the exhalation portion of the respiratory cycle.

when the target is outside the target volume. This is demonstrated in Figure 16-12. With the linear accelerator being turned on and off, the length of time required to deliver the treatment will increase significantly.[25]

How can the location of a moving anatomic target be known when the patient is on the treatment table? At this point in time, there are no delivery systems that treat and image at the same instant in time. There are different commercial devices that can provide the external respiratory signal. They are all surrogate methods, in that an external device is used to track the internal target motion. Perhaps the most widely discussed such device is the Varian Real-time Position Management (RPM) system, in which an infrared reflective plastic box is placed on the patient's upper anterior abdominal surface. Motion is tracked by in-treatment room cameras, which detect the reflective markers. This device can be used for monitoring respiratory motion during both imaging and treatment. This approach is based on the assumption that this device, which is placed on the patient's upper abdomen, is appropriately tracking the motion of the target in the patient's lung. Other vendors have their own approaches to gating their treatment devices.

A completely different approach for both interfraction and infrafraction motion management involves the implantation of an electromagnetic transponder in or near the treatment site. (A transponder is a radio transmitter and receiver that is activated for transmission by the reception of a predetermined signal.) The electromagnetic transponders, glass-encapsulated circuits 8.5 mm in length and 1.85 mm in diameter, are placed in the target using an invasive technique. The position of the target can be determined based on signals received from the transponders, using an electromagnetic array localization system that is placed above the patient. This is shown in Figure 16-13. Real-time feedback is provided, because the target isocenter can be monitored up to 10 times per second. Litzenberg et al.[16] reported on the use of this approach for prostate localization using a commercial system. The use of this technology for other treatment sites is under development.

STEREOTACTIC RADIATION THERAPY

Cranial **stereotactic** treatments have become a routine treatment approach over the past several decades. The stereotactic approach,

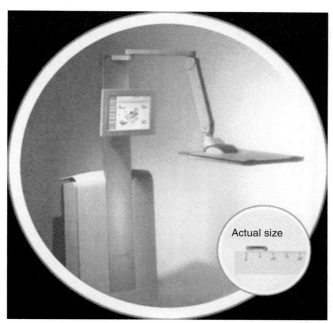

Figure 16-13. An electromagnetic array localization system, which can be used to determine the position of a transponder, which is shown in the *inset*. The photon radiation beam passes through this system. (Courtesy Calypso Medical Technologies, Inc.)

first reported in 1951, has led to the development of dedicated treatment units (e.g., the Gamma knife, which contains more than 200 individual cobalt-60 sources that are focused on a single point). Such a unit is shown in Figure 16-14. Both malignant and nonmalignant conditions, such as arteriovenous malformations, have been managed with this approach.

How does a stereotactic treatment differ from a normal treatment? Stereotaxis is a method, which is used in neurosurgery,

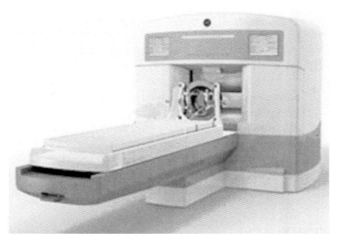

Figure 16-14. A Gamma knife without a patient on the treatment table. The dose is delivered through a series of spots. When the patient is to be treated, the shielding doors open and the patient is moved to a position such that the focused sources irradiate a small volume in the patient's head. The patient is then moved out of the beam and the shielding doors close. A new spot is defined on the frame and the process repeats itself.

neurologic research, and radiation oncology, for locating points within the brain, using an external 3D frame of reference, usually based on the *X, Y, Z* Cartesian coordinate system. The position of the target in the brain is correlated with an external **fiducial** system. (*Fiducials* are a standard of reference in a number of disciplines, including surveying. *Fiduciary,* a term in general use, relates to the holding of something in trust for another or a system of ranking in the field of view of an optical instrument that is used as a reference point or measuring scale.) In radiation therapy, fiducials are used to define a coordinate system in the treatment planning and delivery process, which can be the basis to target the tumor using an external 3D frame of reference. Stereotactic radiation therapy can be thought of as a high-precision targeting technique, which can be used in conjunction with 3D treatment approaches to produce a focused dose distribution with rapid dose falloff. Cranial stereotactic radiation therapy generally involves the invasive fixation of the fiducial system to the skull followed by imaging, treatment planning, and treatment delivery. The fiducial system remains on the patient for this entire process, which may last for 3 to 8 hours.

The management of brain metastases using stereotactic radiation therapy generally involves a single fraction and is called *stereotactic radiosurgery (SRS)*. Fractionated stereotactic treatments are generally called *stereotactic radiation therapy (SRT)*.

Stereotactic body radiation therapy (SBRT) has been defined as a "radiation therapy treatment method to deliver a high dose of radiation to the target, utilizing either a single dose or a small number of fractions with a high degree of precision within the body."[19] The goal of SRT is to deliver the treatment encompassing the target with great accuracy and with rapid dose falloff to spare surrounding tissue.

After approximately 50 years of experience with cranial stereotactic treatments, this approach was expanded to extracranial sites. Why did this development of a highly focused, precise, limited treatment field treatment approach for targets in the body take such a long time? Several important technologic advances were required to permit body stereotactic treatments. One advance is image guidance. The extent of the target needs to be precisely defined to lower the possibility of geometric misses. In addition, the patient needs to be set up using images taken with the patient in the treatment position. Another technologic advance is motion management. Large treatment fields treated using a single fraction result in significant acute and long-term side effects. For stereotactic treatments, the target should be mostly the tumor, and its motion must be well controlled, because the patient will be on the treatment table for a period of time that is much longer than that for routine treatments.

To take advantage of the stereotactic precision in the targeting and treatment delivery, the reference frame and the patient must be properly registered. There are a number of different approaches to register the patient with the frame, including the use of an invasive frame and vacuum-based patient immobilization system. The frame of reference is present for patient simulation, planning, and treatment. The location of target isocenter, which uses the coordinates defined by the frame of reference, can be defined in the planning process and used in treatment delivery. The stereotactic technique evolved from the dedicated unit to the common linear accelerator, using the same basic concepts of stereotactic frame–based, high-precision small-field treatments. One early approach to increasing the accuracy of linac-based stereotactic treatments involved a separate support device for the patient's head, which was independent of the treatment couch. With the advent of high-quality in-room imaging, as described previously, and tighter mechanical specifications for the accelerators, the need for such elaborate patient supporting devices has been lessened. The American College of Radiology has published a practice guideline for the performance of SBRT.[1] This guideline states that the radiation therapy delivery treatment should have mechanical tolerances for radiation therapy of ±2 mm. Section II of this document describes the qualifications and responsibilities of personnel participating in these procedures, including the radiation oncologist, the qualified medical physicist, and the radiation therapist. This guideline states that the responsibilities of the radiation therapist shall be clearly defined and may include assisting the treatment team with patient positioning and immobilization and operating the treatment unit after approval of the clinical and technical aspects by the radiation oncologist and medical physicist.

The Cyberknife is another radiosurgery system that is designed to treat anywhere in the body with high accuracy using a nonisocentric treatment approach. This is an integrated system that combines an accelerator on an industrial robot and two ceiling-mounted x-ray tubes (Figure 16-15). The robot moves the accelerator to predefined positions and delivers relatively small field radiation beams. Image guidance is obtained in almost real time, using a combination of external infrared fiducial markers and radiographs. Fiducial-free spine and lung tracking is being offered. It is reported that treatments can be conducted within 30 to 90 minutes after the patient is first brought into the treatment room. Yu et al.[26] reported that for the treatment of relatively stationary spinal lesions, which are targeted with fiducial tracking, this system is capable of submillimeter accuracy. This system positions itself in the marketplace as an alternative to surgery for many different clinical situations.

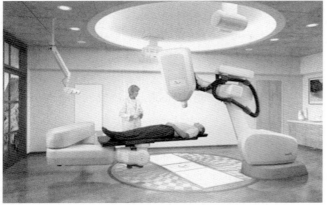

Figure 16-15. An accelerator on a robotic arm. The two ceiling-mounted x-ray tubes are clearly shown.

A well-established application for stereotactic extracranial treatments is the management of metastasis to the spine. The University of Pittsburgh reported their experience with radiosurgery for 500 cases of spinal metastases.[10] Long-term tumor control was obtained in 90% of the lesions treated with radiosurgery as a primary treatment modality using a mean intratumoral dose of 20 Gy. Many other institutions are also offering this important palliative therapy.

There is substantial interest in hypofractionated stereotatic treatments for cancer of the lung, as well as for primary and secondary liver tumors. Some lung cancer patients with early stage lung disease are medically inoperable. Timmerman et al.[22] reported a phase I three-fraction–regimen dose-escalation study in which patients were enrolled in three different groups, based on tumor size. For the smaller tumors, less than 5 cm, greater than 90% local control was observed using a 20 Gy × 3 fraction regimen. Patients who receive this treatment course are at risk for adverse events, including fatal toxicities. However, there are also substantial benefits to be gained, including short treatments with high local control. To state the obvious, SBRT treatments must be simulated, planned, and delivered with great care.

The Radiation Therapy Oncology Group (RTOG) is conducting or planning a number of protocols to study this stereotactic treatment approach, especially for lung tumors. The studies include centrally located lung tumors in inoperable patients and patients with tumors that can be approached surgically. These protocols require the use of a fixed 3D coordinate system defined by fiducial markers. The position of the target within the patient is defined using this coordinate system. A number of different fiducial systems are permitted in these protocols, including metallic seeds, which are invasively placed in the lung near the tumor. Typical doses being studied by such protocols are 45 to 60 Gy, which is delivered in 5 fractions over a 2-week period. Well-defined normal tissue dose-volume limits are required by such a treatment approach. These protocols require that the effect of internal organ motion, due to breathing, be accounted for and that localization images be obtained with the patient on the treatment couch for each fraction. The potential exists that this treatment approach will offer patients high local control with less toxicity than traditional treatments. This treatment approach may increase the number of patients receiving radiation to manage their early-stage lung cancers.

The evolution of radiation oncology toward greater precision in target definition and in patient positioning, including internal organ motion, raises the question of greater precision in dose distributions. IMRT is one approach to obtaining this greater precision. Another approach is heavy charged particles, such as protons.

PROTON TREATMENTS

Protons are heavy charged particles. Electrons are also charged particles, but are approximately 2000 times lighter than protons. The range of the proton beam can be defined to within 1 mm in a water phantom. In addition to the limited range, protons have a very sharp falloff, which is a great clinical

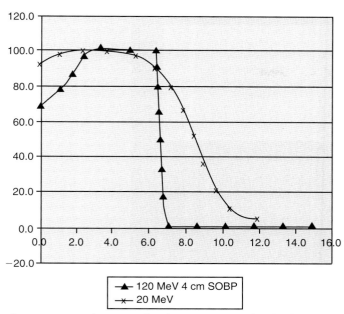

Figure 16-16. The central axis percentage depth dose of a 120-MeV proton beam with a 4-cm spread-out Bragg peak (SOBP) and a 20-MeV electron beam in water. The distal 90% dose is the same for both beams. Note that the 90% to 10% falloff of dose requires several millimeters for a proton beam and several centimeters for an electron beam.

advantage of protons. This is demonstrated in Figure 16-16. The limited range/sharp falloff has the potential of being a major pitfall. The allure of protons is the ability to deposit the dose in the target and to spare normal tissue that is located distally from the target. Consider a target volume in a patient, the spinal cord in a patient with meduloblastoma that is to be treated with a posterior radiation beam. A posterior photon beam will treat the target but exit through the patient's chest and abdomen. A posterior proton beam will stop at the end of range. If the maximum depth of the target is 5.0 cm and the proton beam stops at 5.3 cm, then the patient is well served. If, however, the maximum depth of the target is 5.0 cm and the proton beam stops at 4.7 cm, then the patient is not well served. Proton therapy requires a greater dedication to managing the details of patient simulation, treatment planning, and treatment delivery than photon therapy. DeLaney and Kooy[8] provide a comprehensive review of proton radiotherapy.

Protons have been used in radiation oncology for decades. There is a 1957 article in *Cancer* reporting on the irradiation of the pituitary gland with protons.[15a] The number of institutions offering protons has increased, with more than five institutions offering this type of treatment in the United States at the end of 2007. The number of institutions that offer the use of protons or other heavy particles is expected to grow dramatically in the next decade. Proton facilities are expensive to build, on the order of 10 or more times more expensive than a photon unit, and expensive to maintain, on the order of 10 times more expensive than a photon unit. The clinical conditions that may benefit from this expensive and demanding delivery therapy are being defined. Clearly, the conditions include pediatric patients who are receiving radiation therapy and possibly patients for whom

the acute and long-term toxicities limit the therapeutic options available to them.

The current design of proton facilities has one proton accelerator for three to five treatment beamlines or treatment rooms. After acceleration to the desired energy, the protons are extracted from the accelerator and directed to the treatment rooms using electromagnets, which can be turned on or off. The proton beam that exits from the accelerator is monoenergetic and is described as having a pristine Bragg peak. Most beamlines today use a passive scattering technique to modulate the proton beam—spread out the proton beam along the direction that the beam is traveling. For passive modulation, a rotating modulation wheel or similar device is used to absorb energy, and thus a spread-out Bragg peak (SOBP) is produced. Typically, the widths of the SOBPs can be varied, such as from 2 to 16 cm. Scanning proton beam treatments will soon be available at multiple institutions. Scanning beam treatments will paint the dose distribution by changing the location of the beam spot and the beam energy. Changing the location of the beam spot is easy to do, given the fact that protons are charged particles and can be magnetically steered. Changing the energy of the proton beam, and thus its range, may be relatively easy to do, using a modern proton clinical accelerator.

The proton treatment room has much in common with a photon treatment room. For example, there is a gantry that can rotate 360 degrees, a patient treatment couch, and various in-room imaging systems to define the patient treatment position. The gantry supports the beam nozzle, which contains beam-scattering foils and the rotating modulation wheel, both of which are used for passive modulation. The nozzle also contains the transmission ion chamber and a system that is designed to hold the aperture; the custom block or aperture, which defines the treatment field; and the compensator, a low–atomic number device that compensates for the fact that the patient has air spaces and bones. Tissue heterogeneities affect the range of protons in the patient.

Proton therapy is image-guided therapy. After positioning the patient on the treatment couch, the therapists will produce a set of perpendicular radiographs. The oncologists and the therapists review these images and adjust the patient position appropriately. Just as with photon therapy, reference images can be downloaded from the electronic medical record and used for comparison with the daily images. The daily in-treatment room images can be uploaded to the electronic medical record. Some proton treatment nozzles do not have light fields or reticules, which are traditionally used in photon therapy for aiding in the patient setup.

Retinoblastoma is an uncommon tumor (approximately 200 cases per year) that occurs in very young children. There is substantial experience in the management of this disease with external beam radiation therapy, despite the known sequelae. Protons have been used at Massachusetts General Hospital for several decades.[14] Massachusetts General Hospital is treating these patients under a protocol that is designed to study both local control and adverse effects from the radiation. The ability to stop the proton from entering the brain should limit the consequences of the radiation treatment. This is demonstrated in Figure 16-17.

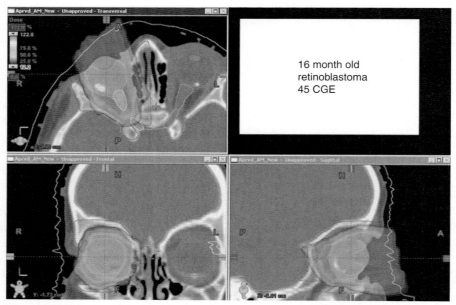

Figure 16-17. A proton dose distribution for a 16-month-old patient with retinoblastoma. Note the limited dose to normal tissue, such as the brain. *CGE,* Cobalt Gray equivalent. (See Color Plate 4.)

SUMMARY

- Radiation is an effective modality in the management of many different types of cancer.
- Radiation is not selective—it can damage both the malignant tissue and the normal tissue.
- The maturation of radiation oncology as a therapeutic modality has included better targeting through improved diagnostic studies, in-treatment room imaging, motion management, and stereotactic techniques.
- This maturation has also included more conformal treatment delivery through the use of intensity-modulated radiation therapy, which in the past decade has become a standard treatment technique. This has also included the expanded use of protons.
- Intensity-modulated radiation therapy appears to be developing as a standard treatment technique in the next decade.

Review Questions

Multiple Choice

1. Modern photon radiation treatment units may:
   a. be one device on the hospital network receiving treatment-specific information
   b. have both kV and MV imaging capabilities
   c. be controlled by multiple computer systems
   d. be designed to deliver nonisocentric treatments
   e. all of the above
2. Image-guided radiation therapy:
   a. has been available only in the 21st Century
   b. permits a faster patient positioning process
   c. must use registered images of the treatment position with the simulation position
   d. requires an x-ray tube mounted on the accelerator C-arm
3. MV images differ from kV images in that MV images have:
   a. better soft tissue contrast
   b. higher spatial resolution
   c. smaller amounts of metal artifacts
   d. lower radiation dose to the patient
4. Four-dimensional CT:
   a. requires the patient to hold his or her breath
   b. can be used to define the extent of respiratory motion
   c. would not display the target motion during the respiratory cycle
   d. images an anatomic location in the patient only once
5. Cone beam CT differs from regular CT in that cone beam CT:
   a. uses a two-dimensional x-ray detector
   b. must use a kV source of x-rays below 10 kV to reduce scattering
   c. produces images that have a smaller amount of scatter
   d. must be produced with a megavoltage source
6. The respiratory cycle of a normal resting adult is approximately:
   a. 1 second
   b. 4 seconds
   c. 10 seconds
   d. 15 seconds
   e. 20 seconds
7. Stereotactic treatments require:
   a. a dedicated treatment unit, such as a Gamma knife
   b. that the site of treatment be in the brain

c. a frame of reference that is used for imaging and treatment

d. a large-dose, single-fraction treatment

8. Managing the patient's respiratory motion can be accomplished by:
   a. asking the patient to hold his or her breath for more than 1 minute
   b. using vacuum bags to position the patient on the treatment table
   c. abdominal compression
   d. respiratory gating
   e. both c and d

9. One significant advantage of protons compared with photons is that:
   a. protons are less expensive to produce than photons
   b. energy is deposited only to malignant tissue and not to normal tissue
   c. protons have limited range in the patient
   d. image guidance is not required

10. An advantage of fiducial marker–guided treatments is that fiducial markers:
    a. emit electromagnetic waves
    b. are easily imaged with ultrasound
    c. contain radioactive material and can be located with a Geiger counter
    d. may be easy to track with x-rays

The answers to the Review Questions can be found by logging on to our website at: *http://evolve.elsevier.com/Washington+Leaver/principles*

Questions to Ponder

1. What are the most important hardware characteristics of an external beam treatment delivery system to facilitate accurate and precise treatments?
2. What are the most important software characteristics for an external beam treatment delivery system to facilitate accurate and precise treatments?
3. What are the advantages of dedicated treatment units over general purpose treatment units?
4. What are the disadvantages of dedicated treatment units over general purpose treatment units?
5. What will the radiation therapy treatment unit of 2020 be like?

REFERENCES

1. American College of Radiology: *ACR practice guideline for the performance of stereotactic body radiation therapy,* Reston, Va, 2006, American College of Radiology, pp 1-8.
2. Barker JL Jr, et al: Quantification of volumetric and geometric changes occurring during fractionated radiotherapy for head and neck cancer using an integrated CT/linear accelerator system, *Int J Radiat Oncol Biol Phys* 59:960-970, 2004.
3. Boyer AL, et al: A review of electronic portal imaging devices (EPIDs), *Med Phys* 19:1-16, 1992.
4. Brock KK, et al: Feasibility of a novel deformable image registration technique to facilitate classification, targeting and monitoring of tumor and normal tissue, *Int J Radiat Oncol Biol Phys* 64:1245-1254, 2006.
5. Chandra A, et al: Experience of ultrasound-based daily prostate localization, *Int J Radiat Oncol Biol Phys* 56:436-447, 2003.
6. Chang EL, et al: Phase I clinical evaluation of near-simultaneous computed tomographic image-guided stereotactic body radiotherapy for spinal metastases, *Int J Radiat Oncol Biol Phys* 59:1288-1294, 2004.
7. Court L, et al: Evaluation of mechanical precision and alignment uncertainties for an integrated CT/LINAC system, *Med Phys* 30:1198-1210, 2000.
8. Delaney TF, Kooy HM, editors: *Proton and charged particle radiotherapy,* Philadelphia, 2008, Lippincott Williams & Wilkins.
9. Ekberg L, et al: What margins should be added to the clinical target volume in radiotherapy treatment planning for lung cancer? *Radiother Oncol* 48:71-77, 1998.
10. Gerszten PC, et al: Radiosurgery for spinal metastases: clinical experience in 500 cases from a single institution, *Spine* 32:193-199, 2007.
11. Hajnal JV, Hill DLG, Hawkes DJ, editors: *Medical image registration,* Boca Raton, Fla, 2001, CRC Press.
12. Jaffray DA, et al: Flat-panel cone-beam computed tomography for image-guided radiation therapy, *Int J Radiat Oncol Biol Phys* 53:1337-1349, 2005.
13. Keall PJ, et al: The management of respiratory motion in radiation oncology report of AAPM Task Group 76, *Med Phys* 33:3874-3900, 2006.
14. Krengli M, et al: Proton radiation therapy for retinoblastoma: comparison of various intraocular tumor locations and beam arrangements, *Int J Radiat Oncol Biol Phys* 61:583-593, 2005.
15. Langen KM, et al: Evaluation of ultrasound-based prostate localization for image-guided radiotherapy, *Int J Radiat Oncol Biol Phys* 57:635-644, 2003.
15a. Lawrence JH: Proton irradiation of the pituitary, *Cancer* 10:795–798, 1957.
16. Litzenberg DW, et al: Positional stability of electromagnetic transponders used for prostate localization and continuous, real-time tracking, *Int J Radiat Oncol Biol Phys* 68:1199-1206, 2007.
17. Mackie TR, et al: The utility of megavoltage computed tomography images from a helical tomotherapy system for setup verification purposes, *Int J Radiat Oncol Biol Phys* 60:1639-1644, 2004.
18. Negoro Y, et al: The effectiveness of an immobilization device in conformal radiotherapy for lung tumors: reduction of respiratory tumor movement and evaluation of daily setup accuracy, *Int J Radiat Oncol Biol Phys* 50:889-898, 2001.
19. Potters L, et al: American Society for Therapeutic Radiology and Oncology and American College of Radiology practice guidelines for the performance of stereotactic body radiation therapy, *Int J Radiat Oncol Biol Phys* 60:1026-1032, 2004.
20. Serago CF, et al: Initial experience with ultrasound localization for positioning prostate cancer patients for external beam radiotherapy, *Int J Radiat Oncol Biol Phys* 53:1130-1138, 2002.
21. Stevens CW, et al: Respiratory-driven lung tumor motion is independent of tumor size, tumor location, and pulmonary function, *Int J Radiat Oncol Biol Phys* 51:62-68, 2001.
22. Timmerman R, et al: Extracranial stereotactic radioablation: results of a phase I study in medically inoperable state 1 non-small cell lung cancer patients, *Chest* 125:1946-1955, 2006.
23. Uematsu M, et al: A dual computed tomography linear accelerator unit for stereotactic radiation therapy: a new approach without cranially fixated stereotactic frames, *Int J Radiat Oncol Biol Phys* 35:587-592, 1996.
24. Wong JR, et al: Image-guided radiotherapy for prostate cancer by CT-linear accelerator combination: prostate movements and dosimetric considerations, *Int J Radiat Oncol Biol Phys* 61:561-569, 2005.
25. Yorke E, et al: Interfactional anatomic variation in patients treated with respiration-gate radiotherapy, *J Appl Clin Med Phys* 6:19-32, 2005.
26. Yu C, et al: An anthropomorphic phantom study of the accuracy of Cyberknife spinal radiosurgery, *Neurosurgery* 55:1138-1149, 2004.

Intensity-Modulated Radiation Therapy

Ronnie G. Lozano

Outline

Key Terms

Beam's eye view (BEV)
Conformal radiation therapy
Dose escalation
Fluence pattern
Forward planning
Homogeneous radiation beam
Inverse treatment planning
Iteration
Optimization
Segment
Sliding window
Step-and-shoot, or segmental, MLC (SMLC)

Objectives

- Define *intensity-modulated radiation therapy (IMRT)*.
- Describe the differences between conventional radiation therapy and IMRT.
- Compare and contrast the difference between forward planning and inverse planning.

- List and describe the types of IMRT delivery systems.
- Discuss the advances and benefits that IMRT provides compared with conventional radiation therapy.

The goal of radiation therapy is to deliver a dose high enough to destroy the cancer cells and at the same time spare normal tissue structures. Often, this is a difficult task. As the dose to a treatment area increases, the probability of tumor control also increases. However, as the dose to a treatment area increases, the probability of inducing normal tissue damage also increases. The process by which external beams of radiation are designed and used to selectively and exclusively irradiate only tumor-bearing sites is called *three-dimensional conformal radiation therapy (3D CRT)*.[12] Intensity-modulated radiation therapy (IMRT) is an advanced form of 3D CRT. The challenge involved in treatment planning is to shape the dose around the tumor volume while sparing dose to any organs at risk (OARs) located near the tumor volume. IMRT attempts to deliver a more sophisticated (conformal) dose to the tumor volume by varying the beam intensity of each of the treatment fields through computer-controlled beam delivery systems. In conventional forms of 3D CRT, the beam intensity is much different. It is nearly uniform for each treatment field delivered.

HISTORIC PERSPECTIVE

Advances in three-dimensional (3D) imaging, such as computed tomography (CT), magnetic resonance imaging (MRI), and positron emission tomography (PET), have provided the necessary data for more

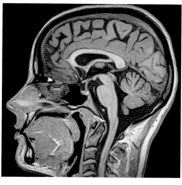 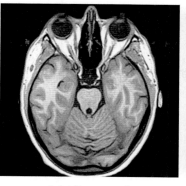 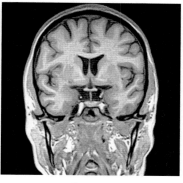

Sagittal   Axial (transverse)   Coronal

Figure 17-1. Multiple images from a magnetic resonance image displaying details of brain anatomy in a sagittal, transverse, and coronal plane. (From Kelley LL, Peterson CM: *Sectional anatomy for imaging professionals*, St. Louis, 2007, Elsevier Mosby.)

advanced radiation therapy treatment planning that may include IMRT. Breakthroughs in medical imaging have provided a way to look at anatomic data in three dimensions. With both the invention of CT in the 1970s and the later addition of MRI and PET, radiation therapy treatment planning can now be accomplished more accurately and with greater precision. In treatment planning, CT and MRI data allow the physician to distinguish between soft tissue structures better than conventional x-ray images and provide important data on the attenuation of the x-ray beam as it passes through the body from hundreds of different angles. The computer sorts huge amounts of x-ray attenuation data and reconstructs images of the human body in several anatomic planes, such as transverse, coronal, and sagittal (Figure 17-1). This allows the physician and dosimetrist to view dose distributions generated by the treatment planning computer to be viewed in several anatomic planes. It is the reformatting of the digital data (from CT and MRI), which may use several post-processing techniques, that provides important information for the radiation oncologist and treatment planning team.

Many treatment planning comparison studies have demonstrated advantages in using 3D CRT, especially its advanced form of IMRT. Early results have shown improvements of local tumor control for prostate cancer and head and neck cancer.[17] Historically, conformal therapy techniques were noticeable as early as the 1960s and 1970s.

A group of researchers at the Harvard Medical School implemented a computer-controlled conformal radiation therapy technique in the mid-1970s for the treatment of more advanced cervical cancer involving paraaortic lymph nodes. The computer controlled the mechanical aspects of treatment delivery such as gantry, dose rate, and couch movements. As the gantry rotated around the patient and the *X* and *Y* collimators moved, the table moved in a number of directions, including left and right, in and out, and/or up and down, in an effort to conform the dose to the target area and spare as much normal tissue as possible, especially in and around the paraaortic nodal area, where the small bowel and spinal cord limited the dose. The workers at Harvard's Joint Center for Radiation Therapy (JCRT) established a method of what is now called *dynamic conformal therapy*.[3,7]

With the research and development that has been accomplished within the past 10 years, radiation therapy has experienced a rapid rate of change in the practice of treatment delivery. The number of publications on IMRT has grown from only two or three a year, in years prior to the mid-1990s, to 353 publications available in 2004.[16] The *International Journal of Radiation Physics and Biology* published 132 articles in 2006 and part of 2007 alone. A 2008 search, using PubMed, a service of the U.S. National Library of Medicine and the National Institutes of Health, yielded 1925 publications on IMRT. Table 17-1 provides a brief chronologic description of the technologic developments in radiation therapy dose delivery.

GENERAL INTENSITY-MODULATED RADIATION THERAPY PRINCIPLES

Three-dimensional CRT and IMRT work together to deliver a beam optimized to the tumor volume. **Conformal radiation therapy** is a radiation therapy technique that uses 3D images of

Table 17-1	Technologic Developments in Radiation Therapy Dose Delivery	
Period	**Issues and Advances**	**Technology**
1940s and before	Nonuniform doses, skin toxicity	Up to 400 kV x-ray
1950s	Improved sparing of normal tissue, target dose uniformity	Cobalt, 4- to 8-MV linear accelerator, 20- to 30-MeV betatron
1960s-1970s	Linear accelerators provided better use of computerized treatment planning, required more physics support	Simulators, multimodality linear accelerators
1970s-1990s	Improved dose computations and targeting, reduction of tissue complications	Three-dimensional treatment planning with CT scanning
1990s to present	Dose escalation with intensity-modulated radiation therapy, improved tumor control, continued reduction of tissue complications	Computer-controlled dynamic treatments, three-dimensional imaging: MRI, PET/CT, CT simulation

CT, Computed tomography; *MeV,* megaelectron volt; *MRI,* magnetic resonance imaging; *MV,* megavolt; *PET,* positron emission tomography.

the tumor so that multiple radiation beams can be shaped exactly (conform) to the contour of the tumor volume. The use of 3D CRT makes every effort to optimize the dose to the contour of the tumor. A general definition of **optimization** is a procedure to make a system as effective as possible. In pharmacy applications, drug dose optimization attempts to establish the best dose of a drug that provides the best results most efficiently. For example, multiple doses of lower-strength medications may be replaced with a single dose of higher-strength medications. Taking these medications once a day in higher strengths instead of multiple lower doses results in the same daily dose and can result in potential cost savings of up to 50% per refill. In the same way, a dose of radiation may be prescribed to deliver a total dose to the tumor in a variety of ways, such as multiple beam angles, shapes, and beam intensities.

For years, beam compensators such as wedges and other forms of customized compensators were used to attenuate the beam in an effort to produce a more **homogeneous radiation beam** within the patient. Producing a homogeneous beam attempts to deliver the same dose throughout a defined volume of tissue through multiple treatment angles and beam intensities. Factors that call for a compensator may include treating tissues of varying densities or thicknesses. A treatment volume that includes a variation in tissue thickness may be a field that extends from the middle of the face and nose to the outer corner of the orbit for example. Another example is a field that includes the natural variance in the thickness and shape of the female breast tissue. These applications require some type of added device to adjust the beam's strength or intensity and deliver the same dose throughout the treatment volume that may include a significant variation in tissue density or thickness. IMRT can accomplish this by varying the intensity of the dose to the tumor volume of each of the treatment fields through computer-controlled beam delivery systems.

Adjusting Beam Shape

The role of multileaf collimation is to produce a beam shape consistent with the 3D volume of the tumor (Figure 17-2). In other words, the beam's shape or geometry projected from the gantry head of the linear accelerator matches some irregular shape of a tumor similar to a puzzle's piece that fits snuggly into an outlined area. In comparison, traditional radiation therapy delivers a beam only in a rectangular shape. A customized shielding block must be inserted into the collimator to create an irregular shape. In the most general terms, by using multileaf collimation, a beam that conforms to a tumor volume or matches the tumor outline tightly like a puzzle piece, minimizes the unnecessary exposure of radiation to normal organs and tissue near the tumor volume. A **segment** refers to the shape that the mechanical aperture (multileaf collimator [MLC]) creates during part of the total dose delivered. A single aperture opening with a designated MLC shape is one of a number of shapes created in dynamic collimator IMRT (Figure 17-3). By changing the beam shape with a predetermined dose, through the use of multiple segments, an intensity-modulated field is produced. Producing a specifically shaped beam that includes the tumor but excludes normal tissue allows the radiation oncologist to prescribe a higher dose to the smaller treatment volume than possible with conventional radiation therapy. Sophisticated real-time imaging systems allow the radiation therapist to confirm beam placement.

Adjusting Dose Delivered

MLC-IMRT uses the collimators as a physical filter to modify the beam the same way a compensator may be used in conventional radiation therapy. An example of a compensator, as explained previously, is a brass or copper wedge. Radiation dose can be adjusted to vary tissue density across a field. IMRT can produce a beam that varies the radiation intensity delivered

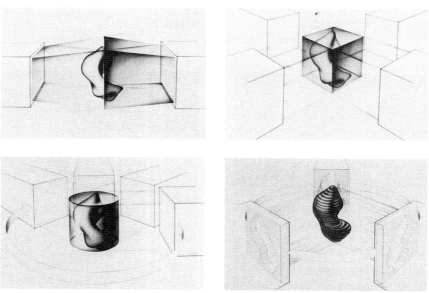

Figure 17-2. Beam shaping using multileaf collimation. (Courtesy Dr. Alan Lichter, University of Michigan, Ann Arbor, Mich.)

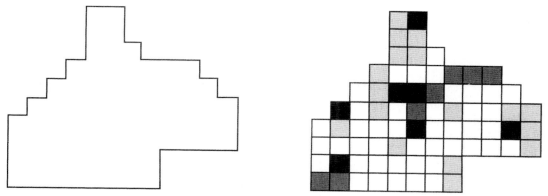

Figure 17-3. Two examples of conformal radiation therapy (CRT). **A,** A CRT field geometrically shaped by a device such as a multileaf collimator. **B,** A CRT field using intensity-modulated radiation therapy (IMRT). Note that each beam segment has varying intensity dose levels, in which the darker shaded segments represent higher dose levels than the lighter segments. Theoretically, any type of pattern is possible with IMRT. (From Leaver D: Intensity modulated radiation therapy: part I, *Radiat Ther* 11:106-124, 2002.)

to the tumor volume. A highly conformal treatment plan typically includes multiple beams shaped by the MLCs. Dynamic multileaf collimation allows changing the beam, using MLCs while the beam is on, to affect beam shape and dose distribution.[1] In this way, the MLC has evolved from merely a replacement for cut blocks to a system capable of beam-intensity modulation.

The total prescribed dose has, in the past, been limited by normal tissue tolerance of radiation, preventing the delivery of a tumorcidal dose in some cases. If a higher dose could be delivered to the tumor volume, then there would be a higher probability of tumor control in most cases. At the same time, without a reduction of the dose to normal tissue, a higher probability of short- and long-term side effects would also be expected. A higher dose may maximize tumor control through the use of IMRT.[17] In many situations, a smaller treatment volume provided by a tightly conformed IMRT treatment plan allows the delivery of a higher dose to the tumor. **Dose escalation** refers to the delivery of higher than traditional doses to a treatment volume. Dose escalation has shown good tumor control with a reduction of complications to normal tissue and organs at risk due to their proximity to the tumor site.[1,13,17,18]

 The limiting factor to achieve full tumor control in conventional treatment has been dose-limiting normal tissue surrounding the tumor.

IMAGE ACQUISITION AND SIMULATION

The simulation process begins with the patient set up in the treatment position, using a CT simulator. Imaging for radiation therapy simulation has included CT imaging, MRI, PET, and other functional imaging studies, which have improved target and tumor volume definitions. Target and nontarget structures are

delineated on a computer display of CT, MRI, or PET images. Delineating structures by outlining their anatomic borders is a means of defining their volume. This is also referred to as *contouring*. Treatment portals are then designed using the perspective, as if seeing out of the lens of the radiation beam; this is referred to as **beam's eye view (BEV).** Current imaging technology allows the visualization of tumor volume with the 3D perspective of the BEV. The reference to the BEV implies that the target volume is visualized as it is treated, in a 3D plane. The 3D BEV of tumor volume and critical normal anatomy allows treatment alternatives with non-coplanar field arrangements. This method of treatment delivery breaks away from the conventional treatments where most fields are treated in the same plane, as parallel opposed pair fields (POP fields). POP fields are defined as fields with a hinge angle of 180 degrees. The hinge angle is the angle at the isocenter of two radiation fields. Non-coplanar fields may have hinge angles of varying degrees. Computerized imaging also provides tissue density data, an added piece of information helpful in treatment planning.

Biologic imaging, in contrast to anatomic imaging, has evolved into a frequently used modality for staging and treatment planning. Dose optimization or dose sculpting is best established with the anatomic fusion of PET and magnetic resonance spectroscopy imaging (MRSI) with CT and MRI. These imaging modalities provide metabolic, physiologic, functional, and molecular information related to the tumor. Treatment planning factors may include tumor hypoxia or tumor burden. Imaging that provides factors influencing radiosensitivity such as hypoxia may be referred to as radiobiologic images.[10,19]

The effectiveness of biologic imaging using PET lies in the metabolic information from PET scanning using fluorodeoxyglucose radiolabeled with [18]F (FDG). Active malignant development is indicated by an enhanced uptake of FDG due to the increased glucose metabolism of cancer cells. This important characteristic has made PET a valuable tool to improve detection, staging, treatment planning, and evaluation. The usefulness of FDG-PET in diagnosing and staging thoracic lesions is now well established by a large number of clinical studies.[8,10] Many studies show that CT is inadequate in defining the gross target volume for lung cancer, indicating that PET is needed to define the entire tumor accurately.[10]

Using MRSI, molecules that can be studied include water, lipids, choline, citrate, lactate, and creatine. MRSI has been used with IMRT treatment planning to deliver a higher dose to those regions with a higher than normal choline/citrate ratio. Based on MRSI-IMRT treatment planning, intraprostatic lesions have received a planned dose of 90 Gy while the entire prostate was treated to 73.8 Gy and the dose to the rectum and bladder was limited to below the specified tolerance.[10,18] The total dose to the prostate using conventional external beam is 70.2 Gy.

MRSI data can also be used to identify and localize regions of high Gleason scores.

The radioactive contrast used in PET includes glucose. Because active tumor cells have a higher metabolism, they take up the radioactive glucose readily. This results in the enhanced imaging based on a biologic process.

Immobilization

Fabrication of custom-designed body molds and immobilization devices are usually part of the simulation and planning process. Several types of immobilization devices are available. The choice will depend on the anatomic site and preference of the radiation oncologist and radiation therapist. Materials commonly used for immobilization include thermoplastics, polyurethane-foaming agents, and vacuum-forming molds. Because small positional errors may affect the treatment outcome more with IMRT than with convention radiation therapy, special attention is needed in the construction and positioning of such devices in an effort to increase treatment reproducibility. Image-guided radiation therapy (IGRT) has helped identify positional errors before the delivery of a daily prescribed dose of radiation therapy.[3,7,17] Usually, orthogonal or cone beam CT images are taken before treatment. The images are evaluated and compared with a "master" digital reconstructed radiograph (DRR) and then adjustments to the patient's position are made before treatment. The use of real-time monitoring of the tumor location, as is the case with respiratory gating, has been a useful method of improving treatment delivery accuracy. The combination of high doses, multiple fields, smaller field volume, and a higher dose rate to subfield segments has made electronic portal imaging devices (EPIDs) and IGRT important and sometimes necessary elements for quality assurance (QA) with IMRT.

As with conventional treatment, the patient should be set up in a position that is stable, consistently reproducible, and as comfortable as possible. We know that treatment positions and treatment tables are not comfortable. A warm, relaxed, and confident patient will maintain the required position longer. It should be emphasized that IMRT treatments are highly conformal and often involve delivering high doses to fields abutting critical structures or another field. The importance of accurate

and consistent positioning and immobilization is paramount. Numerous noninvasive immobilization techniques provide a higher degree of precision. Devices include thermoplastic immobilization products, customized polyurethane cradles, extended head to shoulder/upper thorax immobilization, longer head boards extending from the head to the upper thorax for additional support of the head and shoulders, vacuum cradles, and plaster casts, among other custom-made devices. More elaborate devices such as a stereotactic body frame that achieves accuracy similar to that of stereotactic radiosurgery has been used. Using scales and indexing to record and reproduce the precise position of immobilization devices has evolved for several anatomic sites. It is common today to have three frames of reference for exact positioning—a table reference, an immobilization device reference, and a reference on the patient's skin may be used.

TREATMENT PLANNING

Treatment planning, at one time, was done by hand for conventional radiation therapy treatment, using beam profiles overlaid on the external contour of the patient. Today there are two approaches to treatment planning used in radiation therapy: forward and inverse planning. We will examine each of these methods in more detail and evaluate their effect on developing and delivering an IMRT treatment plan.

Forward planning is a type of trial-and-error method of treatment planning and has been used in radiation therapy for many decades. The more experienced the planner, the less time is needed and more suitable the final treatment plan will be. Typically, the planner may use the following process for conventional or 3D CRT[7]:

- Defining the anatomy as it relates to the target volumes.
- Creating the plan, which may include beam energy, beam arrangement, number of beams, beam weights, and the addition of beam modifiers such as wedges or compensators.
- Calculating the dose according to beam selection and arrangements.
- Evaluating the dose distribution using isodose lines relative to anatomy and (in more recent years) by calculating dose-volume histograms (DVHs) (Figure 17-4).
- Iterative plan optimization is performed if the plan is not adequate or if the planner desires to improve the plan. Each attempt (iterative) to improve the plan involves modifying the plan, performing a new dose calculation, and then reevaluating the plan.
- Completing the plan involves input from the planner and physician. Monitor units (MUs) for treatment are calculated, DRRs are constructed, and the plan is transferred electronically to the treatment delivery system.
- A verification process on the treatment machine, including shifts in the isocenter, is performed and the treatment plan is evaluated visually to check beam angles and possible collision points between the gantry, collimator, and treatment couch. Portal images are taken to compare with the original DRRs and evaluated for accuracy in covering the target volumes.

Treatment plan evaluation relies on knowledge and understanding of dose distributions and DVHs. Data include information in the form of dose distribution displays, graphs showing

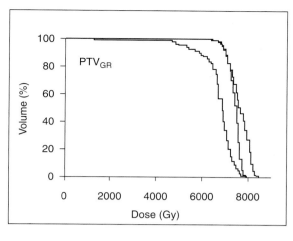 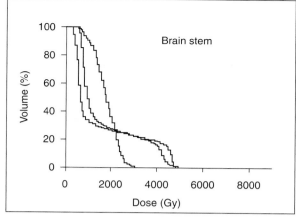

------ Traditional   ------ 3D CRT   ------ IMRT

Figure 17-4. Dose-volume histograms comparing the intensity-modulated radiation therapy, three-dimensional conformal radiation therapy, and traditional plans for the treatment plans. *PTV_{GR}*, Planning target volume. (From Sloan-Kettering Group, editors: *A practical guide to intensity-modulated radiation therapy*, Madison, Wis., 2003, Medical Physics Publishing.)

relationships between the volume of tissue irradiated in terms of specifically defined critical structures, tumor, and unit of absorbed dose. The DVH provides relevant dose data in a 3D format as a function of organ or tumor volume. With this 3D information, it has become possible to define partial volume constraints, such as no more than 25 Gy to 25% of the lung. Upon accepting the treatment plan, all planning data on beam configurations are transferred to the linear accelerator via a computer network, electronic chart, or record and verify system for treatment delivery.[1]

Inverse treatment planning systems work with the defined target dose and programmed normal tissue tolerance doses to create a number of beam portals and beam-intensity patterns within each portal. Rather than trying plans and evaluating what kind of dose distribution is achieved, as in forward planning, the basic concept of inverse planning is to decide up front what the dose distribution should look like and then allow the computer to decide the beam arrangement, beam intensity, gantry angle, and so on. This is done by selecting the optimal dose (goal) desired to control the tumor and specifying a dose limit to any OARs. For example, a patient with head and neck cancer is treated to a dose of 6400 cGy to the gross tumor volume (GTV) and at the same time dose is limited to specific OARs such as the spinal cord, parotid glands, and brain stem (Figure 17-5). The physician selects the dose to the target volumes using some constraints (minimum and maximum dose to that volume) and places limits on the dose to OARs.

Based on these specifications, the inverse treatment planning system adjusts beam shapes and intensities so as to best meet these dose criteria. Computer iterations of beams are performed to establish optimization. The computer program may perform thousands of iterations during this inverse treatment planning process in less time than a human could perform a few iterations. An **iteration**, in terms of computing, refers to a series of repetitions following a sequence of instructions in a computer program, making slight adjustments to each treatment plan until the best

result is achieved according to the criteria selected by the physician and planner. Treatment fields may be divided up into hundreds of tiny separate beamlets, or intensity "bixels." An intensity pattern showing these beam elements is depicted in Figure 17-6.

Inverse planning is approached much differently than forward planning. Typically, the planner may use the following process for IMRT[7]:

- Defining the anatomy as it relates to the target volumes. Inverse planning requires additional attention in defining all anatomic structures that must be considered by the treatment planning system.
- Creating the plan, which may include determining beam energy and directions, designating the beam shape, and dividing the beam into beamlets (intensity bixels).
- Calculating the dose according to beam selection, arrangement, and each beamlet.
- Defining the optimization method according to the "cost function" for the inverse plan. This is defined individually for each patient and is the most critical decision involved in determining what kind of IMRT plan will result from the optimization process.
- Iterative plan optimization is performed using the selected cost functions. The optimization search for the best IMRT plan will continue until predefined stopping criteria are reached.
- Evaluating and reoptimizing the IMRT plan is performed by the physician and planner to evaluate the plan, dose distribution, cost function results, and other relevant information. If the plan is not acceptable, then it is necessary to make changes in the cost function to drive the plan toward different results.
- Completing the plan involves input from the planner and physician. For a beamlet-optimized IMRT plan, this may include leaf sequencing: the preparation of the MLC leaf trajectories (dynamic multileaf collimation delivery) or MLC segment shapes (static multileaf collimation delivery)

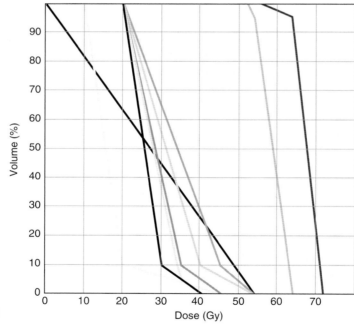

Target Name		Type		Goal (Gy)	Vol Below Goal (%)	Min (Gy)	Max (Gy)	I
GTV-target		Basic		64.0	5	54.0	72.0	
CTV1-target		Basic		54.0	5	52.0	64.0	

Sensitive Structure Name		Type		Limit (Gy)	Vol Above Limit (%)	Min (Gy)	Max (Gy)	I
Tissue		Basic Tissue		54.0	0	0.0	54.0	
Spinal Cord		Basic Structure		35.0	5	20.0	40.0	
LT-Parotid		BU Structure		20.0	10	10.0	45.0	
RT-Parotid		BU Structure		20.0	10	10.0	45.0	
Other 1		Basic Structure		45.0	10	20.0	54.0	
LT-Eye		Basic Structure		45.0	10	20.0	54.0	
Brain-Stem		Basic Structure		35.0	10	20.0	45.0	
LT_TMJ		Basic Structure		30.0	10	20.0	40.0	
RT_TMJ		Basic Structure		30.0	10	20.0	40.0	
Mandible		Basic Structure		40.0	10	20.0	54.0	

A

B

Figure 17-5. A, Example of a dose-volume histogram (DVH)-dose constraints for a commercial inverse planning system (Corvus; 4.0 NOMOS Corporation, Sewichley, Penn). **B**, Simplified DVH based on three-point constraints. (See Color Plate 5.) (From Leibel SA, Phillips TL: *Textbook of radiation oncology*, ed 2, Philadelphia, 2004, Saunders.)

that will create the desired beamlet distribution. In addition, MUs for treatment are calculated, DRRs are constructed, and the plan is transferred electronically to the treatment delivery system.

- A verification process on the treatment machine may include shifts in the isocenter, and the treatment plan is evaluated visually to check beam angles, and possible collision points between the gantry, collimator, and

treatment couch. Portal images are taken to compare with the original DRRs and evaluated for accurate coverage of the target volumes.

Applications of Forward Planning

IMRT plans may be created with conventional 3D CRT treatment planning systems as a form of forward planning. After beam parameters are specified by the dosimetrist, the computer

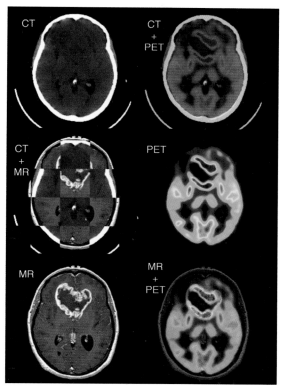

Color Plate 1. Registered or fused images of a brain tumor. Multiplanar reconstruction (side-by-side, checkerboard, and colorwash modes) of computed tomography (CT), magnetic resonance imaging (MRI), and positron emission tomography (PET) of the same patient after spatial registration. (See Figure 6-33.) (From Leibel SA, Phillips TL: *Textbook of radiation oncology*, ed 2, Philadelphia, 2004, Saunders.)

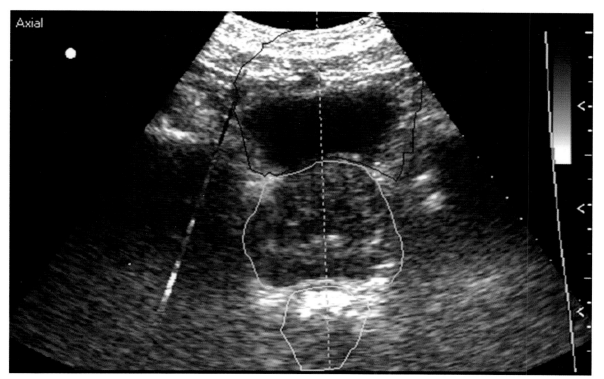

Color Plate 2. Axial ultrasound image with contours of the bladder, prostate, and rectum, which were generated in treatment planning. (See Figure 16-5.)

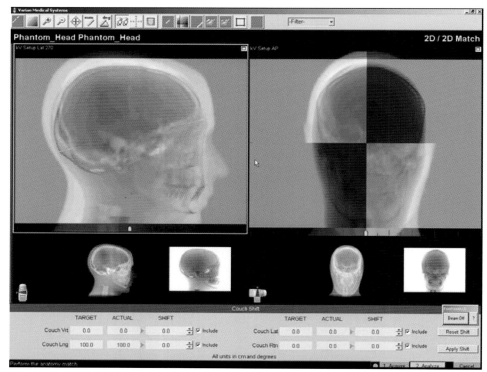

Color Plate 3. Two dimensional reference images (anteroposterior and lateral) and daily images have been registered and fused. The couch shifts, which are designed to bring these two data sets into better alignment is about to be calculated. (See Figure 16-11.)

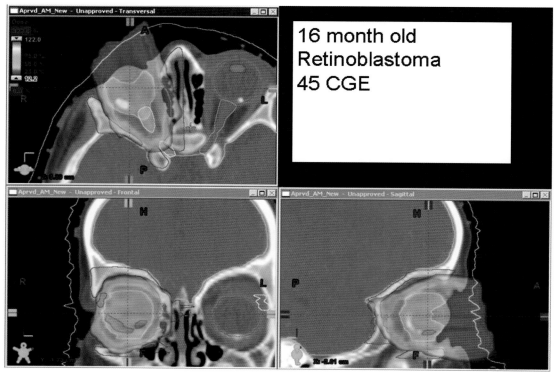

16 month old
Retinoblastoma
45 CGE

Color Plate 4. A proton dose distribution for a 16-month-old patient with retinoblastoma. Note the limited dose to normal tissue, such as the brain. *CGE,* Cobalt gray equivalent. (See Figure 16-17.)

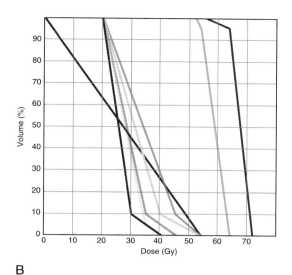

Target Name	Type	Goal (Gy)	Vol Below Goal (%)	Min (Gy)	Max (Gy)	I
GTV-target	Basic	64.0	5	54.0	72.0	
CTV1-target	Basic	54.0	5	52.0	64.0	

Sensitive Structure Name	Type	Limit (Gy)	Vol Above Limit (%)	Min (Gy)	Max (Gy)	I
Tissue	Basic Tissue	54.0	0	0.0	54.0	
Spinal Cord	Basic Structure	35.0	5	20.0	40.0	
LT-Parotid	BU Structure	20.0	10	10.0	45.0	
RT-Parotid	BU Structure	20.0	10	10.0	45.0	
Other 1	Basic Structure	45.0	10	20.0	54.0	
LT-Eye	Basic Structure	45.0	10	20.0	54.0	
Brain-Stem	Basic Structure	35.0	10	20.0	45.0	
LT_TMJ	Basic Structure	30.0	10	20.0	40.0	
RT_TMJ	Basic Structure	30.0	10	20.0	40.0	
Mandible	Basic Structure	40.0	10	20.0	54.0	

A

B

Color Plate 5. A, Example of a dose-volume histogram (DVH)-dose constraints for a commercial inverse planning system (Corvus; 4.0 NOMOS Corporation, Sewichley, Penn). **B**, Simplified DVH based on three-point constraints. (See Figure 17-5.) (From Leibel SA, Phillips TL: *Textbook of radiation oncology*, ed 2, Philadelphia, 2004, Saunders.)

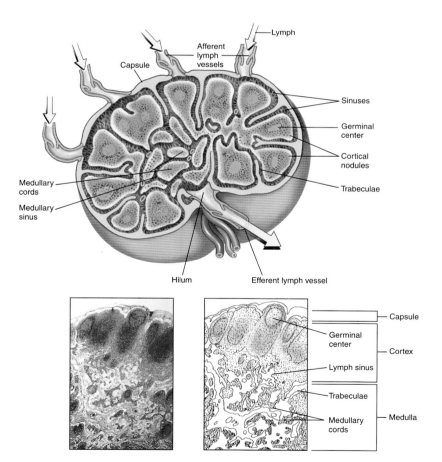

Color Plate 6. Lymph node. *Arrows* indicate the direction of lymph flow. The germinal centers are sites of lymphocyte production. As lymph moves through the lymph sinuses, macrophages remove foreign substances. (See Figure 20-11.) (From Lymphatic system. In Thibodeau GA, Patton KT, editors: *Anatomy and physiology,* ed 6, St. Louis, 2007, Mosby. Photo courtesy of Dennis Strete.)

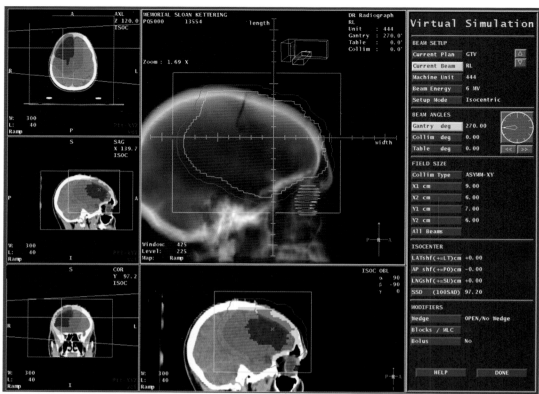

Color Plate 7. Example of CT simulation display (AcqSim, Philips Medical Systems, Andover, Mass). *Upper right* image is a beam's eye view (BEV) digitally reconstructed radiograph (DRR) with planning target volume outlined in yellow and treatment field aperture in blue. *Right panel* shows simulated beam set-up controls. (See Figure 21-24.) (From Leibel SA, Phillips TL: *Textbook of radiation oncology,* ed 2, Philadelphia, 2004, Saunders.)

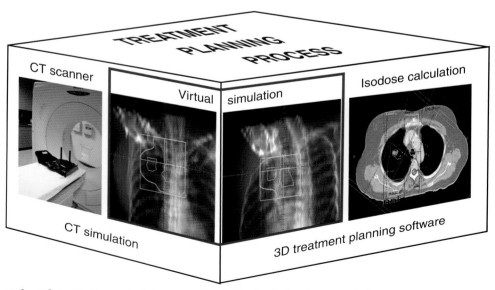

Color Plate 8. Computed tomography (CT) simulation is part of the treatment planning process and includes both the actual CT scanner and the virtual simulation workstation. The treatment planning system includes the virtual simulation workstation and dosage calculation computer. Virtual simulation is defined as the simulation process without the patient actually present. Data are collected from the CT scanning process and then manipulated with the help of the treatment planning software. (See Figure 23-2.)

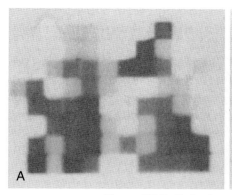 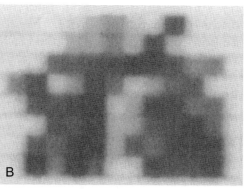 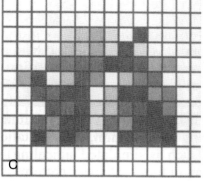

Figure 17-6. A, An intensity pattern from a patient plan delivered to a film with a total of 5 monitor units (MU) at 400 MU/min. **B,** The same intensity pattern delivered with a total of 96 MU at 400 MU/min. **C,** The expected intensity pattern from the planning system. (From Van Dyk J: *The modern technology of radiation oncology: a compendium for medical physicists and radiation oncologists,* vol 2, Madison, Wis., 2005, Medical Physics Publishing.)

calculates the resulting dose distribution. The dose distribution is compared with the desired dose specified by the radiation oncologist. This process may be repeated (manual iterations) if desired specifications are not met. The usefulness and efficiency of this method rests on the experience and intuition of the medical dosimetrist.

Forward planning is an acceptable method for tumors of simpler shape and locations. Complex tumor volumes and geometries in areas that may be in close proximity to critical structures are not cases suitable for forward planning. Some institutions frequently use forward IMRT planning for the treatment of prostate cancer.[10,19]

 In forward planning, the planner specifies beam directions, weighting, and so on. The process of manual iteration of beam intensities, shapes, and direction is a form of manual plan optimization.

Aperture-Based Inverse Planning

The term *aperture* refers to an opening in an instrument, much like an optical instrument that lets only a certain amount of light in or out. A camera, telescope, or adjustable pen flashlight are examples of instruments with apertures. In this context, the term *aperture-based* is used to refer to the specific beam shape for one or a few segments of a beam. Because the dosimetrist designs one or more of the treatment segments for each beam direction, aperture-based inverse planning (ABIP) is considered the middle ground between forward planning and full inverse planning. After designing one or more beam segments, the dosimetrist evaluates computer optimization of the intensities (weights) for each segment.[8,15,19,20]

Applications of Aperture-Based Inverse Planning.

This treatment planning method is often used for breast cancer treatment. The method produces relatively simple IMRT plans with fewer beam segments and fewer MUs than full inverse planning. The segments are designed based on specific beam angles, projections of the target, and critical structures in a BEV. This is considered, in terms of optimization criteria, intuitive despite computer optimization, because some segments are defined on a functional basis, one or more segments having been

manually designed, based on a clinical objective, on the basis of a dose limit to produce the resulting intensity patterns.

 Computer optimization involves the evaluation of many intensity iterations for several subfield segments. This is repeated countless times until an acceptable intensity profile is established, meeting the desire dose constraints.

Pixel-Based (Full) Inverse Planning

The term *pixel-based inverse planning* is derived from the fact that the computer optimizer first divides each beam into many pixels, beamlets, or pencil beams and then adjusts the relative weight of each pixel. The dosimetrist does not directly attempt to optimize or adjust beam intensities. The dosimetrist specifies desired dose limits or constraints (cost functions) for the target and sensitive structures after defining orientation and energy of the beams. Computer optimization then defines the intensity fluences for each selected beam that yields a dose distribution that meets the desired dose constraints. The term **fluence pattern** (*fluent,* as in "flowing") refers to an intensity pattern of the IMRT beam. This may be described as the sequence and progression of dose delivered per beam, as a product of several segments. In a summative effect, each beam angle consists of a series of several segments with different MLC shapes. These subfields (segments) provide the overall intensity-modulated effect produced by the fluence pattern. The complexity of an intensity pattern depends on the number of intensity levels desired.

Plan Evaluation

Dose distributions and DVHs are analyzed during the plan evaluation process.

A score defined by a cost function (an objective function) evaluates the quality of the plan. The cost function has been defined as a mathematical definition of the "goodness" of a treatment plan. The plan is scored on how well it meets the objectives specified by the dosimetrist or physician in terms of dose to the target volume, dose limits to critical structures, and the like. This is referred to as a dose-based objective function where optimization is measured in terms of dose limits and dose-volume limits.

Biologically based objective functions use a calculated radiobiologic response as a measure of the merit of a plan. This type of evaluation is based on the predicted biologic response via a calculation model that relates dose plus volume of irradiated tissue. This type of cost function or objective function is defined by the predicted response for tumor control probabilities or tissue complications. This is characteristic of forward planning in which intensity is manually adjusted based on a predicted radiobiologic response to dose. This was previously described in aperture-based planning.

A dose-based objective function is in the form of a weighted average of differences between delivered and prescribed doses for all voxels (volume elements) in every tissue defined in a treatment plan.[6] This is characteristic of a full inverse planning system. This relationship between dose and tissue voxel is graphically illustrated using a DVH. Figure 17-7 shows how IMRT can spare the brain stem. Beams aimed directly at the brain stem can be assigned with lower dose intensity to the brain stem while still delivering dose to the planned tumor volume.

 Computer optimization is defined by a cost function also referred to as an objective dose-based function. This characterizes inverse planning. Forward planning is characterized by a biologically based objective function because the planner manually sets the parameters based on the expected radiobiologic response as a measure of merit of the plan.

Figure 17-8 illustrates the dose distributions comparing traditional radiation therapy, 3D CRT, and IMRT for treatment of the nasopharynx.

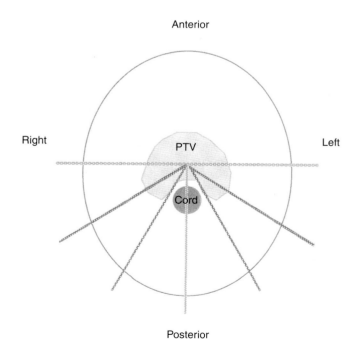

Figure 17-7. A seven-field beam arrangement used for intensity-modulated radiation therapy treatment of a concave-shaped nasopharyngeal tumor in close proximity to the brain stem and spinal cord. *PTV,* Planning target volume. (From Sloan-Kettering Group, editors: *A practical guide to intensity-modulated radiation therapy,* Madison, Wis., 2003, Medical Physics Publishing.)

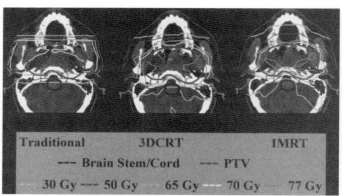

Figure 17-8. Axial dose distributions through the nasopharynx for the intensity-modulated radiation therapy, three-dimensional conformal radiation therapy, and traditional treatment plans. Note the relatively poor coverage of the skull base using the traditional plan and the improved conformality of the intensity-modulated radiation therapy dose. *PTV,* Planning target volume. (From Sloan-Kettering Group, editors: *A practical guide to intensity-modulated radiation therapy,* Madison, Wis., 2003, Medical Physics Publishing.)

INTENSITY-MODULATED RADIATION THERAPY DELIVERY METHODS

Some IMRT delivery systems work with MLCs frequently, but IMRT may also be achieved using different types of technologies. This section describes the different modes of IMRT delivery, including physical modulators, MLC-IMRT, intensity-modulated arc therapy, fan beam intensity modulation, and TomoTherapy.

Intensity-Modulated Radiation Therapy with Physical Modulators

This technique has been described as the simplest method of IMRT. An acrylic resin, metal, or plastic compensator is fabricated with a computer-controlled milling machine. A compensator for each beam serves as the beam-intensity modulator. The compensator must be changed for every field, which requires increased time to deliver the IMRT treatment depending on the number of modulators used for the treatment plan. This technique requires the simplest QA due to the lack of moving collimators.[9] No MLCs are used with physical modulators. The University of North Carolina has treated approximately 1200 patients using compensator-IMRT since 1996 and has used both MLCs and physical compensators for IMRT delivery since multileaf collimation became available in 2001.[5] Mail-order compensator services in the United States are gaining more acceptance and popularity, especially among smaller radiation therapy centers. Some mail-order services provide quality, easy-to-use, and quick-turnaround customized IMRT compensator services.

In principle, a compensator can be designed to produce almost any high-resolution intensity map used in IMRT. Computer-controlled milling machines are used to fabricate either a solid brass compensator directly or a negative Styrofoam mold. The mold is then sealed and filled with compensator material, metal granules, or liquid Cerrobend to form the IMRT compensator. One of the benefits of the physical modulator system is that older accelerators or even a cobolt-60 teletherapy treatment unit can be used without multileaf collimation. The physical modulator fits into a separate slot in the collimator assembly above the block tray.[5]

Multileaf Collimator Intensity-Modulated Radiation Therapy

MLC-IMRT uses the collimators as a physical filter to modify the beam the same way a compensator may be used in conventional radiation therapy. MLC-based IMRT can be a static or dynamic treatment. Figure 17-9 illustrates MLCs. Figure 17-10 illustrates a head and neck treatment showing a conformal beam shape.

Static MLC-IMRT uses conventional MLCs with leaves that are not moved while the beam is on. This technique is similar to conventional treatment, but each field is treated using a combination of segments or subfields where the collimated field is changed. These segments provide the overall intensity-modulated effect produced by the fluence intensity pattern as described in Pixel-Based (Full) Inverse Planning. Static IMRT does not require control of individual leaf speed, and the field

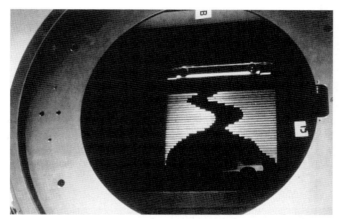

Figure 17-9. Multileaf collimators mounted on the treatment head. (Courtesy Siemens Medical Systems, Concord, Calif.)

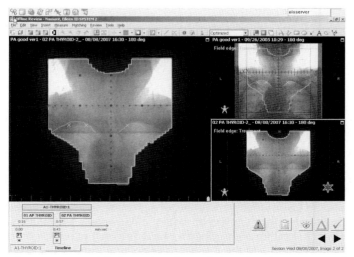

Figure 17-10. Digital overlay view of the planning computed tomography (CT) volume and the cone beam CT volume acquired at treatment. (Copyright ©2007, Varian Medical Systems, Inc. All rights reserved.)

dose is easily verified. It is this simple concept that has made this a very popular treatment technique.

> *The fluence pattern, also referred to an intensity profile, refers to the overall intensity-modulated effect, the cumulative effect of differently collimated segments.*

Dynamic MLC (DMLC) IMRT uses moving MLCs during active treatment while the beam is on. IMRT using DMLCs continuously change the beam shape as the individual leaves move. A continuously varied intensity fluence results in an intensity-modulated field. The fluence pattern may be referred to as the intensity profile. This intensity profile is created by the inverse treatment planning system. DMLCs can deliver a gradually varying intensity profile more accurately and efficiently compared with static IMRT. The system's mechanism is complicated, requiring leaf speed and dose rate modulation. The continuous beam requires comparatively more monitor units to deliver the same intensity pattern as static MLC-IMRT.[3,17] It also requires a more complicated QA.

Step-and-shoot, or segmental, multileaf collimation refers to a technique describing the sequence of leaves moving for repositioning, then coming to rest while the beam is delivered in multiple segments at each gantry angle. This repeated sequence of the MLCs changing position (stepping) and beaming on (shooting) is used with the **Step-and-shoot, or segmental, MLC (SMLC)** IMRT system. The SMLC usually involves 3 to 20 segments per gantry angle where the beam is switched off and on between each segment. Segmental multileaf collimation is typically only a small step away from CRT and is much less labor intensive and easier to deliver. For most anatomic treatment sites, segmental multileaf collimation will add an increase in daily treatment time as compared with CRT. This is usually a result of the increased number of treatment fields used, the total number of monitor units delivered, and the complexity of the treatment plan. Figure 17-6 shows intensity patterns delivered with a step-and-shoot technique.

> *Step and shoot refers to a technique describing the leaves changing position, coming to rest, then delivering a dose of radiation. The leaves move only when the beam is off.*

The **sliding window** technique describes the movement of the MLC from one side of the field to the other within a narrow opening while the beam is on. This technique is used with DMLC systems to generate a continuously varying intensity profile. The leaf movement during treatment must be accurate, and radiation leakage and transmission through or between the MLC must be taken into consideration (Figure 17-11).

Intensity-Modulated Arc Therapy

Intensity-modulated arc therapy (IMAT) technique has been investigated for clinical use in recent years as an alternative to TomoTherapy, a special type of IMAT. It combines gantry rotation with a DMLC system. A linear accelerator is programmed for arc treatment, and the MLC dynamically steps through a sequence of field shapes while the source of radiation rotates around the patient. Each segment is formed with the use of MLC leaves, as well as the backup jaws in the X and Y directions.

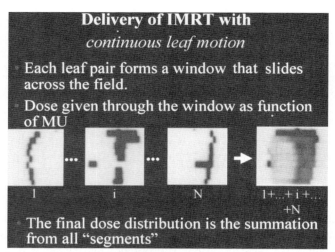

Figure 17-11. Use of an electronic portal imaging device (EPID) system to monitor the delivery of an intensity-modulated radiation therapy (IMRT) treatment. At any instant in time, the IMRT field is an irregular slit (panels 1 to 3 on the *left*), as recorded by a transmission EPID image. The total dose from the beam is the summation of all segments, as indicated in gray scale (white = low dose, black = high dose) in the *rightmost panel*. (From Sloan-Kettering Group, editors: *A practical guide to intensity-modulated radiation therapy*, Madison, Wis., 2003, Medical Physics Publishing.)

In some systems, the dose intensity is modulated by a variable dose rate, a variable gantry speed (a combination of both), or dose delivery over a number of gantry arcs.

Leaf Sequence Files, Intensity Pattern, and Monitor Units

IMRT intensity patterns are complex and may be difficult to understand. Keep in mind that their various graphs, shapes, shades of color, or forms communicate either a position of a leaf—opened, closed, or somewhere in between; a dose pattern related to the positions of the leaves for a specific segment of a field; or a resulting dose to tissue. To gain a better understanding, see Figures 17-21 and 17-22, depicting intensity profiles and dose distributions.

A leaf sequence file is a description of each leaf position (multileaf collimation) as a function of cumulative MUs. The file divides the two-dimensional intensity distributions into a number of one-dimensional intensity profiles, with each profile being delivered by one pair of leaves. Figure 17-12, A, illustrates the relationship for a pair of MLC leaves for the simple intensity pattern shown in Figure 17-12, B. The pattern depicts the leaf movement from right to left. Movement of leaves requires both leaf speed modulation and dose rate modulation. In leaf speed modulation, the leaf speed of movement for each MLC leaf is controlled and varies but is constant for each segment. In dose rate modulation, a maximum dose rate is used whenever it is possible to achieve efficient delivery.[19]

Figure 17-13 illustrates intensity profiles for five IMRT photon beams in relief map format. Note the decrease in beam intensity in the center of the posterior field designed to reduce dose to the rectum (patient is prone) and the scalloping of the

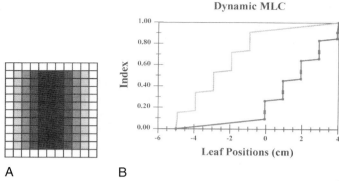

Figure 17-12. A, For a simple intensity pattern displayed in **(B)** trajectories of a pair of leaf positions as a function of monitor units when delivered using dynamic multileaf collimator with the sliding window method. (From Van Dyk J: *The modern technology of radiation oncology: a compendium for medical physicists and radiation oncologists*, vol 2, Madison, Wis., 2005, Medical Physics Publishing with permission of Xia P, Chuang CF, Verhey LJL: Communication and sampling rate limitations in IMRT delivery with a dynamic multileaf collimator system, *Med Phys* 29:412-423, 2002.)

high isodose contours in the posterior portions of the prostate closest to the rectal wall.

Fan Beam Intensity Modulation

Fan beam intensity modulation may be referred to as Tomo-Therapy. The beam is collimated to a narrow slit with modulation of the beam intensity as the gantry rotates. Treatment may consist of a continuous spiral beam covering the treatment volume or may be sequential. This method is similar in concept to the spiral

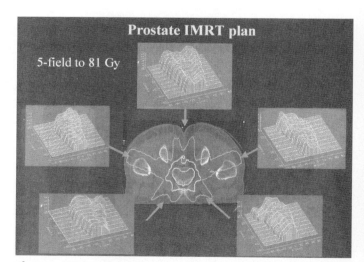

Figure 17-13. Five intensity-modulated radiation therapy photon beams for the treatment of a prostate showing intensity profiles in relief map format. Note the decrease in beam intensity in the center of the posterior field designed to reduce dose to the rectum and the resulting scalloping of the high isodose contours in the posterior portions of the prostate closest to the rectal wall. (From Sloan-Kettering Group, editors: *A practical guide to intensity-modulated radiation therapy*, Madison, Wis., 2003, Medical Physics Publishing.)

nature of a CT scanner. TomoTherapy involves a rotating fan beam that is intensity modulated with a bimodal MLC. The bimodal MLC has multiple leaf pairs similar to a more conventional MLC but differs in that each leaf pair has only two positions, completely open or completely closed. Beam intensity is modulated every 5 or 10 degrees of gantry rotation by moving leaves into and out of the beam. The slit or fan beam is 1.0 to 2.0 cm in beam width (superior to inferior) and spans broadly (transversely).

One system design uses a conventional linear accelerator with a custom-designed MLC system. Treatment is delivered by the axial "stepping" of the treatment couch as the narrow x-ray beam rotates around the patient. This is a sequential treatment technique. The NOMOS Corporation has designed and marketed the Peacock multileaf intensity-modulating collimator (MIMiC). With the NOMOS system, the x-ray beam (commonly 6 MV) is formed by a slot collimator that rotates around the patient and treats a transverse section of the patient 2 cm thick. After one section of the patient is treated, the patient is translated 2 cm and the next continuous transverse section is treated. The process is repeated until the entire target volume has been treated. The mechanical motions of this type of system are identical to second-generation rotate-translate CT scanners.[2]

A more highly dedicated TomoTherapy system is designed with the donut shape of a CT scanner. The linear accelerator produces a 6-MV fan x-ray beam that rotates and modulates by the opening and closing of an MLC system. Treatment progresses as the treatment couch moves through the treatment gantry opening, the beam rotates, and the MLC system provides beam intensity modulation. The system produces a continuous spiral beam as the photon fan beam rotates in synchrony with a translating treatment couch. This results in the delivery of a 3D intensity-modulated beam.

QUALITY ASSURANCE

General Principles

QA evolves as manufactures improve hardware for IMRT treatment delivery. Because a major objective of IMRT is to accurately deliver gradations of low doses to distinctive regions, it follows that QA focuses on mechanical accuracy of hardware to a finely tuned degree and dosimetric accuracy for low MU fields and small field sizes. In addition, patient-related QA involves treatment setup, positioning, and immobilization factors. Specific QA tests should be performed to check the accuracy of each patient's IMRT treatment field. This includes verification that all field and file names are correct and that the proper DMLC leaf motion files or sequence of static MLC segments has been downloaded to the linear accelerator. Before patient treatment, the shapes and intensity patterns of each treatment field should be verified (Figure 17-14).

Leakage

An intensity-modulated field is composed of a collection of subfields with variable intensity patterns referred to as *fluence pattern*. With static MLC-IMRT, these may be referred to as *segments*, each with uniform intensity. The delivery of radiation in this manner is inefficient because the output for each small field adds up to a larger amount than a conventional treatment technique. The total MUs for a typical IMRT treatment using an

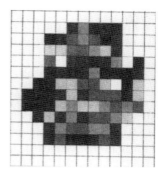 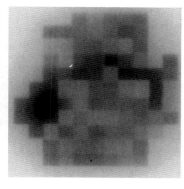

Print Out   EDR Film

Figure 17-14. Comparison between a radiographic film (EDR2; Kodak, Rochester, NY) mounted and exposed in the blocking tray of the linear accelerator and an intensity pattern calculated by the treatment planning computer. (From Xia P, Amols HI, Ling CC: Three-dimensional conformal radiotherapy and intensity modulated radiotherapy. In Leibel SA, Phillips TL, editors: *Textbook of radiation oncology*, ed 2, Philadelphia, 2004, Elsevier Saunders.)

MLC system can be up to 10 times greater than conventional radiation therapy treatment. This corresponds to greater radiation leakage from the treatment head. Leakage through the MLCs also contributes to increased patient exposure.

 The interaction of photons at energies above 10 MV with high Z material results in photodisintegration. This is the basis of neutron production and scattered dose to the patient.

Tongue-and-Groove Effects

Adjacent MLC leaves slide against each other via a tongue-and-groove design, which reduces radiation leakage. When two adjacent leaves have different degrees of extension, the tongue side of the more extended leaf protrudes out and produces an underdose region near the leaf edge. This phenomenon is referred to as the *tongue-and-groove effect*. The magnitude of dose reductions along match lines have been reported to range from 14% to 33% for Siemens, Varian, and Elekta in increasing order.[19]

 A typical IMRT treatment using MLCs requires 10 times more monitor units than conventional treatment due to the inefficiency of segmented treatment. The output for each small field adds up to a larger amount than a field treated conventionally. Potential leakage is greater.

Treatment Planning Factors

Beam data such as output factors and beam profiles are input into the IMRT planning system like in other 3D planning systems. Special measurements include penumbra, head scatter factors, radiation transmission through the MLC leaves, and leaf offset factor to correct discrepancies between the light field and the radiation field. The accuracy of the leaf sequencer that translates an optimal intensity fluence to a deliverable fluence should be verified for a pixel-based inverse planning system. It has been reported that MLC leakage and head scatter in IMRT can contribute more than 5% mean dosimetric error to the planning target volume (PTV).[11,19,21]

Small-Field Dose Calculations

MLC-based IMRT often treats small, off-axis, and irregular fields. The pronounced affect of small fields in dosimetry lies in the basis that the dose delivered per MU varies with the collimator setting and decreases sharply for field sizes smaller than 3×3 cm.[4] This is enhanced with higher energies where electronic equilibrium is more difficult to achieve. Dose deviations with small field size settings have a large effect on the resulting output. The effect of the resulting output intensifies with smaller field sizes and higher energies. A 2-mm deviation changes the resulting dose per MU by 2% and 3% for a 2- × 2-cm field for 6-MV and 18-MV energies, respectively. The same 2-mm deviation for a 1- × 1-cm field changes the resulting dose per MU by 15% and 16% for 6 MV and 18 MV, respectively.[14]

Precision of Leaf Positioning

Precise leaf positioning is of great importance for both DMLC-IMRT and MLC delivery. The dose delivered is directly related to the gap widths between pairs of opposing leaves. A systematic positional error of 1 mm for one leaf may result in a 10% dose error for the corresponding strip of tissue covered by that leaf.[11] Manufacturers provide recommendations and software for mechanical calibration of leaf positions. Routine QA should include a coincidence verification machine readout and actual radiation beam field size produced. A QA study by LoSasso, Chen-Shou, and Ling[11] for DMLC-IMRT includes comprehensive content in these procedures. Leaf position QA verification may be conducted using commercially available MLC test patterns specifically designed to test for small errors in DMLC leaf positions. This testing method can detect positioning errors smaller than 1 mm.

In some IMRT systems, leaf position is monitored during treatment by the control computer every 55 msec. If a leaf deviates from a preset tolerance, an interlock system will activate a "beam hold off" status until all leaves have regained acceptable position. It is reported that clinical field tests show that deviations greater than 1 mm occur less than 1% of the treatment delivery time. The preset tolerance level serves mainly to ensure against a "stuck" leaf. A comprehensive QA program should include the checks listed on Table 17-2. It is noted that the tests should be used for new treatment sites and software and for period spot-checks.[11]

Dose Linearity

The concept that radiation doses are cumulative and may be added is one that radiation therapists easily relate with as reflected in the patient's treatment record or file. Dose linearity is a principle that follows that same principle of adding a continuous, cumulating amount of radiation in an even and proportional magnitude. One may describe radiation doses as linear and additive. As the radiation beam is turned on and off, an "end effect" associated with the beam's interruption may disrupt the linearity. Dose linearity may be verified by comparing the dose

Table 17-2	Important Elements for DMLC Quality Assurance	
	Check	**Objective**
1	Periodic dosimetric verification of IM fields	To ensure accuracy of dose patterns and fluence
2	Biweekly coincidence check of predesigned fields using film image patterns	To provide a visual assessment of the DMLC function
3	Monthly ion chamber and diode array measurements at different gantry and collimator angles	To ensure a constant DMLC output and to track long-term stability
4	Ion chamber measurements in a solid phantom for patient fields	To provide a direct, independent check of MU calculations
5	Film dosimetry with sufficient spatial resolution for IM patterns	Efficiently compares the delivered and the planned dose distributions

DMLC, Dynamic multileaf collimator; *IM*, intensity-modulated; *MU*, monitor units.

measured when delivering 200 MU once with a dose achieved by delivering 50 MU four times. The difference between these two measurements defines the end effects for delivering 50 MU four times. The effects of the step-and-shoot technique on dose linearity is a result of many small dose segments with low MUs. An effective dose linearity check should duplicate the conditions of the step-and-shoot technique with small MU segments.

Symmetry and Flatness

For conventional treatment units, flatness and symmetry are monitored by multiple internal ionization chambers through feedback circuits that run from the ionization chambers to the bending magnet's steering coil. Beam profiles are also measured at various field sizes as a quality check for flatness and symmetry with conventional units. With segments using a small number of MUs, an ionization chamber may be used to measure point doses at several symmetric locations within a square intensity-modulated field to check the field symmetry and flatness.

Contouring

The computer optimization process in inverse planning depends greatly on the accuracy of delineated target volume and critical structures ultimately affecting the quality of treatment. The accuracy of planning and treatment delivery begins with accurate delineation of target volume and critical structures. At some institutions, the radiation oncologists contour the tumor volume directly on the treatment planning station while the medical dosimetrists contour the other structures involved. The entire work is verified by the radiation oncologists.

Dosimetric Verification

A dosimetric check at multiple specific points in a phantom ensures that each IMRT treatment plan is correct. A patient-specific phantom plan is created within the treatment planning system using the beam configurations of the patient plan but recalculated with the phantom geometry. The phantom plan can be measured using ionization chambers with diodes, thermoluminescent dosimetry, and/or film. Independent computer programs provide dosimetric QA checks as an alternative to the in-phantom dosimetry measurements that entail recalculating the dose in a phantom plus time-consuming physical measurements. Verification of absolute dose to specific points within each IMRT field must be performed either with an independent computer program or via in-phantom dosimetry measurements.

Treatment Information Routing

Treatment data including beam configuration and patient information may be routed via a local area network from a treatment planning system to a record and verify system. Verification of accuracy plays an important role to ensure that data have not been lost or modified during the data transfer process. Transferred data may be lost or altered because of incorrect default settings in some record and verify systems.[19] An enormous amount of data must be transferred from the treatment planning system to the linear accelerator and MLC computers, much more data than can be transferred manually, and much more data than can be checked manually. Confidence issues include having to trust one computer to check another computer. An ongoing comprehensive physics QA program is emphasized by much of the literature. This is stressed as one author from the Memorial Sloan-Kettering professional group eloquently states, "using the MLC control computer to monitor its own performance is akin to asking the fox to guard the chicken coop."[1] Commercially available systems integrate several systems used within the planning process to create a centralized treatment management system for easy access by all team members.

Verification of Patient Setup

Patient setup verification serves to accurately corroborate and document the initial CT isocenter relative to the treatment isocenter. Some institutions obtain a second set of orthogonal images using the treatment isocenter. The orthogonal pair is compared with the orthogonal DRRs produced by the treatment planning system or from the CT simulator to ensure the accuracy of the newly shifted isocenter. The treatment isocenter is verified again on the treatment table on day 1 of treatment. It is verified at least weekly thereafter. Commercially available verification systems are designed for combining treatment planning simulation images and motion data for verifying patient plans. High-resolution imaging capability is emphasized with modern equipment and treatment techniques. The systems support the verification of 3D treatment plans with automatic setup of 3D fields and verification using dynamic digital radiographs. Checks for dynamic IMRT before the first treatment should include the outer boundary of the treatment field and the intensity pattern. Verification may be done with radiographic film or with EPIDs.

CLINICAL APPLICATIONS

Cases are adapted from Van Dyk J: *The modern technology of radiation oncology: a compendium for medical physicists and radiation oncologists,* vol 2, Madison, Wis., 2005, Medical Physics Publishing.)

Prostate Cancer

One IMRT case for prostate cancer was planned using the forward planning method to simultaneously boost portions of the prostate gland referred to as the *dominant intraprostatic lesions (DILs)* to a high dose of 90 Gy while treating the remaining prostate gland to a conventional dose of 75.6 Gy. One DIL is located at the most distal portion of the gland on the right, and the other is located at the most proximal portion of the glad on the left. Seven coplanar gantry angles with multiple segments in each field are used in the plan, combined with the use of dynamic wedges in some fields. The shapes of these segments are designed manually in such a way that the adjacent critical structures are partially shielded from the radiation while the DILs receive full dose and the normal lobe of the prostate receives a lower conventional dose. Typically, a total of 18 MLC segments are used in these 7 beams. Figure 17-15 shows 3 MLC segments in the BEV of the right anterior oblique field for a prostate case containing two DILs. As shown, the first segment **(A)** exposes the entire tumor volume with a normal margin; the second segment **(B)** shields the rectal wall and exposes the rest of the tumor volume. The third segment **(C)** irradiates only the two DIL regions. Figure 17-16 shows the dose distributions, displayed in transverse (axial), coronal, and sagittal views. The isodose lines are displayed on an absolute dose scale ranging from 30 to 90 Gy. The contour of one of the DILs, located at the right apex, is shown in solid orange, and the PTV is shown as a pink line. Compared with inverse planned IMRT with two delivery methods, SMLC, and sequential TomoTherapy,[10] this forward planning method is able to achieve similar dose constraints for the rectal wall and bladder while maintaining similar dose coverage to the target. The biggest advantage of this forward planning method is its delivery efficiency, resulting in a treatment of approximately 7 minutes versus 15 minutes for the inverse planned IMRT plan, using a Siemens linear accelerator with an autosequence delivery system.

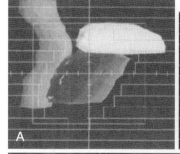
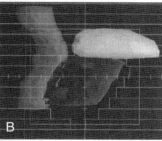
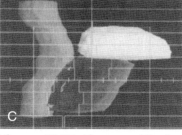

Figure 17-15. Three multileaf collimator segments in the beam's eye view of the right anterior oblique field for a prostate case containing two dominant intraprostatic lesions (DILs). The two DILs are contoured in blue, the rectum in brown, and the bladder in yellow. (From *Int J Radiat Oncol Biol Phys*, vol 48, pp. 1559-1568. Copyright 2000, and *The Modern Technology of Radiation Oncology*, Volume 2, Copyright 2003, with permission of Elsevier and Medical Physics Publishing.)

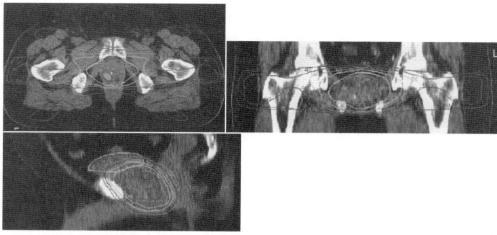

Figure 17-16. The dose distributions for a prostate case using the forward planning method, displayed in axial, coronal, and sagittal images. (From Van Dyk J: *The modern technology of radiation oncology: a compendium for medical physicists and radiation oncologists,* vol 2, Madison, Wis., 2005, Medical Physics Publishing.)

CASE II

Breast Cancer

The aperture-based planning method was used in this case to treat breast cancer. Although the conventional treatment technique using opposed tangential fields with wedging on one or both sides can create reasonably uniform dose distributions to the intact breast, an aperture-based plan without any wedges can improve dose uniformity and reduce the dose to the lung.[6,15] In the aperture-based plan, the 3D dose distribution is first calculated using equally weighted, open conventional tangential fields, and then multiple segments are constructed to conform to selected isodose surfaces (such as 110%, 105%, and so forth) projected on the BEV plane, as shown in Figure 17-17. Additional MLC segments that conform to the lung tissue in the fields are also constructed to reduce dose to the lung. This tool has been made available in commercial treatment planning systems. The relative weights of these segments can be adjusted manually or optimized by the computer using multiple sampling dose points randomly added in the entire target volume to achieve the most uniform dose to the target volume. Compared with the conventional wedge field technique, this aperture-based IMRT plan results in smaller hot spots and a lower maximum dose while maintaining similar coverage of the treatment volume. Treatment time (including patient setup) is approximately 8 to 10 minutes, and the typical planning time is 60 minutes.

CASE III

Head and Neck Cancer

The pixel-based IMRT planning method is effectively used in the treatment of head and neck cancer. Optimal use of this planning method is with nasopharyngeal cancer because of its difficult tumor location with many nearby sensitive structures. Seven to 10 coplanar beam directions are used as shown in Figure 17-18, which shows a typical isodose distribution displayed in transverse, coronal, and sagittal views. Three different treatment techniques, dependent on patient-specific clinical criteria, are described for IMRT of the nasopharynx. The first technique uses IMRT to treat only the primary tumor, with the IMRT fields matched to conventional opposed lateral fields, which are then matched to an anteroposterior supraclavicular field.

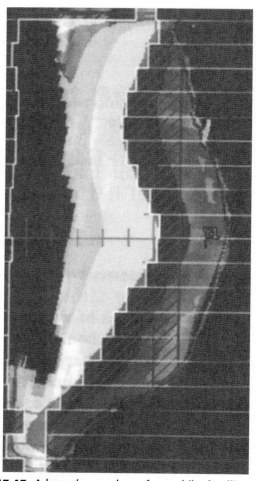

Figure 17-17. A beam's eye view of a multileaf collimator segment for tangential breast field with block corresponding to the 105% open-field isodose surface (the image demonstrates a two-dimensional central-axis reconstruction of the isodose surfaces). (From *Int J Radiat Oncol Biol Phys,* vol 48, pp. 1559-1568. Copyright 2000, and *The Modern Technology of Radiation Oncology,* Volume 2, Copyright 2003, with permission of Elsevier and Medical Physics Publishing.)

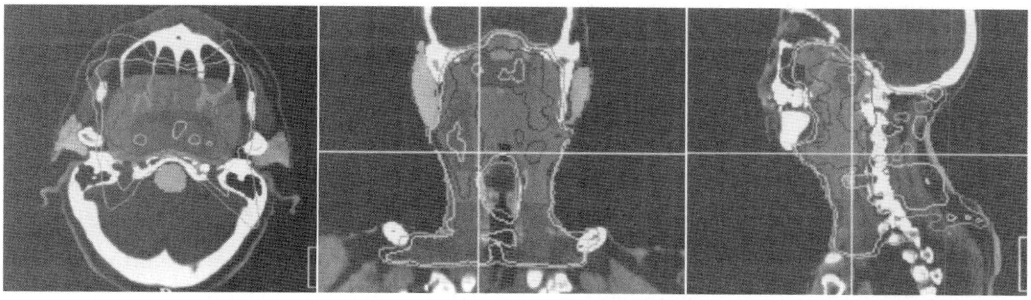

Figure 17-18. Typical isodose distributions for a nasopharyngeal case, displayed in axial, coronal, and sagittal images. (From Van Dyk J: *The modern technology of radiation oncology: a compendium for medical physicists and radiation oncologists,* vol 2, Madison, Wis., 2005, Medical Physics Publishing.)

The second technique treats the primary tumor and upper neck nodes with IMRT fields, which are matched to a conventional supraclavicular field. The third technique treats the entire PTV with IMRT. Two sets of planning dose constraint templates have been established, one for patients with early-stage nasopharyngeal tumors, and the other for those with advanced-stage tumors. The treatment goal in either case is to deliver 70 Gy at 2.12 Gy per fraction to more than 95% of the GTV and simultaneously deliver 59.4 Gy at 1.8 Gy per fraction to more than 95% of the PTV. For early-stage nasopharyngeal cancer, the maximum doses to the spinal cord, brain stem, chiasm, and optic nerves are limited to 38, 51, 28, and 24 Gy, respectively. For advanced-stage nasopharyngeal cancer, where the increased size of the PTV renders such conservative dose limits unrealistic, the maximum normal tissue doses for the spinal cord, brain stem, chiasm, and optic nerves are relaxed slightly to 43, 55, 43, and 42 Gy, respectively. The mean doses to parotid glands, temporomandibular joints, and middle/inner ears are limited to 28, 38, and 50 Gy, respectively.

The treatment planning for a nasopharynx may incorporate FDG-PET or MRI studies after the planning CT. The images are registered with the planning CT for improved tumor/normal tissue delineation over CT alone. This is done conveniently with the recent development of PET/CT units. MRI shows the tumor extent much better than CT alone. The fusion of MRI and PET images with CT images aids in tumor localization and improves planning. Figure 17-19 shows registered CT, MRI, and PET images for a patient with advanced nasopharyngeal cancer. The treatment planning CT scan shows a

very large area of abnormality that could represent either tumor or post-obstruction sinus/nasal changes depending on the area. The PET image reveals increased uptake in the bilateral retropharyngeal lymph nodes, indicating gross involvement at this level in contrast to the remaining cervical nodes. The MRI was superior to CT for evaluating the intracranial extension, due to its superior soft tissue resolution. The use of MRI in this setting increases the certainty of covering the full extent of tumor while minimizing exposure to healthy brain tissue.[4]

CASE IV

Nasopharynx

The following nasopharynx case splits a field due to the limitation of the DMLC field size on the equipment. The total intensity required in the overlap is distributed between the two subfields, creating a feathered region. Ten DMLC fields are delivered from seven gantry directions. Beam directions and intensity profiles for the intensity-modulated field approximately 16 cm wide and its split subfield are illustrated in Figures 17-20 and 17-21. The dose distributions and DVHs are shows in Figure 17-22. A prescription dose of 70 Gy is delivered to gross disease (PTV) and 54 Gy to the elective nodal regions (PTV). The spinal cord and brain stem received 45 Gy, the average mean dose

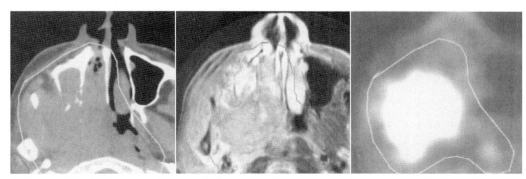

Figure 17-19. Computed tomography, magnetic resonance imaging, and ^{18}F-fluorodeoxyglucose positron emission tomography images for a patient with primary nasopharynx cancer. (From Sloan-Kettering Group, editors: *A practical guide to intensity-modulated radiation therapy,* Madison, Wis., 2003, Medical Physics Publishing.)

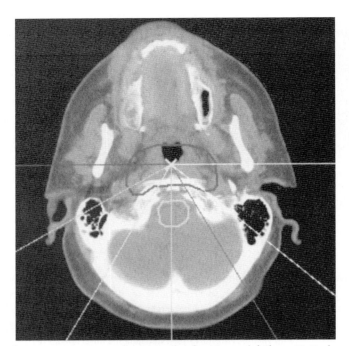

Figure 17-20. Beam directions for the Memorial Sloan-Kettering Cancer Center intensity-modulated radiation therapy nasopharynx technique. Typically, 10 treatment fields directed from seven gantry angles are used. (From Sloan-Kettering Group, editors: *A practical guide to intensity-modulated radiation therapy*, Madison, Wis., 2003, Medical Physics Publishing.)

to the parotid glands is 27 Gy, and the cochleae received an average maximum dose of 64 Gy. The supraclavicular nodes are treated with a single anterior lower neck field, the superior edge, which is matched to the IMRT fields.[4]

RECENT ADVANCES

Positon Emission Tomography/Computed Tomography Simulation

The development of the PET/CT simulator has been the next upgrade from the CT simulator. Combination PET/CT units housed in a common gantry is a desired feature among centers to allow patients to be scanned in the same position and imaging session. This is noted to improve the registration quality of PET and CT images, improving the fused planning images.

Low-Dose/High-Resolution Kilovoltage X-ray Imaging

The evolution of new technology in computerization, plasma viewing, medical imaging, and beam production is making the integration of complex systems into one gantry possible. The focus in targeting and tracking a tumor during treatment delivery as part of IGRT continues to evolve. Systems combine technologies to produce more sophistication in tracking and definition. Low-dose, high-resolution kilovoltage x-ray imaging and integrated software have been developed to verify all treatment parameters. One system has incorporated a unique 150-kV x-ray tube designed for generating precise, high-resolution CT-quality images from a moving gantry.

Another system that combines high and low energies for treatment delivery is referred to as *adaptive radiation therapy (ART)*. The system provides both kilovoltage and megavoltage imaging capabilities by providing a separate radiation source and imaging panel for each energy range. Each energy range is then used to provide the images necessary for dose-guided radiation therapy. The arrangement of the sources and imaging panels are 180 degrees (in-line) from one another, which allows imaging of both the patient and the treatment at the same time. In addition, this provides synchronized image and dose monitoring, quality cone beam information correlated with the treatment plan, and both entrance and exit treatment ports.

Four-Dimensional TomoTherapy Treatment Technique

A four-dimensional TomoTherapy technique with improved motion control and patient tolerance has been investigated. The technique used achieved a dose distribution on the moving target similar to that of conventional treatment for a static target. Breathing synchronization successfully delivered a feasible four-dimensional TomoTherapy treatment technique.[22]

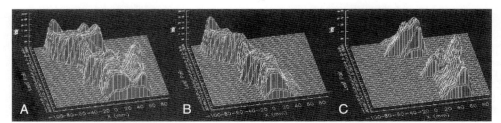

Figure 17-21. Intensity profiles for a left lateral nasopharynx field before (**A**) and after (**B** and **C**) field splitting to overcome the dynamic multileaf collimator maximum field width limitation. (From Sloan-Kettering Group, editors: *A practical guide to intensity-modulated radiation therapy*, Madison, Wis., 2003, Medical Physics Publishing.)

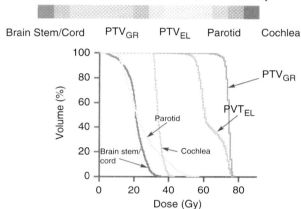

Figure 17-22. Axial dose distributions through the nasopharynx and neck for a seven-field intensity-modulated radiation therapy plan. (From Sloan-Kettering Group, editors: *A practical guide to intensity-modulated radiation therapy*, Madison, Wis., 2003, Medical Physics Publishing.)

SUMMARY

- Multileaf collimator intensity-modulated radiation therapy (MLC-IMRT) uses the collimators as a physical filter to modify the beam the same way a compensator may be used in conventional radiation therapy. IMRT works by adjusting two beam properties: beam shape and dose delivered. A segment refers to the shape that the mechanical aperture, the MLCs, create within a sequence of collimator patterns. By changing the beam shape, through the use of multiple segments, an intensity-modulated field is produced.
- A basic difference regarding treatment planning is that of forward planning using a predicted dose response to tissue for conventional radiation therapy versus inverse planning. Another difference involves manual portal design, specifically in regard to shielding. In terms of treatment delivery, conventional treatment design produces radiation in a rectangular form that requires the use of customized blocks to deliver an irregular beam shape. Even with the use of an MLC system, shielding serves the sole purpose of collimation system. IMRT involves sophisticated treatment planning systems to optimize treatment delivery using fluence patterns as a product of several segmented treatment shapes to affect beam intensity.

- Forward planning is typical of standard three-dimensional conformal radiation therapy (3D CRT), in which an individual specifies beam directions, weighting, and so on. After beam parameters are specified by the dosimetrist, the computer calculates the resulting dose distribution.
- In full inverse planning, the dosimetrist does not directly attempt to optimize or adjust beam intensities. The dosimetrist specifies desired dose limits or constraints for the target and sensitive structures after defining orientation and energy of the beams. Computer optimization then defines the intensity fluences for each selected beam that yields a dose distribution that meets the desired dose constraints.
- Linac-based IMRT with physical modulators uses milled compensating filters, which are constructed from various attenuation materials such as brass or Cerrobend.

Review Questions

Multiple Choice

1. The role of multileaf collimation is to produce a beam shape consistent with the 3D volume of the _____, referred to as beam sculpting.
   a. normal tissue
   b. tumor and surrounding tissue
   c. tumor
   d. field
2. The role of IMRT is to produce a beam that varies the radiation intensity delivered to the tumor volume producing changes in dose delivered as a function of _____ within the field and tumor status. This forms the basis of the DVH.
   a. tissue volume
   b. monitor units
   c. critical structures
   d. total dose
3. In inverse treatment planning, the planner _____ MLC settings.
   a. specifies
   b. does not specify
4. In inverse treatment planning, desired doses _____ to the tumor, as well as to normal tissues.
   a. are specified
   b. are not specified
5. Treatment portals are designed using the perspective of a:
   a. medical physicist
   b. oncology certified nurse
   c. certified dosimetrist
   d. beam's eye view
6. Computer iterations are performed to establish:
   a. dose patterns
   b. leaf movement files
   c. optimization
   d. field placement
7. Plan evaluation for IMRT relies on analysis of dose distribution to assess dose to designated normal tissue. One item of study includes the:
   a. dose-volume histogram
   b. port film

c. electronic portal imaging detector

d. record and verify system

8. PET is an effective modality of biologic imaging, useful for tumor delineation because:

a. the magnetic frequency highlights tumor

b. photon emission has been shown to define active cellular proliferation

c. protons are attracted to the tumor

d. glucose metabolism of cancer cells take up the ^{18}F-fluorodeoxyglucose

9. The step-and-shoot IMRT delivery systems are of higher complexity than dynamic systems requiring complicated leaf speed and dose rate modulation.

a. true

b. false

10. A fluence pattern may also be referred to as a(n):

a. intensity profile

b. beam direction pattern

c. wedged pattern

d. filter profile

The answers to the Review Questions can be found by logging on to our website at: *http://evolve.elsevier.com/Washington+Leaver/principles*

Questions to Ponder

1. Today's mass communication industry has marketed the term *high definition* (HD) in various forms that appeal to the human senses. Draw a parallel with HD and the trend toward high resolution ability in radiation therapy. Do they both enhance visual acuity and our perspectives, making new things possible?

2. Wedges, boluses, and customized compensators have traditionally been used to "trick the beam," accounting for an abrupt change within the treated field. The objective was to modify the beam, creating a more homogenous distribution. What is meant by IMRT using anatomy/physiology as a guide for beam optimization?

3. Computer optimization uses a cost function in the inverse planning process. Explain the process involving computer iterations, beam weights, a dose-based objective function, and the final score to evaluate the final treatment plan.

4. Explain why the total MUs for a typical IMRT treatment using an MLC system can be up to 10 times greater than a conventional treatment system.

5. One of the principal radiation interactions with matter is responsible for the production of neutrons, resulting in a scattered dose to the patient. Name the interaction, the minimum energy level of occurrence, and the connection to IMRT.

REFERENCES

1. Amos HI, Ling CC, Leibel SA: Overview of the IMRT process. In Sloan-Kettering Group, editors: *A practical guide to intensity-modulated radiation therapy*, Madison, Wis, 2003, Medical Physics Publishing.

2. Boyer AL: Intensity-modulated radiation therapy. In Kahn FM: *Treatment planning in radiation oncology*, ed 2, Philadelphia, 2007, Lippincott Williams & Wilkins.

3. Chin L, et al: A computer-controlled radiation therapy machine for pelvic and paraaortic nodal areas, *Int J Radiat Oncol Biol Phys* 7:61-70, 1981.

4. Chong LM, Hunt MA: IMRT for head and neck cancer. In Sloan-Kettering Group, editors: *A practical guide to intensity-modulated radiation therapy*, Madison, Wis, 2003, Medical Physics Publishing.

5. Compensator IMRT (website): www.touchbriefings.com/pdf/2460/chang.pdf. Accessed January 21, 2008.

6. Evans PM, et al: The delivery of intensity modulated radiation therapy to the breast using multiple static fields, *Radiother Oncol* 5:79-89, 2000.

7. Fraass BA, Eisbruch A: Conformal therapy: treatment planning, treatment delivery, and clinical results. In Gunderson LL, Tepper JE, editors: *Clinical radiation oncology*, ed 2, Philadelphia, 2007, Elsevier Churchill Livingstone.

8. Kistin LL, et al: Intensity modulation to improve dose uniformity with tangential breast radiation therapy: initial clinical experience, *Int J Radiat Oncol Biol Phys* 48:1559-1568, 2000.

9. Leaver DL: Intensity modulated radiation therapy: Part 1, *J Radiat Oncol Sci Radiat Ther* 11:115, 2002.

10. Ling CC, et al: Imaging for IMRT. In Sloan-Kettering Group, editors: *A practical guide to intensity-modulated radiation therapy*, Madison, Wis, 2003, Medical Physics Publishing.

11. LoSasso T, Chen-Shou C, Ling C: Comprehensive quality assurance for the delivery of intensity modulated radiation therapy with a multileaf collimator used in the dynamic mode, *Med Phys* 28:2209-2219, 2001.

12. Prado KL, Starkschall G, Mohan R: Three-dimensional conformal therapy. In Kahn FM: *Treatment planning in radiation oncology*, ed 2, Philadelphia, 2007, Lippincott Williams & Wilkins.

13. Santanam L, et al: Intensity modulated neutron radiotherapy for the treatment of adenocarcinoma of the prostate, *Int J Radiat Oncol Biol Phys* 68:1546-1556, 2007.

14. Sharp MB, et al: Monitor unit setting for intensity modulated beams delivered using a step-and-shoot approach, *Med Phys* 27:2719-2725, 2000.

15. Shepard DM, et al: Direct aperture optimization: a turnkey solution for step-and-shoot IMRT, *Med Phys* 29:1007-1018, 2000.

16. Van Dyk J: Advances in modern radiation therapy. In Van Dyk J, editor: *The modern technology of radiation oncology: a compendium for medical physicists and radiation oncologists*, vol 2, Madison, Wis, 2005, Medical Physics Publishing.

17. Xia P, Amols HI, Ling CC: Three-dimensional conformal radiotherapy and intensity modulated radiotherapy. In Leibel SA, Phillips TL, editors: *Textbook of radiation oncology*, ed 2, Philadelphia, 2004, WB Saunders.

18. Xia, P, et al: Forward or inversely planned segmental multileaf collimator IMRT and sequential tomotherapy to treat multiple dominant intraprostatic lesions of prostate cancer to 90 Gy, *Int J Radiat Oncol Biol Phys* 51:244-254, 2001.

19. Xia P, Verhey LJ: Intensity modulated radiation therapy. In Van Dyk J, editor: *The modern technology of radiation oncology: a compendium for medical physicists and radiation oncologists*, vol 2, Madison, Wis, 2005, Medical Physics Publishing.

20. Xiao YJ, et al: An optimized forward-planning technique for intensity modulated radiation therapy, *Med Phys* 27:2093-2099, 2002.

21. Yang Y, Xing L: Incorporating leaf transmission and head scatter corrections into step-and-shoot leaf sequences for IMRT, *Int J Radiat Oncol Biol Phys* 55:1121-1134, 2003.

22. Zhang T, et al: Breathing-synchronized delivery: a potential four-dimensional tomotherapy treatment technique, *Int J Radiat Oncol Biol Phys* 68:1572-1578, 2007.

BIBLIOGRAPHY

Khan FM: Introduction: process, equipment, and personnel. In Khan FM, editor: *Treatment planning in radiation oncology*, ed 2, Philadelphia, 2007, Lippincott Williams & Wilkins.

Sloan-Kettering Group, editors: *A practical guide to intensity-modulated radiation therapy*, Madison, Wis, 2003, Medical Physics Publishing.

Van Dyk J, editor: *The modern technology of radiation oncology: a compendium for medical physicists and radiation oncologists*, vol 2, Madison, Wis, 2005, Medical Physics Publishing.

Radiation Safety and Protection

Joseph S. Blinick, Elizabeth G. Quate

Outline

Objectives

- Identify the types and sources of radiation emitted during radioactive decay.
- List the units used with various radiation quantities.
- Understand the operation of instruments used to measure radiation, and determine which one is best suited for a particular measurement.
- List the risks associated with exposure to radiation.

- List and give examples of the three principal means of minimizing radiation exposure.
- Discuss the information needed to perform radiation shielding design for therapy equipment.
- Identify the equipment needed to ensure safe operation of a radiation therapy department.
- Identify the equipment needed to ensure safe performance of brachytherapy procedures.

Key Terms

The levels of radiation **exposure** in a radiation therapy department can be quite high. Thus, it is important to consider the principles of radiation protection to avoid unnecessary exposure to patients, operators, and the public.

In this chapter, we discuss types of radiation and their sources, as well as the detection and measurement of levels of radiation in the environment of a therapy department. We also discuss the risks of exposure to **ionizing radiation** (radiation with sufficient energy to separate an electron from its atom), the regulatory requirements for limits of exposure to radiation for various groups, and practical methods for individual radiation protection.

DETECTION AND MEASUREMENT

Types of Radiation

Within a radiation therapy department, there are two major groups of radiation sources. The first comprises external beam therapy machines, such as cobalt teletherapy units or linear accelerators. These use gamma rays, x-rays, and sometimes, electrons. The second group comprises brachytherapy sources, which use gamma rays and x-rays from sources such as cesium-137 (^{137}Cs), iridium-192 (^{192}Ir), and iodine-125 (^{125}I). Sources in this group may also emit alpha and beta particles. Table 18-1 summarizes types of ionizing radiation and some of their characteristics.

Alpha particles. **Alpha particles** consist of two protons and two neutrons and are therefore simply helium nuclei. They are emitted from unstable heavy nuclei such as radium or radon during the decay process. Because of their charge and relatively heavy mass, alpha particles can travel only short distances (most can be stopped by a sheet of paper), but they produce intense ionization and are therefore high **linear energy transfer (LET)** radiation (see Chapter 4 for a discussion of LET). Thus, they are extremely hazardous if ingested or inhaled but are less dangerous if the exposure is external. Alpha particles emitted by radium and radon are easily stopped by the material used to encapsulate the sources. If the integrity of

Table 18-1	Types of Ionizing Radiation			
Type of Radiation	**Charge Number**	**Atomic Mass**	**Origin**	
Alpha particles (α)	+2	4	Nucleus	
Beta particles				
Negatron (β⁻)	−1	0	Nucleus	
Positron (β⁺)	+1	0	Nucleus	
Neutrinos (ν)	0	0	Nucleus	
X-rays	0	0	Electron shells	
Gamma rays (γ)	0	0	Nucleus	

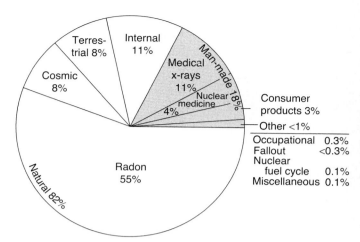

Figure 18-1. The total average effective dose equivalent for the U.S. population results from many sources of both natural and man-made radiation. This diagram illustrates the percentage that each of these sources contributes to the effective dose equivalent. (From National Council on Radiation Protection & Measurements: *Report No. 93, Ionizing radiation exposure of the population of the United States,* Bethesda, Md, 1987, NCRP Publications.)

the capsule is compromised, however, exposure to alpha particles is possible.

Beta particles. Beta particles are electrons emitted by the nucleus. They may be either negatively charged (negatron or β⁻) or positively charged (positron or β⁺). Positrons are not stable and may exist for only very short periods of time. Whenever beta particles are emitted, they are accompanied by a small, massless, chargeless particle known as the *neutrino* (see Chapter 14). Both types of beta particles have the same rest mass as an electron and are usually emitted from the nucleus with high velocities. Beta particles and energetic electrons are more penetrating than alpha particles and may pose both an external and an internal threat. High-energy (1 MeV) beta particles may have a range as long as 2 cm within soft tissue. Metals may be used for shielding, but bremsstrahlung radiation may result. The probability of bremsstrahlung x-ray production is directly proportional to the square of the atomic number of the absorber and inversely proportional to the square of the mass of the incident particle.[1] Thus, bremsstrahlung radiation is much more likely to occur with beta particles than with alpha particles. It is often more suitable to shield beta particles with low–atomic number materials, such as plastics or glass, than with metals, such as lead or steel.

X-rays and gamma rays. X-rays and gamma rays are both forms of electromagnetic radiation (photons). **Photons** have no mass and no charge. **Gamma rays** are photons emitted from a nucleus. **X-rays** are extranuclear and result from rearrangements within the electron shells or from bremsstrahlung radiation. Except for their origin, there is no difference between x-rays and gamma rays. X-rays and gamma rays may be more penetrating than either alpha or beta particles, and substantial shielding may be required, depending on the energy of the photon.

 X-rays, gamma rays, and electrons are the most common types of ionizing radiation used in radiation therapy.

Sources of Radiation

People have been exposed to naturally occurring ionizing radiation since the beginning of time. However, it was not until the beginning of the 20th century that the general public had any exposure to man-made sources of radiation. In fact, even today, it is estimated that 82% of the radiation exposure of

the U.S. population comes from natural background sources[5] (Figure 18-1).

Natural background radiation comes from three sources: cosmic rays that bombard the earth, terrestrial radiation that emanates from radioactive materials naturally occurring in the earth, and internal deposits of radionuclides in our bodies:

1. *Cosmic rays.* Cosmic rays originate from nuclear reactions in space or from our own sun. Although the earth's atmosphere acts as a protective shield against much of the initial bombardment, the primary cosmic rays interact with molecules in the atmosphere to create other reactive agents, known as *secondary particles.* These include neutrons, protons, and pions (short-lived subnuclear particles), which go on to produce energetic electrons, muons (another subnuclear particle), and photons. The average annual effective dose equivalent at sea level in the United States from cosmic rays is approximately 0.26 millisieverts (mSv) (26 millirems [mrem]). The exposure from cosmic rays varies with solar sunspot cycles, latitude, and altitude. The magnetic nature of the earth accounts for the variation in dose resulting from latitude. The charged particles incident on the earth are drawn along the magnetic field lines, which are directed toward the poles. Thus, exposure is higher at the polar regions than at the equator. Latitude, solar cycles, and other factors may account for a variation of 10% in exposure. The intensity varies even more with increasing elevation. The dose approximately doubles with each 2000 meter (m) increase in altitude in the lower atmosphere, because there is less atmosphere to absorb the incident rays. People in Denver (elevation 1600 m) receive approximately 0.5 mSv (50 mrem) from cosmic rays.[5]

2. *Terrestrial radiation.* The earth is made up of hundreds of materials, many of which are naturally radioactive because of the presence of small amounts of long-lived isotopes of uranium, thorium, and radium, among others. This is the source of terrestrial radiation. The distribution of these materials varies with geographic location and the composition of the soil in the area. In the United States, the average annual effective dose equivalent is 0.16 mSv (16 mrem) along the Eastern Seaboard but may be as high as 0.63 mSv (63 mrem) in the Rocky Mountains.[5] Additional exposure to the public occurs because many materials used in construction contain these radioactive elements. The largest exposure to terrestrial radiation involves radon. Radon may be particularly harmful because it is an easily inhaled gas and it and its many progeny emit alpha and beta particles, as well as gamma rays. Lung tissue can be damaged as deposited products decay. Radon concentration in houses varies greatly with the makeup of the soil, the design of the building, and the degree to which the building is airtight. The average radon concentration in the United States is 37 millibecquerel/L (1 pCi/L), which yields approximately 2 mSv (200 mrem) to the bronchial epithelium per year.[2] The Environmental Protection Agency (EPA) estimates that radon exposure is the second leading cause of lung cancer in the United States (following smoking).[8]

3. *Internal exposure.* Internal exposure results from the radioactive materials that are normally present in our bodies. These include carbon-14, hydrogen-3, strontium-90, potassium-40, and very small amounts of uranium and thorium. Potassium-40 delivers the highest dose to the body (0.2 mSv/yr or 20 mrem/yr). Again, concentrations of these radioactive materials in the body depend on geographic location.

The average annual *effective dose equivalent* in the United States resulting from natural background radiation is estimated to be approximately 1.0 mSv (100 mrem) from all sources except radon. When radon is taken into consideration, the average increases to approximately 3.0 mSv (300 mrem).[5] These values can vary greatly. In the Kerala region of India, for example, the annual dose may be as great as 13 mSv (1300 mrem).[2]

Man-made sources also contribute to the annual dose to individuals. These sources include medical x-rays, nuclear medicine procedures, consumer products such as televisions and tobacco products, nuclear reactors, and the fuel cycle and fallout from above-ground nuclear weapons testing. These sources emit a broad spectrum of alpha and beta particles, electrons, x-rays, and gamma rays. The average annual effective dose equivalent from these sources to an exposed individual is approximately 0.60 mSv (60 mrem). Medical procedures contribute approximately 0.50 mSv (50 mrem) of that total, and consumer products contribute another 0.11 mSv (11 mrem).[5] The other sources together contribute less than 1% of the dose from man-made sources. However, the potential for much higher radiation exposure from these nuclear sources is evident in light of the atomic bomb explosions at Hiroshima and Nagasaki, Japan, in 1945 and the Chernobyl power plant incident in the Soviet Union in 1986. The other significant dose from man-made sources is from

tobacco products. Smokers inhale radioactive materials that are present naturally in tobacco (primarily polonium-210) and may receive an additional annual effective dose equivalent of 13 mSv (1300 mrem).[5]

Most of the radiation to which the general population is exposed comes from natural background radiation, smokers excluded. It is not possible to effectively protect the entire population from these sources. That is why it is important to do all we can to minimize the radiation exposures from man-made sources, and why we strive to develop and implement valid radiation protection practices.

Units

Exposure is defined as the amount of ionization produced by photons in air per unit mass of air. The traditional unit for exposure is the Roentgen. One Roentgen (R) of exposure creates 2.58×10^{-4} Coulomb (C) of charge per kilogram (kg) of air. The Système Internationale (SI) unit for exposure is C/kg of air (see Table 18-2 for conversions between traditional units and SI units). Exposure is defined only for ionization produced by photons interacting with air. For practical reasons, exposure is limited to photons whose energy is less than 3 MeV.

Absorbed dose is defined as the energy absorbed per unit mass of any material. The traditional unit for absorbed dose is the rad, defined as 100 ergs of energy absorbed per gram of absorbing material. The comparable SI unit is the gray (Gy), which is defined as 1 joule of energy absorbed per kilogram of absorbing material (1 Gy = 100 cGy = 100 rad). For interactions between photons and soft tissue (i.e., most tissue other than bone), the numeric values for absorbed dose in rad and the exposure in R will be the same to within 10%. This difference may be ignored for radiation protection purposes but is significant when therapeutic doses to patients are being calculated or measured.

Dose equivalent takes into account the fact that different types of radiation produce different amounts of biologic damage. Alpha particles and neutrons, for example, are high-LET radiation and therefore have a greater biologic effect than x-rays. Thus, a 0.2-Gy (20-cGy) absorbed dose of alpha particles would be more damaging to a given mass of human tissue than a 0.2-Gy absorbed dose of x-rays. To account for these differences in biologic response, each type of radiation is assigned a quality factor (QF). Table 18-3 lists certain types of radiation and their QF, or weighting factor. The traditional unit, rem, is defined as the product of the absorbed dose in rads multiplied by the QF. The SI unit is the sievert (Sv), and it is defined as the absorbed dose in gray multiplied by the QF. For photons and most electrons, the QF is taken to be 1, so the numerical values

Table 18-2	Traditional and SI Unit Equivalents	
	Traditional Units	**SI Units**
Exposure	1 roentgen	2.58×10^{-4} C/kg
Absorbed dose	100 rad	1 Gy
	1 rad	1 cGy
Dose equivalent	100 rem	1 Sv
Activity	1 Ci	3.7×10^{10} Bq

Table 18-3	Quality Factors (QFs) for Various Ionizing Radiations	
Type of Radiation		**QF**
X-rays and gamma rays (γ)		1
Beta particles, positrons, and muons		1
High-energy external protons		1
Protons, other than recoil protons and energy >2 MeV		2
Thermal neutrons		5
Fast neutrons		20
Alpha particles		20
Fission fragments, other heavy nuclei		20

Adapted from NCRP: *Report No. 116: Limitation of exposure to ionizing radiation,* Bethesda, Md, 1993.

of the dose equivalent in sievert or rem and the absorbed dose in gray are the same.

Effective dose equivalent takes into account the effect of irradiation of only part of the body or the effect of nonuniform irradiation of the body. The dose to each significant organ is multiplied by a weighting factor for that organ, and the sum is taken. The resultant value provides a measure of the risk to the individual that a uniform exposure to the entire body of the same value would have. The units for effective dose equivalent are also the sievert and the rem.

Activity is the rate at which a radioactive isotope undergoes nuclear decay. The traditional unit of activity is the curie (Ci), which is defined as 3.7×10^{10} disintegrations per second. The SI unit is the becquerel (Bq), which is 1 disintegration per second.

1 Ci = 1000 mCi; 1 mCi = 1000 μCi

Measurement Devices

Many instruments and devices can be used to detect radiation, and several find use within the radiation oncology department. An instrument designed to calibrate the radiation output of a therapy machine will not necessarily be suitable for measuring low levels of radioactive contamination. It is important to understand the characteristics of each measuring device and the applications for which each is used.

Gas-Filled Detectors.   One type of device is the gas-filled detector. This instrument has a chamber filled with a gas that is ionized in part or whole when radiation is present. Either the total quantity of electrical charge is measured or the rate at which charge is produced is measured. Two kinds of gas-filled detectors may be found in a radiation therapy department. These are the ionization chamber and the Geiger-Müller (G-M) detector. The simplest of these, the ionization chamber, consists of two electrodes within a gas-filled chamber, an applied voltage across the electrodes, and electronics and a meter to amplify and measure the electrical signal (Figure 18-2). The sensitivity of the chamber (smallest amount of radiation detectable) depends on the mass of gas within the chamber (chamber volume). The response of the chamber also depends on the applied voltage (Figure 18-3). If there is no voltage, the positive and negative

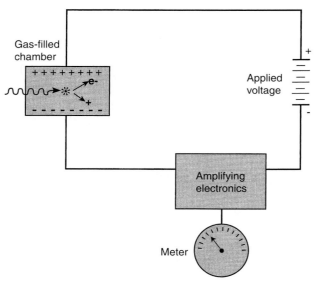

Figure 18-2. An ionization chamber that consists of two electrodes within a gas-filled chamber. A voltage is applied across the electrodes. Electronics and a meter are used to amplify and measure the electrical signal.

ions produced in the gas by the radiation will recombine instead of migrating to either of the electrodes. As the voltage across the electrodes is increased, more and more of the ions produced in the chamber will be collected on the electrodes; positive ions migrate to the cathode and negative ions to the anode. Ideally, ionization chambers should be operated at a voltage at which all of the ion pairs are collected and none recombine. Such a voltage (typically 100 to 300 volts) is said to produce saturation. When a positive ion reaches the cathode, it combines with one of the negative charges to form a neutral atom. This leaves a negative charge vacancy on the cathode, which is filled by a negative charge (electron) from the battery. The electrometer detects either the total charge that flows or the rate of charge flow and displays the value on the meter. The calibration can be set to read milliRoentgen (mR) or mR/hour.

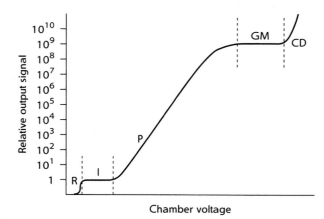

Figure 18-3. The signal output from a gas-filled chamber depends on applied voltage. The stages of the chamber response are *R,* recombination region; *I,* ionization region; *P,* proportional region; *GM,* Geiger-Müller region; *CD,* region of continuous discharge. (From Bushong SC: *Radiologic science for technologists: physics, biology, and protection,* ed 7, St. Louis, 2000, Mosby.)

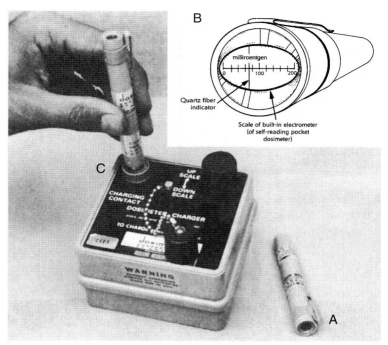

Figure 18-4. Pocket ionization chamber. **A**, The pocket ionization chamber, or pocket dosimeter, resembles a fountain pen. **B**, The quartz fiber indicator of the built-in electrometer of the self-reading pocket dosimeter generally used in radiology indicates exposures of 0 to 5.2 × 10^{-5} C/kg (0 to 200 milliRoentgens). **C**, Before use, the pocket dosimeter must be charged to a predetermined voltage by a special charging unit so that the charges of the positive and negative electrodes will be balanced and the quartz fiber indicator reads zero. (Courtesy Dosimeter Corporation of America, Cincinnati, Ohio.)

When ionization chambers are properly calibrated, their accuracy approaches 2%, which makes them suitable for measurement of the radiation output of therapy equipment. Ionization chambers with large air volumes are also suitable for environmental surveys around therapy rooms.

A form of ionization chamber, the pocket dosimeter, is used for personnel monitoring (Figure 18-4). In this chamber, the electrodes are arranged concentrically—that is, one electrode is in the form of a thin rod and the other is a cylinder around it. When fully charged, a thin filament within the unit is displaced by static electricity to one end of a scale that can be viewed by holding the dosimeter up to a light. As radiation ionizes the air within the chamber, the ions deplete the charges on the electrodes and the filament is not displaced as far. The instrument is calibrated so that the position of the filament indicates the amount of exposure received by the chamber.

Because ionization chambers are not very sensitive, they are not suitable for the detection of very low levels of radiation or radiation contamination.

If the chamber voltage is increased beyond that of the saturation region, the primary ions are energetic enough to produce additional ionizations, or secondary ions, in the gas. The G-M region is reached as the voltage of the chamber is increased even further. An avalanche of secondary ions is produced for each primary ionization that occurs, so individual events can be detected. This makes the G-M counter a very sensitive instrument and appropriate for detecting low levels of radiation or

radioactive contamination (Figure 18-5). G-M detectors tend to be strongly energy dependent, which means they respond differently to different photon energies. In addition, if a G-M detector is placed in a high-level radiation field, it may produce a reading of zero because of overloading of the gas-filled detector. Increasing the voltage beyond the G-M range causes the gas insulation to break down. Electrical arcing occurs, and a continuous electrical discharge is produced. There is no useful reason for a detector to operate in this range, and damage to the chamber may result.

 Because of their sensitivity, G-M detectors are best for finding contamination and other low levels of radiation.

Thermoluminescent Dosimeters. Because of their small size, **thermoluminescent dosimeters (TLDs)** are widely used to measure radiation in a number of applications (Figure 18-6). As the name implies, thermoluminescent materials give off light when heated. Whenever a crystalline material is irradiated, electrons are released from bound states in the valence band and become free to migrate in the conduction band. An energy gap separates these two regions, and it is this energy gap that must be overcome by the energy of the incoming radiation. In most materials, electrons immediately drop back from the conduction band to the valence band with the emission of characteristic photons. However, in some materials such as lithium fluoride (LiF) with some impurities deliberately introduced into the

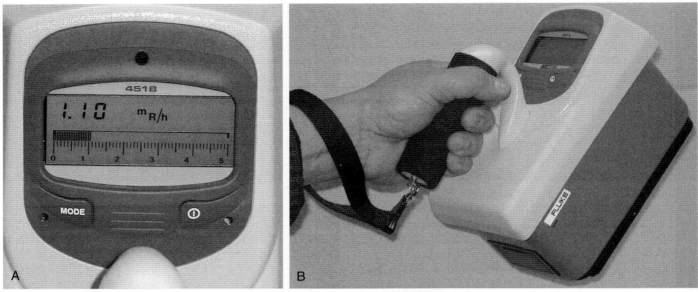

Figure 18-5. A Victoreen ion chamber survey meter. (Courtesy Fluke Biomedical, Cleveland, OH.)

crystal structure, traps appear in the energy gap, and some of the electrons that would otherwise drop back to the valence band get caught in the traps. At a later time, if the crystal is heated to 100° to 200° C, the electrons will receive enough thermal energy to move back into the conduction band. Most of them immediately fall back to the valence band with the release of the characteristic photons. In the case of LiF (and other thermoluminescent materials), these characteristic photons are within the visible light range. In general, the more radiation absorbed by the crystal, the more electrons will be in traps, and the more characteristic photons will be released when the crystal

is heated later. Thus, the amount of light is a measure of the dose received by the crystal.

The atomic number of LiF is close to that of tissue (Li has an atomic number of 3, and F has an atomic number of 9), so LiF mimics tissue closely and is therefore useful as a patient or phantom dosimeter. If proper care is taken, doses can be measured with an accuracy of approximately 5%. TLDs are also used for mailed intercomparison of therapy unit calibration, in ring badges used for personnel monitoring, and for measurements of environmental levels of radiation. In these applications, TLDs have the advantage that the dose information can be stored for hours, days,

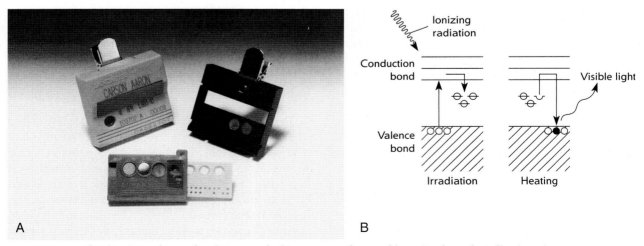

Figure 18-6. Thermoluminescent dosimeters may be used in a number of applications in a radiation therapy department. **A,** A badge containing chips may be used for personnel monitoring. **B,** Electron transitions occurring when thermoluminescent lithium fluoride is irradiated and heated. (**A,** Courtesy Landauer, Inc, Glenwood, Ill; **B,** From Bushong SC: *Radiologic science for technologists: physics, biology, and protection,* ed 7, St. Louis, 2000, Mosby.)

or even weeks, until the dosimeter is heated. However, the readings may diminish with time because some of the electrons spontaneously leak out of the traps. In addition, if the dosimeter is heated in transit, all the information may be lost. Despite this potential disadvantage, thermoluminescent dosimetry is a well-established technique for the measurement of radiation.

Film. After development, x-ray film exposed to radiation turns black. The amount of blackness is called the *optical density,* and the optical density is related to the amount of radiation received by the film. The actual relationship is not linear and depends on the type of film, the type and energy of the radiation, and the details of processing the film.

However, once calibrated, film is a convenient and inexpensive way to provide information about the doses received by individuals working in or visiting areas where radiation may be present.

A typical **film badge** has a slot in which the film (in its protective paper cover) may be placed and several thin metal filters that surround portions of the film (Figure 18-7). The filters allow discrimination between different types and energies of radiation. Low-energy radiation will not penetrate any of the filters but can reach the film in the area where no filters are present. Medium-energy radiation will penetrate the no-filter and tin filter areas but will not get through the lead filter. High-energy radiation penetrates all areas. This discrimination is necessary because of the strong energy dependence of film. The response at high energies (1 MeV) may be up to 20 times lower than the response at low energies (30 keV).

REGULATIONS AND REGULATORY AGENCIES

Advisory and Regulatory Agencies

The primary task of **advisory agencies** is to analyze the existing data related to radiation exposure and to assess the radiobiologic risks associated with those exposures. These agencies can then develop recommendations for dose limits. Some of these agencies include the National Council on Radiation Protection & Measurement (NCRP), the International Commission on Radiation Protection (ICRP), the United Nations Scientific Committee on the Effects of Atomic Radiation (UNSCEAR), and the National Academy of Sciences Advisory Committee on the Biological Effects of Ionizing Radiation (NAS-BEIR). The recommendations may be acted on by Congress or state governments and made into law.

It is the role of the **regulatory agencies** to license users of radioactive materials and radiation-producing equipment, inspect such users, and enforce the appropriate laws. One of the leading federal regulatory agencies in the United States is the Nuclear Regulatory Commission (NRC), which oversees the use of isotopes produced in nuclear reactors. These isotopes are commonly used in nuclear medicine departments, in laboratories, and as sources for teletherapy (external beam radiation) and brachytherapy (internal implants). Many states have entered into agreements concerning licensing, inspection, and enforcement with the NRC and have become "agreement" states. As part of the agreement, states must maintain a certain level of compatibility with NRC regulations.

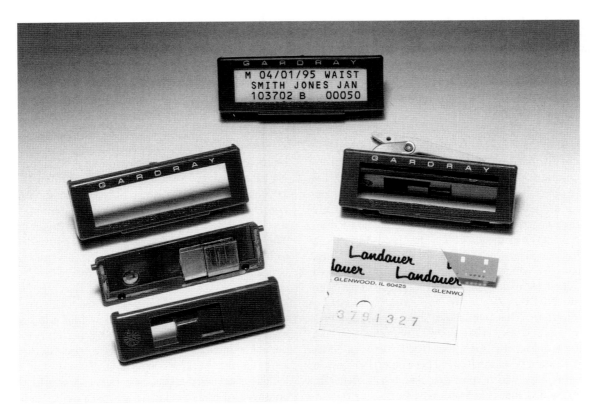

Figure 18-7. Film badge. It consists of sensitive film, several thin metal filters, and a plastic holder. (Courtesy Landauer, Inc, Glenwood, Ill.)

Transportation of radioactive materials is primarily the concern of the Department of Transportation (DOT) and the NRC. The use of machines that produce ionizing radiation, such as x-ray units and linear accelerators, falls under the jurisdiction of the Food and Drug Administration (FDA) and state agencies. The EPA and the Occupational Safety and Health Administration (OSHA) also have regulations that relate to the use of radiation.

Risk Estimates

Estimating the risks of exposure to ionizing radiation is an extremely complex and difficult process. Although we probably know more about the effects of radiation on humans than is known about any other chemical or biologic hazard, our knowledge is far from complete. Information about the risks of radiation has come from many sources, including victims of the bombs at Hiroshima and Nagasaki, at the end of World War II, people who received radiation for ankylosing spondylitis, women who received multiple fluoroscopic examinations for tuberculosis, and children treated with radiation for nonmalignant thymus and thyroid diseases.

In all of these cases, individual doses are not known precisely. In addition, individual variations are known to occur for any given radiation dose. Because there are no special effects attributable to ionizing radiation, the many effects that occur at low levels may be indistinguishable from those resulting from normal background levels.

We have a far greater knowledge of the effects of high doses of radiation than those of low doses. In sufficiently high quantities, radiation can be lethal. A single whole-body exposure of approximately 4.5 Gy (450 rads) is lethal for 50% of the exposed population within 30 days of the event. This is termed the $LD_{50/30}$.

Even at levels below the lethal dose, there are significant long-term effects related to exposure to radiation. These fall into two general classifications: nonstochastic and stochastic. Nonstochastic effects are those for which a threshold exists and for which the severity of the effect increases with dose. Examples of such effects are erythema (skin reddening), epilation (loss of hair), cataract formation, and infertility. The threshold doses for these effects are relatively high, which is reflected in the higher permitted doses to the specific organs involved. Stochastic effects are those that have no threshold and for which the probability of occurrence is a function of dose. In this case, the severity of the effect is not a function of the dose. Either the effect occurs or it does not. Examples of stochastic effects are cancer induction, genetic effects, and embryologic and teratogenic effects. Because of the lack of a threshold dose, these effects are of more concern at low levels of radiation exposure. The mechanisms by which these effects occur are discussed in Chapter 4. Risk estimates for stochastic effects have been compiled by the NCRP in *Report No. 115: Risk Estimates for Radiation Protection*.[6] This publication assesses reports prepared by the UNSCEAR (1988), the Committee on the Biological Effects of Ionizing Radiations (BEIR V) (NAS/NRC, 1990), and Publication 60 of the ICRP. These reports discuss in length the methods by which risks associated with radiation exposure are estimated and what those risks are.

Cancer Risks. The survivors of the atomic bomb explosions at both Hiroshima and Nagasaki are the primary source for

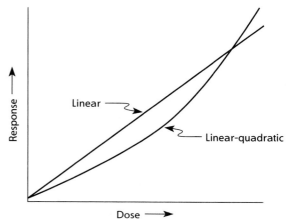

Figure 18-8. Linear and linear-quadratic dose-response curves. These are used for estimation of risks from exposure to ionizing radiation. (From Bushong SC: *Radiologic science for technologists: physics, biology, and protection,* ed 7, St. Louis, 2000, Mosby.)

estimating the cancer risks associated with ionizing radiation in NCRP Report No. 115, although data from other studies were considered. A linear-quadratic response for leukemias and a linear response for solid cancers were used in the estimation process (Figure 18-8). No distinction was made between high-dose-rate and low-dose-rate exposures. The estimate for lifetime cancer risks for acute whole-body exposure to low-LET radiation is approximately 8 in 100 per Sv (8 in 10,000 per rem).[6]

Genetic Risks. There are large uncertainties in assessing genetic risks. In part, the uncertainties occur because the effects mutations have on life-threatening illnesses such as cancer and heart disease are unknown. As a model for radiation protection guidelines, a risk of 1 in 100 per Sv (1 in 10,000 per rem) has been assigned for the occurrence of severe hereditary effects for the general population by the reporting agencies, based on animal data only.[6]

Embryologic and Teratogenic Effects. The effects of exposure to ionizing radiation on the embryo and fetus are discussed in Chapter 4. NCRP Report No. 115 primarily addresses the probability of radiation effects on the fetal brain and the possible induction of childhood cancer. The NCRP assigned an overall risk estimate of 4 in 10 per Gy (4 in 1000 per rem). Both linear and linear-quadratic responses were considered in forming this estimate. In addition, there may be threshold doses below which these effects will not be observed. The thresholds are related to gestational age and are estimated to be 0.12 to 0.23 Gy (12 to 23 rem) for 8 to 16 weeks after conception and 0.23 Gy (23 rem) for 16 to 25 weeks after conception.[6]

The NCRP further estimates that the total detriment from all causes resulting from exposure to low-LET radiation is approximately 7 in 100 per Sv (7 in 10,000 per rem) for the general population and approximately 6 in 100 per Sv (6 in 10,000 per rem) for the working population. This overall risk estimate includes fatal and nonfatal cancers, severe hereditary effects, and nonspecific life shortening.[6] These risks are higher than the previous estimates discussed in NCRP *Report No. 91: Recommendations on Limits for Exposure to Ionizing Radiation,*[4] which assigned a nominal lifetime somatic risk of 1 in 100 per Sv (1 in 10,000 per rem) for adults. It is likely that these estimates will change again as more data become available.

 The overall risk of exposure to radiation is approximately 7 in 10,000 persons per rem.

There are many uncertainties in assigning risk estimates for the effect of ionizing radiation on humans. These include difficulties in assigning individual doses, choice of appropriate control groups, choice of an appropriate extrapolation model, determination of differences between effects at low dose rates compared with effects at high dose rates, and difficulties with the transfer of risk estimates from one population to another. However, these projections are necessary to develop recommendations for radiation protection standards.

Regulatory Concepts

As Low as Reasonably Achievable (ALARA). Regardless of which models are used to estimate the risks of radiation exposure, it is universally agreed that the less radiation received, the lower the risk. For this reason, it is considered prudent to attempt to maintain exposures **as low as reasonably achievable (ALARA)**, in keeping with economic and social factors. In practice, this means that measures should be taken, whenever possible, to reduce individual exposures well below regulatory limits.

Comparable Risk. The NCRP believes that a radiation worker should be at no higher risk of death from his or her employment than a worker in other "safe" industries. A "safe" industry is defined as one in which the annual accidental fatality rate is approximately 10^{-4} (or 1 in 10,000 per year). The NCRP has made an attempt to compare injuries, illnesses, and accidental death rates in various work places with the risks of ionizing radiation, specifically; cancer induction; and severe hereditary effects. This is a difficult task, in part because of the latent nature of these effects. The effective dose equivalent limits specified by the NCRP reflect the average annual doses received by radiation workers and the risks associated with those doses that we have already discussed.

Genetically Significant Dose. The **genetically significant dose (GSD)** is a measure of the genetic risk to a population as a whole from exposure to ionizing radiation of some or all members of that population. It is the effective dose equivalent to the gonads weighted for age and sex distribution. The GSD is the gonadal dose that, if received by every member of the population, would be expected to result in the same total genetic effect on the population as the sum of the individual doses actually received. Everyone does not contribute equally to the GSD. For example, the dose received by a 60-year-old postmenopausal woman would have no effect on the genetic future of a given population. The weighting factor for that person would be zero. The dose received by a teenager would have a much higher effect, because there is a long reproductive life ahead for that person. The weighting factor assigned to the dose for the teenager would reflect the number of children he or she would likely produce. All sources of natural and man-made ionizing radiation contribute some dose to the GSD. NCRP Report No. 93[5]

(Ionizing Radiation Exposure of the Population of the United States) reports the GSD for the United States circa 1980 to 1982 was 1.3 mSv (130 mrem), of which 1.0 mSv (100 mrem) results from natural sources.

Dose Limits

The recommended effective dose equivalent limits for radiation workers and the general public are contained in NCRP Report No. 91[4] and have been adopted by the NRC and most states. These limits are summarized in Table 18-4.* There are two important points to note about these values: (1) the limits are exclusive of medical exposures for both radiation workers and the general public and (2) the limits are a summation of both internal and external exposures.

Radiation Workers. It can be seen from Table 18-4 that the effective dose equivalent (whole body) limit for radiation workers is more than that for the general public. There are relatively few radiation workers, and it is thought that a slightly increased risk to this group is worth the benefits of radiation to society at large. The same situation occurs in other occupations, such as nursing, driving a truck, or doing construction work, where the amount of risk is similar or even higher.

The effective dose equivalent, which is the limit for stochastic effects, is 50 mSv (5 rem) per year. Nonstochastic limits are set at 150 mSv (15 rem) for the lens of the eye and 500 mSv (50 rem) for all other tissues and organs, including extremities. There are special guidelines for planned special exposures and emergency situations. In general, if the limit for the whole-body dose is met by adherence to radiation safety standards at a medical facility, then the nonstochastic limits will also be met.

General Public. The NCRP recommends that the annual effective dose equivalent limit for this population be 1 mSv (0.1 rem) for persons who are exposed continuously or frequently and 5 mSv (0.5 rem) for persons who are infrequently exposed. These limits do not include doses from natural background radiation or medical procedures, which in most cases cannot be controlled.

Embryo/Fetus. The total dose equivalent for an embryo or a fetus is 5 mSv (0.5 rem) during the gestational period. It is recommended that the exposure be distributed uniformly with respect to time and should not exceed 0.5 mSv (0.05 rem) in any month.

Personnel Monitoring

Monitoring of the radiation dose received by individual radiation workers serves several purposes: (1) it allows the worker to know how much radiation he or she is receiving (at least in the area where the monitor is kept or worn), (2) it allows the facility safety officer and administration to determine whether certain areas or workers are receiving more radiation than expected, and (3) it provides a permanent record of radiation received if questions arise at a later time. The NRC and most state regulatory

---

*The NCRP has published a more recent report (NCRP Report No. 116: *Limitation of Exposure to Ionizing Radiation*, Bethesda, Md, 1993), which has some minor changes in the methodology and recommendations compared with NCRP Report No. 91.

Table 18-4	Summary of NCRP Recommendations*		
A. Occupational exposures (annual)[†]			
1. Effective dose equivalent limit (stochastic effects)		50 mSv	(5 rem)
2. Dose equivalent limits for tissues and organs (nonstochastic effects)			
a. Lens of eye		150 mSv	(15 rem)
b. All others (e.g., red bone marrow, breast, lung, gonads, skin, and extremities)		500 mSv	(50 rem)
3. Guidance: cumulative exposure		10 mSv × age in years	(1 rem × age in years)
B. Planned special occupational exposure, effective dose equivalent limit[†]			
C. Guidance for emergency occupational exposure[†]			
D. Public exposures (annual)			
1. Effective dose equivalent limit, continuous or frequent exposure[†]		1 mSv	(0.1 rem)
2. Effective dose equivalent limit, infrequent exposure[†]		5 mSv	(0.5 rem)
3. Remedial action recommended when:			
a. Effective dose equivalent[‡]		>5 mSv	(>0.5 rem)
b. Exposure to radon and its decay products[§]		>0.007 Jhm^{-3}	(>2 WLM)
4. Dose equivalent limits for lens of eye, skin, and extremities[†]		50 mSv	(5 rem)
E. Education and training exposures (annual)[†]			
1. Effective dose equivalent limit		1 mSv	(0.1 rem)
2. Dose equivalent limit for lens of eye, skin, and extremities		50 mSv	(5 rem)
F. Embryo-fetus exposures[†]			
1. Total dose equivalent limit		5 mSv	(0.5 rem)
2. Dose equivalent in a month		0.5 mSv	(0.05 rem)
G. Negligible individual risk level (annual)[†]			
Effective dose equivalent per source or practice		0.01 mSv	(0.001 rem)

From National Council on Radiation Protection and Measurements: *Report No. 116: Limitation of exposure to ionizing radiation,* Bethesda, Md, 1993.
*Excluding medical exposures.
[†]Sum of external and internal exposures.
[‡]Including background but excluding internal exposures.
[§]WLM stands for working level month and refers to a cumulative exposure for a working month (170 hr). As applied to radon and its daughter products, 1 WLM represents the cumulative exposure experienced in a 170-hour period caused by a radon concentration of 100 pCi/L. The occupational limit for miners is 4 WLM/yr, which results in an absorbed dose equivalent of approximately 0.15 Sv (15 rem) per year.
*Jhm^{-3}, Joule-hours per cubic meter.

agencies require individuals to be monitored if it is expected that 10% of the effective dose equivalent limit will be exceeded.

To be effective, devices used for personnel monitoring must be reasonably accurate, inexpensive, and easy to use. Four examples of such devices are the film badge dosimeter, the TLD, the optically stimulated luminescence (OSL) dosimeter, and the pocket ionization chamber (pocket dosimeter). The methods by which these devices work were described earlier in this chapter and are described subsequently.

A film badge is still a commonly used personnel monitoring device in medical facilities, especially if only one monitor is to be used. It is relatively inexpensive and is easy to use. The filters within the film holder allow energy discrimination to be made, which in turn allows estimates to be made of the doses received at different tissue depths. In particular, film badge readings may be used to estimate the deep dose equivalent (the dose received at a depth of 1 cm), the eye dose equivalent (that received at the depth of the lens of the eye, taken to be 0.3 cm), and the shallow dose equivalent (that received at a depth of 0.007 cm). The overall accuracy of the film badge is approximately ±20%, and erroneous readings can result if the badge is not read for a long period of time or if the film is exposed to heat and/or humidity. In addition, for most facilities the film badges cannot be read immediately on site and must be sent out, so there is always a lag between the time of exposure and the receipt of the readings.

TLDs trap electrons in their internal crystal structure when exposed to radiation. When they are heated at a later time, light is given off as the crystals rearrange themselves. The amount of light emitted is proportional to the amount of radiation absorbed. TLDs respond to radiation more like tissue than film does, which results in readings that are potentially more accurate. However, it is not possible to estimate the energy (or energy components) of the radiation beam. The TLD is less susceptible to the effects of temperature and humidity compared with film, but the individual dosimeters are more expensive than film. TLDs are primarily used in ring and wrist badges because of their small size. Like film, TLDs are usually sent out to be read, with a waiting period for receipt of the results.

Dosimeters using OSL technology are rapidly becoming the standard for use in medical facilities (Figure 18-9). This type of device uses laser light to stimulate rearrangement of electrons trapped in aluminum oxide (Al_2O_3) when it is irradiated. OSL dosimeters are more sensitive than film (minimum reading 1 mrem compared with 10 mrem for film) and, through the use of filters, can also distinguish energies allowing determination of deep, eye, and shallow doses. As is the case with both film and TLD, the dosimeters are usually sent out to be read but have the advantage of having the capability of being restimulated numerous times to confirm the accuracy of the measurement.

Optically stimulated luminescence (OSL) dosimeters have largely replaced film badge dosimeters for personnel monitoring.

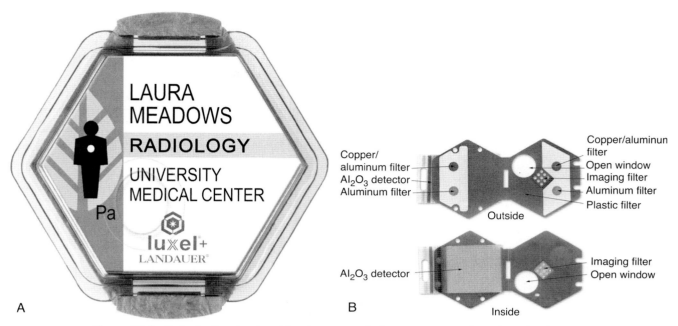

Figure 18-9. A, Optically stimulated luminescence dosimeter. **B,** It consists of an aluminum oxide strip, filters, and a welded plastic cover. (Courtesy Landauer, Inc, Glenwood, Ill.)

When the dosimeter is analyzed, it is stimulated with laser light at a selected frequency. This causes the aluminum oxide to give off light in direct proportion to the amount of radiation exposure, with accuracy as low as 1 mrem and precision of ±1 mrem. For pregnant employees and those working in low-level radiation environments, this new degree of sensitivity is an improvement over the film badge system. The Luxel dosimeter, developed by Landauer, is hexagonal in shape; comes preloaded with the aluminum oxide strip, which measures approximately 1.5 cm × 2.0 cm; and is placed between a plastic holder that incorporates three separate filters. One filter is unique in that it appears as a small metal grid of approximately 25 small holes that allow for differentiation of a single exposure or continuous exposure over days or weeks. All of these components are factory sealed within the plastic hexagonal radiation dosimeter used for x-ray, gamma-ray, and beta-ray radiation.

Pocket ionization chambers (pocket dosimeters) can be read immediately, which is a significant benefit, but they are subject to erroneous readings if exposed to humidity or mechanical shock. Their initial cost is high, but once obtained, the operating cost is low, so use of pocket dosimeters over a long period can be cost-effective when compared with the use of film or OSL badges.

PRACTICAL RADIATION PROTECTION: EXTERNAL BEAM

The radiation beams produced by radiation therapy equipment, such as linear accelerators, betatrons, and even cobalt-60 units, are much more intense than those produced by conventional x-ray units. In addition, the energy of the beams is much higher, and thus the radiation is more penetrating. For these reasons, extra care must be taken by facility designers and operators to be sure that the radiation exposure to patients, personnel in the department, and the general public is kept ALARA. The time-honored methods of radiation protection are time, distance, and shielding. In addition, there are several safety devices that contribute to the safe operation of radiation therapy facilities.

Time

As expected, the less time one is exposed to radiation, the less dose is acquired. From a practical point of view, there is little opportunity to use this method in a radiation therapy department, because all personnel are outside the therapy room when the equipment is operated. However, cobalt-60 units continuously emit small amounts of radiation even when the source is in the off position (by regulation, the maximum level cannot exceed 10 mR/hr at any point 1 m from the source, and the average level cannot exceed 2 mR/hr at 1 m from the source). Therefore it is prudent to spend as little time near the head of a cobalt-60 unit as practicable, consistent with the need to properly position the patient and any accessories. Brachytherapy patients also emit radiation after the sources have been implanted, so the time spent near such patients should be minimized.

Distance

Increasing the distance from a source of radiation can drastically reduce the radiation exposure. If the source is small, the inverse square law applies, and doubling the distance from the source reduces the exposure to one fourth its original level (Figure 18-10). If the distance is tripled, the reduction factor is 9. Even if the source is relatively large, the radiation level will fall off with distance. Again, the major applications of this method of protection are around cobalt-60 units and brachytherapy patients, because for all other therapy units the operator will be outside the treatment room during operation of the unit.

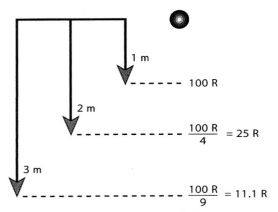

Figure 18-10. Radiation exposure. Radiation exposure from a small source is dependent on the inverse square of the distance from the source. For example, if the distance is doubled, the exposure is reduced to one fourth of its original value.

Shielding

Shielding is the most important method for protection of operators and members of the general public in a radiation therapy department. The shielding requirements for superficial x-ray therapy units are similar to those for conventional x-ray units, because the energies are similar. However, all other external beam therapy units produce radiation beams of higher energy, and the shielding requirements are consequentially greater. The choice of shielding material depends on the energy of the beam. Lead is the preferred material for superficial units because it is more effective than concrete or steel at stopping photons at these low energies, at which photoelectric collisions dominate. At higher energies, at which Compton interactions dominate (which includes cobalt-60 units, linear accelerators, and betatrons), all materials attenuate radiation equally gram for gram, and the choice of material is usually based on economic and space factors. Stated another way, a given wall may be shielded by equal masses of concrete, steel, or lead. Because of the different densities of these materials, the thickness required will be different for each material. Half-value layers for several materials at different energies are listed in Table 18-5. For cobalt-60 radiation, a 1-m (3.28-ft) thick wall of concrete may be replaced by 0.30 m (1.0 ft) of iron or 0.21 m (8.2 inches) of lead (Figure 18-11). If space is at a premium (e.g., when an existing room is being upgraded), lead or steel may be preferred, even though they are usually much more expensive than concrete. On the other hand, for new construction, concrete is usually the material of choice because of its relatively low cost.

In calculating the shielding requirements for any radiation-producing machine, several factors must be taken into account. These include the workload (W) of the machine (how many patients will be treated per week and how much radiation will be given to each one), the primary beam use factor (U) for each wall (the fraction of time of use the beam will be aimed at the wall), the occupancy factor (T) for each area adjacent to the therapy room (the fraction of time the area will be occupied), the distance (d) from the source of radiation to the occupied area, and the effective dose equivalent limit (P) for the occupied area (radiation worker or general public). Table 18-6 summarizes

Table 18-5	Half-Value Layers: Approximate Values Obtained at High Attenuation for the Indicated Peak Voltage Values Under Broad Beam Conditions*

	Attenuation Material HVL		
Peak Voltage (kV)	Lead (mm)	Concrete (cm)	Iron (cm)
50	0.06	0.43	
100	0.27	1.6	
300	1.47	3.1	
500	3.6	3.6	
1000	7.9	4.4	
6000	16.9	10.4	3.0
10,000	16.6	11.9	3.2
Cesium-137	6.5	4.8	1.6
Cobalt-60	12.0	6.2	2.1
Radium	16.6	6.9	2.2

Data obtained from National Council on Radiation Protection & Measurements: *Report No. 49: Structural shielding design and evaluation for medical use of x-rays and gamma rays of energies up to 10 MeV,* Bethesda, Md, 1976, NCRP Publications.
HVL, Half-value layer.
*Note: With low attenuation, these values will be significantly less.

the parameters that must be considered in shielding design. Consideration must be given to scatter radiation from the patient and leakage radiation from the head, as well as to the primary beam. If the primary beam is intercepted by a beamstopper, the transmission through the beamstopper must be taken into account. Consideration must also be given to the special requirements of techniques such as Cyberknife and intensity-modulated radiation therapy (IMRT), in which many small beams and oblique angles are used.

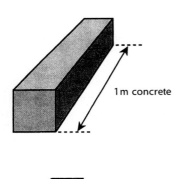
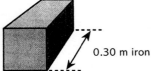
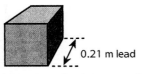

Figure 18-11. Thicknesses of various materials. These thicknesses provide equal attenuation for a cobalt-60 source.

Table 18-6	Summary of Shielding Parameters
Workload (W)	Number of patients per week × Amount of radiation for each
Primary beam use factor for each wall (U)	Fraction of time the beam is aimed at a particular wall
Occupancy factor (T)	Fraction of time area will be occupied
Distance (d)	Distance from the source of radiation to occupied area
Effective dose	Limit for occupied area; radiation worker equivalent limit or general public

 Optimizing time, distance, and shielding are the fundamental techniques for radiation protection.

Workload. Workloads for superficial and orthovoltage x-ray units are usually specified in milliamp-minutes per week (mA-min/week) and may be determined from an estimate of the beam-on time for each patient, the mA used, and the number of treatments per week. For cobalt-60 units and other high-energy units, the workload is usually specified in centigray per week at the isocenter. This number can be determined from the number of treatments given per week and the dose delivered to the isocenter for each one. For a typical linear accelerator, 200 patients may be treated per week (40 per day) and the isocenter dose may be 300 cGy, which yields a workload figure of 60,000 cGy per week at isocenter. If IMRT will be used, the workload may be significantly greater.[7]

Use Factor. In conventional x-ray rooms, the equipment is pointed down most of the time, and, except in diagnostic chest rooms, the primary beam is rarely aimed at the walls and almost never at the ceiling. Even in fluoroscopy rooms when the beam is aimed up, the beam must be intercepted by a barrier so that no radiation reaches the ceiling. In radiation therapy rooms, on the other hand, the situation is very different. During anteroposterior or posteroanterior (AP/PA) treatments, for example, the primary beam is alternately aimed down and up. Furthermore, many treatments are given with lateral, oblique, and even rotational beams, so radiation may be aimed at the floor, ceiling, and at least two of the four walls within the room. For these reasons, the **use factors** for therapy differ from those used with conventional x-rays. Ideally, the use factors (which can range from 0 to 1) should be determined from knowledge about how the equipment is actually used. However, if these values are not known, the use factors recommended by the NCRP in either Report No. 49,[3] *Structural Shielding Design and Evaluation for Medical Use of X-Rays and Gamma Rays of Energies Up to 10 MeV,* or Report No. 151,[7] *Structural Shielding Design and Evaluation for Megavoltage X- and Gamma-Ray Radiotherapy Facilities,* may be used. It should also be noted that these use factors apply to the primary beam. Both scatter and leakage radiation strike all surfaces of the room, so the use factor for these sources of radiation is always 1.

Occupancy Factor. If the area on the other side of a treatment room wall were totally unoccupied (e.g., if it were below grade and the earth extended for a distance of many meters), no shielding would be required. Similarly, an area that will be occupied all the time the machine is in operation would require considerable shielding. The **occupancy factor** is the fraction of time an area adjacent to the therapy room is occupied. Values can range from 0 to 1. Again, the best occupancy factors are those derived from knowledge about the occupancy of surrounding areas (including allowance for changes in the future). In the absence of such knowledge the recommendations of NCRP Report No. 151 may be used.[7] Some examples are 1 for offices, control areas, nurses' stations, and so forth; ½ for adjacent treatment and examination rooms; ⅕ for corridors and staff lounges; ⅛ for treatment vault doors; 1/20 for storage areas and unattended waiting rooms; and 1/40 for outdoor areas, and the like.[7]

Distance. As already mentioned, the greater the distance a person is from a source of radiation, the less radiation that is received. Thus, adjacent areas that are far from the sources of radiation in a treatment room will receive less radiation than those that are closer, and less shielding will be required. The primary beam distance is measured from the source to the appropriate surface when the machine is pointed toward that surface. For scatter radiation, both the distance from the source to the patient and the distance from the patient to the appropriate surface must be considered. In addition, the fraction of the radiation incident on the patient that is scattered must also be considered. This fraction depends on the incident beam energy and the scatter angle. Values are tabulated in NCRP Report No. 49.[3] For leakage radiation, the most appropriate distance is the distance from the source to the appropriate wall, when the head of the machine is closest to that surface.

Effective dose equivalent limits. As discussed earlier, radiation workers have different effective dose equivalent limits than members of the general public. In general, the shielding requirements for areas that will be frequented only by radiation workers or areas under positive control by a radiation worker (restricted areas) will not require as much shielding as areas accessible to the general public (unrestricted areas). However, in many cases the shielding design for restricted areas is based on the limits for unrestricted areas in the name of ALARA.

The application of the values obtained for each of the factors already discussed to determine actual thicknesses of shielding materials is a complex process for which training, experience, and judgment are required. In the case of shielding designs for cobalt-60 units, the person performing the design must be approved by the NRC or an agreement state. Similarly, shielding designs for linear accelerators must be performed, in most cases, by persons approved by the state.

Partly as a result of the recent reductions in the effective dose equivalent limit for the general public, several groups have reexamined the conservative assumptions that have been made in obtaining values for workloads, use factors, and occupancy factors, and changes in the methodology for performing shielding calculations may be published in the near future.

Safety Equipment

Because of the high levels of radiation that exist within the treatment room, no one but the patient is allowed to be in the room during the treatment. The NRC and virtually all states have additional regulations designed to protect both the operator of the equipment and the patient.

Warning Signs. Entrance doors to therapy rooms must be posted with signs to warn anyone about to enter the room that radiation might be present. Because the levels in the room can exceed 1 mSv (100 mrem) in 1 hour, the room must have a sign posted that says "Caution, High Radiation Area." In some cases, the radiation levels may be in excess of 5 Gy (500 cGy) in 1 hour, in which case the sign is supposed to read, "Grave Danger, Very High Radiation Area."

Warning Lights. Beam-on light indicators are required on the control panel, at the entrance door, and on the treatment unit itself. These lights should be illuminated whenever the therapy unit is energized to alert personnel that the beam is on. In the case of cobalt-60 units, a mechanical indication that the source is in the on position is also required on the head of the unit.

Door Interlocks. Entrance doors to therapy rooms must be equipped with an interlock that will shut off the machine (or in the case of a cobalt-60 unit, return the source to the off position) if the door is opened during treatment. The circuit design must be such that the unit will not produce radiation again when the door is closed unless the operator deliberately turns the machine back on. In addition, it is common to have interlocks on access doors to the machine stands so that if someone is working on the unit it cannot be accidentally energized.

Visual and Aural Communication. It is necessary for the radiation therapist to be able to see the patient throughout the treatment. If the patient moves or shows signs of distress, the therapist can turn off the unit and enter the room. For superficial and orthovoltage units, visual monitoring may be by means of a leaded glass window. However, for high-energy machines, the thickness of glass required usually makes this method impractical. In these cases, monitoring is usually done by means of closed-circuit television systems. Care must be taken to position the camera so that the patient is in view no matter what the position of the gantry. Often, two separate television systems are used. Regulations require that visual communication be available at all times, so if only one system is used and it fails, the treatment room cannot be used until the television system is repaired. Regulations also require the availability of aural communication between therapist and patient. Again, this is primarily a safety measure for the patient, because it allows the patient to notify the therapist if he or she is in distress.

"Beam-On" Monitors. High-energy therapy units are required to have an independent beam-on monitor in the room to alert the therapist if he or she enters the room when the beam is on. This monitor must not be connected to the therapy machine in any way and must have provision for battery operation in the event of an electrical failure.

Emergency Off Controls. In the unlikely event that a high-energy therapy machine may be energized when a therapist is in the room, emergency push buttons are located at several points within the room and on the machine itself that will remove all power to the unit when pressed. The circuits are designed so that the machine will not be energized when the buttons are released unless the therapist proceeds through the normal start procedure at the control panel. In the case of cobalt-60 units, means and instructions are also provided to therapists so that they can mechanically return the source to the off position should it become stuck. This is also an unlikely event. In all cases, the therapist must be concerned first with the care of the patient and next with his or her own welfare. The dose received by a therapist standing 1 m to the side of a patient being treated at 300 cGy/min will be approximately 0.5 cGy/min. Although all unnecessary radiation is to be avoided, the few seconds required to move the table to remove the patient from the beam if it cannot be shut off will be unlikely to deliver a dose to the therapist in excess of the effective dose equivalent limit.

Quality Assurance. No safety device is effective if it is not working, so frequent testing of the devices on a regular basis is necessary. Such tests are required either by regulation or by recognized protocols. The visual and aural communication systems are easy to test daily. Testing of emergency off buttons may cause harm to the treatment unit, so manufacturer's recommendations should be followed carefully. Testing of beam-on monitors can be done either by turning the television camera to visualize the monitor or by using a mirror so that an image of the monitor can be seen by the television camera.

 Safety equipment must be tested frequently to ensure that it operates properly when needed.

PRACTICAL RADIATION PROTECTION: BRACHYTHERAPY

The sources used for implants require special consideration, because, like cobalt-60, they are always on. A license from either the NRC or an agreement state is required to receive, possess, and use such sources. Sources may be obtained only from facilities or firms licensed to distribute them. Sources must be stored in heavily shielded "safes" in an area secure from theft or loss, in keeping with the increasingly stringent requirements of the Department of Homeland Security.

Written Directives and Inventory

Before an implant is prepared, a written directive must be completed by the requesting physician, and certification must be made that the implant was assembled in accordance with the directive. A careful inventory must be maintained of all sources, and any time sources are removed or returned, a log entry must be made and a complete inventory performed. Inventories are also required at least weekly, even if no sources have been removed from or returned to the safe.

Transportation

If sources must be transported within the hospital, shielded carriers must be used. In most cases, the required shielding makes the carriers too heavy to carry by hand, and wheeled carriers are necessary. Whenever sources are moved within the hospital—either in carriers or already implanted within a patient who is being moved—the route should be chosen to minimize exposure to other hospital personnel or members of the general public.

Patient Rooms

The room used by a patient with a radioactive implant also requires special consideration. A private room with a bath (if the patient will be allowed to use the bath) should be provided. Placement of the patient's bed should be such that a patient in an adjoining room will not receive a dose in excess of the effective dose equivalent limit for the general public. This usually implies that the bed be placed by a wall adjacent to a stairway or other little occupied area. In some cases, shielding may be required on the wall. Radiation exposure to the areas above and below the patient's room should also be considered.

Training of Personnel

All personnel who may care for the patient with an implant must be thoroughly instructed in radiation safety procedures and the actions to take if the implant is dislodged or other emergencies occur. Nurses should use personnel monitors. Ancillary personnel such as dietary aides, maintenance personnel, and housekeeping personnel also need to receive instruction about radiation safety at a level commensurate with their risk. Personnel monitors are usually not required for such personnel.

Warning Signs and Surveys

The entrance door to the patient's room must be posted with a caution sign, and visiting periods should be limited (typically to 20 minutes per visitor per day), with the visitor remaining behind a line established by the radiation safety officer. Radiation warning signs are also placed on the patient's wrist, bed, and chart to ensure that no one will be inadvertently exposed because he or she was not aware that the patient contained radioactive materials. After the patient returns to his or her room and/or after placement of the radioactive material in the patient, a survey must be performed of the contents of the patient's room. After removal of the implant, a survey must again be performed to ensure that no sources have been inadvertently left behind. Nothing should be removed from the patient's room, nor should the patient be discharged, until this survey is performed.

Leak Tests

Because it is possible for the material encapsulating the radioactive material in implant sources to sustain damage and leak, brachytherapy sources must be leak tested at intervals not to exceed 6 months. The method used must be sensitive enough to detect removable contamination at a level of 0.005 μCi (11,100 disintegrations per minute [dpm]). Leak tests must also be performed on cobalt-60 units every 6 months. In this case, however, the limit for removable contamination is 0.05 μCi.

High-Dose-Rate Brachytherapy

Conventional low-dose-rate brachytherapy procedures require the patient to be hospitalized for 24 to 72 hours. High-dose-rate units have become available that allow the treatment time to be shortened. The sources in these units have considerably greater activity than those used in low-dose implants (10 Ci iridium-192 versus 65 mCi cesium-137) and therefore cannot be handled manually. This implies less exposure for those who would normally prepare and insert low-dose-rate implants. However, it also implies the need for computer control of the position and dwell time of the sources and the possibility of error or the loss of control of the source. For these reasons, special procedures are required to ensure the safe operation of such devices.

SUMMARY

- There are two major sources of radiation exposure in the radiation therapy department: megavoltage treatment machines (linear accelerators) and brachytherapy sources.
- Regardless of which models are used to estimate the risks of radiation exposure, it is universally agreed that the less radiation received, the lower the risk.
- In keeping with the ALARA concept, every means should be taken to reduce individual exposure.
- Practical radiation protection from external beam radiation should include the time-honored methods of time, distance, and shielding.
- A resurgence in the use of brachytherapy sources requires the radiation therapy practitioner to be prepared to demonstrate a comprehensive knowledge of its uses in terms of radiation safety and protection.

Review Questions

Multiple Choice

1. Activity is defined as:
   a. rest mass is same as an electron but has a positive charge
   b. product of absorbed dose and QF
   c. rate of nuclear decay
   d. ionization per unit mass of air by photons
2. The source of ionizing radiation that contributes the most to exposure of the general population in the United States is:
   a. medical procedures
   b. nuclear power plants
   c. natural background radiation
   d. above-ground nuclear testing
3. Which type of device is best suited for output measurements of radiation therapy equipment?
   a. TLD
   b. ionization chamber
   c. G-M detector
   d. x-ray film
4. Stochastic, or nonthreshold, effects of radiation exposure do not include:
   a. cancer induction
   b. cataract formation
   c. genetic effects
   d. birth defects
5. Exposure of which of the following people would contribute the most to the genetically significant dose?
   a. 50-year-old woman
   b. 70-year-old man
   c. 20-year-old woman
   d. all contribute equally
6. The annual effective dose equivalent limit for radiation workers is:
   a. 0.5 mSv
   b. 5 mSv
   c. 50 mSv
   d. 500 mSv

7. A G-M detector is 2 m from a small brachytherapy source and measures an exposure rate of 10 mR/hr. What exposure rate would you expect to measure if the detector were moved to 4 m from the source?
   a. 5 mR/hr
   b. 20 mR/hr
   c. 2.5 mR/hr
   d. 1 mR/hr
8. Absorbed dose is defined as:
   a. rest mass of an electron but has a positive charge
   b. product of absorbed dose and QF
   c. ionization per unit mass of air by photons
   d. energy absorbed per unit mass
9. Exposure is defined as:
   a. rest mass of an electron but has a positive charge
   b. product of absorbed dose and QF
   c. rate of nuclear decay
   d. ionization per unit mass of air by photons
10. An alpha particle is best defined as:
   a. produced by electron rearrangement
   b. produced during nuclear decay; has no charge or mass
   c. short-range, relatively heavy-mass, high-LET particle
   d. rest mass is same as an electron but has a positive charge

The answers to the Review Questions can be found by logging on to our website at: *http://evolve.elsevier.com/Washington+Leaver/principles*

Questions to Ponder

1. What are some of the sources of natural background radiation? Is it possible or reasonable to attempt to shield or protect the general population from these sources?
2. What are the factors that must be considered in designing the shielding for a linear accelerator facility?
3. Why is it important that regulatory agencies such as the NRC or state agencies oversee the operation of radiation therapy facilities?
4. What are the primary reasons for implementing a radiation protection program? How does the concept of ALARA affect the development of such a program?
5. What are some of the specific challenges associated with many of the newer technologies in radiation therapy, such as IMRT and high-dose-rate brachytherapy?

REFERENCES

1. Bushberg JT, et al: *The essential physics of medical imaging,* Baltimore, 1994, Williams & Wilkins.
2. Hall EJ: *Radiobiology for the radiologist,* ed 5, Philadelphia, 2000, Lippincott Williams & Wilkins.
3. National Council on Radiation Protection & Measurements (NCRP): *Report No. 49: Structural shielding design and evaluation for medical use of x-rays and gamma rays of energies up to 10 MeV,* Washington, DC, 1976, NCRP Publications.
4. National Council on Radiation Protection & Measurements (NCRP): *Report No. 91: Recommendations on limits for exposure to ionizing radiation,* Bethesda, Md, 1987, NCRP Publications.
5. National Council on Radiation Protection & Measurements (NCRP): *Report No. 93: Ionizing radiation exposure of the population of the United States,* Bethesda, Md, 1987, NCRP Publications.
6. National Council on Radiation Protection & Measurements (NCRP): *Report No. 115: Risk estimates for radiation protection,* Bethesda, Md, 1993, NCRP Publications.
7. National Council on Radiation Protection & Measurements (NCRP): *Report No. 151: Structural shielding design and evaluation for megavoltage X- and gamma-ray radiotherapy facilities,* Bethesda, Md, 2005, NCRP Publications.
8. Statkiewicz-Sherer MA, Visconti PJ, Ritenour ER: *Radiation protection in medical radiography,* ed 2, St. Louis, 1993, Mosby.

Quality Improvement in Radiation Oncology

Judith M. Schneider

Outline

Evolution of quality improvement
  Radiation measurement
  Hospital oversight and
    accreditation
Regulating agencies
  Federal agencies
  State agencies

Professional organizations
Definitions
Components of quality
  improvement
  Quality improvement team
  Development of a quality
    improvement plan

Quality improvement process
  Continuous quality improvement
    methodologies
  Quality control in treatment
    planning and delivery
  Assessment of the data
  Summary

Key Terms

Aspect of care
Continuous quality
  improvement (CQI)
Flowchart
Health care
  organizations
Lean
Outcomes
Peer review
Quality assessment
Quality assurance
Quality audit
Quality control
Quality improvement
  (QI)
Quality indicators
Radiation oncology
  team
Six Sigma
The Joint Commission
  (TJC)
Total quality
  management (TQM)

Objectives

- Define *quality improvement in health care* and list some synonymous terms.
- Explain Dr. W. F. Deming's principles of management as they relate to continuous quality improvement (CQI).
- Discuss the evolution and purpose of quality improvement in radiation oncology.
- Describe the significant roles of both accreditation and regulatory agencies, as well as professional organizations, in the development of a quality improvement plan for radiation oncology.

- Delineate the responsibilities of the quality improvement team members in radiation oncology.
- Differentiate between quality control, quality assurance, and quality management.
- Discuss the CQI methodologies of Lean and Six Sigma.
- Analyze the major components of a quality improvement plan in radiation oncology.
- Explain the role of data assessment in a quality improvement plan.

Quality improvement (QI) in health care is "an approach to the continuous study and improvement of the processes of providing health care services to meet the needs of patients and others. Synonymous terms include continuous quality improvement (CQI), continuous improvement (CI), and total quality management (TQM)."[6, 21] It is premised on Dr. W. E. Deming's 14 principles of management, which were first introduced in Japan's industry after World War II and into the United States' health care industry in the early 1980s. The Deming principles of management emphasize CQI in a product (service) through proactive employee participation in a "customer-responsive" environment.[24,25,27,34] According to Deming, quality is not only achieved but maintained by the following[25,27]:

1. Delineate the health care organization's mission and goals, so that there is a reason for improving.
2. Instead of setting thresholds, which are expected levels of compliance, always strive for improvement no matter how good the product (service).
3. Improve the process rather than "inspect for errors."
4. Plan for the future by analyzing "long-term costs" and "appropriateness of product (service)."
5. Allow the employee to contribute to the improvement process.
6. Encourage and support employees through education.
7. Ensure qualified leaders for the improvement system.
8. Eliminate fear by encouraging employees to offer suggestions.
9. Eliminate staffing barriers by helping employees understand the needs of other departments or sections.
10. Require management to always keep employees informed of what is happening.
11. Emphasize quality first rather than quantity.

12. Promote and encourage teamwork versus individual performance.
13. Encourage and support an employee's educational and self-improvement program.
14. Support and train all employees in the "transformation process."

Today's **health care organizations** are facing the same dilemmas as industry did many years ago involving quality control and cost containment. Appropriate use of CQI assists the health care organization in responding to the problems of "increased competition," "escalating costs," "quality concerns," and "demands for increased accountability."[27] Participation in CQI has been demonstrated to decrease costs, increase customer satisfaction, and ensure quality throughout the health care organization.[24,25]

Traditionally, quality assurance activities were used by health care organizations to systematically analyze the quality of health care services rendered and to meet the criteria for accreditation by **The Joint Commission (TJC)**, formally known as the Joint Commission on the Accreditation of Healthcare Organizations (JCAHO), an independent, not-for-profit organization dedicated to improving the quality of care in health care settings.[21] Quality assurance focuses on performance measurement, which is based on the comparison of processes with **outcomes** to quality indicators, the measurable dimension of quality that defines what is to be monitored.[11,24] It stresses control and assessment of performance, hence the terms *quality control,* providing standards of measurement, and *quality assessment,* involving the systematic collection and review of quality assurance data.

A **continuous quality improvement (CQI)** plan integrates quality assurance, quality control, and assessment into a complex, systemwide improvement program revolving around the health care organization's mission and goals.[24] It eliminates duplication of quality assurance and quality improvement efforts but still provides assurance that services are of high quality.[34]

In recent years, with the increase in complexity of radiation treatment planning and delivery, it has become imperative that a radiation oncology center, regardless of its size, develop and implement a well-defined, structured, and functional quality improvement plan. This plan should encompass all aspects of the radiation therapy treatment process from patient consultation through and including follow-up care.

Quality improvement in radiation oncology involves ongoing activities encompassing administrative, clinical, physical, and technical aspects of the radiation oncology process as defined by the American College of Radiology (ACR) and the American Association of Physicists in Medicine (AAPM).[23,26] Each of these aspects, which are influenced by their own structure and process, are relevant to the outcomes of the radiation oncology process and should be monitored in a quality improvement plan. (Figure 19-1 contains a fishbone diagram indicating the major process and structure elements of the clinical aspects of the radiation therapy process.[9]) The quality improvement plan includes a quality control program to measure the radiation output; mechanical integrity of the treatment and simulation units and brachytherapy sources and equipment; and quality assessment programs to measure all aspects of the treatment planning, delivery, and patient care process. A **peer review** and audit mechanism is an integral part of the plan.

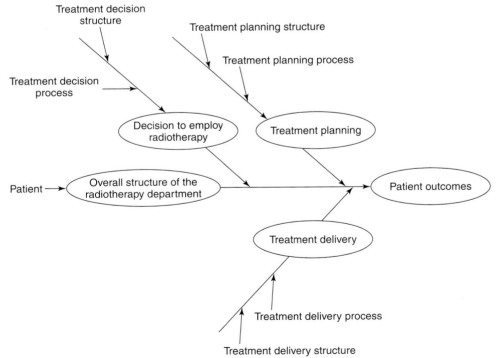

Figure 19-1. A "fishbone" diagram showing the major structure and process elements of the clinical radiation therapy program. (Used with permission from Brundage MD, Dixon PF, MacKillop WJ, et al: A real-time audit of radiation therapy in a regional cancer center, *Int J Radiat Oncol Biol Phys* 43:121, 1999.)

EVOLUTION OF QUALITY IMPROVEMENT
Radiation Measurement

Before the process of quality improvement can be implemented, standards must be developed by which one can compare, evaluate, and establish quality control.[37] From the time of the discovery of the x-ray, standards for its measurement have been proposed, starting with the original erythema dose as the unit of measurement and evolving into exact scientific standards for the measurement of the gray (Gy) as specified by national and international agencies. During the Second International Congress of Radiology held in Stockholm, Sweden, in July 1928, several recommendations were made, including that an "international unit of x-radiation" be adopted and that the unit be called the *Roentgen*. The complete recommendations were published in the report entitled "Recommendations of the International X-Ray Unit Committee," published in 1929.[38] This marked the beginning of quality control in radiation measurements, although it was not defined as such. As technology advanced in radiation oncology, the number of governing regulations increased. There is no comparison between this simple two-page document and the volumes of regulations that currently exist. With the advent of the unit of measure came the standardization of equipment performance with an increased emphasis on quality control. Thus quality improvement in radiation oncology was initially focused on the physical aspect of treatment equipment performance.

Hospital Oversight and Accreditation

The oversight of patient care in hospitals began in 1917 when the American College of Surgeons (ACS) established the Hospital Standardization Program, and in 1919 the concept of "minimum standards" was developed. From 1917 until 1951 the ACS worked to improve the hospital-based practice of medicine. In 1952, the Joint Commission on Accreditation of Hospitals (JCAH) was formed through the efforts of the ACS, the American Medical Association (AMA), the American Hospital Association (AHA), the American College of Physicians (ACP), and the Canadian Medical Association (CMA). With the passage of Medicare in 1965, JCAH accreditation of hospitals increased in importance when the U.S. Congress determined that JCAH-accredited facilities would be recognized for purposes of Medicare reimbursement. In 1988, the name of the JCAH was changed to JCAHO to broaden its scope to include ambulatory centers, group practices, health maintenance organizations, community health centers, emergency and urgent care centers, and hospital-based practices under its accreditation umbrella.

Although the original mission of the JCAH was to ensure safety in hospitals, that mission has evolved and expanded to include quality improvement based on the measurement of patient outcomes. Initially, JCAHO standards for radiation oncology were included in those for the radiology departments, because most radiation therapy departments came under the auspices of that department, but rarely were the radiation therapy facilities visited. In 1987, however, the JCAHO developed separate standards for radiation oncology, and a dedicated quality improvement plan is now required for each department. The original emphasis was on the quality control aspects of radiation oncology and concentrated on the treatment units themselves and the process used to deliver patient care. Now the emphasis is on "doing the right thing" and "doing the right thing well" as it relates to the facility's organization-wide performance versus specific departmental performance.[20] Doing the right thing refers to delivering effective and appropriate treatment, and doing the right thing well refers to providing patient care effectively, accurately, in a timely manner, and with respect and caring for the patient.

REGULATING AGENCIES

Today there are a multitude of national, state, and professional agencies with regulations and standards that must be adhered to by the radiation oncology facility to ensure high-quality patient care and safety. These standards and regulations provide the cornerstones for the radiation oncology facility's quality improvement plan. It is imperative that a radiation oncology facility become familiar with all national, state, and professional regulations that affect the facility's operation. This is an ongoing process, because along with the development and use of new equipment and treatment techniques comes new guidelines and practice standards that must be followed.

Federal and state government and professional and accreditation agencies mandate standards to ensure not only that equipment is functional and operates within acceptable limits but also that operators of this equipment are truly qualified individuals.

Federal Agencies

The U.S. Nuclear Regulatory Commission (NRC) was created in 1974 as a result of Congress passing legislation to divide the Atomic Energy Commission that, since 1954, had been managing the nation's atomic energy programs. The Atomic Energy Commission was separated into the Energy Research and Development Administration and the NRC. The mission of the NRC is to "ensure adequate protection of the public health and safety, the common defense and security, and the environment in the use of nuclear materials in the United States." The NRC's scope of responsibility includes regulation of commercial nuclear power reactors; nonpower research, test, and training reactors; fuel cycle facilities; medical, academic, and industrial uses of nuclear materials; and the transport, storage, and disposal of nuclear materials and waste. Its regulations are issued under the U.S. Code of Federal Regulations (CFR) Title 10, Chapter 1.[28,29] Use of radioisotopes in brachytherapy and the cobalt for external treatments falls under the regulation of the NRC.

Although the NRC is the major federal regulating agency for ensuring adequate protection of public health and safety in the use of radioactive materials, other federal agencies assist the NRC in fulfilling its mission. One such agency is the U.S. Environmental Protection Agency (EPA). The EPA was established in 1970 to consolidate into one agency a variety of federal research, monitoring, standard-setting, and enforcement activities to guarantee protection of the environment. The EPA's mission is "to protect human health and safeguard the natural environment—air, water, and land—upon which life depends."[12] Therefore, the EPA is involved with regulation of the disposal, storage, and handling of nuclear waste materials as it relates to environmental protection issues.

The transportation of hazardous materials is monitored and regulated through the Department of Transportation (DOT), another federal agency assisting the NRC in carrying out its mission. The DOT's effort is coordinated through the Office of Hazardous Materials (OHM), which is responsible for overseeing a national safety program for transporting hazardous materials by air, rail, highway, and water.[31,36]

In 1968, Congress passed the Radiation Control for Health and Safety Act, which provided for the development and administration of standards that would reduce human exposure to radiation from electronic products. Implementation of this act was carried out through the Bureau of Radiologic Health (BRH), which is now called the *Center for Devices and Radiologic Health (CDRH)*. This Act is now incorporated into the Federal Food, Drug, and Cosmetic Act (FFDCA), as Chapter V, Subchapter 3, Electronic Product Radiation Control. This Act regulates both medical and nonmedical electronic products such as diagnostic x-ray or ultrasound imaging devices, microwave or ultrasound diathermy devices, x-ray or electron accelerators, sunlamps, microwave ovens, television receivers and monitors, entertainment lasers, industrial x-ray systems, and cordless and cellular telephones.[13]

Provisions of this Act require the manufacturers of these products that emit radiation to keep records in reference to quality testing of their products and communications to the dealers, distributors, and purchasers of these products as it relates to radiation safety issues.

The FFDCA holds the manufacturers responsible in the reporting of safety issues regarding radiation-producing electronic products and also facilities who uses these products. The Safe Medical Devices Act of 1990 (SMDA) requires medical facilities to report to the FDA any medical device that has caused death or injury of a patient or an employee.[13,28] Failure to report such incidences can result in civil penalties to the medical facility, as well as to the health care professional.

To ensure safe and healthful working conditions for working men and women, the U.S. Congress passed the Occupational Safety and Health Act of 1970. By provisions of this Act, the Occupational Safety and Health Administration (OSHA) was created "to save lives, prevent injuries, and protect the health of America's workers."[7,30]

In the mid-1980s, OSHA mandated a policy on bloodborne pathogens, which stated that an exposure control plan must be in place for all industries in which workers may come in contact with blood and other infectious materials. This plan must contain precautionary procedures, educational programs for employees, and proper disposal procedures.[30,33] The policy on bloodborne pathogens is part of the radiation oncology facility's policy and procedures manual.

OSHA also set standards for exposure to cadmium and lead, which primarily covers industrial work environments, but these standards would apply to mold rooms, where Cerrobend (shielding) block is constructed, in radiation oncology facilities.[30] It is important for the personnel working in mold rooms to be aware of and to follow the safety standards outlined by OSHA.

State Agencies

Section 274b of the Atomic Energy Act of 1954 provides a basis for the NRC to relinquish to the states portions of its regulatory authority relating to licensing and regulating by-product materials (radioisotopes), source materials (uranium and thorium), and

certain quantities of special nuclear materials. The first agreement state was established in 1962. Currently, 34 states have entered into agreements with the NRC[32] (Figure 19-2). In such agreements, the NRC provides assistance to the states through reviewing of the agreement request, conducting training courses and workshops, and evaluating technical licensing and inspection issues. The NRC is highly involved with the agreement states keeping all chains of communication open in a variety of areas.

Professional Organizations

Several professional organizations provide practice standards to guide appropriately educated professionals within their organizations. Professional practice standards establish the role of the practitioner and create criteria to be used to evaluate performance. The ACR, with more than 30,000 members, is the primary professional organization of radiologists, radiation oncologists, and clinical medical physicists in the United States. The ACR creates standards in the hopes of producing high-quality radiologic care. It has developed specific standards for brachytherapy and external beam therapy.[5]

The AAPM, a professional organization for medical physicists, has been a forerunner in the development of minimum standards to guide medical physicists in the development of a quality assurance program as it relates to treatment planning and delivery. Several reports have been produced by special task groups of the AAPM relating to the development of a comprehensive quality assurance program in radiation oncology, such as the AAPM Task Group 40 report and, more recently, the AAPM Task Group 53 report, which outlined a comprehensive quality assurance program for radiation therapy treatment planning.[1,2,5]

In 1995, the professional organization for radiation therapists, the American Society of Radiologic Technologists (ASRT), developed practice standards for radiation therapists. The professional practice standards are divided into three sections: clinical performance standards, which define activities related to the care of patients and the delivery of procedures and treatments; quality performance standards, which include the activities of the practitioner in the technical areas of performance involving equipment safety and TQM; and professional performance standards, which define activities in the areas of education, interpersonal relationships, personal and professional self-assessment, and ethical behavior.[8] To be effective, the quality improvement plan must incorporate all practice standards for each member of the quality improvement team.

The radiation therapist may keep current with the regulations and guidelines created by various relevant agencies by visiting the following:
National: NRC at http://www.nrc.gov
FFDCA at http://www.fda.gov
DOT at http://www.dot.gov
OSHA at http://www.osha.gov
EPA at http://www.epa.gov
State: NRC agreement states at http://nrc-stp.ornl.gov
Professional: ACR at http://www.acr.org
AAPM at http://www.aapm.org
ASRT at http://www.asrt.org
Accrediting: TJC at http://www.jointcommission.org

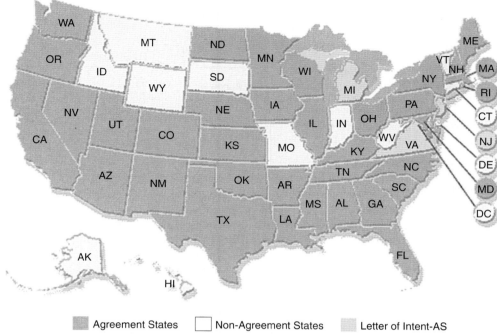

Figure 19-2. A map of the NRC agreement states. (Retrieved December 26, 2007, from the NRC website: http://nrc-stp.ornl.gov/rulemaking.html.)

DEFINITIONS

Multiple definitions exist regarding the various components of quality improvement; the definitions used throughout the rest of this chapter are those developed by the International Standards Organization (ISO)[18] and accepted as the American national standard.[1]

Quality, in reference to radiation oncology, is defined as "the totality of features and characteristics of a radiation therapy process that bear on its ability to satisfy stated or implied needs of the patient."[18] To determine whether quality standards are met, each feature or characteristic of the radiation therapy process must be identified and measured and the results analyzed.

Quality assurance is defined as "all those planned or systematic actions necessary to provide adequate confidence that a product or service will satisfy given requirements for quality."[18] The term is used to refer to the planned and systematic actions to ensure that a radiation therapy facility consistently delivers high-quality care in the treatment of patients leading to the best outcomes with the least amount of side effects. All aspects of the radiation therapy process must be routinely and continuously measured, the results analyzed, and corrective action taken as required to ensure quality patient care. This type of review is referred to as a **quality audit**.[11,28]

Quality control is defined as "the operational techniques and activities used to fulfill requirements for quality."[18] The term is typically used to refer to those procedures and techniques used to monitor or test and maintain the components of the radiation therapy quality improvement program, such as the tests performed to measure the mechanical integrity of the treatment units.

Measurement of patient outcomes is now required by the TJC. This measurement includes not only areas such as morbidity,

mortality, recurrence of disease, and survival rates but also patient satisfaction and quality of life. As part of its "Agenda for Change," TJC created the Joint Commission's Indicator Measurement System (IM system), which provides a continuous evaluation of performance as part of the accreditation process to help health care organizations measure and improve their quality of care through the use of common **quality indicators**. Every quarter, organizations participating in this system are required to send their data electronically to the system's national database, which then prepares a comparative report for each indicator. The IM system focuses primarily on acute inpatient care, although the indicators may be relevant to some outpatient surgical settings. Currently, 130 participants are part of the IM system, with the number submitting data steadily increasing.[22] Having an adequate computerized data analysis system is an essential component for CQI.

The TJC has replaced the term *quality assurance* with terms such as **quality assessment** or *quality improvement,* because the emphasis is now on the ongoing evaluation of all aspects of care for the purpose of determining areas where improvement is needed. The key word is "ongoing"; hence, this program is often referred to as CQI or **total quality management (TQM)**.

COMPONENTS OF QUALITY IMPROVEMENT

Quality Improvement Team

The quality improvement team is composed of all personnel in the radiation oncology department who interact with the patient and family. Each individual makes a contribution to the quality of care and level of patient satisfaction. Only through continuous evaluation of all aspects of the radiation therapy process can the ultimate goal to deliver quality radiation and patient

Table 19-1	Responsibilities of Members of the Quality Improvement (QI) Committee		
QI Activity	**Goals**	**Frequency**	**Reporting Mechanism**
Develop and monitor a CQI program	Oversee departmental peer-review activities	Ongoing	QI committee meeting minutes
Collect and evaluate data	Develop and implement new policies and procedures as needed	Monthly meetings	Chart rounds reports
Determine areas for improvement	Oversee implementation of and adherence to departmental policies and procedures		Policies and procedures
Implement change as necessary			Incident reports
Evaluate results of actions taken			

CQI, Continuous quality improvement.

care be achieved. However, this is not accomplished without the cooperative efforts and commitment to quality of each member of the **radiation oncology team**.[16,23]

Common practice is for the medical director of a radiation oncology center to be responsible for the establishment and continuation of a quality improvement program.[16] The director may appoint a quality improvement committee to develop and monitor the program, collect and evaluate the data, determine areas for improvement, implement changes when areas for improvement have been identified, and evaluate the results of the actions taken. Table 19-1 delineates the responsibilities of the quality improvement committee.

It is also the responsibility of the director to ensure that all employees are qualified for their jobs. Job descriptions must clearly state the qualifications, the credentials or license required, continuing education requirements, and the scope of practice for each position. Institutional requirements regarding maintenance of qualifications in cardiopulmonary resuscitation attendance at infectious disease, fire, and safety seminars; and observance of all radiation safety standards are to be strictly adhered to.

Staff physicians are required to actively participate in departmental quality improvement activities, and documentation of participation is reviewed as part of the medical staff recredentialing process. The radiation oncologists participate in these activities during chart review, morbidity and mortality conferences, review and development of departmental policies and procedures, portal film review, patient and family education, and the completion and review of incident reports.

Members of the physics division (physicists, dosimetrists, and engineers) develop and carry out the quality control program to meet the needs of the department and to be in compliance with national, state, and professionally accepted or mandated standards. They also conduct weekly and final physics reviews of the treatment records.

The radiation therapists perform warm-up procedures on the treatment units, perform quality control tests on the simulation and treatment units, verify the presence of completed and signed prescription and consent forms, review the prescription and treatment plan on each patient before the initiation of treatment, deliver accurate treatment adhering to the prescription, accurately record treatment delivered, take initial and weekly portal films, evaluate the health status of the patient daily before treatment delivery to ensure there are no adverse reactions to treatment or other impending physical or psychological

problems that require assistance, participate in patient and family education, and provide care and comfort to meet the needs of the patient.[3]

The oncology nurses perform a nursing assessment on each new patient to determine overall physical and psychological status; evaluate the educational needs of each patient and family to determine any barriers to education; develop an educational program to meet the needs of the patient and family; evaluate the effectiveness of the entire educational program, including the education given to the patient by the radiation oncologist, nurses, and radiation therapists; monitor the patient's health status on a routine or as-needed basis throughout the course of treatment; and order, evaluate, and record blood counts and weights according to departmental policy.

The departmental support staff gathers pertinent information and prepares the treatment chart before the patient's initial visit; contacts the patient and/or family to set up appointments and give instructions regarding information or diagnostic studies to be brought with the patient; greets and assists the patient and family daily; informs the radiation oncologists, nurses, and/or radiation therapists of the patient's arrival; answers the patient's questions and gives assistance whenever possible or refers the patient to an individual who can help; completes and files treatment records; and sets the tone for the entire radiation therapy treatment encounter.

Development of a Quality Improvement Plan

A quality improvement plan or program lists the organizational structure, responsibilities, procedures, processes, and resources for implementing a comprehensive quality system. Included in the plan is an audit mechanism to document measurement and evaluation activities to verify that all aspects of the radiation oncology process meet national, state, institutional, and/or departmental quality standards and a mechanism to institute change when quality standards are not met. It requires access to a computerized data acquisition and analysis system.[19]

The plan may be developed and overseen by a departmental quality improvement committee. The objectives of the program are as follows:

1. Establish a program that promotes an ongoing collection of information about important aspects of care
2. Use the information gathered to substantiate that high standards of care are being met or to identify opportunities to improve patient care

3. Implement action as necessary to modify and improve the quality of patient care
4. Assess the effectiveness of actions taken to improve the quality of patient care
5. Report quality assessment activities to the radiation oncology staff, hospital quality improvement department, and other departments or committees as requested

Refer to Box 19-1 for a summary of the elements in a quality improvement plan.

The first step in the development of such a plan is to identify all aspects of departmental activities that affect the patient's care. This process might be facilitated by the use of a **flow-chart**, which is a pictorial representation of the steps necessary in a process. Flowcharts use ovals to identify the beginning or end of a process, rectangles to indicate an action to be taken, and diamonds to represent a decision. By following the patient's progress, or flow, through the department, areas for improvement can be identified. Quality indicators may then be developed for each important **aspect of care**. As stated previously, indicators are tools used to measure, over time, a department's performance of functions, processes, and outcomes.[21] Well-defined and measurable indicators help focus attention on opportunities for improved patient care. Refer to Table 19-2 for some identifiable quality indicators correlated to specific aspects of care in the radiation therapy process.

QUALITY IMPROVEMENT PROCESS

It is the responsibility of each individual radiation oncology center to formulate and implement quality improvement standards, based on its own "strengths and needs, in accordance with previously developed national, state, and professional guidelines."[23,26] Because of the variations in the "strengths and needs" of each individual radiation oncology center, this chapter does not address the step-by-step technical procedures for specific quality improvement processes but instead refers the reader to reports generated by various professional and national organizations such as the ACR, AAPM, the American College of Medical Physics (ACMP), and the NRC.[1,4,5,23]

Continuous Quality Improvement Methodologies

There are several process improvement methodologies that a health care organization may adopt to assist in improving quality and reducing costs. One such process improvement methodology is called Lean. **Lean** is a system-wide set of methods and

Table 19-2	Quality Indicators in the Radiation Therapy Process
Aspect of Care	**Indicators**
Consultation and informed consent	History and physical report in treatment record
	Pathology report in treatment record
	Consent form signed by patient or legal guardian
	Consent form signed by radiation oncologist
Treatment planning	Quality control program for simulator, imaging processing equipment, immobilization devices, and accessory equipment
	Quality control program for treatment planning computer systems
	Adherence to departmental policies and procedures
	Target volume indicated on planning films
	Setup information, diagrams, and photographs in treatment record
	Calculations and graphic plans double-checked
Treatment delivery	Quality control program for treatment unit, imaging processing equipment, immobilization devices, accessory equipment, and safety equipment
	Written and signed prescription
	Approved treatment plan
	Comparison of portal films with simulation films
	Weekly review of portal films by radiation therapist
	Initial and weekly portal films signed by radiation oncologist
Documentation of treatment delivery	Adherence to the prescription
	Documentation of weekly physics review
	Adherence to professional and departmental standards
	Completeness of treatment record
	Incident/unusual occurrence reports
Patient outcomes	Completion notes/treatment summary filed in chart
	Follow-up notes filed in chart
	Documentation of treatment outcomes, including:
	Morbidity
	Mortality
	Recurrence
	Survival
	Patient satisfaction
	Quality of survival

Box 19-1	Components of a Continuous Quality Improvement Plan

- Evaluation of both quality and appropriateness of care
- Evaluation of patterns or trends
- Assessment of individual clinical events
- Action to be taken to resolve identified problems
- Identification of important aspects of care for assessment
- Identification of indicators to monitor and acceptable thresholds
- Methods of data collection
- Annual review of quality improvement plan for effectiveness

tools for improving a process by emphasizing speed and efficiency.[10,14,15] It was first used in the early days of mass production of automobiles (circa 1910). It focuses on time and waste in a process. The Lean technique is very simplistic and easy to implement. **Six Sigma** is another process improvement method. It focuses on improving the process through precision and accuracy, with the elimination of defects in the process.

It was originally formulated by Bill Smith for the Motorola Corporation in 1986. This method is more complex to implement, requiring extensive training of all participants. Six Sigma incorporates the martial arts ranking terminology to define key leadership roles. (For example, black belts are project leaders who help coach, develop, lead, and advise management and employees to achieves their goals; they devote 75% of their time to a project. Green belts help ensure the success of Six Sigma techniques. They lead improvement projects on a smaller scale. They devote 50% of their time to a project. Yellow belts have a solid basic knowledge of the Six Sigma methodology. They do not handle projects.) Because of the different emphasis between these two methodologies, they are often used together and referred to as *Lean Six Sigma.*

Continuous quality improvement is important to the operation of a radiation oncology facility. Health care organizations are seeking various methodologies to assist them in achieving quality outcomes. To find more information about CQI methodologies, visit the American Society for Quality at http://www.asq.org.

Quality Control in Treatment Planning and Delivery

A major component of the quality improvement plan focuses on quality control procedures that are routinely performed, documented, and evaluated on the simulator, image processing equipment, immobilization devices, accessory equipment, treatment planning computer systems, and treatment units. Safety equipment such as emergency switches, door interlocks, and communication devices are included in the quality control checks.[16,24] This is to ensure that all is in proper working order according to manufacturer, department, and national specifications. Instrumentation that is used in performing these quality control checks, such as calibration equipment (ionization chamber and electrometer), scanning equipment, dosimetry accessories (solid phantom materials, thermometer, barometer), and miscellaneous dosimetry devices such as the thermoluminescent dosimeter (TLD) system and film, must also be periodically tested. Each radiation oncology center determines the frequency of these quality control checks based on the stability of equipment performance. Unstable equipment performance requires more frequent checks until the equipment performance has stabilized, and then the frequency may be reduced. Regular intervals such as daily, weekly, monthly, or annually are usually established for the quality control procedures. To reduce the risk of the patient being simulated or treated with faulty equipment, it is best to perform the daily quality checks in the morning before the first patient is simulated or treated.[16,24] The quality control procedures and tolerances are established and managed by the physicist; however, the radiation therapist plays a major role in obtaining this information. This is due to the therapist's familiarity with and knowledge of the equipment. Therefore it is imperative that the therapist be familiar with commonly performed quality control procedures and recommended tolerances for both the conventional and computed tomography simulator, cobalt-60 unit, and medical accelerator (Tables 19-3 through 19-7).

Table 19-3	QA of Simulators	
Frequency	**Procedure**	**Tolerance***
Daily	Localizing lasers	2 mm
	Distance indicator (ODI)	2 mm
Monthly	Field size indicator	2 mm
	Gantry/collimator angle indicators	1 degree
	Cross-hair centering	2 mm diameter
	Focal spot-axis indicator	2 mm
	Fluoroscopic image quality	Baseline
	Emergency/collision avoidance	Functional
	Light/radiation field coincidence	2 mm or 1%
	Film processor sensitometry	Baseline
Annually	**Mechanical checks**	
	Collimator rotation isocenter	2 mm diameter
	Gantry rotation isocenter	2 mm diameter
	Couch rotation isocenter	2 mm diameter
	Coincidence of collimator, gantry, couch axes, and isocenter	2 mm diameter
	Table top sag	2 mm
	Vertical travel of couch	2 mm
	Radiographic checks	
	Exposure rate	Baseline
	Table top exposure with fluoroscopy	Baseline
	Kilovolt peak and milliamperage calibration	Baseline
	High and low contrast resolution	Baseline

*The tolerances mean that the parameter exceeds the tabulated value (e.g., the measured isocenter under gantry rotation exceeds 2 mm diameter).
From AAPM: Comprehensive QA for radiation oncology: report of AAPM Radiation Therapy Committee Task Group 40, *Med Phys* 21:518-616, 1994.

However, quality control procedures and tolerances should be developed for any new treatment planning and delivery system that is used in the radiation therapy process. Documentation of quality control testing is an important aspect for determining equipment performance over a period of time. All results should be recorded in a logbook or kept on a computerized data collection system, along with actions that were taken to correct any deviations beyond the tolerance limits and the results of any necessary retesting. This documentation is a legal record and should be kept for the life of the equipment or as long as it is used in the radiation therapy process.[12,19]

ASSESSMENT OF THE DATA

An integral part of implementing the quality improvement process in radiation oncology is a continual statistical assessment of the data collected. Having a computerized data analysis system is mandatory.[35]

The TJC has developed its own indicator-based performance system (IM system) that organizations may use to provide a continuous evaluation of performance data, which is

Table 19-4	Commonly Performed Quality Control Procedures and Recommended Tolerances for the CT Simulator (as Established by the AAPM)	
Procedures	**Tolerances (±)**	
I. DAILY		
Alignment of gantry lasers with center of imaging plane	2 mm	
II. MONTHLY and after laser adjustments		
Orientation of gantry lasers with respect to the imaging plane	2 mm over the length of laser projection	
Spacing of lateral wall lasers with respect to lateral gantry lasers	2 mm and scan plane	
Orientation of wall lasers with respect to the imaging plane	2 mm over the length of laser projection	
Orientation of the ceiling laser with respect to the imaging plane	2 mm over the length of laser projection	
A. MONTHLY or when daily laser QA tests reveal rotational problems		
Orientation of the CT scanner tabletop with respect to the imaging plane	2 mm over the length and width of the tabletop	
B. MONTHLY		
Table vertical and longitudinal motion	1 mm over the range of table motion	
III. SEMI-ANNUALLY		
Sensitivity profile width	1 mm of nominal value	
IV. ANNUALLY		
Table indexing and position	1 mm over the scan range	
Gantry tilt accuracy	1 degree over the gantry tilt range	
Gantry tilt position accuracy	1 degree or 1 mm from nominal position	
Scan localization	1 mm over the scan range	
Radiation profile width	Manufacturer specification	
V. After replacement of major generator components		
Generator tests	Manufacturer specification or AAPM Report 39 recommendations	

From AAPM: Quality assurance for computed-tomography simulators and the computed-tomography-simulation process: Report of AAPM Radiation Therapy Committee Task Group 66, *Med Phys* 30:2765, 2003.
CT, Computed tomography; *QA,* quality assurance.

Table 19-5	Commonly Performed Quality Control Procedures and Recommended Tolerances for Image Performance Evaluation of the CT Simulator (as Established by the AAPM)	
Procedures	**Tolerances (±)**	
I. DAILY		
CT number accuracy for water	0-5 HU	
Image noise	Manufacturer specifications	
In plane spatial integrity X or Y direction	1 mm	
II. MONTHLY		
CT number accuracy for 4-5 different materials	5 HU	
In plane spatial integrity for both X and Y directions	1 mm	
Field uniformity: most commonly used kVp	5 HU	
III. ANNUALLY		
CT number accuracy with an electron density phantom	5 HU	
Field uniformity utilizing other kVp settings	5 HU	
Electron density to CT number conversion	Consistent with commissioning results and test phantom, manufacturer specifications	
Spatial resolution	Manufacturer specifications	
Contrast resolution	Manufacturer specifications	

From AAPM: Quality assurance for computed-tomography simulators and the computed-tomography-simulation process: Report of AAPM Radiation Therapy Committee Task Group 66, *Med Phys* 30:2766, 2003.
CT, Computed tomography; *HU,* Hounsfield unit; *kVp,* kilovoltage peak.

Table 19-6	QA of Cobalt-60 Units	
Frequency	**Procedure**	**Tolerance***
Daily	**Safety**	
	Door interlock	Functional
	Radiation room monitor	Functional
	Audiovisual monitor	Functional
	Mechanical	
	Lasers	2 mm
	Distance indicator (ODI)	2 mm
Weekly	Check of source positioning	3 mm
Monthly	**Dosimetry**	2%
	Output constancy	
	Mechanical checks	
	Light/radiation field coincidence	3 mm
	Field size indicator (collimator setting)	2 mm
	Gantry and collimator angle indicator	1 degree
	Cross-hair centering	1 mm
	Latching of wedges, trays	Functional
	Safety interlocks	
	Emergency off	Functional
	Wedge interlocks	Functional
Annually	**Dosimetry**	
	Output constancy	2%
	Field size dependence and output constancy	2%
	Central axis dosimetry parameter constancy (PDD/TAR)	2%
	Transmission factor consistency for all standard accessories	2%
	Wedge transmission factor consistency	2%
	Timer linearity and error	1%
	Output constancy versus gantry angle	2%
	Beam uniformity versus gantry angle	3%
	Safety interlocks	
	Follow test procedures of manufacturers	Functional
	Mechanical checks	
	Collimator rotation isocenter	2 mm diameter
	Gantry rotation isocenter	2 mm diameter
	Couch rotation isocenter	2 mm diameter
	Coincidence of collimator, gantry, couch axis with isocenter	2 mm diameter
	Coincidence of radiation and mechanical isocenter	2 mm diameter
	Table top sag	2 mm
	Vertical travel of table	2 mm
	Field light intensity	Functional

ODI, Optional distance indicator.

*The tolerances listed in the tables should be interpreted to mean that if a parameter either: (1) exceeds the tabulated value (e.g., the measured isocenter under gantry rotation exceeds 2 mm diameter); or (2) that the change in the parameter exceeds the nominal value (e.g., the output changes by more than 2%), then an action is required. The distinction is emphasized by the use of the term constancy for the latter case. Moreover, for constancy, percent values are ± the deviation of the parameter with respect to its nominal value; distances are referenced to the isocenter or nominal SSD.

From AAPM: Comprehensive QA for radiation oncology: Report of AAPM Radiation Therapy Committee Task Group 40, *Med Phys* 21:518-616, 1994.

then used in the accreditation process. Although currently focusing on acute care hospitals only, it is expected that the IM system's scope will be further expanded to include a broader group of health care organization in the future.[31]

Each of the aspects of care delineated under the quality improvement process discretely collects data through the use of check sheets, data sheets, and checklists. These data should then be statistically analyzed against internal and external customer satisfaction and placed in a meaningful format such as charts, graphs, and histograms with distribution to all employees.[24,25,27]

The selection of the appropriate solution or response should be substantiated by the data analysis. This task may be appropriately delegated to the quality improvement committee. However,

in a large health care facility/organization, this might necessitate the procurement of assistance from other "organization-wide systems such as strategic planning, performance management, measurement, budgetary, and management information." By doing that, the health care organization becomes a true "quality organization which continues to improve."[24]

Statistical analysis of the data collected in assessment of a quality improvement process is vital to the selection of the appropriate solution or response. These data should be organized in a format that is easy to understand. Learn more about different types of charts or graphs that may be used to display data by visiting the American Society for Quality at http://www.asq.org.

Table 19-7	QA of Medical Accelerators	
Frequency	**Procedure**	**Tolerance**[a]
Daily	**Dosimetry**	
	X-ray output constancy	3%
	Electron output constancy[b]	3%
	Mechanical	
	Localizing lasers	2 mm
	Distance indicator (ODI)	2 mm
	Safety	
	Door interlock	Functional
	Audiovisual monitor	Functional
Monthly	**Dosimetry**	
	X-ray output constancy[c]	2%
	Electron output constancy[c]	2%
	Backup monitor constancy	2%
	X-ray central axis dosimetry parameter (PDD, TAR) constancy	2%
	Electron central axis dosimetry parameter constancy (PDD)	2 mm @ therapeutic depth
	X-ray beam flatness constancy	2%
	Electron beam flatness constancy	3%
	X-ray and electron symmetry	3%
	Safety interlocks	
	Emergency off switches	Functional
	Wedge, electron cone interlocks	Functional
	Mechanical checks	
	Light/radiation field coincidence	2 mm or 1% on side[d]
	Gantry/collimator angle indicators	1 degree
	Wedge position	2 mm (or 2% change in transmission factor)
	Tray position	2 mm
	Applicator position	2 mm
	Field size indicators	2 mm
	Cross-hair centering	2 mm diameter
	Treatment couch position indicators	2 mm/1 degree
	Latching of wedges, blocking tray	Functional
	Jaw symmetry[e]	2 mm
	Field light intensity	Functional
Annually	**Dosimetry**	
	X-ray/electron output calibration constancy	2%
	Field size dependence of x-ray output constancy	2%
	Output factor constancy for electron applicators	2%
	Central axis parameter constancy (PDD, TAR)	2%
	Off-axis factor constancy	2%
	Transmission factor constancy for all treatment accessories	2%
	Wedge transmission factor constancy[f]	2%
	Monitor chamber linearity	1%
	X-ray output constancy versus gantry angle	2%
	Electron output constancy versus gantry angle	2%
	Off-axis factor constancy versus gantry angle	2%
	Arc mode	Manufacturer's specifications
	Safety interlocks	
	Follow manufacturer's test procedures	Functional
	Mechanical checks	
	Collimator rotation isocenter	2 mm diameter
	Gantry rotation isocenter	2 mm diameter
	Couch rotation isocenter	2 mm diameter
	Coincidence of collimator, gantry, and couch axes with isocenter	2 mm diameter
	Coincidence of radiation and mechanical isocenter	2 mm diameter
	Table top sag	2 mm
	Vertical travel of table	2 mm

[a]The tolerances listed in the tables should be interpreted to mean that if a parameter either: (1) exceeds the tabulated value (e.g., the measured isocenter under gantry rotation exceeds 2 mm diameter); or (2) that the change in the parameter exceeds the nominal value (e.g., the output changes by more than 2%), then an action is required. The distinction is emphasized by the use of the term constancy for the latter case. Moreover, for constancy, percent values are ± the deviation of the parameter with the respect to its nominal value; distances are referenced to the isocenter or nominal SSD.

[b]All electron energies need not be checked daily, but all electron energies are to be checked at least twice weekly.

[c]A constancy check with a field instrument using temperature/pressure corrections.

[d]Whichever is greater. Should also be checked after change in light field source.

[e]Jaw symmetry is defined as difference in distance of each jaw from the isocenter.

[f]Most wedges' transmission factors are field size and depth dependent.

From AAPM: Comprehensive QA for radiation oncology: report of AAPM Radiation Therapy Committee Task Group 40, *Med Phys* 21:518-616, 1994.

SUMMARY

- Quality improvement (QI) in health care is a systematic approach to the continuous study and improvement of the process of providing health care services to meet the needs of patients and others. Synonymous terms include continuous quality improvement (CQI) and total quality management (TQM). It is premised on Dr. W. E. Deming's 14 principles of management. These principles emphasize CQI through proactive employee participation in a "customer-responsive" environment. It involves doing things right and doing things well.

- Regulatory and accreditation agencies, along with professional organizations, establish standards to which a radiation oncology facility must adhere. These standards are the foundation of a QI plan.

- A QI plan lists the organizational structure, responsibilities, procedures, processes, and resources for implementing a comprehensive quality system. The quality improvement team members assist in the documentation and collection of data.

- The QI team consists of all personnel in the radiation oncology facility who interact with the patient and family. After the data are collected, they must be systematically analyzed to substantiate an appropriate solution or response. This task may be delegated to the QI committee.

- Because of the diversity of health care organizations, they may choose to use a variety of management methods to implement the CQI plan. This may include the adoption of system-wide programs such as Lean, Six Sigma, or Lean Six Sigma.

- A successful QI plan is the end result of total commitment and involvement from all health care providers at all times. Linked to cost containment, increased quality of care, professional practice standards, and the TJC criteria, CQI has become routine practice in the delivery of health care.

- It is the responsibility of the radiation therapist and every other radiation oncology team member to become educated about QI. They will undoubtedly be involved in many aspects of CQI in their professional careers, with the ultimate benefit going to our customers, especially our patients.

Review Questions

Multiple Choice

1. What is the recommended frequency of checking audio and video monitors in treatment rooms?
   a. daily
   b. weekly
   c. monthly
   d. yearly
2. Quality improvement is specifically:
   a. a proactive means to ensure quality patient care
   b. the operational techniques and activities used to fulfill quality requirements
   c. both a and b
   d. neither a nor b

3. Ongoing evaluation of all aspects of care for the purpose of determining areas where improvement is needed is known as:
   a. total quality management
   b. quality assessment
   c. quality assurance
   d. quality control
4. An assessment of an aspect of a plan of action by those with the same job title and responsibilities is known as:
   a. quality control
   b. peer review
   c. quality indicator
   d. flowcharting
5. The operational techniques and activities used to fulfill requirements of quality are called:
   a. quality audit
   b. quality control
   c. quality management
   d. quality assessment
6. Members of a quality improvement team in radiation oncology include:
   a. all personnel in radiation oncology who come in contact with the patient and family
   b. clinical physicists and dosimetrists only
   c. personnel appointed by the medical director
   d. only the medical director, physicists, and lead therapist
7. An information analysis tool that may be used to identify specific steps in a process is called a:
   a. cause-and-effect diagram
   b. control chart
   c. flowchart
   d. histogram
8. The Indicator Measurement (IM) system, created by The Joint Commission, evaluates the quality of care among health care organizations through the comparison of common quality:
   a. assurance techniques
   b. audits
   c. indicators
   d. surveys
9. The radiation oncology quality improvement plan:
   a. identifies the responsibilities, procedures, processes, and resources for implementing the CQI plan
   b. includes verification that the radiation oncology process meets only the national standards
   c. is basically concerned with machine measurements
   d. is monitored solely by the physicists
10. Statistical analysis of the quality improvement data:
    a. is insignificant to implementing the quality improvement plan
    b. is a voluntary step in the quality improvement process
    c. is applied to only a select number of the collected data sets
    d. may help substantiate an appropriate solution to an outcome

The answers to the Review Questions can be found by logging on to our website at: *http://evolve.elsevier.com/Washington+Leaver/principles*

Questions to Ponder

1. Explain why the phrase "If it ain't broke, don't fix it" cannot be applied in a quality improvement program.
2. An initial step in improving a process is defining those activities used in completing the process. Develop a flowchart outlining the steps necessary to complete a double-exposure portal film in the radiation oncology department.
3. Referring to Deming's principles of management, what suggestions would you give a co-worker who consistently complains about a specific problem relating to the treatment delivery process in radiation oncology?
4. Describe how information collected for quality assessment should be used in a quality management plan.
5. Explain the differences between quality assurance and quality management.

REFERENCES

1. American Association of Physicists in Medicine: Comprehensive QA for radiation oncology: report of AAPM Radiation Therapy Committee Task Group 40, *Med Phys* 21:518-616, 1994.
2. American Association of Physicists in Medicine: *Quality assurance for clinical radiotherapy treatment planning: report of AAPM Radiation Therapy Committee Task Group 53,* College Park, Md, 1998, The American Association of Physicists in Medicine.
3. American Association of Physicists in Medicine: *Clinical use of electronic portal imaging: report of AAPM Radiation Therapy Committee Task Group 58,* College Park, Md, 2001, The American Association of Physicists in Medicine.
4. American College of Medical Physics: *Radiation control and quality assurance in radiation oncology: a suggested protocol, Report No. 2,* Reston, Va, 1986, American College of Medical Physics.
5. American College of Radiology: *Standards* (website): http://www.acr.org/SecondaryMainMenuCategories/quality_safety/guidelines.aspx. Accessed November 14, 2008.
6. American Society for Quality Organization. (website): http://www.asq.org/learn-about-quality/continuous-improvement/overview/overview.html.
7. American Society of Radiologic Technologists: Government relations section: *OSHA updates facility consultation regulations* (website): http://www.asrt.org/asrt.htm. Accessed April 10, 2003.
8. American Society of Radiologic Technologists: Professional development section: *Practice standards for medical imaging and radiation therapy* (website): http://www.asrt.org/asrt.htm. Accessed July 10, 2007.
9. Brundage MD, et al: A real-time audit of radiation therapy in a regional cancer center, *Int J Radiat Oncol Biol Phys* 43:121, 1999.
10. Decarlo N, Gygi G, Williams B: *The complete idiot's guide to Lean Six Sigma,* New York, 2007, Penguin Group (USA).
11. Earp KA, Gates L: A model QA program in radiation oncology, *Radiol Tech* 61:297-304, 1990.
12. Environmental Protection Agency: *Timeline* (website): http://www.epa.gov/history/timeline/index.htm. Accessed July 10, 2007.
13. Food and Drug Administration: *Accidental radiation occurrences and radiation incidents.* (website): http://www.accessdata.fda.gov/scripts/cdnh/cfdocs/cfcfr/CFRSearch.cfm?FR=1002.20. Accessed November 14, 2008.
14. George ML: *Lean Six Sigma for service,* New York, 2003, McGraw-Hill Companies.
15. George ML, et al: *The Lean Six Sigma pocket toolbook: a quick reference guide to 100 tools for improving quality and speed,* New York, 2005, George Group.
16. Hendee WR, Ibbott GS: *Radiation therapy physics,* ed 3, Hoboken, NJ, 2004, Wiley & Sons.
17. Industrial Security Clearance Review Office Subcommittee: *Radiation oncology in integrated cancer management,* Blue Book, December 1991.
18. International Standards Organization: International Standards Organization Report ISO-8402-1986, Netherlands, Springer, 1986.
19. Joint Commission on Accreditation of Healthcare Organizations: *Improving organization performance*: comprehensive accreditation manual for hospitals, update 3, Oakbrook Terrace, Ill, August 1998, The Author.
20. Joint Commission on Accreditation of Healthcare Organizations: *1994 Accreditation manual for hospitals,* Oakbrook Terrace, Ill, 1994, The Author.
21. Joint Commission on Accreditation of Healthcare Organizations: *1995 Accreditation manual for hospitals,* Oakbrook Terrace, Ill, 1995, The Author.
22. Joint Commission on Accreditation of Healthcare Organizations: *The IM system: leading the way to performance measurement—comprehensive accreditation manual for hospitals, update 3,* Oakbrook Terrace, Ill, August 1997, The Author.
23. Khan FM: *The physics of radiation therapy,* ed 3, Philadelphia, 2003, Lippincott Williams & Wilkins.
24. Kirk R: The big picture: total quality management and continuous quality improvement, *J Nurs Admin* 24:37-41, 1994.
25. Lapresti J, Whetstone WR: Total quality management: doing things right, *Nurs Manage* 24:34-36, 1993.
26. Levitte SH, Khan F: Quality assurance in radiation oncology, *Cancer* 74(suppl 9):2642-2646, 1994.
27. Nelson MT: Continuous quality improvement (CQI) in radiology: an overview, *Appl Radiol* 23:11-16, 1994.
28. Norris TG: Quality assurance in radiation therapy, *Radiat Ther* 9:161-184, 2000.
29. Nuclear Regulatory Commission: *Mission* (website): http://www.nrc.gov/about-nrc.html. Accessed November 14, 2008.
30. Occupational Safety and Health Administration: US Department of Labor (website): http://www.osha-slc.gov/index.html. Accessed July 10, 2007.
31. Office of Hazardous Materials: *Mission* (website): http://www.phmsa.dot.gov/hazmat/about. Accessed November 14, 2008.
32. Office of State and Tribal Programs (website): http://www.nrc.gov/about-nrc./state-tribal.html. Accessed November 14, 2008.
33. Papp J: *Quality management in the imaging sciences,* St. Louis, 2006, Mosby, pp 1-31.
34. Sherman J, Malkmus MA: Integrating quality assurance and total quality management/quality improvement, *J Nurs Admin* 24:37-41, 1994.
35. Thwaites D, Scolliet P, Leer JW: Quality assurance in radiotherapy, *Radiother Oncol* 35:61-73, 1995.
36. US Department of Transportation: *Quality assurance* (website): http://www.dot.gov/safety.html. Accessed July 10, 2007.
37. Van der Schueren E, Hariot JC, Leunens G: Quality assurance in cancer treatment, *Eur J Cancer* 29A:172-181, 1993.
38. Wambersie A: The role of the ICRU in quality assurance in radiation therapy, *Int J Radiat Oncol Biol Phys* 10(suppl 1):81-86, 1984.

BIBLIOGRAPHY

American Association of Physicists in Medicine: *Acceptance testing and quality control of photostimulable storage phosphor imaging systems: report of AAPM Task Group 10, Report No. 93,* College Park, Md, 2006, The American Association of Physicists in Medicine.

American Association of Physicists in Medicine: Guidance document on delivery, treatment planning, and clinical implementation of IMRT: Report of the IMRT Subcommittee of the AAPM Radiation Therapy Committee, *Med Phys* 30(8), 2003.

American Association of Physicists in Medicine: Quality assurance for computed-tomography simulators and the computed-tomography simulation process: report of the AAPM Radiation Therapy Committed Task Group 66, *Med Phys* 30, 2003.

Khan F: *Treatment planning in radiation oncology,* ed 2, Philiadelphia, 2007, Lippincott Williams & Wilkins.

Stevens AT: *Quality management for radiographic imaging: a guide for technologists,* New York, 2001, McGraw-Hill Companies.

20 CHAPTER

Surface and Sectional Anatomy

Charles M. Washington

Outline

Key Terms

Objectives

1. Relate the importance and use of imaging modalities in radiation therapy.
2. Compare and contrast aspects of anatomic positioning, anatomy features and organ/tissue location used by the radiation oncology team for treatment planning and delivery.
3. Understand the components and function of the lymphatic system and its role in treatment field design.
4. Correlate superficial anatomic landmarks and cross-sectional perspectives to deeply seated internal anatomy.

Radiation therapy practice requires all team members to demonstrate keen knowledge of human anatomy and physiology. The radiation therapist learns early in the educational curriculum that he or she must have a comprehensive understanding of surface and cross-sectional anatomy. Knowledge of human anatomy is essential in simulation, treatment planning, and accurate daily treatment delivery. This chapter focuses on the surface and sectional anatomy used in simulation and treatment delivery performed by the radiation therapist. Surface anatomy will be related to deep-seated structures within the human body. An overview of the diagnostic tools used to visualize internal structures is presented, along with a review of lymphatic physiology. This is included because the lymphatics play a major role in treatment field design and disease management. A brief review of skeletal anatomy is presented to ensure a common basis for understanding important spatial relationships. Surface and sectional, along with topographic, landmarks are presented in practical radiation therapy applications.

PERSPECTIVE

The primary objective in managing cancer with radiation therapy is to deposit enough dose to result in cancer cell death while minimizing the effect on the surrounding normal tissues. The challenge is to define a patient-specific therapy plan that localizes the tumor and surrounding dose-limiting tissues, such as the spinal cord, kidney, and eyes. In addition, the radiation therapist must maintain the integrity of the plan throughout its administration. Surface anatomy has changed very little over the past 40 years. Clinical application is essential in understanding of a disease process on anatomic grounds, corresponding surface location of internal structures, and the appearance of internal imaged structures.[12]

Visual, palpable, and imaged anatomy forms the basis of clinical examination.[11] This is the case in radiation therapy. Surface and sectional anatomy provides the foundation that the radiation therapist needs to be effective in simulation, treatment planning, and the daily administration of therapy treatments. Without this foundation, it would be like traveling from Texas to Maine for the first time, without any planning. We know the general direction of where we want to go, but we would not know the most efficient way to get there. Sectional anatomy emphasizes the physical relationship between internal structures.[10] The radiation therapist must have a complete understanding of imaging modalities that enable tumor visualization, identification of pertinent lymphatic anatomy, and the site-by-site relationship of surface and sectional anatomy. A systematic approach to this information will allow the radiation therapist to link vital classroom information to its clinical application.

RELATED IMAGING MODALITIES USED IN SIMULATION AND TUMOR LOCALIZATION

More than any other innovation, the ability to painlessly visualize the interior of the living human body has governed the practice of medicine during the 20th century.[2] In recent years, advancements in medical imaging techniques allow for effective ways to diagnose and localize pathologic disorders. The medical imaging modalities used in simulation and tumor localization fit into two categories: ionizing and nonionizing imaging studies. Ionizing imaging studies use ionizing radiation to produce images that demonstrate anatomy. Examples of ionizing imaging studies include conventional radiography; computed tomography (CT); and nuclear medicine imaging, particualry positron emission tomography (PET) and the fusion of PET and CT. Nonionizing imaging studies use alternative means of imaging the body, such as magnetic fields in magnetic resonance imaging (MRI) and echoed sound waves in ultrasonography.

Conventional Radiography

A radiograph provides a two-dimensional image of the interior of the body. Computerized radiography (CR) and digital radiography (DR) can also be used to visualize internal anatomy without exposing a physical film. In either case, photostimulable plates or detectors capture the latent images for visualization on

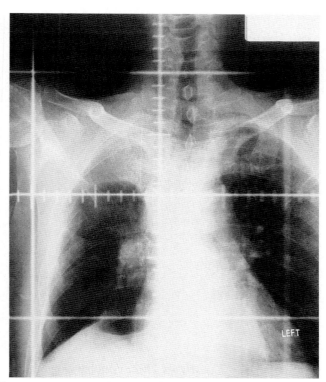

Figure 20-1. Typical thorax conventional simulation film. Note how bony anatomy is distinguishable from cartilage and soft tissue.

computer screens. The latent images produced demonstrate the differences in tissue densities of the body; however, x-rays do not always distinguish subtle differences in tissue density. Figure 20-1 demonstrates a conventional chest radiograph produced by a radiation therapy simulator. The pertinent anatomy can be distinguished and outlined for practical application. Any anomaly, a variation from the standard, is recognizable on the image, as is any structure considered to be dose limiting.

Radiation therapy uses an extensive amount of diagnostic imaging in its daily practice. Simulators use specialized diagnostic x-ray equipment to localize the treatment area and reproduce the geometry of the therapeutic beam before treatment. Radiographic localization, once the most common method used to localize tumor volumes, is still a prominent way to capture treatment planning information. Other techniques also aid in visualization of human anatomy. Although used less often today, **lymphangiography**, a specialized technique that uses injected dyes to help visualize the lymphatic system, may still be used in some cases. Figure 20-2 shows a radiograph that uses lymphangiography. The lymphatic channels are the white areas of higher density. Filling defects, lymphatic channels that are not completely visible or appear frothy, can demonstrate the presence of pathologic changes. These all provide valuable information for patient treatment planning. Overall, conventional radiology is still an important component in radiation therapy.

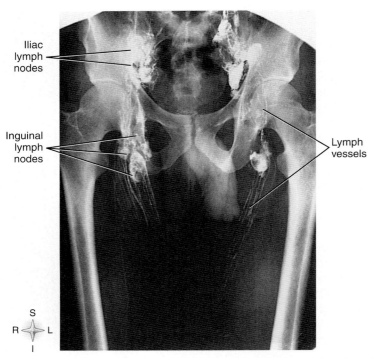

Iliac lymph nodes

Inguinal lymph nodes

Lymph vessels

S
R — L
I

Figure 20-2. Lymphangiogram. The lymphatic channels can be imaged and used to assess the status of the lymphatics. (From Ballinger PW, Frank ED: *Merrill's atlas of radiographic positions and radiologic procedures,* ed 10, vol 2, St. Louis, 2003, Mosby.)

Computed Tomography

In modern radiation therapy treatment planning and delivery, the use of CT imaging has become the most common means of data capture. The translation of three-dimensional information is essential to the complex treatment delivery systems used today, such as intensity-modulated radiation therapy (IMRT), stereotactic radiosurgery (SRS), and all image-guided radiation therapies (IGRTs).

CT is an ionizing radiation–based technique in which x-rays interact with a scintillation crystal that is more sensitive than x-ray film.[1] CT scanning combines x-ray principles and advanced computer technologies. The x-ray source moves in an arc around the body part being scanned and continually sends out beams of radiation. As the beams pass through the body, the tissues absorb small amounts of radiation, depending on their densities. The beams are converted to signals that are projected onto a computer screen. These images look like radiographs of slices through the body. They are typically perpendicular to the long axis of the patient's body. The CT scan provides important anatomic and spatial relationships at a glance. A series of scans allows the examination of section after section of a patient's anatomy.

The entire CT process takes only seconds for each slice, and it is completely painless. The detail of the images produced is approximately 10 to 20 times the detail of conventional radiography. Display of CT images reflects the differences among four basic densities: air (black), fat (dark/gray), water/blood (gray/light), and bone/metal (white).[1] CT demonstrates bone detail well. Radiation therapy treatment planning commonly uses CT images, particularly with three-dimensional and conformal treatment plans and virtual simulation techniques.

Four-dimensional CT (4D CT): *With the implementation of 4D CT, physicists are able to track the movement of a moving tumor (e.g., in the lung), throughout the entire breathing cycle, so physicians can follow exactly where the tumor is located at all points of the cycle. The same technology is used as for gated breathing techniques: a box with indicating markers is placed on the patients' abdomen/chest during the simulation. This enables physicians to determine whether treatment with the gated breathing technique (where radiation is given only during a specific portion of the patient's breathing cycle) would allow the planner to minimize the amount of normal tissue in the field.*

Nuclear Medicine Imaging

The branch of medicine that uses radioisotopes in the diagnosis and treatment of disease is known as *nuclear medicine.* Nuclear medicine imaging uses ionizing radiation to provide information about physiology, as well as anatomic structure. This is typically useful in noted abnormalities secondary to tumor activity, specifically metastatic disease.[16] Sensitive radiation detection devices display images of radioactive drugs taken through the body and their uptake in tissues. Although this imaging technique plays an important role in tumor imaging, it detects disease dissemination more than primary tumors. Bone and liver metastases are localized using nuclear medicine scans. These scans are relatively safe and can provide valuable information. The radionuclide bone scan is the procedure of choice for skeletal scanning. Figure 20-3 shows a bone scan.

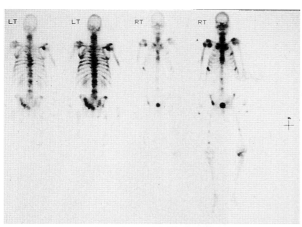

Figure 20-3. Radionuclide bone scan. Multiple focal lesions in bone of patient with prostate cancer.

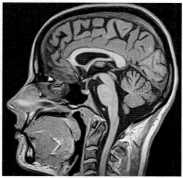

Sagittal

Figure 20-4. Sagittal magnetic resonance image section through the head. (From Kelley LL, Peterson CM: *Sectional anatomy for imaging professionals*, ed 2, St. Louis, 2007, Elsevier Mosby.)

Areas of increased uptake, the dark spots, demonstrate high-activity areas that correspond to pathologic changes (uptake in the urinary bladder is normal). The radionuclide liver scan is the initial scan of choice for liver metastasis. Gallium scans localize areas of inflammation and tumor activity in patients with lymphoma. They are useful in monitoring changes in tumor size. Radiation safety procedures are important in nuclear medicine scanning. In both intravenous application and ingestion of radioactive isotopes, care in monitoring patient exposure to ionizing radiation is important. The elimination of isotopes that have run through the body (through urination) also requires careful monitoring and precautions.

PET scanning uses short-lived radioisotopes such as carbon-11, nitrogen-13, or oxygen-15 in a solution commonly injected into a patient. The radioisotope circulates through the body and emits positively charged electrons, called *positrons*. These positrons collide with conventional electrons in body tissues, causing the release of gamma rays. These rays are detected and recorded. The computer creates a colored PET scan that demonstrates function rather than structure. It can detect blood flow through organs such as the brain and heart, diagnose coronary artery disease, and identify the extent of stroke or heart attack damage. PET is useful in diagnosing many different cancers. In that way, the physician can prescribe the appropriate treatment regimen early. In addition, PET images are being used more and more to outline specific areas of anatomy and are then correlated to other imaging studies such as CT and magnetic resonance (MR) in treatment planning. The role of PET/CT is increasing not only as an oncologic staging tool but also as an effective means of providing additional information for more effective treatment planning. With both anatomic and physiologic information, the potential to visualize extension of disease not always seen on CT (due to size) can direct the radiation oncology team to make sure that the treatment field covers all diseased areas. This in itself can translate into better overall treatment results.

Magnetic Resonance Imaging

MRI records data that are based on the magnetic properties of the hydrogen nuclei, which can be thought of as tiny magnets

spinning in random directions. These hydrogen nuclei (magnets) interact with neighboring atoms and with all applied magnetic fields.[1] In this imaging modality, a strong uniform magnetic energy is applied to small magnetic fields that lie parallel to the direction of the external magnet. The patient is pulsed with radiowaves, which causes the nuclei to send out a weak radio signal that is detected and reworked into a planar image of the body. The images, which indicate cellular activity, look similar to a CT scan. Figure 20-4 shows a sagittal MRI scan of the head.

MRI has a diagnostic advantage over CT in that it provides information about chemicals in an organ or tissue. In this way, MRI can perform a noninvasive (one not involving puncture or incision of the skin or insertion of a foreign object into the body) biopsy on tumors. The disadvantages of MRI are the expensive magnetic shielding requirements, low throughput (the number of patients an hour a machine can serve) when compared with CT, and increased cost in comparison with CT. MRI scans can be indexed, registered, and fused with CT scans and used in the treatment planning process. In these cases, the best of both imaging modalities are used to outline tumors for better conformal treatment planning.

Ultrasound

Ultrasound (US) uses high-frequency sound waves, which are not heard by the human ear. These waves travel forward and continue to move until they make contact with an object; at that point, a certain amount of the sound bounces back. Submarines use this principle to find other underwater vessels, as well as the depth of the ocean floor. US remains a less expensive and less hazardous alternative to the earlier studies.[16] A transducer, a handheld instrument, generates high-frequency sound waves. It moves over the body part being examined. The transducer also picks up the returning sound waves. Normal and abnormal tissues exhibit varying densities that reflect sound differently. The resultant image is processed onto a screen and is called a *sonogram*. The images can be a still two-dimensional, cross-sectioned image or a moving image, such as the heart of a fetus.

US offers no exposure to ionizing radiation, is noninvasive and painless, and requires no contrast media. However, it does

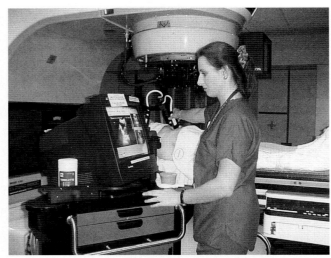

Figure 20-5. Therapist obtaining ultrasound information for intensity-modulated radiation therapy (IMRT) prostate treatment.

not effectively penetrate bone or air-filled spaces. It is therefore not useful in imaging the skull, lungs, or intestines. In radiation therapy, the use of US continues to increase. It is very helpful in noninvasively determining internal organ location as evidenced in the increasing use of US to locate and guide brachytherapy implants, locating tumors within the eye, and increasing positioning efficiency during conformal prostate treatment delivery with IMRT applications. Figure 20-5 shows a radiation therapist obtaining US localization information for a patient about to be treated for prostate cancer.

Modern imaging modalities provide important information to the radiation therapy team for tumor localization. Cross-sectional images are very valuable. They provide views within the patient and display organs with their normal shape and orientation, typically in treatment position. The direct relationships allow for accurate treatment planning. We can relate the patient's surface anatomy to the inner structure. In addition to displaying organs with their normal living shape, normal anatomic relationships can be observed. In particular, the study of sectional images allows the radiation therapy practitioner to develop an excellent three-dimensional concept of anatomy.[10] These modalities provide the basic information necessary to develop critical thinking skills in surface and sectional anatomy that is essential in the role of the radiation therapist.

ANATOMIC POSITIONING

Radiation therapy requires daily reproducible positioning for effective treatment delivery. The radiation therapist uses various terms to describe the relationship of anatomic parts, planes, and sections that serve as the foundation in understanding the body's structural plan.

Definition of Terms

When using terms that reference human body position, it is assumed that the body is in the anatomic position; this allows for clear reference of directional relationships. The **anatomic position** is one in which the subject stands upright, with feet together flat on the floor, toes pointed forward, arms straight

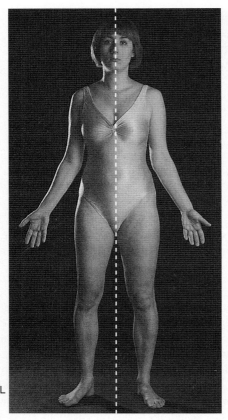

Figure 20-6. Anatomic position and bilateral symmetry. In the anatomical position, the body is in an erect, or standing, posture with the arms at the sides and palms forward. The head and feet are also pointing forward. The dotted line shows the body's bilateral symmetry. As a result of this organizational feature, the right and left sides of the body are mirror images of each other. (From The body as a whole. In Thibodeau GA, Patton KT, editors: *Anatomy and physiology*, ed 2, St. Louis, 1993, Mosby. Courtesy Joan M. Beck.)

down by the sides of the body with palms facing forward, fingers extended, and thumbs pointing away from the body.[11] Figure 20-6 demonstrates this position.

Directional terms explain the location of various body structures in relation to each other. These terms are precise and avoid the use of unnecessary words and paint a clear picture for the radiation therapist. *Superior* means toward the head; *inferior,* toward the feet; *medial,* toward the midline of the body; and *lateral,* toward one side or the other. *Anterior* relates to anatomy nearer to the front of the body; *posterior,* nearer to or at the back of the body. *Ipsilateral* refers to a body component on the same side of the body, whereas *contralateral* refers to the opposite side of the body. *Supine* means lying face up; *prone* means lying face down. Table 20-1 outlines the directional terms commonly used by the radiation therapy team.

Planes and Sections

The human body may also be examined with respect to planes, which are imaginary flat surfaces that pass through it. Figure 20-7 illustrates the standard anatomic planes. The *sagittal plane* divides the body vertically into right or left sides. The *median sagittal plane,* also called the *midsagittal plane,* divides

Table 20-1	**Directional Terms**	
Term	**Definition**	**Example**
Superior	Toward the head or upper part of a structure	The manubrium is superior to the body of the sternum.
Inferior	Away from the head or lower part of a structure	The stomach is inferior to the lung.
Anterior	Toward or nearer to the front	The trachea is anterior to the esophagus, which is anterior to the spinal cord.
Posterior	Nearer to the back	The esophagus is posterior to the trachea.
Medial	Nearer to the midline; the midline is an imaginary vertical line that divides the body into equal right and left components	The ulna is on the medial side of the forearm.
Lateral	Farther from the midline or to the side	The pleural cavities are lateral to the pericardial cavity.
Ipsilateral	On the same side	The ascending colon and appendix are ipsilateral.
Contralateral	On the opposite side	The ascending colon and descending colon are contralateral.
Proximal	Nearer to the point of origin or attachment	The humerus is proximal to the radius.
Distal	Farther from the point of origin or attachment	The phalanges are distal to the carpals.
Superficial	On or near the body surface	The skin is superficial to the thoracic viscera.
Deep	Away from the body surface	The ribs are deep to the skin of the chest.

Modified from Tortora G, Anagnostakos N, editors: *Principles of anatomy and physiology,* ed 6. Copyright © 1990 by Biological Sciences Textbooks, Inc., A & P Textbooks, Inc., and Elia-Sparta, Inc. Reprinted by permission of Harper Collins Publishers, Inc.

the body into two symmetric right and left sides. There is only one median sagittal plane. A *parasagittal plane* is a vertical plane that is parallel to the median sagittal plane and divides the body into unequal components, both right and left. A *coronal* or *frontal plane* is perpendicular (at right angles) to the sagittal plane and vertically divides the body into anterior and posterior sections. A *horizontal* or *transverse plane* is perpendicular to the midsagittal, parasagittal, and coronal planes and divides the

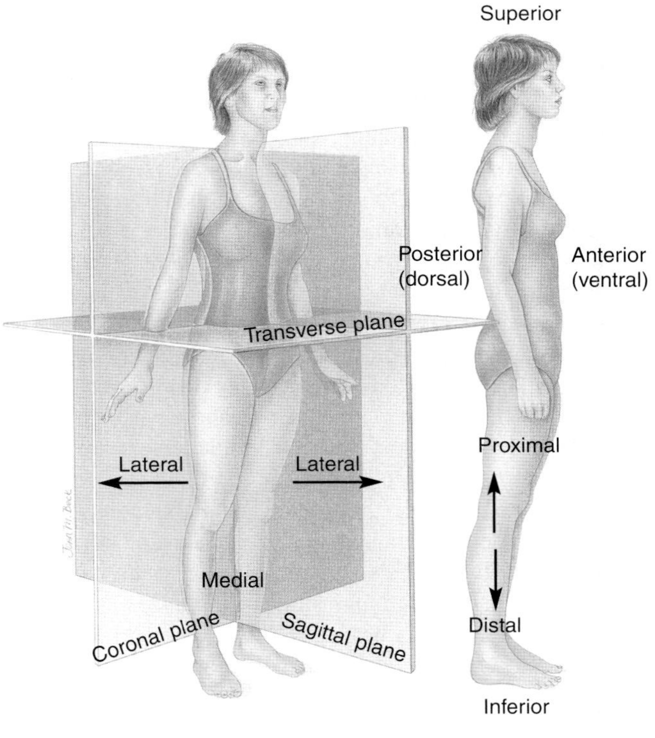

Figure 20-7. Directions and planes of the body. These planes provide a standardized reference for the radiation therapist. (From Organization of the body. In Thibodeau GA, Patton KT, editors: *Anatomy and physiology,* ed 2, St. Louis, 1993, Mosby. Courtesy Joan M. Beck.)

human body into superior and inferior parts. When a health care professional views a body structure, that structure is often seen in a sectional view. A sectional view looks at a flat surface resulting from a cut made through the three-dimensional structure.

Surface and cross-sectional anatomy in radiation therapy are not solely a set of definitions or a listing of body parts. The practitioner must relate the body's physical perspective to its overall function. The standardized anatomic terms presented will assist in accurately realizing those relationships.

BODY CAVITIES

The spaces within the body that contain internal organs are called **body cavities** (Figure 20-8). The two main cavities are the posterior, or dorsal, and the anterior, or ventral, cavities. The dorsal cavity can be further divided into (1) the spinal or vertebral cavity, protected by the vertebrae, which contains the spinal cord, and (2) the cranial cavity, which contains the brain.

The anterior cavity is subdivided by a horizontal muscle, called the *diaphragm,* into the thoracic cavity and the abdominopelvic cavity. The thoracic cavity is further divided into a pericardial cavity, which contains the heart and two pleural cavities, including the right and left lungs.

The abdominopelvic cavity has two sections: the upper abdominal cavity and the lower pelvic cavity. There is no intervening partition between the two. The principal structures located in the abdominal cavity are the peritoneum, liver, gallbladder, pancreas, spleen, stomach, and most of the large and small intestines. The pelvic section contains the rest of the large intestine, rectum, urinary bladder, and internal reproductive system.

The abdominopelvic cavity is large and is divided into four quadrants by placing a transverse plane across the midsagittal plane at the point of the umbilicus (navel). The four quadrants are the right upper, left upper, right lower, and left lower. The abdominal cavity can also be sectioned into a number of regions. Figure 20-9 shows the quadrants and regions of the abdomen and pelvis. Table 20-2 outlines the regions of the abdominal cavity.

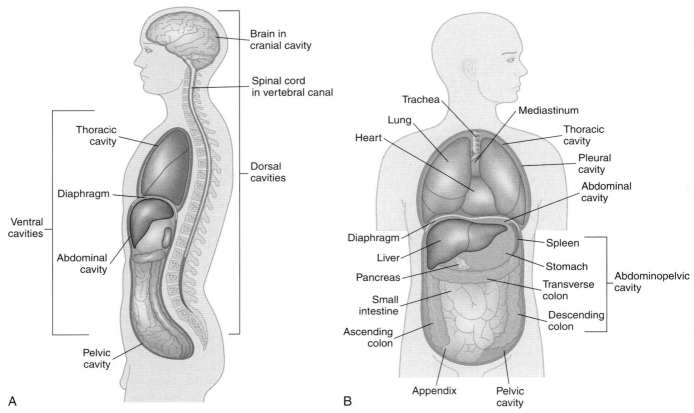

Figure 20-8. Major body cavities. **A**, Sagittal view. **B**, Anterior view. (From Kelley LL, Peterson CM: *Sectional anatomy for imaging professionals*, ed 2, St. Louis, 2007, Mosby.)

The surface markings and locations of all structures are approximations and generalizations.[10] However, knowledge of the varying body types will provide the radiation therapist with practical information. If the therapist has an idea of where the internal structures are, especially during a simulation, he or she can locate the placement of the treatment portal sooner and more accurately. This equates to less time on the conventional simulation table for the patient and lower fluoroscopic exposure times, because the simulation will not require as much location time.

BODY HABITUS

Roentgen's discovery of the x-ray allowed scientists at the turn of the 19th century to revolutionize the medical field, both diagnostically and therapeutically.[2] These early radiographs showed differences in the location of internal anatomy from one person to the next. Although everyone had the same organs, the organs were not necessarily in the exact same place. It was agreed that humans are a variable species with regard to structural characteristics, and it is evident that variety in general physique corresponds to great variation in visceral form, position, and motility. There is consistency between certain physiques and certain types of visceral form and arrangement. It is obvious that a thorax of certain dimensions can house lungs of only a certain form. The same is true for the abdomen. Knowing this can greatly assist the radiation therapist in relating internal anatomy to varying body types.

The physique, or **body habitus**, of an individual can be classified into four groups. The *hypersthenic habitus* represents approximately 5% of the population. This body type exhibits a short, wide trunk; great body weight; and a heavy skeletal framework. The abdomen is long with great capacity, the alimentary tract is high, and the stomach is almost thoracic. The pelvic cavity is small. When a chest film of this body type is being taken, it may be necessary to turn the cassette crosswise to image the entire chest.

The *sthenic habitus* resembles the hypersthenic habitus. These individuals make up close to half (approximately 48%) of the population. They are of considerable weight with a heavy skeletal framework. The alimentary tract is high but not as high as in the hypersthenic habitus. Most stout, well-built persons are sthenics.

The *hyposthenic habitus,* entailing approximately 35% of the population, has a slender physique. This habitus demonstrates many of the sthenic characteristics but appears to be frailer. The abdominal cavity falls between the sthenic and the asthenic.

The *asthenic habitus* demonstrates a more slender physique, light body weight, and a lighter skeletal framework. It is found in 10% to 12% of the population. The thorax has long, narrow lung fields with its widest portion in the upper zones. The heart is commonly pendent in form. The asthenic has an abdomen longer than the hypersthenic and is typically accompanied by a pelvis with great capacity. The alimentary tract is lowest of all types mentioned. Figure 20-10 compares the various body habitus. Although the internal components are the same in all

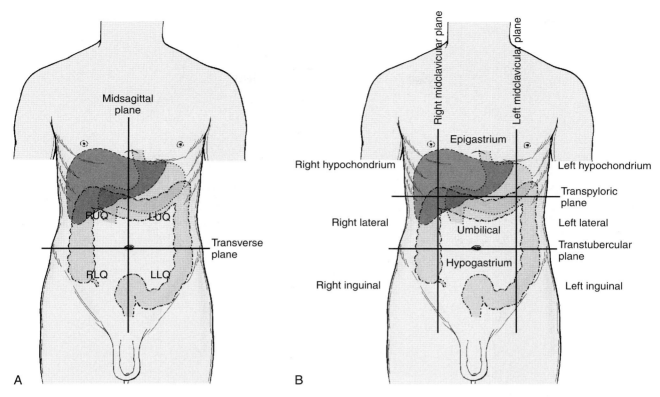

Figure 20-9. Abdomen. **A**, Division of the abdomen into four quarters. Diagram shows relationship of internal organs to the abdominopelvic quadrants. *RUQ*, Right upper quadrant; *LUQ*, left upper quadrant; *RLQ*, right lower quadrant; *LLQ*, left lower quadrant. **B**, Nine abdominopelvic regions showing the most superficial organs. (From Kelley LL, Peterson CM: *Sectional anatomy for imaging professionals*, ed 2, St. Louis, 2007, Mosby.)

body types, the locations vary. These categories can help standardize the variances demonstrated from person to person.

LYMPHATIC SYSTEM

Knowledge of the **lymphatic system** is very important in radiation therapy. For local and regional control of malignant disease processes to be achieved, the anatomy of the lymphatic system must be considered. Many tumors spread through this system; often, areas of tumor spread are predicted based solely on that knowledge. For example, in a head and neck treatment plan the

Table 20-2	Regions of the Abdominal Cavity
Region	**Description**
Umbilical	Centrally located around the navel
Lumbar	Regions to the right and left of the navel; lumbar refers to the lower back, which is located here
Epigastric	Central region superior to the umbilical region
Hypochondriac	Regions to the right and left of the epigastric region and inferior to the cartilage of the rib cage
Hypogastric	Central region inferior to the umbilical region
Iliac	Regions to the right and left of the hypogastric region; iliac refers to the hip bones, which are located here

supraclavicular fossa (SCF) is commonly treated even if there is no clinical evidence of tumor present (prophylactic treatment). This is important because the lymphatic drainage of the head and neck eventually drains to that area, which is the location of the right and left lymphatic ducts. This increases the potential for dissemination of disease to other parts of the body. In any examination of surface and cross-sectional anatomy specific to radiation therapy, the lymphatic system is very important.

The lymphatic system consists of lymphatic vessels; lymphatic organs; and the fluid that circulates through it, called *lymph*. The system is closely associated with the cardiovascular system and is composed of specialized connective tissue that contains a large quantity of lymphocytes. Lymphatic tissue is found throughout the body.

The lymphatic system has three main functions. First, lymphatic vessels drain tissue spaces of interstitial fluid that escapes from blood capillaries and loose connective tissues, filters it, and returns it to the bloodstream, an essential part of maintaining the overall fluid levels in the body. This function of draining and transporting interstitial fluid is the most important system role.[8] Second, the lymphatic system absorbs fats and transports them to the bloodstream. Third, this intricate system plays a major role in the body's defense and immunity. **Immunity** is the ability of the body to defend itself against infectious organisms and foreign bodies. Specifically, lymphocytes and macrophages protect the body by recognizing and responding to the foreign matter.

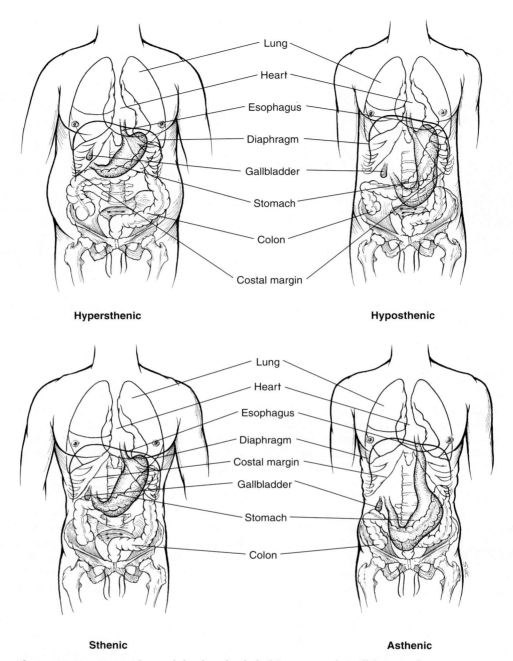

Lung
Heart
Esophagus
Diaphragm
Gallbladder
Stomach
Colon
Costal margin

Hypersthenic

Hyposthenic

Lung
Heart
Esophagus
Diaphragm
Costal margin
Gallbladder
Stomach
Colon

Sthenic

Asthenic

Figure 20-10. Comparison of the four body habitus. Note that all feature the same structures. However, the internal viscera vary in position from one physique to another.

Lymphatic Vessels

Lymphatic vessels contain lymph. Lymph is excessive tissue fluid consisting mostly of water and plasma proteins from capillaries. It differs from blood by the absence of formed elements in it. Lymphatic vessels start in spaces between cells; at that point they are referred to as *lymphatic capillaries.* These lymphatic vessels are extensive; virtually every region of the body that has a blood supply is richly supplied with these capillaries. It stands to reason that those areas that are avascular do not demonstrate the same number of vessels. Examples of these avascular areas are the central nervous system and bone marrow. These lymphatic capillaries are more permeable for substances to enter than are associated blood capillaries. Cellular debris, sloughed off cells, and foreign substances that occur in the intercellular spaces are more readily collected through these lymphatic pathways and transported away for filtration. They start blindly in the interstitial spaces and flow in only one direction.

Lymphedema, also known as lymphatic obstruction, *is a condition of localized fluid retention caused by a compromised lymphatic system. This often becomes a problem in the field of radiation therapy when dealing with patients with breast cancer. When performing surgery to remove and stage breast cancer, surgeons often take out many axillary lymph nodes to see whether the cancer has begun to spread. In doing this, the natural flow of lymph through the arm is disrupted, and without rehabilitation, lymphedema can occur. In these patients, the arm swells, often reducing circulation, and there is the danger of developing an infection of that limb. Lymphedema can usually be controlled by wearing compression bandages and through therapeutic exercises. Surgeons have also begun using a technique known as the* sentinel node biopsy *in hopes of reducing the risk of lymphedema development by reducing the number of lymph nodes removed during surgery.*

The lymphatic capillaries join to form larger lymphatic vessels. Lymphatic vessels resemble veins in structure but have thinner walls and more valves that promote the one-way flow. These larger vessels follow veins and arteries and eventually empty into one of two ducts in the upper thorax—the **thoracic duct** or the **right lymphatic duct**—which then flow into the subclavian veins.

Fluid movement in the lymphatic system depends on hydrostatic and osmotic pressures that increase through skeletal muscle contraction. As the muscles around the vessels contract, the lymph is moved past a one-way valve that closes. This prevents the lymph from flowing backward. Respiratory movements create a pressure gradient between two ends of the lymphatic system. Fluid flows from high-pressure areas, such as the abdomen, to low-pressure areas, such as the thorax, where pressure falls as each inhalation occurs.

Lymph Nodes

Along the paths of the lymph vessels are lymph nodes. These nodes vary in size from 2 to 30 mm in length, and they often occur in groups.[8] A lymph node contains both afferent and efferent lymphatic vessels. **Afferent lymphatic vessels** enter the lymph node at several points along the convex surface. They contain one-way valves that open into the node, bringing the lymph into it. On the other side of the node are efferent vessels. The **efferent lymphatic vessels** are overall smaller in diameter than the afferent vessels; their valves open away from the node, again facilitating one-way flow.[8] There are more afferent vessels coming into a node than efferent vessels coming out of it, slowing the flow through the nodes. This is similar to driving along a four-lane highway during rush hour and getting to a point of road construction that restricts traffic flow to one lane. You can go in only one direction and must wait your turn to move through the area. This slowing of the lymph through the node permits the nodes to effectively filter the lymph, and, through

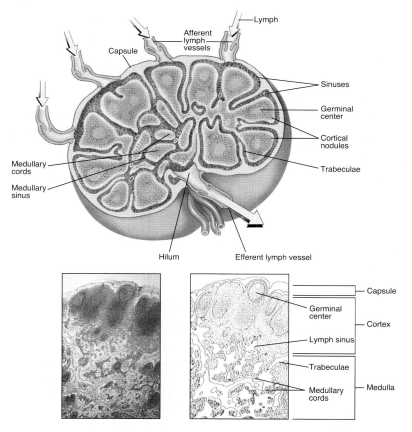

Figure 20-11. Lymph node. *Arrows* indicate the direction of lymph flow. The germinal centers are sites of lymphocyte production. As lymph moves through the lymph sinuses, macrophages remove foreign substances. (See Color Plate 6.) (From Lymphatic system. In Thibodeau GA, Patton KT, editors: *Anatomy and physiology*, ed 6, St. Louis, 2007, Mosby. Photo courtesy of Dennis Strete.)

phagocytosis, the endothelial cells of the node engulf, devitalize, and remove contaminants. Figure 20-11 demonstrates the components of a typical lymph node. The substances can be trapped inside the reticular fibers and pathways throughout the node, causing edema. Edema is an excessive accumulation of fluid in a tissue, producing swelling. This can occur when excessive foreign bodies, lymph, and debris are being engulfed in the node. This is evident when a person has a cold or the flu. The subdigastric nodes, located in the neck just below the angle of the mandible, become swollen and tender because of the heightened phagocytic activity in that area to rid the body of the trapped contaminants. The swelling goes down as the pathogen is devitalized. Edema also occurs when altered lymphatic pathways cause more than normal amounts of lymph filtration. This is commonly seen in postmastectomy patients. The arm on the side of the surgery is often swollen because of the altered natural lymphatic pathways after the operation. The same amount of lymph is redirected through alternate routes, causing the slowdown of lymphatic flow.

Lymphatic Organs

The spleen is the largest mass of lymphatic tissue in the body. It is located posterior to and to the left of the stomach in the abdominal cavity, between the fundus of the stomach and the diaphragm. It is roughly 12 cm in length and actively filters blood, removes old red blood cells, manufactures lymphocytes (particularly B cells, which develop into antibody-producing plasma cells) for immunity surveillance, and stores blood. Because the spleen has no afferent lymphatic vessels, it does not filter lymph. However, the spleen is often thought of as a large lymph node for the blood. During a *laparotomy,* which is surgical inspection of the abdominal cavity, in patients with lymphoma, this organ is often removed for biopsy and staging purposes. In this case, the bone marrow and liver then assume the functions of the spleen.

The thymus is located along the trachea superior to the heart and posterior to the sternum in the upper thorax. This gland is larger in children than in adults and more active in pediatric immunity. The gland serves as a site where T lymphocytes can mature.

The tonsils are series of lymphatic nodules embedded in a mucous membrane. They are located at the junction of the oral cavity and pharynx. These collections of lymphoid tissue protect against foreign body infiltration by producing lymphocytes. The *pharyngeal tonsils,* or *adenoids,* are in the nasopharynx; *the palatine tonsils* are in the posterior lateral wall of the oropharynx; the *lingual tonsils* are at the base of the tongue in the oropharynx.

The *thoracic duct* is on the left side of the body and is typically larger than the right lymphatic duct. It serves the lower extremities, abdomen, left arm, and left side of the head and neck and drains into the left subclavian vein. This duct is approximately 35 to 45 cm in length and begins in front of the second lumbar vertebra (L2) where it is called the *cisterna chyli.* As lymph travels through the lower extremities to the cisterna chyli, it continues its upward trek to the thoracic duct. As it passes through the mediastinum, it bypasses many of the mediastinal node stations. Because of this anatomic fact, pedal lymphangiography, a technique used to visualize nodal status by injecting dye into lymphatic outlets in the feet, cannot be used to visualize mediastinal disease. The *right lymphatic duct* serves only the right arm and right side of the head and neck and drains into

Box 20-1	Lymphatic Flow Overview

Tissue fluid leaves the cellular interstitial spaces and becomes
Lymph; as it enters a
Lymphatic capillary, it merges with other capillaries to form an
Afferent lymphatic vessel, which enters a
Lymph node where lymph is filtered. It then leaves the node via an
Efferent lymphatic vessel, which travels to other nodes, then merges with other vessels to form a
Lymphatic trunk, which merges with other trunks and joins a
Collecting duct, either the right lymphatic or the thoracic, which empties into a
Subclavian vein, where lymph is returned to the bloodstream.

the right subclavian vein. This duct is approximately 1 to 2 cm in length. These ducts drain into the right and left subclavian veins, which in turn drain to the heart by way of the superior vena cava. Box 20-1 reviews the flow of lymph through the lymphatic system.

Knowledge of the location of the lymph nodes and direction of lymph flow is important in the diagnosis and prognosis of the spread of metastatic disease. Cancer cells, especially carcinomas from epithelial tissues, often spread through the lymphatic system. Metastatic disease sites are predictable by their lymphatic flow from the primary site.[15] Inadequate knowledge of the lymphatic system often translates into ineffective treatment delivery.

AXIAL SKELETON: SKULL, VERTEBRAL COLUMN, AND THORAX

Most imaging modalities provide valuable information through visualization of differences in anatomic densities. The denser a component, the whiter it appears on a radiograph. The axial skeleton provides the radiation therapist with a wealth of information used to reference the location of internal anatomy. The following sections briefly review axial skeleton anatomy and provide the reader with a reference necessary in relating internal structures to surface anatomy.

Skull

There are approximately 29 bones in the skull, and these are mostly joined by sutures, joints held together by connective tissue, which limits movement. The mandible and ossicles, which are bones in the middle ear, are the only bones in the skull not joined by sutures.

The frontal, parietal, temporal, sphenoid, and occipital bones all form the lateral aspect of the skull vault. The first two meet in the midline at the *bregma,* the roof of the skull, often referred to as the "soft spot," and the last two meet at the lambda. The facial skeleton, or visceral cranium, includes the 14 bones of the face. It consists of two maxillary bones, two zygomatic bones, two nasal bones, two lacrimal bones, two palatine bones, two inferior conchae, and one mandible.

Sutures

There are four prominent sutures in the skull. These sutures, or fibrous joints, allow little or no movement between them, which makes the transitions between bones of the skull smooth and stable. The *coronal suture* lies between the frontal bone and the two parietal bones. On either side of the skull, it begins at the bregma and ends at the temporal bone. The *sagittal suture* lies between the two parietal bones and runs from the bregma to the lambda. The *lambdoidal suture* is in the posterior portion of the skull and lies between the parietal and occipital bones. Finally, the *squamosal suture,* one on each side of the skull, is located near the ear and lies between the parietal and temporal bones. Identification of these sutures radiographically can assist the radiation therapist in locating corresponding underlying structures. Figure 20-12 shows the bones of the skull and sutures.

Paranasal Sinuses

The bones of the skull and face contain the **paranasal sinuses**, which are air spaces lined by mucous membranes that reduce the weight of the skull and give a resonant sound to the voice. When a person has sinusitis, an inflammation and blockage of the sinus cavities, the voice often has a "stuffed up" tone (loss of resonance). The paired sinuses are air-filled spaces within the frontal, maxillary, sphenoid, and ethmoid bones. They are lined with mucous membranes and are relatively small at birth. They enlarge during development of the permanent teeth and reach adult size shortly after puberty.[10] The paranasal sinuses are easily seen on plain x-ray, CT, and MRI. Cross sections are an excellent tool to study

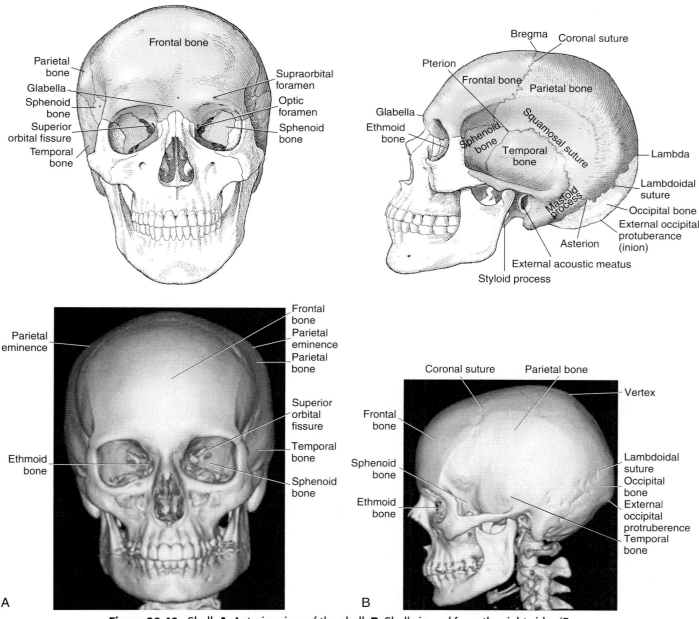

Figure 20-12. Skull. **A**, Anterior view of the skull. **B**, Skull viewed from the right side. (From Kelley LL, Peterson CM: *Sectional anatomy for imaging professionals*, ed 2, St. Louis, 2007, Mosby.)

the surface relations in these areas.[15] Figure 20-13 demonstrates the paranasal sinuses in cross section.

The *maxillary sinus* is a pyramid-shaped cavity that is enclosed in the maxilla. It is the largest of the paranasal sinuses. The roof of the sinus forms the floor of the orbit. The *frontal sinus* lies in the frontal bone above the orbit. It may be located on the surface by a triangle between the following three points: the nasion, a point 3 cm above the nasion, and the junction of the medial and middle thirds of the superior orbital margin (SOM). The *sphenoid sinus* lies posterior and superior to the nasopharynx enclosed in the body of the sphenoid bone at the level of the zygomatic arch. Superiorly the sinus is related to the sella turcica (which is approximately 2 cm anterior and 2 cm superior to the external auditory meatus) and the pituitary. The pituitary may be surgically removed through a transsphenoidal approach, one that goes through the nasal cavity. The *ethmoid sinus* is bilateral but consists of a honeycomb of air cells lying between the middle wall of the orbit and the upper lateral wall of the nose.

Vertebral Column

The vertebral column, located in the midsagittal plane of the posterior cavity, extends from the skull to the pelvis. It consists of separate bones, the vertebrae, which appear as rectangular densities on radiographs.[10] There are 33 bones in the adult vertebral column, as shown in Figure 20-14, which also indicates the number of bones in each section. There are 7 cervical,

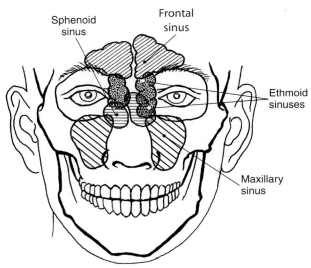

Figure 20-13. The paranasal sinuses. The anterior view shows the anatomic relationship of the paranasal sinuses to each other and to the nasal cavity. (From Kelley LL, Peterson CM: *Sectional anatomy for imaging professionals*, ed 2, St. Louis, 2007, Mosby.)

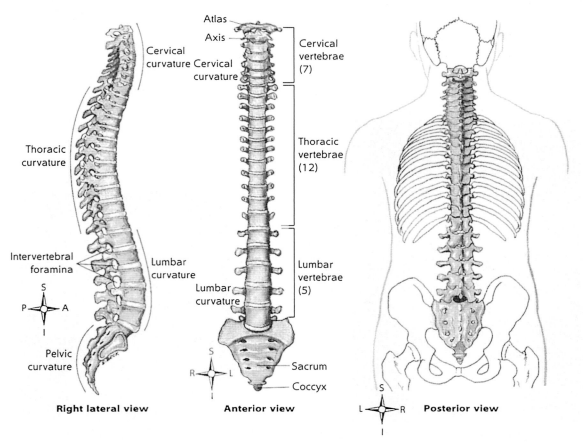

Figure 20-14. The vertebral column (three views). (From Support and movement. In Thibodeau GA, Patton KT, editors: *Anatomy and physiology*, ed 2, St. Louis, 1993, Mosby.)

12 thoracic, 5 lumbar, 5 sacral, and 4 coccygeal vertebrae. At the inferior aspect of the column, the sacrum has 5 fused bones, whereas the coccyx is composed of 4 fused bones.

The sacrum supports the rest of the vertebral column and thus provides the support necessary for the human body's erectness. The vertebrae are separated by radiolucent fibrocartilage called *intervertebral disks.* In the cervical and thoracic spine, the disks are of similar thickness. In the lumbar spine, the height increases progressively down the column.[10,13,14]

The vertebral column is also very flexible. Although there is limited motion between any two neighboring vertebrae, the vertebral column is capable of substantial motion. The column also protects the spinal cord and provides points of attachment for the skull, thorax, and extremities.

Vertebral Characteristics. Most vertebrae share several common characteristics. They have a body that is attached to a posterior vertebral arch. These two components border the *vertebral foramen,* the passage through which the spinal cord passes. There are spinous and transverse processes that allow for muscle attachments. The *spinous process* is posterior and forms where two laminae meet. These laminae are often palpated in aligning spinal treatment fields. The *transverse processes* are lateral projections where a pedicle joins a lamina. Figure 20-15 exhibits a typical vertebra with its prominent features labeled.

The first two vertebrae, C1 and C2, are atypical from all others. C1, the *atlas,* serves the specialized function of supporting the skull and allowing the head to tilt in the "yes" motion. It has no vertebral body. C2, the *axis,* has an odontoid process that extends into the ring of the atlas. When the head turns from side to side, it pivots on this process. These two vertebrae are shown in Figure 20-16.

Vertebral Column Curvatures. The vertebral column demonstrates several curvatures that develop at different levels.[10] These curvatures can be classified as either primary or compensatory (secondary) curvatures. **Primary vertebral curves** are developed in utero as the fetus develops in the C-shaped fetal position, and they are present at birth. **Compensatory** or **secondary vertebral curves** develop after birth as the child learns to sit up and walk. Muscular development and coordination influence the rate of secondary curvature development.

The *cervical curve* extends from the first cervical to the second thoracic vertebrae (C1 to T2). It is convex anteriorly and develops as the child learns to hold his or her head up and sits alone at approximately 4 months of age. This curve is a secondary curvature. The *thoracic curve* extends from T2 to T12 and is concave anteriorly. This is one of the primary curves of the vertebral column. The *lumbar curve* runs from T12 to the anterior surface of L5. This convex forward curve develops when the child learns to walk at approximately 1 year of age. The *pelvic curve* is concave anteriorly and inferiorly and extends from the anterior surfaces of the sacrum and coccyx. This is the other primary curve. The thorax can also have a slightly right or left lateral curve that is influenced by the child's predominate use of his or her right or left hand during childhood and adolescence.

The cervical, thoracic, lumbar, and pelvic curves are demonstrated in the normal human vertebral column. There are also three abnormal curvatures that are present both clinically and radiographically. *Kyphosis* is an excessive curvature of the vertebral column that is convex posteriorly. These curves can develop with degenerative vertebral changes. *Scoliosis* is an abnormal lateral curvature of the vertebral column with excessive right or left curvature in the thoracic region. This abnormal curvature can develop if only one side (half) of the vertebral bodies are irradiated in pediatric patients, as in the case of patients treated for Wilms' tumor. The radiation slows vertebral body growth on one side while the contralateral side grows at a normal rate, thus creating scoliotic changes. *Lordosis* is an excessive convexity of the lumbar curve of the spine.

Thorax

The illustration in Figure 20-17 shows the full thorax made up of the bony cage formed by the sternum, costal cartilage, ribs, and thoracic vertebrae to which they are attached.[11,17] The **thorax** encloses and protects the organs in the thoracic cavity and upper abdomen. It also provides support for the pectoral girdle and upper extremities.

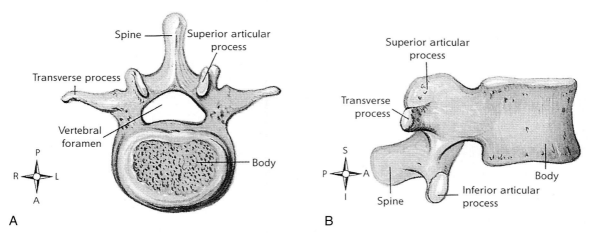

Figure 20-15. Lumbar vertebrae. **A**, Third lumbar vertebra viewed from above (superior). **B**, Third lumbar vertebra viewed from the side (lateral). (From The skeletal system. In Thibodeau GA, Patton KT, editors: *Anatomy and physiology*, ed 2, St. Louis, 1993, Mosby.)

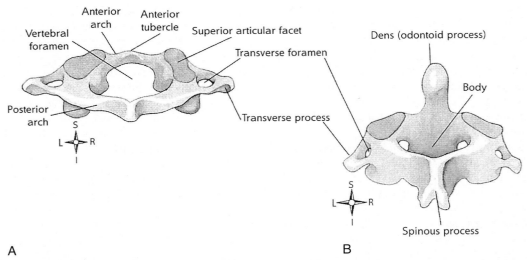

Figure 20-16. Cervical vertebra. **A**, First cervical vertebra (atlas) viewed from behind (posterior). **B**, Second cervical vertebra (axis) viewed from behind (posterior). (From The skeletal system. In Thibodeau GA, Patton KT, editors: *Anatomy and physiology*, ed 2, St. Louis, 1993, Mosby.)

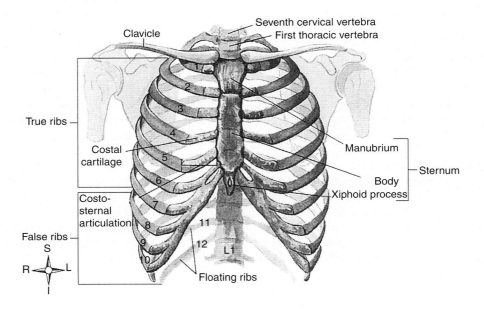

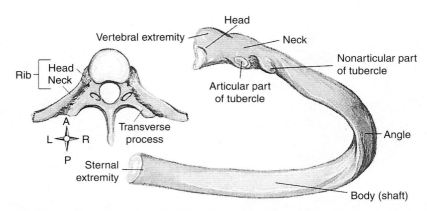

Figure 20-17. The bony framework of the thorax provides many useful landmarks. (From Support and movement. In Thibodeau GA, Patton KT, editors: *Anatomy and physiology*, ed 2, St. Louis, 1993, Mosby.)

Sternum and Ribs. The sternum, or breastbone, comprises three parts: the *manubrium,* which is the superior portion; *the body,* the middle and largest portion; and the *xiphoid process,* which is the inferior projection that serves as ligament and muscle attachments. The manubrium has a depression called the suprasternal notch (SSN), which occurs at the level of T2 and articulates with the medial ends of the clavicles. This point may be used in measuring the angle of chin tilt in patients with head and neck cancer when thermoplastic immobilization masks are not used. It also serves as a palpable landmark when setting up a SCF field. The manubrium also articulates with the first two ribs. The junction of the manubrium and the body form the *sternal angle,* also called the *angle of Louis;* it occurs at the level of T4.

The body of the sternum articulates with the second through tenth ribs. There are 12 pairs of ribs, of which the superior 7 pairs are considered true ribs. They are easily seen in the asthenic body habitus and palpable in most others.[9] They articulate posteriorly with the vertebrae and anteriorly with the sternum directly through a cartilaginous joint. These are known as the *vertebrosternal ribs.* The next three pairs join with the vertebrae posteriorly and anteriorly with the cartilage of the immediately anterior rib. These ribs are classified as *vertebrochondral ribs.* The next (last) pairs articulate only with the vertebrae and do not connect with the sternum in any way; they are called *floating ribs.*

The axial skeleton is easily seen with most imaging techniques used in radiation therapy. A thorough working knowledge of these components serves the radiation therapist in overall daily operations. This information is used in relating the surface and cross-sectional anatomy, as well as the palpable bony landmarks that are used in field placement and treatment planning.

SURFACE AND SECTIONAL ANATOMY AND LANDMARKS OF THE HEAD AND NECK

The human head demonstrates various anatomic features that are both interesting and useful to the radiation therapist. These structures are rich in bony, moveable soft tissue landmarks and lymphatics commonly used in field placement, position locations, and so forth. The bony landmarks are very stable and are typically used as reference points, as in the case of locating a positioning or central axis tattoo. Soft tissue landmarks can also be extremely useful. However, they tend to be more mobile and provide a less reliable reference than the bony landmarks.

Bony Landmarks—Anterior and Lateral Skull

Figures 20-18 and 20-19 outline the locations of the following anterior and lateral bony structures.

The *frontal bone* is the area of maximum convexity on the forehead and articulates with the frontal process of the maxillary bone on the medial side of the orbit.[10,11] Together with the lacrimal bones, it protects the lacrimal duct and glands.

The *glabella* is the slight elevation directly between the two orbits in the frontal bone. It is just above the base of the nose. This palpable landmark is more prominent in some individuals than in others.

The *nasion* is the central depression at the base of the nose. It is formed by the point at which the frontal and nasal bones join.

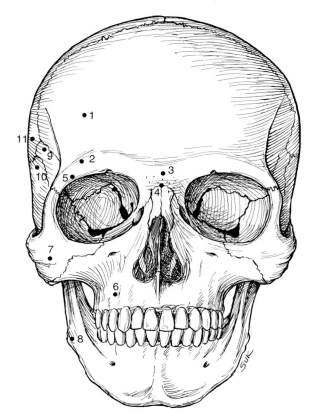

Figure 20-18. Bony landmarks of the anterior skull. *1,* Frontal bone; *2,* superciliary arch; *3,* glabella; *4,* nasion; *5,* superior orbital margin (SOM); *6,* maxilla; *7,* zygomatic bone; *8,* angle of mandible; *9,* sphenoid bone (greater wing); *10,* temporal bone; *11,* parietal bone.

The *superciliary* arch starts at the glabella and moves superiorly and laterally above the central portion of the eyebrow. The central part lies superficially to the frontal sinuses on either side and forms the brow of the skull.

The superior orbital margin (SOM) rests just inferior to the eyebrow and is more pronounced on its lateral aspect. The SOM forms the roof of the orbit and serves as one of the points used to delineate the inferior border of whole brain fields (along with the tragus and mastoid tip). By ensuring that part of the SOM is in the treatment field, the frontal part of the brain will also be in the field.

The *maxilla* is the bone felt between the ala (lateral soft tissue prominence) of the nose and the prominence of the cheek. This bone houses the largest of the paranasal sinuses. The inferior alveolar ridge of the maxilla houses the teeth sockets.

The *zygomatic bone* forms part of the lateral aspect of the orbit and the prominence of the cheek. The articulation between the frontal process of the zygomatic bone and the zygomatic process of the frontal bone can be palpated in the lateral orbital margin (LOM). The *mid-zygoma point,* a point midway between the external auditory meatus (EAM) and the lateral canthus, lies roughly at the floor of the sphenoid sinus and the roof of the nasopharynx. One centimeter superior to that point corresponds to the floor of

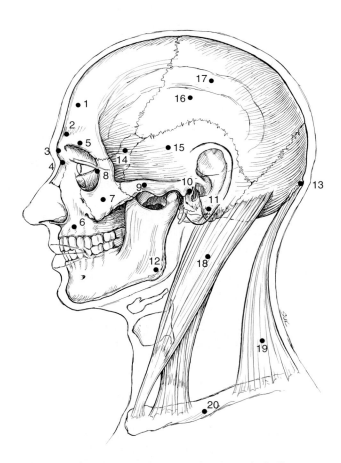

Figure 20-19. Bony landmarks of the lateral skull. *1,* Frontal bone; *2,* superciliary arch; *3,* glabella; *4,* nasion; *5,* superior orbital margin (SOM); *6,* maxilla; *7,* zygomatic bone; *8,* lateral canthus; *9,* mid-zygoma point; *10,* external acoustic meatus (EAM); *11,* mastoid process; *12,* angle of mandible; *13,* external occipital protuberance (EOP) or inion; *14,* greater wing of sphenoid; *15,* temporal bone; *16,* parietal bone; *17,* parietal eminence; *18,* sternocleidomastoid muscle; *19,* trapezius muscle; *20,* clavicle.

the sella turcica, and 1.5 cm superior to the point corresponds to the pituitary gland.

The *mastoid process* is an extension of the mastoid portion of the temporal bone at the level of the ear lobe. It is commonly used to delineate the posterior point of the inferior whole brain border (imaginary line that extends from the SOM to the mastoid tip, commonly going through the tragus of the ear).

The *external occipital protuberance* (EOP or inion) is the prominence in the posterolateral aspect of the occipital bone of the skull.

The *angle of the mandible* is the point at which the muscles used for chewing are attached. In addition, there are several lymph node groups located inferior and medial to that point, and it is also a classic landmark for the tonsils.

Landmarks Around the Eye

Whenever practical, the landmarks used around the eye should be the bony landmarks. They are radiographically visible and are easily checked if a second course of treatment is necessary

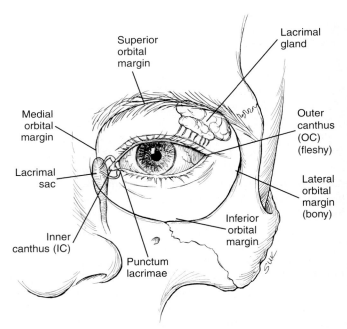

Figure 20-20. Landmarks around the eye and orbit.

in the same or neighboring area. The soft tissue landmarks often change with age, weight, and surgical changes. They are open to variable interpretation and misinterpretation because of the extreme flexibility of the skin. Figure 20-20 illustrates these landmarks. The following outlines the important landmarks about the eye.

The *superior orbital margin* forms the upper border of the orbit.

The *inferior orbital margin* (IOM) forms the lower border of the bony orbit.

The *lateral orbital margin* (LOM) is a bony landmark that forms the lateral border of the bony orbit.

The *medial orbital margin* is extremely difficult to palpate and therefore is not clinically useful as an anatomic landmark. It does have some usefulness radiographically.

The *inner canthus* (IC) is a soft tissue landmark that is formed at the junction of the upper and lower eyelids at the medial aspect of the eye.

The *outer canthus* (OC) is a soft tissue landmark that is formed at the junction of the upper and lower eyelid at the lateral aspect of the eye.

The *punctum lacrimae* is a soft tissue landmark that can be used as a point of reference in the surface anatomy of the eye. This white-appearing section of the eye lies just next to the IC on the lower eyelid. Tears are drained through this duct into the lacrimal duct. This opening can become blocked by fibrotic changes secondary to ionizing radiation administered to the area, causing constant tearing. Extreme caution should be exercised to avoid this occurrence, particularly when treating the anterior maxillary sinus field arrangement.

Landmarks Around the Nose

As in the case of the eye, the landmarks used around the nose should be the bony landmarks. Soft tissue landmarks often

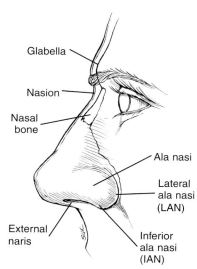

Figure 20-21. Landmarks around the nose.

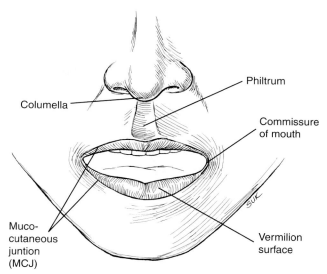

Figure 20-22. Landmarks around the mouth.

change with age, weight, and surgical changes and are open to variable interpretation and misinterpretation because of the extreme flexibility of the skin. Figure 20-21 illustrates these landmarks. The following outlines the landmarks around the nose, some being reiterated from previous sections.

The *lateral ala nasi* (LAN) is a soft tissue landmark formed by the lateral attachment of the ala nasi with the cheek. The *inferior ala nasi* (IAN) is a soft tissue landmark formed by the inferior attachment of the ala nasi with the cheek. Both of these landmarks are prominent in most people and can be very useful landmarks when measuring in any direction, such as superior to inferior, medial to lateral, and anterior to posterior.

The *nasion* is the depression of the nose where it joins the forehead at the level of the SOM. It is a very useful landmark if it is deep and pronounced and coincides with the crease of the nose. If it is shallow, it is more open to variable interpretation.

The *glabella* is the bony prominence in the forehead at the level just superior to the SOM. As in the case of the nasion, it is useful if it is prominent and sharp. It is not useful if it is flat or extremely curved, where it, too, would be open to misinterpretation.

The ala nasi, dorsum of the nose, and external nares are useful as checkpoints in the surface anatomy of the nose and useful in the positioning of radiation treatment portals.

Landmarks Around the Mouth

Landmarks around the mouth are generally not very accurate because of the extreme flexibility in the area. Every effort should be made to document these landmarks with reference to more stable anatomic points, if possible. If these landmarks are used, it is important to note the position of the mouth, as well as any positioning or immobilization devices used, such as a cork, oral stent, or similar devices. Figure 20-22 illustrates the landmarks around the mouth.

The *commissure of the mouth* is formed at the junction of the upper and lower lip. This landmark is extremely mobile.

The *mucocutaneous junction* (MCJ) is located at the junction of the vermilion border of the lip with the skin of the face.

The *columella* is located at the junction of the skin of the nose with the skin of the face at the superior end of the philtrum.

Landmarks Around the Ear

The external ear consists of the auricle or pinna, which is formed from a number of irregularly shaped pieces of fibrocartilage covered by skin. It has a dependent lobule, or ear lobe, and an anterior tragus, commonly used as anatomic references.[7,11,16] Parts of the ear are labeled in Figure 20-23.

The *tragus* is made up of a fairly stable cartilage that partially covers the external auditory meatus in the external ear and is often used in radiation therapy during initial positioning. A pair of optical lasers, coincident with each other, can be focused on the tragus on both sides of the patient. Doing this places the patient's head in a relatively nontilted position, because their locations are typically symmetrical. Just anterior to the tragus corresponds to the posterior wall of the nasopharynx. The posterior limit of many head and neck off-cord fields lies at this point.

The *tragal notch* is the semicircular notch in the ear immediately inferior to the tragus. The *superior tragal notch* (STN) makes up the superior margin of the tragal notch. The inferior tragal notch (ITN) defines the inferior margin of the tragal notch. The *anterior tragal notch* (ATN) makes up the anterior margin of the tragal notch.

Landmarks and Anatomy Around the Neck

The boundaries of the anterior aspect of the neck are the body and angles of the mandible superiorly and the superior border and SSN of the sternum and the clavicles. The posterior aspect of the neck is bound superiorly by the EOP and laterally by the mastoid processes. The posterior inferior border ends at approximately the level of the seventh cervical vertebra to the first thoracic vertebra (C7-T1).[10] Figure 20-24 illustrates the features of the neck anatomy.

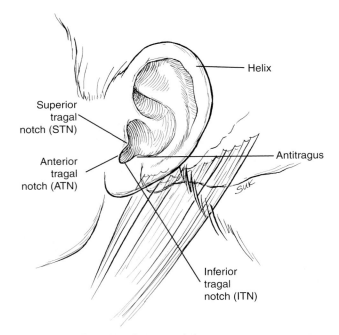

Figure 20-23. Landmarks around the ear.

The upper cervical vertebrae are not easily palpated; the last cervical and first thoracic vertebrae are the most obvious. The hyoid bone lies opposite the superior border of C4. When the head is in the anatomic position, the hyoid bone may be moved from side to side between the thumb and middle finger, approximately 1 cm below the level of the angle of the mandible, C2-3. Table 20-3 relates the location of the cervical bony landmarks to other associated anatomic features.

Pharynx

The pharynx is a membranous tube that extends from the base of the skull to the esophagus. It connects the nasal and oral cavities with the larynx and esophagus. It is divided into the nasopharynx, oropharynx, and laryngopharynx, shown in Figure 20-25. Note that in looking at the low neck in a sectional view, the therapist can easily remember how to distinguish the order of the spinal cord, esophagus, and trachea. If looking from

Table 20-3	Cervical Neck Landmarks and Associated Anatomy
Cervical Spine	**Associated Anatomy**
C1	Transverse process lies just inferior to the mastoid process; may be palpated in the hollow inferior to the ear
C2-3	Level with the angle of the mandible; lies 5 to 7 cm below the external occipital protuberance
C4	Located just superior to the hyoid bone of the neck; serves as a point of muscle attachment
C4	Level with the superior portion of the thyroid cartilage and marks the beginning of the larynx
C6	Level with the cricoid cartilage; location of the junction of the larynx to trachea and pharynx to esophagus
C7	First prominent spinous process in the posterior neck

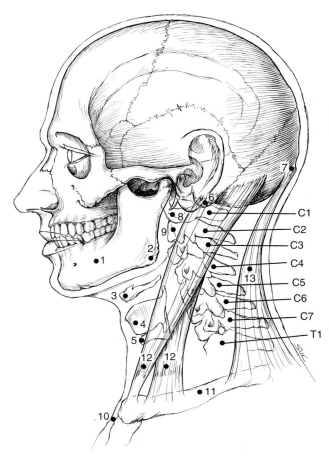

Figure 20-24. The neck demonstrates many useful anatomic landmarks that can assist the radiation therapist. Relating surface structures to deeper anatomy is essential in the practice of radiation therapy. *1*, Body of mandible; *2*, angle of mandible; *3*, hyoid bone; *4*, thyroid cartilage; *5*, cricoid cartilage; *6*, mastoid process; *7*, external occipital protuberance (EOP); *8*, atlas; *9*, axis; *10*, suprasternal notch; *11*, clavicle; *12*, sternocleidomastoid muscle; *13*, trapezius muscle.

a posterior to anterior perspective, the order is always **SET** up: S—spinal cord, E—esophagus, and T—trachea:

1. The *nasopharynx*, or *epipharynx*, communicates with the nasal cavity and provides a passageway for air during breathing.
2. The *oropharynx*, or *mesopharynx*, opens behind the soft palate into the nasopharynx and functions as a passageway for food moving down from the mouth, as well as for air moving in and out of the nasal cavity.
3. The *laryngopharynx*, or *hypopharynx*, is located inferior to the oropharynx and opens into the larynx and esophagus.

Larynx

The larynx connects to the lower portion of the pharynx above it and is connected with the trachea below it. It extends from the tip of the epiglottis at the level of the junction of C3 and C4 to the lower portion of the cricoid cartilage at the level of the C6 vertebra.[7] The larynx is subdivided into three anatomic regions: the supraglottis, glottis, and subglottis. Figure 20-26 illustrates sectional views of the larynx. The larynx is actually an enlargement in the airway at the top of the trachea and below

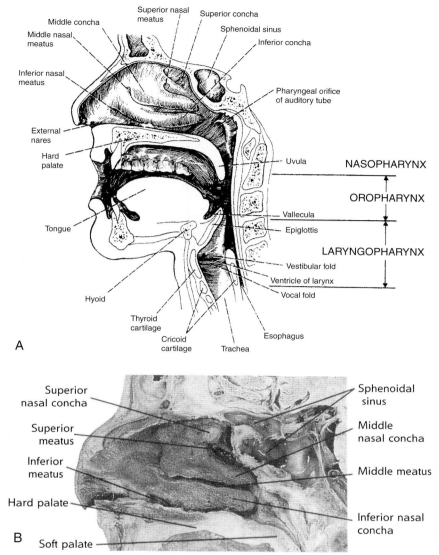

Figure 20-25. Nasal cavity and pharynx. **A,** Sagittal section through the nasal cavity and pharynx viewed from the medial side. **B,** Photograph of a sagittal section of the nasal cavity. (**A** is from Bomford CK, Kunkler IH: *Walter and Miller's textbook of radiotherapy,* ed 6, St. Louis, 2003, Churchill Livingstone, and **B** is from The lymphatic system and immunity. In Seeley RR, Stephens TD, Tate P, editors: *Essentials of anatomy and physiology,* St. Louis, 1991, Mosby.)

the pharynx. It serves as a passageway for air moving in and out of the trachea and functions to prevent foreign objects from entering the trachea.

The *thyroid cartilage* forms a midline prominence, the laryngeal prominence or Adam's apple, which is more obvious in the adult male. The vocal cords are attached to the posterior part of this prominence. The *cricoid cartilage* serves as the lower border of the larynx and is the only complete ring of cartilage in the respiratory passage; the others are open posteriorly. It is palpable as a narrow horizontal bar inferior to the thyroid cartilage and is at the level of the C6 vertebra.

Nasal and Oral Cavities

The nasal cavity opens to the external environment through the nostrils. Posteriorly the nostrils are continuous with the nasopharynx and are lined with a ciliated mucous membrane.

The oral cavity has a vestibule, which is the space between the cheeks and teeth and the oral cavity proper that opens posteriorly into the oropharynx and houses the soft palate, hard palate, uvula, anterior tongue, and floor of the mouth.

Surface Anatomy of the Neck

Anatomic landmarks around the neck are mainly used as checkpoints and reference points that can establish the patient's position or the anatomic position of the treatment field. The most commonly used landmarks of the neck are as follows:
1. Skin profile
2. Sternocleidomastoid muscle—attached to the mastoid and occipital bones superiorly and sternal and clavicular heads inferiorly. These muscles form the V shape in the neck and are associated with a great number of lymph nodes.

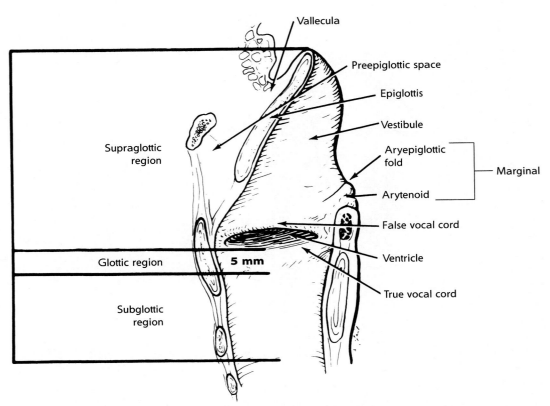

Figure 20-26. Posterior view of the base of the tongue, larynx, and hypopharynx. Note the pyriform sinus, pharyngeal wall, and postcricoid area. (From Cox JD, editor: *Moss' radiation oncology: rationale, technique, results,* ed 7, St. Louis, 1994, Mosby.)

3. Clavicle
4. Thyroid notch
5. Mastoid tip
6. EOP
7. Spinous processes

These surface neck landmarks assist the radiation therapist in referencing locations of treatment fields and dose-limiting structures. They are illustrated in Figure 20-27.

Lymphatic Drainage of the Head and Neck

The lymphatic drainage of the head and neck is through deep and superficial lymphatic channels, around the base of the skull, and deep and superficial lymph chains. The head and neck area is very rich in lymphatics. Enlarged cervical lymph nodes are the most common adenopathy seen in clinical practice.[11] They are typically associated with upper respiratory tract infections but may also be the site of metastatic disease from the head and neck, lungs, or breast or primary lymphoreticular disease such as Hodgkin's disease. The lymph nodes of the head and neck are outlined in the following section. Figures 20-28 and 20-29 demonstrate the lymphatic chains and nodes in the head and neck.

The *occipital lymph nodes,* typically one to three in number, are located on the back of the head, close to the margin of the trapezius muscle attachment on the occipital bone. These nodes provide efferent flow to the superior deep cervical nodes.

The *retroauricular lymph nodes,* usually two in number, are situated on the mastoid insertion of the sternocleidomastoid muscle deep to the posterior auricular muscle. They drain the posterior temporooccipital region of the scalp, auricle, and external auditory meatus. They provide efferent drainage to the superior deep cervical nodes.

The *deep parotid lymph nodes* are arranged into two groups. The first group is embedded in the parotid gland, whose superior border is the temporomandibular joint (TMJ); posterior border, the mastoid process; inferior border, the angle of the mandible; and anterior border, the anterior ramus. The second group—the subparotid nodes—are located deep to the gland and lie on the lateral wall of the pharynx. Both drain the nose, eyelid, frontotemporal scalp, EAM, and palate. They provide efferent flow to the superior deep cervical nodes.

The *submaxillary lymph nodes* are facial nodes that are scattered over the infraorbital region. They span from the groove between the nose and cheek to the zygomatic arch. The *buccal lymph nodes* are scattered over the buccinator muscle. These nodes drain the eyelids, nose, and cheek and supply efferent flow to the submandibular nodes. The *submandibular lymph nodes* lie on the outer surface of the mandible. They drain the scalp; nose; cheek; floor of the mouth; anterior two thirds of the tongue; gums; teeth; lips; and frontal, ethmoid, and maxillary sinuses. They provide efferent drainage to the superior deep cervical nodes.

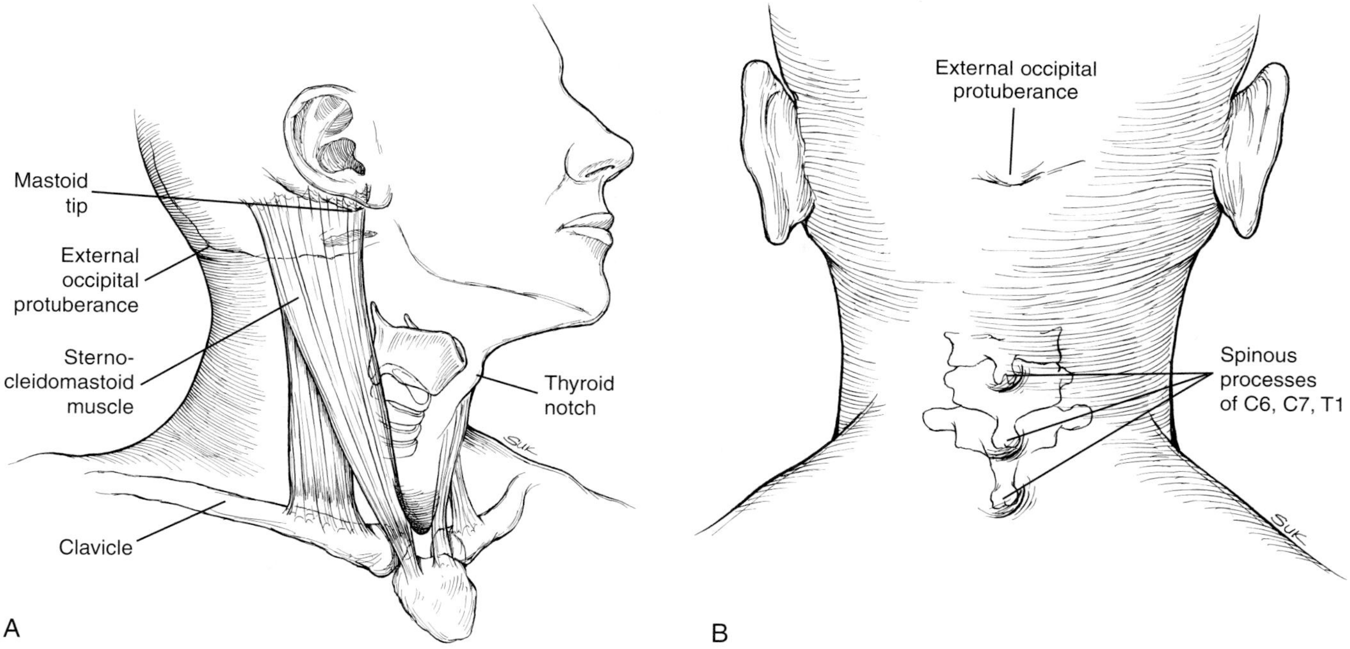

Figure 20-27 labels:

Mastoid tip

External occipital protuberance

Sterno-cleidomastoid muscle

Clavicle

Thyroid notch

A

External occipital protuberance

Spinous processes of C6, C7, T1

B

Figure 20-27. Surface anatomy of the neck. **A**, Anterolateral view. **B**, Posterior view.

The *retropharyngeal lymph nodes,* one to three in number, lie in the buccopharyngeal fossa, behind the upper part of the pharynx and anterior to the arch of the atlas. These nodes are commonly involved in nasopharyngeal tumors and subsequently are included in the treatment fields.

The *submental lymph nodes* are found in the submental triangle of the digastric muscles, lower gums and lips, tongue, central floor of the mouth, and skin of the chin. These nodes provide efferent drainage to the submandibular nodes.

The *superficial cervical lymph nodes* form a group of nodes located below the hyoid bone and in front of the larynx, trachea, and thyroid gland.

The *deep cervical lymph nodes* form a chain of 20 to 30 nodes along the carotid sheath and around the internal jugular

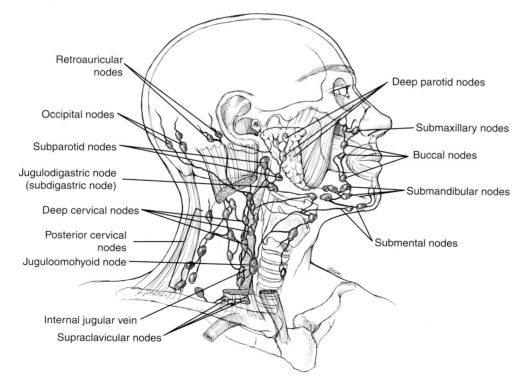

Figure 20-28 labels:

Retroauricular nodes

Occipital nodes

Subparotid nodes

Jugulodigastric node (subdigastric node)

Deep cervical nodes

Posterior cervical nodes

Juguloomohyoid node

Internal jugular vein

Supraclavicular nodes

Deep parotid nodes

Submaxillary nodes

Buccal nodes

Submandibular nodes

Submental nodes

Figure 20-28. Topographic view of head and neck lymph nodes.

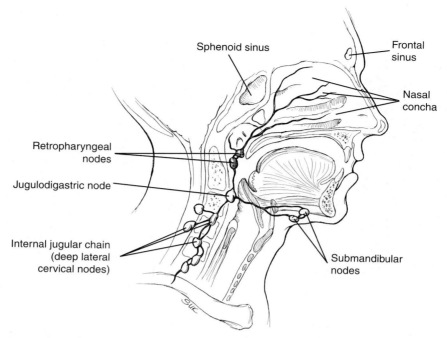

Figure 20-29. Sagittal view of deep lymph nodes in the head and neck in relation to underlying structures.

chain along the sternocleidomastoid muscle. The *jugulodigastric lymph node,* at times called the *subdigastric node,* is typically located superior to the angle of the mandible and drains the tonsils and the tongue. Inferiorly, the chain spreads out into the subclavian triangle. One of the nodes in this group lies in the omohyoid tendon and is known as the *juguloomohyoid lymph node.*[10,11] When these two nodes are enlarged, it may signal carcinoma of the tongue, because enlarged neck nodes may be the only sign of the disease. These vessels supply efferent flow to form the jugular trunk, which drains to the thoracic or right lymphatic duct, both in the SCF. The cervical lymph nodes are typically included in the treatment fields of most head and neck cancers that spread through the lymphatics, which include most of these cancers. The fields that encompass the group are commonly called *posterior cervical strips.*

SURFACE AND SECTIONAL ANATOMY AND LANDMARKS OF THE THORAX AND BREAST

Various malignant diseases manifest themselves in the human thorax. Cancers of the lung, breast, and mediastinal lymphatics require the radiation therapist to have a working knowledge of the surface and sectional anatomy of the thorax. The human thorax demonstrates various anatomic features that are commonly used in field placement, position locations, and so forth. The thorax extends from the clavicles superiorly to the costal margin inferiorly.

Anterior Thoracic Landmarks

The clavicles are visible throughout their entire length in the anterior thorax, especially in the asthenic body habitus. The clavicles are easily palpable. The radiation therapist uses the clavicles when outlining a SCF field to treat the lower neck and upper

chest lymphatics. The supraclavicular lymph nodes are located superior to the clavicles; they are often treated prophylactically in head and neck, as well as lung, cancers. In addition, the brachial plexus, a network of nerves located at the medial section of the clavicle and often involved in superior sulcus (Pancoast) tumors of the lung, can be referenced to this point.

The musculature of the anterior chest wall includes the pectoralis major, pectoralis minor, and deltoid. The pectoralis major is medially attached to the clavicle and superior five costal cartilages. It passes laterally to the axilla. The inferior border of the muscle is not as visible in the female, because it is covered by the breast.[10,11] The pectoralis minor is overlapped by the pectoralis major. The deltoid muscle forms the rounded portion of the shoulder.

The Breast and Its Landmarks

The male breast remains poorly developed throughout life, whereas the female breast develops to a variable degree during puberty. Although the sizes of the female breasts vary, they typically lie between the second rib superiorly and the sixth rib inferiorly. The female breast is shown in Figure 20-30. The medial border is the lateral aspect of the sternum, and the lateral border corresponds to the midaxilla. The breast tissue is teardrop shaped; the round, drop portion is situated medially, and the upper outer portion, called the *tail of Spence,* extends into the axilla. The upper limits of tangential treatment fields are typically high near the SSN, to include the entire breast and tail of Spence when the SCF is not treated.

The breast can be divided into quadrants: upper outer, upper inner, lower outer, and lower inner. Most tumors are located in the upper outer quadrant of the breast. Tumor location is important in associating the tumor spread patterns. If the breast tumor is located in an inner quadrant, the medially located

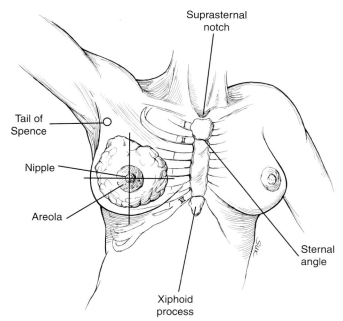

Figure 20-30. Surface anatomy of the female breast. This gland is teardrop shaped with a portion extending from the anterior chest wall into the axilla.

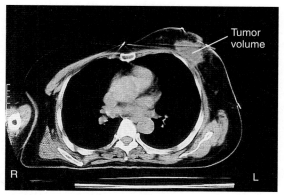

Figure 20-31. Computed tomography view of the female breast and thorax. The contour of the breast and chest wall from images like this greatly enhance accuracy of treatment planning. Note how tumor volume can easily be related to other internal anatomy.

nodes, such as the internal mammary nodes, may be involved. If the tumor is located in an outer quadrant, the axillary nodes need to be examined for possible involvement. This information is particularly important to the therapist because tumor location and extension dictate field parameters.

Other surface anatomy of the breast includes the nipple, areola, and inframammary sulcus. The nipple projects just below the center of the breast. In the male, the nipple lies over the fourth intercostal space; the location varies in the female. The areola is the area that surrounds the nipple. Its coloration changes with varying hormonal levels, as seen in pregnancy. The inframammary sulcus, the inferior point of breast attachment, varies from person to person. In females with large breasts, the breast overhangs this point of attachment and causes considerable concern during its external beam treatment because the breast can bolus itself in these cases.

Radiographically, the breast produces shadows that are easily seen on conventional radiographs. Figure 20-31 shows a CT slice through a section of the thorax and breast. Note how the patient's internal anatomy can be related to the contour of the breast. This information is very useful in treatment planning.

Posterior Thoracic Landmarks

The posterior thorax is formed by the structures commonly referred to as the *back*. On initial inspection, the back is made up of various muscles and bony landmarks. The major musculature includes the trapezius, teres major, and latissimus dorsi. The *trapezius muscle* is a flat triangular muscle that produces a trapezoid shape with the lateral angles at the shoulders and the superior angle at the EOP. The inferior angle is at the level of T12. The *teres major* is a band of muscle between the inferior angle of the scapula and the humerus and forms the posterior wall of the axilla. The *latissimus dorsi* is the broad muscle on either

side of the back that spans from the iliac crest of the pelvic bones to the posterior axilla.[4,5,10,11] Figure 20-32 demonstrates the surface anatomy of the posterior thorax.

The spines of the thoracic vertebrae slope inferiorly; the tips lie more inferior than the corresponding vertebral bodies and are easily palpable. The scapula, the large posterior bone associated with the pectoral girdle, is easily palpated on the back. The spine of the scapula is located at the level of T3. The inferior angle of the scapula is located at the level of T7.

The lower back has a few bony landmarks that serve the radiation therapist well. *The crest of the ilium* is located at the level of L4. This point is important in locating the subarachnoid space, the point at which lumbar punctures are commonly made. The *posterosuperior iliac spine* (PSIS) is approximately 5 cm from midline, is easily palpable, and lies at the level of S2.

Internal and Sectional Anatomy of the Thorax

Bone detail can easily be visualized sectionally with CT. MRI demonstrates soft tissue anatomy not clearly seen with conventional x-ray equipment. Fascial planes are identified, allowing separation of organ systems, vascular supply, muscles, bone, and lymphatic system.[1,3,6] The thorax provides a lot of anatomic information that the radiation therapist uses in the daily administration of ionizing radiation.

The *trachea* is the part of the airway that begins at the inferior cricoid cartilage, at the level of C6. It is approximately 10 cm long and extends to a point of bifurcation, called the *carina,* at the level of T4-5. Topically, it corresponds to the angle of Louis and is demonstrated in Figure 20-33. The bifurcation forms the beginning of the right and left main bronchi. This can assist the therapist in locating the initial location of treatment field borders, especially lung cancer fields whose inferior border commonly lies a few centimeters below this anatomic reference point.

The diaphragm is the dome-shaped muscle that separates the thorax and abdomen. It is important in respiration and lies between T10 and T11. The esophagus and inferior vena cava pass through the diaphragm at the level of T8-9, whereas the descending aorta goes through at the level of T11-12. These features are shown in cross section in Figure 20-34.

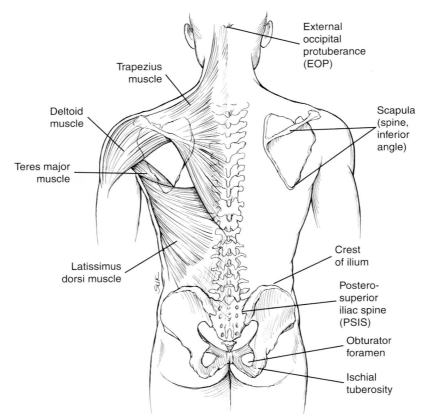

Figure 20-32. Surface anatomy of the posterior thorax.

The pleural cavity extends superiorly 3 cm above the middle third of the clavicle. The anterior border of the pleural cavity reaches the midline of the sternal angle. The pleura is more extensive in the peripheral regions around the outer chest wall. The diaphragm bulges up into each pleural cavity from below. The pleura marks the limit of expansion of the lungs.[10,11]

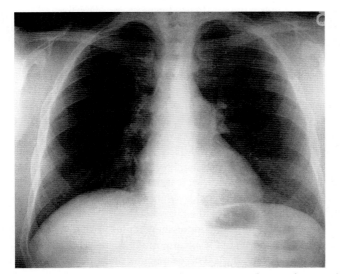

Figure 20-33. This x-ray image demonstrates the trachea and its distal bifurcation, the carina. The branching typically occurs at T3-4.

The lungs correspond closely with the pleura, except in the inferior aspect, where they do not extend down into the lateral recesses. The anterior border of the right lung corresponds to the right junction of the costal and mediastinal pleura down to the level of the sixth chondrosternal joint. The anterior border of the left lung curves away laterally from the line of pleural reflection. The surface projection of the lung and pleura is noted in Figure 20-35.

The heart rests directly on the diaphragm in the pericardial cavity and is covered anteriorly by the body of the sternum. The base of the heart lies at the level of T4. A cardiac shadow can clearly be seen in a radiograph of the chest.

Associated with the thorax and heart are an abundance of arteries and veins—the great vessels. The aorta has ascending and descending components. The ascending aorta runs from the aortic orifice at the medial end of the third left intercostal space up to the second right chondrosternal joint. This arch continues above the right side of the sternal angle and then turns down behind the second left costal cartilage. The descending aorta runs down behind this cartilage, gradually moving across to reach a point just to the left of midline, approximately 9 cm below the xiphisternal joint where it enters the abdomen. This aortic arch has the innominate, left common carotid, and left subclavian arteries extending from it. The superior vena cava is located at the level of T4. It runs down through the pericardium, where it enters the heart. The inferior vena cava does not extend a great distance in the thorax; it lies in the right

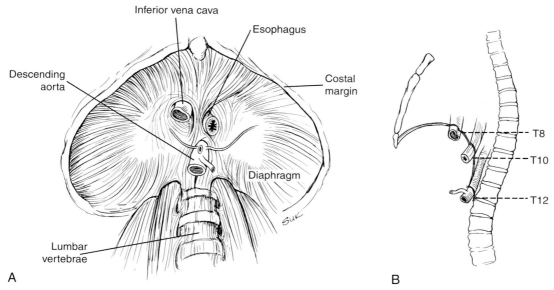

Figure 20-34. Cross section of the lower thorax showing esophagus and inferior vena cava passing through the diaphragm. **A,** Inferior surface of the diaphragm. **B,** Sagittal view of the diaphragm.

cardiodiaphragmatic angle and enters the heart behind the sixth right costal cartilage.

Lymphatics of the Breast and Thorax

The lymphatic drainage of the thorax and breast is very important to the radiation therapist. The thorax is very rich in lymphatic vessels. The lymphatics of the axilla, SCF, and mediastinum play a major role in radiation therapy field arrangement of breast, head and neck, lung, and lymphatic cancers. The lymph nodes of the thorax are divided into nodes that drain the thoracic wall and breast and those that drain the thoracic viscera.

Breast Lymphatics. There are three lymphatic pathways associated with the breast: the axillary, transpectoral, and internal mammary pathways. These pathways are the major routes of

lymphatic drainage for the breast. There are specific lymph node groups associated with each pathway that are shown in Figure 20-36.

The **axillary lymphatic pathway** comes from trunks of the upper and lower half of the breast. Lymph is collected in lobules that follow ducts, which anastomose behind the areola of the breast; from that point they drain to the axilla. This pathway is also referred to as the *principal pathway*. The nodes of this pathway drain the lateral half of the breast. It is important to note these nodes in invasive breast cancers: axillary nodes are commonly biopsied to assess disease spread. The axillary lymph nodes are commonly at the level of the second to third intercostal spaces and can be divided into low, mid, and apical axillary nodes.

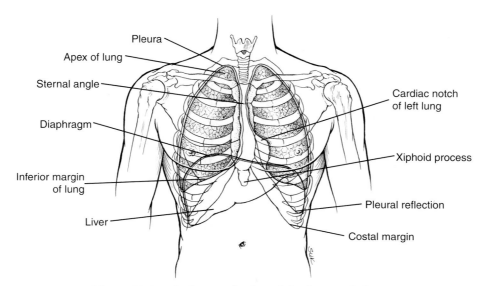

Figure 20-35. Surface projection of the lung and pleura.

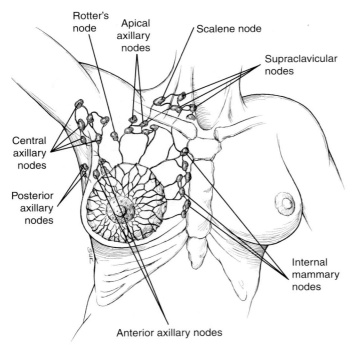

Figure 20-36. The lymphatic pathways associated with the breast: axillary, transpectoral, and internal mammary.

The **transpectoral lymphatic pathway** passes through the pectoralis major muscle and provides efferent drainage to the supraclavicular and infraclavicular fossa nodes. One of the intermediate nodes in the infraclavicular fossa worth noting is Rotter's node. Nodes of the SCF and low neck, generally 1 to 3 cm deep, are often treated when there is involvement of the transpectoral pathway. The scalene node, found in the low neck/SCF, is often biopsied to note disease spread.

The **internal mammary lymphatic pathway** runs toward the midline and passes through the pectoralis major and intercostal muscles close to the body of the sternum (T4 to T9). Associated with this pathway are the internal mammary nodes. These nodes are more commonly involved with primary breast cancers that are located in the inner breast quadrants and when there are positive axillary nodes. These nodes are generally 2.5 cm from midline (with variations from 0 to 5 cm) and approximately 2.5 cm deep (with variations from 1 to 5 cm). CT scans are extremely helpful to the radiation oncology team in assessing the location of these nodes. The lateral location and depth assist in determining the field width and treatment energy, respectively.

Breast lymphatic flow is also important from a surgical standpoint. With radical breast surgery, lymphatic flow is often compromised. As the channels of flow are altered because of surgical intervention, the lymph has fewer drainage paths back to the cardiovascular system. This slowed drainage causes edema that is sometimes seen in the arm of patients who have received radical breast surgery. Exercise and elevation of the limb help drain stagnant lymph. This complication has led the cancer management team to use less radical surgery when possible, along with other modalities.

Thoracic Lymphatics. The mediastinum demonstrates a rich intercommunicating network of lymphatics. The most important nodes to note are the lymphatics of the thoracic viscera and pulmonary veins. They are commonly involved in Hodgkin's disease and in lung cancers, in which they can be radiographically demonstrated as a widened mediastinum. The lymphatics of the lung and mediastinum are shown in Figure 20-37.

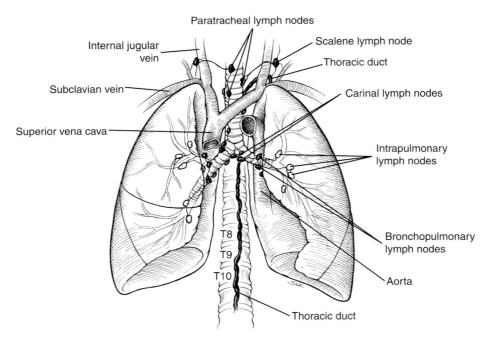

Figure 20-37. The mediastinum demonstrates a large number of lymph nodes.

The *superior mediastinal nodes* are located in the superior mediastinum. They lie anterior to the brachiocephalic veins, the aortic arch, and the large arterial trunks that arise from the aorta. They receive lymphatic vessels from the thymus, heart, pericardium, mediastinal pleura, and anterior hilum. The *tracheal nodes* extend along both sides of the thoracic trachea. They are also called the *paratracheal nodes.* The *superior tracheobronchial nodes* are located on each side of the trachea. They are superior and lateral to the angle at which the trachea bifurcates into the two primary bronchi.

The *inferior mediastinal nodes* are located in the inferior mediastinum. The inferior tracheobronchial nodes lie in the angle below the bifurcation of the trachea. They are also called the *carinal nodes.* The *bronchopulmonary nodes,* often called the *hilar nodes,* are found at the hilus of each lung, at the site of the division of the main bronchi and pulmonary vessels into the lobular bronchi and vessels. These nodes are involved in most lung cancer cases. The *pulmonary nodes,* also known as the *intrapulmonary nodes,* are found in the lung parenchyma along the secondary and tertiary bronchi.

In the right lung, all three lobes drain to the intrapulmonary and hilar nodes. They then flow to the carinal nodes and then to the paratracheal nodes before they reach the brachiocephalic vein through the scalene node and right lymphatic duct. In the left lung, the upper lobe drains to the pulmonary and hilar nodes, carinal nodes, left superior paratracheal nodes, and then the brachiocephalic vein through the thoracic duct. The left lower lobe drains to the pulmonary and hilar nodes, then to the right paratracheal nodes, where it follows the path outlined for the right lung. This is important when designing the treatment field of a patient with lung cancer.

SURFACE AND SECTIONAL ANATOMY AND LANDMARKS OF THE ABDOMEN AND PELVIS

The abdomen and pelvis house many organs that are treated for malignant disease. Their management presents treatment planning challenges for the radiation therapist and medical dosimetrist because of the abundance of radiosensitive structures within the abdominal and pelvic cavities. Treating a colorectal cancer to a dose of ≥ 60 Gy can be difficult when the neighboring anatomy tolerates much less. Knowledge of surface and cross-sectional anatomy of the abdomen and pelvis is essential in radiation therapy. The radiation therapist must be able to bridge knowledge of surface and sectional anatomy with various body habitus to visualize internal anatomy. However, relating internal structures to the topography of the area is not without certain challenges, particularly in the anterior abdomen. When compared with the head, neck, and thorax, the anterior abdomen does not demonstrate as many bony landmarks to reference. However, there are stable bony landmarks in the pelvis that are commonly referenced.

Anterior Abdominal Wall

The *anterior abdominal wall* is bordered superiorly by the inferior costal margin and inferiorly by the symphysis pubis, inguinal ligament, anterosuperior iliac spine (ASIS), and iliac crest. The anterior aspect of the wall is formed by sheets of interlacing muscles that provide stability and form to the abdomen.

The major muscles that help form the anterior abdominal wall include the rectus abdominis, transverse abdominis, internal oblique, and external oblique.

The *external oblique muscle* extends from the lower eight ribs to an insertion point that spans from the iliac crest to the midline aponeurosis, a sheetlike tendon that joins one muscle to another. It extends from the outer lateral body to the midline.

The *internal oblique muscle* spans from the iliac crest and inguinal ligament to the cartilage of the last four ribs. It runs in a midline to an outer, lateral perspective.

The *transverse abdominis muscle* runs from the iliac crest, inguinal ligament, and last six rib cartilages to the xiphoid process, linea alba (a tough fibrous band that extends from the xiphoid process to the symphysis pubis), and pubis on both sides. Thus this muscle runs from side to side.

The *rectus abdominis muscle* is commonly called the "six pack" by sports buffs. This muscle runs from the symphysis pubis to the xiphoid process and has three transverse fibrous bands that separate the muscle into six sections that are prominent in individuals with pronounced muscular tone.

These muscles work together in providing structure to the anterior abdominal wall. Figure 20-38 shows the interrelated nature of these muscles.

A number of structures can be palpated in the abdomen. The xiphoid process lies in the epigastric region at the level of T9. This bony landmark is very stable. The radiation therapist typically uses this structure and the SSN in making sure that a patient is lying straight on the treatment couch. If both landmarks are in line with the projection of a sagittal laser, the thorax is usually straight. The xiphoid can also be used in conjunction with the symphysis pubis or associated soft tissue landmarks to ensure that the lower body is straight. The cartilages of the seventh to tenth ribs form the costal margin. This forms the inferior border of the rib cage. The umbilicus, also known as the *navel* or *belly button,* is an inconsistent, mobile landmark on the anterior abdomen. It is typically at the level of L4 when an individual is in a recumbent position. When standing, in the infant, and in the pendulous abdomen, it lies at a lower level.

Posterior Abdominal Wall (Trunk)

In the posterior wall, the lower ribs, lumbar spines, PSIS, and iliac crest are palpable. A line, called the *intercristal line,* can be drawn between the iliac crests.[11] This line will typically pass between the spines of the third and fourth lumbar vertebrae, a location important when performing lumbar punctures.

Landmarks of the Anterior Pelvis

The anterior pelvis exhibits several bony and soft tissue landmarks that are useful to the radiation therapist. They are outlined in the following section and demonstrated in Figure 20-39.

The *iliac crest* extends from the ASIS to the PSIS. The ASIS is palpable, and measurements may be taken from it in the superoinferior or mediolateral direction. It is often used in referencing the location of the femur. The *lateral iliac crest*

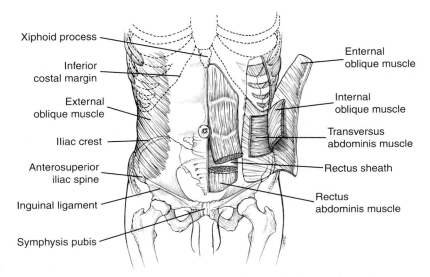

Figure 20-38. The muscles of the anterior and lateral abdominal wall work in unison to provide structure and stability to the torso.

is also easily palpable and, being on the lateral pelvic wall, may be used as a transverse level on either the anterior or the posterior pelvis. The *lateral iliac crest level* is the line joining the right and left lateral iliac crests. These crests are the most superior margin of the ilium on the lateral pelvic wall. Measurements may be taken from this level in the superoinferior direction.

The head of the femur and greater trochanter, although not direct components of the true pelvis, are important to note when considering the lateral pelvic anatomy. The *head of the femur* articulates with the hip at the acetabulum. If irradiated beyond tolerance, fibrotic changes can occur, causing painful and/or limited motion of the joint. Usually this joint is shielded in moderate to large pelvic portals to limit this occurrence. The *greater trochanter* is the only part of the proximal femur that can be palpated; therefore its relationship to bony points of the hip bone is important.[8] The radiation therapist uses the greater trochanter when aligning patients during simulation to alleviate pelvis rotation. The patient should be horizontally level when the greater trochanters are at the same height from the tabletop.

The radiation therapist can measure this using a ruler and optical lasers.

The symphysis pubis appears as the 5-mm midline gap between the inferior parts of the pelvic bones.[10] The *upper border pubis* is the palpable upper border of the midline pubic bone. It is fairly easy to palpate, except in extremely obese patients. When palpating it, care should be taken to allow for overlying tissue. The *lower border pubis* is the palpable lower border of the pubic bone in midline. It is not as easily palpable as the upper border pubis, because it lies more inferiorly and posteriorly. All of these can be accurately located radiographically. The radiation therapist uses these components when setting the anterior border of lateral prostate fields (the prostate lies immediately posterior to the symphysis pubis).

The ischial tuberosities are located in the inferior portion of the pelvis. This corresponds to the lower region of the buttock. When a person sits down, the ischial tuberosities bear the weight of the body. Many radiation oncologists use the ischial tuberosities as the inferior border of the anterior and posterior prostate treatment portals.

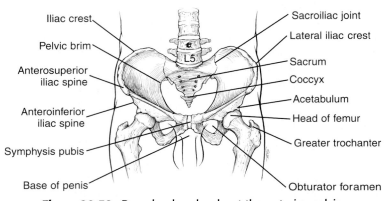

Figure 20-39. Bony landmarks about the anterior pelvis.

When pelvic irradiation is indicated, the radiation therapist can use the anatomy of the perineum, the diamond-shaped area bounded laterally by the ischial tuberosities, anteriorly by the symphysis pubis, and posteriorly by the coccyx, to assist in portal location. Treatment lines in these areas commonly fade because of perspiration and garment rubbing.[8] Knowledge of the area can thus provide a practical means of field verification. Both male and female anatomy demonstrates useful landmarks.

The *anterior commissure of the labia majora* is easily distinguishable in the female. It is an important soft tissue landmark, because it is used as a reference point from which the upper or lower border pubis is measured. Thus checking back to this soft tissue landmark may eliminate variations in the palpation of the pubic bone.

The *base of the penis* is taken as being the line joining the anterior skin of the penis with the skin of the anterior pelvic wall. This level is used as a reference point from which the upper or lower border pubis is measured in the male.

A therapist may measure changes in the lateral position of prostate fields by referencing appropriate measurements from the base of the penis.

Landmarks of the Posterior Pelvis

The most commonly used bony surface landmarks of the posterior pelvis are the PSISs, the coccyx, the iliac crests, and the lateral iliac crests. Because the latter two were also mentioned in the previous section, only the PSIS is discussed here. The PSISs are indicated by dimples above and medial to the buttock, approximately 5 to 6 cm from the midline. They are palpable, and measurements may be taken in the superoinferior or mediolateral direction. The coccyx lies deep to the natal cleft with its inferior end approximately 1 cm from the anus.

Abdominopelvic Viscera

The organs of the abdomen and pelvis can be visualized by various means. Radiographs, CT, MRI, and US are commonly used to provide information concerning organ location. It is worth noting that the location of any organ in the abdomen and pelvis can vary with respiration, anatomic position, and level of fullness. This is why it is extremely important to place radiation therapy patients in a reproducible position that limits movement daily. As observed earlier, body habitus affects the location of internal organs. This holds true for the abdomen and pelvis, as well. This section examines the location of the abdominal and pelvic viscera.

Location of the Alimentary Organs

The esophagus begins at the lower border of the cricoid cartilage in the neck and travels through the diaphragm to the cardiac sphincter, the entrance to the stomach, at the level of T10 approximately 2 to 3 cm to the left of midline. To visualize the esophagus radiographically, the patient commonly is instructed to swallow a radiopaque substance such as barium before examination.

The duodenum, a C-shaped section of the small bowel approximately 25 cm in length, starts to the right of midline at the edge of the epigastric region. The stomach lies between the duodenum and the distal esophagus and is of variable size and location,

partly covered by the left rib cage and filling the epigastric region. The root of the small gut mesentery, made up of sections called the *jejunum* and *ileum*, extends from the duodenum to the inlet to the large bowel.[10,11]

The start of the large bowel is the cecum. It lies in the right iliac region at the level of L4. The ascending colon (15 cm in length) and hepatic flexure of the colon on the right side and the splenic flexure and descending colon (25 cm in length) on the left side are largely retroperitoneal structures, whereas the transverse and sigmoid colon have a mesentery and vary in their position from one person to the next.[10,11] However, similarities are demonstrated within common body habitus. The rectum starts at the level of S3 and ends approximately 4 cm from the anus. It is one of the dose-limiting structures when prostate treatment fields are outlined. Rectal visualization is thus important during the simulation process.

Figure 20-40 delineates the surface projections of the alimentary tract in the abdomen and pelvis.

Location of Nonalimentary Organs

The radiation therapist benefits from a working knowledge of the nonalimentary organs of the abdomen and pelvis. Many times these organs are involved in malignant processes and must be included in the patient's treatment scheme. Figure 20-41 demonstrates the surface projections of the organs outlined here.

The liver is an irregularly shaped organ located in the right hypochondriac region of the abdomen above the costal margin. The superior margin of the liver, which bulges into the diaphragm, is at the level of T7-8. The liver is commonly imaged with CT, US, and nuclear medicine studies.

The gallbladder is located below the lower border of the liver and contacts the anterior abdominal wall where the right lateral border of the rectus abdominis crosses the ninth costal cartilage. This location is called the *transpyloric plane*. Again, US is useful in distinguishing biliary obstructions, as well as gallstones.

The spleen, mentioned earlier as a lymph node for the blood, is located posteriorly approximately 5 cm to the left of midline at the level of T10-11. The normal organ lies beneath the ninth through eleventh ribs on the left side of the body. This organ is often examined surgically in patients with lymphoma to determine disease extension. If the organ is removed for biopsy, the splenic pedicle, the point of attachment of the organ to its vascular and lymphatic connections, is included in the abdominal treatment field for Hodgkin's disease.

Three components, the head, body, and tail, compose the pancreas. The head of the pancreas is located in the C section of the duodenum. The body extends slightly superiorly to the left across midline, at the level of L1. The tail of the pancreas passes into the hilum, a concave point of an organ that has vascular inlets and outlets, of the spleen.

Location of the Urinary Tract Organs

The kidneys lie on the posterior abdominal wall in the retroperitoneal space. The hilum of the right kidney is at the level of L2, whereas the hilum of the left is at the level of L1. The right kidney lies lower than the left because of the presence of the adjacent liver. Superior and medial to each kidney are the adrenal glands. The kidneys are generally not fixed to the abdominal wall; they can move as much as 2 cm with respiration. When the radiation

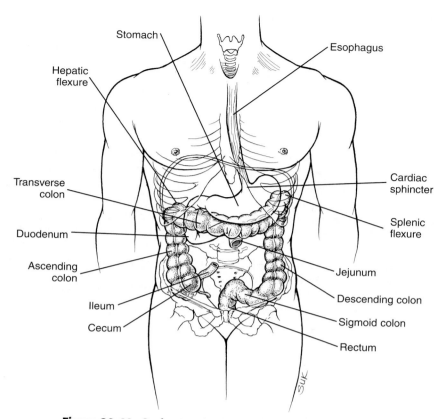

Figure 20-40. Surface projection of the alimentary organs.

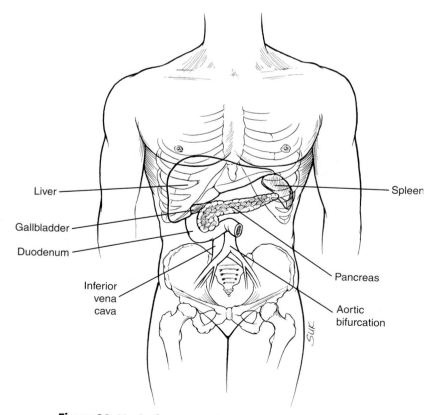

Figure 20-41. Surface projection of nonalimentary organs.

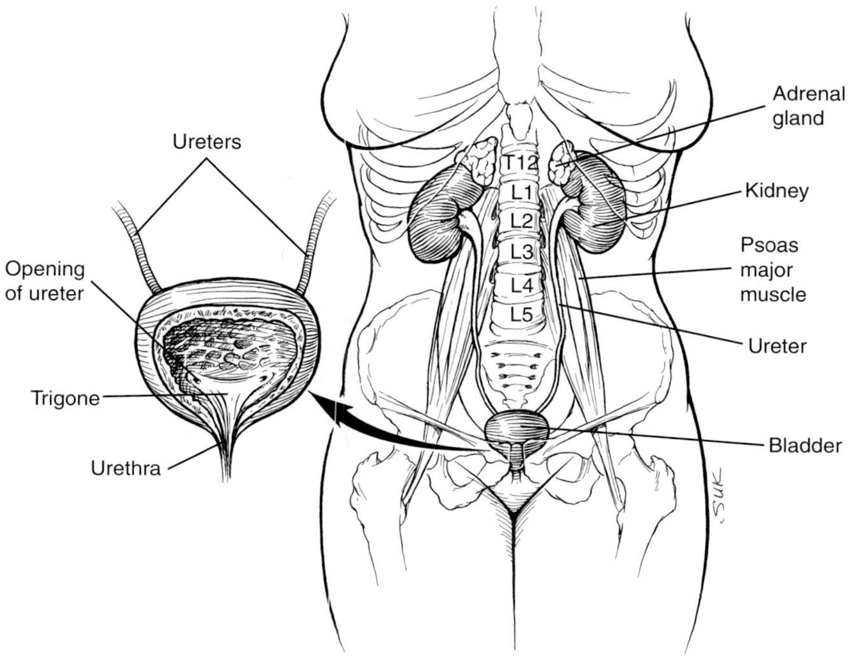

Figure 20-42. Surface projection of the urinary tract and adrenal glands.

therapist outlines the location of these radiation-sensitive structures, it is important to take this into account.

The ureters are tubular structures that transport urine from the kidneys to the urinary bladder. They run anterior to the psoas muscles and enter the pelvis lateral to the sacroiliac (SI) joint. The ureters, as well as the kidneys, are commonly imaged with CT, US, and intravenous and retrograde studies.

The urinary bladder is located in the pelvis. The neck of the bladder lies posterior to the symphysis pubis and anterior to the rectum. This organ also lies immediately superior to the prostate in the male. The urinary bladder is a dose-limiting structure in the treatment of prostatic cancer. It is commonly visualized with contrast agents during the simulation process.

The topographic relations of the urinary tract organs are shown in Figure 20-42.

Lymphatics of the Abdomen and Pelvis

The lymphatic drainage routes for the abdomen and pelvis are very important to the radiation therapist. There is an abundance of lymphatic vessels in this section of the body. Those of the retroperitoneum and pelvis play a major role in radiation therapy field arrangement of gynecologic, genitourinary, and lymphatic cancers. Figures 20-43 and 20-44 show the nodes and nodal groups outlined here.

The lymphatic pathways and nodes of the abdomen are often referred to as the *visceral nodes* because they are closely associated with the abdominal organs. The three principal groups of nodes of the abdomen that drain the corresponding viscera before entering the cisterna chyli or the thoracic duct are the celiac, superior mesenteric, and inferior mesenteric groups, also called the *preaortic nodes.*

The *celiac nodes* include the nodes that drain the stomach, greater omentum, liver, gallbladder, and spleen, as well as most of the lymph from the pancreas and duodenum. The *superior*

mesenteric nodes drain part of the head of the pancreas; a portion of the duodenum; the entire jejunum, ileum, appendix, cecum, and ascending colon; and most of the transverse colon. The *inferior mesenteric nodes* drain the descending colon, the left side of the mesentery, the sigmoid colon, and the rectum.

The posterior abdominal wall demonstrates a rich network of lymphatic vessels. The paraaortic nodes provide efferent drainage to the cisterna chyli, which is the beginning of the

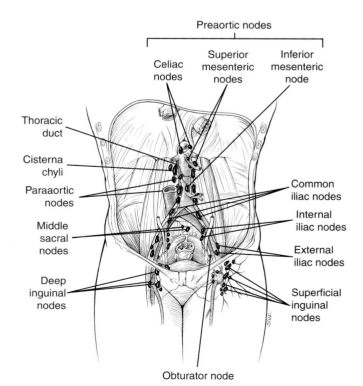

Figure 20-43. Abdominal lymph nodes.

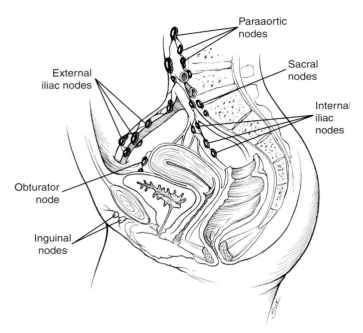

Figure 20-44. Lymphatics of the pelvis.

thoracic duct. These nodes run adjacent to the abdominal aorta from T12 to L4. This major section of the lymphatic system eventually receives lymph from most of the lower regions of the body. The *paraaortics* directly drain the uterus, ovary, kidneys, and testicles. It is interesting to note that embryonically the testes develop near the kidneys and descend into the scrotum after birth. As they descend, they take the vascular and lymphatic vessels with them as direct means for blood and lymph flow.

The *common iliac nodes* lie at the bifurcation of the abdominal aorta at the level of L4. These nodes directly drain the urinary bladder, prostate, cervix, and vagina. This chain moves laterally and breaks up into the external and internal iliac nodes. The *external iliac nodes* drain the urinary bladder, prostate, cervix, testes, vagina, and ovaries. The *internal iliac nodes,* also known as the *hypogastric nodes,* drain the vagina, cervix, prostate, and urinary bladder. These nodes are more medial and posterior to the external iliac nodes previously mentioned.

The *inguinal nodes* are more superficial than the previously mentioned nodes. These nodes directly drain the vulva, uterus, ovaries, and vagina. These nodes are commonly treated with electrons because of their superficial location.

APPLIED TECHNOLOGY

Practical application of the material presented in this chapter is very important. To enhance the comprehensive understanding of the relationships presented, the last section of this chapter presents diagrams that relate structures to vertebral body levels and CT scans through the head, neck, thorax, abdomen, and pelvis. The appropriate structures pertinent to the radiation oncology practitioner are demostrated. Figures 20-45 through 20-49 show these diagrams and scans.

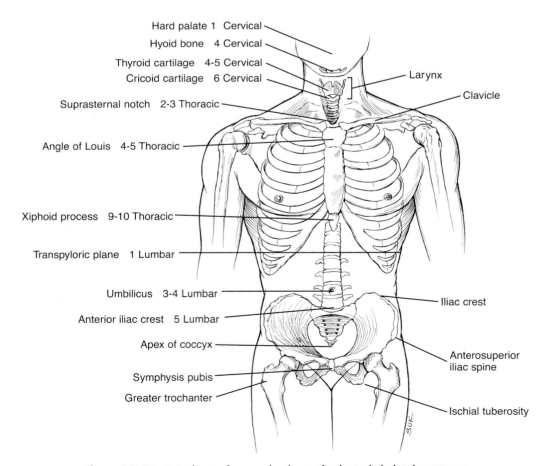

Figure 20-45. Anterior surface projections of selected skeletal anatomy.

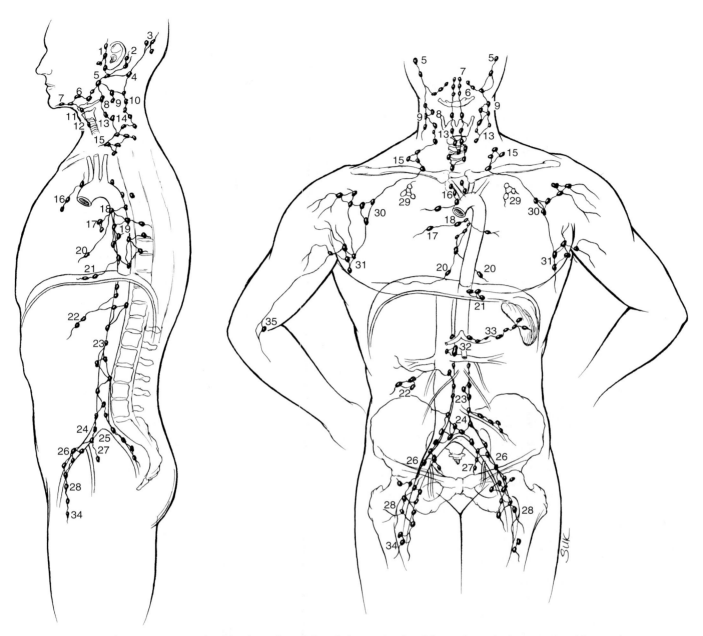

Figure 20-46. Major lymph nodes of the abdomen and pelvis. *1*, Preauricular; *2*, mastoid; *3*, occipital; *4*, upper cervical; *5*, parotid; *6*, submaxillary; *7*, submental; *8*, jugulodigastric; *9*, upper deep cervical; *10*, spinal accessory chain; *11*, infrahyoid; *12*, pretracheal; *13*, jugu-loomohyoid; *14*, lower deep cervical; *15*, supraclavicular; *16*, mediastinal; *17*, interlobar; *18*, intertracheal; *19*, posterior mediastinal; *20*, lateral pericardial; *21*, diaphragmatic; *22*, mesenteric; *23*, paraaortic; *24*, common iliac; *25*, lateral sacral; *26*, external iliac; *27*, hypogastric; *28*, inguinal; *29*, interpectoral; *30*, axillary apex; *31*, axillary; *32*, cisterna chyli; *33*, splenic; *34*, femoral; *35*, epitrochlear.

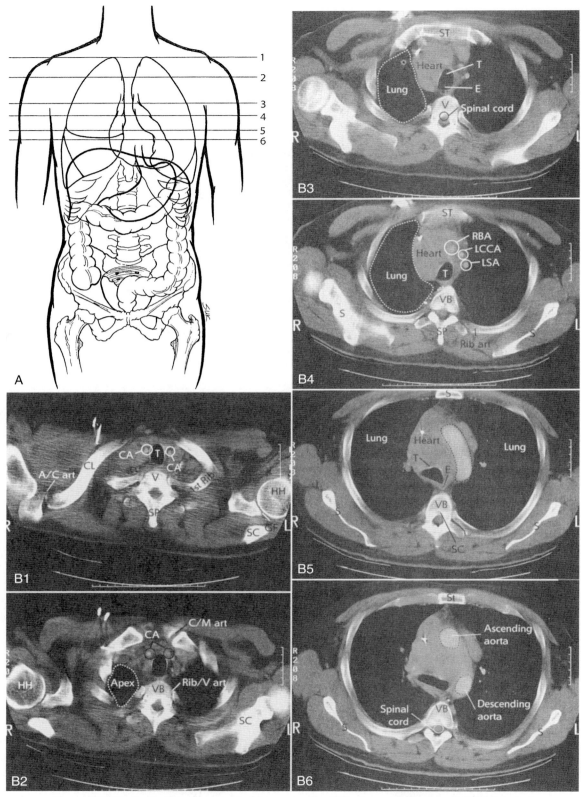

Figure 20-47. A, Sectional computed tomography (CT) views of the thorax with labeled anatomy **(B).** *ACA,* Ascending aorta; *A/C art,* acromial clavicular articulation; *CA,* carotid artery; *CL,* clavicle; *C/M art,* clavicular macrobial articular; *DCA,* descending aorta; *E,* esophagus; *GF,* glenoid fossa; *HH,* humeral head; *LCCA,* left common carotid artery; *LSA,* left subclavian artery; *RBA,* right bronchocephalic artery; *Rib/V art,* rib/vertebral artery; *SC,* scapula; *SP,* spinous; *ST,* sternum; *T,* trachea; *V,* vein; *VB,* vertebral body.

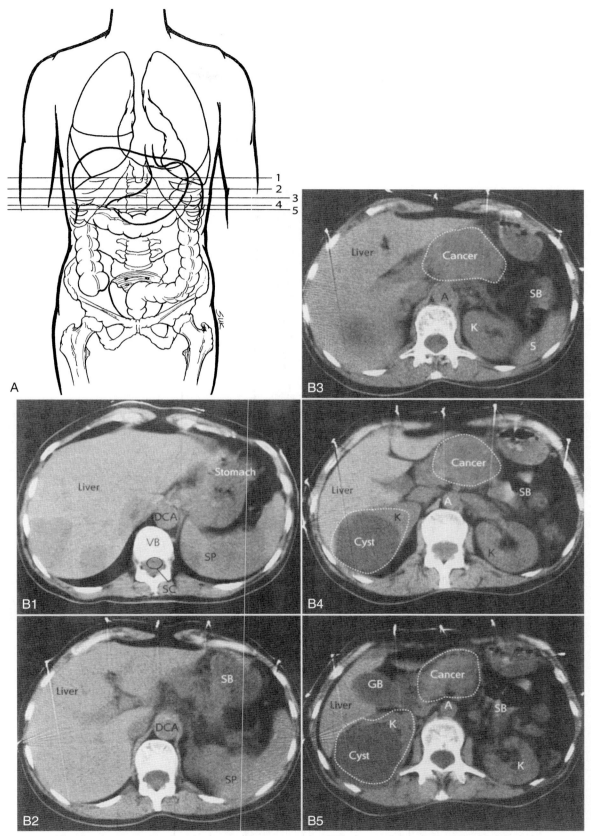

Figure 20-48. A, Sectional computed tomography (CT) views of the abdomen with labeled anatomy **(B)**. *A,* Aorta; *DCA,* descending aorta; *GB,* gallbladder; *K,* kidney; *L,* liver; *S,* spleen; *SB,* small bowel; *SC,* spinal cord; *SP,* spinous process; *VB,* vertebral body.

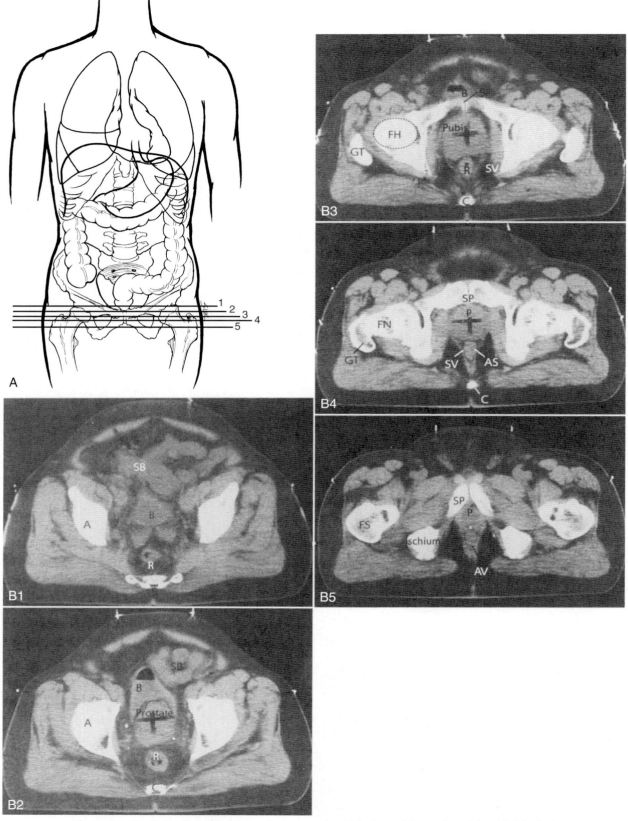

Figure 20-49. **A**, Sectional computed tomography (CT) view of the male pelvis with labeled anatomy **(B)**. *A*, Acetabulum; *AS*, axial sphincter; *AV,* anal verge; *B*, bladder; *C*, coccyx; *FH,* femoral head; *FN*, femoral neck; *FS,* femoral shaft; *GT*, greater tuberosity; *I*, ischium; *P,* prostate; *R*, rectum; *S*, sacrum; *SB,* small bowel; *SP,* symphysis pubis; *SV,* seminal vesicles.

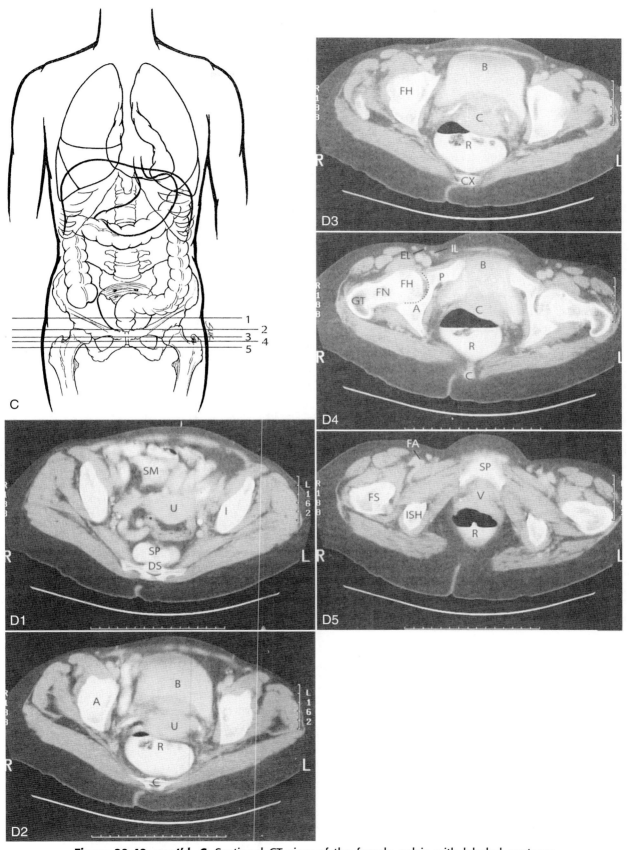

Figure 20-49—cont'd. C, Sectional CT view of the female pelvis with labeled anatomy **(D)**. *A*, Acetabulum; *B*, bladder; *C*, cervix; *CX*, coccyx; *DS*, descending sigmoid; *EL*, external iliac; *FA*, femoral artery; *FH,* femoral head; *FN*, femoral neck; *FS*, femoral shaft; *GT*, greater tuberosity; *I*, ilium; *IL*, internal iliac; *ISH*, ishium; *P*, pubis; *R*, rectum; *SM*, small intestine; *SP*, symphasis pubis; *U*, uterus; *V*, vagina.

SUMMARY

- Radiation therapy requires its practitioners to demonstrate more than a passing acquaintance with surface and sectional anatomy.
- The complex simulation procedures and planning used in patient treatment mandates strict attention to detail.
- The radiation therapist must use information provided by several imaging modalities to achieve its ultimate goal: to administer a tumoricidal dose of radiation to the tumor and tumor bed while sparing as much normal tissue as possible.
- The lymphatic vessels play a major role in treatment field delineation and disease management.
- The complexity of radiation therapy requires the radiation therapist to use all available means to function effectively. Each therapist should review his or her practical skills in surface and sectional anatomy, because it is crucial for accurate treatment planning and delivery.
- For patients to completely benefit from the new technology in radiation therapy, the radiation therapist must have a strong anatomic base that will allow effective treatment delivery.
- Medical imaging greatly assists not only in localizing tumors and areas of related interest, it also promotes greater treatment delivery options through more precise and exacting means.
- Body habitus knowledge helps the radiation therapist quickly locate treatment areas and relate internal structure location as related to body type. Knowing how the human body varies is essential to effective practice.
- The lymphatic system and its related components depict possible routes of tumor spread. The system's one-way flow makes the spread patterns predictable. Closely associated with neighboring structures and the cardiovascular system, the lymphatic channels and extent of their involvement in a cancer diagnosis are essential in the radiation treatment field design and delivery.
- Anatomic landmarks are important tools in locating and recalling treatment areas. There are two types of landmarks to consider: bony and soft tissue. Although all provide useful information, the bony landmarks are more stable and more predictably referenced. Soft tissue landmarks are useful in locating general areas but may not be as exact in comparison.

Review Questions

Multiple Choice

1. Which plane goes through the middle of the body from the front to back through the sagittal suture of the skull that divides the body into two equal parts?
   a. midsagittal
   b. coronal
   c. horizontal
   d. superior

2. Which muscle partitions the anterior cavity into the thoracic and abdominal portions?
   a. diaphragm
   b. rectus abdominus

   c. trapezius
   d. pectoralis major

3. Which vessel returns lymph from the entire body back into the bloodstream, with the exception of the upper right limb and the right side of the thorax, head, and neck?
   a. cisterna chyli
   b. thoracic duct
   c. right lymphatic duct
   d. superior vena cava

4. The angle of the mandible is generally located at which vertebra number level?
   a. C1
   b. C4
   c. T1
   d. T4

5. Which structures run anterior to the psoas stripes (muscles) and enters the pelvis lateral to the sacroiliac joint? Tumors in these structures are very rare.
   a. kidneys
   b. urethra
   c. ureters
   d. adrenal glands

6. If the punctum lacrimae of the eye is overirradiated, fibrotic changes can occur. If this happens, what would be the clinical signs?
   a. dry eye
   b. constantly tearing eye
   c. cataracts
   d. ocular muscle atrophy

7. In the lower neck, the esophagus lies:
   a. anterior to the trachea and posterior to the spinal cord
   b. anterior to the spinal cord and posterior to the trachea
   c. anterior to the trachea and inferior to the spinal cord
   d. inferior to the spinal cord and posterior to the trachea

8. Which of the following are examples of primary curves?
   I. thoracic
   II. lateral
   III. pelvic
   a. I and II
   b. I and III
   c. II and III
   d. I, II, and III

9. The trachea is a hollow tube approximately 10 cm in length that extends from the larynx to a bifurcation called the:
   a. bronchus
   b. carina
   c. bronchiole
   d. lung

10. Which of the following are commonly used soft tissue landmarks of the anterior pelvis?
    a. umbilicus
    b. base of penis
    c. both a and b
    d. neither a nor b

The answers to the Review Questions can be found by logging on to our website at: *http://evolve.elsevier.com/Washington+Leaver/principles*

Questions to Ponder

1. Examine the process of how lymph is transported through the lymphatic system.
2. Describe how the directional flow of lymph is facilitated through the lymphatic system.
3. Describe events that can occur if lymphatic channels are compromised through either surgical or radiation damage.
4. Why are landmarks about the mouth, as well as other soft tissue landmarks, not very accurate? What would we have to do to use them accurately?
5. How could a therapist locate the pituitary gland by using only topographic landmarks?
6. How can body habitus affect abdominal organ location?
7. What is the significance of including a portion of lung tissue in the tangential fields of the patient treated for breast cancer?
8. Analyze the relationship of surface anatomy knowledge with performance of effective simulation procedures. How can this knowledge also affect daily treatment administrations?

REFERENCES

1. Barrett CP, et al: *Primer of sectional anatomy with MRI and CT correlation,* Philadelphia, 1994, Lippincott Williams & Wilkins.
2. Bentel GC: *Radiation therapy planning,* ed 2, New York, 1995, McGraw-Hill.
3. Collins JD, et al: Anatomy of the abdomen, back, and pelvis as displayed by magnetic resonance imaging: part one, *J Natl Med Assoc* 81:680-684, 1989.
4. Collins JD, et al: Anatomy of the abdomen, back, and pelvis as displayed by magnetic resonance imaging: part two, *J Natl Med Assoc* 81:809-813, 1989.
5. Collins JD, et al: Anatomy of the abdomen, back, and pelvis as displayed by magnetic resonance imaging: part three, *J Natl Med Assoc* 81:857-861, 1989.
6. Collins JD, et al: Magnetic resonance imaging of chest wall lesions, *J Natl Med Assoc* 83:352-360, 1991.
7. Cox JD, Ang KK, editors: *Radiation oncology: rationale, techniques, results,* ed 8, St. Louis, 2003, Mosby.
8. Foldi M, Strosenreuther R: *Foundations of manual lymph drainage,* St. Louis, 2003, Mosby.
9. Kelley LL, Peterson CM: *Sectional anatomy for imaging professionals,* ed 2, St. Louis, 2007, Mosby.
10. Keogh B, Ebbs S: *Normal surface anatomy,* Philadelphia, 1984, Lippincott.
11. Lumley JSP: *Surface anatomy: the anatomical basis of clinical examination,* ed 3, London, 2002, Churchill Livingstone.
12. Novelline RA, Squire LF: *Living anatomy: a working atlas using computed tomography, magnetic resonance and angiography images,* Philadelphia, 1987, Hanley & Belfus.
13. Panjabi MM, et al: Human lumbar vertebrae, *Spine* 17:299-302, 1992.
14. Panjabi MM, et al: Thoracic human vertebrae, *Spine* 16:888-901, 1991.
15. Philippou M, et al: Cross-sectional anatomy of the nose and paranasal sinuses, *Rhinology* 28:221-230, 1990.
16. Rubin P: *Clinical oncology: a multidisciplinary approach for physicians and students,* ed 8, Philadelphia, 2001, WB Saunders.
17. Tortora GJ, Grabowski SR: *Principles of human anatomy and physiology,* ed 10, New Jersey, 2002, John Wiley & Sons.

BIBLIOGRAPHY

Stanton R, Stinson D: *An introduction to radiation oncology physics,* Madison, Wis, 1992, Medical Physics Publishing.
Stewart GS: Trends in radiation therapy for the treatment of lung cancer, *Nurs Clin North Am* 27:643-651, 1992.
Vann AM, Dasher BG, Chestnut SK, Wiggers NH: *Portal design in radiation therapy,* Columbia, SC, 2006, RL Bryan Company.
Wechsler RJ, Steiner RM: Cross-sectional imaging of the chest wall, *J Thorac Imag* 4:29-40, 1989.

Simulator Design

Dennis Leaver, Nora Uricchio, Patton Griggs

Outline

Objectives

- Compare and contrast the theory of conventional, computed tomography (CT), and virtual simulation.
- Describe, as though you were educating an interested patient, the purpose of the isocenter.
- List and describe the components and the operation of a simulator, including the radiographic, fluoroscopic, and CT units.
- Explain the purpose of each of the components within the head of the gantry of a conventional simulator.

- Describe the use of multislice detectors in CT image formation.
- Explain the application of Hounsfield units in CT image formation and their use in treatment planning.
- Discuss why variable slice thickness and spacing are extremely important in obtaining CT studies beneficial to producing high-quality digitally reconstructed radiographs.
- Explain why the design of a simulator room should involve the expertise of numerous professionals.

Key Terms

The effective use of the simulator is important in achieving the goal of delivering a dose of radiation to the target volume and at the same time reducing the dose to the normal surrounding tissue. This is the goal of radiation therapy. In most cases, this requires a high degree of precision and accuracy. It is the right combination of high-technology equipment, such as the simulator, and the involvement of dedicated professionals that can sometimes make the difference between a geographic miss and curing the patient of cancer. The primary purpose of the simulator is to assist the physician and other members of the radiation therapy team in the treatment planning process by establishing and documenting the appropriate volume to be treated and identifying the normal structures within or adjacent to this volume.

Simulation may involve computed tomography (CT) scans or other imaging studies to help the radiation oncologist plan how to direct the radiation. The areas receiving radiation are marked with either a temporary or a permanent marker, which may consist of small marks or a tiny "tattoo," approximately the size of a freckle, showing where the radiation will be aimed. These small marks are also used to determine the exact site of the initial treatments. An effective simulation procedure should determine optimal patient positioning, beam entry points, and other points helpful in patient positioning and field localization.[2]

There are a number of approaches to the simulation process: conventional simulation and CT simulation. The development of commercially available CT simulators has fused the process of patient scanning, tumor and target localization, treatment planning, and treatment field verification into a single integrated operation.[27] CT simulation differs from conventional simulation in a number of ways. During conventional simulation, patient data are obtained using fluoroscopy, radiography, and physical measurements of the patient (Figure 21-1). This information is then entered into the treatment planning computer. With CT simulation, patient data are gathered using detailed CT images, usually in the transverse plane. The captured data are then processed to produce **digitally reconstructed radiographs (DRRs)**, which are produced by recording the x-ray source of the CT scanning information through

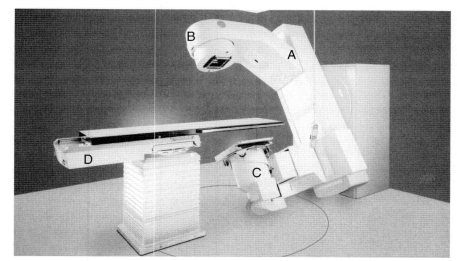

Figure 21-1. Components and motions of a radiation therapy simulator. These include the gantry *(A)* (including the collimator head *[B]* and image intensifier *[C]*) and patient support assembly *(D)* (treatment couch). (Courtesy Siemens Medical Solutions. From Leibel SA, Phillips TL: *Textbook of radiation oncology,* ed 2, Philadelphia, 2004, Saunders.)

a three-dimentional model of the patient. A laser alignment system documents the simulation process before patient data are transferred electronically through a computer link to the treatment planning computer (Figure 21-2). In the following sections, both the conventional and the CT simulator design are discussed along with information related to the historic perspective of the simulation process (Box 21-1).

HISTORIC PERSPECTIVE

Historically, radiation oncology began as a subsection of diagnostic radiology. The simulation process also has its roots in diagnostic radiology (remember, the conventional simulator uses an x-ray tube as one of its primary components). Before the widespread commercial availability of the simulator, most patients' treatment planning occurred on the cobalt unit,

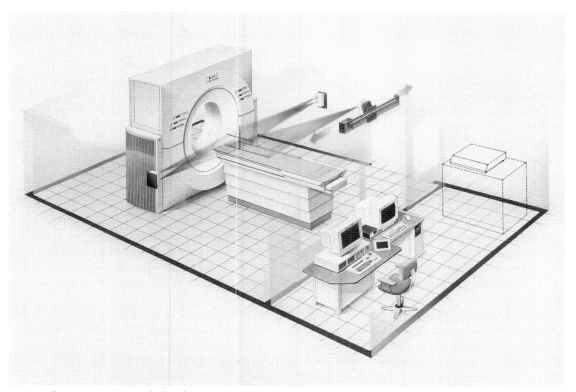

Figure 21-2. Virtual simulation. This technique uses a computed tomography (CT)-based simulator linked into a treatment planning computer. The laser light system delineates field borders once a plan has been completed. (Used with permission from Picker International, Cleveland, Ohio.)

"Radiation oncology, together with surgical and medical oncology, are the three primary disciplines involved in cancer treatment. Radiation oncology with either curative or palliative intent is used to treat up to sixty percent (60%) of all cancer patients. The use of radiation therapy requires detailed attention to personnel, equipment, patient and personnel safety, and continuing staff education." The American College of Radiology (ACR) states, under the equipment section, that "high-energy and electron beams, a computer-based treatment planning system, simulation, dosimetry with direct participation of a qualified medical physicist, brachytherapy and ability to fabricate treatment aids must be available to patients in all facilities, either on site or through arrangements with another center." Regular maintenance and repair of equipment is mandatory and is also recommended as part of the ACR Standards for Radiation Oncology.[2]

Radiation oncology equipment should include the following:

1. Megavoltage radiation therapy equipment for external beam therapy (e.g., a linear accelerator or cobalt-60 teletherapy unit). If the cobalt-60 unit is the only megavoltage unit, it must have a treatment distance of 80 cm or more.
2. Electron beam or x-ray equipment for the treatment of skin lesions or superficial lesions.
3. Simulator capable of duplicating the setups of any megavoltage unit and producing radiographs of the fields to be treated. Fluoroscopic capability is highly recommended.
4. Appropriate brachytherapy equipment for intracavitary and interstitial treatment (or arrangements for referral to appropriate facilities).
5. Computer dosimetry equipment capable of providing external beam isodose curves as well as brachytherapy isodose curves.
6. Physics calibration devices for all equipment.
7. Beam-shaping devices.
8. Immobilization devices.

betatron, or linear accelerator. Competition for space and capital budget requests within the radiology department contributed to this initial approach (in the early days) of setting up new patients on the treatment unit.

In the past, a "simulation time" was scheduled on the treatment unit or a conventional diagnostic x-ray unit to "set up" new patients.[6,7,18,20] There were several problems associated with this type of procedure. First, it took time away from treating patients. "Room simulations" (treatment room) required a fair amount of time to adequately estimate the target volume and provide some parameters to ensure reproducibility on subsequent days of treatment. Second, the quality of the planning radiographs (which were a type of port film) was very poor. High-energy x-rays and gamma rays do not produce good-quality images. In addition, the initial estimates of the target volume (without the aid of fluoroscopy and/or CT images) depended to a large degree on the radiation therapy team's

understanding and application of topographic anatomy. Figure 21-3 illustrates the difference between a conventional simulation radiograph and a portal image. The simulation radiograph (Figure 21-3, A), which is exposed using x-rays in the diagnostic range (70 to 120 kVp), demonstrates overall improved contrast and visibility of detail compared with the corresponding portal localization image (Figure 21-3, B), which was produced using a 6-MV x-ray beam.

The development of the conventional radiation therapy simulator was prompted by the introduction of linear accelerators and other high-energy treatment units. It was thought that if a machine could be built that duplicated the mechanical and geometric features of a treatment unit, then the treatment unit could be used for its original purpose—to deliver a prescribed dose of radiation to the patient (Figure 21-4). Initially, it was thought that the cobalt unit, betatron, and linear accelerator deserved most of the credit for curing or effectively palliating a patient's cancer. It was not long before the benefits of the conventional simulator were also established.

During a conventional simulation procedure, time could be scheduled to position, immobilize, and align the target volume with the simulator's isocenter, providing more accurate data and lessoning the burden on the treatment unit. Images created on the conventional simulator, with the aid of fluoroscopy and diagnostic-quality images, greatly improved the simulation process. Until recently, most simulation procedures were performed on the conventional fluoroscopy-based simulator. Computer-aided simulation using CT images and computer software of the patient in the treatment position to perform simulation without a conventional simulator has gained more widespread acceptance.[9] Sherouse first used the term *virtual simulation* to describe the combination of computer simulation techniques, CT simulation, and DRRs.[1,32]

It has taken many years, since CT became available in the 1970s, to realize the full potential that CT can have on the radiation therapy simulation and treatment planning process. Much of the delay can be attributed to the time it has taken the medical and computer industries to develop faster scanning capabilities and very rapid computer processing speed.[1,3,5] Today, CT simulation can be used to describe several types of radiation therapy localization procedures, including the following[9,13,20,21,30]:

- **Conventional simulator with a CT mode**, which can provide an external contour of the patient and additional information on the location, size, and thickness of internal structures. Essentially, this is a conventional simulator, which has special capabilities to rotate 360 degrees, capturing patient data and displaying those data in transverse sections.
- A **conventional simulator** session, followed by a CT scan on a second diagnostic CT scanner, perhaps located in the radiology department.
- **CT simulation**, which may acquire CT data, outline the target volume and critical structures, and project treatment beams onto the patient, establishing external reference marks used for treatment setup purposes. This is done with the patient present.

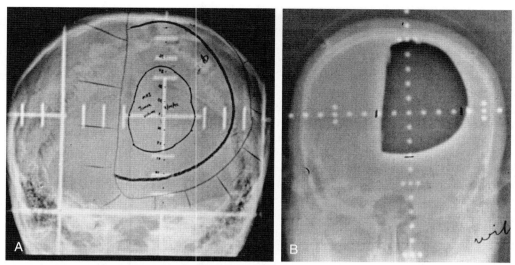

Figure 21-3. Simulation radiograph. **A**, Exposure using x-rays in the diagnostic range (70 to 120 kVp) demonstartes overall improved contrast and visibility of detail as compared with the corresponding portal localization radiograph **(B)**, which was produced using phtons in the 4- to 32-MV range. Higher contrast in **A** is due to the increased amount of the photoelectric effect observed with lower-energy (kilovoltage) exposures. The poorer contrast in **B** is a result of greater Compton's effect, observed with exposures in the energy range (megavoltage). (From Bourland J: Radiation oncology physics. In Gunderson LL, Tepper JE, editors: *Clinical radiation oncology,* ed 2, Philadelphia, 2007, Churchill Livingstone.)

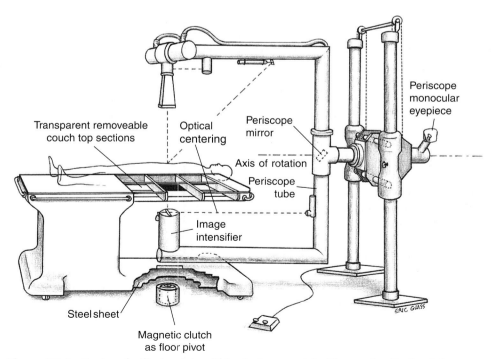

Figure 21-4. Custom-built simulator. This device, used in Newcastle, England, in 1955, shows isocentric capabilities and a periscope system for imaging purposes. (Redrawn with permission from Farmer ET, Fowler JF, Haggith JW: Megavoltage treatment planning and the use of xeroradiography, *Br J Radiol* 36:426-435, 1963.)

- **Virtual simulation**, where the simulation is performed on a volumetric image of the patient (usually a CT image), not the patient—hence, the name "virtual simulation." Virtual simulation may include the addition of data from magnetic resonance imaging (MRI) and positron emission tomography (PET) scans of the patient in the treatment position. This takes place within the computer where the proposed treatment geometry is designed and viewed on screen, using numerous software tools.[9] The patient need not be present during a virtual simulation process.

The simulation process has evolved rapidly in recent years, especially as three-dimensional treatment planning has expanded, demanding the visualization of anatomy in three dimensions. Simulation procedures now have the capabilities to position, immobilize, and align the target volume with reference points in or on the patient, using fluoroscopy, CT, MRI, and PET images.[30] The simulation process is entering a new era in radiation therapy simulation and treatment planning. It has become much more demanding and requires increased accuracy and precision in identifying the tumor and surrounding critical structures than it did 25 years ago. Will the virtual simulator equipment replace the conventional simulator?

CONVENTIONAL SIMULATOR DESIGN

Conventional simulators are designed to simulate the mechanical, geometric, and optical conditions of a variety of treatment units.[4,26,30] This is their basic purpose. It is critical that the mechanical parameters and geometric characteristics of the simulator match those of the treatment unit.

To ensure that the critical mechanical parameters of the simulator match the geometry of the treatment unit, each department should establish a comprehensive quality assurance program. The purpose of a quality assurance program is to objectively and systematically monitor the quality and appropriateness of the simulation process as it relates to patient care. The British Standards Institution, which represents the United Kingdom's view on standards in Europe and at the international level, has published a guide to functional performance values for the conventional radiation therapy simulator.[10] The guide, which is based on International Electrotechnical Commission (IEC) standards for the safety of medical electrical equipment,* may be useful in establishing specific elements for a quality assurance program.

To create some uniformity in the design of a simulator, certain criteria and specifications should be followed by the manufacturer. Specific design features and performance specifications of the simulator are also outlined in the *British Journal of Radiology* Supplement.[7] Table 21-1 summarizes the simulator performance specifications in *British Journal of Radiology* Supplement 23.[8]

Mechanical Components

The mechanical components of the conventional simulator include the gantry, treatment couch, and controls. An introduction to the essential components of the radiation therapy simulator will

*IEC 601-1: 1988, from BSI Medical Electrical Equipment—Part 1: General requirements for safety, and Amendment 1, 1991. In addition, IEC 601-1 is supplemented by IEC 1168: 1993, Radiotherapy simulators—Functional performance characteristics.

Table 21-1	A Summary of the Conventional Simulator Specifications	
	Specification	**Description**
GANTRY		
Height of isocenter above the floor	≤115 cm	
Angle of rotation at ≤100 cm SAD	>360°	0.03-1.0 rpm
Angle of rotation at >100 cm SAD	±90°	
Isocenter accuracy, diameter	2 mm	
Clearance between gantry and isocenter	≤110 cm	
X-RAY HEAD AND COLLIMATOR		
Source-axis distance	80-100 cm*	0.5-5 cm sec⁻¹
Beam-limiting diaphragms at 100 cm	50 cm × 50 cm max	
Diaphragm rotation	>220°	0.01 rpm
Beam-delineating wires at 100 cm	50 cm × 50 cm max	
Source-skin distance indicator	60-150 cm	
X-RAY TUBE AND GENERATOR		
Focal spot size	0.3 mm × 0.3 mm	
Target angle	≥20°	
Continuous rating of target	500 HU sec⁻¹	
Generator	Three phase	
Radiographic output (minimum)	500 mA, 90 kV	
Fluoroscopic output (minimum)	6 mA, 125 kV	
IMAGING DEVICE		
Film cassette and grid	≥35 cm²	Manual rotation
Image intensifier	12 inch	
Scanning movements of the image intensifier	±20 cm	3 cm sec⁻¹
Radial movements of the image intensifier	210-260 cm	3 cm sec⁻¹
COUCH		
Couch top	220 cm × 45 cm	
Rotation about couch support	360°	Manual rotation
Rotation about isocenter	±100°	0.003-0.05 rpm
Vertical movement	+2 to 250 cm	0.1-3.0 cm sec⁻¹
Minimum couch movement	<50 cm	
Longitudinal movement	230 to +100 cm	Manual, 2 cm sec⁻¹
Lateral movement	±20 cm	Manual, 2 cm sec⁻¹

Used with permission from Bomford CK, Dawes PJDK, Lillicrap SC, et al: Treatment simulators, *Br J Radiol* suppl 23, 1989.
HU, Hounsfield units; *SAD*, source-axis distance.
*Extending to 175-cm source-couch distance when the beam is vertical.

reveal many similarities, especially in their mechanical functions. This may include the gantry, treatment couch, controls, and other ancillary devices and safety features. Each of these components is discussed separately in this section.

Gantry. The gantry arm is the rigid C-shaped structural support of the gantry. It provides support for both the x-ray tube, located within the head of the gantry at one end of the open part of the C, and the image-intensifying/film holder system, located at the opposite end. These components of the gantry should be constructed in such a way that their alignment with the central axis of the beam can be maintained over the life of the simulator.[8] Figure 21-1 illustrates the three gantry components, including the gantry arm, gantry head, and image intensifier/film holder. Through 360-degree rotation, the gantry can potentially direct the beam toward the patient from any angle. In addition, the head of the gantry moves in a radial direction, or up and down, much like the periscope on a submarine.

Before looking at each of the components of the gantry in more detail, an explanation and description of the motions of the conventional simulator, as illustrated in Figures 21-5 and 21-6, may be helpful. Table 21-2 describes each of the motions of the simulator illustrated in Figure 21-5.

Isocenter. The gantry rotates around a fixed point in space, called the *isocenter*. The isocentric method, proposed by Howard-Flanders and Newbery in 1950, is still used today in radiation oncology.[15] This is an abstract concept. The **isocenter** should be considered as a reference point in space, a fixed distance (80 to 100 cm) from the focal spot on the anode. If the isocenter is placed either on the surface of the patient (fixed source-skin distance [SSD] treatment, also referred to as target-skin distance [TSD]) or at some location within the patient (isocentric source-axis distance [SAD] treatment, also referred to as target-axis

Table 21-2	**Mechanical Motions of the Simulator**		
Location*	**Motion**	**Major Component**	**Description**
A	Collimator rotation	Gantry head	
B	Gantry rotation	Gantry arm	Variable speed
C	SAD adjustment	Gantry arm	
D	Vertical movement	Patient support assembly	
E	Lateral movement	Patient support assembly	
F	Pedestal rotation	Patient support assembly	Not found on all simulators
G	Longitudinal movement	Patient support assembly	
H	Radial movement	Image intensifier	
I	Lateral movement	Image intensifier	Scanning ability
J	Longitudinal movement	Image intensifier	Scanning ability
K	Rotation about isocenter	Patient support assembly	

SAD, Source-axis distance.
*Each letter (A to J) corresponds to the components illustrated in Figure 21-5.

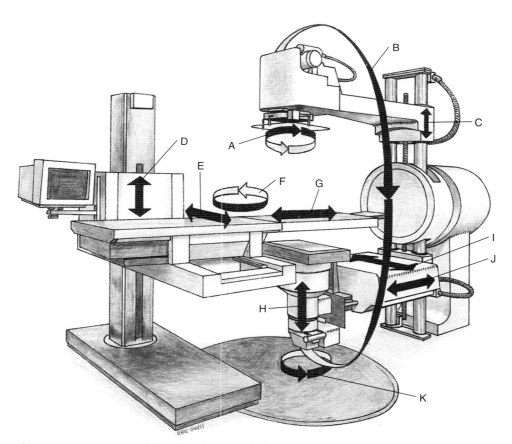

Figure 21-5. Motions of the simulator. Each letter corresponds to 1 of the 11 motions described in Table 21-2.

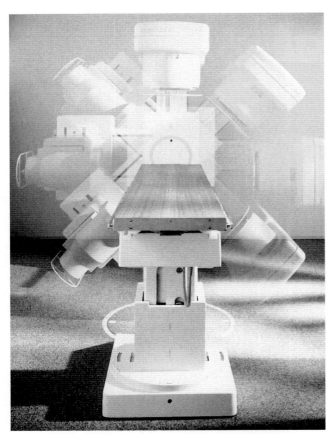

Figure 21-6. Radiation therapy simulator movements. (Used by permission from Philips Medical Systems, Shelton, Conn.)

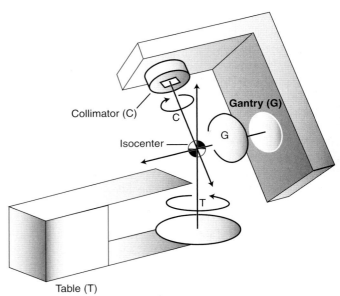

Figure 21-7. The isocenter is a reference point in space where three axes of rotation from the collimator, gantry, and table intersect on the conventional simulator and linear accelerator treatment unit. (From Bourland J: Radiation oncology physics. In Gunderson LL, Tepper JE, editors: *Clinical radiation oncology*, ed 2, Philadelphia, 2007, Churchill Livingstone.)

distance [TAD]) in the simulator room, then it can also be reproduced on or within the patient in the treatment room.

In searching for this invisible point in the simulator or treatment room, it would take some understanding to locate it. It could be measured. The isocenter is generally located 80 to 100 cm from the focal spot and between 100 and 130 cm above the floor, depending on the manufacturer's specifications. The distance from the isocenter to the source of x-ray production (focal spot) is the same from any gantry angle.

The treatment couch, sometimes mounted on a turntable, allows rotation about a fixed axis that passes through the isocenter (Figure 21-7). Thus, there are three axes of rotation—the central axis of the beam, the axis of rotation of the gantry, and the treatment couch axis—that all meet at a point known as the isocenter.[15] The **central axis** is the central portion of the beam emanating from the target. It is the only part of the beam that is not divergent. In a treatment plan with multiple fields, the central axes of each beam are directed toward the isocenter.

Each part of the gantry revolves around the isocenter. It is like the axle of a bicycle wheel. All the spokes of the wheel have a relationship with the axle. The head of the gantry is always, like the spokes of the wheel, the same distance from the isocenter regardless of its position in space.

The **protractor** (gantry angle scale), located at the central point of rotation of the gantry arm, is an instrument in the shape of a graduated circular device. It is used to measure the gantry angle, which may range from 0 to 360 degrees. Because of a lack of agreement among manufacturers of simulators and treatment equipment on the angular specifications of the protractor, some simulators and treatment units do not correspond in this area. One unit may indicate a 0-degree reading when the gantry is in the vertical position, and another may read 360 degrees. The IEC has developed recommendations for linear and angular scale placement and 0-degree location on the protractor for treatment units, as well as simulators.[23] A conversion chart, located near the simulator work area, may be helpful in matching gantry angle readouts.

Gantry Head. The gantry also provides stability for the collimator assembly, optical distance indicator (ODI), x-ray tube, field-defining wires, beam-restricting diaphragm (also called *x-ray shutters blades,* or *collimators*), and accessory holder. Figure 21-8 illustrates the components of the gantry head. Each of these features is discussed in this section.

Design features of the collimator assembly allow it to provide support for the x-ray tube aperture, field-defining wires, light field indicator, beam-limiting diaphragms, and an accessory holder. Essentially, the collimator assembly comprises most of the gantry head, except for an optical beam–directing device mounted at the head of the gantry. The **optical distance indicator (ODI)**, sometimes called a *rangefinder*, projects a scale onto the patient's skin, which corresponds to the SSD (Figure 21-9). This is generally mounted near the collimator. The motorized collimator assembly should rotate around the central axis of the x-ray beam through at least a 220-degree collimator rotation angle.[7,8] For example, this allows a 10- × 10-cm square-shaped field projected on the

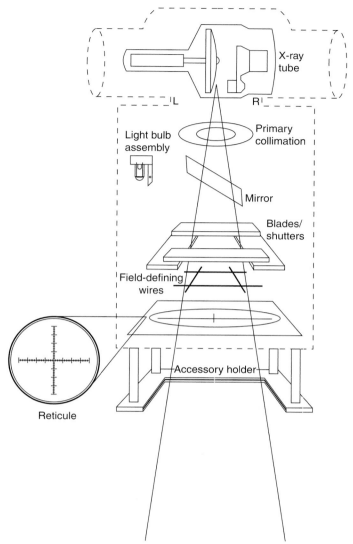

Figure 21-8. Components of the gantry head. These include the port of the x-ray tube housing, the field light mirror, collimator blades (shutters), field-defining wires, central axis crosshairs, and the accessory holder.

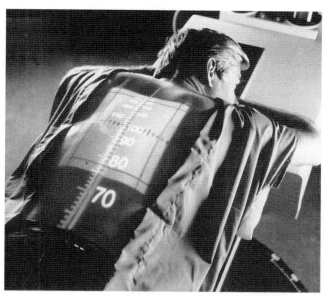

Figure 21-9. Use of the optical distance indicator (ODI). It projects a graduated light beam, in centimeters, on the patient's skin, which allows for accurate measurements of source-skin distance (SSD). (Courtesy Oldelft Corp, Fairfax, VA.)

patient's skin to become a 10- × 10-cm diamond-shaped field, if the collimator is rotated 45 degrees. The **collimator assembly** also directs the path of the x-ray beam toward the patient, after it emerges from the x-ray tube.

Mounting the simulator's x-ray tube onto the diaphragm system is recommended. When or if the x-ray tube must be replaced, the alignment of the geometric axis of the diaphragm system is made easier if it is mounted onto the gantry and not the x-ray tube.[7,8] The x-ray tube used for simulation must have a large and a small focal spot; preferably, the small focal spot should be no greater than 0.6 mm. To obtain a sharp image of the 0.5-mm-diameter field-defining wires that are located in the collimator assembly, a small focal spot is necessary. For this reason and others, careful selection of the x-ray tube and generator is significant.

Field-defining wires are located in the collimator assembly. It is recommended that the remote and locally controlled

field-defining wires (also called delineators) simulate a maximum field size up to 40 × 40 cm at 100 cm SSD on any treatment unit available. The wires represent the edge of the treatment field within the larger image that is defined by the beam-limiting diaphragms (see Figure 21-3, A). To simulate a variety of field sizes from 0 to 40 × 40 cm (or larger) at 100 cm, the four extremely narrow wires, each representing a field border, must move symmetrically within tolerance. The scale indicating the range of field sizes at this distance should be displayed accurately within 2 mm inside the simulator room and remotely at the control panel.[8] Some simulators provide independent motorized movement of each of the field-defining wires and beam-limiting diaphragms. This allows for the simulation of half-field blocks and asymmetric beams. One can understand the strict tolerance and routine quality assurance that are necessary if one is to depend on this definition of the beam edge.

Also located within the collimator assembly are the **beam-restricting diaphragms**, which are made of 2 to 3 mm of lead. They are an important part of the simulator because the diaphragms define both the size and the axis of the x-ray beam.[7,8] Beam-restricting diaphragms operate much the same way as the field-defining wires. These thin blades of lead define the simulator's x-ray beam during fluoroscopy or during a radiograph by limiting the area exposed. To minimize the amount of unwanted scatter reaching the film or image intensifier, the irradiated field must be kept as small as possible. The diaphragms serve this purpose. Every image should show evidence of **collimation** (restricting the beam with the diaphragms) by displaying a 1- to 2-cm clear border of unexposed film. Primarily, the beam-restricting diaphragms restrict the coverage of the x-ray field.

A secondary purpose of the beam-restricting diaphragms is to optically indicate the coverage of the x-ray field. The field light represents the radiation field, so one can see on the patient's skin where the x-ray field will be directed. It does this much the same way it restricts the x-ray field on a radiograph. In addition to restricting the radiation on an image, it restricts a light field on the patient's skin. A special light bulb (usually a quartz-iodine projector lamp), located within the collimator assembly, is used for this purpose.[15] An angled mirror, located above the field-defining wires and beam-restricting diaphragms, projects an image from the filament of the light bulb through the diaphragms and onto the patient, as demonstrated in Figures 21-9 and 21-10. Critical care should be taken when replacing this bulb. In fact, each time a field light bulb is replaced (both on the conventional simulator and on the treatment unit), a special test is performed called a *light field/radiation field coincidence test.* This type of quality assurance test evaluates the maximum distance between the light field edge and the x-ray field edge. At the normal treatment distance for field sizes 5 × 5 cm to 20 × 20 cm, the coincidence should be 1 mm or 0.5% for field sizes greater than 20 × 20 cm.[8] It is only through careful evaluation that one can be certain that the light field actually represents the x-ray field.

Fiducial Plate. Plexiglas or plastic trays imbedded with lead markers at regular intervals are called **fiducial plates** or *beaded trays.*[33] These trays, sometimes referred to as a *reticule,* are positioned in the head of the gantry between the field-defining wires and the accessory holder. Because the lead markers, which may be shaped like BBs or small lines, are spaced to represent the geometry of the field at the treatment distance, a separate tray is necessary on most simulators to represent 80- and 100-cm SSD treatments. Other trays are also available from some manufacturers. Tray selection should be checked before each simulation procedure to ensure accurate geometric representation of the treatment unit (if the simulator supports multiple treatment units with different treatment distances). Magnification can be determined using this type of tray system, because the hash marks or lead beads represent 1 or 2 cm at the isocenter. On some simulators, the fiducial tray serves a second purpose. The tray not only helps to document the field size on the simulation radiograph but also protects the delicate tungsten wire crosshairs (see Figure 21-10), which are located within the collimator assembly and mark the center of the field radiographically.

Accessory Holder. On most simulators, an adjustable accessory holder is mounted on the collimator or gantry head. It appears to hang down (when the gantry is positioned vertically) from the head of the gantry (Figure 21-11). The accessory holder may serve two or three purposes: a block tray holder; an electron cone adapter; or, on some simulators, a device for checking multileaf collimator (MLC) fields on the patient before treatment.

A specific block tray distance must be set on the simulator for each treatment unit to provide geometric duplication of

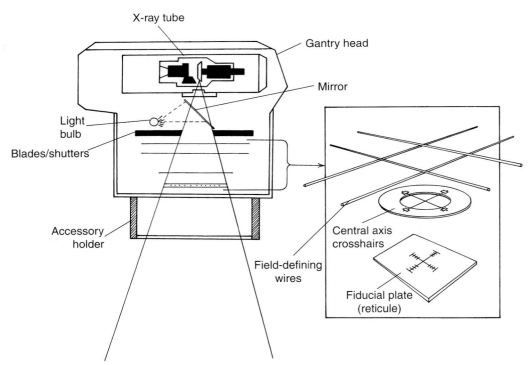

Figure 21-10. X-ray field coverage. An angled mirror, located above the field-defining wires and beam-restricting diaphragms, projects an image from the filament of the light bulb through the diaphragms, field-defining wires, and central axis crosshairs and onto the patient.

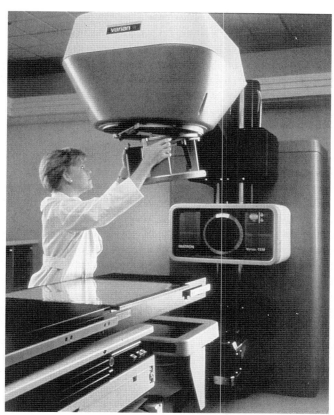

Figure 21-11. Removable accessory holder. This can be mounted on the collimator head of the gantry to accommodate custom blocks or an electron cone. (Courtesy Varian Medical Systems, Palo Alto, Calif.)

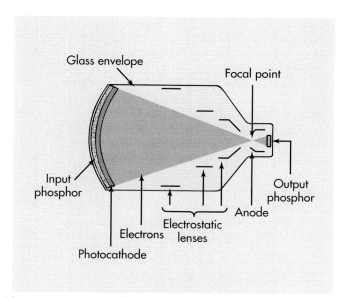

Figure 21-12. Image intensifier. This device is made up of a glass envelope containing an input screen (input phosphor), photocathode, electrostatic lenses, anode, and output screen (output phosphor). (From Bushong S: *Radiologic science for technologists: physics, biology, and protection,* ed 8, St. Louis, 2004, Mosby.)

shielding blocks. This distance generally ranges from 40 to 60 cm. It is adjustable to accommodate a number of different treatment units within a single department.

An accessory holder should also support the weight of various electron cones because it may be necessary to simulate electron setups for the treatment unit. This can easily be accomplished on the simulator if the accessory holder can support the weight of an electron cone and reproduce the geometry of the desired treatment field.

Image Intensifier System. Another valuable component, located at the opposite end of the gantry arm, is the **image intensifier** (Figure 21-12). This complex device receives and processes the created image, which is a result of radiation interacting with the patient, field-defining wires, beam-restricting diaphragms, crosshairs, and accessory holder.

A typical image intensifier system contains four major components: the film holder, image intensifier, television camera, and video monitor. As illustrated in Figure 21-5, the image intensifier system can scan in several directions. In addition to its scanning design during fluoroscopy, the image intensifier also provides mechanical support as a film holder in the radiography mode.

The image intensifier has a frame mounted onto it, which can accommodate a 35- × 43-cm radiographic cassette. The cassette slides into a groove in the film holder, which supports it at right angles to the central axis of the x-ray beam, regardless of

the gantry position. This is an important feature that reduces distortion (elongation and foreshortening) in the production of radiographs. Some film holders provide 180-degree rotation of the 35- × 43-cm (14- × 17-inch) cassette. This is a feature found on some simulators so that the cassette may be positioned crosswise instead of lengthwise, if necessary, during a radiographic exposure. In most European countries, 35- × 35-cm cassettes are commonly used.

The image intensifier also reduces *object-image receptor distance (OID),* also referred to as *object-film distance (OFD).* It should be remembered that the image intensifier can move radially (closer to and away from the gantry head, like a periscope on a submarine). In doing so, OID is reduced to a minimum during fluoroscopy or for a radiographic exposure. Figure 21-13 illustrates two radiographs, taken at 100 cm TSD and the same radiographic exposure technique. However, the source-image receptor distance (SID), thus the OID, has been increased for radiograph B. Note two things as a result. The image in radiograph B is somewhat larger because of magnification from the increased OID (examine the size of the central square made by the field-defining wires). Also note that the overall density of radiograph B is decreased (lighter) because of the inverse square law (the same amount of radiation has been spread out over a larger area).

The image intensifier is a useful tool during fluoroscopy because it converts an x-ray image into a visible image on a television monitor. There are several design components that enable it to accomplish this task. Structurally, it is made up of a glass envelope containing an input screen, photocathode, electrostatic lenses, anode, and output screen, as shown in Figure 21-12. It amplifies the brightness of an image, usually between 500 and 8000 times.[12] The ultimate purpose of an

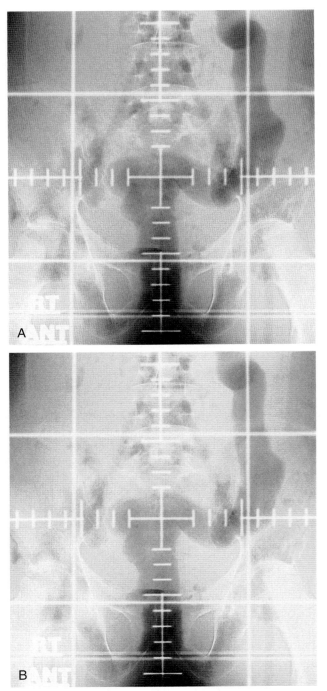

Figure 21-13. Effect of increasing object-image receptor distance (OID). These two radiographs, **A** and **B**, were taken at 100 cm target-skin distance (TSD) and with the same radiographic exposure technique. The source-image receptor distance (SID), thus the OID, has been increased for radiograph **B** from 140 to 155 cm TSD. Note two things as a result. The image in radiograph **B** is considerably larger because of magnification from the increased OID. Also note that the overall density of radiograph **B** is decreased as a result of the inverse square law (the same amount of radiation has been spread out over a larger area).

image intensifier is to convert the x-ray image into a video image, which is then viewed on a television monitor. Let us examine that process in more detail.

The primary x-ray beam exiting the patient passes through the tabletop and strikes the input screen of the image intensifier. A fluorescent screen, which is built into the image intensifier as the input screen, absorbs x-ray photons. It can range in size up to 35 cm in diameter. The larger the diameter, the less scanning that is required during fluoroscopy. During fluoroscopy, light photons, emitted by the input screen (much like the photons emitted from an intensifying screen in a radiographic cassette), are then absorbed by the photocathode. Electrostatic lenses, positioned inside the perimeter of the unit, focus and accelerate the converted electrons. As the electrons are focused, they gain more speed as they near the end of their journey through this vacuum tube containing the cathode and anode. The focusing lens helps direct the electrons toward the anode at the opposite end of the image intensifier tube. As the electrons accelerate and focus toward the anode, their energy increases, as does their ability to emit light at the output screen. The output is significantly greater than the input. For example, one 50-keV photon striking the input screen may produce 200,000 light photons at the output screen.[12] Light photons produced at the output screen are then processed electronically through a video system. In a small shielded area of the simulator room, the video image appears on a television monitor. The image intensification process simply changes the quantity of photons and electrons representing the image at each stage of the process.

During fluoroscopy, the x-ray tube current is usually less than 10 mA. This is in contrast to the 100 to 500 mA used for producing radiographs. The kilovoltage (or kVp) used during fluoroscopy depends on the body section examined. Most image intensifiers have an automatic brightness system maintained by varying the kilovoltage or milliamperes (mA) automatically during fluoroscopy. Such features may be referred to by different names, such as *automatic brightness control (ABC), automatic brightness stabilization (ABS), automatic exposure control (AEC),* or *automatic gain control (AGC).*[11]

The image intensifying system must have a collision avoidance system. This may take the form of a mechanical touchbar/microswitch system, which will prevent the image intensifier from colliding with the patient or treatment couch. A combination of electronic position sensors and some type of computer logic may accomplish the same objective. A computer, integrated with the simulator, can prevent the collision of gantry or image intensifier with the floor or treatment couch by plotting and constantly evaluating the position of each component. Some simulators also come equipped with audio alarms as part of their collision avoidance system.

Digital Fluoroscopy. The digital fluoroscopy system of displaying the x-ray image is conducted much the same way as conventional fluoroscopy. The equipment may look similar, but one noticeable difference is the addition of a computer between the television camera (located at the base of the image intensifier) and the television monitor (Figure 21-14). It is the addition of a charge-coupled device (CCD), which was developed in the 1970s for military purposes, that provides the digital link.

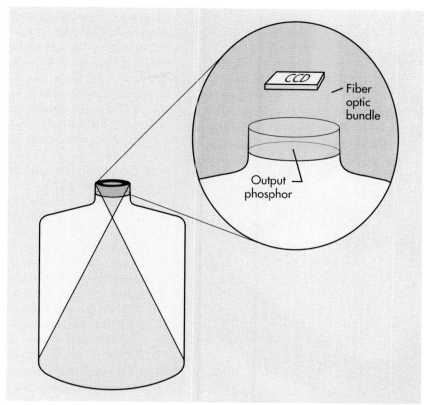

Figure 21-14. The charge-coupled device (CCD) can be added to the image intensifier tube in place of a video camera. (From Bushong S: *Radiologic science for technologists: physics, biology, and protection,* ed 8, St. Louis, 2004, Mosby.)

In today's market, CCDs are used in camcorders, commercial television, security surveillance, and astronomy. The key component of a CCD is a layer of crystalline silicon. When the silicon is illuminated, an electrical charge is generated, which is then sampled pixel by pixel and manipulated to produce a digital image. Digital imaging is adapting rapidly in the medical community. Images, which can be stored, manipulated, and transferred to various workstations, are produced from fluoroscopy, CT, MRI, sonography, and converted (digitized) x-ray images from film.[11]

Patient Tabletop (Couch). The device in which a patient is positioned during treatment or simulation may be called a treatment couch or patient **tabletop** (see Figure 21-1, D). It is essential that the patient tabletop on the simulator provides support identical to that of the patient tabletop on the treatment unit to maintain reproducibility. Some tabletops can support up to 159 kg (350 lb) and range in width from 45 to 50 cm. If the couch width in the simulator is not similar to that of the treatment unit, then reproducibility may become a problem, especially with larger patients.

It is desirable for the tabletop to be a hard flat surface that minimally attenuates the x-ray beam. Part of the table should enable the therapist to view the patient through the tabletop when the beam is directed up vertically through the table. This is important in recording posterior and posterior oblique SSDs. Some simulators provide a tabletop with a segment that can be

removed and a section of more supportive transparent material substituted in its place. This may be a square or rectangular section of plastic or a frame with strings, similar to a tennis or racquetball racquet woven tightly together (Figure 21-15). After extended use, this tennis racquet section should be restrung to provide more patient support and reduce the amount of sag during simulation. The tennis racquet insert, if used on the simulator, may more accurately represent the potential for sag during actual treatment conditions, when a similar insert can be used. This process may reduce the number of discrepancies between simulation and treatment. Tabletop manufacturers have developed some models that are hard, flat, and radiolucent and come without metal supports. These tabletops are mostly constructed out of a carbon fiber material.

What is carbon fiber material? The material used for radiologic purposes, such as tabletops and cassettes, is made by binding a fabric of pure carbon fiber with a resin. The result is a material that is extremely supportive with a low density and low x-ray absorption. It also has a high **tensile strength** (resistance in lengthwise stress, measured in weight per unit area), which reduces table sag when a patient is positioned at the end of the couch. Carbon fiber is used in tabletops as the outside support around a plastic foam center.[22]

There are several unique features of the simulator couch, which allows the tabletop its mobility. A standard feature allows the tabletop to mechanically move in a horizontal and

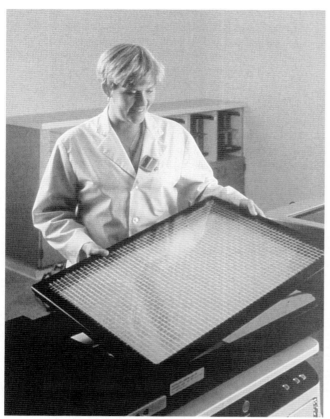

Figure 21-15. Couch top accessory. This may include a square or rectangular frame with strings, similar to a tennis or racquetball racquet, woven tightly together. After extended use, the tennis racquet section should be restrung to provide more patient support and reduce the amount of sag during simulation. (Courtesy Varian Medical Systems.)

lengthwise direction. It must do this smoothly and accurately with a patient in the treatment position. This permits the precise and exact positioning of the isocenter during simulation. Some tabletops may provide the opportunity through rotation of the couch for patient positioning in two additional directions. One direction allows the tabletop to be rotated horizontally (laterally) 90 degrees in either direction. For example, if the tabletop were the big hand of a watch at the 6 o'clock position, it could be rotated to either the 3 or the 9 o'clock position, while maintaining the same isocenter. This type of positioning limits gantry rotation to approximately 30 degrees from vertical because of the possible collision of the image intensifier with the couch. The amount of gantry rotation depends on the thickness of the patient and the level of the isocenter. A second motion on some models also allows the couch to extract the patient from the C-shaped opening in the gantry by rotating the patient on another axis. This other axis is located several meters from the isocenter within the couch. Experimenting with the various motions of the couch will demonstrate its versatility and range of motion.

In addition, a set of local controls may be located on the couch. These can mimic those of the treatment units as a **pendant** (handheld control) suspended from the ceiling or

attached to the treatment couch. These controls should allow access to the mechanical movements and optical features of the simulator, allowing the operator easy control of the simulator's mechanical functions, ODI, and room lights.

Simulator Controls. Control of simulator movements should be possible through local control within the simulator room and through remote control, usually located behind a separately shielded area. Local and remote control of the mechanical simulator functions should provide for all motor-driven motions, specifically the field-defining wires, beam-restricting diaphragms, collimator rotation, radial movement of the gantry head, and linear and rotation movements of the couch. Scanning and radial movements of the image intensifier should also be located within the simulator room. Activation of the optical features of the simulator, such as the field light, ODI, positional lasers, and room lights, should be available along with several emergency off switches, positioned strategically throughout the simulator room.

Remote controls, located in the shielded control room, should duplicate those within the simulator room. This includes all of the optical features and motor-driven movements of the simulator along with digital indicators for field size, TAD, TSD, gantry, and collimator angle. Familiarity with all of the simulator's features will allow for efficient and accurate treatment planning. This can become more critical, especially when simulating pediatric patients, those with dyspnea, and palliative cases in which the patient is experiencing severe pain.

Control Area. Within the shielded control area, several components are strategically positioned (Figure 21-16). This includes the x-ray generator (along with a circuit breaker for the incoming voltage), a television monitor, the remote control panel, and an observation window. It is important that this room be large enough to hold several members of the radiation therapy team, students, and other interested observers.

An observation window, installed along the wall facing the simulator, allows the radiation therapist and others involved in the simulation process to view the patient and the mechanical motions of the equipment. Whether the window is made of thick plate glass or lead glass depends on the distance it is located from the simulator and/or whether it is inclined to be irradiated by the primary beam. A 0.7- × 1.5-m (2.3- × 5-ft) size is recommended.[8] Usually, larger sizes can adapt to additional staff and students without overcrowding. The control panel should be located close enough to the observation window so that the radiation therapist can observe the patient while the simulator is moving.

In addition, a video monitor positioned near the control panel provides ready access to the fluoroscopic image during the simulation process. A dimmer switch, which can control the lighting level in the simulator and control area, is also necessary. Monitoring a fluoroscopic video image without the distraction of overhead lighting is more efficient. It might be compared with watching television in a dark room (sometimes while watching television, the image may appear sharper and more detailed when the room lighting is kept low or turned off). X-ray view boxes or large liquid crystal display (LCD) monitors

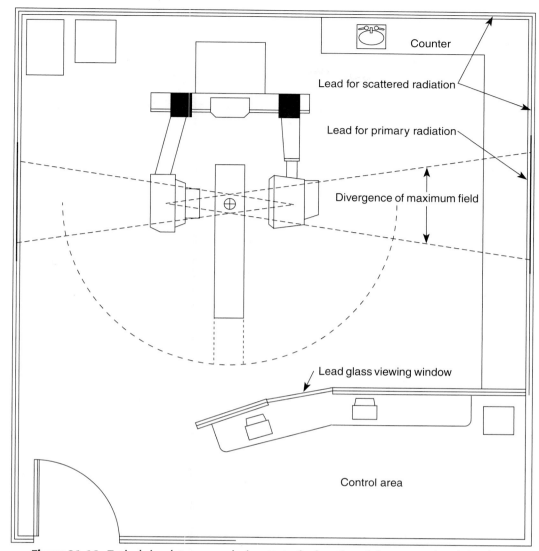

Figure 21-16. Typical simulator room design. Note the location of the conventional simulator in relationship to the primary barriers and control area with lead glass window.

mounted in the control room are helpful in comparing images or scans during the simulation process. In addition, other video monitors may be used for patient data storage and retrieval.

The x-ray generator is another important component, which provides radiographic and fluoroscopic control of the simulator. Exposure reproducibility, which should be maintained within 5%, is an important consideration for guaranteeing image quality.[34] The *British Journal of Radiology* Supplement 23[8] recommends that the tube and generator ratings be 8 to 10 times greater than for general diagnostic radiography. In part, this may be because of the increased distance used in radiation therapy simulation (70 cm in diagnostic imaging to between 130 and 200 cm on the simulator). A three-phase generator is recommended. It should be capable of radiographic outputs of up to 500 mA at 90 kVp, 300 mA at 150 kVp, and 6 mA at 125 kVp for fluoroscopy.[8] A single-phase generator may limit the higher exposure factors needed for some examinations, especially a large lateral pelvis—a most challenging body part to image effectively.

Kilovoltage and milliamperage exposure factors are controlled by the radiation therapist at the operating console. By adjusting the voltage and current of the x-ray generator, exposure factors can be selected. It may appear intimidating to the novice at first, with its many buttons and control knobs, although some systems are equipped with anatomically programmed radiography (APR). Bushong[11] describes the process from a diagnostic radiography perspective: "Rather than have the radiologic technologist (radiographer) select a desired kVp and mAs, graphics on the control panel guide the technologist. To produce an image the technologist simply touches a picture or a written description of the anatomy to be imaged and another indication of body habitus. The microprocessor selects the appropriate kVp and mAs automatically. The whole process is phototimed, resulting in near-flawless radiographs...."

It is easy to see why the control room should be large enough to accommodate several members of the radiation therapy team along with students and other interested observers. Field size, gantry angle, exposure technique, and several other important parameters can be manipulated from within the shielded walls of the control room. If the components within the control room are well positioned and accessible, the entire simulation process is more efficient. Detail to room design is a wise investment that will provide many dividends, especially during peak times of the simulator's use.

COMPUTED TOMOGRAPHY SIMULATOR DESIGN

When referring to CT simulation, two types of machines may actually produce CT images: one may be an actual CT scanner adapted for simulation and the other a conventional simulator with a CT mode. They both can provide an external contour of the patient and additional information on the location, size, and thickness of internal structures. This advanced method of simulation, using CT images, has replaced conventional simulation in many instances and will continue to grow in popularity. CT provides the most useful information for treatment planning purposes because the scans can produce a three-dimensional representation of the patient and external structures, which is adapted more easily in today's digital treatment planning process.[25]

Simulators with a Computed Tomography Mode

Simulators with a CT mode incorporate the conventional benefits of a simulator with the added benefits of cross-sectional information obtained during the simulation process. In contrast, conventional simulators provide information from **orthogonal** projections (two radiographs taken at right angles). To produce a reconstructed image similar to a conventional CT image, the imaging device (x-ray tube and receptor) on the simulator must record information while the gantry rotates. This recorded information consists of transmitted beam intensities that correspond to tissue densities (Figure 21-17).

The cost, compared with purchasing a conventional CT scanner for this purpose, is an advantage with this type of simulator. Disadvantages include poor image quality compared with that of a conventional CT scanner, increased amount of time to simulate a patient, and the limitation that the x-ray tube can tolerate only a specific amount of heat (each scan generates more heat units than a conventional x-ray, so delays may be encountered waiting for the tube to cool down). The differences in image quality between a conventional CT scanner and a simulator with a CT mode are very noticeable. Note the differences in image quality in Figure 21-17, A and B. More detail is visible using a conventional diagnostic CT scanner, as demonstrated in Figure 21-17, B. However, the geometry produced with a simulator using a CT mode is not restricted by the conventional CT aperture opening (the opening through which the patient passes through the scanner) and is more representative of the treatment unit geometry.

Computed Tomography Simulator

The components needed to construct a CT imaging system were available to medical physicists 20 years before Godfrey Hounsfield first demonstrated the technique in 1970. Hounsfield, who was a British physicist/engineer at the time, shared the 1979 Nobel Peace Prize in physics with Alan Cormack,

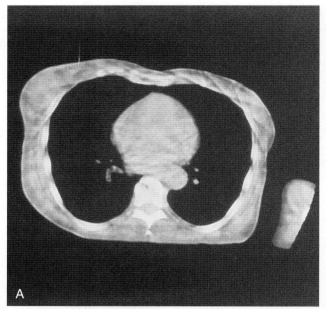

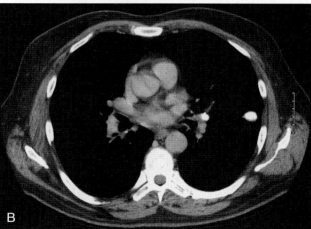

Figure 21-17. Planning computed tomography (CT) image. **A,** This CT image of the thorax, generated by a conventional simulator with a CT mode, is used for treatment planning purposes. (Courtesy Varian Medical Systems.) **B,** This CT image of the thorax, generated by a diagnostic CT scanner, provides better image quality and increased visibility of detail. (From Eisenberg RL, Johnson NM: *Comprehensive radiographic pathology,* ed 4, Philadelphia, 2007, Mosby.)

a Tufts University medical physicist, who had earlier developed the mathematics now used to reconstruct CT images.[11,29] This medical imaging tool has transformed the way we diagnose disease!

In terms of data acquisition for CT, there are two major methods used in today's scanners—the slice-by-slice and volumetric approaches. Using the slice-by-slice approach, one can create an image using a fanlike beam to image a specific thickness of the patient in the transverse plane (Figure 21-18). If a loaf of bread were used to represent the patient, the slice-by-slice approach simply alters the thickness of the slice from as little as 0.4 mm to as much as 1.0 cm.[16] Most CT scanners today are third-generation imaging systems, which means the x-ray

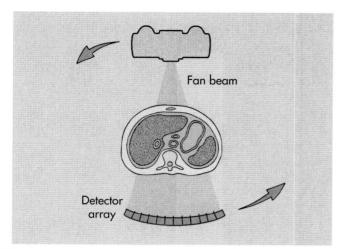

Figure 21-18. Third-generation computed tomography (CT) scanners operate in the rotate-only mode with a fan x-ray beam and a multiple detector array revolving concentrically around the patient. (From Bushong S: *Radiologic science for technologists: physics, biology, and protection,* ed 8, St. Louis, 2004, Mosby.)

Gantry

The gantry includes the x-ray tube, the detector array, the high-voltage generator, the couch, and the mechanical support devices for each. These subsystems receive electronic commands from the operating console and transmit data to the computer, where image production takes place.[11]

X-ray Tubes. X-ray tubes used for CT imaging are similar in design to those used in the conventional simulator, diagnostic x-ray, and angiography, with a few special features. Because there is a great deal of stress placed on the CT x-ray tube, the tube must be able to withstand large amounts of heat from multiple exposures over a short period of time on numerous patients scheduled each day. Heat may be dissipated by using a large-diameter, thick anode disk, rotating at up to 10,000 rpm. Cooling oil, circulated around the x-ray tube; small fans; and, in some cases, a heat exchanger, may be used to reduce the amount of heat buildup around the x-ray tube. Manufacturers will usually list the anode heat capacity in **MHU (million heat units)** and

source and detector array rotate around the patient, or fourth-generation systems, where the x-ray source rotates and the detectors are stationary.[11,36] The x-ray tube and detector can continue to rotate around the patient without concern of cables becoming tangled because of slip rings. A **slip ring** is a metal strip carrying electronic signals and power that is swept up by special brushes made of metal. The use of a slip ring can be equated to the metal on the ceiling of a bumper car ride. The power to the bumper car comes from the metal bar attached to the car rising to the ceiling.[35] Some of these systems have millisecond imaging times and can accommodate variable slice thicknesses, which is necessary for radiation therapy applications.[11,19] Modern diagnostic scanners, according to Geoffrey Rubin, MD, chief of cardiovascular imaging at Stanford University, can produce an image using 1.25-mm-thick axial sections in less than 30 seconds.[16]

During an axial scan, the patient is positioned at a fixed point and the x-ray tube rotates 360 degrees around the patient (translation). With the volumetric approach or **spiral CT**, the patient is positioned at a fixed point, and, while the x-ray tube is rotating, the patient moves into the aperture to create a scan pattern that resembles a "slinky" or coiled spring (Figure 21-19). **Aperture size** (the diameter of the hole into which the patient is positioned) is an important factor in radiation oncology. Ideally, the aperture would be 80 cm or greater to accommodate a variety of patient setups, especially breast simulations and wide body sections such as the pelvis.[15,17,24] However, as aperture size increases, so do the number of detectors, the patient dose, and time to scan the patient. The exact treatment position may not always be produced on a scanner with the small aperture that is found on some units.[27] Table 21-3 compares aperture size and many other important variables offered through several vendors who manufacture CT scanners for radiology and radiation oncology.

There are three major system components incorporated in all CT scanners—the gantry, couch, and computer control system. We will examine each of these components and their subsystems.

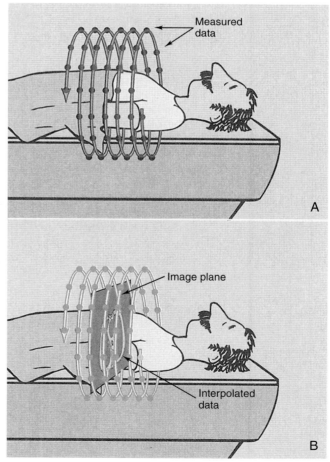

Figure 21-19. A, During spiral computed tomography (CT), image data are continuously sampled. **B,** Interpolation of data is performed to reconstruct the image in any transverse plane. (Used by permission from Bushong SC: *Radiologic science for technologists: physics, biology, and protection,* ed 8, St. Louis, 2004, Mosby.)

Table 21-3	Aperture Size and Other Important Variables Offered through Several Vendors Who Manufacture Computed Tomography Scanners for Radiology and Radiation Oncology					
Company Name	**Product Name**	**FDA Approved**	**DICOM Compliant**	System	**Gantry Size (cm, unless otherwise noted)**	**Gantry Weight (lb)**
GE Healthcare	BrightSpeed Edge	Yes	Yes		$193 \times 206 \times 102$	3902
GE Healthcare	BrightSpeed Elite	Yes	Yes		$193 \times 206 \times 102$	3902
GE Healthcare	BrightSpeed Excel	Yes	Yes		$193 \times 206 \times 102$	3902
GE Healthcare	LightSpeed RT	Yes	Yes		$189 \times 223 \times 101$	3894
GE Healthcare	LightSpeed RT 16	Yes	Yes		$189 \times 223 \times 101$	3894
GE Healthcare	LightSpeed VCT	Yes	Yes		$189 \times 223 \times 101$	4193
GE Healthcare	LightSpeed VCT Select	Yes	Yes		$189 \times 223 \times 101$	4193
GE Healthcare	LightSpeed VCT XT	Yes	Yes		$189 \times 223 \times 101$	4193
GE Healthcare	LightSpeed VCT Standard	Yes	Yes		$189 \times 223 \times 101$	4193
GE Healthcare	LightSpeed Xtra	Yes	Yes		$189 \times 223 \times 101$	3894
NeuroLogica Corp.	CereTom CT NL3000 - Portable Head/Neck	Yes	Yes, PACS ready, modality worklist		$133 \times 72 \times 153$	700 (on wheels)
Philips Medical Systems	Brilliance CT big-bore oncology configuration	Yes	Yes, uses DICOM 3.0 Interface		$199 \times 251 \times 97$	3888.95
Philips Medical Systems	Brilliance CT big-bore radiology configuration	Yes	Yes		$199 \times 251 \times 97$	3888.95
Philips Medical Systems	Brilliance CT, 16-slice configuration	Yes	Yes		$203 \times 239 \times 94$	3888.95
Philips Medical Systems	Brilliance CT, 40-channel configuration	Yes	Yes		$203 \times 239 \times 94$	4279.17
Philips Medical Systems	Brilliance CT, 64-channel configuration	Yes	Yes		$203 \times 239 \times 94$	4279.17
Siemens Medical Solutions	SOMATOM Definition	Yes	Yes		1990 mm $\times$ 940 mm $\times$ 2280 mm	5940
Siemens Medical Solutions	SOMATOM Emotion	Yes	Yes		1780 mm $\times$ 790 mm $\times$ 2320 mm	1200
Siemens Medical Solutions	SOMATOM Sensation	Yes	Yes		1990 mm $\times$ 940 mm $\times$ 2280 mm	4400
Toshiba America Medical Systems	Aquilion 32	Yes	Yes		$195 \times 233 \times 96$	3857
Toshiba America Medical Systems	Aquilion 64	Yes	Yes		$195 \times 233 \times 96$	3857
Toshiba America Medical Systems	Aquilion 64 CFX	Yes	Yes		$195 \times 233 \times 96$	3857
Toshiba America Medical Systems	Aquilion LB (large-bore)	Yes	Yes		$210 \times 230 \times 101$	4189

Modified from CT Data Sheet, *RT Image*, 20(19), 2007, Valley Forge, PA. Used by permission. *GOS*, Gadolinium oxysulfide; *PACS*, Picture Archiving and Communications System.

antry iameter (cm)	No. of Detectors	Type of Detector	No. of Detection Channels	Patient Table Weight Limit (lb)
)	16 × 912, 14,592	HiLight ceramic	8 × 912, 7296	450
)	16 × 912, 14,592	HiLight ceramic	16 × 912, 14,592	450
)	16 × 912, 14,592	HiLight ceramic	4 × 912, 3648	450
)	24 × 912, 21,888	HiLight ceramic	4 × 912, 3648	450
)	24 × 912, 21,888	HiLight ceramic	24 × 912, 21,888	500
)	64 × 912, 58,368	HiLight ceramic	64 × 912, 58,368	500
)	64 × 912, 58,368	HiLight ceramic	32 × 912, 29,184	500
)	64 × 912, 58,368	HiLight ceramic	64 × 912, 58,368	500
)	64 × 912, 58,368	HiLight ceramic	64 × 912, 58,368	500
)	64 × 912, 58,368	HiLight ceramic	64 × 912, 58,368	500
2	>3200	Solid-state crystal scintillator	8 Slice	Unlimited
5	19,584	Solid-state GOS	TBD	Standard: 204 kg with full accuracy Optional: 295 kg
5	19,584	Solid-state GOS	19,584	Standard: 204 kg with full accuracy Optional: 295 kg
)	16,128	Solid-state GOS	16,128	Standard: 204 kg with full accuracy Optional: 295 kg
)	34,944	Solid-state GOS	34,944	Standard: 204 kg with full accuracy Optional: 295 kg
)	43,008	Solid-state GOS	43,008	Standard: 204 kg with full accuracy Optional: 295 kg
8	21,504 and 11,264	Ultrafast ceramic	32,768	220
)	1344; 11,776; or 17,664	Ultrafast ceramic	—	200
)	43,008 or 26,880	Ultrafast ceramic	43,008 for 64-slice configuration 26,880 for 40-slice and open configurations	450 standard, 615 optional
2	32/64 rows	Solid-state	32/64 896 channels × 64 rows, 57,344 elements	450
2	64 rows	Solid-state Gd(2)O(2)S	896 channels × 64 rows	450
2	64 rows	Solid-state Gd(2)O(2)S	896 channels × 64 rows, 57,344 elements	450
0	40 rows	Solid-state Gd(2)O(2)S	994 channels × 40 rows, solid-state, 39,760 elements	450

the maximum anode heat dissipation (how quickly the heat is removed from the tube assembly) rate in KHU (thousand heat units). With spiral CT, greater thermal demands are placed on the x-ray tube, because the tube may be energized continuously up to 60 seconds. High heat capacity and high cooling rates are trademarks of x-ray tubes designed for spiral CT.[11]

Detectors. The gantry of a CT scanner, which contains the rotating x-ray tube, is essentially the circular "doughnut" in which the patient is inserted during the scan (Figure 21-20). Solid-state **detectors** are designed to convert radiation to light (see Figure 21-18). Then photodiode assemblies convert light to an electronic signal that receives and measures the attenuated beam from a rotating x-ray tube. Spacing of the detectors varies depending on the design; however, generally 1 to 8 detectors/cm or 1 to 5 detectors/degree are available. Ninety percent of the incident x-ray is absorbed and contributes to the output. Because of the spacing of the detectors, the net output is near 90%.

Multislice detector arrays were introduced in the early 1990s (Figure 21-21). The advantages were shorter imaging times per scan or the ability to image more anatomy in the same time.[11] A single-slice detector is 2 cm long. If you have an eight-slice CT scanner, the 2-cm-long detector is divided into eight parts of 2.5 mm each. These detectors can be combined to also produce four 5-mm slices or two 1-cm slices. The smaller the detector size, the better is the spatial resolution.

Computed Tomography Numbers. The composition of a CT image is represented by varying shades of gray. Structures represented on the scan may range from black to white, depending on the density of the structure and the amount of information received by the detectors. This is one of the advantages CT simulation has compared with fluoroscopy-based simulation.

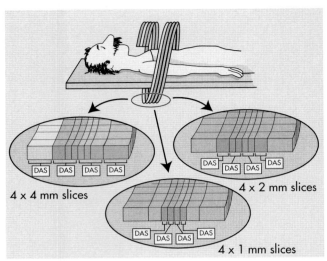

Figure 21-21. This multidetector device has an asymmetric eight-detector array, which provides a choice of slice thickness by switching the data acquisition system (DAS). (From Bushong S: *Radiologic science for technologists: physics, biology, and protection,* ed 8, St. Louis, 2004, Mosby.)

CT can differentiate between soft tissue structures, such as the pancreas and stomach, much better than can radiographic images. As the beam is attenuated by the patient, varying degrees of absorption of the x-ray beam occur, depending on how much tissue (patient thickness) the beam travels through and the density of that tissue. The detectors will register more of the x-ray beam as it passes through lung tissue in the thorax than when the x-ray beam passes through the soft tissue of the abdomen. Tissue density of an object is directly related to its *atomic number,* or how many protons and neutrons are packed in the nucleus of an atom. The more protons and neutrons in the nucleus, the higher is the atomic number and the greater chance there is for the x-ray beam to be absorbed or attenuated through the photoelectric effect and Compton scattering. Bone and metal (such as surgical clips, fiducial markers, or dental fillings) have the greatest chance of absorbing or attenuating the x-ray beam and appear as whiter areas on the scan. Black areas on the CT scan represent low-density objects such as gas in the stomach or air in the lungs.

$$CT\ number = k(u_t - u_w)/(u_w)$$

where u_t is the attenuation coefficient of the tissue in the pixel under analysis, u_w is the x-ray attenuation coefficient of water, and k is a constant that determines the scale factor for the range of CT numbers. When k is 1000, the CT numbers are called Hounsfield units.[11]

Each small square on a CT image is called a **pixel** (**p**icture **element**), which is a two-dimensional representation of a corresponding tissue volume or **voxel** (**vo**lume **element**). Figure 6-28 illustrates how pixels and voxels are used in viewing an image for CT scanning application. On your home computer monitor, you might increase the amount of detail you are able to view by

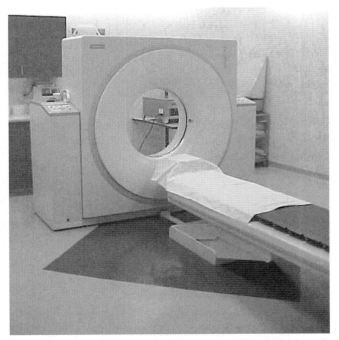

Figure 21-20. Spiral computed tomography (CT) imaging system showing the circular gantry and patient couch.

increasing the number of pixels from 512×512 to 1024×1024, which is called the *matrix size*. The image looks better as pixel size increases, because you are able to see more detail because there are more pixels to represent image information. In CT scanning, the small cell or pixel is assigned a value called a *CT number* or *Hounsfield unit,* which represents the density of the tissue and is directly related to the x-ray linear attenuation coefficient (u) for the tissue in that voxel. The linear attenuation coefficient is a function of both electron density and atomic number of the tissue within the pixel.[13]

 The tissue volume is known as a voxel, and it is calculated by multiplying the pixel size by the thickness of the CT slice.

Hounsfield units (HU) are named after Sir Godfrey Hounsfield, an English engineer who invented CT. After his initial scans on a preserved human brain, then a fresh cow brain, he allowed a scan of his own brain to further document one of the greatest medical breakthroughs in imaging. He assigned values from +1000 for dense bone to −1000 for air and represented water as "0." Structures with a beam attenuation of less than 0 are represented by a negative number, and structures with an attenuation greater than 0 have a positive HU. These units have an important application in treatment planning, because the representative densities or HU of a CT scan are very useful in calculating the dose for a specific treatment plan. Table 21-4 provides information regarding HU of various tissues and linear attenuation coefficients for several kVp x-ray values. Notice the small differences in approximate CT numbers for muscle, gray matter, cerebrospinal fluid, and water. This information is also useful in producing DRRs.

Table 21-4	Computed Tomography (CT) Number for Various Tissues and X-ray Linear Attenuation Coefficients (cm⁻¹) at 3 kVp Values			
	Approximate	Linear Attenuation Coefficient (cm⁻¹)		
Tissue	CT Number	100 kVp	125 kVp	150 kVp
Dense bone	1000	0.528	0.460	0.410
Muscle	50	0.237	0.208	0.184
White matter	45	0.213	0.187	0.166
Gray matter	40	0.212	0.184	0.163
Blood	20	0.208	0.182	0.163
Cerebrospinal fluid	15	0.207	0.181	0.160
Water	0	0.206	0.180	0.160
Fat	−100	0.185	0.162	0.144
Lungs	200	0.093	0.081	0.072
Air	1000	0.0004	0.0003	0.0002

Hounsfield units of various tissues and linear attenuation coefficients for several kVp x-ray values are listed. Notice the small differences in approximate CT numbers for muscle, gray matter, cerebrospinal fluid, and water. CT numbers range from +1000 to −1000.

From Bushong SC: *Radiologic science for technologists: physics, biology, and protection,* ed 8, St. Louis, 2004, Mosby Elsevier.

Patient Treatment Couch

The **couch** (see Figure 21-20) is similar to that of a conventional simulator in that it is capable of translation and made of low Z material such as carbon fiber. If the scanner has a curved couch top, an insert should be purchased to provide a flat surface for scanning patients in the treatment position. Some couches come with predrilled holes or notches along the lateral edge of the couch to provide a suitable locking location to register immobilization devices such as headholders, prone pelvis immobilization devices, and breast boards. This becomes an important feature with the increased use of three-dimensional conformal therapy and intensity-modulated radiation therapy (Figure 21-22).

The patient positioning couch must be very accurate in terms of mechanical positioning. Precise patient positioning is essential, especially when indexing the patient to a specific position within the gantry opening. Special flat tabletop inserts made of carbon fiber are used in radiation therapy CT scanners. Carbon fiber provides little attenuation of the x-ray beam and at the same time provides good longitudinal support of the patient, especially when the patient is extended out away from the central support of the couch assembly into the gantry opening.

Computer Control Station

As computer technology increases with faster processors and larger memory, scan time and image reconstruction time are reduced. Depending on the image format, as many as 250,000 equations must be solved simultaneously, requiring a large-capacity computer to process the images.[11] **Reconstruction time**, the time it takes the computer to analyze and process the information received from the detectors and display it on a TV monitor, is an important variable in the application of CT simulation. With the use of special array processors, image reconstruction can be accomplished in less than 1 second.[11] The results are seen at the control station on one or more video monitors and can also be copied on x-ray film as a DRR. One of the important benefits of CT simulation compared with conventional simulation is the production of high-quality DRRs.

The original concept of a DRR was developed by Sherouse et al.,[32] indicating that the DRR is determined by recording the x-ray source of the CT scanning information through a three-dimensional model of the patient, which is made up of voxels. These voxels can then be manipulated by separating out the photoelectron and Compton components of the beam using various types of filters to change the appearance of the image. In this case, the filter refers to a mathematic formula and not a metal device used to harden an x-ray beam. One filter can simulate a 60- to 80-kVp radiograph similar to a conventional simulator radiograph. Another can simulate a high-energy MV beam, similar to a portal image produced on the linear accelerator. Other filters produce DRRs that customize the image for special circumstances such as depth control or depth shading, used to identify a region of interest or target volume identified by the user.[1,32]

The quality of a DRR depends on multiple factors, such as window level selection, spatial resolution, and noise. The technique called **windowing** allows the radiation therapist to change

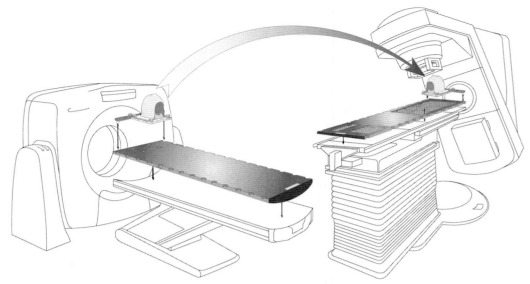

Figure 21-22. A CT simulator and linear accelerator both demonstrate a thermoplastic mask used primarily to immobilize the head and neck area, indexed to the simulator and treatment couch. Note the small notches along the lateral edge of each tabletop used for indexing the immobilization device. (Courtesy MED-TEC, Orange City, Iowa.)

the appearance of the image after it has been acquired by the CT scanner. Two characteristics of the window are *window level* and *window width*. These options allow the image to be manipulated for viewing a specific type of tissue by adding or subtracting contrast and/or density. For example, a window level of 50 can be used for abdominal imaging, and a window level of −500 demonstrates good lung detail in the thorax[11] (Figure 21-23). Spatial resolution is limited by the size of the pixel matrix (typically 512×512 for CT) and the field of view (FOV). As the FOV is increased, as might be necessary with a large-bore (85-cm) aperture, and matrix size remains constant, pixel size increases and special resolution decreases.

To compensate for a reduction in spatial resolution, matrix size must increase, which describes the number of pixels in an image. Noise is considered any undesirable characteristic detracting from image quality. For example, streaklike patterns appearing near the diaphragm may be due to motion from respiratory movement during the scan time. Metal, such as dental fillings or a hip prosthesis, gives rise to streak and star-shaped artifacts on the image. Manufacturers of CT imaging systems are continually working to reduce image noise and improve image quality. An improvement in image quality usually translates into additional cost.

Variable slice thickness and spacing are extremely important criteria in obtaining CT studies beneficial to producing high-quality DRRs. Some scanners provide limited slice thickness settings (e.g., 2 or 5 mm) and slice spacing (e.g., 2, 3, or 5 mm) during the actual scan.[25] Other manufacturers allow the operator to select slice thickness from 1 to 10 mm, with some units providing slice thickness as low as 0.4 mm.[16] For optimal image reconstruction in producing a high-quality DRR, slice thickness and slice spacing should be evaluated for each anatomic region. Mutic et al.[27] recommend thin-slice CT scans

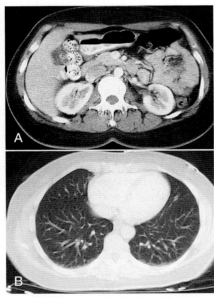

Figure 21-23. The selection of window level depends on the anatomy imaged. **A**, Soft tissue of the abdomen requires a low window level (level 50). **B**, The lung fields require a negative window level (level −500). (From Bushong S: *Radiologic science for technologists: physics, biology and protection,* ed 8, St. Louis, 2004, Mosby.)

with no more than 5-mm spacing to reduce the problem of volume averaging while accurately representing the target in three-dimensional space. To maximize the useful resolution on the DRR when performing CT simulation of the head and neck, Martin[25] recommends acquiring 1-mm slices at 1-mm spacing through the region containing the tumor and 3-mm slices at 3-mm spacing through peripheral areas of the treatment volume.

Slice thickness and spacing are important in producing useful DRRs, and they also affect storage and communication components within the computer system. Variable slice thickness and spacing, along with other important variables, are selected at the time of the scan at the control console.

Controls Associated with the Virtual Simulator Workstation

The workstation associated with CT simulation may appear complex and cumbersome with multiple monitors, controls for the CT console, hardware necessary to produce high-quality DRRs, and a virtual simulation workstation to perform target volume definition and dose calculation. Learning to use the equipment properly takes time and patience. Numerous hardware configurations are possible, depending on the type of equipment and needs of the department. Figure 21-2 demonstrates the physical layout and possible hardware configuration of a virtual simulation room.

Two main components of a CT simulator workstation are a target localization routine that allows the target to be defined and transfers the appropriate marks to the patient skin surface and a virtual simulation package that generates DRRs, which

are used to evaluate and simulate the case.[27] The DRRs become the "master" to compare subsequent portal images with during the treatment verification process (Figure 21-24).

Located within a properly shielded environment and with viewing access to the patient, the CT console allow for the selection of radiographic technical factors (such as kVp, mA, and scan time); mechanical movements of the gantry and couch; and computer commands for manipulating, reconstructing, and storing of the CT slices. The operator's console usually has two monitors. One to indicate patient data and provide information for each scan (number and thickness of slices, radiographic technique, and couch position) and the other to view and manipulate the reconstructed images before storing or transfer to external devices, such as a virtual simulation workstation.

The virtual simulation workstation is essentially a computer and monitor with huge amounts of storage capacity, memory, and processing capability. With conventional simulation, the field locations are determined first, the target is defined, and then the fields are shaped to treat the target. In virtual simulation, the target is defined first, and then the fields are shaped to conform to the target.[27] To accomplish this goal, the virtual simulation workstation needs access to vast amounts of data,

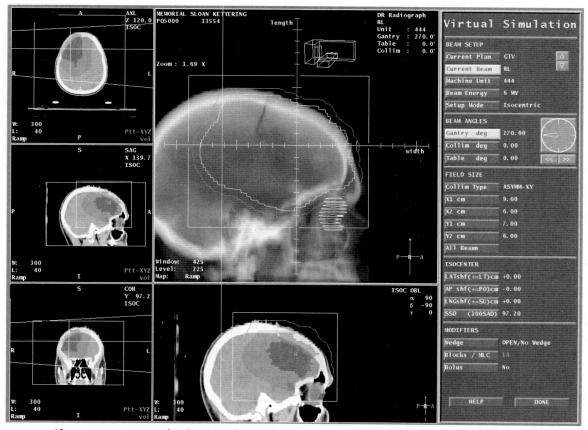

Figure 21-24. Example of CT simulation display (AcqSim, Philips Medical Systems, Andover, Mass). *Upper right* image is a beam's eye view (BEV) digitally reconstructed radiograph (DRR) with planning target volume outlined in yellow and treatment field aperture in blue. *Right panel* shows simulated beam setup controls. (See Color Plate 7.) (From Leibel SA, Phillips TL: *Textbook of radiation oncology,* ed 2, Philadelphia, 2004, Saunders.)

which may include the following[25]: CT study, DRRs, field parameters, patient information, treatment plan information, and estimated dose grids.

If the virtual simulation workstation is used to perform target volume definition, virtual simulation, DRR production, and treatment planning, a single station may easily become overused. Additional virtual simulation stations should be considered in the design of a CT simulation system.[25] Just as a busy retail store may need numerous computer terminals to adequately process customer purchases, additional virtual simulation workstations may help streamline treatment planning in a busy radiation therapy department.

Patient Marking System

Either isocenter or field edge marking systems are available for CT simulation. In conventional simulation, side lasers and an overhead laser are used to triangulate three reference points on the patient. After the target is defined and the fields are shaped to treat the target, the patient's isocenter is tattooed or otherwise marked. With CT simulation, the patient is temporarily marked with reference points before scanning. After the target volume has been determined, the computer calculates the isocenter, with reference to the temporary marks and the lasers and/or couch adjusted automatically. Movable lasers can be used for all three reference points. Field edge marking systems are available with some CT scanners used to control the position of lasers that identify on the patient's skin the superior, inferior, and lateral field borders and/or isocenter.[27,31]

Gammex has developed a CT positional laser system that consists of a robotic laser tracking system, which has two side-wall cross lasers with a movable horizontal line and one overhead laser with a movable sagittal line. These lasers provide movement in two dimensions, and the CT tabletop (couch) movement provides the third dimension. The lasers can be controlled through most treatment planning systems, with the Gammex CT Simulation software or with the remote handheld pendant. Lasers can accept exported coordinates from treatment planning systems, allowing easy and accurate movement to the marking location. Diode lasers are available in green or red. Not only does the integrated green laser enhance contrast on various skin tones, especially dark skin tones, its unique design incorporates power-stabilizing circuitry that extends diode life.[14]

 A CT simulation laser system consists of a single overhead laser line that moves to project the sagittal plane, two vertical moving lateral lasers to project the coronal plane, and fixed lasers to project the transverse plane. Most systems can be supplied with red or green lasers.

ROOM DESIGN

The design of a simulator room is a process that must involve the expertise of numerous professionals, including an architect, an engineer, and a radiologic physicist. Input should also be encouraged from the therapists and the radiation oncologists in the department. Before designing the room, the site must be chosen. The ideal location is close to the treatment machines.

This facilitates communication among all parties involved in the patient's treatment.

Space Allocations

The simulator room should be of sufficient size to accommodate not only the machine and all of its components but also its full range of motions. The equipment will have a longer life if sufficient space is provided. It will also be a more pleasant work area if personnel have room to comfortably perform their duties, such as preparing the patient for simulation, constructing immobilization devices, and preparing contrast media.

Space must also be allocated for a good-sized counter that should include a sink and a work space and writing area. The work space should be of sufficient size to allow for the manufacture of various immobilization devices used in radiation therapy. Cabinets and drawer space for the storage of simulation equipment and spare simulator parts are necessary in any simulator room. In addition, storage space should be available for routine immobilization devices and other related equipment such as a breast board, belly board, wingboard, and especially a hot water tank used in the construction of thermoplastic immobilization devices.

The control area is normally set in one corner of the room, usually near the entrance. This area is designed to protect the operators from radiation and to house the simulator's controls, treatment planning equipment if a CT simulator is used, and x-ray generator. It must be large enough for several pieces of equipment, which might include a record and verify system and one or more LCD monitors, work area, and numerous personnel. It is important that the operator have full visual and aural contact with the patient at all times. A lead glass window may be installed for patient visualization. Figure 21-16 illustrates a typical conventional simulator room design.

Other Considerations

There are several other considerations worth mentioning concerning the simulator. Simulator manufacturers have very specific requirements for ventilation of the room. They reserve the right to negate the warranty if these requirements are not met. The lighting system is also important. The intensity must be adjustable, with independent control of the room and the control area. For conventional simulation, visualization of the light field is easier in low light, as is the fluoroscopy image. On the other hand, certain simulation duties need maximum light, such as recording pertinent information, preparing contrast materials, or constructing an immobilization device. Task lighting in certain areas, such as under cabinets, is very beneficial.

Conventional simulator positioning lasers, which project a small red or green beam of light toward the patient during the simulation process, must be installed. There are several types available, and the department personnel must choose the style they believe best suits their needs. Side lasers are more stable if they are recessed in the wall to prevent inadvertent collisions. A third overhead laser is installed and represents the anterior central axis or midsagittal plane when the gantry is rotated from its vertical position. These lasers provide the therapist several external reference points in relationship to the position of the isocenter. Daily checks, which provide strict quality control of the positional lasers, are a must.

Shielding Requirements

As with all radiation equipment, room shielding is an important consideration. Radiation rooms are most commonly shielded with lead or concrete or a combination of the two. Lead is the denser of the two, and less is needed to stop an equal amount of radiation. Lead is also more expensive than concrete and very difficult to support structurally. This is the reason many diagnostic and radiation therapy departments are located in the basements of hospitals. Shielding costs are reduced significantly by the surrounding earth, and precious space is gained when thick concrete walls need not be built.

Not all walls may have the same amount of shielding. Primary walls are those at which the radiation will be aimed directly, and therefore they need more shielding than secondary walls, which have only scattered radiation impinging on them.

Several factors are taken into consideration in determining the required wall thickness. The time the machine is normally aimed at a wall or ceiling is called the *use factor (U)*. A standard use factor for a simulator's primary walls and ceilings is ¼. Floors are usually 1 because more exposures are made with the simulator in the vertical position. An occupancy factor (T) takes into consideration how an area on the other side of an irradiated wall is going to be used. An office where someone could be sitting for 40 hours a week would require more shielding in the wall than a storage closet where workers would spend 10 minutes once or twice a week.

Another important factor is workload. Workload (W) for a simulator is defined as the current (mA) multiplied by the time (minutes) a department expects to run the machine in a normal week. These estimates are always on the high side to calculate the largest possible scenario. A value in units of mA-min is used to describe workloads of diagnostic machines.

The weekly permissible dose (P) is 10 times higher (under normal conditions) for people who have chosen a career in the radiation field (radiation workers) compared with members of the general public. The most recent recommendations are 1 mSv/week for the occupationally exposed and 0.02 mSv/week for the general public.[28] Controlled areas are made off limits to members of the general public for this reason. Uncontrolled areas (areas where access is not limited) will have a lower P value and therefore need more shielding.

The calculation of barrier thickness is much more complicated than is shown here, but the following formula is the basis of most shielding calculations:

$$B = P(d)^2/WUT$$

The distance (in meters) from the source to the opposite side of the barrier is symbolized by *d*. The transmission of radiation through the barrier required to meet the weekly permissible dose is shown as *B*. This value is then used as a reference (to a graph or chart) to determine the barrier thickness relative to the maximum photon energy and the type of shielding that will be used.

Many of the factors used in consideration of the simulator room design, such as space allocations, equipment motions, and shielding design, provide for more efficient use of this essential piece of equipment. Because the time invested during the simulation process can seriously affect the outcome of a patient's treatment plan, a thorough knowledge of the simulator, its use, and its limitations is necessary if the simulator's maximum potential is to be reached.

The educational community continues to debate as to how CT simulation education must evolve as therapists are physically required to do less in the planning process and more in treatment planning work. The role of the CT simulator will probably expand as the demand for conventional simulation decreases. However, it must be remembered that not all cases requiring radiation therapy are suitable for CT simulation. The conventional simulator may actually be more suitable in some unique cases.

SUMMARY

- The primary purpose of the simulator is to assist the physician and other members of the radiation therapy team in the treatment planning process by establishing the appropriate volume to be treated and identifying the normal structures within or adjacent to this volume.
- Simulation is of two types: conventional and computed tomography (CT).
- The type of simulator purchased should be considered based on the department's needs, such as types of treatment (radical or palliative) and number of patients and fields treated each day, with special consideration given to the type and complexity of treatment.
- Conventional simulators are designed to simulate the mechanical, geometric, and optical conditions of a variety of treatment units.
- The mechanical components of the conventional simulator include the gantry, treatment couch, and controls.
- CT simulation can describe several types of radiation therapy localization procedures, including a conventional simulator with a CT mode, a conventional simulator session, followed by a CT scan on a second diagnostic CT scanner, CT simulation, and virtual simulation.
- The gantry of a CT scanner includes the x-ray tube, the detector array, the high-voltage generator, the couch, and the mechanical support devices for each.
- In terms of data acquisition for CT, there are two major methods used in today's scanners—the slice-by-slice approach and the volumetric approach.
- In CT scanning, the small cell or pixel is assigned a value called a CT number or Hounsfield unit, which represents the density of the tissue and is directly related to the x-ray linear attenuation coefficient (u) for the tissue.
- With the evolution of the simulator design from more conventional simulators using radiography and fluoroscopy to applications of CT simulation and digitally reconstructed radiographs, there has been a shift in responsibility and effort from the simulator equipment to the treatment planning computer.
- The simulator equipment will have a longer life if sufficient space is provided. Space should be provided to comfortably perform all the simulation duties, such as preparing the patient for simulation, constructing immobilization devices, and preparing contrast media.

Review Questions

Multiple Choice

1. The device that projects a scale onto the patient's skin, corresponding to the SSD, is called a(n):
   a. couch
   b. gantry
   c. ODI
   d. collimator assembly

2. To control scatter radiation during fluoroscopy, the _____ _____ should be adjusted.
   a. isocenter
   b. treatment couch
   c. field-defining wires
   d. beam-restricting diaphragms

3. All of the following are optical devices used during the conventional simulation process *except:*
   a. patient tabletop
   b. ODI
   c. light field
   d. lasers

4. Black areas on the CT scan represent _____ objects such as gas in the stomach or air in the lungs.
   a. low-density
   b. medium-density
   c. high-density
   d. none of the above

5. Which of the following factors are *not* taken into consideration when determining shielding requirements for a simulator?
   a. use factor (U)
   b. occupancy factor (T)
   c. workload (W)
   d. inverse scattering intensity (I)

6. Which of the following involve three-dimensional treatment planning?
   I. virtual simulation
   II. AP images
   III. CT simulators
   IV. portal images
      a. I and II only
      b. I and III only
      c. II and III only
      d. II and IV only

7. CT and MRI scans provide the most useful information for treatment planning purposes because:
   a. they are the most cost-effective method
   b. they are the least cost-effective method
   c. the scans can produce a three-dimensional representation of the patient and external structures
   d. the images are essential in comparing with port film taken during treatment

8. All of the following are considered drawbacks to CT simulation *except:*
   a. the size of the aperture may be too small to accommodate all treatment positions
   b. the verification and use of certain beam-shaping devices and treatment accessories are limited
   c. treatment planning data can be obtained in three dimensions
   d. the digitally reconstructed radiographs, which are used as "masters" to compare with the portal images, are of poorer quality compared with conventional simulation radiographs

9. Which of the following steps in the radiation therapy process immediately *proceeds* the actual treatment of a patient?
   a. simulation and treatment planning
   b. diagnosis
   c. consultation
   d. biopsy of the tumor

10. The major difference between a conventional simulator and a CT simulator is the:
    a. image intensifier
    b. collection of anatomic patient data
    c. room shielding requirements
    d. production of scatter radiation

The answers to the Review Questions can be found by logging on to our website at: *http://evolve.elsevier.com/Washington+Leaver/principles*

Questions to Ponder

1. Discuss the importance of tumor localization.
2. Describe, as though you were educating an interested patient, the purpose of the isocenter.
3. Explain the purpose of each of the components within the head of the gantry of a conventional simulator.
4. How do the couch and the additional movements of the simulator provide an accurate representation of the treatment plan?
5. Discuss the process of tumor localization and treatment planning using CT simulation.
6. What are the advantages and disadvantages of CT simulation versus conventional simulation?

REFERENCES

1. Aird EGA, Conway J: CT simulation for radiotherapy treatment planning, *Br J Radiol* 75:937-949, 2002.
2. American College of Radiology: *ACR standards for radiation oncology,* pp 466-488, Reston, Va, 2002, American College of Radiology.
3. Baker GR: Localization: conventional and CT simulation, *Br J Radiol* 79(1):S36-S49, 2006.
4. Bentel CG: *Radiation therapy planning,* New York, 1993, McGraw-Hill.
5. Bidault LM, et al: Imaging in radiation oncology. In Leibel SA, Phillips TL, editors: *Textbook of radiation oncology,* Philadelphia, 2004, WB Saunders.
6. Bomford CK, et al: Treatment simulators, *Br J Radiol* special report No. 10, 1976.
7. Bomford CK, et al: Treatment simulators, *Br J Radiol* suppl 16, 1981.
8. Bomford CK, et al: Treatment simulators, *Br J Radiol* suppl 23, 1989.
9. Bourland J: Radiation oncology physics. In Gunderson LL, Tepper JE, editors: *Clinical radiation oncology,* Philadelphia, 2007, Churchill Livingstone.
10. British Standards Institution: *Medical electrical equipment, part 3. Particular requirements for performance, section 3.129. Methods of declaring functional performance characteristics of radiotherapy simulators, Supplement 1. Guide to function performance values* (pp 1-14), London, 1994, Author.
11. Bushong SC: *Radiologic science for technologists: physics, biology, and protection,* ed 8, St. Louis, 2004, Mosby.
12. Carlton RR, McKenna-Adler A: *Principles of radiographic imaging,* Albany, NY, 2000, Delmar Publishing.

13. Chen GTY, Pelizzari CA, Rietzel ERM: Imaging in radiotherapy. In Kahn FM, editor: *Treatment planning in radiation oncology,* ed 2, Philadelphia, 2007, Lippincott Williams & Wilkins.

14. CT simulator lasers (website): www.gammex.com. Accessed January 5, 2008.

15. Day MJ, Harrison RM: Cross-sectional information/treatment simulation. In Bleehen NM, Glatstein E, Haybittle JL, editors: *Radiation therapy planning,* New York, 1983, Marcel Dekker.

16. Diagnostic imaging (website): www.diagnosticimaging.com/thinslicect. Accessed January 5, 2008.

17. Dickson S, et al: CT simulation in a large department using SOMATOM Emotion Duo scanner, *Electromedia* 71:28-35, 2003.

18. Farmer ET, Fowler JF, Haggith JW: Megavoltage treatment planning and the use of xeroradiography, *Br J Radiol* 36:426-435, 1963.

19. Fielding JR, Burke M, Jewells VS: Imaging in oncology. In Genderson LL, Tepper JE, editors: *Clinical radiation oncology,* ed 2, Philadelphia, 2007, Churchill Livingstone.

20. Haddad P, et al: Computerized tomographic simulation compared with clinical mark-up in palliative radiotherapy: a prospective study, *Int J Radiat Oncol Biol Phys* 65:824-829, 2006.

21. Hendee WR, Ibbott GS, Hendee EG: *Radiation therapy physics,* Hoboken, NJ, 2005, John Wiley and Sons.

22. Hufton AP, et al: Low attenuation material for table tops, cassettes, and grids: a review, *Radiography* 53:17-18, 1987.

23. International Electrotechnical Commission: *CEI/IEC 976 medical electron accelerators in the range 1-50 MeV—functional performance characteristics,* Geneva, 1989, Author.

24. Karzmark CJ, Nunan CS, Tanabe E: *Medical linear accelerators,* Princeton, NJ, 1993, McGraw-Hill.

25. Martin EE: CT simulation hardware. In Purdy JA, Starkschall G, editors: *Three-dimensional planning and conformal radiation therapy,* Madison, Wis, 1999, Advanced Medical Publishers.

26. Meetens H, Bijhold J, Strachee J: A method for the measurement of field placement errors in digital portal images, *Phys Med Biol* 35:299, 1990.

27. Mutic S, et al: Simulation process in determination and definition of treatment volume and treatment planning. In Leavitt SH, et al, editors: *Technical basis for radiation therapy: practical clinical applications,* New York, 2006, Springer.

28. National Council of Radiation Protection and Measurements: *NCRP Report #16: limitation of exposure to ionizing radiation,* Bethesda, Md, 1993, NCRP.

29. Nobel peace prize (website): http://nobelprize.org/nobel_prizes/medicine/laureates/1979/hounsfield-lecture.html. Accessed December 3, 2007.

30. Purdy JA: Principles of radiologic physics, dosimetry and treatment planning. In Halperin EC, Perez CA, Brady LW, editors: *Principles and practice of radiation oncology,* Philadelphia, 2008, Lippincott Williams & Wilkins.

31. Ragan DP, et al: CT-based simulation with laser patient marking, *Med Phys* 20:379-380, 1993.

32. Sherouse GW, Novins KL, Chaney EL: Computation of digitally reconstructed radiographs for use in radiotherapy treatment design, *Int J Radiat Oncol Biol Phys* 18:651-658, 1990.

33. Stanton R, Stinson D, Shahabi S: *Applied physics for radiation oncology,* Madison, Wis, 2000, Medical Physics Publishing.

34. Van Dyk J, Mah K: Simulation and imaging for radiation therapy planning. In Williams JR, Thaites DI, editors: *Radiotherapy physics in practice,* Oxford, 2000, Oxford University Press.

35. Wolbarst A: *Physics of radiology,* Madison, Wis, 2000, Medical Physics Publishing.

36. Zimeras S: *Virtual simulation for radiotherapy treatment using CT medical data,* Brussels, 2003, Marie Curie Industry Host Fellowship Grant No. HPMI-CT-1999-00005.

Conventional (Fluoroscopy-Based) Simulation Procedures

Dennis Leaver, Rosann Keller, Nora Uricchio

Outline

Nomenclature
    Acronyms
Tumor and normal tissue
    localization
    Anatomic body planes
    Computed tomography imaging
    Fluoroscopy-based simulation
        localization methods
Fluoroscopy-based simulation
    procedure

Presimulation planning
Patient positioning
Patient immobilization
Preparing the room
Explanation of
    simulation procedure
Operating fluoroscopy-based
    conventional simulator
    controls
Setting field parameters

Producing quality radiographic
    images
    Documenting pertinent data
Contour devices
Treatment verification
Emergency procedures
Rationale of fluoroscopy-based
    simulation procedures
Summary

Objectives

- Define common acronyms used during a conventional fluoroscopy-based simulation procedure.
- Compare and contrast the use of various body planes in determining tumor and normal tissue localization.
- Describe the evolution of the radiation therapy simulation process from a historic prospective.
- Describe the difference between fluoroscopy-based simulation and CT simulation.
- Provide a general description of the following steps in the fluoroscopy-based simulation process: presimulation planning, patient positioning, patient

immobilization, preparing the room, explanation of simulation procedure, operating fluoroscopy-based conventional simulator controls, setting field parameters, producing quality radiographic images, and documenting pertinent data.
- Compare several contour methods, including computed tomography, solder, plaster, and thermoplastic.
- Discuss the importance of the treatment verification process.
- List and describe two emergency procedures that may be encountered during the simulation process.

Key Terms

Bite block
Body habitus
Caliper
Clinical target
    volume (CTV)
Complex
    immobilization
    devices
Contour
Contrast media
CT imaging
Digitally reconstructed
    radiographs (DRRs)
Field size
Fluoroscopy-based
    simulation
Four-dimensional
Gross tumor volume
    (GTV)
Immobilization
Interfraction
Intrafraction
Irradiated volume
Isocentric technique
Localization
Organ at risk (OAR)
Orthogonal films
Patient
    positioning aids
PET scanner
Planning target
    volume (PTV)
Radiopaque marker
Separation
Simple immobilization
    devices
Simulation
Target volume
Treatment volume
Vac-Lok
Verification
Verification simulation

I n this chapter, the complexities of fluoroscopy-based simulation and target volume localization are discussed. This includes nomenclature (definitions) and the importance of patient assessment and education before the simulation procedure. A description of tumor and normal tissue localization methods, patient immobilization, and types of contours and an outline of the steps involved in the conventional simulation procedure and treatment verification process are also included. Simulation procedures have been divided into two separate chapters. In this chapter, conventional fluoroscopy-based simulation techniques are discussed. Specifics regarding computed tomography (CT) simulation are examined in Chapter 23.

Patients treated with radiation therapy, either for cure or for palliation, will be involved in numerous processes ranging from diagnosis to ongoing patient follow-up. There are various steps that a patient will experience as part of the entire process of external beam radiation therapy. The actual planning process (Figure 22-1) of a prescribed dose of radiation, although important, is a small part of the whole process. Before treatment can begin, a simulation procedure is necessary in almost all cases. In many cases, the ultimate success of treatment is directly related to the effectiveness of the simulation procedure. This procedure helps in determining the size and shape of the treatment volume relative to important normal tissues.[20] Not every step in the radiation therapy process may be needed for every patient, nor will the steps always occur in sequence. The process varies for each patient, depending on the department's protocol, the patient's condition, and the type and/or extent of disease.

The simulation process (patient positioning and imaging as indicated in Figure 22-1) involves the participation of several team members, each with a variety of unique skills. Both simulation and treatment require a solid foundation in the theory and application of radiation oncology techniques. In addition, effective patient care skills are essential to provide comfort and care for the patient throughout the simulation process. It is the team approach, involving each member, that can provide effective planning, as well as localization and documentation of the patient's disease in relationship to normal tissue structures. Table 22-1 identifies key staff functions in the radiation therapy process from diagnosis to patient follow-up.

DIAGNOSIS

- screening
- cancer imaging
- pathology
- staging

THERAPEUTIC DECISIONS

- cure
- palliation
- benign
- surgery/radiation/chemotherapy
- patient interview

SIMULATION

- fluoroscopy-based
- CT simulation (virtual)
- patient positioning
- immobilization devices
- digitally reconstructed radiographs (DRRs)

TREATMENT PLANNING

- identifying planning target volume
- identifying critical structures
- selection of treatment technique
- isodose distribution
- calculation of treatment beams
- optimization

TREATMENT

- treatment verification and imaging
- dosimetry checks
- treatment delivery and monitoring
- patient assessment
- record keeping

PATIENT FOLLOW-UP

- patient assessment
- normal tissue response
- tumor control

Figure 22-1. The various steps involved in the process of external beam treatment. The process may vary somewhat depending on the treatment goal. It is the team approach, involving each member, that usually provides effective planning. (Adapted from Van Dyk J, Mah K: Simulators and CT scanners. In Williams JR, Thwaites DI, editors: *Radiotherapy physics in practice*, Oxford, 2000, Oxford University Press.)

Table 22-1	Key Staff Functions in the Radiation Therapy Process
Function	**Team Member(s)**
Diagnosis	Pathologist
	Referring physician
	Radiation oncologist
Therapeutic decisions	Radiation oncologist
	Referring physician
Target volume localization	Radiation oncologist
	Radiation therapist
	Dosimetrist
	Physicist
Simulation and treatment planning	Radiation oncologist
	Radiation therapist
	Physicist
	Dosimetrist
Fabrication of treatment aids	Dosimetrist
	Radiation therapist
	Mold room assistant
Treatment	Radiation therapist
	Physicist
	Dosimetrist
	Radiation oncologist
Patient evaluation during treatment	Radiation oncologist
	Radiation therapist
	Oncology nurse
Patient follow-up	Radiation oncologist
	Oncology nurse

A simulator can take various forms, ranging from a simple diagnostic radiographic unit with fluoroscopy and/or CT capabilities to a stand-alone CT simulator. Conventional simulation, also referred to as **fluoroscopy-based simulation**, implies the use of a piece of x-ray equipment capable of the same mechanical movements of a treatment unit. It can mimic gantry angles and table angles and display a representation of the treatment field on the patient's skin. Regardless of the method of simulation that is used, the outcome should define the anatomic area to be treated so that it is reproducible for daily treatment. An elaborate and complicated simulation is of no value unless it is reproducible on the treatment unit.

In recent years, CT simulation has become more popular and effective in covering the clinical tumor volume with greater accuracy and sparing greater volumes of normal tissue than conventional/fluoroscopy-based simulation. The incorporation of computer software, used with CT simulation and three-dimensional (3D) treatment planning, has been a critical step forward in defining tumor volumes and sparing normal tissue structures. This is CT simulation's greatest advantage over fluoroscopy-based simulation. Although fluoroscopy-based simulation is still available in many clinical facilities, CT simulation has become a mainstay of most radiation therapy departments. CT simulation units are now included as part of the overall plan for new clinical construction.

The development of cross-sectional imaging modalities such as magnetic resonance imaging (MRI) and positron emission tomography (PET) has provided valuable information that is often incorporated into the simulation software by a complex process of image fusion. Some challenges remain, especially in localizing moving anatomic structures. Breath-holding and gated respiration techniques, still under investigation, have produced **four-dimensional** (3D treatment planning + time = 4D) data sets that can be used to reduce margins or to minimize dose to normal tissue or organs at risk. In addition, image-guided radiation therapy (IGRT) has proved to be effective in addressing the **interfraction** motion (the change in target position from one fraction to another) or **intrafraction** motion (the change in target position during treatment delivery as might occur in the thorax with respirations) of both target volumes and critical normal structures. Whichever method of localization and simulation is adopted, the role of quality control is important for the overall accuracy of the patient's treatment.[2]

Four historical developments occurred in the early 1990s that greatly affected radiation treatment planning and the simulation process:
1. *Virtual simulation was introduced, which provided the ability to use a diagnostic-type scanner to take multiple images.*
2. *CT images on a conventional treatment simulator were dramatically improved, which allowed them to be used for planning purposes.*
3. *Treatment planning computers were developed that could carry out 3D treatment planning.*
4. *A true virtual simulator provided the ability to generate high-resolution DRRs.*

A state-of-the-art CT simulator, specifically designed for the radiation therapy department, included a high-performance CT scanner with laser and patient marking systems and a virtual simulator (see Chapter 23).

CT simulation will undoubtedly meet the demands of modern radiation therapy planning better than conventional simulation. Radiation oncologists are now required to define the target volume more precisely, not just in two dimensions, but also in three dimensions and sometimes four dimensions. With the introduction of intensity-modulated radiation therapy (IMRT) and IGRT, it is possible and in many situations advantageous to escalate the dose to the tumor volume. Because CT simulation allows visualization of anatomy in three dimensions, better than conventional fluoroscopy-based simulation, this enables the treatment planner to conform the dose around the target volume irradiating the tumor to as high a dose as possible, and at the same time sparing the normal tissues.[2]

Fluoroscopy-based simulation, along with a CT scan performed after the initial conventional simulation process and then integrated into the treatment planning process, can accomplish some of the same goals of CT simulation, but it is not without difficulties and increased input from several of the staff members, such as the physician, radiation therapist, and dosimetrist. Conventional fluoroscopy-based simulation may be the only simulation equipment in some radiation therapy departments or it may supplement one or two CT simulators in a busy department. Conventional simulation is still considered a valuable tool in the radiation therapy planning process.

NOMENCLATURE

Before a discussion of exactly what fluoroscopy-based simulation is, a review of several key definitions and acronyms, designed to provide a foundation in simulation procedures, is helpful.

Simulation (a single- or multiple-step process) is carried out by the radiation therapist under the supervision of the radiation oncologist. It is the precise mockup of a patient treatment with radiographic documentation of the treatment portals.[9] The term *simulation* may take on different meanings, depending on the institution and the individual. First, it is a general term describing the mockup process, which can also include the selection of immobilization devices, radiographic documentation of treatment ports, measurement of the patient, construction of patient contours, and shaping of fields.[9] Second, it may be a more specific term in which the simulator artificially duplicates the actual treatment conditions (verification) by confirming measurements, verifying treatment, and confirming shields.[20] Third, it may involve a virtual simulation workstation, equipped with a CT scanner, software to perform target volume definition and treatment planning dose calculation, and the production of **digitally reconstructed radiographs (DRRs)**.

Localization means geometric definition of the position and extent of the tumor or anatomic structures by reference of surface marks that can be used for treatment setup purposes.[20] The radiation oncologist and radiation therapist, along with other team members, localize the tumor volume and critical normal structures using clinical; radiographic; and/or CT, MRI, and PET image information.

Verification is a final check that each of the planned treatment beams does cover the tumor or **target volume** and does not irradiate critical normal structures.[20] This is usually done as the second part of a two-step process on the simulator or treatment unit. Some radiation therapists may refer to it as "part B" or "part 2" of the simulation process. Verification involves taking radiographic images or portal images of each of the treatment beams using external marks and other immobilization devices intended for treatment reproducibility. It is an essential process that provides verification of the treatment plan.

Radiopaque marker refers to a material with a high atomic number. It is usually made of lead, copper, or solder wire. Frequently, it is used on the surface of a patient or appropriately placed in a body cavity. This is done to delineate special points of interest for calculation purposes or to mark critical structures requiring visualization during treatment planning. Small radiopaque markers are often used to mark specific points on a patient during the CT acquisition phase of the simulation procedure.

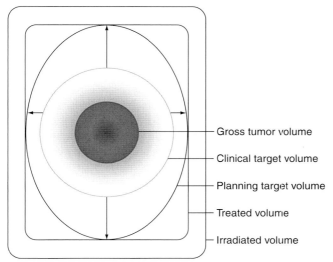

Gross tumor volume

Clinical target volume

Planning target volume

Treated volume

Irradiated volume

Figure 22-2. International Commission on Radiation Units and Measurements (ICRU) Report 50 defining target volumes used in radiation therapy. (From Cox JD, Ang KK, editors: *Radiation oncology: rationale, technique, results*, ed 8, St. Louis, 2003, Mosby.)

Contrast media is a compound or agent used as an aid in visualizing internal structures, because it has the ability to enhance the differences in adjacent anatomic structures. Barium (atomic number of 56) and iodine (atomic number of 53) are compounds commonly used to visualize anatomic structures with x-rays.

Separation refers to the measurement of the thickness of a patient along the central axis (CA) or at any other specified point within the irradiated volume. Separations are helpful in calculating the amount of tissue in front of, behind, or

around a tumor. A **caliper**, which is a graduated ruled instrument with one sliding leg and one that is stationary, is used to determine the patient's thickness. A patient's separation is also referred to as the *intrafield distance*, or sometimes the *innerfield distance (IFD)*.

Field size involves the dimensions of a treatment field at the isocenter, which are represented by width × length. This measurement, determined by the field-defining wires on the fluoroscopy-based simulator and collimator opening on the treatment unit, defines the dimensions of the treatment portal at the isocenter.

There are several definitions related to the patient planning process provided by the International Commission on Radiation Units and Measurements (ICRU) in an effort to standardize radiation therapy terminology.[8] Figure 22-2 illustrates several target volumes described by ICRU Report 50.[8] Uniform application of these terms when radiation treatments are prescribed, recorded, and reported helps with the comparison of treatment results from different centers.[3] Three specific target volumes are further defined (Figure 22-3); gross tumor volume (GTV), clinical target volume (CTV), and planning target volume (PTV).[8] ICRU Report 62[8a] updates ICRU Report 50 regarding a further defining of **organs at risk (OAR)**, which are critical structures that may limit the amount of radiation delivered to the tumor volume.

Gross tumor volume (GTV) indicates the gross palpable or visible tumor.

Clinical target volume (CTV) indicates the gross palpable or visible tumor (GTV) and a surrounding volume of tissue that may contain subclinical or microscopic disease.

Planning target volume (PTV) indicates the CTV plus margins for geometric uncertainties, such as patient motion, beam penumbra, and treatment setup differences.

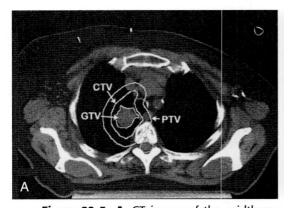
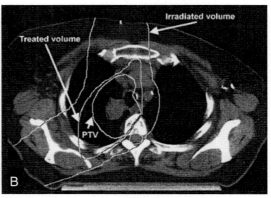

Figure 22-3. A, CT image of the midthorax showing a cancer of the lung. The obvious tumor mass is outlined as the GTV. The CTV and PTV are also shown. **B**, The same CT image as in **A**, showing the PTV, the treated volume, and the irradiated volume. A two-field technique was used, with anterior and posterior oblique fields of 6-MV x-rays. (Used by permission from Van Dyk JV, Mah K: Simulation and imaging for radiation therapy planning. In Williams JR, Thwaites DI, editors: *Radiotherapy physics in practice*, Oxford, 2000, Oxford University Press.)

ICRU Report 62[8a]

One of the important factors that has contributed to the success of the current 3D treatment planning process is the standardization of nomenclature published in 1993 in ICRU Report 50[8], which provided the radiation oncology community a language and methodology for image-based 3D planning for defining the volumes of known tumor, suspected microscopic spread, and marginal volumes necessary to account for setup variations and organ and patient motion. ICRU Report 62[8a] was published in 1999 as a supplement to Report 50 to formulate more accurately some of the definitions, to take into account the consequences of the advances made in recent years, and to address perceived limitations of Report 50, perhaps the most criticized of which being that it does not account for OAR positional uncertainties.[1] (See www.icru.org for additional information.)

Acronyms

Acronyms are commonly used in any highly technical work environment. A common language evolves in communicating thoughts and ideas between team members. An introduction to several more important acronyms used during simulation procedures will be helpful. Many of the useful acronyms are illustrated in Figure 22-4 and defined in Table 22-2.

TUMOR AND NORMAL TISSUE LOCALIZATION

The primary function of the simulator is to localize the tumor volume in three dimensions. The fluoroscopy-based simulator is not used exclusively or in total isolation for the localization of most tumors but together with other imaging modalities such as CT, MRI, PET, and single-photon emission computed tomography (SPECT).[20] However, some simulation procedures may be done exclusively on the simulator radiographically, fluoroscopically, or using a CT scanner with or without the aid of contrast media. In this section, several aspects of tumor localization are discussed. These include anatomic body planes, CT, source-skin distance/source-axis distance (SSD/SAD) localization methods, fluoroscopy and radiography, and the use of contrast media to aid in tumor and normal tissue localization.

One of the greatest challenges for the medical-physics community is the ability to combine imaging modalities such as CT, MRI, PET, and SPECT so that data can be correlated accurately in the planning and verification stages of radiation therapy.[20] This process of overlaying one image study onto another

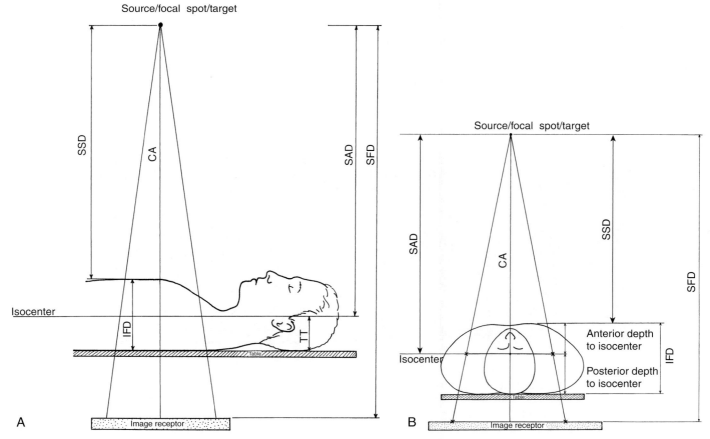

Figure 22-4. A list of common acronyms used in radiation therapy: **(A)** a lateral view and **(B)** a superior view illustrating terms in a transverse plane.

Table 22-2	Acronyms Used During Radiation Therapy Treatment and Fluoroscopy-Based Simulation Procedures
Acromym	**Definition**
CA (CAX)	Central axis is a line perpendicular to the cross section of the simulation or treatment field. It is the only imaginary line emanating from the source (focal spot) of radiation that is not divergent.
Film	Unexposed recording medium used to capture the x-ray image and store it until processing.
IFD	Intrafield distance (also called *separation*) is a measurement used for treatment planning purposes to determine the thickness of a body part from entrance point to exit point, often measured along the CA.
Image	Any process used to capture the x-ray, MRI, or sonographic information, including film, electronic, or DRR.
Isocenter	Point in space where radiation beams intersect from any of the 360-degree gantry angles. It is similar to the spokes of a bicycle wheel intersecting at the axle.
SAD	Source-axis distance is the distance from the source of radiation to the axis of the radiation beam or isocenter (also referred to as *TAD [target-axis distance]*).
SFD	Source-film distance is the distance from the source of radiation to the film (also referred to as *TID [target-image receptor distance]*).
SSD	Source-skin distance is the distance from the source of radiation to the skin surface of the patient (also referred to as *TSD [target-source distance]*).
Source/focal spot	Geometric point or area where the radiation beam emerges and fans out or diverges as it moves farther from the source, target, or focal spot.
TT	Tabletop distance is the distance from the tabletop to the isocenter.

Other acronyms are used by the radiation therapy team during the simulation and treatment process. The more common ones are listed as a reference.

provides more information during the planning process and enhances the strength of each individual imaging modality through a synergistic effect. More research is needed to study and examine computerized image correlation (fusion). This method is commonly used with CT simulation.

 Image fusion is the digital overlaying of data, voxel by voxel, from two or more different imaging modalities: CT, MRI, SPECT, and PET. Currently, most 3D fusion images are composed of PET images superimposed on CT or MRI. Image fusion techniques primarily take advantage of blending the 3D anatomic information gained from CT or MRI with the physiologic measurement from nuclear medicine scans such as PET or SPECT.

Anatomic Body Planes

A review of the three major body planes helps in understanding the nature of 3D localization. As illustrated in Figure 22-5, the body can be described in three planes: the coronal, sagittal, and axial planes. An anteroposterior (AP) radiograph displays anatomy in the coronal plane, showing structures in the

inferior/superior and left/right direction (two dimensions only). This radiographic view provides information for planning purposes in only one plane. The depth of the tumor volume cannot be found on a conventional simulator without the aid of a lateral radiograph (Figure 22-6). This view shows anatomic information in the sagittal plane, displaying structures in the inferior/superior and AP direction. Axial images can be obtained only through CT and MRI modalities (see Chapter 20).

Computed Tomography Imaging

Applications and advantages of CT, PET, PET/CT, and MRI in radiation therapy treatment planning have been documented.[2,11,13,17,20] Radiation therapy CT planning procedures are distinctly different from conventional diagnostic procedures. For example, unlike CT scans done for diagnostic purposes, in which a curved couch top is used, a flat insert is required when scanning for radiation therapy planning purposes. Flat couch tops are standard for radiation therapy simulators. It is important to scan the patient in the treatment position. If the treatment position is supine on a flat couch, then the patient should be scanned supine on a flat surface. In addition, positional lasers incorporated into the design of the CT scanner will aid in the reproducibility of the simulation process.[20]

Some studies have shown modifications in 30% to 80% of a select number of conventional non-CT treatment plans because of the additional information provided by CT. In addition, some 10% to 40% of all radiation therapy patients might benefit from CT scanning for radiation therapy treatment planning. Cross-sectional information provided by MRI and **CT imaging** contributes considerable information to the radiation oncologist in four major areas: diagnosis, tumor and normal tissue localization, tissue density data for dose calculations, and follow-up treatment monitoring.[20] The demands of modern radiation therapy planning are quite different from those 20 years ago. Radiation oncologists are now required to define the target volume more precisely, not just in two dimensions but in three dimensions. It has therefore become more common to visualize anatomy in three dimensions, which is easier with CT scanning technology. This enables treatment planning to conform to the dose around the target volume in order to irradiate the tumor to as high a dose as possible and at the same time spare normal surrounding tissues.[2]

There are two types of applications involving CT imaging in radiation therapy. One provides detailed diagnostic information used by the radiologist and radiation oncologist to evaluate the extent of the disease. This is conventional CT (usually performed outside the radiation therapy department). A newer technique, also performed outside the radiation therapy department, uses the combination of a **PET scanner**, which is a nuclear medicine procedure that has become useful in oncology to examine the biochemical or physiologic (functional) aspects of a tumor, along with a CT scanner in a single device called a *PET/CT scanner*.

The second application of CT imaging is designed solely for radiation therapy treatment planning. Concerning the second application, some manufacturers have introduced simulators that can reconstruct information analogous to conventional CT images. Others have developed software in which the radiation

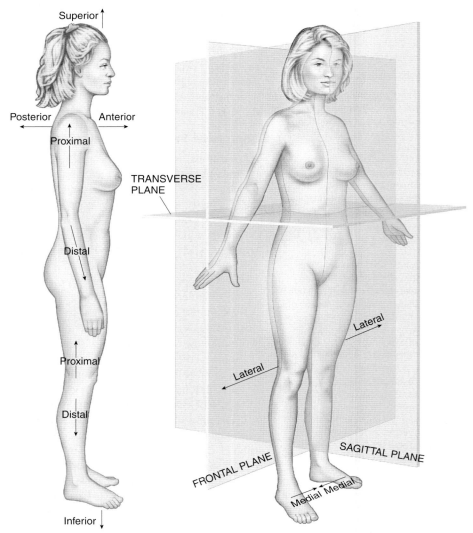

Figure 22-5. The body described in three planes: the coronal, sagittal, and axial planes. (From Thibodeau GA, Patton KT: *Anatomy and physiology*, ed 6, St. Louis, 2007, Mosby.)

therapy beam can be displayed in coronal, sagittal, and axial planes. A CT simulator can provide several advanced image manipulation and viewing advantages such as beam's eye view (BEV) display, which allows the anatomy to be viewed from the perspective of the radiation beams and allows field shaping electronically at the computer workstation.[17] A BEV allows the possibility of virtual simulation. By outlining target volumes on each image, irregular field shapes can be determined and a special laser device used to outline this field shape directly on the patient's skin.[20] (See Chapter 23 for more information about CT simulation and BEV.) Some authors predict that conventional or fluoroscopy-based simulators will soon be rendered obsolete by the CT simulator, although some developmental work still remains, such as larger scan tunnel, improved image segmentation, and correlation software.[17]

In addition, some CT scanners are used in the treatment room and aligned "on rails" to verify the patient's position in the treatment position just before treatment on the linear accelerator. This method of image guidance provides data on daily treatment

position, which can then be adjusted each day just before treatment delivery.

Fluoroscopy-Based Simulation Localization Methods

Most treatment planning on the fluoroscopy-based simulator is divided into two types of procedures: SAD and SSD setups. Both methods may use fluoroscopy to initially view the area. In each case, radiographs document what has been done during the simulation process. These radiographs are considered part of the patient's medical record. They are routinely used as "masters" when comparing subsequent imaging films from the treatment unit.

The decision to use one setup method over the other may be decided by many factors, including the nature and extent of the patient's disease and the goals and expected outcome of the treatment (cure or palliation). Other factors that are considered include the type of equipment available and department protocol.

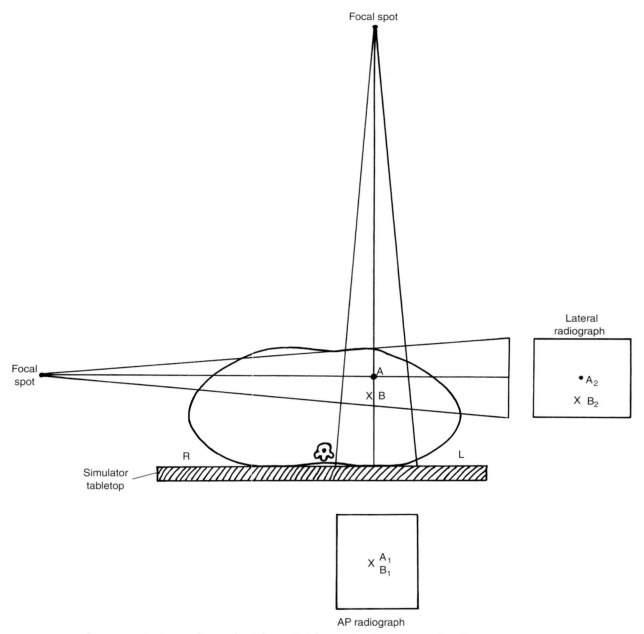

Figure 22-6. Two radiographs taken at right angles to one another (orthogonal radiographs) are often obtained to aid in the treatment planning process. Note in this schematic that points *A* and *B* cannot be distinguished from one another, except on the lateral radiograph.

The SSD approach positions a fixed treatment distance of 80 or 100 cm or greater on the patient's skin for each field (Figure 22-7, A). There may be some unique circumstances where an extended distance, beyond 100 cm, is needed to cover a larger area on the patient. The SSD method requires repositioning the patient for each field before treatment. Usually this approach uses a single field, two laterals or an AP/posteroanterior (PA) treatment approach (sometimes called *parallel opposed [POP] fields* because the central axes of each field oppose each other). This field arrangement requires tumor localization in two dimensions only, because all tissues within these fields are treated.[3]

Note that in Figure 22-7, A, the field size is defined (at 100 cm) on the patient's skin.

The SAD approach is also called the **isocentric technique** (Figure 22-7, B). It provides tumor localization in three dimensions. Using the SAD strategy, the isocenter is placed within the target volume with the aid of fluoroscopy and other imaging modalities. Here, as illustrated in Figure 22-7, B, the field size is defined at the isocenter within the patient (100 cm). In both situations the field size is defined at 100 cm. The only difference is where that distance is located (on the skin surface or within the patient). Once the isocenter has been located,

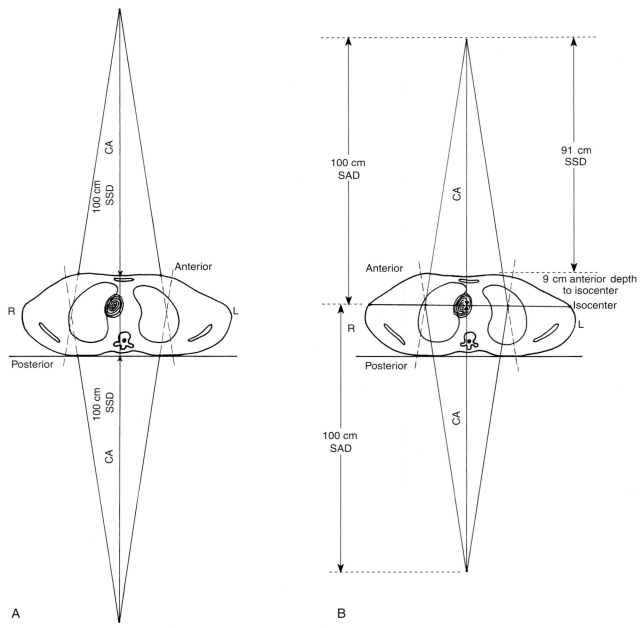

Figure 22-7. Differences between a source-skin distance (SSD) approach **(A)**, where the field size is defined on the surface, and source-axis distance (SAD) approach **(B)**, where the field size is defined at a depth calculated within the patient, are demonstrated. Both methods used in the planning and delivery of a prescribed course of radiation therapy require careful documentation.

orthogonal films may be taken. **Orthogonal films** are two radiographs taken at right angles to one another. They are often obtained to aid in the treatment planning process. Usually an AP and lateral projections are used to obtain information on the treatment depth and to establish an anterior setup distance as a reference point (see Figure 22-6).

With the isocentric approach, the reading on the patient's skin varies from field to field. It depends on several factors. It will not be 80 or 100 cm, as happens with the SSD approach. Rather, the distance will vary for each field (Figure 22-8),

depending on the thickness or separation of the patient. It may also depend on the depth of the tumor from the AP, PA, oblique, or lateral skin surface.

Contrast Media. To help in localizing the tumor volume and normal critical structures, contrast media may be needed during the simulation procedure. Contrast media, used in radiographic or fluoroscopic studies, visually enhance anatomic structures that would normally be more difficult to see. Commonly used contrast media include barium sulfate, iodinated contrast materials, and negative contrast agents such as air.

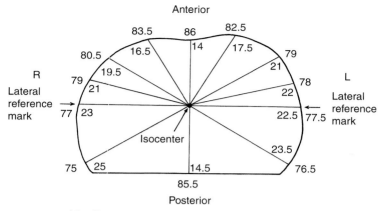

Figure 22-8. Source-skin distance (SSD) varies with the patient's separation when an isocentric technique is used. Note that, using a combination of SSD measurements, a patient's separation can be calculated. In this example, the anterior SSD through the central axis (CA) is 86 cm (depth of 14 cm) and the posterior SSD is 85.5 cm (depth of 14.5 cm). The IFD can be calculated by adding the two depths (14 + 14.5 = 28.5 cm).

Before the administration of any contrast medium, a careful evaluation of the patient should be performed. Severe allergic reactions to some contrast agents, requiring emergency intervention, have been observed. In addition, barium sulfate, which is administered orally or rectally, may be contraindicated with a suspected bowel perforation or obstruction. The proper selection and administration of the contrast medium should be evaluated before the simulation procedure.

Barium sulfate, which is not absorbed by the gastrointestinal (GI) tract when administered, outlines the GI tract. Before its administration, barium sulfate is prepared as a suspension in water to obtain the desired concentration or consistency. It is commonly used to visualize the esophagus, stomach, small bowel, colon, or oral cavity. Depending on the patient's condition, amount of barium, and its application, the patient should be advised as to the use of a laxative. Patients who had a small dab of barium paste placed inside the cheek to help localize a tonsillar lesion would be advised differently from someone who drank a 12-oz cup of barium to evaluate the amount of small bowel in a pelvic treatment field.

Iodinated contrast materials used in radiation therapy are usually of two types: aqueous ionic contrast medium and nonionic contrast medium.[4] Although their actions are different, both provide positive contrast (a white area on the image) of a vessel or an organ. Iodinated contrast materials are commonly used to help localize the kidneys, bladder, and prostate, and they are sometimes used in the GI tract when barium is contraindicated. Except for the GI tract, sterile procedures must be followed when administering iodinated contrast material. For example, contrast medium may be used intravenously to document the location of the kidneys (for an abdominal field) or through a bladder catheterization to assist in localizing the prostate.

Negative contrast agents, which include substances such as carbon dioxide, oxygen, and air, have a low atomic number and appear as dark areas on a radiograph. Examples of their use include a small amount of air introduced (with or without

barium) into the rectum to help define its location or the use of normal gas exchange in the thorax, which helps define some lung tumors. Another example might include a Foley catheter balloon filled with 5 to 10 mL of air within the bladder. This is used to define the inferior extent of the bladder in reference to the prostate gland.

The primary function of the fluoroscopy-based simulator is to localize the tumor volume relative to normal tissue structures. The use of contrast agents, fluoroscopy, and radiography together with other imaging modalities, such as PET, CT, and MRI, greatly enhances the ability to localize and pinpoint the tumor volume. Many of these tools are available to the radiation oncologist and radiation therapist. However, their use and application may vary from patient to patient and institution to institution. The actual process of simulating a patient on a fluoroscopy-based simulator, which is discussed in the next section, varies less.

FLUOROSCOPY-BASED SIMULATION PROCEDURE

The use of fluoroscopy-based simulators during tumor and normal tissue localization is well documented.[5,9,19] The localization of a treatment field during simulation must reflect precisely what will happen in the treatment room. Patient position, beam alignment, and field size must be the same at the end of simulation and the beginning of treatment. In this section, the simulation procedure is discussed in detail. Box 22-1 outlines the common components involved in a conventional fluoroscopy-based simulation procedure.

Presimulation Planning

An assessment of all relevant patient information and an evaluation of possible treatment approaches before the patient arrives are ideal. This is especially true for difficult cases involving patients who have had previous treatment or have extensive disease.[13] In many institutions, this may be done as

1. Presimulation planning
2. Room preparation
3. Explanation of procedure
4. Patient positioning and immobilization
5. Operation of simulator controls
6. Setting field size parameters
7. Exposure factors
8. Radiographic exposure and image processing
9. Documenting pertinent data
10. Final procedures

part of a morning conference, where the discussion of specific cases occurs among the radiation therapy team members. The discussion during these meetings should relate to treatment planning, simulation, and concerns for those patients under treatment, although, because of busy schedules or a late addition to the day's schedule, this is not always possible. Minimally, the patient's history and physical examination notes should be reviewed by the radiation oncologist and radiation therapist, using other available pertinent information such as radiographs; PET, CT, and MRI scans; pathology reports; and operating reports.

The importance of the therapist and physician consultation before the actual simulation cannot be overemphasized. Radiation oncologists, even within the same institution, vary in their approach to simulation and treatment. For example, one physician may prefer to use a small amount of barium in the rectum for all endometrial cases, whereas another physician may use flexible beaded tubing to identify the rectum radiographically. In addition, the physician may be called away from the simulation area during the procedure and may not be immediately available to answer questions. Therefore, a plan should be established before beginning the simulation procedure if at all possible.[18]

Additional attention in the presimulation planning process will involve determining patient positioning and the selection or preparation of immobilization devices.

Patient Positioning

One of the weakest links in treatment planning is patient positioning.[4] If the patient is not comfortable and does not remain still during treatment administration, then sophisticated treatment plans and elaborate immobilization devices are not as effective. If a stable position cannot be maintained and reproduced daily, the result is either a geometric miss of the target volume or irradiation of greater amounts of uninvolved normal tissue.[11]

For most simulation procedures, the patient is positioned supine or prone. Occasionally, other positions are used. On rare occasions, a sitting position may be necessary because of the patient's medical condition. For example, a patient may need to be positioned in an erect or a semierect position (sitting on the end of the treatment table) because of an advanced lung mass that has compromised the patient's breathing and the return of blood through the superior vena cava.

Daily reproducibility is essential. The positioning of the patient for treatment is usually depicted by a patient alignment system (Figure 22-9). Three-directional lasers accomplish this through the transverse and sagittal planes. A patient's age, weight, and general health, as well as the anatomic area to be simulated, can affect the patient's position. Usually, India ink tattoos, visual skin marks, or references to topographic anatomy are used to delineate the treatment area. Immobilization devices improve the accuracy and reproducibility of a planned course of treatment. To achieve this, the integrity of a patient's position must be maintained throughout the course of treatment. As little as one or two patient positioning errors can increase the possibility of missing the treatment volume. This can reduce the dose to the tumor volume considerably, as well as treat areas that do not need treatment. Thus, daily reproduction of the prescribed, planned, and simulated treatment is essential to its outcome. Also important is prohibiting patient movement during simulation, treatment setup, and treatment delivery.[10,11] Effective immobilization is essential to achieving this goal.

Traditional positioning, immobilization, and alignment using modern head and neck practice techniques includes conventional thermoplastic masking, baseplate fixation to the treatment couch, three-point laser alignment, and weekly portal film evaluation. This may not be suitable for intensity-modulated radiation therapy (IMRT), in which highly conformal treatment techniques commonly establish steep dose gradients between tumor and avoidance structures.[7] Additional attention to immobilization may be necessary for patients receiving IMRT.

Patient Immobilization

Accuracy and reproducibility of daily setup are essential to reducing possible treatment complications. Once the threshold dose for tumor response has been reached, small increases in the absorbed dose may make large differences in tumor control. In a similar manner, once the threshold for normal tissue injury has been reached, small increases in dose may greatly increase the risk of complications.[15] Thus, the need for accurate patient positioning and the maintenance of that positioning by immobilization is evident.

Although the need for immobilization is apparent, achieving it is not always simple or easy. Effective immobilization devices constrain the patient from moving during treatment and do the following:
- Aid in daily treatment setup and reproducibility
- Provide immobilization of the patient or treatment area with minimal discomfort to the patient
- Support the conditions prescribed in the treatment plan
- Increase precision and accuracy of treatment

It is also important that immobilization devices provide the following benefits:
- Are rigid and durable enough to withstand an entire course of treatment
- Facilitate the patient's condition and treatment unit limitations

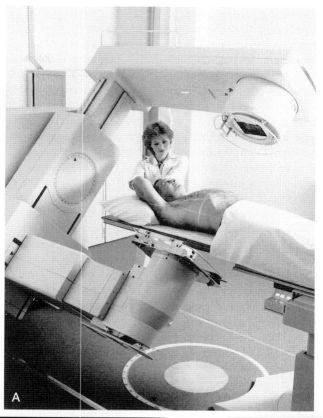

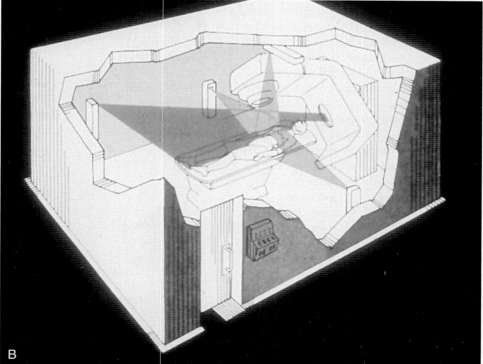

Figure 22-9. Usually two side lasers and an overhead laser are used to accurately define the location of the isocenter during simulation **(A)**, which demonstrates an oblique setup on a Philips SLS Conventional Simulator, and **(B)** treatment delivery, which shows the THER-A-CROSS system. The directional lasers correspond to external reference marks on the patient. (A, Courtesy Philips Medical Systems, Shelton, Conn. B, Courtesy Gammex RMI, Milwaukee, Wis.)

In addition, immobilization and positioning aids that can be adapted for many patients with minimal modification and that are cost-effective are desirable. They can usually be broadly divided into three categories: positioning aids, simple immobilization, and complex immobilization.[20] **Patient positioning aids** are devices designed to place the patient in a particular position for treatment. There is generally very little structure in these devices to ensure that the patient does not move. Simple immobilization devices restrict some movement but usually require the patient's voluntary cooperation. **Complex immobilization devices** are individualized immobilizers that restrict patient movement and ensure reproducibility in positioning.

Positioning aids are the most commonly used devices in patient setup. In general, they are widely available and easy to use and may be used for more than one patient, thus making them convenient and inexpensive. Head holders are probably the most commonly used positioning aids. They are usually made of formed plastic or molded polyurethane foam. They come in a variety of heights and neck contours. The different heights and contours allow for the desired head and neck angulation (flexion or extension) to achieve the best treatment position. Patients who must be treated in prone position may use different versions of a support device, which elevates the face from the tabletop and supports the head or chin. There are also devices that support the patient's chin while the patient is in the prone position. This device typically may be angled to have the patient in the desired position but the face and forehead are left virtually free from pressure.

A variety of sponge pillows and foam cushions are available. Various sizes and shapes are useful in different treatment positions. Foam neck rolls assist in proper chin extension, and other shapes and sizes are particularly useful in positioning extremities. Foam cushions and pillows also tend to make patients more comfortable on hard treatment and simulation tables. Comfortable patients are more likely to be cooperative and are better able to maintain treatment position, both of which contribute to setup reproducibility and treatment accuracy.

The positioning devices mentioned in this chapter are widely used in radiation oncology departments. They assist the therapist in positioning the patient for treatment. Most are designed to be comfortable for the patient, which encourages him or her to maintain proper treatment position. These devices will not, however, prevent patient movement during treatment. The patient must be cooperative and fully understand the importance of not moving during setup or treatment in order for the devices to be effective.

Simple immobilization devices are commonly used in addition to positioning aids. They typically provide some restriction of movement and stability of treatment position in cooperative patients. However, patients who insist on moving will not be entirely deterred by these devices.

The least complex and most readily available simple immobilization tool is tape. Masking tape or paper tape is a standard supply in almost every treatment room. Plastic or cloth straps with Velcro at the ends can sometimes be substituted for tape.

Another very simple and accessible immobilization device is the rubber band. Large rubber bands, approximately 1 to 2 cm in thickness, can be used to bind the patient's feet together when he or she is in supine position. This helps ensure that the legs and feet are consistently in a reproducible position by limiting hip motion.

A number of devices are available to restrict patient movement for treatment of the head and neck area. With some slight variation, most consist of a head frame and/or a bite block. The head frame can be used for many different patients. Each patient will require his or her own bite block. The bite block serves two purposes. It helps the patient maintain the position of the chin, and it moves the tongue out of the treatment area. Bite blocks can be made of cork, Aquaplast pellets, or dental wax.

Immobilization of the shoulders, arms, and legs can be accomplished using several methods, including using arm-to-foot straps and a fully adjustable carbon fiber shoulder depression system that is designed to increase setup reproducibility and reduce patient motion without requiring a large sheet of thermoplastic covering the shoulders (Figure 22-10). The primary purpose is to move the patient's shoulders out of lateral head and neck fields.

Simple immobilization devices are easy to use and generally cost-effective. Items such as tape and rubber bands are inexpensive. Some devices may be used by several patients over time, which reduces cost. In choosing to use any simple

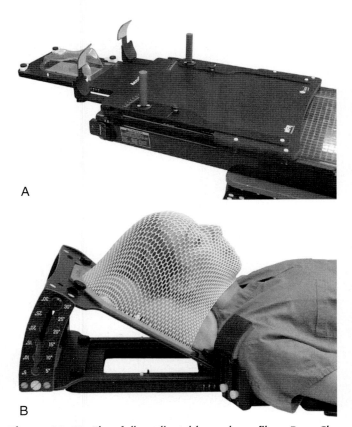

A

B

Figure 22-10. The fully adjustable carbon fiber Bear-Claw (WFR/Aquaplast) shoulder depression system **(A)** is designed to increase setup reproducibility and reduce patient motion without requiring a large sheet of thermoplastic covering the shoulders. An adjustable device **(B)** is also available for the treatment of pituitary adenomas and other tumors. (Courtesy WFR/Aquaplast Corp, Wyckoff, NJ.)

immobilization device, the radiation therapist must keep the patient in mind. Patients must understand the importance of holding still during treatment and must cooperate with the radiation therapist; otherwise, any simple immobilization device will be ineffective.

Complex immobilization devices are becoming increasingly popular because there are many new products available and the use of complex 3D and 4D treatment planning techniques, which demand rigid immobilization, has increased. Because each device is individualized, they tend to be more costly. However, the advantages are that unusual patient positions can be achieved, and, in many cases, portal markings can be made on the device, thus alleviating the need for patients to keep skin markings. Complex immobilization devices can be made of a number of different products, such as plaster, carbon fiber, plastic, and Styrofoam. The materials used will depend on the treatment area, availability of materials, and individual practitioner preference.

The earliest complex immobilization devices were constructed of plaster of paris. Plaster is still used today in some radiation oncology centers. The plaster is used to make a cast of the body part to be treated. Preparing a plaster cast is fairly easy. A thin piece of cloth or plastic wrap is placed over the part to be immobilized. Plaster of paris strips are prepared and applied. A number of strips must be used for the cast to be thick and strong enough so that it will maintain its shape and not break during the course of treatment. Care must also be taken to allow the strips to dry thoroughly before removing the cast because failure to do so will jeopardize the cast's integrity.

Foaming agents, such as Alpha Cradle (Smithers Medical Products, Inc.), have become widely used immobilization devices (Figure 22-11). It is popular because it can be used to immobilize practically any anatomic part, such as the head and neck area, the thorax, and the extremities. Before being made for the individualized patient, a shell with a plastic bag or other protective sheeting and a set of foam agents are set aside. When the foaming agents are combined and placed in the plastic-covered shell, they begin to expand. When a patient is positioned in the shell, the foam automatically contours or molds around the patient. After approximately 10 minutes, the foam will have hardened and the cradle is complete and ready to use. Making the cradle takes very little time on the therapist's part. The chemical reaction of the foaming agents produces a small amount of heat, which most patients do not find uncomfortable. One concern in the making this type of immobilization device is the safe use of the foaming agents. Inappropriate use of the agents and inaccurate disposal of their containers after use could lead to environmental problems and/or hazardous situations.[19]

Another immobilization device that is currently available is called **Vac-Lok** (CIVCO, Inc.) (Figure 22-12). This device consists of a cushion and a vacuum compression pump. The patient is placed into treatment position on a partially inflated cushion. The cushion is partially evacuated until it is semirigid, and the therapist molds it around the area to be immobilized. Once the shape is established, the vacuum procedure is completed until the cushion is completely rigid. Cushions are available in several shapes and sizes to accommodate most anatomic sites. The advantage to using this system is that the cushions can be deflated, cleaned, and reused after a patient has completed his or her treatment course.[14]

Thermoplastic molds (WFR/Aquaplast Corp) is yet another commonly used immobilization device (Figure 22-13). The thermoplastic becomes pliable when warmed in a hot water bath. When pliable, it can be molded around the patient. The material comes in sheets, perforated or unperforated. It is lightweight and easy to use in making immobilization devices and is very popular for immobilization for head and neck treatment. Using an Aquaplast mask requires the addition of a headrest and some type of frame to secure the mask on the patient and to the table during setup and treatment. **Bite blocks** made of cork, Aquaplast pellets, or dental wax may also be used with a mask to position the chin and move the tongue out of the treatment area. Although thermoplastic molds have traditionally been used for immobilization of the head, other uses include the head and shoulders (Figure 22-13, B), pelvic immobilization, full body molds, and supports for large breasts (Figure 22-14).

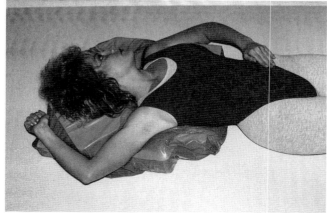

Figure 22-11. Alpha Cradle. (Courtesy Smithers Medical Products, Inc, Akron, Ohio.)

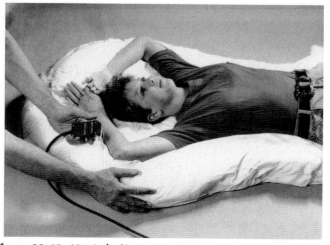

Figure 22-12. Vac-Lok. (Courtesy CIVCO, Inc, Orange City, Iowa.)

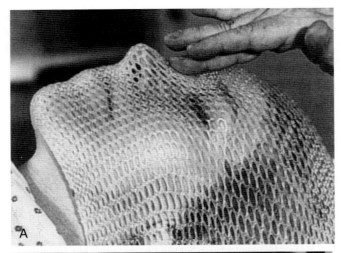

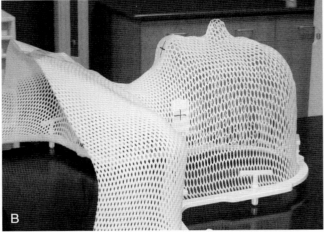

Figure 22-13. A, Aquaplast mask. **B**, Thermoplastic immobilization device for head and shoulders. (A, Courtesy WFR/Aquaplast Corp, Wyckoff, NJ. B, Courtesy Paula Keogh, Maine Medical Center, Portland, Me.)

There are several advantages to using a thermoplastic immobilizer. Patient markings can be made directly on the mask or on tape placed on the mask. The perforated plastic also helps patients feel more comfortable because they can breath and see through the perforations.[21] The casts may be cut to further increase patient comfort, especially if the mask is tight around the eyes and forehead or if a patient feels claustrophobic. The treatment field may also be cut out to reduce beam attenuation, thus minimizing possibility of skin reactions with lower beam energies. It should be noted, however, that excessive cutting reduces the integrity of this immobilizer. In addition, modifications in the mask to accommodate weight loss or reduction in swelling can be made on a completed mask at any time during the course of treatment. A heat gun may be used to heat the problem area until it is pliable, and then changes may be made.

In addition, other important immobilization devices used to set up and position specific treatment areas, such as for breast and pelvic treatments, are available. A traditional breast board (see Figure 22-14) may be used to abduct the affected arm and shoulder away from the chestwall and at the same time elevate the patient on an adjustable angle board for patient positioning and daily reproducibility. A "wingboard" (Figure 22-15) is more commonly used to abduct both arms above the patient's head and may be preferred for CT simulation. A "belly board" (Figure 22-16) is commonly used to treat pelvic malignancies with the patient in the prone position. It has adjustable inserts to accommodate a variety of patients and provides a means of reducing the amount of small bowel in the treatment field. A large, angled, prone headrest (Figure 22-16) allows more comfort for the patient's upper chest and head area.

Although complex immobilization devices are somewhat time-consuming and costly to make, they allow for customized patient positioning options. They typically provide more

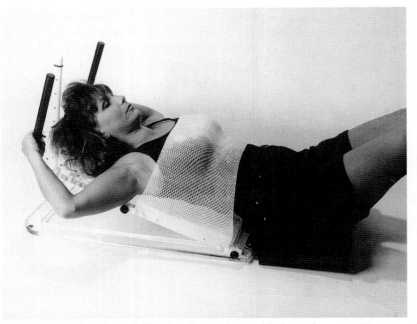

Figure 22-14. Aquaplast immobilization for patient with large breasts. (Courtesy WFR/ Aqaplast Corp, Wyckoff, NJ.)

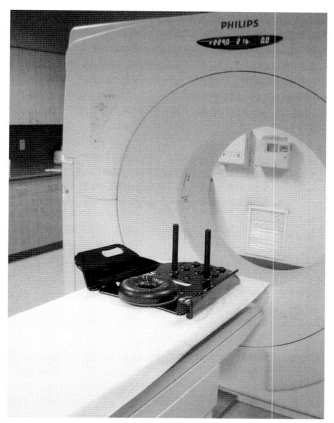

Figure 22-15. A "wingboard" is used to abduct both arms above the patient's head and may be preferred for CT simulation. (Courtesy Paula Keogh, Maine Medical Center, Portland, Me.)

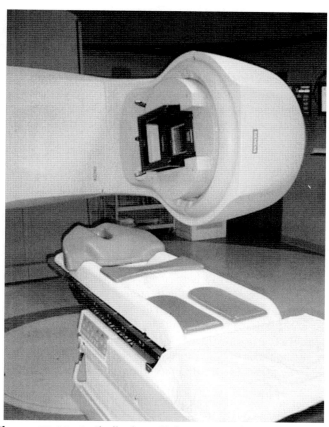

Figure 22-16. A "belly board" is commonly used to treat patients in the prone position. (Courtesy Paula Keogh, Maine Medical Center, Portland, Me.)

stability and prevent patient movement and usually save time in daily treatment procedures, thus justifying the cost for many practitioners.

With the use of record and verify systems, tolerances may be set on many of the treatment unit's positions, such as couch height and couch positions in the left/right and inferior/superior directions. If this is a consideration, indexing complex immobilization devices, such as thermoplastic immobilization devices and foaming agent devices to the treatment couch, may provide for "tighter" tolerance settings. Specific points may be marked during the simulation process on the immobilization device and will correspond to the relative position of the device located on the treatment couch. In some situations, the immobilization device is secured to the same spot, through perhaps predrilled holes along the lateral length of the tabletop, on both the simulator and treatment couch. During the treatment setup process, the immobilization device is indexed or positioned on the treatment couch in the same position it was in during simulation.

Over the years, a number of immobilization devices have been developed and used to improve the treatment outcome for radiation therapy patients. Some of the devices are simple yet effective in immobilizing patients. Others are more complex and are made individually for the particular patient. The choice of immobilization devices depends on many considerations,

including the condition of the patient, the area to treated, and the availability and cost of materials. Radiation therapists must be prepared to recommend and use the appropriate device for a particular patient to ensure the best possible treatment outcome for that patient.

Certain accommodations for unique cases and an assessment of whether the simulation procedure is simple, intermediate, or complex should also be made. It is important to consider the patient's fears and anxieties, especially when performing simulations on small children and others with special needs. For all cases, if a clear treatment approach is known at the beginning of the simulation, the procedure will go more efficiently and accurately, enhancing the patient's confidence in the entire process and reducing the time needed to complete it.[13]

Preparing the Room

Effective use of time on the simulator is essential. Proper room preparation can aid in the effective use of that time. A review of all the pertinent information needed for the simulation procedure allows the therapist to prepare the simulation room in advance. The time demands on the simulator can be pressing, bearing in mind that one fluoroscopy-based simulator can serve two or three treatment units. A typical fluoroscopy-based simulation day involves simulating 3 to 12 cases, depending on the complexity of the treatment plan, the number of treatment units in the department, the total number of new patients seen at the institution each year, and other factors. To explain the specific needs concerning the simulator's room preparation, three examples are provided.

Head and Neck. The room is first cleaned from the simulation before this patient. If a thermoplastic mask is used, the temperature in the water tank is checked. A clean sheet or paper sheet is placed on the simulator couch. A headrest (which can range from A to F and will be either transparent plastic or a solid foamlike material) selected for the simulation procedure is related to the patient's anatomy. Often this simulation requires a C or D headrest. This should elevate the chin and isolate the treatment area (neck).

If the patient requires a stent, bite block, or special mouthpiece, this is made before the simulation begins. Wires help the therapist visualize a surgical scar or any other pertinent anatomic areas. Pull straps or some kind of mechanism should be available (if needed) to pull or push the top of the shoulders down inferiorly and out of the treatment field. Tape should be readily available, possibly placed at the head of the couch. This is useful for drawing any marks on the thermoplastic mask (if used) or securing a wire on the patient's skin. A cloth or paper towels should be available to dry the excess water from the thermoplastic mask. The **treatment volume** may have already been decided during the presimulation session with the physician, making the simulation more accurate and time efficient.

Thorax. Because the patient generally receives part of the treatment through the treatment couch from a direct posterior field or posterior oblique portal, a table pad is not recommended. The simulation must duplicate the treatment setup in all aspects. A cushion on the table may interfere with reproducibility. If the patient is in severe pain, accommodations required for a pad or cushion during treatment and simulation can be calculated. The B headrest, which positions the head in a neutral position, may be appropriate when the treatment portal will not cover the cervical lymph nodes. If the cervical lymph nodes must be encompassed in the treatment volume, a C headrest may be used to elevate the chin more, thus isolating the neck lymph nodes.

Depending on the patient's arm position, an Alpha Cradle can be constructed or the **Vac-Lok** used to provide patient **immobilization**. This increases the stability of the patient's arms (especially if they are positioned above the head) and increases reproducibility during treatment. An appropriate field size is set, positioning the collimator with no rotation.

If a CT scan is needed for treatment planning purposes, the radiation therapist must arrange this ahead of time. This will involve additional time for the patient and therapist. This may be performed on the conventional simulator if it is equipped with a CT mode or may be scheduled on a conventional CT scanner in the radiology department. If the scan is performed on a conventional CT scanner, the therapist must accompany the patient to ensure the patient is in the same treatment position when scanned. Radiopaque markers may also be needed to obtain accurate CT data for treatment planning purposes. BBs, wires, arrows, or another type of radiopaque material is necessary to visualize specific points of interest on a radiograph and/or CT scan. This is done to help the dosimetrist transfer these anatomic points to the treatment planning computer. For example, a cross-table lateral film may be taken to provide data for a dose calculation to the spinal cord. A chain or wire is taped to the patient's posterior surface before the simulation begins.

Pelvis. The room is cleaned from the simulation before this patient. If an Alpha Cradle is used to immobilize the lower extremities, it is constructed first with the patient in the supine treatment position. A rubber band may be secured around the metatarsal area to immobilize the patient's lower extremities during the construction of the Alpha Cradle. A comfortable headrest is selected along with an appropriate "foam ring" or suitable device to secure the hands on the upper thorax.

Any contrast agents used to visualize the bladder or rectum are prepared ahead of time and are administered by the physician before fluoroscopy. This may require a sterile tray to catherize the male penis for prostate localization.

If a CT scan is needed for treatment planning purposes, the therapist must arrange this ahead of time. This may be performed on a conventional CT scanner in the radiology department. If the scan is performed on a conventional CT scanner, the therapist must accompany the patient to ensure the patient is in the same treatment position when scanned. Radiopaque markers may also be needed to obtain accurate CT data for treatment planning purposes.

Details concerning the preparation of the room become more important with a busy schedule. Establishing a definite treatment approach at the beginning of the simulation procedure allows the process to proceed more efficiently and accurately. The patient gains confidence in the radiation therapy staff if one of the first impressions of the department is positive. This can be enhanced if the simulation procedure is accurate, organized, and not rushed. It also provides an opportunity to educate the patient and answer questions concerning the treatment process, side effects, and skin care.

Explanation of Simulation Procedure

Assessment. The therapist must assess the patient's needs, recognize cultural differences, respond to nonverbal communication, and then attempt to communicate therapeutically and effectively with the patient.

In the conventional simulator, the radiation therapist should assess the patient's physical condition and emotional state. The therapist should determine whether the patient is nervous, fearful, or withdrawn. If a patient requires oxygen or medications or has difficulty standing, sitting, or walking, the therapist can try to make the patient more comfortable. If a patient has difficulty hearing or speaking, provisions can also be made. Good observation and listening skills are essential to proper patient assessment.

Communication. Our entire health care system is based on effective communication. Miscommunication can have a major effect on the patient's care. The radiation therapist should also establish an environment conducive to communication. If there are distractions in the area, such as unwanted noises or the usual distractions of a radiation oncology department, it may be preferable to retreat to a private area to communicate with the patient (the simulator room is much better for this than a busy waiting room). Radiation therapists must establish an environment where they can facilitate the communication clearly, effectively, and therapeutically. Prior to the simulation procedure, the therapist should explain the procedure appropriate to the patient's level of understanding and inform the patient what will be required of him or her during the procedure. This should be done in a professionally responsible and compassionate manner.

Educating the Patient and Family. Professionally, the radiation therapist is obligated to educate the patient not only about the physical aspects of radiation therapy that the patient can see and feel but also about the emotional aspects of radiation therapy. The simulation treatment procedure should be explained in detail. This explanation should be done slowly and clearly, using all therapeutic communication techniques. The equipment must be explained to the patient. It is helpful to mention that the simulation is not an actual treatment and that the conventional simulator is an x-ray machine not a therapeutic treatment machine. The patient should be shown where he or she will lie on the table, which way the head should be placed, whether the patient will be supine or prone, and whether he or she will be on a belly board or on a wingboard with the arms above the head. Basic patient positioning should be communicated along with an explanation of why that position is needed. This facilitates patient cooperation.

The patient should also be given an explanation of what procedures to follow after the simulation. This might include instructions on how to take care of the skin marks, as well as the skin itself, before the treatments begin and while under treatment. When special orders are needed before the patient is to receive treatment, such as arriving for treatment with a full or empty bladder, this should be communicated at this time. When barium (oral or rectal) is used during the simulation, follow-up instructions are needed. An appointment time for the first treatment should be discussed, providing the therapist's name and department number in case communication is necessary before the next appointment.

Operating Fluoroscopy-Based Conventional Simulator Controls

Accurate patient positioning requires an understanding of how the mechanical, optical, and radiographic components of the fluoroscopy-based simulator work. An understanding of their use is important. Mechanical components of the simulator include the motions of gantry rotation, collimator movements, and treatment couch. Optical components may include the laser system, optical distance indicator (ODI), and field light indicator.

Previous background in radiography is helpful, but not essential, in understanding the radiographic components of the conventional simulator. State regulations may require the use of technique charts, which include guidelines for selecting kVp, mA, and time factors used in deciding radiographic exposure techniques. In some institutions, in an attempt to increase familiarity with conventional simulation procedures, certain therapists will perform most of the simulation procedures.

This means they rotate less frequently, if at all, through other (treatment) areas of the department.

It is also important to know the limits of the mechanical, optical, and radiographic components. For example, it is important to know the limits of gantry rotation with the use of specific immobilization devices or table angles. This is helpful in avoiding possible collisions on the treatment unit. In addition, it is important to know how to handle a burned-out ODI light bulb partway through a simulation procedure. Can the simulation procedure be completed or should it be interrupted? This will depend on when during the simulation process the ODI fails.

Radiographically, obtaining good-quality lateral pelvic images may require the use of a double- or triple-exposure technique with some x-ray generators. This may be caused by heat limits on the x-ray tube. Two shorter exposures, instead of one longer one, may produce a better-quality image and less overall heat units on the x-ray tube. A lateral view of the pelvis can be a most challenging image to produce for the radiation therapist.

Setting Field Parameters

Familiarity with both the controls in the simulator room and those located on the control console is essential for a smooth, accurate, and efficient simulation procedure. Once the patient has been oriented to the simulation procedure and positioned on the simulator couch, the actual localization process can begin.

Establishing the field parameters may be done in one or more conventional simulation session(s), depending on the complexity of the case. It is the complex cases that often require more than one session. In these situations, the target volume may not be visible on routine radiographs. It may be close to sensitive structures. Sometimes previous diagnostic studies identifying the location of the target volume were obtained with the patient in a different position from that of the simulation. In those cases, the primary purpose of the first simulation is to establish a frame of reference between the data obtained during conventional simulation and previously obtained diagnostic information, such as a CT scan.[13,20]

Field parameters such as width, length, gantry angle, collimator angle, and position of the isocenter should be established for both the SSD and SAD (isocentric) setup. Initially, an estimate of the tumor volume may be established before fluoroscopy. This may be done by positioning the isocenter and setting a field width and length. The isocenter is positioned at the CA (middle of the treatment field) on the patient's skin for a SSD approach and within the patient for a SAD technique. The locations of the CA and field edges are then more accurately localized, usually with the aid of fluoroscopy.

Orthogonal films and a contour, which provide 3D information, may be used with the isocentric technique. For example, several fields may be used in an attempt to control esophageal cancer and at the same time limit dose to surrounding normal tissues. Here the patient's isocenter may be established using oral contrast and documented with an orthogonal pair of radiographs. At this point, two radiographs have been taken to document the position of the isocenter. The primary purpose of the first simulation is to establish a frame of reference. A CT scan is then performed with the patient in the treatment position (perhaps in the radiology department). A shift in the isocenter may be necessary based on information about the tumor volume obtained from the CT scan. Any shifts can be measured from the original isocenter (first simulation) on the first day of treatment or verified on the simulator during a second session.

There is no one universally accepted approach to establishing the field parameters. For simple parallel opposed treatment fields, a short simulation session may be all that is necessary. More complex cases can be simulated using various approaches. A longer single simulation session can be used to document the isocenter, field width, and length along with other setup parameters in more complex cases. Multiple conventional simulation sessions can also be used, incorporating orthogonal films and/or CT treatment planning. Even longer sessions may be required if using a virtual simulation technique.[20] Whatever approach is used, it is necessary to document the treatment fields with radiographs. Whenever possible, a radiograph should be taken for each treatment portal.

PRODUCING QUALITY RADIOGRAPHIC IMAGES

Radiographic images taken at the time of simulation document the treatment portals. Not only do they serve as part of the patient's medical record but they are also used as masters to compare with portal images (taken on the treatment unit). Quality is important. Several aspects of producing good-quality radiographs are discussed in this section, including selecting exposure techniques, orienting the film, processing the film, and documenting the radiographic images (see Chapter 6 for additional information on exposure techniques).

Selecting appropriate radiographic exposure techniques is a complex process. Several important details contribute to choosing the best technical factors. The use of critical thinking skills aids in producing good-quality radiographs. This happens especially when those skills are applied to the four main technical factors (kVp, mA, time, and distance) in the right combination. Students should also be aware that exposure techniques will vary from one clinical site to the next and from one simulator to another.

Categorizing patients into a specific **body habitus** (general physical appearance and body build—see Chapter 20) is helpful in selecting adequate exposure factors. Attenuation of the x-rays will vary, depending on the patient's thickness and, to a lesser degree, the body's composition. The composition of the patient's tissues can also change because of a specific disease process. For example, it is easier to penetrate the chest without the presence of pneumonia or atelectasis. Both pathologic conditions result in increased radiation absorption. Knowing when to deviate from average exposure factors displays evidence of good critical thinking skills and is often necessary in producing useful images, especially in systems without automatic exposure control.

Before the technical factors are selected, several elements concerning the type and orientation of the film must be considered. Will a grid be used? Some departments may have the option of using a grid or various cassettes with different screen and film combinations. Other departments may use a

photostimulable plate to obtain digital images during a conventional simulation procedure (see Chapter 6 for more information). The use of a fast screen and film combination may be used in obtaining a good-quality lateral radiograph of the pelvis. Other factors to consider before exposure include centering the film, reducing the size of the diaphragm opening, and setting an appropriate source-film distance. Some conventional simulators will not allow an exposure unless the image intensifier is centered in relationship to the CA. Evidence of collimation, by reducing the diaphragm opening on the radiograph, should appear as a clear 1- to 2-cm border on the processed film. This not only makes it easier to visualize the **irradiated volume** and some surrounding anatomy but also reduces the amount of unwanted scatter radiation from reaching the film. Reducing scatter radiation generally improves radiographic contrast and the visibility of detail. Source-film distance should be recorded to document the magnification factor. This information may be needed for multileaf collimator calculations or fabricating custom shielding blocks.

Quality control experts agree that the radiographic film processor is the most sensitive variable factor in the production of a radiograph.[5] It may be the therapist's responsibility, especially in smaller satellite facilities and freestanding clinics, to monitor the quality control of the processor. This may be done through film sensitometry using a densitometer. The whole process adds a few minutes to the morning warm-up procedure on the simulator.

Documenting Pertinent Data

Information gathered during the simulation procedure needs accurate documentation. This information is essential to accurately reproduce the geometry of the setup on the treatment unit (Box 22-2). It is also used to maintain accurate medical records and to aid in the treatment planning and dose calculation processes. Documentation of pertinent information involves both marking the patient and documenting information in the patient's paper and/or electronic chart. Some institutions make use of a simulation worksheet designed to guide the therapist in documenting all of the patient's field parameters and measurements. Photographs or digital images may be taken of the patient's setup and marked with pertinent information.

One of the most important measurements obtained during the conventional simulation process is the patient's IFD or separation. This measurement directly influences the dose to both the tumor and normal tissues. Therefore it is important to use a caliper correctly in determining the patient's IFD. If the treatment area is relatively flat, then one IFD measurement is generally taken at the CA. If the treatment area is sloped, as is often the case in the thorax, then multiple IFD measurements are obtained (superior, center, and inferior field edges). Caution must be used when obtaining an IFD value in an area where there may be an air gap, as is common in the cervical and lumbar regions. Here the lordotic curve is more pronounced. Accurate IFD measurements translate into accurate dose calculations. If a CT scan is obtained as part of the simulation procedure, patient thicknesses (IFDs) can be obtained from the CT data.

There are two schools of thought in documenting and communicating the location of treatment fields. One method involves

<table>
<tr><td colspan="2">

Box 22-2   **Documentation of Treatment Field Location**

</td></tr>
</table>

• Machine parameters
• Anterior setup distance
• Treatment SSD, TSD
• Tabletop-to-isocenter distance
• Collimator width
• Collimator length
• Gantry angle
• Couch angle
• Collimator angle
• Multileaf collimator
• Electron cone
• Patient's position
• Supine/prone/other
• Arm position
• Leg position
• Head support
• Table pad/egg crate
• Immobilization devices
• Index position for immobilization device(s)
• Other special devices
• Shifts from isocenter
• Diagram of field arrangement
• Schematic diagram for field arrangement
• Shielded field diagram
• Location of central axis
• Location of field edges
• Location of tattoos
• Reference to bony anatomy
• Wedge position/orientation
• Other pertinent data
• Bolus
• Tissue compensator
• Special instructions
• Setup photographs

TSD, Target-source distance.

establishing marks on the patient's skin. The other method references bony landmarks in and around the treatment area.

Using bony landmarks, the treatment field's CA and field edge(s) are referenced to specific anatomic landmarks. For example, in the treatment of head and neck cancer, the patient's CA might be referenced 2 cm inferior and 1.3 cm posterior to the external auditory meatus. Gerbi,[6] in describing the location of the treatment field using bony landmarks, lists several advantages over the use of skin marks: (1) skin marks are highly mobile, especially for obese patients, whereas the location of the target volume remains essentially constant with respect to bony structures; (2) a resimulation is not required if the skin marks are lost; and (3) the treatment field can be easily reconstructed long after the current course of therapy.

External skin marks or permanent tattoos can also be used to reference the patient's treatment position. Small tattoos on the patient's skin may be used to reference the position of the treatment field's CA or field edges. They are applied at the time of simulation using India ink with a small-gauge needle. Semipermanent marks, applied with felt-tipped markers or carfusion (a silver nitrate–based solution effective in "staining"

the skin), also help to reference the treatment area on the patient's skin but is less accurate. A small tattoo less than 1 mm in size provides more accuracy than skin marks for laser alignment. However, tattoos must be used with caution in certain circumstances, especially in cases of obesity, weight loss, and change in tumor size, in which the skin can shift in relation to the internal anatomy.[3] Some institutions use a combination of both methods, depending on the individual case.

 If on-board imaging (OBI) devices, such as a kV x-ray tube mounted on the linear accelerator, are available, they can provide image data that are correlated with simulation and treatment planning information to ensure patient reproducibility of the setup each day. An x-ray, a fluoroscopic image, or a type of CT scan called cone beam CT can be obtained while rotating the gantry using OBI. Whichever imaging modality is used, it verifies daily patient positioning and minimizes setup errors using skin marks, tattoos, or radiographic anatomy.

Information documented in the treatment chart to aid in the daily setup of the patient may be organized in several ways and is usually institutionally dependent (Figure 22-17). This may be accomplished with a "paper" chart or, more commonly, with an electronic chart. Pertinent information should include machine parameters such as SSD (target-surface distance [TSD]); table-top-to-isocenter distance; collimator width and length (field size); and gantry, couch, and collimator angles. Any indicated shifts from the isocenter should also be documented. A description of the patient's position, along with any immobilization and support devices used in reproducing the patient's position, should be documented. Included in the setup instructions is a schematic diagram of the field arrangement. There should also be an area for setup photographs (if used); an area for a face photo; and an area describing bolus, wedges, and tissue compensator.

CONTOUR DEVICES

A **contour** is a reproduction of an external body shape, usually taken through the transverse plane of the CA of the treatment beam (or center of the treatment volume). Contours may be taken through other planes of interest in the treatment volume to provide more information about the overall dose distribution. The most accurate and common method of obtaining contour information is with CT. Manual contours are rarely performed today with the wide availability of CT data. There are instances in which it is necessary to obtain a contour by hand.

The purpose of a contour is to provide the therapist and dosimetrist with the most precise replica of the patient's body shape so that accurate information may be gathered concerning the dose distribution within the patient. The treatment volume and internal structures (tumor volume, critical organs) are transposed within the contour using data from the simulation images and/or CT or MRI films.

Manual production of an accurate contour, using solder wire, a thermoplastic tube, or a plaster strip, takes time (Figure 22-18). Often the contour is the last step in the simulation procedure, and accuracy may be compromised by the pressure to hurry and finish as a result of patient physical or

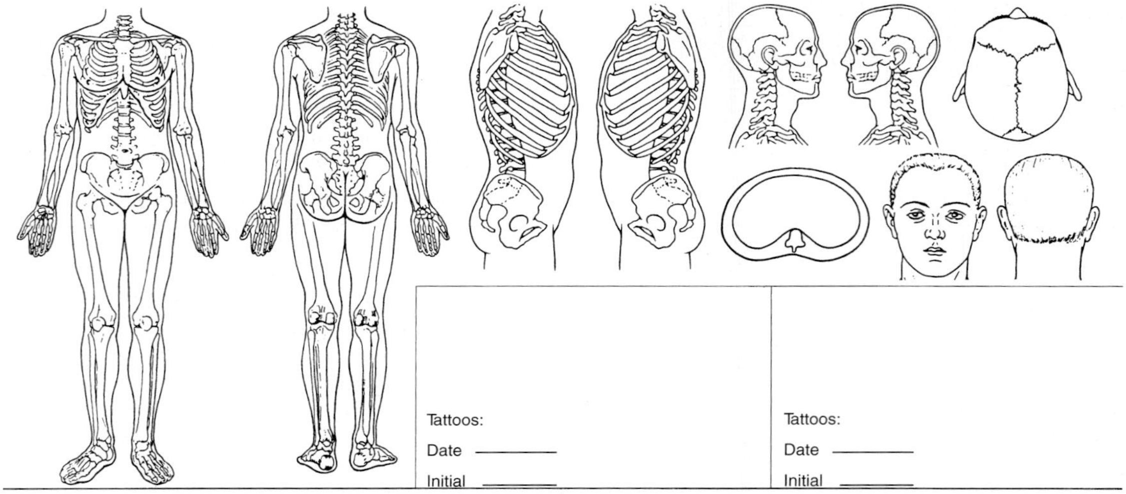

INSTRUCTIONS: Field Number(s):   Treatment Field Order

Patient position: ☐ Supine ☐ Prone ☐ Reverse on table ☐ Safety strap ☐ Full table pad
Head and neck support: _____ Pillow ↓ Head ☐ Head immobilizer ___ Neck rest ☐ Face rest ☐ Prone pillow ☐ Other_____
Leg support: ☐ Lg pillow ↓ knees ☐ Sm rd ↓ knees ☐ Lg pillow ↓ ankles ☐ No support ☐ Toe strap
Hand and arm position: ☐ Hands on chest ☐ Hands on abdomen ☐ Arms along side ☐ Arms above head ☐ Mantle position ___ Armboard ☐ Breast board ___ Arm ___ Head
Accessory devices: ☐ Tongue cork or blade ☐ Dental rolls ☐ Carriers or prosthesis ☐ Jump rope ☐ Aquaplast _____ Shims ☐ Alpha cradle ☐ Foot holder
Table position: ☐ Window ☐ Spline ☐ F.T.T. ☐ Decubitus board ☐ Lexan table extension ☐ CNS board

Special instructions

_____
_____
_____
_____
_____
_____
_____
_____
_____
_____
_____

INSTRUCTIONS: Field Number(s):   Treatment Field Order

Patient position: ☐ Supine ☐ Prone ☐ Reverse on table ☐ Safety strap ☐ Full table pad
Head and neck support: _____ Pillow ↓ Head ☐ Head immobilizer ___ Neck rest ☐ Face rest ☐ Prone pillow ☐ Other_____
Leg support: ☐ Lg pillow ↓ knees ☐ Sm rd ↓ knees ☐ Lg pillow ↓ ankles ☐ No support ☐ Toe strap
Hand and arm position: ☐ Hands on chest ☐ Hands on abdomen ☐ Arms along side ☐ Arms above head ☐ Mantle position ___ Armboard ☐ Breast board ___ Arm ___ Head
Accessory devices: ☐ Tongue cork or blade ☐ Dental rolls ☐ Carriers or prosthesis ☐ Jump rope ☐ Aquaplast _____ Shims ☐ Alpha cradle ☐ Foot holder
Table position: ☐ Window ☐ Spline ☐ F.T.T. ☐ Decubitus board ☐ Lexan table extension ☐ CNS board

Special instructions

_____
_____
_____
_____
_____
_____
_____
_____
_____
_____
_____

Figure 22-17. The treatment portion of the patient's paper chart is used to document the patient's setup parameters. (Courtesy of Mayo Clinic, Rochester, Minn.)

department schedule concerns. If a contour is inaccurate, adequate treatment planning may be compromised. The setup distances may not correspond to the actual treatment distances encountered during patient positioning.

CT-generated contours are the most accurate of all transverse contouring methods, because there is no hand molding or manipulation to introduce significant error. An important point to note is that the patient must be in the exact treatment position on the scanner with a flat tabletop comparable with the simulator and treatment tables. Also, a large-diameter CT aperture (85 cm) should be used to allow patient positioning in the CT scanner that exactly matches simulation and treatment. Patient immobilization devices should be used that will not cause image artifacts.[11] Sometimes the total contour of the patient is missing from the field of view, especially on large patients, which would cause errors in the accuracy of the information. The external

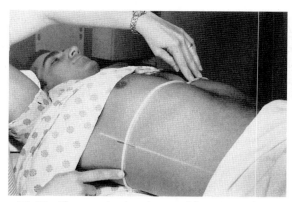

Figure 22-18. Thermoplastic tube used for contouring.

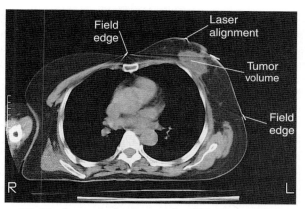

Figure 22-19. Computed tomography (CT) slice used for treatment planning. Note how the radiopaque markers on this paitent with breast cancer are seen on the outer portion of the patient's contour. This provides useful information for the treatment planning team (tumor volume is marked).

alignment marks on the patient should be marked with plastic radiopaque catheters so that they can be delineated on the CT scan for reference (Figure 22-19).

Many different materials and devices are used in the production of contours, each having both advantages and disadvantages. Each department must assess its own needs in deciding which means are to be used. Although CT is the mainstay of patient contouring, many materials and methods can be used effectively. Table 22-3 summarizes the advantages of several methods.

TREATMENT VERIFICATION

As discussed earlier in the chapter, *simulation* can have more than one meaning. First, it is a general term describing the mockup process. This can include the selection of immobilization devices, radiographic documentation of treatment ports, measurement of the patient, construction of patient contours, and shaping of fields.[9] For most cases in most institutions, the word *simulation* is applied to this type of procedure. However, it can also refer to a type of treatment verification. This may be a more specific term, in which the simulator artificially duplicates the actual treatment conditions by confirming measurements and verifying treatment.[20]

Verification simulation is a final check that each of the planned treatment beams covers the tumor or target volume and does not irradiate critical normal structures.[20] This is usually done as the second part of a two-step process on the simulator (it may also be performed on the treatment unit during the first

day of treatment using portal images — a type of "part B" simulation procedure). It involves taking images of each of the treatment beams using external marks and other immobilization devices intended for treatment reproducibility. An example should help further explain this idea.

A patient with cancer involving the head of the pancreas might benefit from external beam radiation therapy. Two simulation procedures are necessary. The first simulation is performed to establish a point of reference for the radiation oncologist and treatment planning staff (part A of the simulation procedure). This is accomplished through fluoroscopy and orthogonal films. An isocenter is located in the patient and then documented by reference to external landmarks or tattoos. At the end of the first simulation, a target volume has not been established. A field size may not have been selected. Before the second simulation (in this case called *treatment verification* or *part B* of the simulation procedure), additional treatment planning must be done.

Often the patient's tumor volume is drawn on the contour or planned with the aid of a CT or MRI scan with the patient in the treatment position. The information from the CT scan or contour is transferred to the treatment planning computer, where a new isocenter may be determined based on the extent of disease. Usually only a slight shift, if any, from the original isocenter is needed. The second simulation or verification is done as a

Table 22-3	Advantages and Disadvantages of Contouring Materials/Methods		
Material/Method	**Advantage**		**Disadvantage**
Solder wire	Reusability, pliability		Pliability (distortions)
Plaster strips	Inexpensive, transferability of surface ink markings		Drying time, messy, not reusable
Aquaplast contour tubes	Inexpensive, reusable, shapes well		Drying time, not well-suited for intricate areas
Pantograph contouring device	Time-saving operation, reproduces detail well		Cost, size, storage space required
CT	Accurate transverse views		Cost of interface
MRI	Accurate transverse, coronal, and sagittal contours		Cost of interface
Sonography	Discernible transverse correlation of internal structures		Poor quality of imaged deep structures

CT, Computed tomography; *MRI*, magnetic resonance imaging.

final check. Does each of the treatment beams cover the target volume? Are any critical structures such as the spinal cord affected? Radiographic or portal images of each of the treatment beams using external marks and other immobilization devices are taken to complete the verification process.

Treatment verification, which captures images electronically or with film, are produced in the radiation therapy treatment room on the first day of treatment and provides assurance that the correct area is irradiated. Ideally, portal images or DRRs of each treatment are compared with the simulation images before treatment. Greater differences between the simulation images and portal images as compared with differences between one portal image and the next have been documented.[6,16] Extra time should be scheduled the first day of treatment to evaluate the patient's position and verify the treatment plan. Errors and setup inaccuracies are more common during the transfer of information from the simulator to the treatment unit. This stresses the importance of verification on the first day of treatment.

EMERGENCY PROCEDURES

Any sudden, unexpected situation requiring immediate attention is an emergency. Fortunately the radiation oncology department generally does not experience this often. There are, of course, emergencies in which a patient may need immediate treatment because of the sudden onset of symptoms. Examples of this include treatment for spinal cord compression, excessive bleeding from endometrial cancer, or a life-threatening obstruction caused by the unchecked growth of the tumor. Even in these situations, there is some time for planning. The simulation procedure can be discussed and a plan developed for the

patient's treatment. This plan may be as simple as several large fractions of radiation to a single field.

Other situations may arise during a conventional simulation procedure that may require immediate attention. Certification in cardiopulmonary resuscitation equips the therapist to respond to specific medical conditions involving an obstructed airway or heart attack. In addition, a "crash cart" should be available. Usually the cart contains specific drugs and equipment needed to respond to certain emergencies, such as cardiac arrest or anaphylactic shock. The most common cause of anaphylactic shock during a simulation procedure is an allergic reaction to the contrast medium.

In any case, there should be access to a nearby phone to initiate a response. Many hospitals have specific procedures to initiate a rapid response, such as "code 99" or "code blue." Knowing what to do before an emergency occurs can sometimes make the difference between life and death.

The mechanical operations of the simulator equipment can create a potential hazard to the patient and medical personnel. Knowing the location of "emergency off" switches is vital. These switches, which cut the power to the mechanical motions of the gantry and treatment couch, are generally incorporated into the room design and strategically located on the walls. It is also important to know the location of the main circuit breaker for the simulator. The circuit breaker generally controls power to both the mechanical components and the x-ray generator. Emergency switches are also incorporated into the simulator controls, both in the room and remotely in the shielded control area. An observation window allows the radiation therapist and others involved in the simulation process to view the patient and

Table 22-4	Anatomic Landmarks of the Head and Neck Region	
Landmark	**Description**
Superior orbital margin (SOM)	Roof of the orbit
Inferior orbital margin (IOM)	Forms the lateral margin of the bony orbit
External occipital protuberance (EOP)	Central prominence in the occipital bone
Mastoid process	Most lateral and inferior extension of the temporal bone
Zygomatic arch	Bony prominence of the cheek
Glabella	Located between the orbits
Nasion	The depression at the base of the nose
Inner canthus (IC)	Located at the medial aspect of the eye where the upper and lower eyelids meet
Outer canthus (OC)	Located at the outer aspect of the eye where the upper and lower eyelids meet
Tragus	Located near the external auditory meatus
Commissure of the mouth	Located at the junction of the upper and lower lip
C1	Lies inferior to the mastoid process
C2	Located at the level of the angle of the mandible
C3-4	Lies at the level of the hyoid bone
C4	Corresponds to the level of the thyroid cartilage
C6	Located at the level of the cricoid cartilage
C7	First prominent process of the cervical vertebrae
Sternocleidomastoid muscle	Thick band of muscle in the neck, originating at the level of the sternum and clavicle and inserting at the mastoid process of the temporal bone

mechanical motions of the equipment. It is made of thick plate glass or leaded glass and installed in the control area along the wall facing the simulator. Anticollision devices, mounted on the collimator head and image intensifier of a conventional simulator, may prevent a potential collision by terminating the power and/or sounding an audio alarm. Some simulators are equipped with an integrated computer circuitry that prevents collisions by monitoring each component through a type of internal surveillance. In addition, some simulation rooms are equipped with cameras and monitors similar to those found in the treatment rooms.

The response to any sudden, unexpected situation requiring immediate attention during the simulation procedure should be well thought out in advance. Many potential emergency situations are minimized through careful planning of the procedure and observation of the equipment.

RATIONALE OF FLOUROSCOPY-BASED SIMULATION PROCEDURES

Patients treated with radiation therapy, either for cure or for palliation, will be involved in various procedures, including simulation. It helps in figuring out the location and extent of the patient's disease and the location of sensitive normal structures. The fluoroscopy-based simulation process may include presimulation planning, room preparation, patient positioning and immobilization, operation of controls, setting field parameters, radiographic exposure, documenting pertinent data, treatment verification, and emergency procedures.

The outcome of the simulation procedure should define the anatomic area so that it is reproducible for daily treatment. Landmarks may be used to document and position the CA and field edges during a simulation procedure (Table 22-4). A complicated simulation is of little value unless it is reproducible. This means the ultimate success or failure of treatment may be directly related to the effectiveness of the simulation process.

Achieving ideal results in radiation therapy depends on delivering an appropriate dose to a well-defined region and at the same time reducing the dose to normal critical structures. Accomplishing this task demands a high degree of precision and accuracy in delivering the dose. In addition, a systematic and logical approach to the treatment of the particular disease is necessary. The use of the simulator is essential in achieving this goal.[13]

SUMMARY

- Nomenclature plays an important role in radiation therapy, including acronyms and specific terms related to simulation.
- There are three anatomic body planes used in the simulation process. They are the sagittal, coronal, and transverse planes.
- A simulator can take various forms, ranging from a simple diagnostic radiographic unit with fluoroscopy and/or computed tomography (CT) capabilities to a stand-alone CT simulator.
- Conventional simulation, also referred to as *fluoroscopy-based simulation,* implies the use of a piece of x-ray equipment capable of the same mechanical movements of a treatment unit.

- Fluoroscopy-based simulation localization procedures include the following steps: presimulation planning, patient positioning, patient immobilization, preparing the room, explanation of simulation procedure, operating fluoroscopy-based conventional simulator controls, setting field parameters, producing quality radiographic images, and documenting pertinent data.
- The incorporation of computer software, used with CT simulation and 3D treatment planning, has been a major advance in defining tumor volumes and sparing normal tissue structures.
- Several volumes used for treatment planning are defined by ICRU Report 50 and are defined as follows:
  - Gross tumor volume (GTV) indicates the gross palpable or visible tumor.
  - Clinical target volume (CTV) indicates the gross palpable or visible tumor (GTV) and a surrounding volume of tissue that may contain subclinical or microscopic disease.
  - Planning target volume (PTV) indicates the CTV plus margins for geometric uncertainties, such as patient motion, beam penumbra, and treatment setup differences.
- Verification simulation is usually done as the second part of a two-step process on the simulator (it may also be performed on the treatment unit during the first day of treatment using portal images — a type of "part B" simulation procedure). It involves taking radiographic images or portal images of each of the treatment beams.

Review Questions

Multiple Choice

1. A patient's separation = 25 cm. If the posterior SSD = 89 cm, what will be the anterior SSD measure?
   a. 87.5 cm
   b. 89 cm
   c. 88.25 cm
   d. 86 cm
2. Presimulation planning is important because it:
   a. will involve determining patient positioning and the selection or preparation of immobilization devices
   b. will help determine the patient's separation
   c. will be helpful in determining any radiographic exposure technique used during simulation
   d. will involve the patient and his or her family in the treatment process
3. The GTV treatment volume will contain:
   a. tumor
   b. involved lymphatics
   c. normal tissue
   d. all of the above
4. _____ is the initial phase of treatment planning in which actual visualization of the treatment volume is documented before treatment.
   a. Initial consultation
   b. Simulation
   c. Brachytherapy
   d. Radiation treatment

5. The distance from a source of radiation to a radiograph is:
   a. SAD
   b. SFD
   c. SSD
   d. all of the above

6. The distance from a source of radiation to the patient's skin is:
   a. SAD
   b. SSD
   c. SDD
   d. SFD

7. Historically, all of the following were critical steps in the evolution of 3D CT-based simulation *except:*
   a. virtual simulation was introduced, which provided the ability to use a diagnostic-type scanner to take multiple images
   b. CT images on a standard treatment simulator were dramatically improved, which allowed them to be used for planning purposes
   c. treatment planning computers were developed that could carry out 3D treatment planning
   d. target volumes were no longer needed to define the treatment area

8. The second part of the two-step conventional simulation process is called:
   a. CT simulation
   b. treatment
   c. verification
   d. immobilization

9. Which of the following is *not* a desirable quality of an effective and useful immobilization device?
   a. ensures immobilization with minimal patient discomfort
   b. requires additional setup time
   c. is durable enough to withstand the entire treatment plan
   d. achieves conditions prescribed in treatment plan

10. Patient immobilization is important because:
    a. sophisticated treatment planning techniques allow more accurate delivery of treatment
    b. missing the tumor once or twice in a treatment course can reduce the planned dose by 10% or more
    c. daily reproduction of the planned treatment is essential to treatment outcomes
    d. all of the above

The answers to the Review Questions can be found by logging on to our website at: *http://evolve.elsevier.com/Washington+Leaver/ principles*

Questions to Ponder

1. Discuss the importance of the presimulation consultation among radiation team members.
2. Explain the differences between GTV, CTV, and PTV.
3. While in the middle of a simulation, the SAD is inadvertently changed from 100 cm to 110 cm. How much will the field size change? How can the simulation therapist detect this change?
4. Discuss the difference between fluoroscopy-based simulation and CT simulation.
5. Write out an appropriate explanation for a patient about to have a simulation for lung cancer.
6. Describe at least six treatment parameters documented during a simulation procedure and discuss their importance.
7. Describe the importance of immobilization devices in radiation therapy.
8. Describe the differences between patient positioning and immobilization devices.

REFERENCES

1. American Association of Medical Physicists in Medicine (website): www.aapm.org. Accessed October 2, 2007.
2. Benedick FA, Eisbruch A: Conformal therapy: treatment planning, treatment delivery, and clinical results. In Gunderson LL, Tepper JE, editors: *Clinical radiation oncology,* Philadelphia, 2007, Elsevier Churchill Livingstone.
3. Bentel GC: *Patient positioning and immobilization in radiation oncology,* New York, 1999, McGraw-Hill.
4. Bushong SC: *Radiologic science for technologists: physics, biology, and protection,* ed 8, St. Louis, 2004, Elsevier Mosby.
5. Carlton RR, McKenna-Adler A: *Principles of radiographic imaging,* Albany, NY, 2005, Thompson Delmar Learning.
6. Gerbi BJ: The simulation process in the determination and definition of treatment volume and treatment planning. In Levitt SH, Khan FM, Potish, RA, Perez CA, editors: *Levitt and Tapley's technological basis of radiation therapy: clinical application,* ed 3, Philadelphia, 1999, Lippincott Williams & Wilkins.
7. Hong TS, et al: The impact of daily setup variations on head-and-neck intensity-modulated radiation therapy, *Int J Radiat Oncol Biol Phys* 61:779-788, 2005.
8. ICRU Report 50. *Prescribing, recording, and reporting photon beam therapy,* Bethesda, Md, 1993, International Commission on Radiation Units and Measurements.
8a. ICRU Report 62. *Prescribing, recording and reporting photon beam therapy,* Bethesda, Md, 1999, International Commission on Radiation Units and Measurement.
9. Inter-Society Council for Radiation Oncology: *Radiation oncology in integrated cancer management,* Philadelphia, 1991, American College of Radiology.
10. Karzmark CJ, Nunan CS, Tanabe E: *Medical linear accelerators,* New York, 1993, McGraw-Hill.
11. Khan FM: *The physics of radiation therapy,* ed 3, Baltimore, 2003, Lippincott Williams & Wilkins.
12. Leaver D, Keller R, Uricchio, N: Simulation procedures. In Washington CM, Leaver D, editors: *Principles and practice of radiation therapy,* ed 2, St. Louis, 2004, Mosby.
13. Levitt LH, et al: *Technical basis of radiation therapy: practical clinical applications,* New York, 2006, Springer.
14. Med-Tec, Inc, Orange City, Iowa, personal communication, March 2002.
15. O'Connor-Hartsell S, Hartsell W: Minimizing errors in patient positioning, *Radiat Ther* 3:15-19, 1994.
16. Perez CA, et al: *Principles and practice of radiation oncology,* ed 4, Philadelphia, 2004, Lippincott Williams & Wilkins.
17. Purdy JA: Principles of radiologic physics, dosimetry and treatment planning. In Perez CA, et al, editors: *Principles and practice of radiation oncology,* ed 4, Philadelphia, 2004, Lippincott Williams & Wilkins.
18. Redpath AT, McNee SG: Treatment planning for external beam therapy: advanced techniques. In Williams JR, Thwaites DI, editors: *Radiotherapy physics in practice,* Oxford, 2000, Oxford University Press.
19. Smithers Medical Products, Inc, Tallmadge, Ohio, personal communication, March 2002.
20. Van Dyk JV, Mah K: Simulation and imaging for radiation therapy planning. In Williams JR, Thwaites DI, editors: *Radiotherapy physics in practice,* Oxford, 2000, Oxford University Press.
21. WFR/Aquaplast Corp, Wyckoff, NJ, personal communication, April 2003.

23

Computed Tomography Simulation

Nora Uricchio

Outline

History
Principles of operation
  Computed tomography
    simulation
  Benefits of computed
    tomography simulation
  Considerations and limitations
    of computed tomography
    simulation
Computed tomography
  simulation procedures
  Presimulation planning
  Contrast agents

Room preparation
Explanation of procedure
Patient positioning and
  immobilization
Computed tomography data
  acquisition
Virtual simulation of treatment
  fields
Generation of dose
  distributions
Documenting data
Image quality
  Spatial resolution

Image contrast
Noise
Dose
Artifacts
Computed tomography image
  processing controls
Quality assurance
Integration with treatment planning
Respiratory gating with computed
  tomography simulation
Summary

Objectives

- List the historical facts and contributors that led to the development of computed tomography (CT).
- Discuss the basic concepts of how a CT image is created.
- Describe considerations and limitations of CT simulation.
- Compare and contrast the benefits and contraindications of contrast agents used with CT simulation.

- Discuss image quality factors for CT.
- Describe common artifacts that occur on CT and how to minimize these artifacts.
- Discuss radiation safety, dose associated with CT, and quality assurance procedures in CT.

Key Terms

Artifacts
Contrast
Field of view
Filtered back projection
Hounsfield units
Image matrix
Interpolation
Noise
Osmolality
Pitch
Pixel
Projections
Reconstructed field of
  view
Scan field of view
Spatial resolution
Translation
Virtual simulation
Voxel
Window level
Window width (WW)

O ver the past three decades, medical imaging has revolutionized how we simulate and calculate radiation therapy treatments.[2,15] With the rapid computer technology progression, imaging modalities such as computed tomography (CT), magnetic resonance imaging (MRI), and positron emission tomography (PET) have become an essential part of the radiation therapy department, providing detailed information for accurate treatment planning in the transverse, coronal, and sagittal planes. In the past, patients were contoured only at the central axis using solder or plaster contouring methods. Treatments were often simple anteroposterior (AP)/posteroanterior (PA) or four-field techniques delivered to a large area because the localization process was vague. Advances in imaging have facilitated more accurate treatment delivery. Research is aimed at giving tumors higher doses with the hope of controlling a larger percentage of the disease. This has also led to an increased interest in treating moving targets.[15] This chapter will discuss the history, basic principles, and operation of the CT simulator and its importance in radiation therapy.

HISTORY

In the early 1970s, an imaging technology was introduced to clinical medicine that has drastically changed the way anatomy is viewed. Godfrey Hounsfield, a physicist/engineer working for the British company EMI, first demonstrated CT imaging in 1973.[4] This head scanner was designed with a water bath positioned around the superior part of the head during scanning (Figure 23-1). Alan Cormack, a Tufts University medical physicist, developed the mathematics used to reconstruct the CT images. As a result, Cormack and Hounsfield shared the 1979 Nobel Prize in physics for their

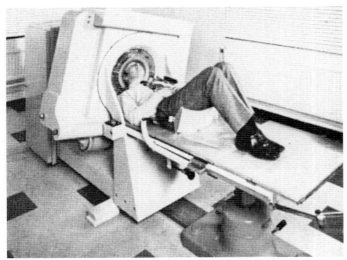

Figure 23-1. First-generation model of a computed tomography (CT) head scanner. (Courtesy Thorn EMI, London, England. In Seeram E: *Computed tomography: physical principles, clinical applications, and quality control,* ed 2, Philadelphia, 2001, Saunders.)

developments in CT.[4] Since then, four generations of CT scanners have been developed, each improving the scanning technique from the previous generation. Today, there are tens of thousands of CT scanners installed in hospitals and medical centers throughout the world. In the 1990s, a separate CT unit was developed specifically for radiation therapy simulation, in some departments replacing the fluoroscopy-based conventional simulator.

 For more information about Godfrey Hounsfield and the history of the CT scanner, visit http://nobelprize.org/nobel_prizes/medicine/laureates/1979/hounsfield-autobio.html.

CT scanning has been used in radiation therapy almost as long as the CT scanner has been in existence, providing information necessary for the planning of the patient's treatment. A study published in 1977 by Munzenrider and Pilepich[23] compared the use of CT data and the absence of CT data in the radiation therapy treatment planning process. These data demonstrated the benefits of CT in radiation therapy treatment planning. The CT data were judged to be essential in 55%, helpful in 31%, and not necessary in 14% of the patients in the study. Although CT proved to be beneficial, the technology was lacking in regard to facilitating the transfer of the CT information to the treatment planning system. In many cases, this was a difficult transition.

In the late 1970s and early 1980s, Hunt and Coia[13] attempted to market a type of CT scanner specifically for radiation therapy simulation. This failed for two reasons: the lack of high-quality digitally reconstructed radiographs (DRRs) and a limited treatment planning system that did not allow for interactive definition of target volumes and dose calculations. Four developments occurred in the early 1990s that greatly affected radiation treatment planning and allowed for more sophisticated integration of computer software:

1. Virtual simulation was introduced, which provided the ability to design the fields without a conventional simulator with better visualization of internal structures using three-dimensional (3D) images on the computer.
2. CT images produced on a conventional simulator were dramatically improved, which allowed them to be used for planning purposes.
3. Treatment planning computers were developed with more sophisticated algorithms and faster computer speed that could carry out 3D treatment planning.
4. A true virtual simulator provided the ability to generate high-resolution DRRs.

Today, all major manufacturers offer a CT scanner that can be used for radiation therapy. A state-of-the-art CT simulator, specifically designed for the radiation therapy department, should include a high-performance CT scanner with laser and patient marking systems and virtual simulation.[13] The localization and verification of a treatment field during CT simulation must reflect precisely what will happen in the treatment room when a prescribed dose of radiation therapy is delivered. CT simulation is part of the treatment planning process and includes both the actual CT scanner and the virtual simulation workstation. The treatment planning system includes the virtual simulation workstation and dosage calculation computer (Figure 23-2).

PRINCIPLES OF OPERATION

The essential components of a CT scanner are as follows: monitor, keyboard, intercom, tower cabinet, array processor, high-voltage generator, gantry, and couch.

Located in the external part of the gantry are the controls for couch movements, gantry tilt, emergency off buttons, and localizer lasers. Located in the internal aspect of the gantry are the detector array and x-ray tube. CT scanners are designed with a finely collimated x-ray fan beam and a detector array (group of detectors) that rotate around the patient in a continuous fashion (Figure 23-3). The finely collimated beam is created by the prepatient collimator via metal plates attached to the x-ray tube. Collimation absorbs photons that would enter the patient's body at several angles producing unwanted scatter radiation[24] (Figure 23-4). This prepatient collimation in a conventional (single-slice) CT scanner determines the slice thickness. As the x-ray tube and opposing detector make one complete rotation (360 degrees) around the patient, thousands of x-ray transmission measurements are recorded by the detectors.[14] CT information is generally recorded by a group of solid-state image detectors or gas-filled detectors.[30]

 Prepatient collimation determines slice thickness and patient dose.

To understand data acquisition in CT, consider the first and simplest of CT systems. An x-ray tube and detector assembly moving across the patient in a straight line completes a **translation**.[27,30] After the first translation, the tube and detector rotate 1 degree and complete another translation. This continues until at least 180 degrees of data have been collected.[27]

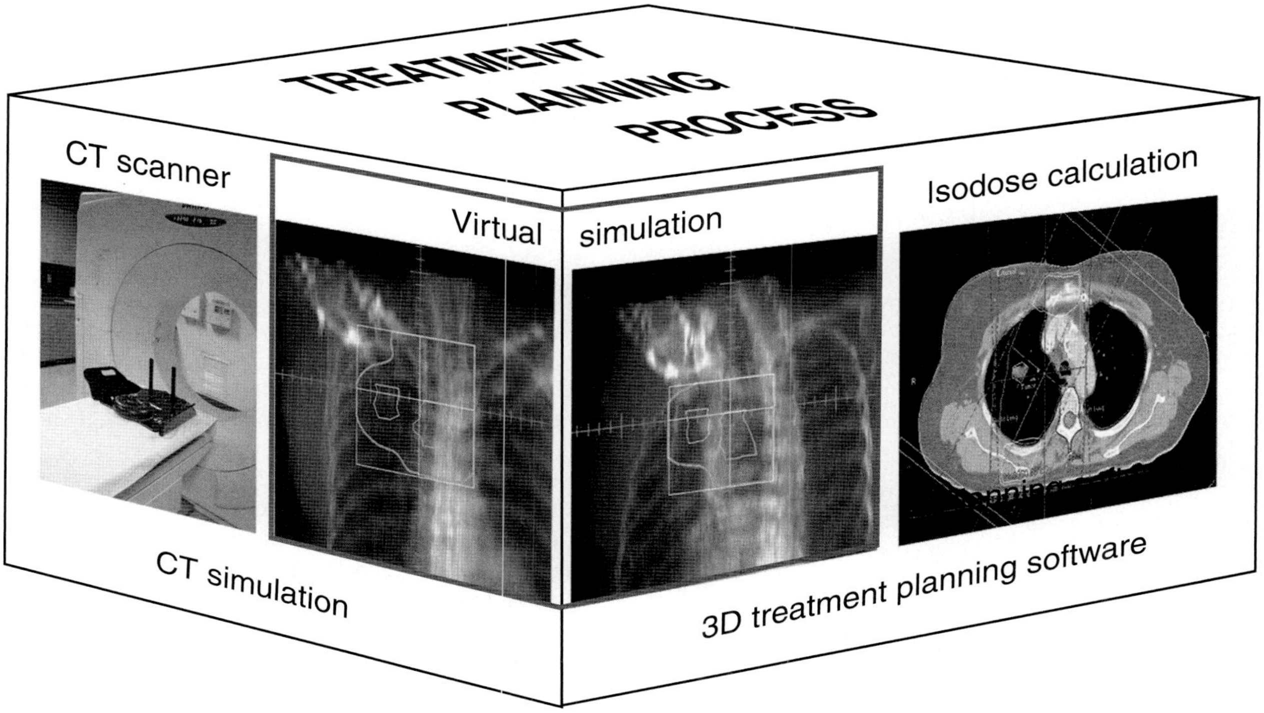

Figure 23-2. Computed tomography (CT) simulation is part of the treatment planning process and includes both the actual CT scanner and the virtual simulation workstation. The treatment planning system includes the virtual simulation workstation and dosage calculation computer. Virtual simulation is defined as the simulation process without the patient actually present. Data are collected from the CT scanning process and then manipulated with the help of the treatment planning software. (See Color plate 8.)

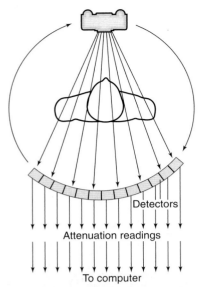

Figure 23-3. During scanning, the x-ray tube and detectors rotate around the patient to collect views. (From Seeram E: *Computed tomography: physical principles, clinical applications, and quality control*, ed 2, Philadelphia, 2001, Saunders.)

The intensity of radiation detected varies based on the density and effective atomic number of structures in the beam. The part of the beam that falls on one detector is called a *ray*. One complete translation of rays is called a *view*, which generates a *profile*[27] (Figure 23-5). The numerous intensity profiles or **projections** are created and stored in digital form in the computer as raw data.[4] The signal is analyzed by the computer and reconstructed on a monitor, giving a transverse cross section of the body. Images seen on the screen are a display of cells in rows and columns, called the **image matrix**. Matrix size can be selected. However, 512×512 is commonly used in CT. In a 512×512 matrix, there are a total of 262,144 pixels of information! Each

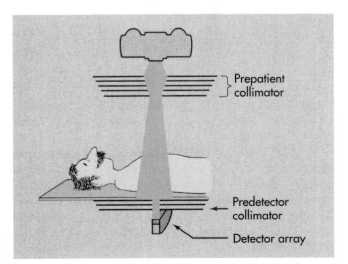

Figure 23-4. Computed tomography imaging systems incorporate both a prepatient collimator and a predetector collimator. (From Bushong S: *Radiologic science for technologists: physics, biology, and protection*, ed 8, St. Louis, 2004, Mosby.)

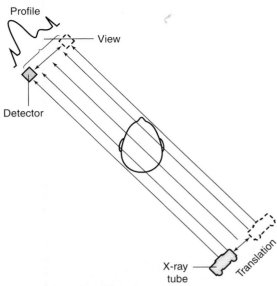

Figure 23-5. In computed tomography (CT), a ray is the part of the x-ray beam that falls onto one detector. A view is a collection of these rays for one translation across the object. The view generates an electrical signal called a profile or projection. (From Seeram E: *Computed tomography: physical principles, clinical applications, and quality control*, ed 2, Philadelphia, 2001, Saunders.)

cell on the image matrix is called a **pixel** (picture element). Each pixel and the slice thickness or volume is called a **voxel** (volume element) (Figure 23-6).

Filtered back projection, also called the *summation method*, is a commonly used method of reconstructing CT data.[27] The term *filter* here refers to a mathematic function, not a metal filter. A simple example may help explain how it works. Imagine a square box with two holes cut from each side divided into four cells labeled a, b, c, and d (Figure 23-7). There is a butterfly in cell "c". If the box is covered and one looks through the four sets of holes, the location of the butterfly can be determined. Let "1" represent the presence of the butterfly for each viewing. If the butterfly cannot be seen, this is represented with "0". Examining all possibilities of the paths:

$$a + b = 0$$
$$c + d = 1$$
$$a + c = 1$$
$$b + d = 0$$

Four equations result, and if solved simultaneously the solution is c = 1, which represents the location of the butterfly. In CT, there are more than 250,000 simultaneous equations requiring solutions.[4] For each projection, a value is given to each pixel. The average linear attenuation coefficient of each projection per pixel results in an exact density assigned to each pixel.[8] Attenuation rates displayed as pixels of different shades of gray are called **Hounsfield units** (HUs)[30] (Figure 23-8). Hounsfield units, which correspond to the electron density of a specific tissue such as lung, soft tissue, and bone, are set at −1000 for air (zero density), 0 for water (unit density), 15 for cerebrospinal fluid (CSF), 20 for blood, 40 for gray matter, 50 for muscle, and 1000 for dense bone.[10,26]

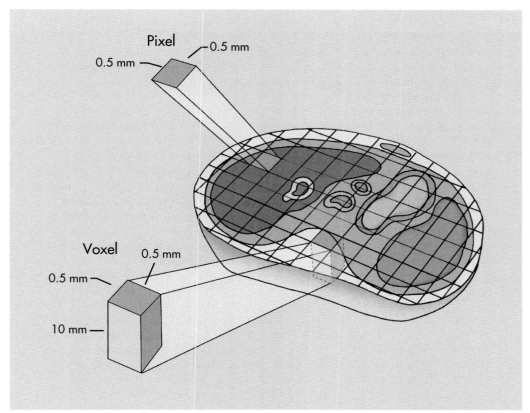

Figure 23-6. Each cell in a computed tomography image matrix is a two-dimensional representation (pixel) of a volume of tissue (voxel). (From Bushong S: *Radiologic science for technologists: physics, biology, and protection, ed 8*, St. Louis, 2004, Mosby.)

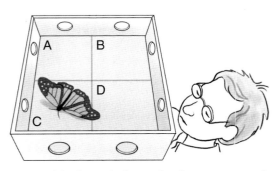

Figure 23-7. This four-pixel matrix demonstrates the back projection method for reconstructing a computed tomography (CT) image. (Redrawn from Bushong S: *Radiologic science for technologists: physics, biology, and protection,* ed 8, St. Louis, 2004, Mosby.)

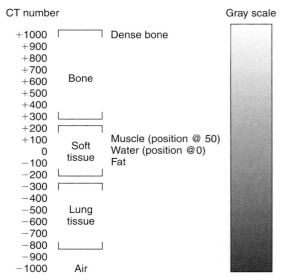

Figure 23-8. The relationship between computed tomography (CT) number and brightness level. (From Seeram E: *Computed tomography: physical principles, clinical applications, and quality control,* ed 2, Philadelphia, 2001, Saunders.)

Computed Tomography Simulation

A state-of-the-art CT simulator, specifically designed for the radiation therapy department, may include a high-performance CT scanner with laser and patient marking systems. A CT scanner located in the radiation oncology department may be either a conventional (slice-by-slice) CT or a helical/spiral (volume) CT scanner. With a conventional CT scanner, the tube rotates once around a stationary table, producing a "slice" of data. The table is moved a small increment and the tube rotates again, producing another "slice" of data. In helical or spiral CT scanning, the gantry rotates continuously in one direction while the table moves inward as the gantry is scanning (Figure 23-9). The advantage of helical scanning is that it is faster and produces less heat.

The localization and verification of a treatment field during CT simulation must reflect precisely what will happen in the treatment room. Patient position, beam alignment, and the planning volume must be the same at the end of treatment planning and the beginning of treatment[27] (Table 23-1). Policies and procedures should be developed within the radiation therapy department related to the unique issues involved in CT and virtual simulation procedures. Before introducing the many steps involved in the CT simulation process (Box 23-1), some of the benefits, considerations, and limitations are discussed. [2,13,25,28]

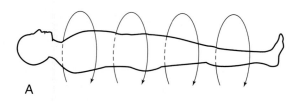
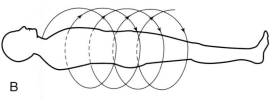

Figure 23-9. A, Conventional slice-by-slice scanning. **B,** Volume scanning. (From Seeram E: *Computed tomography: physical principles, clinical applications, and quality control,* ed 2, Philadelphia, 2001, Saunders.)

Table 23-1	Summary of CT Simulation Major Steps	
With a Dedicated CT Simulator		**Without a Dedicated CT Simulator**

With a Dedicated CT Simulator	Without a Dedicated CT Simulator
DURING SIMULATION PLANNING	**DURING SIMULATION PLANNING**
• Explanation of procedure	• Explanation of procedure
• Straighten patient	• Straighten patient
• Immobilization and positioning	• Immobilization and positioning
• Administration of contrast	• Administration of contrast
↓	↓
• Mark reference point on patient using laser system	• Localize area of interest
• Scout or pilot film (preliminary image)	↓
• Physician selects area to scan	• Mark reference point on patient using laser system
↓	↓
CT SCAN IS PERFORMED	• Scout or pilot film
• CT scan completed using specific department protocol	**PHYSICIAN DETERMINES AREA TO BE SCANNED**
• Transfer reconstructed image to virtual simulation station	• The patient is aligned to reference points
↓	• Patient marks are beginning point for CT scan; CT is "zeroed out"
VIRTUAL SIMULATION STATION	• CT scan is transferred to treatment planning system to optimize plan
• Contouring	↓
• Localize tumor and target volumes and normal structures	• If no DRRs can be created, the patient is brought to the conventional simulator to document treatment portals
↓	
• Determination of target isocenter and transfer to patient using laser system	
• Patient is marked, patient leaves	
↓	
• Transfer CT data to treatment planning system	

CT, Computed tomography; *DRRs,* digitally reconstructed radiographs.

<table>
<tr><td colspan="2">

Box 23-1   **Procedure Outline for Computed Tomography (CT) Simulation**

1. Presimulation planning
2. Room preparation
3. Explanation of procedure
4. Patient positioning and immobilization
5. CT data acquisition
5. Target and normal tissue localization
6. Virtual simulation of treatment fields
7. Generation of dose distributions
8. Documentation of pertinent data

</td></tr>
</table>

Benefits of Computed Tomography Simulation

CT simulation provides the following[18]:
1. The ability to outline critical structures and view these structures in three dimensions.
2. The ability to delineate the target volume and lymph nodes in the patient's treatment position.
3. Optimal beam placement.
4. Cone down or boost fields can be accomplished without the patient present (virtual simulation).
5. Beam's eye view (BEV) display allows anatomy to be viewed from the perspective of the radiation beam.
6. CT simulation allows field shaping electronically at the graphic display station.
7. Virtual simulation allows comparison of beams and construction of DRRs without the patient present.
8. The calculation of dose distribution.

Considerations and Limitations of Computed Tomography Simulation

1. The size of the aperture of the CT scanner must be large enough to accommodate patients in the treatment position with complex immobilization devices.
2. Patient couch must simulate treatment couch, including the width and shape of the couch.
3. Laser system to localize isocenter must be present.
4. The time between the start of CT acquisition and patient marking must be minimized to avoid potential patient movement and localization errors.
5. Careful consideration must be taken when using CT numbers for dose inhomogeneity corrections during dosage calculations.
6. Machine setup parameters, beam-shaping devices, and treatment accessories such as block verification are unable to be verified on the CT scanner.
7. Scanning and display fields of view must be large enough so that the patient's entire external contour can be visualized.

Virtual simulation mimics fluoroscopy in conventional simulation. Once scans are completed through the area of interest, the information is transferred to the treatment planning computer via a local area network. **Virtual simulation** is defined as the simulation process without the patient actually present. Data are collected from the CT scanning process and then manipulated with the help of the treatment planning software to create a treatment plan for the patient after the patient has left the department. A boost field can be developed and prescribed, based on the patient's reference marks, without the patient present; thus, the term *virtual simulation* is used. At a separate computer workstation, physicians working with radiation therapists can delineate tumor and other critical structures (see Figure 23-2). Some departments will complete the virtual simulation and mark the patient after the target volume is delineated. The scans are then transferred to the treatment planning station, at which time critical structures are outlined and a treatment plan is developed. Once the treatment planning is finalized, DRRs are generated.

COMPUTED TOMOGRAPHY SIMULATION PROCEDURES

In the following section, CT simulation procedures are discussed in detail. The CT simulation process consists of consultation with the patient, fabrication and registration of immobilization devices, CT data acquisition, target and normal tissue localization, virtual simulation of treatment fields, generation of dose distributions, marking of the patient with planned fields, and production of images for treatment verification (DRRs).[29] Consultation of the patient occurs in the same manner as in conventional simulation. Tumor localization, isodose planning, and shielding design take on new dimensions with CT simulation. These occur using virtual simulation techniques.

Presimulation Planning

The presimulation planning for CT simulation is similar to that for conventional simulation. The physician and therapist need to be aware of the limitations of the CT scanner, especially with regard to immobilization and patient positioning. Discussion with the patient should also include the time involved for the procedure, patient positioning, and the use of contrast.

Contrast Agents

When performing CT, contrast media may be used to help differentiate anatomic structures or highlight an abnormality. Contrast can be administered into the body via four methods: intravascularly (intravenously), orally, intrathecally, or intraarticularly.[24] The most common methods of administration contrast during CT simulation are orally and intravenously.

Medical History. Prior to injecting any contrast media into the patient, a thorough medical history must be obtained to evaluate the possibility of an adverse reaction to contrast media.[12] Patients receiving contrast media usually complete a questionnaire or are asked several questions to determine whether they have a rare allergy to the contrast agent and are at risk for any side effects, some of which may be minor and some of which may be life-threatening (Box 23-2).

A common agent used to localize the gastrointestinal tract is barium sulfate. Barium is not water soluble. Therefore, patients with a high risk of gastrointestinal perforation would not receive barium sulfate and instead would receive an aqueous iodinated agent such as Gastrograffin. Both can be administered orally or rectally. Table 23-2 lists the factors that increase the risk for an adverse reaction to contrast agents.[1]

Risk factors for receiving intravenous (IV) contrast are patients who are over 50, are diabetic, have impaired kidney function, have cardiovascular disease, or have had a reaction to contrast in the past. Patients at high risk may need to receive blood work to evaluate kidney function, prior to their simulation session. Baseline blood urea nitrogen (BUN) and creatinine levels are obtained to assess the patient's kidney function. If the patient's creatinine is near an unsafe level, the amount of contrast that is necessary would be decreased or not given to the patient. In some patients, the administration of iodinated contrast media can cause kidney damage and require temporary or permanent dialysis. This may be more likely in patients with an elevated creatinine level. The risk may be reduced in some patients by using a low-osmolality contrast medium.

IV contrast can be ionic iodine or nonionic iodine. Ionic iodine contrast media have a high **osmolality**, which is a measure of the total number of particles in solution per kilogram of water.[1] When a contrast medium is injected into the blood vessel, the ionic contrast medium has an effect of displacing water in the body. Through osmosis, water moves from the body cells into the vascular system, causing hypervolemia and vessel dilation. The high osmolality of contrast media attracts water to move into blood vessels. This produces pain and discomfort and may cause a decrease in blood pressure because of the vessel dilation or may increase blood pressure because of hypervolemia.[1] If a patient is dehydrated, the decreased body cell volume can result in shock. Using a lower-osmolality substance such as nonionic iodine decreases the risk of these side effects. Adverse reactions have rarely been seen when nonionic substances are used. However, a careful medical history needs to be taken.[12] A list of patient history factors is given in Table 23-3.[1]

IV contrast is usually an iodine-based solution injected into the vein using a power-assisted injector, or it may simply be hand injected using a syringe. A power injector (Figure 23-10) allows the contrast to be delivered at a rapid rate during the CT scan. The nonionic contrast often comes in prefilled vials specifically made for the power injector. Injecting a contrast medium at a rapid rate can be painful for the patient due to the viscosity (thickness of substance) of the contrast medium concentration and the size of

Table 23-2	Patient History Factors in Barium Sulfate Examinations
Factor	**Importance**
Age	Ability to communicate, hear, and follow directions
	↑ Risk of colon perforation caused by loss of tissue tone
Diverticulitis or ulcerative colitis	↑ Difficulty in holding an enema
	↑ Risk of colon perforation
Long-term steroid therapy	↑ Risk of colon perforation
Colon biopsy within previous 2 wks	Lower gastrointestinal series contraindicated
Pregnancy	Inform radiation oncologist before proceeding with examination
Mental retardation, confusion, or dizziness	↑ Risk of aspiration during upper gastrointestinal series
Recent onset of constipation or diarrhea	↑ Risk of colon perforation or tumor rupture
Nausea and vomiting	↑ Risk of aspiration during upper gastrointestinal series

↑, Increased.

From Adler AM, Carlton RR: *Introduction to radiologic sciences and patient care*, ed 4, St. Louis, 2007, Saunders/Elsevier.

the molecule. Heating the contrast medium to body temperature in a warmer reduces viscosity and facilitates rapid injection.[1] Keeping the unused contrast medium does reduce the shelf-life. Some departments will discard the contrast medium if it has been in the warmer for up to 30 days and has not been used. Box 23-3 lists the steps necessary to connect the power injector.

Once the iodine-based liquid is injected, it causes many organs and structures, such as the kidneys and blood vessels, to become much more visible on the CT scan. As CT images are acquired, the beam of radiation is attenuated or absorbed as it passes through the blood vessels and organs filled with the high-density contrast agent. This causes the blood vessels and organs containing the contrast to "enhance" and show up as white areas on the CT images.

Contrast media are often manufactured specifically for CT. High–atomic number contrast media can create star artifacts on the CT scans (artifacts are discussed later in the chapter). Usually between 30 and 100 mL of contrast is used for a CT simulation examination, depending mostly on the patient's age and weight. Some centers may use a chart based on the patient's weight to determine a more specific dose. For example, smaller patients may receive 75 mL and larger patients may receive 150 mL of the iodinated contrast for their examination. Once the contrast medium is administered, patients should be monitored for side effects. Seventy percent of adverse reactions occur within 5 minutes; most others occur within 30 minutes.[1] High-risk patients should be monitored for longer than 30 minutes. The most common reaction is a feeling of warmth and discomfort at the injection site. Box 23-4 lists categories of reactions, and Box 23-5 details the management of acute reactions.

Contrast is often used to enhance structures in patients with a specific pathology, such as head and neck, lung, brain, abdominal, and pelvis tumors.

Box 23-2	Administration of Intravenous Contrast Sample Questionnaire

- Have you ever received iodinated contrast media before?
- Have you ever had a reaction to iodinated contrast media?
- Do you have any allergies to food or medications?
- Do you have any of the following conditions?
  - Allergies
  - Kidney problems
  - Cardiac disease
  - Diabetes
  - High blood pressure
  - Sickle cell anemia
  - Multiple myeloma
  - Pheochromocytoma
- Is there any chance that you are pregnant?
- Have you had anything to eat or drink within the last 4 hours?

Table 23-3	Patitent History Factors in Water-Soluble Iodine Contrast Examinations	
FACTORS	**IMPORTANCE**	
Age	↑ Risk with increased age	
Allergies or asthma	↑ Risk of allergic-like reactions	
Diabetes	Insulin usually given before procedure; these patients should be scheduled before others	
Coronary artery disease	↑ Risk of tachycardia, bradycardia, hypertension, myocardial infarction (heart attack)	
Hypertension	Hypertension with tachycardia	
Renal disease	Inform radiation oncologist if creatinine level is greater than 1.4 mg/dL	
Multiple myeloma	Abnormal protein binds with contrast and can cause renal failure Patients must be hydrated	
Confusion or dizziness	Blood-brain barrier effects	
Sickle cell anemia or family history of chronic obstructive pulmonary disease	↑ Risk of blood clots ↑ Risk of dyspnea (difficulty in breathing)	
Previous iodine contrast examinations	Did the patient have difficulties with procedure?	
Pregnancy	Inform radiation oncologist before proceeding	
History of blood clots	↑ Risk of blood clots	
Use of beta blockers	↑ Risk of anaphylactoid reaction	
Use of calcium channel blockers	↑ Risk of heart block	
Use of metformin (Glucophage)	↑ Risk of lactic acidosis if renal failure occurs	

↑, Increased.
From Adler AM, Carlton RR: *Introduction to radiologic sciences and patient care,* ed 4, St. Louis, 2007, Saunders/Elsevier.

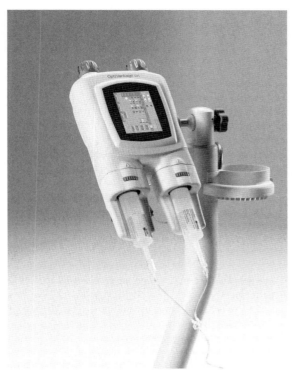

Figure 23-10. Power injector used to inject contrast during computed tomography (CT) scans. (Courtesy Couidien Imaging Solutions.)

Timing of the contrast injection is critical. It may be injected before the scan or during the scan depending on what area of the body must be visualized. The following section discusses sites where contrast is most commonly administered during CT simulation, the contrast used, and how and when it is administered:

Head and Neck and Lung. In patients with head and neck cancer and lung tumors, contrast may be administered with a power injector often seconds prior to the scan. The purpose of the contrast is to highlight the vessels and distinguish them from lymph nodes. Injecting just prior to the scan allows the images to be captured when the contrast is in the vessels.

Liver. The power injector may also be used if the physician would like to enhance some of the blood vessels the liver, which has dual blood supply from both the portal vein and the hepatic artery. Scanning that occurs approximately 20 to 40 seconds after the initiation of the injection will visualize the hepatic arterial phase. The venous phase occurs from 60 to 90 seconds after the start of the injection. If scanning occurs after the portal venous phase, then many hepatic tumors may not be visualized on the images.[24]

Pelvis. In some patients with prostate tumors, a delayed scan may be required. IV contrast would be administered prior to the scan through an IV push. Allowing a minimum of 15 minutes' after the injection will allow the contrast to filter through the heart and blood vessels to the bladder for better visualization of the pelvic anatomy.[24] To visualize the rectum and/or the vagina, a marker can be placed in or near these structures.

Brain. IV contrast is administered 10 to 30 minutes prior to the scan through an IV push. Because tumors are usually more vascular than normal anatomy, contrast media will highlight the tumor more than the normal structures.

Gastrointestinal Tumors. A barium paste can be used to coat the esophagus. Dilute barium sulfate solution, if there is no concern of perforation, will highlight the stomach or small bowel during an abdominal CT scan. If the physician would like to see the small bowel, the patient is given the barium at a minimum of 30 minutes prior to the simulation.

When scanning a patient for treatment planning, some radiation oncologists prefer to minimize the use of contrast agents, because the image of the contrast on the scan may alter dose calculations. Inaccurate dose calculations could occur because some treatment planning systems may interpret the area of contrast, registering a high HU similar to bone, that would attenuate the beam more than it would the actual soft tissue that is highlighted by the contrast. If contrast is used, then the dosimetrist, at the direction of the physician, will contour the structures outlined by the contrast and change the HU to one for that structure.

Box 23-3	Steps for Using a Power Injector

1. Check to be sure the patient questionnaire was completed. Note any precautions as stated by nurse or physician.
2. Have anaphylactic kit on hand.
3. Retrieve appropriate contrast medium from warmer.
4. Check expiration date of contrast to be injected. Do not use if expired.
5. Place syringe in power injector according to manufacturer specifications.
   a. Remove covering of syringe. The tip of the syringe is sterile. Connect tubing to syringe using sterile technique.
   b. Remove air in syringe and IV line.
   c. Connect to patient's IV site.
6. Position and immobilize patient.
7. Select protocol for rate and amount of contrast to be injected. These are often preset based on the protocol for the department.
   a. If a smaller needle was used in the patient, the rate of administration is decreased.
8. Prepare scanner. Do not begin scan yet.
9. Begin power injection.
   a. Depending on what needs to be visualized, the scan will begin as dictated by the physician.
   b. Some departments will not inject the contrast unless a physician or nurse is present.

Box 23-4	Categories of Reactions to Contrast Media

MILD

Nausea, vomiting
Altered taste
Sweats
Cough
Itching
Rash, hives
Warmth
Pallor
Nasal stuffiness
Headache
Flushing
Swelling: eyes, face
Dizziness
Chills
Anxiety
Shaking
Signs and symptoms appear self-limited without evidence of progression (e.g., limited urticaria with mild pruritis, transient nausea, one episode of emesis).
Treatment: Requires observation to confirm resolution and/or lack of progression but usually no treatment. Patient reassurance is usually helpful.

MODERATE

Moderate degree of clinically evident focal or systemic signs or symptoms including:
Tachycardia/bradycardia
Hypotension
Bronchospasm, wheezing
Hypertension
Dyspnea
Laryngeal edema
Pronounced cutaneous reaction
Treatment: Clinical findings should be considered as indications for immediate treatment.
These situations require close, careful observation for possible progression to a life-threatening event.

SEVERE

Life-threatening with more severe signs or symptoms, including:
Laryngeal edema
Profound hypotension
Unresponsiveness
Convulsions
Clinically manifest arrhythmias
Cardiopulmonary arrest
Treatment: Requires *prompt* recognition and treatment; almost always requires hospitalization.

Contrast media and markers must have a low atomic number to reduce the effects of unwanted artifacts on the image. There are many commercially available contrast media and markers made specifically for CT scanning. A summary of contrast materials used is listed in Table 23-4.

Room Preparation

The room preparation for CT simulation is similar to that for conventional simulation. Special attention to the fabrication and registration of immobilization devices should be given careful thought because of the aperture (bore) size of the scanner. A large-diameter (85-cm) CT aperture should be used if available to allow patient positioning that exactly matches the treatment position. Patient immobilization devices should be used that will minimize image artifacts.[14]

Explanation of Procedure

Patients are instructed on how to change and to remove all metallic objects including jewelry, dentures, eyeglasses, and hair accessories from the area of interest. Patients are often told to hold still and breathe normally during the scanning process. Depending on the area that is treated, patients may be asked to hold their breath during a scan. Scans may be done at full inhalation and at full exhalation. Simulation time may also vary depending on the institution and the needs of the patient. It is possible to complete the patient portion of the simulation (data acquisition and marking) in 15 to 60 minutes. Patients should be told the purpose of the procedure, to hold still and breathe

Box 23-5	Management of Acute Reactions to Contrast Media in Adults

URTICARIA

1. Discontinue injection if not completed.
2. No treatment needed in most cases.
3. Give histamine (H_1)-receptor blocker: diphenhydramine (Benadryl) PO/IM/IV 25-50 mg

   If severe or widely disseminated: α-agonist (arteriolar and venous constriction)

   Epinephrine SC (1:1000) 0.1-0.3 mL (0.1-0.3 mg) (if no cardiac contraindications)

FACIAL OR LARYNGEAL EDEMA

1. Give α-agonist (arteriolar and venous constriction): epinephrine SC or IM (1:1000) 0.1-0.3 mL (0.1-0.3 mg) or, if hypotension evident, epinephrine (1:10,000) slowly IV 1 mL (0.1 mg). Repeat as needed up to a maximum of 1 mg.
2. Give O_2 6-10 L/min (via mask).

If not responsive to therapy or if there is obvious acute laryngeal edema, seek appropriate assistance (e.g., cardiopulmonary arrest response team).

BRONCHOSPASM

1. Give O_2 6-10 L/min (via mask). Monitor electrocardiogram, O_2 saturation (pulse oximeter), and blood pressure.
2. Give β-agonist inhalers (bronchiolar dilators, such as metaproterenol [Alupent], terbutaline [Brethaire], or albuterol [Proventil, Ventolin]) 2-3 puffs; repeat prn. If unresponsive to inhalers, use SC, IM, or IV epinephrine.
3. Give epinephrine SC or IM (1:1000) 0.1-0.3 mL (0.1-0.3 mg) or, if hypotension evident, epinephrine (1:10,000) slowly IV 1 mL (0.1 mg). Repeat as needed up to a maximum of 1 mg.

Call for assistance (e.g., cardiopulmonary arrest response team) for severe bronchospasm or if O_2 saturation <88% persists.

HYPOTENSION WITH TACHYCARDIA

1. Ensure legs elevated 60° or more (preferred) or Trendelenburg position.
2. Monitor electrocardiogram, pulse oximeter, and blood pressure.
3. Give O_2 6-10 L/min (via mask).
4. Rapid IV administration of large volumes of isotonic lactated Ringer's or normal saline.

If poorly responsive: Epinephrine (1:10,000) slowly IV 1 mL (0.1 mg) Repeat as needed up to a maximum of 1 mg.
If still poorly responsive, seek appropriate assistance (e.g., cardiopulmonary arrest response team).

HYPOTENSION WITH BRADYCARDIA (VAGAL REACTION)

1. Monitor vital signs.
2. Ensure legs elevated 60° or more (preferred) or Trendelenburg position.
3. Secure airway: give O_2 6-10 L/min (via mask).
4. Secure IV access: rapid administration of lactated Ringer's or normal saline.
5. Give atropine 0.6-1 mg IV slowly if patient does not respond quickly to steps 2 through 4.
6. Repeat atropine up to a total dose of 0.04 mg/kg (2-3 mg) in adult.
7. Ensure complete resolution of hypotension and bradycardia prior to discharge.

HYPERTENSION, SEVERE

1. Give O_2 6-10 L/min (via mask).
2. Monitor electrocardiogram, pulse oximeter, and blood pressure.
3. Give nitroglycerin 0.4-mg tablet, sublingual (may repeat ×3), or topical 2% ointment, apply 1-inch strip.
4. If no response, consider labetalol 20 mg IV, then 20-80 mg IV q10min up to 300 mg.
5. Transfer to intensive care unit or emergency department.
6. For pheochromocytoma: phentolamine 5 mg IV. (May use labetalol for pheochromocytoma if phentolamine is not available.)

SEIZURES OR CONVULSIONS

1. Give O_2 6-10 L/min (via mask).
2. Consider diazepam (Valium) 5 mg IV (or more, as appropriate) or midazolam (Versed) 0.5-1 mg IV.
3. If longer effect needed, obtain consultation; consider phenytoin (Dilantin) infusion 15-18 mg/kg at 50 mg/min.
4. Careful monitoring of vital signs required, particularly of PO_2 because of risk of respiratory depression with benzodiazepine administration.
5. Consider using cardiopulmonary arrest response team for intubation if needed.

PULMONARY EDEMA

1. Elevate torso.
2. Give O_2 6-10 L/min (via mask).
3. Give diuretics: furosemide (Lasix) 20-40 mg IV, slow push.
4. Consider giving morphine (1-3 mg IV).
5. Transfer to intensive care unit or emergency department.

IM, Intramuscular; *IV,* intravenous; *PO,* orally; *PO_2,* partial pressure of oxygen; *prn,* as needed; *q10min,* every 10 minutes; *SC,* subcutaneous.
From American College of Radiology (ACR). *Manual on Contrast Media,* 6.0 edition. American College of Radiology; 2008. Reprinted with permission of the American College of Radiology. No other representation of this material is authorized without expressed, written permission from the American College of Radiology.

normally, and to be assured that there is visible and audible monitoring during the scanning process. They should also be told that the table will move during the procedure and, if contrast is administered, they may experience a metallic taste in their mouth and/or a warm, flushing sensation in their body. Reassure patients that they are constantly monitored even though the therapist is not in the room.

Patient Positioning and Immobilization

Many of the same considerations used with conventional simulation are appropriate for CT simulation. Some CT tables may be curved (this is rare). If so, then a flat table needs to be mounted on the couch to simulate the treatment table. Immobilization devices are also fabricated. The CT scanner may have limitations on the number and type of immobilization

Table 23-4	Summary of Use of Contrast Media			
Area	**Contrast**	**Method of Administration**	**Patient Preparation**	**Timing of Administration**
Lung, head and neck	Ionic or nonionic	IV	NPO 4 hours prior to exam	Seconds prior to scan
Pelvis	Markers	Placed in rectum/vagina	None	Placed in orifice prior to scan
	Barium	Oral		
Brain	Ionic or nonionic	IV	NPO 4 hours prior to exam	10–30 minutes prior to scan
Prostate	Ionic or nonionic	IV	NPO 4 hours prior to exam	
GI visualization	Diluted barium	Oral	Drink 30 minutes prior to scan	

GI, Gastrointestinal; *IV,* intravenous; *NPO,* nothing by mouth.

devices it can accommodate, depending on the size of the aperture. Before beginning the scan, the therapist should check that the devices and the patient will fit into the aperture (bore) of the CT scanner. For example, a patient treated for breast cancer with a steep slope may need an angle board for treatment. Depending on the type and angle of breast board, the patient position, and the device used, the patient may not fit into the scanner.

Optimizing the patient position and immobilization device depends on several factors, including the patient's medical condition and treatment technique.[13] The transfer of information, such as the exact location of immobilization devices from simulation to the treatment machine, is improved when devices are referenced or indexed to the treatment table (Figure 23-11). The patient and immobilization device are then "locked" into place on the treatment table using a system of numbered or lettered holes, or notches, along the lateral edge of the carbon fiber tabletop. This should reduce the possibility of movement and increase daily reproducibility of the treatment setup.[17] Initially, the patient should be clinically straightened, using a line between the sternal notch and xiphoid process if the patient is supine, and marked before scanning. This process also provides temporary reference marks that may be used later in the simulation process. A scout or pilot scan is performed to check patient alignment and view the anatomy in the area of interest.

Computed Tomography Data Acquisition

When scanning a patient in CT, the patient is not positioned at isocenter as is the case during a conventional simulation procedure. The patient is positioned in the center of the bore so that the patient's contour is not cut off laterally. Otherwise, it is possible that the patient's anatomy will not be visible in the diameter of the scanning window or **field of view (FOV)**. The area for which projection data are collected for a CT scan is determined by the **scan field of view**. The external alignment marks on the patient should be marked with radiopaque catheters or markers so that they can be delineated on the CT scan for reference.[29] It is also recommended to not only include the anatomy in the scan field of view, but also the immobilization devices and tabletop index location. This will allow treatment planning personnel to provide a tabletop index position for

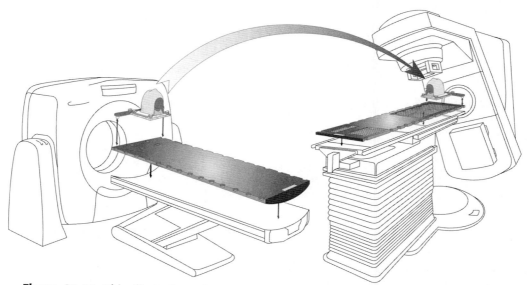

Figure 23-11. This illustration of a computed tomography (CT) simulator and linear accelerator shows a thermoplastic mask used primarily to immobilize the head and neck area, indexed to both the simulator and treatment couch. (Courtesy MED-TEC, Orange City, Iowa.)

setup information and also to calculate the dose with the immobilization devices included in the calculation if requested. The **reconstructed field of view** is the diameter or the area of a CT scan that is displayed on the computer. This needs to be large enough to display the entire contour.

The CT process begins with a scout or localizer image.[8] This is accomplished by scanning the patient quickly in the inferior/superior dimension to obtain data used to reconstruct an image that looks similar to a radiograph (Figure 23-12). CT scanners often record these in the AP (if patient is supine) and lateral views. During the acquisition of these images, the x-ray tube is stationary and the table moves through the gantry. With some manufacturers' multislice spiral scanners, both AP and lateral views may be acquired on the same scan. The image is used to select the area to be scanned. Departmental protocol may identify the number of cuts, thickness of cuts, and in some circumstances, the space between cuts. These protocols are often preset in the newer scanners. In a helical CT scanner, the distance traveled by the couch during an x-ray tube rotation, called the **pitch**, needs to be determined. Pitch determines the closeness of the helix[30] (Figure 23-13). The formula for calculating pitch for a single-slice helical scanner as follows:

$$\text{Pitch} = \frac{\text{Couch movement in the } z \text{ direction during 1 rotation of the tube}}{\text{Slice thickness}}$$

Example: Pitch 1 = 10-mm couch movement/10-mm slice 1:1 ratio.

A pitch of less than 1 results in overlapping images. A pitch larger than 1 increases the volume that can be imaged in a

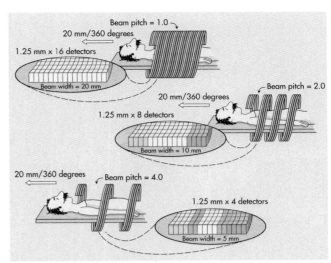

Figure 23-13. Beam pitch is the patient couch movement divided by x-ray cone beam width. (From Bushong S: *Radiologic science for technologists: physics, biology, and protection*, ed 8, St. Louis, 2004, Mosby.)

given time and decreases patient dose, which are advantages of helical CT.

Pitch is expressed as a ratio:
0.5:1 results in overlapping images,
2:1 ratio results in reduced patient dose and more anatomy scanned in a shorter amount of time.

Because helical scanners collect data in a spiral fashion, the data must be interpreted to construct the data to create a transverse (axial) plane (Figure 23-14). This mathematic process called **interpolation** estimates attenuation between two known points[4] (Figure 23-15). Interpolation is completed prior to reconstruction of an image. A pitch larger than 2 will lead to errors such as missed pathology or anatomy.

Based on the physician's orders, the therapist must select inferior and superior anatomic reference borders, indicating to the computer the volume of tissue to be scanned in the superior/inferior direction. Care must be taken to scan enough slices above and below the treatment area to account for non-coplanar beams and for image fusion. Data acquisition generates huge volumes of data and heat units on the x-ray tube, so the therapist must be sure to scan only what is necessary. If heat units can be minimized during the scan, the life of the x-ray tube will be extended. Depending on the type of scan used with spiral CT and thickness of slice, the actual scan time may be 1 to 3 minutes.

Slice thickness and spacing are important criteria in obtaining CT studies beneficial to producing high-quality DRRs. For optimal image reconstruction needed to produce a high-quality DRR, slice thickness and slice spacing should be evaluated for each anatomic region. Gerbi[10] recommends thin CT scans with no more than 5-mm spacing to reduce the problem of volume averaging while accurately representing the target in 3D space. To maximize the useful resolution on the DRR when performing CT simulation of the head and neck, Martin[20] recommends

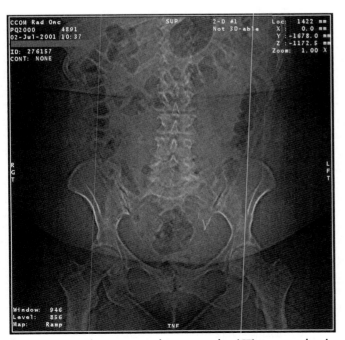

Figure 23-12. The computed tomography (CT) process begins with a scout or pilot image. This is accomplished by scanning the patient quickly in the inferior/superior dimension to obtain information needed to reconstruct a digitally reconstructed radiograph (DRR) image that looks similar to a radiograph.

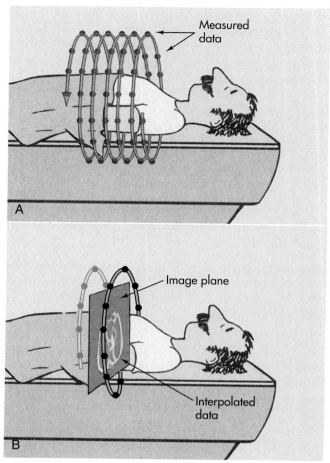

Figure 23-14. A, During spiral computed tomography, image data are continuously sampled. **B**, Interpolation of data is performed to reconstruct the image in any transverse plane. (From Bushong S: *Radiologic science for technologists: physics, biology, and protection*, ed 8, St. Louis, 2004, Mosby.)

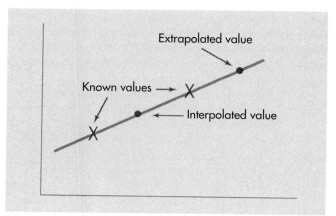

Figure 23-15. Interpolation estimates a value between two known values. Extrapolation estimates a value beyond known values. (From Bushong S: *Radiologic science for technologists: physics, biology, and protection*, ed 8, St. Louis, 2004, Mosby.)

acquiring 1-mm slices at 1-mm spacing through the region containing tumor and 3-mm slices at 3-mm spacing through peripheral areas of the treatment volume. Not only are slice thickness and spacing important in producing useful DRRs, but they also affect storage and communication components within the computer system. Common practice is to scan with a slice thickness of 2 to 3 mm. This provides a balance between creating good DRRs and minimizing the storage within the computer. When using a helical scanner, the images can be reconstructed at any increment because the raw data correspond to the helix. Data for the transverse cuts will be interpolated between adjacent sections.

Target and Normal Tissue Localization. Once data generated from the CT scanner have been reconstructed and transferred to the virtual simulation workstation or the treatment planning system, target and normal tissue localization can begin. If the intent is to mark and delineate the isocenter for the patient during a single CT simulation session, simultaneous and fast network transfer of data between the CT console and the virtual simulation workstation is essential to help minimize patient motion between scanning and field marking. The physician

must localize the target volume of interest (VOI) and identify critical normal tissue structures on each of the high-resolution two-dimensional CT images obtained during the scanning process. This is probably the most labor-intensive step in CT simulation. Attention to detail is a must. The sophisticated treatment planning software available today provides a number of options for the user to localize and draw volumes on each scan (see Figure 21-24).

Virtual Simulation of Treatment Fields

The field size for each treatment field is established at the virtual simulation station or using the treatment planning system after the target and normal tissue localization process has been completed. Unlike conventional simulation, the fields can be designed, if desired, after the patient has left the CT scanner.

The physician must communicate preferences for beam arrangements to the treatment planner. The virtual simulation process determines the isocenter in reference to marks placed on the patient earlier in the simulation process. Treatment planning computers can display the sectional images or give a BEV of the fields created. Two commonly used planning techniques are forward planning and inverse planning. In forward planning, the planner selects the number, direction, and shape of beams including beam-modifying devices such as wedges. Once the plan is optimized, the computer calculates the dose distribution. This type of planning is used on conventional and conformal treatments. With inverse planning, used for intensity-modulated radiation therapy (IMRT), one begins with an end in mind. The planner may specify the desired dose limits for the tumor volume and the critical structures. The computer produces a plan that modulates the intensity of the beams to optimize the dose to the tumor volume and minimize the dose to the normal structures. A dose-volume histogram (DVH) is also created, showing the dose distribution in relation to the VOI and critical structures (Figure 23-16).

Generation of Dose Distributions

Dose distributions, calculated by the treatment planning system, are based on the target drawings on each CT slice transferred to

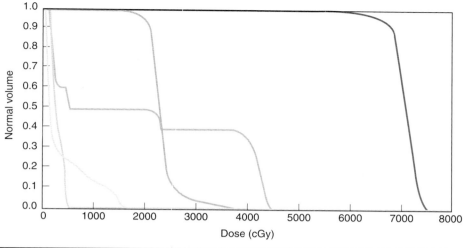

Figure 23-16. Dose volume histogram picture of treatment plan. (From Leibel SA, Phillips TL: *Textbook of radiation oncology*, ed 2, Philadelphia, 2004, Saunders.)

Current	Region of interest	Trial	Beam	Color	Dash color	% Outside grid	% > Max
◇	tumor volume	Trial_1	All beams/sources	red	No dash	0.00%	0.00%
◇	chiasm	Trial_1	All beams/sources	green	No dash	0.00%	0.00%
◇	cord	Trial_1	All beams/sources	forest	yellowgre	53.61%	0.00%
◇	left parotid	Trial_1	All beams/sources	lightblue	No dash	0.00%	0.00%
◇	brainstem	Trial_1	All beams/sources	slateblue	No dash	0.00%	0.00%
◇	rt inner ear	KD2	All beams/sources	yellowgre	No dash	0.00%	0.00%
◇	rt eye	KD2	All beams/sources	blue	tomato	0.00%	0.00%

the system. Dose distribution is also based on information gained from the patient's external contour, the outlined targets to be irradiated, and any internal organ at risk.[13] Treatment planning systems allow dose computation from CT (Hounsfield) numbers. Dose calculation algorithms that use electron density values derived from CT images are complex and require computer processing. One type of algorithm, which can produce greater accuracy at the expense of increased computational time, is the Monte Carlo technique. This calculation technique predicts dose distribution from a beam of radiation passing through a patient by simulating the behavior of a large number of photons that make up the beam.[26]

Documenting Data

Information documented in the treatment chart to aid in the daily setup of the patient may be organized in several ways and is usually institutionally dependent. Patient position and immobilization devices must be documented. A digital camera can capture the patient's position and immobilization devices as they appeared during the simulation process. This information can then be transferred to the electronic medical record for use

during treatment. With CT simulation, the exact field size, gantry position, shielding, and sometimes isocenter are often determined when the treatment plan is completed. If the target volume has been determined, CT simulators have applications allowing the computer to calculate the isocenter, with reference to the temporary marks or starting point, and the lasers and/or couch are adjusted automatically. Movable lasers can be used for all three reference points. Field edge marking systems are available with some CT scanners used to control the position of lasers that identify on the patient's skin the superior, inferior, and lateral field borders and/or isocenter.[28] If the treatment unit is equipped with a verification and record system, patient setup data can be captured and transferred.

IMAGE QUALITY

The four most desired qualities of CT images are spatial resolution, image contrast, low noise, and low dose.[30] **Spatial resolution** refers to the clarity or the measure of detail in a CT image. Image **contrast** refers to the ability to see differences in the shades of gray in tissue. **Noise** is the grainy appearance of an image. Parameters, such as mAs, kVp, slice thickness, table increment, pitch reconstruction interval, FOV, matrix size, and reconstruction filter affect the desired quality of the image.[24]

Spatial Resolution

Factors that are inherent to the equipment are focal spot size, detector aperture size, focal spot–to–patient distance, and patient-to-detector distance. Factors that the therapist has control over are pixel size, slice thickness, and the reconstruction filter used. A small pixel size creates better spatial resolution; however, the image is noisy. The FOV and the matrix size (Figure 23-17) affect the pixel size and, in turn, spatial resolution.

$$Spatial\ resolution = FOV/Matrix$$

 Keeping the same field of view, a larger image matrix will result in better spatial resolution.

A commonly used matrix size in CT is 512 × 512. If there is a 40 × 40 FOV, the pixel size is 0.8 × 0.8 mm. If there is a 20 × 20 FOV, the pixel size is 0.4 × 0.4 mm.[8] Using the same FOV, resolution will be improved with a larger image matrix[4] (Figure 23-18).

Thinner slices allow for better spatial resolution. The HU assigned is the average of attenuation coefficients of a voxel. If the slice thickness includes a rapid change in the tissue density, such as the lung and liver area, it may create an artifact called *partial volume*.

Reconstruction filters are applied to the raw data. Two basic options are a smooth filter or a sharp filter. A smooth filter is used to improve the contrast between soft tissues. It may help but may also decrease the finer structural details. A sharp filter used for musculoskeletal examinations may improve the resolution but will increase noise.[24]

Image Contrast

Image contrast, as in radiography, is not affected by mAs. However, it is affected by kVp. kVp in the 120 to 140 range is often used for the CT beam energy.[30] The sharp reconstruction

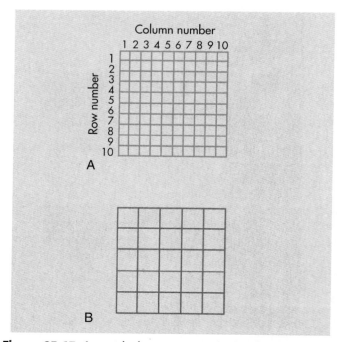

Figure 23-17. A matrix is an arrangement of columns and rows. Two matrices are shown. **A**, A 10 × 10 matrix of cells. **B**, A 5 × 5 matrix of cells. (From Bushong S: *Radiologic science for technologists: physics, biology, and protection*, ed 8, St. Louis, 2004, Mosby.)

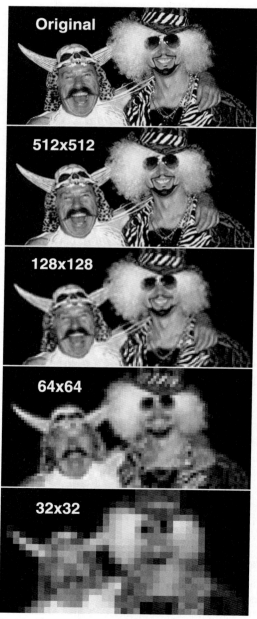

Figure 23-18. The 512 × 512 matrix is an acceptable rendition of the original. At a 32 × 32 matrix, the image demonstrates poor resolution. (From Bushong S: *Radiologic science for technologists: physics, biology, and protection*, ed 8, St. Louis, 2004, Mosby.)

filters also decrease contrast. Image contrast is inherent in the various tissue densities such as soft tissue, air in the lungs, and bony anatomy. CT is superior in displaying better image contrast compared with a conventional radiographic image. For example, the liver on a CT scan can be differentiated from other soft tissue structures in the abdomen much better than a conventional AP radiographic image of the abdomen.

Noise

If a homogeneous medium such as water is scanned, each pixel should have a value of zero. This naturally occurring variability is known as *scan noise*. The level of noise depends on several factors: mAs, kVp, filtration, pixel size, slice thickness, detector efficiency, and patient dose. An increase in kVp and mAs decreases noise. The more photons are detected by the image receptor, the less noisy is the image. A sharper construction filter increases noise. An increase in image matrix increases noise because the smaller the pixel size, the fewer photons there are per image receptor. Increased FOV and slice thickness decrease noise.[24]

Dose

Dose delivered to a patient in a single CT slice at the skin surface is in the range of 1 to 6 cGy, which is considerably greater than other imaging modalities. Methods for reducing dose are always of interest, especially in children.[30] Dose to the patient increases with an increase in mAs. A thicker slice and a greater pitch may decrease the dose to the patient.[3] In scanning a smaller region of anatomy, the dose to the patient will decrease. Last, minimizing repeat scans by reducing motion artifacts will help reduce the dose.[24]

The smaller the pixel size, the greater is the spatial resolution, but the greater is the noise. To reduce noise, a higher mAs can be used. However, that would also contribute to a higher patient dose. A balance must be achieved between spatial resolution, noise, and patient dose.[4]

 The smaller the pixels are, the better the spatial resolution and the larger the noise. Reducing the noise would require a higher technique (kVp and mAs), which would lead to a higher dose administered to the patient.

Artifacts

CT artifacts are unwanted image abnormalities that can be caused by patient motion, anatomy, design of the scanner, or system failure. Common CT **artifacts** that can gravely degrade the quality of the images, sometimes to the point of making them diagnostically unusable, are beam hardening, partial volume effect, star artifact, ring artifact, and motion and helical artifacts.

Some CT imaging artifacts can be avoided with careful planning and the use of critical thinking skills by the radiation therapist. Beam hardening artifacts (Figure 23-19) can be seen as dark bands often near bone. To minimize these artifacts, thin slices should be used and extremely dense contrast media should be avoided. Partial volume artifacts (Figure 23-20) occur when thick slices are obtained. Star artifacts (Figure 23-21) can occur from surgical clips or other metallic objects within

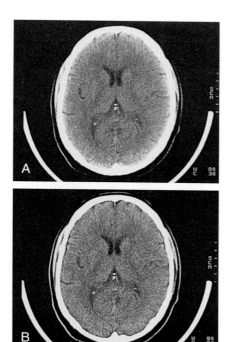

Figure 23-19. The effect of beam hardening on the appearance of the computed tomography (CT) image. **A,** The cupping artifact is visible. **B,** The cupping artifact is reduced through software. (Courtesy Siemens Medical Systems; Iselin, NJ. In Seeram E: *Computed tomography: physical principles, clinical applications, and quality control,* ed 2, Philadelphia, 2001, Saunders.)

the patient. Avoiding the metal object within the FOV if possible, would be the only way to avoid this type of artifact. A ring artifact (Figure 23-22) can occur if a detector is not working properly and may be more common in third-generation CT scanners. Artifacts similar to the ring artifact occurring in a helical scanner appear as an arc. Motion artifacts (Figure 23-23) appear as streaks or less resolution, commonly seen in and around the diaphragm when the abdomen and thorax are scanned. Faster scanners help reduce motion artifacts, especially when patients can hold their breath during a scan.[30] Helical scanning of the thorax and abdomen can lead to object shape distortion.[5] Careful patient positioning prior to scanning and proper selection of scanning parameters are the most important factors in avoiding CT artifacts.

COMPUTED TOMOGRAPHY IMAGE PROCESSING CONTROLS

After images have been reconstructed, adjustments can be made to the images seen on the computer screen. This is known as *windowing* and *leveling* and allows the manipulation of contrast on the visible image. HUs cover a range of 2000 units (−1000 to 1000). A computer monitor can display only 256 gray levels, of which only approximately 80 are visually discernible to the human eye.[7,11] The display can be optimized by changing how the HUs are displayed on the screen. This can be related to the brightness and contrast of a television screen.[24] **Window width (WW)** is the range of numbers displayed or the contrast

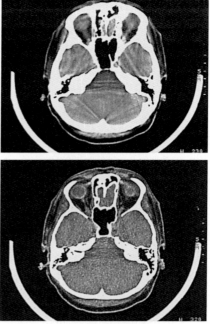

Figure 23-20. Partial volume artifacts appear as streaks across the petrous and occipital protuberances in these two CT slices. (Courtesy Siemens Medical Systems; Iselin, NJ. In Seeram E: *Computed tomography: physical principles, clinical applications, and quality control,* ed 2, Philadelphia, 2001, Saunders.)

on a CT image. If WW is narrowed, greater contrast or sharper changes in the shades of gray result. This is useful in visualizing tissues with similar densities.[24] A clinically useful gray scale is achieved by setting the window level (WL) and WW on the computer console to a suitable range of HUs, depending on the tissue examined. The term **window level**

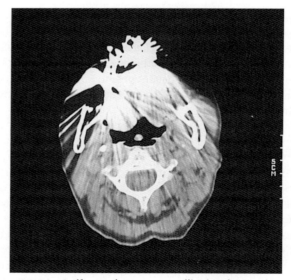

Figure 23-21. Artifacts due to metallic implants. (Courtesy Siemens Medical Systems; Iselin, NJ. In Seeram E: *Computed tomography: physical principles, clinical applications, and quality control,* ed 2, Philadelphia, 2001, Saunders.)

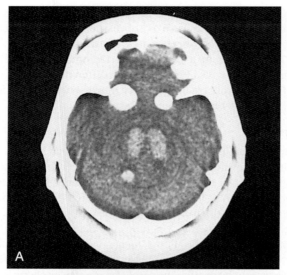

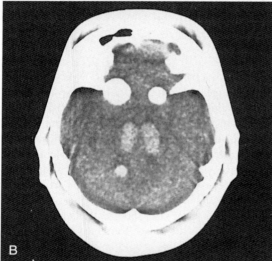

Figure 23-22. The ring artifact **(A)** and correction using the balancing algorithm **(B)**. (Courtesy Siemens Medical Systems; Iselin, NJ. In Seeram E: *Computed tomography: physical principles, clinical applications, and quality control,* ed 2, Philadelphia, 2001, Saunders.)

represents the central HU of all the CT numbers within the WW. The WW covers the HU of all the tissues of interest, and these are displayed as various shades of gray. Tissues with CT numbers outside this range are displayed as either black or white. Both the WL and WW can be set independently on the computer console by the radiation therapist. Their respective settings affect the final displayed image[7] (Figure 23-24). Figure 23-25, column A, demonstrates the anatomy represented by the Hounsfield numbers. In Figure 23-25, column B, the WW is 200. Those numbers between +100 and −100 are shades of gray. All Hounsfield numbers greater than 100 appear white and those less than −100 appear black. The same holds true for columns C and D with a different WW.[27] The effect of a wide window will decrease contrast and a narrow WW will increase contrast, as seen in Figure 23-26.[27]

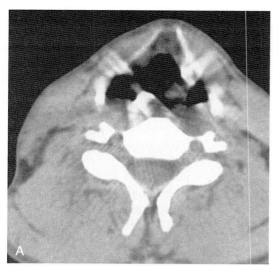

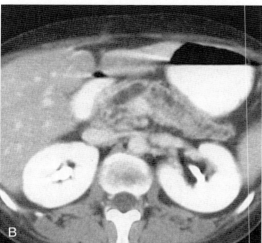

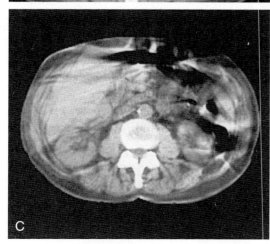

Figure 23-23. Motion artifacts due to swallowing **(A)**, peristalsis **(B)**, and patient movement **(C)**. (Courtesy Siemens Medical Systems; Iselin, NJ. In Seeram E: *Computed tomography: physical principles, clinical applications, and quality control,* ed 2, Philadelphia, 2001, Saunders.)

QUALITY ASSURANCE

CT scanners used for radiation therapy simulation should have similar mechanical checks as linear accelerators, because they are meant to simulate the geometry of the treatment beam.[16] Both mechanical checks and image-quality performance checks should be evaluated according to the guidelines in the 2003 report of the AAPM Radiation Therapy Committee Task Group No. 66,[23a] which outlines quality assurance for CT simulators and the CT simulation process. These guidelines (Tables 23-5 and 23-6) can be used to establish a department-specific quality assurance program based on the amount of CT simulation experience and departmental goals.

Daily warm-up procedures for the CT simulator include warming up the x-ray tube according to the manufacturer's specifications, checking the laser system, and scanning a water phantom. The water phantom scan checks noise levels by comparing the Hounsfield number of water at various areas of the phantom (Figure 23-27). These levels should be within ±3 from zero. The scan should have a large enough region of interest. If scanning air, the Hounsfield number should read −1000 with ±5 variance allowed.[3] The quality of the beam must be checked yearly including spatial resolution, contrast resolution, and correlation of Hounsfield numbers with electron density.[3,16] Monthly tests include CT (Hounsfield) number/electron density verification, reconstruction slice location, image transfer protocols, left/right registration, and distance between known points in the image.[9]

  For more information regarding quality assurance for radiation therapy CT simulators, see the American Association of Physicists in Medicine website at http://www.aapm.org/pubs/reports/.
Report No. 83—Quality assurance for computed-tomography simulators and the computed-tomography-simulation process: report of the AAPM Radiation Therapy Committee Task Group No. 66—is available for review.

INTEGRATION WITH TREATMENT PLANNING

Once the CT scan for treatment planning has been completed, the digital data must be transferred to the treatment planning system. This can be accomplished by magnetic tape, optical disk, or electronic network.[15] DICOM (Digital Imaging and Communications in Medicine) is the standard image format to transfer information between the imaging devices and the treatment planning computer[15] (see Chapter 27). When creating a treatment plan using CT simulation, gantry limits, collimator limits, and table angle limits must be kept in mind. It is possible to create a treatment plan that cannot be executed in the treatment room.

Multiple image studies of the same patient are often used to produce all the information needed for accurate identification of target volume and critical organs.[15] Image registration and correlation or image fusion are used in identifying preoperative volume and transfer to postoperative scans, fusing MRI and PET scans, which are useful in determining the extent of the tumor.[15]

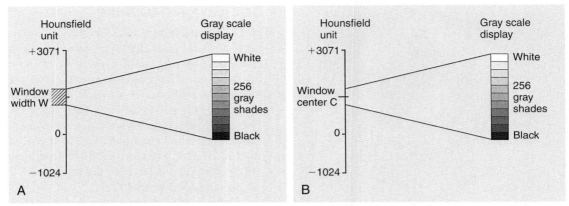

Figure 23-24. The concept of window width **(A)** and window level **(B)** in computed tomography (CT) windowing. (Courtesy Siemens Medical Systems; Iselin, NJ. In Seeram E: *Computed tomography: physical principles, clinical applications, and quality control*, ed 2, Philadelphia, 2001, Saunders.)

For example, a patient with a nasopharyngeal tumor may have had both MRI and CT diagnostic scans that showed bony invasion on the CT, while the high-intensity areas on MRI showed the extent of soft tissue tumor localization. This information is important when designing tumor volumes.[6] Maurer and Fitzpatrick[21] define registration as "the determination of a one-to-one mapping between two coordinates in one space and those in another, such that points in the two spaces which correspond to the same anatomical point are mapped to each other." The process of image registration begins with two sets of images. The treatment planner locates image features on both

sets that are the same. These features can include a bony prominence or a soft tissue ventricle of the brain. A manual match mode allows the treatment planner to select three points on both scans. In addition to the points selected, scans can be overlaid and the dosimetrist is able to rotate the scans to get the best match. One of the challenges with image registration is that often the patients are not in the same position or the modalities are different, making it difficult to fuse the two images. Once the physician approves the fused images, outlines of treatment volumes and critical structures can take into account all the information of the fused images (Figure 23-28).

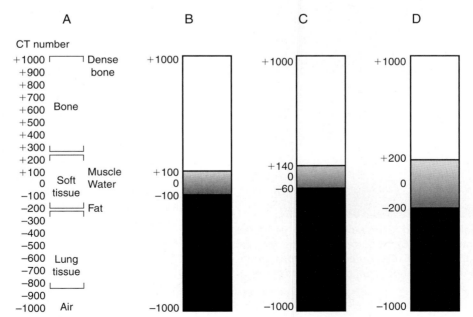

Figure 23-25. Graphic illustration of the effect of different window width and window level settings on the appearance of the computed tomography (CT) image. (From Seeram E: *Computed tomography: physical principles, clinical applications, and quality control*, ed 2, Philadelphia, 2001, Saunders.)

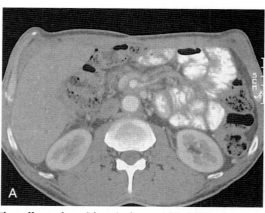 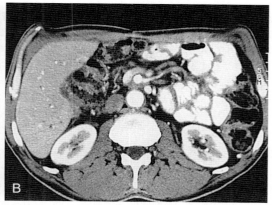

Figure 23-26. The effect of a wide window width **(A)** and a narrow window width **(B)** on the appearance of the computed tomography (CT) image. (From Seeram E: *Computed tomography: physical principles, clinical applications, and quality control,* ed 2, Philadelphia, 2001, Saunders.)

Table 23-5	Test Specifications for Electromechanical Components of a CT Simulator from Report No. 83 of the AAPM Radiation Therapy Committee Task Group No. 66 on Quality Assurance for Computed-Tomography Simulators and the Computed-Tomography-Simulation Process*		
Performance Parameter	**Test Objective**	**Frequency**	**Tolerance Limits**
Alignment of gantry lasers with the center of imaging plane	To verify proper identification of scan plane with gantry lasers	Daily	±2 mm
Orientation of gantry lasers with respect to imaging plane	To verify that gantry lasers are parallel to and orthogonal with the imaging plane over the full length of laser projection	Monthly and after laser adjustments	±2 mm over the length of laser projection
Spacing of lateral wall lasers with respect to lateral gantry lasers and scan plane	To verify that lateral wall lasers are accurately spaced from the scan plane This distance is used for patient localization marking	Monthly and after laser adjustments	±2 mm
Orientation of wall lasers with respect to imaging plane	To verify that the wall lasers are parallel to and orthogonal with the imaging plane over the full length of laser projection	Monthly and after laser adjustments	±2 mm over the length of laser projection
Orientation of the ceiling laser with respect to imaging plane	To verify that the ceiling laser is orthogonal with imaging plane	Monthly and after laser adjustments	±2 mm over the length of laser projection
Orientation of the CT scanner tabletop with respect to imaging plane	To verify that the CT scanner tabletop is level and orthogonal with imaging plane	Monthly or when daily laser QA tests reveal rotational problems	±2 mm over the length and width of the tabletop
Table vertical and longitudinal motion	To verify that the table longitudinal motion according to digital indicators is accurate and reproducible	Monthly	±1 mm over the range of table motion
Table indexing and position	To verify table indexing and position accuracy under scanner control	Annually	±1 mm over the scan range
Gantry tilt accuracy	To verify accuracy of gantry tilt indicators	Annually	±1° over the gantry tilt range
Gantry tilt position accuracy	To verify that the gantry accurately returns to nominal position after tilting	Annually	±1° or ±1 mm from nominal position
Scan localization	To verify accuracy of scan localization from pilot images	Annually	±1 mm over the scan range
Radiation profile width	To verify that the radiation profile width meets manufacturer specification	Annually (optional if the CTDI accuracy has been verified)	Manufacturer specifications
Sensitivity profile width	To verify that the sensitivity profile width meets manufacturer specification	Semiannually	±1 mm of nominal value
Generator tests	To verify proper operation of the x-ray generator	After replacement of major generator component	Manufacturer specifications or AAPM Report No. 39 recommendations

From Mutic S, et al: *Med Phys* 30(10): 2762-2792, 2003.
AAPM, American Association of Physicists in Medice; *CTDI,* computed tomography dose index; *QA,* quality assurance.
*Depending on the goals and prior clinical experience of a particular CT simulation program, these tests, frequencies, and tolerances may be modified by the medical physicist.

Table 23-6	Test Specifications for Imaging Performance of a CT Simulator from Report No. 83 of the AAPM Radiation Therapy Committee Task Group No. 66 on Quality Assurance for Computed-Tomography Simulators and the Computed-Tomography-Simulation Process*		
Performance Parameter	**Frequency**		**Tolerance Limits**
CT number accuracy	Daily—CT number for water Monthly—4 to 5 different materials Annually—Electron density phantom		For water, ±5 HU
Image noise	Daily		Manufacturer specifications
In-plane spatial integrity	Daily—x or y direction Monthly—both directions		±1 mm
Field uniformity	Monthly—most commonly used kVp Annually—other used kVp settings		Within ±5 HU
Electron density to CT number conversion	Annually—or after scanner calibration		Consistent with commissioning results and test phantom manufacturer specifications
Spatial resolution	Annually		Manufacturer specifications
Contrast resolution	Annually		Manufacturer specifications

From Mutic S, et al: *Med Phys* 30(10): 2762-2792, 2003.

*Depending on the goals and prior clinical experience of a particular CT simulation program, these tests, frequencies, and tolerances may be modified by the medical physicist.

RESPIRATORY GATING WITH COMPUTED TOMOGRAPHY SIMULATION

For many years, motion artifacts have been recognized with CT scanning. With the advancements in tumor localization in radiation therapy, breathing motion remains a challenge in localizing thorax and upper abdomen tumors.[19,22] Organs can move up to several centimeters in a few seconds.[5] One method to overcome breathing motion artifacts is to have the patient hold their breath during the scan, often at full inhalation

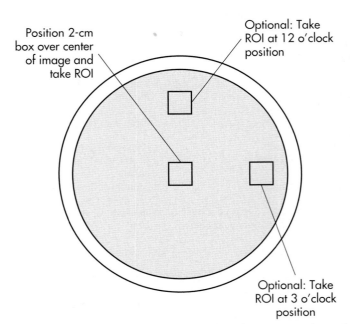

Figure 23-27. Test for noise and uniformity. *ROI,* Region of interest. (From Papp J: *Quality management in the imaging sciences,* ed 3, St. Louis, 2006, Mosby.)

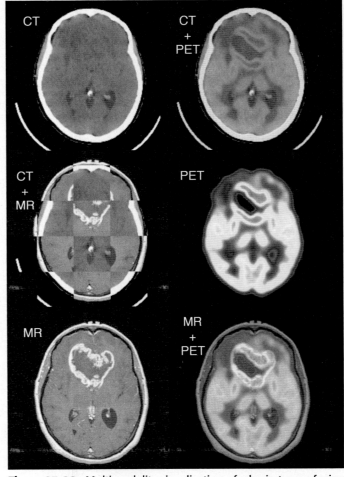

Figure 23-28. Multimodality visualization of a brain tumor fusing a computed tomography (CT) scan, magnetic resonance (MR) image, and positron emission tomography (PET) scan of the same patient. (From Leibel SA, Phillips TL: *Textbook of radiation oncology,* ed 2, Philadelphia, 2004, Saunders.)

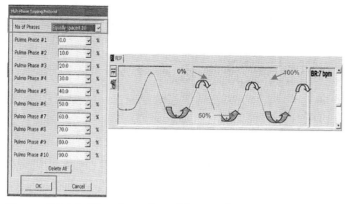

Figure 23-29. Waveform breathing cycle. (Courtesy Philips Medical Systems.)

or full exhalation.[19] However, many patients cannot hold their breath. These challenges have led to the development of four-dimensional scanning, which captures the organ motion during all cycles of the respiratory phase. In order to perform four-dimensional CT scanning, a method to measure the respiratory phase is needed. This can be accomplished by using a spirometer (a machine that measures various lung volumes, such as tidal volume, inspiratory reserve volume, and vital capacity of the lungs) or a measurement of the motion of the abdomen, which usually consists of a device strapped to the abdomen that records the breathing cycle. The patient's breathing waveform will be recorded and the pitch is set according to the breath rate (Figure 23-29). A very slow pitch such as 0.5:1 is common, which allows for very thin slices and multiple scans per couch position, recording the anatomy at the various phases of the breathing cycle.[9] This scan creates approximately 1500 slices of image data that will then be placed into tidal volume bins according to their phase of the breathing. The resulting scan can have 10 CT slices at each phase of breathing from full inhalation to full exhalation per couch position.[19] Once these data are acquired, the physician will decide what information will be used. If respiratory gating will be used with the treatment machine, the physician may select only a few phases to create a plan. This will allow a plan to be created with a smaller tumor volume and will be treated only at the planning phase of the respiratory cycle. If respiratory gating will not be used, an MIP (maximum intensity projection) can be created. This takes the scans at full inhalation and the scans at full exhalation and fuses them together. This fused scan shows the maximum amount of tumor movement during the respiratory cycle. Treatment planning can occur based on the motion of the tumor. The advantage to this method is the ability to spare normal lung and ensure maximum dose coverage to the tumor.

SUMMARY

- The use of computed tomography (CT) simulation has become the primary method of simulation over the last several years. CT simulation provides more complete anatomic patient data, which allows for better treatment planning.

- CT scanners record radiation attenuated through a series of detectors that are stored in a digital "raw" format. These data are reconstructed to create an image.
- Attenuation profile summaries are displayed as pixels of different shades of gray and are measured in Hounsfield units.
- Benefits of CT simulation include the ability to view all critical structures, which allows for more accurate treatment planning.
- CT image data can be used for radiation therapy dose calculations.
- Because the CT scanner does not reflect the geometry of the linear accelerator, careful simulation must occur to ensure the ability to treat the patient as planned.
- Contrast media are most commonly used to enhance structures in patients with a specific pathology, such as head and neck, lung, brain, and abdominal and pelvis tumors.
- The most common contrast agents are barium given orally or placed in the rectum and ionic or nonionic iodinated contrast, which is given through an IV line. A patient questionnaire must be completed prior to administering contrast media.
- Communicating with and reassuring the patient are key to performing a successful simulation.
- When scanning a patient, the lasers are not necessarily placed at isocenter. The patient needs to be in the center of the field of view so that the patient's contour is not cut off.
- Spatial resolution, image contrast, low noise, and low dose are associated with image quality. The smaller the pixel size, the greater is the spatial resolution. However, the greater is the noise. To reduce noise, a higher mAs value can be used, which would contribute to a higher patient dose.
- Common artifacts in CT scanning are beam hardening artifacts, partial volume artifacts, star artifacts, ring artifacts, and motion artifacts.
- More sophisticated computers allow various modalities to be fused together, such as CT and MRI. Respiratory gating can be used during simulation. These benefits result in better treatment planning, resulting in better patient care.
- Sophisticated computers and methods of imaging will continue to improve, resulting in better patient care. It is important to have an understanding of conventional simulation techniques to apply the principles to CT simulation.

Review Questions

Multiple Choice

1. A projection is defined as:
   a. an intensity pattern created from the linear attenuation coefficient
   b. the x-ray tube and detector completing one revolution around the patient
   c. the raw data recorded from the CT scan
   d. part of the equipment of the CT scanner

2. The average linear attenuation coefficient per pixel is called:
   a. Hounsfield units
   b. CT number
   c. image matrix
   d. filtered back projection

3. Contrast media may be given to patients with a brain tumor:
   a. 10 minutes prior to scan
   b. immediately before the scan
   c. the day before the scan
   d. time does not matter

4. If the field of view for CT scanning is larger using the same image matrix, the:
   a. spatial resolution is better
   b. spatial resolution is worse
   c. slices are thinner
   d. image contrast is better

5. Which of the following will reduce image noise?
   I. sharper image filter
   II. increase kVP and mAs
   III. larger pixel size
   IV. increased FOV
   a. III only
   b. II and III
   c. I and IV
   d. II, III, and IV

6. CT artifacts created from motion during the scan are called:
   a. beam hardening artifacts
   b. partial volume artifacts
   c. star artifacts
   d. ring artifacts

7. To increase contrast when viewing a DRR, one would:
   a. narrow the window width range to be displayed
   b. widen the window width range to be displayed
   c. increase the window level
   d. decrease the window level

8. A pitch of 0.5 will:
   a. increase patient dose
   b. lead to interpolation errors
   c. move the table faster through the scanner
   d. determine the slice thickness

9. Daily quality assurance checks for the CT simulator include:
   I. laser position verification
   II. electron density verification
   III. water phantom scan
   a. I only
   b. II and III
   c. I and III
   d. I, II, and III

10. Respiratory gating used during CT simulation consists of recording the patient's breathing pattern and scanning:
    a. at full exhalation
    b. with a fast pitch during the entire breathing pattern
    c. at full inhalation
    d. with a slow pitch during the entire breathing pattern

The answers to the Review Questions can be found by logging on to our website at: *http://evolve.elsevier.com/Washington+Leaver/ principles*

Questions to Ponder

1. Discuss the importance of contrast agents used in CT simulation.
2. Describe, as though you were educating an interested patient, the purpose of the CT simulation procedure.
3. Explain the purpose of each of the components of the CT simulator.
4. Discuss the role each of the following have on CT image quality: spatial resolution, image contrast, noise, dose, and artifacts.
5. Discuss the process of tumor localization and treatment planning using CT simulation.
6. What are the advantages and disadvantages of CT simulation versus conventional simulation?

REFERENCES

1. Adler A, Carlton R: *Introduction to radiographic sciences and patient care*, Philadelphia, 2007, WB Saunders.
2. Aird EGA, Conway J: CT simulation for radiotherapy treatment planning, *Br J Radiol* 75: 937-949, 2002.
3. Bushong SC: *Computed tomography*, New York, 2000, McGraw-Hill.
4. Bushong S: *Radiologic science for technologist: physics, biology, and protection*, ed 8, St. Louis, 2004, Mosby.
5. Chen G, Kung J, Beaudette K: Artifacts in computed tomography scanning of moving objects, *Semin Radiat Oncol* 14:19-26, 2004.
6. Chen GT, Pelizzari CA: Image correlation: applications in nuclear medicine and beyond, *J Nucl Med* 35:1781, 1994.
7. CT physics. Retrieved January 2008 from http://intl.elsevierhealth.com/e-books/pdf/940.pdf.
8. Fleckenstein P, Tranum-Jensen J: *Anatomy in diagnostic imaging*, ed 2, Copenhagen, Denmark, 2001, Blackwell Publishing.
9. Ford E, Mageras G: Respiration correlated spiral CT: a method of measuring respiratory induced anatomic motion for radiation treatment planning, *Med Phys* 30:88-97, 2003.
10. Gerbi BJ: The simulation process in the determination and definition of treatment volume and treatment planning. In Levitt SH, Khan FM, Potish RA, Perez CA, editors: *Levitt and Tapley's technological basis of radiation therapy*, ed 3, Philadelphia, 1999, Lippincott Williams & Wilkins.
11. Goldman L: Personal communication, June 20, 2007.
12. Hofer M: *CT teaching manual: a systematic approach to CT reading*, Stuttgart, 2005, Georg Thieme Verlag.
13. Hunt M, Coia L: The treatment planning process. In Purdy JA, Starkschall G, editors: *3D planning and conformal radiation therapy*, Madison, Wis, 1999, Advanced Medical Publishers.
14. Khan FM: *The physics of radiation therapy*, ed 2, Baltimore, 2003, Lippincott Williams & Wilkins.
15. Khan F: *Treatment planning in radiation oncology*, ed 2, Philadelphia, 2007, Lippincott Williams & Wilkins.
16. Kutcher TG, et al: Comprehensive QA for radiation oncology, *Med Phys* 21(4): 581-618, 1994.
17. Leaver DT: IMRT: Part 2, *Radiat Ther* 11:17-32, 2003.
18. Leibel S, Phillips T: *Textbook of radiation oncology*, Philadelphia, 2004, WB Saunders.
19. Low D, Nystrom M: A method for reconstruction of four-dimensional synchronized CT scans acquired during free breathing, *Med Phys* 30: 1254-1263, 2003.
20. Martin EE: CT simulation hardware. In Purdy JA, Starkschall G, editors: *3D planning and conformal radiation therapy*, Madison, Wis, 1999, Advanced Medical Publishers.

21. Maurer C, Fitzpatrick J: A review of medical image registration. In Maciunas RJ, *editor: Interactive image guided neurosurgery (pp 17-44), American Association of Neurological Surgeons, 1993, Park Ridge, Ill.*

22. Morin O, Gillis A: Megavoltage cone-beam CT: system description and clinical applications, *Med Dosimetry* 31:51-61, 2006.

23. Munzenrider J, Pilepich M: Use of body scanner in radiotherapy treatment planning, *Cancer* 40:170-179, 1977.

23a. Mutic S, et al: Quality assurance dor computed-tomography simulators and the computed-tomography-simulation process: report of the AAPM Radiation Therapy Committee Task Group No. 66, *Med Phys* 30(10): 2762-2792, 2003.

24. Nielsen C, Kaiser D, Femano P: *The CT CrossTrainer,* Clifton, NJ, 2005, Medical Imaging Consultant, Inc.

25. Purdy JA: Principles of radiologic physics, dosimetry and treatment planning. In Perez CA, Brady LW editors: *Principles and practice of radiation oncology,* ed 4, Philadelphia, 2004, Lippincott Williams & Wilkins.

26. Redpath AT, McNee SC: Treatment planning for external beam therapy: advanced techniques. In Williams JR, Thwaites DI, editors: *Radiotherapy physics in practice,* Oxford, 2000, Oxford University Press.

27. Seeram E: *Computed tomography: physical principles, clinical applications, and quality control,* Philadelphia, 2001, WB Saunders.

28. VanDyk JV, Mah K: Simulation and imaging for radiation therapy planning. In Willams JR, Thwaites DI, editors: *Radiotherapy physics in practice,* Oxford, 2000, Oxford University Press.

29. Washinton CM, Leaver D: *Principles and practice of radiation therapy,* ed 2, St. Louis, 2004, Mosby.

30. Wolbarst A: *Physics of radiology,* ed 2, Madison, Wis, 2005, Medical Physics Publishing.

BIBLIOGRAPHY

Coia LR, Schultheiss TE: *A practical guide to CT simulation,* Madison, Wis, 1995, Medical Physics Publishing.

Golman LW, Fowlkes JB: *Medical CT and ultrasound* (website): www.AAMP.org. Accessed 1995.

Shirish KJ: *CT simulation for radiotherapy,* Madison, Wis, 1993, Medical Physics Publishing.

Photon Dosimetry Concepts and Calculations

Julius Armstrong, Charles M. Washington

Outline

Key Terms

Objectives

- Identify and accurately apply the information in a radiation therapy prescription to calculate the treatment time (i.e., monitor unit or minute setting).
- Define the terms used in radiation therapy to calculate the monitor unit setting and/or minute setting and the dose to selected points of interest.
- Define *machine output* in terms of *dose rate*.
- Identify the major data tables required to perform a radiation treatment time calculation.
- Calculate an equivalent square of a rectangular field using Sterling's formula.
- Analyze the need for percentage depth dose, tissue-air ratio, tissue-phantom ratio, and tissue-maximum ratio tables.
- Identify the differences in calculation models used for nonisocentric versus isocentric calculations.

- Apply the correct calculation model to calculate the monitor unit setting and doses to points of interest.
- Explain the effect on the treatment time calculation when using wedge filters, compensating filters, and/or a block tray.
- Calculate changes in dose rate as a function of distance from the target using the inverse square law.
- Describe the effect of the inverse square law on the monitor unit setting.
- Calculate the monitor unit setting for a given patient treatment.
- Calculate the dose to points of interest such as the dose to the cord and the dose to the depth of maximum equilibrium.

The administration of ionizing radiation for cancer treatment requires knowledge of anatomy, physics, and biologic responses. The success or failure of a radiation therapy course depends on precise and accurate administration of radiation to a localized site outlined by a radiation oncologist. The treatment planning team has to quantify the overall prescribed dose of radiation and determine how much dose will be delivered over the time frame outlined. There are many parameters of photon beam dose calculation that must be addressed; the radiation therapist and medical dosimetrist must be able to determine treatment machine settings to deliver the prescribed dose through manual and computerized methods.

Today, there is greater emphasis on computer calculation models, and many oncology departments use programmed calculators to verify the **monitor units (MUs)** calculated by the computer. In addition, with three-dimensional (3D) treatment planning more importance is placed on determining the dose delivery to volumes of tissues, such as the clinical target volume. In this chapter, the emphasis is placed on calculating the MU setting for a dose prescribed to a single point and for calculating the dose to other points such as cord doses and doses to the depth of maximum equilibrium (D_{max}). Understanding these newer concepts still requires a basic understanding of the factors that affect dose delivery and a comfort level with MU and point-dose calculations. It is not possible to cover every established method of performing dose calculations, because most clinical settings have site-specific methods for calculating dose, normally determined by a medical radiation physicist. This chapter provides clinical examples of dose calculations, both MU and time, and examples that encompass components used in treatment planning. This will allow the treatment planning and delivery team to use the principles presented with the calculation methods used in any radiation therapy center.

It is important to mention that this chapter was written with the beginning practitioner in mind. A brief review of basic terminology and concepts provides a basic overview, starting with basic calculations and then moving toward the more advanced calculations.

RADIATION THERAPY PRESCRIPTION

When a patient requires medicine to address an ailment, the physician writes a medical prescription. That prescription is a communication tool between the physician and the pharmacist. The medical prescription provides the pharmacist the name of the medication, as well as its dose, route, and quantity, and must also state how often and how long the patient should take the medicine. The pharmacist must also be familiar with the effects of the drug or combination of drugs prescribed.

The **radiation therapy prescription** is a communication tool between the radiation oncologist and the treatment planning and delivery team, particularly the radiation therapist and medical dosimetrist. The prescription, whether in written or electronic format, provides the information required to administer the appropriate radiation treatment. This legal document defines the treatment volume, intended tumor dose (TD), number of treatments, dose per treatment, and frequency of treatment.[2] The prescription also states the type and energy of radiation, beam-shaping devices such as wedges and compensators, and any other appropriate factors. The radiation therapist must be able to discuss with the patient the treatment procedure, function of the devices, and treatment side effects. In practice, there is no standard radiation therapy prescription. The organization and detail of prescriptions vary from one radiation oncology center to another. It is very important that the radiation prescription be clear, precise, and complete. For example, if a thorax is to be treated using anterior and posterior opposed fields, the prescription commonly sets a spinal cord limit not to exceed 4500 cGy. This instruction should be clear and exact;

there should be no instruction that is open to interpretation. Every parameter and phase of the treatment must be clearly defined in the radiation therapy prescription.

The radiation oncologist will commonly define the region to be treated, technique, treatment machine, energy, fractionation, and daily and total doses within a radiation prescription form. All of the necessary parameters may be located in one or more areas of the treatment record. Most oncology centers use some type of computerized patient management systems. The patient treatment instructions may be found on one screen, whereas the field sizes and gantry, collimator, and couch angles may be found on another screen. Nearly all patients have a computerized isodose or 3D treatment plan that is also part of the patient's record. The computerized plans (e.g., isodose plan, 3D) should show field sizes, machine angles, doses, beam weighting, wedges, compensators, or multileaf collimator (MLC) setting or customized blocks. These plans are considered part of the radiation therapy prescription and should always be dated and signed by the radiation oncologist.

The radiation therapist and medical dosimetrist must make sure that all parts of the prescription match before treatment. For example, the doses, treatment machines, and so forth should be the same on the prescription form and the computerized plan.

CONCEPTS USED IN PHOTON BEAM DOSE CALCULATIONS

When ionizing radiation is administered to a patient, there are many factors that must be identified. As noted earlier, beam energy, distance from the source of radiation, and field size are just a few of the variables that must be addressed to accurately calculate a **treatment time** (length of time a unit is physically left on to deliver a measured dose) or MU setting. [Note: the MU is the treatment "time" for a linear accelerator. Some older technologies, such as cobalt-60 treatment machines, required an actual treatment time, which is set in minutes.] The radiation physicist uses mathematics, computers, and specialized equipment to develop dose calculation data used by the medical dosimetrist and radiation therapist. Many of the data are organized in tables to provide quick reference for these calculations. Before any attempt at performing a dose calculation is made, a number of terms used must be defined. It is important to be consistent in the use and understanding of these terms. The nomenclature used outlines the parameters necessary for accurate treatment delivery. It is important to remember that there are different approaches, methods, and terms used for dose and MU calculations. The radiation therapist and medical dosimetrist must ensure that the appropriate information for each individual application is used.

Dose

Everyone involved with treatment planning and delivery must have a clear idea of what is meant by dose. The *dose,* or **absorbed dose**, is measured at a specific point in a medium (typically a patient or phantom) and refers to the energy deposited at that point. Dose is commonly measured in Gray (Gy), which is defined so that 1 Gy equals 1 J/kg.[1,2] Note: before the Gy, the rad was the unit of absorbed dose—100 rad equals 1 Gy and 1 rad equals 1 cGy.

Depth

Depth is the distance beneath the skin surface where the prescribed dose is to be delivered. Sometimes the radiation oncologist will specify the depth of calculation. For example, when an area is treated with a single treatment field, the radiation oncologist will state the exact point, or depth, for the calculation. Using a posterior field for treatment of vertebral body metastasis, the radiation therapy prescription may state that a dose of 3 Gy to a depth of 5.0 cm is to be delivered. For opposed fields, the patient's midplane is often used for the depth of calculation. Most multiple field arrangements use the isocenter, or intersection of the beams, for the calculation depth. Treatment techniques such as stereotactic also require that the dose is prescribed to a volume, whereas intensity-modulated radiation therapy techniques require that doses are specified to a number of volumes. Computed tomography (CT) scans, which provide visual information on the patient's shape (contour) and location of organs and other anatomic structures, are useful in determining the point of calculation.

The depth of the calculation affects measurements of dose attenuation.

Separation

Separation is a measurement of the patient's thickness from the point of beam entry to the point of beam exit (Figure 24-1). When calculating a treatment time or MU setting, the separation is normally measured along the beam's central axis. The separation can be measured directly using calipers, measured indirectly using the readings supplied by optical distance indicators (ODIs) located on the treatment units, or measured it from the treatment plan. Often, for parallel opposed treatment fields (two fields focused at a point of specification directed 180 degrees apart), the calculation is done to deliver the prescribed dose at the patient's midplane or midseparation. To find the midseparation, the total separation is divided by 2. For example, if the treatment prescription requires delivery of 2 Gy per fraction at midseparation using opposed fields, the patient's separation at the central axis would be measured. If the separation were measured as 20 cm, the midseparation (midplane) would be 10 cm. In that case, a depth of 10 cm would be used for the MU calculation.

Source-Skin Distance

Source-skin distance (SSD) is the distance from the source or target of the treatment machine to the surface of the patient or

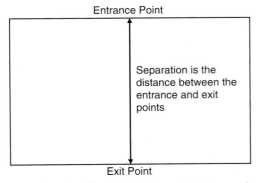

Figure 24-1. Diagram demonstrating patient separation as the distance between the beam entrance and exit points.

phantom (a volume of tissue equivalent material). The SSD is normally measured using an ODI. This device projects a distance scale onto the patient's skin (Figure 24-2, A). The number read is the distance from the source of photons to the patient's skin surface.

 Setting and verifying the appropriate SSD on a daily basis is crucial to the accurate delivery of the radiation treatment plan. Most radiation treatment centers ensure that the radiation therapist is doing so by requiring weekly documentation of the SSD of all fields. Because of the nature of the disease and the side effects of various treatments the patient is enduring, there is a high tendency for weight loss specifically in the head and neck region, as well as lung and abdomen. By verifying and documenting weekly SSDs, dosimetrists can take into account change and account for it by decreasing MUs or altering the plan. If the SSD changes significantly, the patient may need to be resimulated and immobilization devices modified.

Source-Axis Distance and Isocenter

The **source-axis distance (SAD)** is the distance from the source of photons to the isocenter of the treatment machine (see Figure 24-2, B). The **isocenter** is the intersection of the axis of rotation of the gantry and the axis of rotation of the collimator for the treatment unit. This is usually a point in space at a specified distance from the source or target that the gantry rotates around. Cobalt-60 treatment machines typically have a SAD of 80 cm, whereas the SAD for most modern linear accelerators is 100 cm. When the gantry rotates around the patient, the SSD will continually change; however, the SAD and isocenter are at a fixed distance and therefore do not change. In a isocentric treatment, the isocenter is established inside the patient. The treatment machines are designed so that the gantry will rotate around this reference point.

Field Size

Field size refers to the physical dimensions set on the collimators of the therapy unit that determine the size of the treatment field at a reference distance. Depending on the type of machine this is the setting for the X and Y jaws or the upper and lower jaws. The field size is normally defined at the machine's isocenter. For example, when a field size of 10 × 10 cm is set on the treatment unit (*x* and *y* digital readouts), the square treatment field measures 10 × 10 cm at the isocentric distance for that particular machine. On most linear accelerators, that distance would be at 100 cm. On a cobalt-60 machine, the distance would be at 80 cm.

Field size changes with distance from the source of radiation because of divergence. The 10 × 10 cm field size would measure smaller at distances shorter than the isocentric distance and larger at distances greater than the isocentric distance. In an isocentric patient treatment, the field size set would be inside the patient at the isocenter distance. This is called an *SAD treatment*. The physical size measured on the patient's surface at that point would be smaller, because it would be at a distance shorter than the isocenter. In the nonisocentric (SSD) patient treatment, the field size set on the collimator would be the same

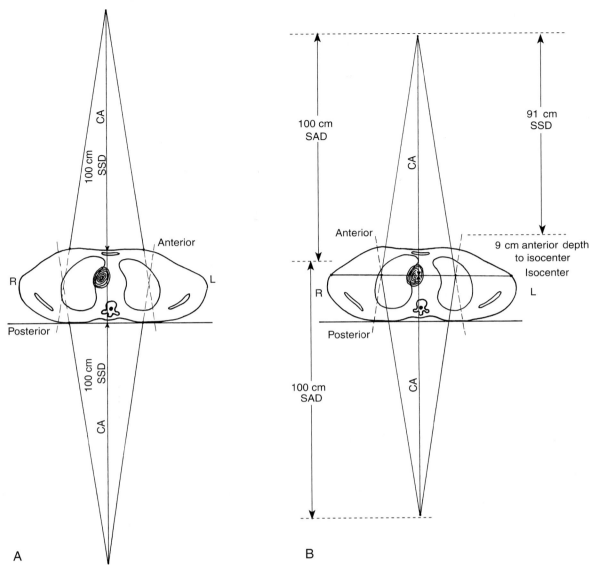

Figure 24-2. Differences between a source-skin distance (SSD) approach **(A)**, where the field size is defined on the surface, and source-axis distance (SAD) approach **(B)**, where the field size is defined at a depth calculated within the patient, are demonstrated. Both methods used in the planning and delivery of a prescribed course of radiation therapy require careful documentation.

as measured on the skin surface, because the isocentric distance is set at the skin surface in this instance. For an extended distance treatment (greater than 100 cm to the skin), the field size on the skin will be greater than the field size at the isocenter due to the increased distance.

Scatter

The radiation treatment beam is composed of both primary and scatter radiation. Any interaction of the primary radiation may result in scatter. When the primary beam interacts with matter, the result is scatter radiation made up of photons or electrons. There is a change of direction associated with scatter radiation. When an electron interacts with the target in the linear accelerator, photons are produced. These photons are the primary beam.

As the primary photons travel to the patient, they will interact with the flattening filter, and then some of them will interact with the collimator. When the primary photon interacts with the collimator, the photon beam may also be deflected back toward the patient. The deflected photons are considered scatter radiation. When the photons reach the patient and travel through the patient, they will interact mostly with the electrons. Many of these photons will change direction with each electron interaction and thus create scatter radiation within the patient. Radiation that is scattered back toward the surface of the patient is given a special name and is called *backscatter* (this will be covered in more detail later in this chapter). The absorbed dose received by the patient results from secondary radiation caused by interactions in which the primary and scattered photons impart energy to the electrons. Then the electron undergoes tens of thousands of collisions while giving up some energy at each collision. Most of the absorbed dose that is received by the patient results from the collisions of the scattered electrons with other electrons.

Depth of Maximum Equilibrium (D_{max})

The depth of maximum equilibrium, also known as D_{max}, is the depth at which electronic equilibrium occurs for photon beams. D_{max} is the point where the maximum absorbed dose occurs for single-field photon beams and mainly depends on the energy of the beam. The depth of maximum ionization increases as the energy of the photon beam increases. D_{max} occurs at the surface for low-energy photon beams and beneath the surface for megavoltage photon beams. Other factors such as field size and distance may influence the depth at which maximum ionization occurs. Table 24-1 lists the approximate depth of D_{max} for various photon beam energies. When the depth of D_{max} occurs at a significant depth (1.0 to 4.0 cm) below the skin, the dose to the skin is reduced. This principle is known as *skin sparing* and is a very important concept.

There are times when it is important to know what the dose is at D_{max}. When a patient is treated using a single field, the dose at D_{max} should be calculated and recorded because the dose at D_{max} will be higher than the prescribed dose. The dose at D_{max} is also greater than the prescribed dose when opposed treatment fields are used to treat the patient and will be greater than the dose delivered to the patient's midplane. The dose at D_{max} will be slightly greater than the midplane dose for high-energy treatment beams and for patients with a small separation. When low-energy treatment beams (cobalt-60, 4 MV, and 6 MV) are used, the dose at D_{max} can be significantly higher than the midplane dose. This is especially true for large patient separations. When megavoltage photon beams are used, it may not be necessary to calculate the dose at D_{max} when using multiple field arrangements to treat the patient. By using many fields, the dose at D_{max} will normally be less than the prescribed dose.

Output

The **output** can be referred to as the dose rate of the machine and, in the past, has been measured in the absence of a scattering phantom and in tissue equivalent material.[1] Today, the dose rate is normally measured in phantom. It is the amount of radiation "exposure" produced by a treatment machine or source as specified at a reference field size and at a specified reference distance. The reference field size and distance are used so that we may relate standardized measurements to those that vary from the standards. Changing the field size, distance, or attenuating medium will change the dose rate. **Dose rate** increases with increased field size. Remember that a therapeutic beam of radiation is made up of primary and scatter radiation and measured at a point of reference. If the field size is increased on a treatment machine, the primary component would remain the same. However, the increased area would cause increased scatter, which would add to the output (all other parameters remaining constant). If the distance from the source of radiation to the point of measurement increases, the dose rate would decrease because of the inverse square law. An example of output on a cobalt-60 unit may be 100 cGy/min, whereas a linear accelerator reference output may be 1.0 cGy/MU at the reference field size and distance.

Output Factor

The **output factor** is the ratio of the dose rate of a given field size to the dose rate of the reference field size. The output factor allows for the change in scatter as the collimator setting changes. The output factor is usually normalized or referenced to a 10 × 10 cm field size. This means that the output factor for a 10 × 10 cm field size is 1.00 for the linear accelerator or cobalt-60 unit. The output factor will be greater than 1.00 for field sizes larger than 10 × 10 cm because of an increase in scatter as the collimator setting is increased. The output factor will be less than 1.00 for field sizes smaller than 10 × 10 cm because of a decrease in scatter as the collimator setting is decreased.

The term *output factor* may be a generic term. Many institutions use other terminology, such as *relative output factor, collimator scatter factor, field size correction factor,* and *phantom scatter factor.* Khan[4] defines measured values for collimator scatter factor and total scatter factors and a derived value for phantom scatter factor. We will use the conventions defined by Kahn in this chapter (Sc [collimator scatter factor]; Sp [phantom or patient scatter factor]; and Sc, p for combined collimator and phantom scatter).

Output factors relate the dose rate of a given collimator setting to the dose rate of the reference field size and are very useful and practical for calculations involving linear accelerators and cobalt-60 treatment machines. The reference dose rate (RDR) for the cobalt-60 treatment machine is constantly changing due to the decaying of the cobalt-60 radioisotope used as the source of gamma-ray emissions in these machines. Usually, the RDR is updated monthly. Even though the RDR is changed every month, the output factors do not change. Therefore by using output factors, only the RDR must be changed. Normally the RDR is 1.0 cGy/MU for linear accelerators. The RDR does not normally change for linear accelerators. This means that in some centers the output factor is the dose rate for that field size (any number multiplied by 1 does not change). For example, let us say that the RDR is 1.0 cGy/MU for a 10 × 10 cm field size measured at 100 cm from the target in free space. Let us also say that the output factor for the 15 × 15 cm collimator setting is 1.02 (larger than

Table 24-1	Approximate Depths of D_{max}	
Beam Energy	**Depth of D_{max} (cm)**
200 kV	0.0
1.25 MV	0.5
4 MV	1.0
6 MV	1.5
10 MV	2.5
18 MV	3.5
24 MV	4.0

1.00 because the field size is greater than the reference). The dose rate for the 15×15 cm collimator setting can be calculated as follows:

$$\text{Dose rate}_{\text{(Given field size)}} = \text{Dose rate}_{\text{(Reference field size)}}$$
$$\times \text{Output factor}_{\text{(Given field size)}}$$
$$\text{Dose rate}_{\text{(Given field size)}} = 1.0 \text{ cGy/MU} \times 1.02$$
$$\text{Dose rate}_{\text{(Given field size)}} = 1.02 \text{ cGy/MU}$$

Today, some treatment centers use more than one output factor. For example, some calculation models require the use of a collimator scatter factor (Sc) and a phantom scatter factor (Sp). Sc is used to determine the scatter, usually measured in air, from the collimators (or head scatter, which is defined later) and Sp is used to determine the scatter from the patient. Later in the chapter, we will see that using both Sc and Sp can simplify the MU calculation.

Another term is *head scatter*. Historically, the scatter that is generated in the treatment head is called *collimator scatter*. However, scatter is generated in both the collimator and the flattening filter. The combination of scatter generated in the flattening filter and collimator is known as *head scatter*. When the primary beam passes through the flattening filter, some photons are absorbed, some pass through, and some are scattered. These scattered photons are spread out spatially across the flattening filter. In essence, the flattening filter acts as a second source of photons that is broader than the primary source. If you imagine looking from the patient back to the x-ray target, you will see the entire flattening filter if the collimators are wide enough. If the collimators are then partially closed, part of the filter will be blocked from your view. Thus, as the field size changes, the amount of scatter from the flattening filter that reaches the patient will change.

Inverse Square Law

The inverse square law is a mathematic relationship that describes the change in beam intensity caused by the divergence of the beam. As the beam of radiation diverges or spreads out, there is a decrease in the intensity. Therefore, as the distance from the source of radiation increases, the intensity will decrease. For example, a photon beam that is made up of 400 photons is administered in a field size of 10×10 cm at a distance of 100 cm. The area of the beam is 100 cm^2 (given by the formula, width $\times$ length). If the photon coverage is uniform, there is an intensity of 4 photons/cm^2. At a distance of 200 cm, the field size will double to dimensions of 20×20 cm. The area of this field would then be 400 cm^2. There are still only 400 photons to cover this larger area. Now if the photon coverage is uniform, there will be 1 photon/cm^2. By doubling the distance, the intensity or number of photons per square centimeter has decreased to one fourth of the original intensity.

One practical application of the inverse square law is its effect on the output or dose rate of the treatment machine. The dose rate is commonly measured at the isocenter of the treatment machine. For linear accelerators, the dose rate at the isocenter for a 10×10 cm field is often 1.0 cGy/MU. When the MUs are calculated for treatment at distances greater than the standard, the inverse square law is used to account for the decrease in dose rate at distances beyond the isocenter.

The dose rate of the beam is inversely proportional to the square of the distance. This means that even a small change in distance can have a large effect on the dose rate. For example, if the dose rate is 1.0 cGy/MU at 100 cm, then the dose rate is 0.64 cGy/MU at 125 cm (see below for the method used to calculate the change in dose rate).

The equation commonly used for the inverse square law is as follows:

$$\frac{I_1}{I_2} = \frac{(d_2)^2}{(d_1)^2}$$

This equation may be used to find the change in dose rate with a change in distance (note that we are replacing the general term *I*, intensity, with a more specific term, dose rate at distance). We will use the following equation to calculate the dose rate at distances other than the reference (isocenter) distance:

$$\frac{\text{Dose rate at distance}_1}{\text{Dose rate at distance}_2} = \frac{(\text{Distance}_2)^2}{(\text{Distance}_1)^2}$$

Example: Distance$_1$ is defined as 125 cm for this example. Rearranging the previous equation, we get the following:

$$\text{Dose rate at distance}_1 = \text{Dose rate at distance}_2 \times \frac{(\text{Distance}_2)^2}{(\text{Distance}_1)^2}$$

Substituting the values in our example, we have the following:

$$\text{Dose rate at 125 cm} = \text{Dose rate at 100 cm} \times \frac{(100 \text{ cm})^2}{(125 \text{ cm})^2}$$

$$\text{Dose rate at 125 cm} = 1.0 \text{ cGy/MU} \times \frac{(100 \text{ cm})^2}{(125 \text{ cm})^2}$$

$$\text{Dose rate at 125 cm} = 0.64 \text{ cGy/MU}$$

The following is a second example for calculating the dose rate at a different distance using the inverse square law:

Example: The dose rate of a linear accelerator is 1.0 cGy/MU at a distance of 100 cm. Calculate the dose rate at 90 cm.

Distance$_1$ is defined as 90 cm for this example. Rearranging the previous equation, we get the following:

$$\text{Dose rate at distance}_1 = \text{Dose rate at distance}_2 \times \frac{(\text{Distance}_2)^2}{(\text{Distance}_1)^2}$$

Substituting the values in our example, we have the following:

$$\text{Dose rate at 90 cm} = \text{Dose rate at 100 cm} \times \frac{(100 \text{ cm})^2}{(90 \text{ cm})^2}$$

$$\text{Dose rate at 90 cm} = 1.0 \text{ cGy/MU} \times \frac{(100 \text{ cm})^2}{(90 \text{ cm})^2}$$

$$\text{Dose rate at 90 cm} = 1.235 \text{ cGy/MU}$$

Note: In this chapter, the correction for distance in the MU and dose calculations is referred to as the *inverse square correction factor (ISCF)*. Some clinics may refer to this correction as the *distance correction factor*.

Equivalent Squares of Rectangular Fields

A square field is a field that has equal dimensions for the field width and length, such as a 10×10 cm field. A rectangular field has a field width and length that are different, as is the case with a 10×15 cm field. In a clinical setting, most patients are treated with rectangular fields of different sizes. Treatment calculation tables use field size as a qualifying parameter. Using different rectangular field sizes would require extensive tables with thousands of number combinations. Because of this, a method was needed to make the amount of data and number of tables manageable. The method devised was to take different rectangular field sizes and compare them with square fields that demonstrate the same measurable scattering and attenuation characteristics, known as an **equivalent square of rectangular fields (ESRF)** or, simply, **equivalent square**.

A formula may be used to calculate the equivalent square of a rectangular field. One formula, Sterling's formula, is commonly called the $4 \times$ Area $\div$ Perimeter method. Using this formula, the area and perimeter of the rectangular field are calculated. The area is divided by the perimeter, and the result is then multiplied by 4. The number derived would be one side of the square field that has approximately the same measurable scattering and attenuation characteristics as the original rectangular field. This essentially takes field shape into account. This formula is an approximation and should be used when an ESRF

table is not available. In general, if the ratio of width or length exceeds 2, for example a 16×4 cm field, the use of standardized tables of equivalent squares is recommended. Table 24-2 demonstrates an example of a chart showing ESRF. Although a formula or equation may appear to be an exact calculation, Sterling's formula does not always account for the loss of scatter back to the central point (e.g., central axis, isocenter). Using the formula, mathematically the equivalent square will increase as either the field width or length increases. However, there is a point (distance) where the scatter created may not reach the point of interest. Therefore, because one dimension of the field may be much greater than the other dimension, the scatter to the central axis may be overestimated by the formula. Thus, the ESRF table will provide a more accurate result. For example, using the formula, we obtain the following results for a 12.0×16.0 cm field size and a 7.0×40.0 cm field size: 13.7 cm and 11.9 cm, respectively. However, if we refer to the equivalent square table, we see that the equivalent square of the fields are 13.7 and 10.7. Thus, for the field where both the width and length are similar, the formula and the table produce the same or similar results. However, when one dimension of the field is much greater than the other dimension, the formula and table produce two very different results. The table "based on measurements" actually provides a more accurate result than Sterling's formula.

Table 24-2	Sample Equivalent Squares of Rectangular Fields Chart												
Long Axis (cm)	**0.5**	**1.0**	**2.0**	**3.0**	**4.0**	**5.0**	**6.0**	**7.0**	**8.0**	**9.0**	**10.0**	**11.0**	**12.0**
0.5	0.5												
1	0.7	1.0											
2	0.9	1.4	2.0										
3	1.0	1.6	2.4	3.0									
4	1.1	1.7	2.7	3.4	4.0								
5	1.2	1.8	2.9	3.8	4.5	5.0							
6	1.2	1.9	3.1	4.1	4.8	5.5	6.0						
7	1.2	2.0	3.3	4.3	5.1	5.8	6.5	7.0					
8	1.2	2.1	3.4	4.5	5.4	6.2	6.9	7.5	8.0				
9	1.2	2.1	3.5	4.6	5.6	6.5	7.2	7.9	8.5	9.0			
10	1.3	2.2	3.6	4.8	5.8	6.7	7.5	8.2	8.9	9.5	10.0		
11	1.3	2.2	3.7	4.9	6.0	6.9	7.8	8.5	9.3	9.9	10.5	11.0	
12	1.3	2.2	3.7	5.0	6.1	7.1	8.0	8.8	9.6	10.3	10.9	11.5	12.0
13	1.3	2.2	3.8	5.1	6.2	7.2	8.2	9.1	9.9	10.6	11.3	11.9	12.5
14	1.3	2.3	3.8	5.1	6.3	7.4	8.4	9.3	10.1	10.9	11.6	12.3	12.9
15	1.3	2.3	3.9	5.2	6.4	7.5	8.5	9.5	10.3	11.2	11.9	12.6	13.3
16	1.3	2.3	3.9	5.3	6.5	7.6	8.6	9.6	10.5	11.4	12.2	12.9	13.7
17	1.3	2.3	3.9	5.3	6.5	7.7	8.8	9.8	10.7	11.6	12.4	13.2	14.0
18	1.3	2.3	3.9	5.3	6.6	7.8	8.9	9.9	10.9	11.8	12.6	13.5	14.3
19	1.4	2.3	4.0	5.4	6.6	7.8	8.9	10.0	11.0	11.9	12.8	13.7	14.5
20	1.4	2.3	4.0	5.4	6.7	7.9	9.0	10.1	11.1	12.1	13.0	13.9	14.7
40	1.4	2.4	4.1	5.6	7.0	8.3	9.5	10.7	11.9	13.0	14.1	15.2	16.3

Example: Sterling's formula calculation for a field of dimensions 10 cm × 20 cm:

$$\text{Equivalent square (ES)} = 4 \text{ (Area/Perimeter)}$$
$$\text{ES} = 4 \ (10 \times 20)/([10 \times 2] + [20 \times 2])$$
$$\text{ES} = 4 \ (200)/60$$
$$\text{ES} = 13.3$$

ESRF tables are used to find the output, output factor, and tissue absorption factors. Most radiation beam data tables are constructed so that the ESRF must be known to use the table. For example, to look up the output factor for a collimator setting of 7 × 19 cm, converting the rectangular field to a square field is required. The equivalent square is found to be 10 × 10 cm.[8] The output factor for a 10 × 10 cm field would be used, because it is effectively the same as that of a 7 × 19 cm field, all other parameters remaining unchanged. The output factor for a 10 × 10 cm field is 1.000. Therefore, the output factor for a 7 × 19 cm field is also 1.000.

When MLCs or blocks are used to customize the shape of the treatment area, two portions of the field are created. The first is the area being shielded, and the second is the area being treated. When looking at the area being treated, its dimensions must be determined. This derived field size is called the **effective field size (EFS)** or *blocked field size (BFS)*, which is the equivalent rectangular field dimension of the open or treated area within the collimator field dimensions. Usually some method of approximation is used to determine the EFS (a square or rectangular field that approximates the same physical volume as the blocked shape). The EFS is normally smaller than the collimator field size, although it may be larger for some extended distance treatments. The general rules for measuring EFS are as follows:

1. Basic field shape should be maintained for the effective field (a field that looks like an elongated rectangle should retain a rectangular shape after measurement).
2. One should visualize the closest rectangular area that can be adapted to the irregular field.
3. The rectangular field is converted to an equivalent square.

The actual collimator setting equivalent square may be used to determine the collimator scatter factor (Sc). The EFS equivalent square is normally used to determine the phantom scatter factor (Sp) and **tissue absorption factors**, such as the percentage depth dose (PDD), tissue-air ratio (TAR), tissue-phantom ratio (TPR), or tissue-maximum ratio (TMR), which are discussed in the following section. (*Special note:* Whether to use the actual equivalent square or EFS may be based on the construction of the linear accelerator used in your clinic. Some manufacturers construct the treatment head so that the MLC is on the proximal side of the x and y jaws. Other manufacturers have the MLC on the distal side of the jaws.)

TISSUE ABSORPTION FACTORS

As the beam of radiation travels through the body, it gives up energy. The more tissue the beam traverses, the more it is attenuated (the more energy it gives up). A number of different methods have been used for measuring the attenuation of the beam as it travels through tissue. In historical order, they are **percentage depth dose (PDD)**, **tissue-air ratio (TAR)**, **tissue-maximum ratio (TMR)**, and **tissue-phantom ratio (TPR)**. The first of these methods used in a treatment setting was PDD. It may be helpful to remember that in the early days of radiation therapy, the patients were treated using an SSD technique, which will be referred to as a *nonisocentric treatment* in this chapter. PDD was primarily developed for SSD treatments. Using appropriate corrections, any of the four methods (PDD, TAR, TPR, and TMR) may be used for SSD or SAD treatments. However, PDD works best with SSD (nonisocentric) treatments, whereas TAR, TMR, and TPR work very well with SAD (isocentric) treatments.

As previously stated, when a photon beam is directed it immediately begins to release its energy. Because of this, a dose is released from the point of beam entry into the body and continues on, also depositing some exit dose as it leaves the body; therefore the dose must be modified to ensure that the tolerance dose of any surrounding structures is not exceeded.

The characteristics of a proton beam are dramatically different. With proton therapy, the physician can predict and control the exact depth at which the beam is deposited in the patient. The position that the physician picks to deposit the dose is called the Bragg peak. After the beam reaches the Bragg peak, the dose is deposited and then there is quick falloff of the beam in order to eliminate exit dose. This allows the physician to increase the tumoricidal dose delivered to the patient because there is minimal effect on surrounding critical structures, reducing toxicity and increasing chances of tumor control.

Percentage Depth Dose

PDD is the ratio, expressed as a percentage, of the absorbed dose at a given depth to the absorbed dose at a fixed reference depth, usually D_{max},[7,8] (Figure 24-3) as follows:

$$\text{PDD} = \frac{\text{Absorbed dose at depth}}{\text{Absorbed dose at } D_{max}} \times 100\%$$

Normally, the depth of D_{max} is used for the fixed reference depth. PDD is dependent on four factors: energy, depth, field size, and SSD. PDD increases as the energy, field size, and SSD increase. This is a direct relationship. Higher energies are more penetrating, so a greater percentage of dose is available at a specific depth compared with a lower energy. As field size increases, more scatter is added to the deposited beam, thus increasing PDD. As the distance from the source of radiation to the patient (phantom) surface increases, the PDD increases.

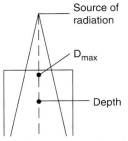

Figure 24-3. Diagram of percentage depth dose (PDD). PDD measures the dose along the central ray at depth as it compares with the dose at maximum equilibrium (D_{max}).

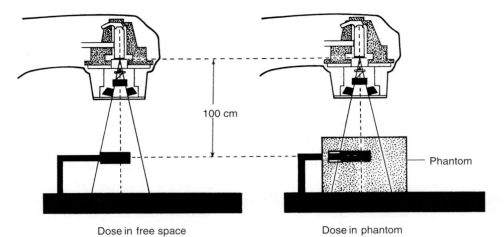

100 cm

Phantom

Dose in free space   Dose in phantom

Figure 24-4. Diagram of tissue-air ratio (TAR). TAR compares the dose in tissue at a specific depth with the dose in air at the same distance from the source (at the isocenter). When the depth in tissue corresponds to the level of D_{max}, the TAR is known as the backscatter or peak/phantom scatter factor.

The increase in PDD is based on a mathematic relationship and will be discussed in the section for the Mayneord "F" factor. PDD decreases as the depth in tissue increases (inverse relationship), because dose is deposited in tissue as it traverses it; thus a smaller percentage is available at greater depths.

Tissue-Air Ratio

TAR is the ratio of the absorbed dose at a given depth in phantom to the absorbed dose at the same point in free space (Figure 24-4):

$$TAR = \frac{Dose \ in \ tissue}{Dose \ in \ air}$$

Free space (in air) is a term used for measurements using a build-up cap or miniphantom (a small volume of tissue equivalent material that does not include full scatter). A maxiphantom (phantom) is a large volume of tissue equivalent material that produces "full scatter." It may not be possible to take a true air measurement. A build-up cap is a device made of acrylic or other phantom material that is placed over an ionization chamber to produce conditions of electronic equilibrium, which allows for a more accurate measurement. The miniphantom is a sphere of tissue equivalent material surrounding a point of interest. There is just enough material to produce build-up at the center (depth of D_{max}).[4] The ionization chamber then measures the flow of electrons and eventually the dose rate of the treatment machine (Figure 24-5).

When determining the TAR, the dose is measured at a reference distance from the target but within two sets of conditions. The first measurement is in free space (build-up cap or miniphantom), and the second measurement is in phantom (the point of measurement does not change between the two measurements). The amount of phantom material used for the second measurement corresponds to the depth of interest.

TAR depends on energy, field size, and depth.[4] TAR increases as the energy and field size increase and decreases as the depth increases. These characteristics are consistent with PDD. However, TAR is independent of SSD (distance) because both of the measurements for the "ratio" are measured at the same

distance from the source of radiation. TAR is normally used to perform calculations for SAD treatments involving low-energy treatment units such as a cobalt-60 or 4-MV linear accelerator. Some treatment centers use TAR for energies greater than 4 MV.

Scatter-Air Ratio

The absorbed dose of radiation used to treat cancer is made up of two distinct components as it is measured along the central ray of the beam at the point of calculation: primary radiation that is emitted from the treatment unit and scatter radiation from the surrounding irradiated tissue. Several noted physicists (e.g., Clarkson, Cunningham) contributed greatly to this concept of primary and scatter radiation making up the therapeutic beam. The primary part of total absorbed dose is represented by the zero-area (zero field size) TAR. This zero-area TAR cannot be measured directly. The difference between the TAR for a field of definite area and that for a zero area would be a measure of the contribution from scattered radiation. The contribution of scatter to points of calculation in the irradiated tissue, along the central ray and points off axis, is particularly important as the irregular shapes of the treatment fields are considered.

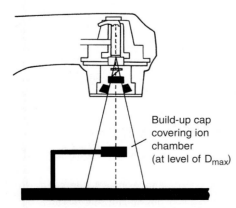

Build-up cap covering ion chamber (at level of D_{max})

Dose rate measured in free space (air)

Figure 24-5. Dose rate measured in air. There is a build-up cap over the ionization measuring chamber to allow for maximum scatter component to be accounted for.

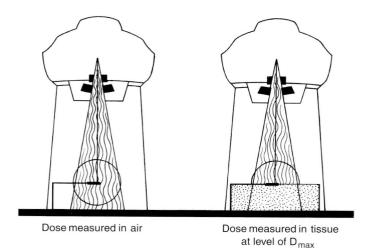

Dose measured in air | Dose measured in tissue at level of D_{max}

Figure 24-6. Backscatter or peak/phantom scatter factor relates dose in tissue to dose in air at the level of maximum equilibrium.

Off-axis point doses can also be calculated to good approximation by entering the appropriate SSD and depth, with allowance for off-axis output profile in determining the primary dose contribution. In their use, they are added back to adjusted SAR values to calculate an effective TAR for a specific field geometry, so the result is not sensitive to what model was used, provided the same one is used to derive the SAR. Virtually all modern treatment planning computer systems include irregular field algorithms to accurately calculate treatment doses for shaped fields.[3,5]

Backscatter Factor and Peak Scatter Factor

The **backscatter factor (BSF)** or **peak scatter factor (PSF)** is the ratio of the dose rate with a scattering medium (water or phantom) to the dose rate at the same point without a scattering medium (air) at the depth (level) of maximum equilibrium.[1-4,6,7] Backscatter is then a TAR at the depth (level) of D_{max}. The BSF is measured at the surface for orthovoltage and other low-energy x-ray treatment machines (energies less than 400 kV) (Figure 24-6). The BSF is measured at the depth of D_{max} for megavoltage photon beams. The preferred terminology is to use BSF for low-energy beams and PSF for high-energy beams (greater than 4 MV). The PSF is sometimes normalized to a reference field size, usually 10×10 cm, for energies of 4 MV and higher.[1]

Tissue-Phantom Ratio and Tissue-Maximum Ratio

TPR is the ratio of the absorbed dose at a given depth in phantom to the absorbed dose at the same point at a reference depth in phantom as follows:

$$TPR = \frac{\text{Dose in tissue}}{\text{Dose in phantom}}$$

The reference depth may be any depth, for example, 5.0 cm. If the reference depth is chosen to be the depth of D_{max}, then the TPR is referred to as the TMR, as seen in Figure 24-7:

$$TMR = \frac{\text{Dose in tissue}}{\text{Dose in phantom } (D_{max})}$$

The TMR is related to the TAR by the formula: TAR = TMR × BSF for low-energy beam, or TAR = TMR × PSF for high-energy beams.

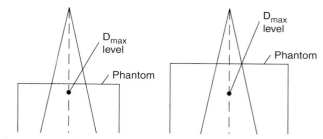

Figure 24-7. Tissue-maximum ratio compares dose at the depth of D_{max} with dose at the depth where the distance from the source to each point is the same. If another point of reference is used instead of D_{max}, the relationship is known as tissue-phantom ratio.

TMR and TPR were developed because of difficulties in measuring the TAR for high-energy beams. TAR is measured using some form of a build-up cap (small volume tissue equivalent material). With high-energy beams, a large build-up cap would be required to accurately measure it. As the build-up cap becomes increasingly larger, phantom scatter is introduced into the "free space" of the TAR. A build-up cap is not needed for measuring TPR or TMR, because both measurements are done in phantom. Thus, TMR overcame the problem of getting a true free space measurement.

Because the depth of D_{max} depends on field size, the reference depths for TMR change with field size accordingly. One advantage of a TPR over a TMR is that the reference depth will not change with field size. By using a reference depth of D_{max} for the 10×10 cm field size, the dependence of the depth of D_{max} with field size has been eliminated with the use of TPR.

When determining the TMR and TPR, the dose is measured at one distance from the target but at two different depths under phantom-specific conditions. The first measurement is at the depth of D_{max} or another established standard, and the second measurement is at the desired depth. The point of measurement does not change between the two measurements. The amount of phantom material used for the second measurement is determined by the depth of interest. The value of TMR is never greater than 1.00, and the value of TPR has no upper limit. The deeper the reference depth, the greater the TPR.[7]

Summary of Tissue Absorption Factors
Percentage depth dose (PDD) was commonly used for (and can still be used for) nonisocentric treatment calculations.
Tissue-air ratio (TAR) was one of the first methods used for isocentric treatment calculations.
Tissue-maximum ratio (TMR) and tissue-phantom ratio (TPR) are two methods currently used for isocentric and nonisocentric calculations.

Dose Rate Modification Factors

Any device placed in the path of the radiation beam will attenuate some of it. The transmission factor is the ratio of the radiation dose with the device to the radiation dose without the device and accounts for the material in the beam's path. Examples of such factors include tray transmission, wedge, and compensating filter factors.

Tray Transmission Factor

Most modern linear accelerators have MLCs and, for most situations, have eliminated the need for blocks that are mounted onto or placed on a block tray. Most block trays are made of a plastic derivative. When a tray is used, some of the beam is absorbed by the tray and the MU setting must be increased to ensure that the prescribed dose is delivered. The *tray transmission factor* (tray factor) defines how much of the radiation is transmitted through a block tray. The medical physicist takes two measurements: the first measurement is with the tray in the path of the beam, and the second measurement is without the tray in the path of the beam. The ratio of these two measurements is known as the tray transmission factor. For example, if a dose with the tray in place is measured as 97 cGy and the dose without the tray is 100 cGy, the ratio of the two doses, $^{97}/_{100}$, will yield a tray transmission factor of 0.97. This means that 97% of the radiation is transmitted through the tray, and 3% of the radiation is attenuated. Tray factors vary with beam energy. As energy increases, the effect of the material in the beam's path is lessened because of the increased penetrating power of the higher energy. Thus, departments may use the same trays on different treatment units (Figure 24-8) and simply use an appropriate tray factor for the energy with which it is used.

To deliver the correct dose to the patient, the radiation attenuated by the tray must be taken into consideration. This is normally done by having the tray transmission factor as a dose rate modifier. When the tray transmission factor is handled in this manner, it should always be represented by a number less than 1.00. Although this is the method used in this chapter, some therapy departments may multiply the MU or time setting by a tray factor that is greater than 1.00. For example, if the calculated MU setting before taking the tray into account is 100 MU and the tray factor is 1.03 (denoting a 3% attenuation), by multiplying the 100 MU by 1.03, a corrected MU setting of 103 would be obtained. When the tray factor is greater than 1.00, it is not a tray transmission factor and cannot be multiplied by the

dose rate to account for the attenuation. In these cases, the machine setting must be increased by this factor.

Wedge and Compensator Filter Transmission Factors

The wedge transmission factor (wedge factor) depicts the amount of the radiation transmitted through a physical wedge placed in the beam to shape the beam delivery. A wedge is made of a dense material, usually lead or steel, that attenuates the radiation beam progressively across a field. The thinner side of the wedge attenuates less of the beam than does the thicker side, resulting in an alteration of the beam isodose patterns.[1,2] The physicist takes several measurements and defines the wedge transmission factor, which is specific for each beam energy with which it is used. If a wedge has a wedge transmission factor of 0.67, this means that 67% of the radiation is transmitted through the wedge and 33% of the radiation is attenuated. To deliver the correct dose to the patient, a correction must be made for this amount of beam attenuation.

The compensator filter transmission factor is measured in the same manner as the wedge transmission factor. A compensator filter alters the isodose patterns just as in the wedge (Figure 24-9). However, the compensator filter is individually produced for each patient and alters the patterns so that they are at maximum efficiency for that patient. Both factors are normally multiplied into the dose rate when doing a treatment unit calculation. Examples of treatment unit calculations involving physical wedges and compensators can be found in the section on applications. An important fact to remember is that anytime a tray, wedge, or compensating filter is used, the MU setting must be adjusted upward to account for the radiation that is absorbed by one of these accessory devices.

PRACTICAL APPLICATIONS OF PHOTON BEAM DOSE CALCULATIONS

Having a clear understanding of the factors that affect radiation treatment delivery is extremely important to the radiation oncology team. Small changes in parameters can change the dose administered to the patient. A field size set incorrectly will change the machine output in reference to the patient. A sagging tabletop that inaccurately sets the patient at a wrong distance can have the same effect. With all this in mind and continuing to focus on the relationships presented, this section presents practical applications of treatment unit calculations. Tables needed for the calculations are located at the end of the chapter.

Treatment Unit Calculations General Equation

When attempting to perform treatment unit calculations, a number of variables must be accounted for. Field size variations, energy changes, and modifiers in the beam's path can alter the amount of radiation received by a patient, as either an underdose or an overdose. Although the complexity of each calculation varies within these parameters, there is one basic equation that addresses virtually every scenario. The general equation for performing MU or treatment time calculation can be represented as follows:

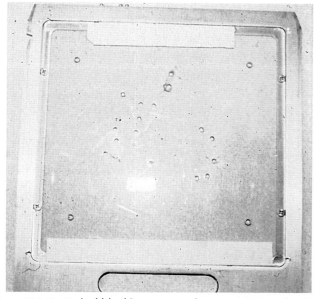

Figure 24-8. Typical blocking tray used to support standardized or custom shielding blocks.

$$\text{MU, or time, setting} = \frac{\text{Dose at a point}}{\text{Dose rate at that point}}$$

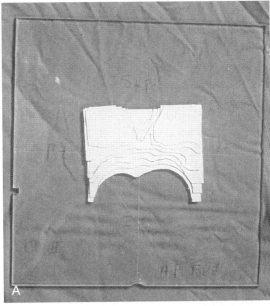
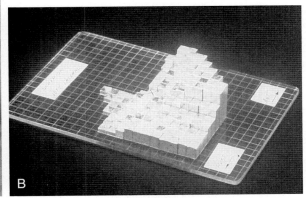

Figure 24-9. Compensator filters. **A,** Lead sheet compensator filter. **B,** Aluminum cube compensator filter. These filters attenuate the beam so that topographic variances are accounted for. Through this process, the distribution of dose at depths below the surface is even.

The MU setting represents the setting to be used on a linear accelerator, and the time setting represents the minutes for a cobalt-60 treatment unit. The dose at a point represents the prescribed dose as determined by the radiation oncologist. The dose rate at that point represents the dose rate of the treatment unit at the point of calculation (depth or point as identified in the prescription). There are three general points necessary when performing a treatment calculation: (1) one must know the dose at a point, (2) one must know the dose rate at that point, and (3) the dose and dose rate must be in the same medium (usually tissue).

Normally the dose and dose rate will be expressed in air or tissue. If the dose is expressed in tissue and the dose rate in air, then we have an "apple and orange" situation. As a rule for simplifying these calculations, it is desirable to have the dose rate expressed in air when using TAR for the megavoltage setting calculation. It is also desirable to have the dose rate expressed in tissue when using PDD, TPR, or TMR for the MU setting calculation.

SOURCE-SKIN DISTANCE (NONISOCENTRIC) TREATMENT CALCULATIONS

An SSD treatment occurs when the patient's skin surface is set up at the reference distance (or isocenter distance). Therefore, in an SSD treatment, the field size is defined on the patient's skin. It is important to know the reference (isocenter) distance because the distance can vary for treatment unit type: cobalt-60 is typically 80 cm and linear accelerators are 100 cm, and these will be the respective distances used in this chapter. The output or dose rate of the machine for SSD treatments should be expressed at the depth of D_{max}; the field size will be defined at the skin surface, and the dose rate will be measured in tissue at the depth of D_{max}.

To perform nonisocentric SSD treatment calculations, a six-step process can be used:

Step 1. Determine the equivalent square of the collimator setting (used for the collimator scatter factor [Sc]).

Step 2. Determine the EFS equivalent square of the treated area used for phantom or patient scatter Sp and the PDD if applicable.

Step 3. Determine the appropriate table.

Step 4. Determine the prescribed dose.

Step 5. Look up the factors using the appropriate data tables (located at the end of the chapter).

Step 6. Use the appropriate equation to determine the treatment unit setting.

These six steps will be used in all the examples for calculating the minute setting for a cobalt-60 treatment machine or the MU setting for a linear accelerator treatment machine.

Six-Step Process

1. Determine the equivalent square for the collimator setting.
   a. Used to determine Sc
2. Determine the effective field size.
   a. Used to determine both Sp and the tissue absorption factor
3. Determine the appropriate tissue absorption table.
   a. PDD, TAR, TMR, or TPR
4. Determine the prescribed dose.
   a. Usually from the radiation therapy prescription
5. Look up the factors using the appropriate data tables:
   a. Reference dose rate, Sc, Sp, other factors (tray factor, wedge factor, etc.)
6. Use the appropriate equation to calculate the minute or monitor unit setting.

The advantages of using PDD for calculations are as follows:

The PDD is normalized to the depth of D_{max}; the PDD at D_{max} is 100%. Therefore, it is easy to calculate doses at various depths because the PDD at each depth is the percentage of the D_{max} dose or percentage. For example, the PDD at a depth of 5 cm is 85.0. Therefore, the dose delivered to a depth of 5 cm is 85% of the dose at D_{max}. Thus, if the D_{max} dose is 200 cGy, then the dose at a depth of 5 cm is equal to 85% of 200, or 170 cGy.

The field size on the surface (skin) is used to look up the PDD at each depth. (*Note:* Later we will see that for TAR, TMR, and TPR, the field size changes at each depth and a field size correction must be calculated.)

As long as the patient is treated at the reference distance, there is no inverse square correction required.

The disadvantage to using PDD for calculations is that if the patient is treated at any distance other than the reference distance, the PDD must be recalculated for the new distance and an inverse square correction factor must be applied.

When using PDD, the ISCF is (Reference SSD + depth of D_{max})^2/(Treatment SSD + depth of D_{max})^2.

PDD Inverse Square Correction Factor

The reference distance for cobalt-60 is 80 cm and the depth of D_{max} is 0.5 cm. Therefore, 80.5 cm is used for cobalt-60 calculations using PDD.

The reference distance for a 6-MV linear accelerator is 100 cm and the depth of D_{max} is 1.5 cm. Therefore, 101.5 cm is used for 6-MV linear accelerator calculations using PDD.

Equations Used for SSD Calculations

CALCULATING THE MINUTE SETTING FOR COBALT-60 TREATMENTS USING PDD:

$$\text{Minute Setting} = \frac{\text{Prescribed Dose}}{\text{RDR} \times \text{ISCF} \times \text{Sc} \times \text{Sp} \times (\text{PDD}/100) \times \text{Other Factors}}$$

CALCULATING THE MONITOR UNIT SETTING USING PDD:

$$\text{MU Setting} = \frac{\text{Prescribed Dose}}{\text{RDR} \times \text{ISCF} \times \text{Sc} \times \text{Sp} \times (\text{PDD}/100) \times \text{Other Factors}}$$

CALCULATING THE DOSE TO A POINT USING PDD: RATIO METHOD:

$$\frac{\text{Dose}_A}{\text{PDD}_A} = \frac{\text{Dose}_B}{\text{PDD}_B}$$

CALCULATING THE DOSE TO A POINT USING PDD: SPECIAL EQUATIONS:

$$\text{Given Dose} = \frac{\text{TD}}{\text{PDD}_{TD}} \times 100$$

$$\text{Tumor Dose} = \frac{\text{Given Dose} \times \text{PDD}_{TD}}{100}$$

The following two examples are for cobalt-60 treatment units. Although most radiation oncology departments no longer have this type of treatment unit, the methods for the calculations will, for the most part, be identical to those for linear accelerator calculations.

Example 1: A patient is treated on the cobalt-60 treatment machine at 80 cm SSD to his thoracic spine. The patient is prone and will be treated through a single treatment field. The collimator setting is 10×10 cm. There is no blocking used for this treatment. The prescription states that a dose of 3000 cGy is to be delivered to a depth of 5 cm in 10 fractions. Calculate the treatment time.

This is the most basic calculation and involves only the RDR, scatter factors (Sc and Sp), and PDD. Because there is no blocking used, the equivalent square for the collimator setting or actual field size is used to look up Sc, Sp, and PDD.

Step 1. Determine the equivalent square of the collimator setting.

The equivalent square of a 10×10 cm field is 10×10 cm, or 10 cm^2.

Step 2. Determine the EFS equivalent square.

There is no blocking in this field. Therefore, the EFS is the same as the collimator equivalent square (i.e., 10 cm^2).

Step 3. Determine the appropriate tissue absorption factor table.

The patient is treated using nonisocentric treatment. Therefore, PDD will be used for the calculation.

Step 4. Determine the prescribed dose.

From the prescription, the total prescribed dose to a depth of 5 cm is 3000 cGy. This dose is to be delivered in 10 fractions. Therefore, the dose per fraction is 300 cGy.

To obtain the dose per fraction, divide the total dose by the number of fractions as follows:

$$\text{Dose per fraction} = \frac{\text{Total prescribed dose}}{\text{Number of fractions}}$$

$$\text{Dose per fraction} = \frac{3000 \text{ cGy}}{10 \text{ fractions}}$$

$$\text{Dose per fraction} = 300 \text{ cGy}$$

$$\text{Dose per treatment field} = \frac{\text{Dose per fraction}}{\text{Number of fields}}$$

$$\text{Dose per treatment field} = \frac{300 \text{ cGy}}{1}$$

$$\text{Dose per treatment field} = 300 \text{ cGy}$$

Step 5. Look up the factors using the appropriate data tables.

The factors for the dose rate at a point are 1, reference dose rate; 2, collimator scatter; 3, phantom scatter factor; and 4, tissue absorption factor—in this case, PDD. The following information can be obtained in the data tables located at the end of the chapter (Tables 24-3 through 24-10):

Reference dose rate = 51.7 cGy/min (Table 24-3)
Sc for (10×10 cm) = 1.000 (Table 24-4, Sc)
Sp for (10×10 cm) = 1.000 (Table 24-4, Sp)
PDD (5,10,80) = 78.3 (Table 24-5)

Step 6. Use the appropriate equation for determining the treatment setting.

$$\text{Time setting} = \frac{\text{Dose at point}}{\text{Dose rate at that point}}$$

therefore

$$\text{Time setting} = \frac{\text{Prescribed dose}}{\text{RDR} \times \text{ISCF} \times \text{Sc} \times \text{Sp} \times \frac{\text{PDD}}{100}}$$

$$\text{Time setting} = \frac{300 \text{ cGy}}{51.7 \text{ cGy/min} \times (80.5/80.5)^2 \times 1.00 \times 1.0 \times \frac{78.3}{100}}$$

$$\text{Time setting} = \frac{300 \text{ cGy}}{40.4811 \text{ cGy/min}}$$

Time setting = 7.41 minutes

The treatment unit would have to be set for 7.41 minutes to treat a 10 × 10 cm field size at 80 cm SSD to deliver 300 cGy to a depth of 5 cm.

Again, the previous six-step process will be used throughout this chapter for cobalt-60 treatment time and linear accelerator MU setting calculations.

Example 2: A patient is treated on the cobalt-60 treatment machine at 80 cm SSD. The patient is prone and will be treated through a single treatment field. The collimator setting is 15 × 15 cm. There is no blocking used for this treatment. The prescription states that a dose of 3000 cGy is to be delivered to a depth of 5 cm in 10 fractions.

Example 2 is essentially the same treatment as example 1. The only difference is that the **collimator** setting has changed. In this setting, the RDR, is still the rate for a 10 × 10 cm field; however, Sc, Sp, and PDD will change because of the different field size.

1. Determine the equivalent square for the collimator setting. Equivalent square is 15.
2. Determine the EFS. EFS is 15.
3. Determine the appropriate tissue absorption table. PDD
4. Determine the prescribed dose. 300 cGy per fraction
5. Look up the factors using the appropriate data tables:

The factors for the dose rate at a point are RDR, Sc, Sp, and PDD as follows:

Reference dose rate = 51.7 cGy/min (Table 24-3)
Sc (15 × 15 cm) = 1.030 (Table 24-4)
Sp (15 × 15 cm) = 1.016 (Table 24-4)
PDD (5,15,80) = 80.7 (Table 24-5)

Note that the reference dose rate is the same in both examples. This is because the reference dose rate is always the dose rate for the 10 × 10 cm collimator setting. The reference dose rate is multiplied by Sc of the actual collimator setting to correct for the variance from the standard. This takes the different amount of scatter into account. Also note that both Sp and the PDD have increased in example 2 because of increased scatter from the larger collimator surface and larger volume of tissue treated.

Use the appropriate equation to calculate the minute or MU setting.

$$\text{Time setting} = \frac{\text{Prescribed dose}}{\text{RDR} \times \text{ISCF} \times \text{Sc} \times \text{Sp} \times \frac{\text{PDD}}{100}}$$

$$\text{Time setting} = \frac{300 \text{ cGy}}{51.7 \text{ cGy/min} \times (80.5/80.5)^2 \times 1.030 \times 1.016 \times \frac{80.7}{100}}$$

$$\text{Time setting} = \frac{300 \text{ cGy}}{43.66 \text{ cGy/min}}$$

Time setting = 6.87 minutes

The time setting calculated for example 2 has decreased from example 1 because of the increased scatter, which raises the dose rate at the point of calculation. Because the dose rate has increased, the time necessary to deliver the dose will decrease. This is similar to driving a car. If a person must travel 300 miles and drives at 50 miles per hour, the trip will take 6 hours. However, if the driving speed is increased to 60 miles per hour, the driving time will be reduced to 5 hours.

The treatment time for the cobalt-60 machine is given in real-time (i.e., minutes). The dose rate for the cobalt-60 machine is defined in centigray per minute. Real-time is used with the cobalt-60 machine because the dose rate is caused by the radioactive decay of the isotope source. The half-life of cobalt-60 is approximately 5.3 years. This means that after 5.3 years, the dose rate of the unit will be half of its original dose rate. For example, if the dose rate is 50 cGy/min today, then the dose rate will be 25 cGy/min 5.3 years from today. As the dose rate decreases, the time it takes to deliver the prescribed dose increases.

Because the rate of decay for the cobalt-60 machine is relatively slow, it can be assumed that the dose rate is constant over a short period of time. The time frame for this constant dose rate is 1 month. This means that every month the minute settings used to treat the patient with the cobalt-60 machine must be adjusted. The rate of adjustment is approximately 1.1% each month. The following equation can be used to make the monthly adjustment in the minute setting for patients who are already on treatment:

New minute setting = Old minute setting × 1.01

If it takes 2.00 minutes to deliver 100 cGy on January 1, then it will take 2.02 minutes to deliver 100 cGy on February 1. Also, because of the slow decay or long half-life, the dose rate of the cobalt-60 machine is considered constant for a given treatment.

LINEAR ACCELERATOR NONISOCENTRIC MONITOR UNIT SETTING CALCULATIONS

The major difference in the time setting calculation for the cobalt-60 machine and the MU setting calculation for the linear accelerator is in the measurement of the reference dose rate. The reference dose rate for the cobalt-60 treatment machine is measured in centigray per minute, whereas the reference dose rate for the linear accelerator is measured in centigray per MU.

In looking at the dose rate for the linear accelerator, it might be helpful to look at a simple time, distance, and speed calculation. The following formula can be used to calculate the time it takes to drive a given distance:

$$\text{Time} = \frac{\text{Distance}}{\text{Speed}}$$

If a driver makes a 450-mile trip, driving the entire distance at exactly 50 miles per hour, it will take exactly 9 hours to complete the trip:

$$\text{Time} = \frac{450 \text{ miles}}{50 \text{ miles/hr}}$$

$$\text{Time} = 9 \text{ hours}$$

No matter how many times this trip is made, it will take 9 hours as long as a constant speed of 50 miles per hour is maintained. This type of constant speed (dose rate) happens in the cobalt-60 machine and is the principle behind the time setting calculation. In the linear accelerator, the dose rate varies slightly from one moment to the next. If the dose from the linear accelerator were measured using real-time, the dose could be different each time. Therefore real-time cannot be used to deliver the prescribed dose with a linear accelerator. Instead, a different system of time called *MU* is used. From our example, we need to travel 450 miles each trip regardless of the speed. Depending on traffic conditions, the time it takes to go 450 miles will change at each day. The MU setting ensures that the same dose is delivered at each treatment regardless of the "real-time" conditions. Normally the dose rate for the linear accelerator is 1.0 cGy/MU for a 10×10 cm field size defined at the isocenter.

Linear Accelerator Nonisocentric Calculations

The parameters for examples 1 and 2 of cobalt-60 will be repeated for the linear accelerator. The same trends seen between the cobalt-60 calculations will be noted in the linear accelerator calculations.

Example 3: A patient is treated on the 6-MV linear accelerator at 100 cm SSD. The collimator setting is 10×10 cm. There is no blocking used for this treatment. The prescription states that a dose of 3000 cGy is to be delivered to a depth of 5 cm in 10 fractions. Calculate the MU setting.

Step 1. Determine the equivalent square for the collimator setting: 10.
Step 2. Determine the EFS: no blocks and therefore the EFS is also 10.
Step 3. Determine the appropriate tissue absorption factor: nonisocentric treatment, therefore PDD.
Step 4. Determine the prescribed dose: 300 cGy per fraction.
Step 5. Look up the factors: the factors for the dose rate at a point are RDR, Sc, Sp, and PDD:

Reference dose rate = 0.993 cGy/MU (Table 24-3)
Sc (10×10 cm) = 1.000 (Table 24-4)
Sp (10×10 cm) = 1.000 (Table 24-4)
PDD (5,10,100) = 87.1 (Table 24-6)

$$\text{MU setting} = \frac{\text{Prescribed dose}}{\text{RDR} \times \text{ISCF} \times \text{Sc} \times \text{Sp} \times \frac{\text{PDD}}{100}}$$

$$\text{MU setting} = \frac{300 \text{ cGy}}{0.993 \text{ cGy/MU} \times (101.5/101.5)^2 \times 1.00 \times 1.0 \times \frac{87.1}{100}}$$

$$\text{MU setting} = \frac{300 \text{ cGy}}{0.8649 \text{ cGy/MU}}$$

$$\text{MU setting} = 347 \text{ MU}$$

If the collimator setting is changed from 10×10 cm to 15×15 cm would the MU setting be greater than or less than 347 MU? (See example 4.)
Both the scatter (Sc and Sp) and PDD will increase with the increased collimator setting. Therefore, the MU setting will be less than 347 MU.

Example 4: A patient is treated on the 6-MV linear accelerator at 100 cm SSD. The collimator setting is 15×15 cm. There is no blocking used for this treatment. The prescription states that a dose of 3000 cGy is to be delivered to a depth of 5 cm in 10 fractions. Calculate the MU setting.

Reference dose rate = 0.993 cGy/MU (Table 24-3)
Sc (15×15 cm) = 1.021 (Table 24-4)
Sp (15×15 cm) = 1.014 (Table 24-4)
PDD (5,15,100) = 87.9 (Table 24-6)

$$\text{MU setting} = \frac{\text{Prescribed dose}}{\text{RDR} \times \text{ISCF} \times \text{Sc} \times \text{Sp} \times \frac{\text{PDD}}{100}}$$

$$\text{MU setting} = \frac{300 \text{ cGy}}{0.993 \times (101.5/101.5)^2 \times 1.021 \times 1.014 \times \frac{87.9}{100}}$$

$$\text{MU setting} = \frac{300 \text{ cGy}}{0.0937}$$

$$\text{MU setting} = 332 \text{ MU}$$

Example 5: A patient is treated on the 6-MV linear accelerator at 100 cm SSD. The collimator setting is 15×15 cm. The field is blocked to an EFS of an 8×8 cm equivalent square. A 5-mm solid plastic tray is used to hold the blocks. The prescription states that a dose of 3000 cGy is to be delivered to a depth of 5 cm in 10 fractions.

(*Note:* The six-step process will be used; however, it will no longer be outlined step by step.)

The prescribed dose is 300 cGy per fraction.
The factors for the dose rate at a point are RDR, Sc, Sp, and PDD:

Reference dose rate = 0.993 cGy/MU (Table 24-3)
Sc (15×15 cm) = 1.021 (Table 24-4)
Sp (8×8 cm) = 0.992 (Table 24-4)
PDD (5,8,100) = 86.8 (Table 24-6)
Tray factor = 0.97 (Table 24-10)

$$\text{MU setting} = \frac{\text{Prescribed dose}}{\text{RDR} \times \text{ISCF} \times \text{Sc } (15 \times 15) \times \text{Sp } (8 \times 8) \times \frac{\text{PDD}}{100} \times \text{Tray factor}}$$

$$\text{MU setting} = \frac{300 \text{ cGy}}{0.993 \text{ cGy/MU} \times (101.5/101.5)^2 \times 1.021 \times 0.992 \times \frac{86.8}{100} \times 0.97}$$

$$\text{MU setting} = \frac{300 \text{ cGy}}{0.8468 \text{ cGy/MU}}$$

$$\text{MU setting} = 354 \text{ MU}$$

Note that the blocks created a smaller treated volume and thus there was a reduction in the Sp and PDD compared with example 4. In addition, a tray was used, which further reduced the dose rate. To compensate for the reductions in Sp and PDD and use of the tray, the MU setting needs to be increased for example 5. The MU setting for example 4 was 332 MU, and the setting in example 5 was 354 MU. Again, it is important to notice that smaller field sizes require higher MU settings than do larger field sizes. In addition, fields that have any device such as a block tray wedge or compensator will also require higher MU settings than fields that do not have these devices.

EXTENDED DISTANCE CALCULATIONS USING PERCENTAGE DEPTH DOSE AND SOURCE-SKIN DISTANCE TREATMENT

There are occasions when areas of a patient's body must be treated that are larger than the collimator areas achievable by conventional radiation therapy treatment units. This is the case in total body and total skin irradiation techniques and some mantle field arrangements. In these cases, larger field areas are possible by extending the distance of the treatment area. Because of divergence, as the distance from the source increases, the field size increases. In this manner, very large areas can be treated in a single field. The alternative would be to split the treatment fields up into areas that could be accommodated at conventional distances with the challenge of accurately matching divergent fields. To avoid this challenge, extended distances are commonly used. For example, the isocenter on a linear accelerator is 100 cm. In a standard SSD treatment, the patient is treated at 100 cm SSD. However, to set up a larger field, the patient may be set up at 125 cm SSD. To reiterate, an extended distance treatment is one in which the patient is set up at a distance beyond the isocenter or reference distance.[7]

In performing this type of calculation, several points must be considered. PDD is used for the calculation because its arrangement is nonisocentric. PDD depends on four factors: energy, field size, depth, and SSD. If any of these factors change, the PDD changes. If the energy is increased from cobalt-60 (1.25 MeV) to 6 MV, the PDD increases because of increased penetrating power. If the field size, at a given energy, changes from 10×10 cm to 15×15 cm, the PDD increases because of an increase in scatter. If the depth is increased from 6 cm to 10 cm, the PDD will

decrease, because more attenuation and beam absorption occur. As the SSD is increased, the PDD will increase because of a change in the inverse square law with a change in distance and because of an increase in scatter. As a result of these changes, special considerations must be used to calculate treatment times and MUs at extended distance treatment when using PDD.

Mayneord Factor

The Mayneord factor is a special application of the inverse square law. There are many forms of the Mayneord factor cited by different authorities. If it is understood where the numbers for the Mayneord factor are derived from, the likelihood of applying the numbers correctly is increased, resulting in no real need to memorize what appears to be a complex equation.

Reference or standard distance PDD values are determined from direct measurement. When patients are treated at an extended distance, the distance from the source of radiation to the depth of D_{max} and the depth of the calculation point also changes. Note that it is the distances that change and not the specified depth of treatment. If a patient is treated on a 6-MV linear accelerator with a 10×10 cm field size at 100 SSD to a depth of 8 cm and the distance is extended to 125 SSD, the depth of D_{max} and the point of calculation remain the same; the depths are 1.5 cm and 8 cm, respectively. However, the distance to these points for a 125-cm SSD treatment will be 126.5 cm (125.0 + 1.5 cm) and 133 cm (125.0 + 8.0 cm), respectively (Figure 24-10).

There are other factors to consider. The energy of the treatment machine is the same in the standard and extended distance treatment. A 6-MV accelerator has the same energy at 125 cm as it does at 100 cm. If the field size was 10×10 cm in both cases and the depth of calculation is 8 cm for both treatments, these factors should have little or no effect on the calculation. Because the 10×10 cm field was defined on the skin in both treatments, the field size at the calculation point will be slightly different because of divergence. This would slightly change the amount of scatter. The major change will result from the change in distance. The original distances from source to D_{max} and depth were 101.5 and 108 cm, respectively. These distances

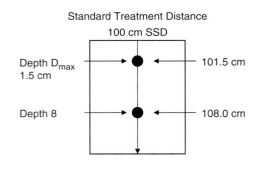

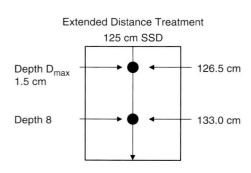

$$F = \frac{(108.0)^2}{(101.5)^2} \times \frac{(126.5)^2}{(133.0)^2}$$

Figure 24-10. Diagram demonstrating the Mayneord factor.

should be removed from the measured PDD by multiplying by the inverse as follows:

$$\frac{(108)^2}{(101.5)^2}$$

Then the correct distance is used in the calculation by multiplying by the square of the ratio of the new distances:

$$\frac{(126.5)^2}{(133)^2}$$

This allows for the correct attenuation of the beam for the new distances. These derived correction factors are then multiplied by the PDD referenced from the table, the result being the new PDD for the extended distances.

The Mayneord factor can be calculated using these distances. Note that the depth of D_{max} is 1.5 cm for a 6-MV linear accelerator and is reflected in the numbers. The PDD (8,10,100) is 75.1%.

The original distances were 101.5 cm and 108 cm. The new distances are 126.5 cm and 133 cm:

$$\text{New PDD}_{(8,10,125)} = 75.1\% \times \frac{(108)^2}{(101.5)^2} \times \frac{(126.5)^2}{(133)^2}$$

$$\text{New PDD} = 76.9\%$$

Again, the Mayneord factor is an inverse square correction of the PDD. It can also be used in shortened treatment distances. It should be noted that the Mayneord factor does not account for changes in scatter because of a change in beam divergence. Therefore, the Mayneord factor gives us the approximate value for the new PDD. To obtain the exact value for the new PDD, actual beam measurements using an ionization chamber or other appropriate devices would be necessary.

The following example uses the Mayneord factor in the calculation of a MU setting for a 6-MV accelerator.

Example 6: A patient is treated on the 6-MV treatment unit at an extended distance of 125 cm. The collimator setting is 20×20 cm, and the field size on the patient's skin is 25×25 cm. The prescription states that a dose of 3000 cGy is to be delivered to a depth of 5 cm in 10 fractions using a single posterior treatment field arrangement. Calculate the MU setting.

We can use a similar process for extended distance
 calculations. We will use the same five steps discussed
 earlier and add a sixth step for the Mayneord factor.
The collimator setting is 20×20 cm, which is conveniently
 the equivalent square.
The field size at the treatment SSD of 125 cm is 25×25 cm.
 Therefore, the EFS equivalent square is 25^2 cm.

$$\text{Reference dose rate} = 0.993 \text{ cGy/MU}$$
$$\text{Sc } (20 \times 20 \text{ cm}) = 1.038$$
$$\text{Sp } (25 \times 25 \text{cm}) = 1.028$$
$$\text{PDD } (5,25,100) = 88.9$$

The prescribed dose is 3000 cGy in 10 fractions. Therefore,
 the daily prescribed dose is 300 cGy/fraction.
The original distances when the PDD was measured were
 101.5 cm to the depth of D_{max} and 105 cm to a depth of
 5 cm. Therefore, the inverse of these distances are 105/101.5.

The patient is treated at 125 cm SSD. Therefore, the distances to the depth of D_{max} and the depth of calculation are 126.5 and 130, respectively (125.0 + 1.5 = 126.5 and 125.0 + 5.0 = 130.0).

Calculate the New Percentage Depth Dose Using the Mayneord Factor. Determine the PDD at a depth of 5 cm:

$$\text{New PDD}_{(5,25,100)} = 88.9\% \times \frac{(105)^2}{(101.5)^2} \times \frac{(126.5)^2}{(131)^2}$$

$$\text{New PDD} = 90.08\%$$

The equation to be used is, again, a variation of dose divided by dose rate. The dose rate is affected by the factors mentioned in the problem. Because the treatment is at an extended distance, the intensity of the beam is affected by the inverse square law. While the PDD increased due to the extended distance, the intensity (dose rate) of the beam would decrease because of the increased distance. The correction relates the distance from the source to the point of treatment unit calibration (where referenced data were measured) and the treatment SSD plus D_{max}. The inverse square correction would then be included as a dose rate correction in the denominator of the equation. It may be written as follows:

$$\text{Inverse square correction} = \frac{(\text{Reference source calibration distance})^2}{(\text{Treatment SSD} + D_{max})^2 \times \frac{\text{PDD}}{100}}$$

The treatment time can now be calculated, as follows:

$$\text{MU setting} = \frac{\text{Prescribed dose}}{\text{RDR} \times \text{Inverse square correction} \times \text{Sc} \times \text{Sp} \times \text{PDD}}$$

$$\text{MU setting} = \frac{300 \text{ cGy}}{0.993 \text{ cGy/MU} \times \left(\frac{101.5}{126.5}\right)^2 \times 1.038 \times 1.028 \times \frac{90.08}{100}}$$

$$\text{MU setting} = \frac{300 \text{ cGy}}{0.6145 \text{ cGy/MU}}$$

$$\text{MU setting} = 488 \text{ MU}$$

Again, notice that as the treatment distance increases the MU setting increases to offset the loss of intensity due to the increased distance.

Calculating the Given Dose for an Source-Skin Distance Treatment Using Percentage Depth Dose

Often, it is important to know the dose to points other than the prescription point. Dose-limiting and critical structures are anatomic sites that cannot withstand the same amount of exposure as neighboring tissues without damage. The spinal cord, bowel, and lens of the eye are examples of dose-limiting structures that are commonly monitored. The anatomy to be monitored will be determined chiefly by the region of the body being irradiated.

SSD calculations are often done at D_{max}. When a single field is used to treat a patient, such as a posterior spine field, the dose at D_{max} is known as the *given dose*. Other names for the given dose are *applied dose, entrance dose, peak absorbed dose,* or *D_{max} dose.* This is the point where the PDD is equal to 100%. As the depth increases from that point, the PDD will decrease. If a prescription calls for the administration of 300 cGy to a certain depth below D_{max} through a single field, the given dose will have to be more than the 300 cGy based on these concepts. The dose at depth is also called the *TD*. This is done for cobalt-60, as well as linear accelerators. Each treatment field has its own given dose. Calculating the given dose can be accomplished by using the ratio of the prescribed dose for the field and the PDD at the depth of the prescribed dose as follows:

$$\text{Given dose} = \frac{TD}{PDD} \times 100$$

When writing the PDD, the following convention will be used: PDD (d,s,SSD), indicating that this refers to the PDD at depth (d), for equivalent square (s), at the treatment distance (SSD). If the PDD at a depth of 5 cm for a 10×10 cm field treatment at 80 cm SSD is 78.3%, the convention for writing this information is PDD (5,10,80) = 78.3%.

There is a direct relationship between the dose and the PDD at a point. Thus a ratio or direct proportion can be established as follows:

$$\frac{\text{Dose}_A}{PDD_A} = \frac{\text{Dose}_B}{PDD_B}$$

Note that the above equation can be used to calculate the dose to any point of interest (on the central axis) when using PDD. In this chapter, this equation is referred to as the *ratio method* for calculating the dose.

The following example calculates the given dose.

Example 7: A patient is treated on the cobalt-60 treatment machine at 80 cm SSD. The collimator setting is 10×10 cm. There is no blocking or MLC used for this treatment. The prescription states that a dose of 3000 cGy is to be delivered to a depth of 5 cm in 10 fractions (the dose per fraction is 300 cGy). Calculate the given dose:

$$\text{Given dose} = \frac{TD}{PDD} \times 100$$

$$\text{Given dose} = \frac{300 \text{ cGy}}{78.3} \times 100$$

$$\text{Given dose} = 383.1 \text{ cGy}$$

Again, it should be noted that, in this case, to deliver 300 cGy to a depth of 5 cm with a 10×10 cm field at 80 cm SSD, a dose of 383.1 cGy is delivered to D_{max}. This calculation would be done exactly the same for any linear accelerator.

The given dose formula can be rearranged to solve for the TD if the given dose is known. The following example demonstrates this. Before any calculations, it should be noted that the TD should be less than the given dose in a single-field calculation because the TD will be located at a depth greater than the level of D_{max}.

Example 8: A patient is treated on the 6-MV linear accelerator at 100 cm SSD. The collimator setting is 15×15 cm. There is no blocking or MLC used for this treatment. The prescription states that a dose of 300 cGy per fraction is to be delivered at

D_{max} (given dose). What is the dose delivered at a depth of 5 cm?

From data given in Table 24-7, the PDD (5,15,100) is 87.9.

$$\text{TD} = \text{Given dose} \times \frac{\text{PDD at depth of calculation}}{100}$$

$$\text{TD} = 300 \text{ cGy} \times \frac{87.9}{100}$$

$$\text{TD} = 263.7 \text{ cGy}$$

As expected, the TD is lower than the given dose.

Any other point along the central axis can be found if the depth and PDD are known. If a dose at a depth of 3 cm was sought in the preceding example, it would be somewhere between the dose at D_{max} and the dose at 5 cm. By looking up the PDD at the desired depth, the information can be derived.

In earlier years of radiation therapy, the use of lower-energy machines and the resultant higher given doses presented problems. To treat tumors at depth, it was necessary to give the superficial tissues higher doses. Coupled with the use of lower-energy therapy machines that had a shallower D_{max}, heightened skin reactions were common and sometimes limited the administration of radiation therapy.

There are times when nonisocentric treatments are done for parallel opposed fields. At those times, it may be beneficial to the radiation oncology team to note the total dose at D_{max}. In this case, the given dose is added to the exit dose. The exit dose is the dose absorbed by a point that is located at the depth of D_{max} at the exit of the beam. For example, the depth of D_{max} for a 6-MV photon beam is approximately 1.5 cm. If a patient is treated using parallel opposed anterior and posterior photon beams and the patient's central axis separation is 20 cm, the total D_{max} dose can be calculated. The given dose would be calculated at a depth of 1.5 cm and the exit dose at a depth of 18.5 cm (20 cm − 1.5 cm). The following example calculates the total D_{max} dose and cord dose using a linear accelerator. Each field contributes to the total dose of each.

Example 9: A patient is treated on the 6-MV linear accelerator at 100 cm SSD. The collimator setting is 15×15 cm. The field is blocked to an 8×8 cm EFS. A 5-mm solid plastic tray is used to hold the blocks. The prescription states that a dose of 4000 cGy is to be delivered to a depth of 10 cm in 20 fractions using an anterior and posterior (AP:PA) treatment field arrangement. The patient's central axis separation is 20 cm. The cord lies 3.0 cm beneath the posterior skin surface. Calculate the total D_{max} dose and the cord dose.

We see that, in this arrangement, the cord calculation point lies 3.0 cm from the posterior surface and 17.0 cm from the anterior surface. It is important to note here that all points of calculation are along the central axis. To obtain the anterior depth of the cord, the posterior depth of the cord should be subtracted from the patient's total separation (20.0 cm − 3.0 cm = 17.0 cm). The depth of D_{max} for the 6-MV linear accelerator is 1.5 cm. The depth of the posterior field exit point is 18.5 cm (20.0 cm − 1.5 cm).

The factors required for this calculation are as follows:

PDD (1.5,8,100) = 100.0 (PDD at the depth of D_{max})

PDD (3,8,100) = 95.0 (PDD at depth of 3 cm for posterior cord dose)

PDD (10,8,100) = 66.7 (PDD at depth of 10 cm for midplane dose)

PDD (17,8,100) = 45.2 (PDD at depth of 17 cm for anterior cord dose)

PDD (18.5,8,100) = 41.6 (PDD at depth of 18.5 cm, which represents the exit dose)

Determining Total D_{max} Dose

A. Calculate the anterior dose contribution to D_{max} (given dose). In this problem, the direct proportion formula is used as follows:

$$\frac{\text{Dose at point A}}{\text{PDD at point A}} = \frac{\text{Dose at point B}}{\text{PDD at point B}}$$

$$\frac{\text{Dose}_{1.5\,cm}}{\text{PDD}_{1.5\,cm}} = \frac{\text{Dose}_{10\,cm}}{\text{PDD}_{10\,cm}}$$

$$\frac{\text{Dose}_{1.5\,cm}}{100} = \frac{100\,\text{cGy}}{66.7}$$

$$\text{Dose}_{1.5\,cm} = 149.9\,\text{cGy}$$

B. Calculate the posterior dose contribution to D_{max} (exit dose). Using the exit point (A) and D_{max} point (B), we have depths of 18.5 cm and 1.5 cm, respectively:

$$\frac{\text{Dose}_{1.5\,cm}}{\text{PDD}_{1.5\,cm}} = \frac{\text{Dose}_{18.5\,cm}}{\text{PDD}_{18.5\,cm}}$$

$$\frac{149.9\,\text{cGy}}{100} = \frac{\text{Dose}_{18.5\,cm}}{41.6}$$

$$\text{Dose}_{18.5\,cm} = 62.4\,\text{cGy}$$

C. Add the anterior and posterior dose contributions to obtain total D_{max} dose.

$$D_{max}\,\text{dose (total)} = D_{max}\,\text{dose (anterior)} + D_{max}\,\text{dose (posterior)}$$
$$D_{max}\,\text{dose (total)} = 149.9\,\text{cGy} + 62.4\,\text{cGy}$$
$$D_{max}\,\text{dose (total)} = 212.3\,\text{cGy}$$

Determining Cord Dose (Contribution from Both Fields)

A. Calculate the anterior dose contribution to the cord. Using the cord point (A) and D_{max} (B), we have depths of 17.0 cm and 1.5 cm, respectively:

$$\frac{\text{Dose}_{1.5\,cm}}{\text{PDD}_{1.5\,cm}} = \frac{\text{Dose}_{17\,cm}}{\text{PDD}_{17\,cm}}$$

$$\frac{\text{Dose}_{17\,cm}}{45.2} = \frac{149.9\,\text{cGy}}{100}$$

$$\text{Dose}_{17\,cm} = 68.8\,\text{cGy}$$

B. Calculate the posterior dose contribution to the cord. Using the cord point (A) and D_{max} point (B), we have depths of 3.0 cm and 1.5 cm, respectively:

$$\frac{\text{Dose}_{3\,cm}}{\text{PDD}_{3\,cm}} = \frac{\text{Dose}_{1.5\,cm}}{\text{PDD}_{1.5\,cm}}$$

$$\frac{\text{Dose}_{3\,cm}}{95.0} = \frac{149.9\,\text{cGy}}{100}$$

$$\text{Dose}_{3\,cm} = 142.4\,\text{cGy}$$

C. Add the anterior and posterior dose contributions to obtain the total cord dose.

$$\text{Cord dose (total)} = \text{Cord dose (anterior)} + \text{Cord dose (posterior)}$$
$$\text{Cord dose (total)} = 67.8\,\text{cGy} + 142.4\,\text{cGy}$$
$$\text{Cord dose (total)} = 210.2\,\text{cGy}$$

If this calculation were done on a cobalt-60 treatment machine (1.25 MeV) and compared with the preceding calculation, the following chart could be built:

Point of Calculation	Cobalt-60	6 MV	% Difference
Total dose at D_{max}	232.5	212.3	9.5
Total cord dose	218.9	211.2	3.7
Total dose to midplane	200.0	200.0	0.0

Although the midplane dose is constant in both cases, the total doses to D_{max} and the cord are different for the two energies. The data demonstrate that the total dose at D_{max} and the cord dose are less for higher treatment energies. Both doses will be even less for energies of 18 MV or greater. One of the advantages of using higher-energy beams, especially for parallel opposed treatment field arrangements, is that the total dose at D_{max} will be significantly less. In this case, the patient will receive approximately 3.7% less dose to the cord if a 6-MV beam is used instead of the cobalt-60 beam.

SOURCE-AXIS DISTANCE (ISOCENTRIC) CALCULATIONS

An SAD or isocentric treatment occurs when the treatment machine's isocenter is established at some reference point within the patient. When this is established, it can also be referred to as an *isocentric technique*. Because the field size is defined at the isocenter, the collimated field matches the field size setting inside the patient at the isocenter and not on the skin surface as seen in the nonisocentric SSD treatment.

One advantage that SAD treatment techniques have over SSD techniques is that when the patient has been properly positioned and the isocenter for the treatment has been established, there is usually no movement of the patient relative to the treatment isocenter for each of the subsequent treatment fields. For example, a patient is treated using an anterior and posterior treatment field arrangement on a 6-MV, 100-cm isocentric linear accelerator. The patient's central axis separation is 20 cm, and the dose is calculated at the patient's midplane (equal distance established from both anterior and posterior skin surfaces). If we were to treat this arrangement with an SSD technique, the anterior field would be established at 100 cm to the anterior skin surface. After, the anterior field was treated, the gantry would be rotated 180 degree to treat the posterior field. However, the treatment table would have to be raised until the ODI reads 100 cm on the patient's posterior skin surface.

In treating the same patient with an SAD (isocentric) technique, the anterior SSD would be established at 90 cm. The isocenter is positioned 10 cm beneath the anterior skin surface and 10 cm beneath the posterior skin surface, making it midplane as prescribed. (Note that the 10-cm anterior depth and 10-cm posterior depth add up to the 20-cm central axis separation.) The SAD is 100 cm (90 cm SSD + 10 cm depth). After the anterior field was treated, the gantry would be rotated 180 degrees to treat the posterior field. However, in an isocentric technique, the gantry is rotating about the isocenter, which has been established inside the patient. Therefore the patient is at the correct posterior SSD of 90 cm without raising or lowering the treatment table. Less movement between treatment fields lowers the chance of having treatment errors because of positioning variations that occur during patient movement.

To calculate the MU setting and/or doses to specific points, TAR, TMR, and TPR work very well for isocentric techniques. PDD can also be used for isocentric treatment techniques. However, there are two main differences from PDD that will affect calculations using TAR, TMR, or TPR. Both are caused by the way PDD and TAR, TMR, and TPR are calculated. PDD is calculated from two measurements at two different points in space. TAR, TMR, and TPR are calculated using two measurements at the same point in space. This affects the beam geometry (field divergence) and application of the inverse square law.

First, when TAR is used for calculations, the field size at the point of calculation must be used. Under some conditions, the field size at the point of interest must be determined. One example would be when trying to determine a dose delivered to points other than the isocenter along the central axis. In this case, the treatment field size at the alternate point would change because of beam divergence and would need to be calculated. Another effect on the calculation involves the application of the inverse square law. An inverse square correction will be needed when the dose to a point other than the isocenter is being calculated. These points are covered in greater detail in the example problems.

ISOCENTRIC CALCULATION PROCESS

Equations Used for SSD Calculations

CALCULATING THE MONITOR UNIT SETTING

TAR CALCULATIONS:

$$\text{MU Setting} = \frac{\text{Prescribed Dose}}{\text{RDR} \times \text{ISCF} \times \text{Sc} \times \text{TAR} \times \text{Other Factors}}$$

TMR CALCULATIONS:

$$\text{MU Setting} = \frac{\text{Prescribed Dose}}{\text{RDR} \times \text{ISCF} \times \text{Sc} \times \text{Sp} \times \text{TMR} \times \text{Other Factors}}$$

TPR CALCULATIONS:

$$\text{MU Setting} = \frac{\text{Prescribed Dose}}{\text{RDR} \times \text{ISCF} \times \text{Sc} \times \text{Sp} \times \text{TPR} \times \text{Other Factors}}$$

CALCULATING CHANGES IN FIELD SIZE WITH DISTANCE

$$\frac{\text{Field Size}_A}{\text{Distance}_A} = \frac{\text{Field Size}_B}{\text{Distance}_B}$$

CALCULATING DOSE TO A POINT USING TAR, TMR, AND TPR

$$\text{Dose}_A = \frac{\text{Dose}_B}{\text{TAR}_B} \times \frac{(\text{SCPD}_B)^2}{(\text{SCPD}_A)^2} \times \text{TAR}_A$$

$$\text{Dose}_A = \frac{\text{Dose}_B}{\text{TMR}_B} \times \frac{(\text{SCPD}_B)^2}{(\text{SCPD}_A)^2} \times \text{TMR}_A$$

$$\text{Dose}_A = \frac{\text{Dose}_B}{\text{TPR}_B} \times \frac{(\text{SCPD}_B)^2}{(\text{SCPD}_A)^2} \times \text{TPR}_A$$

The same basic six-step process described earlier in the section on nonisocentric calculations involving PDD will be used with these isocentric technique calculations:

Step 1. Determine the equivalent square of the collimator setting (used for Sc).
Step 2. Determine the equivalent square of the EFS (used for TAR, TMR, or TPR and Sp when appropriate).
Step 3. Determine the appropriate tissue absorption table.
Step 4. Determine the prescribed dose.
Step 5. Look up the factors using the appropriate data tables.
Step 6. Use the appropriate equation for determining the MU setting.

Example 10: A patient is treated on the 6-MV linear accelerator treatment machine at 100 cm SAD. The treatment SSD is 95 cm. The collimator setting is 15×15 cm. The field is blocked to an 8×8 cm EFS. A 5-mm solid plastic tray is used to hold the blocks. The prescription states that a dose of 3000 cGy is to be delivered to a depth of 5 cm in 10 fractions through a single field. Calculate the MU setting using TAR.

Step 1. The collimator equivalent square is 15.0.
Step 2. The EFS is 8.0.
Step 3. TAR will be used for the calculation (reminder: when using TAR, only Sc is used, because Sp is "built into" the TAR table).
Step 4. The prescribed dose is 300 cGy per fraction (3000 cGy/10 fractions).
Step 5. The factors for the dose rate at a point are RDR, Sc, TAR, and tray factor:

Reference dose rate = 1.0 cGy/MU (Table 24-3)
Sc (15×15 cm) = 1.021 (Table 24-4)
TAR (5,8) = 0.941 (Table 24-8)
Tray factor = 0.97 (Table 24-10)

Step 6. Use the appropriate equation to determine the MU setting:

$$\text{MU setting} = \frac{\text{Prescribed dose}}{\text{RDR} \times \text{ISCF} \times \text{Sc}_{(CS)} \times \text{TAR}_{(EFS)} \times \text{Tray factor}}$$

$$\text{MU setting} = \frac{300 \text{ cGy}}{1.0 \text{ cGy/MU} \times (100/100)^2 \times 1.021 \times 0.941 \times 0.97}$$

$$\text{MU setting} = 322 \text{ MU}$$

ISCF is the inverse square correction factor. SCPD is the source–to–calculation point distance. CS stands for collimator setting.

Note: The ISCF used for isocentric calculations (using TAR, TMR, or TPR) can be determined using the following:

$$\text{ISCF} = (\text{Reference Distance/SCPD})^2$$

A patient is treated at 100 cm SAD. The SSD is 90 cm and therefore the isocenter is located at a depth of 10 cm.

Determine the ISCF for a depth of 10 cm and a depth of 15 cm.

$$\text{ISCF (for a depth of 10 cm)} = (100 \text{ cm}/100 \text{ cm})^2$$
$$\text{ISCF (for a depth of 15 cm)} = (100 \text{ cm}/105 \text{ cm})^2$$

In both cases the reference distance is 100 cm (isocenter distance). The SCPD at a depth of 10 cm is equal to the 90 cm SSD + the 10 cm depth (100 cm). The SCPD at a depth of 15 cm is equal to the 90 cm SSD + 15 cm depth (105 cm).

Example 11: A patient is treated on the 6-MV linear accelerator treatment machine at 100 cm SAD. The treatment SSD is 90 cm. The collimator setting is 15×15 cm. The field is blocked to an 8×8 cm EFS. A 5-mm solid plastic tray is used to hold the blocks. The prescription states that a dose of 4000 cGy is to be delivered to a depth of 10 cm in 20 fractions using an anterior and posterior (AP/PA) treatment field arrangement. Calculate the MU setting using TAR.

The factors for the dose rate:

$$\text{Reference dose rate} = 1.0 \text{ cGy/MU}$$
$$\text{Sc } (15 \times 15 \text{ cm}) = 1.021$$
$$\text{TAR } (10,8) = 0.787$$
$$\text{Tray factor} = 0.97$$
$$\text{Prescribed dose} = 100 \text{ cGy/field}$$

$$\text{MU setting} = \frac{\text{Prescribed dose}}{\text{RDR} \times \text{ISCF} \times \text{Sc}_{(CS)} \times \text{TAR}_{(EFS)} \times \text{TF}}$$

$$\text{MU setting} = \frac{100 \text{ cGy}}{1.0 \text{ cGy/MU} \times (100/100)^2 \times 1.021 \times 0.787 \times 0.97}$$

$$\text{MU setting} = \frac{100 \text{ cGy}}{0.7794 \text{ cGy/MU}}$$

$$\text{MU setting} = 128 \text{ MU/field}$$

Today, TMR and/or TPR have replaced TAR as the method of hand-calculations for obtaining the MU setting and/or dose to a point.

When TMR or TPR is used for dose calculation, the output for the 10×10 cm field size is normally 1.0 cGy/MU. In the TMR calculations presented in this chapter, two scatter factors are used. One of the scatter factors corrects for collimator scatter (Sc). The other scatter factor corrects for patient scatter (Sp). The total scatter factor is obtained by multiplying Sc by Sp.

For the following examples, we will use TMR. However, because the depth of D_{max} changes slightly with changes in field size, many centers now use TPR, which is independent of the change in depth of D_{max} with changes in field size. When TPR is used, any depth may be chosen as the reference depth. This includes the depth of D_{max} for a 10×10 cm field. In other words, a 6-MV TMR table can become a TPR table by choosing the reference depth of 1.5 cm.

Example 12: A patient is treated on the 6-MV linear accelerator treatment machine at 100 cm SAD. The treatment SSD is 95 cm. The collimator setting is 15×15 cm. No blocks are used for this treatment. The prescription states that a dose of 3000 cGy is to be delivered to a depth of 5 cm in 10 fractions through a single field. Calculate the MU setting using TMR. The factors for the dose rate at a point are RDR, Sc, Sp, and TMR:

$$\text{Reference dose rate} = 1.0 \text{ cGy/MU}$$
$$\text{Sc } (15 \times 15 \text{ cm}) = 1.021$$
$$\text{Sp } (15 \times 15 \text{ cm}) = 1.014$$
$$\text{TMR } (5,15) = 0.937 \text{ (Table 24-9)}$$
$$\text{Prescribed dose} = 300 \text{ cGy}$$

$$\text{MU setting} = \frac{\text{Prescribed dose}}{\text{RDR} \times \text{Sc}_{(CS)} \times \text{Sp}_{(EFS)} \times \text{TMR}_{(EFS)}}$$

$$\text{MU setting} = \frac{300 \text{ cGy}}{1.0 \text{ cGy/MU} \times 1.021 \times 1.014 \times 0.937}$$

$$\text{MU setting} = \frac{300 \text{ cGy}}{0.9701 \text{ cGy/MU}}$$

$$\text{MU setting} = 309 \text{ MU}$$

Example 13: A patient is treated on the 6-MV linear accelerator treatment machine at 100 cm SAD. The treatment SSD is 90 cm. The collimator setting is 15×15 cm. MLCs are used to create a 12×12 cm EFS. The prescription states that a dose of 4000 cGy is to be delivered to a depth of 10 cm in 20 fractions using an anterior and posterior (AP/PA) treatment field arrangement. Calculate the MU setting using TMR. The factors for the dose rate:

$$\text{Reference dose rate} = 1.0 \text{ cGy/MU}$$
$$\text{Sc } (15 \times 15 \text{ cm}) = 1.021$$
$$\text{Sp } (12 \times 12 \text{ cm}) = 1.006$$
$$\text{TMR } (10,12) = 0.797$$
$$\text{Prescribed dose} = 100 \text{ cGy/port}$$

$$\text{MU setting} = \frac{\text{Prescribed dose}}{\text{RDR} \times \text{ISCF} \times \text{Sc}_{(CS)} \times \text{Sp}_{(EFS)} \times \text{TMR}_{(EFS)}}$$

$$\text{MU setting} = \frac{100 \text{ cGy}}{1.0 \text{ cGy/MU} \times (100/100)^2 \times 1.021 \times 1.006 \times 0.797}$$

$$\text{MU setting} = \frac{100 \text{ cGy}}{0.8186 \text{ cGy/MU}}$$

$$\text{MU setting} = 122 \text{ MU}$$

Deriving Given Dose and Dose to Points of Interest for Isocentric Problems

The given dose is the dose delivered at the depth of D_{max} for a single treatment field. In this example problem, each treatment field has its own given dose. Calculating the given dose using TAR, TMR, or TPR is more complex than when using PDD. To calculate the given dose using TMR for this example, the prescribed dose for the field, the SCPD, and the TMR at the depth of the prescribed dose must be known.

As discussed earlier, both measurements for the TMR are made at the same distance from the source. The field size increases because of divergence as the distance from the source increases. Therefore, when TMR (or TAR or TPR) is used, the field size at the point of calculation must be known. To find the field size at any distance, the following relationship, based on similar triangles, can be used:

$$\frac{\text{Field Size}_A}{\text{Distance}_A} = \frac{\text{Field Size}_B}{\text{Distance}_B}$$

In practice, the equivalent square of the rectangular field is used in place of the actual field size. For example, if the field size is 20×10 cm, its equivalent square of 13.0 would be used for the field size. To calculate the given dose using TMR/TPR, the following equation is used:

$$\text{Dose}_A = \frac{\text{Dose}_B}{\text{TMR}_B} \times \frac{(\text{SCPD}_B)^2}{(\text{SCPD}_A)^2} \times \text{TMR}_A$$

where:
Dose_A = Dose at point A
Dose_B = Dose at point B
TMR_A = TMR at point A
TMR_B = TMR at point B
SCPD_A = Source-to–calculation point distance for point A
SCPD_B = Source-to–calculation point distance for point B

Note that the ratio of SCPD_B and SCPD_A is the application of the inverse square law. SCPD is found by adding the depth to the SSD for that point. The following table assists in the organization of data when calculating the dose to points using TAR, TMR, and TPR.

Chart for Organizing Data

Point	SSD	Depth	SCPD	Equivalent Square	TMR	Dose
A						
B						
C						
D						

Example 13a: A patient is treated on the 6-MV linear accelerator treatment machine at 100 cm SAD. The treatment SSD is 90 cm. The collimator setting is 15×15 cm. MLCs are used to create a 12×12 cm EFS. The prescription states that a dose of 4000 cGy is to be delivered to a depth of 10 cm in 20 fractions using an anterior and posterior (AP/PA) treatment field arrangement. Calculate the total dose to the depth of D_{max}, and the total dose to the cord. For this example, the cord lies at a depth of 5 cm beneath the patient's posterior skin surface.

In Example 13a, the total dose delivered to two points, at D_{max} and at the level of the spinal cord, must be calculated. There is a dose contributed to each point from both the anterior and posterior treatment fields (obtained by adding the dose delivered by the anterior field to the dose delivered by the posterior field). Deriving this information is explained in the next series of steps. It should be noted that deriving this information can be done with TMR, TPR, and TAR.

Part 1. Calculate the dose to points from the anterior field. Point A represents the depth of D_{max} beneath the skin surface. Point B represents the isocentric point, in this case at a depth of 10 cm at midplane. Point C represents the depth of the cord beneath the anterior skin surface. The cord depth below the skin surface is found by subtracting the depth of the cord beneath the posterior surface (5 cm) from the patient's total central axis separation. With that we have the following.

Point	SSD	Depth	SCPD	Equivalent Square	TMR	Dose
A	90	1.5	91.5			
B	90	10	100	12.0	0.797	100 cGy (Rx dose to midplane)
C	90	15	105			
D	90	18.5	108.5			

With this the equivalent square and TMR for points A, C, and D can be found:

Field size at point A:

$$\frac{\text{Field size}_A}{91.5 \text{ cm}} = \frac{12.0 \text{ cm}}{100 \text{ cm}}, \text{ therefore 11.0 (10.98 rounded off) cm}$$

Now the TMR (1.5,100) can be found. Note that the exact numbers are not directly listed in the tables. Interpolation can be used to derive the exact numbers. In this case, TMR (1.5,100) = 1.000. (*Note:* If 6-MV TMR is used and the reference depth of the TMR is set to 1.5 cm depth, then the TMR at a depth of 1.5 cm is equal to 1.000 for all field sizes.)

Field size at point C:

$$\frac{\text{Field size}_C}{105 \text{ cm}} = \frac{12.0 \text{ cm}}{100 \text{ cm}}, \text{ therefore 12.6 cm;}$$

$$\text{TPR (15,12.6)} = 0.6672$$

Field size at point D:

$$\frac{\text{Field size}_D}{108.5 \text{ cm}} = \frac{12.0 \text{ cm}}{100.\text{cm}}$$

$$\text{Field size}_D = 13.0$$

At this point, there is enough information to calculate the dose from the anterior field to points A, C, and D.

The TMR at depth of D_{max} is 1.000.
The TMR at a depth of 10 cm is 0.7970.
The TMR at a depth of 15 cm is 0.6672.
The TMR at a depth of 18.5 cm is 0.5880.

Further completing the chart:

Point	SSD	Depth	SCPD	Equivalent Square	TMR	Dose
A	90	1.5	91.5	11.0	1.000	
B	90	10	100	12.0	0.797	100 cGy (Rx dose to midplane)
C	90	15	105	12.6	0.6672	
D	90	18.5	108.5	13.0	0.5880	

We know the midplane dose (depth 10 cm) is 100 cGy per field. Using the previous information, we can calculate the dose to points A, C, and D from the anterior field.

Dose to point A (from anterior field):

$$\text{Dose}_A = \frac{\text{Dose}_B}{\text{TMR}_B} \times \frac{(\text{SCPD}_B)^2}{(\text{SCPD}_A)^2} \times \text{TMR}_A$$

$$\text{Dose}_A = \frac{100 \text{ cGy}}{0.797} \times \frac{(100 \text{ cm})^2}{(91.5 \text{ cm})^2} \times 1.000$$

$$\text{Dose}_A = 149.9 \text{ cGy}$$

Dose to point C (from anterior field):

$$\text{Dose}_C = \frac{\text{Dose}_B}{\text{TMR}_B} \times \frac{(\text{SCPD}_B)^2}{(\text{SCPD}_C)^2} \times \text{TMR}_C$$

$$\text{Dose}_C = \frac{100 \text{ cGy}}{0.797} \times \frac{(100 \text{ cm})^2}{(105 \text{ cm})^2} \times 0.6672$$

$$\text{Dose}_C = 75.9 \text{ cGy}$$

Dose to point D (from anterior field):

$$\text{Dose}_D = \frac{\text{Dose}_B}{\text{TMR}_B} \times \frac{\text{SCPD}_B}{\text{SCPD}_D} \times \text{TMR}_D$$

$$\text{Dose}_D = \frac{100 \text{ cGy}}{0.797} \times \frac{(100 \text{ cm})^2}{(108.5 \text{ cm})^2} \times 0.5880$$

$$\text{Dose}_D = 62.7 \text{ cGy}$$

At this point, the table for the anterior perspective can be completed.

Point	SSD	Depth	SCPD	Equivalent Square	TMR	Dose
A	90	1.5	91.5	11.0	1.000	149.9 cGy
B	90	10	100	12.0	0.797	100 cGy (Rx dose to midplane)
C	90	15	105	12.6	0.6672	75.9 cGy
D	90	18.5	108.5	13.0	0.5880	62.7 cGy

At this point, note the confirmation of trends discussed earlier in the chapter. As the depth of calculation increases, the TMR decreases (because of more attenuation). In addition, the dose is greater closer to the skin surface.

Part 2. Calculate the dose to points from the posterior field.

Again, point A represents the depth of D_{max} beneath the anterior skin surface. Point B represents the isocentric point, in this case at a depth of 10 cm at midplane. Point C represents the depth of the cord beneath the anterior skin surface. However, these points are now measured with respect to the posterior surface. Another grid can be produced. Due to the symmetry of the doses for parallel opposed treatment fields, the dose at the depth of D_{max} from the posterior field (point D) is the same as the dose at the depth of D_{max} from the anterior field (point A). The same relationship exists for the doses at the depth of 18.5 cm. Therefore, the only calculation that is required from the posterior field is the dose to the depth of 5 cm.

Dose to point C (from posterior):

$$\text{Dose}_C = \frac{100 \text{ cGy}}{0.797} \times \frac{100 \text{ (cm)}^2}{95 \text{ (cm)}^2} \times .9308$$

$$\text{Dose}_C = 129.4 \text{ cGy}$$

Point	SSD	Depth	SCPD	Equivalent Square	TMR	Dose
A	90	18.5	108.5	13.0	5880	62.7 cGy
B	90	10	100	12.0	0.797	100 cGy (Rx dose to midplane)
C	90	5	95	11.4	0.9308	129.4 cGy
D	90	1.5	91.5	11.0	1.000	149.9 cGy

Part 3. Add the doses to the points from the anterior and posterior fields to finalize the problem.

Point	Anterior	Posterior	Total
A	149.9	62.7	212.6
B	100	100	200.0
C	75.9	129.4	205.3
D	62.7	149.9	212.6

This technique gives a perspective of the doses received at points other than the isocenter for SAD calculations. If calculations for several energies were performed for the parameters just given, a pattern would definitely be noted. Lower energies would deposit a higher dose at the outer aspects of the treatment volume. In other words, the D_{max} doses would be higher for the lower energies, all other parameters remaining the same. Conversely, as energy increases, the superficial doses would be lower. In all cases, the dose to isocenter would be the same. The higher-energy beams exhibit more skin sparing (less superficial dose) and are therefore deemed to be better suited for treatment of deep-seated tumors.

Extended Distance Treatment

Example 14: A patient is treated on the 6-MV linear accelerator at 144 cm SSD. The collimator setting (field size at 100 cm) is 10 × 10 cm. The prescription states for a dose of 100 cGy to be administered to a depth of 6 cm using a single anterior field.

In this example, the patient is being treated at an "extended" distance. To calculate the MU setting, a correction must be made for the loss of intensity due to the increased distance. Therefore, an ISCF will be applied.

The field size at the isocenter is 10 × 10 cm. However, the point of calculation is 150 cm (144 cm SSD + 6 cm depth). Using similar triangles, the field size at 150 cm is 15 × 15 cm. Also in this calculation, the collimator scatter is based on the field size at 100 cm. Therefore, we will use Sc for a 10 × 10 cm field. In addition, Sp will be calculated for a 15 × 15 cm field size (field size at the calculation depth). (*Note:* There are other techniques for determining Sp for extended distance calculations.)

$$\text{Reference dose rate} = 1.0 \text{ cGy/MU}$$
$$\text{Sc} = 1.000$$
$$\text{Sp} = 1.014$$
$$\text{TMR} (6,15) = 0.913$$
$$\text{ISCF} = (100/150)^2, \text{ which equals } 0.4444$$

$$\text{MU setting} = \frac{\text{Prescribed dose}}{\text{RDP} \times \text{ISCF} \times \text{Sc} \times \text{Sp} \times \text{TMR}}$$

$$\text{MU setting} = \frac{100 \text{ cGy}}{1.0 \text{ cGy/MU} \times (100/150)^2 \times 1.00 \times 1.014 \times 0.913}$$

$$\text{MU setting} = \frac{100 \text{ cGy}}{0.4115 \text{ cGy/MU}}$$

MU setting = 243 MU

Note the large increase in the MU setting required to administer 100 cGy at the increased distance (150 cm).

UNEQUAL BEAM WEIGHTING

Some radiation therapy cases use parallel opposed or multiple-beam arrangements, with different doses delivered to the treatment portals. This is commonly done when the tumor volume lies closer to the skin surface but would still benefit from multiportal treatment. The result is a greater dose near the entrance of the favored field and a lower dose in the tissue near the entrance of the opposing field.[1,2] Although uneven doses are administered in the outer tissues, the doses to the point of specification should remain consistent with the prescription. In other words, the isocenter in an SAD technique still receives the overall prescribed dose.

Look at the basic dose calculation equation:

$$\text{Treatment setting} = \frac{\text{Dose}}{\text{Dose rate}}$$

The component that is affected directly by the field weighting is the prescribed dose per port. If a prescription is written to deliver 200 cGy through two ports and the fields are equally weighted, each port would deliver 100 cGy to the prescription point. However, if the prescription describes a treatment to be delivered from an AP/PA perspective and specifies that the AP field is to receive twice the amount of the PA field (written as 2 to 1 or 2:1), a different dose must be delivered through each field.

The total dose to be delivered through all ports (in this case, two) should be divided by the sum of the weighting. In this case, the weighting sum is 3 (2 + 1), and the total dose is divided by this number: 200 cGy/3 = 66.7 cGy. This defines the amount of each dose component. Then this component is multiplied by the weighting for each port; this provides the appropriate dosage to be delivered through each port as follows:

AP dose = 66.7 cGy × 2 = 133.4 cGy
PA dose = 66.7 cGy × 1 = 66.7 cGy

These numbers would be used in the dose calculation to find the time or MU setting for each treatment portal. A quick check for accuracy would be to add the individual port doses; they should be equal (or very close because of rounding off numbers) to the original dose prescribed.

This method can be used for any number of treatment ports and beam arrangements and can be used in all treatment calculations. Weighting does not affect the dose rate, only the dose to be administered through each port.

Example 15: A patient is treated on the 6-MV linear accelerator treatment machine at 100 cm SAD. The treatment SSD is 90 cm. The collimator setting is 15 × 15 cm. The EFS is 12 × 12. The prescription states that a dose of 180 cGy/fraction is to be delivered to a depth of 10 cm using an AP/PA treatment field arrangement. The fields are weighted 2:1 AP/PA. Calculate the MU setting using TMR.

The total dose is 180 cGy and the total weights are 3 (2 + 1). Dividing 180 cGy by a total weight of 3 results in a dose of 60 cGy for a weight of 1. Therefore, for a weight of 2, the dose is 60 cGy × 2, which equals 120 cGy. The next step is to calculate the MU setting for 120 cGy and 60 cGy.

$$\text{MU setting} = \frac{\text{Prescribed dose}}{\text{RDR} \times \text{ISCF} \times \text{Sc} \times \text{Sp} \times \text{TMR} \times \text{Other factors}}$$

$$\text{Anterior field MU setting} = \frac{120 \text{ cGy}}{1.0 \text{ cGy/MU} \times (100/100)^2 \times 1.021 \times 1.006 \times 0.797}$$

$$\text{Anterior field MU setting} = \frac{120 \text{ cGy}}{0.8186 \text{ cGy/MU}}$$

Anterior field MU setting = 147 MU

$$\text{Posterior field MU setting} = \frac{60 \text{ cGy}}{1.0 \text{ cGy/MU} \times (100/100)^2 \times 1.021 \times 1.006 \times 0.797}$$

$$\text{Posterior field MU setting} = \frac{60 \text{ cGy}}{0.8186 \text{ cGy/MU}}$$

Posterior field MU setting = 73 MU

SEPARATION OF ADJACENT FIELDS

Many treatment techniques involve the junction of fields with the adjoining margins either abutted or separated depending on various circumstances. This may be due to the need to break what would be a very large, irregularly shaped field into two or more fields, which would be better managed. It may also be needed because of the need to use different beam energies over a large area that needs to also be continuous. Because of rapid "falloff" of the dose near the edge of each field, a small change in the relative spacing of the field borders can produce a large change in the dose distribution in the junction volume.

The hazard of having a "gap" or junction area may be a dose that (1) exceeds normal tissue tolerance or (2) is inadequate to therapeutically treat the tumor.

Fields may be abutted or have a gap between them:
1. *Abutted fields*—If the adjacent fields are abutted on the surface, the fields overlap to an increasing degree with depth because of divergence.
2. *Separated fields*—The theory behind this is that one can abut the field edges at depth as opposed to on the skin surface. In this way, one can spare a tissue at depth and prevent an overdose because of overlapping fields. One would have them abut at a desired depth, leaving a gap on the skin surface.

Examples of abutting fields would include lateral head and neck and supraclavicular fossa fields or tangential breast and supraclavicular fossa arrangements. Examples of separated fields are evident in craniospinal irradiation or mantle and para-aortic fields in lymphoma cases. In either case of abutting or separated fields, the medical dosimetrist and radiation therapist must be able to make sure that the area of overlap (or nonoverlap) occurs where it is intended.

There are several common methods of obtaining dose uniformity across field junctions, including dosimetric isodose matching, junction shifts, half-beam blocking, and geometric matching:

Dosimetric isodose matching—With the availability of modern treatment planning computers, separation of fields can easily be calculated and plotted for maximum dose uniformity. The hot and cold spots can easily be seen and compensated for. The accuracy of dosimetric isodose matching depends on the accuracy of the individual field isodose curves.

Junction shift—Fields that abut on the skin surface can be moved during the course of treatment so that any hot or cold spot inherently present can be spread, or feathered, over a distance. This technique calls for a shift in field sizes for the abutting fields. The fields are shifted one or more times during the course of the patient's treatment to move the areas of overlap. In this way, the overall dose in any areas of overlap is spread out over a greater volume and allows for a better opportunity of lowering side effects in that area.

Half-beam blocking—Specific shielding blocks can be designed to block out one side of a treatment field to produce a field that has no divergence along one side, most commonly along the central ray of the beam where there is no divergence. Two abutting fields can then be used to match field borders on the phantom surface and have no divergence at depth. Asymmetric jawed fields or MLCs can also accomplish this on modern treatment units.

Geometric matching—It is possible to achieve dose uniformity at the junction of two fields at depth through geometric means (Figure 24-11). This is possible because the geometric boundary of each abutting field is defined by the 50% decrement line (at the edge of all fields, the dose to the very edge falls off to 50% of the dose at the central ray). By knowing the field sizes of adjacent fields, the treatment SSD, and the depths, the size of the gap on the patient can be calculated to ensure that the fields abut at the correct depth. Note that it is possible to have fields at different depths; the important aspect is that the fields abut at a depth and that the gap measurement on the skin surface can be calculated with the following equation:

$$\text{Gap} = \left(\frac{L_1}{2} \times \frac{d}{SSD_1} \right) \times \left(\frac{L_2}{2} \times \frac{d}{SSD_2} \right)$$

where:
L_1 = Length of the first field
SSD_1 = Treatment source-skin distance of the first field
L_2 = Length of the second field
SSD_2 = Treatment source-skin distance of the second field
Depth = Depth of abutment

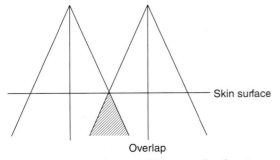

Figure 24-11. Geometric matching at depth. Because of divergence, a gap on the patient's skin between two adjacent fields converges at a depth within the patient.

The following example demonstrates the calculation of a field gap.

Example 16: A patient is treated using two adjacent fields. The collimator setting for field 1 is 8 cm width × 12 cm length. The collimator setting for field 2 is 10 cm width × 20 cm length. Both fields are set up at 100 cm SSD. Calculate the gap on the skin surface for the fields to abut at 5 cm depth.

The geometric gap calculation is based on the principles of similar triangles. A very important consideration when performing a gap calculation is to make sure that the field size (L) is corrected for the SSD. In this example, the field size is defined at the skin surface that is 100 cm SSD. Therefore the field size is the same as the collimator setting. A second consideration is that the depth must be the same for both fields:

$$\text{Gap} = \frac{12 \text{ cm}}{2} \times \frac{5 \text{ cm}}{100 \text{ cm}} + \frac{20 \text{ cm}}{2} \times \frac{5 \text{ cm}}{100 \text{ cm}}$$
$$\text{Gap} = 0.3 \text{ cm} + 0.5 \text{ cm}$$
$$\text{Gap} = 0.8 \text{ cm}$$

The 0.8 cm calculated is the minimal skin gap between the two fields. This means that the distance between the inferior border of field 1 and superior border of field 2 must be at least 0.8 cm. Often, the gap is made slightly larger to allow for variations in the day-to-day setup.

Example 17: A patient is treated using two adjacent fields. The collimator setting for field 1 is 8 cm width × 16 cm length. The collimator setting for field 2 is 10 cm width × 26 cm length. Field 1 is set up at 95 cm SSD and field 2 is set up at 90 cm SSD. Calculate the gap on the skin surface for the fields to abut at 5 cm depth.

Because the collimator setting is the field size at 100 cm, we must adjust the field sizes to the appropriate SSD. For field 1, this is 15.2 cm, and for field 2, it is 23.4 cm:

$$\text{Gap} = \frac{15.2 \text{ cm}}{2} \times \frac{5 \text{ cm}}{95.0 \text{ cm}} + \frac{23.4 \text{ cm}}{2} \times \frac{5 \text{ cm}}{90.0 \text{ cm}}$$
$$\text{Gap} = 0.400 \text{ cm} + 0.65 \text{ cm}$$
$$\text{Gap} = 1.05 \text{ cm}$$

Again, 1.063 cm is the minimum gap, and the treatment team would probably round up and measure 1.10 on the skin.

Table 24-3	Reference Dose Rate	
Treatment Machine	**Dose Rate Specified**	**Reference Dose Rate for a 10 × 10 cm Collimator Setting**
Cobalt-60	SSD/PDD	51.7 cGy/min at depth of D_{max}
Cobalt-60	SAD/TAR	50.6 cGy/min in air at 80 cm
6 MV	SSD/PDD	0.993 cGy/MU at depth of D_{max}
6 MV	SAD/TAR	1.000 cGy/MU in air at 100 cm
6 MV	SAD/TMR/TPR	1.000 cGy/MU in air at 100 cm

PDD, Percentage depth dose; *SAD*, source-axis distance; *SSD*, source-skin distance; *TAR*, tissue-air ratio; *TMR*, tissue-maximum ratio; *TPR*, tissue-phantom ratio.

Table 24-4	Scatter Factors

SCATTER FACTOR/COMBINED SCATTER (Sc, Sp)

Mach/Eq Sq	4.0	5.0	6.0	7.0	8.0	9.0	10.0	11.0	12.0	13.0	14.0	15.0	16.0	17.0	18.0	19.0	20.0	22.0	24.0	26.0	28.0	30.0	32.0	35.0
Cobalt-60	0.928	0.945	0.962	0.971	0.980	0.990	1.000	1.009	1.019	1.028	1.037	1.046	1.053	1.060	1.067	1.074	1.081	1.089	1.096	1.102	1.105	1.109		
6 MV	0.927	0.940	0.954	0.967	0.979	0.990	1.000	1.007	1.014	1.021	1.028	1.035	1.039	1.044	1.049	1.053	1.058	1.065	1.072	1.079	1.084	1.088	1.092	1.098
10 MV	0.925	0.938	0.953	0.967	0.979	0.990	1.000	1.005	1.011	1.016	1.022	1.027	1.032	1.037	1.041	1.046	1.051	1.058	1.065	1.069	1.071	1.073	1.077	1.081
18 MV	0.904	0.922	0.941	0.961	0.976	0.988	1.000	1.007	1.014	1.021	1.028	1.036	1.041	1.046	1.051	1.056	1.060	1.067	1.073	1.079	1.084	1.087	1.090	1.093

SCATTER FACTOR FOR COLLIMATOR SCATTER (Sc) (USED WITH PDD, TAR, TMR/TPR)

Mach/Eq Sq	4.0	5.0	6.0	7.0	8.0	9.0	10.0	11.0	12.0	13.0	14.0	15.0	16.0	17.0	18.0	19.0	20.0	22.0	24.0	26.0	28.0	30.0	32.0	35.0
Cobalt-60	0.946	0.961	0.975	0.981	0.987	0.993	1.000	1.006	1.012	1.018	1.024	1.030	1.035	1.039	1.044	1.048	1.053	1.057	1.061	1.063	1.063	1.063		
6 MV	0.948	0.961	0.970	0.979	0.987	0.994	1.000	1.004	1.008	1.013	1.017	1.021	1.024	1.028	1.031	1.035	1.038	1.041	1.045	1.048	1.051	1.052	1.053	1.055
10 MV	0.938	0.951	0.962	0.973	0.982	0.991	1.000	1.005	1.009	1.014	1.018	1.023	1.026	1.030	1.033	1.037	1.040	1.044	1.048	1.051	1.052	1.054	1.057	1.061
18 MV	0.914	0.931	0.948	0.965	0.978	0.989	1.000	1.006	1.012	1.017	1.023	1.029	1.032	1.036	1.039	1.043	1.046	1.052	1.057	1.063	1.066	1.067	1.069	1.070

SCATTER FACTOR FOR PHANTOM SCATTER (Sp) (USED WITH PDD, TMR/TPR)

Mach/Eq Sq	4.0	5.0	6.0	7.0	8.0	9.0	10.0	11.0	12.0	13.0	14.0	15.0	16.0	17.0	18.0	19.0	20.0	22.0	24.0	26.0	28.0	30.0	32.0	35.0
Cobalt-60	0.981	0.983	0.987	0.990	0.993	0.997	1.000	1.003	1.007	1.010	1.013	1.016	1.017	1.020	1.022	1.025	1.027	1.030	1.033	1.037	1.040	1.043		
6 MV	0.978	0.978	0.984	0.988	0.992	0.996	1.000	1.003	1.006	1.008	1.011	1.014	1.015	1.016	1.017	1.017	1.019	1.023	1.026	1.030	1.031	1.034	1.037	1.041
10 MV	0.986	0.986	0.991	0.994	0.997	0.999	1.000	1.000	1.002	1.002	1.004	1.004	1.006	1.007	1.008	1.009	1.011	1.013	1.016	1.017	1.018	1.018	1.019	1.019
18 MV	0.989	0.990	0.993	0.996	0.998	0.999	1.000	1.001	1.002	1.004	1.005	1.007	1.009	1.010	1.012	1.012	1.013	1.014	1.015	1.015	1.017	1.019	1.020	1.021

PDD, Percent depth dose; TAR, tissue-air ratio; TMR, tissue-maximum ratio; TPR, tissue-phantom ratio.

Table 24-5   Percentage Depth Dose Table Cobalt-60 at 80 cm SSD

Eq Sq Depth (cm)	0.0	4.0	5.0	6.0	7.0	8.0	9.0	10.0	11.0	12.0	13.0	14.0	15.0	16.0	17.0	18.0	19.0	20.0	22.0	24.0	26.0	28.0	30.0
0.0	14.9	15.0	17.4	19.8	21.7	23.6	25.5	27.4	28.1	28.8	29.5	30.1	30.8	32.3	33.7	35.2	36.7	38.1	41.2	44.3	47.4	50.4	53.4
0.5	100.0	100.0	100.0	100.0	100.0	100.0	100.0	100.0	100.0	100.0	100.0	100.0	100.0	100.0	100.0	100.0	100.0	100.0	100.0	100.0	100.0	100.0	100.0
1.0	95.6	96.4	96.6	96.8	96.9	97.0	97.0	97.1	97.1	97.1	97.2	97.2	97.2	97.3	97.3	97.4	97.4	97.5	97.7	97.8	98.0	98.1	98.2
2.0	87.4	90.2	90.7	91.3	91.6	92.0	92.3	92.6	92.8	92.9	93.1	93.3	93.5	93.6	93.7	93.8	93.9	94.0	94.1	94.2	94.3	94.4	94.4
3.0	80.1	84.2	85.1	85.8	86.4	87.0	87.4	87.8	88.1	88.5	88.8	89.1	89.3	89.5	89.7	89.9	90.1	90.1	90.2	90.3	90.4	90.5	90.4
4.0	73.2	78.4	79.4	80.4	81.2	81.9	82.6	83.1	83.5	84.0	84.4	84.8	85.1	85.3	85.5	85.8	86.0	86.0	86.1	86.2	86.4	86.5	86.3
5.0	67.1	72.9	74.0	75.1	76.0	76.9	77.7	78.3	78.8	79.4	79.9	80.4	80.7	81.0	81.3	81.6	81.9	81.9	82.0	82.1	82.2	82.3	82.1
6.0	61.4	67.7	68.9	70.1	71.1	72.0	72.9	73.6	74.2	74.8	75.4	76.0	76.3	76.7	77.0	77.3	77.5	77.6	77.7	77.9	78.1	78.2	78.0
7.0	56.2	62.7	64.0	65.3	66.4	67.4	68.3	69.0	69.7	70.3	71.0	71.6	71.9	72.3	72.7	73.1	73.3	73.4	73.6	73.7	73.9	74.0	73.8
8.0	51.5	58.0	59.4	60.7	61.9	62.9	63.9	64.6	65.3	66.1	66.8	67.4	67.8	68.2	68.6	69.1	69.2	69.3	69.5	69.7	69.9	69.9	69.7
9.0	47.3	53.7	55.1	56.4	57.5	58.6	59.6	60.4	61.1	61.9	62.6	63.2	63.6	64.1	64.5	65.0	65.1	65.2	65.4	65.7	65.9	65.9	65.8
10.0	43.3	49.7	51.0	52.3	53.5	54.5	55.6	56.3	57.1	57.9	58.6	59.2	59.7	60.2	60.6	61.1	61.2	61.3	61.6	61.9	62.1	62.1	61.9
11.0	39.8	45.9	47.2	48.5	49.7	50.7	51.7	52.5	53.3	54.1	54.9	55.4	55.9	56.4	56.9	57.3	57.4	57.5	57.8	58.1	58.4	58.4	58.2
12.0	36.4	42.4	43.7	45.0	46.2	47.2	48.1	48.9	49.7	50.5	51.3	51.8	52.3	52.8	53.3	53.6	53.8	53.9	54.3	54.6	55.0	54.8	54.7
13.0	33.4	39.2	40.5	41.6	42.8	43.8	44.7	45.5	46.3	47.1	47.8	48.3	48.8	49.4	49.9	50.1	50.3	50.5	50.9	51.2	51.6	51.4	51.3
14.0	30.7	36.1	37.4	38.6	39.6	40.6	41.5	42.3	43.1	43.9	44.6	45.1	45.6	46.1	46.7	46.8	47.0	47.2	47.6	48.0	48.3	48.1	48.0
15.0	28.1	33.4	34.6	35.7	36.7	37.7	38.5	39.3	40.0	40.8	41.5	42.0	42.5	43.1	43.6	43.8	43.9	44.1	44.6	45.0	45.2	54.1	44.9
16.0	25.9	30.8	31.9	33.0	34.0	34.9	35.7	36.4	37.2	38.0	38.6	39.1	39.6	40.2	40.6	40.8	41.0	41.2	41.6	42.1	42.2	42.1	42.0
17.0	23.8	28.4	29.5	30.5	31.4	32.3	33.1	33.8	34.6	35.3	35.9	36.4	36.9	37.5	37.8	38.0	38.3	38.5	38.9	39.4	39.5	39.3	39.2
18.0	21.8	26.2	27.2	28.2	29.1	30.0	30.7	31.4	32.1	32.8	33.4	33.9	34.4	34.9	35.2	35.4	35.6	35.9	36.3	36.8	36.8	36.7	36.6
19.0	20.0	24.2	25.1	26.0	26.9	27.7	28.4	29.1	29.8	30.5	31.0	31.5	32.0	32.5	32.8	33.0	33.2	33.5	33.9	34.4	34.4	34.3	34.2
20.0	18.4	22.3	23.2	24.1	24.9	25.7	26.3	27.0	27.6	28.3	28.8	29.3	29.8	30.3	30.5	30.7	30.9	31.2	31.7	32.2	32.1	32.0	31.9
21.0	17.0	20.6	21.5	22.3	23.1	23.8	24.4	25.0	25.7	26.3	26.8	27.2	27.7	28.1	28.4	28.6	28.8	29.1	29.6	30.0	29.9	29.8	29.7
22.0	15.6	19.0	19.8	20.6	21.3	22.0	22.6	23.2	23.8	24.3	24.8	25.3	25.7	26.1	26.3	26.6	26.8	27.0	27.5	27.9	27.8	27.7	27.6
23.0	14.3	17.5	18.3	19.0	19.7	20.4	20.9	21.5	22.1	22.6	23.1	23.5	23.9	24.3	24.5	24.7	25.0	25.2	25.7	26.0	25.9	25.8	25.7
24.0	13.1	16.1	16.8	17.5	18.2	18.8	19.3	19.9	20.4	20.9	21.4	21.8	22.2	22.5	22.7	23.0	23.2	23.4	23.9	24.1	24.1	24.0	23.9
25.0	12.1	14.9	15.6	16.2	16.8	17.4	17.9	18.5	19.0	19.5	19.9	20.3	20.7	20.9	21.2	21.4	21.6	21.8	22.3	22.5	22.4	22.3	22.3

26.0	11.1	13.7	14.3	14.9	15.5	16.1	16.6	17.1	17.6	18.0	18.4	18.8	19.2	19.4	19.6	19.8	20.1	20.3	20.8	20.9	20.8	20.7	20.7
27.0	10.2	12.7	13.3	13.8	14.4	14.9	15.4	15.8	16.3	16.7	17.1	17.5	17.8	18.1	18.3	18.5	18.7	18.9	19.4	19.4	19.4	19.3	19.2
28.0	9.4	11.7	12.2	12.8	13.3	13.7	14.2	14.6	15.1	15.5	15.8	16.2	16.5	16.7	17.0	17.2	17.4	17.6	18.0	18.0	18.0	17.9	17.9
29.0	8.7	10.8	11.3	11.8	12.3	12.7	13.1	13.6	14.0	14.4	14.7	15.1	15.4	15.6	15.8	16.0	16.2	16.4	16.8	16.7	16.7	16.6	16.6
30.0	8.0	9.9	10.4	10.9	11.3	11.7	12.1	12.5	12.9	13.3	13.6	13.9	14.2	14.4	14.6	14.8	15.0	15.2	15.6	15.5	15.5	15.4	15.4
BSF/ PSF	1.000	1.015	1.018	1.021	1.025	1.028	1.032	1.035	1.038	1.041	1.045	1.048	1.051	1.053	1.056	1.058	1.061	1.063	1.066	1.070	1.073	1.077	1.080

BSF, Backscatter factor; *PDD,* percentage depth dose; *PSF,* peak scatter factor.

Table 24-6   6-MV Percentage Depth Dose at 100 cm SSD

Eq Sq Depth (cm)	0.0	4.0	5.0	6.0	7.0	8.0	9.0	10.0	11.0	12.0	13.0	14.0	15.0	16.0	17.0	18.0	19.0	20.0	22.0	24.0	26.0	28.0	30.0	32.0	35.0
0.0	19.2	19.2	19.2	20.5	21.8	23.0	24.3	25.6	26.7	27.9	29.1	30.2	31.4	32.6	33.8	35.1	36.3	37.5	39.0	40.4	41.9	43.2	44.5	45.7	47.6
1.0	96.8	96.9	96.9	97.0	97.0	97.0	97.1	97.1	97.2	97.2	97.3	97.3	97.4	97.4	97.5	97.5	97.6	97.6	97.7	97.8	98.0	98.1	98.1	98.2	98.3
1.5	100.0	100.0	100.0	100.0	100.0	100.0	100.0	100.0	100.0	100.0	100.0	100.0	100.0	100.0	100.0	100.0	100.0	100.0	100.0	100.0	100.0	100.0	100.0	100.0	100.0
2.0	97.4	98.2	98.4	98.4	98.5	98.5	98.6	98.6	98.6	98.6	98.6	98.6	98.6	98.6	98.6	98.7	98.7	98.7	98.7	98.7	98.7	98.7	98.7	98.7	98.7
3.0	91.1	93.8	94.4	94.7	94.9	95.0	95.0	95.1	95.1	95.1	95.2	95.2	95.2	95.3	95.3	95.4	95.4	95.5	95.5	95.6	95.6	95.6	95.6	95.6	95.5
4.0	85.3	89.6	90.6	90.9	91.3	91.4	91.5	91.5	91.5	91.6	91.6	91.7	91.7	91.8	91.9	92.0	92.1	92.2	92.2	92.3	92.4	92.3	92.3	92.3	92.2
5.0	79.9	84.5	85.6	86.1	86.6	86.8	87.0	87.1	87.3	87.5	87.7	87.8	87.9	88.1	88.2	88.3	88.5	88.6	88.7	88.8	89.0	89.0	89.0	89.0	88.9
6.0	74.8	79.7	80.9	81.5	82.1	82.4	82.7	83.0	83.2	83.5	83.8	84.0	84.1	84.3	84.5	84.7	84.8	85.0	85.2	85.4	85.6	85.6	85.7	85.8	85.7
7.0	70.1	75.1	76.3	77.1	77.8	78.3	78.7	79.0	79.3	79.6	79.9	80.3	80.4	80.6	80.8	81.0	81.2	81.4	81.7	82.0	82.2	82.3	82.4	82.5	82.3
8.0	65.7	70.8	72.1	72.9	73.7	74.2	74.7	75.1	75.5	75.9	76.2	76.6	76.8	77.0	77.3	77.5	77.8	77.9	78.3	78.6	78.8	78.9	79.0	79.1	79.0
9.0	61.5	66.7	68.0	68.9	69.8	70.4	71.0	71.4	71.8	72.2	72.6	73.0	73.2	73.5	73.8	74.1	74.3	74.5	74.9	75.3	75.5	75.6	75.8	76.0	75.7
10.0	57.7	62.8	64.1	65.1	66.1	66.7	67.4	67.8	68.3	68.8	69.2	69.6	69.8	70.1	70.5	70.8	71.0	71.2	71.6	72.0	72.3	72.5	72.7	72.8	72.6
11.0	54.0	59.2	60.4	61.5	62.4	63.1	63.8	64.2	64.8	65.3	65.8	66.1	66.4	66.8	67.1	67.5	67.7	67.9	68.4	68.8	69.0	69.2	69.4	69.6	69.3
12.0	50.7	55.7	57.0	58.0	58.9	59.7	60.4	60.9	61.4	61.9	62.4	62.8	63.1	63.5	63.9	64.3	64.5	64.8	65.3	65.8	66.0	66.2	66.4	66.5	66.2
13.0	47.5	52.4	53.6	54.6	55.6	56.4	57.2	57.7	58.2	58.8	59.3	59.7	60.0	60.4	60.8	61.2	61.5	61.7	62.2	62.7	63.0	63.2	63.4	63.5	63.3
14.0	44.6	49.4	50.6	51.6	52.5	53.3	54.1	54.6	55.1	55.7	56.3	56.6	57.0	57.4	57.8	58.2	58.5	58.8	59.4	59.9	60.1	60.3	60.6	60.6	60.4
15.0	41.8	46.6	47.8	48.7	49.6	50.5	51.2	51.7	52.3	52.9	53.5	53.9	54.2	54.7	55.1	55.5	55.8	56.1	56.6	57.1	57.4	57.6	57.9	57.8	57.6

Continued

Table 24-6   6-MV Percentage Depth Dose at 100 cm SSD—cont'd

Eq Sq Depth (cm)	0.0	4.0	5.0	6.0	7.0	8.0	9.0	10.0	11.0	12.0	13.0	14.0	15.0	16.0	17.0	18.0	19.0	20.0	22.0	24.0	26.0	28.0	30.0	32.0	35.0
16.0	39.2	43.9	45.1	46.0	46.9	47.8	48.5	49.1	49.7	50.3	50.9	51.2	51.6	52.0	52.5	52.8	53.1	53.4	54.0	54.5	54.8	55.1	55.4	55.2	55.1
17.0	36.8	41.4	42.5	43.5	44.3	45.2	45.9	46.4	47.1	47.7	48.2	48.6	49.0	49.4	49.9	50.2	50.6	50.9	51.5	52.0	52.3	52.6	52.9	52.7	52.6
18.0	34.5	39.0	40.1	41.0	41.9	42.7	43.4	44.0	44.6	45.3	45.8	46.2	46.6	47.0	47.5	47.8	48.2	48.5	49.1	49.6	49.9	50.2	50.5	50.3	50.2
19.0	32.4	36.8	37.8	38.7	39.6	40.5	41.1	41.7	42.3	43.0	43.5	43.9	44.3	44.7	45.1	45.5	45.8	46.1	46.8	47.2	47.6	48.0	48.2	48.0	47.9
20.0	30.4	34.6	35.7	36.6	37.4	38.2	38.9	39.5	40.1	40.7	41.2	41.6	42.0	42.5	42.9	43.2	43.6	43.9	44.6	45.0	45.4	45.7	45.9	45.8	45.6
21.0	28.6	32.7	33.7	34.5	35.3	36.1	36.8	37.4	38.0	38.6	39.1	39.5	39.9	40.3	40.7	41.1	41.4	41.8	42.4	42.9	43.2	43.6	43.7	43.6	43.5
22.0	26.8	30.8	31.8	32.6	33.4	34.2	34.8	35.4	36.0	36.9	37.1	37.5	37.9	38.3	38.7	39.1	39.4	39.8	40.4	40.8	41.2	41.6	41.7	41.6	41.5
23.0	25.2	29.1	30.0	30.8	31.6	32.4	33.0	33.6	34.2	34.8	35.2	35.6	36.0	36.4	36.8	37.2	37.5	37.9	38.5	38.9	39.3	39.7	39.8	39.6	39.5
24.0	23.6	27.5	28.4	29.1	29.9	30.6	31.2	31.8	32.4	32.9	33.4	33.7	34.1	34.6	35.0	35.3	35.7	36.0	36.7	37.1	37.5	37.9	37.8	37.7	37.6
25.0	22.2	26.0	26.8	27.6	28.3	29.0	29.6	30.1	30.7	31.3	31.7	32.0	32.4	32.9	33.2	33.6	33.9	34.3	34.9	35.3	35.7	36.1	36.0	35.9	35.8
26.0	20.9	24.5	25.3	26.0	26.7	27.4	27.9	28.5	29.1	29.6	30.0	30.4	30.8	31.2	31.5	31.9	32.2	32.6	33.2	33.6	34.0	34.4	34.3	34.2	34.1
27.0	19.6	23.2	24.0	24.7	25.3	26.0	26.5	27.0	27.6	28.1	28.4	28.8	29.2	29.6	30.0	30.3	30.7	31.0	31.6	32.0	32.4	32.7	32.6	32.6	32.4
28.0	18.4	21.9	22.6	23.3	24.0	24.6	25.1	25.6	26.1	26.6	26.9	27.3	27.7	28.1	28.4	28.8	29.2	29.5	30.1	30.5	30.9	31.1	31.1	31.0	30.9
29.0	17.3	20.7	21.4	22.0	22.7	23.3	23.7	24.2	24.7	25.2	25.6	25.9	26.3	26.7	27.0	27.4	27.7	28.1	28.6	29.0	29.4	29.6	29.5	29.5	29.4
30.0	16.2	19.5	20.2	20.8	21.4	22.0	22.4	22.9	23.4	23.8	24.2	24.6	24.9	25.3	25.7	26.0	26.4	26.7	27.2	27.6	28.0	28.1	28.0	28.0	27.9
PSF	1.000	1.002	1.003	1.007	1.012	1.016	1.021	1.025	1.028	1.031	1.033	1.036	1.039	1.040	1.041	1.043	1.044	1.045	1.048	1.051	1.054	1.057	1.060	1.063	1.067

PDD, Percentage depth dose; PSF, peak scatter factor.

Table 24-7   18-MV Percentage Depth Dose at 100 cm SSD

Eq Sq	0.0	4.0	5.0	6.0	7.0	8.0	9.0	10.0	11.0	12.0	13.0	14.0	15.0	16.0	17.0	18.0	19.0	20.0	22.0	24.0	26.0	28.0	30.0	32.0
0.0	10.0	10.0	10.1	11.7	13.4	15.4	17.6	19.8	21.3	22.8	24.3	25.8	27.3	28.7	30.1	31.5	32.9	34.4	36.2	38.0	39.3	41.2	42.0	42.9
1.0	77.8	77.8	77.8	78.3	78.7	79.3	80.0	80.6	80.9	81.2	81.6	81.9	82.2	82.7	83.2	83.7	84.2	84.7	85.2	85.7	86.2	86.5	86.8	87.0
2.0	95.4	95.5	95.5	95.6	95.7	95.8	96.0	96.2	96.2	96.2	96.2	96.2	96.3	96.5	96.7	96.9	97.2	97.4	97.5	97.7	97.8	97.9	98.0	98.0
3.0	98.3	98.4	98.4	98.4	98.4	98.5	98.6	98.6	98.6	98.6	98.6	98.6	98.7	98.7	98.8	98.9	99.0	99.0	99.1	99.1	99.2	99.2	99.3	99.3
3.5	100.0	100.0	100.0	100.0	100.0	100.0	100.0	100.0	100.0	100.0	100.0	100.0	100.0	100.0	100.0	100.0	100.0	100.0	100.0	100.0	100.0	100.0	100.0	100.0
4.0	98.1	98.8	98.9	98.9	98.9	98.9	98.9	98.9	98.8	98.8	98.8	98.8	98.8	98.8	98.8	98.8	98.8	98.8	98.8	98.7	98.7	98.8	98.8	98.8
5.0	93.5	95.8	96.3	96.3	96.2	96.2	96.1	96.1	96.1	96.0	96.0	96.0	95.9	95.9	95.9	95.8	95.8	95.7	95.7	95.7	95.7	95.7	95.7	95.8

6.0	89.0	92.8	93.4	93.4	93.4	93.3	93.3	93.3	93.2	93.2	93.2	93.1	93.1	93.0	93.0	92.9	92.9	92.8	92.8	92.8	92.8	92.9	92.9	93.0
7.0	84.9	89.0	89.8	89.9	89.9	89.8	89.8	89.8	89.8	89.8	89.8	89.8	89.8	89.7	89.7	89.6	89.6	89.6	89.6	89.6	89.7	89.7	89.8	89.8
8.0	81.0	85.4	86.2	86.3	86.4	86.4	86.5	86.6	86.5	86.6	86.7	86.6	86.6	86.5	86.5	86.4	86.4	86.4	86.4	86.5	86.6	86.7	86.7	86.8
9.0	77.2	81.8	82.6	82.9	83.1	83.0	83.1	83.2	83.2	83.3	83.4	83.4	83.4	83.4	83.4	83.3	83.3	83.3	83.4	83.4	83.6	83.7	83.8	83.9
10.0	73.6	78.3	79.1	79.5	79.7	79.9	79.9	80.0	80.1	80.3	80.3	80.3	80.3	80.3	80.3	80.2	80.3	80.3	80.4	80.4	80.6	80.8	81.0	81.1
11.0	70.2	74.9	75.7	76.1	76.4	76.5	76.6	76.7	76.9	77.0	77.1	77.2	77.3	77.3	77.3	77.3	77.3	77.4	77.5	77.7	77.9	78.0	78.0	78.1
12.0	67.0	71.7	72.5	72.9	73.2	73.3	73.5	73.6	73.8	73.9	74.1	74.2	74.3	74.4	74.4	74.4	74.4	74.5	74.6	74.9	75.0	75.0	75.2	75.2
13.0	64.0	68.7	69.4	69.8	70.1	70.3	70.5	70.7	70.9	71.0	71.2	71.3	71.4	71.6	71.6	71.6	71.6	71.7	71.9	72.1	72.3	72.4	72.4	72.5
14.0	61.0	65.7	66.4	66.8	67.1	67.4	67.7	67.9	68.0	68.2	68.3	68.5	68.6	68.9	68.9	68.9	69.0	69.1	69.3	69.5	69.7	69.8	69.8	69.8
15.0	58.3	62.8	63.6	64.0	64.4	64.7	64.9	65.1	65.3	65.5	65.7	65.9	66.0	66.3	66.3	66.3	66.4	66.6	66.8	67.0	67.2	67.4	67.4	67.4
16.0	55.6	60.2	60.9	61.4	61.7	62.1	62.4	62.6	62.8	63.0	63.2	63.4	63.5	63.7	63.8	63.9	64.0	64.2	64.4	64.7	64.9	64.9	65.0	65.0
17.0	53.1	57.6	58.3	58.8	59.1	59.5	59.8	60.0	60.3	60.5	60.8	61.0	61.1	61.4	61.5	61.5	61.6	61.8	62.1	62.3	62.5	62.7	62.8	62.7
18.0	50.7	55.1	55.8	56.4	56.7	57.1	57.4	57.7	58.0	58.2	58.5	58.7	58.8	59.1	59.2	59.3	59.6	59.6	59.8	60.1	60.3	60.3	60.5	60.4
19.0	48.4	52.8	53.5	54.0	54.4	54.7	55.0	55.3	55.6	56.0	56.2	56.4	56.6	56.8	56.9	57.0	57.1	57.3	57.6	57.9	58.2	58.3	58.3	58.2
20.0	46.3	50.5	51.2	51.7	52.1	52.4	52.8	53.1	53.4	53.7	54.0	54.2	54.3	54.6	54.7	54.8	54.9	55.2	55.5	55.9	56.1	56.1	56.2	56.1
21.0	44.2	48.3	49.0	49.6	49.9	50.3	50.6	51.0	51.3	51.7	51.9	52.1	52.2	52.5	52.6	52.7	52.9	53.2	53.5	53.9	54.1	54.1	54.2	54.1
22.0	42.3	46.3	46.9	47.5	47.8	48.2	48.6	48.9	49.3	49.6	49.9	50.0	50.2	50.5	50.6	50.7	50.9	51.3	51.6	51.9	52.2	52.3	52.3	52.2
23.0	40.4	44.3	45.0	45.5	45.9	46.3	46.6	47.0	47.3	47.7	47.9	48.1	48.3	48.4	48.5	48.7	48.8	49.0	49.4	49.7	50.0	50.3	50.3	50.2
24.0	38.6	42.4	43.1	43.7	44.0	44.4	44.7	45.1	45.4	45.8	46.0	46.2	46.4	46.6	46.9	47.0	47.2	47.5	47.8	48.2	48.4	48.5	48.4	48.4
25.0	36.9	40.7	41.3	41.9	42.2	42.6	42.9	43.3	43.6	44.0	44.2	44.4	44.6	44.9	45.1	45.2	45.4	45.8	46.1	46.4	46.7	46.7	46.6	46.6
26.0	35.3	38.9	39.6	40.2	40.5	40.9	41.2	41.6	41.9	42.2	42.5	42.7	42.9	43.1	43.2	43.4	43.5	43.7	44.0	44.4	44.7	44.9	44.9	44.8
27.0	33.7	37.3	38.0	38.5	38.9	39.2	39.6	39.9	40.3	40.6	40.8	41.0	41.3	41.5	41.6	41.7	41.9	42.0	42.4	42.7	43.0	43.3	43.2	43.1
28.0	32.2	35.7	36.4	36.9	37.3	37.7	38.0	38.3	38.7	39.0	39.2	39.5	39.7	39.9	40.0	40.1	40.3	40.4	40.8	41.1	41.5	41.6	41.6	41.5
29.0	30.9	34.3	34.9	35.4	35.8	36.1	36.5	36.8	37.1	37.4	37.7	37.9	38.2	38.4	38.5	38.6	38.7	38.9	39.3	39.6	39.9	40.1	40.0	40.0
30.0	29.5	32.9	33.5	34.0	34.3	34.7	35.0	35.3	35.6	35.9	36.2	36.4	36.7	36.9	37.0	37.1	37.3	37.4	37.8	38.1	38.5	38.6	38.5	38.5
PSF	1.000	1.002	1.003	1.006	1.009	1.011	1.012	1.013	1.014	1.015	1.017	1.018	1.019	1.021	1.022	1.024	1.025	1.027	1.028	1.028	1.029	1.030	1.031	1.033

PDD, Percentage depth dose; *PSF*, peak scatter factor.

Table 24-8   6-MV Tissue-Air Ratio

Eq Sq Depth (cm)	0.0	4.0	5.0	6.0	7.0	8.0	9.0	10.0	11.0	12.0	13.0	14.0	15.0	16.0	17.0	18.0	19.0	20.0	22.0	24.0	26.0	28.0	30.0	32.0	35.0
0.0	0.186	0.187	0.187	0.200	0.213	0.227	0.240	0.254	0.266	0.279	0.291	0.304	0.316	0.329	0.342	0.354	0.367	0.380	0.396	0.412	0.428	0.443	0.457	0.471	0.492
1.0	0.957	0.960	0.961	0.965	0.970	0.974	0.979	0.984	0.987	0.990	0.994	0.997	1.000	1.002	1.003	1.005	1.006	1.008	1.012	1.017	1.021	1.025	1.028	1.032	1.037
1.5	1.000	1.002	1.003	1.007	1.012	1.016	1.021	1.025	1.028	1.031	1.033	1.036	1.039	1.040	1.041	1.043	1.044	1.045	1.048	1.051	1.054	1.057	1.060	1.063	1.067
2.0	0.982	0.992	0.994	0.999	1.004	1.009	1.014	1.018	1.021	1.024	1.027	1.030	1.032	1.034	1.035	1.037	1.038	1.039	1.043	1.046	1.049	1.052	1.055	1.057	1.061
3.0	0.936	0.966	0.973	0.979	0.986	0.991	0.996	1.001	1.004	1.007	1.010	1.013	1.016	1.018	1.020	1.021	1.023	1.025	1.028	1.032	1.035	1.038	1.041	1.043	1.047
4.0	0.894	0.940	0.951	0.959	0.966	0.972	0.977	0.982	0.985	0.988	0.991	0.994	0.997	0.999	1.001	1.004	1.006	1.008	1.012	1.015	1.019	1.022	1.025	1.027	1.031
5.0	0.853	0.903	0.915	0.924	0.933	0.941	0.946	0.952	0.956	0.961	0.965	0.970	0.974	0.977	0.979	0.982	0.984	0.987	0.991	0.996	1.000	1.003	1.006	1.009	1.013
6.0	0.814	0.867	0.880	0.890	0.900	0.909	0.916	0.923	0.928	0.933	0.939	0.944	0.949	0.952	0.955	0.958	0.961	0.964	0.969	0.974	0.979	0.984	0.987	0.990	0.995
7.0	0.777	0.831	0.845	0.857	0.868	0.878	0.886	0.894	0.900	0.906	0.911	0.917	0.923	0.926	0.930	0.933	0.937	0.940	0.946	0.951	0.957	0.962	0.965	0.969	0.974
8.0	0.742	0.798	0.812	0.824	0.837	0.847	0.856	0.865	0.871	0.878	0.884	0.891	0.897	0.901	0.905	0.908	0.912	0.916	0.922	0.928	0.934	0.939	0.943	0.946	0.952
9.0	0.708	0.765	0.779	0.792	0.805	0.817	0.826	0.836	0.843	0.850	0.856	0.863	0.870	0.874	0.878	0.883	0.887	0.891	0.898	0.904	0.911	0.916	0.920	0.924	0.930
10.0	0.676	0.733	0.747	0.761	0.775	0.787	0.798	0.808	0.815	0.822	0.830	0.837	0.844	0.848	0.853	0.857	0.862	0.866	0.873	0.880	0.887	0.892	0.897	0.901	0.908
11.0	0.645	0.702	0.716	0.730	0.744	0.756	0.767	0.778	0.786	0.793	0.801	0.808	0.816	0.821	0.826	0.830	0.835	0.840	0.847	0.854	0.861	0.867	0.872	0.876	0.883
12.0	0.616	0.672	0.686	0.700	0.714	0.727	0.738	0.749	0.757	0.765	0.772	0.780	0.788	0.793	0.798	0.804	0.809	0.814	0.822	0.829	0.837	0.843	0.848	0.852	0.859
13.0	0.588	0.643	0.657	0.671	0.684	0.697	0.709	0.721	0.729	0.737	0.745	0.753	0.761	0.766	0.772	0.777	0.783	0.788	0.796	0.804	0.812	0.818	0.823	0.828	0.835
14.0	0.561	0.616	0.630	0.643	0.656	0.669	0.681	0.693	0.701	0.709	0.718	0.726	0.734	0.740	0.745	0.751	0.756	0.762	0.771	0.779	0.788	0.794	0.799	0.804	0.811
15.0	0.536	0.590	0.604	0.617	0.630	0.642	0.655	0.667	0.675	0.684	0.692	0.701	0.709	0.715	0.721	0.726	0.732	0.738	0.747	0.755	0.764	0.771	0.776	0.781	0.788
16.0	0.511	0.565	0.579	0.592	0.605	0.617	0.630	0.642	0.651	0.659	0.668	0.676	0.685	0.691	0.697	0.702	0.708	0.714	0.723	0.732	0.741	0.748	0.753	0.758	0.766
17.0	0.488	0.542	0.555	0.568	0.581	0.593	0.605	0.617	0.626	0.634	0.643	0.651	0.660	0.666	0.672	0.678	0.684	0.690	0.699	0.708	0.717	0.725	0.730	0.736	0.744
18.0	0.466	0.518	0.531	0.544	0.557	0.569	0.581	0.593	0.602	0.611	0.619	0.628	0.637	0.643	0.649	0.655	0.661	0.667	0.676	0.686	0.695	0.703	0.708	0.714	0.722
19.0	0.445	0.496	0.509	0.521	0.534	0.546	0.558	0.570	0.579	0.588	0.596	0.605	0.614	0.620	0.626	0.632	0.638	0.644	0.653	0.663	0.672	0.680	0.686	0.692	0.701
20.0	0.424	0.474	0.478	0.499	0.512	0.524	0.535	0.547	0.556	0.565	0.573	0.582	0.591	0.597	0.603	0.609	0.615	0.621	0.631	0.640	0.650	0.658	0.664	0.670	0.679

21.0	0.405	0.455	0.467	0.479	0.490	0.502	0.513	0.525	0.534	0.543	0.551	0.560	0.569	0.575	0.581	0.587	0.593	0.599	0.609	0.618	0.628	0.636	0.642	0.649	0.658
22.0	0.387	0.435	0.447	0.459	0.470	0.482	0.493	0.504	0.513	0.522	0.530	0.539	0.548	0.554	0.560	0.566	0.572	0.578	0.588	0.597	0.607	0.615	0.622	0.628	0.638
23.0	0.370	0.417	0.429	0.440	0.451	0.463	0.474	0.485	0.493	0.502	0.510	0.519	0.528	0.534	0.539	0.546	0.552	0.558	0.567	0.577	0.587	0.595	0.602	0.608	0.618
24.0	0.352	0.399	0.411	0.422	0.433	0.443	0.454	0.465	0.473	0.482	0.490	0.499	0.507	0.513	0.519	0.525	0.531	0.537	0.547	0.557	0.567	0.575	0.582	0.588	0.598
25.0	0.337	0.383	0.394	0.405	0.415	0.426	0.436	0.447	0.455	0.463	0.471	0.480	0.488	0.494	0.500	0.506	0.512	0.518	0.528	0.538	0.548	0.556	0.562	0.569	0.579
26.0	0.321	0.366	0.377	0.387	0.398	0.408	0.418	0.428	0.436	0.444	0.453	0.461	0.469	0.475	0.481	0.486	0.492	0.498	0.508	0.518	0.528	0.536	0.543	0.549	0.559
27.0	0.307	0.351	0.362	0.372	0.382	0.392	0.402	0.412	0.419	0.427	0.435	0.443	0.451	0.457	0.462	0.468	0.474	0.480	0.490	0.500	0.510	0.518	0.525	0.531	0.541
28.0	0.292	0.336	0.347	0.357	0.366	0.376	0.385	0.395	0.403	0.410	0.418	0.425	0.433	0.439	0.444	0.450	0.455	0.461	0.471	0.482	0.492	0.500	0.507	0.513	0.523
29.0	0.279	0.322	0.333	0.342	0.351	0.361	0.370	0.379	0.386	0.394	0.401	0.409	0.416	0.422	0.427	0.433	0.438	0.444	0.454	0.464	0.474	0.483	0.489	0.495	0.505
30.0	0.266	0.308	0.318	0.327	0.336	0.345	0.354	0.363	0.370	0.377	0.385	0.392	0.399	0.405	0.410	0.416	0.421	0.427	0.437	0.447	0.457	0.465	0.471	0.478	0.487

TAR, Tissue-air ratio.

Table 24-9	6-MV Tissue-Maximum Ratio																								
Eq Sq Depth (cm)	0.0	4.0	5.0	6.0	7.0	8.0	9.0	10.0	11.0	12.0	13.0	14.0	15.0	16.0	17.0	18.0	19.0	20.0	22.0	24.0	26.0	28.0	30.0	32.0	35.0
0.0	0.186	0.187	0.186	0.199	0.210	0.223	0.235	0.248	0.259	0.271	0.282	0.293	0.304	0.316	0.329	0.339	0.352	0.364	0.378	0.392	0.406	0.419	0.431	0.443	0.461
1.0	0.957	0.958	0.958	0.958	0.958	0.959	0.959	0.960	0.960	0.960	0.962	0.962	0.962	0.963	0.963	0.964	0.964	0.965	0.966	0.968	0.969	0.970	0.970	0.971	0.972
1.5	1.000	1.000	1.000	1.000	1.000	1.000	1.000	1.000	1.000	1.000	1.000	1.000	1.000	1.000	1.000	1.000	1.000	1.000	1.000	1.000	1.000	1.000	1.000	1.000	1.000
2.0	0.982	0.990	0.991	0.992	0.992	0.993	0.993	0.993	0.993	0.993	0.994	0.994	0.993	7.692	0.994	0.994	0.994	0.994	0.995	0.995	0.995	0.995	0.994	0.994	0.994
3.0	0.936	0.964	0.970	0.972	0.974	0.975	0.976	0.977	0.977	0.977	0.978	0.978	0.978	7.692	0.980	0.979	0.980	0.981	0.981	0.982	0.982	0.982	0.982	0.981	0.981
4.0	0.894	0.938	0.948	0.952	0.955	0.957	0.957	0.958	0.958	0.958	0.959	0.960	0.960	7.692	0.962	0.963	0.964	0.965	0.966	0.966	0.967	0.967	0.966	0.966	0.966
5.0	0.853	0.901	0.912	0.918	0.922	0.926	0.927	0.929	0.930	0.932	0.934	0.936	0.937	7.692	0.940	0.942	0.943	0.944	0.946	0.948	0.949	0.949	0.949	0.949	0.949
6.0	0.814	0.865	0.877	0.884	0.889	0.895	0.897	0.900	0.903	0.905	0.909	0.911	0.913	7.692	0.917	0.556	0.920	0.922	0.925	0.927	0.929	0.931	0.931	0.931	0.933
7.0	0.777	0.829	0.842	0.851	0.858	0.864	0.868	0.872	0.875	0.879	0.882	0.885	0.888	7.692	0.893	0.895	0.898	0.900	0.903	0.905	0.908	0.910	0.910	0.912	0.913
8.0	0.742	0.796	0.810	0.818	0.827	0.834	0.838	0.844	0.847	0.852	0.856	0.860	0.863	7.692	0.869	0.871	0.874	0.877	0.880	0.883	0.886	0.888	0.890	0.890	0.892
9.0	0.708	0.763	0.777	0.786	0.795	0.804	0.809	0.816	0.820	0.824	0.829	0.833	0.837	7.692	0.843	0.847	0.850	0.853	0.857	0.860	0.864	0.867	0.868	0.869	0.872
10.0	0.676	0.732	0.745	0.756	0.766	0.775	0.782	0.788	0.793	0.797	0.803	0.808	0.812	7.692	0.819	0.822	0.826	0.829	0.833	0.837	0.842	0.844	0.846	0.848	0.851
11.0	0.645	0.701	0.714	0.725	0.735	0.744	0.751	0.759	0.765	0.769	0.775	0.780	0.785	7.692	0.793	0.796	0.800	0.804	0.808	0.813	0.817	0.820	0.820	0.824	0.828
12.0	0.616	0.671	0.684	0.695	0.706	0.716	0.723	0.731	0.736	0.742	0.747	0.753	0.758	7.692	0.767	0.771	0.775	0.779	0.784	0.789	0.794	0.798	0.800	0.802	0.805
13.0	0.588	0.642	0.655	0.666	0.676	0.686	0.694	0.703	0.709	0.715	0.721	0.727	0.732	7.692	0.742	0.745	0.750	0.754	0.760	0.765	0.770	0.774	0.776	0.779	0.783

Continued

Table 24-9 6-MV Tissue Maximum Ratio—cont'd

Eq Sq Depth (cm)	0.0	4.0	5.0	6.0	7.0	8.0	9.0	10.0	11.0	12.0	13.0	14.0	15.0	16.0	17.0	18.0	19.0	20.0	22.0	24.0	26.0	28.0	30.0	32.0	35.0
14.0	0.561	0.615	0.628	0.639	0.648	0.658	0.667	0.676	0.682	0.688	0.695	0.701	0.706	7.692	0.716	0.720	0.724	0.729	0.736	0.741	0.748	0.751	0.754	0.756	0.760
15.0	0.536	0.589	0.602	0.613	0.623	0.620	0.642	0.651	0.657	0.663	0.670	0.677	0.682	7.692	0.693	0.696	0.701	0.706	0.713	0.718	0.725	0.729	0.732	0.735	0.739
16.0	0.511	0.564	0.577	0.588	0.598	0.607	0.617	0.626	0.633	0.639	0.647	0.653	0.659	7.692	0.670	0.673	0.678	0.683	0.690	0.696	0.703	0.708	0.710	0.713	0.718
17.0	0.488	0.541	0.553	0.564	0.574	0.584	0.593	0.602	0.609	0.615	0.622	0.628	0.635	7.692	0.646	0.650	0.655	0.660	0.667	0.674	0.680	0.686	0.689	0.692	0.697
18.0	0.466	0.517	0.529	0.540	0.550	0.560	0.569	0.579	0.586	0.593	0.599	0.606	0.613	7.692	0.623	0.628	0.633	0.638	0.645	0.653	0.659	0.665	0.668	0.672	0.677
19.0	0.445	0.495	0.507	0.517	0.528	0.537	0.547	0.556	0.563	0.570	0.577	0.584	0.591	7.692	0.601	0.606	0.611	0.616	0.623	0.631	0.638	0.643	0.647	0.651	0.657
20.0	0.424	0.473	0.486	0.496	0.506	0.516	0.524	0.534	0.541	0.548	0.555	0.562	0.569	7.692	0.579	0.584	0.589	0.594	0.602	0.609	0.617	0.623	0.626	0.630	0.636
21.0	0.405	0.454	0.466	0.476	0.484	0.494	0.502	0.512	0.519	0.527	0.533	0.541	0.548	7.692	0.558	0.563	0.568	0.573	0.581	0.588	0.596	0.602	0.606	0.611	0.616
22.0	0.387	0.434	0.446	0.456	0.464	0.474	0.483	0.492	0.499	0.506	0.513	0.520	0.527	7.692	0.538	0.543	0.548	0.553	0.561	0.568	0.576	0.582	0.587	0.591	0.598
23.0	0.370	0.416	0.428	0.437	0.446	0.456	0.464	0.473	0.480	0.487	0.494	0.501	0.508	7.692	0.518	0.523	0.529	0.534	0.541	0.549	0.557	0.563	0.568	0.572	0.579
24.0	0.352	0.398	0.410	0.419	0.428	0.436	0.445	0.454	0.460	0.468	0.474	0.482	0.488	7.692	0.499	0.503	0.509	0.514	0.522	0.530	0.538	0.544	0.549	0.553	0.560
25.0	0.337	0.382	0.393	0.402	0.410	0.419	0.427	0.436	0.443	0.449	0.456	0.463	0.470	7.692	0.480	0.485	0.490	0.496	0.504	0.512	0.520	0.526	0.530	0.535	0.543
26.0	0.321	0.365	0.376	0.384	0.393	0.402	0.409	0.418	0.424	0.431	0.439	0.445	0.451	7.692	0.462	0.466	0.471	0.477	0.485	0.493	0.501	0.507	0.512	0.516	0.524
27.0	0.307	0.350	0.361	0.369	0.377	0.386	0.394	0.402	0.408	0.414	0.421	0.428	0.434	7.692	0.444	0.449	0.454	0.459	0.468	0.476	0.484	0.490	0.495	0.500	0.507
28.0	0.292	0.335	0.346	0.355	0.362	0.370	0.377	0.385	0.392	0.398	0.405	0.410	0.417	7.692	0.427	0.431	0.436	0.441	0.449	0.459	0.467	0.473	0.478	0.483	0.490
29.0	0.279	0.321	0.332	0.340	0.344	0.355	0.362	0.370	0.375	0.382	0.388	0.395	0.400	7.692	0.410	0.415	0.420	0.425	0.433	0.441	0.450	0.457	0.461	0.466	0.473
30.0	0.266	0.307	0.317	0.325	0.332	0.340	0.347	0.354	0.360	0.366	0.373	0.378	0.384	7.692	0.394	0.399	0.403	0.409	0.417	0.425	0.434	0.440	0.444	0.450	0.456

Table 24-10	Tray, Wedge, and Compensator Factors					
	Tray	**Factor**	**Wedge**	**Factor**	**Brass Compensator**	**Factor**
Cobalt-60	5 mm solid	0.96	15 degree	0.828	1 mm	0.956
	5 mm slotted	0.97	30 degree	0.744	2 mm	0.914
			45 degree	0.653	3 mm	0.874
			60 degree	0.424	4 mm	0.835
6 MV	5 mm solid	0.97	15 degree	0.828	1 mm	0.965
	5 mm slotted	0.98	30 degree	0.714	2 mm	0.931
			45 degree	0.580	3 mm	0.899
			60 degree	0.424	4 mm	0.867
18 MV	5 mm solid	0.98	15 degree	0.866	1 mm	0.945
	5 mm slotted	0.99	30 degree	0.775	2 mm	0.927
			45 degree	0.656	3 mm	0.918
			60 degree	0.449	4 mm	0.892

SUMMARY

- The methods used in most therapy centers will reflect that treatment team's philosophy, as developed by the medical physics team and the radiation oncologists.
- The output of every treatment unit used to deliver a dose of radiation to a patient is the amount of radiation exposure that is produced by a treatment unit as defined by a reference field size and at a specified reference distance.
- Each time there is a variation from a standard used to measure the reference beam, a "correction" is made with various output factors.
- Each time any item, be it a wedge, shielding tray, or compensating filter, is used, it must be accounted for in the beam calculation with a modifier that considers the attenuation of the beam through it.
- The time or number of monitor units used to deliver a prescribed dose, no matter how complex treatment is, can be found by dividing dose by dose rate. The key is to understand all of the components that modify each one.
- This material should provide the radiation therapist and medical dosimetrist with a good basis on which to further explore dosage treatment factors and concepts of treatment planning in radiation therapy.

Review Questions

Multiple Choice

1. Percentage depth dose increases with increasing:
   - I. energy
   - II. depth
   - III. field size
   - a. I and II
   - b. I and III
   - c. II and III
   - d. I, II, and III

2. Tissue-air ratio decreases with decreasing:
   - I. field size
   - II. depth
   - III. SSD
   - a. I
   - b. II
   - c. III
   - d. I, II, and III

3. When blocking is used in a treatment calculation, the area of the collimator is used in determining:
   - I. TMR
   - II. Sc
   - III. PDD
   - a. I
   - b. II
   - c. III
   - d. I, II, and III

4. Which of the following central axis depth dose quantities would most likely be used to compute an accurate monitor unit setting on an 18-MV unit for an isocentric treatment?
   - a. percentage depth dose
   - b. backscatter factor
   - c. tissue-maximum ratio
   - d. all of the above

5. Two parallel opposed equally weighted cobalt-60 fields are separated by 20 cm of tissue and treated with an SSD technique. The maximum dose will occur:
   - a. directly on the skin surface
   - b. at the midline of the patient
   - c. 0.5 cm under the skin surface
   - d. 5 cm under the skin surface

6. The advantage(s) of using parallel opposed isocentric fields for treatment delivery is(are) (compared with non-isocentric):
   a. less opportunity for movement error
   b. less overall dose to the skin surface
   c. both a and b
   d. neither a nor b

7. A wedge filter _____ the output of the beam and thus must be taken into account in the treatment calculations.
   a. increases
   b. decreases
   c. does not affect
   d. not enough information given

8. The Mayneord factor is used to convert:
   a. PDD with a change in SSD from the standard
   b. TAR with a change in SSD from the standard
   c. exposure rate with a change in SSD from the standard
   d. an exposure in roentgens to cGy

9. Any time an object is placed in the path of a therapeutic beam of radiation, it must be corrected for in the dose calculation to account for beam absorption.
   a. true
   b. false

10. A therapeutic radiation beam is composed of the TAR for a 20×10 cm field size plus the scatter component.
    a. true
    b. false

The answers to the Review Questions can be found by logging on to our website at *http://evolve.elsevier.com/Washington+Leaver/principles*

Questions to Ponder

1. Analyze how the collimator or field size can affect the output of a linear accelerator.
2. Describe how the source-skin distance causes percentage depth dose to vary.
3. A patient's larynx is to be treated using an isocentric technique on a linear accelerator; the patient's separation at the central axis is 9 cm and will be treated to midplane.

The treatment will use parallel opposed right and left lateral fields. The isocenter of the machine is established at 100 cm.
   a. What is the SSD on the patient's skin?
   b. If a field size of 6×6 cm is set on the collimator, what is the field size on the skin surface?

4. Explain the relationship between beam quality (energy) and TMR.

5. A 20-cm thick patient is to be treated on a cobalt-60 unit at 80 cm SAD. Two opposed 15×15 cm ports are used to deliver a treatment dose of 180 cGy per day to the midline (midplane). Determine the treatment time per port.

6. A patient is to receive 5040 cGy to his lung in 28 fractions. The treatment will use 15×11 cm opposed 6-MV photons to midplane at 100 cm SAD. The separation is 21 cm. The field is blocked to an 11×11 cm equivalent field. A 5-mm solid tray is used to support the blocks. Find the MU for each port each day.

7. Calculate the MU setting to deliver 300 cGy to a depth of 12 cm on a 6-MV unit using a single beam at 100 cm SSD using a field size of 15×8 cm. With this information, determine what the dose would be at a depth of 6 cm.

8. Compare and contrast the factors that influence percentage depth dose and tissue-phantom ratio.

REFERENCES

1. Bentel GC: *Radiation therapy planning,* ed 2, New York, 1996, McGraw-Hill.
2. Bentel GC, Nelson CE, Noell KT: *Treatment planning and dose calculations in radiation oncology,* ed 4, Elmsford, NY, 1989, Pergamon Press.
3. Johns H, Cunningham J: *The physics of radiology,* ed 4, Springfield, Ill, 1983, Charles C Thomas.
4. Khan FM: *The physics of radiation therapy,* ed 3, Philadelphia, 2003, Lippincott Williams & Wilkins.
5. Khan FM: *Treatment planning in radiation oncology,* ed 2, Philadelphia, 2007, Lippincott Williams & Wilkins.
6. Selman J: *The basic physics of radiation therapy,* ed 3, Springfield, Ill, 1990, Charles C Thomas.
7. Shahabi S: *Blackburn's introduction to clinical radiation therapy physics,* Madison, Wis, 1989, Medical Physics Publishing.
8. Stanton R, Stinson D: *Applied physics for radiation oncology,* Madison, Wis, 1996, Medical Physics Publishing.

Photon Dose Distributions

Karl L. Prado, Charlotte M. Prado

Outline

Objectives

- Describe the nature and characteristics of isodose distributions of single-photon fields.
- Discuss the combination of multiple fields used to produce cumulative isodose distributions.
- Compare and contrast corrections made to isodose distributions to account for contour irregularities and tissue heterogeneities.
- Analyze the principles and types of algorithms used for photon dose calculations and treatment planning.
- Discuss the rationale for three-dimensional conformal radiation therapy.

- List and explain treatment planning concepts and definitions for target volumes, critical structures, and margins to account for uncertainties.
- Describe the tools currently available for modern treatment planning and how these tools are used.
- Compare methods of quantitative treatment plan evaluation.
- Explain the treatment plan verification process needed before actual implementation.

Key Terms

The patient will benefit from a course of radiation therapy.

Thus begins the treatment planning process. Radiation will be used to treat the patient. How is the patient best treated? What are the goals and constraints of treatment? Does the attained dose distribution meet these goals? **Treatment planning** can be defined as the process by which dose delivery is optimized for a given patient and clinical situation. The radiation therapy planning and delivery process is intricate. Radiation dose deposition and distribution methods must be properly understood and planned to ensure disease is treated and normal structures are spared. The clinical picture is often variable and decision making is complex. The treatment planning method must be an effective tool in the decision-making process. It should simplify the definition of specific treatment goals and facilitate their implementation. In this chapter, clinical radiation dose distributions produced by external beams of photons are discussed, and photon beam treatment planning methods are reviewed.

PHOTON DOSE DISTRIBUTIONS

Single-Field Isodose Distributions

Dose distributions are spatial representations of the magnitude of the dose produced by a source of radiation. They describe the variation of dose with position within an irradiated volume. The percentage depth dose (PDD) curve (Figure 25-1) is an example of a one-dimensional representation of the variation of dose. Percent depth dose curves, explained in a previous chapter, describe dose variation with depth along the central axis of a beam. **Isodose distributions**, on the other hand, are two-dimensional (2D) spatial representations of dose. Typical isodose distributions illustrate dose variation both along and across the direction of a beam of radiation. These are illustrated in greater detail in later sections of the chapter.

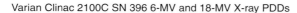

Varian Clinac 2100C SN 396 6-MV and 18-MV X-ray PDDs

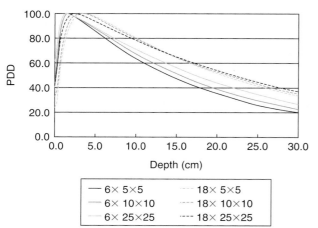

— 6× 5×5	···· 18× 5×5
— 6× 10×10	---- 18× 10×10
— 6× 25×25	---- 18× 25×25

Figure 25-1. Percentage depth dose (PDD) curves are typically plotted as a function of depth and are normalized to the PDD at the depth of maximum dose. Here are shown 6-MV and 18-MV x-ray depth dose curves. Note the variation of PDD with energy and field size. Note also the shift of the depth of maximum dose and the difference in PDD field size variation between 6- and 18-MV x-rays.

Treatment planning attempts dose distribution optimization for a given clinical goal in a given clinical situation. Treatment fields are used in ways that produce adequate tumor dose and minimal normal tissue dose. It is, hence, necessary to understand how dose distributions are both produced and then used. The discussion begins with simple, single fields and then progresses to more complex multiple-field arrangements.

Open Fields: Profiles. A beam profile is another one-dimensional spatial representation of the variation of beam intensity. A profile describes radiation intensity as a function of position across the beam at a given depth. It depicts the beam's intensity in a direction perpendicular to the beam's direction. The concept of beam-intensity variation as a function of position within the beam is best understood if one thinks about the response of a small radiation detector moving within a tank of water that is being irradiated. Figure 25-2 illustrates this process—a common method of measuring clinical beam data. As the radiation detector moves across the beam at some depth in the phantom, beam intensity (detector response) is plotted as a function of position within the beam. The resulting intensity curve as a function of position within the beam is called a **profile**. The intensity curves shown in Figure 25-2 are typical of photon field profiles. They are characterized by a rapid increase in intensity (as the radiation detector enters the beam), followed by a region of relatively uniform intensity (characterizing the central portion of the beam), then ending with a rapid decrease in intensity (as the detector exits the beam).

The shape of a beam's profile is a function of depth. At shallow depths, because scatter is less of a contributor to the total intensity of the beam than it is at deeper depths, the beam's profile better characterizes the beam's "primary" intensity. The D_{max} profile, shown in Figure 25-3, illustrates the influence of the accelerator's flattening filter on the beam. Flattening filters are introduced into photon beams to reduce the increased photon intensity existing in the center of the beam. Evidence for this effect is the somewhat reduced intensity shown in the center of the beam compared with that existing away from the central axis. The flattening filter is designed to produce a "flat" intensity pattern at some predefined depth (normally 10 cm). Box 25-1 expands on this thought. Note the flatter shape of the 10-cm depth profile of Figure 25-3 compared with the D_{max} profile. At deeper depths, scatter becomes a more significant

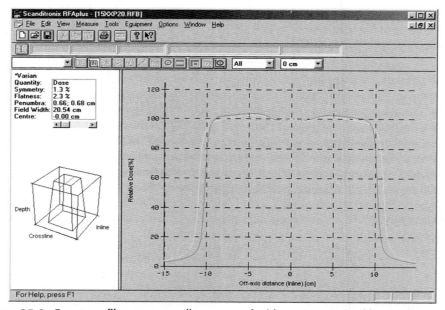

Figure 25-2. Beam profiles are normally measured with a computerized beam-data acquisition system that includes a water tank, radiation detector, and specialized software designed for radiation beam measurement and analysis. Note the beam-data acquisition geometry shown on the bottom-left portion of the screen showing the direction of ionization-chamber travel within the water tank. Two "in-plane" scans were acquired and the resulting profiles are displayed. (See Color Plate 9.)

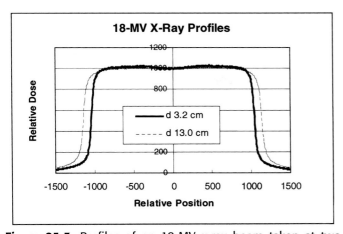

Figure 25-3. Profiles of an 18-MV x-ray beam taken at two depths, D_{max} and 13.0 cm. Note the differences in shape and size. The deeper profile is wider because the field diverges and its size increases with depth. The deeper profile is also "flatter" than the shallower profile because the accelerator's flattening filter is designed to produce flat beams at a depth of approximately 10 cm (see Box 25-1).

Box 25-1 Photon Beam Shape Specifications

It is often necessary to analyze profiles quantitatively to characterize the shape of photon beams. When profiles are measured along a direction parallel to the direction of electron motion along the accelerator's waveguide (parallel to the treatment couch), the profile is often termed a radial or "in-plane" profile. A profile measured along a direction perpendicular to the direction of the electron travel (perpendicular to the treatment couch), is often called a transverse or "cross-plane" profile.

Accelerator manufacturers provide specifications of the flatness and symmetry of photon beams. These specifications ensure that the accelerator produces beams possessing characteristics suitable for clinical use. The flatness and symmetry of clinical beams are checked periodically as a part of the accelerator's ongoing quality assurance program. A common way to define **flatness** is by noting the difference between the maximum and minimum intensity of the central 80% of the profile and specifying this difference as a percentage of the central axis intensity:

$$\text{Flatness}_{(\%)} = 100 \times [(I_{max} - I_{min})/I_{CAX}]$$

In this previous equation, I_{max} and I_{min} are the maximum and minimum intensities of the central 80% of the profile, respectively, and I_{CAX} is the intensity of the profile on its central axis. **Symmetry** can also be quantified in a similar fashion by noting profile intensities on either side of the central axis:

$$\text{Symmetry}_{(\%)} = 100 \times [(I_{+x} - L_{-x})_{max}/I_{xo}]$$

In this equation, I_{+X} and L_{-X} are corresponding profile intensities at a distance x on either side of the profile's central axis, and I_{X0} is the central axis intensity. A common definition of symmetry specifies the maximum point-to-point difference. As before, symmetry is defined in the central 80% of the profile.

---

component of dose, and a greater amount of scattered radiation exists along the center of the beam than along the periphery. This offsets the shape of the beam's primary profile, producing a relatively flat dose distribution.

Open Fields: Isodose Distributions. Isodose distributions consist of a series of isodose curves. The traditional **isodose curve** is a 2D representation of how dose varies with position within a beam along directions both parallel and perpendicular to the beam's direction. It is a collection of points, all having the same dose (hence the term *iso*dose). Figure 25-4 presents typical isodose distributions produced by photon beams of different energies.[9] The numerical values of the lines represent percentages of the dose existing at a point along the central axis at the depth of D_{max}. Thus, the 90% isodose contains all points within the plane of presentation where the dose is equal to 90% of the dose at D_{max}. The dose at points between isodose curves will lie between the doses represented by the curves.

Isodose distributions combine both the depth-dose and off-axis-profile characteristics of the beam. The numerical value of the isodose line along the central (depth) axis of the isodose curves is equal to the PDD at that depth. The shape of the isodose curve along a direction perpendicular to the central axis describes the off-axis characteristics of the beam. Isodose distributions will vary with beam energy, source-skin distance (SSD), and field size. Note also from Figure 25-4 that beams produced by accelerators are, in general, flatter than cobalt-60 or low-energy x-ray beams. As mentioned previously, this is due to the introduction of flattening filters used in linear accelerators. Note the shape of the 90% isodose curve of the 4-MV beam shown in Figure 25-4, C. The flattening filter causes the "dip" in the central region of the curve.

 In its simplest form, a given beam's isodose curve combines dose variation versus depth (percent-depth dose) with dose variation across the beam (profile) in a single two-dimensional graphic representation.

Wedged Fields: Isodose Distributions. It is often desirable to produce beams of nonuniform intensity across the field. Introducing an attenuator of varying thickness in the beam can produce the desired difference in intensity. As a consequence of its shape, this variable-thickness attenuator is called a **wedge**. When a wedge is introduced into a beam, differential attenuation along the varying thickness of the wedge produces a dose gradient along the wedged dimension of the beam; that is, less dose exists under thicker portions of the wedge than exists along less thick portions. At a given depth within a wedged beam, and in a direction toward the toe or thinner portion of the wedge, the dose increases with distance from the central axis of the beam. Similarly, the values of isodoses toward the heel or thicker portion of the wedge decrease with increasing distance from the central axis.

Examples of wedged-field isodose distributions are shown in Figure 25-5.[3] Note that wedged-field isodose lines are now "tilted"—a given-valued isodose penetrates to a greater depth along thinner portions of the wedge. The amount of incline of the isodose curves depends on the shape of the wedge.

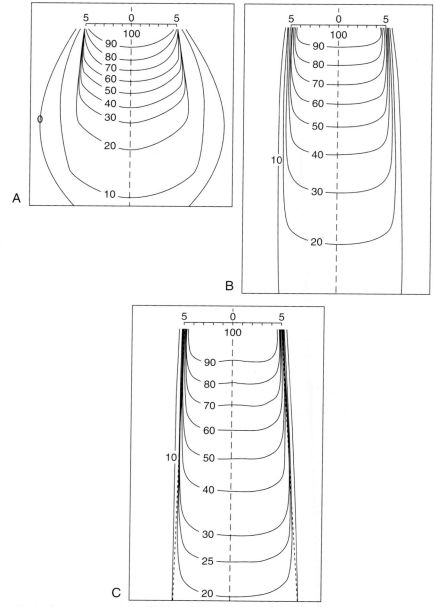

Figure 25-4. Open, 10 × 10 cm fields of different energies. **A**, 200 kVp, 1 mm Cu half-value layer (HVL), source-skin distance (SSD) 50 cm; **B**, cobalt-60 SSD 80 cm; and **C**, 4-MV 100 SSD. (Redrawn from Khan FM: *The physics of radiation therapy*, ed 2, Baltimore, 1994, Williams & Wilkins.)

Wedges with a greater variation in thickness from heel to toe will produce more inclined isodoses. The angle between the slanted isodose line and a line perpendicular to the central axis of the beam is called the **wedge angle**. Wedges are designed to produce certain discrete wedge angles. Traditionally, wedges supplied with the treatment machine are fabricated to produce discrete wedge angles of 15 degrees, 30 degrees, 45 degrees, and 60 degrees. Because, for any given wedge, the tilt of isodose lines varies slightly with depth (again because of the relative influence of scatter), either the depth of the 80% depth dose or a depth of 10 cm is often chosen for wedge-angle measurement and subsequent wedge attenuator design.[6,8]

Wedged-field isodoses demonstrate similar dependencies on beam energy, SSD, and field size as do open-field isodoses. Because of the presence of the wedge attenuator in the beam, on the other hand, the energy spectrum of wedged fields differs slightly from that of its nonwedged counterpart. This results in slight differences between open- and wedged-field PDD. The effect is more pronounced at lower beam energies and larger wedge angles. Table 25-1 shows data that illustrate this effect. The PDD at 20 cm depth in a 6-MV, 15 × 15 cm photon field increases by 4% when a 45-degree wedge is introduced; an 18-MV photon beam shows a 2% increase in depth dose under similar circumstances.

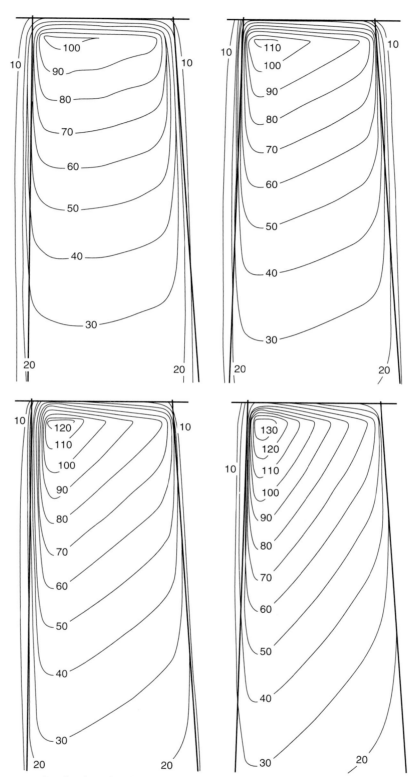

Figure 25-5. The tilt of wedged-field isodose curves are dependent on the particular wedge filter used. This figure shows typical isodose distributions produced by conventional 15-degree, 30-degree, 45-degree, and 60-degree conventional wedge filters. (Redrawn from Bentel GC: *Radiation therapy planning,* ed 2, New York, 1996, McGraw-Hill.)

Table 25-1	6- and 18-MV Open- and Wedged-Field Percent Depth Dose Data*			
Percentage Depth Dose	6-MV Open	6-MV 45-Degree Wedge	18-MV Open	18-MV 45-Degree Wedge
Depth 10 cm	69.3	70.5	79.1	80.7
Depth 20 cm	41.8	43.5	53.7	54.7

*Data for a Varian Clinac 2100C, 15 × 15 cm fields, 100 cm source-skin distance (SSD).

Wedged-field isodose distributions can also be produced without the use of wedge attenuators. If a collimator jaw is allowed to move across the beam during irradiation, a variation in intensity across the beam similar to that produced by a wedge can be achieved. The use of a moving collimator jaw to produce a wedged field is often termed **dynamic wedge**. Often, jaw movements during production of dynamic wedge fields are controlled to produce only fields equivalent to those produced by conventional wedges—15-degree, 30-degree, 45-degree, and 60-degree wedged fields. More recently, dynamic wedge capability has been extended to produce a wider range of wedged fields not limited to the conventional wedge angles. This capability has been called *enhanced dynamic wedge*.[16]

Clinical use of dynamic wedges has far-reaching dosimetric consequences beyond the scope of this chapter. The traditional "wedge attenuation factor" no longer exists as such because the wedging function is no longer produced by differential attenuation through an attenuator. Dynamic wedge factors are more related to field-size–dependent output factors because wedging is now a function of collimator jaw positions. In addition, because wedge attenuators are not used, the PDD of dynamic wedge fields is the same as that of their open-field counterparts.

Isodose distributions that are even more complex can be achieved by varying the field aperture with the unit's multileaf collimator during irradiation. Fields produced in this fashion are often termed intensity modulated. *Although this is not commonly done, the term* intensity modulated *could also be used to describe the effect of wedging an otherwise open field.*

Multiple-Field Isodose Distributions

Combined-Field Isodose Distributions: Open Fields.
Except for a few clinical situations in which the treatment depth is shallow, such as the treatment of supraclavicular nodes or portions of the spinal column, single-photon fields are rarely used solely. Very often, multiple fields are used in combination to take advantage of the improved dose distribution that results from aiming multiple fields from different directions at a common target area. Multiple fields convergent on a shared target result in a concentrated dose in the common target area.

The most common combined-field geometry is the **parallel-opposed field set**. In this field geometry, two treatment fields share common central axes, 180 degrees apart. A second field equal in size but mirrored in shape but opposite in direction compensates for the falloff in dose with depth from the first field.

Parallel-opposed fields are often used to treat regions near the middle of the treatment area. Examples of clinical parallel-opposed fields are anteroposterior (AP) and posteroanterior (PA) thoracic fields and right- and left-lateral head and neck fields.

Parallel-opposed fields work best in situations in which beam energy and patient thickness can be matched to allow for a uniform dose within the irradiated volume. With proper selection of energy and under favorable patient-thickness conditions, parallel-opposed fields can be used to deliver reasonably uniform doses. This can be seen in Figure 25-6.[9] In this figure, the doses at all points along the central axes of parallel-opposed beams 25 cm apart are shown for beams of different energies. (This figure is best understood if one thinks of the parallel-opposed beams as entering from the left and right of the figure.) Note that as beam energy increases, the dose along the central axes of the beams becomes more uniform. Lower-energy beams, because of their decreased penetrating ability, produce higher doses at their respective entrance depths, producing a less uniform dose distribution as a function of depth. A similar situation occurs as patient thickness increases and the entrance-to-midline dose ratio becomes unacceptably high. This is shown in Figure 25-7 where, for example, approximately 15% more dose exists at the entrance of 4-MV beams in a 25-cm-thick patient than at the patient's midline.[9] Under these circumstances, other beam combinations may be more appropriate.

Multiple convergent beams are often used in situations in which parallel-opposed beams cannot produce acceptable dose distributions or when it may be desirable to further restrict the high-dose region of the dose distribution. This is demonstrated in Figure 25-8 where the dose distributions resulting from the use of a parallel-opposed field set, a three-field arrangement, and a four-field arrangement are contrasted. Note that as supplementary fields are added, the high-dose region conforms to the

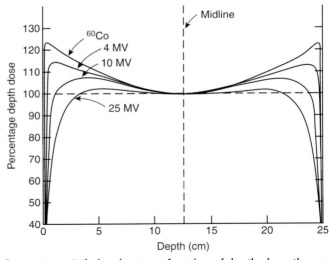

Figure 25-6. Relative dose as a function of depth along the central axis of parallel-opposed fields incident on a patient 25 cm thick. Curves, showing dose relative to the dose existing at mid-depth, are representative of the dose produced by 10 × 10 cm² treatment fields of energies cobalt-60, 4 MV, 10 MV, and 25 MV. (Redrawn from Khan FM: *The physics of radiation therapy*, ed 2, Baltimore, 1994, Williams & Wilkins.)

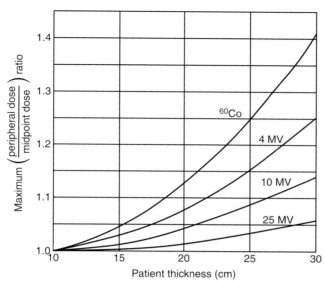

Figure 25-7. A patient is treated with parallel-opposed fields. This figure shows the maximum dose along the central axes of the fields expressed as a ratio of dose at the patient's midline. The curves, plotted as a function of patient thickness, are representative of cobalt-60, 4-MV, 10-MV, and 25-MV 10 × 10 cm², 100-cm source-skin distance (SSD) fields. Note that, for a patient 25 cm thick, parallel-opposed cobalt-60 fields produce a maximum dose along the central axis 25% greater than that produced at the patient's midline. (Redrawn from Khan FM: *The physics of radiation therapy,* ed 2, Baltimore, 1994, Williams & Wilkins.)

intersection of the beams and that the relative dose outside the beams' intersection decreases. Note also that, as a consequence of the equal angles between the fields, the dose distribution is relatively uniform within the region of the beams' intersection.

Combined-Field Isodose Distributions: Wedged Fields. Not uncommonly, there are clinical situations in which parallel-opposed or equally angled beams are not appropriate for the particular treatment scenario. An example is the treatment of disease in one side of the brain where sparing of the opposite hemisphere is desired. In this situation, a pair of wedged beams can be used to produce a region of reasonably uniform dose. Recall that the isodoses of wedged fields are tilted at an angle characterized by the wedge angle. A region of uniform dose can be achieved in the area common to two wedged fields if the angles of the central axes of the fields bear an appropriate relationship to the wedge angles of the beams. If ø is the angle between the beams' central axes, called the **hinge angle**, and θ is the wedge angle of the beams, then the relationship between the hinge and wedge angles that produces a uniform dose distribution is as follows:

$$\theta = 180° - 2\theta \text{ or } \theta = 90° - \theta/2$$

The previous relationship applies to pairs of wedged fields. The hinge angle can be adjusted slightly to accommodate clinical restraints such as protection of normal structures for instance. Wedged-field combinations are not limited to only pairs of wedged fields. Wedged fields can be used with open or other wedged fields in other fashions. Figure 25-9 shows examples of

the use of wedged fields to achieve more uniform dose distributions under normal-structure–sparing constraints.

Corrections to Isodose Distributions

Beam data for treatment planning systems are almost always obtained from measurements acquired in water phantoms. The data represent dose distributions obtained when a flat-surfaced homogenous (water) medium is irradiated. When actual irradiation conditions differ from those under which standard isodose distributions were obtained, corrections must be applied. Corrections for beam incidence onto surfaces other than flat surfaces and for angles of incidence other than 90 degrees ("normal" incidence) are called **obliquity** or **contour corrections**. Corrections that account for the presence of irradiated media other than water are called **heterogeneity corrections**.

Obliquity/Contour Corrections. The effective SSD method is a graphic contour-correction method that uses an isodose chart (a set of isodose curves). It entails "sliding" the isodose chart along the irregular contour such that its surface line is at the contour surface at a vertical line above the given point of interest. The PDD value at the point of interest is read and then corrected using an inverse square correction. Referring to Figure 25-10, the isodose chart is shifted from its position at the central axis (surface $S'' – S''$) to a position on the contour above the point A.[9] The PDD value (P) at point A is read off the chart and is then corrected by multiplying it by an inverse square factor to give the corrected PDD value (P'). The inverse square correction factor (CF) to be applied is as follows:

$$P' = P \times \left(\frac{SSD + d_m}{SSD + d_m + h} \right)^2$$

where, h is the tissue deficit or excess (either plus or minus) above the point of interest relative to the central axis.

Example: Suppose that (in Figure 25-10) point A was located at a depth of 5 cm in a 10 × 10 cm field and that the gap above point A was 3 cm. A 10 × 10 cm isodose curve would be slid down until the horizontal line representing the surface intersects the surface of the contour directly above the point of interest (i.e., point A). Suppose the isodose value now read *(solid line)* at P is 78%. This isodose value is corrected using the previously shown inverse square correction to yield the resultant depth dose:

$$P' = P \times \left(\frac{SSD + d_m}{SSD + d_m + h} \right)^2 = 78\% \times \left(\frac{100 + 1.5}{100 + 1.5 + 3} \right)^2 = 73.6\%$$

The dose at point A is 73.6% of the dose at the (preshift) D_{max} point.

The tissue-air ratio (TAR) (or tissue-maximum ratio [TMR]) method assumes that the tissue deficit (h) mentioned previously is filled with tissue-like material. In this method, again using Figure 25-10, the isodose curve is placed on the central axis at the surface $S'' – S''$ and the *(dashed curve)* isodose value (P) at point A is read as if a flat surface existed at $S''–S''$. Because the

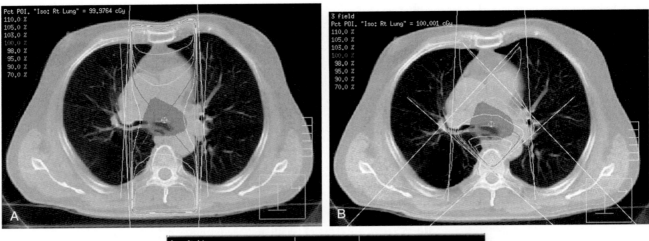

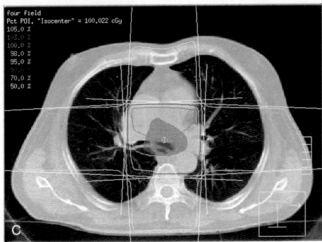

Figure 25-8. Thorax isodose distributions produced by a parallel-opposed field arrangement **(A)**, a three-field arrangement **(B)**, and a four-field arrangement **(C)**. The shaded area in the center of the computed tomography (CT) image represents the target volume. The numeric values of the isodoses represent percentages of the dose at the isocenter of the fields. (See Color Plate 10.)

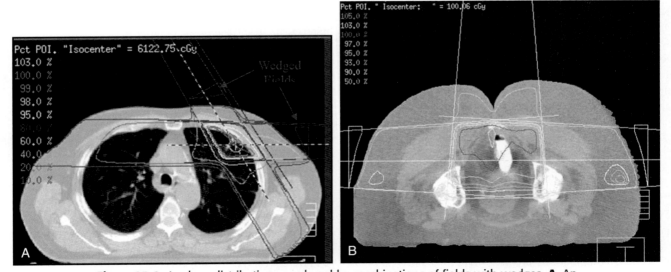

Figure 25-9. Isodose distributions produced by combinations of fields with wedges. **A,** An angled wedge pair. **B,** A combination of a posterior open field with two lateral wedged fields. (See Color Plate 11.)

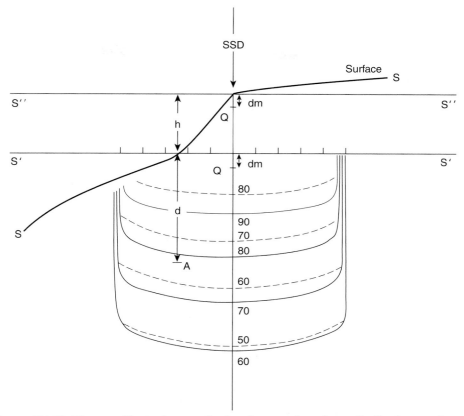

Figure 25-10 Diagram illustrating methods of correcting dose distribution under an irregular surface such as $S - S$. The *solid* curves are from an isodose chart that assumes a flat surface located at $S' - S'$. The *dashed* isodose curves assume a flat surface at $S'' - S''$ without any air gap. (Redrawn from Khan FM: *The physics of radiation therapy*, ed 2, Baltimore, 1994, Williams & Wilkins.)

isodose value has been underestimated by assuming that a depth of $h + d$ rather than d exists at point A, the isodose value P is corrected using the TAR (or TMR) ratio:

$$P' = P \times [\text{TAR}(d)/\text{TAR}(d + h)]$$

The TAR method can be illustrated, again using Figure 25-10 and the numeric assumptions of the previous example. Suppose that the PDD value at point A (when the isodose chart is placed at $S''- S''$) is 64.0%. Because this value assumes a depth of $5 + 3 = 8$ cm, it is corrected using the TAR ratio:

$$\left(\frac{\text{TAR}(5)}{\text{TAR}(8)}\right) = \left(\frac{0.905}{0.787}\right) = 1.15$$

$$P' = 64.0\% \times 1.15 = 73.6\%$$

Heterogeneity Corrections. Standard isodose charts and depth dose tables assume homogeneous, unit density (water) media. However, within a patient are fat, bone, muscle, and air, which attenuate and scatter the beam differently than does water. Boundary interfaces can present additional (transitional zone) problems (i.e., near bone, air cavities, metal prostheses, and so forth).

In the megavoltage range of x-ray energies, common in radiation oncology, the Compton effect is the predominant mode of

interaction[5,6] and thus the attenuation of the beam in any medium is a function, mostly, of the electron density of the medium (number of electrons per cm^3). To explain some of the methods used to account for the presence of some material that is not water equivalent, we use the schematic representation shown in Figure 25-11.[9]

Assume that dose is to be calculated at a point P at a depth d in a heterogeneous phantom. The radiation beam first traverses a depth d_1 of water-equivalent material, then through some other material (inhomogeneity) having a depth d_2, and then again through a depth d_3 of water-equivalent material. If ρ represents the density of the heterogeneous material relative to water, then the total (uncorrected) depth d and the effective (corrected) depth d_{eff} are each given by the following equations:

$$d = d_1 + d_2 + d_3$$

$$d_{eff} = d_1 + \rho_e d_2 + d_3$$

The effective SSD method assumes that the corrected PDD is equal to the PDD for the effective depth d_{eff} multiplied by an inverse square correction. The effective depth is the equivalent radiologic path length, d_{eff}, previously:

PDD (FS, SSD, d) corrected =

$$\text{PDD (F, SSD, } d_{eff}) \times (\text{SSD} + d_{eff}/\text{SSD} + d)^2$$

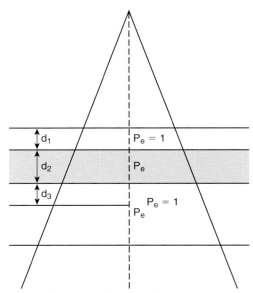

Figure 25-11. Schematic diagram showing a water-equivalent phantom containing an inhomogeneity of electron density P_e relative to that of water. *P* is the point of dose calculation. (From Khan FM: *The physics of radiation therapy*, ed 2, Baltimore, 1994, Williams & Wilkins.)

The TAR or TMR method applies an attenuation correction to the use of a TAR (or TMR) that is based on the physical depth as opposed to the effective or radiologic depth:

$$CF = \frac{TAR(d_{eff},r_d)}{TAR(d,r_d)} \ or \ \frac{TMR(d_{eff},r_d)}{TMR(d,r_d)}$$

where *d* is the actual, physical depth to the point *P*; d_{eff} is the effective water depth taking into account the relative electron densities of the materials ($d_{eff} = d_1 + \rho_e d_2 + d_3$); and r_d is the field size at the depth of calculation. The dose at point *P* (achieved assuming water-equivalent depths) is multiplied by the CF to get the inhomogeneity-corrected dose. Note that TMRs can also be used in the same fashion as TARs.

Example: Consider the following as an illustration of the TAR method for heterogeneity corrections and refer to Figure 25-11. Assume the phantom of Figure 25-11 is irradiated with a 10 × 10 cm, 80-cm SSD, cobalt-60 field. Further assume that $d_1 = 5$ cm, $d_2 = 10$ cm, and $d_3 = 3$ cm and that the density ρ_e of the 10-cm thick medium relative to water is 0.3. Under those assumptions, $d_{actual} = 5 + 10 + 3 = 18$ cm, and $d_{eff} = (5 \times 1) + (10 \times 0.3) + (3 \times 1) = 11$ cm. The distance to the point *P* is 80 + 18 = 98 cm, and the field size at *P* is (98/80) × 10 = 12.25 × 12.25 cm. The CF to be applied is as follows:

CF = TAR (11,12.25)/TAR (18,12.25) = 0.704/0.487 = 1.45

The dose at *P*, considering the presence of the heterogeneity, is 1.45 times the dose computed ignoring the presence of the heterogeneity. [Note that the previous correction produces the "effective" TAR that results as a consequence of the presence of the heterogeneity. The effective TAR at *P* = 0.487 × 1.45 = 0.487 × (0.704/0.487) = 0.704.]

The heterogeneity correction methods explained up to this point assume infinite slabs of heterogeneous media and do not take into account the relative location of the heterogeneity with respect to the point of calculation. As such, these methods yield only rough approximations of the effects of heterogeneities on dose calculations performed under assumptions of homogeneous media. More sophisticated calculations take these effects into account to varying degrees of accuracy.[18] Some of these methods are as follows:

1. *Power law TAR method*—a TAR correction method that accounts for the relative location of the point of calculation with respect to the inhomogeneity.
2. *Generalized Batho correction*—a generalization of the power law method to allow for dose calculations at points within the heterogeneity.
3. *Equivalent TAR method*—a method that considers the effects of heterogeneities on scatter, as well as on primary. In this method, both the field size and the depth are "scaled" to account for the presence of heterogeneities.
4. *Delta volume method*—in this method, primary and scatter are separated. The irradiated volume is broken into volume elements and scatter is computed from a weighted summation of the scatter from each of the volume elements. This scatter is then added to the primary.

Typical Heterogeneity Corrections. Tables 25-2 and 25-3, modified from Anderson,[1] can be useful in estimating the dose or correction to the dose beyond a given inhomogeneity.

Example (refer again to Figure 25-11): Assume that this phantom is irradiated with a single beam of 4-MV photons and that the dose is calculated at a point *P* assuming homogeneous media. The point *P* is located at a total physical depth of 6 cm. It is located beyond an inhomogeneity 2 cm thick. The homogenous dose at *P* from the single 4-MV beam is 100 cGy. If the inhomogeneity has a relative density of healthy lung (0.25), what is the radiologic depth and what is the heterogeneity-corrected dose at *P*? If the inhomogeneity has a relative density of bone (1.65), what is the radiologic depth and what is the heterogeneity-corrected dose at *P*?

The physical depth is 6 cm, of which 2 cm consists of the inhomogeneity. Thus, the radiologic (or effective) depth of the point *P* is 4 + (0.25 × 2.0) = 4.5 cm (assuming healthy lung), and 4 + (1.65 × 2.0) = 7.3 cm (assuming bone). The dose at *P* assuming a lung heterogeneity is approximately 100 cGy + (100 × 0.03 × 2) = 106 cGy (an increase in dose of 3% per cm of lung). The dose at *P* assuming a bone heterogeneity is approximately: 100 cGy − (100 × 0.03 × 2) = 94 cGy (a decrease in dose of 3% per cm of bone).

Table 25-2	Increase in Dose to Tissues Beyond Healthy Lung*
Beam Quality	**Correction Factor**
Orthovoltage	+10%/cm of lung
Cobalt-60	+4%/cm of lung
4 MV	+3%/cm of lung
10 MV	+2%/cm of lung
25 MV	+1%/cm of lung

*TAR method and $\rho_{e\ lung}$ = 0.25.

Table 25-3	Reduction of Dose Beyond 1 cm of Hard Bone*
Beam Quality	**Correction Factor**
1 mm Cu HVL	−15%
3 mm Cu HVL	−7%
Cobalt-60	−3.5%
4 MV	−3%
10 MV	−2%

Cu, Copper; *HVL,* half-value layer.
*TAR method and $\rho_{e\ bone} = 1.65$.

 The previously described isodose-distribution corrections have been presented here to illustrate the fundamental processes underlying these corrections. In state-of-the-art treatment planning systems, modern dose calculation algorithms take into account tissue heterogeneities and contour irregularities explicitly.

TREATMENT PLANNING ESSENTIALS

The treatment planning process has changed significantly over the past few years. Treatment planning systems, capable of handling large three-dimensional (3D) anatomy data sets, accurately modeling treatment unit capabilities, and offering very useful visualization tools, have now taken on the role of virtual patient simulators. Treatment planning tools allow for greater dose delivery precision. The accuracy of dose calculations has increased considerably. Optimization techniques permit more homogenous tumor volume irradiation while providing increased normal tissue protection.

This section provides an overview of current treatment planning capabilities and methods. Although both three-dimensional conformal radiation therapy (3D-CRT) and intensity-modulated radiation therapy (IMRT) are addressed, the characteristics common to both techniques are pointed out. Treatment planning fundamentals including basic concepts, treatment planning algorithms, and the treatment planning process are emphasized.

Rationale for Three-Dimensional Conformal Radiation Therapy

It is well known in radiation oncology that radiation dose affects both tumor-bearing and normal tissues. The degree of biologic effect is dependent on several factors, among them the magnitude of the dose and the radiosensitivity of the tissue. The desired outcome in radiation oncology is a high degree of tumor control with very little deleterious side effects. This is often achievable only to a certain degree.

Figure 25-12 is often used to explain the compromise between probability of tumor control and the incidence of normal tissue complications.[13] Both tumor-control probability and normal tissue complication incidence increase with dose. When tumors are more radiosensitive than their surrounding normal tissues, a relatively high degree of tumor control may be achievable, at some given dose, with a reasonably low normal tissue complication probability. This is the case shown in Figure 25-12, A-C. When tissues of equivalent radiosensitivity surround tumors, any dose producing a reasonable tumor-control probability will

also induce normal tissue complications with an equal probability. This is the case illustrated by Figure 25-12, A, where the dose producing a reasonable tumor-control probability also produces a high complication rate.

Greater tumor-control probability and lower normal tissue complication probability can be achieved simultaneously if tumor doses are maximized while normal tissue doses are maintained

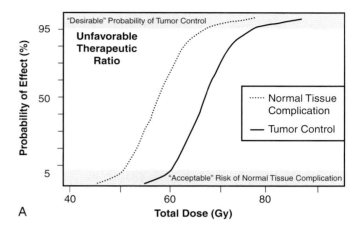

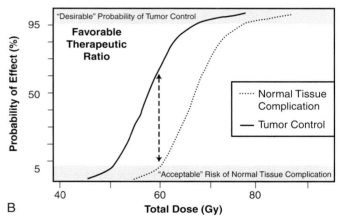

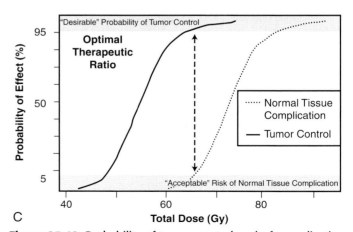

Figure 25-12 Probability of tumor control and of complication incidence as a function of dose. **A,** the ratio is unfavorable because the tissue tolerance does is less than the tumor control dose. **B,** the ratio is favorable because the tolerance does is greater than the tumor control dose. **C,** this is the optimal ratio that predicts low complication as shown by the curve separation. (From Gunderson LL, Tepper JE: *Clinical radiation oncology,* Philadelphia, 2007, Churchill Livingstone.)

at a minimum. This is the rationale for conformal radiation therapy. In **three-dimensional conformal radiation therapy (3D-CRT)**, 3D image visualization and treatment planning tools are used to conform isodose distributions to only target volumes while excluding normal tissues as much as possible. This section discusses the tools and processes used during 3D-CRT.

Three-Dimensional Treatment Planning and Delivery Methods. Three-dimensional treatment planning (3DTP) is the process by which 3D visualization, dose calculation, and plan-evaluation tools are used to produce optimized treatment-field arrangements. Planning is image based, and patient anatomy is represented by computed tomography (CT) data sets. Tumor volumes and critical structures are identified using image-contouring tools that enhance their visualization. Margins are established around tumor volumes to include disease microinvasion and allow for tumor volume and patient motion. Beams are arranged to target tumor volumes and to avoid critical structures. Treatment plans are then objectively evaluated based on their volume-dose relationships.

Current 3DTP methods include both conventional 3D-CRT and IMRT. In both methods, target volumes and critical structures are defined and beams are arranged in an attempt to maximize the dose to targets while minimizing the dose to critical structures. Intensity-modulation techniques allow for the modification of the distribution of intensity within a treatment beam to achieve the stated goal.

There are several types of IMRT delivery systems; most use multileaf collimators (MLCs). A "step-and-shoot" system will have the gantry in a fixed position with an initial MLC pattern. A portion of the dose is delivered through this leaf pattern or segment. (Beam is delivered *after* the MLC has achieved the shape corresponding to its appropriate segment.) With the gantry in the same position, the beam is automatically interrupted and the leaf pattern changes to that corresponding to the second segment. The beam is then turned on for the second segment. This may occur several times to produce the desired intensity map. During dynamic MLC (DMLC) treatment delivery techniques, the leaves of the MLC move during the delivery of the dose ("sliding window" technique). After the dose of the first beam is delivered for either of these two types of IMRT techniques (segmental MLC and dynamic MLC), the gantry is moved to the next position and the treatment is delivered in the same way for the next beam.

IMRT is often "inverse planned." IMRT **inverse planning** systems calculate dose distributions and create MLC patterns based on initial dose delivery and avoidance parameters. The intensity of the beams is then altered, by opening and closing the MLC, to achieve the requested doses. Beam arrangements are set up by the planner. The planning system then computes alternative intensity patterns until the best possible solution is determined.

The 3D-CRT uses conventional **forward planning**. Forward planning requires that dose-altering parameters and beam modifiers be entered into the treatment plan by the planner. After the initial dose calculation is completed, the planner evaluates the dose distribution and edits the modifiers or other parameters to produce an improved plan. This process is repeated until an acceptable plan is achieved.

Treatment Planning Algorithms

Treatment planning algorithms are the planning systems' dose calculation processes. They consist of a series of mathematical equations, and their associated input parameters, that produce values of dose as a function of position within the **dose calculation matrix**—a grid of points at which dose is computed and subsequently displayed.

Treatment planning algorithms can be categorized on the basis of their dose calculation methodology.[14] Data-driven algorithms compute dose mainly from interpolations between measured beam data—depth dose data, off-axis profiles, and so forth. CFs are applied to account for differences between the measurement geometry and the geometry of the patient. Examples of data-driven algorithms are the Bentley-Milan algorithm and the scatter integration algorithm. Data-driven algorithms are now seldom used in modern planning systems.

Model-driven algorithms mainly use equations, "fit" to measured data, that are intended to predict the variation of dose with changes in parameters such as depth, distance off axis, and proximity to field edges. Patient dose is computed by simulating the actual physics of the radiation transport process—the beam is produced in the target of the accelerator, is transported through the head of the machine, and is incident on the patient where it is attenuated and absorbed. An example of a modern model-driven algorithm is the convolution algorithm (such as the one used by the ADAC Pinnacle[3] treatment planning system).

Treatment planning algorithms can also be classified according to the dimensionality of the calculation methodology. A common classification is 2D and 3D algorithms. Although descriptions of 2D and 3D algorithms often differ, several distinguishing traits are salient. Some of the features of 2D and 3D systems are shown in Table 25-4. The 3D algorithms make use of entire CT data sets that are treated as one comprehensive CT volume; 2D algorithms often treat CT data as a series of independent CT planar contours. This is of particular importance during the dose calculation phase. The 3D algorithms use the entire data set when estimating scatter to each point in the volume; 2D algorithms assume that all CT image planes are of equal size, shape, and composition as the current calculation plane and compute scatter under that (inaccurate) presumption. Because of the availability of volume information, 3D algorithms also permit evaluations of plan quality using a tool called the *dose-volume histogram (DVH)*. The DVH is discussed later in the chapter.

Treatment planning algorithms can be evaluated based on several criteria. Algorithms differ in their ability to properly model beam intensities under different irradiation conditions. An ideal algorithm will properly represent a beam's depth dose

Table 25-4	Characteristics of 2D versus 3D Calculation Algorithms	
3D Algorithms		**2D Algorithms**
3D data set		Independent contours
Comprehensive anatomy		Limited anatomy
3D dose corrections		In-plane corrections only
Volumetric evaluation (DVH)		Limited evaluation tools

2D, Two-dimensional; *3D,* three-dimensional; *DVH,* dose-volume histogram.

and off-axis intensity. It will properly characterize the irradiation geometry (gantry, collimator, and couch angles) and the effects of beam modifiers such as independent jaws, MLCs, wedges, compensators, and bolus. Treatment planning algorithms should also properly model patient data sets such as CT and magnetic resonance imaging (MRI) data. Dose calculation accuracy and speed are yet other considerations.

Calculation Algorithms—Scatter Integration. To simplify the explanation of the dose calculation process, it is often useful to consider dose as consisting of primary and scatter components.[1] In basic terms, at all points in the irradiated volume, dose from primary radiation is computed first, then the dose from scattered radiation is added. A scatter-integration–like algorithm may use an equation similar to the schematic formula that is shown in the following:

$$D(f,r,d,x) = D_{ref} \times OF_{pri} \times ISF(f+d) \times OAF(x,d) \times T(r)$$
$$\times OF_{scat}(r) \times [TPR(0,d) + SPR_{avg}(r,d)]$$

where:

$D(f,r,d,x)$ = dose at some point P at a depth d, source-surface distance f, field size r, and off-axis distance x

D_{ref} = a known reference dose, for example, dose at D_{max}, 100 cm SSD, 10×10 cm field

OF_{pri} = an output factor describing the change in primary output as a function of collimator setting (akin to Khan's Sc)[9]

$ISF(f+d)$ = an inverse square correction

$OAF(x,d)$ = an off-axis factor that models the beam's profile

$T(r)$ = beam transmission through wedges, trays, and other possible beam modifiers

OF_{scat} = an output factor describing the change in scatter contribution as a function of field size and shape (akin to Khan's Sp)

$TPR(0,d)$ = the primary (0×0 field) TPR or TMR

$SPR_{avg}(r,d)$ = the average scatter-phantom (or scatter-maximum) ratio, a function of field size and shape, that is added to the primary TPR (or TMR) to produce an effective TPR (or TMR)

The product of $D_{ref} \times OF_{pri} \times ISF(f+d) \times OAF(x,d) \times T(r)$ describes the primary radiation intensity that is available at P. The remaining parameters OF_{scat}, $TPR(0,d)$, and $SPR_{avg}(r,d)$ are a function of the conditions within the attenuating media.

Example: The previous equation may seem complex, but in reality it is not. The perceived complexity is due to the large number of variables and parameters that require definition. To illustrate the calculation method, consider the following situation: Suppose that a phantom is irradiated with a 12×12 cm field; the SSD is 90 cm and dose is to be computed to a point P that is 10 cm deep. If the accelerator is calibrated so that 1 cGy/MU (D_{ref}) exists at D_{max}, 100 cm SSD, for a 10×10 cm field, then the dose at P is 1 cGy/MU $\times$ the output factors for a 12×12 cm field (OF_{pri}) and (OF_{scat}) $\times$ an inverse square correction for possible differences between calibration and calculation distances [$ISF(f+d)$] $\times$ the appropriate TMR [$TPR(r,d)$] and tray transmission factors [$T(r)$]. Remaining variables [such as $SPR_{avg}(r,d)$ and $OAF(x,d)$] are used when needed to account for situations such as irregular blocking or dose to points away from the central axis.

Calculation Algorithms—Convolution Algorithm. Newer algorithms, such as the convolution algorithms used in 3D planning systems, work in a similar way. Primary and scatter contributions are computed separately and then are summed. A 3D convolution algorithm[11] may use a calculation methodology described by the following:

$$D(r) = \int \frac{\mu}{\rho}(r) \times \Psi(r) \times K(r' \to r) dV$$

Here, $D(r)$ represents the dose at some point r. The primary fluence, $\psi(r)$, describes the primary dose that exists at the point r. It is the in-air fluence that exits the head of the treatment unit, is moderated by beam modifiers, and is then attenuated by the patient. The $\psi(r)$ term contains all primary radiation output, inverse square, off-axis, and beam-modifier corrections. [It is analogous to the product $D_{ref} \times OF_{pri} \times ISF(f+d) \times OAF(x,d) \times T(r) \times TPR(0,d)$ used in the description of the scatter-integration algorithm.]

The product of $\psi(r)$ and $\mu/\rho(r)$ produces a quantity that represents the total radiation energy released at the point r. The incident fluence is projected onto the patient's CT data set and is attenuated.

The result is a matrix of radiation energy that is available for dose deposition.

The dose-spread kernel, $K(r' \to r)$, represents the energy distribution from the primary interaction site throughout the irradiated volume. $K(r' \to r)$ is a description of how dose is deposited in the vicinity of a primary interaction site. $K(r' \to r)$ can be thought of as describing the dose at r that is produced at all contributing interaction sites r'. [It is, in some ways, analogous to the terms OF_{scat} and $SPR_{avg}(r,d)$ used to compute scattered dose in the scatter-integration algorithm.]

Because the total dose at the point r is dependent on the total radiation energy released at all points r', the total dose at r is the "superposition" (a "fluence and attenuation coefficient-weighted summation") of the function $\psi(r) \times \mu/\rho(r)$ and the dose-spread function $K(r' \to r)$. The integration sign, $\int$, represents the summation process.

Although the mathematical description of dose-calculation algorithms may seem intimidating, the concepts are relatively straightforward. The dose to all points from primary radiation is computed, and then scattered radiation from these primary dose depositions is added to obtain the total dose. The effects of contour irregularities and tissue heterogeneities are taken into account, as appropriate, in each step.

Treatment Planning Concepts and Tools

Treatment planning algorithms constitute the calculation engine of the treatment planning process. Calculation algrithms are only one piece of the entire 3D planning process. Before dose is calculated, treatment beams must be established in a way that achieves the intent of radiation therapy—maximization of tumor, or target, dose and minimization of normal tissue dose.

Planning Volume and Margin Concepts. Because the 3D-CRT process seeks to conform dose to specific target volumes, it is imperative that these volumes be accurately defined. The International Commission on Radiation Units and Measurements (ICRU) has recommended the use of specifically defined volumes[7]:

Gross tumor volume (GTV) is the gross palpable, visible, and/or demonstrable extent and location of malignant growth. It is the volume of known disease. Disease that is visible on CT is a common example of a GTV.

Clinical target volume (CTV) is a tissue volume containing the GTV and/or subclinical microscopic malignant disease. The CTV includes gross visible or palpable disease *plus* any possible microscopic extensions of disease that may not be visible or palpable. The CTV is the volume that must always be enclosed by the treatment isodose. Untreated portions of the CTV could lead to local failure of therapy.

Planning target volume (PTV) is a geometric volume; it has dimensions believed to always contain the CTV, taking into account all possible geometric uncertainties such as setup uncertainties and patient and/or organ motion.

Treated volume is the volume enclosed by the isodose surface selected as being appropriate to achieve the purpose of treatment (i.e., the volume enclosed by the prescription isodose surface).

These volumes are shown schematically in Figure 25-13.[7]

Margins are created around the CTV and PTV to ensure appropriate beam targeting. As previously stated, the margin surrounding the GTV is devised to account for the uncertainties existing in the precise definition of disease. The PTV includes a margin around the CTV to ensure that the CTV is always contained within the PTV. The exact definitions of these margins are evolving as newer technologies are introduced (Box 25-2). The GTV to CTV margin is mostly pathology driven. The margin of the PTV around the CTV is designed to make certain that the CTV is always contained within the treated volume. Note that the PTV margin around the CTV is not necessarily symmetric. The PTV allows for target motion and uncertainty in positioning.[17] Greater spatial uncertainties in the position of the target volume may exist in one dimension than in another. For example, it is generally believed that prostate motion in the AP direction may exceed lateral prostate motion.[2] Thus, the PTV margin around the CTV should be designed to account for these types of uncertainties.

Newer target volume and margin descriptions have been introduced to better account for the specific uncertainties in target definition caused by motion. An internal margin (IM) is added around the CTV to account for the CTV's internal motion within the patient. The result is an internal target volume (ITV): ITV = CTV + IM. A setup margin (SM) is added around the ITV to account for the uncertainty in patient position. The final result is now the PTV: PTV = ITV + SM.

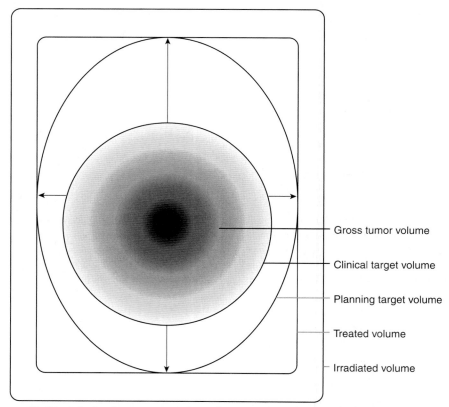

Gross tumor volume
Clinical target volume
Planning target volume
Treated volume
Irradiated volume

Figure 25-13. Schematic representation of treatment volume relationships. The clinical target volume contains the gross tumor volume, as well as volumes with possible (subclinical) disease. The planning target volume is designed to always contain the clinical target volume under all treatment conditions. See text for details. (Reprinted with permission from International Commission on Radiation Units and Measurements: *Prescribing, recording, and reporting photon beam therapy,* ICRU Report 50. Bethesda, Md, 1993, The Commission.)

Precise definitions of the CTV and PTV have become areas of much recent attention and focus. If one is to treat disease while sparing normal structures, GTVs should be expanded to CTVs and then to PTVs in insightful ways.

Molecular and functional imaging are now being used to better define diseased anatomy that was previously only suspected of containing disease. Positron emission tomography (PET) with ^{18}FDG (fluoro-2-deoxy-D-glucose), for example, is now commonly used to stage non–small cell lung cancer, due to its increased sensitivity to the metabolic activity associated with tumor cell proliferation. The figure below clearly demonstrates an increased concentration of ^{18}FDG in a mediastinal lymph node that could have been otherwise undetected in CT. Using advanced functional imaging techniques such as this, population-based traditional expansions of GTVs to CTVs could be reduced.

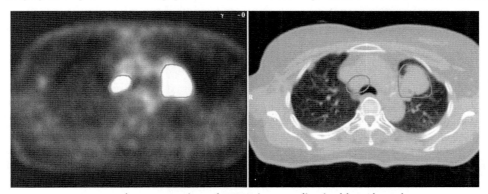

Increased concentration of ^{18}FDG in a mediastinal lymph node.
(See Color Plate 12.)

Image-guided radiotherapy (IGRT) techniques seek to further reduce expansions of target volumes by decreasing the uncertainty associated with daily patient positioning. If images of a patient's target volume are taken daily, and the patient position is suitably adjusted, the CTV to PTV expansion can be fittingly modified. In the figure below, the GTV as seen on an image of a daily CT taken with an in-room CT scanner *(Daily)*, is compared with the GTV defined on the treatment planning CT *(Ref)*; by properly aligning the target volumes of both image sets, corrections to the patient's position can be made, thus decreasing the uncertainty in patient position.

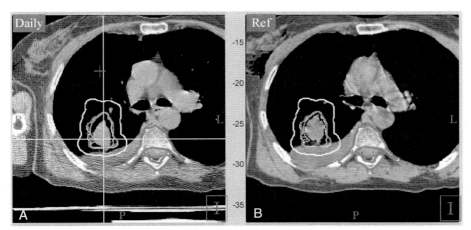

GTV as seen on an image of a daily CT taken with **(A)** an in-room CT scanner *(Daily)*, and compared with **(B)** the GTV defined on the treatment planning CT *(Ref)*. (See Color Plate 13.)

Prescriptions are commonly formulated based on isodose surfaces, generated by the treatment planning system, relative to the PTV. The PTV should be enclosed by an isodose surface within an accepted percentage range of the prescribed dose. (For example, dose could be prescribed to the isocenter based on the fact that the PTV is enclosed by a 95% to 98% isodose surface.) This process will ensure that the CTV will always receive a dose that has been deemed adequate within an acceptable dose range.

Treatment fields are often designed from **beam's eye views (BEVs)** of PTVs. (BEVs are images reconstructed from CT data that represent the patient's anatomy and defined volumes from the perspective of the treatment beam. BEVs are discussed in more detail in the next section). BEV-designed treatment fields should include a margin that allows for full dose coverage of the PTV and accounts for beam penumbral effects—the distance from the 50% to the 90% profile level. Although this margin will account, primarily, for possible lateral radiation-transport equilibrium losses, it should also allow for exclusion of critical structures.[12] Figure 25-14 illustrates the volume and margin concepts that have just been discussed.

Treatment Planning Tools. **Virtual simulation** is a process by which treatment fields are defined using patient CT image data and treatment-unit geometric information.[4] Specialized software is used to contour patient anatomy, set up the treatment beam arrangement, identify the location of patient markings, and design blocking for the treatment fields (Figure 25-15). Most of the simulation process is completed without the presence of the patient. Because the virtual simulator software contains treatment machine parameters, the limitations of conventional simulators, such as the presence of image intensifiers and possible differences between simulator and treatment-unit geometry, do not interfere with the field arrangements. Clinicians are better able to make decisions on the field arrangement. They also have more information available to use in virtual simulation. The patient's cross-sectional CT anatomy can be used to view the path of the beam through possible sensitive structures. Field shape and position can be edited to avoid critical structures.

Treatment planning systems have drawing tools that allow the planner to outline structures and planning volumes. The process of identifying structures, target volumes, or normal tissues by creating contours around them is often called **organ segmentation**. Segmented structures can be displayed graphically as outlines surrounding the structure or can be filled to create a solid volume. Segmented structures are commonly used to assist in field shaping and positioning and in isodose evaluation.

Anatomy that is to be identified for treatment planning may be better defined using other imaging modalities in addition to CT. Because of the physical principles underlying their image production, MRI and positron emission tomography (PET) scans show anatomy differently than does CT. Both MRI and PET incorporate physiology in the production of images. This can be used to better differentiate between diseased and normal tissues. Treatment planning systems are often capable of combining the images from the different modalities with the CT image. The process of combining the images is often called **image fusion** or image registration. Properly fused images can combine the enhanced imaging capabilities of MRI and/or PET with the spatial accuracy of CT. Anatomy can be defined on any of the image data sets and can then be displayed on the CT image (Figure 25-16).

Once a beam has been created, the clinician can view the patient as seen through the opening of the beam. As stated previously, this particular view of the patient anatomy from the perspective of the treatment field is called a *BEV*. The BEV changes in shape and size the same way the radiation beam diverges through the patient. Field size and blocking can be demonstrated according to their size and shape in relation to the plane of the body being viewed. When a BEV is reconstructed such that diverge-corrected patient anatomy from the CT data set is also included in an image that imitates a radiograph, the resulting image is called a **digitally reconstructed radiograph (DRR)**. A typical DRR is shown in Figure 25-17.

A **room's eye view** demonstrates the geometric relationship of the treatment machine to the patient. The room's eye view

allows clear visualization of the entrance and exit of the beam through the patient. This view may also help prevent possible orientations of the equipment that could result in collisions with the patient or treatment table.

Other image-rendering techniques allow visualization of anatomic structures that have been highlighted. The skeleton of the body or the skin can be distinguished by choosing image-visualization techniques that display the specific ranges of CT density. Skin rendering allows the planner to see markers that were placed on the skin during the CT scan. Room lasers and field and block outlines can be displayed on the patient's skin (Figure 25-18). This technique is similar to looking at the field light on the patient in a conventional simulator.

The 3D treatment plans can be objectively evaluated using dose and volume information. An extremely useful evaluation tool is the **dose-volume histogram (DVH)**. Lawrence et al.[10] have explained the fundamentals of DVHs and their clinical interpretations in detail. The DVH is a plot of target or normal structure volume as a function of dose. It is, in essence, a frequency distribution of the number of target or normal structure voxels (volume elements) receiving a certain dose. In its most common form (the "cumulative" DVH), it is a plot of volume versus the minimum dose absorbed within that volume. Figure 25-19 presents a cumulative DVH for a hypothetical PTV, CTV, and GTV. The characteristics of an optimal target volume DVH are (1) high percentage volume at prescribed target dose (adequate target volume coverage) and (2) rapid decrease in volume beyond the prescribed dose (dose uniformity within target).

Interpretation of normal tissue DVHs is somewhat more complex. Clearly, a desired trait of a normal tissue DVH is large volumes maintained at lower doses. This is often not attainable, and DVHs such as those shown in Figure 25-20 result.[15] Depending on their response to radiation, tissues can be characterized as either serial response tissues or parallel response tissues. The overall function of organs consisting of **serial response tissues** can be affected by the incapacitation of only one element. The spinal cord is such an organ. The high-dose region of a serial tissue DVH is of particular importance. The overall function of organs consisting of **parallel response tissues**, on the other hand, is affected by the injury of a number of elements of that organ above a certain minimum "reserve." The liver is an example of such an organ. Interpretation of DVHs of organs of parallel response tissue is less clear.

Site-specific DVH-based criteria are now commonly used for the evaluation of critical structures in treatment plans. In thoracic radiation therapy, for instance, a DVH-based constraint used for normal lung is $V_{20} < 40\%$ (meaning less than 40% of normal lung should receive a dose in excess of 20 Gy). Another thoracic constraint is $V_{50} < 50\%$ for the heart.

The Three-Dimensional Treatment Planning Process

Imaging and Anatomy Differentiation. The treatment planning process begins at the time of patient CT imaging. The area to be imaged is identified. It is important to include enough anatomy to identify anatomic landmarks for treatment setup confirmation. Setting the CT slice thickness and table indexing

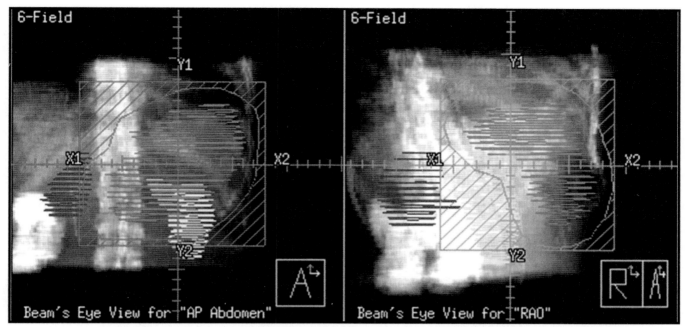

Figure 25-14. Use of the beam's eye view (BEV) tool for treatment-field design and placement. Note the differences between the anteroposterior (AP) and right anterior oblique (RAO) fields. The shape and spatial relationships of the tumor and the kidney volumes change as a function of gantry angle, allowing more favorable tumor volume targeting. (See Color Plate 14.)

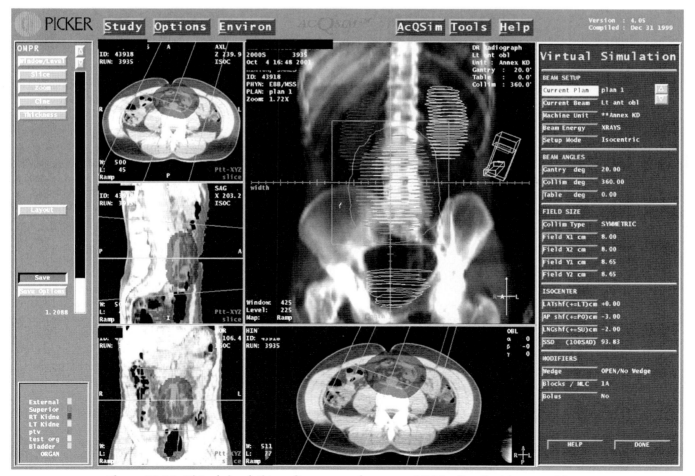

Figure 25-15. Virtual simulation software sample screen. A "virtual" patient is created from computed tomography (CT) data. The software supports normal tissue and target volume definition and identification; treatment fields can then be designed and placed. (See Color Plate 15.)

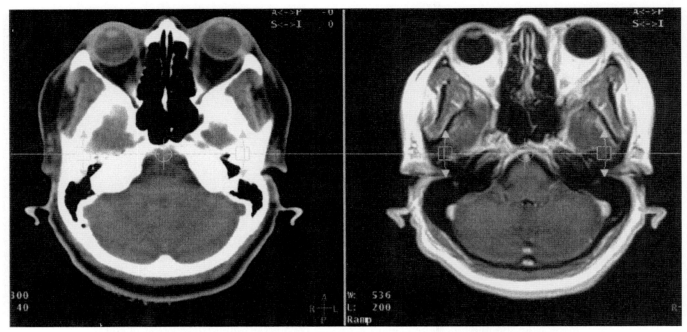

Figure 25-16. Computed tomography (CT) and magnetic resonance imaging (MRI) image fusion. The superior soft tissue imaging ability of the MRI image on the *right* can be combined with the superior spatial accuracy of the CT image on the *left* to produce a composite, correlated image. In the fusion process, common anatomic features are identified in each image, and these common features are then used to "link" the data sets so that they form a composite set. From that point on, features identified on an image of one modality are shown on its corresponding second-modality image.

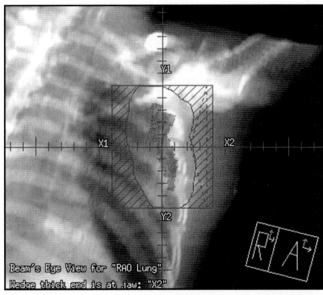

Figure 25-17. Digitally reconstructed radiograph (DRR). A DRR is a two-dimensional radiograph-like image that is reconstructed from a computed tomography (CT) data set. The image of this figure was reconstructed from a thoracic data set to produce a view equivalent to that obtained if a radiographic image were obtained from the patient's right anterior side. Superimposed on the image is the projection of the contoured clinical target volume and the treatment field designed to cover the volume with a 2-cm margin. (See Color Plate 16.)

to small increments will increase the quality of radiographs created from the CT data sets. The patient is set up on the CT scanner in treatment position. Immobilization devices are made and used during the scan. Once the patient is positioned on the table, the center of the volume to be scanned is placed at the intersection of the transverse, sagittal, and coronal positioning lasers. Preliminary marks are made on the patient, and radiopaque markers are placed to identify the location of patient marks on the CT images. These marks will be used later as the reference position for final isocenter localization following the virtual simulation (Figure 25-21).

CT images are reconstructed and sent to the planning system. The images in the planning system can be viewed either three-dimensionally or through different anatomic planes, the most common being transverse, sagittal, and coronal views. Important anatomic areas are defined in the course of organ segmentation. Target areas are identified on the patient's CT data set. Tumor-bearing regions classified and contoured as GTVs, CTVs, and PTVs are defined. The minimum dose acceptable for target structures is identified, as well as the acceptable homogeneity of the dose throughout the target. Within the volume to be irradiated, there may be critical structures requiring that a specified volume be limited to a certain maximum dose. These significant anatomic structures are outlined in the treatment planning system, as well. Normal tissue volumes and their dose limits are generally determined by clinical criteria.

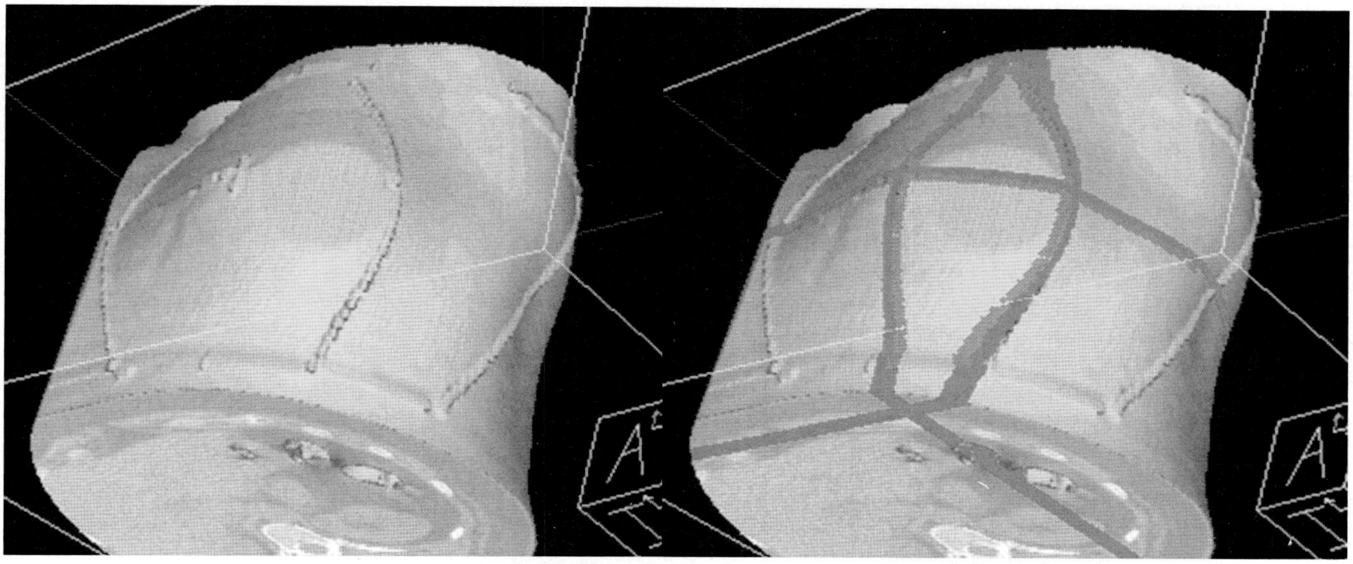

Figure 25-18. Use of image-visualization tools to aid in treatment-field placement during virtual simulation and treatment planning. The computed tomography (CT) data set can be visualized using an image-rendering technique that emphasizes the patient's skin and any markers placed on the skin. In this figure, beams have been placed such that the lasers that indicate their isocenter coincide with catheters placed on the patient before CT. (See Color Plate 17.)

Treatment-Field Definition. After target and anatomy definition, the orientation of treatment beams is arranged. Beam location is referenced to the marks previously made on the patient. In the planning system, the location of patient marks becomes the origin or starting point of the plan. To identify the origin, the transverse CT image containing the radiopaque markers is used. Alignment tools are used to find the point where lines through the markers would intersect. The origin point is placed at this intersection. Beam coordinates can now be referenced to this point to define the isocenter position. The center of the PTV is a recommended starting point for the placement of isocenter. Some treatment planning systems can automatically set the isocenter to the center of the PTV. If manual means are necessary for isocenter positioning, coronal, transverse, and sagittal views can be used to set the position of the isocenter to the center of the PTV.

Using both 2D and 3D viewing techniques, the angles of the gantry and couch are adjusted to include the PTV in the beam while excluding critical structures out of the path of the beam. The collimator size and rotation can be adjusted also to exclude structures from the beam. The shape of the treatment field can be fashioned using an MLC or conventional blocking. Autofielding, a technique used to set an open area around the PTV from the perspective of the BEV, can be used to shape the field following the contour of the PTV. The autofield should include a margin around the PTV that allows for beam penumbra and block edge effects. The margin should be sufficient to allow isodose lines of 90% or greater to cover the PTV. A blocking technique called *autoblocking* can be used to create a block or an MLC shield to decrease dose to critical structures. These structures can be covered with the block plus a margin of extra blocking if deemed necessary.

Several beams are commonly created to deliver dose to the PTV. Once the beams have been set up, the amount of dose to be delivered from each beam is determined. Beam weighting is used to set dose limits for each beam. A point inside of the area to be treated is chosen to receive 100% of the dose. This normalization point is usually the beams' isocenter. If the isocenter of any of the beams is close to a block or near the surface of the patient, another point of normalization can be chosen. Each beam is then assigned a percentage of the total dose to be delivered. When the plan is "normalized," numerical values of isodoses are equal to fractions of the dose existing at the point of normalization.

Treatment Plan Evaluation and Implementation. The plan is evaluated after the dose calculations are completed. Each treatment plan is assessed to determine whether it can be used to deliver the prescribed dose within target dose homogeneity and normal tissue protection constraints that have been established. Multiple plans can be compared using DVHs as bases for the comparison. Dose distributions can be displayed as isodose lines on 2D planes or as clouds of dose for 3D viewing (Figure 25-22). The 3D isodose clouds allow the planner to select an isodose value and then rotate the 3D image of the PTV to view the distribution of dose around it. This technique will show if any portion of the PTV extends outside of the isodose cloud and is not covered properly.

The complexity of the treatment plan is also reviewed. The number of fields used and the viability of the field arrangement are considered. Time of treatment delivery, setup reproducibility and complexity, and plan-verification feasibility are important plan-evaluation criteria, as well.

Once the plan is approved, documentation is produced and filed in the patient's treatment record to clearly communicate

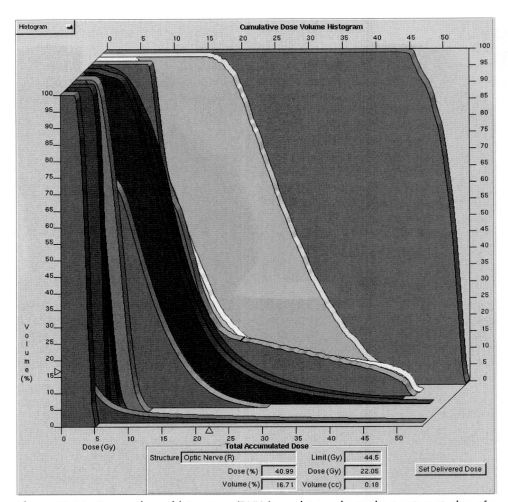

Figure 25-19. Dose-volume histograms (DVHs) used to evaluate the treatment plan of a patient. This figure shows a composite plot of the DVHs of the target volume and of critical structures within the irradiated volume. Dose is represented on the *x*-axis of the plots, and the *y*-axis represents the percentage of total volume enclosed by that dose level. To illustrate, note the *x,y* value of the target DVH on the upper-right corner of the figure. It appears that 100% of the target volume will be receiving a dose of 45 Gy or greater. Moving a little farther to the right on the target DVH shows that approximately 80% of the target volume will be receiving a dose of approximately 50 Gy or greater. (See Color Plate 18.)

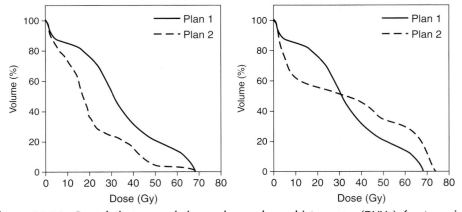

Figure 25-20. Cumulative normal tissue dose-volume histograms (DVHs) for two rival treatment plans. *Left*, plan 2 is superior to plan 1 over the complete dose range; *right*, the superior plan will depend on how the organ responds to radiation damage. (Redrawn from Purdy JA, Starkschall G, editors: *A practical guide to 3-D planning and conformal radiation therapy,* Madison, Wis, 1999, Advanced Medical Publishing.)

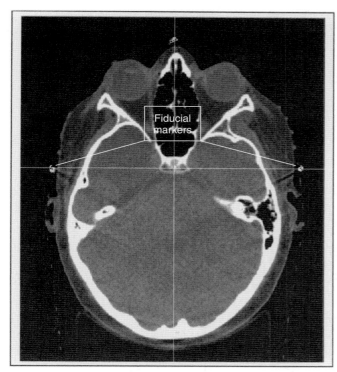

Figure 25-21. Establishment of treatment plan coordinate-system origin. External radiopaque markers, placed on the patient before computed tomography (CT), are routinely used to register the origin of the coordinate system of the treatment plan. This origin corresponds with the skin marks made on the patient. In this figure, markers placed on the immobilization mask of a patient are used to register the position of the plan origin. Any possible isocenter displacement from this point is noted as an "isocenter shift."

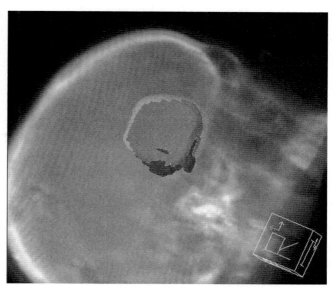

Figure 25-22. An isodose "cloud" enclosing a target volume. The prescription isodose level can be demonstrated in a three-dimensional (3D) visualization called an *isodose cloud*. If the cloud is shown semitransparent, the coverage of the target volume can be assessed. In this figure, a semitransparent isodose cloud produced by a three-field beam arrangement is superimposed on a hypothetical pituitary target volume. Shown are target areas not covered by the prescribed dose. (See Color Plate 19.)

plan parameters. Isodose distributions in transverse, coronal, and sagittal planes are printed. These should show the approved isodose distribution and the magnitude and location of hot spots. The use of heterogeneity corrections is documented. BEVs or, preferably, DRRs for each field are printed along with the corresponding MLC information if applicable. An orthogonal pair of DRRs can be printed to be used as a reference of the location of isocenter. Applicable DVHs should also be included in the documentation. Patient setup instructions should be clearly documented so that the position of the beams' isocenter and its relationship to patient markings are evident. If the patient is to be set up to original markings and the isocenter is to be shifted to a new position, shift instructions should be clearly specified and properly verified. It is highly recommended that a record and verify system be used, because 3D treatment plans are often complex and commonly have multiple beams with varying combinations of couch, gantry, and collimator positions.

The treatment plans of new patients should be verified as they are implemented clinically for the first time. Treatment initiation is an extremely important last step of the planning process. Before delivery of the treatment, each field should be checked to ensure that there are no collisions between the machine and the treatment table or the patient. Beam paths are examined to ensure

that the treatment couch does not adversely interfere with either beam delivery or port filming. Any delivery or filming limitations should be identified and approved. Each field's blocks or MLC patterns are examined. DRRs should be used for comparisons with port films. Patient SSDs are checked. The relationships between field blocking, collimator settings, and planned wedge orientations are also assessed. All documentation is reviewed to ensure consistent adherence to the plan. The treatment planning phase ends only when there is certainty that the plan can be consistently delivered accurately.

SUMMARY

The treatment planning process pulls together the entire radiation oncology team—both clinical and technical staffs. The sciences of radiation oncology, biology, therapy, dosimetry, and physics collaborate to optimize a patient's treatment. This chapter discussed the role of physics and dosimetry in the treatment planning process. The fundamental principles of photon-beam treatment planning and the basics of the treatment planning process were described. Specifically addressed were the following points:

- Isodose distributions describe, in graphic form, how radiation dose is deposited in an absorbing medium. In its simplest form, an isodose distribution describes the absorbed dose delivered to a rectangular phantom of water-equivalent material.
- Isodose distributions in a water phantom can be, and are, used to evaluate the characteristics of single beams of radiation. The effects of beam modifiers, such as wedges, can also be discerned.

- Combinations of multiple beams are also well characterized using isodose distributions.
- Corrections can be made to water-phantom–based isodose distributions to account for the effects of patients' contour irregularities and heterogeneous composition. These corrected dose distributions are then used to evaluate the appropriateness of a patient's treatment plan.
- Treatment planning has evolved from a simple two-dimensional review of dose distributions to a process of identifying three-dimensional target structures and organs at risk and then evaluating the three-dimensional dose to these volumes.
- This new treatment planning paradigm, called *three-dimensional conformal radiation therapy*, has been made possible by the increased efficiency of three-dimensional dose calculation algorithms and by the increased capabilities of modern computer planning systems.
- Planning volumes have been precisely defined by the International Commission on Radiation Units and Measurements.
- Improved visualization tools are now available to the treatment planner to assist in better target definition and coverage and in sparing of normal tissue.
- These visualization tools have been packaged into software products collectively known as *virtual simulation tools*.
- Virtual simulation is the process by which a patient's treatment plan can be developed using the patient's CT data set—the "virtual patient." Targets and organs at risk are defined and visualized, and three-dimensional dose is evaluated.
- Treatment plan appropriateness is commonly evaluated using a tool known as the *dose-volume histogram*. The dose-volume histogram correlates target or organ volume to the dose received by that volume.

Review Questions

Multiple Choice

1. Isodose distributions are _____-dimensional representations of the spatial distribution of dose.
   a. one
   b. two
   c. three
   d. four
2. Wedged-field isodose distributions are characterized by increased radiation intensity under the _____ of the wedge.
   a. heal (thicker portion)
   b. toe (thinner portion)
   c. both a and b
   d. neither a nor b
3. Use of parallel-opposed fields only is contraindicated as beam energy _____ and patient thickness _____.
   a. decreases, decreases
   b. increases, increases
   c. decreases, increases
   d. increases, decreases

4. _____ corrections account for the dose effects produced by the presence of materials of density different from water or unit density.
   a. Homogeneity
   b. Heterogeneity
   c. Isocentric
   d. none of the above
5. In treatment planning, when dose delivery parameters are computed based on target dose–delivery and normal tissue–avoidance criteria, the process is termed _____ planning.
   a. forward
   b. inverse
   c. reciprocal
   d. reverse
6. IMRT is a treatment planning and delivery process that seeks to achieve treatment plan optimization by varying the _____ of treatment beams in addition to their position.
   a. field size
   b. intensity
   c. area
   d. energy
7. The CTV is a treatment planning volume that includes gross visible and/or palpable disease and _____ disease.
   a. microscopic
   b. subclinical
   c. both a and b
   d. neither a nor b
8. Image _____ is a process by which images produced by different modalities can be combined to use the best features of each modality.
   a. production
   b. fusion
   c. manipulation
   d. none of the above
9. The quality of DRRs can be improved by _____ the thickness of CT slices.
   a. increasing
   b. decreasing
   c. rotating
   d. multiplying
10. A plan-evaluation tool that simultaneously presents dose and volume information in a graphic form allowing objective plan assessment is the dose-volume histogram.
    a. true
    b. false

The answers to the Review Questions can be found by logging on to our website at: *http://evolve.com/Washington+Leaver/ principles*

Questions to Ponder

1. The use of heterogeneity corrections in dose calculations is becoming more commonplace because these calculations are more accurate. Most of our clinical outcome data, on the

other hand, are based on homogeneous dose calculations. What are the challenges associated with clinical heterogeneity-correction implementation, if existing clinical outcomes data are to be preserved?

2. It is clear that use of the newer technology that has become available in the field of radiation oncology produces superior radiation dose distributions. It is also becoming apparent, however, that this technology comes at an increased cost in terms of resources needed per patient. How are these two apparently conflicting patient-treatment perspectives to be reconciled?

3. It is often necessary, in treatment planning, to make compromises between tumor control and normal tissue complication probabilities. What are the factors that need to be considered when making these determinations?

4. Multimodality image fusion is becoming the "standard of care" for the definition of target volumes in specific disease sites. In what disease sites is multimodality fusion becoming the norm? What imaging modalities are commonly used, and why? Does the use of multimodality fusion affect traditional GTV to CTV expansions (margins)? Why?

5. Discuss the necessary features of an appropriate quality assurance review of a patient's treatment plan before initiation of treatment. Address in the discussion the specifics of ensuring that the prescription is fulfilled: dose to targets and normal structures, appropriate transfer of information to the treatment unit, verification of position of anatomy, and so forth.

REFERENCES

1. Anderson DW: *Absorption of ionizing radiation,* Baltimore, 1984, University Park Press.
2. Antolak JA, et al: Prostate target volume variations during a course of radiotherapy, *Int J Radiat Oncol Biol Phys* 42:661-672, 1998.
3. Bentel GC: *Radiation therapy planning,* ed 2, New York, 1996, McGraw-Hill.
4. Coia LR, Schultheiss TE, Hanks GE: *A practical guide to CT simulation,* Madison, Wis, 1995, Advanced Medical Publishing.
5. Hendee WR: *Medical radiation physics,* St. Louis, 1970, Mosby.
6. International Commission on Radiation Units and Measurements (ICRU) Report 24: *Determination of absorbed dose in a patient irradiated by beams of x or gamma rays in radiotherapy procedures,* Bethesda, Md, 1976, International Commission on Radiation Units and Measurements.
7. International Commission on Radiation Units and Measurements (ICRU) Report 50: *Prescribing, recording, and reporting photon beam therapy,* Bethesda, Md, 1993, International Commission on Radiation Units and Measurements.
8. International Electrotechnical Commission (IEC) Performance Standard 976: *Medical electron accelerators—functional performance characteristics,* Geneva, 1989, International Electrotechnical Commission.
9. Khan FM: *The physics of radiation therapy,* ed 2, Baltimore, 1994, Williams & Wilkins.
10. Lawrence TS, et al: Clinical interpretation of dose-volume histograms: the basis for normal tissue preservation and tumor dose escalation. In Meyer JL, Purdy JA, editors: *3-D conformal radiotherapy,* Basel, Switzerland, 1996, Karger.
11. Mackie TR, Liu HH, McCulough EC: Model-based photon dose calculation algorithms. In Khan FM, Potish RA, editors: *Treatment planning in radiation oncology,* Baltimore, 1998, Williams & Wilkins.
12. Mohan R, et al: Three-dimensional conformal radiotherapy. In Khan FM, Potish RA, editors: *Treatment planning in radiation oncology,* Baltimore, 1998, Williams & Wilkins.
13. Perez CA, Brady LW: *Principles and practice of radiation oncology,* Philadelphia, 1998, Lippincott-Raven Publishers.
14. Starkschall G, Hogstrom KR: Dose-calculation algorithms used in 3-D radiation therapy treatment planning. In Purdy JA, Starkschall G, editors: *A practical guide to 3-D planning and conformal radiation therapy,* Madison, Wis, 1999, Advanced Medical Publishing.
15. Ten Haken RK, Kessler ML: 3-D RTP plan evaluation. In Purdy JA, Starkschall G, editors: *A practical guide to 3D planning and conformal radiation therapy,* Madison, Wis, 1999, Advanced Medical Publishing.
16. Varian Medical Systems: *C-Series Clinac: enhanced dynamic wedge implementation guide,* Palo Alto, Calif, 1996, Varian Medical Systems.
17. Verhey L, Bentel G: Patient immobilization. In Van Dyk J, editor: *The modern technology of radiation oncology,* Madison, Wis, 1999, Medical Physics Publishing.
18. Wong JW, Purdy JA: On methods of inhomogeneity corrections for photon transport, *Med Phys* 17:807-814, 1990.

Electron Beams in Radiation Therapy

Adam F. Kempa

Outline

Key Terms

Objectives

- List the characteristics of an electron versus a photon that lead to an increased probability of electrons' interaction with matter.
- Identify the predominant mechanism of interaction and loss of energy of electron beams with low-atomic-number materials in the range of electron beam energies used in clinical radiation therapy.
- Identify the two variables that affect the energy spectrum of an electron beam in the patient.
- List two methods of producing clinically useful electron beams for use in clinical radiation therapy.
- Describe the characteristics of a clinically useful electron beam in terms of treatment of superficial lesions and dose to deep underlying tissues.
- Given the depth of the 50% isodose line in centimeters, determine the mean energy of an electron beam.
- Given the mean energy of an electron beam, determine the treatment depth (depth of the 80% isodose line) in centimeters.
- Given the mean energy of an electron beam, determine the practical range in tissue in centimeters.
- State the relationship between increasing energy of electron beams and the percent depth dose.

- State the relationship between increasing energy of electron beams and the surface dose.
- Describe the dependence of the width of the 80% isodose curve on the energy of an electron beam.
- Illustrate how the width of the of 80% isodose curve in a 16-MeV electron beam may effect the selection of field size.
- Indicate the distance limitation beyond standard source-skin distance for electron beam treatments recommended by the American Association of Physicists in Medicine (AAPM) Task Group 25 for the use of distance correction factors.
- When considering the effects of irregular-shaped electron treatment fields on dose, identify one general rule that may indicate when closer investigation of the dose delivered by an irregular field is needed.
- Describe the result at depth of abutting the edges of two electron fields at the surface.
- Describe the result of placing a gap at the surface between the edges of two electron fields.
- Discuss one method used to decrease the amount that the dose will vary to a particular anatomic location when two adjacent electron beams are used for a treatment course.

The goal of this chapter is to provide an accurate overview of electron beam therapy at the student level. To accomplish this goal, concepts dealing with the physics of electrons and electron beams are dealt with in a general manner. Often, important issues become obscured by intricacy and detail. A more detailed treatment of electron beam therapy may be found in the references listed at the end of the chapter.

The art of radiation therapy treatment planning may be described as making use of the unique physical properties of various sources of radiation to optimize and individualize a patient's treatment. Electron beams are a good example of this concept. Selection of the energy of an electron beam allows the choice of depth of treatment and the dose to tissues deep to the treatment volume. Basic rules of thumb may be used to understand how the energy of an electron beam is defined and to provide a basis for the selection of an electron beam energy for treatment.

REVIEW OF THE PHYSICS OF ELECTRON BEAMS

Interactions of Electron Beams with Matter

Before a meaningful discussion of electron beam dosimetry can take place, the physical differences between electron beams and photon beams must be considered. A photon has no charge or mass. An electron has a negative charge and a mass approximately 2000 times smaller than that of a proton.

Electron beams' interactions with matter differ from those of photon beams largely because of these two characteristics. Because the electron has mass, the probability of an interaction between the electron and an atom is greater than that of a photon, which has no mass. Similarly, the probability of a negatively charged electron interacting with an atom's Coulomb forces is greater than that of a photon with no charge.

Collisional and Radiation Interactions

Electron beams interact with matter by a combination of collisional processes and radiation processes.[5] The energy loss of these two processes is expressed in terms of mass stopping powers. The **mass stopping power** *(S/p)* is the rate of energy loss per unit length *(S)*, divided by the density of the medium *(p)*.[5] The total mass stopping power is the sum of all energy losses. This includes both losses caused by collisions of electrons with atomic electrons *(S/p)$_{col}$* and radiation losses or **bremsstrahlung** production *(S/p)$_{rad}$*. Bremsstrahlung (German for "braking radiation") is caused by electron decelerations when passing through the field of atomic nuclei. The expression for the total mass stopping power *(S/p)$_{tot}$* is as follows[5]:

$$(S/p)_{tot} = (S/p)_{col} + (S/p)_{rad}$$

The contribution of each of these processes is affected by the energy of the electron beam and the atomic (Z) number of the irradiated material.[7]

A refinement of the total mass stopping power is the **restricted mass collisional stopping power**. The restricted mass collisional stopping power better describes the absorbed dose by accounting for energy transferred by delta rays. Delta rays are electrons scattered with enough energy to cause further ionization and excitations in other atoms.[2] All of the energy loss resulting from the interactions of the delta rays may not be deposited locally. Energy transfer by collisions of delta rays is restricted by specification of an energy below which energy losses are counted as part of the restricted collisional mass stopping power.[15] Energy losses considered as part of the restricted collisional mass stopping power relate to local absorption of dose.[15] Above this specified energy, the energy losses are not counted as part of the restricted collisional mass stopping power.[15] By this mechanism, a more accurate representation of absorbed dose is obtained. In the American Association of Physicists in Medicine (AAPM) Task Group 21, the stopping power ratios were determined for monoenergetic electron beams. A further refinement of restricted mass collisional stopping powers has been incorporated in the AAPM Task Group 51 protocol.[1] The Task Group 51 protocol uses stopping power ratios for "realistic electron beams." These values reflect a spectrum of electron beam energies leading to a more precise representation of dose.

In collisional losses, the predominant interaction may be described as an incident electron interacting with the electron of an atom. Low Z number materials have a greater **electron density** (number of electrons per unit mass) than do high Z number materials.[15] As one would expect, collisional interactions are the predominant process by which electrons lose energy in low Z number materials. Radiation or bremsstrahlung losses occur when an incident electron interacts with the Coulomb forces of the nucleus of an atom.[15] The probability of the occurrence of energy loss resulting from the radiation process increases with increasing energy or increasing Z number of the absorbing material.[7]

Energy Dependence of Electron Interactions

"For water, energy loss by collision is approximately 2 MeV/cm in the energy range of 1 to 100 MeV."[15] Radiation losses vary from 0.01 to 0.4 MeV/cm in the 1- to 20-MeV energy range.[15] A crude comparison of these values demonstrates that collisional interactions occur several times more often than radiation interactions in low Z number materials. In clinical radiation therapy in the energy range from 1 to 20 MeV, the predominant mechanism by which an electron beam loses energy is by collisional interactions in tissues because of the low Z number of tissue.[7]

Electron Beam Energy Spectrum Dependence on Depth

An electron beam emerges from the accelerator guide of the linear accelerator at a point called the *accelerator window*. Before the electron beam moves through the accelerator window, the energy spectrum is very narrow.[5] The electron beam then moves through various components of the linear accelerator, the accelerator window, scattering foils, ionization monitor chambers, and the air between the patient and treatment machine to the patient surface. The spectrum of the beam at the patient surface is decreased and broadened in energy because of interactions with the accelerator components.[5] As the electron beam passes into the patient, it undergoes a decrease in energy and broadening of the energy spectrum.[7] The energy spectrum of the electron beam in the patient depends on the depth in the patient and the energy spectrum at the surface of the patient.[5]

Production of Clinically Useful Electron Beams

Electron beams are most commonly produced by linear accelerators in current practice. There are several modifications of the linear accelerator required for electron beam production. The first is to remove the "target" and flattening filter used to produce x-rays from the path of the electron beam. The second is to decrease the "electron gun" current to lower the dose rate of the electron beam to clinically acceptable ranges. The reason for the reduction in the current becomes apparent when one considers the amount of current used in x-ray mode compared with that used in electron mode. "In normal electron therapy mode operation, the beam current through the electron window is on the order of 1/1000 of the beam current at the x-ray target for x-ray therapy mode."[6] Without a reduction of the current at the electron gun window, unwieldy dose rates in the thousands of centigrays per second could result.[6] A narrow electron beam commonly referred to as a *pencil beam* is produced by the linear accelerator. This pencil beam of electrons may be widened for clinical use by two methods: the use of a scattering foil or the use of a scanning electron beam.

Scattering Foils

The most common method of producing a beam wide enough for clinical use is to use a scattering foil.[6] A scattering foil is a thin sheet of a material that has a high Z number placed in the path of the pencil beam of electrons. A second scattering foil may be added to create a "dual scattering foil" arrangement. The first scattering foil is used to widen the beam; the second is used to improve the flatness of the beam.[6] Often, the x-ray field flattening filter and scattering foil are mounted on a carousel arrangement (Figure 26-1). This allows for a simple switch from photon to electron mode of operation.

Scanning Beams

Scanning electron beams are the second way that a beam wide enough for clinical purposes may be produced. The narrow pencil beam of electrons is scanned by magnetic fields across the treatment area. This constantly moving pencil beam distributes the dose evenly throughout the field. **Scanning beams** are especially useful above 25 MeV, when the thickness of the required scattering foils would result in difficulties with their mechanical size and would cause problems with electron contamination.[6]

Advantages and Disadvantages of Scattering Foils versus Scanning Beams

A drawback of the use of scattering foils is the production of bremsstrahlung contamination by the electron beam's interaction with the **scattering foil**. An advantage of the use of scattering foils is that they are relatively simple and reliable when compared with the scanning beam method. An advantage of the scanning beam method is that there is none of the bremsstrahlung contamination caused by the interaction of the electron beam and the scattering foil. However, x-ray contamination from the collimators, ionization chambers, and intervening air

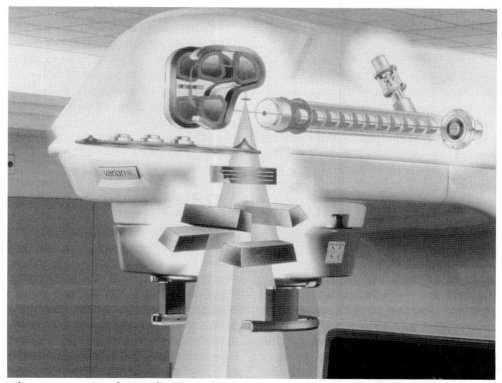

Figure 26-1. Up to four or five scattering foils mounted in a "carousel" arrangement within the head of a modern linear accelerator. (Courtesy Varian Medical Systems, Palo Alto, Calif.)

is still present.[6] A disadvantage of the scanning beam method is the maintenance of complex electronic systems. Failures of the scanning beam mechanism could allow the entire dose to be delivered in one small area of the patient with disastrous results.[15]

CHARACTERISTICS OF THERAPEUTIC ELECTRON BEAMS

Dosage Gradients of Clinically Useful Electron Beams

Electron beam therapy offers the ability to treat superficially located lesions with almost no dose to the deep underlying tissues. This is illustrated by Figure 26-2, A. The darkened high-dose area is followed by a narrow lighter low-dose area and a white area indicating negligible dose. The implication for treatment planning is that organs and structures deep to the darkened area will receive minimal dose. This results from rapid falloff of percent depth dose with increasing depth and is characteristic of electron beams less than 15 MeV.[13]

Figure 26-2, B, numerically demonstrates this rapid falloff of dose with depth. The rate of change of a value (dose) with a change in position is termed a **gradient**. Although the relative distances between the surface to 80% and from 80% to 10% isodose curves are approximately equal, the rates of change of isodose values are not. In the first half of the distance, there is a 20% change compared with a 70% change in isodose values in the second half of the distance. This advantageous dosage gradient may be manipulated by varying the energy of the electron beam.

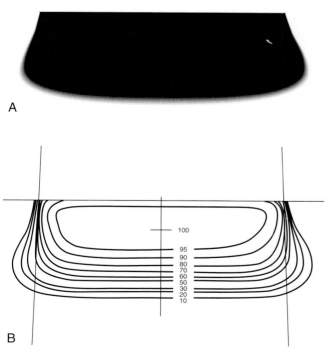

A

B

Figure 26-2. A, Film of a 12-MeV 14 × 8 cm electron beam used for obtaining isodose curves. **B,** Isodensity curves from the 12-MeV electron beam. (From Khan F: *The physics of radiation therapy,* Baltimore, 1984, Lippincott Williams & Wilkins.)

Table 26-1	Comparison of Percent Depth Dose Data for Varying Electron Beam Energies		
Nominal Beam Energy (MeV)	**Percent Depth Dose/Depth (cm)**		
10.6	100%/1.9	80%/3.5	10%/5.2
15	100%/2.9	80%/4.9	10%/7.1
30	100%/3.7	80%/8.7	10%/14.6

This may be demonstrated by a comparison of percent depth dose data in the following example (Table 26-1). The 80% isodose value is commonly used to describe the treatment depth of an electron beam. As the nominal energy of the electron beam is increased, the depth of the 80% isodose value increases from 3.5 cm at 10.6 MeV, to 4.9 cm at 15 MeV. At the nominal energy of 30 MeV, the rapid falloff of dose with increasing depth is greatly diminished. The 80% isodose value is at a depth of 9 cm, and, at approximately 15 cm, 10% of the dose remains. "The clinically advantageous shape cut-off to the percentage depth dose achieved with low-energy electron beams of 10 to 15 MeV is lost at very high energies, and consequently there is no real clinical advantage in using electron beams of energies higher than about 20 MeV."[13] Restated simply, high-energy electron beams begin to approximate the depth dose characteristics of low-energy photon beams with the disadvantage of having no "true" skin-sparing effect.

Shape of the Plot of Percentage Depth Dose versus Depth

The characteristic shape of the plot of dose versus depth for an electron beam is demonstrated in Figure 26-3. The dose at the surface begins at approximately 85% of maximum and builds up to 100% in the first few centimeters below the surface. Beyond the 80% to 90% depth dose in Figure 26-3, the falloff dose with increasing depth is rapid. The curve does not reach 0 but "flattens out" at a value of a few percent. The dose in this end region is composed of bremsstrahlung-produced x-ray contamination from the interaction of the electron beam with scattering foils, ionization chambers, collimators, and air between the patient and the treatment unit.[5] Although this dose is clinically insignificant in most cases, caution is warranted when large areas are treated, as in total-body electron treatments for mycosis fungoides (cutaneous T-cell lymphoma).[7] An interesting use of this x-ray contamination has been to obtain port film radiographs of electron beam treatments.[3]

Shape of Electron Beam Isodose Curves

Electron beam isodose curves have a characteristic shape, which is described as a lateral bulge or ballooning of the isodose curves. "As the beam penetrates a medium, the beam expands rapidly below the surface due to scattering."[15] This is evident in Figure 26-2, B, where the 10%, 20%, 30%, and 50% isodose curves balloon or bulge beyond the edge of the field. The lateral scattering or ballooning of the electron beam decreases with increasing electron beam energy.[7]

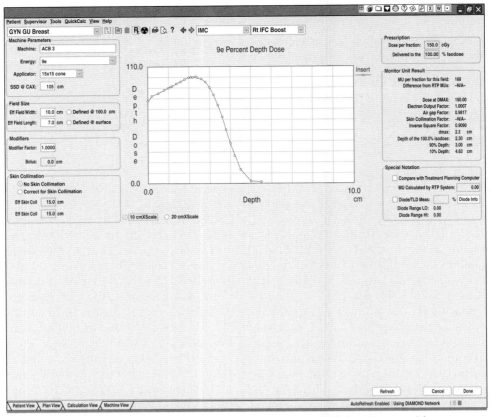

Figure 26-3. Central axis depth dose distribution measured in water. Incident energy, 13 MeV; 8 × 10 cm cone; effective source-skin distance (SSD) is 68 cm.

TREATMENT PLANNING OF ELECTRON BEAM THERAPY

Electron Beam Rules of Thumb

Treatment planning using electron beams may be explained using several relationships or rules of thumb that provide estimates of several aspects of electron beams. The resulting information gained by application of the rules of thumb clarifies the use of a particular electron beam for a specific treatment application.

Mean energy of the electron beam in MeV at surface [(depth in centimeters of 50% isodose line) × (2.4)]: The first of these relationships is used to determine the energy of an electron beam. As an electron beam passes through matter, it decreases both in intensity and in energy with increasing depth. For this reason, the measurement of an electron beam's energy depends on the depth of the electron beam in the phantom or patient. Although there are several methods of determining the energy of an electron beam, one method is widely used because of its practicality in the clinical setting. Simply stated, the depth of the 50% dose in centimeters (R_{50}) is multiplied by a constant (C_4). The resulting product is the mean energy of the electron (E_o) beam stated in MeV at the phantom surface[10] as follows:

$$E_o = C_4 R_{50}$$

The value of the constant C_4 has varied slightly from 2.33 MeV in the American Association of Physicists in Medicine (AAPM) Task Group 21 to 2.4 MeV in Task Group 25.[10] There is little difference between the final value determined by the use of either number for the constant C4. For this reason, it is recommended that physicists select one of the two values along with other parameters and use it consistently in the calibration protocol.[10]

The second of these relationships deals with the reduction of the energy of an electron beam as it moves through matter. The energy of an electron beam at a given depth in water may be approximated based on the following relationship. The rate at which an electron beam loses energy is approximately 2 MeV/cm in water.[2] For example, an electron beam with an energy of 10 MeV incident on the phantom surface will have an energy of 6 MeV at a depth of 2 cm in water.

The practical range in centimeters in tissue (mean energy at surface/2): The third relationship deals with the practical range (E_r) in centimeters of an electron beam in tissue. The practical range of an electron beam is determined by dividing the energy of the electron beam in MeV by 2 as follows:

$$E_r = MeV/2$$

Past the practical range within the patient, dosage drops off quickly with depth to a value of several percent. The dosage does not reach zero because of the bremsstrahlung radiation produced by the interaction of the beam with collimators, the intervening air, and the patient.

The practical range is a helpful guide in treatment planning. This simple relationship demonstrates clearly that a lesion at a depth of 4 cm is beyond the range of a 7-MeV electron beam. In a similar manner, this relationship can be used in the selection of the energy of an electron beam so that critical structures receive a minimal dose.

The depth of the 80% isodose line in centimeters in tissue (mean energy at surface/3): The fourth relationship is directly related to the choice of an electron beam energy for a specific treatment depth. The depth of the 80% isodose value is often specified as treatment depth. Treatment depth may be determined by dividing the energy of the electron beam in MeV by 3 as follows:

$$80\% \text{ Isodose} = \text{MeV}/3$$

In a similar manner, the depth of the 90% isodose curve may be found by dividing the energy of the electron beam in MeV by 4 as follows:

$$90\% \text{ Isodose} = \text{MeV}/4$$

Use of these simple relationships gives insight into a particular treatment. For example, a patient treated with a 10-MeV electron beam will have the following: an 80% isodose at a depth of 3.3 cm, a 90% isodose line at a depth of 2.5 cm, and a range within the patient of approximately 5 cm. Structures deeper than 5 cm receive a minimal dose.

The relationships for the depth of the 80% and 90% isodose lines and the dose to deep structures are for homogeneous treatment volumes of tissue-equivalent material. If the treatment area overlies an air cavity such as a lung, the choice of the isodose line for treatment must take into account the increased transmission through the lung tissue. Selection of the isodose line for treatment may vary from the 70% to the 80% isodose line in an attempt to minimize the dose to the lung.[9]

Electron Beam Characteristics at the Surface

Difficulties in measuring the dose at the phantom's surface have caused the AAPM Task Group 25 to specify the surface dose as the dose at 0.5 cm on the central axis of the electron beam.[10] Surface dose values for electron beams in the 6- to 20-MeV range vary from 80% to 100%. In megavoltage photon beams, increased energy of the treatment beam results in a decrease in surface dose. With electron beams, the reverse is true. As the energy of the electron beam increases, the surface dose and percent depth dose also increase.[8]

 Megavoltage electron beams in the 6- to 20-MeV energy range have varying degrees of dose reduction at the skin surface. Variables that affect the surface dose include the scattering system, atomic number of the absorber, beam energy, field size, and beam collimation. Of these variables, only the last three may be manipulated for treatment planning purposes.

There is little effect of field size on both surface dose and percent depth dose of electron beams, provided the fields are of sufficient size.[5] The rule is that the electron beam's diameter (field size) in centimeters should not be less than the practical range. This rule is extended to include field sizes that are less than the practical range in either dimension.[15] For example,

a 10-MeV electron beam's percent depth dose characteristics will not vary significantly as long as the diameter (field size) is 5 cm or greater ($R_p = 10$ MeV/2 = 5). "The field size dependence of the depth dose curves increases as the energy of the electron beam increases."[16] The surface dose depends on the field size in a similar manner. In general, "the smaller the diameter the larger the surface dose."[16] Increased dose produced by increasing field size continues until the diameter of the electron beam equals the practical range of the electron beam. Additional increases in field size where the diameter of the field is greater than the practical range of the electrons will not result in a significant change in dose.[17]

 The actual absorbed dose at the surface of a water-equivalent medium usually is approximately 0.85 of the maximum in the absence of contamination of the beam.[5]

Electron Beam Characteristics in the Build-up Region

The region from the surface to the depth of maximum dose is at risk for being underdosed in many clinical situations. This is most true for lower-energy electron beams (less than 12 MeV). A bolus may be used to increase the dose to the surface, much as in megavoltage beams. However, the use of bolus materials in electron beam therapy is somewhat more complicated than in photon beam therapy. It is possible to decrease the dose in an electron beam setup by use of a bolus. For this reason, "a partial bolus should never be used with electrons."[14] The dose under a small (1 × 1 cm) bolus placed in the middle of a small treatment field may decrease the surface dose by 10% to 15%.[14] Another problem, sometimes called an *edge effect,* results from the use of a large bolus with an edge perpendicular to the surface, across a portion of a treatment field. Areas of increased dose and decreased dose of 20% to 30% may be produced.[4] Near the border between bolused and unbolused portions of the field, areas under the bolus have decreased dose and the unbolused areas have increased dose. In an attempt to reduce the areas of increased and decreased dose, the edge of the partial bolus may be beveled so that it forms a 45-degree angle with the surface. Although this eliminates the area of decreased dose near the surface, the area of increased dose remains.[14]

The use of bolus materials in electron beam therapy is not limited to increasing the dose to the surface. Hogstrom[4] identifies two other uses for bolus material in electron beam therapy: as a tissue compensator for irregular surfaces or air cavities and to shape isodose distributions to better conform to the treatment volume or decrease the dose to critical structures at depth. "A simple rule of thumb for bolus—that utilization of bolus to make the patient anatomy present itself as a water phantom results in a more uniform dose distribution."[4]

Energy Dependence of the Width of the 80% Isodose Curve

With increasing electron beam energy, the ballooning of the isodose lines decreases. As always, this should be based on a careful evaluation of measured data specific to the treatment machine, beam energy, and treatment cone used. It should also be noted that there is a similar constriction of the 90% isodose line for electron beams in this energy range.

 "At approximately 15 MeV, the phenomenon of lateral constriction of the higher isodose values, such as at the 80% line, occurs."[15] To cover an area at depth with the 80% isodose line, a larger area must be treated on the skin surface. "A good standard is to leave a margin of at least 1 cm between the lateral edge of the target volume and the projected edge of the collimator."[4]

Distance Correction Factors for Electron Beam Treatments

Anatomic restrictions most often require the use of electron beams at an extended source-skin distance (SSD).[10] In the AAPM Task Group 25 report, extended SSD is defined as treatments that are not more than 15 cm beyond standard SSD. This constraint will apply to the following discussion of extended SSD treatments.[10] "The use of an extended treatment distance has only minimal effect on the central-axis depth dose and the off-axis ratios."[10] For this reason, it is suggested that the use of standard depth dose curves will give an approximation that is within a millimeter at extended distances.[10] However, factors such as the output of an electron beam and the beam penumbra change dramatically with a change in treatment distance.[10]

Clinical electron beams are created by scanning a narrow pencil-width beam across the treatment area or by use of a scattering foil. In either case, there is no simple point source of the electron beam from which changes in distance may be calculated. This may be resolved in two different ways: by determining an "effective point source" or by determining the position of the "virtual source." Two methods of correction of the output of electron beams relate to these methods.

Effective Point Source Method

The effective point source is defined "such that the dose varies in accordance with the inverse square law with distance from this source."[8] This method allows for use of an inverse square correction factor with the following factors[10]:

D'_{max} = Dose to D_{max} at extended distance
D_{max} = Dose to D_{max} at nominal or normal distance
SSD = Nominal or normal SSD
SSD' = Extended SSD
SSD_{eff} = Effective SSD
d_{max} = Depth of maximum dose on central axis
g = Difference between the extended SSD and the nominal SSD ($SSD' - SSD$)

The formula is as follows:

$$D'_{max} = \frac{D_{max}\left(SSD_{eff} + d_{max}\right)^2}{\left(SSD_{eff} + g + d_{max}\right)^2}$$

Conditions such as large air gaps, small treatment field sizes, or low-energy beams may require additional modification of this formula or a new calibration measurement specific for the individual set of treatment conditions.

Virtual Source Method

One method of finding the position of a virtual point source is by "back-projection" of the 50% width of the beam profiles from several distances.[8] The point at which these back-projections intersect is termed the *virtual source position*.[8] The parameters for the virtual SSD output correction factor are identical to those of the effective point source method, with the following exceptions:

SSD_{vir} is virtual SSD for calibration
f_{air} is air gap correction factor

$$D'_{max} = \left(D_{max}\right)\frac{\left(SSD_{vir} + d_{max}\right)^2}{\left(f_{air}\right)\left(SSD_{vir} + g + d_{max}\right)^2}$$

In the virtual SSD method, the variation in the inverse square law for small field sizes, low beam energy, and large air gaps is corrected by the factor f_{air}. The factor f_{air} depends on the energy, field size, and extent of the air gap.[8]

IRREGULAR FIELDS AND ELECTRON BEAMS

Shielding Dependence on Electron Beam Energy

Various methods have been used to shape electron beams for clinical purposes. These include lead strips, cutouts, or masks placed directly on the patient's skin or at the end of the treatment cone or collimator. Low-melting-point shields that insert into the end of the treatment cone (Figure 26-4) have also been used. The thickness of the shielding material required increases with increasing beam energy and field size. In the measurement of the transmission of shielding material, two approaches are used to address the effect of field size on the thickness of material needed. The first approach is to measure the transmission with large field sizes; this will provide a shield thickness that is appropriate to any smaller fields used.[10] A second method relates to the use of internal shields where the thickness of the shielding device is limited by the internal space available within

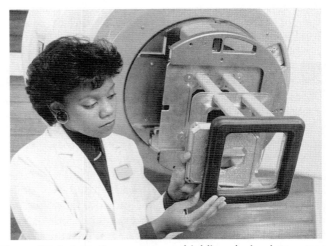

Figure 26-4. Inserting a custom shielding device into a treatment cone. (Courtesy Varian Medical Systems, Palo Alto, Calif.)

the patient. In the case of internal shielding devices, a calibration measurement under actual conditions specific to the individual patient's treatment is recommended.[10]

A rule of thumb may be used to approximate the thickness of shielding material needed in external beam treatments. "The thickness of lead in millimeters required for shielding is approximately given by the energy in MeV divided by two"[10] as follows:

$$MeV/2 = Shield\ thickness\ in\ millimeters\ of\ lead$$

Khan[9] suggests that an additional millimeter of lead be added to the amount indicated by the rule of thumb method to provide an "extra safety margin." Use of lead or alloys for shielding may result in an increase in dose if the thickness of the shielding material is not sufficient to reduce the dose to less than 5% of the total dose.[7] The thickness of Lipowitz alloy (Cerrobend) required may be obtained by multiplying the thickness in lead indicated by the rule of thumb by 1.2.[10]

Internal Shielding

In some cases, it is appropriate to place shielding devices within the oral cavity or under the eyelids. The objective is to shield the electron beam as it exits from the volume of tissue to be treated before it reaches normal tissue. A danger in the use of internal shielding devices is that the dose to the tissues directly in front of the shield may be increased by 30% to 70% because of the electron backscatter from the shield.[7] This problem may be minimized by placing a low Z number material between the shield and the tissue. Caution should be used in the selection of the thickness of low Z number material, which should be greater than the range of the backscattered electrons. Dental acrylic is commonly used to surround the lead shield, separating it from the oral cavity and reducing electron backscatter.[7] In the case of internal eye shields, there may not be sufficient space to allow adequate thickness of both lead and low atomic Z number material to absorb the electron backscatter produced by the lead shield.[7] Lead shields thick enough to reduce dosage to "acceptable levels" may be coated "with a thin film of wax or dental acrylic (to absorb very low energy electrons)."[7]

Effects of Irregularly Shaped Electron Fields on Dose

An in-depth discussion of the calculation of irregular electron fields is beyond the scope of this chapter. However, situations that result in changes of dose will be identified. "Field shaping affects the output factor as well as depth dose distribution in a complex manner."[7] Variables encountered in field shaping that affect dose include the field size, the thickness of shielding material, the amount of blocking, and the treatment distance.[7] The dose rate or output factor of a clinical electron beam has a greater dependence on field size than that of a clinical photon beam.[12] The dose at any point in the patient is composed of primary and scatter radiation. The greater dependence on field size of clinical electron beams than that of photon beams results from the amount of scatter radiation that contributes to the total dose. In photon beams, approximately 10% to 30% of the dose results from scatter radiation. In electron beams, almost all the absorbed dose results from electrons that have been scattered.[12]

Lateral equilibrium of these scattered electrons is an important feature in electron beam dosimetry. Lateral equilibrium is reached when the number of electrons entering an area equals the number of electrons leaving the area. This condition is met when the diameter of the field size exceeds that of the practical range of the electron beam.[12] When the diameter of the electron beam field is less than the practical range, there is a decrease in dose. The smaller the diameter of the electron beam, the greater is the change in the dose because of the lack of electronic equilibrium. For this reason, changes in dose associated with irregularly shaped electron fields may be anticipated if the dimensions of any portion of the treatment field are less than the practical range (MeV/2) of the electron beam.[17] Field shaping or blocking causes changes in the output of an electron beam. The size of the change in output depends on the percentage of the area of the total treatment field that is shielded or blocked. The higher the percentage of the field that is blocked, the greater is the change in output. If greater than 25% of the treatment area is blocked, measurement of the output factor for that specific treatment is recommended.[7] The effect of the electron beam energy on the output factor increases with increasing electron beam energy when blocking is used.[14] For example, at extended treatment distances (110 cm SSD), field blocking causes a large change in the output of an electron beam, which may also require measurement of the output. Olch et al.[14] state that "for SSD at 110 cm, almost any blockage severely changes the output factor."

The use of irregularly shaped electron beams should be approached with caution. Although it has been suggested that the output factor, depth dose, and isodose distribution should be measured for any irregularly shaped electron field, this is not practical.[7] A more reasonable approach is to investigate cases of irregularly shaped electron fields in which the field edges are not greater than the practical range.[4] Computerized treatment planning of irregularly shaped electron fields by pencil-beam algorithms may resolve the uncertainties in their use. It has been demonstrated that, by using treatment planning computers with computed tomography (CT) scans, both irregular fields at nonstandard air gaps and dosage behind inhomogeneities may be calculated that are in agreement with measured data.[4] However, Hogstrom[4] indicates that careful evaluation of treatment planning computer programs used to calculate irregularly shaped electron fields is necessary. It should be noted that the treatment planning computer represents only half of the tools required.[17] CT images of the treatment area with the patient in treatment position can be used to obtain calculation data that are not otherwise readily available.

Tissue Heterogeneities and Their Effects on Electron Beams

"The sensitivity of high-energy electron dose distribution to the presence of tissue heterogeneities makes it essential to consider these effects in treatment planning and selection of technique."[10] The change in the dose distribution "depends on the shape, size, electron density (number of electrons/cm[3]) and the effective atomic number of the heterogeneity."[11] The methods of calculating dose distributions are beyond the scope of this chapter; however, changes in the dose distributions as the result of tissue heterogeneity are described.

Small heterogeneities cause local disturbances in the dose distribution.[7] Difficulties in determining the dose distribution around small heterogeneities result from enhanced scattering effects.[11] The dose to tissues behind small bones is decreased, as might be expected, because of the shielding effect of the bone. The dose to tissues lateral to the bone is increased because of lateral scattering of the electron beam.[11] The effect of a small air cavity surrounded by tissues is somewhat different. As might be expected, the dose to tissues beyond the air cavity is increased as a result of decreased scattering of the electrons as they pass through the air cavity. Similarly, the dose to tissues lateral to the air cavity is not increased, as in the case of a bone surrounded by tissue. This results from the decreased scattering of the electrons when passing through the air cavity. The dose to tissues beyond the air cavity is also increased because of additional electron scattering from surrounding tissues.[11] Changes in dose range from a 20% underdose behind bone to a 15% to 35% overdose behind air cavities.[11]

The situation for large tissue heterogeneities of uniform density differs from that of small heterogeneities.[11] The major factor responsible for changes in the dose distribution of large tissue heterogeneities of uniform density is absorption.[11] The determination of actual dose distribution resulting from a large heterogeneity depends on the complex interrelationships of several factors. However, the effect of large heterogeneities may be discussed in a general sense.[5]

At the boundary where the electron beam leaves the bone and enters tissue, there is a small increase in dose because of increased scattering of the electrons interacting in the bone.[11] Tissues beyond the boundary of large high-density heterogeneities such as bone receive a lower dose.[5] This results in the dose distribution being moved toward the surface.[5,11] Tissues beyond low-density heterogeneities, such as lung, receive a greater dose because of the reduced absorption of the lung tissue. "This results in the dose distribution being moved toward greater depth. In the lung, the range of the electrons is increased by a factor of 3, with an associated increase in dose to the lung and the tissue beyond the lung."[11,15] An additional concern with large heterogeneities involves areas of increased and decreased dose, or "hot and cold spots," which may appear at the lateral edges of the heterogeneity.[5]

Gaps in Electron Beam Therapy

The use of combinations of two or more electron beams or electron beams and photon beams should be undertaken with great care. As previously stated, electron beam isodose curves have a characteristic shape (see Figure 26-2, B), which is described as a lateral bulge or ballooning of the isodose curves. Because of this characteristic shape, electron fields with adjacent treatment areas that abut each other on the surface will result in an overlap at depth.[7] Separating the treatment fields or placing a "gap" on the patient's or phantom's surface results in an underdose or cold spot on the surface.[14] This is demonstrated in Figure 26-5, which shows isodose distributions for adjacent electron fields. Note that the lowest dose to surface and superficial tissues results from the largest gap (1.5 cm). Similarly, the highest dose at depth results from the smallest gap on the surface (0.5 cm). "In a clinical situation, the

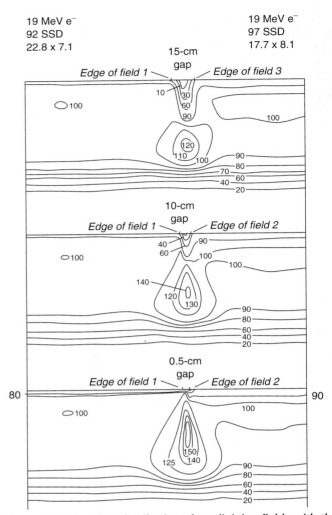

Figure 26-5. Isodose distributions for adjoining fields with the same electron beam energy with different gap widths between fields. (From Tapley N, Almond PR, editors: *Clinical applications of the electron beam,* New York, 1976, Wiley.)

decision as to whether the fields should be abutted or separated should be based upon the uniformity of the combined dose distribution across the target volume."[9] To decrease the amount that the dose will vary to a particular anatomic location, the abutment line may be moved two or three times during the patient's treatment course.[4] Treatments delivered in this fashion ensure that no one anatomic area will receive all of the increased or decreased dose.

CLINICAL APPLICATIONS OF ELECTRON BEAMS IN RADIATION THERAPY

In the next section, three cases are presented representing the clinical application of electron beams in radiation therapy. Various principles of treatment planning covered in the preceding portion of this chapter are demonstrated. The clinical cases are followed by a summary of the cases, which is meant to underscore the treatment planning principles outlined in each case.

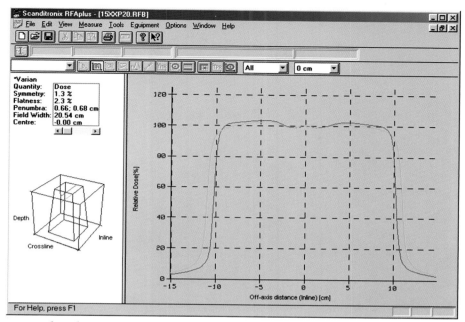

Color Plate 9. Beam profiles are normally measured with a computerized beam-data acquisition system that includes a water tank, radiation detector, and specialized software designed for radiation beam measurement and analysis. Note the beam-data acquisition geometry shown on the bottom-left portion of the screen showing the direction of ionization-chamber travel within the water tank. Two "in-plane" scans were acquired and the resulting profiles are displayed. (See Figure 25-2.)

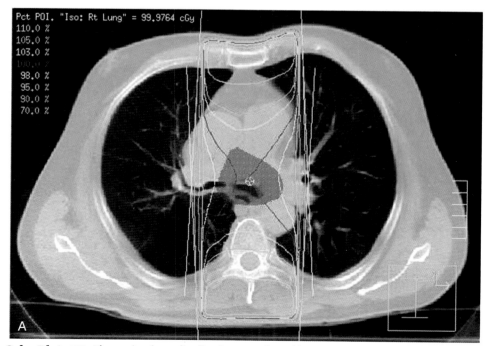

Color Plate 10. Thorax isodose distributions produced by a parallel-opposed field arrangement **(A)**, a three-field arrangement

Continued

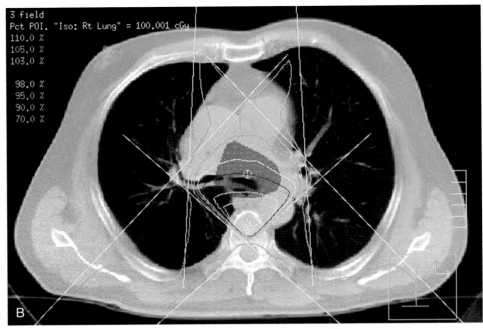

3 field
Pct POI. "Iso: Rt Lung" = 100.001 cGy
110.0 %
105.0 %
103.0 %

98.0 %
95.0 %
90.0 %
70.0 %

B

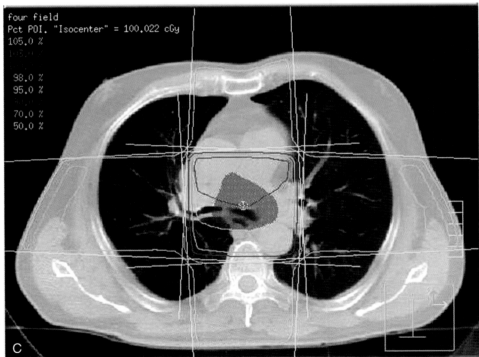

four field
Pct POI. "Isocenter" = 100.022 cGy
105.0 %

98.0 %
95.0 %

70.0 %
50.0 %

C

Color Plate 10. Cont'd (B), and a four-field arrangement **(C)**. The shaded area in the center of the computed tomography (CT) image represents the target volume. The numeric values of the isodoses represent percentages of the dose at the isocenter of the fields. (See Figure 25-8.)

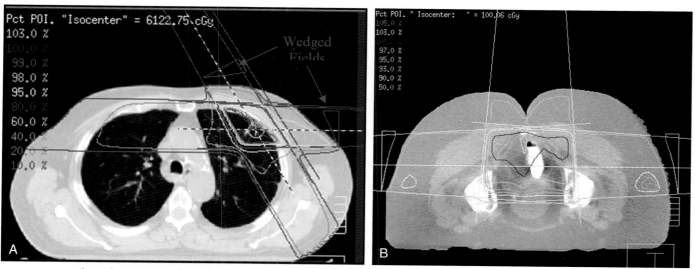

Color Plate 11. Isodose distributions produced by combinations of fields with wedges. **A**, An angled wedge pair. **B**, A combination of a posterior open field with two lateral wedged fields. (See Figure 25-9.)

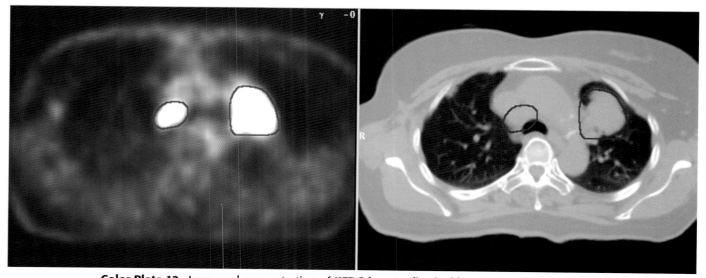

Color Plate 12. Increased concentration of ^{18}FDG in a mediastinal lymph node. (See pg. 541.)

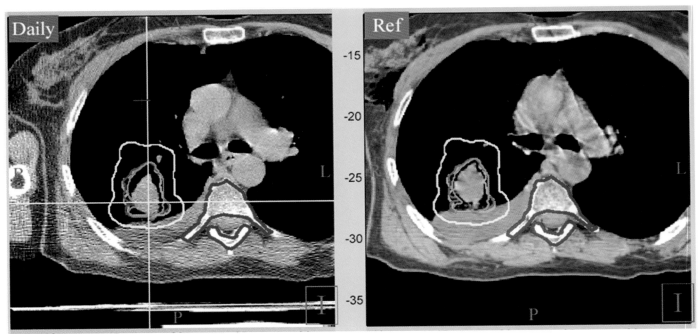

Color Plate 13. GTV as seen an an image of a daily CT taken with **(A)** an in-room scanner *(Daily)*, and compared with **(B)** the GTV defined on the treatment-planning CT *(Ref)*. (See pg. 541.)

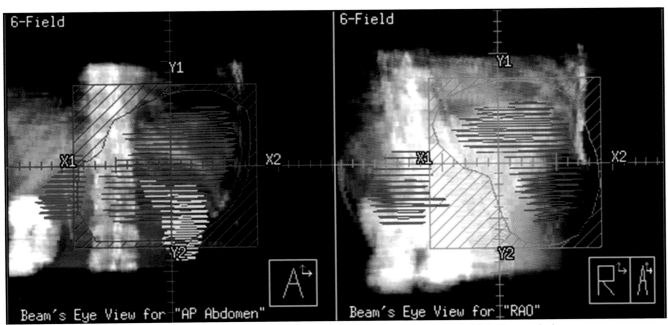

Color Plate 14. Use of the beam's eye view (BEV) tool for treatment-field design and placement. Note the differences between the anteroposterior (AP) and right anterior oblique (RAO) fields. The shape and spatial relationships of the tumor and the kidney volumes change as function of gantry angle, allowing more favorable tumor volume targeting. (See Figure 25-14.)

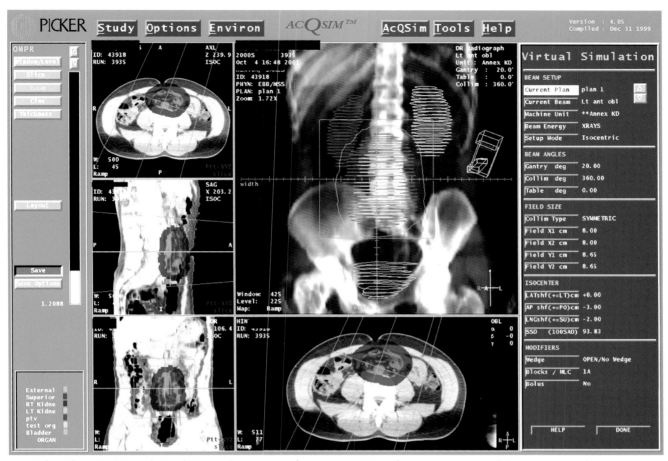

Color Plate 15. Virtual simulation software sample screen. A "virtual" patient is created from computed tomography (CT) data. The software supports normal tissue and target volume definition and identification; treatment fields can then be designed and placed. (See Figure 25-15.)

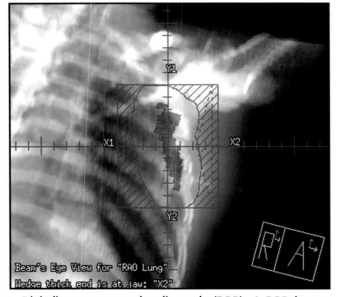

Color Plate 16. Digitally reconstructed radiograph (DRR). A DRR is a two-dimensional radiograph-like image that is reconstructed from a computed tomography (CT) data set. The image of this figure was reconstructed from a thoracic data set to produce a view equivalent to that obtained if a radiographic image were obtained from the patient's right anterior side. Superimposed on the image is the projection of the contoured clinical target volume and of the treatment field designed to cover the volume with a 2-cm margin. (See Figure 25-17.)

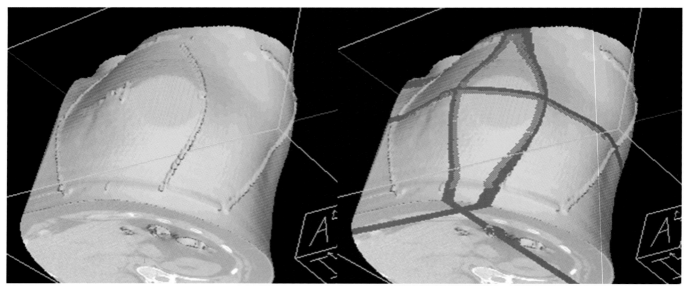

Color Plate 17. Use of image-visualization tools to aid in treatment-field placement during virtual simulation and treatment planning. The computed tomography (CT) data set can be visualized using an image-rendering technique that emphasizes the patient's skin and any markers placed on the skin. In this figure, beams have been placed such that the lasers that indicate their isocenter coincide with catheters placed on the patient before CT. (See Figure 25-18.)

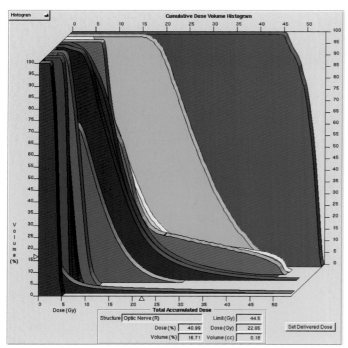

Color Plate 18. Dose-volume histograms (DVHs) used to evaluate the treatment plan of a patient. This figure shows a composite plot of the DVHs of the target volume and of critical structures within the irradiated volume. Dose is represented on the x-axis of the plots, and the y-axis represents percent of total volume enclosed by that dose level. To illustrate, note the x,y value of the target DVH on the upper-right corner of the figure. It appears that 100% of the target volume will be receiving a dose of 45 Gy or greater. Moving a little farther to the right on the target DVH shows that approximately 80% of the target volume will be receiving a dose of about 50 Gy or greater. (See Figure 25-19.)

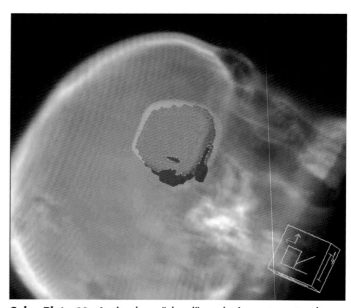

Color Plate 19. An isodose "cloud" enclosing a target volume. The prescription isodose level can be demonstrated in a three-dimensional (3D) visualization called an *isodose cloud*. If the cloud is shown semitransparent, the coverage of the target volume can be assessed. In this figure, a semitransparent isodose cloud produced by a three-field beam arrangement is superimposed on a hypothetical pituitary target volume. Shown are target areas not covered by the prescribed dose. (See Figure 25-22.)

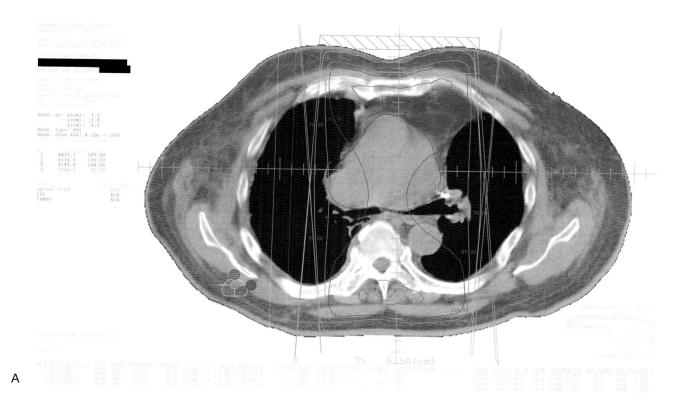

A

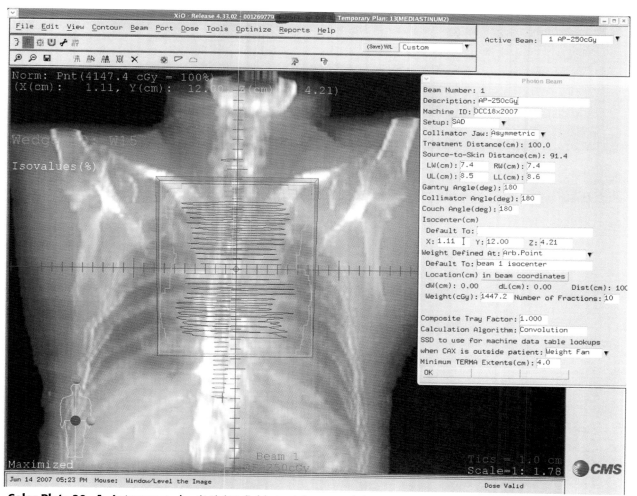

B

Color Plate 20. A, Anteroposterior (AP)/AP fields to right upper lobe and mediastinum. **B,** Beam's eye view of AP field.

Continued

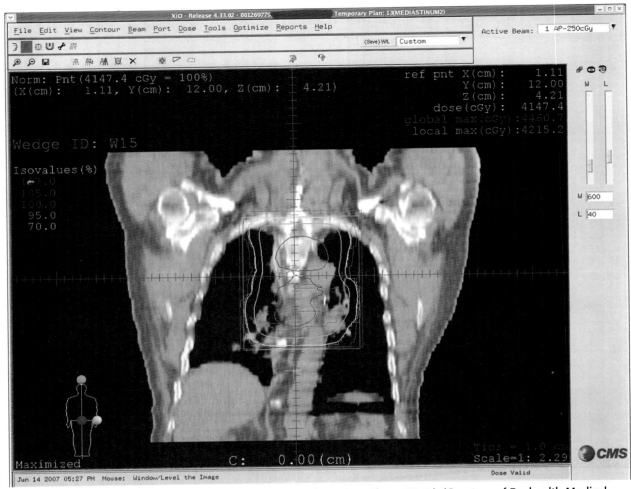

C

Color Plate 20. cont'd C, Beam's eye view of isodose values. (See Figure 32-9.) (Courtesy of Bayhealth Medical Center at Kent General Hospital, Dover, Del.)

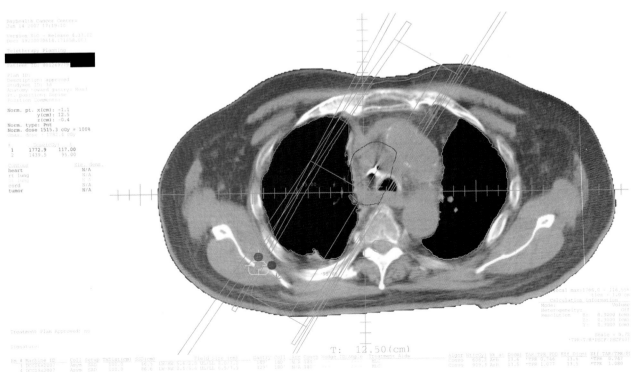

Color Plate 21. Reduced fields with parallel-opposed off-cord obliques. (See Figure 32-10.) (Courtesy of Bayhealth Medical Center at Kent General Hospital, Dover, Del.)

CASE I

Chest Wall Electron Treatment Considerations

Correen Fraser

A 46-year-old woman with a history of bilateral cystic breasts noticed an increase in the size of a left breast mass. Subsequent workup revealed a poorly differentiated invasive ductal carcinoma, ER/PR and HER-2/neu positive, stage IIB, T3 N0 M0. Following neoadjuvant chemotherapy plus paclitaxel (Taxol) and trastuzumab (Herceptin), the patient received a left modified radical mastectomy. In addition to the primary, pathology revealed a DCIS component and 0/10 lymph nodes positive. Family history of cancer was significant for mother, maternal grandmother, and maternal aunt with breast cancer.

The patient was simulated for a definitive course of chest wall radiation therapy. After mastectomy, the average thickness of the chest wall was 1.6 cm. The major characteristics of electron beam therapy are rapid falloff, superficial dose distribution, and a skin dose of 80% to 100%, depending on the beam energy. With many critical structures such as heart, lungs, and spinal cord underlying the chest wall, these beam qualities made electron therapy an excellent option for this patient. A CT simulation was obtained with the patient in the supine position on a breast board with the left arm raised above the head. Before the CT scan, the physician placed wires to map the area of chest wall to be treated. A Varian 2100 CD 6/18x linear accelerator with electron ranging from 6 MeV to 20 MeV was used for the radiation treatment. For this case, a dual scattering foil 6-MeV beam was prescribed based on the chest wall thickness, underlying critical structures, and skin surface dose needed. A beam angle perpendicular/enface to the chest wall at 100 SSD was designed using an electron cone with custom alloy block to define the treatment area. Planning calculations were completed to display isodose distributions in three dimensions (Figure 26-6).

The 20-cm electron cone was used with an 18 × 18 cm custom alloy block coinciding with the physician-placed wires (Figure 26-7). A prescribed dose

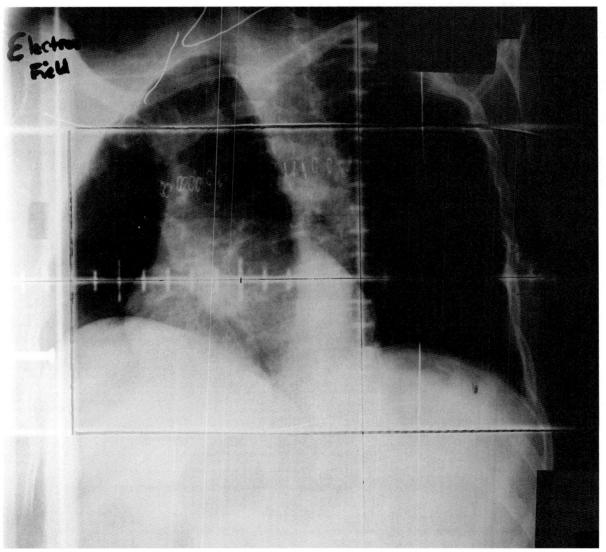

Figure 26-6. Simulator verification film of the treatment volume for chest wall irradiation. The metal clips designate the mastectomy scar and the site of possible residual disease.

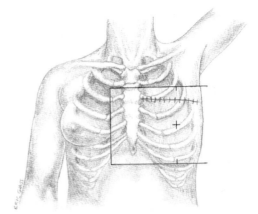

Figure 26-7. Electron chest wall field that is to be treated.

of 5000 cGy was delivered to the chest wall in 25 fractions, 200 cGy/day to the 90% isodose line. The 90% depth dose for the 6-MeV beam is 1.7 cm. No bolus was necessary to improve skin dose or shift the dose distribution to limit dose to the underlying critical structures. A boost of 1000 cGy in 5 fractions, 200 cGy/day to the 90% isodose line will be given using a 2-cm block margin around the surgical scar.

CASE II

Complementing Dose Delivery with Electrons

Ahmad Hammoud

A 37-year-old African American woman had recent history of a stage T3 N0 M0 infiltrating ductal carcinoma of the left breast that was initially noticed as a palpable lump through self-examination. Her initial

mammogram was done, which demonstrated a 5-cm density in the left breast. She subsequently had a sonography-guided biopsy of this lesion. The pathology from that biopsy came back positive for an invasive ductal carcinoma, high grade, with associated DCIS with comedonecrosis. Her tumor was ER/PR negative, HER-2/neu negative.

As part of her staging evaluation, she had a CT scan of the chest, abdomen, and pelvis. CT scanning of the chest confirmed the mass in the left breast, as well as several enlarged axillary lymph nodes. No radiographic evidence of metastatic disease in the pelvis or abdomen was present.

The patient then underwent a sentinel lymph node excision in which a total of three sentinel lymph nodes were removed, and all results came back negative for metastatic disease. Thereafter, the patient started neoadjuvant chemotherapy, which consisted of four cycles of doxorubicin (Adriamycin) cyclophophamide (Cytoxan)–based chemotherapy followed by four cycles of Taxol. One month after the completion of the chemotherapy regimen, the patient underwent a needle localization lumpectomy for which the pathology came back positive for poorly differentiated infiltrating ductal carcinoma measuring 2.5 cm in size. Margins were widely negative.

The patient was referred to radiation oncology for an adjuvant course of radiation therapy. The patient was prescribed 5000 cGy (200 cGy/fraction) to the entire left breast. This course was to be followed by an electron boost of 1000 cGy (200 cGy/fraction) to the scar and lumpectomy site. Three-dimensional simulation was performed for the patient, and treatment planning was performed using the Varian Eclipse TPS version 7.3.

The initial course was planned using two shallow tangential 6-MV photon beams with "field-in-field" compensation to achieve a homogeneous dose distribution, along with a single 12-MeV electron field that matched, on the patient's skin, along the posterior border of the medial photon field (Figure 26-8). By using this beam/modality arrangement as opposed to the standard two-field tangent beam arrangement, a substantial amount of heart and lung was able to be spared. The electron beam was able to treat the medial aspect of the breast tissue and rapidly drop off before reaching the heart. The patient completed treatment with a 15-MeV electron 1000-cGy boost to the scar and lumpectomy site.

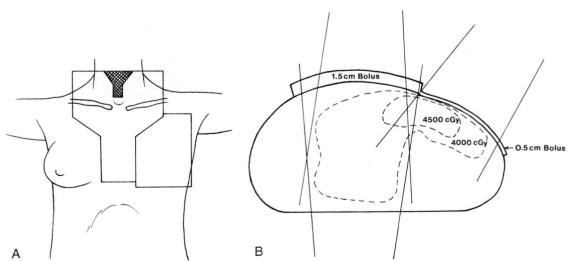

Figure 26-8. A, Anteroposterior/posteroanterior (AP/PA) 15-MV photon field used to treat mediastinum, left internal mammary, and bilateral supraclavicular areas and the oblique 12-MeV electron beam used. **B,** Cross-sectional view showing orientation of the AP/PA photon fields, oblique electron field, and bolus materials.

CASE III

Head and Neck Node Treatment with Electrons

Valerie Marable

A 52-year-old African American male had a 1-month history of sore throat, hoarse voice, and hemoptysis. He was treated unsuccessfully with antibiotics. Triple endoscopy revealed prominent exophytic lesions involving the left false cord, extending to the epiglottis, and encroaching on the entire border of the left ventricular fold. CT scans were also obtained. He was diagnosed with a T3 N0 M0 squamous cell carcinoma of the larynx.

The patient adamantly refused surgical treatment, but he agreed to a definitive course of radiation therapy. He was simulated supine with his arms in a reproducible position, and triangulation setup marks were tattooed. Measurements were taken from stable landmarks for each tattoo, as well as the chin-to-suprasternal notch distance for proper head angulation. Isodistance photographs were taken for the construction of three-dimensional compensators to maximize the homogeneity of dose with the initial larger photon ports. All fields were shaped with custom Cerrobend blocks.

A hyperfractionated approach was used with 100 cGy/fraction delivered twice per day and a 6- to 8-hour interval between fractions. Bilateral 6 MV (Figure 26-9, A) were treated to provide a homogeneous dose to the entire target volume, which included the primary tumor plus lymphatics. At 3960 cGy, the photon ports were modified (Figure 26-9, B) to exclude the dose-limiting spinal cord. Spinal cord tolerance is generally accepted as 4500 to 5000 cGy. This amount will vary with certain circumstances, such as the patient's overall condition, the length of the spinal cord irradiated, the dose per fraction, the number of fractions per day, and the use of chemotherapy. This patient was hyperfractionated and was tentatively scheduled to receive chemotherapy at the end of the radiation course. With this in mind, his spinal cord dose for the initial photon field was kept just below 4000 cGy.

The posterior neck nodes were matched to the off-cord photon fields and treatment continued twice per day at the same dose using 7-MeV electrons up to 5500 cGy. The dose was normalized to a depth of 1.6 cm, which was the

maximum buildup for the energy. This energy was selected to provide an adequate dose to the nodes while delivering a minimal percentage to the spinal cord. The primary site was central and anterior to the spinal cord (Figure 26-9, C). It was boosted with bilateral 6 MV fields, which were also given at 100 cGy/fraction twice a day to a total dose of 6600 cGy delivered in 6 weeks.

Summary of the Clinical Cases

Case I details the use of an electron beam to treat a patient's chest wall after mastectomy. The goal of this treatment is to deliver a sufficient dose to the chest wall while preserving the lungs and pericardium located just a few centimeters below the skin surface. In this case, it was determined that a bolus was not needed to increase the surface dose to the patient or shape the dose distribution at depth. CT simulation was performed with the patient in treatment position, and the thickness of the chest wall was determined so that the selection of and the treatment energy of the electron beam could be made. A 6-MeV electron beam was selected to deliver a dose of 5000 cGy to the chest wall. An additional boost dose of 1000 cGy to the surgical scar was planned.

Case II describes the use of electron beams and photon beams to treat a patient's entire left breast after lumpectomy. The goal of this treatment is to deliver a sufficient dose to the intact breast and lymphatics while preserving the lungs and heart. Use of opposed tangential beams typically is associated with irradiation of a large amount of lung and heart. By use of an electron beam to treat the medial portion of the patient, a significant amount of lung and heart may be spared. The entire left breast was to receive 5000 cGy via this combination of photon and electron beams. An additional 1000-cGy boost to the scar and lumpectomy site was delivered with a 15-MeV electron beam.

Case III describes a form of electron beam treatment that is being replaced with intensity-modulated radiation therapy. The goal of treatment was to deliver 5500 cGy to the lymph nodes

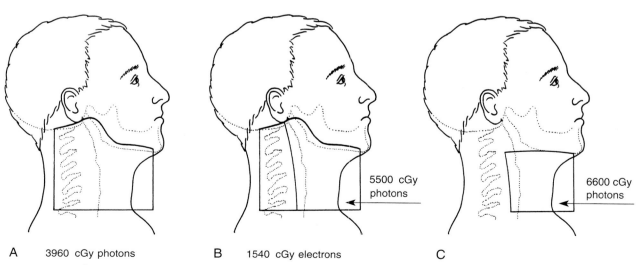

A 3960 cGy photons	B 1540 cGy electrons	C

Figure 26-9. A, Treatment port used to deliver 3960 cGy with 6 MV photons. **B,** Modified treatment ports. Anterior port treated to 5500 cGy with 6 MV photons; posterior port treated to 1540 cGy with 7-MeV electrons. **C,** Primary site boosted to 6600 cGy with 6 MV photons.

of the patient's neck and 6600 cGy to the primary tumor. The parallel-opposed 6 MV photons were used to provide a homogenous dose to the lymph nodes of the neck. If continued for the entire treatment course, this would exceed the limit of spinal cord tolerance. A combination of electron and photon beams were used to overcome this problem. 6 MV photons were used for the entire treatment course and electron beams were used at the end of the treatment course to treat the lymph nodes in the neck. This combination of cobalt-60 photons and electrons accomplished the goal of delivering 5500 cGy to the lymph nodes in the neck while limiting the dose to the spinal cord. In addition, the use of the 6 MV photons for the majority of the treatment course limited the dose to the patient's skin because of the skin-sparing effect of the megavoltage photon beam. To achieve the goal of delivering 6600 cGy to the primary tumor, the treatment field was reduced in size as treatment progressed.

SUMMARY

- Photons do not have charge or mass. Electrons have charge and mass, which increases the probability of an electron interacting with matter.
- Collisional interactions are the predominate mechanism by which electron beams interact with low-atomic-number materials and lose energy in clinical radiation therapy.
- The electron beam spectrum in the patient depends on the depth in the patient and the energy spectrum at the patient surface.
- Two methods for producing clinically useful electron beams are scattering foils and scanning beams.
- Electron beam characteristics are such that superficially located lesions may be treated with almost no dose to the underlying tissues deep to the superficial tissues treated.
- The mean energy of an electron beam may be determined by the product of depth of the 50% isodose line in centimeters (R_{50}), multiplied by a constant (C_4).
- The treatment depth (depth of the 80% isodose line) in centimeters is equal to the mean energy of an electron beam divided by 3.
- The practical range in tissue in centimeters of an electron beam is equal to the mean energy of an electron beam divided by 2.
- As the energy of an electron beam increases, both the surface dose and percent depth dose increase.
- As the energy of an electron beam reaches approximately 15 MeV, the width of the 80% isodose curve is decreased.
- A 1-cm margin between the lateral edge of the target volume and edge of the treatment field should be used for a 16-MeV, electron beam.
- Extended source-skin distance for electron beams is defined in the AAPM Task Group 25 report as 15 cm beyond standard source-skin distance.
- If the dimensions of any portion of an irregularly shaped electron field are not greater than the practical range of the electron beam, a closer investigation of the dose (measurement) is needed.
- When the edges of two electron fields are abutted at the surface, an overlap of the two electron beams will occur at depth.

- An underdose on the surface will be the result of placing a gap at the surface between the edges of two electron fields.
- To decrease the amount that the dose will vary to a particular anatomic location when two adjacent electron beams are used for a treatment course, the area where the two beams meet may be moved two or three times during the patient's treatment course.

Review Questions

1. What is the predominant mode of electron beam interaction or scattering in the 1- to 20-MeV energy range used in radiation therapy?
   a. collisional
   b. radiation
   c. bremssrahlung
2. An advantage of the use of scattering foils in electron beam therapy is
   a. decreased bremssrahlung contamination
   b. scattering foils are simple and reliable in use
   c. precision treatment with the use of low-maintenance complex electronic systems
3. A patient is to be treated with a 16-MeV electron beam. Calculate the depth of the 80% and 90% isodose lines.
   a. 3 cm and 4 cm
   b. 4 cm and 5 cm
   c. 5 cm and 4 cm
   d. 8 cm and 5 cm
4. A patient has a tumor at a depth of 4 cm. What energy of electron beam should be used so that the 80% isodose line encompasses the tumor?
   a. 8 MeV
   b. 10 MeV
   c. 12 MeV
   d. 14 MeV
5. What is the range in tissue for a 12-MeV electron beam?
   a. 3 cm
   b. 4 cm
   c. 6 cm
   d. 8 cm
6. Which of the following are treatment planning considerations in the use of bolus in an electron beam used for radiation treatments?
   I. an underdose in the region from surface to maximum dose
   II. a decrease in surface dose of 10% to 15%
   III. an edge effect causing an increase of 20% to 30%
   a. I
   b. I and II
   c. I and III
   d. I, II, and III
7. Using the value of 2.4 for the constant C_4, determine the mean energy of an electron beam at the surface, whose 50% isodose value is at a depth of 5 cm.
   a. 8 MeV
   b. 10 MeV
   c. 12 MeV
   d. 14 MeV

8. A patient is to be treated with a 7-MeV electron beam. How thick (in centimeters) should a lead shield be to reduce the dose to less than 5% of the useful beam?
   a. 3.0 cm
   b. 3.5 cm
   c. 4.0 cm
   d. 4.5 cm

9. Two electron beams adjoin or abut each other on the patient's skin surface. How does this affect the dose to the patient at depth below the point where the fields abut?
   a. the dose at depth is increased
   b. the dose at depth is decreased
   c. there is no change to the dose at depth

10. A 12-MeV electron beam is used to deliver a dose to a 4 × 4 cm field size. What should be considered for this particular treatment?
    a. the source-skin distance should be decreased 5 cm
    b. the source-skin distance should be increased 5 cm
    c. the dose rate or output factor should be measured

11. A patient is to be treated with a 15-MeV electron beam to a treatment volume that measures 10 cm in width and length at depth. Select the best field size for this treatment.
    a. 10 x 10 cm
    b. 11 x 11 cm
    c. 12 x 12 cm
    d. 13 x 13 cm

The answers to the Review Questions can be found by logging on to our website at: *http://evolve.elsevier.com/Washington+Leaver/ principles*

Questions to Ponder

1. Compare and contrast the use of 1- to 20-MeV electron beams with that of photon beams in radiation therapy.
2. Discuss the situations in which a special calibration of an electron beam may be required.
3. Describe two specific clinical situations in which electron beam therapy is useful.
4. Compare and contrast the relationship between electron beam energy and the depth of maximum dose with that of photon beams.

REFERENCES

1. Almond PR, Biggs PJ, Coursey BM, et al: AAPM's TG-51 protocol for clinical reference dosimetry of high-energy photon and electron beams, *Med Phys* 26:1847-1870, 1999.
2. Cunningham R, Johns HE: *The physics of radiobiology*, ed 4, Springfield, Ill, 1983, Charles C Thomas.
3. Grimm DF, et al: Electron beam port films, *Med Dosim* 14:31-33, 1989.
4. Hogstrom KR: Treatment planning in electron beam therapy. In Vaeth JB, Meyer JL, editors: *Frontiers of radiation therapy and oncology*, vol 25, *The role of high energy electrons in the treatment of cancer*, New York, 1991, Karger.
5. International Commission on Radiation Units and Measurements: *Radiation dosimetry: electrons with initial energies between 1 and 50 MeV*, report no. 21, Washington, DC, 1972, The Commission.
6. Karzmark CJ, Nunan CS, Tanabe E: *Medical electron accelerators*, New York, 1993, McGraw-Hill.
7. Khan FM: *The physics of radiation therapy*, Baltimore, 1984, Williams & Wilkins.
8. Khan FM: Basic physics of electron beam therapy. In Vaeth JB, Meyer JL, editors: *Frontiers of radiation therapy and oncology*, vol 25, *The role of high energy electrons in the treatment of cancer*, New York, 1991, Karger.
9. Khan FM: *The physics of radiation therapy*, ed 3, Baltimore, 2003, Lippincott Williams & Wilkins.
10. Khan FM, Doppke KP, Hogstrom KR, et al: Clinical electron-beam dosimetry: report of AAPM Radiation Therapy Committee Task Group No. 25, *Med Phys* 18:73-109, 1991.
11. Klevenhagen SC: *Physics of electron beam therapy, medical physics handbooks*, Bristol, UK, 1985, Adam Hilger.
12. McPharland BJ: Methods of calculating the output factors of rectangular electron fields, *Med Dosim* 14:17, 1989.
13. Mould RF: *Radiotherapy treatment planning*, Bristol, UK, 1981, Adam Hilger.
14. Olch A, et al: External beam electron therapy: pitfalls in treatment planning and deliverance. In Vaeth JB, Meyer JL, editors: *Frontiers of radiation therapy and oncology*, vol 25, The *role of high energy electrons in the treatment of cancer*, New York, 1991, Karger.
15. Perez CA, Brady LW, Halperin EC, Schmidt-Ullrich RK: *Principles and practice of radiation oncology*, ed 4, Philadelphia, 2004, Lippincott Williams & Wilkins.
16. Rustgi SN, Working KR: Dosimetry of small field electron beams, *Med Dosim* 17:107-108, 1992.
17. Tapley N duV: *Clinical applications for the electron beam*, New York, 1976, Wiley.

Electronic Charting and Image Management

Annette M. Coleman, Cara Zeidman

Outline

The radiation oncology electronic medical record
  Workflow management
Computerization of patient records
  Input methods
  Data types
  Image data
  Presentation

Connectivity and interoperability
  Proprietary interfaces
  Standards-based interfaces
  Health level 7
  Digital imaging and communications in medicine
Information systems
  Networking
  Security and privacy

Considerations for implementation and continuing education
Data compilation
Decision making
Public health
Cancer registry
Summary

Objectives

- Define *electronic medical record (EMR)*.
- Identify the role of nonclinical information to the EMR.
- Describe unique aspects of radiation oncology prompting development of a specialty EMR.
- Define *workflow* and its role in the EMR.
- Differentiate between data entry, data types, and data presentation.
- Differentiate between proprietary and open standard communication protocols.

- Identify roles and responsibilities of the information systems staff.
- Identify systems on which EMRs may be operated and the necessity for mechanisms securing system privacy, security, and stability.
- State three potential goals of the collation of multiple patient records.

Key Terms

Abstracting
Algorithms
Application service providers (ASPs)
Biometric technology
Computerized physician on-line order entry (CPOE)
Digital imaging and communications in medicine (DICOM)
Evidence-based care
Health Insurance Portability and Accountability Act of 1996 (HIPAA)
Health level 7 (HL7)
Hospital information system (HIS)
Local area network (LAN)
Medical informatics
Medical information system (MIS)
Medical records
Network
User interface
Wide area network (WAN)
Wireless local area networks (WLANs)

Medical records consolidate, organize, and document an individual's health care experience. These data take the form of a sequentially recorded narrative describing the patient's medical history, medications, any test findings, treatment plans, and communication between the provider and outside consultants and between the provider and the patient. The term *medical records* reflects the plural nature of these critical documents because they are independently created and maintained by each practice or institution providing care to the individual.

In specialty care clinics such as radiation oncology, facility management systems, including demographic, scheduling, and billing systems, have long leveraged the benefits of computerization. The awareness of efficiencies gained through the implementation of these systems and universality of much of the data across health care made practice management systems a logical starting place for the generation of the electronic medical record (EMR) for clinical care. For radiation oncology, complex treatment planning and treatment delivery requirements necessitated the integration of computers and have been in its practice for several decades. Knowledge regarding cancer, an individual's diagnosis, and options for care and documentation requirements for treatment is growing exponentially. The convergence of these evolutions make radiation oncology an intensely data-driven environment. Now that immediate access to ever-increasing quantities of information is a standard expectation, just collecting the data becomes insufficient; a user expects the information to be presented appropriately. The goal of the EMR is to provide not only collection and storage of information but also facilitation of the patient encounter by providing the clinician with the most relevant information for the specific task at hand.

The EMR forms a comprehensive hub for information management in the modern radiation oncology department. Primarily referral based, radiation oncology depends on data exchange with external and internal sources. The clinic itself must resourcefully manage operating processes to provide modern services to as large a population as possible. Treatment planning and delivery systems incorporate rapidly changing technology to increase tumor effects while reducing normal tissue damage. The complexity of linear accelerators increasingly necessitates the integration of verifiy and record (V & R) systems to guide and monitor the physical settings required for the delivery of complex treatment plans. Specialized systems are leveraged to optimize some of these functions, yet each remains dependent on core primary information about the patient—information identifying the individual, their illness, comprehensive intervention plan, and response to care. Centralization of patient medical history in the EMR provides the foundation for improved safety and efficiency resulting from fully informed decision making.

THE RADIATION ONCOLOGY ELECTRONIC MEDICAL RECORD

Well-documented medical records demonstrate clear reasoning for a course of treatment and attention to patient response. Caregivers follow professional guidelines to ensure that medical record keeping maintains community standards of quality and accuracy. Quality in charting requires entries to be made as soon after a patient encounter as possible to ensure accuracy and completion. Errors or poor documentation are potential sources of harm; therefore, each caregiver is responsible for the character of the record. When corrections are required, they must be dated, initialed, and entered legibly, without masking the original error.[9] It would seem that with everyone working toward the same standards, one clinic's medical records would be organized exactly the same as those of any other clinic. In actual practice, however, clinical workflow within a practice or institution steers medical records toward a format that best suits that team's needs. Within a radiation oncology department, the patient's chart is used by many clinical and administrative staff members. These may include physicians, radiation therapists, physicists, medical dosimetrists, nurses, tumor registrars, and administrative staff. Each team member gathers patient information critical to her or his role so that she or he can provide efficient and effective patient care. The compilation of each team member's contribution comprises a radiation oncology record documenting the rationale, plan, delivery, and follow-up care given the patient in the specialty clinic. The radiation oncology record is independent of a patient's other medical records, including those of the hospital or other departments where radiation oncology is part of a larger organization.

Classically dependent on printed documentation, bound collections of printed materials from diverse sources, handwritten, clinical notations entered in a diary-like chronologic sequence, paper records offer static presentation accessible to one caregiver at a time. Transcribed reports from internal and external sources are organized in more or less chronologic order; and copies of any outbound documents are maintained. Although logical for recording information, retrieval requirements do not follow this same sequential pattern—manual searching for relevant information is required during the patient encounter. More energy is expended on the search than in the application of information.

In contrast, the EMR captures, aggregates, and presents information relevant to patient care in digital form. Information is collected from many sources, including external physicians or facilities such as laboratories or pharmacies, and in many forms, such as images or text.[4] Once data are collected, record accessibility for caregivers and administration is limited only by the nature of the system installed by a facility. Data can be selectively presented to clinicians, organizing complex information with a clinical focus, to answer questions specific to a task. It may be that workflow management is the most defining feature of the specialty EMR.

Workflow Management

Workflow can be defined as an assembly of tasks performed to accomplish a goal. The tasks range from the very high level, such as the general path a patient takes moving through the clinic, to the very specific procedures defining when the therapist tattoos a patient. Workflows may be simple, involving few steps or decisions, or very complex, with changing pathways as each decision is made. They may involve one individual or team working at the same time or may require information being passed between individuals who are separated by time or location.

Looking specifically at a patient who has been referred to radiation oncology, the typical series of events includes consultation, decision to treat, simulation, verification of treatment plan, treatment delivery, monitoring of response, and follow-up (Figure 27-1). Each event is further supported by many complex processes involving information shared between a diverse care team (Figure 27-2). On consultation, the oncology nurse performs an initial functional assessment including vital signs and weight. The radiation oncologist, possibly with the assistance of a resident, a physician's assistant, or nurse practitioner, follows with an examination. The assessments of all specialists contributing to patient care must be equally accessible to the care team. Nutritionists and social workers may conduct and document baseline interviews at the initiation of treatment, often continuing supportive assessment and interventions throughout the course of treatment. Conclusions, interventions, and patient response to treatment are included in the medical record using views and forms designed by the institution or individual professional.

Although this general pathway is followed at radiation oncology clinics worldwide, how each event is executed will meet the specific needs of the facility and change over time. Traditional records are static in nature and not easily responsive to changing workflows. Electronic charts increasingly provide flexibility to rapidly adapt to evolving workflow and information needs. Changing technology changes process, the EMR's goal is not to replicate past practice—it is to optimize efficiency and accuracy through process formalization and single point of data entry.

Process formalization is demonstrated in **computerized physician on-line order entry (CPOE)**. CPOE is on-line management of the entire order tracking and documentation process from order entry to return of results and is a standard workflow component of an electronic chart. Laboratory orders, radiology examinations, and medications have specific ordering

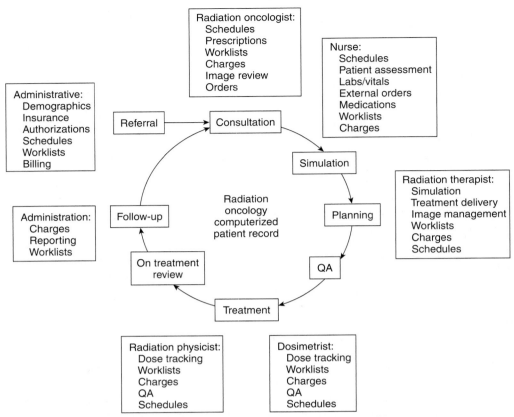

Figure 27-1. Patient flow in radiation oncology. *QA,* Quality assurance.

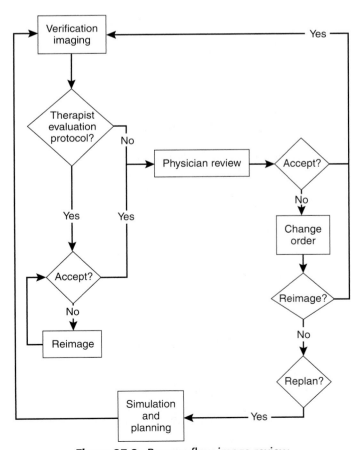

Figure 27-2. Process flow image review.

requirements that are commonly shared among hospitals or independent providers; the radiation oncology EMR may offer complete CPOE functionality or integrate with hospital systems. A relatively linear process, one action follows another—the physician enters an order, another team member executes the order, and results are recorded.

Treatment machine settings are an example of the efficiencies and accuracy gained through single-point data entry where the same information may be required in different forms by different members of the care team. The radiation therapist is interested in enabling accurate and fast treatment setup and delivery as provided through the V & R process. The physicist is interested in accurate transfer of these same settings from the treatment planning to the delivery system and confirmation that they were applied at treatment. The physician, although not generally requiring the actual machine settings, must have ready access to the summary of dose delivered having used those settings (Figures 27-3 and 27-4).

COMPUTERIZATION OF PATIENT RECORDS

Electronic charts leverage a broad spectrum of computing capabilities. Biomedical computing brings together computing, biology, medicine, and supporting activities such as image analysis and treatment planning. Medical informatics encompasses these elements in an evolving discipline involving the storage, retrieval, and optimal use of biomedical data, information, and knowledge for problem solving and decision making.[1] The radiation oncology EMR manages information from a variety of

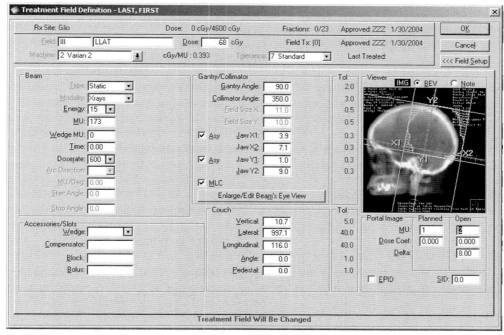

Figure 27-3. Treatment field details.

sources and a wide range of applications from word processing to the algorithms used to calculate treatment plans and storage and display of medical images to biometric devices. The integration of these is a necessity yet one of the greatest challenges of creating a comprehensive EMR.

Input Methods

Because the data that the computer system must manage are of such a wide variety, the means used to input this data is also very varied. The most widely used mechanism for data entry has been and continues to be the keyboard and mouse. In general, familiarity with these devices makes them a ready default for data entry. However, skillful use is not universal and alternatives must be available for individuals' special needs and for entering extended narratives or other complex information.

Extended narratives can be supported by speech recognition systems (also called *voice recognition programs*). This software translates verbal communication into text and enters it,

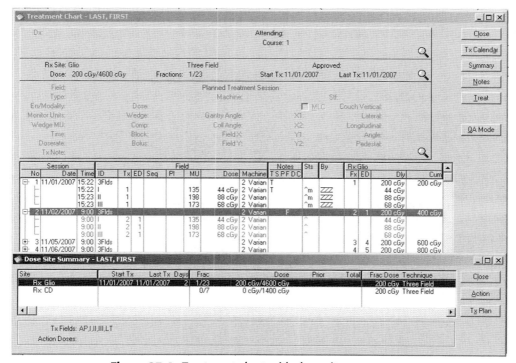

Figure 27-4. Treatment chart with dose site summary.

facilitating rapid entry of lengthy narratives. Accuracy of voice recognition systems can vary widely along with the ability to adapt to medical terminology—even pronunciation variations and regional accents of speakers.

Peripheral devices offer rapid and mobile data entry options. Bar codes offer an alternative method of entering repetitive data; keystrokes encoded in bar codes are read with a variety of hardware devices. Biometric devices measure physical characteristics such as fingerprint or retinal scanners and may be used to identify individuals or enter signatory authorization in an electronic format. Cameras and scanners also generate a wide variety of image information. Electronic completion devices, such as signature pads, are commonly being used to document consent for treatment, because they allow the establishment of a direct link between a digitized handwritten signature and a specific document.

Not all information is directly entered. Some portion of patient information may be gathered in its completed form from an outside source (Figure 27-5). Reports ranging from physician referrals to laboratory to imaging examination reports are collected on receipt of a patient referral to the radiation oncology department.

These may be in electronic formats, but often traditional media must be scanned or otherwise manually entered into the chart by clinic staff. Later in this chapter, electronic interfaces for these information sources will be discussed.

Regardless of the mechanism of entry, data must be organized at the time of collection. Consistency in data entry and completion of procedures are facilitated through the development of a variety of forms and templates designed for clinicians to directly enter responses and prompting completion of tasks and data entry (Figure 27-6).

Narrative observations dictated by the physician may be transcribed into written documentation in the form of reports or letters to outside physicians or to the patients themselves. Ultimately, the clinician prefers flexible options for entering and retrieving patient information. Communications integrating information from the patient record with free text for observations or comments can be among the most flexible options for recording patient encounters. Word processing has supported templating of routine documents for a very long time. EMRs' ability to insert information from their database into transcribed documents streamlines their creation and ensures consistency.

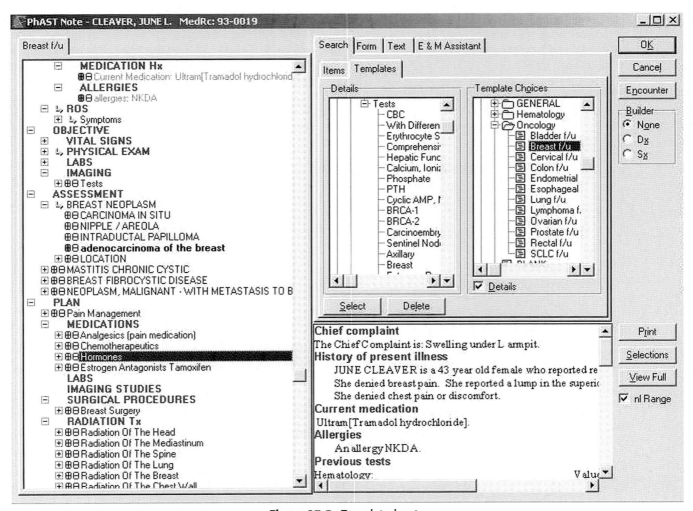

Figure 27-5. Templated note.

Patient: {PatientNameFL}
DOB: (Admin.Birth_Date}
ID#: {Patient.SS_Number}
Visit Date: {Object.Encounter_Date}
Referred by Dr. {Admin.Ref_MD_ID*PnP NameFL}

Radiation Oncology–Completion Note

Patient Info: {Patient.First_Name} {Patient.Last_Name},
                      {Admin.Age}yo{Admin.Gender@L}

Disease: **{Admin.Adm_Diag*Topog.ICDO_Code}**
                      {Admin.Adm_Diag*Topog.Description}

{Site.Summary}

Tolerance: The patient tolerated treatment fairly well.

F/U Plans: Patient will be followed.

Electronically {Object Status} by {Admin.Attending_MD_ID*
PnP.NameFL},MD/Transcribed by
{Object.Trans_ID*PnP.NameLFI}

{CClist}

A

Patient: FIRST LAST
DOB: 1/04/1948
ID#:
Visit Date: 11/03/2007
Referred by

Radiation Oncology–Completion Note

Patient Info: FIRST LAST, 59 yo female

Disease: {Admin.Adm_Diag*Topog.ICDO_Code} Parietal lobe

Treatment Summary:

Radiation Oncology–Course: 1 Protocol:						
Treatment site	Current dose	Modality	From	To	Elapsed days	Fx.
Glio	4600	x15	8/6/2007	9/5/2007	31	23

Tolerance: The patient tolerated treatment fairly well.

F/U Plans: Patient will be followed.

Electronically Pending by Transcribed
by Z, Z Z

cc:

B

Figure 27-6. A, Templated database insertions. **B,** Postinsertion integration.

Data Types

Information may be selected from predefined lists or typed in as free text response in forms displayed to the user. The benefit of predefined lists is consistency in data entry and later in compilation or comparisons of records. Predefined lists can be defined using external standards or can be unique to a given practice.

An example of an organization standardizing clinical information in oncology is the World Health Organization (WHO),

which publishes diagnosis and morphology codes classifying diseases, including cancer, and a wide variety of signs, symptoms, abnormal findings, complaints, social circumstances, and external causes of injury or disease. When the WHO was established after World War II, it took charge of publishing mortality classifications. The *International Statistical Classification of Diseases, Injuries, and Causes of Death (ICD)*[17] was published in 1948, and soon WHO began to code and tabulate mortality and morbidity data. In the early years of nomenclature and coding of neoplasms (1950s and 1960s), the principal system for classifying diseases was the *ICD* series published by WHO. Eventually, *ICD* was used to code and tabulate the diagnoses on medical records for the purpose of storage and retrieval. The morphology code for cancer records the type of cell that has become neoplastic and its biologic activity. Every health condition can be assigned to a unique category and given a code. These codes are revised periodically, and the publication is currently in its 10th edition. The benefit of following such a standard is ease of compilation of data. Becausee everyone (ostensibly) is using the rating system the same way, data from multiple centers can be easily combined and compared.

The morphology codes published by WHO record the kind of tumor that has developed and how it behaves. There are three parts to a complete morphology code:
  4 digits for cell type (histology)
  1 digit for behavior
  1 digit for grade, differentiation, or phenotype
In ICD-O morphology codes, a common root codes the cell type of a given tumor, and an additional digit codes the behavior. The grade, differentiation, or phenotype code provides supplementary information about the tumor.[17] For more information, see http://training.seer. cancer.gov/module_coding_primary/unit01_hist_ bkgrnd01.html.

Alternatively, a department may create its own list of standard responses to a given question. Defining acceptable entries can be quite challenging, because opinions vary among individuals within an organization on format and granularity requirements. For example, pain could be measured in multiple ways. One might quantify on a scale of 0 to 10 or 1 to 5 where 0 is equal to "no pain" and 5 or 10 is equal to "unbearable pain." Alternatively, a series of qualitative statements to describe pain level (none, minor, moderate, severe, unbearable) may be listed. Once agreed on and in use, results can be compared over time for an individual patient or across many patients within the practice (Figure 27-7).

Not all findings can be easily translated into a predefined list. Physical findings such as dimensions of a tumor or number of involved lymph nodes may vary significantly and require direct text fields for data entry. An electronic system can easily accommodate the entry of this information, but a large amount of data entered as free text leads to compilation issues. One of the greatest obstacles to merging information is the lack of a commonly accepted vocabulary. Free text cannot be easily organized into bundles that might illuminate or demonstrate patterns, yet this merging is critical to decrease variances in practice patterns and improve outcomes across geographic and practice boundaries.

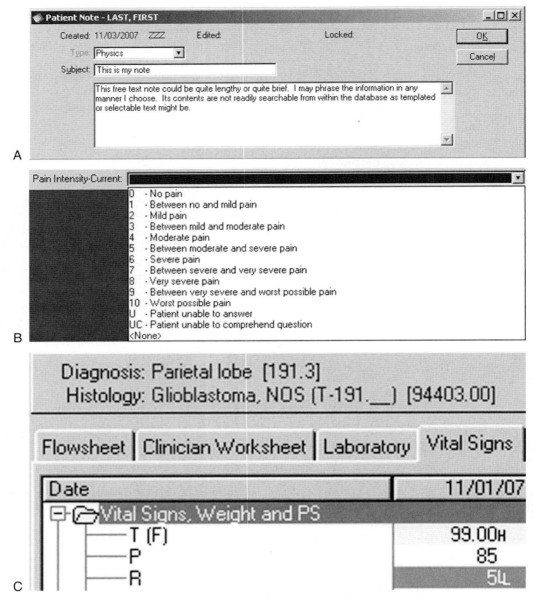

Figure 27-7. A, Free text. **B**, Multiple choice selections. **C**, Alerts.

Every piece of information displayed does not require independent entry. Data can also be generated automatically as a result of simply interacting with the electronic chart. Date and time of the entry or any other record are easily automated in electronic systems. User name and password combinations ensure signatures are unique, and evidence of which operator viewed or otherwise interacted with the system is readily recorded in addition to constraining access to information.

Algorithms (finite sets of instructions used by computers to compute a desired result) might be applied to pieces of information to determine another value. For example, diagnosis code and tumor size, node, and metastatic state (TNM) data can be used to calculate disease stage, saving the clinician from manual determination and entry. This can be especially useful as changes to the usual measure are made and a user must transition to a new formula. Automating this process

can confirm that the same formula is being applied as of a given date.

Other algorithms may compare information such as prescribed medications with patient allergies or other drug incompatibilities. The algorithm could be as simple as providing an alert when a patient over the age of 65 is prescribed a given medication up to having the system automate a page to an outside physician if three of five warning signs are triggered. The complexity of the algorithm to run, as well as the resulting action by the software, is limited only by the imagination of the person developing the code in combination with the ability of the software to support the actions.

Order entry for the radiation prescription is uniquely within the domain of the radiation oncology EMR and can illustrate a variety of entry requirements using a combination of the aforementioned types of data entry (Figure 27-8).

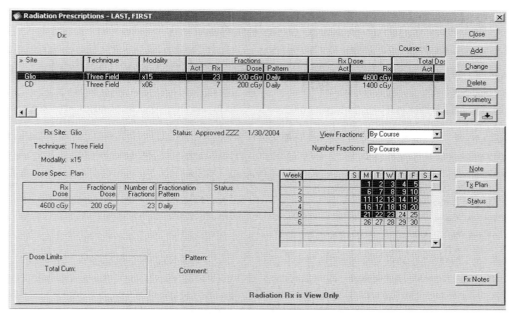

Figure 27-8. Radiation prescription.

Information requirements include diverse descriptions of treatment volumes and techniques, total dose to be delivered, fraction size, pattern, and sequencing.

Image Data

The EMR in radiation oncology would be incomplete without images. From identification photographs to treatment planning CT scans to verification imaging, the role of standard and medical image management is essential to patient care and the medical record. In addition, task management tools necessary to coordinate activities to be performed is incorporated. The electronic chart contains information such as the patient's identification, ordered and planned procedures, and treatment machine data, which are needed by multiple peripheral systems such as simulators or treatment planning systems. Collected from sources ranging from digital cameras to digital scanners to treatment planning systems to medical imaging devices themselves, images may be stored once and made selectively available for everyone from the front desk to the clinical staff delivering care. When included, images and textual information may be integrated to facilitate planning and create a more robust perspective on the history of care.

The EMR system provides image access at all times and in all places and facilitates image-centric workflows. For example, the EMR system, using filtered lists of treatment images in need of review, may provide alerts at the time of treatment delivery to ensure proper actions can be pursued. Workflows as basic as those mimicking the traditional film and lightbox evaluation of planar verification imaging are standard expectations of the radiation oncology EMR. Today, with the insurgence of image-guided and adaptive radiation therapy techniques, expectations are rapidly evolving to include three- and four-dimensional imaging visualization, increased transfer of images between systems, and an exponential increase in computing and storage demands.

Images created in one system may be required in several others. A central database with the ability to share or refer to a single master copy of an image being used by connected systems can provide a distinct advantage over multiple duplications.

Replication of image data through the multiple systems using it in radiation oncology is rapidly recognized as a challenge. Radiology has long addressed issues with access and portability of diagnostic images through the use of picture archiving and communications systems (PACS). Conceived in the mid-1980s and introduced commercially in the early 1990s, these systems replace hard copy medical images with electronic images and are dedicated to storage, retrieval, distribution, and presentation of these medical images throughout the health care enterprise.

Although the basic need to manage electronic imaging in radiation oncology may appear to mimic that of radiology, data, workflows, and connected systems are distinctly different. Treatment course descriptions add layers to the organization and relationship of image studies to one another, and treatment history is tightly interwoven with verification imaging. Repeated verification imaging, particularly the growing use of cone beam computed tomography (CBCT), is producing large volumes of data. Often one image must be sent to several places, multiple times, over many days or weeks. One computed tomography (CT) scan might be produced by a diagnostic system or virtual simulator, sent to the EMR, then sent to treatment planning and imaging verification systems, and returned with corresponding verification images and annotations, all of which must be shareable back to treatment planning for assessment of response and potential replanning, against which more verification imaging will proceed. So, just as diagnostic radiology staff realized early the need to integrate with radiology information systems (RIS) to manage patient data and workflow, so, too, radiation oncology staff increasingly finds the need to access PACS that meet their unique information and workflow needs. Integration with the radiation oncology EMR provides the context and details of radiation treatment courses to manage and organize treatment-related imaging.

Presentation

The **user interface** of the EMR refers to the graphic, textual, and auditory information the program presents to the user and the input methods (as described previously in this chapter) the user employs to control the program. It is, quite simply, what it looks and feels like. In the case where two systems may have the same functional capabilities, often it is the user interface that sways a clinician to prefer one over the other.

The design of a user interface affects the amount of effort the user must expend to input information into the system, interpret the output of the system, and learn how to do both of these things. It describes how well a product can be used for its intended purpose by its target users with efficiency, effectiveness, and satisfaction, also taking into account the requirements from its context of use. Usability is the degree to which the design of a particular user interface takes into account how that piece of the software fits into the overall patient visit and the logic that is required by the user to figure out how to use it. The extent that usability is taken into account in the design of the system will have a huge effect on how effective, efficient, and satisfying the user will "feel" about the software.

Selective presentation of information is a primary challenge in the design of the EMR. Too much information clutters without improving decisions, whereas too little slows completion of a process as answers are sought. Safety and efficiency are improved by reducing the effort expended distinguishing information required for a specific task from the general clinical picture. Software can be written to review data entered and selectively display and even highlight notable values, similar to spell-check functions in word processing. Information entered in one context can be viewed and acted upon in other contexts. For example, the physician enters a complete description of the patient's diagnosis; the radiation treatment chart typically displays only the disease name and stage but can allow for immediate access to the detailed view. Presentation of information may be designed for a work group (i.e., a nursing view, a physician view), a procedure, or even an individual's preferences. Alternatively, views may be designed around the process (image review, for example). Summary data can be readily collated, then presented in tables or graphs to aid interpretation of repeated findings. With continuous access, the documentation and communication among members of the care team are optimized.

Computerization of processes often begins as an in-house project to meet very specific needs. Eventually these custom systems may evolve into commercial products with features generalized to allow their implementation in a wider variety of settings. So, although a commercial system provides a more economic solution to a larger market, features may be counterintuitive to those using the program or require undesired changes in procedures. Within radiation oncology, the EMR is maturing and coming full circle on this path. Systems available today are increasingly configurable to meet the information needs of the various clinical and administrative constituencies they serve

rather than presenting information in one format that everyone must use.

CONNECTIVITY AND INTEROPERABILITY

Historically, as a specific need in health care arose, a solution directly targeted to that need developed, one specific problem producing one specific solution. Yet overlaps and redundancies between systems grow and questions arise as to why information cannot be shared between them. Linking of systems can clearly improve information reliability and safety by eliminating the need to duplicate data entry, but this process is more complicated than might seem at initial evaluation.

An interface is the handshake that allows data to pass from one system to another. In an ideal scenario, one piece of information would smoothly transfer from one place to another without loss of integrity; the reality is that existing transfer mechanisms are subject to interpretation and translation. Although two systems may include the same pieces of data, they may not store or present them the same way. Whereas a caregiver can intuitively interpret information presented in slightly different formats, computers require instructions to equate and transfer like information. In a simple example, couch values from one linear accelerator might be recorded in millimeters and reported in the sequence of vertical, lateral, longitudinal, whereas another may record in centimeters and report the sequence as vertical, longitudinal, lateral. The EMR must map the inbound messages to its own recording and presentation format. Interfaces explicitly define file formats that can be created and read between systems. Several types of interface formats are widely used to build the radiation oncology EMR.

Proprietary Interfaces

Proprietary communication protocols are developed and owned by private or commercial entities. In the absence of national or international standards, proprietary protocols and interfaces can provide much needed tools for sharing information across diverse data sources. In radiation oncology, the demands of connecting treatment planning systems, imaging, and delivery systems advanced much more rapidly than the evolution of standard protocols. Proprietary protocols develop to meet community needs and may become or provide a basis for industry standards. Drawbacks of proprietary protocols include duplication of effort when solving common problems in unique ways. Proprietary systems can be wasteful of time and resources during development and can add difficulty for users who must understand the variety of capabilities and operating procedures of resulting systems. These systems also offer little progress toward solving the overriding problem of universal access. As standards-based interfaces have become available, commercial manufacturers are increasingly transitioning, yet proprietary interfaces remain widely in use in radiation therapy, particularly for connectivity to linear accelerators.

Standards-Based Interfaces

Nonproprietary communication standards are developed by national and international committees accredited by organizations such as the American National Standards Institute (ANSI) or the International Standards Organization (ISO).

Wide representation from the industry for which interoperability standards are being designed is included. As such, agreement can be a long process, and latitude in interpretation exists. Standards are subsequently published in the public domain and commercial providers use them to create interfaces. Interface solutions may require compliance statements describing in detail how their system adheres to the published standard.

Often referred to as *open systems development*, compliance with nonproprietary standards for interfaces is desirable for vendors and consumers. Just as the standardization of electrical outlets in a home supports development for any household device, so can standardization facilitate connectivity of system components in the radiation center. Independent system components can be developed with greatly reduced coordination of effort between manufacturers. Data are not trapped within a given system, and components of a larger system can be more readily interchanged. As choices for clinics increase, competition drives continual improvement of commercial offerings and maintains clinics' abilities to choose the best solutions for their organization.

Two communication standards routinely applied in radiation therapy EMRs are **health level 7 (HL7)** and **digital imaging and communications in medicine (DICOM)**.

Health Level 7

HL7 interfaces enable sharing of information useful across the entire health care facility. HL7 is an ANSI-accredited organization developing standards for exchanging clinical and administrative data. Specifically, HL7 defines standards for "the exchange, management and integration of data that supports clinical patient care and the management, delivery and evaluation of health care services."[7] Moreover, on an ongoing basis, HL7 develops a set of protocols on the fastest possible track that is both responsive and responsible to its members. The group addresses the unique requirements of already installed hospital and departmental systems, some of which use mature technologies.[7]

Patient information includes admission, discharge, and transfer (ADT) data such as demographics; financial information for billing; scheduling information; clinical documents such as transcriptions, orders, laboratory results, and medications; and other data. By using HL7 interfaces, clinical and administrative information may be entered only once yet used in any specialty department's record. This avoids wasted time and reduces error produced by multiple entries of data. Updates and corrections may be propagated through the same interface, allowing a single point of entry to disseminate corrections throughout the organization.

The Clinical Context Object Workgroup (CCOW) is another HL7 standard promoted to increase efficiency. CCOW intends to automate multiple application log-ins and synchronize patient record selection through a single point.[7] Users of multiple applications that complement the work process are assisted when working on a single patient's records even though the information is managed by multiple databases.

Digital Imaging and Communications in Medicine

Whereas HL7 facilitates transfer of general clinical and administrative patient data, DICOM standards are specific to the needs of image and information transfer in radiology and radiation oncology. DICOM standards are produced by a joint committee of the National Electrical Manufacturers Association (NEMA) and the American College of Radiology (ACR) that is affiliated with several international agencies.[5] This committee was formed to provide communication standards for sharing image information regardless of manufacturer facilitating the use of PACS distribution of diagnostic images. DICOM has been expanded to include radiation therapy imaging and treatment information. DICOM RT enables radiation therapy manufacturers to concentrate on a single internationally accepted format for interoperability between their system and others in the industry.

DICOM 3 refers to the third part of the base standards and describes each type of information that may be transferred. These information types are called *information object definitions (IODs)*. IODs may describe formats for the exchange of image or textual information. Several IODs expressly describe radiation therapy information:

- Radiation therapy (RT) image—conventional and virtual simulation images, digitally reconstructed radiographs (DRRs) or portal images
- RT dose—dose distributions, isodose lines, dose-volume histograms (DVHs)
- RT structure set—contours drawn on images, that is, CT
- RT plan—text information describing treatment plans including prescriptions and fractionation, beam definitions, and so forth
- RT beams and RT brachytherapy—treatment session reports for external beam or brachytherapy, may be used as part of a V&R system
- RT treatment summary—cumulative summary information, may be used after treatment to send information to a hospital EMR[6]

In theory, information transfer should be seamless, but connectivity in itself does not guarantee ease of use between systems with different purposes. An effort to evolve basic connectivity to functional interoperability is the goal of yet another initiative. The Integrating the Healthcare Enterprise (IHE) initiative was formed in the late 1990s to improve interoperability between computerized systems in diagnostic radiology. In 2004, the IHE for Radiation Oncology (IHE-RO) was formed. Composed of leading radiation oncology professionals, international standards organizations, and industry representatives, clinical workflows and technical requirements are defined for sharing data between disparate yet critical component systems such as CT to treatment planning to the EMR. Using standards such as HL7 and DICOM, manufacturers build solutions to meet the requirements defined by the clinical community and gather in meetings called "Connectathons," where they test and refine interoperability. Once a solution is successfully validated, approved vendors are then entitled to participate in demonstrations for the clinical community, typically held at major clinical association meetings.

 See the following websites for more information on HL7 (http://www.hl7.org), IHE (http://www.ihe.net), and DICOMRT (http://medical.nema.org).

INFORMATION SYSTEMS

Patient safety and legal requirements necessitate that access to patient information be secure, stable, and dependable. When the patient record is maintained electronically and critical systems such as a V&R system are integrated, its availability is required to provide radiation oncology care. The complexity and criticality of the EMR's functions and the technical infrastructure to support it necessitate information systems (IS) expertise. **Medical** or **hospital information system (MIS or HIS)** departments may use several specialists in areas ranging from systems analysts to hardware and network specialists. These professionals manage the array of requirements from supporting the system infrastructure to ensuring that it is used efficiently by clinicians and staff.

Systems analysts are members of the IS team and may be included in the selection and implementation process of introducing an EMR. The systems analyst is generally a resource skilled at evaluating patterns of information use and providing objective insight. The systems analyst coordinates resources and often remains with the organization throughout the entire change process to manage purchases, installations, and workspace layouts; to produce new policies and procedures; and to measure results.[11] The EMR itself is only a tool to facilitate the process of patient care, without a detailed understanding of this process the transition will be fraught with obstacles and challenges.[12] Systems analysts perform the complex task of analyzing activities in an organization to precisely determine what must be accomplished and how it must be accomplished. Radiation oncology is a dynamic environment and management of the EMR reflects the complexities of care. The systems analyst may supervise or even have primary responsibility for system management, designing, implementing, and maintaining software configuration settings or configurable components.

 For more information on Healthcare Information Management Systems Society, see http://www.himss. org/ASP/index.asp.

Networking

One of the key features of the EMR is its centralization of information with distributable access. The demand for sharing data is the result of a desire to improve care through access to information and increasing efficiency. Informed decision making is best supported by presenting all the information available regarding a patient to all clinicians when and where they need it. Access to the electronic chart is limited only by the network on which it is operated.

The most common platform for the EMR is the client/server configuration. The database and program executables reside on a central computer, the *file server*, and are accessed from distributed terminals or computers, known as *clients*. Such systems run on networks. A computer **network** is a system of independent, interconnected computers or terminals communicating with one another over a shared medium, consisting of hardware and communication protocols. The most common network protocol is the Ethernet protocol (Figure 27-9). Ethernets require special hardware, including cards within the computers and particular cables.

A **local area network (LAN)** is geographically confined to an area in which a common communication service may be used. **Wireless local area networks (WLANs)** are increasingly popular in clinical settings because they facilitate the use of wireless personal digital assistants (PDAs), laptops, and other pervasive computing devices at the point of care. However, because of the relative immaturity of wireless network technology and evolving standards, WLANs, improperly configured, can present significant security risks. Understanding the security limitations of the technology and available fixes can help minimize the risks of clinical data loss and maintain compliance with federal guidelines.[2] For larger geographic areas or when multiple LANs are to be connected, a **wide area network (WAN)** may be used. WANs use a variety of communication services including telephone dial-up, T1 or T3 lines, or even the Internet to communicate over long or short distances.

Alternatively, web-based EMRs use the Internet to gain controlled access to servers maintained by **application service providers (ASPs)**. Applications and data are stored off-site and maintained by the ASP provider. Users access servers through secure and private Internet connections, reducing information system maintenance and making charts accessible wherever an Internet connection exists.

Regardless of the location of the system, file servers must have backup systems in place for database protection. Backup systems might be as simple as tapes recording copies of files or as complex as servers using multiple hard drives recording duplicate information should one fail. Regardless of type of equipment used, backups must be performed on a regular basis, usually daily. File restoration must be periodically tested, and full backups should be rotated to off-site storage so potential catastrophes such as fire, flood, and so forth will not result in permanent loss of patient records.

Security and Privacy

Computerizing patient records has the potential to make private information accessible to unauthorized viewers, risking patient harm should it be used to make unfair employment, insurance coverage, or other decisions. Access to view and enter data must be restricted to qualified and authorized individuals. Passwords are currently the most common method of restricting access to the electronic chart and in conjunction with security privileges; individuals may be assigned access to only portions of the chart necessary to performance in their role. Password security guidelines are designed to enforce sufficient uniqueness and complexity to avoid improper impersonation and may be extended to include **biometric technology** such as fingerprint or retinal scanning for further security. Although the ability to transfer large amounts of electronic data from one system to another holds great promise for streamlining health care and supporting clinical decision making, transferred data must be secured during transfer and accurately assigned in the receiving system.

To facilitate the proper exchange of information while restricting access to necessary personnel, the U.S. Congress passed the **Health Insurance Portability and Accountability Act of 1996 (HIPAA)**. HIPAA guidelines and regulations require security precautions to not only restrict access but also

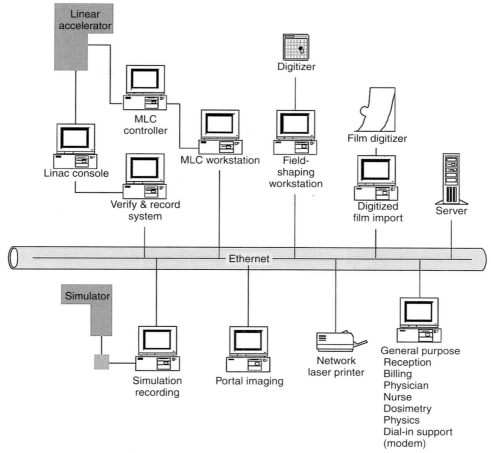

Figure 27-9. Radiation oncology network diagram. *MLC,* Multileaf collimator.

keep records of who is accessing information. To this end, regulations are developed under the provisions of this act to standardize information sets for health care reimbursement and to restrict access to the minimum needed to provide care.[13,14] By providing standards for communicating information necessary to achieve health care reimbursement, providers are assisted in the complex process of obtaining payment for their services without endangering their patients' right to privacy.[14] In general, access to information that is identifiable to an individual is restricted except to those caregivers to whom the patient has given consent. Full disclosure is extended when the purpose of disclosure is to provide treatment decision making. Certain exceptions are included in the regulations for public health needs, certain law enforcement activities, general oversight of care (i.e., quality assurance procedures), and some research activities.[10,13]

Considerations for Implementation and Continuing Education

The most effective method to maximize benefits is the education of the staff. No matter how robust software is, if it is not used the benefits will be lost. Universal acceptance of the EMR is in its early years. The radiation therapist may find himself or herself working in facilities at various stages of acceptance, which certainly affects workflow and department interactions.

As with adoption of any new technology that will be experienced over one's career, the radiation therapist will have a role and responsibility to adoption. Strategies for success in any change endeavor have common concepts. Formation of a team of champions who can establish and promote a long-range vision aligned with the goals of various constituencies and those of the organization is the first step of implementation. This team should be truly cross-functional, representing each role in the department, and thoroughly investigate current critical processes and develop expertise in the new technology to produce transition plans that fit with the organization. The team should examine barriers with the goal of diminishing their effect, commit to bidirectional communication of plans and concerns, and provide and accept as much training as possible.

Education needs to occur before the initial use of the software and then continue over time. Staff development is typically included with the purchase of complex systems and may be delivered through a variety of methods. Manuals can pass along a preset catalog of information but do not answer each person's individual questions and are not always accessible. Help menus often explain specific information about software functionality but are not always sensitive to the nuances of the information sought by the user.

It must be remembered that continuing education is needed to optimally use any electronic system. With time, the most common training method can become "I've seen." "I've seen" is similar to the child's game of "whisper down the lane." One person may learn from a primary source. He or she then shares this information with a coworker. This coworker shares it with the next and so on. Although this method is positive in that the information and processes are shared, the degeneration or telescoping of the information over time must be considered. Software updates and enhancements not withstanding, staff turnover and department changes such as treatment standards and staff will affect how any chart is used.

DATA COMPILATION

Medical informatics is the organization, analysis, management, and use of information in health care, and the EMR enables medical informatics. Challenges to individual patient care, analysis of patterns of care, and outcomes across the population are integral to the ongoing development of the EMR.

The explosion of information available today for clinical decision making requires complex management tools. For example, a series of test results in a single chart may require manual transcription of values to a graph to visualize rates of change over time or, as in abstracting for cancer registry, details from many, many charts must be transferred into other systems to accurately describe patterns of disease presentation, treatment, and outcomes.

Decision Making

The medical record charts the decisions, actions, and responses for an individual. Options and decisions for care are based on historical knowledge of the natural history of the disease and current understanding of available treatment interventions. As treatment choices evolve, new information feeds continual improvement in care. The ability to review information across large populations can lead to in-depth analysis. Therefore, a course of care for an individual has the potential to improve our collective knowledge for future patients.

Standards of care derive from compiling the customs and behavior of the members of the profession. These are then developed and reflect a consensus of how the profession is to be practiced. Standards cannot be fixed but must adapt to incorporate newly determined therapies and may define acceptable scales for judging individual variations.

Optimal clinical and business decision making depends on accessible and accurate data for evaluation. The analysis process generates a thorough understanding of existing procedures along with performance measurements that can be referenced when determining response to the improvement plan. Problems are defined; goals and plans for achieving those goals are formulated; and a program is executed. Continual refinements are targeted by repeating this process using understanding gained from earlier efforts.

Practitioners commonly base clinical decision making on their knowledge and experience, patient preference, and clinical circumstances. **Evidence-based care** combines this information with scientific evidence. This combination is the optimal method for defining the clinical care of individual patients.[16]

As the knowledge base for cancer management grows, accessibility to information becomes increasingly critical to the decision-making process of defining an individual course of treatment. The EMR may also extend its scope by providing links to research groups and literature sources, accessing empiric evidence published in an increasing range of journals and other forums. As recommendations are applied to an individual treatment plan, specific risks and response norms could be flagged for attention should the patient's response be inconsistent with expectations.

Public Health

In addition to the advantages to individuals, the emergence of the computerized patient record provides the framework to compile and analyze data from large populations to aid the epidemiologist's goals for improving overall public health. Population-based data reporting is much more readily accomplished with computerized systems than through retrospective medical chart review.

The history of public health is the history of how people have tried to understand the causes of disease and what can be done to reduce disease and improve health. The Department of Health and Human Services (DHHS) is the principal agency that the U.S. federal government uses to protect the health of all Americans and to provide essential human services, especially for those who are least able to help themselves. Three of the most readily recognizable public health service organizations are the following:

National Institutes of Health (NIH)—The NIH is the world's premier medical research organization, supporting more than 35,000 research projects nationwide involving diseases such as cancer, Alzheimer's disease, diabetes, arthritis, heart ailments, and acquired immunodeficiency syndrome (AIDS).

Food and Drug Administration (FDA)—The FDA ensures the safety of foods and cosmetics and the safety and efficacy of pharmaceuticals, biologic products, and medical devices.

Centers for Disease Control and Prevention (CDC)—Working with states and other partners, the CDC provides a system of health surveillance to monitor and prevent disease outbreaks (including bioterrorism), implement disease-prevention strategies, and maintain national health statistics.[15]

Federal law requires that diagnosis and treatment information be collected and maintained for the lifetime of any cancer patient. Only a limited amount of funding can be applied to address health issues. When trends can be established, decisions can be made regarding the allocation of that funding. These trends are determined as each patient's medical history and treatment are measured and patterns of care and outcomes are evaluated among the general population. This information must be gathered not only within a single department but also across all similar treatment centers to see trends that currently exist and paths to quality improvement. Designed to ensure quality care for the patient whose history and treatment is described, the medical record is also a source of data for measuring and evaluating patterns of care and outcomes among the general population. The data-gathering process in cancer registry is termed **abstracting**. Where an EMR is in use, data entry and abstracting may be assisted by interfacing with the cancer registry system.

Cancer Registry

A cancer registry is an information system designed for the collection, management, and analysis of data on persons with the diagnosis of a malignant or neoplastic disease (cancer).[3] Cancer registries are valuable research tools for those interested in the etiology, diagnosis, and treatment of cancer. Fundamental research of cancer epidemiology is initiated using accumulated data. Multiple agencies use collected data to make public health decisions aimed at maximizing the effectiveness of limited public health funds, such as the placement of screening programs. An electronic repository of this information allows for a more efficient method of evaluating the data.

Cancer registries can be classified into three general types:

Health care institution registry—Also known as hospital-based. These registries focus on all patients who are diagnosed and/or treated for cancer within a specific cancer center. These do not distinguish where the patient is from; the institution must follow everyone who passes through its doors. This tracking is required by law to be passed up to a state or central registry.

Central registries—These are the compilations of all the health care institution registries that are then broken down by specific geographic areas. The generated data show larger-scale trends than the individual cancer center.

Special purpose registries—A registry to maintain data regarding a particular type of cancer, such as brain tumors, can be established if initial data at either the institutional or central level point toward potential trends.

SUMMARY

- The electronic medical record (EMR) captures, aggregates, and presents information relevant to patient care in digital form.
- The EMR should incorporate process flow and the unique charting needs for a given patient population and various caregivers. To be useful in the complex medical environment, it must be flexible and configurable yet provide codified data that can be easily sorted and reported on.
- Nonclinical information such as demographics, scheduling, and reimbursement information is integral to the comprehensive medical record. Integration of systems leverage the benefits of centralization; shared information advances reliability and accuracy resulting from single point of entry.
- Data are entered into the EMR through a growing variety of human and electronic interfaces ranging from simple keyboard entry to electronic communications to biometric devices.
- The complexity and criticality of the EMR's functions and the technical infrastructure to support it necessitate information systems expertise.
- Whereas computerization is not new to treatment planning or delivery, its application to the medical record has been accepted only recently as a primary instrument in radiation oncology. With their potential for improved collection and organization of data, EMRs provide multiple caregivers simultaneously access to charted information, ensuring availability when and where it is needed. As the workflow engine, the EMR selectively presents information relevant to tasks or examinations at hand, and when further enabled with portals to research and other decision-making tools, the electronic environment becomes ideal for ensuring individual patient care plans are made with current information.

- The exchange of information between systems in radiation oncology is enabled through extensive use of interfaces. Interfaces improve efficiency and accuracy by reducing redundant data entry and resulting errors. Many options exist for designing interface systems including custom, proprietary, and standard formats. Proprietary interfaces are designed and owned by commercial entities. Nonproprietary standards designed by professional organizations (HL7, DICOM) are part of the public domain; these public standards are highly desirable yet can be the hardest to integrate and make available for use.
- With all its potential benefits, implementation of an EMR is not without challenge. Software selection must balance privacy, security, and accessibility. Although information must be available to authorized individuals, it must be protected from loss or unsanctioned viewing.
- Software operation is dependent on the system on which it is installed. Most commonly installed on networked client/server systems (networks), a radiation oncology department may depend on other departments to ensure network stability and apply disaster recovery programs to safeguard loss of data. Software and the network it is run over must be sufficiently robust to have minimal downtime.
- Streamlining the flow of medical information between systems and among caregivers holds great promise for improving health care. Full access to the patient's medical history is invaluable to diagnosis and treatment of illnesses, and streamlining administrative processes enables better use of resources. Data from many patients can be more readily compiled, providing more accurate profiles of illness and response to treatment choices.
- Universal introduction and acceptance represents a complex undertaking that places new demands on computer systems management and security and clinical practice procedures. As technical limitations are addressed, the key to successful introduction of these systems will be practitioners' ability to successfully reengineer department processes, making them safer, more secure, and more efficient. Yet despite these challenges, all indications are that stakeholders at all levels of health care, from patients to providers to legislators, remain strongly committed to advancing health information technology and integrating it more fully into health care delivery.[8]

Review Questions

Multiple Choice

1. EMRs provide:
   I. workflow management
   II. one central record
   III. retrospective data analysis
   a. I and II
   b. I and III
   c. II and III
   d. I, II, and III

2. EMRs expedite the process of extracting data from individual patient records for evaluation of patterns of care and outcomes. This is called:
   a. analysis
   b. compiling
   c. interfacing
   d. abstracting
3. Of the following, which would *not* generally be considered an aspect of the user interface?
   a. data input methods
   b. screen layout
   c. interface protocols
   d. selection of information displayed
4. The Southern Radiation Center backs up their data to tape every night. Each week they should carefully put this backup tape:
   a. in a shipment to an off-site storage location
   b. in the back of the director's desk
   c. in a fireproof box near the treatment machine
   d. back in the machine that runs the backup
5. HIPAA regulations provide requirements for:
   a. computerization of patient records
   b. tracking of all individuals accessing patient information
   c. government regulation of treatment methods
   d. password access to patient records
6. Nonproprietary data communication standards in medicine include:
   I. HL7
   II. PACS
   III. DICOM
   a. I and II
   b. I and III
   c. II and III
   d. I, II, and III
7. Radiation oncology EMRs are most commonly installed on a(an):
   a. WAN
   b. ASP server
   c. WLAN
   d. LAN
8. Data gathering and interpretation is *not* facilitated by the use of:
   a. templates
   b. radio button selections
   c. free text
   d. drop lists
9. Standards of care are:
   a. fixed compilation of the customs and behaviors of a professional group
   b. dynamic
   c. an assumed activity that any person would demonstrate in a given situation
   d. the result of improved treatment outcomes
10. Which of the following information has a role in the radiation oncology EMR?
    I. patient schedule
    II. PET scans
    III. letters to the patient
    a. I and II
    b. I and III
    c. II and III
    d. I, II, and III

The answers to the Review Questions can be found by logging on to our website at: *http://evolve.elsevier.com/Washington+Leaver/principles*

Questions to Ponder

1. What are unique characteristics of radiation oncology practice that encourage implementation of a specialty EMR in addition to the general EMR used in the hospital?
2. How does the image review process change between hard copy and electronic environments? Are there other processes for which differences might be foreseen?
3. What do national and international standards organizations contribute to achievement of medical informatics goals through the EMR?
4. Discuss some relative advantages and disadvantages between in-house developed EMRs and commercial systems.
5. Discuss some relative advantages and disadvantages between proprietary and open system interfaces.

REFERENCES

1. Adams RD, Wright DL: Medical informatics, virtual reality and radiation therapy, *Radiat Ther* 10:73-76, 2001.
2. Bergeron BP: Wireless local area network security, *J Med Pract Manage* 20:138-142, 2004.
3. Cancer Registry Field: *What is a cancer registry?* (website): http://www.ncra-usa.org/about/index.htm#sub2. Accessed September 2007.
4. Carter JH: *Electronic medical records, a guide for clinicians and administrators,* Philadelphia, 2001, American College of Physicians–American Society of Internal Medicine.
5. *Digital Imaging and Communications in Medicine (DICOM) part 1: information objects definitions,* Rosslyn, Va, 2001, National Electrical Manufacturers Association (website): http://medical.nema.org. Accessed May 2002.
6. *Digital Imaging and Communications in Medicine (DICOM) part 3: information objects definitions,* Rosslyn, Va, 2001, National Electrical Manufacturers Association (website): http://medical.nema.org. Accessed May 2002.
7. *HL7 health level 7* (website): www.HL7.org. Accessed July 7, 2008.
8. Kunkler T: *Don't believe the hype,* Oncology Net Guide 8(7), 11, 2007.
9. Midwest Medical Insurance Company Risk Management Committee: Medical record documentation: is yours a help or a hindrance in a lawsuit? *SDJ Med* 51(2): 51–52, 1998.
10. Norris TG: Quality assurance in radiation therapy, *Radiat Ther* 9:161-184, 2000.
11. Silver GA, Silver ML: *Computers and information processing,* New York, 1993, HarperCollins.
12. Smith D, Mancini-Newell L: A physician's perspective: deploying the EMR, *J Health Care Inf Manage* 16(2): 71-79, 2002.
13. US Department of Health and Human Services: *HHS fact sheet: protecting the privacy of patients' health information: summary of the final regulation,* Washington, DC, December 20, 2000, DHHS.
14. US Department of Health and Human Services: *HHS fact sheet: administrative simplification under HIPAA: national standards for transactions, security and privacy,* Washington, DC, January 22, 2002, DHHS.
15. US Department of Health and Human Services: *HHS: What we do,* Washington, 2007, US Department of Health and Human Services (website): http://www.hhs.gov/about/whatwedo.html. Accessed September 2007.
16. *What is EBM?* (website): www.cebm.utoronto.ca/intro/whatis.htm. Accessed September 2007.
17. World Health Organization: *International statistical classification of diseases, injuries, and causes of death (ICD)* (website): www.training.seer.cancer.gov/module_coding_primary/unit01_hist_bkgrnd01.html. Accessed December 2007.

Practical Applications

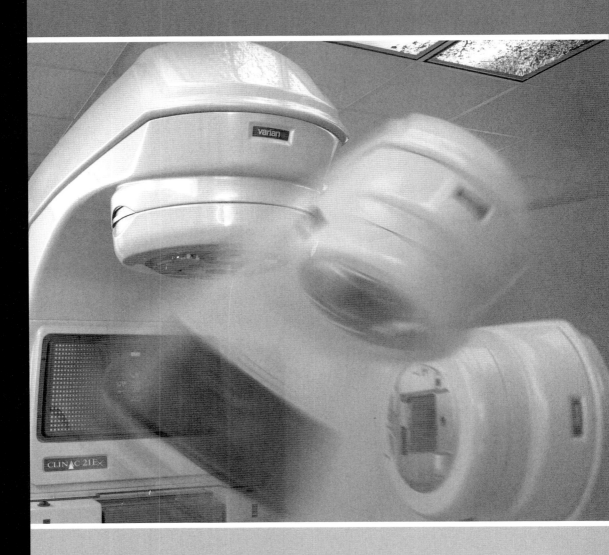

Bone, Cartilage, and Soft Tissue Sarcomas

Lisa Bartenhagen, Jana Koth

Outline

Objectives

- Recall epidemiologic trends associated with bone and soft tissue sarcomas.
- Sketch appropriate anatomy of bone and connective tissue.
- Discuss various pathology, staging, and grading systems for bone and soft tissue sarcomas.
- Identify the treatments of choice for a variety of bone and soft tissue sarcomas.
- Compare and contrast current procedures available for detection and diagnosis of diseases in this category.

- Support the idea that the degree of differentiation and aggression of tumor growth greatly affects the patient's prognosis.
- Recall generally accepted doses of radiation for various bone and soft tissue sarcomas.
- Simulate a bone or soft tissue sarcoma patient as part of the cancer care team.
- Apply knowledge of radiobiology to educate patients on possible side effects of treatment.
- Discuss emerging treatments and technology for the management and cure of bone and soft tissue sarcomas.

Key Terms

DISEASE MANAGEMENT PROFILE

Cancer of the bone and cancer of the soft tissue are challenging for the cancer care team due to their unique character, the infrequency of occurrence, and the difficulties in predicting outcomes. Connective tissue tumors represent one of the most morphologically heterogeneous classifications in human pathology. To date, clinical outcomes for bone and soft tissue tumors have been somewhat discouraging. The evolution of a **multidisciplinary approach** of surgery, radiation therapy, and chemotherapy to planning and treating these diseases has improved over the past 30 years, and clinical trials involving gene therapy are currently under way. As radiation therapists, a comprehensive knowledge of this multifaceted disease is necessary to provide the best quality care possible.

BONE AND CARTILAGE TUMORS

Natural History

The skeletal system is composed of bones or osseous and cartilaginous tissues. These tissues give the body its shape, form, and ability to move. Bones and cartilage possess the exceptional ability to support and protect softer tissues in the body. Bones also serve as a reservoir for fats, minerals, and other substances vital to blood cell production. The extraskeletal connective tissues include all those soft tissues that provide connection, support, and locomotion. Although bone tumors refer to malignancies involving the bone, they frequently may also include tumors of a collective group of tissues such as cartilage, joints, and blood vessels surrounding the bone. Bone marrow, responsible for blood cell production, is not spared from the attack of malignant cells. Soft tissue tumors are limited to those sarcomas arising in the extraskeletal, connective tissues and are found throughout the human body.

The two types of bone tumors examined in this chapter are primary and metastatic. Malignant primary bone tumors do not constitute a major health hazard compared with other neoplastic disorders. In 2008, an estimated 2380 new cases of primary bone cancer were reported, with approximately 1470 deaths resulting from this disease.[1] Although the number of primary bone cancer cases has decreased over recent years, the number of metastatic bone cancers remains high.[1]

This chapter focuses on bone tumors, as well as soft tissue sarcomas. Tumors of the primary bone include osteosarcoma, chondrosarcoma, fibrosarcoma, malignant histiocytoma, malignant giant cell tumors, multiple myeloma, and metastatic bone disease. Fibrosarcomas and malignant histiocytomas have been reclassified to be included in a group of tumors known as *malignant fibrous histiocytoma (MFH)*. These tumors, along with Ewing's sarcoma, are unique among connective tissue cancers in that they affect both bone and soft tissue.

 See the website www.bonetumor.org for additional information. It provides information on bone tumors and learning resources including cases studies, reviews, and games.

Epidemiology

Osteosarcoma, the most common osseous malignant bone tumor, comprises an estimated 35% of all primary skeletal malignancies. Approximately 85% of osteosarcomas occur in patients younger than 35 years with peak incidence in young adults aged 20 to 30 years.[47] Male-to-female ratio among children younger than 15 years is approximately 1:1. This ratio increases to 2:1 for males to females in all patients older than the age of 15.[17,47] Osteosarcoma is more prevalent in tall individuals. Table 28-1 and Figure 28-1 depict the prevalence of various bone tumors.

The next most common type of bone tumor is *chondrosarcoma,* which accounts for 26% of all bone tumors.[1,21] The majority of chondrosarcomas are diagnosed in adults between the ages of 30 and 60.[47] Overall incidence among men and women has been reported as being equal, or a slight 2:1 male-to-female incidence has been documented.[17]

Fibrosarcoma is a bone malignancy that also may occur in soft tissue. Now included in MFH classifications, these tumors account for less than approximately 6% of primary bone tumors.[1,47] The majority of cases are diagnosed in patients between the ages of 30 and 70. A slight male predominance is reported in MFH cases.[47]

Ewing's sarcoma accounts for approximately 16% of bone tumors and approximately 3% of childhood cancers.[1,15] This disease can affect anyone from the age of 5 months to 60 years, peaking in children from 10 to 20 years of age. Occurrence in children younger than 5 years of age is rare. It is also unusual for this tumor to affect Asian or African children.[15] This disease appears to be more predominant in males than in females.[17]

Multiple myeloma is a malignant disease of the plasma cells.[17] Abnormal resorption of bone causes painful osseous lesions.[71] Arising in the B-cell lymphocytes of the bone marrow, this disease process makes up approximately 10% of all hematologic malignancies.[64] Multiple myeloma is usually seen in middle-aged and older adults, peaking in the seventh decade.[20] It is more common in men than women, with a ratio of 1.5:1.[64]

Giant cell tumors of the bone (GCTB) account for approximately 5% of primary bone tumors.[11] Only approximately 10% of cases are malignant.[1] GCTB arises in the metaphysis or epiphysis of long bones in young adults and have a high propensity for recurrence.[47]

Metastatic bone disease accounts for the majority of malignant bone lesions.[1] These lesions occur most often in the spine and pelvis and are less common farther from the trunk. Common primary sites that tend to metastasize are the prostate, breast, lung, kidney, and thyroid, with lung being the most common site.[17]

Etiology

Although the exact cause cannot be identified, there are several possible causes of primary bone tumors. Genetics play a role, with two common suppressor genes being RB1 and TP53. There seems to be an association between these genes and the development of osteosarcoma.[53,63]

Areas of prolonged growth or overstimulated metabolism appear to have a direct link with the site of the neoplasm. This is seen in adult tissues affected by metabolic stimulation from the following:

Paget's disease—a condition characterized by excessive and abnormal bone resorption and formation

Table 28-1	Malignant Bone Tumors				
Tumor	**Age (years)**	**Sex Ratio (M/F)**	**Treatment (5-year Survival Rate)**	**Bones Commonly Involved**	**Location**
Osteosarcoma	10-25	2:1	SC (60%)	Metaphysis	Long bones of extremities (knee joint), jaws
Chondrosarcoma	35-60	2:1	S (variable, 45%-90%)	Diaphysis or metaphysis	Pelvis, ribs, vertebrae, long bones (proximal part)
Ewing's sarcoma	10-20	2:1	CS (45%)	Diaphysis	Long bones; may be multiple
Giant cell tumor	20-40	1:1	S (95%)	Epiphysis	Long bones (knee joint)

C, Chemotherapy; *S,* surgery.
From Damjanov I: *Pathology for the health professions,* ed 3, St. Louis, 2006, Saunders.

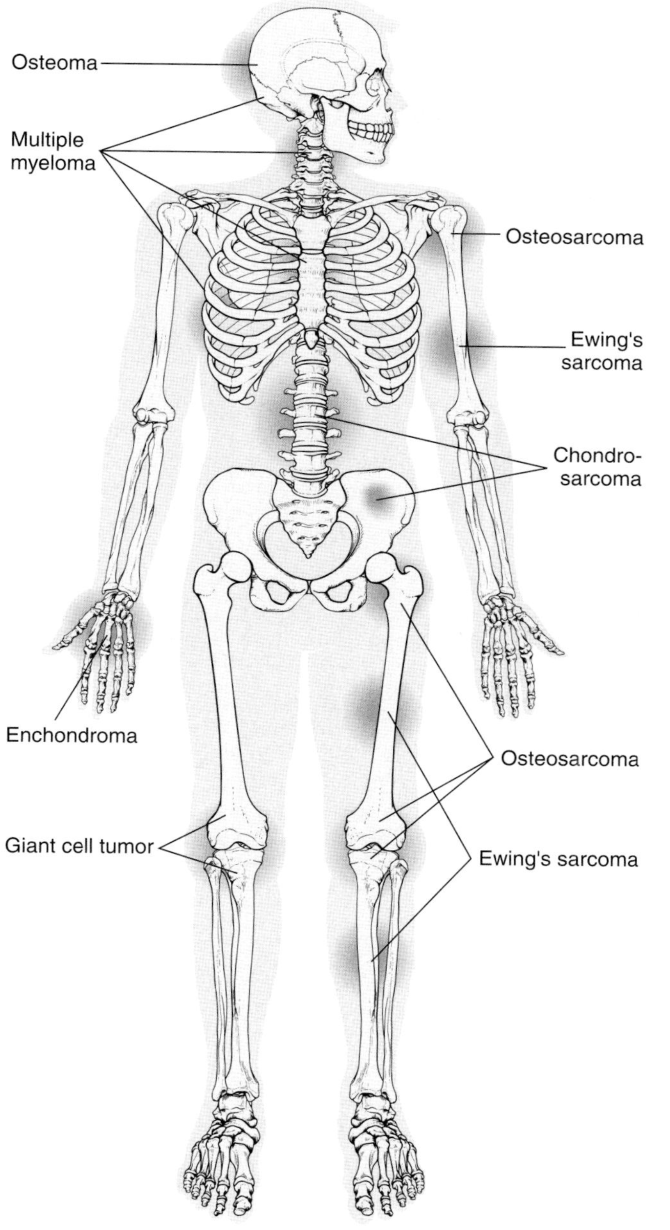

Figure 28-1. A schematic representation of common sites of origin for primary bone tumors. (From Damjanov I: *Pathology for the health professions,* ed 3, St. Louis, 2006, Saunders.)

Hyperparathyroidism—a condition caused by an abnormal parathyroid gland, resulting in a loss of calcium from the bones

Osteomyelitis—an infection of the bone or bone marrow

Additional causes include old bone infarcts and fracture callus.[53] Cells that are proliferating or rapidly dividing also tend to be more prone to a malignant transformation.

Radiation is another **etiologic factor** linked to the formation of osteosarcomas, chondrosarcomas, and fibrosarcomas. Exposure to radioisotopes from occupational and medicinal uses may contribute to the formation of these tumors. Based on laboratory observations, another suggestion is that the role of

infectious agents in bone cancers (particularly osteosarcomas) has been indicated.[53]

Although no single cause of Ewing's sarcoma has been identified, there is a strong association with chromosomal translocation. In most cases, patients with Ewing's sarcoma have been found to have a translocation affecting chromosomes 11 and 22.[8]

General Anatomy and Physiology, Including Pertinent Lymphatic Considerations

Bone tumors have their embryologic origin in the mesoderm, the primitive mesenchyme, and/or the ectoderm cells, which give rise to the common connective tissues (Figure 28-2).

The high incidence rate of bone tumors in children supports the assumption that these neoplasms arise in areas of rapid growth. The most common site of a primary bone sarcoma is near the growth plate. A typical long bone, as illustrated in Figure 28-3, consists of the **diaphysis** (the main shaft of the bone), two **epiphyses** (the knoblike portions at either end of the bone), the cartilage cap (covers the articular surface), and the **periosteum** (the hard, dense covering of the bone). The growth plate is the area in long bones where rapid cell proliferation and remodeling activity takes place.[17] Because they possess large growth plates, the distal femur and proximal tibia are the two most common locations for bone tumors.[53]

Osteosarcomas are most commonly found in the distal femur or proximal tibia. The third most common site is the proximal humerus. Lesions appear in other areas, such as the proximal femur, distal tibia, and fibula, with rare occurrences in the vertebrae, ileum, facial bones, and mandible. In a study of patients 24 years or older, 41% of the lesions were found in flat bones associated with Paget's disease.[47]

Chondrosarcomas are typically found in the femur, although they can also involve the shoulder girdle and proximal humerus. Like osteosarcomas, chondrosarcomas are rarely found in the distal extremities.[47]

Fibrosarcomas (MFH) and GCTB often arise in long, tubular bones. These bones usually include the femur and tibia.[47]

Ewing's sarcoma can be present in virtually any bone but is most frequently seen in the lower half of the body. It can occur in any part of the bone but is most commonly seen in the diaphysis. Metaphyseal involvement occurs less often, and epiphyseal involvement is rare.[40] For treatment purposes, the entire medullary cavity (the cavity of the bone that contains fats or yellow marrow) of the affected bones should be considered. In general, extension occurs through the bony cortex into the soft tissue, giving rise to a large, soft tissue component. In axial lesions, the soft tissue mass is often larger than the intraosseous component.[16]

Multiple myeloma can occur in any bone and is characterized by **lytic** (areas of bone destruction) lesions demonstrated on diagnostic radiographs. However, the vertebral pedicles are rarely involved in patients who have multiple myeloma, compared with patients with metastatic carcinoma.[66]

Metastatic bone disease most often involves the vertebral bodies, pelvic bones, and ribs. However, with widespread metastases, lesions are sometimes found in the humerus, femur,

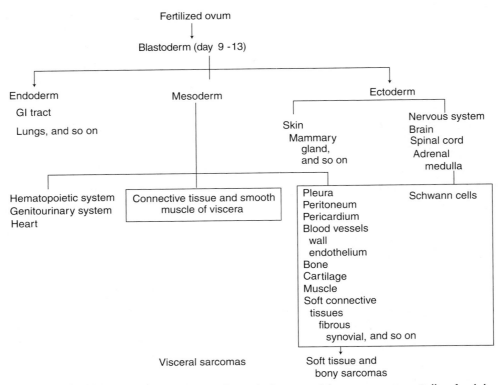

Figure 28-2. Embryonic derivation of the soft tissue and bony sarcomas. Cells of origin determine designations as particular types of soft tissue sarcomas. (From Rosenberg SA, Suit HA, Baker LH: Sarcomas of soft tissues. In DeVita VT, Hellman S, Rosenberg SA, editors: *Cancer: principles and practice of oncology,* vol 2, ed 2, Philadelphia, 1982, JB Lippincott.)

scapula, sternum, skull, or clavicle. Although the distal extremities are often spared from metastatic disease, lesions in the foot are more common than lesions in the hand and usually result from a primary lung carcinoma.[16]

Clinical Presentation

The most common presenting symptom with bone tumors is pain in the affected area.[1] Some swelling and locally engorged veins in instances of neglect may accompany this. Patients with osteosarcoma usually complain of nonspecific pain and swelling in the involved area that begins insidiously and progresses over a few months.[9] Weight loss and symptoms related to anemia are also late complaints. Pathologic fractures are not commonly seen in patients with osteosarcoma.[47] Chondrosarcomas, fibrosarcomas (MFH), and GCTB have symptoms similar to those of osteosarcomas, although the duration of the symptoms may be somewhat longer. Pain usually correlates with the degree of histologic aggressiveness of the disease, and rapid worsening of symptoms may indicate the histologic grade or cell type. Pathologic fractures are common in fibrosarcomas (MFH). Also seen are neurologic abnormalities in vertebral lesions, a decreased range of motion of the involved extremity, and muscular atrophy.[47]

Patients with Ewing's sarcoma also complain of pain and swelling in the affected area. The symptoms are frequently present for several months before a diagnosis is made. Patients with axial lesions especially have a prolonged duration of symptoms.

In most patients, a palpable mass is evident, demonstrating the propensity for this tumor to break through the cortex and involve surrounding tissue. Other symptoms include a fever, weight loss, and generalized fatigue. Occasionally, the presence of lung metastases may cause symptoms that encourage the patient to seek medical treatment early.[15]

Patients with multiple myeloma typically present with painful bony lesions, caused by bone loss. This loss of bone is caused by a disruption in the process of bone formation and resorption.[30,71] Patients may also have pathologic fractures and hypercalcemia, which sets this disease apart from the other primary bone tumors.[70]

Detection and Diagnosis

Patients generally have pain that tends not to be activity related and may be worse at night. A complete history of the patient is important to determine the exact duration of the symptoms. In addition, an indication of a previous carcinoma may suggest a new metastatic lesion of a bone. It is important to consider that a sarcoma may develop in a previously irradiated area. A long history (usually lasting years) of symptoms from a long bone lesion may indicate a benign condition, whereas symptoms that rapidly progress over weeks or a few months usually signify a higher likelihood of a malignant process.[48,53]

Primary bone tumors are rare. This low incidence is a contributing factor in making early detection extremely difficult.

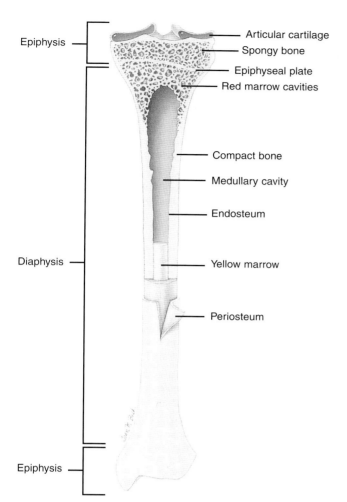

Epiphysis

— Articular cartilage
— Spongy bone
— Epiphyseal plate
— Red marrow cavities

— Compact bone

— Medullary cavity

— Endosteum

Diaphysis

— Yellow marrow

— Periosteum

Epiphysis

Figure 28-3. A longitudinal section of long bone showing diaphysis, epiphyses, and articular cartilage. (From Thibodeau GA, Patton KT: *Anatomy and physiology*, ed 3, St. Louis, 1996, Mosby. Courtesy Joan M. Beck.)

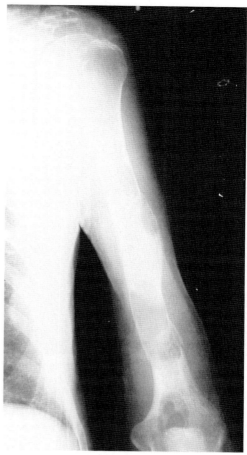

Figure 28-4. Several lytic lesions are present throughout the humerus of this patient with metastatic renal cell carcinoma. Note the destruction of the periosteum along the mid-portion and lower portion of the shaft.

Usually, only persistent pain in a bone initiates a physician's investigation. Because pain is present early in the course of malignant lesions and they usually progress rapidly, incidental discoveries of these lesions are rare.[53]

An important tool for a diagnosis and prognosis of a bone tumor is the radiograph. A variety of parameters are associated in accurately diagnosing a bone lesion. Some of these parameters are the permeative pattern, the sunburst periosteal reaction, the onionskin periosteal reaction, and whether the lesion is osteolytic or **osteoblastic** (pertaining to bone-forming cells). All of these indicate a bone lesion's level of advancement, its aggressiveness, and its rate of growth. Figure 28-4 illustrates several lytic lesions of the humerus caused by metastatic renal cell carcinoma, and Figure 28-5 shows the presence of a Ewing's sarcoma of the upper humerus.

Computed tomography (CT) has been extremely helpful in establishing the extent of the tumor in the bone and determining the presence or absence of soft tissue masses. However, magnetic resonance imaging (MRI) has replaced CT in many instances (Figure 28-6). MRI is used particularly in instances of

highly malignant bone tumors because of the accurate detail it exhibits concerning the relationship of normal tissues and neurovascular structures with the tumor tissue. This is essential in planning a surgical biopsy and treatment. MRI demonstrates with high sensitivity the reactive zone of the tumor in the bone and differentiates any marrow edema adjacent to tumor tissue.

Bone scans using technetium-99m have played an important role in bone tumor evaluation. Figure 28-7 demonstrates a bone scan of a patient with osteosarcoma. This modality is useful, as with this case, to rule out distant metastases.

Bone scans are extremely sensitive and can detect tumor foci in bone that are not yet visualized on diagnostic radiographs. Therefore, the extent of the tumor in the bone and the presence of skip metastases can be demonstrated accurately. Bone scans can also identify distant bony metastases even though they are uncommon in primary bone tumors. For multiple myeloma, however, bone scan results are often negative and may underestimate the extent of the disease.[66]

The diagnosis of primary bone tumors requires many diagnostic and some surgical procedures. The most important of these is the surgical **biopsy**. This procedure should be sufficient to confirm a pathologic diagnosis. The biopsy site and approach must be discussed with the surgeon and radiation oncologist

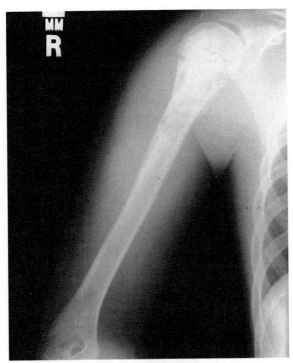

Figure 28-5. Ewing's sarcoma of the upper right humerus. Note the diffuse permeative destruction of the bone, with periosteal reaction involving the proximal portion of the humerus.

before the procedure is performed. If the biopsy incision is poorly placed, the delivery of optimal radiation therapy may be technically impossible. Many patients have a considerable associated soft tissue mass; they can undergo a soft tissue biopsy rather than a biopsy of intraosseous tissue. A soft tissue biopsy avoids further weakening of the bone, the integrity of which is already compromised by the tumor. This is especially true in

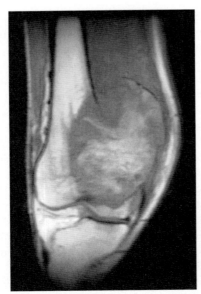

Figure 28-6. A magnetic resonance image of an osteosarcoma of the distal femur. (With permission from *Applied Radiology* (website): www.appliedradiology.com/documents/cases/images/Ly-Figure 2. Accessed May 8, 2007.)

patients who have lesions in weight-bearing bones, which have increased potential for pathologic fracture.

Increasing pain that develops gradually over a few weeks or months is the most frequent symptom associated with bone metastases (Figure 28-8). The pain becomes localized and progressively severe during this time and may be worse at night. For this reason, a complete metastatic workup is necessary to accurately assess the extent of the disease. This workup may include CT and MRI scans, blood tests, and diagnostic radiographs. The areas most frequently involved include the vertebral bodies, pelvic bones, and ribs. In patients with widespread disease, lesions in the humerus, femur, scapula, sternum, skull, or clavicle are not uncommon. Radiographs are also necessary to rule out a pathologic fracture and determine whether surgical intervention is necessary.

Pain may also be positional and relieved simply by shifting weight from the involved area. Bone involvement may also cause pain by nerve entrapment resulting from tumor expansion and pressure on the nerve by the direct destruction of bone. This type of pain occurs in patients with vertebral involvement or sacral metastases caused by the radicular nature of the pain. A careful and extensive neurologic workup is necessary because vertebral destruction is often associated with extradural spine disease, which can result in spinal cord compression. Early treatment of a partial or complete spinal cord blockage is crucial to prevent paralysis and sensory loss. This is one of the few emergency procedures encountered in radiation oncology.[53]

The radiographic appearance of bony metastases takes on different aspects according to the type of lesion. Osteolytic lesions have ragged margins and may appear as a granular, mottled-looking area on an x-ray film.[53] If the margins are smooth, a benign process must be considered. In comparing Figures 28-9 and 28-10, a difference is evident between the ragged and smooth borders of the tumor, generally indicating a benign or malignant process.

Multiple myeloma, as well as breast, kidney, and thyroid carcinomas, commonly produce lytic lesions. The loss of outline of one or more pedicles may be the earliest indication of vertebral body involvement in the spine. If a patient has multiple bone lesions without a known primary tumor site, multiple myeloma must be considered.

Pathology

Osteosarcomas are generally classified as poorly differentiated tumors. Less than 1% of these tumors are diagnosed as a grade 1 (grade ranges from 1 to 4), with 85% categorized as a grade 3 or 4.[47] Predominant histologic subtypes of osteosarcomas are osteoblastic, chondroblastic, fibroblastic, or mixed chondroblastic.[45]

Chondrosarcomas arise from mesenchymal elements of the bone. The degree of cellularity and rate of mitosis are important in establishing a grade for chondrosarcomas, which range from 1 to 3. Histologic examples of low-grade chondrosarcomas are clear cell and juxtacortical chondrosarcomas. Mesenchymal chondrosarcomas are usually undifferentiated and associated with a higher grade.[47]

Fibrosarcomas originate in mesenchymal tissue and often have the appearance of normal fibroblasts but are malignant.

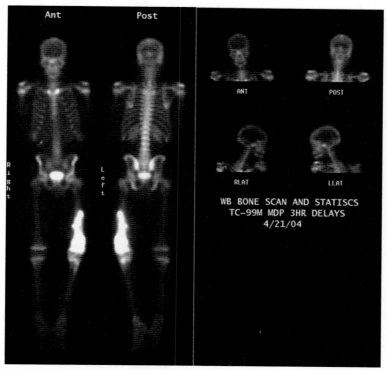

Figure 28-7. This bone scan demonstrates a large osteosarcoma in the left femur while ruling out the presence of distant metastases.

Improvements in histologic classification have categorized low-grade fibrosarcomas as low-grade myxofibrosarcoma, low-grade fibromyxoid sarcoma (FMS), hyalinizing spindle cell tumor with giant collagen rosettes (HST), and sclerosing epithelioid fibrosarcoma (SEF).[28]

The cell of origin for MFH is the histiocyte or the macrophage. MFH is an undifferentiated pleomorphic sarcoma with histiocytic and fibroblastic differentiation.[47]

GCTB are histologically composed of round or spindle-shaped mononuclear cells uniformly incorporated in with multi-nucleated giant cells.[69] Grading for this type of tumor is not prognostically reliable.

Ewing's sarcoma is composed of populations of small, blue, round cells with a high nuclear-to-cytoplasmic ratio. These cells are arrayed in sheets.[8] Approximately 90% to 95% of Ewing's tumors have a cytogenetic translocation between the *EWS* gene on chromosome 22 and the *FLI1* gene on chromosome 11.[40] These alterations make a diagnosis of Ewing's sarcoma definitive.

Plasma cells originate from B-cell lymphocytes. They develop from stem cells found in all tissues of the body, making it possible for plasma cell tumors to manifest in any organ or tissue of the body.[54] Multiple myeloma is characterized by neoplastic proliferation of a single clone of plasma cells. These cells produce a monoclonal protein that, along with the proliferation of plasma cells, leads to the destruction of bone.[34]

Staging

Pathologic staging and grading of primary bone tumors are intimately associated with current anatomic staging systems. **Grade** is determined to be either low (G1) or high (G2) grade

and is nearly synonymous with early (I and II) or late (IIB and III) stage. No universally accepted staging system exists for primary bone sarcomas. The Enneking staging system classifies tumors according to the grade (G), local extent of the disease (T), determined to be either intracompartmental (T1) or extra-compartmental (T2), and presence or absence of distant metastases (M). Box 28-1 shows this staging system.[48]

Spread Patterns

The tendency for almost all sarcomas, especially high-grade tumors, is to metastasize hematologically to the lungs, particularly the periphery of the lung.[19] Occasionally, osteosarcoma, MFH, and chondrosarcoma will metastasize to other sites, including bone, liver, and brain.[31] Lung metastases tends to occur in approximately 80% of patients with osteosarcoma within 1 to 2 years after the initial diagnosis.[47] Low-grade tumors are locally invasive and do not tend to metastasize readily, making them easier to control. Local recurrence is common with low-grade tumors. When this occurs, growth continues and the tumor eventually evolves into a high-grade tumor. **Skip metastases** are another pattern of spread in osteosarcomas.[47] A skip metastasis is a second, smaller focus of osteosarcoma in the same bone or a second bone lesion on the opposing side of a joint space. This phenomenon is attributed to the extensive spread by the lesion into the marrow cavity of the bone. The overall aggressiveness of bone tumors makes control difficult. Lymphatic spread of most bone tumors is not of great concern unless the tumor arises in the trunk of the body. There the lymph vessels and nodes are more prominent and a greater chance exists of the tumor invading the lymph system. If this occurs,

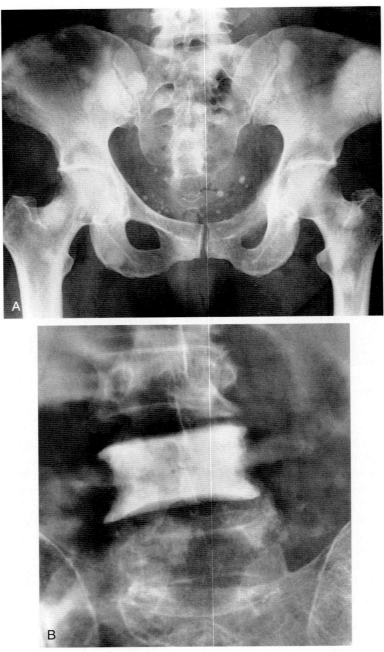

Figure 28-8. A, Osteoblastic metastases from bladder cancer (areas of increased density) involving the pelvis and proximal femurs. **B**, Osteoblastic lesion of L4 metastatic from prostate cancer. (From Eisenberg RL, Dennis CA: *Comprehensive radiographic pathology*, ed 2, St. Louis, 1995, Mosby.)

the microscopic tumor cells can be carried to other parts of the body through the lymphatic system.

Treatment Considerations

In the following sections, specific treatment techniques are discussed regarding osteosarcoma, chondrosarcoma, fibrosarcoma (MFH), giant cell tumors, multiple myeloma, Ewing's sarcoma, and metastatic bone disease. The role of surgery, chemotherapy, and radiation therapy will be discussed.

Osteosarcoma. The presence or absence of metastases at the time of diagnosis is the most important prognostic indicator for this neoplasm. Approximately 17% of patients are determined to have distant metastasis at presentation.[47] Other factors include age, gender, tumor size and location, grade of the tumor, duration of symptoms, and the interval between chemotherapy and surgery.[19] Male gender, duration of symptoms less than 6 months, and patient age younger than 10 years are factors associated with a worse prognosis.[47] Patients with fewer of

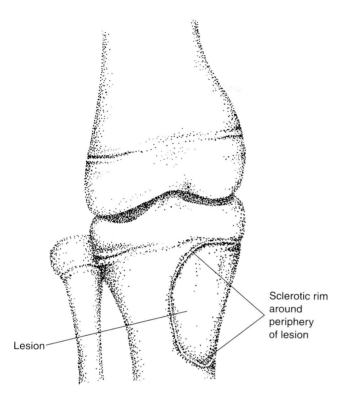

Figure 28-9. Benign appearance of bone tumors demonstrating a sclerotic rim around the periphery of the lesion.

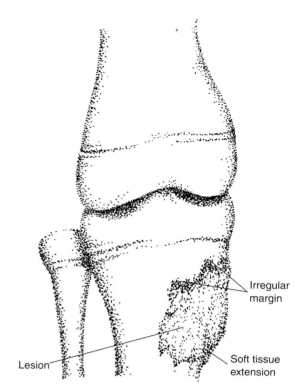

Figure 28-10. Malignant appearance of bone tumors demonstrating an irregular margin with soft tissue extension.

these indictors may respond well to aggressive surgical and chemotherapeutic treatment. Reason dictates that the smaller and less aggressive the tumor, the more easily it can be surgically removed and the less chance it has to metastasize. In addition, lesions that occur in the extremities, predominantly the lower extremity, rather than in axial primaries are more favorable. This has to do with the easy accessibility for surgical removal of the tumor to obtain local control.

The treatment of osteosarcoma requires a multidisciplinary approach. Because this tumor is relatively chemosensitive and radioresistant, the management of the primary tumor consists of neoadjuvant, multiagent chemotherapy combined with resection of the primary tumor.[63] Adjuvant chemotherapy is also often used.[37]

Historically, treatment for the primary lesion was amputation. This achieved excellent local control, but quality of life and functionality were unsatisfactory. Approximately one third of patients are still treated by amputation because of inoperability or the inability for surgeons to obtain clear margins.[19] The evolution of new chemotherapy regimens has greatly affected the shift from amputation to **limb-sparing surgery (LSS)**. Along with improved surgical techniques, neoadjuvant chemotherapy has yielded reports of complete or subtotal tumor localization ranging from 28% to 50%.[3]

LSS has been used in patients who have osteosarcoma to reduce the functional and psychological morbidity of amputation. In this procedure, the bone involved with the tumor is removed and reconstructed with an implant. Rotational and free flap techniques are being used during surgery to aid in soft tissue coverage of the reconstruction. The improved handling of soft tissue and use of implants rather than allograft bone have decreased the incidence of complications, which include wound necrosis, infection, and fracture.[47] Disease-free survival rates of patients with LSS are much the same as those for patients who have undergone an amputation as long as the margins of resection are not compromised.[47]

Radiation therapy is not a treatment of choice for patients with osteosarcomas. These tumors are **radioresistant**, and doses required for a clinical response often result in tissue damage and subsequent amputation. When radiation is used as a single modality, controlling the primary tumor and preventing pulmonary metastases have been unsuccessful. However, radiation has been used preoperatively, along with chemotherapy, and in patients for whom surgery is not feasible. Doses of radiation therapy that are commonly delivered can include 55 to 60 Gy for close but negative margins; 60 to 68 Gy for microscopically positive margins; and for those with gross disease remaining after surgery, doses of 68 Gy or higher can be delivered.[18]

Palliative radiation therapy can be beneficial for pain control or the temporary control of metastases. When treating an osteosarcoma, it is important to include the surgical scar in the treatment field to eradicate any microscopic disease and to spare 1 to 3 cm of skin to avoid distal edema and constrictive fibrosis.[47] The use of CT and MRI is important in the treatment planning process. **Intraoperative radiation therapy (IORT)** is also used in the treatment of sarcomas. This technique is primarily used for lesions of the extremities. The tumor is resected and the surgical bed is treated with electrons. When IORT is given in conjunction with external beam radiation, a single dose

Box 28-1	Enneking Staging System for Bone Sarcomas

GRADE

LOW GRADE (G1)
- Parosteal osteosarcoma
- Endosteal osteosarcoma
- Secondary chondrosarcoma
- Fibrosarcoma, low grade
- Atypical malignant fibrous histiocytoma
- Giant cell tumor
- Adamantinoma

HIGH GRADE (G2)
- Classic osteosarcoma
- Radiation-induced sarcoma
- Paget's sarcoma
- Primary chondrosarcoma
- Fibrosarcoma, high grade
- Giant cell sarcoma

LOCAL EXTENT
INTRACOMPARTMENTAL (T1)
- Intraosseous
- Parosseous
- Intrafascial

EXTRACOMPARTMENTAL (T2)
- Soft tissue extension
- Extrafascial or deep fascial extension

DISTANT METASTASES
M0: no distant metastases
M1: distant metastases present

STAGE GROUPING

STAGE	G	T	M
1A	G1	T1	M0
1B	G1	T2	M0
IIA	G2	T1	M0
IIB	G2	T2	M0
III	G1 or G2	T1 or T2	M1

Modified from Moss WT: *Radiation oncology*, ed 6, St. Louis, 1989, Mosby.

of 16 Gy is given, whereas doses of 50 to 60 Gy in a single fraction may be delivered if no other radiation is planned.[47] The addition of chemotherapy to the treatment repertoire has shown promise for control of osteosarcoma.

An advantage of IORT treatments is that normal tissue and critical structures in the vicinity of the tumor bed may be moved out of the field. This allows the delivery of high doses for radiation.

Before 1972, chemotherapy for osteosarcoma was ineffective. In 1972, however, doxorubicin or high doses of methotrexate were shown to produce significant tumor regression. Since then, other agents such as cisplatin, epidoxorubicin, ifosfamide, cyclophosphamide, etoposide (VP-16), and bleomycin have been the basis for adjuvant chemotherapy.[19,37,47] Dincbas et al.[19] performed a study on patients with nonmetastatic high-grade osteosarcomas. Patients were treated with neoadjuvant cisplatin, epidoxorubicin, ifosfamide, and methotrexate regimens. Preoperative radiation therapy was delivered to doses of 35 Gy in 10 fractions or 46 Gy in 23 fractions using parallel opposed ports. Definitive limb-sparing surgery was performed after the third course of chemotherapy, and then six courses of postsurgery chemotherapy were administered.[19] Results from this multidisciplinary approach showed a tumor necrosis rate of 90% or greater in 87% of patients. The 5-year local control and overall survival rates were 97.5% and 48.4%, respectively. Four percent of patients had local failures and 56% developed distant metastasis.[19] The conclusion from this study is that local control of osteosarcoma is improving using a multimodality approach, but overall cure and prevention of metastases remain dilemmas.

The most common metastases from osteosarcoma occur in the lungs and, less commonly, bone.[31] This seems to occur in approximately 80% of patients within 1 to 2 years after the initial diagnosis.[47] Another issue to consider in the treatment of any malignancy is the increasing incidence of acquiring a secondary malignancy. Osteosarcoma is the most common postradiation sarcoma of bone.[36] Unlike primary osteosarcomas, postradiation-induced osteosarcomas do not respond as well to chemotherapy. Median survival for this type of tumor is 23 months.[36]

Other complications from treatment of osteosarcoma include hematological spread, nephrotoxicity, and neurotoxicities from chemotherapy. Side effects of radiation are site dependent and may include skin reaction, reduction in blood counts, and pathologic fractures.[19,47] It is noteworthy to recall that it is normal to experience more side effects when several modalities are used in a combined sequence.

Therapeutic approaches currently being investigated include the use of tumor suppressor gene therapy. This therapy focuses to restore the functionality of a tumor suppressor gene that is inactivated in cancer cells.[63] Mutations in the *p53* gene are increasing in frequency with osteosarcoma cases, and researchers are optimistic that adenovirus-mediated *p53* tumor suppressor gene therapy will increase clinical benefits for patients with osteosarcoma.

Chondrosarcoma. Chondrosarcomas are malignant mesenchymal neoplasms that produce cartilage, but no osteoid, and may occur in any cartilage-forming bone[33] (Figure 28-11). The prognosis of patients with chondrosarcomas and benign chordomas depends on two factors. One factor is the histologic grade of the tumor. Lesions are graded on a scale of 1 to 3, with 3 being the most anaplastic (exhibiting a loss of cell differentiation). Low-grade tumors are locally invasive and do not tend to metastasize, making them easier to control. High-grade tumors, in contrast, often metastasize, particularly to the lungs, giving the patient a poorer prognosis and making tumor control more difficult. The other prognostic indicator is the tumor's location. If the tumor is located peripherally, it is more surgically accessible; however, if it appears in the pelvis, sacral area, or head and neck, surgery may not be possible or the tumor may be unable to be completely resected.

Surgical resection is the primary method of treatment for chondrosarcomas and chordomas, the benign condition, which includes removal of the entire mass, with adequate bone and soft tissue margins. External beam radiation therapy (EBRT) does not usually play a role in treating these patients because of

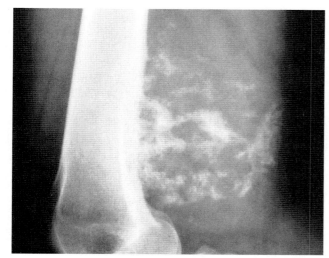

Figure 28-11. Large chondrosarcoma located in the area of the distal femur. Note the prominent dense calcification of the lesion. (From Eisenberg RL, Dennis CA: *Comprehensive radiographic pathology*, ed 2, St. Louis, 1995, Mosby.)

the radioresistant qualities of this type of tumor. However, radiation therapy is used definitively when the tumor cannot be completely removed due to proximity of critical structures such as the brain stem, cranial nerves, and major blood vessels. Doses of 40 to 55 Gy and, in some cases, 70 Gy can be delivered to achieve local control.[33,47] Recently, photon-based radiosurgery or charged particle radiotherapy has been used to improve tumor control rates. In a study performed at the Mayo Clinic, 29 patients with chondrosarcoma or chordoma underwent stereotactic radiosurgery. Nineteen patients had adjuvant EBRT to doses of 45 to 54 Gy. The range of stereotactic radiosurgery doses was 10 to 20 Gy, and the patients were followed for 4.5 years. Seventy-five percent of all patients and 100% of patients with chondrosarcoma had tumor shrinkage or control. Reports of 89% and 32% actuarial tumor control were documented at 2 and 5 years, respectively.[33] Patients who underwent radiosurgery alone had no radiotoxicity, and those who had combined EBRT experienced complications including cranial nerve deficits, radiation necrosis, and pituitary dysfunction. This study shows that treatment of chondrosarcomas is still very challenging, and to date, chemotherapy agents do not appear to have any substantial effect on the disease.

 A lead wire, or radiopaque marker, outlining the incision that must be treated is helpful when treatment ports are designed. It is important to remember that the marker gives information at the skin surface only and not at depth. Care must be taken if angled fields are planned.[7]

Fibrosarcomas. Treatment for fibrosarcomas involving bone consists of an aggressive surgical procedure using wide or radical excision. Because these tumors have a high incidence rate of recurrence, even with aggressive surgery, postoperative radiation is now recommended. Fibrosarcomas are not highly radiosensitive, but irradiation is recommended for inoperable tumors, postoperative residual disease, and palliation. Doses of

66 to 70 Gy using a shrinking-field technique are recommended if radiation therapy is prescribed to control a skeletal fibrosarcoma.[47] The prognostic indicators for fibrosarcomas include the histologic grade, the location in the bone (medullary or periosteal), and whether the lesions arise de novo (anew) or are secondary to a preexisting bony condition.[47]

Malignant Fibrous Histiocytoma. Treatment for MFH is similar to that of many bone tumors. Obtaining a complete local excision will maximize the chances for prolonged relapse-free survival.[45] Skin grafts, amputation, and disarticulation (separation of bone at the joint) are common methods of treatment, as well.[9] Preoperative and postoperative chemotherapy clinical trials in conjunction with surgery to investigate limited surgical approaches are under way. Radiation therapy may be used as a definitive treatment for inoperable lesions, as well as being administered palliatively. Doses of 46 to 66 Gy may be delivered using external beam radiation and single fractions of 15 to 30 Gy given using an IORT technique.[47] MFH of the bone carries a poorer prognosis than does MFH of soft tissue. The disease is extremely aggressive and overall entails a poor prognosis for most patients with the disease.[47]

Giant Cell Tumors. GCTB are treated locally because of their low propensity to metastasize. Current management of this disease is dependent on the anatomic site of the tumor and how much bone destruction has occurred. For the majority of tumors, surgical curettage is the treatment of choice. However, the local control rate for curettage alone is approximately 61%, so additional therapies such as intracavitary high-speed burr drilling and locally applied liquid nitrogen, phenol, or hydrogen peroxide are often used.[11] If a patient is a candidate for local excision, local control rates as high as 91% can be achieved with no additional treatment.[11]

Radiation therapy is reserved for GCTB that occur in areas where complete surgical excision is not possible, as in the case of large or axially located tumors.[47] Recommended doses of radiation to the tumor range from 45 to 55 Gy protracted over 5 to 6 weeks. The University of Texas M. D. Anderson Cancer Center treated 25 patients for management of GCTB. Radiation doses of 25 to 65 Gy were delivered. The actuarial local control rate was 62% and 57% at 5 and 10 years, respectively, and the overall survival rates were 91% and 84%, respectively.[11] Twelve patients had recurrence and were successfully treated with additional therapy; four treatments included interferon-α2b therapy. The action of interferon is to inhibit tumor angiogenesis; continued research in this area is being performed. The M. D. Anderson data suggested that radiation therapy can be administered adjuvantly with surgery or as an alternative treatment when resection is not a viable option. The risk of a benign tumor transforming into a malignant giant cell tumor after radiation is a possibility, although reports show this occurring more often in patients who were treated with low-dose orthovoltage units.[5]

Multiple Myeloma. Myeloma is a low-growth fraction tumor with only a small percentage of tumor cells in cycle at any time (Figure 28-12). This means that the time before patients need treatment can range from 1 to 3 years, with the actual time of treatment ranging from 1 to 10 years or longer.[66]

Patients who have advanced renal disease in addition to multiple myeloma have a poorer prognosis. Other findings

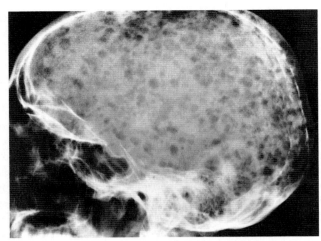

Figure 28-12. Abundance of lytic lesions scattered throughout the skull in this patient with multiple myeloma. Flat bones (such as the skull, vertebrae, ribs, and pelvis) tend to be more affected. (From Eisenberg RL, Dennis CA: *Comprehensive radiographic pathology*, ed 2, St. Louis, 1995, Mosby.)

associated with shortened median survival times or remission durations include age older than 65 years, severe anemia , hypercalcemia, elevated blood urea nitrogen (BUN), elevated M protein, hypoalbuminemia, and a high tumor cell burden. In addition, patients responding rapidly to treatment have shorter median survival time and shorter remission duration than do patients responding more slowly. Patients diagnosed early in the disease process are much more likely to have a longer survival or remission duration.[66]

The treatment that is typically used for patients with multiple myeloma is a combination of chemotherapy and radiation therapy. EBRT is effective in controlling the pain from a bony lesion, whereas chemotherapy is given with a curative intent. Survival can be increased from 1 to 4 years with new chemotherapy agents.[4] Common chemotherapy agents include melphalan and cyclophosphamide.[64]

Autologous stem cell transplantation following high-dose chemotherapy is also becoming a common treatment regimen.[51] This is currently the preferred treatment for patients younger than the age of 60 years.[64]

Radiation therapy plays an important role in the management of patients with multiple myeloma. Most commonly, patients present with pain at the lesion site. A dose of 30 Gy is effective in controlling the pain in most of these patients.[71] With the use of irradiation to treat localized lesions, the field must be planned carefully so that the entire lesion is treated. In addition, generous margins should be used in the treatment of osteolytic lesions of the long bones. For these reasons, MRI has been supportive in guiding the location, planning, and treatment portals for a lesion. The objective should be to treat the entire lesion but spare as much normal tissue as possible. Figure 28-13 shows a single posterior treatment field for disease in the sacrum and lumbar vertebrae.

Total-body irradiation has been used in instances when patients have failed to respond to all alkylating chemotherapeutic agents. This mode of treatment is a last resort to treat unresponsive patients. In addition, these patients already have blood-forming

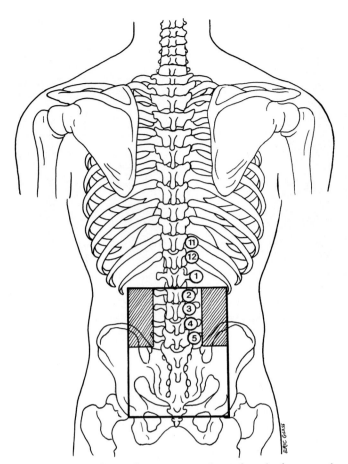

Figure 28-13. Schematic representation of a single posterior treatment field for metastatic disease in the sacrum and lumbar vertebrae. Shaded areas represent shielding blocks used to spare normal tissue. Circled numbers correspond to thoracic and lumbar vertebrae.

systems and immune systems compromised by chemotherapy and probably would not tolerate total-body irradiation.

The use of **radionuclides** in conjunction with proteasome inhibitors is becoming more common. Proteasome inhibitors, such as bortezomib, inhibit growth of myeloma cells and decrease drug resistance.[12,34] A study by Goel et al.[27] showed promising results with the use of bortezomib and radionuclides to treat multiple myeloma. They found that this combination was effective in slowing myeloma cell growth. One major reason for this is that bortezomib is considered a radiosensitizer.

Surgery does not play an important role in the treatment of multiple myeloma but is used in certain instances. If a patient has a pending pathologic fracture, it may be appropriate to stabilize the bone before initiating radiation therapy. In addition, for paraspinal masses, which can be extremely large and can cause paralysis and pain, debulking the tumor before radiation therapy is initiated may be advised.

Supportive intervention for these patients is extremely important and should not be forgotten. This type of care includes treatment for anemia, hypercalcemia, azotemia (abnormal levels of urea, creatinine, body waste compounds, and other nitrogen-rich compounds in the blood), and frequent infections. These patients cannot be cured, so in addition to palliative therapies for the relief of pain, support care is necessary to sustain a desirable quality of life.

Ewing's Sarcoma. Treatment of Ewing's bone sarcoma includes surgery, chemotherapy, and radiation therapy. A combination of the three modalities is most effective in achieving local control and improving long-term survival.[72] Overall survival rates of 50% or greater may be achieved with the use of these modalities.[8]

Surgery is now becoming one of the main treatment options for Ewing's sarcoma, simply because of advanced surgical procedures. At one time, surgical resection caused great morbidity to the patient, especially those with bulky tumors. Amputation was more common years ago than it is now.[35] Surgical reconstruction may be an option for young patients who want to avoid less-than-satisfactory cosmetic results. Although there are several types of techniques used, the decision greatly depends on the patient's age, tumor location, and where additional therapies will be used.[8]

Ewing's sarcoma is sensitive to chemotherapy, and newer agents have become more effective in increasing overall survival rates. Before the use of these agents, survival rates did not reach 10%.[8] Common chemotherapy agents include vincristine, doxorubicin (Adriamycin), cyclophosphamide, ifosfamide, and etoposide.[35] Chemotherapy can be useful in reducing the need for radical surgery or high-dose, large-volume irradiation. Another option is to administer chemotherapy before surgery to shrink the tumor for easier removal. The ultimate goal for patients with Ewing's bone sarcoma is the eradication of the entire tumor and the preservation of as much function as possible at the same time.

Most patients with Ewing's sarcoma will undergo surgery and chemotherapy. However, there is a demand for radiation therapy, especially for patients with unresectable tumors. Pelvis and spine tumors are typically more aggressive, and the use of surgery can be limited.[35] In these cases, achieving local control with radiation therapy becomes important. In patients in whom surgery is performed, radiation therapy is used postoperatively to treat positive surgical margins. It is possible to achieve local control rates of 93% with surgery and external beam therapy.[32]

A treatment volume includes a 2-cm margin around the soft tissue component and the entire bone, to doses of 55 to 60 Gy for definitive cases. Preoperative and postoperative cases typically require a lower dose. In postoperative patients with residual disease, a 3-cm margin is treated in addition to the tumor.[35] Important considerations include the treatment of the surgical scar to eradicate any cancer cells present and the shaping of fields to maintain lymphatic drainage and avoid fluid buildup in the extremity.[15]

Bone marrow transplantation (BMT) may be a promising treatment for patients whose prognosis is poor. Studies are under way that use BMT in the hope of gaining positive results for patients with metastases at the time of the diagnosis.

Prognostic indicators in patients who have Ewing's bone sarcoma include the location of the tumor, the amount of extension at diagnosis, and the patient's age at diagnosis. Pelvic tumors carry a poorer prognosis because of the greater incidence of extraosseous extension.[40]

The most important prognostic factor listed for Ewing's bone sarcoma is the extent of the disease at the time of the diagnosis. Several variables are directly or indirectly related to this factor. Patients who have grossly metastatic disease at the time of the diagnosis usually experience a poor outcome. Early studies have shown that patients with bone or bone marrow involvement did not do as well as patients with limited pulmonary involvement. Another prognostic factor is the extension in the soft tissue component of the primary tumor, producing a less favorable prognosis than that in patients with limited or no soft tissue involvement. In addition, because the bone is involved (>8 cm or <8 cm), the size of the primary tumor may influence the likelihood of a successful outcome. High serum levels of lactic dehydrogenase appear to be associated with a poor outcome, possibly because they reflect the tumor burden or activity of the tumor. A high leukocyte count may also be associated with an increased risk of tumor recurrence.[15]

Another important factor with Ewing's bone sarcoma is the site of the involvement, which is relevant to the success of therapy. The involvement of the pelvis or sacrum is associated with a worse prognosis than that of the proximal extremities (humerus and femur) or central sites such as the ribs and vertebrae. These sites are less favorable than the involvement of a distal extremity site, which makes treatment much easier. The local recurrence rate in the primary site is 15% for children with extremity lesions, 47% for children with rib primaries, and 69% for children with pelvic tumors.[15]

Metastatic Bone Disease. The majority of malignant bone lesions are metastatic. The radiation therapist treats more patients with metastatic bone disease than patients with primary bone lesions. The development of bone metastases in patients with cancer is a common and often catastrophic event. Bone metastases give rise to pain, pathologic fractures, frequent neurologic deficits, and forced immobility, causing a significant decrease in the quality of life for these patients. Patients with breast, prostate, kidney, thyroid, and lung carcinomas are likely to develop bone metastases sometime during the course of their advanced disease.

Metastatic bone disease is not curable; therefore, maintaining a certain quality of life for these patients becomes important. The prognosis for patients who have metastatic bone disease depends on the primary site, histology, and degree of metastases at the time of diagnosis. Relieving the pain, decreasing the need for and amount of narcotic medication, and maintaining ambulation are the first and most vital steps for improving the quality of the patient's life. Patients with metastatic bone cancer may survive for many years with the disease because the lesions are rarely the cause of death; therefore, all aspects of their care should be considered in the initial management plans.[56]

The treatment goal of bone metastases is concentrated on the palliation of pain and the prevention of fractures to weight-bearing bones. To accomplish an effective method of treatment, a careful evaluation of the tumor type, extent of the disease, degree of symptomatology, and physical status of the patient must be completed.[16]

The use of radiation therapy is important in the **local control** of the lesion, relieving pain and preventing the loss of function of the bone or bones involved. However, radiation therapy does not address the systemic disease, which may require hormonal therapy or chemotherapy, depending on the histology of the primary site. Surgery becomes an option for these patients when the stabilization of a weight-bearing bone is needed or when debulking of an extradural mass is necessary to relieve excruciating pain. Radiation therapy is usually introduced after the surgical procedure to obtain local control.[56,65]

Radiation portals need to encompass all involved areas but spare uninvolved tissue when possible. If stabilization has been performed surgically, radiation therapy should be initiated as soon as the wound has healed. The portal should include the fixation device and any micrometastases that may have been dislodged during the surgical procedure. However, a strip of soft tissue should be left unirradiated to preserve lymphatic drainage.[56]

 Often, patients treated for malignancies in the lower extremities may need to be reversed on the treatment couch, with the feet toward the gantry. It is very important that this position is documented clearly in the treatment chart.

The treatment of bone metastases involving the pelvis and vertebrae must be carefully planned. The portal should encompass the area involved with the tumor yet avoid uninvolved bone (to spare bone marrow) and other normal tissue. In the treatment of the spine, the portal should include the symptomatic vertebrae, with a one-vertebral-body margin above and below the involved vertebrae. If necessary, custom-made blocks or multileaf collimation can be used to shield uninvolved bone and reduce the amount of small bowel in the field.[56,65]

The introduction of strontium-89 and samarium-153 has provided excellent results in bone pain relief for patients with prostate and, to a lesser degree, breast cancer that is metastatic to bone. [89]Sr and [153]Sm are radiopharmaceutical agents used for the palliation of metastatic bone pain and may be administered in radiation oncology or nuclear medicine facilities. [89]Sr is a pure beta-emitter that causes minimal irradiation of the normal tissues. This agent localizes to osteoblastic areas or skeletal metastatic lesions from the primary cancer. The radioisotope has a therapeutic half-life of 50.5 days; therefore, its therapeutic effect may last up to 15 months. Approximately 1 to 3 weeks may pass before the patient notices any substantial effect.[64] Radionuclide therapy is generally administered to patients on an outpatient basis. The agent is introduced via a slow intravenous push into a peripheral vein. Patients receiving ^{89}Sr may experience a mild flushing sensation during the administration process, but otherwise they feel nothing.

Because this agent can cause a slight reduction in platelet and white blood cell counts 5 to 6 weeks after treatment, patients must have a complete blood count taken before the administration of [89]Sr. The patient's blood counts are monitored at prescribed regular intervals to ensure that the counts are stabilized.[65]

As with any form of treatment, possible acute and chronic side effects and complications are possible when treating patients with bone tumors. Patients receiving multimodality treatment involving combined radiation therapy and chemotherapy are at higher risk for moderate to severe complications.

This is somewhat normal when more than a single modality is used for treatment.[19] The type and severity of the side effects depend on many factors, such as the type of disease, chemotherapeutic agents, and anatomic site of the radiation therapy portal. Aggressive systemic treatment (chemotherapy) and local treatment (radiation) may cause acute problems, including **erythema**, fever, neutropenia, mucositis, nausea, vomiting, and diarrhea. Late or chronic effects of radiation to bone may lead to growth delays in pediatrics, scoliosis after vertebral irradiation, increased sensitivity to chronic infection, fracture, and necrosis. Radiation-induced malignancies are also sequels of treatment.[47]

At the time of the diagnosis, all of the complications (acute and long term) must be considered before a course of treatment is planned and initiated. Modifications may be necessary for obtaining the best technique while trying to prevent complications. In general, the side effects experienced by patients with primary bone cancer are fairly well tolerated. Because the amputation of a limb is sometimes necessary to control the disease, the use of prosthetic devices allows patients to lead a somewhat normal life. Follow-up care and close monitoring of these patients are extremely important.

CASE I

Fibrous Dysplasia

A 26-year-old African American woman presented with a growth in her hard palate/premaxilla. There is a personal history of smoking and a family history of cancer with her father diagnosed with prostate cancer and osteosarcoma. She reported the lump growing rapidly, having tripled in size in 3 months. On examination, the clinical diagnosis was fibrous dysplasia. Surgical resection was performed with an iliac bone reconstruction.

The final pathology demonstrated a chondroblastic osteosarcoma with positive margins at the left lateral and posterior resection margins.

Are the etiologic factors consistent with this patient's diagnosis?

She received 12 weeks of systemic chemotherapy including ifosfamide and Adriamycin.

A second surgical resection was then performed with less than 50% necrosis of tumor remaining; therefore, an additional three cycles of ifosfamide/ VP-16 and three cycles of ifosfamide/Adriamycin were given.

Why do you think a second resection was performed?

Side effects of chemotherapy included prolonged periods of pancytopenia. The patient enjoyed a remission period of approximately 16 months when a 6-mm recurrence was found on a follow-up CT. She then underwent a maxillectomy and later extraction of teeth in preparation for radiation therapy.

On consultation in radiation oncology, the patient was educated that the role of radiation therapy in osteosarcoma of the head and neck is controversial due to the tumor being relatively radioresistant. Because standard treatment had failed for this patient, radiation therapy seemed reasonable to obtain local control.

What tumor characteristics make this case radioresistant in comparison to other histologies?

A conventional simulation was performed to plan for an intensity-modulated radiation therapy (IMRT) treatment course. The patient was immobilized with an Aquaplast, cervical headrest, and standard bite block. Her arms were on her abdomen, with her hands holding a ring, and there was a sponge under her knees. A right and left lateral film, with field size 5 × 21 cm, was obtained for multileaf intensity modulating collimator (MIMiC), IMRT planning. The dose was prescribed to a total dose of 66 Gy—50 Gy initially and 16 Gy to a boost field in a total of 33 fractions. There were 7 arc fields, using 6-MV photons, prescribed to the 87% and 90% isodose lines, respectively.

The volume treated was confined to the oral cavity and maxillary sinus. Regional lymphatics were not electively irradiated in light of low risk of lymphatic metastasis from well-differentiated osteosarcoma. The dose delivered to the cord was 11.6 Gy.

The patient experienced significant mucositis during and after therapy, with a total weight loss of 20 pounds.

What might you suggest to manage these side effects?

Pain management included a fentanyl (Duragesic) patch, viscous lidocaine, and morphine (MS Contin). The patient also was prescribed fluoxetine (Prozac) for depression. The course of radiation therapy was completed and the patient underwent 40 hyperbaric chamber treatments to aid in the healing of osteoradionecrosis of the right maxilla.

Upon follow-up the patient is disease free, requiring routine adjustments of her facial obturator. She is encouraged to continue mouth-opening exercises and strict oral hygiene. Overall, the patient is doing very well.

CASE II

Osteomyelitis

A 52-year-old white man, with an insignificant medical history, presented with flulike symptoms followed by pain in his right anterior thigh and groin. He was treated with a cortisone injection, but it was not effective.

What conditions might the physician have been trying to treat?

One week later, plain films and MRI were obtained. The studies showed a 7.3 × 7.6 cm destructive process in the subtrochanteric region that could mimic either infection or malignancy. A biopsy was performed, and the final diagnosis showed acute osteomyelitis of the right hip, as well as chondrosarcoma. The osteomyelitis was treated with cefazolin (Ancef) and levofloxacin (Levaquin). The Levaquin was discontinued due to chills and considerable fatigue. His condition was deemed stable, but he could not undergo surgery for resection and reconstruction at that time because of the size of tumor, so neoadjuvant chemotherapy was ordered. The patient received three cycles of Adriamycin, ifosfamide, and mesna with excellent response. A resection and right total hip arthroplasty were then performed. It was noteworthy that the preoperative MRI showed a lesion in the right sacral spine that was thought to be a separate chondrosarcoma primary, but this lesion was surgically unapproachable (Figure 28-14).

After 3 months of healing and rehabilitation, the patient was seen in radiation oncology to treat the right hip surgical bed and give definitive

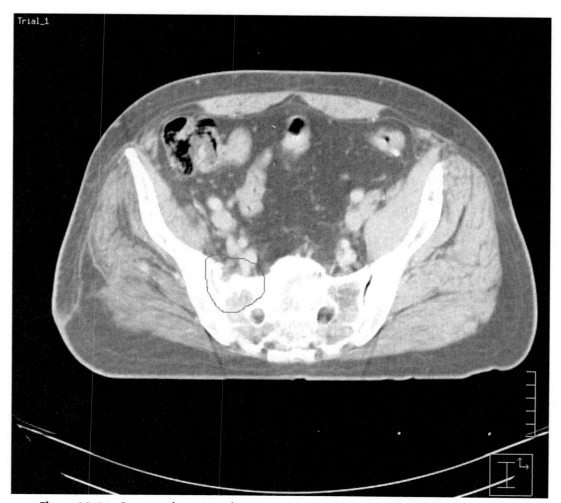

Figure 28-14. Computed tomography treatment planning image denoting sacral mass.

radiation therapy to the sacral lesion. The patient was simulated using CT guidance, positioned supine in a Vac-Lok with two pillows, no knee sponge, and toes together. His arms were on his abdomen, with his hands holding a ring.

What would happen to the isocenter if the patient was treated with a knee sponge, considering the simulation did not include one?

The prescription was written to give 45 Gy in 35 fractions to an anteroposterior/posteroanterior (AP/PA) comprehensive field encompassing the right hip and sacral spine (Figure 28-15); 25-MV photons were used to deliver 1.8 Gy/fraction. A sacral boost was delivered via a six-field conformal technique (right anterior oblique, left anterior oblique, left lateral, left posterior oblique, right posterior oblique, right lateral). Again, 25-MV photons were used to deliver 1.8 Gy/fraction for a dose of 19.8 Gy, bringing the total dose to the sacrum to 64.8 Gy. The patient tolerated treatment well with no interruptions.

Approximately 16 months postradiation, the patient shows no evidence of disease. He states that he has a slight clicking in his thigh due to the prosthesis but can carry out most activities with minimal limitations. Otherwise, he is doing well.

SOFT TISSUE SARCOMAS

Soft tissue sarcomas (STS) are a class of malignant tumors occurring in the extraskeletal connective tissue. Primarily, these lesions arise from mesenchymal origins. These tissues include all those that provide connection, support, and locomotion. They are grouped together because they share similarities in appearance pathologically, as well as in clinical presentation and behaviors. Although in many respects they resemble bone tumors and are often associated with primary bone cancer, they may also occur in any anatomic structure containing connective tissue such as blood vessel walls and viscera.

This section of the chapter presents fundamental information critical to understanding the nature of this disease, including its etiology, tissue derivation, histology, staging, grading, and patterns of spread. Factors affecting treatment decision making and options in radiation therapy treatment planning and modalities are addressed.

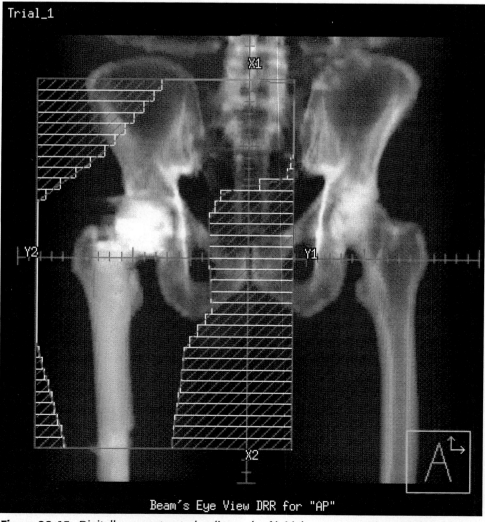

Figure 28-15. Digitally reconstructed radiograph of initial anteroposterior sacral and femur field.

Natural History

The natural history of STS is highly dependent on the site of the initial neoplasm and its grade. The local growth pattern of STS follows the lines of least resistance in the longitudinal axis of the **primary site compartment**. The primary site compartment consists of the natural anatomic boundaries surrounding the STS primary. It is composed of common fascia plane(s) of muscles, bone, joint, skin, subcutaneous tissues, and major neurovascular structures.[53]

As a tumor progresses and grows, it pushes away other structures and forms a **pseudocapsule** that is made of compressed normal and fibrotic tissue. Trunk and head and neck primaries are generally high grade and tend to invade adjacent muscle groups, whereas extremity tumors spread along the longitudinal axis of muscular compartments.[42] The likelihood of regional lymph node involvement is low at approximately 2% to 10%.[43] Intermediate- and high-grade lesions typically undergo hematogenous metastases, primarily to the lungs. Retroperitoneal primaries also have a high potential for lung metastases but also spread to the liver and other abdominal structures.

Epidemiology

In comparison with other malignancies, the incidence of STS is fairly low. There are approximately 10,000 new cases of STS diagnosed each year, accounting for 1% of malignancies in adults.[1,50] Although the prevalence is low, the overall mortality rate is considerably high at approximately 3500 deaths per year.[67]

The male-to-female ratio for STS is roughly equal at approximately 1.5:1.[1,44] STS are diagnosed most often in the fifth and sixth decades of life, although diagnosis can be made at any age.[38,52] Rhabdomysarcoma, a form of STS, is most common in children, with the peak incidence in the first two decades of life and median age at diagnosis of approximately 5 years old.[60,61] As previously stated, STS can occur anywhere in the body, with the extremities accounting for 60%, followed by the retroperitoneum at 19%. Fifteen percent originate in the abdominal/thoracic wall, and approximately 6% originate in the head and neck region.[46] Of the STS found in the extremities, most occur in the lower extremity, especially the thigh.

The overall incidence of STS has been increasing over the past 50 years. Some literature attributes the increase to the increase in Kaposi's sarcoma, which is often associated with acquired immunodeficiency syndrome (AIDS).[13] Improved methods of detecting and diagnosing the disease may also correlate with increased incidence. Rates of STS are generally highest in African Americans, and no geographic location significance has been identified.[42]

Etiology

The etiology of STS is unidentifiable, although there is an association with a variety of genetic and environmental factors. Certain viral infections, such as the Epstein-Barr virus in those with AIDS, have shown an increased incidence of leiomyosarcoma.[41] Radiation exposure is potentially an etiologic agent for sarcoma. Historically, radiation therapy for benign conditions such as tuberculosis and thyroid disease gave rise to sarcomas. Therapeutic irradiation for lymphoma, cervical and testicular cancer, or breast cancer has increased the risk of a secondary malignancy 3 to 15 years post–radiation therapy.[13] The benefits of radiation in such circumstances, however, outweigh the potential risk. A rare complication of breast cancer treatment called Stewart-Treves syndrome (a chronic lymphedema) may increase the risk of developing angiosarcomas.[13] Several genetic conditions are associated with an increased risk of STS. The most common is neurofibromatosis type 1. It carries a 10% lifetime risk of malignant peripheral-nerve sheath tumors.[13] Germline mutations in the *RB1* tumor suppressor gene of children with hereditary retinoblastoma place them at an exceptionally high risk of STS and osteosarcoma.[13,42] Patients with Li-Fraumeni syndrome (an unusual intraabdominal desmoid tumor) also have a 30-fold increase of developing a sarcoma at 45 years of age or younger.[10] Industrial toxins such as 2,3,7,8-tetrachlorodibenzo-*p*-dioxin are implemented as etiologic agents for sarcomas but are controversial, as is the concept of those exposed to the dioxane-containing Agent Orange.[10]

General Anatomy and Physiology, Including Pertinent Lymphatic Considerations

The embryonic ancestry of STS begins in the primitive **mesoderm**. The loosely formed network of cells in the mesoderm, the primitive mesenchyme, and the ectoderm give rise to the most common connective tissues, such as the pleura, peritoneum, pericardium, walls and endothelium of blood vessels, bone, cartilage, muscles, and soft connective tissue. Visceral connective tissue, similar muscle organs, and smooth muscle organs (e.g., the kidney, ureters, uterus, gonads, heart, and a variety of hematopoietic tissues) all derive from the remainder of the primitive mesoderm. Refer back to Figure 28-2 for a schematic representation of tissue origin.

Skeletal muscle is composed of striated muscle fibers varying from very large in size to extremely small. Fibers of normal muscle can be found in Figure 28-16. Muscle cells are specialized, with their primary function being contraction. This allows the body to move, breathe, and maintain posture.[17] Lymphatic drainage is site specific and plays little role in the management of STS. Skeletal muscle has a limited capacity to respond to tumor formation, so once symptoms present, diagnosis can be fairly straightforward.

Clinical Presentation

Symptoms of STS are often nonspecific. Most patients initially present with a painless, gradually enlarging mass. Average time from onset to diagnosis is reported at 4 to 6 months.[43] The size of the tumor at diagnosis is site dependent. Head and neck and distal extremities are likely to be diagnosed earlier than are thigh or retroperitoneal tumors. Other presenting symptoms of site-specific STS are weakness, increased pressure such as paresthesia, distal edema, or presence of warmth or distended vascularity when fixed to other structures.[13,57]

 Although soft tissue sarcomas spread readily through hematopoietic pathways, spread locally along muscle planes, tendinous attachments, and the tissue compartments from which they originate is possible.

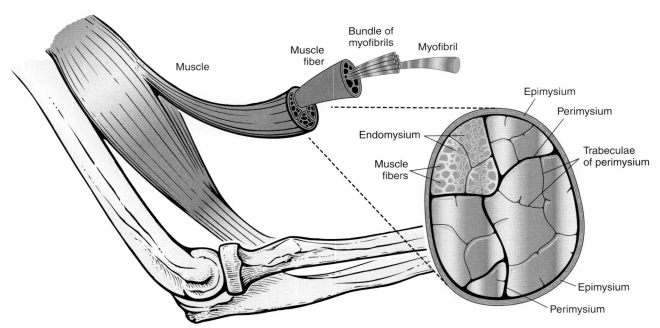

Figure 28-16. Normal muscle anatomy. (From Damjanov I: *Pathology for the health professions*, ed 3, St. Louis, 2006, Saunders.)

Detection and Diagnosis

Once the patient has consulted a physician, a detailed history and physical examination, including diagnostic imaging, are needed. MRI has been adopted as the modality of choice for STS detection because of its exceptional soft tissue contrast and specificity[50,57] (Figures 28-17 and 28-18). CT is still widely used in STS imaging. Positron emission tomography (PET) is quickly becoming an essential part of the workup in seeking metastases, additional lesions, or lymph node extensions.[38] Chest radiographs and CT scans of the chest, in indicated cases, should be performed for complete staging, because most STS metastasize to the lungs.[23] Bone scans may be used to look for other metastatic disease.

After localization of the tumor, a biopsy to obtain viable tumor tissue is essential to identify the histology of the tumor and provide information in determining the treatment protocol. There are various methods of biopsy. An open biopsy has a relatively high risk of complications but a small likelihood of misdiagnosis, whereas needle biopsies will have fewer complications but are sometimes less definitive and accurate.[38,39] The open biopsy should be performed with consideration of subsequent definitive operative procedures, because the biopsy site

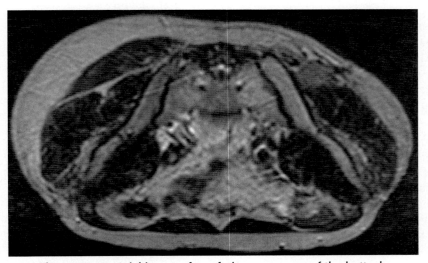

Figure 28-17. Axial image of a soft tissue sarcoma of the buttock.

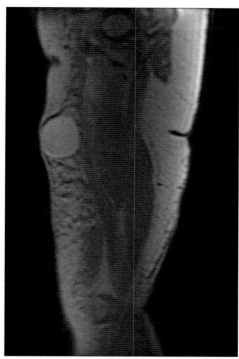

Figure 28-18. Magnetic resonance imaging coronal view of soft tissue sarcoma in the lower extremity.

and tissue that may be contaminated will need to be entirely removed during resection. Inadequately performed biopsies will lead to increased extent of resection and increased volume to be treated with radiation.[42]

As stated previously, the needle biopsy results in fewer complications. Two methods of needle biopsy are fine-needle biopsy and core biopsy. It is important to acquire enough tissue for a pathologic diagnosis, and with needle biopsies, this may be a concern if the tumor is not easily accessible. Surgeons advocate for both types of procedures, but with the core-needle biopsy determining 80% of the subtype and grade of a tumor and having qualified pathologists with a diagnostic accuracy of greater than 95%, open biopsies are becoming a less common practice.[13]

Pathology

Sarcomas are classified histologically and named according to the tissues in which they arise. Currently there are more than 50 histologic types of STS. The most common in adults are MFH (which can be classified as both a tumor of the bone and as a tumor of the soft tissue) at 28%, leiomyosarcoma (12%), liposarcoma (15%), synovial sarcoma (10%), and malignant peripheral nerve sheath tumors (6%).[46] Rhabdomyosarcoma is the most common histology in the pediatric population.[61] The histologic distinction will aid in the staging of STS.

Staging

Staging is essential for treatment planning and prognosis. There are two primary systems for staging STS—the **Musculoskeletal Tumor Society (MSTS)** and **American Joint Commission on Cancer (AJCC)**.[2]

The MSTS system has three components including the grade of the tumor (G1 being a low-grade tumor and G2 representing high-grade), anatomic location (T1 being compartmentalized and T2 being extracompartmental), and presence or absence of metastases (M1 and M0, respectively).[38] Tumors are then defined as follows:

Stage IA	G1, T1, M0
Stage IB	G1, T2, M0
Stage IIA	G2, T1, M0
Stage IIB	G2, T2, M0
Stage III	M1 with any G or T

The second system set forth by the AJCC looks at the tumor's grade, size of primary tumor, regional lymph node involvement, and metastasis. These categories are listed in Box 28-2.

With both systems, higher grades and an increasing anatomic extent of the disease readily correlate to an advanced stage. In all but a few specific histopathologic tumors (synovial sarcomas and rhabdomyosarcomas), lymph node involvement is rare. However, when it is present, it is considered equivalent to metastasis and becomes more important than grade in determining the stage.[53]

Spread Patterns

STS initially invade aggressively along local, anatomically defined planes composed of neurovascular structures, fascia, and muscle bundles (Figure 28-19). Lymphatic extension is not common. Hematologic pathways are the primary routes of spread; the lung is the most common site of metastasis, followed much less commonly by the bones, liver, and skin.

Retroperitoneal sarcomas (RPS) have a 50% or greater local recurrence rate over 10 years, whereas extremity and truncal lesions recur at 20% during the same time interval.[10] On the other hand, the metastatic rate for visceral and high-grade extremity STS is approximately 50%. This emphasizes that death from STS is more likely to be due to systemic failure when the primary is a visceral or extremity lesion and more likely a consequence of local progression for lesions in the retroperitoneum.[10]

Treatment Considerations

Improved imaging procedures have resulted in better demonstration of tumor localization and metastatic extension. This improvement, in addition to radical wide-margin surgical techniques, sophisticated radiation therapy treatments, and effective antineoplastic agents, has helped the general management of STS progress to a multidisciplinary team approach. Treatment protocols are influenced by many factors, including size and site of the tumor, histologic stage and grade, its proximity to neurovascular or visceral structures, the patient's age and general health status, presence of metastases, and the desires of the patient and the patient's family.[38]

Surgery. Surgical resection with negative histologic margins used alone or with radiation and/or chemotherapy remains the standard of treatment for STS. However, its approach has changed drastically over the past 30 years.[67] In the 1970s, 50% of patients with limb STS underwent amputation, and even though local recurrence rates were less than 15%, a large number of patients died of metastatic disease. LSS with radiation therapy and chemotherapy obtain the same overall survival rates as for those undergoing amputation while conserving limb function. In contrast to those diagnosed with extremity STS, patients with retroperitoneal STS die of locally recurrent disease without distant metastasis.[46] This reiterates the importance of complete resection at presentation. Tumors of the head and neck region are also optimally treated with surgery.

Surgical procedures can be categorized several ways. Intralesional is resection within the tumor, often leaving gross tumor. A marginal technique involves cutting through the surrounding fibrous membrane, often leaving microscopic foci of tumor. Wide excision is cutting outside the membrane and compartment, leaving no other tumor than skip metastases, and

a radical procedure most likely involves amputation of the entire limb including the entire compartment in which the tumor was located.[38] When possible, most oncologic surgeons prefer to achieve a wide margin for high-grade sarcomas with a 1- to 2-cm margin of normal tissue.[46] Care must be taken during the procedure to avoid the zone of reactive tissue containing microscopic extensions, called the *pseudocapsule,* because this is a prime site for local recurrence.[67] Including the prior biopsy scar, excision scar, and/or drain site scar in the resection is also important to the procedure.[25]

Radiation Therapy. Based on the careful evaluation of individual patients, radiation therapy may be delivered by external beam radiation (including photon, electron, proton, and heavy particle beams), brachytherapy, IORT, or a combination of these modalities. Except for a few extremely small superficial tumors or when surgery is not medically recommended, adjuvant radiation therapy is combined with surgery and, in some cases, with chemotherapy for patients with large intermediate- and high-grade lesions, to increase local control rates. It is also for patients with incomplete resection, with tumors in close proximity to critical structures, or with locally advanced or recurrent disease.

There are proponents for both **preoperative** and **postoperative** radiation therapy, with studies reporting that both techniques achieve similar levels of local control with no significant difference in long-term survival.[49] Advantages associated with preoperative radiation therapy include the following[14,50]:
1. Better oxygenation of an undisturbed tumor bed might enhance the effects of radiation, necessitating a lower dose of radiation.
2. Preoperative radiation fields are smaller, irradiating less tissue, which may result in less morbidity from fracture, edema, and fibrosis.
3. By shrinking the tumor, surgical resection may be simplified, allowing for clear margins of resection.
4. Postoperative boosts may still be administered if close to positive margins because the tissue has not received a maximum dose of radiation.

The main drawbacks of preoperative radiation are the increased difficulty in pathologically assessing surgical margins after irradiation and the risk of complications in wound healing. Preoperative radiation therapy shows a 35% complication rate versus a 17% complication rate with postoperative radiation.[49] The implantation of fibroblasts into previously irradiated skin to help with wound healing is currently being studied, and if found effective, could be significant for patients receiving preoperative radiation therapy.

When preoperative radiation therapy is chosen, a total dose of approximately 50 Gy is delivered once or twice daily over a 5-week period. Postoperative doses range from 60 to 66 Gy.[59] These doses are needed for maximum cell kill to hypoxic tumor cells and are higher than what is needed for the oxygenated, undisturbed preoperative tumor beds.[13] An AP/PA parallel opposed field technique is most commonly used for treatment. Obliques are sometimes used for retroperitoneal lesions (RPS) to avoid critical structures such as the spinal cord and kidneys, and laterals are typically used in head and neck cases.[68] Due to

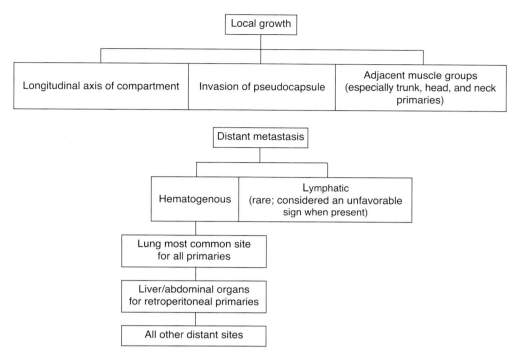

Figure 28-19. Patterns of soft tissue sarcoma (STS) spread. STS metastatic patterns progress from local invasion to the early hematogenous extension to the lung, liver, abdominal organs, and all other distant sites. Lymphatic spread is rare.

frequently large field sizes needed for RPS, doses may need to be limited to 45 to 50 Gy to minimize the dose to the bowel.

 When treating an upper extremity, it is important to extend the arm away from the body to minimize scatter radiation to the body and allow for any possible beam angle.[7]

Postoperative radiation therapy usually includes an original volume including the entire compartment and margins of 3 to 6 cm. The final volume, or boost volume, is the primary tumor volume plus a 2- to 3-cm margin. The scar should receive the full dose by inclusion tangentially or boosted with bolus or electrons. No regional lymph nodes, except for rhabdomyosarcomas, synovial sarcomas, and epithelioid sarcomas, are included with radiation therapy techniques. Total circumferential radiation of extremities must be avoided by leaving at least a 1- to 3-cm strip of skin and soft tissue to avoid future excessive fibrosis and edema.[42] Figure 28-20 illustrates a treatment setup for a lower extremity.

In cases of STS in the head and neck when surgery is not possible, IMRT or proton beam therapy may be used to escalate the dose while minimizing doses to normal tissue. Proton beams accomplish this because they deposit little of their energy in tissue until then end of their range, and that energy is deposited over a short distance. The result is a steep rise in absorbed dose known as the *Bragg peak*.[18] Several Bragg peaks of decreasing energies are superimposed on each other to achieve an optimal dose distribution. Doses of 74.4 to 81.6 Gy may be delivered in cases using proton beam therapy and IMRT.[43] Other charged particles being used for treatment of STS include neon, carbon, and

fast neutrons. These particles have a high linear energy transfer, which affects the biologic effectiveness and has less reliance on cell cycle, DNA repair, and oxygen enhancement ratio (OER) than other forms of radiation. Late normal tissue effects are currently a concern with this modality of treatment.[18]

Brachytherapy may be delivered as the only form of radiation following surgery or supplemental to external beam radiation. Management of STS with brachytherapy involves placement of after-loading catheters intraoperatively in the tumor bed approximately 1 cm apart. The catheters are loaded 4 to 7 days after surgery to allow for initial wound healing. Doses delivered are generally 46 Gy to a distance of 0.5 to 1 cm from the implant plane or 30 to 40 Gy if given as a boost.[18] Isotopes used in brachytherapy are ^{192}Ir and occasionally ^{125}I for select RPS and head and neck patients.[26]

IORT is another adjunctive modality for selected patients. This technique affords the delivery of a high dose to areas at risk with the advantage of sparing normal adjacent tissues. Typical electron energies used in IORT range from 9 to 15 MeV with doses of 10 to 20 Gy being delivered.[68] Doses of 15 Gy are often given for patients with microscopic disease, and patients having gross residual disease receive 20 Gy normalized to the 90% isodose line. IORT is advantageous for RPS and pelvic sarcomas because the tolerance doses for surrounding structures, which may be moved out of the treatment field, often constrain the dose that can be delivered to the tumor. Neuropathy is the major complication reported in 10% of patients undergoing IORT when nerves cannot be moved out of the treatment field.[68]

Overall, STS require fairly high doses of radiation to achieve local control and long-term survival. With the technologic

Radiation of anterior compartment of thigh

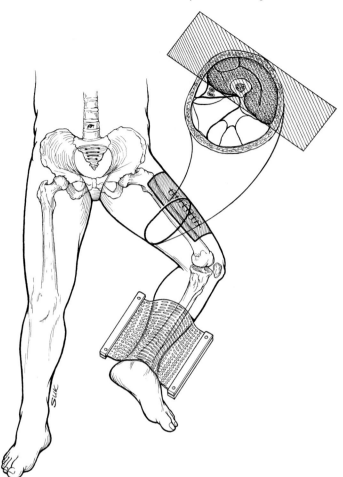

Figure 28-20. Appropriate treatment position demonstrating access to the tumor compartment.

advances of conformal therapy and IMRT, boost fields of 75 Gy are being reached.[18] These capabilities have had a positive influence on outcomes of long-term survival and limited morbidity from treatment.

Chemotherapy. The role of chemotherapy in the treatment of STS is controversial. Use of the modality is generally limited to patients with advanced, high-risk, recurrent, or metastatic tumors. When chemotherapy is administered, it is usually given adjuvantly or neoadjuvantly. Traditional chemotherapy approaches did not take into consideration the heterogeneity of STS. Chemosensitivity of a tumor depends on the tumor subtype. The likelihood a tumor will respond to chemotherapy and result in improved survival is further influenced by the grade of the tumor, the patient's age, performance status, and evidence of metastases. For example, a particularly aggressive uterine leiomyosarcoma may respond to high-dose gemcitabine with docetaxel, whereas paclitaxel and taxanes are more useful in treating scalp angiosarcomas.[22,29] Palliation is the primary role for patients with unresectable or metastatic disease. Ifosfamide and doxorubicin are generally used for these.

The Sarcoma Meta-analysis Collaboration studied 1568 patients receiving doxorubicin-based adjuvant therapy from 14 clinical trials, looking for improvements in overall survival, recurrence-free survival, and recurrence. Analysis showed a 10-year absolute benefit of 6% for local control, 10% for distant control, and 10% for recurrence-free survival; however, the overall survival rate for this 10-year period was only 4%.[55]

One area in which chemotherapy has shown positive outcomes is in the treatment of adolescents with Ewing's soft tissue sarcoma and rhabdosarcoma. For these patients, multiagent chemotherapy combined with radiation therapy in necessary. During the past 30 years, survival rates have improved from 25% to more than 70% in many cases of rhabdomyosarcoma and from 10% to more than 60% for Ewing's soft tissue sarcoma.[13,60] Acceptable cytotoxic agents for these subtypes of STS are vincristine, cyclophosphamide, dactinomycin, etoposide, cisplatin, ifosfamide, and doxorubicin.

Despite the mixed views of the role of chemotherapy, progress is being made. New chemotherapy agents and dosing regimens paired with radiation therapy are supplementing surgical approaches for the treatment of STS.

Role of Radiation Therapist

An understanding of the academic and scientific aspects of connective tissue sarcomas is important, and having the ability to apply that information with meaningful caregiving skills is the therapist's comprehensive responsibility to the patient. Simulation and treatment techniques may require critical thinking to position and immobilize the patient in a comfortable way following extensive surgery. Precision during treatment is important to maintain the lymphatic drainage needed for the extremity or minimizing dose to the spine and kidneys for a retroperitoneal lesion. The predilection for bone malignancies and STS to occur in younger populations in anatomic sites where disfigurement is often a threat may require educational and communication techniques unique to children, teenagers, young adults, and middle-aged patients. Bony metastases may occur in elderly patients, who also require specific communication skills. The therapist's relationship with the patient is based on trust, professionalism, and knowledge of the disease. Because everyone involved in the care of the patient must fully understand the importance of daily treatments and the nature and severity of expected side effects, an assessment of the patient's physical, emotional, and coping status is essential in daily interactions with patients and their families. In this section, several roles of the radiation therapist are discussed, including the following: education, communication, assessment, and management of accessory medical equipment.

Education. Knowledge is power. Studies indicate patients often feel dissatisfied with the information received about their treatment and care. When given appropriate information about health care procedures, reports of anxiety, pain, distressing side effects, and length of hospital stay are generally reduced.[58]

Taenzer and Fisher's study [62] indicated that providing patient education is one of the skills that radiation therapists use most often. The educator role of the radiation therapist extends beyond dispensing information. It is an ongoing, integral part of the treatment process that includes the patient, family, and other health care team professionals. Teaching tools include the use of appropriate print materials written in terms easily understood by the patient and family, videos, DVDs, and support groups sharing information.

Just as it is important for some patients to be offered a lot of information about their treatment, others may not benefit from this information. Radiation therapists are responsible for making professional evaluations and judgments concerning what and how much education is appropriate for each patient and family.

Communication. Disfigurement, loss of limbs, decreased motor functions, or a threat of any of these leads to heightened emotional responses typically described by patients with cancer as feelings of denial, frustration, anger, depression, fear, grief, bereavement, rejection, and loss of control. Although Taenzer and Fisher indicated that therapists reported offering emotional support and referrals to other professionals as nontechnical skills used frequently, they also indicated that these skills were among the most difficult to acquire and use effectively.[62] Patients and families face many issues when dealing with cancer treatment. Various issues include fear of treatment, a loss of control, changes in body image and treatment-related side effects, changes in family roles, and financial implications of treatment.[24]

Listening, attending, touching, and questioning skills provide the basis for effective communication with the patient. Therapists can enhance their communication with their patients by asking open-ended questions such as, "What are you feeling?" rather than "How are you feeling?"[58] Openness and assertiveness offer the patient a comfortable invitation to talk. This is generally not different for patients with a diagnosis of bone cancer or STS and can be accomplished by the therapist on a daily basis, as well as by appropriate referrals to support groups or other health professionals as needed.

> *Stability is important to the patient during treatment. Try to keep scheduled treatment times as prompt as possible and not continuously reschedule the patient. Although it may seem minute, that time slot is his or hers and provides the patient with a small amount of control over the situation.*

Assessment. Appraising and evaluating the patient's condition before, during, and after daily treatment are important for good cancer management of bone and STS tumors. In the treatment of patients with bone metastases, care must be taken to observe and evaluate the condition for further spread of the disease. Patient assessment and interventions obviously include the patient's pathophysiologic and emotional status. The cancercidal doses administered to achieve local control require a regular assessment of the skin's integrity. Monitoring of the anticipated erythema and dry and/or moist desquamation may necessitate a decision to withhold treatment until the radiation oncologist verifies confirmation to proceed. Many patients with bone tumors or STS are immunocompromised because of concomitant chemotherapy, so they are at higher risk for infection, especially at the surgical site.[6] Close observation for symptoms of infection and regular notation of blood values with appropriate interventions described by institutional policy are the therapist's responsibility. An evaluation of the patient's

nutritional status and performance rating may also indicate the need for an intervention referral. Recognition of and responding to medical emergencies such as allergic reactions, adverse drug interactions, medical disorders, and cardiac arrest are included in the radiation therapist's purview of professional obligations.

Monitoring Medical Equipment. Patients treated for connective tissue cancers may range from the very old (those with metastatic bone disease) to the extremely young (those with Ewing's sarcoma). The needs of these patients and the accessory medical equipment may include intravenous fluids, oxygen, urinary catheter, chest tubes, or shunts. In the case of pediatric and adolescent patients with these primaries, they may be recovering from radical surgery such as amputation and/or undergoing adjuvant chemotherapy demanding appropriate observation, evaluation, and interventions. Patients treated under sedation may require additional intense monitoring and observation, (e.g., a pulse oximeter). Attention to placement of these devices during the setup and positioning of the treatment equipment and monitoring of the patient during treatment are important for patient safety and accurate radiation dose delivery.

The radiation therapist's broad-based patient care responsibilities include the knowledge and understanding of connective tissue sarcomas as malignant processes and treatment delivery competency. The therapist is the patient's advocate in coordination of referrals for all aspects of conditions relevant to the patient's disease status and treatment.

CASE III

Metastatic Lesion

A 70-year-old white woman had swelling in her right forearm for several months' duration and then felt a palpable mass. The patient has a family history indicative of cancer with a mother having colon cancer, a paternal uncle with metastatic liver disease, a paternal aunt with breast cancer, and a paternal grandmother who had an unknown type of cancer. The patient herself has a history of uterine leiomyosarcoma, in which at diagnosis there were approximately 35 to 40 tumors noted studding the peritoneum, mesentery, and pelvic cul-de-sac. The uterus was enlarged to 12 weeks' gestational size with a tumor erupting from the uterus. At that point, the patient underwent a total abdominal hysterectomy and bilateral salpingo-oophorectomy with resection of the pelvic and abdominal tumor nodules. A segmental jejunum resection with anastomosis and appendectomy was also performed. Following surgery, there was gross residual disease, so the patient received six cycles of Adriamycin chemotherapy.

The patient went without evidence of disease until the symptoms of swelling, pain, and weakness in her arm made her seek medical attention. MRI revealed a mass involving the medial proximal forearm in the flexor muscle group measuring 4 × 3.2 × 5.2 cm. A pelvic CT scan done during patient assessment also revealed a mass located to the left of the rectosigmoid colon measuring 3.2 × 2.2 cm. Physicians believed the mass in the forearm to be metastatic disease versus a new primary and the pelvic lesion to be a recurrence. It was recommended that the patient have preoperative radiation therapy to the forearm and address the pelvic mass at a later date.

Knowing the characteristics of STS, why is the assumption that the forearm mass was a metastatic lesion reasonable?

The patient was simulated in the supine position, B headrest, left arm at her side, and her affected right arm above her head. A sponge was placed under her knees. The treatment fields consisted of an AP and right anterior oblique. The prescription stated to deliver 50 Gy, 2.5 Gy/fraction for 25 fractions. Multileaf collimation was used for field shaping, and a 0.5-cm bolus was placed over the biopsy incision on the AP field. Wedge-in and wedge-out monitor units were given to produce an approximate 55-degree wedge, heels together for both fields. The patient's discomfort during treatment was managed with medication. She did experience some mild erythema and swelling in the treatment field but completed the treatments without interruption.

One month post radiation the patient underwent surgical resection of the tumor and IORT. At the time of resection, the median nerve and ulnar nerve were visualized in the tumor bed. The median nerve was retracted with a Penrose drain and shielded with a strip of lead. The ulnar nerve was also shielded with a lead strip. A 6-cm round intraoperative electron cone was docked under aseptic conditions. A dose of 15 Gy was delivered using 6-MeV electrons prescribed to the 90% isodose line with a 0.5-cm bolus covering the treatment field. After the 5 minute procedure, the placement of the cone and shielding was verified and then removed. A small area of the median nerve, measuring less than 1 cm, may have been exposed during irradiation.

What long-term complications could arise from this?

Two months following treatment for the leiomyosarcoma of the forearm, the patient's pelvic mass was reassessed. Over a period of 6 months, the tumor appeared to be 1 mm larger. Because the mass had been fairly stable, it was decided to let the patient further recuperate for her surgery. Three years after treatment, the patient continues to struggle with metastatic disease. The lesion near her sigmoid colon has grown to 7.3 × 7.1 cm, and there are additional masses in the right gluteus maximus muscle and left posterior ileum, both measuring greater than 3 cm. The patient was told she is not a candidate for further surgery, so she is being followed at her hometown physician for pain control.

CASE IV

Alveolar Rhabdomyosarcoma

An 8-year-old African American boy had bilateral lower quadrant pain and decreased appetite. A large abdominal mass was palpated by his primary care physician, and a CT of the abdomen was obtained. The CT revealed a right-sided abdominal mass measuring 12 cm in greatest dimension. Also noted were enlarged periaortic lymph nodes. The patient underwent a CT-guided biopsy of the periaortic lymph node the following day, and pathology confirmed a diagnosis of alveolar rhabdomyosarcoma.

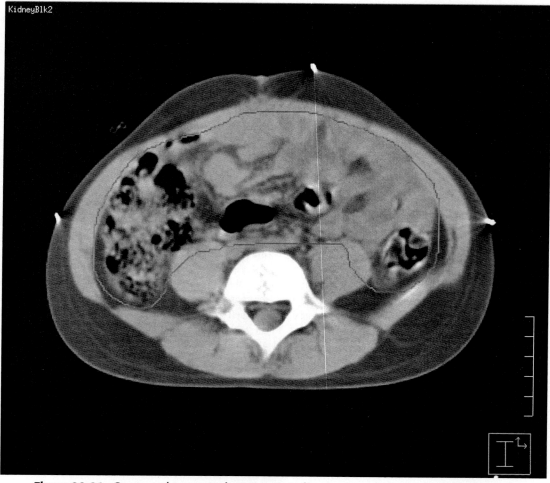

Figure 28-21. Computed tomography treatment planning image contouring the retroperitoneum, including large amounts of bowel.

Past medical history is unremarkable for this patient; however, he was born at 27 weeks' gestation. There is no family history of malignancies, and the patient has a healthy mother, father, and brother. The patient's parents both smoke cigarettes.

Immediately following his diagnosis, the patient was started on a chemotherapy treatment protocol, specifically for rhabdomyosarcomas. Weekly treatments included vincristine, cyclophosphamide, dactinomycin, and topotecan. He received 12 weeks of chemotherapy, followed by an exploratory laparotomy. Although the patient had a significant response to chemotherapy, residual disease was found (Figure 28-21). The surgeon resected several 3×3 cm nodules surrounding the umbilical arteries, primarily right-sided. An additional mass in the right lower quadrant, measuring 1×3 cm, was also removed. Upon examining the omentum, multiple nodules were found. A fine-needle aspiration was performed and confirmed these nodules to be residual rhabdomyosarcoma.

Because of the extent of this patient's disease, consolidative radiation therapy was suggested. The parents were informed about the benefits, risks, and acute and long-term side effects. Possible complications associated with abdominal treatment include damage to the small bowel, kidneys, and liver. There is also a risk of acquiring a second malignancy.

What might be done in the planning process to minimize dose to critical structures?

The patient received whole abdominal radiation, with a total dose of 24 Gy in 16 fractions. The course of treatment was given through an opposing AP technique using 6-MV photons. Renal blocks were added after a prescribed dose of 13.5 Gy (Figure 28-22). A boost was not given because of the diffuse peritoneal involvement. The patient tolerated the treatments well with no interruptions. Upon completion, he had no clinical evidence of disease progression.

SUMMARY

- Osteosarcoma is the most common osseous bone tumor, occurring most often in patients 20 to 30 years of age. Chondrosarcomas and fibrosarcomas affect adults 30 to 70 years old, whereas Ewing's sarcoma is primarily a pediatric tumor, occurring in adolescents aged 10 to 20 years. Multiple myeloma tends to affect the middle-age and elderly population, peaking in the seventh decade.
- The incidence of STS is fairly low. It is diagnosed most often in the fifth and sixth decades of life.

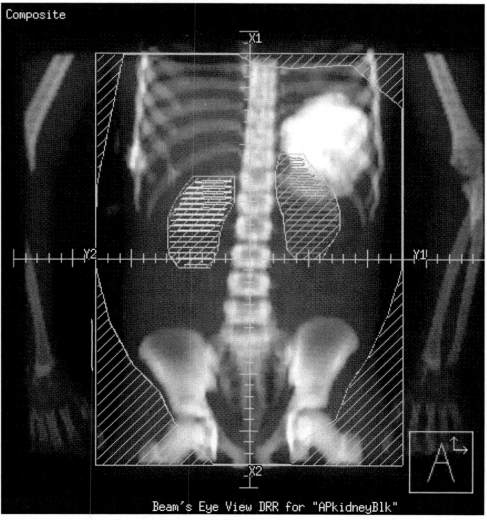

Figure 28-22. Digitally reconstructed radiograph of anteroposterior abdomen field with kidney blocks.

Rhabdomysarcoma, a form of STS, is most common in children, with the peak incidence in the first two decades of life and median age at diagnosis of approximately 5 years old.

- A typical long bone consists of the diaphysis, two epiphyses, and the cartilage cap. A muscle is composed of the perimysium, epimysium, endomysium, and muscle fibers.
- Osteosarcomas are generally classified as poorly differentiated tumors. Chondrosarcomas arise from mesenchymal elements of the bone and are usually undifferentiated and associated with a higher grade. Fibrosarcomas originate in mesenchymal tissue. The cell of origin for malignant fibrous histiocytoma is the histiocyte or the macrophage. Giant cell tumors of the bone are histologically composed of round or spindle-shaped mononuclear cells uniformly incorporated in with multinucleated giant cells. Ewing's sarcoma is composed of populations of small, blue, round cells. Plasma cells associated with multiple myeloma originate from B-cell lymphocytes. No universally accepted staging system exists for primary bone sarcomas. Grade is determined to be either low or high grade.
- The standard treatment for bone and soft tissue sarcomas is surgery. With advancements in treatment options, chemotherapy and radiation therapy may become more widely used in some cases.
- Athough the radiograph serves as a common detection method, CT and MRI are becoming more widely used to detect bone and soft tissue sarcomas. Nuclear medicine scans, especially bone scans, are beneficial in detecting bone metastases. A biopsy must be performed to determine the diagnosis.
- The patient's prognosis is affected by the differentiation and aggression of the tumor. The more differentiated, the better is the prognosis. Less-aggressive tumors carry a better prognosis. Less-differentiated, more-aggressive tumors are associated with a worse prognosis.
- Average doses of radiation for most bone and soft tissue sarcomas are 50 to 60 Gy. However, in patients with gross disease doses may go as high as 70 Gy to achieve local control. Intraoperative therapy may be used in conjunction with external beam therapy, to give an additional dose of approximately 15 Gy in a single fraction. Patients with multiple myeloma require a lower total dose for pain control. Doses around 30 Gy are typically effective.
- The simulation process is extremely important to ensure proper treatment of bone and soft tissue sarcomas. The therapist must be sure the patient is in a reproducible position, while keeping the patient as comfortable as possible. It is also important to work efficiently, because these patients may be in pain.
- Most bone tumors are radioresistant because of their high mitotic activity. It is important for the therapist to understand that these tumors are not sensitive to radiation therapy, making them difficult to treat. This is primarily why sarcomas are treated with surgery.
- Emerging treatments include limb-sparing surgery, intraoperative radiation therapy, tumor suppressor gene therapy, new chemotherapy agents, stem cell transplantation, and the use of radionuclides.

Review Questions

Multiple Choice

1. The incidence rate of bone cancer is highest during:
   a. infancy
   b. adulthood
   c. adolescence
   d. equal for all ages

2. A nonosseous malignant tumor of the marrow is a(an):
   a. fibrosarcoma
   b. chondrosarcoma
   c. osteosarcoma
   d. multiple myeloma

3. A bone lesion resulting from primary sites elsewhere in the body is a(n):
   a. osteosarcoma
   b. multiple myeloma
   c. metastatic disease
   d. chondrosarcoma

4. The most common site of a primary bone sarcoma is:
   a. epiphyseal
   b. metaphyseal
   c. diaphyseal
   d. shaft

5. Prognostic indicators for patients with primary bone cancer include all of the following *except:*
   a. age
   b. gender
   c. location
   d. weight

6. The most common site of metastasis from primary bone cancer is:
   a. brain
   b. bowel
   c. lung
   d. distal extremities

7. _____ is most commonly used in treating metastatic bone disease resulting from primary prostate or breast cancer.
   a. Technetium-99 m
   b. Iodine-131 m
   c. Strontium-89 m
   d. Iodine-125 m

8. Although the exact cause of STS is unknown, a factor that has been implicated is:
   a. prior sun exposure
   b. appearance as a second primary 5 to 15 years after high-dose radiation therapy for other cancers
   c. predisposition of Paget's disease
   d. tobacco use

9. Factors or clinical signs that are incorporated in the staging systems and considered appropriate as general prognostic indicators for STS include:
   I. histology
   II. size
   III. gender
   a. I and II

b. I and III
c. II and III
d. I, II, and III

10. Regional lymph nodes are generally not included in the treatment portals for STS. Which of the following are exceptions for this statement?
    I. rhabdomyosarcoma
    II. synovial sarcoma
    III. leiomyosarcoma
    a. I and II
    b. I and III
    c. II and III
    d. I, II, and III

11. The rationale for leaving a 1- to 3-cm strip of skin and soft tissue rather than total circumferential irradiation of an extremity being treated for STS is that it:
    a. decreases excessive erythema
    b. promotes healing of the incision scar
    c. avoids future excessive fibrosis and edema
    d. increases future mobility for the treated limb

12. Advantages of preoperative radiation therapy for STS include:
    a. decreased difficulty with postirradiation surgical wound healing
    b. availability of the precise extent and description of the tumor
    c. possibility of a larger treatment volume
    d. possibility of less aggressive surgery because of tumor regression

13. Intraoperative electron beam radiation usually involves energies ranging from 9 to 15 MeV with doses to the range of:
    a. 10 to 20 Gy
    b. 20 to 25 Gy
    c. 25 to 30 Gy
    d. 30 to 40 Gy

14. The estimated number of new cases of primary bone cancers diagnosed each year is approximately:
    a. 1000 to 1800
    b. 2300 to 2800
    c. 3000 to 3600
    d. 3800 to 4000

15. Radiation therapy doses for postoperative STS are generally in the range of:
    a. 60 to 66 Gy
    b. 50 to 55 Gy
    c. 40 to 48 Gy
    d. 36 to 40 Gy

The answers to the Review Questions can be found by logging on to our website at: *http://evolve.elsevier.com/Washington+Leaver/ principles*

Questions to Ponder

1. Explain why patients with Ewing's sarcoma of the pelvis carry a poorer prognosis than patients with the same tumor of an extremity.

2. Define *skip metastases* and explain how radiation therapy can be used to treat these lesions.

3. Explain the techniques involved in detecting primary bone tumors and the challenges associated with obtaining diagnoses of them.

4. Despite the evidence that lymphatic involvement of STS is rare, the radiation therapy technique selected for rhabdomyosarcomas, synovial sarcomas, and epithelioid sarcomas often includes the regional lymph nodes. Explain the rationale for this exception.

5. Why is a boost with bolus or electrons to the scar often required during radiation to bone and STS?

REFERENCES

1. American Cancer Society (website): http://www.cancer.org. Accessed November 22, 2008.
2. American Joint Committee on Cancer: Soft tissue sarcoma. In Greene FL, editor: *AJCC cancer staging manual,* ed 6, New York, 2002, Springer.
3. Bacci G, et al: Long-term outcome for patients with nonmetastatic osteosarcoma of the extremity treated at the Istituto Ortopedico Rizzoli according to the Istituto Ortopedico Rizzoli/osteosarcoma-2 protocol: an updated report, *J Clin Oncol* 18:4016-4027, 2000.
4. Bataille R, Harousseau JL: Multiple myeloma, *N Engl J Med* 336:1657, 1997.
5. Bell RS, et al: Supervoltage radiotherapy in the treatment of difficult giant cell tumor of bone, *Clin Orthop* 174:208, 1983.
6. Bennett MV: Cancers of the bone. In Varricchio CG, editor: *American Cancer Society professional education publication: a cancer source book for nurses,* ed 7, Atlanta, 1997, Jones & Bartlett.
7. Bentel GC: Treatment planning: miscellaneous treatments. In Wonsiewicz M, Navozov M, editors: *Radiation therapy planning,* ed 2, New York, 1996, McGraw-Hill.
8. Bernstein M, et al: Ewing's sarcoma family of tumors: current management, *Oncologist* 11:503-519, 2006.
9. Bose AC, et al: Primary cutaneous malignant fibrous histiocytoma: a case report, *Med Sci Monit* 12:CS61-C63, 2006.
10. Brennan MF: Soft tissue sarcoma: advances in understanding and management, *Surgeon* 3:216-223, 2005.
11. Caudell JJ, et al: Radiotherapy in the management of giant cell tumor of bone, *Int J Radiat Oncol Biol Phys* 57:158-165, 2003.
12. Chatterjee M, Chakraborty T, Tassone P: Multiple myeloma: monoclonal antibodies-based immunotherapeutic strategies and targeted radiotherapy, *Eur J Cancer* 42:1640-1652, 2006.
13. Clark MA, et al: Soft tissue sarcomas in adults, *N Engl J Med* 353:701-711, 2005.
14. Clarkson R, Ferguson PC: Primary multidisciplinary management of extremity soft tissue sarcomas, *Curr Treat Options Oncol* 5:451-462, 2004.
15. Constine LS, et al: Pediatric solid tumors. In Rubin P, editor: *Clinical oncology: a multidisciplinary approach for physicians and students,* ed 8, Philadelphia, 2001, WB Saunders.
16. Cordon-Cardo C: Sarcomas of the soft tissues and bone. In DeVita VT, Hellman S, Rosenberg SA, editors: *Cancer: principles and practice of oncology,* ed 5, Philadelphia, 1997, Lippincott-Raven.
17. Damjanov I: *Pathology for the health professions,* ed 3, St. Louis, 2006, Elsevier Saunders.
18. DeLaney TF, et al: Radiotherapy for local control of osteosarcoma, *Int J Radiat Oncol Biol Phys* 61:492-498, 2005.
19. Dincbas FO, et al: The role of preoperative radiotherapy in nonmetastatic high-grade osteosarcoma of the extremities for limb-sparing surgery, *Int J Radiat Oncol Biol Phys* 62:820-828, 2005.
20. Dispenzieri A, Kyle RA: Multiple myeloma: clinical features and indications for therapy, *Best Pract Res Clin Haematol* 18:553-568, 2005.
21. Evans RG: The bone. In Cox JD, editor: *Moss' radiation oncology: rationale, technique, results,* ed 7, St. Louis, 1994, Mosby.
22. Fata R, et al: Paclitaxel in the treatment of patients with angiosarcoma of the scalp or face, *Cancer* 86:2034-2037, 1999.

23. Fenstermacher MJ: Imaging evaluation of patients with soft tissue sarcoma, *Surg Oncol Clin North Am* 12:305-332, 2003.
24. Ferszt GG, Waldman RC: Psychosocial responses to disease and treatment. In Varricchio, editor: *American Cancer Society professional education publication: a cancer source book for nurses,* ed 7, Atlanta, 1997, Jones & Bartlett.
25. Flugstad DL, et al: Importance of surgical resection in the successful management of soft tissue sarcoma, *Arch Surg* 134:856-861, 1999.
26. Glutin PH, et al: Brachytherapy of recurrent tumors of the base of skull and spine with I-125 sources, *Neurosurgery* 20:938-945, 1987.
27. Goel A, et al: PS-341-mediated selective targeting of multiple myeloma cells by synergistic increase in ionizing radiation-induced apoptosis, *Exp Hematol* 33:784-795, 2005.
28. Hansen T, et al: Low-grade fibrosarcoma: report on 39 not otherwise specified cases and comparison with defined low-grade fibrosarcoma types, *Histopathology* 49:152-160, 2006.
29. Hensley ML, et al: Gemcitabine and docetaxel in patients with unresectable leiomyosarcoma: results of a phase II trial, *J Clin Oncol* 20: 2824-2831: 2002.
30. Hoppe RT, Constine LS, Qazi R: Hodgkin's disease and the lymphomas. In Rubin P, editor: *Clinical oncology: a multidisciplinary approach for physicians and students,* ed 8, Philadelphia, 2001, WB Saunders.
31. Kempf-Bielack B, et al: Osteosarcoma relapse after combined modality therapy: an analysis of unselected patients in the Cooperative Osteosarcoma Study Group (COSS), *J Clin Oncol* 23:559-568, 2005.
32. Koontz BF, Clough RW, Halperin EC: Palliative radiation therapy for metastatic Ewing sarcoma, *Cancer* 106:1790-1793, 2006.
33. Krishnan S, et al: Radiosurgery for cranial base chordomas and chondrosarcomas, *Neurosurgery* 56:777-784, 2005.
34. Kyle RA, Rajkumar V: Treatment of multiple myeloma: an emphasis on new developments, *Ann Med* 38:111-115, 2006.
35. La TH, et al: Radiation therapy for Ewing's sarcoma: results from Memorial Sloan-Kettering in the modern era, *Int J Radiat Biol Phys* 64:544-550, 2006.
36. Lewis VO, et al: Outcome of postradiation osteosarcoma does not correlate with chemotherapy response, *Clin Orthop Relat Res* 450:60-66, 2006.
37. Machak GN, et al: Neoadjuvant chemotherapy and local radiotherapy for high-grade osteosarcoma of the extremities, *Mayo Clin Proc* 78: 147-155, 2003.
38. Mankin HJ, Hornicek FJ: Diagnosis, classification and management of soft tissue sarcomas, *Cancer Control* 12:5-21, 2005.
39. Mankin HJ, Mankin CJ, Simon MA: The hazards of the biopsy, revisited. Members of the Musculoskeletal Tumor Society, *J Bone Joint Surg Am* 78:656-663, 1996.
40. Marcus RB: Ewing's sarcoma. In Perez CA, Brady LW, Halperin EC, et al, editors: *Principles and practice of radiation oncology,* ed 4, Philadelphia, 2004, Lippincott Williams & Wilkins.
41. McClain KL, et al: Association of Epstein-Barr virus with leiomyosarcomas in young people with AIDS, *N Engl J Med* 332:12-18, 1995.
42. McGinn CJ: Soft tissue sarcomas (excluding retroperitoneum). In Perez CA, Brady LW, Halperin EC, et al, editors: *Principles and practice of radiation oncology,* ed 4, Philadelphia, 2004, Lippincott Williams & Wilkins.
43. Mendenhall WM, et al: Adult head and neck soft tissue sarcomas, *Head Neck* 916-922, 2005.
44. Mendenhall WM, et al: Retroperitoneal soft tissue sarcoma, *Cancer* 104:669-675, 2005.
45. Minard-Colin V, et al: Outcome of flat bone sarcomas (other than Ewing's) in children and adolescents: a study of 25 cases, *Br J Cancer* 90:613-619, 2004.
46. Mocellin S, et al: Adult soft tissue sarcomas: conventional therapies and molecularly targeted approaches, *Cancer Treat Rev* 32: 9-27, 2006.
47. Montemaggi P, Brady LW, Horowitz SM: Bone. In Perez CA, Brady LW, Halperin EC, et al, editors: *Principles and practice of radiation oncology,* ed 4, Philadelphia, 2004, Lippincott Williams & Wilkins.
48. Moss WT: *Radiation oncology,* ed 6, St. Louis, 1989, Mosby.
49. O'Sullivan B, et al: Preoperative versus postoperative radiotherapy in soft-tissue sarcoma of the limbs: a randomized trial, *Lancet* 359:2235-2241, 2002.
50. Palesty AJ, Kraybill WG: Developments in the management of extremity soft tissue sarcomas, *Cancer Invest* 23:692-699, 2005.
51. Qazilbash MH, et al: Risk factors for relapse after complete remission with high-dose therapy for multiple myeloma, *Leuk Lymph* 47:1360-1364, 2006.
52. Raut CP, Pisters PWT: Retroperitoneal sarcomas: combined modality treatment approaches, *J Surg Oncol* 94:81-87, 2006.
53. Rosier RN, O'Keefe RJ, Sahasrabudhe DM: Bone tumors. In Rubin P, editor: *Clinical oncology: a multidisciplinary approach for physicians and students,* ed 8, Philadelphia, 2001, WB Saunders.
54. Ruiz-Arguelles GJ, San Miguel JE: Cell surface markers in multiple myeloma, *Mayo Clin Proc* 69:684-690, 1994.
55. Sarcoma Meta-analysis Collaboration: Adjuvant chemotherapy for localized respectable soft-tissue sarcoma of adults: meta-analysis of individual data, *Lancet* 350(9092): 1647-1654, 1997.
56. Scarantino CW, Ornitz RD, Woodard SA: Metastases and disseminated disease. In Rubin P, editor: *Clinical oncology: a multidisciplinary approach for physicians and students,* ed 8, Philadelphia, 2001, WB Saunders.
57. Scoggins CR, Pollock RE: Extremity soft tissue sarcoma: evidence-based multidisciplinary management, *J Surg Oncol* 90:10-13, 2005.
58. Shell JA, Kirsch S: Psychosocial issues, outcomes and quality of life. In Otto SE, editor: *Oncology nursing,* ed 4, St. Louis, 2001, Mosby.
59. Spiro IJ, et al: Soft tissue sarcaroma. In Rubin P, editor: *Clinical oncology: a multidisciplinary approach for physicians and students,* ed 8, Philadelphia, 2001, WB Saunders.
60. Stevens MCG: Treatment for childhood rhabdomyosarcoma: the cost of cure, *Lancet Oncol* 6:77-84, 2005.
61. Stevens MCG, et al: Treatment of nonmetastatic rhabdomyosarcoma in childhood and adolescence: third study of the International Society of Paediatric Oncology—SIOP malignant mesenchymal tumor 89, *J Clin Oncol* 23:2618-2628, 2005.
62. Taenzer P, Fisher P: Psychological issues in radiation therapy, *Can J Med Radiat Technol* 20:81, 1989.
63. Ternovoi VV, et al: Adenovirus-mediated p53 tumor suppressor gene therapy of osteosarcoma, *Lab Invest* 86:748-766, 2006.
64. Tosi P, Gamberi B, Giuliani N: Biology and treatment of multiple myeloma, *Biol Blood Marrow Transplant* 12:81-86, 2006.
65. Vaneerat R, Powers WE, Temple HT: Palliation of bone metastases. In Perez CA, Brady LW, Halperin EC, et al, editors: *Principles and practice of radiation oncology,* ed 4, Philadelphia, 2004, Lippincott Williams & Wilkins.
66. Wasserman TH: Myeloma and plasmacytomas. In Perez CA, Brady LW, Halperin EC, et al, editors: *Principles and practice of radiation oncology,* ed 4, Philadelphia, 2004, Lippincott Williams & Wilkins.
67. Wells G, et al: Soft tissue sarcoma of the extremity and trunk: issues for the general surgeon, *Am Surg* 72:665-671, 2006.
68. Willett CG, et al: Intraoperative electron beam radiation therapy for retroperitoneal soft tissue sarcoma, *Cancer* 68:278-283, 1991.
69. Wulling M, et al: The nature of giant cell tumor of bone, *J Cancer Res Clin Oncol* 127:467-474, 2001.
70. Yeh HS, Berenson JR: Myeloma bone disease and treatment options, *Eur J Cancer* 42:1554-1563, 2006.
71. Yeh HS, Berenson JR: Treatment for myeloma bone disease, *Clin Cancer Res* 12:6279-6284, 2006.
72. Yock TI, et al: Local control in pelvic Ewing sarcoma: analysis from INT-0091—a report from the Children's Oncology Group, *J Clin Oncol* 24:3838-3843, 2006.

BIBLIOGRAPHY

American Cancer Society (website): www.cancer.org.
Bentel GC: Treatment planning: miscellaneous treatments. In Wonsiewicz M, Navozov M, editors: *Radiation therapy planning,* ed 2, New York, 1996, McGraw-Hill.
Bernstein M, et al: Ewing's sarcoma family of tumors: current management, *Oncologist* 11:503-519, 2006.
Clarkson R, Ferguson PC: Primary multidisciplinary management of extremity soft tissue sarcomas, *Curr Treat Options Oncol* 5:451-462, 2004.

Dincbas FO, et al: The role of preoperative radiotherapy in nonmetastatic high-grade osteosarcoma of the extremities for limb-sparing surgery, *Int J Radiat Oncol Biol Phys* 62:820-828, 2005.

Mankin HJ, Hornicek FJ: Diagnosis, classification and management of soft tissue sarcomas, *Cancer Control* 12:5-21, 2005.

Montemaggi P, Brady LW, Horowitz SM: Bone. In Perez CA, Brady LW, Halperin EC, et al, editors: *Principles and practice of radiation oncology,* ed 4, Philadelphia, 2004, Lippincott Williams & Wilkins.

Palesty AJ, Kraybill WG: Developments in the management of extremity soft tissue sarcomas, *Cancer Invest* 23:692-699, 2005.

Rosier RN, O'Keefe RJ, Sahasrabudhe DM: Bone tumors. In Rubin P, editor: *Clinical oncology: a multidisciplinary approach for physicians and students,* ed 8, Philadelphia, 2001, WB Saunders.

Tosi P, Gamberi B, Giuliani N: Biology and treatment of multiple myeloma, *Biol Blood Marrow Transplant* 12: 81-86, 2006.

Yeh HS, Berenson JR: Treatment for myeloma bone disease, *Clin Cancer Res* 12:6279-6284, 2006.

Lymphoreticular System Tumors

Sally Green

Outline

Key Terms

Objectives

- Compare and contrast characteristics of Hodgkin's lymphoma and non-Hodgkin's lymphoma.
- Identify lymph node regions most commonly involved in Hodgkin's lymphoma.
- Explain the "B" symptoms and the role they play in Hodgkin's lymphoma.
- Identify the staging system used for Hodgkin's lymphoma and explain the differences in the four stages.
- Discuss the common methods of treatment for Hodgkin's lymphoma.
- Identify the risk factors for non-Hodgkin's lymphomas.
- Compare and contrast follicular lymphomas with diffuse lymphomas.
- Identify the three categories of lymphomas in the REAL/WHO classification system.
- Explain the role of chemotherapy and radiation therapy in the treatment of non-Hodgkin's lymphomas.
- Compare and contrast the survival rates of patients with Hodgkin's lymphoma and those with non-Hodgkin's lymphoma.

Lymphomas are the predominant cancers of the lymphoreticular system. The two main categories of lymphomas are Hodgkin's lymphoma (Hodgkin's disease) and non-Hodgkin's lymphoma (NHL). Hodgkin's lymphoma was the first lymphoma identified in 1832 as a disease distinct from inflammation. Later in that century, pathologists determined Hodgkin's lymphoma to be a separate disease entity from the lymphomas and leukemias.

HODGKIN'S LYMPHOMA

Hodgkin's lymphoma is treated as a separate category of lymphomas because of the presence of the **Reed-Sternberg cell** (Figure 29-1) in the lymph nodes of patients with Hodgkin's lymphoma and because Hodgkin's spreads in a predictable, systematic, or contiguous pattern through the lymph system. The Reed-Sternberg cell is a giant connective tissue cell containing one or two large nuclei. The presence of this cell determines whether the diagnosis is Hodgkin's lymphoma or NHL.

Epidemiology

The National Cancer Institute estimates that approximately 8220 individuals will be diagnosed with Hodgkin's lymphoma in 2008, and approximately 1350 individuals will die of Hodgkin's lymphoma in 2008.[15] Hodgkin's lymphoma accounts for less than 1% of the newly diagnosed cancers per year. Approximately 1000 more cases occur in men than in women, indicating a slight male predominance. Worldwide, the incidence of Hodgkin's is more common in developed countries than in undeveloped countries. To date, no explanation exists to account for this phenomenon.

Approximately one half of Hodgkin's lymphomas are diagnosed in patients younger than 40 years of age, with the median age of 38 years at the time of the diagnosis. Hodgkin's lymphoma is rare in children younger than 10 years.[15]

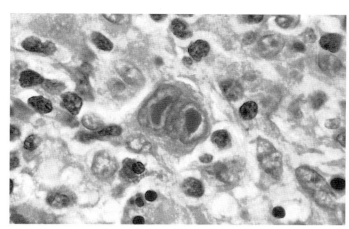

Figure 29-1. Reed-Sternberg cell is a giant connective tissue cell. It is characterized by one or two large nuclei. (Courtesy of Dr. Robert W. McKenna, Department of Pathology, University of Texas Southwestern Medical School, Dallas, Texas. In Kumar V, et al: *Robbins basic pathology*, ed 8, Philadelphia, 2007, Saunders.)

Prevalence is a statistic of primary interest in public health because it identifies the level of burden of disease or health-related events on the population and health care system. Prevalence represents new and preexisting patients alive on a certain date, in contrast to incidence, which reflects new cases of a condition diagnosed during a given period of time. Prevalence is a function of both the incidence of the disease and survival. For example, on January 1, 2005, in the United States there were approximately 156,172 men and women alive who had a history of Hodgkin's lymphoma—80,386 men and 75,786 women. This includes any person alive on January 1, 2005 who had been diagnosed with Hodgkin's lymphoma at any point before January 1, 2005 and includes persons with active disease; those who are cured of their disease can also be expressed as a percentage.[15]

Etiology

Specific causes of Hodgkin's lymphoma remain elusive to researchers. Other than defective T-cell functioning, no conclusive evidence linking Hodgkin's to environmental or occupational exposure or to genetic predisposition has been identified. Occasionally, clusters of patients with Hodgkin's lymphoma occur in some communities; however, the data have been insufficient to determine the specific origin of the disease in such cases. There are, however, components of the Epstein-Barr virus genome in the cellular deoxyribonucleic acid (DNA) of the Reed-Sternberg cells that are present in this disease. The link between a prior infection with the Epstein-Barr virus and Hodgkin's lymphoma has been investigated, but most cases in the United States are not Eptstein-Barr virus related.[12]

No one knows what causes Hodgkin's disease; however, several factors have been identified to be associated with Hodgkin's disease. It is important to note that these factors may increase the risk of developing Hodgkin's disease, but that most people with these conditions still do not develop Hodgkin's disease. Infection with the Epstein-Barr virus may play a role in the development of certain types of Hodgkin's disease. Epstein-Barr virus also causes mono-nucleosis, which is known as mono or kissing disease.[14]

Prognostic Indicators

The stage of Hodgkin's lymphoma has the greatest effect on the prognosis of the patient, with the histology of the specific category of Hodgkin's having the least effect. In other words, the later the stage, the worse is the prognosis. The risk of a relapse after treatment is greater in the later stages because there is increased bulky disease.

More males than females are diagnosed with Hodgkin's lymphoma, and the prognosis is also slightly worse for males. Gender may also influence the choice of treatment, based on a consideration of toxicities to the reproductive system. Fertility may be preserved in most men through the use of radiation therapy but not with alkylating agents (chemotherapy). In women, the ovaries cannot be completely protected during radiation therapy to the pelvic area, and some women experience menopause after radiation therapy. Youth is a favorable prognostic factor, with younger patients (those in their teens to twenties) doing better than older patients, who have more difficulty tolerating aggressive treatments. The extent of the disease, the presence of "B" symptoms (to be discussed later), the number of sites of involvement, the presence of the disease in the lower abdomen, splenic involvement, and an elevation of serum markers (such as erythrocyte sedimentation rate) are all factors influencing the natural history of the disease.

Anatomy and Lymphatics

The primary function of the lymph nodes is the production of lymphocytes and the filtration of foreign particles and cellular debris from the lymph before it is returned to the circulatory system. A review of the lymphatic system is important for understanding the nature of Hodgkin's lymphoma and NHLs. Please see Chapter 20 for a detailed discussion. The major lymph node regions are of particular importance in treating Hodgkin's lymphomas. The major lymph nodes (Figure 29-2) are as follows:

1. Waldeyer's ring (tonsillar lymphatic tissue surrounding the nasopharynx and oropharynx) and cervical, preauricular, and occipital lymph nodes
2. Supraclavicular and infraclavicular lymph nodes
3. Axillary lymph nodes
4. Thorax (includes hilar and mediastinal nodes)
5. Abdominal cavity (includes para-aortic nodes)
6. Pelvic cavity (includes iliac nodes)
7. Inguinal and femoral lymph nodes

The thymus and spleen are lymphatic organs whose functions are closely related to the lymph nodes. The thymus contains large numbers of lymphocytes (called *thymocytes*), most of which remain inactive. However, some thymocytes develop into T lymphocytes, which play a part in the immune process.

The spleen is the largest lymphatic organ. It resembles a large lymph node in its structure, but its cavities are filled with blood instead of lymph. The spleen filters the blood similar to the way that lymph nodes filter lymphatic fluid; however, through the action of its phagocytes, the spleen destroys damaged red blood cells and the remains of ruptured cells carried in the blood. The splenic lymphocytes help in the body's defense against infection.

Clinical Presentation

Hodgkin's lymphoma usually appears as a painless mass that the patient discovers. The most common sites of presentation

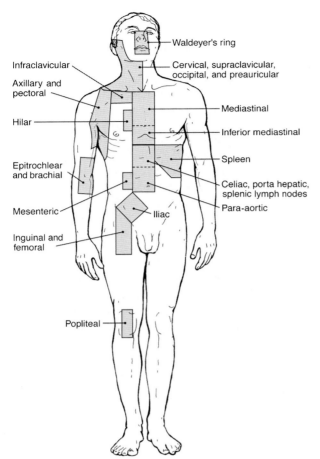

Figure 29-2. Major lymphatic regions of the body. These regions play a significant role in the staging and treatment planning of Hodgkin's lymphoma. After the lymphatic regions of known involvement are determined, the regions at risk for subclinical disease due to contiguous spread may then be established. Identification of both the primary lymphatic region of involvement and the contiguous lymph node regions at risk are essential in treatment planning. (From Gunderson LL, Tepper JE: *Clinical radiation oncology*, Philadelphia, 2000, Churchill Livingstone.)

are in the neck and supraclavicular regions. Mediastinal masses are usually detected on a radiograph of the chest. Most patients have the disease above the diaphragm.

Approximately one third of the patients also experience the following systemic symptoms: unexplained fevers (higher than 38° C, or 100.4° F), drenching night sweats, and weight loss of 10% of their body weight in 6 months. These are referred to as **B symptoms**. Generalized **pruritus** (severe itching) and/or alcohol-induced pain in the disease-involved tissues may also be included as B symptoms, but they are present only in some instances.

Sometimes Hodgkin's is discovered during pregnancy, but pregnancy per se has no effect on the natural history. Pregnancy is merely coincidental because of the age-group of the patients. Patients testing positive for the human immunodeficiency virus (HIV) are not at a greater risk than the general population for developing Hodgkin's. However, if an HIV-infected patient contracts Hodgkin's, the disease appears at a more advanced stage. Treatment for these patients is a challenge because of

their poor tolerance for chemotherapy and the occurrence of opportunistic infections.

Detection and Diagnosis

Enlarged lymph nodes in the neck, clavicular, or axilla regions are usually the first indication of Hodgkin's lymphoma. As mentioned previously, a mediastinal mass is usually discovered on a routine chest radiograph. Occasionally, these patients experience a cough, shortness of breath, or chest discomfort. The enlarged node may be the only symptom a patient experiences. However, approximately one third of patients have B symptoms.[3] An enlarged spleen or abdomen, bony tenderness, and pleural effusion indicate a later stage of Hodgkin's disease. Enlarged groin nodes can be an early symptom, although Hodgkin's rarely originates in the groin.

The diagnostic workup includes a complete history and physical examination. Standard laboratory studies should include a complete blood cell and platelet count, liver and renal function tests, and blood chemistry and thyroid function tests. Occasionally, patients display anemia, leukopenia, lymphopenia, or thrombocytosis, which may be indicative of bone marrow involvement. A serum alkaline phosphatase level is a nonspecific marker of tumor activity, hepatic bone marrow disease, or bone disease.

Radiographic studies should include a chest x-ray examination, computed tomography (CT), magnetic resonance imaging (MRI), or positron emission tomography (PET)/CT for disease detection and treatment planning. A PET/CT with FDG is extremely useful in reducing the target volumes treatment planning. A bone marrow biopsy should be restricted to patients with B symptoms or subdiaphragmatic disease. There is only a 5% chance of bone marrow involvement in patients who have Hodgkin's lymphoma.

The spleen is usually involved when the high para-aortic nodes are involved. It is also at risk with lymphocyte depletion or mixed cellularity histologies. A liver biopsy should be done when splenic involvement occurs, but the liver is rarely involved if the spleen is not.

Pathology

Hodgkin's is identified pathologically by the presence of the Reed-Sternberg cell. The current system used for histologic classification is the World Health Organization (WHO) modification of the Revised European-American Lymphoma (REAL) classification.[9] It divides Hodgkin's into two categories and four subcategories:

1. Nodular lymphocyte predominant Hodgkin's lymphoma (NLPHL)
2. Classic Hodgkin's lymphoma (CHL)
   a. Lymphocyte-rich Hodgkin's lymphoma (LRHL)
   b. Nodular sclerosing Hodgkin's lymphoma (NSHL)
   c. Mixed cellularity Hodgkin's lymphoma (MCHL)
   d. Lymphocyte-depleted Hodgkin's lymphoma (LDHL)

Nodular lymphocyte predominant has a B-cell origin, which distinguishes it from classic Hodgkin's lymphoma, and it is the most favorable of the categories. The median age for NLPHL is the mid 30s, and there is a 3:1 male predominance. In general, the cervical or inguinal lymph nodes are involved but not the mediastinal. Eighty percent of these patients have stage I or II disease. Fewer than 10% of these patients experience any of the symptoms, and there is a 90% survival at 10 years posttreatment.[9]

Patients with classic Hodgkin's lymphoma generally lack bulky disease, mediastinal disease, and B symptoms. CHL is characterized by the presence of typical, diagnostic Reed-Sternberg cells. There are four subcategories of CHL: lymphocyte rich, nodular sclerosing, mixed cellularity, and lymphocyte depleted.

- Like NLPHL, classic Hodgkin's has a male predominance, but unlike classic Hodgkin's, there is an older median age of onset.
- Nodular sclerosing Hodgkin's lymphoma is the most common subtype in developed countries, accounting for 60% to 80% of all cases.[9] NSHL is the type that occurs most commonly in adolescents and young adults. The mediastinum and supradiaphragmatic sites are most often involved in NSHL, and approximately one third of the patients experience B symptoms.
- Mixed cellularity Hodgkin's's lymphoma accounts for 15% to 30% of all Hodgkin's lymphomas. It can occur at any age and lacks the early adult peak of NSHL. Abdominal lymph nodes and splenic involvement are more common in MCHL.
- Lymphocyte-depleted Hodgkin's lymphoma is the least common subtype (less than 1%) in the United States. It occurs in older patients and HIV-infected patients. It usually presents with advanced disease such as spleen, liver, and bone marrow involvement and B symptoms. As a result, LDHL carries the worst prognosis of the four subtypes.

Staging

The **Ann Arbor staging system** has been the accepted method of classification for Hodgkin's disease since 1971 (Box 29-1).

These stages can be subdivided into A or B groups. An "A" indicates the lack of general symptoms. For example, stage IIA may indicate that two or more node regions are involved in the thorax and that the patient has not experienced any symptoms, such as fever, night sweats, and weight loss. A "B" next to the stage number (e.g., stage IB) indicates the presence of these symptoms. The presence of B symptoms usually indicates a worse prognosis.

Routes of Spread

Hodgkin's disease has a predictable pattern of spread, and 90% of the patients have **contiguous** spread. In other words, the cancer will spread to the adjacent node or region. The rapidity of the growth and spread of the disease, however, is not predictable.

Spread to the viscera occurs after spread to the adjacent lymph nodes. Obviously, visceral spread indicates a higher stage and worse prognosis.

The spleen becomes involved in late stages, and the likelihood of disseminated disease increases with splenic involvement. The liver and/or bone marrow is at increased risk with

---

Box 29-1	American Joint Committee on Cancer Staging Classification for Lymphoid Neoplasms

ANN ARBOR STAGING

Stage I: Involvement of a single lymph node region (I) or localized involvement of a single extralymphatic organ or site in the absence of any lymph node involvement (IE) (rare in Hodgkin's lymphoma).

Stage II: Involvement of two or more lymph node regions on the same side of the diaphragm (II), or localized involvement of a single extralymphatic organ or site in association with regional lymph node involvement with or without involvement of other lymph node regions on the same side of the diaphragm (IIE). The number of regions involved may be indicated by a subscript, for example II_3.

Stage III: Involvement of lymph node regions on both sides of the diaphragm (III), which also may be accompanied by extralymphatic extension in association with adjacent lymph node involvement (IIIE) or by involvement of the spleen (III_S) or both ($IIIE_S$).

Stage IV: Diffuse or disseminated involvement of one or more extralymphatic organs, with or without associated lymph node involvement; or isolated extralymphatic organ involvement in the absence of adjacent regional lymph node involvement, but in conjunction with disease in distant site(s). Any involvement of the liver or bone marrow, or nodular involvement of the lung(s). The location of stage IV disease is identified further by designating the specific site.

Greene FL, et al: *AJCC cancer staging of manual,* ed 6, New York, 2002, Springer-Verlag.

---

splenic involvement. Hodgkin's disease can also spread to the lungs and skeletal system in the late stages. It rarely involves the organ systems of the upper aerodigestive tract, central nervous system (CNS), skin, gastrointestinal (GI) tract, Waldeyer's ring, or Peyer's patches.

Treatment Techniques

Stages I and II. Before the 1960s, there were no effective methods of treating Hodgkin's lymphoma. Surgery was done only for biopsy, to determine the pathology and stage of disease, or to debulk large tumors. Chemotherapy agents used at that time were extremely toxic and caused subsequent leukemia in the patients. The breakthrough in Hodgkin's treatment was the development of **total-nodal irradiation** for the treatment of stages I and II disease. In this method of treatment, the contiguous lymphatic chains are irradiated with a cancericidal dose. The patients are treated with anterior and posterior fields to the supradiaphragmatic lymph nodes in a **mantle field** (Figure 29-3) followed by anteroposterior (AP)/posteroanterior (PA) radiation to the subdiaphragmatic lymph nodes, including the para-aortic nodes and the spleen (or the splenic pedicle if the spleen had been removed). The combination of mantle field and para-aortic fields is referred to as **extended-field irradiation** (Figure 29-4). The mantle and para-aortic fields are most commonly treated sequentially with a break in treatment occurring between fields to enable the patient to recover from the side effects of treatment. Total-nodal irradiation (see Figure 29-4) refers to the treatment

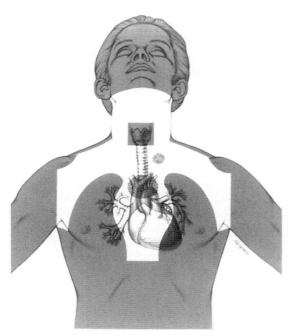

Figure 29-3. A typical mantle field for the treatment of Hodgkin's disease. Note the blocking of healthy lung tissue and humeral heads. An anterior larynx block and posterior cervical spine block are optional, depending on the location of the affected nodes. The treatment is with parallel opposed anterior and posterior fields. (From Cox JD: *Moss' radiation oncology*, ed 7, St. Louis, 1994, Mosby.)

of the pelvic, retroperitoneal, and inguinal nodes in addition to the supradiaphragmatic and subdiaphragmatic nodes. These nodes were included in treatment if the disease originated inferior to the diaphragm or in the inguinal nodes. The delivery of these adjacent large treatment fields required meticulous treatment planning and simulation and frequent verification films.

With the total dose of 35 to 44 Gy delivered by 6- to 10-MV photons to both the mantle and para-aortic fields, this treatment was very successful and produced high cure rates in patients with early-stage Hodgkin's disease. Using radiation therapy alone with either the total-nodal or extended field technique reduces the acute and late drug-related toxicities and avoids drug resistance, so chemotherapy may be used as a salvage treatment in the case of recurrence. From the 1960s to the mid-1990s, chemotherapy was reserved for use in patients with unfavorable stages I and II (A and B) and stages III and IV disease. This was because the standard of care, the MOPP regimen (mechlorethamine, vincristine [Oncovin], prednisone, and procarbazine), was extremely toxic and induced leukemia as a late-term side effect.

Radiation is not without toxicities. Total-nodal and extended-field radiation increase the risk of second solid malignancies of the lung, GI tract, and breast.[5] Remembering that patients with Hodgkin's disease tend to be younger than 40 years of age and are very curable, these late-term complications are cause for concern. Fortunately, less toxic chemotherapy agents have been developed and are currently the primary method of treating early-stage Hodgkin's lymphoma. The ABVD chemotherapy

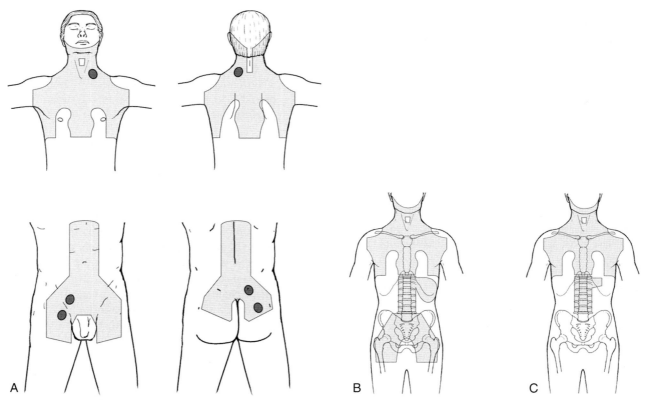

Figure 29-4. A, Extended fields include treatment of contiguous lymph node regions. **B**, Total-nodal irradiation; standard fields treat all lymph node areas typically involved by Hodgkin's lymphoma. **C**, Subtotal or modified total-nodal irradiation, which excludes only the pelvic nodes. (Drawings by Louis Clark. In Gunderson LL, Tepper JE: *Clinical radiation oncology*, Philadelphia, 2000, Churchill Livingstone.)

regimen is composed of doxorubicin (Adriamycin), bleomycin, vincristine, and dacarbazine.

Today, the standard of treatment for stages I and II Hodgkin's lymphoma is the ABVD regimen alone or in combination with radiation (30 to 36 Gy) to the involved lymph node region, termed **involved-field irradiation** (Figure 29-5). When there is bulky disease, the combined therapy of chemotherapy plus involved-field irradiation reduces the risk of relapse.[13]

Treatment Field Design and Techniques: Mantle Field.
A mantle field is illustrated in Figure 29-3. It includes all major lymph node regions above the diaphragm: submandibular, occipital, cervical, supraclavicular, infraclavicular, axillary,

hilar, and mediastinal. Anteriorly, the superior border is at the inferior portion of the mandible, and the inferior border is at the level of the insertion of the diaphragm (usually around T10). Posteriorly, the superior border includes the occipital nodes, and the inferior border is the same as it is anteriorly (approximately T10). Laterally, the axillary nodes are included. Precise blocking is extremely important in this field. As much healthy lung as possible should be spared by blocking the lungs anteriorly and posteriorly; however, adequate margins need to be designed around sites of involvement. Some lung will be radiated because the mediastinal and hilar nodes must be included in this field. Humeral head blocks are also important to prevent future bone

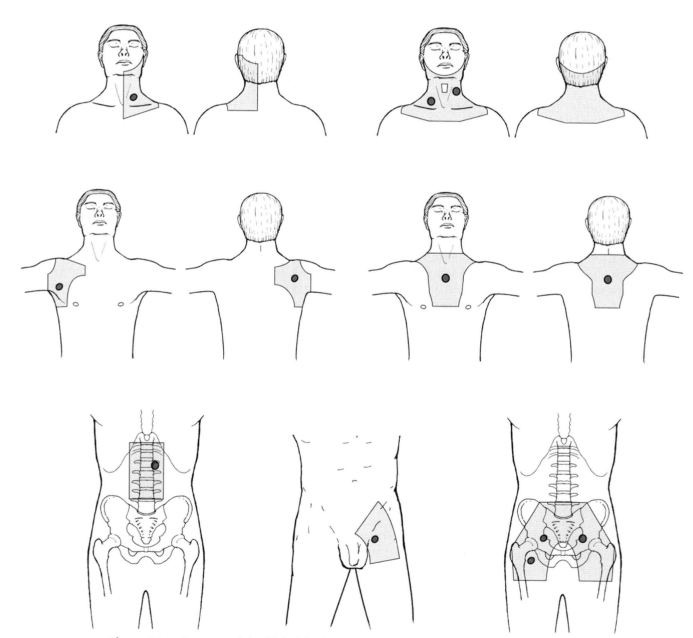

Figure 29-5. Because of the high risk of subclinical involvement in adjacent lymph nodes within a region, the involved-field treatment is the minimum field size typically used in radiation therapy for Hodgkin's lymphomas. (Drawings by Louis Clark. In Gunderson LL, Tepper JE: *Clinical radiation oncology*, Philadelphia, 2000, Churchill Livingstone.)

destruction, and a larynx block should be included anteriorly unless bulky disease is adjacent to the larynx. Posteriorly, a cord block may be needed, depending on the total dose. A posterior cord block may be used from the outset of treatment or added at 40 Gy, unless it is contraindicated by the location of the primary tumor.

The cardiac silhouette is irradiated to a dose of 15 Gy, but then a block shielding the apex of the heart should be added. After 30 to 35 Gy, a subcarinal block (5 cm inferior to the carina) should also be added to shield more of the pericardium and heart.

For the treatment of the mantle field, the patient lies supine (for anterior) with the arms **akimbo** (elbows bent) and hands on the hips or with hands placed above the head. The chin must be extended as much as possible to prevent exposure to the mouth, particularly from the exit dose of the posterior field. Treatment in the prone position for the posterior field forces the chin superiorly and eliminates the exit dose to the oral cavity. Body molds are helpful in reducing body movement and increasing the patient's comfort.

Subdiaphragmatic Fields. The most common treatment of the subdiaphragmatic fields is the treatment of the para-aortic nodes and the spleen or splenic pedicle when no evidence of subdiaphragmatic disease is present. The inferior border of the mantle field determines the superior border, with a gap between to avoid overdosing of the spinal cord. The inferior border is typically L4 or L5 or below the bifurcation of the aorta (see Figure 29-3).

Total-Nodal Irradiation. The classic total-nodal irradiation technique includes an inverted Y field. Included in the inverted Y field are the retroperitoneal, common iliac, and inguinal lymph nodes. The full inverted Y is seldom treated as a prophylactic measure, but it is treated for subdiaphragmatic disease. Sometimes it is also used for stage IB or IIB disease. If the pelvis is not included in the treatment fields, the radiation method is referred to as *subtotal lymphoid irradiation*.

Blocking in the subdiaphragmatic fields is also extremely important because of the presence of the liver, kidneys, and bone marrow–containing pelvic bones and reproductive organs. A low dose to the liver is delivered with partial transmission blocks of 50% to deliver 20 to 22 Gy if (1) the spleen is involved, (2) radiation alone is used as a primary treatment, or (3) the liver is involved.

The ovaries are located over the iliac lymph nodes; therefore, an **oophoropexy** can be performed to reduce the risk of infertility. During this procedure, the ovaries are clipped behind the uterus. A midline block of 10 half-value layer (HVL) may then be placed to shield the gonads. In male patients, no special blocking is used to protect the testes unless the inguinal and femoral nodes are irradiated. In such instances, the dose to the testes may be as high as 10%. This dose can be reduced to 0.75% to 3% with the use of a 10-HVL midline block. The inguinal and femoral nodes are treated only if disease appears in these nodes or adjacent to them.

The involved-field radiation includes only the affected lymph node region such as the supraclavicular, ipsilateral cervical, or inguinal nodes. Adjuvant chemotherapy is always used before irradiation of involved fields. See Figure 29-5 for examples of involved-field radiation.

Stages III and IV. Advanced stages of Hodgkin's disease (stages IIIA, IIIB, and IV) are usually treated with chemotherapy with or without radiation therapy. Chemotherapy is also used for patients who relapse after radiation therapy; this is referred to as *salvage therapy*. ABVD chemotherapy is the most common chemotherapeutic regimen used. Other drug combinations currently in clinical trials are a MOP-BAP (mechlorethamine, Oncovin, prednisone, bleomycin, Adriamycin, and procarbazine) hybrid or an ABVD with MOPP/ABV.[13]

The debate continues on the role of adjuvant radiation therapy for advanced-stage Hodgkin's lymphoma. Patients receiving chemotherapy tend to relapse at the original site of the disease. When involved-field radiation therapy is used following chemotherapy, there is a lowered risk of local relapse.[14] To further the argument for radiation therapy, 20% of patients with stages III and IV disease fail to enter a complete remission after their initial chemotherapy. Clinical trial outcomes indicate that patients with late-stage disease who received consolidative irradiation after chemotherapy obtained an 82% to 85% disease-free survival rate.[14] Unfortunately, patients treated with radiation after chemotherapy experienced more deaths from causes other than Hodgkin's than those who received additional chemotherapy. It is therefore generally recommended that only stage III patients with NSHL and bulky nodal involvement receive adjuvant radiation therapy.[14]

Autologous bone marrow stem cell transplants and peripheral blood stem cell transplants have been used when Hodgkin's disease becomes resistant to standard treatment with chemotherapy and radiation. Experience has proved that it is best to perform the autologous stem cell transplant soon after the first treatments fail. However, if the patient remains in remission for a long period after the first treatment, a second course of either radiation or chemotherapy is recommended.[15] In preparation for the bone marrow transplant, low-dose total-body irradiation (TBI) may be used to deplete the bone marrow function of the patient.

Radiation may also be used for palliation to prolong survival and provide symptomatic relief. It may be used to alleviate pain, to decrease the tumor mass to eliminate obstructions, and to improve the overall quality of life.

Because the initial doses of radiation range from 25 to 40 Gy, additional treatment with radiation to affected sites is entirely possible. Twice-a-day treatment may be necessary for a rapidly growing, chemotherapy-resistant tumor.[14]

Pediatric Treatments. Children and adolescents may be treated with chemotherapy alone or in combination with involved-field radiation therapy. High-dose, extended-field radiation therapy is seldom used in childhood cases because of the long-term effects on the growth process, cardiac toxicities, and the occurrence of second malignancies (particularly lung, breast, and GI tract). Likewise, systemic therapy alone has undesirable side effects: myelosuppression, gonadal injury, and secondary acute myelogenous leukemia (AML). Researchers have achieved excellent treatment outcomes and reduced treatment side effects with combined modality treatments that use lower does and smaller volumes of radiation therapy and fewer cycles of less toxic chemotherapy. Involved-field radiation may be reduced to as low as 15 to 25 cGy, and the chemotherapy regimens of MOPP/ABVD have proved to be highly effective.[11]

Side Effects. Acute side effects of radiation treatment are dependent on the size of the fields treated. The following is a list of side effects for the mantle and para-aortic fields:

- Fatigue
- Occipital hair loss (may be permanent, depending on the dose)
- Skin erythema
- Sore throat (esophagitis)
- Altered taste (especially with preauricular nodes)
- Transient dysphagia from radiation-induced esophagitis
- Dry cough
- Nausea
- Occasional vomiting
- Diarrhea (rare)

Most of the side effects are managed by good nursing care, which may include an antiemetic, the application of nongreasy skin creams, protection from sunlight, additional rest, an altered diet (soft, bland foods and no alcohol), throat lozenges, and diarrhea medication. Because the course of treatment is relatively short for each phase of treatment, patients with Hodgkin's disease usually manage their side effects well.

Late-stage complications depend on the treatment technique, total dose, and irradiated volumes. Most of the complications result from the mantle field treatment. They include the following:

- Mild radiation pneumonitis (depending on the volume of the lung treated) 6 to 12 weeks after the end of treatment
- Hypothyroidism in one third of patients
- Herpes zoster
- Transient xerostomia, which requires careful, permanent dental care
- Increased dental caries
- Radiation carditis, which occurs in fewer than 5% of patients
- L'hermitte's syndrome, which is a transient complication consisting of numbness, tingling, or electric sensations throughout the body caused by the extreme head flexion necessary for a mantle field

Patients are at increased risk for lung, breast, and GI cancers after mantle treatment. In addition, breast cancer in previously irradiated Hodgkin's patients tends to be more aggressive than in normal populations.[8] Treatment-related second malignancies and cardiac complications are the main causes of death other than Hodgkin's disease itself in long-term survivors.[14]

Xerospermia can result in men after pelvic irradiation if no precautions are taken. With precautions, the sperm count diminishes during treatment but returns to normal levels afterward. The MOPP, but not the ABVD, regimen causes sterility in men.

In women older than 30 years, even with oophoropexy and well-planned pelvic irradiation precautions, the scattered dose may be sufficient to decrease ovarian functions and cause menopausal symptoms. Younger women do not experience these menopausal symptoms. Chemotherapy also affects women similarly. Combined chemotherapy and radiation therapy, however, may affect menstrual function and fertility in younger women.

Psychosocial problems that patients with Hodgkin's disease commonly experience include depression (associated with the low energy levels during treatment), marital difficulties, and a decrease in sexual interest. Patients who have recovered from Hodgkin's disease sometimes are denied coverage by insurance providers because of an increased risk of later disease.

Results of Treatment

Stages IA and IIA. Most studies indicate that patients with stage IA disease have a cure rate of approximately 90% with radiation therapy as the only form of treatment.[13] Eighty percent of patients with stage IIA disease achieve a cure with radiation therapy alone. Patients with stages IA and IIA disease with favorable prognostic factors (sedimentation rate of less than 40 to 50 mm/hr, patient age of 40 to 50 or younger, lymphocyte predominant or nodular sclerosing histology, and no bulky adenopathy) have an 80% relapse-free survival rate at 5 to 10 years with mantle field, para-aortic, and splenic radiation therapy and no laparotomy.[13] To date, the treatment of early-stage, favorable disease with ABVD chemotherapy and involved-field or extended-field radiation has proved to be equivalent in overall survival and failure-free survival rates. However, statistics on 15-year survival are not yet available on this group of patients.[13]

Stages IB and IIB. It is recommended that patients with B symptoms receive combination chemotherapy with or without additional radiation therapy, because 25% of these patients relapse after radiation.[13] Patients in this category have similar survival rates to patients with stages IA and IIA. The 10-year relapse-free rate is 78% to 88%. However, the subgroup that experiences fevers and weight loss has a 10-year survival relapse-free rate of 48% to 57%, regardless of the type of therapy.[13]

Stages I and II, with Bulky Mediastinal Involvement. Patients in this group have no difference in survival rates from those with stages IA and IIA, but their relapse rates are as high as 50%. These patients are at special risk for developing complications related to treatment. Usually, chemotherapy is used first to reduce the mediastinal disease and so that less lung tissue is included in the treatment fields.

Subdiaphragmatic Stages I and II. Approximately 10% of patients with Hodgkin's disease have this type of disease. Current practice recommends that patients with subdiaphragmatic presentation should receive chemotherapy and involved-field radiation.[13] This treatment avoids the extended pelvic and abdominal field irradiation of the inverted Y and splenic field techniques, which have serious side effects to the bone marrow.

Stage IIIA. A summary of 11 studies that used combined chemotherapy and radiation showed a 10-year survival rate of approximately 80% to 90%. With radiation alone, the 10-year survival rate declined to 68% to 80%.[14]

Stages IIIB and IV. The 10-year survival rate is 43% to 51% with the use of systemic MOPP or ABVD. Radiation may be added to treat bulky disease, and doing so increases the 5-year disease-free survival rate to as much at 82%.[14]

Treatment for relapse must be individualized. In general, patients who received radiation alone are candidates for chemotherapy. Some researchers recommend the delivery of low-dose radiation (15 to 25 Gy) to the previously treated areas after chemotherapy and 35 to 44 Gy to the previously untreated areas.

Pediatric Treatment Outcomes. Long-term, disease-free survival for pediatric patients with early-stage disease who are treated with combined chemotherapy and radiation therapy ranges from 85% to 96%. Children and adolescents with advanced-stage disease who have received combined modality treatments achieved from 77% to 93% disease-free survival. Treatment results for pediatric patients with Hodgkin's who receive chemotherapy alone range from 60% to 100% for all stages.[11]

Role of Radiation Therapist

For patients who have Hodgkin's disease, the radiation therapist plays a vital role not only in delivering the radiation but also in assisting with side effect management education and offering psychological support during treatment.

The first priority of the therapist is the accurate delivery of the prescribed radiation dose. Positioning the patient consistently is vital for the accuracy of the treatments. When treating a mantle field, the chin is hyperextended, and the use of a thermoplastic mask for head immobilization contributes to consistency and ease of treatment. Leveling marks on the side of the patient's thorax ensure that the patient is lying consistently flat. The use of horizontal marks on the shoulders (in alignment with the central axis) as a positioning guide for the arms is also helpful. If the patient also has a para-aortic field, the gap measurement must be measured precisely and daily to prevent either an overdose or an underdose.

Accuracy in block or multileaf collimator (MLC) placement can mean the difference in shielding disease or in delivering an unnecessary dose to healthy tissue. Complex blocking (either Cerrobend or MLC) is necessary to shield the lungs and heart. Figure 29-6 demonstrates the use of shielding in a mini-mantle field. The use of MLCs simplifies the need for custom blocking; however, because of the complex block arrangements and the limits of the MLCs, additional custom blocks may be necessary. Verification films should be taken at least weekly to ensure accuracy.

Because of the addition of cord blocks, cardiac blocks, and shrinking fields (in mantle treatments), the maintenance of accurate records is critical. Clear and precise notes should be written in the charts, indicating all blocking changes. Verification films should be taken before changes in blocking, especially before the addition of the cord block.

The blood counts require rigorous monitoring because of the radiation and/or chemotherapy effects on the bone marrow. Again, the therapist should pay close attention to the counts and ensure that they are taken as prescribed.

Communication is the second priority of any radiation therapist. The patient must be informed about daily procedures and any additional occurrences, such as portal images or new blocking. As the treatment progresses, the therapist plays an important role in the management of side effects. Often, the therapist is told first of these side effects. According to institution policies, the therapist may advise the patient regarding the way to handle the side effects or refer the patient to a nurse, dietitian, or physician. Communication with the family and other professionals involved with the patient's care regarding the side effects is critical.

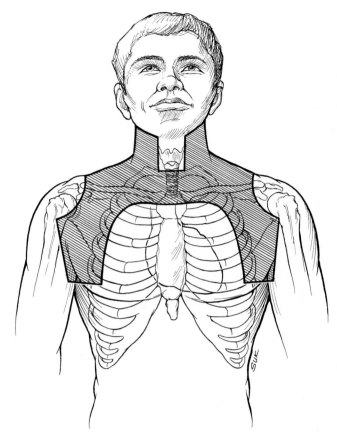

Figure 29-6. A mini-mantle, or supramediastinal mantle field, for disease limited to the cervical, supraclavicular, or axilla regions. Note the use of blocks to shield the lungs. Treatment is delivered anteriorly and posteriorly with parallel opposed portals.

Because of the daily contact with the patient, the therapist is in the position of evaluating the patient's physical and emotional needs. Many times, referral to another agency or individual such as a social worker, support group, or chaplain is appropriate.

CASE I

Nodular Sclerosing Hodgkin's Lymphoma

A 28-year-old white woman had been in good health until 6 weeks before her initial consultation. At that time, she noticed swelling in her lower neck. A biopsy revealed NSHL. Her weight had remained stable, she had no energy loss, and she did not exhibit any B symptoms. At the time of the biopsy, a chest radiograph also revealed mediastinal adenopathy, classifying her disease as stage IIA (more than one involved area on the same side of the diaphragm).

The patient had a tonsillectomy at age 4. Seven years before her diagnosis, the patient had a benign lymph node removed from the high cervical area. She smoked lightly in high school and had an occasional glass of wine. She had no family history of cancer, although her maternal grandmother had a bilateral mastectomy for reasons unknown to the patient.

In addition to the biopsy and chest radiograph, a liver function test and CT scan were performed. The outcomes were negative for any abdominal involvement. Therefore, the conclusion was made that a bone marrow biopsy was unnecessary. During physical examination, the physician did not find any organomegaly, masses, inguinal adenopathy, or epitrochlear lymphadenopathy. The patient was also presented to a tumor board. The tumor board recommended a lymphangiogram to serve as an additional diagnostic procedure and assist in the treatment planning. The consensus of the tumor board was that radiation alone would be the optimal treatment for this patient.

She was treated with parallel opposed mantle fields to 41.4 Gy in 25 fractions (1.8 Gy/day) over 35 elapsed days with 6-MV photons. The mantle field measured 33 × 29.5 cm anteriorly and 31 × 29.5 cm posteriorly, both at 105 cm skin-source distance (SSD). She was treated in the supine position for the anterior field and in the prone position for the posterior field.

After a month break from the completion of the mantle fields, she received radiation therapy to the para-aortic lymph nodes and spleen anteroposteriorly/posteroanteriorly to 39.6 Gy in 22 fractions over 29 elapsed days. This field measured 25 × 17 cm and was treated at 105 cm SSD in a spade field configuration. The superior border was T10, and the inferior border was between S1 and S2.

During the mantle field treatment, the patient experienced severe nausea and vomiting, beginning after the third fraction. Prochlorperazine (Compazine) was given, without much relief, followed by metoclopramide (Reglan) after a dose of 16.2 Gy (9 fractions) was delivered. Metoclopramide brought some minor relief, but on the fifteenth treatment, intramuscular injections of pyridoxine (Pyridoxine) were given and resulted in dramatic improvement. During this time, the patient lost 10 pounds and experienced headaches, a sore throat, and a dry mouth. She also had difficulty swallowing. She was instructed to drink tepid liquids, and she was given throat lozenges and Tylenol No. 3. By the end of the mantle treatment course, she had regained 2 pounds.

The patient tolerated her para-aortic treatments better. When she returned 1 month after the completion of the mantle field, she was feeling better, was eating well, and had good energy levels. At 3060 cGy, she experienced some nausea and vomiting, which were relieved by metoclopramide. Her total weight loss during the last half of treatment less than 4 pounds.

Approximately 1 month after the completion of her treatments, she experienced a herpes outbreak on her right chest wall, which cleared in approximately 1 week. She experienced no other late or chronic side effects.

Three years posttreatment, the patient gave birth to a second child. Her treatment in the late 1980s was the standard of care for that time. Unfortunately, she became one of the Hodgkin's survivors who subsequently developed breast cancer (18 years post–radiation therapy), but she was treated successfully for her breast cancer.

NON-HODGKIN'S LYMPHOMA

NHL may arise anywhere that the lymph travels. It may occur in the lymph nodes, a group of lymph nodes, an organ such as the stomach or lung, or any combination of these. NHLs differ from Hodgkin's disease in several ways, including the following:

1. They occur primarily in older persons; the median age is 67 years.[15]
2. They can originate in the lymph nodes or in extranodal tissue.
3. They are more likely to spread randomly, rather than in an orderly pattern.
4. Multiple sites are often involved and extranodal lesions are common.
5. The prognosis of NHLs is strongly dependent on the specific histology.
6. NHLs encompass a wide variety of diseases, which the experts continue to attempt to classify into appropriate categories.

Epidemiology

The incidence of lymphomas has increased 65% since the 1970s. Projections from the National Cancer Institute's Surveillance Epidemiology and End Results (SEER) Cancer Statistics estimate 66,120 new cases in the United States in 2008 and 19,160 deaths from NHL in 2008.[15] The male-to-female ratio is similar to that of Hodgkin's disease in that there is a slight male predominance. In the United States, white males have a higher incidence than African Americans, Japanese Americans, Chinese Americans, Hispanics, and Native Americans. Worldwide, the incidence of NHL varies greatly from country to country. For example, Burkitt's lymphoma is common in Africa but rare in other countries, although patients with AIDS tend to get this form of lymphoma. Lymphomas are the third most common childhood malignancy, accounting for 10% of all childhood cancers. Two thirds of these childhood lymphomas are NHL.[4]

The median age is 67, but lymphoma incidence actually peaks in the 80- to 84-year-old age group. The incidence has tripled for patients older than 65.5; researchers have yet to explain this increase in incidence.

Etiology

Researchers have discovered that lymphomas are genetic alterations of the B- or T-lymphocyte cells.[4] The exact causes of NHL, however, are largely unknown. However, researchers have identified many risk factors such as exposure to particular infectious agents and reduced immune function. Burkitt's lymphoma is caused by the Epstein-Barr virus. Serologic (blood) studies have shown an association between human T-cell leukemia/lymphoma virus (HTLV-1) and T-cell leukemia/lymphoma. Patients with AIDS have a 165% increased risk of developing NHL in the first 3.5 years after their AIDS diagnosis.[4] Other immunosuppressed patients, such as those having heart and kidney transplants, are also at increased risk.

People exposed to ionizing radiation are at a greater risk of developing lymphomas. There is an increased incidence of lymphomas in atomic bomb survivors who were exposed to 10 Gy or more. Patients who received radiation therapy for ankylosing spondylitis (a chronic inflammatory disease affecting the spine, which was formerly treated with radiation) are at risk for contracting lymphomas. Patients with Hodgkin's disease who were treated with the MOPP chemotherapy are at a 20-fold risk of developing NHL, and patients receiving chemotherapy in general are at a greater risk of developing NHL. There is also an increased incidence in patients who take phenytoin to control seizures, in agricultural workers exposed to herbicides, and in industrial workers exposed to solvents and vinyl chloride. Recent studies have identified higher incidences in women with high dietary intake of *trans*-unsaturated fats[15] and in people who participate in recreational drug use.[4]

In addition to the histology of the disease, age is an important prognostic factor. The younger the patient, the better is the prognosis, in part because older patients have less tolerance to the treatment. Older patients also tend to have more advanced disease at the time of diagnosis. Unfortunately, 50% of patients with NHL are older than 60 years.

Suppression of the immune system is thought to cause increased risk of NHLs. This includes infection with the human immunodeficiency virus (HIV), organ or bone marrow transplant (requiring immune suppression medications), rheumatoid arthritis, and inherited immune deficiencies. The use of pesticides and herbicides was studied by the National Academy of Sciences (NAS) as a risk factor because agricultural workers had higher rates of NHLs. The NAS found a "positive association" between exposure to herbicides and NHL.[14]

Clinical Presentation

The signs and symptoms of NHL are similar to those of Hodgkin's lymphoma: enlarged lymph nodes, fever, night sweats, fatigue, itching, and weight loss. Unlike Hodgkin's lymphoma, however, NHL may arise in a wide variety of sites, most commonly in the lymph nodes, GI tract, and Waldeyer's ring. Lymphomas of the CNS commonly occur in patients with AIDS.

Clinically, lymphomas can appear as enlarged nodes or are discovered when the patient has symptoms related to the site and extent of tumor involvement. For example, shortness of breath or a cough is symptomatic of lung involvement. Abdominal pain or a change in bowel habits may indicate pelvic disease. Symptoms of brain involvement are headaches, vision problems, and seizures. Disease outside the lymph system is more common in intermediate- and high-grade lymphomas. In general, when the lymphoma occurs outside the nodes, such as in the GI tract or CNS, the course of disease is worse. Waldeyer's ring is the least worrisome of all of the extranodal sites.

Systemic symptoms (as seen in patients with in Hodgkin's disease) are rare, occurring in only 10% to 15% of the patients at the time of presentation, and no conclusive evidence exists as to whether the presence of symptoms plays a part in the overall prognosis. Distinguishing the importance of the histology from that of the stage of disease is difficult.

Detection and Diagnosis

The diagnostic workup defines the extent of the disease and assists in the decision on the treatment course. The history and physical examination are, of course, the standard first steps, as are the cytologic evaluations. Included in the blood tests are a complete blood count, an HIV test, a blood chemistry, a urinalysis, serum lactate dehydrogenase (LDH), liver function tests, and serum alkaline phosphatase. A bone marrow biopsy is necessary because bone marrow involvement is common in many lymphomas; however, MRI may be just as sensitive, if not more sensitive, than a biopsy and can also identify CNS involvement.[4] A chest radiograph; a CT of the abdomen, pelvis, neck, and chest; and a bone scan are also part of the first line of diagnostic tests. PET scans have been increasingly used for staging, as well.

Further diagnostic tests may include a gallium whole-body scan and upper GI or small bowel series. A CT scan of the brain may be recommended if previous tests or symptoms indicate possible disease at this site. A lymphangiogram of the pelvis and abdomen is performed if the CT scan shows abnormal results.

Pathology

There are two types of lymphoid tissue: primary (central) lymph tissue and peripheral (secondary) lymph tissue. The primary lymphoid tissue harbors the lymphoid precursor cells, both B and T cells. The peripheral tissue is where the antigen-specific reactions occur. The primary lymphoid tissues are the bone marrow and the thymus. The bone marrow produces the precursor B cells (which make antibodies) and precursor T cells (which are responsible for the regulation of the immune system). Most lymphomas in the United States are of B-cell origin. The immature T-cell precursors must migrate to the thymus in the anterior mediastinum to undergo maturation.

Peripheral lymphoid tissues are the lymph node, the spleen, and mucosa-associated lymphoid tissue (MALT) found in the epithelium of the nasopharynx and oropharynx (Waldeyer's ring), the GI tract, the distal ileum (**Peyer's patches**), the colon, and the rectum. Lymphomas arising out of these mucosa-associated tissues are referred to as *MALT lymphomas.*

Features that best predict the prognosis of lymphomas are size, shape, and pattern of the cells. Small and round or angulated cells are called *cleaved cells.* Other lymphomas may be composed of large cells or combinations of small and large cells. Intermediate-sized lymphocytes with rapidly dividing cells are characteristic of aggressive, high-grade lymphomas.

In the normal lymph nodes are microscopic clusters or follicles of specialized lymphocytes. In lymphomas, some lymphocytes arrange themselves in a similar pattern called a *follicular,* or *nodular, pattern.* These lymphomas and small cell lymphomas tend to be low grade and follow a slower or indolent course with an average survival time for patients of 6 to 12 years.

The more aggressive lymphomas (intermediate and high grade) lose their normal appearance by the diffuse involvement of tumor cells that are usually moderate or large sized.

Lymphomas can be histopathologically classified as follicular (or nodular) and diffuse, with 40% appearing as follicular and 60% as diffuse. The follicular lymphomas are of B-cell origin and tend to run an indolent course with prolonged survival. Although many patients have advanced disease, the median survival for patients with follicular types is 5 to 7 years. Follicular lymphomas usually appear below the diaphragm, and the involvement of the mesenteric lymph nodes is common. Children seldom get follicular lymphomas, and these lymphomas do not commonly involve Waldeyer's ring.

Diffuse lymphomas can be of B- or T-cell origin and run a more aggressive course. Ironically, they usually appear with more localized disease, but they spread quickly to other nodes and extranodal sites. There is also an increase in bone marrow and Waldeyer's ring involvement. The lymphatics are the most common site of recurrence with either type.

Grading. Lymphoma classification systems have continually evolved since the 1950s. The current system commonly used is the Revised European-American Classification of Lymphoid Neoplasms (REAL) that has been combined with the World Health Organization (WHO) classification of hematologic malignancies (Box 29-2). The REAL classification system combines morphology, immunophenotype, genetic features, and clinical features to define disease entities and is a major advancement over the former systems.

| Box 29-2 | Updated European-American Classification of Lymphoid Neoplasms/World Health Organization Classification of Lymphoid Neoplasms (REAL/WHO classification)* |

B-CELL NEOPLASMS

- Precursor B-cell neoplasms
- *Precursor B-lymphoblastic leukemia/lymphoma (B-ALL/LBL)*
- Mature (peripheral) B-cell neoplasms
  - B-cell chronic lymphocytic leukemia/small lymphocytic lymphoma
  - B-cell prolymphocytic leukemia
  - Lymphoplasmacytic lymphoma
  - Splenic marginal zone B-cell lymphoma (±villous lymphocytes)
  - Hairy cell leukemia
  - Plasma cell myeloma/plasmacytoma
- Extranodal marginal zone B-cell lymphoma of MALT type
- Mantle cell lymphoma
- Follicular lymphoma
- Nodal marginal zone B-cell lymphoma (±monocytoid B cells)
- Diffuse large B-cell lymphoma
- Burkitt's lymphoma

T- AND NK-CELL NEOPLASMS

- Precursor T-cell neoplasm
  - Precursor T-lymphoblastic leukemia/lymphoma (T-ALL/LBL)
  - Mature (peripheral) T-cell neoplasms
  - T-cell prolymphocytic leukemia
  - T-cell granular lymphocytic leukemia
  - Aggressive NK-cell leukemia
  - Adult T-cell lymphoma/leukemia (HTLVI+)
  - Extranodal NK/T-cell lymphoma, nasal type
  - Enteropathy-type T-cell lymphoma
  - Hepatosplenic γ δ T-cell lymphoma
  - Subcutaneous panniculitis-like T-cell lymphoma
  - Mycosis fungoides/Sézary syndrome
  - Anaplastic large cell lymphoma, primary cutaneous type
  - *Peripheral T-cell lymphoma, unspecified*
  - *Angioimmunoblastic T-cell lymphoma*
  - *Anaplastic large cell lymphoma, primary systemic type*

HODGKIN'S DISEASE

- Lymphocytic predominance, nodular ± diffuse areas
- Classic Hodgkin's disease
  - Nodular sclerosing
  - Mixed cellularity
  - Lymphocyte depleted
  - Lymphocyte-rich classic Hodgkin's disease

From Harris NL, et al: Lymphoma classification—from controversy to consensus: the R.E.A.L. and WHO classification of lymphoid neoplasms, *Ann Oncol* 11(suppl 1):3-10, 2000.

MALT, Mucosa-associated lymphoid tissue; *NK*, natural killer.
*More common entities are given in italics.

Staging

Categorizing lymphomas into staging systems is as complex as grading them. As research continues, particularly patients with HIV, additional light is shed onto this disease process. Although the Ann Arbor system is most commonly used for the staging

of NHLs, it is not completely satisfactory. In contrast to patients with Hodgkin's lymphoma, many patients with NHL have advanced disease. The Ann Arbor system also fails to account for bulky disease, which plays a significant role in lymphomas because many patients have advanced disease but experience relatively long survival. Although the diaphragm plays an important role in the staging of Hodgkin's disease, it is insignificant in the progression of lymphomas. Therefore, a major factor in the Ann Arbor system is inconsequential in NHLs.

Treatment Techniques

NHLs include a wide variety of clinical diseases, and the treatment choices depend largely on the specific subtype, the extent of the disease, and the patient's age and general health. Choices of treatment fall into five categories[4]:

1. No initial therapy (for indolent, low-grade disease)
2. Chemotherapy
3. Radiation therapy
4. New biologic therapies
5. Stem cell transplants

Surgery is used primarily for diagnostic purposes, because it is ineffective in controlling the progression of the disease. The most common practice is to administer chemotherapy with or without radiation for most patients. The stage and grade, more than the particular treatment regimen, determines the ultimate outcome of treatment.[15]

Localized disease involving only one site or two immediately adjacent sites, with tumors less than 10 cm in diameter and no systemic symptoms, has a high likelihood of cure. This may be true for all subtypes, but most studies have been conducted on diffuse, histologically aggressive lymphomas.

Chemotherapy is administered to treat occult disease and reduce the risk of distant failure. In general, it is given as the sole treatment, depending on the particular lymphoma, or before radiation therapy. The chemotherapy dose can be reduced by half when radiation therapy follows immediately. Likewise, the radiation dose can be reduced when treatment is combined with chemotherapy. Multiagent chemotherapy has proved more effective than single-agent regimens because the multiagent regimens prevent cellular sensitization to any one drug.[4] Formerly, the most common treatment for stage I and nonbulky stage II diffuse, aggressive NHL was the CHOP regimen (cyclophosphamide, hydroxydaunorubicin [doxorubicin] vincristine [Oncovin], and prednisone), given in three or four cycles and followed by radiation therapy to the involved site and adjacent lymph nodes.

Since CHOP was introduced in the 1970s, there has been no apparent change in mortality from lymphomas in the United States.[1] Therefore, new regimens have been developed, including the following[4,6]:

1. CVP (cyclophosphamide, vincristine, prednisone)
2. mBACOD (methotrexate, bleomycin, doxorubicin [Adriamycin], cyclophosphamide, vincristine [Oncovin], dexamethasone)
3. FND (fludarabine, mitoxantrone, and dexamethasone)
4. ProMACE/CytaBOM (prednisone, doxorubicin, [Adriamycin], cyclophosphamide, etoposide, cytarabine, bleomycin, vincristine [Oncovin], methotrexate, leucovorin)

5. PACEBOM (prednisolone, doxorubicin [Adriamycin], cyclophosphamide, etoposide, bleomycin, vincristine [Oncovin], methotrexate)

Cure is rare for patients with disseminated, low-grade NHL. However, patients who are asymptomatic at the time of the diagnosis can be monitored closely without therapy until symptoms occur, and a substantial portion of these patients have spontaneous remissions. If the symptoms can be improved or the patient is unwilling to proceed without therapy, treatment usually includes radiation therapy, single-agent chemotherapy, or a combination chemotherapy regimen with or without radiation therapy. Complete remissions can be achieved in most patients, and the remissions tend to last for extended periods. Interferon has been used successfully in combination with CHOP. Patients receiving this treatment have a longer remission time and a higher rate of survival than those treated with CHOP alone. Monoclonal antibodies, such as rituximab, have proved to be effective in the treatment of relapsed B-cell NHLs.[16]

Autologous bone marrow and stem cell transplants have proved to be very effective (50% 5-year survival) either for treating stages III and IV NHLs or for treating recurring disease.[3,4]

Current data indicate that 60% to 80% of adults with diffuse, aggressive NHL in stage II to IV can achieve complete remissions. Long-term, disease-free survival can be achieved in 30% to 50% of these patients. Larger doses of chemotherapy are given to patients who have histologically aggressive disease.[15]

Patients infected with HIV are particularly prone to NHLs. These lymphomas usually have a B-cell origin, are often associated with the Epstein-Barr viral genome in the tumor, and often occur in unusual extranodal sites such as the brain. Unfortunately, because of their already suppressed immune system, these patients do not tolerate treatment well. If no opportunistic infection occurs, the patients can tolerate some therapy and often respond well to treatment. The choice of chemotherapeutic agents for this population remains controversial.

Radiation Therapy. The role of radiation therapy in the treatment of lymphomas varies substantially from that in the treatment of Hodgkin's lymphoma. Although NHLs are sensitive to radiation, only a small portion of patients obtain a cure if treated with local or regional radiation alone. This is because there is a high probability of disease spread to other lymphatic or organ sites. Therefore, most lymphomas are treated with both radiation to the involved site and chemotherapy for systemic treatment.

Because lymphomas are radiosensitive, they regress quickly; however, radiation does not always alter the natural history of these diseases. In the study of treatment regimens, true survival and disease-free relapse must be distinguished.

Typically, radiation is given to the site of involvement, with coverage to the draining nodal groups on the same side of the diaphragm. Although total-nodal radiation can be used for stages I and II, it is not a common practice in the United States. The reason for this is that, although longer disease-free survival accompanies total-nodal radiation, there is no change in overall survival rates.

Radiation therapy is a standard management for stages I and II low-grade lymphomas, especially for patients younger than 40 years. Doses of 35 to 45 Gy are recommended for local control. Intermediate-grade lymphomas are generally treated with a CHOP regimen followed by 30 to 35 Gy of radiation therapy.[15]

Radiation therapy alone is used to treat stages I and II follicular lymphomas and the low-grade B-cell lymphoma of MALT. Follicular and mantle cell lymphomas can be curatively treated with 30 to 36 Gy with a boost to 36 to 40 Gy to the involved or regional field. The recurrence rate after 10 years is only 10%. MALT lymphomas may be treated with either surgery alone or local or regional radiation therapy of 30 Gy.[4]

Investigation of new treatments for late-stage lymphomas include the use of interferon-α (an antitumor agent) alone, in combination with chemotherapy, or as an adjuvant to chemotherapy; monoclonal antibodies; and high-dose chemotherapy with fractionated total-body radiation followed by bone marrow transplantation.

If a patient relapses, the same chemotherapy is often used. However, two additional agents have proved effective in the treatment of relapses: fludarabine and 2-chlorodeoxyadenosine (2CdA). High-dose-rate chemotherapy, radiation, and bone marrow transplantation are also used for the treatment of relapse in stages I and II. Radiation alone may also be used to reduce bulky disease and/or to relieve pain.

The 5-year survival rate is 90% for patients in stages I and II and 80% for those in stages III and IV. The average survival time for patients with low-grade lymphomas is 6 to 12 years.

Intermediate-grade lymphomas can be divided into favorable and unfavorable tumors. Favorable tumors are those less than 4 to 10 cm in diameter in which the LDH level is normal and no B symptoms are present. For patients with favorable stages I and II disease, treatment options include the following[6]:

1. Chemotherapy alone (CHOP)
2. Chemotherapy and radiation therapy
3. Primary radiation alone to the site, particularly if the patient is unable to tolerate chemotherapy

The 5-year survival rate is 80% to 90% for patients with stage I intermediate-grade lymphomas and 70% to 80% for patients in stage II.[6]

Unfavorable lymphomas in stages I, II, III, and IV are treated with combination chemotherapy. Regimens include CHOP, mBACOD, ProMACE/CytaBOM, and MACOP-B (methotrexate, Adriamycin, cyclophosphamide, vincristine, prednisone, and bleomycin). The survival rate is significantly lower for these patients than it is in the earlier stages. A 5-year survival rate of 40% to 50% is the norm for these patients.[6]

High-grade and lymphoblastic lymphomas usually receive multiagent chemotherapy with prophylactic CNS radiation. Patients in stage IV have extensive disease, usually with bone marrow involvement, and/or CNS involvement along with a high LDH level. In general, these patients have done poorly with conventional therapy and may benefit from intensive chemotherapy and radiation, followed by bone marrow transplantation.

The 5-year survival rate is 80% for patients with limited disease and 20% for patients with extensive disease involving the bone marrow or CNS.

AIDS-associated lymphomas are usually intermediate- and high-grade lymphomas and are highly aggressive. Of course, the condition of the patient dictates the treatment.

If given total-nodal irradiation at high doses, patients with stage III nodular lymphomas achieve a 33% remission rate after 10 years. However, with diffuse lymphomas, only 10% of the patients survive 10 years after total-nodal radiation. Chemotherapy (either a single alkylating agent or a combination of agents) is usually used for this stage.

Unless the disease originates in the mediastinum, mediastinal spread is rare. The mantle technique is commonly used in instances of mediastinal involvement. A mini-mantle or supramediastinal mantle is appropriate if no mediastinal disease or upper abdominal disease is present. Anteriorly, the inferior border for a mini-mantle field should be at the level of the inferior portion of the head of the clavicles; posteriorly, it should be at the inferior surface of the shaft of the clavicles (see Figure 29-6).

Preauricular nodes are often involved in the diffuse lymphomas and are at high risk in patients with cervical adenopathy. In such instances, these nodes should be treated with a prophylactic dose of 3600 cGy, administered in right and left lateral ports over 4 weeks.

Subdiaphragmatic Treatment. Mesenteric lymph node involvement is common with lymphomas occurring inferior to the diaphragm. In such instances, the whole abdomen is treated with the following four-field techniques[15] (Figure 29-7).

1. An AP/PA field extending from the dome of the diaphragm to the iliac crest (unless the tumor is at the level of the iliac crest, and then the field continues to the floor of the pelvis) is treated initially. The lateral portions of the ileum should be blocked to protect the iliac bone marrow, and the right lobe of the liver and the kidneys should also be protected. Over 2 to 3 weeks, 15 Gy should be delivered at a rate of 1.5 Gy/day.

2. After the AP/PA course of treatment, the upper abdomen is treated from lateral fields, based on the initial isocentric setup. If abdominal disease is massive, the pelvic portion may continue with an AP/PA configuration. The posterior margin of these fields should be anterior to the kidneys but should include the para-aortic nodes. Anteriorly, the field should include the anterior abdominal wall. Another 15 Gy over a 2-week period should be given, bringing the total dose to 30 Gy over 4 to 5 weeks. If the disease is on the posterior abdominal wall, the kidneys cannot be shielded. If the kidneys lie in the same plane as the para-aortic nodes, the lateral fields should be omitted.

3. Finally, a wide AP/PA para-aortic field (10 to 12 cm) is treated with kidney blocks, delivering 15 Gy in another 2-week period. The lateral margins of such a field should extend from the lateral margins of one kidney to the lateral margins of the other, with five HVL kidney blocks.

The total dose delivered to the whole abdomen is 45 Gy in 6 to 7 weeks. Pelvic irradiation may continue on an AP/PA basis throughout this period of abdominal irradiation if blood counts permit. Midline blocks should be no higher than the symphysis pubis.

When total-body irradiation is used for palliation in advanced cases of nodular lymphocytic lymphoma or nodular mixed lymphoma, 150 cGy to the midplane should be delivered over 5 weeks. Two or three fractions should be delivered weekly for a total of 30 cGy per week. The major complications of such treatment are thrombocytopenia or leukopenia. The platelet counts must be closely watched, with counts taken before each treatment.

Central Nervous System and Gastric Lymphomas. NHL is approximately 60 times more common in patients with AIDS than in the general population.[2] These patients typically have high-grade and large cell immunoblastic-type lymphomas and Burkitt's lymphoma. These lymphomas commonly occur in the CNS, with two thirds appearing with cerebral disease. Extranodal sites are also common in these patients with lymphoma-AIDS.

Surgery is necessary for a diagnosis, but an excision is not necessarily therapeutic. Radiation therapy improves the median survival time, but only to 15 months. A typical radiation field is a whole-brain field with extension to the upper cervical spinal cord and occasionally the orbit if it is at risk. Doses greater than 50 Gy may lead to longer survival rates. Chemotherapy can be effective if the patient's immune system is not already severely depressed.[15]

Lymphomas of the GI tract are the most common of the extranodal lymphomas. They are most commonly diffuse, large cell lymphomas. They appear with gastric symptoms, and a diagnosis is obtained via an endoscopic biopsy. The regimens recommended for such cancers are surgery and chemotherapy, a biopsy, chemotherapy and radiation therapy, or a biopsy and radiation therapy. One third of the patients have unresectable disease at the time of surgery. Surgery delays chemotherapy administration and causes morbidity from the functional loss of the stomach. A 10% mortality rate accompanies this surgery.[15]

Bone marrow transplants have been conducted increasingly with patients with lymphoma. Allogenic or autologous transplants can be performed. Often, these transplants are performed if the therapy for relapse or primary disease has failed. Typically, bone marrow transplants are done for aggressive cell types.

Side Effects. The side effects of radiation therapy treatment for lymphomas depend on the areas treated. For example, if a patient receives radiation to the mouth and neck, the side effects will be a dry mouth, difficulty swallowing, a loss of appetite, mucositis, mouth sores, a candidal infection, altered taste, redness of the skin, a sore throat, possible hair loss, transient dysphagia from esophagitis, and a dry cough.

Management of these side effects therefore includes eating small, frequent meals and avoiding extremely hot or cold fluids and/or alcohol. Good skin care includes the use of aloe vera or an approved topical application if the skin begins to redden. However, the patient must be cautioned not to have the skin care product on at the time of treatment because of increased skin irritation. For this reason, many centers do not recommend any skin creams until after the radiation therapy. Corn starch, however, is allowed and works effectively at relieving skin irritations.

Abdominal treatment is sure to cause nausea and vomiting. Antiemetics such as prochlorperazine (Compazine) and trimethobenzamide (Tigan) should be taken 30 minutes before the treatment to control the vomiting or nausea. The use of tetrahydrocannabinol (THC) or marijuana (Marinol) is sometimes prescribed to control the nausea and improve the appetite for these

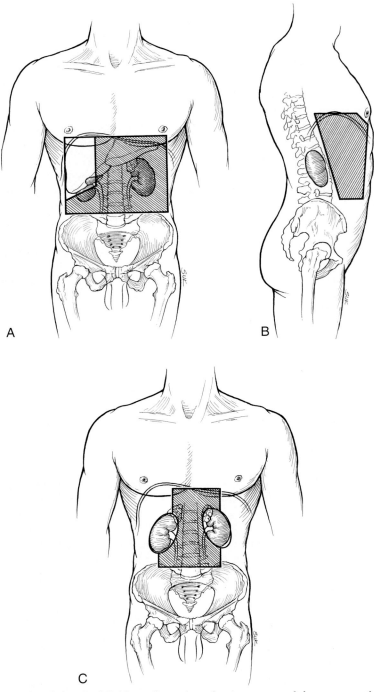

Figure 29-7. The abdominal field configurations for treatment of the para-aortic and mesenteric lymph nodes. **A**, Anteroposterior/posteroanterior (AP/PA) abdominal field. This portion is treated only to 1500 cGy because of exposure to the kidneys. **B**, Lateral fields then follow to spare the kidneys. The total dose to the lateral fields should be 1500 cGy. **C**, AP/PA para-aortic fields with five half-value layer (HVL) kidney blocks. The total dose to all three fields is 4500 cGy.

patients. Fatigue is also common in this group of individuals, and plenty of rest should be encouraged. Patients who work full time should be strongly encouraged to limit their work hours during treatments. In addition, providing help at home in dealing with family stress (e.g., child care, meal preparation) should be investigated.

If the pelvis is treated, diarrhea may occur, depending on the dose. In such instances a low-fiber diet should be recommended, and diarrhea medications may be indicated.

Vomiting and low blood counts are the primary side effects of total-body irradiation. Chronic effects of NHL treatments are caused more by the chemotherapeutic drugs than by the radiation therapy. Alkylating agents used in the treatment of NHL and Hodgkin's disease can cause sterility and the risk of a second cancer (usually leukemia). No risk is involved if the patient is treated by radiation alone to limited fields.

Results of Treatment

Patients with stages I and II follicular lymphomas have excellent survival rates with radiation therapy alone. The patients have an 80% to 100% 5-year survival rate, assuming that no abdominal disease is present.

Patients with localized stages I and II large cell lymphomas typically receive adjuvant chemotherapy after the site of involvement is treated. Some groups use chemotherapy without adjuvant radiation as the primary treatment with good results, but these groups generally experience increased morbidity.

Patients with high-stage, indolent, nonaggressive lymphomas have several options. These options include no treatment, combination chemotherapy, combination chemotherapy and radiation therapy, low-dose total lymph node irradiation (TBI), and chemotherapy with TBI and bone marrow transplantation.

In patients with stage III nodular lymphoma, a 5- to 10-year survival rate exists, with conservative management of patients who do not have symptoms and are feeling well. The treatment for these patients tends to be a small-field, low-dose radiation therapy for symptom relief. Patients who receive intensive chemotherapy have good responses but high rates of relapse.

Patients with nodular mixed lymphomas receive good results (possibly cures) with the C-MOPP (cyclophosphamide, Oncovin, procarbazine, prednisone) regimen.

Total lymphoid radiation for stage III has resulted in a 30% freedom-from-relapse rate at 10 years; results are the same for whole-body radiation. Similar results occur for stage IV, but total-nodal radiation is not considered appropriate for these patients.

For stages III and IV diffuse histology, chemotherapy is the mainstay, with the C-MOPP or BACOP regimens being used. Of the patients in this group, 40% achieve long-term freedom from relapse.

Role of Radiation Therapist

The radiation therapist's role in treating the patient with lymphoma is similar to that for the patient with Hodgkin's disease. Accuracy is the primary concern. If abutting fields are present, the therapist should be careful to match fields or measure gaps with extreme accuracy.

The therapist must be aware of the importance of blocking the critical structures in the fields (i.e., spine, liver, and kidney). Keeping precise records is vital, and clear notes should be written to indicate blocking changes. Portal images should be taken before the onset of blocking changes, particularly in regard to the liver and kidney blocks, because these structures have extremely low tolerances to radiation. (The liver's maximum tolerance is 30 Gy, and the kidney's maximum tolerance is only approximately 23 Gy.) Therefore, precision in block placement is paramount.

Blood counts should be taken regularly for these patients. Monitoring these counts and ensuring that the blood is drawn often become the duty of the therapist.

Because patients with NHL tend to be older than patients with Hodgkin's disease, they may have worse overall health and may rely on the therapist for additional support. As with all patients, communications and instructions must be clear. Communication is critical, not only with the patients but also with their families, especially as side effects require management.

CASE II

Non-Hodgkin's Lymphoma

A 30-year-old woman with intermediate-grade, large cell NHL developed chest pain in September, which worsened until December, when she had a chest x-ray examination. A 10.5-cm mediastinal mass was discovered on the radiograph. A biopsy then revealed the intermediate-grade, large cell lymphoma. At the time of the workup, she experienced superior vena cava syndrome. Chemotherapy began shortly. ProMACE/CytaBOM was delivered in six cycles, the last of which ended in April of the following year. The patient tolerated the chemotherapy well. Chest radiographs and CT scans showed the near-total resolution of the mediastinal mass, and no evidence of tumor involvement existed outside the chest.

She has no family history of carcinoma. She works as an accountant and does not use cigarettes or alcohol. She has not experienced any of the following: headaches, dizzy spells, nausea, vomiting, shortness of breath, coughing, diarrhea, constipation, and abdominal pain. Her appetite and energy level are good. In addition, she does not exhibit cervical, supraclavicular, axillary, or inguinal adenopathy.

Because of the size of the initial mass, limited radiation therapy was given to the involved field only. Over 31 days, 39.6 Gy of 6-MV photons was delivered in 22 fractions to the involved field. The patient experienced fatigue at 10.8 Gy, which was unusual for such a limited field of treatment and after only 6 fractions. However, the fatigue resolved within the week, and the patient felt much better by the 12th fraction. She experienced an unrelated bladder infection, which was cleared up with trimethoprim-sulfamethoxazole (Bactrim DS).

After the completion of the radiation, she was seen in follow-up in August of the same year. To date, she has not experienced any further side effects or any chronic effects. The patient has been disease free since this time.

SUMMARY

New forms of non-Hodgkin's lymphoma (NHL) are being identified as a result of advances in immunologic molecular diagnosis and the use of special techniques. Enteropathy-associated (small intestine disorder) T-cell lymphomas and mantle cell–derived lymphomas are two such diseases.

Further investigation has shown nodular lymphocyte predominant Hodgkin's lymphoma (NLPHL) to be a B-cell proliferation that may progress to a high-grade B-cell NHL. Also, many cases of lymphocyte-depleted Hodgkin's lymphoma (LDHL) have been reclassified as T-cell NHL. The relationship between Hodgkin's disease and non-Hodgkin's large cell anaplastic lymphoma are becoming increasingly blurred. Therefore, current research continues to shed new light on these disease processes, which increasingly are appearing more interrelated.

Treatment advances are also being continually developed. The hope is that the prognosis will improve for patients in all the categories of lymphomas.

- The presence of the Reed-Sternberg cell, a giant connective tissue component, is essential in pathologically distinguishing Hodgkin's from non-Hodgkin's lymphomas.
- Understanding the lymphatic system, its orderly flow, and its components is very important in assessing, and treating lymphomas.
- The major lymph nodes regions are of particular importance in treating Hodgkin's lymphoma. The major nodes include: Waldeyer's Ring, cervical, preauricular, occipital, supraclavicular and infraclavicular, axillary, thorax, abdominal cavity, pelvic cavity, inguinal, and femoral lymph nodes.
- Enlarged lymph nodes, many times painless, are often the first indication of lymphomas.
- The Ann Arbor staging system has been the accepted method of classification of Hodgkin's lymphoma, with the A groups having no symptoms and the B group indicating presence of symptoms. The REAL and WHO systems are commonly used in the grading of Non-Hodgkin's lymphomas.
- Treatment programs for lymphomas often use radiation therapy and chemotherapy in combination. The treatment fields encompass the large lymph node groups above and below the diaphragm as necessary. The Mantle and inverted-Y are examples of large fields used to treat the lymph node chains.
- Treatment fields design and dose regimens used in lymphoma management have demonstrated the complexity of radiation therapy treatment planning, including off-axis calculations.
- The role of the radiation therapist in managing lymphoreticular diseases is very important as a keen understanding of the lymphatic system, treatment set up, and dose delivery can be challenging.

Review Questions

Multiple Choice

1. The _____ lymph nodes are typically treated in a mantle irradiation field.
   a. hilar
   b. para-aortic
   c. inguinal
   d. Waldeyer's ring
2. The following is *not* a B symptom:
   a. fever higher than 38° C
   b. night sweats
   c. itching
   d. weight loss
3. Which subtype of Hodgkin's lymphoma offers the most favorable prognosis?
   a. lymphocytic predominance
   b. nodular sclerosis
   c. mixed cellularity
   d. lymphocytic depletion
4. When treating a posterior mantle field, the superior field border should include the _____ lymph node group.
   a. para-aortic
   b. hilar

   c. occipital
   d. axillary
5. The following may be seen as an acute complication of treatment:
   a. radiation pneumonitis
   b. L'hermitte's syndrome
   c. fatigue
   d. all of the above
6. NHL differs from Hodgkin's disease in which of the following ways?
   I. occurs in older persons
   II. can originate in extralymphatic tissues
   III. is less likely to spread randomly
   a. I and II
   b. I and III
   c. II and III
   d. I, II, and III
7. Subdiaphragmatic field arrangements used in the inverted Y commonly include:
   a. para-aortic nodes
   b. inguinal nodes
   c. both a and b
   d. neither a nor b
8. Chemotherapy treatment regimens have had an increasing role in lymphoma management.
   a. true
   b. false
9. The following radiographic studies are commonly used in the diagnostic workup of lymphoma:
   I. thoracic CT scan
   II. PET scan
   III. MRI
   a. I and II
   b. I and III
   c. II and III
   d. I, II, and III
10. AIDS-associated lymphomas are usually intermediate- and high-grade disease and are highly aggressive.
    a. true
    b. false

The answers to the Review Questions can be found by logging on to our website at: *http://evolve.elsevier.com/Washington+Leaver/ principles*

Questions to Ponder

1. Compare and contrast the differences between Hodgkin's lymphoma and non-Hodgkin's lymphoma, including the causes, clinical presentation, routes of spread, prognosis, and treatment modalities.
2. Why is the Ann Arbor staging system appropriate for Hodgkin's disease but difficult to apply to NHLs?
3. Which is the greater prognostic factor—the stage or the histologic subtype—in Hodgkin's lymphoma? How does this differ in NHLs?
4. For the treatment of a subdiaphragmatic lymphoma with a four-field abdomen technique, which structures need to be blocked or protected?

5. Compare and contrast involved-field radiation with total-nodal radiation and explain when each method is used.
6. What considerations must the therapist keep in mind daily when setting up a patient with Hodgkin's disease for a mantle field and for a para-aortic field?

REFERENCES

1. Armitage JO: Treatment of non-Hodgkin's lymphomas, *N Engl J Med* 328:1023-1029, 1993.
2. Beral V, et al: AIDS-associated non-Hodgkin's lymphoma, *Lancet* 337: 805-809, 1991.
3. Bolwell B: Autologous bone marrow transplantation for Hodgkin's disease and non-Hodgkin's lymphoma, *Semin Oncol* 21(suppl 7):86-96, 1994.
4. DeVita VT, Hellman S, Rosenberg SA, editors: *Cancer: principles and practice of oncology,* ed 6, Philadelphia, 2001, Lippincott Williams & Wilkins.
5. Dietrich PY, et al: Second primary cancers in patients continuously disease-free from Hodgkin's disease: a protective role for the spleen? *Blood* 84:1209-1215, 1994.
6. Dollinger M, Rosenbaum EH, Cable G: *Everyone's guide to cancer therapy,* Kansas City, Mo, 1991, Andrews McMeel.
7. Duhmke E, et al: Low dose radiation is sufficient for the noninvolved extended-field treatment in favorable early-stage Hodgkin's disease: long term results of a randomized trial of radiotherapy alone, *J Clin Oncol* 19: 2905-2914, 2001.
8. Gaffney DK, et al: Breast cancer after mantle irradiation for Hodgkin's disease: correlation of clinical, pathologic and molecular features including loss of heterozygosity at BRCA1 and BRCA2, *Int J Radiat Oncol Biol Phys* 49:539-546, 2001.
9. Harris NL, et al: A revised European American Classification of Lymphoid Neoplasms. A proposal from the International Lymphoma Study Group, *Blood* 84:1361-1392, 1994.
10. Hoane BR, et al: Comparison of initial lymphoma staging using computed tomography (CT) and magnetic resonance (MR) imaging, *Am J Hematol* 47:100-105, 1994.
11. Hudson MM, Donaldson SS: Treatment of pediatric Hodgkin's lymphoma, *Semin Hematol* 36:313-323, 1999.
12. Jarrett R, Mackenzie J: Epstein-Barr virus and other candidate viruses in the pathogenesis of Hodgkin's disease, *Semin Hematol* 36:260-269, 1999.
13. Leibel SA, Phillips TL: *Textbbook of radiation oncology,* ed 2 (pp 1375-1416), Philadelphia, 2004, WB Saunders.
14. National Cancer Institute: Hodgkin's disease (website): http://www.oncolink.com. Accessed August 19, 2008.
15. National Cancer Institute: Surveillance epidemiology and end results (website): http://seer.cancer.gov/statfacts. Accessed April 17, 2007.
16. Ng AK, Mauch PM: Radiation therapy in Hodgkin's lymphoma, *Semin Hematol* 36:290-302, 1999.
17. Perez CA, Brady LW: *Principles and practice of radiation oncology,* ed 3 (pp 1963-2012), Philadelphia, 1998, Lippincott.
18. Wood AM: Rituximab: an innovative therapy for non-Hodgkin's lymphoma, *Am J Health Syst Pharm* 58:215-229, 2001.

BIBLIOGRAPHY

Advani R, Horning S: Treatment of early stage Hodgkin's disease, *Semin Hematol* 36:270-281, 1999.
Armitage JO, et al: Salvage therapy for patients with lymphoma, *Semin Oncol* 21(suppl 7):82-85, 1994.
Bonadonna G: Modern treatment of malignant lymphomas: a multidisciplinary approach, *Ann Oncol* 5(suppl 2):5-16, 1994.
Dasher B, Wiggers N, Vann AM: *Portal design in radiation therapy,* Atlanta, 1994, RL Bryan.
Dreger P, et al: Stem-cell transplantation for chronic lymphocytic leukemia: the 1999 perspective, *Ann Oncol* 11(suppl 1):49, 2000.
Fisher RI: Diffuse large-cell lymphoma, *Ann Oncol* 11(suppl 1):29-33, 2000.
Ghielmini SF, et al: The effect of Rituximab on patients with follicular and mantle-cell lymphoma, *Ann Oncol* 11(suppl 1):123, 2000.
Gladstein E, Kaplan HS: *Determination of tumor extent and tumor localization of Hodgkin's disease and non-Hodgkin's lymphomas: technical basis of radiation therapy practical clinical consideration,* Philadelphia, 1984, Lea and Febiger.
Gonzalez C, Mederios J: Non-Hodgkin's lymphomas and the Working Formulation, part 2, *Contemp Oncol* 43-55, 1993.
Gunderson LL, Tepper JE: *Clinical radiation oncology* (pp 1116-1188), New York, 2000, Churchill Livingstone.
Harris NL, et al: Lymphoma classification: from controversy to consensus—the R.E.A.L. and WHO classification of lymphoid neoplasms, *Ann Oncol* 11(suppl 1):3-10, 2000.
Holleb AI, Fink D, Murphy GP: *American Cancer Society textbook of clinical oncology,* Atlanta, 1991, American Cancer Society.
Horning SJ: Follicular lymphoma: have we made any progress? *Ann Oncol* 11(suppl 1):23-27, 2000.
Horning SJ, et al: The Stanford experience with combined procarbazine, Alkeran and vinblastine (PAVe) and radiotherapy for locally extensive and advanced stage Hodgkin's disease, *Ann Oncol* 3:747-754, 1992.
Kaminski MS, et al: Radioimmunotherapy of B-cell lymphoma with (^{131}I) AntiB (Anti CD-20) antibody, *N Engl J Med* 329:459, 1993.
Khan KM: *The physics of radiation therapy,* Baltimore, 1984, Williams & Wilkins.
Kuniyoshi M, et al: Prevalence of hepatitis B or C virus infection in patients with non-Hodgkin's lymphoma, *J Gastroenterol Hepatol* 2:215-219, 2001.
Linch DC, et al: A randomised British national lymphoma investigation trial of CHOP vs. a weekly multi-agent regimen (PACEBOM) in patients with histologically aggressive non-Hodgkin's lymphoma, *Ann Oncol* 11(suppl 1): 87-90, 2000.
Loeffler M, et al: Meta-analysis of chemotherapy versus combined modality treatment trials in Hodgkin's disease, *J Clin Oncol* 16:818-829, 1998.
Maartenese E, et al: Different age limits for elderly patients with indolent and aggressive non-Hodgkin's lymphoma and the role of relative survival with increasing age, *Cancer* 89:2667-2676, 2000.
Mao Y, Hu J: Non-Hodgkin's lymphoma and occupational exposure to chemicals in Canada, *Ann Oncol* 11(suppl 1):69, 2000.
Mikhaell NG, et al: 18-FDG-PET for the assessment of residual masses on CT following treatment of lymphomas, *Ann Oncol* 11(suppl 1):147, 2000.
Noordijk EM, et al: Combination of radiotherapy and chemotherapy is advisable in all patients with clinical stage I and II Hodgkin's disease—six year results of the EORTC-GPMC controlled clinical trials H7-VF, H-7-F and H7-U, *Int J Radiat Oncol Biol Phys Suppl* 39:173, 1997 (abstract).
Ozsahin M: Early stage Hodgkin's disease: to mantle or not to mantle? *J Clin Oncol* 19:3298, 2001.
Sonneveld P, et al: Full-dose chemotherapy for non-Hodgkin's lymphoma in the elderly, *Semin Hematol* 31(suppl 3):9-12, 1994.
Wirth A, et al: Long term results of mantle field irradiation alone in 261 patients with clinical stage I and II supradiaphragmatic Hodgkin's disease, *Int J Rad Oncol Biol Physics Suppl* 39(2), 1997.

Leukemia

Susan B. Belinsky, Mary Ann McKenney

Key Terms

Auer rods
Diplopia
Ecchymoses
Epistaxis
Leukoencephalopathy
Menorrhagia
Nadir
Papilledema
Petechiae
Pluripotent
Progenitors
Pruritus
Purpura
Stomatitis

Objectives

- Define the key terms in the chapter.
- Differentiate between the acute and chronic leukemias.
- Discuss the hallmarks of diagnosis for each of the four major subtypes of leukemia.
- Describe the systems used to classify the leukemias.

- Identify the critical structures contained within each treatment field for the four major subtypes of leukemia.
- Discuss why total-body irradiation treatments are given and the next line of therapy.
- Describe the different cell lines in the bone marrow.
- Explore the role radiation therapists have in treating the pediatric population with acute lymphocytic leukemia.

NATURAL HISTORY

Leukemia is a heterogeneous group of neoplastic diseases of the hematopoietic system affecting approximately 44,240 persons per year.[17] It is broadly divided into acute and chronic types, based on the disease's natural history. Acute leukemia progresses quickly and is characterized by proliferation of undifferentiated cells in the bone marrow, whereas chronic leukemia is distinguished by a slower progression of disease and the uncontrolled expansion of mature cells. Acute and chronic leukemias are further subdivided into myelogenous leukemias (those arising directly or indirectly from hematopoietic stem cells) and lymphocytic leukemias (those arising from other cells populating the bone marrow). Therefore, consideration of three factors (natural history of the disease, degree of cellular maturation, and dominant cell line) results in the four main subtypes of leukemia (Table 30-1): acute lymphocytic leukemia (ALL); chronic lymphocytic leukemia (CLL); acute myelogenous leukemia (AML, which is sometimes referred to as acute nonlymphocytic leukemia [ANLL]); and chronic myelogenous leukemia (CML).

Leukemia is the general name for four distinct types of blood cancers. Individuals with leukemia are affected and treated differently, depending on which one of the four types of leukemia the patient is diagnosed as having.

HISTORICAL PERSPECTIVE

The first documented description of a case of leukemia appears to be that of Alfred Velpeau, a French surgeon, who in 1827 recorded his observations. Dameshek and Gunz[3] described the case:

His patient, a 63-year-old florist and seller of lemonade, who had abandoned himself to the abuse of spirituous liquor and of women without, however, becoming syphilitic, fell ill in 1825 with a swelling of the

Table 30-1	**Four Main Subtypes of Leukemia**	
Natural History of the Disease	**Lymphocytic**	**Myelogenous**
Acute	ALL	AML
Chronic	CLL	CML

ALL, Acute lymphocytic leukemia; *AML,* acute myelogenous leukemia; *CLL,* chronic lymphocytic leukemia; *CML,* chronic myelogenous leukemia.

abdomen, fever, and weakness. He died soon after admission to the hospital and was at autopsy found to have an enormous liver and spleen, the latter weighing ten pounds. The blood was thick, like gruel … resembling in consistency and color the yeast of red wine.

In 1844, Alfred Donné reported his microscopic observations of leukemia cells in his treatise "Cours de Microscopie." His studies included the examination of a postmortem sample of blood from a woman who had suffered from a large abdominal tumor and diarrhea, as well as samples collected in vivo from other patients. Donné is credited with the first known observation of leukemic cells and the establishment of the disease as a hematologic condition.[5]

In 1845, Rudolf Virchow, a German physician, referred to the blood taken from a patient with splenic enlargement and massive accumulations of white blood cells (WBCs) as *weisses blut* ("white blood"). In 1847, Virchow first used the term *leukemia.* A decade later, Virchow described two types of leukemia: splenic and lymphatic. The advent of staining techniques in microscopy in the late 19th century permitted the morphologic subdivision of the myelogenous and lymphocytic leukemias.[30]

Because of the unique nature of each of the four subtypes of leukemia, they are discussed separately in this chapter.

PERTINENT ANATOMY

Leukemia develops during the formation of the constituent elements of the blood and lymphocytes. The hematopoietic process through which mature erythrocytes, neutrophils, eosinophils, basophils, monocytes, and platelets are formed and the lymphopoietic process through which lymphocytes are formed begin at the most primitive level with the pluripotent stem cells. These cells have a self-renewing capability and generate differentiating cells of multiple lineages. The cells of the **pluripotent** stem cell pool differentiate into either myeloid or lymphoid stem cells (Figure 30-1). The myeloid stem cell pool provides the **progenitors** for the six types of blood cells, whereas the lymphoid pool provides the progenitors for the classes of lymphocytes. In the normal course of differentiation and maturation, these cells eventually become fully mature, functional blood cells and lymphocytes. During leukemic development, the production of the hematopoietic or lymphopoietic progenitors is uncontrolled and greatly accelerated, resulting in incomplete or defective cellular maturation. Acute leukemia involves the rapid proliferation of primitive, undifferentiated stem cells, whereas cellular differentiation is largely preserved in chronic leukemia.

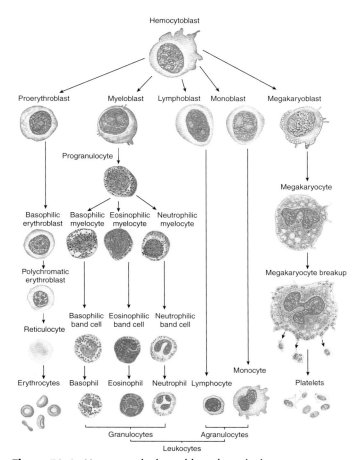

Figure 30-1. Hematopoiesis and lymphopoiesis.

The symptoms of leukemia result from the leukemic cells' interference with normal processes. The leukemic cells accumulate in the bone marrow, impairing the body's normal production of adequate supplies of red blood cells (RBCs), WBCs, and platelets. The decrease in the number of these necessary blood components in the circulating blood results in anemia, thrombocytopenia, neutropenia, and the related symptoms of fatigue, pallor, bleeding, and infection.

> The normal range of blood values for a complete blood count (CBC) are as follows:
> WBCs range from 3.90 to 10.80 thousand/mm³, RBCs range from 3.90 to 5.40 million/mm³, and platelets range from 150 to 424 thousand/mm³.

With the acute leukemia subtypes, the accumulating leukemic cells are immature or have undergone a defect in maturation. ALL is characterized by the invasion of the bone marrow by leukemic lymphoblasts. AML results from the proliferation of defective or incompletely matured cells derived from the pluripotent hematopoietic stem cell pool.

In chronic leukemia, the maturation of the cells is preserved, but unregulated proliferation results in the accumulation of leukemic cells in the bone marrow. CLL is a disorder of morphologically mature, but immunologically less mature, lymphocytes. An increased proliferation of these short- and long-life lymphocytes and the prolonged survival of the long-life lymphocytes results in an enormous accumulation of these cells in the marrow, blood, lymph nodes, liver, and spleen. This causes an enlargement of the involved organs and a decrease in bone marrow function. CML involves the replacement of marrow cells with mature myeloid cells that are insensitive to the normal proliferation control mechanisms.

Facts from the Leukemia and Lymphoma Society regarding leukemia are as follows[10-13]:
* *There are 218,659 people in the United States who are either living with or are in remission from leukemia.*
* *This year, approximately 44,200 people will be diagnosed with leukemia.*
* *This year, approximately 21,800 people will die of leukemia.*
* *Thirty-two percent more males are living with leukemia than females. More males are diagnosed with leukemia and more males die of it than females.*
* *Leukemia causes more deaths than any other cancer among children and young adults younger than the age of 20 years.*

ACUTE LYMPHOCYTIC LEUKEMIA

Epidemiology

The acute subtypes account for approximately 50% of all instances of leukemia in the United States.[1] ALL is the most common of the pediatric malignancies, and approximately 80% of children with acute leukemia have the ALL subtype. There are approximately 5400 estimated new cases a year with an age-adjusted incidence of 1.6 per 100,000.[1,17]

ALL is primarily a disease of children, with its peak incidence between 2 and 3 years old.[16,26] It is relatively uncommon in persons older than the age of 15 years.[16] The incidence of ALL is higher among males than among females.[14] Hispanic children have an increased prevalence of ALL compared with African American children and white children.[16,17] The disease is more common among white children than among African American children.[22] Individuals in higher socioeconomic groups and more developed countries tend to develop the disease more often.[14]

Acute lymphocytic leukemia (ALL) is one of the four types of blood cancer. Other names for ALL are acute lymphoblastic leukemia and acute lymphoid leukemia.[10]

Etiology

The causes of acute leukemia are unknown. Physical and chemical agents have been associated with increased instances of leukemia. The markedly higher incidence of acute leukemia among survivors of the atomic bomb explosions in Japan has suggested that ionizing radiation may play a role in leukemogenesis. Japanese atomic bomb survivors had a 10- to 15-fold increase in the incidence of acute leukemia, with a greater increase in the incidence of ALL than of AML. It is interesting to note that there was no significant increase in leukemia after the 1986 Chernobyl nuclear accident. The atomic bombs from Hiroshima and Nagasaki released neutrons and gamma rays. The accident from Chernobyl resulted in large amounts of radioactive iodine, causing an increase in thyroid cancer.[7] Alkylating agents such as cyclophosphamide have been associated with an increased risk of acute leukemia.[2]

Heredity appears to play a role in the development of acute leukemia. If one identical twin is diagnosed with acute leukemia, the risk of the other twin developing the disease within 1 year is approximately 20%.[2] Down syndrome is associated with a 10- to 30-fold increased risk of acute leukemia.[16]

Naturally occurring retroviruses and the human T-cell lymphotropic virus have been implicated as causative agents in instances of adult ALL but not of childhood ALL.[20]

Prognostic Indicators

More than 75% of patients with ALL can be expected to experience a complete remission, although the duration of the remission and subsequent potential for cure appear to be related to a number of factors, including clinical variables such as age and WBC count at the time of the diagnosis.[14] ALL in children younger than 1 and older than 10 years carries a poor prognosis.[6] In adult ALL, advancing age is an adverse prognostic sign, with patients older than 50 years faring worse than younger patients. An initial leukocyte count of less than 10,000/mm^3 is more favorable than a count of 20,000 to 49,000/mm^3. A WBC count greater than 50,000/mm^3 is the least favorable.[20]

Other features with prognostic value include central nervous system (CNS) leukemia at the time of the diagnosis; a mediastinal mass; massive organomegaly and/or adenopathy; and biologic qualities of the leukemic cells such as the immunophenotype, cytogenetics, and deoxyribonucleic acid (DNA) content. Poor performance status, impaired organ function, and low serum albumin levels are unfavorable prognostic indicators.

Clinical Presentation

The symptoms of ALL at the time of presentation stem from the suppression of the normal blood components, which causes anemia, thrombocytopenia, neutropenia, and associated symptoms. A nonspecific flulike malaise is common, with fatigue and pallor resulting from the anemia. Thrombocytopenia is manifested by oozing gums, **epistaxis** (nose bleeds), **petechiae** (tiny red spots on the skin caused by the escape of small amounts of blood), **ecchymoses** (discoloration of the skin caused by the escape of blood into tissues), **menorrhagia** (excessive menstrual bleeding), and excessive bleeding after dental procedures. Neutropenia causes an increased susceptibility to respiratory, dental, sinus, perirectal, and urinary tract infections. Other common symptoms at the time of presentation are liver, splenic, and testicular enlargement. The disease at times may mimic rheumatoid arthritis with joint swelling, bone pain, and tenderness, often causing a child to limp or refuse to walk. Unlike AML, the symptoms of ALL rarely occur more than 6 weeks before the diagnosis. Vomiting, headaches, **papilledema** (swelling of the optic disc), neck stiffness, and cranial nerve palsy are indicative of CNS involvement.

Detection and Diagnosis

A blood cell count is one indicator for detecting ALL. Thrombocytopenia and anemia occur in most patients (two thirds) at the time of the diagnosis. Leukocyte counts vary from low to high. An abnormal increase in white cells indicates a poor prognosis.

Immunophenotyping includes a morphologic evaluation, special stains, electron microscopic examination, and surface marker studies. It can establish a diagnosis in 90% of patients.[16]

A bone marrow aspiration biopsy is necessary to make a definitive diagnosis. The amount of leukemic blast cells is the determinant for a definitive diagnosis. A biopsy revealing greater than 25% leukoblasts is positive for leukemia.[26]

Other abnormalities may be present at the time of the diagnosis. These include hyperuricemia and several metabolic abnormalities, hyperkalemia, hypomagnesemia, hypocalcemia, and hypercalcemia. Of the patients identified with having ALL, 30% have low serum levels of immunoglobulins at the time of the initial diagnosis.

Leukemic infiltrates of the liver, periosteum, and bone may be present. A mediastinal mass may be present in some high-risk patients. This can be demonstrated on a chest radiograph.

Extramedullary leukemia is important in regard to relapse. The two most common sites for extramedullary leukemia are the CNS and testes (sanctuary sites, because they are "hidden" from most chemotherapy agents). A diagnosis of these two sites is obtained through a cytologic examination and a wedge biopsy, respectively.

Pathology

ALL is characterized by an unregulated proliferation of lymphoblasts. The disease cells limit the production of other healthy cells by overcrowding and inhibiting cell growth and differentiation.[14]

Staging and Classification

The two means to classify ALL are based on the morphologic appearance and immunologic surface markings. The main system in place is the immunologic classification. The French-American-British (FAB) system is a morphologic classification that is not in use for this subtype, but some physicians refer to this system.[15] The FAB classification divides lymphoblastic leukemias into three levels (L1, L2, and L3). These divisions of ALL are based on the cell size, nuclear shape, number, prominence of nuclei, and amount and appearance of cytoplasm. These levels are as follows[21]:

L1—a small cell with a high nucleus; a regular cytoplasm ratio; or a clefted cell and small, inconspicuous nucleoli

L2—larger blast cells with irregular nuclear membranes, one or more prominent nucleoli, and a relative abundance of cytoplasm

L3—large lymphoblasts with round to oval prominent nucleoli and basophilic cytoplasm

Most pediatric ALLs are L1. L3 carries a poor prognosis and is associated with B-cell versus T-cell ALL.

Immunologic classification identifies the surface-marking characteristic of blast cells. Approximately 13% to 15% of patients with ALL are categorized by T-cell markers. About 80% to 85% of the patients are classified by B-cell with 60% to 65% accounting for early pre–B-cell and 20% to 25% for pre–B-cell lineage types.[15] Ninety percent of these cases are identified by the common ALL antigen positive (CALLA⁺). This cell type reacts to an antibody made from a surface antigen generally found in ALL cells.[21]

Treatment Techniques

Treatment techniques used for ALL are radiation therapy, chemotherapy, and bone marrow transplantation. These three modalities are used alone or in combination with each other.

The use of drugs and regimens may vary among institutions. Protocols are frequently updated and changed as new information is discovered.

If radiation therapy is administered, four different techniques may be used for treating ALL. All the treatment techniques and devices discussed in this chapter are those used at Tufts-New England Medical Center's Radiation Oncology Department and Dana-Farber/Brigham and Women's Cancer Center, Department of Radiation Oncology. Most radiation oncology facilities use similar types of treatment techniques; however, Dana-Farber/Brigham and Women's Cancer Center uses two 4-MV linear accelerators simultaneously to treat patients with leukemia.

The New England Medical Center's Radiation Oncology Department Experience. Three main protocols are in use at this facility. The patient may receive total-body radiation with the dose totaling 1200 cGy. For 3 consecutive days, 200 cGy is given two times a day (bid). The patient may receive total-body irradiation (TBI) with the dose totaling 1350 cGy. For 3 consecutive days, 150 cGy is given bid. A mini-TBI fractionation schedule is given over 2 days in which the first day is bid with a total dose of 600 cGy. These doses are used to immunosuppress the patient in combination with a bone marrow transplant.

The dose rate set on the treatment unit is 100 cGy/minute, prescribed at midplane at the central region, the umbilicus. This low dose rate is necessary to spare late-responding tissues. These tissues include all visceral organs. The most common example is the lung.

A helmet field may be used to encompass the meninges. The helmet dose is 1800 cGy, delivered 200 cGy each day for 9 consecutive days.

The CNS technique is a combination of a helmet and spine field. This technique is used to treat positive cells in the cerebral spinal fluid. The helmet field is treated to a total dose of 2400 cGy. The dose is delivered 150 cGy each day for 16 days. This is combined with a field to encompass the entire spine. The spine receives a total of 1500 cGy, with 150 cGy each day for 10 days.

Field design and critical structures. With TBI, the field size used is 40 × 40 cm. This is the largest jaw size that can be set on the treatment unit. The gantry is then placed in the lateral position at 270 degrees. The collimator angle is either 135 or 225 degrees. The patient sits in the diamond-shaped box with the

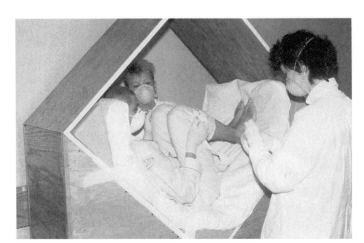

Figure 30-2. New England Medical Center's custom-made immobilization device for total-body irradiation.

knees toward the chest, the arms by the side, and the forearms on the side of the knees (Figure 30-2). The upper arms are wrapped with connected small water bags in this position to act as bolus. This position is necessary to place the entire person in the beam. The diamond-shaped box is about 5 feet from the gantry, so that the light field covers the exact outer rim of the box, ensuring total coverage of the patient. The patient's eyes and face should be looking straight ahead. Compensators are taped to the outside of the blocking tray. The compensators are placed according to their shadow on the patient. A lead attenuator is taped to the inside of the blocking tray covering the whole field. A double Lucite Plexiglas beam spoiler is hung against the TBI box.

Half of the treatment is given in this manner. Then the box, which is on wheels, is rotated 180 degrees. The second half of the treatment is given to the patient's other side. The patient is treated from the right and left lateral positions. After the completion of one lateral treatment field, the box is rotated manually 180 degrees and the other lateral is treated.

Thermoluminescent dosimeters (TLDs) are placed between the patient's ankles, knees, and thighs once during a treatment to check midline doses. To even the dose over the uneven surfaces of the body, lead compensators are placed on a Lucite tray in the beam's path. The compensators are positioned over the thinnest body parts, such as the head and neck area and the foot and ankle areas.

The field design for a helmet field is derived from specific anatomic landmarks; the field size should cover the meninges and C2, with fall-off around the head (Figure 30-3). The patient lies supine on a plastic head cup for stability and comfort. The lenses of the eyes should be blocked with an adjustable block.

The spinal cord is a critical structure for the treatment of the head to the level of C2. (The helmet field is used as described previously.) With spinal cord involvement, there should be a recorded dose for this particular site.

For the treatment of the CNS, the patient is placed in the prone position. Numerous headholders, such as the Smithers or Osborne holders (Figure 30-4), comfortably stabilize the head.

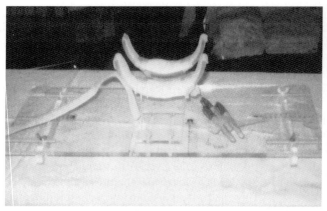

Figure 30-4. A Smither's headholder for total central nervous system treatments.

The patient's chin should be tucked slightly to avoid a crease in the neck (Figure 30-5). This is a critical match area and should be flat with no skinfolds.

The field arrangement is in two volumes. The first field arrangement is the cranial volume, which includes two lateral parallel opposed ports with the helmet field design arrangement. The second volume is the spinal field, which contains the entire spine. To encompass the entire spine, the field may have to be treated in two parts. A gap calculation must be done for the two fields. The match is at the level of the spine. In addition to the gap calculation just mentioned, another is done for the match of the spine and helmet field. The gap calculations are done to ensure coverage of the entire CNS with no cold spots (see Chapter 8).

The field size of these beam arrangements depends on the contour of the patient. The field must include the entire spine and the whole brain, including C2.

Another technique used to ensure that all the meninges are being treated is the feathering technique. With this technique, the junctions are shifted by changing the lengths of all fields. This is done daily with multiple match lines. The marks can be differentiated by different-colored marks drawn on the patient's

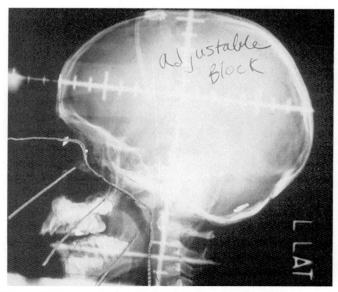

Figure 30-3. Simulation film for a helmet field that covers the meninges encompassing C2.

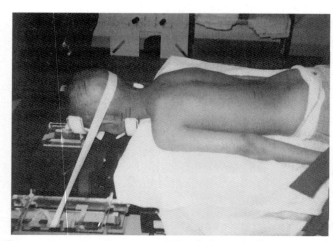

Figure 30-5. A patient immobilized through the use of the Smither's headholder. (Courtesy Tufts-New England Medical Center's Radiation Oncology Department.)

skin. These marks correspond to the same-colored pens used to record information in the treatment chart.

The only border that must remain stable is the posterior border of the spine. A block is positioned at the posterior border of the spine for stability. As the length of the fields shift, the border with the blocked area remains stable.

The critical structures include the lens of the eyes, which can be localized and blocked, and the spinal cord, which must be carefully monitored for the total dose received.

The Dana-Farber/Brigham and Women's Cancer Center Department of Radiation Oncology Experience. There is a one-of-a-kind dedicated TBI unit that has been in place since 1983. It consists of two opposed 4-MV stationary linear accelerators, one mounted in the ceiling and the other in a pit under the floor (Figure 30-6). Patients lie supine on a canvas-covered frame large enough to accommodate the tallest person. The field size at a distance of 205 cm is 75 × 200 cm. Both radiation beams run at the same time. The treatment room is equipped with positive pressure and high-efficiency particulate air (HEPA) filtered air and thoroughly cleaned daily for use by immunosuppressed patients.

The patient has a chest simulation, and customized 85% transmission lung shields are cut and placed anterior to posterior to lower the dose to the lungs to within 5% of the prescribed dose, to decrease the incidence of interstitial pneumonitis. A portal imager verifies lung shield placement.

Fractions range from 150 to 200 cGy per treatment given bid 5 to 6 hours apart to a total dose of 1200 to 1400 cGy. The dose rate has a slight variation depending on the institution-specific formula. Typically, the dose rate is set for an adult at 200 cGy/minute and less for the pediatric population. The dose is calculated to the midline of the patient at the umbilicus, and the average treatment time for a child and an adult is 15 and 20 minutes, respectively. The fractionated irradiation and low dose rate give time for the repair process to take place yet allow destruction of leukemic cells.

For those children in whom anesthesia is indicated, a portable anesthesia machine is set up with television cameras focused on the monitors and the child (Figure 30-7). A team of anesthesiologists delivers propofol (Diprivan), a very quick-acting anesthetic. It can be delivered easily through a central line, and the children recover rapidly and become fully awake posttreatment. They may have clear liquids for an hour or two before they must begin fasting again for their afternoon treatment.

In some situations, a C2 whole brain boost may be treated prophylactically. The daily dose to the brain is in the range of 150 to 200 cGy to a total dose of 750 to 1000 cGy in addition to the TBI.

The dose to the C2 whole brain is delivered by lateral opposed fields. The patient is supine and simulated in a head cup with a thermoplastic mask. The field covers the meninges with C2 fall-off around the head. Custom shielding blocks the face and lenses of the eyes.

Chemotherapy. The chemotherapy treatment techniques used in treating ALL are divided into four groups: remission induction, consolidation, prophylaxis of overt CNS disease, and maintenance or continuation therapy.[16,20,26] Induction therapy typically involves the use of prednisone or dexamethasone,

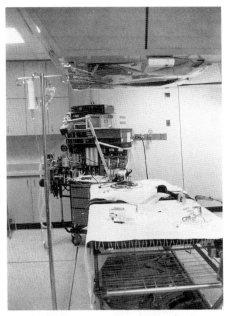

Figure 30-6. A dedicated total-body irradiation unit that has been in place since the early 1980s. It consists of two opposed 4-MV stationary linear accelerators, one mounted in the ceiling and the other in a pit under the floor.

vincristine, and L-asparaginase. These chemotherapeutic agents are given immediately after the diagnosis to eradicate all detectable leukemia. For high-risk patients, an anthracycline, daunorubicin, is added to the regimen. Consolidation therapy uses high-dose intravenous methotrexate, and L-asparaginase begins after remission has been achieved. Maintenance therapy involves the use of intravenous mercaptopurine (6-MP) and systemic methotrexate.[20] The chemotherapeutic agent shown to be most effective in preventing overt CNS disease in several clinical trials is methotrexate. This drug is given either systemically or intrathecally. The duration of chemotherapeutic treatment is based on continuous complete remission for 2 to 3 years.[26]

Bone Marrow Transplantation. Another treatment technique used for ALL is bone marrow transplantation.[25] Bone marrow transplantation, which was considered an experimental procedure until approximately 25 years ago, is the treatment of choice for several diseases, including ALL, AML, and CML. The procedure involves the harvesting of healthy marrow from a suitable donor. For the donor to be suitably matched to the patient, specific human leukocyte antigen (HLA) loci (specific gene location) are required. The loci that are taken into consideration are *HLA-A, HLA-B, HLA-C, HLA-DR,* and *HLA-DQ.* Three of these loci are essential for matching. If the donor is not related to the patient, all but one locus is allowable.[8] The marrow is then infused into a patient whose diseased marrow has been destroyed or ablated by chemotherapy or TBI. The transplanted marrow finds its way into bone marrow cavities and begins supplying the patient with normal, healthy hematopoietic cells.

The most desirable donors are identical twins because they are generally identical to the patient for all transplantation antigens. Allogeneic transplants, available to 20% to 30% of patients, use HLA-histocompatible siblings as donors. In recent years,

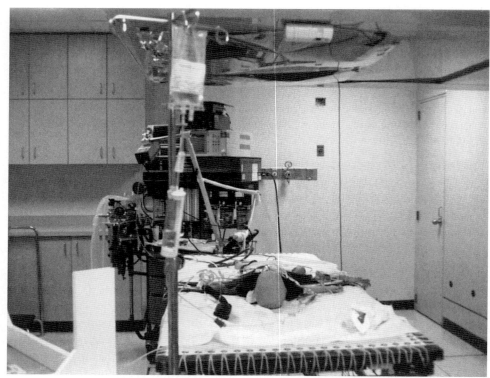

Figure 30-7. A portable anesthesia machine set up with television cameras to monitor a pediatric case, a child in whom anesthesia is indicated.

bone marrow registries have been developed to locate and use nonrelated histocompatible donors. Some success has been achieved with the use of marrow from donors in whom only a partial match of transplantation antigens is present.

For potential bone marrow donors, risks are small and primarily related to anesthesia. The aspiration of bone marrow is a technically simple transplant procedure performed in the operating room under sterile conditions and anesthesia. Multiple aspirations are drawn from the donor's anterior and posterior iliac crests. A small amount of heparin is used to prevent clotting.

The marrow recipient is treated before the transplant with a large dose of cyclophosphamide and TBI or with chemotherapy alone (busulfan and cyclophosphamide).[6] These measures reduce the leukemic cell load and impair the host's ability to reject the donor marrow. After an intravenous injection, the donor marrow cells migrate to the recipient's marrow cavities and begin to produce normal cells in the blood within 2 to 4 weeks.

Autologous bone marrow transplants involve the reinfusion of a patient's own marrow that has been harvested and cryopreserved while the patient was in remission. Leukemic cells are removed from the collected marrow through the use of monoclonal antibodies directed against cell-surface antigens that are expressed on leukemic blasts but not on normal stem cells.

Factors that lead to failure in bone marrow transplants are recurrent leukemia (primarily in autologous donors) and graft-versus-host disease, which occurs in approximately 50% of patients. This condition may exist only as a slight skin rash, or it may progress to a life-threatening syndrome involving the skin, liver, and/or gastrointestinal tract.[26]

Side Effects. Patients receiving TBI experience numerous side effects. The gastrointestinal side effects include nausea, vomiting, diarrhea, anorexia, and malaise. Mucosa of the mouth, pharynx, bladder, and rectum may be affected. Normal secretions are inhibited, and their functions are impaired. The integumentary side effects include skin reactions, itching, tingling, bruising, and dry and inelastic skin that cracks easily. Alopecia can occur, as well as blanching or erythema of the skin and mucous membranes. A respiratory-related side effect is interstitial pneumonitis. These side effects are acute and subside in time.

Chronic side effects include permanent sterility and cataracts of the eyes (easily reversed with surgery). Hepatic fibrosis and radionecrosis of the genital tissue, muscle, and kidney are also chronic side effects.

The side effects for helmet and CNS radiation are skin reactions and hair loss for the integumentary system. The hematopoietic reactions are a decrease in blood counts and **leukoencephalopathy** (demyelinating brain lesions). Nausea and vomiting are the gastrointestinal side effects. The effect on the CNS is somnolence syndrome, characterized by drowsiness and malaise that is self-limiting. Serious injury to the tissue or blood vessels in the brain can lead to lethargy, seizures, spasticity, paresis, difficulty with movements, and L'hermitte's sign.

L'hermitte's sign may develop if the spine receives radiation treatment. This syndrome is characterized by a sensation of an electric shock in the arms, legs, or neck when the patient flexes the neck. These are the acute symptoms of helmet and CNS radiation.

The chronic side effects include neuropsychological deficits, intellectual deficits, and cataract formation. Growth retardation and hypothalamic-pituitary dysfunction are a result of irradiation to the brain and CNS. Hypothalamic-pituitary dysfunction is an abnormality in the hormonal secretions that include growth hormones, thyroid hormones, adrenal hormones, and sex-related hormones. Myelopathy is another side effect causing irreversible injury to the spinal cord. Secondary tumors are also seen as a late effect. These tumors can be benign or malignant.

Chemotherapy has many side effects. The results from the cytotoxicity for each drug are different. The effects of vincristine are anorexia, constipation, and a metallic taste in the mouth. Neurologic effects include jaw pain, diplopia (double vision), vocal cord paresis, impotence, general motor weakness, and loss of deep tendon reflexes. The effects on the skin are alopecia and dermatitis.

Prednisone and dexamethasone are hormones, the effects of which are an exaggeration of normal physiologic action, suppression of immune function, hypertension, hyperglycemia, increased appetite, muscle weakness, diabetes, and fluid retention. Gastric irritation, osteoporosis, cataracts, menstrual irregularity, and a modification of tissue reactions leading to infection or slow tissue healing are other side effects of prednisone and dexamethasone.

L-Asparaginase causes gastrointestinal reactions such as anorexia, nausea, and vomiting. Neurologic reactions such as lethargy, progressive malaise, headaches, and confusion often result from this drug. Immunologic reactions can be seen secondary to a decreased number of lymphoblasts. The blood chemistry as a result of this agent has the following abnormalities: hypoalbuminemia, hyperglycemia, or altered blood-clotting factors. Elevated blood urea levels or pancreatic enzymes are also seen. Fever and chills are common side effects of this drug.

Most side effects for 6-MP are gastrointestinal, including nausea, vomiting, diarrhea, and anorexia. Myelosuppression is commonly seen with the administration of this agent. Hyperpigmentation of the skin is also seen, and hepatotoxicity is considered a major side effect.

Patients treated with methotrexate develop a rapid onset of bone marrow depression, with **nadir** (the lowest point) occurring in 10 to 14 days. Side effects include nausea, vomiting, stomatitis, pharyngitis, diarrhea, and renal dysfunction. Alopecia and a rash with associated erythema and **pruritus** (itching) are integumentary effects. Brown pigmentation of the skin and photosensitivity are other effects. Infertility and congenital malformation may result from this drug.

ACUTE MYELOGENOUS LEUKEMIA

Epidemiology

The incidence rate of AML is approximately 13,290 cases per year.[1] AML typically occurs in patients older than 40 years of age, with a median age of 67 years at time of diagnosis.[11,27] In contrast to ALL (the predominant pediatric leukemia), approximately 80% of adults with acute leukemia have the myelogenous subtype. The incidence of AML is slightly higher among white males, with the gender difference being more obvious in older patients.[2] Jews of Eastern European descent have a higher incidence of AML than other groups.[11]

Etiology

Risk factors for AML are similar to those for ALL. Exposure to ionizing radiation appears to increase a person's risk for developing the disease. An increased incidence of AML has occurred in military personnel at Nevada bomb test sites and in patients treated with radiation for ankylosing spondylitis, menorrhagia, and thymic enlargement. Thorium dioxide 25% (Thorotrast), an intravenous radiocontrast used for angiography procedures between 1928 and 1952, showed an increased risk of AML due to the alpha particles emission.[29] Fanconi's anemia and Bloom syndrome (genetic disorders with a chromosome breakage tendency) and other inherited conditions as well as exposure to benzene and alkylating agents, have been associated with AML risk.[2,11] Tobacco smoke has been implicated in the development of AML.[4]

Prognostic Indicators

Unfavorable prognostic variables of AML are similar to those of ALL. Unfavorable signs include an age older than 60 years, myelodysplastic syndrome, a poor performance status, impaired organ function, and low serum albumin.[23] Children with AML have a poorer prognosis than those with ALL. As with ALL, a WBC count of less than 20,000/mm^3 is more favorable than a WBC count of 20,000 to 49,000/mm^3. A WBC count of greater than 50,000/mm^3 is the least favorable.[21] For AML, age and chromosome status are two major prognostic indicators for treatment decisions.[24]

 The number of patients with acute myelogenous leukemia who enter remission, stay in remission for years, or are cured has increased significantly over the past 30 years.[11]

Clinical Presentation

The onset of AML may be abrupt, although most patients experience a 1- to 6-month prodromal period, during which symptoms are present. As with ALL, symptoms at the time of presentation include nonspecific flulike symptoms. Fatigue, pallor, and dyspnea on exertion are secondary to anemia. Petechiae, **purpura** (hemorrhage under the skin), epistaxis, gingival bleeding, and gastrointestinal or urinary tract bleeding may result from reduced platelet production. Neutropenia may result in a susceptibility to local infections, such as skin abscesses, or systemic infections with accompanying fever, chills, and site-specific symptoms. The sensation of an enlarged spleen may be present.

Detection and Diagnosis

Specific tests for detecting AML include CBCs, differential leukocyte and platelet counts, and blood smears. Abnormal blood counts lead to the detection of AML. Thrombocytopenia, anemia, and an increased leukocyte count should be suspect in patients with these conditions. Another form of detection is that of chromosomal abnormalities, which occur in 30% to 50% of patients with AML.[11,21]

The circulation of **Auer rods** (structures present in the cytoplasm of myeloblasts, myelocytes, and monoblasts) in the leukemic cells is central to the diagnostic finding of AML. A definitive diagnosis is made via a bone marrow aspiration and biopsy. In AML, the bone marrow is hypercellular. The diagnosis is made based on the percentage of blast cells. If more than 30% blast cells are present, acute leukemia is the diagnosis. A staining procedure is the final step to determine a differential diagnosis of AML. In summary, a diagnosis of AML is based on the circulation of Auer rods in leukemic cells, an increase in leukemic blast cells, and a decrease in normal precursors.

Immunophenotyping that includes a morphologic evaluation, special stains, electron microscopic examination, and surface marker studies can establish a diagnosis in 90% of patients with AML.[17] Morphologic evaluations are based on monoclonal antibodies reacting with a surface antigen that is expressed on the membrane of the leukemic cell.

Pathology

AML results from the unregulated proliferation of early precursor cells that have lost the ability to differentiate in response to hormonal signals and cellular interactions. This proliferation or clonal disease involves the hematopoietic stem cells or pluripotent cells. The result is a gradual accumulation of undifferentiated cells in marrow or other organs.

These undifferentiated cells have a decreased proportion of blast cells in the S or M phase of the cell cycle compared with normal bone marrow blast cells. Because of this decrease of blast cells in these specific phases, the cells do not reach maturity or are defective at maturity.

Staging and Classification

For a morphologic evaluation, the FAB system is used. AML is categorized in different maturation states, from M0 (undifferentiated) to M7 (megakaryocytic). They are as follows[4]:

M0—Minimal evidence of maturation exists.

M1—The cells tend to have fine azurophil granules and may have few Auer rods. Minimal evidence exists of differentiation along the rest of the granulocytic or monocytic lineages.

M2—The number of blast cells is greater than 30%, and less than 20% of monocytic precursors have abundant cytoplasm and moderate to marked granularity.

M3—The acute promyelocytic leukemia (APL)–predominant cell is heavily granulated with azurophil granulation. Many cells have bundles of Auer rods whose nucleus is often bilobed or kidney shaped.

M4—The myeloid precursors or other granulocytic precursors are between 20% and 80% of the nonerythroid nucleated cells. The monocytic cells comprise 20% or more of the nonerythroid nucleated cells.

M5—The proportion of granulocyte precursors is less than 20%.

M6—Fewer than 30% of the cells are of myeloid or monocytic lineage, and more than 50% are megaloblastic erythroid precursors.

M7—This state is often associated with extensive marrow fibrosis that has an increase in reticulin or collagen.

Other classifying techniques include cytochemical, immunologic, and chromosomal studies.

Treatment Techniques

The treatment techniques for AML are radiation therapy, chemotherapy, and bone marrow transplantation. These three techniques are used in a combined fashion.

Radiation therapy is administered to the whole body (TBI). It is given bid for 3 days, with a total dose of 1200 cGy. (See the ALL treatment technique section on pp. 631-633 for further details.)

The chemotherapy treatment techniques for treating AML are divided into two groups: remission induction and postremission consolidation/maintenance. The drugs used in remission induction therapy are cytosine arabinoside (Cytarabine) combined with an anthracycline antibiotic such as daunorubicin, doxorubicin, or idarubicin. Cytosine arabinoside is used for consolidation/maintenance therapy.[11] Cytosine arabinoside mimics the natural building blocks of ribonucleic acid (RNA) and DNA to prevent the cell from growing. The other chemicals used in the regimen, the anthracycline antibiotics, impede cell survival by interacting directly with the nuclear DNA.

Bone marrow transplantation is the final treatment technique used in treating AML. (See p. 633 for a description of the bone marrow transplantation procedure.)

Field Design and Critical Structures. The field design and critical structures are described in the section on ALL on p. 631.

Side Effects. Bone marrow depression, which occurs in 4 to 7 days, and immunologic suppression are the hematopoietic side effects of cytosine arabinoside. Nausea, vomiting, esophagitis, stomatitis, diarrhea, and ulceration are common gastrointestinal problems. Renal effects include urinary retention and thrombophlebitis. Rashes and alopecia are skin reactions. In the reproduction system, mutagenic and teratogenic problems arise.

Bone marrow depression also occurs after the use of the anthracycline antibiotics. With these drugs, common gastrointestinal problems are abdominal pain and stomatitis. Myocardial toxicity is the dose-limiting factor for daunorubicin. The integumentary effects are alopecia, hyperpigmentation of the nail beds, and sun sensitivity. Reproductive side effects are teratogenic or mutagenic. The urine turns red after one or two administrations.

CHRONIC LYMPHOCYTIC LEUKEMIA

Epidemiology

CLL affects approximately 15,110 new cases per year and accounts for approximately 30% of the leukemia cases in the United States.[1,2] CLL is nearly twice as common as the chronic myelogenous subtype. The incidence of CLL increases with age, with 65 years as the average age of onset. The disease is rare in persons younger than 40 years. More than half of patients with new cases of CLL are 70 years or older.[1] CLL affects approximately 2.7 per 100,000. The disease affects twice as many males as females and is less common in Asian populations.[12]

Etiology

Heredity appears to play a role in the development of CLL. First-degree relatives of persons with CLL have a two- to sevenfold increase in risk, and the familial clustering of CLL is the most notable of all the leukemias.[2] Immunologic factors such as immunodeficiency syndromes and viruses have been associated with CLL. Several small studies have attempted to determine a suspected link between CLL and chemicals (primarily carbon tetrachloride and carbon disulfide) used in the rubber industry.

CLL is the only leukemia for which an association with radiation exposure has not been established.

 Exposure to high-dose radiation or benzene is not a risk factor for chronic lymphocytic leukemia (CLL), as is the case with other types of leukemia. In some families, more than one blood relative has CLL. However, this is not common. Doctors are studying CLL to understand why the initial change to the lymphocyte takes place. They are also studying why some families have more than one relative with CLL.[12]

Prognostic Indicators

Prognostic factors for CLL include the stage at the time of diagnosis, age, doubling time of the peripheral blood lymphocyte count, and pattern of bone marrow involvement. The T-cell variety of CLL tends to run a more aggressive clinical course and results in shorter survival times.[15]

Clinical Presentation

This subtype is characterized with minimal changes in their blood count.[9] CLL most often occurs as incidental findings on blood tests taken during routine medical visits, with lymphocyte counts often equal to or higher than 10,000/mm³. Patients are often asymptomatic, with abnormalities found only on peripheral blood smears and a bone marrow biopsy. Complaints include fatigue, fever, night sweats, and weight loss. Lymphadenopathy may be present in CLL, and the spleen is almost always enlarged. Complaints of uncomfortable neck masses are common at later stages.

Detection and Diagnosis

Blood tests are used to detect CLL. Patients always exhibit lymphocytosis. Other manifestations of the disease are anemia and thrombocytopenia. Laboratory tests that determine monoclonal surface immunoglobulin and B-cell markers are important to the diagnosis. Phenotyping of leukemic lymphocytes reveals a B-cell origin in 95% of CLL cases.[14]

Other factors leading to the detection and diagnosis of CLL include the enlargement of lymph nodes and the spleen. Of patients with CLL, 50% have chromosomal abnormalities.

Pathology

The origin of CLL may be in the bone marrow lymphoid tissue.[14] A pathologic examination of CLL reveals an increased proliferation of leukemic cells in the bone marrow, blood, lymph nodes, and spleen, with resulting organ enlargement and decreased bone marrow function.[4]

Staging and Classification

One classification system for CLL is the modified Rai staging system.[4] With this system, the three major prognostic groups used to categorize patients are as follows:

Stage 0—low risk
Stages I and II—intermediate risk
Stages III and IV—high risk

These stages are based on the presence of adenopathy, splenomegaly, anemia, and lymphocytosis.[2] Most patients are in the intermediate-risk category, followed by an equal percentage for the other prognostic groups.

The Binet staging system categorizes patients into three stages based on the involvement of five specific anatomic sites: the cervical nodes, axillary nodes, inguinal nodes, spleen, and liver. These stages are as follows[21]:

Stage A—no cytopenia and involvement of up to two sites
Stage B—involvement of three or more sites
Stage C—anemia, thrombocytopenia, or both

Cytochemistry is used to classify CLL according to two subtypes: B-cell CLL and T-cell CLL.[4]

Treatment Techniques

The optimal treatment for CLL is unknown. It is believed that some patients with an early stage of the disease will not benefit from treatment. Chemotherapy is administered for progressive anemia and thrombocytopenia. The drugs used primarily are chlorambucil, an alkylating agent, and prednisone.[12] Chlorambucil prevents the separation of the strands of DNA, which is necessary for cell replication.[12]

Other treatment techniques are radiation therapy and surgery. Palliative radiation therapy is used for localized masses of lymphoid tissue and/or an enlarged spleen. The treatment is given in an anteroposterior/posteroanterior (AP/PA) fashion to a dose of 500 cGy, delivering 100 cGy/day for 5 days.

The surgery used for treating CLL is the splenectomy. An enlarged spleen causes cytopenia, which is the result of accelerated removal or excessive pooling of platelets or RBCs. A splenectomy is used in a situation in which a markedly enlarged spleen produces cytopenia.

Field Design and Critical Structures. The field design for treating a spleen is clinical. The field must encompass the entire spleen with a 1-cm margin around the organ. Field setups are done through palpation or fluoroscopy. CT or conventional simulation can be used to localize the spleen and ensure that the kidney is safely out of the field. Many places use CT alone now with contrast to do this simulation.

Side Effects. Cloramabucil causes bone marrow depression. Gastrointestinal side effects include anorexia, nausea, and vomiting. Dermatitis and urticaria are other side effects. Reproductive side effects include mutagenesis, teratogenesis, and sterility.

Prednisone causes gastrointestinal peptic ulcers and pancreatitis. Metabolic responses include centripetal obesity, hyperlipidemia, hyperosmolar nonketotic coma, and immunosuppression. The neurologic side effect is pseudotumor cerebri. Glaucoma and cataracts may also appear. Hypertension, skin striae, amenorrhea, and impaired wound healing are also side effects.

CHRONIC MYELOGENOUS LEUKEMIA

Epidemiology

CML accounts for approximately 15% of all adult leukemias. The incidence of this disease, which is rare in childhood and uncommon before the age of 35 years, peaks among persons in their mid-60s. A slight predominance of cases exists among males.[2]

Etiology

The cause of CML is unknown. Radiation and benzene exposure have been linked with the development of the disease, but no other environmental or genetic factors have been clearly implicated as causes. The identification of the Philadelphia chromosome by Nowell and Hungerford in 1960 and its presence in 95% of CML patients has led to much interest regarding its possible etiologic role in this disorder.

Prognostic Indicators

The prognosis for patients with CML is affected by numerous factors, including the spleen size, platelet count, hematocrit, gender, and percentage of blood myeloblasts. The disease typically transforms into an acute leukemia after a chronic phase of approximately 3 to 4 years, when the patient enters a blast crisis. A patient in the active phase of the disease has a median survival time of approximately 2 years.[18]

Clinical Presentation

The natural history of CML is divided into three stages: chronic; accelerated; and acute phase, or blast crisis. The early phase of the disease is usually insidious; clinical symptoms are generally mild and nonspecific. Malaise, fatigue, heat intolerance, sweating, and easy bruising are common complaints. Symptoms related to splenic enlargement include vague discomfort in the left upper quadrant (LUQ), early satiety, weight loss, and peripheral leg edema. Within 3 to 4 years, most patients undergo a transformation to a blast crisis. At this stage, all the organs of the body are invaded by leukemic blast cells, and the circulating blood count can reach several hundreds of thousands per cubic millimeter. During the blast crisis, symptoms include fever, bone pain, and more pronounced weight loss.

The active-disease phase of CML, as defined by the Chronic Leukemia Myeloma Task Force, is characterized by weight loss greater than 10% of the body weight in less than 6 months, fever, extreme fatigue, anemia, thrombocytopenia, organ involvement (other than lymph nodes, spleen, bone marrow, and liver), and progressive or painful enlargement of the spleen.

Detection and Diagnosis

The detection and diagnosis of CML are difficult. This disease is insidious and generally not detected, except incidentally. Specific indicators lead to a diagnosis. These abnormal indicators include mild to moderate anemia and leukocytosis. Myeloblasts, promyelocytes, and nucleated RBCs, which indicate CML, are present in the blood. Bone marrow specimens reveal increased granulocytic and often megakaryocytic hyperplasia. Another indicator of CML is a low or absent leukocyte alkaline phosphatase (LAP) score. The most important diagnostic factor for detecting CML is the presence of the Philadelphia chromosome.

Pathology

CML pathogenesis is a result of abnormal hematopoietic stem cells that give rise to progeny that have the Philadelphia chromosome.[14] Because of the abnormal stem cell pool, an increased proliferation of granulocytic and megakaryocytic cells exists. Erythropoiesis is impaired.

Staging and Classification

The three distinct stages of CML are the chronic (or stable) phase, accelerated phase, and acute phase (or blast crisis). (For a further description of stages, see the clinical presentation section.)

Treatment Techniques

The three treatment techniques for treating CML are radiation therapy, chemotherapy, and bone marrow transplantation. Radiation therapy is delivered to the spleen and total body. The treatment technique for the spleen is the same as that for CLL. (See the treatment techniques section for CLL on p. 637.) The treatment technique for TBI is the same as that for ALL.

The drugs used are imatinib mesylate (Gleevec), interferon-α and hydroxyurea. Imatinib mesylate is a monoclonal antibody. It inhibits abnormal protein kinase expressed by the Philadephia chromosome.[19] Interferon-α is an immunotherapeutic drug. It causes a gradual reduction of the leukocyte count toward normal, an increase in the RBC count, and a decrease in the spleen size. Hydroxyurea, a chemotherapeutic agent, blocks DNA synthesis by inhibiting a ribonucleotide reductase.

The final treatment technique for CML is bone marrow transplantation. (See the treatment technique section for ALL on p. 631.) Allogeneic bone marrow transplantation is the only curative treatment for CML. The success rate for patients is lower when they are in the accelerated phase, especially if they have developed a blast transformation.

Field Design and Critical Structures. The spleen field design is explained in the CLL section on p. 637. The TBI field design is explained in the ALL section on p. 631.

Side Effects. The side effects of Gleevel are severe skin reactions, fluid retention and edema, GI disturbances, hemorrhage, anemia, neutropenia, thrombocytopenia, liver toxicities, and potential immunosuppression.[19] Interferon side effects include flulike symptoms: fever, chills, malaise, muscle aches, anorexia, and weight loss.

Hydroxyurea affects the hematopoietic system, with bone marrow depression, rapid leukopenia, and erythrocytic abnormalities. The gastrointestinal side effects are anorexia and diarrhea. Facial erythema and maculopapular rash are integumentary reactions. The reproductive side effect is teratogenic.

Some patients have very high WBC counts at the time the doctor discovers their chronic myelogenous leukemia (CML). This can reduce blood flow to the brain, lungs, eyes, and other places in the body. Leukapheresis is a process whereby patients can have WBCs removed by a machine. A drug called hydroxyurea (Hydrea) may also be used to decrease the WBC count. Leukapheresis can be used for patients diagnosed with CML in the first months of pregnancy, when drug therapy may be harmful to the unborn baby.[13]

ROLE OF RADIATION THERAPIST

Because of the systemic nature of leukemia, chemotherapy is the front-line treatment for the disease. Radiation therapy plays a relatively small, although significant, role in the management of this group of diseases. Therapists who work in health care facilities in which bone marrow transplants are not performed or in which specialized pediatric oncology services are not provided may see few patients with leukemia. Issues relating to scheduling treatments and communicating with and providing support and reassurance for children and their parents must be taken into consideration in departments that routinely treat patients with leukemia. Therapists should work closely with the child life specialist assigned to pediatric oncology patients to gain a better understanding of the patients' and their families' status.

In treating children who have leukemia, therapists must be prepared to communicate with and provide support for the patients and their parents. The radiation oncology experience may evoke fear; the equipment is large and imposing, and the child has most likely undergone numerous painful medical procedures. Sufficient time should be allowed for an explanation of the procedures and the provision of necessary support. Creative methods of eliciting the cooperation of a young child (e.g., stuffed animals and rewards for holding still) and extreme patience may be necessary if anesthesia for daily treatment must be avoided. Exposure of the anatomic areas to be treated may cause emotional concern for a young patient and must be considered and respected by the treatment team. Therapists must be aware of the concerns of the patient's parents, who often have had to subject their child to painful medical procedures and are themselves coping with issues of denial, acceptance, and possible loss.

Last-minute changes and delays in scheduling often accompany the treatment of patients with leukemia. Radiation therapists should be aware of these modifications and realize that the flexibility of daily treatment schedules is often necessary. Children who require anesthesia for their daily treatments not only need extra time and equipment for treatment but also require careful coordination of radiation oncology, anesthesia, and nursing schedules. The radiation oncologist may need to set up treatment fields daily for leukemia patients treated for an enlarged liver or spleen. The radiation oncologist palpates the organ and modifies the field as needed. Onboard imaging (such as portal imaging or CT on rails) can be used for daily setup if available. The physician and therapist are able to verify (check) the fields using image overlay. If the therapist notes a change of size, resimulation may be requested. Modifications may be necessary as the patient responds to treatment. Patients treated for the control of blood counts may need to have blood drawn and blood count results reported before each treatment. Extra time may be required for positioning and precise matching of multiple fields for CNS treatment.

TBI in preparation for bone marrow transplantation requires special attention and consideration by the radiation therapist. As much as 1½ hours must be set aside in the treatment schedule for each of these procedures. If bid treatment is prescribed, major interruptions in the daily treatment schedule can occur, requiring the rescheduling of other patients' appointments. Because the bone marrow transplant patient's immune system is compromised, the treatment room and machine must be scrubbed with disinfectant before the patient's arrival. The treatment team must use reverse isolation techniques (i.e., gown, gloves, and mask). Extra time and patience are required to ensure that the patient is in a position that can be maintained for the actual treatment. Because an extended source-skin distance (SSD) is required to achieve the necessary field size, the actual treatment (beam on) time required to deliver the prescribed dose is often as long as 45 minutes. The patient may experience nausea during treatment. The treatment must then be interrupted, and the patient must be allowed to move and walk around until the nausea subsides. At that time the patient can be repositioned, and the treatment can be resumed.

Present Outcomes

The most exciting outcomes that have taken place in the past 50 years are in the area of pediatric leukemia. The most common form of pediatric leukemia is ALL. Because of the advancement of multidisciplinary therapeutic interventions, children's survival has gone from 4% in 1962 to current 5-year survival rates of 75% to 85%.[17]

Over the years, treatment advances for AML have not improved the remission rates substantially. Adults with AML in the induction phase of therapy go into complete remission approximately 50% to 70% of the time. The overall 5-year survival rate for AML is 21%.[24] It is important to note that the younger the individual is when diagnosed will ultimately result in a better remission rate compared with when the diagnosis is made in the older adult.[21]

Because there is no definitive therapy for cure for CLL, the 5-year survival rate is 74%.[17] This survival rate is determined by the stage of the disease at presentation. Leukemia is not treated in the early stages of CLL. This subtype of leukemia occurs predominately in the senior population. The disease progresses slowly. Oncologists treat CLL in a conservative manner. Typically, no treatment is given in the early stages.

In general, CML has no treatment cure. The survival rates depend on what phase the individual has developed. In the accelerated phase, survival is approximately 1 year or less, and in the more severe phase, after blast transformation, individuals live only a few months.[14] There are longer survival rates for those individuals who are undergoing lymphocytic transformation.[14] Immunotherapy, specifically monoclonal antibodies, is the most recent advance in the treatment of CML. Imatinib mesylate is administered during the chronic phase of the disease. This therapy provides for most patients a long remission period.[13] Clinical trials involving immunotherapy are being investigated with other subtypes of leukemia.

CASE I

Acute Lymphocytic Leukemia

A 12-year-old boy with recurrent ALL is considered for TBI before a bone marrow transplant. At age 3, he exhibited easy bruisability, fatigue, and coughing. Blood work performed at that time revealed a high WBC count, anemia, and thrombocytopenia. A bone marrow aspiration that extracted marrow from the patient's anterior iliac crest was done. A diagnosis of ALL was made at that time. After the diagnosis, a chest x-ray examination was done to check for mediastinal involvement, thymic enlargement, and pleural effusion. No changes were seen.

His first course of treatment was chemotherapy. He received a chemotherapeutic regimen of prednisone, vincristine, and L-asparaginase and was placed in remission.

Approximately 14 months later, the patient exhibited testicular swelling. He received modified chemotherapy and radiation to his testes and remained in remission.

Approximately 10 months later, the patient developed a nonproductive cough and a low-grade fever. These symptoms were treated with antibiotics, and they resolved. Approximately 3 months later, he showed increased fatigue and a nonproductive cough. A CBC at this time was significant for a WBC count of 400,000/mm³ with 19% blasts. He had an immature T-cell, FAB classification of L2. A chest radiograph taken at that time revealed a mediastinal mass. He also exhibited hepatosplenomegaly.

The patient was scheduled to receive a regimen of vincristine, prednisone, and L-asparaginase. His family was tested, and his brother had an HLA match. The patient was enrolled in an in-house protocol for bone marrow transplantation: high-dose cyclophosphamide (Cytoxan) and TBI, followed by a bone marrow transplant.

CASE II

Acute Myelogenous Leukemia

A 41-year-old mother of two was considered TBI followed by bone marrow transplantation. She initially complained of heavy menstrual periods and progressive fatigue. She noted dyspnea on exertion, petechiae, and some gingival bleeding.

Approximately 2 months later, a blood test was performed and the patient was found to have pancytopenia with a WBC of 900/mm³, hematocrit at 17%, and platelet count of 80,000/mm³. A bone marrow aspiration and biopsy showed myeloblasts, and the diagnosis of AML was made.

The patient received induction chemotherapy with cytosine arabinoside and daunorubicin. This treatment was complicated by neutropenia, a fever, and a rash that developed over her body.

She had her first postremission consolidation therapy 1 month later, with cytosine arabinoside combined with hydrocortisone. She tolerated this treatment well. Her maintenance therapy consisted of 6-thioguanine, vincristine, and prednisone. This treatment caused diarrhea, anorexia, and dermatitis.

The patient now awaits her TBI and bone marrow transplant. Her brother is a 5.6 HLA match. She is being prepared for a bone marrow transplant and is having a second cycle of consolidation therapy.

CASE III

Chronic Lymphocytic Leukemia

Mrs. W. is a 68-year-old woman who was diagnosed with CLL 2 years ago. She was treated at a neighborhood health center for a thyroid condition. During a routine blood test, her differential count showed a lymphocytosis of 67% (WBC was 10,800/mm³). Her hematocrit had dropped from an average of 36% to 32.2%. Therefore, she was referred for further evaluation.

The patient's initial history revealed night sweats and a fever. She had chronic sinus congestion and hearing loss. She denied having a cough, shortness of breath, or chest pain, but she did note slight fatigue. Her spleen was enlarged.

Her physical examination showed clear lungs, no hepatomegaly, and no arthritis. Her blood work showed a hemoglobin of 11.6 g/100 mL, a hematocrit of 35.1%, a mean corpuscular volume (MCV) of 90.1 mm³, and unremarkable RBC morphology. Her WBC was 11,700/mm³. These results indicate

that the hemoglobin and hematocrit were at the lower limits of normal. The lymphocytosis was consistent with CLL stage 0. Peripheral blood lymphocyte markers were obtained, revealing 63% B cells. This is also consistent with CLL stage 0.

Approximately 10 months after diagnosis, Mrs. W. developed neuropathy with pain and numbness of her feet. A neurologist examined her and no pathologic changes were identified. A few months later, she developed leg ulcers. At this point, she was started on a treatment of prednisone. Her pain improved, and her ankle ulcers healed.

Mrs. W. is presently asymptomatic, and her prognosis is excellent.

CASE IV

Chronic Myelogenous Leukemia

A 17-year-old girl with CML complained of a 1-month history of fatigue, easy bruising, and the passing of large blood clots during a menstrual period. Blood work was performed and revealed a WBC of 78,000/mm³. A blood smear showed numerous myeloid forms consistent with CML. Her hematocrit was 35%, and her platelet count was 204,000/mm³.

A bone marrow biopsy and aspiration were performed and found to be consistent with CML. Her LAP score was 36. Cytogenetics showed a translocation of the chromosomes 9 and 22. This is consistent with a Philadelphia chromosome.

The patient was first given interferon-α. She tolerated this well, aside from some mild flulike symptoms and diarrhea. Approximately 3 months later, the patient received 500 cGy to her spleen. This was followed by TBI and a bone marrow transplant 1 week later.

SUMMARY

- There are four major subtypes of leukemia, which are divided into acute and chronic types.
- The most common pediatric malignancy is acute lymphocytic leukemia (ALL).
- ALL has been associated with ionizing radiation, physical and chemical agents, and heredity.
- For a definitive diagnosis for ALL, a bone marrow aspiration biopsy is necessary.
- Treatment techniques for ALL are chemotherapy, radiation therapy, and bone marrow transplantation.
- ALL and acute myelogenous leukemia (AML) patients present with nonspecific flu-like symptoms.
- The hallmark for diagnosing AML is the presence of Auer rods.
- The primary classification of AML is based on maturation status.
- AML risk factors are ionizing radiation, certain genetic disorders, exposure to benzene, and alkylating agents.
- Chronic lymphocytic leukemia (CLL) is primarily a geriatric malignancy with the median age of 65 years old.
- CLL and chronic myelogenous leukemia (CML) are typically asymptomatic and are revealed as incidental findings.
- Treatment is not administered in the early stage of CLL; rather, watchful waiting is commonly used.
- The hallmark of diagnosis for CML is the presence of the Philadelphia chromosome.

Review Questions

Multiple Choice

1. Which of the following concerning CLL is *not* true?
   a. It is a disease of children.
   b. It resembles CML but with a malignant lymphoid cell line.
   c. It can be confused with lymphoma.
   d. Therapy is usually reserved until the patient is symptomatic.

2. Which of the following is a specific characteristic of CML?
   a. a disease of children
   b. Philadelphia chromosome
   c. requirement of prophylactic CNS radiation
   d. presentation with an enlarged spleen

3. Which of the following is *not* a common symptom associated with acute leukemia at the time of presentation?
   a. fatigue
   b. easy bleeding and bruisability
   c. nausea and vomiting
   d. fever

4. Which of the following leukemias has *not* been associated with previous radiation exposure?
   a. CML
   b. CLL
   c. AML
   d. ALL

5. Anatomic sites that are potential sanctuaries for leukemic cells are the:
   I. testes
   II. spleen
   III. CNS
   a. I and II
   b. I and III
   c. II and III
   d. I, II, and III

6. Which of the following is *not* one of the main subtypes of leukemia?
   a. ALL
   b. AML
   c. CCL
   d. CLL

7. The primary treatment modality for leukemia is:
   a. surgery
   b. immunotherapy
   c. ionizing radiation
   d. chemotherapy

8. The most documented etiologic factor for leukemia in humans is:
   a. surgery
   b. immunotherapy
   c. ionizing radiation
   d. chemotherapy

9. The type of leukemia that essentially has no cure is:
   a. ALL
   b. AML
   c. CLL
   d. CML

10. Splenomegaly indicates:
    a. an enlargement of the liver
    b. an enlargement of the spleen
    c. an increase in the circulating platelets
    d. a better-than-average prognosis for ALL and CLL

The answers to the Review Questions can be found by logging on to our website at: *http://evolve.elsevier.com/Washington+Leaver/ principles*

Questions to Ponder

1. Discuss the main factors that differentiate the four subtypes of leukemia.

2. Describe the various treatment techniques used for the four main subtypes of leukemia.

3. Evaluate each of the four major subtypes of leukemia for responsiveness to therapy.

4. Differentiate between detection and diagnosis in reference to the specific subtypes of leukemia.

5. Describe the different types of bone marrow transplantation techniques.

REFERENCES

1. American Cancer Society: *Cancer facts and figures 2007* (website): http://www.cancer.org. Accessed November 22, 2008.
2. Brown CK, et al, editors: *Holland-Frei manual of cancer.* Hamilton, Ontario, 2005, BC Decker.
3. Dameshek W, Gunz F: *Leukemia,* ed 2, New York, 1964, Grune & Stratton.
4. DeVita V, Hellman S, Rosenberg S, editors: *Cancer principles and practice of oncology,* Philadelphia, 2005, Lippincott Williams & Wilkins.
5. Freireich E, Lemak N: *Milestones in leukemia research and therapy,* Baltimore, 1991, John Hopkins University Press.
6. Halperin EC, et al: *Pediatric radiation oncology,* ed 4, Philadelphia, 2005, Lippincott Williams & Wilkins.
7. Howe GR: Leukemia following the Chernobyl accident, *Health Phys* 93:512-515, 2007.
8. Kolb E, Gidwani P, Grupp S: Hematopoietic stem cell transplantation (website): http://www.emedicine.com/ped/topic2593.htm. Accessed November 8, 2007.
9. Lenhard R, Osteen R, Gansler T, editors: *Clinical oncology,* Atlanta, 2001, American Cancer Society.
10. Leukemia and Lymphoma Society: Acute lymphocytic leukemia. The Leukemia and Lymphoma Society: Fighting Blood Cancers (website): http://www.leukemia-lymphoma.org/all_page?item_id=7049. Accessed June 1, 2007.
11. Leukemia and Lymphoma Society: Acute myelogenous leukemia. The Leukemia and Lymphoma Society: Fighting Blood Cancers (website): http://www.leukemia-lymphoma.org/all_page?item_id=8459. Accessed June 6, 2007.
12. Leukemia and Lymphoma Society: Chronic lymphocytic leukemia. The Leukemia and Lymphoma Society: Fighting Blood Cancers (website): http://www.leukemia-lymphoma.org/all_page?item_id=7059. Accessed June 8, 2007.
13. Leukemia and Lymphoma Society: Chronic myelogenous leukemia. The Leukemia and Lymphoma Society: Fighting Blood Cancers (website): http://www.leukemia-lymphoma.org/all_page?item_id=8501. Accessed June 8, 2007.
14. Lichtman MA, et al, editors: *Williams hematology,* ed 7, New York, 2006, McGraw-Hill.
15. MedlinePlus. American Cancer Society (website): http://www.cancer.org/docroot/CRI/content/CRI_2_4_3X_How_is_childhood_leukemia_staged_24.asp?sitearea. Accessed November 16, 2007.

16. National Cancer Institute: Childhood acute lymphoblastic leukemia treatment (PDQ). National Cancer Institute (website): http://www.cancer.gov/cancertopics/pdq/treatment/childALL/Patient/page2. Accessed June 5, 2007.

17. National Cancer Institute: Surveillance, epidemiology, and end results. National Cancer Institute (website): http://seer.cancer.gov/statfacts/html. Accessed May 12, 2007.

18. Perez C, et al, editors: *Principles and practice of radiation oncology,* ed 4, Philadelphia, 2004, Lippincott Williams & Wilkins.

19. Physicians' Desk Reference: *Gleevec Tablets (Novartis),* Thomson Micromedex Healthcare Series (website): http://www.thomsonhc.com/hcs. Accessed June 7, 2007.

20. Pui C, Evans W: Treatment of acute lymphoblastic leukemia, *N Engl J Med* 354:166-176, 2006.

21. Scigliano E, et al: The leukemias. In Rubin P, editor: *Clinical oncology: a multidisciplinary approach for physicians and students,* ed 8, Philadelphia, 2001, WB Saunders.

22. St. Jude Children's Research Hospital: Leukemia/lymphoma: acute lymphocytic lymphoma (ALL) (website): http://www.stjude.org. Accessed May 8, 2007.

23. Stock W: Controversies in treatment of AML: case-based discussion, *Hematology* 1:185-191, 2006.

24. Stone R, O'Donnell M, Sekeres M: Acute myeloid leukemia, *Hematology* 1:98-117, 2004.

25. Thomas E: Bone marrow transplantation, *CA J Clin* 37:291-296, 1987.

26. Thomson Micromedex Healthcare Series: Acute lymphoid leukemia—acute (website): http://thomsonhc.com/hcs. Accessed June 1, 2007.

27. Thomson Micromedex Healthcare Series: Acute myeloid leukemia—acute (website): http://www.thomsonhc.com/hsc. Accessed June 1, 2007.

28. University of Virginia Health System: Leukemia: acute lymphoblastic leukemia (website): http://www.med-ed.virginia.edu/courses/path/innes/wed/lymphoid.cfm. Accessed June 8, 2007.

29. Wax PM: *Toxicologic plagues and disasters in history in Goldfrank's toxicologic emergencies,* ed 8 (website): http://online.statref.com.ezproxy.mcphs.edu. Accessed November 11, 2007.

30. Wiernik P, et al, editors: *Neoplastic diseases of the blood,* New York, 1991, Churchill Livingstone.

BIBLIOGRAPHY

Brager B, Yasko J: *Care of the client receiving chemotherapy,* Reston, Va, 1984, Reston Publishing.

Henderson E, Han T: Current therapy of acute and chronic leukemia in adults, *CA J Clin* 36:322-350, 1986.

Tarbel N, Mauch P, Chin L: Total body irradiation. In *JCRT handbook,* Boston, 1994, Joint Center for Radiation Therapy.

Washington C, Leaver D, editors: *Principles and practice of radiation therapy,* St. Louis, 2004, Mosby.

CHAPTER 31

Endocrine System Tumors

Robert D. Adams, Tammy Newell

Outline

Key Terms

Objectives

- Discuss epidemiologic factors of this tumor site.
- Identify, list, and discuss etiologic factors that may be responsible for inducing tumors in this anatomic site.
- Describe the symptoms produced by a malignant tumor in this region
- Discuss the methods of detection and diagnosis for tumors in this anatomic region.
- List the varying histologic types of tumors generic to this region.
- Describe the diagnostic procedures used in the workup and staging for this site.
- Describe in detail the most common routes of tumor spread for this site.
- Differentiate between histologic grading and staging.
- Describe in detail the anatomy and physiology of this anatomic region/organ.
- Identify the treatment(s) of choice for this malignancy.
- Discuss the rationale for treatment with regard to treatment choice, histologic type and stage of the disease.

- Describe in detail the treatment methods available for this diagnosis.
- Describe the differing types of radiation treatments that can be used for treating this tumor site.
- Identify the appropriate tumor lethal dose for various stages of this malignancy.
- Discuss the expected radiation reactions for the area based on time-dose-fractionation schemes.
- Discuss tolerance levels of the vital structures and organs at risk (OAR).
- Describe the instructions that should be given to a patient with regard to skin care, expected reactions and dietary advice.
- Discuss the rationale for using multi-modality treatments for this diagnosis.
- Describe the various treatment planning techniques for this anatomic site including external beam and brachytherapy options.
- Discuss survival statistics and prognosis for various stages for this tumor site.

The endocrine system is composed of multiple glandular organs responsible for complex metabolic regulatory functions. The principal organs of this system include the following glands: pituitary (which resides in the sella turcica at the base of the brain), thyroid, and adrenal. Also included are the parathyroid glands and specialized cells in the pancreas called the islets of Langerhans, which are referred to as the endocrine portions of the pancreas. Each of these organs (or specialized portions of them) produces hormones under complex feedback-control mechanisms that affect various functions to meet ongoing metabolic needs and stresses of the organism. The master regulatory gland of this system is the pituitary. This gland produces many hormones under the influence of the hypothalamus, which directly affects the function of other endocrine organs. This sophisticated mechanism of stimulation and inhibition of endocrine organ function, which is called a **negative feedback** loop, is critical for maintaining metabolic homeostasis (stability) and providing the organism with the ability to respond to various stresses.

Many disorders of the endocrine organs can result in disruption of this complex surveillance and response system. These disorders may be related to benign, congenital, degenerative, traumatic, autoimmune, or infectious processes that may affect the function of one or many organs in the endocrine system. The result can range from minor to potentially life-threatening dysfunction. Probably the most widely recognized endocrine dysfunction is insufficient insulin production by the islet cells of the pancreas, or diabetes mellitus. Although this is a complex multisystem disease, the abnormality in glucose metabolism caused by insulin deficiency can be disastrous. This situation is remedied through the supply of insulin via an injection or oral medication to reestablish homeostasis of glucose metabolism.

The function of the endocrine system may also be affected by neoplastic change in the various glands. Although true primary malignancies of these organs are rare, they are important to consider because of the wide-ranging effects they can have on the organism as a whole. Metabolic function altered by neoplastic change in various endocrine organs can produce clinical syndromes that are often well recognized. These syndromes can lead the clinician to perform various diagnostic studies to confirm the suspicions related to an endocrine gland tumor. This chapter discusses neoplastic lesions of the thyroid, pituitary, and adrenal gland. Pancreatic tumors, which can display endocrine and exocrine function, are discussed in Chapter 35.

THYROID CANCER

Epidemiology

Although thyroid cancers are the most common of the endocrine malignancies (accounting for approximately 94% of all new cases and 63% of deaths), they represent only 2% of all cancers.[13]

Etiology

Unlike other endocrine glands for which the incidence of malignancy is rare, thyroid cancer has several recognized etiologic factors.

External radiation to the thyroid gland, particularly before puberty, is the only well-documented etiologic factor. Approximately 25% of the patients who receive between 2 cGy and several hundred cGy of external radiation to the thyroid gland develop thyroid carcinoma. These carcinomas are usually a low-grade papillary subtype.[12]

Many studies have been conducted on the inhabitants of Nagasaki and Hiroshima after the explosion of the atomic bomb in 1945. Of 20,000 heavily and lightly exposed individuals examined every year since 1959, approximately 0.2% have developed thyroid cancer. Again, most of these cancers have been papillary.[12]

After the radioactive fallout from a nuclear test in the Marshall Islands, the inhabitants have been systematically studied annually and compared with a nonexposed population. According to the results in 1974, 34 of 229 exposed persons developed thyroid lesions. Three of the total number of patients developed cancers. Those irradiated before the age of 20 showed the highest incidence rate of thyroid nodularity.[12]

 The Marshall Islands Program was established in 1954 by the Department of Energy (DOE), following the accidental exposure to people in the Marshall Islands to fallout from the U.S. nuclear test at the Bikini Atoll. More information is available at http://www.eh.doe.gov/health/marshall/marshall.htm.

The Chernobyl incident of 1986 has produced conflicting studies on the increase of thyroid cancer, probably because of the extremely short interval between radiation exposure and tumor occurrence. One study conducted 4½ years after the Chernobyl reactor accident showed no significant difference in thyroid nodularity among persons residing in highly contaminated and control villages.[17] However, another study's data confirm that the neoplasms increasingly diagnosed between 1986 and 1991 among children of the Republic of Belarus were thyroid carcinomas.[8] In the Cancer Registry of Belarus, 101 instances of thyroid cancer in children younger than 15 years had been noted between 1986 and 1991, in contrast to only 9 cases between 1976 and 1985.[8]

External radiation for benign disease, especially in young patients, was a widespread practice in the United States in the 1930s, 1940s, and 1950s. X-rays or radium was used to treat benign conditions such as acne, tonsillitis, hemangiomas, and thymic enlargement. Young patients who received radiation for malignant conditions, such as mantle irradiation for Hodgkin's disease, demonstrated an increased risk of developing thyroid cancer.[12,16]

The latent (time) period between exposure and incidence of abnormalities varies with age. The average **latent period** in infants is 11 years, and in adolescents it is 15 to 30 years. Whether adults develop cancer at a higher rate after exposure is questionable.[12]

Prolonged stimulation of the thyroid gland with a thyroid-stimulating hormone (TSH) in laboratory animals has produced thyroid cancer. However, no human population studies have been done that support this hypothesis.[21]

Some other, less well-defined, factors include the following[3]:
- Long-standing, nontoxic colloid goiter in relation to papillary and anaplastic carcinoma
- The relationship of follicular adenomas as premalignant lesions to follicular carcinomas
- The role of genetics for medullary carcinoma*

Prognostic Indicators

Age, gender, histologic subtype, and capsular invasion are prognostic. Lesions confined to the gland have an overall better prognosis than those demonstrating capsular invasion. Patients with well-differentiated thyroid carcinoma (papillary and follicular) have a better prognosis than do those with undifferentiated carcinoma (anaplastic).

Anatomy

The thyroid gland, consisting of a right and left lobe, lies over the deep structures of the neck; is close to the larynx, trachea,

---

*A large proportion of cases are familial, occurring as part of two complex endocrine syndromes: multiple endocrine neoplasia (MEN) IIa and IIb.

parathyroid glands, and esophagus; and is anterior and medial to the carotid artery, jugular vein, and vagus nerve.[12] (See Figure 31-1 for the anatomy of the thyroid gland and its anatomic relationships to surrounding structures.)

The lateral lobes are approximately 5 cm in length and extend to the level of the midthyroid cartilage superiorly and the sixth tracheal ring inferiorly. These lobes are connected in the midline by the **isthmus** at the level of the second to fourth tracheal rings. The thyroid gland weighs approximately 25 g.[12]

Lymphatic capillaries are arranged throughout the gland and drain to many nodal sites. These sites include the internal jugular chain, Delphian node (anterior cervical node), pretracheal nodes, and paratracheal nodes in the lower neck.[12] Superior mediastinal lymphatics can be considered the lowest part of the cervical lymphatic system. If it is involved, this represents significant regional spread of disease.[12]

Physiology

The thyroid gland produces several hormones, including thyroxine (T_4) and triiodothyronine (T_3), which are responsible for metabolic regulation. Thyroidal function is regulated by pituitary and hypothalamic hormones, which respond to complex systemic negative feedback mechanisms based on metabolic needs. The TSH produced in the pituitary gland causes direct stimulation of thyroid cells to produce and release hormones that are critical for carbohydrate and protein metabolism.

The production of these hormones relies on the thyroid gland's ability to remove iodine from the blood. Without sufficient

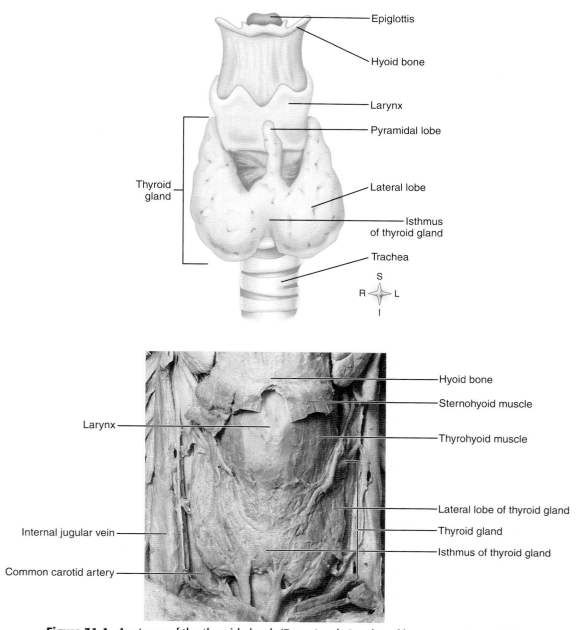

Figure 31-1. Anatomy of the thyroid gland. (From Jacob S: *Atlas of human anatomy,* 2002, St. Louis, Elsevier. In Thibodeau GA, Patton KT: *Anatomy and physiology,* ed 6, St. Louis, 2007, Mosby.)

amounts of iodine, several clinical disorders can be observed from the resultant deficiency in thyroid-hormone production. Functional disorders of the thyroid gland are characterized by hyperactivity (**hyperthyroidism**) or underactivity (**hypothyroidism**).

Disorders from hypothyroidism can include the following[26]:

- **Cretinism**—this disorder appears in infants shortly after birth. Symptoms include stunted growth, abnormal bone formation, retarded mental development, a low body temperature, and sluggishness.
- **Myxedema**—this disorder occurs if hypothyroidism develops after growth. Symptoms include a low metabolic rate, mental slowness, weight gain, and swollen tissues caused by excess body fluid.

Disorders from hyperthyroidism can include the following[26]:

- **Graves' disease**—this disorder is characterized by an elevated metabolic rate, abnormal weight loss, excessive perspiration, muscular weakness, emotional instability, and exophthalmos.
- **Goiter**—this disorder is a physical sign of an enlarged thyroid gland. Overstimulation by TSH causes an enlargement of thyroid cells. If this is associated with increased hormone production, it is referred to as toxic goiter.

In addition, a specialized subgroup of cells exists in the thyroid known as C-cells. These produce calcitonin, which is a hormone involved in calcium metabolism.

Clinical Presentation

Most patients with thyroid cancer have a palpable neck mass, which is often detected during a routine physical examination. Almost 25% of young people with differentiated thyroid carcinoma present because of a palpable cervical lymph node metastasis as a result of occult primary thyroid cancer.[12] These occult, differentiated thyroid cancers can go undetected for years because of their indolent nature. A biopsy should be performed on persistent, enlarged lymph nodes found in children, teenagers, and young adults, with a clinical differential of Hodgkin's disease, benign inflammatory disease, or papillary carcinoma of the thyroid gland.[12]

Lesions in the thyroid gland should arouse suspicion if they exhibit extreme hardness, appear fixed to deep structures or skin, and are associated with recurrent laryngeal nerve paralysis (hoarseness).

Anaplastic carcinomas are usually large, hard, and fixed; grow rapidly; and occur in older patients. Patients can appear with symptoms related to compression and/or invasion of the esophagus, airway, or recurrent laryngeal nerves. Symptoms include pain, dysphagia, dyspnea, stridor, and hoarseness.[12]

Most patients with medullary carcinoma initially have an asymptomatic painless mass.[12] They may appear with systemic symptoms of diarrhea related to vasoactive substances (calcitonin) produced by the tumor. This usually represents an advanced stage of the disease. (See Table 31-1 for clinical symptoms and signs of patients with thyroid carcinoma.)

Table 31-1	Clinical Symptoms and Signs in 106 Patients with Thyroid Carcinoma		
Symptoms and Signs	Patients (n = 66) with Papillary Carcinoma (%)	Patients (n = 33) with Follicular Carcinoma (%)	Patients (n = 7) with Anaplastic Carcinoma (%)
Hoarseness	9	15	55
Dysphagia	11	12	28
Pain and pressure	8	6	28
Dyspnea	3	6	43
Increasing size	56	75	85
Solitary nodule	60	65	14
Multinodular	33	20	70
Found in routine examination	27	30	0

Modified from Ureles AL, et al: Cancer of the endocrine glands. In Rubin P, editor: *Clinical oncology: a multidisciplinary approach for physicians and students*, Philadelphia, 1993, Saunders.

Detection and Diagnosis

Clinical presentation cannot determine a diagnosis of carcinoma. For confirmation of the diagnostic suspicion of cancer, a biopsy (most important), specialized imaging studies, and laboratory testing are necessary.

Laboratory testing includes an analysis of the thyroglobulin and calcitonin levels. Thyroglobulin levels cannot distinguish between a benign tumor and differentiated thyroid cancer.[12,23] Postoperatively, however, elevated levels indicate residual, recurrent, or metastatic differentiated thyroid cancer and can be correlated with iodine-131 (I-131) imaging for the detection of thyroid cancer. As such, thyroglobulin levels may be useful for monitoring patients who have an established diagnosis of thyroid cancer. Calcitonin levels that are elevated preoperatively indicate C-cell hyperplasia and/or medullary thyroid cancer.[9,12] Postoperative elevated levels indicate residual, recurrent, or metastatic medullary thyroid carcinoma.

Imaging studies include radionuclide imaging, sonography, computed tomography (CT), and magnetic resonance imaging (MRI). Each examination can provide useful information for the diagnosis of thyroid cancer.

Radionuclide thyroid imaging is commonly used to evaluate the function and anatomic location of a palpable thyroid nodule through the localization of hot or cold spots in the gland. By this means the detection of occult cancers in high-risk patients can be accomplished. This imaging technique can detect a primary lesion in patients with suspected regional and distant thyroid cancer metastases. In addition, radionuclide imaging can detect local-regional or distant metastases in patients with known thyroid cancer. Patients previously treated for thyroid cancer are typically monitored with repeat scans.

The four radiopharmaceuticals most commonly used for radionuclide imaging of the thyroid are I-131, I-125, I-123, and technetium-99m (Tc-99m). A thyroid nodule can image in three ways: (1) **cold thyroid nodule** (no radionuclide uptake),

(2) **warm thyroid nodule** (slightly higher concentration than the rest of the thyroid gland), and (3) **hot thyroid nodule** (radionuclide uptake much higher than the rest of the thyroid gland).[12] (See Figure 31-2 for abnormal thyroid uptake.) Most cold nodules are thyroid adenomas or colloid cysts, with only 15% to 25% representing thyroid cancers. If multiple cold nodules appear, the incidence of the malignancy drops to 5%.[12]

The incidence rate of cancer with warm or hot nodules is low and usually represents a functioning adenoma or areas of normal tissue in an otherwise diseased gland. Some metastatic, well-differentiated follicular carcinomas accumulate radioiodine. Most metastatic, differentiated thyroid tumors do not accumulate radioiodine until all normal thyroid tissue has been ablated. This happens because normal-functioning thyroid tissue preferentially accumulates iodinated radiopharmaceuticals relative to the tumor.

Sonography can determine whether a nodule is solid or cystic. This technique is used as a complementary test to radionuclide imaging. A nodule found to be solid through sonography has a 30% probability of being a cancer.[12,22]

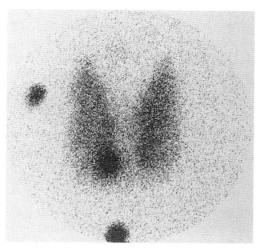
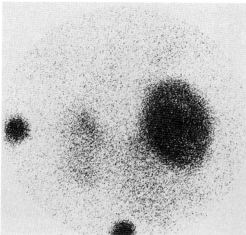

Figure 31-2. Abnormal thyroid imaging with both images demonstrating a hot nodule. (From Christian PE, Waterstram KM: *Nuclear medicine and PET/CT, technology and technique,* St. Louis, 2007, Mosby.)

A CT scan cannot differentiate between a benign or malignant lesion. However, it can show the local and regional extent of advanced or recurrent cancer.[12] CT can also help a radiation oncologist in treatment planning if the use of external beam radiation is anticipated.

MRI can be useful in depicting lesion margins, lesion extent, tissue heterogenicity, cystic or hemorrhagic regions, cervical lymphadenopathy, invasion of adjacent structures, and additional nonpalpable thyroid nodules.[12,15,18]

A needle biopsy in some circumstances can obviate surgery by differentiating malignant from nonmalignant lesions. Two types of needle biopsies are needle aspiration cytology (performed with a small-gauge needle) and core needle biopsy (performed with a large-cutting biopsy needle of the Silverman type).

Both biopsies have a false-negative rate of up to 10%. A needle biopsy is indeterminate for follicular carcinoma because it cannot be diagnosed by cytologic or histologic criteria. However, a needle biopsy may play a role in the management of anaplastic thyroid malignancies and lymphomas because the diagnosis is more obvious.[12]

Pathology

Malignant thyroid neoplasms are divided into four categories: (1) papillary, (2) follicular, (3) medullary, and (4) anaplastic[13]. Rare tumors that account for less than 5% of thyroid malignancies include the following[12]:

- Lymphoma and plasmacytoma
- Squamous cell and mucin-producing carcinoma
- Teratoma and mixed tumors
- Sarcoma, carcinosarcoma, and hemangioendothelioma
- Metastatic carcinoma to the thyroid
- Thyroid cancer at unusual sites, including the median aberrant thyroid gland, lateral aberrant thyroid gland, and struma ovarii

Differentiated thyroid cancers include papillary, mixed papillary-follicular, and follicular carcinomas. These tumors arise from the thyroid follicle cell and can usually be treated with I-131 and thyroid hormone suppression.[12]

Papillary and mixed papillary-follicular cancers are the most common types of thyroid cancer, representing 33% to 73% of all malignant thyroid lesions. As previously mentioned, papillary carcinoma is the type most frequently seen in irradiated individuals. These tumors are slow growing, are nonaggressive, and have an excellent prognosis. This type of cancer is two to four times more common in females than males. The peak for occurrence is in the third to fifth decade of life, although the cancer can occur at any age. In children younger than 15 years, papillary carcinoma accounts for 80% of thyroid cancers.[12]

Follicular carcinoma accounts for 14% to 33% of all thyroid cancers. These tumors have the greatest propensity to concentrate I-131. They are two to three times more common in women than men, with the average age for a diagnosis from 50 to 58 years. They rarely occur in children. Follicular carcinoma has a worse overall prognosis than papillary carcinoma.[12,32]

Medullary thyroid cancer represents 5% to 10% of all thyroid cancers. About 80% of medullary thyroid cancers appear spontaneously, with 20% occurring as part of familial multiple endocrine neoplasia (MEN) syndromes (IIa, IIb, or III). No gender differentiation is seen between spontaneous and familial forms. With regard to age, however, spontaneous forms occur from the fifth decade on, whereas familial forms have been seen in patients younger than 10 and as old as 80 years. Medullary carcinoma has a worse prognosis than papillary, mixed papillary-follicular, and possibly follicular cancers, although it has a better prognosis than anaplastic carcinoma.[12]

Anaplastic carcinoma carries the worst overall prognosis. It is more aggressive than the previously mentioned types, and a patient's life expectancy is usually short after the diagnosis is established. Anaplastic carcinoma represents 10% of all malignant thyroid lesions. The age of occurrence is from 40 to 90 years, with the incidence in women outnumbering that in men by four to one.[12]

Staging

The American Joint Committee on Cancer has staged thyroid cancers according to the histologic type and age of the patient (Box 31-1).

Routes of Spread

Each pathologic classification has its own route of spread, which ranges from slow growing to extremely aggressive.

Papillary and mixed papillary-follicular carcinomas metastasize to regional lymph nodes through lymphatic channels. At the time of operation, 50% to 70% of these carcinomas have cervical lymph node metastases, although the presence of metastases in regional lymph nodes does not significantly worsen the prognosis. Bloodborne metastases can occur.

Follicular cancers have a tendency to invade vascular channels and metastasize hematogenously to distant sites, including the bone, lung, liver, and brain. Lymph node metastases are uncommon.

Medullary thyroid cancer can vary from indolent to rapidly fatal growth patterns. Medullary carcinoma spreads regionally before displaying distant metastases, with up to 50% of patients having regional metastases at the time of the diagnosis. Metastases occur hematogenously and through lymphatic routes involving mainly the cervical nodes, lung, liver, and bone.

Anaplastic carcinoma displays local invasion of structures such as the trachea. Skin invasion is also seen, giving rise to dermal lymphatic metastases on the chest and abdominal walls. Regional neck nodes are often involved, although sometimes the primary tumor is so extensive that the regional node status is difficult to assess.[12]

Treatment Techniques

Surgery. Papillary carcinoma and mixed papillary-follicular carcinomas are rarely invasive and seldom require the resection of the muscles of the neck, internal jugular vein, esophagus, or trachea. Radical neck dissections are warranted only if nodes are grossly involved with metastatic disease. Because papillary and mixed papillary-follicular carcinomas are usually indolent diseases, prophylactic or elective neck dissections are no longer performed. During radical neck dissections, special care is taken to spare the recurrent laryngeal, vagus, spinal accessory,

and phrenic nerves. Care is also taken to preserve the parathyroid glands.[30]

For small, lateralized lesions that do not show extrathyroidal involvement or lymph node metastasis, lobectomy including removal of the isthmus is required. Surgery for mixed papillary-follicular carcinoma is the same as that for papillary carcinoma, unless vascular invasion or bloodborne metastases are present, in which case the lesion is treated as follicular cancer.

For encapsulated follicular carcinoma confined in the thyroid, a lobectomy including the isthmus can often successfully control the disease. In early stages in which the spread to cervical lymph nodes is rare, prophylactic neck dissection is not needed. If a second lesion is present in the contralateral lobe, a total or near-total thyroidectomy is performed, usually with good results.[30] If follicular carcinoma is extrathyroidal or metastatic disease is present, a bilateral total thyroidectomy is mandatory.

For medullary carcinoma that is sporadic and intrathyroidal, a lobectomy plus isthmus removal is required. If the lesion has extended beyond the thyroid to involve lymphatics and/or soft tissue, a radical en bloc resection is required. Because regional lymph nodes occur in 50% of the patients, an elective neck dissection may be advisable.[30] In the familial form, in which the cancer is generally bilateral, a total thyroidectomy is warranted.

For undifferentiated (anaplastic) carcinoma, surgery is effective on only a few occasions. Surgery is often necessary to alleviate a central airway obstruction resulting from extrinsic compression of the larynx and upper trachea caused by this aggressive malignancy. A tracheotomy is usually required to preserve a patient's airway. Radical surgical attempts are not always justified or technically possible because growth into soft tissue and deeper structures of the neck is often present.[12]

For malignancies that metastasize to the thyroid (an extremely rare situation), the treatment varies with primary sites, including the larynx, esophagus, lung, kidney, rectum, and skin. A biopsy is usually needed to differentiate a metastasis from a primary thyroid cancer.

Side effects of surgery can include tumor hemorrhage, damage to parathyroid gland resulting in temporary or permanent hypoparathyroidism, and temporary or permanent vocal cord paralysis.

Radioactive Iodine. Radioactive iodine is used to treat papillary, mixed papillary-follicular, and follicular cancers. Indications for radioactive iodine include the following:

- Inoperable primary tumor
- Thyroid capsular invasion
- Thyroid ablation after a partial or subtotal thyroidectomy
- Postoperative residual disease in the neck and recurrent disease
- Cervical or mediastinal nodal metastasis
- Distant metastasis

The routine use of I-131 after surgery in small, lateralized, well-differentiated cancers is debatable; thyroid suppression therapy alone may be adequate. Because normal thyroid tissue has a greater propensity than differentiated thyroid cancer to absorb iodine, the consensus seems to be that all normal tissue should be ablated to allow residual or metastatic disease to accumulate I-131. An ablation dose administered

Box 31-1 American Joint Committee on Cancer and the International Union Against Cancer Tumor Node Metastasis Classification for Carcinoma of the Thyroid Gland

PRIMARY TUMOR (T)

TX	Primary tumor cannot be assessed
T0	No evidence of primary tumor
T1	Tumor 2 cm or less in greater dimension limited to the thyroid
T2	Tumor more than 2 cm but not more than 4 cm in greatest dimension limited to the thyroid
T3	Tumor more than 4 cm in greatest dimension limited to the thyroid or any tumor with minimal extrathyroid extension (e.g., extension to sternothyroid muscle or perithyroid soft tissues)
T4a	Tumor or any size extending beyond the thyroid capsule to invade subcutaneous soft tissues, larynx, trachea, esophagus, or recurrent laryngeal nerve
T4b	Tumor invades prevertebral fascia or encases carotid artery or mediastinal vessels
	All anaplastic carcinomas are considered T4 tumors.
T4a	Intrathyroidal anaplastic carcinoma—surgically resectable
T4b	Extrathyroidal anaplastic carcinoma—surgically unresectable

REGIONAL LYMPH NODES (N)

Regional lymph nodes are the central compartment, lateral cervical, and upper mediastinal lymph nodes.

NX	Regional lymph nodes cannot be assessed
N0	No regional lymph node metastasis
N1	Regional lymph node metastasis
N1a	Metastasis to level VI (pretracheal, paratracheal, and prelaryngeal/Delphian lymph nodes)
N1b	Metastasis to unilateral, bilateral, or contralateral cervical or superior mediastinal lymph nodes

DISTANT METASTASIS (M)

MX	Distant metastasis cannot be assessed
M0	No distant metastasis
M1	Distant metastasis

STAGE GROUPING

Separate stage groupings are recommended for papillary or follicular, medullary, and anaplastic (undifferentiated) carcinoma.

PAPILLARY OR FOLLICULAR

Age younger than 45 years

I	Any T	Any N	M0
II	Any T	Any N	M1

PAPILLARY OR FOLLICULAR

Age 45 years and older

I	T1	N0	M0
II	T2	N0	M0
III	T3	N0	M0
	T1	N1a	M0
	T2	N1a	M0
	T3	N1a	M0
IVA	T4a	N0	M0
	T4a	N1a	M0
	T1	N1b	M0
	T2	N1b	M0
	T3	N1b	M0
	T4a	N1b	M0
IVB	T4b	Any N	M0
IVC	Any T	Any N	M1

MEDULLARY CARCINOMA

I	T1	N0	M0
II	T2	N0	M0
	T3	N0	M0
III	T1	N1a	M0
	T2	N1a	M0
	T3	N1a	M0
IVA	T4a	N0	M0
	T1	N1b	M0
	T2	N1b	M0
	T3	N1b	M0
	T4a	N1b	M0
IVB	T4b	Any N	M0
IVC	Any T	Any N	M1

ANAPLASTIC CARCINOMA

IVA	T4a	Any N	M0
IVB	T4b	Any N	M0
IVC	Any T	Any N	M1

With permission from American Joint Committee on Cancer (AJCC), Chicago, IL: *AJCC Cancer Staging Manual*, ed 6, New York, 2002, Springer-Verlag.

after a thyroidectomy may vary from 50 to 100 mCi. If a tracer dose of radioiodine reveals persistent thyroid activity after this procedure, a second ablation dose is needed. (See Box 31-2 for guidelines for patients receiving I-131.)

After all normal thyroid tissue is ablated, I-131 (for differentiated thyroid cancers) can be used to treat local and regional disease and distant metastasis. Some of the side effects are listed in Box 31-3.

 Two important thyroid hormones that regulate the metabolism of lipids, proteins, and carbohydrates are thyroxine and triiodothyronine. Thyroxine is also known as T_4 because it contains four atoms of iodine, and triiodothyronine is referred to as T_3 because it contains three atoms of iodine. What would you conclude occurs when radioactive I-131 is administered to a patient with incompletely resected thyroid cancer or distant metastases?

Box 31-2	Guidelines for Patients Receiving Iodine-131 (I-131)

PLANNING

Order I-131 at least 48 hours in advance. Schedule patient for hospital admission.

ROOM PREPARATION

Must cover the following with plastic bags: telephone receiver, telephone, food table, basin faucet handles, nurse call set. Disposable plastic-lined paper next to bed, commode, and shower. Two radiation waste containers in room for laundry and foods/paper. A safety shield must be placed at the head of bed.

PATIENT PREPARATION

Instruct to wear footies when ambulating. Instruct to keep outside door closed and bathroom door open at all times. Obtain vital signs and blood and urine samples before I-131 administration.

ADMINISTRATION

Patient must wear hospital gown with a "chuck" around neck and in lap. Personnel administering I-131 should wear gown, gloves, and mask. Vial containing I-131 should be vented in nuclear medicine hood to allow any volatile I-131 to escape just before administration if possible. During administration, the patient should sit on the side of the bed in front of the I-131, which is in a lead vial on a covered table. Open vial with T-bar, insert drinking straw, put small amount of water in vial (along straw so it does not splash). Patient takes I-131 through straw with additional water placed in lead vial to remove as much I-131 as possible. Swish and swallow several cups of water to rinse I-131 from oral cavity. Do not remove straw from vial; bend it over and carefully place lead cap on.

INITIAL SURVEY

Within 15 minutes, measure the radiation exposure rate at 1 m from the midline of the patient's abdomen in both anteroposterior (AP) and lateral directions. Calculate the average. Patient may be released when same readings show less than 30 mCi of I-131 or less than 5 mR/hour at 1 m, which is usually about 24 to 48 hours after 100 mCi was given but is variable. An inventory or survey form with initial activity and exposure rate, nursing instructions, and decontamination form should be posted on the room door. Do not collect urine unless lead container is available and there is a specific reason.

SAFETY

At <30 mCi I-131, patient can be discharged (or exposure rate of 5 mr/hr at 1 m).

Visiting is discouraged; limit to 0.5 hr/day per visitor, no children younger than 18 years or pregnant women. Visitors should wear gown, gloves, and mask and sit in designated chair across room. If they come close to patient, they should sit behind lead shield. Patients should wear hospital gowns, not personal clothing (I-131 in sweat, breath) and should leave bed only to go to bathroom or designated chair. They should drink copious amounts of water to speed release of unused radioactivity, shower frequently, flush toilet several times after each use. Males should urinate seated. There should be no personal items except those to be disposed of at discharge. After discharge, patients should practice good personal hygiene for 1 to 2 days. Do not hold children closely for 2 to 3 days.

Modified form Grigsby PW and Luk K: Thyroid. In Perez, CA, Brady LW, editors: *Principles and practice of radiation oncology*, Philadelphia, 1998, Lippincott-Raven.

Box 31-3	Side Effects of I-131

- Inflammation of salivary glands
- Nausea
- Vomiting
- Fatigue
- Bone marrow suppression (only after repeated administrations)

Thyroid Hormonal Therapy. Thyroid hormone suppression therapy is routinely given for differentiated thyroid cancers, although its effectiveness remains unproved. Differentiated thyroid carcinoma grows under the stimulation of TSH. Thus, through the lowering of TSH levels, tumor activity should be decreased.[12]

External Beam Radiation. Responsiveness to external beam radiation varies according to histologic type. Among differentiated thyroid cancers, papillary and mixed papillary-follicular carcinomas are more radiosensitive than follicular carcinomas. Medullary thyroid cancer is less radiosensitive than papillary carcinoma. In general, anaplastic carcinomas are not very responsive.

External beam radiation can be used alone or in conjunction with I-131 and surgery. Following are several indications for its use:
- Inoperable lesion
- Patient physically unfit for surgery
- Incomplete surgical removal of thyroid carcinoma
- Superior vena cava syndrome
- Skeletal metastases in which minimal accumulation of I-131 occurred
- Residual disease involving the trachea, larynx, or esophagus

In differentiated thyroid cancer for the curative treatment of inoperable localized disease or in patients with gross residual disease, tumor doses should be 6500 cGy in 7 weeks (180 to 200 cGy daily).[12] The radiation field should include the entire thyroid gland, neck, and superior mediastinum using three-dimensional treatment planning techniques, including intensity-modulated radiation therapy (IMRT). Treatment planning should include the use of CT or MRI to evaluate dose distribution because of the high degree of variability of the body contour involved. IMRT improves the dose to the planning tumor volume and significantly reduces the dose to the spinal cord[13] (Figure 31-3).

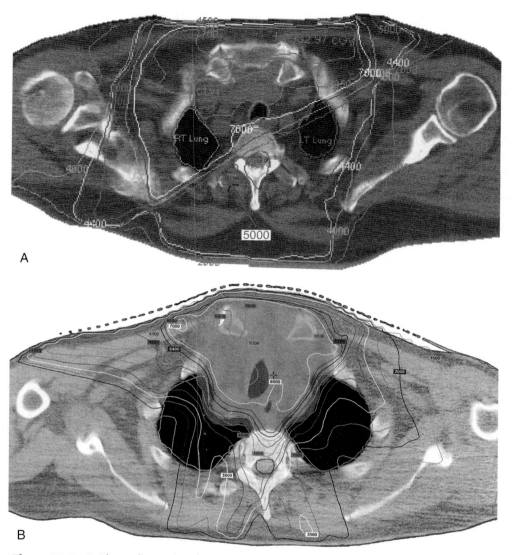

Figure 31-3. A, Three-dimensional treatment planning for a patient with locally recurrent and progressive papillary thyroid cancer. **B**, Intensity-modulated radiation therapy (IMRT) plan for a patient with thyroid cancer using 9 IMRT fields to a total dose of 60 Gy to the low neck and 54 Gy to the lateral upper neck and mediastinum. (From Hay I, Petersen IA: Thyroid cancer. In Gunderson LL, Tepper JE: *Clinical radiation oncology,* Philadelphia, 2007, Churchill Livingstone.)

For metastatic bone involvement, doses of 3500 to 4500 cGy in 3 to 5 weeks are recommended.[12]

For the simulation of a thyroid cancer patient, the head should be extended to avoid exposure to the oral cavity, with the use of an immobilization device for reproducibility. So that adequate tumor coverage is ensured, the tumor volume should be wired out, and a CT scan of the treated area should be obtained for treatment planning. Dose distribution must be considered through this area, especially the cord dose.

For medullary carcinoma that has not extended below the clavicles, radiation therapy can be considered. The recommended dose is 5500 to 6500 cGy in 6 to 7 weeks. The treatment fields should encompass the primary lesion, bilateral cervical node chains, and superior mediastinum.

For residual disease after a surgical resection, a dose of 5000 to 6000 cGy in 5 to 5½ weeks is recommended.

For bone metastasis, radiation therapy is warranted and often effective.

Anaplastic carcinoma is the least radiosensitive of all the thyroid cancers. Tumor control is seldom accomplished, even after a dose of 6000 cGy to the primary lesion, neck, and superior mediastinum.[12]

CASE I

Thyroidectomy

A 34-year-old woman underwent a right hemithyroidectomy about 10 to 12 years ago for benign disease. A needle aspiration biopsy 2 years earlier also showed benign disease, after exhibiting a cold nodule on a thyroid scan. Other than this asymptomatic nodule, the patient had no other symptoms.

Because of its persistence, this left-sided nodule was excised. Pathology showed follicular carcinoma with capsular invasion. No obvious vascular invasion was present. The patient was advised to have a complete lobectomy of the left thyroid gland or an I-131 ablation of the remaining thyroid gland. The patient elected surgical ablation.

Histopathologically, the resected lobe showed focal areas of residual follicular carcinoma with areas of infiltration into the stroma. A careful examination with the patient under anesthesia revealed no evidence of lymph node involvement. A thyroid scan after surgery showed no uptake in the neck. The patient was made hypothyroid for several weeks and then underwent an I-125 scan that showed residual uptake in the left neck, probably corresponding to the previous bed of the left thyroid lobe. No uptake was present on the right side, and there was no cervical lymph node involvement. No other activity was seen on the body scan. The patient was referred for I-131 thyroid treatment of the residual tumor in the left neck.

The acute risks of nausea and potential long-term risks of solid and hematologic cancer induction were discussed with the patient. The precautions to be taken by the patient and her family, with specific regard to exposure to the children, were carefully outlined. The advised procedures were based on the National Council on Radiation Protection (NCRP) recommendations for people ingesting radioactive material for therapeutic purposes.

With her consent, the patient was given 30 mCi of I-131 via a capsule. The dose was relatively low because the patient effectively had a total thyroidectomy and was young. After observation for 1 hour without any nausea or vomiting and with the exposure rate being measured and recorded, the patient was discharged. A 6-month repeat thyroid scan showed no residual uptake in the left neck.

PITUITARY TUMORS

Pituitary tumors are less aggressive than many central nervous system tumors, although pituitary neoplasms still pose problems as a result of local growth causing compressive and destructive effects and endocrine abnormalities caused by pituitary hormone dysfunction. The pituitary is composed of an anterior, a posterior, and an intermediate lobe. Tumors of the posterior and intermediate portion are virtually unknown. This section addresses tumors arising from the anterior pituitary gland, or adenohypophysis.

Epidemiology and Etiology

Pituitary tumors are most always benign, with malignancies accounting for fewer than 1% of all pituitary tumors.[2] These neoplasms represent 10% of all intracranial tumors, although small, asymptomatic adenomas appear in approximately 25% of all pituitary glands examined at autopsy. With the increasing quality of diagnostic studies, these pituitary neoplasms are now estimated to account for 30% of all intracranial tumors.[24]

Pituitary adenomas can be classified as functioning or nonfunctioning, as related to the hormones they produce. Hormone production often serves as a diagnostic and treatment-response marker. Pituitary adenomas categorized as functioning are as follows:

- **Prolactin (PRL)**-secreting tumors are the most common, representing 65% of all functioning pituitary adenomas. These neoplasms grow large and show little tendency toward local invasion.[24,29]
- **Growth hormone (GH)**-secreting tumors represent 15% of all pituitary adenomas and are more likely to be locally invasive.[29]

- **TSH**-secreting tumors represent fewer than 1% of all pituitary adenomas.
- **Adrenocorticotrophic hormone (ACTH)**-secreting tumors are more likely to be invasive compared with the other functioning adenomas.[24]

Chromophobe adenomas, which are nonfunctioning, are usually larger than functioning tumors and tend to exhibit invasive characteristics.[19] Patients usually have visual symptoms caused by the compression of the optic chiasm or a headache, rather than syndromes associated with the hypersecretion of pituitary hormones. These syndromes are listed in Table 31-2.

Pituitary tumors can occur at any age, from infancy to old age, although they are rarely found before puberty and are most commonly diagnosed in middle-aged and older patients.[29] No significant difference exists in the prevalence of adenomas among men and women.

Because of the rarity of malignant pituitary tumors, little knowledge of the etiology exists. Hardy et al.[11] have found an association between PRL-secreting tumors in women and the use of oral contraceptives. However, no clear etiologic link has been determined.

Prognostic Indicators

The prognosis depends on the type of adenoma and a combination of other factors, including the following: (1) the extent of the abnormalities (through mass effect or hormonal alterations), (2) the success of the treatment in normalizing endocrine activity and/or relieving pressure effects, (3) the morbidity caused by the treatment, and (4) the effectiveness of the treatments in preventing a recurrence.

Anatomy

The pituitary gland is 1.3 cm in diameter and located at the base of the brain. Attached to the hypothalamus by a stalklike structure (the **infundibulum**), the pituitary gland lies in the sella turcica of the sphenoid bone. The gland is divided structurally and functionally into an anterior lobe (**adenohypophysis**), a posterior lobe (**neurohypophysis**), and an intermediate lobe. The blood supply to the adenohypophysis is from several superior hypophyseal arteries, and the blood supply to the neurohypophysis is from the inferior hypophyseal arteries.[26] The pituitary gland is close to critical structures of the central nervous system, such as the optic chiasm (superiorly). See Figure 31-4 for the anatomic relationships. Related to topographic anatomy, the pituitary gland is

Table 31-2	Clinical Effects of Excess Secretion of Pituitary Hormones	
Hormones	**Clinical Effects**	
ACTH	Cushing's disease	
GH	Giantism, acromegaly	
Prolactin	Females: infertility	
	Males: impotence, decreased libido	
TSH	Hyperthyroidism	

ACTH, Adrenocorticotrophic hormone; *GH,* growth hormone; *TSH,* thyroid-stimulating hormone.

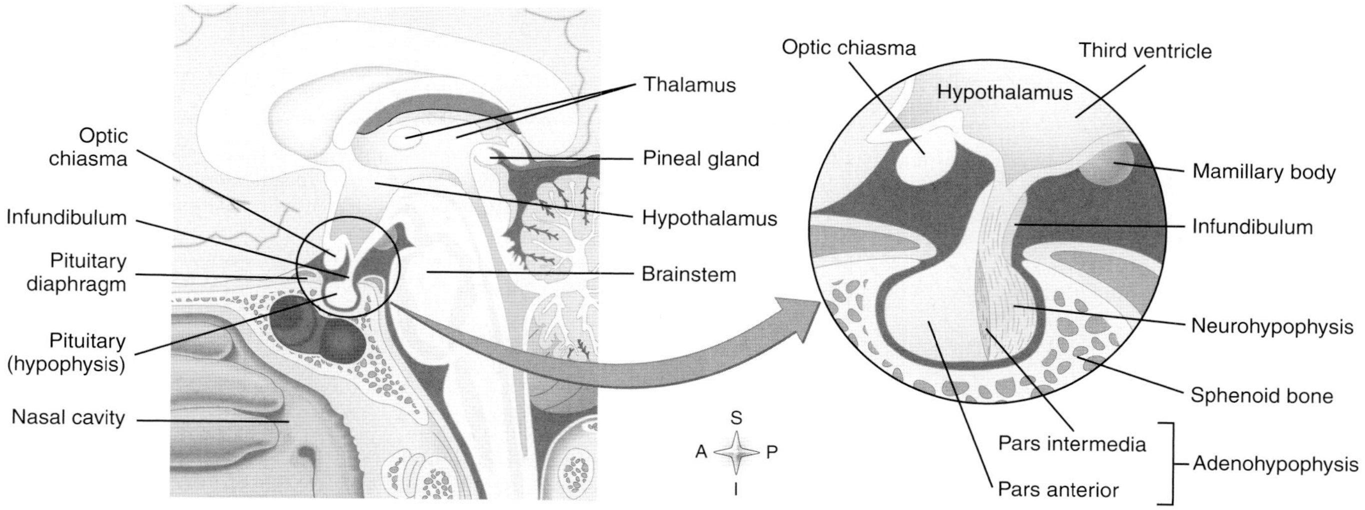

Figure 31-4. The pituitary gland is located within the sella turcica of the skull's sphenoid bone. Note the location of the optic chiasm, superior to the pituitary gland. (From Thibodeau GA, Patton KT: *Anatomy and physiology*, ed 6, St. Louis, 2007, Mosby.)

positioned behind the temporomandibular joint (TMJ) and mid-plane behind the nasal bone (i.e., between the eyes).

Physiology

Derived from the endoderm, the adenohypophysis forms the glandular part of the pituitary. The glandular cells (acidophils and basophils) are responsible for the secretion of seven hormones.

Acidophils secrete the following:

- **GH**—controls body growth
- **PRL**—initiates milk production

Basophils secrete the following:

- **TSH**—controls the thyroid gland
- **Follicle-stimulating hormone (FSH)** —stimulates egg and sperm production
- **Luteinizing hormone (LH)** —stimulates other sexual and reproductive activity
- **Melanocyte-stimulating hormone (MSH)** —relates to skin pigmentation
- **ACTH**—influences the action of the adrenal cortex

The release of these hormones is stimulated or inhibited by the chemical secretions from the hypothalamus, which are called regulatory, or releasing, factors. The posterior lobe or neurohypophysis secretes oxytocin (which causes smooth muscle contractions) and antidiuretic hormone (ADH) or vasopressin, which regulates free water resorption in the kidneys.[26]

> *Patients who have had their pituitary gland removed by surgery (hypophysectomy) or treated by high-dose radiation therapy must be put on hormone replacement for the rest of their lives. Specific hormone deficiencies from the anterior and posterior pituitary gland would include thyroid, adrenal cortical, gonadotropins, prolactin, and antidiuretic and growth hormones.*

Clinical Presentation

Hormonal Effects. Functioning pituitary tumors retain hormone-producing capabilities, although they are unresponsive to regulatory mechanisms and produce hormones regardless of metabolic needs.[24] Hypersecretion of pituitary hormones results in varied clinical presentations, depending on the type of secreting tumor. PRL-secreting tumors produce clinical symptoms such as amenorrhea and galactorrhea, which are detected easier in premenopausal versus postmenopausal women. The hypersecretion of GH produces clinical symptoms such as weight gain; thickening of the bones and soft tissues of the hands, feet and cheeks; and overgrowth of the jaw and tongue. Patients are hypertensive and commonly complain of headaches and lassitude. This clinical syndrome is referred to as acromegaly, if hypersecretion occurs after puberty, and giantism, if it happens before puberty.[28] See Table 31-2 for more hypersecreting syndromes.

In some instances, local compressive effects of the tumor in the pituitary itself may cause deficient production of hormones normally synthesized in the gland. Hormones that have target organs (such as ACTH [adrenals], TSH [thyroid], and FSH [ovaries and testes]) can cause an array of abnormalities that result from a loss of pituitary hormonal action.[7] These clinical manifestations are listed in Table 31-3.

Pressure Effects. The most common manifestation of an expanding pituitary lesion is headache, which occurs in 20% of all patients.[7,24] Local pressure on the lining of the sphenoid sinus and traction on the diaphragma sellae produce these headaches.

Visual acuity and field defects are other clinical manifestations and signify extension beyond the sella. Suprasellar extension of these tumors causes pressure effects on the inferior aspect of the optic chiasm, resulting in visual symptomatology, which is usually progressive. The presentation may be altered

Table 31-3	Clinical Manifestations of Pituitary Hormones	
Hormone	**Target Tissue**	**Clinical Effects**
ACTH	Adrenal cortex	Postural hypotension; impaired tolerance of stress (trauma, surgery); can lead to shock
Prolactin	Gonads	Gonadal atrophy; loss of FSH reproductive function; LH decreased gonadal hormones
TSH	Thyroid	Hypothyroidism (fatigue, slow or slurred speech, bradycardia, decreased reflexes, cold intolerance)
GH	Bones, muscles, organs	Decreased bone growth; lethargy; hypoglycemia

Modified from Donehower MG: Endocrine cancers. In Baird SB, McCorkle R, Grant M, editors: *Cancer nursing: a comprehensive textbook,* Philadelphia, 1991, Saunders.
ACTH, Adrenocorticotrophic hormone; *FSH,* follicle-stimulating hormone; *LH,* luteinizing hormone; *TSH,* thyroid-stimulating hormone; *GH,* growth hormone.

visual acuity, but more commonly, visual field defects are observed. The most common field defect is **bitemporal hemianopsia** (loss of peripheral vision bilaterally). If pressure effects on the optic chiasm persist for significant periods, the result can be permanent visual field defects or blindness. In rare instances, these tumors can extend laterally into the cavernous sinuses (see Figure 31-4) and cause characteristic cranial nerve deficits.

Detection and Diagnosis

Patients with functional tumors have characteristic endocrine abnormalities that are associated with the hypersecretion of hormones. The clinical syndromes from Table 31-2 prompt medical attention. Laboratory testing, which can directly measure hormone levels, can confirm pituitary hormone dysfunction and strongly suggest the diagnosis. The expanding growth of nonfunctioning tumors into the suprasellar area causes pressure symptoms such as headache, visual disturbances, and impairment of various cranial nerves.[29] These symptoms often bring the patient to medical attention and prompt diagnostic studies.

The principal imaging study for the pituitary gland is CT or MRI. MRI is superior to CT in delineating the extent of the tumor process relative to normal critical structures such as the optic chiasm, vascular structures, cranial nerves, and cavernous sinuses just lateral to the pituitary gland (see Figure 31-4). MRI provides detailed anatomic information in transverse, sagittal, and coronal projections. This information is invaluable to the neurosurgeon and radiation oncologist in determining a therapeutic approach.

Pathology

Pituitary tumors are sinusoidal, papillary, or diffuse.[19] Although pituitary tumors appear encapsulated, no true capsule exists. Neoplasms are formed of tightly packed cells that remain separate from normal tissue without a membrane.

Neoplasms are classified according to size. **Microadenomas** are less than 1.0 cm, and **macroadenomas** are greater than 1.0 cm.[19,29] This classification is important because predictions of the prognosis can be made from the tumor size. Larger adenomas are surgically more difficult to remove with complete resections, and recurrence is more common in this group.

Pituitary tumors can also be classified according to their growth patterns (by expansion or invasion) and are separated into intrahypophyseal, intrasellar, diffuse, and invasive adenomas. Intrahypophyseal tumors stay in the pituitary gland, whereas intrasellar lesions grow within the confines of the sella. Diffuse adenomas usually fill the entire sella and can erode its wall. Invasive neoplasms have a more rapid growth rate and tend to erode outside the sella to invade neighboring tissues such as the posterior pituitary gland, sphenoid bone, and cavernous sinus. These neoplasms may even penetrate into the brain and third ventricle. Invasive adenomas are classified as malignant adenomas when metastases are present. Malignant adenomas metastasize via cerebrospinal fluid (CSF) or vascular pathways. This is extremely rare.

Staging

Because most tumors are benign, no true staging exists. However, pituitary tumors have been classified into four grades according to the extent of expansion or erosion of the sella. This system also types tumors into four categories based on suprasellar extension (Box 31-4).

Treatment Techniques

The primary goal of treatment is to normalize pituitary hormonal function or relieve local compressive and/or destructive effects of the tumor. In some instances, both factors must be ameliorated. This can be accomplished surgically, therapeutically with radiation, medically, or with a combination of these modalities. An obvious secondary goal is to prevent recurrence.

Box 31-4	Hardy and Vezina's Pituitary Tumor Classification Grade I—Sella of Normal Size but with Asymmetry

Grade II—Enlarged sella, but with an intact floor
Grade III—Localized erosion or destruction of the sella floor
Grade IV—Diffusely eroded floor
Type A—Tumor bulges into the chiasmatic cistern
Type B—Tumor reaches the floor of the third ventricle
Type C—More voluminous tumor, with extension into the third ventricle up to the foramen of Monro
Type D—Extension into temporal or frontal fossa

Courtesy of Jules Hardy, MD, and Jean L. Vézina, MD.

Surgery. Surgery plays a significant role in the management of pituitary tumors. Before 1970, craniotomies were performed with an associated operative mortality rate of 2% to 25%. Currently, the less invasive transsphenoidal approach is widely used, decreasing the mortality rate to 0.9%. Complications of this surgery are CSF leakage, infection (meningitis), and visual pathway defects, with a combined morbidity rate of about 14%.[29] (See Figure 31-5 for a depiction of the transsphenoidal approach.) In summary, the two main surgical approaches are the transfrontal approach (transfrontal craniotomy) and the transsphenoidal approach, which allows direct access to the pituitary gland without disturbance of the central nervous system structures.

Transsphenoidal surgery is reported to permanently control 70% to 90% of small adenomas. Results with larger adenomas are less satisfactory, although the debulking of large tumors decompresses vital structures.[24] Transsphenoidal surgery results in the improvement of visual field defects in 80% of patients. Only 4% of patients experience worsening of visual field defects with transphenoidal surgery. Results are the same with a craniotomy, with a higher percentage of visual impairment related to the surgical procedure.[27,29]

Characteristic hormonal abnormalities show favorable responses after surgery. If surgical intervention of functioning adenomas is successful, the response in terms of the normalization of hormone levels is almost immediate. Symptomatic relief is seen in 94% of patients with acromegaly, although the recurrence rate after 10 years is 8% to 10%. Results are generally satisfactory for patients with Cushing's syndrome (ACTH-producing adenomas). Although results vary, remission occurs in 80% to 86% of patients, with a recurrence rate over 10 years of 8% to 10%.[29] Similar, excellent results are achieved with PRL-secreting adenomas.

Radiation Therapy. Surgery is often only one part of the overall management for a pituitary adenoma. Although the role of postoperative radiation therapy is controversial, it has been shown in various series to reduce recurrence rates compared with surgery alone. Radiation therapy alone has also been used to control pituitary tumors in patients who refused surgery or those who were medically unfit.

Postoperative radiation therapy is used as an adjunctive modality in the following circumstances:

- An incompletely resected invasive tumor
- Tumors demonstrating suprasellar extension with an associated visual field defect
- Large tumors in which the risk of attempted removal is relatively high
- Persistent hormonal elevation after surgery

Radiation Therapy Techniques. With any treatment technique, a precise target volume must be defined through the use of MRI, CT, surgical, and clinical findings. The treatment volume should be slightly larger than the target volume, allowing for day-to-day variations in the treatment setup. The head must be immobilized to ensure reproducibility and accuracy. The patient's chin is usually tucked to avoid radiation exposure to the eyes. Lead markers on the outer canthus of each eye during simulation documents the eye position with respect to the radiation beam. The use of three tattoos (two lateral and one midline) aids in repositioning. Verification portals should be taken routinely to document the field location. See Figures 31-6 and 31-7 for examples of simulation and portal film.

With high-energy megavoltage linear accelerators (i.e., 10 to 18 MeV) and multiple-field treatment approaches, the dose-volume distribution to the pituitary gland has been greatly enhanced. This results in a more precise dose delivered to the tumor volume, a reduction in the dose to normal central nervous system structures, increased tumor-control probability, and decreased treatment-related morbidity.

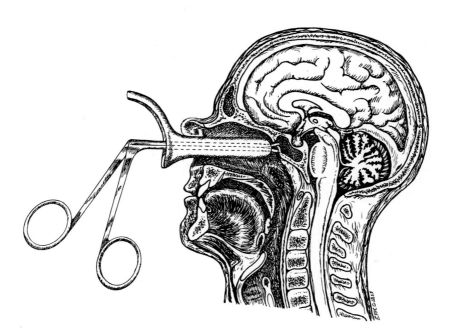

Figure 31-5. Anatomic root for a transsphenoidal hypophysectomy.

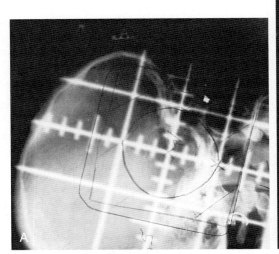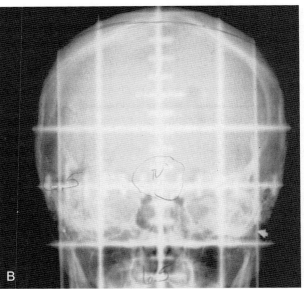

Figure 31-6. A, Lateral simulation film illustrating the portal used for external irradiation of pituitary adenoma. **B,** Anteroposterior (AP) simulation film.

The optimization of dose-volume distribution is illustrated in various treatment plans shown in Figures 31-8, 31-9, and 31-10. These treatment plans show an obvious advantage of high-energy photons and multifield or rotational arrangements to accomplish the goal of optimizing the dose to the target tissue while minimizing the dose to nontarget, normal tissue. This is of paramount importance in the pituitary gland because of the critical normal tissue surrounding it. Image-guided radiation therapy (IGRT) has useful in targeting daily treatments, especially with numerous organs at risk in the head and neck area, such as the parotid glands, lens of the eye, optic nerves and optic chiasma.

Other strategies not widely available are used to treat pituitary adenomas. These strategies include proton beam therapy and stereotactic radiosurgery (see Chapter 16).

Proton Beam Therapy. Because of the proton beam's physical characteristics (i.e., a **Bragg peak** with a rapid dose fall-off at depth), the dose can be precisely delivered within millimeters of a defined target directly related to the beam's energy. This is a particularly attractive feature for treatment near critical structures such as the optic chiasm and the temporal lobe, areas in which an excessive radiation dose can produce devastating clinical consequences.

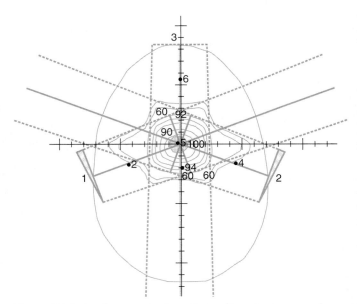

Figure 31-8. Isodose curves for a 2-cm-diameter tumor volume, with the use of a 15-MV linear accelerator and three portal arrangement: an open vertex and two 110-degree posterior oblique, 30-degree wedge fields.

Figure 31-7. Lateral verification film (portal image) on a therapy machine.

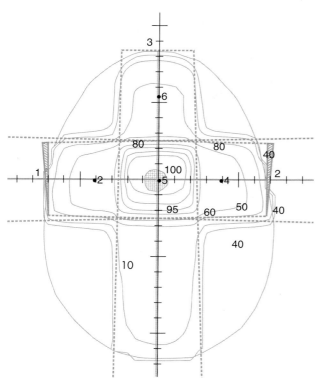

Figure 31-9. Isodose curves for a 2-cm-diameter tumor volume, with the use of a 15-MV linear accelerator and three portal arrangement: open vertex and two lateral 15-degree wedge fields.

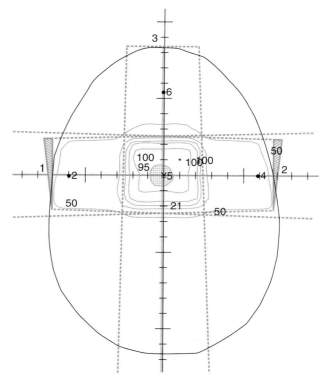

Figure 31-10. Isodose curves for a 2-cm-diameter tumor volume, with the use of a 6-MV linear accelerator and three portal arrangement: open vertex and two lateral 30-degree wedge fields.

 Protons are a valuable tool for clinical use for the following reasons: (1) they are precision controlled; (2) scattering is minimal compared with that from x-rays, neutrons, and cobalt radiation; (3) they have a characteristic distribution of dose with depth; and (4) most of their energy is deposited near the end of their range, where the dose peaks to a high value and then drops rapidly to zero. This sudden change in dose distribution with depth is called the Bragg peak. More information about proton therapy in the United States can be found at:

- *http://www.mdanderson.org/care_centers/radiationonco/ptc/*
- *http://www.massgeneral.org/cancer/about/providers/radiation/proton/whatis.asp*
- *http://www.floridaproton.org/*

Stereotactic Radiosurgery. Stereotactic radiosurgery uses a high-energy photon beam with multiple ports of entry convergent on the target tissue. This is typically done as a single, large fraction of treatment with the patient immobilized in a stereotactic head frame. After being rigidly positioned, the patient undergoes a planning CT scan to define the tumor volume and determine the multiports of entry. With the patient immobilized the entire time, this procedure takes several hours and requires several images on the treatment unit to ensure accuracy.

This technique may not be an optimal approach to this particular disease because pituitary neoplasms are benign and high single-fraction treatment can produce significant normal-tissue morbidity if an uncertainty exists regarding the target volume treated. With improved technology, stereotactic radiation may be delivered as fractionated treatment, making it more desirable in this circumstance.

Results of Treatment

The treatment of pituitary adenomas shows results that are favorable. Surgery for microadenomas is generally curative. Series with radiation therapy alone have demonstrated excellent disease-free survival rates of up to 85% at 5 and 10 years. A direct comparison between the results of different treatment approaches is difficult to make because of the various criteria used to select the optimal treatment, as previously described. However, surgery and radiation therapy alone or in combination clearly produce excellent results.

CASE II

Pituitary Macroadenoma

A 32-year-old woman came to the emergency department with a history of headaches. During examination, the patient demonstrated features of acromegaly. She had a 2-year history of progressively enlarging hands and feet and pain in the joints of the upper extremities. She noted that her shoe size had increased from an 8 to a 10 over this period. She complained of amenorrhea for approximately the past year but denied any visual symptoms.

As part of the initial workup, brain MRI scan showed findings consistent with a pituitary macroadenoma measuring about 1.5 cm in diameter and extending into the suprasellar cistern anterior to the optic chiasm. A slight elevation of the optic chiasm was present. The cavernous sinuses appeared free of tumor extension. The floor of the sella was eroded, and the tumor appeared to extend partially into the sphenoid sinus. The GH was 150 ng/ml (normal range, 1 to 10 ng/ml), and a transsphenoidal hypophysectomy was advised.

After surgery, the patient had a remarkable reduction in the GH level and a reversal of some of the clinical findings of acromegaly. However, with the persistent elevation of GH and radiographic (erosion of sella) and surgical findings (involving the sphenoid sinus), the patient was at an extremely high risk for recurrence of her adenoma. A course of radiation therapy directed at the pituitary fossa, sphenoid sinus, and cavernous sinus region was recommended to improve the probability of local control and normalization of the GH level.

In a supine, immobilized position, the patient was treated via a three-field technique through the use of 6-cm-diameter circular fields with 10-MV photons. Right and left lateral opposed fields in combination with a superior vertex field angled 15 degrees off the horizontal were used. CT and MRI scans were performed through the treatment volume to aid in the treatment planning. This three-field arrangement was treated at 180 cGy/fraction. Equal weighting was provided from each field for 25 treatment fractions to accomplish 4500 cGy to the pituitary fossa, which included the sphenoid sinus.

The patient tolerated the therapy well but still complained of headaches and fatigue at the completion of the therapy. About 3 months after the external beam radiation therapy, the patient continued to show regression of her acral changes. This regression was characterized by thinning facial characteristics, smaller hands, and smaller feet. An MRI scan at that time showed no evidence of a tumor. During subsequent follow-up visits, the patient continued

to do well, with decreasing GH levels. Approximately 2 years after the therapy, the patient's GH level was 3.0 ng/ml.

ADRENAL CORTEX TUMORS

Neoplasms of the adrenal glands are rare, with malignant tumors accounting for only 0.04% of all cancers.[4] Tumors arising in the adrenal glands are classified according to the portion of the gland from which they arise. This includes tumors arising from the **cortex** (outer portion of the gland) and those from the **medulla** (inner portion of the gland). The cortex and the medulla, which make up the adrenal gland (Figure 31-11), have distinct histologic features and physiologic functions. In general, the cortex manufactures steroid hormones that are critical in metabolic regulation, and the medulla produces epinephrine (Adrenalin) under the regulation of the autonomic nervous system.

Epidemiology and Etiology

Adrenocortical tumors are extremely rare, with only 150 to 300 instances in the United states per year (of which approximately 10% are malignant).[31] Men and women are affected equally, although hyperfunctioning malignancies are more common in women. Tumors arise more commonly in the left gland than the right. Although the median age is 50 years, the ages in two series ranged from 1 to 80 years.[4,6]

Adrenal adenomas are benign neoplasms that can be found in 2% of all adults, according to an autopsy series.[26] These adenomas are rarely associated with serious medical illness.

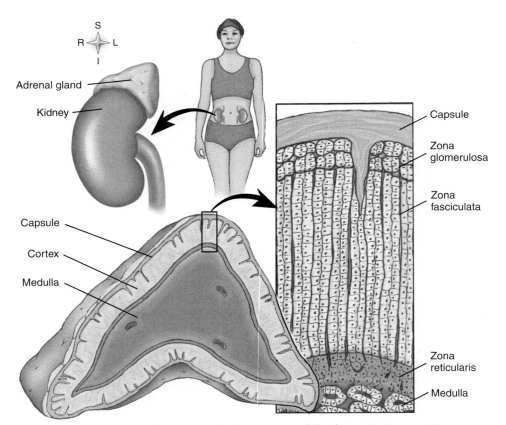

Figure 31-11. Anatomy of the adrenal gland. (From Thibodeau GA, Patton KT: *Anatomy and physiology*, ed 6, St. Louis, 2007, Mosby.)

However, in some circumstances these can cause hypersecretion of normally produced steroid hormones, giving rise to various clinical syndromes. Many adrenal masses represent metastatic disease typically from lung cancer.

Prognostic Indicators

The stage of the disease at the time of diagnosis closely parallels survival rates. Most patients have advanced disease at the time of presentation. Only 30% of patients have a tumor confined to the adrenal gland.[4]

The ability of the surgeon to achieve curative resection is another prognostic factor because surgery is the only modality that has demonstrated a significant effect on survival rates. All patients should have close postoperative surveillance for the detection of abdominal and distant metastases while they are still resectable.

A young age at the time of diagnosis is a favorable prognostic factor.

Anatomy

The adrenal glands are paired organs located on the superior pole of the kidneys. These glands have a yellow cortex and dark brown medulla. They derive their blood supply from the adrenal branches of the inferior phrenic artery, aorta, and renal artery.[4] The lymphatic drainage is to the paraaortic nodes. The normal adrenal gland weighs approximately 20 g.

Physiology

The adrenal cortex produces steroid hormones, including glucocorticoids, mineralocorticoids, and sex hormones, which are responsible for metabolic regulation. These hormones include cortisol, aldosterone, estrogen, and androgen. The cells of the adrenal cortex that manufacture these hormones are regulated by the ongoing stresses and needs of an individual's metabolism. The normal functioning adrenal cortex can respond instantaneously to meet metabolic demands and maintain homeostasis.

Clinical Presentation

Because of the location of adrenal cortex tumors in the abdomen and the inaccessibility for physical examination, many patients develop symptoms of pain from advanced cancer. Alternatively, clinical manifestations of symptoms related to excess hormone production may prompt medical attention. Well-described syndromes are associated with the excessive production of hormones from the adrenal cortex. These are listed in Table 31-4.

In a series of 47 patients with adrenocortical carcinoma reported by Cohn et al.,[5] symptoms relating to a nonfunctioning tumor included an abdominal mass in 77% of the patients, weight loss in 46%, fever in 15%, and distant metastases in 15%. Many patients have more than one symptom at the time of diagnosis. In the same series, symptoms relating to functional tumors included Cushing's syndrome in 26% of the patients, mixed Cushing's syndrome and virilization in 24%, virilization in 15%, and feminization in 9%.

Detection and Diagnosis

Patients may exhibit functioning or nonfunctioning tumors. With functioning tumors, the clinical syndromes from Table 31-4 often lead to the diagnosis and can be easily confirmed with laboratory testing. In nonfunctioning tumors, pain is the presenting symptom and is often associated with locally advanced disease.

The principal imaging study for the adrenal gland is CT or MRI. These scans often suggest the diagnosis of an adrenal neoplasm and demonstrate the local and regional extent of the disease. (See Figure 31-12 for an abdominal CT scan of a suspected adrenal neoplasm.) A definite tissue diagnosis requires a needle biopsy under CT guidance.

Pathology

Adrenocortical tumors are usually large, single, rounded masses of yellow-orange adrenocortical tissue. Because they are usually large at the time of diagnosis, they have considerable hemorrhage, necrosis, and calcification.[4]

In a series of 38 patients conducted by Karakousis et al.,[13] tumors were graded according to the cells' resemblance to normal adrenal cortical cells. Well-differentiated (grade I) tumors were distinguished from adenomas by the presence of capsular and vascular invasion and abnormal mitoses. The survival rate for patients with grade I or II tumors is significantly greater than that for patients with grade III tumors.

Table 31-4	Clinical Manifestations of Adrenocortical Hormone Excess	

Hormone	Syndrome	Clinical Manifestations
Aldosterone	Conn's syndrome (aldosteronism)	Hypernatremia, hypokalemia, hypertension, neuromuscular weakness and paresthesias, electrocardiographic and renal function abnormalities
Cortisol (ACTH)	Cushing's syndrome	Acid-base imbalance, hypertension, obesity, osteoporosis, hyperglycemia, psychoses, excessive bruising, renal calculi
Sex hormones (testosterone, estrogen, and progesterone)	Virilization (in women)	Male pattern baldness, hirsutism, deepening voice, breast atrophy, decreased libido, oligomenorrhea
	Feminization (in men)	Gynecomastia, breast tenderness, testicular atrophy, decreased libido

From Donehower MG: Endocrine cancers. In Baird SB, McCorkle R, Grant M, editors: *Cancer nursing: a comprehensive textbook*, Philadelphia, 1991, Saunders.
ACTH, Adrenocorticotrophic hormone.

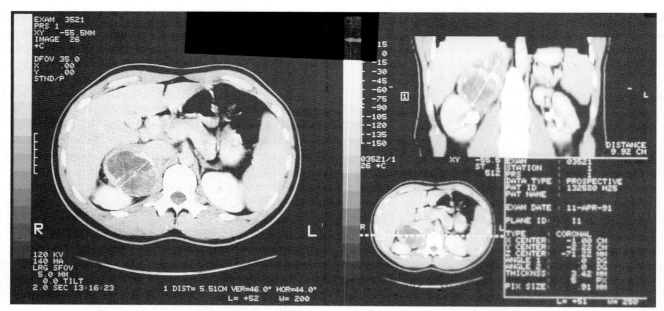

Figure 31-12. An abdominal computed tomography (CT) scan of a suspected adrenal neoplasm.

Staging

No true staging system exists because so few cases are reported. However, an example of a conventional staging system for adrenocortical carcinoma is presented in Box 31-5. This system stages according to the size of the tumor and the extent to which it has advanced locally or distantly.

Box 31-5	Staging System for Adrenocortical Carcinoma

T = EXTENT OF THE PRIMARY TUMOR
1 = <5 cm and confined to the adrenal gland
2 = >5 cm but <10 cm or adherence to the kidney
3 = >10 cm or invasion of surrounding structures including the renal vein

M = PRESENCE AND TYPE OF METASTASES
0 = No demonstrable metastases
1 = Regional lymphatics
2 = Distant metastases, (e.g., liver, lung, bone)

R = TISSUE REMAINING AFTER RESECTION
0 = Tumor completely excised
1 = Tumor entered at operation
2 = Tumor tissue remaining after resection

D = DEGREE OF HISTOLOGIC DIFFERENTIATION
1 = Differentiated, no capsular or vascular invasion
2 = Moderately undifferentiated, capsular or vascular invasion
3 = Anaplastic, capsular and vascular invasion
Stage 1 = ≤3 (e.g., T1 M0 R0 D1)
Stage 2 = 4 or 5 (e.g., T2 M0 R1 D2)
Stage 3 = 6 or 7 (e.g., T3 M1 R1 D2)
Stage 4 = ≥8 (e.g., T3 M2 R2 D3)

Modified from Bradley EL: Primary and adjunctive therapy in carcinoma of the adrenal cortex, *Surg Gynecol Obstet* 141:507, 1995.

Routes of Spread

Adrenocortical carcinomas can grow locally into surrounding tissues. However, these carcinomas may also spread to regional paraaortic nodes, lung, liver, and brain.[1,4]

Local invasion or distant metastases are often present at the time of diagnosis. Tumors on the right side involve the kidney, liver, and vena cava (often by direct extension of the tumor). Tumors on the left side often involve the kidney, pancreas, and diaphragm.

Treatment Techniques

Surgery is the treatment of choice. A complete resection is not always feasible because of invasion to adjacent vital structures such as the spleen, kidney, and parts of the pancreas. Although the resection of adrenal carcinomas is not always for cure, debulking results in decreased pain. Radiation therapy has a limited role, but it may be used as an adjunct to surgery to improve local control and for the palliative treatment of metastatic disease.

The use of systemic treatment in the management of adrenocortical cancer has been disappointing. Most reported series have evaluated patients with locally advanced or metastatic disease. Mitotane is an adrenolytic drug that has demonstrated limited but favorable responses. About a 40% response rate is observed in patients with advanced disease. Some studies have suggested that patients who receive mitotane as adjuvant treatment after surgical resection (i.e., without obvious evidence of metastatic disease) may realize significantly improved disease-free survival.[25] Whether this confers a true overall survival benefit or a delay in the development of metastatic disease is not clear.

Because of the rarity of this malignancy, cytotoxic chemotherapy has not been widely studied. However, some evidence suggests that agents having activity alone or in combination against adrenocortical carcinoma include doxorubicin

(Adriamycin), cisplatin, etoposide (VP-16), cyclophosphamide (Cytoxan), and 5-fluorouracil (5-FU). The role of these agents in an adjuvant setting is far from clear.[10]

ADRENAL MEDULLA TUMORS

Epidemiology and Etiology

Approximately 400 medullary tumors are diagnosed in the United States per year. These are called pheochromocytomas, and only 10% of these have cytologic features that are malignant.[31] The peak incidence of this tumor is in the fifth decade of life, but it can be seen at any age. These tumors may be bilateral in various familial syndromes and can be associated with MEN syndromes. In addition, this type of tumor has been observed in patients with von Recklinghausen's disease (type I neurofibromatosis).

Anatomy

The anatomy of adrenal medulla tumors is discussed in the section on adrenal cortex tumors.

Clinical Presentation

A well-recognized clinical syndrome is associated with pheochromocytomas. The symptoms include hypertension, severe headache, nervousness, palpitations, excessive perspiration, angina, blurred vision, and abdominal and chest pain. These are mediated by the excessive production of epinephrine associated with these tumors. Symptoms vary little among benign and malignant tumors and are often sporadic.[4]

Detection and Diagnosis

These tumors are suspected based on the clinical presentation. CT or MRI scans are used to assess the extent of disease. Laboratory testing, which measures urinary or plasma catecholamines (vanillylmandelic acid [VMA] and precursors of epinephrine), can help confirm the diagnosis. A needle biopsy can establish a tissue diagnosis but may not be necessary if the clinical, radiographic, and laboratory findings support the diagnosis.

Pathology and Staging

Adrenal medulla tumors are well-delineated, circumscribed tumors ranging from dark red, through gelatinous pink, to gray-brown or gray. The tumor size varies from 1 cm to 30 cm, with areas of hemorrhage and necrosis.[20]

Routes of Spread

The metastatic pattern of malignant pheochromocytomas is similar to that of adrenocortical carcinoma. These tumors can grow locally into surrounding tissues and may also spread to regional lymph nodes, lung, liver, and brain.[1,4]

Treatment Techniques

Surgery is the treatment of choice for these tumors. Malignant tumors may grow extensively into surrounding structures, making a complete resection impossible. Persistent elevation of blood pressure indicates residual tumor or metastatic disease.[20]

The surgical resection of benign pheochromocytomas results in a normal life expectancy, and patients with malignant pheochromocytomas can be maintained for many years. Patients with extraadrenal malignancy have a poorer prognosis.

Results of Treatment

Adrenocortical Carcinoma. The outcome for patients treated with this disease is poor. The 5-year survival rates for all stages range between 25% and 40%. The stage at diagnosis and ability to resect the disease have a significant effect on its outcome. Because most patients (65% to 75%) have advanced-stage disease, the ability to accomplish a curative resection is minimized and survival rates decrease.[5]

Adrenal Medulla-Pheochromocytoma. Because the majority of these tumors are benign and the surgical resection is often complete, results of treatment are excellent. Most patients live a normal life span.

CASE III

Adrenocortical Carcinoma

A 26-year-old man was in a normal state of health until approximately 2 months before presentation, at which time he experienced right flank pain and sought medical attention. His past medical history was unremarkable, except that 7 years before, he had sustained a blunt, right-sided chest wall and flank injury. A physical examination demonstrated no evidence of cushingoid changes, hyperaldosteronism, or virilism (signs of a functioning tumor). His blood pressure was normal, and he denied having flushing, sweats, palpitations, and diarrhea.

As part of the initial workup, an intravenous pyelogram (IVP) showed partially calcified mass above the right kidney that was pushing the kidney inferiorly and posteriorly. A CT scan was performed and showed a 10-cm mass that appeared to be involving the right adrenal gland with obvious extrinsic compression of the right kidney. No direct invasion of the inferior vena cava was evident. Obvious hypodense regions and calcified areas were present in this tumor mass. Neither adenopathy nor liver abnormalities were obvious. For a determination of the vascular supply of the tumor before surgery, an arteriogram was performed. It showed a single vessel with a trifurcate artery coming off the aorta serving this tumor mass. The venous phase of the arteriogram showed no gross invasion of the vena cava. Preoperative urinary VMAs and metanephrines (laboratory testing done to rule out pheochromocytoma) values were normal. A preoperative chest x-ray examination was unremarkable.

At the time of surgery, a rock-hard mass was encountered in the upper quadrant above the kidney overlying the entire right renal vein and inferior vena cava. This mass appeared to be involved with peritumoral inflammation and fibrosis. This was an extremely arduous resection secondary to the fibrous adherence to the local structures. A clear cleavage plane was established between the kidney and mass. However, dense adherence was encountered over the inferior vena cava, requiring a resection of a portion of the cava to remove the mass. A lymph node overlying the right renal vein was encountered and surgically resected. At the completion of the procedure, induration that spread in a sheetlike manner was behind the cava. The consensus was that additional resection was not possible.

The patient had an uneventful surgical recovery. Histologically, this proved to be a high-grade adrenocortical carcinoma. Because of concern for a residual tumor overlying the vena cava and in the retroperitoneal space behind the cava, the patient was sent for a radiation oncology consultation.

The radiation oncologist thought that, because there was gross residual disease, the patient was indeed at risk for local regional recurrence and that postoperative external beam treatment was indicated to secure the optimal probability of local control.

The patient was treated in the supine position with combined proton beam and megavoltage (10-MV photon) radiation therapy. The patient received a total dose of 6000 cGy. The photon portion of the treatment included the delivery of 3280 cGy via a parallel-opposed AP/PA pair of using multileaf collimator (MLC)-shaped fields, weighted with a ratio of 1:1. Subsequently, 720 cGy in four fractions were given via a parallel-opposed lateral wedge pair of MLC-shaped fields, weighted with a ratio of 2R:1L. The patient then received 2000 cGy from proton beam therapy. The characteristic properties of the proton beam allow a maximum target dose while limiting radiation exposure to surrounding structures. A high-resolution, contrast-enhanced CT scan with the patient in the treatment position was performed to delineate the primary target volume and neighboring critical dose-limiting structures. The dose to the spinal cord was 4600 cGy; the cauda equina received 4500 cGy, 30% of the right kidney received less than 4000 cGy, and the left kidney received less than 5 Gy.

Other than mild fatigue and mild intermittent nausea, the patient tolerated the treatment well. The patient was sent to a medical oncologist to discuss an adjuvant chemotherapy program. The patient received four cycles of adjuvant chemotherapy with cisplatin and doxorubicin over a 4-month period. Other than minimal weight loss and fatigue, the patient tolerated this treatment well.

Approximately 30 months have passed since the completion of the postoperative external beam radiation therapy. Since that time the patient has undergone a complete radiographic staging with a CT scan of the thorax, abdomen, and pelvis. There is no evidence of recurrence.

ROLE OF RADIATION THERAPIST

Education of the patient and family members during radiation therapy is aimed at helping the patient understand the goals and importance of treatment and the potential side effects. Symptoms experienced during treatment are often difficult to endure and affect the patient's ability to consent to the completion of treatments. However, with the support of family and health care professionals and with information for controlling side effects, the patient can successfully complete a course of therapy. Open communication between the patient and supporting staff members (nursing, dietary, and social services) is of utmost importance in abating and controlling symptoms during and after a course of treatment.

The following are some potential side effects patients can experience while receiving radiation to glands of the endocrine system:

1. Fatigue is a common side effect of most patients receiving radiation therapy. Daily treatments and biologic effects of the disease and radiation can cause fatigue. Poor nutrition, depression, and family and financial worries are all contributing factors. Scheduling appointments around rest or meal times can aid in combating fatigue. The therapist should discuss the daily activity level with the patient to assess potential problems, and family members should be encouraged to assist in daily activities (e.g., meal preparation) to allow for rest time.
   Appointments with the social services department can reduce financial worries and aid in emotional support.

The therapist should encourage patients and family members to discuss their concerns and fears with each other.

2. Skin reactions can be painful and irritating to the patient. The therapist should advise the patient to avoid harsh creams, soaps, and lotions in the irradiated area. Hot water and sun exposure to the treated area should also be avoided. After a reaction starts, the therapist should communicate with the physician, and depending on the degree of desquamation (dry or moist), a treatment break may be warranted.
   For patients who may have a tracheostomy, a plastic cannula should replace a metal one, allowing it to stay in place during treatments. This will aid in preventing the enhancement of a skin reaction at the tracheostomy site. Loose-fitting clothes, especially cotton, should be worn to prevent rubbing and further irritation.

3. Hair loss (**alopecia**) can occur in the irradiated field as a result of the radiosensitivity of hair follicles. High-dose radiation may cause alopecia or delayed hair regrowth. The therapist should try to give the patient and family an appraisal for the potential and degree of hair loss and a time frame for its approximate occurrence. The therapist should inform patients to use mild shampoo and avoid excessive hair washing, which only dries and irritates the skin. In addition, the therapist should inform the patient and family that the new hair may have a different quality, texture, and color. If hair loss becomes significant, the use of a wig or turban may be indicated. Therapists should inform patients of national programs (e.g., "Look … Feel Better") that promote positive feelings and attitudes.

4. **Dysphagia** (difficulty swallowing) is often present in thyroid patients before the start of treatments as a result of the disease process. Early in the treatment, the patient may describe the feeling of "a lump in the throat." The therapist should encourage the patient to eat frequent meals consisting of high-protein and caloric foods. Eggnog, frappes, Ensure, Sustecal, and shakes supply high-protein and caloric intake and are soothing and easy to swallow. The patient should be advised to avoid commercial mouthwash, hot food and drinks, smoking, spicy food, and alcoholic beverages. If available, a dietary consultation should be scheduled within 1 week of the start of treatments.

Visual changes resulting from the disease can also cause a patient to be depressed. Simple pleasures such as reading or watching television can no longer be enjoyed. Unfortunately, little can be done to alter these effects caused by damage to the optic nerve; even treatment may not reverse the damage already inflicted on the nerve. However, audiotapes of best-selling books are available and may offer some enjoyment to the patient. The therapist can also encourage a family member to take time out to read the daily paper or a novel to the patient. The therapist should try to encourage family participation so that the patient does not feel left out.

Endocrine neoplasms can cause an array of previously discussed hormonal upsets, which can result in changes in emotions, appearance, and abilities. An altered body image can lower a patient's self-esteem. Patients with hair loss, hormonal syndromes, or acromegalic features may have misconceived notions of the way others perceive them. The therapist should be alert to these changes, allowing patients to express their feelings, promoting support from family members, and offering support to the family. Illness not only affects the patient but also the family because aggression and anger is often directed toward the family members.

The therapist should offer outside counseling (e.g., "I Can Cope") that is aimed at supporting families and patients through difficult times. Seeing other patients in similar circumstances lets patients know that they are not alone, their feelings are normal, and help is available.

Before the initiation of radiation therapy, the therapist should discuss the treatment process with the patient and family. The therapist should inform them that holding still is of the utmost importance for the delivery of proper treatment. In addition, the therapist should assure them that, although alone in the room, the patient is being carefully monitored. The therapist should take them into the room, explain positioning procedures, show them the monitors and intercom, and clearly explain that the machine will stop and someone will come in if help is needed. The therapist must give them a sense of control. The more they understand, the less anxiety they will feel, making the overall treatment process more tolerable.

Before educating patients and their families, therapists should educate themselves. Therapists should read the consultation, know the basics, and be prepared to address any specific questions or concerns a patient may wish to discuss. The patient must feel comfortable and confident in the therapist, allowing for open communication and trust throughout the duration of the treatment. A lack of trust can inhibit communication and cause undue stress for the patient and family.

Therapists must present themselves in a professional manner. After all, patients are entrusting themselves to the therapist, with little understanding and with much apprehension for what is before them.

SUMMARY

- Endocrine tumors have a wide variety of epidemiologic factors. Thyroid cancers are the most common of the endocrine malignancies, which account for approximately 94% of all new cases
- Thyroid cancer has several recognized etiologic factors, including the following:
  - External radiation to the thyroid gland, particularly before puberty, is the only well-documented etiologic factor. Treatment for benign conditions included; acne, tonsillitis, hemangiomas, and thymic enlargement.
  - Thyroid cancer is more prevalent among inhabitants of Nagasaki and Hiroshima that were present after the explosion of the atomic bomb in 1945.
  - Fallout from a nuclear test in the Marshall Islands in the 1950s led to studies that showed a higher incidence in thyroid changes, including cancer, in those exposed to the radioactive fallout.
  - The Chernobyl incident of 1986 has produced conflicting studies on the increase of thyroid cancer,

probably because of the extremely short interval between radiation exposure and tumor occurrence.
- Malignant thyroid neoplasms are divided into four categories: (1) papillary, (2) follicular, (3) medullary, and (4) anaplastic.
- Detection and diagnosis for tumors for endocrine tumors rely heavily on laboratory test results, the physical examination, diagnostic x-ray studies, and biopsy results. In addition, radionuclide thyroid imaging is commonly used to evaluate the function and anatomic location of a palpable thyroid nodule through the localization of hot or cold spots in the gland.
- Pituitary adenomas can be classified as functioning or nonfunctioning, as related to the hormones they produce. Hormone production often serves as a diagnostic and treatment-response marker. Pituitary adenomas categorized as functioning include the following hormones: prolactin, growth hormone, thyroid-stimulating hormone, and adrenocorticotrophic hormone.
- The rationale for treatment, regarding treatment choice, histologic subtype, and stage of the disease, varies for thyroid, pituitary, and adrenal gland tumors. Thyroid tumors are generally treated with surgery and radioactive I-131. Treatment for pituitary adenomas is controversial and may include surgery and external beam treatment, including intensity-modulated radiation therapy, proton treatment, or radiosurgery. Surgery is the treatment of choice for adrenal gland tumors.
- Radiation reactions for the treatment of tumors of the endocrine system include the following:
  - Fatigue is a common side effect of most patients receiving radiation therapy.
  - Skin reactions can be painful and irritating to the patient. The therapist should advise the patient to avoid harsh creams, soaps, and lotions in the irradiated area. Hot water and sun exposure to the treated area should also be avoided.
  - Hair loss (alopecia) can occur in the irradiated field as a result of the radiosensitivity of hair follicles.
  - Dysphagia (difficulty swallowing) is often present in thyroid patients before the start of treatments as a result of the disease process.
- Organs at risk for external beam radiation therapy include the lung and spinal cord for thyroid cancers and the optic chiasma, optic nerve, lens of the eye, and parotid glands for pituitary adenomas. Dose to these critical structures depends on the type of external beam treatment plan and the total dose given.

Review Questions

Multiple Choice

1. The cancers that are the most common of the endocrine malignancies are:
   a. thyroid
   b. pituitary

c. adrenal gland

d. parathyroid

2. Radioactive iodine-131 is used in the treatment of _____ tumors.
   a. thyroid
   b. pituitary
   c. adrenal gland
   d. parathyroid

3. Of all functioning pituitary adenomas, prolactin-secreting tumors affect the _____ as a target organ.
   a. thyroid
   b. pancreas
   c. breast
   d. uterus

4. The anatomic structure located just superiorly to the pituitary gland is:
   a. sphenoid sinus
   b. maxillary sinus
   c. optic chiasm
   d. occipital lobe of the brain

5. Which of the following is an indication for the use of radioactive iodine?
   a. inoperable primary tumor
   b. thyroid capsular invasion
   c. distant metastasis
   d. all the above

6. The pituitary tumors that remain within the pituitary are:
   a. intrasellar
   b. diffuse
   c. intrahypophyseal
   d. invasive

7. Which of the following would *not* be considered an endocrine-type tumor?
   a. breast
   b. thyroid
   c. adrenal gland
   d. pituitary

8. Which of the following is *not* a hormone secreted by the pituitary gland?
   a. ZH
   b. TSH
   c. FSH
   d. ACTH

9. Proton beams are sometimes used in the treatment of _____ tumors.
   a. breast
   b. thyroid
   c. adrenal gland
   d. pituitary

10. Which of the following does *not* belong in this group?
    a. medulla
    b. cortex
    c. follicular
    d. mineralocorticoids, glucocorticoids

The answers to the Review Questions can be found by logging on to our website at: *http://evolve.elsevier.com/Washington+Leaver/ principles*

Questions to Ponder

1. Discuss the diagnostic tests for a patient suspected of having a low-grade, early-stage malignancy.

2. Discuss the role of I-131 in the management of a patient with papillary or follicular cancer. Why is this iodine-based pharmaceutical useful in thyroid cancer?

3. Discuss the clinical syndromes that can be associated with adrenocortical carcinoma and the factors mediating these symptoms.

4. Explain which imaging studies should be suggested for a patient suspected of having an adrenal neoplasm.

5. Describe the critical structures in proximity to the pituitary gland and the effect of the tumor mass and pressure on these structures. Discuss the presenting symptoms related to the tumor mass and pressure on these structures.

6. Explain for a pituitary adenoma the criteria for postoperative radiation therapy management and the various radiation treatment techniques.

7. As a radiation therapist, discuss the way you would help a patient deal with the physical and emotional changes brought about by an endocrine malignancy. List some of the resources available to patients and their families.

REFERENCES

1. Alkire KT: Cancer of the pancreas, hepatobiliary and endocrine system. In Baird SB, et al, editors: *A cancer source book for nurses*, Atlanta, 1991, American Society Professional Education Publication.

2. Arafah B, Brodkey J, Pearson O: Acromegaly. In Santen R, Manni A, editors: *Diagnosis and management of endocrine related tumors*, Boston, 1984, Martinus Nijhoff.

3. Block MA, et al: Clinical characteristics distinguishing heredity from sporadic medullary thyroid carcinoma, *Arch Surg* 115:142, 1980.

4. Brennan MF: Cancer of the endocrine system. In DeVita VT Jr, Hellman S, Rosenberg SA, editors: *Cancer principles and practice of oncology*, ed 7, Philadelphia, 2004, Lippincott Wiilaims & Wilkins.

5. Cohn K, Gottesman L, Brennan M: Adrenocortical carcinoma. Presented at the seventh annual meeting of the American Association of Endocrine Surgeons, Rochester, Minnesota, April 14-15, 1986.

6. DeAtkine AB, Dunnick NR: The adrenal glands, *Semin Oncol* 118: 131-139, 1991.

7. Donehower MG: Endocrine cancers. In Baird SB, McCorkle R, Grant M, editors: *Cancer nursing: a comprehensive textbook,* Philadelphia, 1991, WB Saunders.

8. Furmanchuk AW, et al: Pathomorphological findings in thyroid cancers of children from the Republic of Belarus: a study of 86 cases occurring between 1986 (Ôpost-Chernobyl') and 1991, *Histopathology* 21:401-408, 1992.

9. Graze K, et al: Natural history of familial medullary carcinoma: effects of program for early diagnosis, *N Engl J Med* 299:980, 1985.

10. Hajjar RA, Hickey RC, Samaan NA: Adrenal cortical carcinoma: a study of 32 patients, *Cancer* 35:549, 1975.

11. Hardy J, Beauregard H, Robert F: Prolactin secreting pituitary adenoma: transsphenoidal microsurgical treatment. In Robyn C, Garter M, editors: *Progress in prolactin physiology and pathology*, Amsterdam, 1978, North Holland Biomedical Press.

12. Hay I, Petersen IA: Thyroid cancer. In Gunderson S, Tepper J, editors: *Clinical radiation oncology*, Philadelphia, 2000, Churchill Livingston.

13. Hay I, Petersen IA: Thyroid cancer. In Gunderson S, Tepper J, editors: *Clinical radiation oncology*, Philadelphia, 2007, Churchill Livingston.

14. Karakousis CP, Rao U, Moore R: Adenocarcinomas: histologic grading and survival, *J Surg Oncol* 29:105-111, 1985.

15. Kroop SA, et al: Evaluation of thyroid masses by MR imaging. Presented at the Radiological Society of North America 71st scientific assembly annual meeting, Chicago, November 17-22, 1985.

16. Mazzaferri EL, et al: Papillary thyroid carcinoma: the impact of therapy in 576 patients, *Medicine* 56:171, 1977.

17. Mettler FA, et al: Thyroid nodules in the population living around Chernobyl, *JAMA* 268:616-619, 1992.

18. Mountz JM, Glazer GM, Sissom JC: Evaluation of thyroid disease using MR imaging and scintigraphy. Presented at the Radiological Society of North American 71st scientific assembly annual meeting, Chicago, November, 1985.

19. Murali R: Tumors of the nervous system. In Nealon TF Jr, editor: *Management of the patient with cancer*, Philadelphia, 1986, WB Saunders.

20. Newsome HH Jr, Kay S, Lawrence W Jr: The adrenal gland. In Nealon TF, editor: *Management of the patient with cancer*, ed 3, Philadelphia, 1986, WB Saunders.

21. Sambade MC, et al: High relative frequency of thyroid papillary carcinoma in northern Portugal, *Cancer* 51:1754, 1983.

22. Scheilbe W, Leopold GR, Woo VL: High resolution real-time ultrasonography of thyroid nodules, *Radiology* 13:413, 1979.

23. Schneider AB, et al: Plasma thyroglobulin in detecting thyroid carcinoma after childhood head and neck irradiation, *Ann Intern Med* 86:29, 1977.

24. Schreiber NW: Endocrine malignancies. In Groenwald SL, editor: *Cancer nursing principle and practice,* Boston, 1987, Jones & Bartlett.

25. Schteingart DE, et al: Treatment of adrenal carcinoma, *Arch Surg* 117:1142-1146, 1982.

26. Thibodeau G, Patton K: *Anatomy and physiology,* ed 6, New York, 2007, Mosby.

27. Trautmann JC, Law ER Jr: Visual status after transsphenoidal surgery at the Mayo Clinic, 1971-1982, *Am J Ophthalmol* 96:200-208, 1983.

28. Varia MA, et al: Pituitary tumors. In Gunderson S, Tepper J, editors: *Clinical radiation oncology*, Philadelphia, 2007, Churchill Livingston.

29. Varia MA: Pituitary tumors. In Tepper J, Gunderson S, editors: *Clinical radiation oncology*, Philadelphia, 2000, Churchill Livingston.

30. Wang Chi-an: Thyroid cancer. In Wang CC, editor: *Clinical radiation oncology: indications, techniques and results,* Littleton, MA, 1988, PBG Publishing.

31. Wittes RE: *Manual of oncologic therapeutics* 1989/1990, Philadelphia, 1989, JB Lippincott.

32. Wool MS: Management of papillary and follicular cancer. In Greenfield LD, editor: *Thyroid cancer*, Boca Raton, FA, 1978, CRC Press.

BIBLIOGRAPHY

Cady B, et al: The effect of thyroid hormone administration upon survival in patients with differentiated thyroid carcinoma, *Surgery* 6:978-983, 1983.

Denny JD, Marty R, Van Herle AJ: Serum thyroglobulin: a sensitive indicator of metastatic well differentiated thyroid carcinoma. Society of Nuclear Medicine Western Regional Meeting II, Las Vegas, 1977.

Hardy J, Vezina JL: Transsphenoidal neurosurgery of intracranial neoplasm. In Thompson RA, Green JR, editors: *Advances in neurology*, vol 15, New York 1976, Raven Press.

Van Herle AJ: Pathophysiology of thyroid cancer. In Greenfield LD, editor: *Thyroid cancer*, Boca Raton, FA, 1976, CRC Press.

Respiratory System Tumors

Donna Stinson, Paul E. Wallner

Outline

Objectives

- Describe how age, gender, lifestyle, and occupational exposure play roles in the development of lung cancer and how each is related to prognosis.
- List the three most common causes of lung cancer in the United States.
- Define Karnofsky Performance Scale and explain its relevance in lung cancer.
- Describe how lung cancer is detected and the process of diagnosis.
- List two anatomical and radiographic features of the carina and explain why it is important in the treatment of lung cancer.

- Explain the importance of the hilum and its role in the spread of lung cancer.
- Describe lung cancer's direct, hematogenic, and lymphatic routes of spread.
- List five or more anatomic sites to which lung cancer commonly metastasizes.
- State the signs and symptoms of lung cancer.
- Describe the roles of surgery, chemotherapy, and radiation therapy in the treatment of lung cancer.

Key Terms

Boost fields
Bronchogenic carcinoma
Bronchoscope
Carina
Conventional fractionation
Hilum
Horner's syndrome
Karnofsky Performance Scale
Mediastinoscopy
Mesothelioma
Kyphosis
Orthogonal images
Pancoast tumors
Paraneoplastic syndromes
Scoliosis
Superior vena cava syndrome

This chapter focuses on bronchogenic carcinoma, although mesothelioma is covered in a limited fashion. Technically, **bronchogenic carcinomas** are primary tumors of the lung that arise in the bronchi. Frequently, however, the term is used to refer to lung cancers collectively, including those that arise in pulmonary alveoli or pleural surfaces. Lung cancers are the most common invasive malignancies in the United States and the most common cause is tobacco exposure. Tumors are classified into two general classes—small cell and non–small cell carcinomas—with small cell carcinomas more likely to metastasize early.

Lung cancer spreads by local extension to other parts of the lung, ribs, heart, and other structures; through primary lymphatics in the thoracic cavity and lymphatic channels in the pleural surfaces; and via the circulatory system at the thoracic duct and aorta.

Radiation therapy is generally used in combination with chemotherapy and/or surgery.

Positron emission tomography (PET)–computed tomography (CT) is used to define extent of non–small cell carcinomas. External beam therapy, especially intensity-modulated radiation therapy (IMRT), is considered standard care with respiratory gating emerging as a treatment option as technology evolves. Critical structures are major life-supporting organs, including heart, lung, and spinal cord. Superior vena cava syndrome may require emergency radiation therapy.

CANCER OF THE RESPIRATORY SYSTEM

Natural History

Prognosis. Although numerous factors affect prognosis, the most significant variables include the following: (1) stage—extent of the disease (Box 32-1), (2) clinical performance status—measured by scales such as the **Karnofsky Performance Scale**[30] (Box 32-2), and (3) weight loss[5]—especially greater than 5% of the total body weight over 3 months. Multiple studies have clearly demonstrated the independent nature of each of these variables in determining the prognosis.[18,21] This effect is so marked

Box 32-1 American Joint Committee on Cancer Staging System for Lung Cancer

PRIMARY TUMOR (T)

TX   Primary tumor cannot be assessed, or tumor proven by presence of malignant cells in sputum or bronchial washings but not visualized by imaging or bronchoscopy

T0   No evidence of primary tumor

Tis   Carcinoma in situ

T1   Tumor 3 cm or less in greatest dimension, surrounded by lung or visceral pleura, without bronchoscopic evidence of invasion more proximal than the lobar bronchus

T2   Tumor with any of the following features of size or extent: More than 3 cm in greatest dimension
- Involves main bronchus, 2 cm or more distal to the carina
- Invades the visceral pleura
- Associated with atelectasis or obstructive pneumonitis that extends to the hilar region but does not involve the entire lung

T3   Tumor of any size that directly invades any of the following: chest wall (including superior sulcus tumors), diaphragm, mediastinal pleura, parietal pericardium; or tumor in the main bronchus less than 2 cm distal to the carina but without involvement of the carina; or associated atelectasis or obstructive pneumonitis of the entire lung

T4   Tumor of any size that invades any of the following: mediastinum, heart, great vessels, trachea, esophagus, vertebral body, carina; or separate tumor nodules in the same lobe, or tumor with a malignant pleural effusion

REGIONAL LYMPH NODES (N)

NX   Regional lymph nodes cannot be assessed

N0   No regional lymph node metastasis

N1   Metastasis in ipsilateral peribronchial and/or ipsilateral hilar lymph nodes, and intrapulmonary nodes including involvement by direct extension of the primary tumor

N2   Metastasis in ipsilateral mediastinal and/or subcarinal lymph node(s)

N3   Metastasis in contralateral mediastinal, contralateral hilar, ipsilateral or contralateral scalene, or supraclavicular lymph node(s)

DISTANT METASTASIS (M)

MX   Presence of distant metastasis cannot be assessed

M0   No distant metastasis

M1   Distant metastasis present

STAGE GROUPING

Occult carcinoma	TX	N0	M0
0	Tis	N0	M0
IA	T1	N0	M0
IB	T2	N0	M0
IIA	T1	N1	M0
IIB	T2	N1	M0
	T3	N0	M0
IIIA	T1	N2	M0
	T2	N2	M0
	T3	N1	M0
	T3	N2	M0
IIIB	Any T	N3	M0
	T4	Any N	M0
IV	Any T	Any N	M1

With permission from American Joint Committee on Cancer (AJCC), Chicago, IL: *AJCC Cancer Staging Manual,* ed 6, New York, 2002, Springer-Verlag.

Box 32-2 Karnofsky Performance Scale

100	Normal; no complaints; no evidence of disease
90	Ability to carry on normal activity; minor signs or symptoms of disease
80	Normal activity with effort; some signs or symptoms of disease
70	Self-care; inability to carry on normal activity or do active work
60	Requirement of occasional assistance, but ability to care for most personal needs
50	Requirement of considerable assistance and frequent medical care
40	Disability; requirement of special care and assistance
30	Severe disability; hospitalization indicated, although death not imminent
20	Extreme sickness; hospitalization necessary; active support treatment necessary
10	Moribund; rapid progression of fatal processes
0	Dead

Modified from Macleod CM, editor: *Evaluation of chemotherapeutic agents,* New York, 1949, Columbia University Press.

that prospective clinical trials for definitive disease management frequently exclude patients who are in an advanced clinical stage (although the disease is apparently limited to the chest), patients with a Karnofsky Performance Scale score of less than 70, or patients with weight loss greater than 5% measured from baseline over a 4- to 6-month period. Individuals with advanced intrathoracic disease, extrathoracic extension, a Karnofsky score below 70, or weight loss greater than 5% rarely survive longer than 2 years regardless of therapy.

Malignant **mesothelioma** of the pleural surfaces has been increasing at a greater rate than other types of lung cancers, presumably related to the long latent period existing between carcinogenic exposure and development of the disease. Although the incidence in the United States is only 3,000 to 4,000 new cases per year,[4] approximately 8 million individuals have been exposed to significant levels of asbestos (the primary etiologic agent), and estimates suggest that by 2030, perhaps 300,000 new cases per year may be evident. Because asbestos exposure had previously occurred in primarily male-dominated industries, the incidence of mesothelioma is seen overwhelmingly in men. Nonoccupational asbestosis and asbestos-related mesothelioma may occur in women.[40]

Asbestos fibers inhaled in industries such as mining, asbestos-material manufacturing and insulation, railroads, shipyards, pipe insulation, and gas mask producers are primarily associated with the production of mesotheliomas. Many types of asbestos particles exist, all of which have potential risks, but the longer and thinner strands produce more chemical reactivity and greater carcinogenesis.

Because metastatic disease to the lung represents a common occurrence for other primary tumor sites, the definitive establishment of the lung disease as primary or secondary is appropriate in most instances. This determination usually has significant implications for subsequent decisions regarding additional evaluation, management, and prognosis.

Epidemiology

Cancers of the bronchial tree, lung, and pleural surfaces represent the most common invasive malignancies in the United States. According to the American Cancer Society, approximately 232,270 new cases will be diagnosed and 166,280 deaths will be caused by the disease in 2008.[2] Considered as a group, these malignancies represent 15% of all new cancers in the United States and 29% of all cancer deaths.[2]

Over the past six decades, there has generally been an absolute increase in new cancers with some leveling of the increase, especially in white males, over the past decade. In 1950, the male/female ratio was approximately 6:1; however, an increase in female incidence has now produced a ratio approaching 1:1.[1,10] In 1987, lung cancer surpassed breast cancer as the leading cause of cancer-related deaths in women.[11]

Etiology

The most common cause of lung cancer is significant tobacco exposure, which is generally defined as more than one pack of cigarettes per day. Although tobacco product manufacturers have consistently denied absolute proof of the link, epidemiologic data strongly suggest an unequivocal causal relationship. Also, an apparent dose-response consistency is related to a higher incidence of lung cancers with (1) an increased duration of smoking, (2) an increased use of unfiltered cigarettes, and (3) an increased number of cigarettes consumed. The use of chewing tobacco, cigars, and pipes, including hookahs, is generally associated with a higher incidence of malignancies in the upper aerodigestive tract rather than the lung. The American Cancer Society reports that 87% of lung cancer cases are a result of smoking tobacco. Second-hand smoke is another cause of lung cancer, with a 30% greater risk of developing lung cancer for spouses of smokers compared with nonsmokers.[2] Increasing incidence of lung cancer among nonsmokers and never-smokers, frequently presenting with an adenocarcinoma cell type, has also become a public health concern.[63]

Of particular concern are younger smokers who become addicted to nicotine in high school, or occasionally earlier, and continue the habit throughout adulthood. The American Cancer Society reported that smoking among high school students declined from 1997 to 2003 due to higher prices on cigarettes, campaigns to restrict smoking in public spaces, and counter advertising, but individuals who smoke more than one pack of cigarettes per day usually acquire their habit before the age of 18. The decrease may have leveled off between 2003 and 2006.[2]

Lung cancer can also be related to occupational exposure. Causative factors include fumes from coal tar, nickel, chromium, and arsenic and exposure to various radioactive materials. Especially dangerous are agents with alpha emissions in their various daughter products, such as uranium and radon. The Environmental Protection Agency estimates that radon is the second leading cause of lung cancer in the United States and has recommended guidelines for various levels of radon exposure. Radon may be present in various levels in soil. Also, depending on the type of home construction, ventilation, insulation, and size, radon may be found in high quantities inside parts of a home.[61]

Pollution and genetic factors may be synergistic in their causative effect, adding to the risk above and beyond the various exposures indicated. However, these relationships are somewhat more difficult to prove.

General Anatomy and Physiology

Organs of the system. The respiratory system consists of the nose, pharynx, larynx, trachea, and both lungs. Air is conducted from the nose; through the pharynx, larynx, and trachea; and into the lungs. Because cancers of the upper respiratory system (nose, pharynx, and larynx) are discussed in Chapter 33; only the anatomy of the trachea and lungs are included in this section.

The lower respiratory system consists of the trachea and lungs. The trachea is the major airway in the thoracic cavity. The wall is composed of rings of cartilage, smooth muscle, and connective tissue. Epithelial cells line the trachea. The trachea begins at the inferior border of the larynx and ends at the level of the fifth thoracic vertebra (T5), where it bifurcates.[60] This bifurcation is called the **carina**, the area in which the trachea divides into two branches. Anatomically and radiographically, the carina corresponds to the level of the fourth and fifth thoracic vertebrae (T4 and T5). At the bifurcation, the trachea divides into the right and left primary bronchi. These bronchi begin a branching process that is similar to the structure of a tree (the bronchial tree). The primary bronchi are also called the right and left mainstem bronchi. The primary bronchi form branches of decreasing size until finally reaching the microscopic level, where gases are exchanged. First, the mainstem bronchi form branches called the secondary bronchi. These lobar bronchi continue to divide into smaller, tertiary bronchi. Also called the segmental bronchi, these tertiary bronchi divide into smaller branches known as bronchioles. Bronchioles are microscopic structures that further divide into alveolar ducts. Many capillaries supply the alveolar ducts. Gases diffuse across the alveolar-capillary membranes. Oxygen and carbon dioxide exchanges take place at this microscopic level.[60]

The **hilum** of the lung is the area in which the blood, lymphatic vessels, and nerves enter and exit each lung. The mediastinum refers to the anatomy between the lungs including the heart, thymus, great vessels, and other structures that help position the lungs on either side of the midline.

Important anatomical structures include lung hila and the carina, as these are the structures where tumor cells gain access to the circulatory system.

Ventilation. Ventilation is the term for oxygen and carbon dioxide exchange to the external environment (i.e., breathing). The physiology of the respiratory system begins as air is inhaled into the body. Air moves inferiorly along the trachea and enters the lungs at the mainstem bronchi. The bronchi divide into many branches. As the branching increases, the cartilage decreases and the amount of smooth muscle in the structures increases.

A respiratory unit is composed of the bronchioli, alveolar ducts, and alveoli. Gas exchange takes place from these units into the lung capillaries and is called external respiration. Oxygenated blood moves from these capillaries and major vessels in the lungs to the heart, where it is pumped throughout the body. Oxygenated blood is carried in the arteries and then exchanged in cells throughout the body for deoxygenated blood. From the capillaries, further exchanges take place through the interstitial fluid to the cells. This is known as internal respiration, a process in which oxygen and carbon dioxide exchanges take place at the cellular level as a result of changes in pressure. Thus, carbon dioxide is removed from the cells, returned through the venous system to the capillaries in the lungs, and finally exhaled through the respiratory units in the following order: (1) alveoli, (2) alveolar ducts, and (3) bronchioli to the external environment.[60]

Blood Supply and Lymphatics. The lymphatic system is important in lung cancer because it is one of the principal routes of regional spread. Lymph nodes and channels permeate the respiratory system. At many points, the lymphatics anastomose (connect) with pulmonary arteries and veins. Lymphatics of the lungs are classified in several ways. They are grouped anatomically according to the tumor, node, metastases (TNM) staging system into mediastinal and intrapulmonic nodes[3] (Box 32-3).

Flow between the mediastinal nodes is complicated and difficult to predict. As an example, mediastinal nodes connect directly with the subcarinal, pretracheal, and diaphragmatic channels. Lymphatic flow is influenced by lung pressures, the diaphragm, movements of the chest wall, and motions of other local organs and vessels.[26]

Mediastinal nodes are subdivided into those in the superior mediastinum and inferior mediastinum, and further classified by number and location. The superior mediastinal nodes include (1) highest mediastinal, (2) upper paratracheal, (3) pretracheal and retrotracheal, and (4) lower paratracheal (including azygos nodes). Inferior mediastinal nodes include (1) subcarinal, (2) paraesophageal (below the carina), and (3) pulmonary ligament.[3]

Box 32-3	Respiratory System Lymphatics

Mediastinal nodes
1. Superior mediastinal
2. Tracheal
3. Aortic
4. Carinal and subcarinal
5. Pulmonary ligaments

Intrapulmonic (hilar, bronchopulmonic) nodes
1. Mainstem bronchus
2. Interlobar
3. Lobar

The other major groups of lymph nodes include (1) aortic, (2) subaortic (A-P window), (3) paraaortic (ascending aortic or phrenic), (4) hilar, (5) intralobar, (6) lobar, (7) segmental, and (8) subsegmental.[3]

The blood supply of the respiratory system is similar to that of the lymphatics. Many of the vessels have similar names. For example, the vessels that supply the trachea are called the tracheal veins and arteries.

The location of the lungs in relation to the circulatory system is important. In fact, the two systems are linked. The lymph channels that drain the heart flow into the mediastinal nodes at the level of the carina.[26] Lymphatic drainage of the lungs meets with the cardiac flow of the lymph at the carina. From this region of the bifurcation of the trachea, access to the circulatory system occurs as the flow enters the thoracic duct and aorta.

In addition, the lymph nodes have arterial and venous blood supplies. Cancer cells trapped in the lymph nodes form emboli that can leave the node through its own blood vessels.[26]

When bronchogenic carcinoma of the lung is treated with radiation, the fields generally include the tumor and draining blood and lymph vessels. A simple field design, such as a mediastinum, includes all the lymphatics and blood vessels that flow in the area of the carina. Structures such as the hilum of each lung, aorta, thoracic duct, esophagus, vertebral bodies, and others are included in fields of this nature. The lungs, mechanics of respiration, blood, and lymphatic supplies are considered in planning a course of radiation therapy for patients with lung cancer.

Clinical Presentation

The signs and symptoms of lung cancer are often insidious and especially difficult to differentiate from the symptoms of chronic obstructive pulmonary disease that often occur. Presenting features are associated with (1) local disease in the bronchopulmonary tissues, (2) regional extension to the lymph nodes, chest wall and/or neurologic structures, and (3) distant dissemination.[12]

Local Disease. Symptoms related to local disease extent are generally among the earliest complaints, with evidence of a cough in approximately 75% of patients. This cough may be severe and unremitting in 40% of the patients. Hemoptysis (blood associated with the cough) may be present in up to 60% of patients and may be the first sign of disease in up to 5% of patients. Approximately 15% of patients complain of a recent onset of dyspnea (shortness of breath), and a similar percentage exhibit chest pain.[12]

Regional Disease. Regional extension of disease (usually to the central mediastinal, paratracheal, parahilar, and subcarinal lymph nodes) may produce pain, coughing, dyspnea, and occasionally an abscess formation secondary to an obstructive pneumonia. Disease extension into the mediastinum may be manifested as dysphagia (difficulty swallowing) because of esophageal compression. Compression of the superior vena cava, especially in lesions of the right lobe extending into the mediastinum, may produce a **superior vena cava syndrome** associated with increasing dyspnea; facial, neck, and arm edema; orthopnea (an inability to lie flat); and cyanosis (a blue tinge to the lips). Hoarseness may occur as a result of compression or invasion of the recurrent laryngeal nerve, especially on the left side, where the nerve takes a somewhat longer course.

Dyspnea may occur secondary to phrenic nerve involvement, producing diaphragmatic paralysis.

Less common are apex tumors of the lung. Apical tumors may be Pancoast tumors, but certain criteria other than anatomic location must be met. A patient with a true **Pancoast tumor** has a tumor in the superior sulcus and a clinical presentation that includes (1) pain around the shoulder and down the arm, (2) atrophy of the hand muscles, (3) Horner's syndrome, and (4) bone erosion of the ribs and sometimes the vertebrae.[33,45] Pancoast tumors involve the cervical sympathetic nerves that cause Horner's syndrome. Classically, **Horner's syndrome** includes an ipsilateral (same-side) miosis (contracted pupil), ptosis (drooping eyelid), enophthalmos (recession of the eyeball into the orbit), and anhydrosis (loss of facial sweating). Arm and shoulder pain is caused by brachial plexus involvement, and these tumors may extend upward into the neck. Erosion of the first and second ribs may cause arm pain. Not all apical tumors are Pancoast tumors.

Metastatic Disease. Distant metastasis is generally associated with anorexia (loss of appetite), weight loss, and fatigue. Approximately 2% of patients with lung cancer may demonstrate **paraneoplastic syndromes** that are thought to represent distant manifestations of the effect of chemicals or hormones produced by these tumors.[27] Typically, symptoms of paraneoplastic syndromes may affect nerves, muscles, and endocrine glands. These symptoms may be improved but rarely controlled for significant periods in the absence of primary tumor control. A frequently seen phenomenon associated with lung cancer is hypertrophic pulmonary osteoarthropathy, which is manifested by clubbing of the distal phalanges of the fingers (Figure 32-1). Although this finding is most frequently associated with benign, long-standing chronic obstructive pulmonary disease, it may be seen as a presenting sign of lung cancer.

Individuals at high risk for the development of lung cancer because of habits such as tobacco consumption, occupational exposures, and/or significant exposure to passive smoke are often encouraged to consider routine chest x-ray screenings. A number of trials have been attempted with the use of annual chest x-ray screenings alone or with the addition of annual sputum cytologies. Most of these attempts to diagnose disease at an earlier stage have not been associated with significant improvement in long-term survival rates; however, further research is ongoing.[28]

Detection and Diagnosis

Radiographic Imaging. Conventional chest x-ray examinations using posteroanterior (PA) and lateral projections remain the principal method of lung cancer detection, although estimates show that approximately 75% of the natural history of the disease has occurred at the time of first radiographic appearance.[50] Conventional CT scans may be suggestive of malignant disease, but the diagnosis is frequently not definitive, although some improvement may be obtained with a contrast-enhanced study, demonstrating variations in blood flow. Low-dose spiral CT may be effective in detecting tumors as small as 6 to 10 mm. Studies are under way to evaluate the use of this modality for screening of high-risk populations. One study completed in the United States, demonstrated findings positive for tumor in 2.7% of screened individuals versus 0.7% detected by conventional chest radiograph. Unfortunately, the high rate of false-positivity

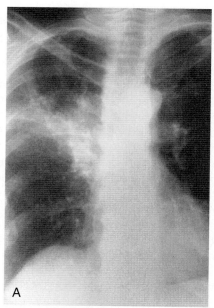

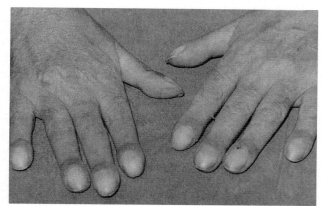

Figure 32-1. Hypertrophic pulmonary osteoarthropathy (clubbing).

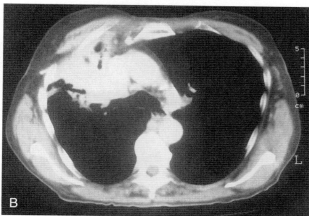

Figure 32-2. A, Posteroanterior (PA) chest radiograph showing a right upper lobe tumor. **B,** Computed tomography (CT) scan demonstrates the involvement of the chest wall.

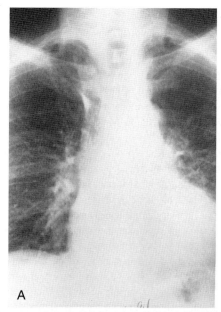

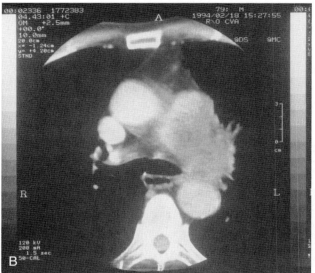

Figure 32-3. A, Posteroanterior (PA) chest radiograph showing midline disease. **B**, Computed tomography (CT) scan demonstrates the involvement of the mediastinum.

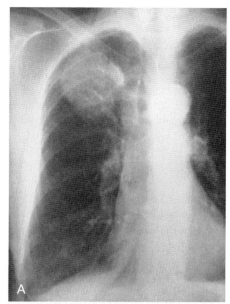

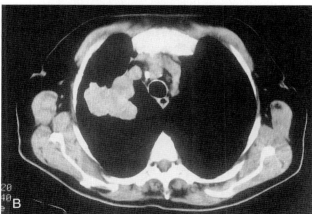

Figure 32-4. A, Posteroanterior (PA) chest radiograph showing a right upper lobe tumor. **B**, Computed tomography (CT) scan demonstrates the involvement of midline structures.

presents a significant drawback to this approach, in both cost and morbidity.[56]

Figure 32-2 shows a radiograph of an abnormal anterior chest, whereas the CT scan demonstrates that the tumor has already invaded the chest wall anteriorly.

At the initial presentation, the most frequent findings include a solitary soft tissue lesion, mediastinal widening secondary to lymphatic extension, parabronchial or parahilar lymphadenopathy, and pleural effusion (Figure 32-3). Obstructive pneumonias may occur with endobronchial extension sufficient to produce bronchial obstruction. Solitary lesions are frequently irregular in contour and marginal distinctness. These lesions, if connected to a bronchus, may eventually break down to produce a thick-walled abscess with an air-fluid level. Long-standing obstructive pneumonias may also lead to abscess formation.

Chest radiographs that are suspicious for lung cancer must lead to other diagnostic interventions. Because a histologic (or cytologic) diagnosis is essential for appropriate management decisions, the next steps in evaluation frequently include CT of the chest to evaluate the following: (1) the primary finding itself, (2) the possibility of other pulmonary lesions, (3) the involvement of mediastinal and paramediastinal structures, and (4) pleural or extrapleural thoracic involvement. Figure 32-4 demonstrates a right upper lobe tumor that has invaded the midline structures, whereas the CT scan shows mediastinal extension.

CT examinations are often crucial in selecting sites for a biopsy. CT examinations should involve the upper abdomen for an evaluation of the liver and adrenal glands, which are frequent sites of metastatic spread. CT scans have become an invaluable aid in the preoperative determination of resectability.

Patients in whom lesions are too peripheral for bronchoscopy or for whom bronchoscopy has failed to demonstrate endobronchial disease may be candidates for a CT-directed percutaneous fine needle aspiration (PFNA). This procedure is highly effective and associated with a small risk of pneumothorax. PFNA is frequently carried out on an outpatient basis with post-procedure time for monitoring of the respiratory status and blood pressure.

MRI studies have been helpful in evaluation of mediastinal and paravertebral disease, and PET scans have become a frequently used tool for determining if peripheral nodular lesions are benign or malignant. Incidentally detected pulmonary nodules in asymptomatic patients may be categorized on the basis PET positivity as probably malignant (Figure 32-5). ^{18}F-2-Deoxy-D-glucose (FDG) PET is accurate in more than 90% of patients with lesions as small as 10 mm. Additional uses for PET scanning include staging, especially for evaluation of normal-sized nodes; determining extent of primary tumor and small adrenal metastases; evaluating recurrent lung cancer (postoperative/radiation fibrosis versus active tumor), and evaluating therapeutic response and prognostic potential.[46]

Laboratory Studies. Pulmonary function studies are beneficial primarily for determining a patient's ability to withstand various types of treatment, especially because many of these patients have preexisting compromised pulmonary function from their chronic pulmonary disease.

Sputum cytology may be positive in up to 75% of patients with lung cancer. These cytologies are of limited use, however, because of the difficulty in determining the precise sites of disease based on expectorated sputum and because specific tissue subtyping may be difficult.[19]

Bone marrow biopsies are of limited value except in individuals who have small cell, undifferentiated carcinoma of the lung in which up to a 40% incidence of bone marrow involvement exists.

A histologic evaluation is generally sought and usually obtained through interventional routes that include surgery.

Hematologic and serum chemical evaluations of the blood are important and should include a complete blood count (CBC), serum calcium, alkaline phosphatase, lactic dehydrogenase (LDH), and serum glutamic oxaloacetic transaminase (SGOT). Serum calcium elevation is indicative of osseous disease. Alkaline phosphatase, LDH, and SGOT may be indicative of liver or bone involvement.

Surgery. Tumor histology is most frequently obtained through a fiberoptic bronchoscopy because up to 75% of lesions may be visible in this fashion. The flexible **bronchoscope**, which is a long flexible tube, has almost completely supplanted the rigid bronchoscope in the diagnosis and management of lung cancer and is used to examine the bronchial tree, to obtain a specimen for biopsy, or in some cases to remove a foreign body. Endobronchial brushing and endobronchial biopsy or a transbronchial biopsy provides a true-positive diagnosis in more than 90% of patients with visible lesions. The patency of bronchi and sites of bleeding can also be established.[49]

A pleural biopsy is used most frequently for pleural-based diseases such as mesothelioma. Thoracentesis (removal of fluid from the chest) or a pleural biopsy may be invaluable in the presence of pleural effusion because malignant effusion adversely affects the prognosis.

CT-directed percutaneous needle biopsy can confirm malignancy in 90% to 95% of lesions greater than 2 cm and in approximately 60% of smaller lesions.[46]

Video-assisted thoracoscopy is used routinely in diagnosis and management of small pulmonary nodules. The procedure

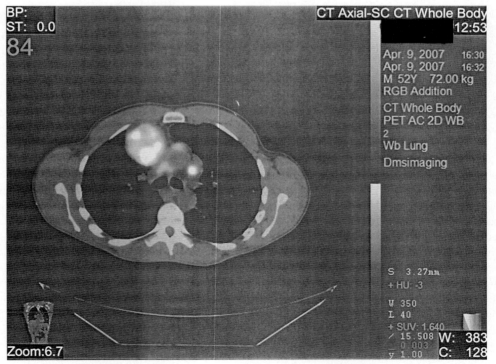

Figure 32-5. Positron emission tomography (PET)-computed tomography (CT) with positive contralateral hilar mass. (Courtesy of Bayhealth Medical Center at Kent General Hospital, Dover, Del.)

involves the insertion of a tube into the chest and visualization of intrathoracic contents on a television monitor. Video-assisted thoracoscopy may be especially beneficial with pleural-based disease or if no dominant masses are demonstrated. The procedure may also assist in staging.[46]

A **mediastinoscopy**, which also uses a small flexible tube, is frequently used for the evaluation of the superior mediastinal extent of disease. If surgical intervention is anticipated, a formal, open mediastinotomy may also be used for visual and pathological evaluation of the mediastinum.

Advanced Disease. CT scanning of the brain prior to initiation of definitive therapy is used primarily for small cell, undifferentiated carcinomas and adenocarcinomas of the lung. Both of these have a high risk for central nervous system metastasis.

The use of formal thoracotomy for diagnosing and staging has generally been abandoned because of the availability of less-invasive interventional studies.

Pathology

Histologic Cell Types. The World Health Organization (WHO) has established a histologic classification of lung cancer that includes 12 primary tumor types with additional subtypes[8] (Box 32-4). Although little question exists whether these categories are distinct pathologically, they are somewhat cumbersome from a clinical perspective, and more frequently the nomenclature of small cell lung cancer (SCLC) and non–small cell lung cancer (NSCLC) are used. This breakdown is appropriate because of the distinct clinical differences between the small cell anaplastic carcinoma and the group of non–small cell lesions, including adenocarcinoma, large cell carcinoma, and epidermoid (squamous cell) carcinoma, which act in a similar fashion clinically. Mesothelioma of the lung remains a distinct, although less frequent, category.[25,40]

Location. Squamous cell (epidermoid) carcinoma is usually associated with tobacco consumption, occurs most frequently in men, and is often located centrally in proximal bronchi.

This lesion represented the most common form of primary pulmonary malignancy until the recent rise in the incidence of adenocarcinomas, which now account for approximately 40% of lung cancers in North America.[55] Adenocarcinomas are less frequently associated with tobacco consumption, occur most often in women, and are frequently more peripheral in location, arising in bronchioles or alveoli. Small cell carcinomas and large cell carcinomas each represent approximately 20% of the remaining lesions, with small cell lesions tending to occur more centrally and large cell lesions appearing more peripherally. SCLC is prone to early spread, and fewer than 10% of these patients have diagnoses of limited stage disease.

Prognosis. Because of its predisposition for early metastasis, the prognosis of SCLC is poor with only 10% to 15% of patients surviving 3 years. NSCLC has a better prognosis with 15% to 20% of patients surviving 5 or more years. Survival is significantly better in early-stage disease when surgery is undertaken for curative intent, with 5-year survival rates approaching 60% or higher for clinical stages IA and IB.[16,42,58]

Staging

The use of clinical and pathologic staging represents an attempt to compare similar cases with regard to the effectiveness of treatment and the prognosis. Before the 1970s, conventional chest x-ray examinations, radioisotope scanning, and serum chemistry analyses were routinely used as the basis for clinical staging. Subsequent evidence has indicated the unreliability of these procedures for accurate evaluation of disease extent.

The advent of CT in the 1970s enhanced the ability to determine resectability before formal thoracotomy by enabling greater definition of the mediastinum, lymph nodes, and chest wall invasion. In many instances the presence of these factors was thought to be a contraindication to curative resection, and during the 1970s and 1980s the frequency of surgical intervention in lung cancer declined.

Box 32-4	**World Health Organization Histologic Classification of Lung Cancer**

I. Epidermoid carcinoma
II. Small cell anaplastic carcinoma
   1. Fusiform cell type
   2. Polygonal cell type
   3. Lymphocyte-like (oat cell) type
III. Adenocarcinoma
   1. Bronchogenic
      a. Acinar, with or without mucin formation
      b. Papillary
   2. Bronchoalveolar
IV. Large cell carcinoma
   1. Solid tumors with mucin-like content
   2. Solid tumors without mucin-like content
   3. Giant cell carcinoma
   4. Clear cell carcinoma
V. Combined epidermoid and adenocarcinoma
VI. Carcinoid tumors

VII. Bronchial gland tumors
   1. Cylindromas
   2. Mucoepidermoid tumors
   3. Others
VIII. Papillary tumors of the surface epithelium
   1. Epidermoid
   2. Epidermoid with goblet cells
   3. Others
IX. Mixed tumors and carcinomas
   1. Mixed tumors
   2. Carcinosarcoma of the embryonal type (blastoma)
   3. Other carcinosarcomas
X. Sarcomas
XI. Unclassified
XII. Mesotheliomas
   1. Localized
   2. Diffuse

Modified from Brambilla WD, et al: The new World Health Organization classification of lung tumours, *Eur Respir J* 18:1059-1068, 2001.

Improvements in local control and systemic chemotherapy have increased the interest in surgical intervention, even in the presence of mediastinal lymph node involvement. This intervention has necessitated a greater use of pathologic staging. A frequently used system is the TNM system, which has been accepted by the American Joint Committee on Cancer[3] (see Box 32-1).

Spread Patterns

Direct. As tumor cells continue to reproduce, the size of the mass increases. The mass itself may grow into surrounding structures. This is called local extension.[47] Tumors of the lungs are most likely to extend to other parts of the lungs, the ribs, heart, esophagus, and vertebral column.[15] They may grow silently for long periods. Patients may seek medical attention for pain related to local extension.

Tumors that are not encapsulated have an ability to invade and attach themselves to local structures such as the chest wall, diaphragm, pleura, and pericardium. When tumors are continuous with local structures, they are called fixed, an ominous prognostic sign. In lung cancer, direct invasion constitutes a T3 tumor (i.e., a minimum of stage III).[3]

Direct extension can occur through the visceral pleura into the pleural cavity. A malignant pleural effusion may occur as fluid in the pleural cavity accumulates. Another possible route of local extension is through the hilum. A tumor at or near the midline may grow directly into the hilum of the opposite lung.

Lymphatic. Cancer cells can break from the tumor mass and enter the lymphatics through two known routes. First, the cells can be trapped in the nodes as the lymphatic fluid is filtered. The cells continue to colonize in the nodes and eventually pass from one node to the next. This lymphatic spread is also called regional extension.[47] Second, cancer cells may grow through the lymph node and gain access to the circulatory system through blood vessels supplying the node.

The primary lymphatics that drain the lungs are the mediastinal and intrapulmonic channels (see Box 32-3). The lymphatics of the other organs in the thoracic cavity play an important role in the spread of lung cancer. The diaphragm, esophagus, pleural cavity, and heart are all in intimate relationship to the lungs.

The drainage pattern of the diaphragm runs through the muscle to the aorta, inferior vena cava, and esophagus. Lymph nodes and channels surrounding the esophagus (periesophageal lymphatics) connect to the cardiac lymphatics because the heart lymph flows in the direction of the periesophageal nodes. From there the flow is toward the thoracic duct. Some of the nodes of the diaphragm drain toward the stomach and pancreas.[26] Drainage continues to the right lymphatic duct.

The pleural surfaces are rich in lymphatic channels. These superficial channels drain into the hilum and connect to the veins and arteries at the bronchioles. Also, the intercostal nodes (between the ribs) have many anastomoses. Drainage flows from the nodes between the ribs to the parasternal, paravertebral, and internal mammary nodes[6] and then to the thoracic duct.

Lymphatics that drain the heart meet at the bifurcation of the trachea. Lymphatics from the left coronary and pulmonary arteries also connect to the cardiac nodes.[20] Thus, channels from the heart and lungs meet in the area of the carina.

Hematogenous. The circulatory system plays a major role in the distant spread of disease.[47] At the bifurcation of the trachea, the lymphatic drainage from the lungs, diaphragm, esophagus, pleural cavity, heart, stomach, and pancreas converges.[26] The drainage then has access to the entire body through the circulatory system at the thoracic duct and aorta.

The thoracic duct drains the left side of the body. The lymph moves medially and superiorly from the lungs into the thoracic duct. After moving through the thoracic duct, the lymph enters the circulatory system at the left subclavian vein. From the right side of the body, the lymph moves superiorly and medially into the right lymphatic duct. From the right lymphatic duct, the lymph flows into the right subclavian vein.[60]

Tumors also gain access to the circulatory system through blood vessels feeding the local lymphatic structures. In addition, spread occurs when malignant cells pass into blood vessels that supply the tumor.[27] Therefore, lung cancer has access to the circulatory system from a variety of directions.

Common Sites for Metastasis. After gaining access to the circulatory system, tumors of the lung set up colonies in virtually any site. These metastases, or secondary growths, occur most commonly in the cervical lymph nodes, liver, brain, bones, adrenal glands, kidneys, and contralateral (opposite) lung.[3]

Contralateral spread from hilum to hilum occurs as cells break away from the tumor and move to the area of the carina. Pressure changes as a result of respiration or gravity may transport the cell into the other hilum and then eventually into a resting place in the other lung. A "new" tumor may then begin to grow.

Treatment Considerations

The primary purpose of clinical and pathologic staging of lung cancer is to guide decision making regarding treatment goals and to understand and communicate issues regarding prognosis to patients and care givers. In the absence of demonstrable extrathoracic extension and despite poor long-term survival probability, patients should be considered as candidates for definitive or curative therapy and treatment programs designed with this intent should be proposed. Individuals with extrathoracic metastasis, severe chronic obstructive pulmonary disease, or other limiting underlying medical problems may be candidates for palliative therapy or supportive care alone. After these decisions are made, despite the fact that lung cancer has been evaluated in clinical trials for decades, an extraordinary degree of controversy exists regarding appropriate management.

All conventional modalities (i.e., surgery, radiation, and chemotherapy) alone or in combination have been studied extensively. Newer modalities such as immunotherapy, agents targeting the cancer cell growth and development pathways, and radiolabeled monoclonal antibodies are also being investigated. Recent reports regarding molecular profiling of lung cancers and targeting of specific cell pathways hold promise for future benefit.[64] Even in circumstances in which combined modalities appear to be advantageous, uncertainty remains concerning the most appropriate tactics of sequencing and dose modifications. However, practice guidelines are routinely updated and available online from the National Comprehensive

Cancer Network and are particularly useful in multidisciplinary settings to determine the most current consensus on treatment pathways.[43,44]

Surgery. Patients who are able to tolerate surgery and have intrathoracic disease of a limited nature, without pleural effusion or evidence of mediastinal extension, should be considered for definitive surgical intervention. Even with CT or PET scanning and careful attention to the mediastinum and paramediastinal tissues, only approximately 20% of all patients with lung cancer may be considered candidates for definitive surgery. Of those lung cancers, up to 90% may be resectable. Patients with complete resections (i.e., no evidence of a tumor at the resection margin and no evidence of regional lymphatic extension) have a 60% to 70% five-year survival rate for clinical stage IA disease; a 50% to 60% five-year survival rate for clinical stage IB disease; and a 50% to 60% five-year survival rate for clinical stage IIA disease. Increasing stage, based on tumor extent or lymph node involvement, significantly reduces 5-year survival and decreases the potential for total excision.[22,58,59] Careful analysis of recurrence patterns following apparently total excision have led to increased interest in postoperative adjuvant therapy and neoadjuvant preoperative therapies to potentially increase resection rates.[31,54]

Although limited wedge resections using video-assisted thoracoscopy (VAT) have been associated with good results for limited-stage disease, if feasible, a lobectomy with regional lymph node sampling is the preferred minimal procedure. Lesions that are central and involve a mainstem bronchus may require a total pneumonectomy. In this situation, careful attention must be given to preoperative and postoperative pulmonary function. If surgery is to be considered as primary therapy, there has been significant interest in the addition of radiation in a preoperative or postoperative setting. Although preoperative radiation had been used frequently, especially for apical tumors, most studies have failed to demonstrate a significant improvement in survival or increased resectability.[9,16,42] Studies combining radiation and chemotherapy in the preoperative and postoperative setting are ongoing.[65]

Surgery may be used occasionally for palliative purposes, but indications in this regard are relatively limited.

Chemotherapy. Although many bronchogenic cancers will respond to single-agent chemotherapy, these responses are rarely complete and are typically short-lived. Numerous trials have demonstrated improvements in response using combined multiple-agent drug programs over single-agent regimens, but issues related to increasing intensity and diversity of drug therapy remain unproved. The most effective single-agent drug remains cisplatin with newer agents such as paclitaxel, docetaxel, vinorelbine, gemcitabine, and irinotecan,[9] all demonstrating moderate (20% to 50%) response as single agents, and improvement in response including 5-year survival, when used in combination with cisplatin or carboplatin. Phase III trials comparing combined-modality chemotherapy and radiation have demonstrated improvements in survival from 13% at 2 years, and 6% at 5 years, up to 26% at 2 years, and 17% at 5 years for appropriate combinations. Recent studies have begun to include molecular targeting agents in the conventional chemotherapy regimens.[64]

SCLC may respond dramatically to chemotherapy if combinations such as cisplatin and etoposide (VP-16) are used in combination with radiation for intrathoracic disease and alone for extensive disease.[16,38,42,48]

Radiation. There is little evidence to suggest that postoperative radiation improves local control and/or survival in the absence of local residual disease or mediastinal-paramediastinal lymphadenopathy. A number of studies have suggested an improvement in 3- and 5-year survival with postoperative radiation if lymph nodes are positive and there is residual local disease. In addition, studies have demonstrated a reduction in local-regional failure.[17,24,34]

The evidence of improvement in local-regional control and survival with the addition of systemic chemotherapy to external radiation now suggests that this combination of modalities represents the standard of care for patients with local residual disease postoperatively or for unresectable disease patients in whom radiation fields can encompass known disease and who are not candidates for surgical intervention. The precise timing of chemotherapy and radiation, for example, sequential or concurrent, remains controversial; the precise definition of radiation fields and time-dose relationship also is unproved.

The Cancer and Acute Leukemia Group B (CALGB) have studied hyperfractionation techniques of 120 cGy twice daily to a total of 6960 cGy, which did not demonstrate improvement of results above and beyond those of conventional radiation. Studies of hyperfractionated accelerated radiation (360 cGy at 150 cGy three times daily for 12 days to a total of 5400 cGy) demonstrated a slight improvement in local regional control, but similar studies carried out by the Radiation Therapy Oncology Group, with concurrent chemotherapy, failed to demonstrate improvement and did produce significant toxicity.

Current standard therapy would generally include concurrent, sequential, or alternating chemotherapy and radiation, using radiation tumor doses between 4500 and 5400 cGy at 180 to 200 cGy per fraction, one fraction per day and five fractions per week.[14,16,23,65]

Recent literature has suggested that increasing doses and reduced morbidity are possible using three-dimensional planning with CT simulators and conformal radiation, or IMRT.[15,2,53] Although dose escalation has been achievable without a concomitant increase in morbidity, improvements in local control and/or survival have not as yet been demonstrated. There is also increasing interest and investigation of image-guided radiation therapy (IGRT) with consideration of and correction for respiratory motion.[62]

Advanced Disease. Palliative radiation is effective and commonly used for control of osseous and brain metastases. Skeletal pain can be relieved for extended periods in up to 90% of patients treated. If architectural bone disruption occurs, as in the case of vertebral body compression or pathologic fracture, the probability of pain relief is reduced. Generally, doses between 3000 and 4000 cGy in 200 to 300 cGy daily dose fractions are sufficient for pain relief and bone healing although recent reports have suggested comparable results with shorter courses of treatment and higher daily dose fractions. Some investigators have proposed using a single dose fraction of 800 cGy, These patients experienced satisfactory relief of pain but required more frequent re-treatment.[1] In those instances in which a pathologic fracture has occurred or evidence exists of impending fracture based on the loss of bone calcium (based on empirical observations rather than specific measurement), consideration should be given to internal fixation before radiation. If internal fixation is carried out, palliative radiation can begin within several days if the surgical incision can be avoided. If the incision is within the treatment field, initiation of radiation should be delayed for 7 to 10 days, providing for satisfactory wound healing. Many patients treated for palliation of osseous metastases will have received previous systemic chemotherapy, and careful attention must be paid to the stability of blood counts.

Patients developing brain metastases may present with seizures, headaches, focal or motor sensory deficits, gait disturbance, visual or speech changes, changes in memory, or personality alteration. Patients with seizure activity should receive antiseizure medication such as phenytoin (Dilantin) and moderate- to high-dose corticosteroids such as dexamethasone or prednisone. In the absence of seizure activity, there has been no demonstrated benefit to antiseizure therapy. Patients in whom significant intracranial edema is demonstrated on CT or MRI studies may note a rapid relief of symptoms with immediate initiation of high-dose corticosteroids, but these agents generally provide only short-term symptomatic relief. Radiation doses of 3000 to 4000 cGy in 10 to 15 fractions produce symptomatic relief in 35% to 75% of treated individuals. Patients in generally good clinical condition with apparent solitary intracranial metastases may benefit from surgical excision followed by radiation. The role of high-dose, short-course stereotactic radiosurgery (SRS) either alone or in combination with surgery and/or whole brain radiation continues to evolve. There is no evidence that the treatment modality used for SRS delivery impacts results.[41]

Signs and symptoms related to partial or complete obstruction of the superior vena cava may be evident in up to 5% of all lung cancer patients and may be secondary to extrinsic pressure on the vena cava or direct tumor extension into the vessel. Superior vena cava syndrome is considered an oncologic emergency requiring immediate initiation of palliative external beam radiation therapy, frequently in combination with high-dose corticosteroid therapy. Usual radiation techniques include three to four fractions of 300 to 400 cGy, followed by a reduction of the daily dose to 180 to 250 cGy. Because of the emergent nature of treatment initiation, sophisticated treatment planning and delivery techniques are often delayed so treatment can begin swiftly. Depending on the patient's general clinical status, extent of disease, and intent of therapy, the total dose is usually 4500 to 5000 cGy. Approximately 85% of patients treated for vena cava obstruction will experience some relief of symptoms within 2 to 3 weeks, but long-term survival is rare.

For control of hemoptysis, radiation doses of 3000 to 4000 cGy in 2 to 3 weeks using a small field are generally sufficient if the site of bleeding can be well localized. Hemoptysis secondary to a small endobronchial lesions or obstruction may be improved or relieved entirely using endoscopic laser fulguration in conjunction with external radiation, conventional low-dose rate brachytherapy, or high-dose rate afterloading brachytherapy.

Side Effects. Common acute side effects that occur during radiation therapy are dermatitis, erythema, and esophagitis. Routine departmental skin care is recommended. Dysphagia associated with inflammation of the esophagus occurs at approximately 3000 cGy (with conventional fractionation and in the absence of concurrent chemotherapy). Esophagitis can be relieved by medication or diet. Oral medications include liquid antacids and mucosal anesthetics such as lidocaine hydrochloride.[47] Occasionally, narcotic or non-narcotic analgesics may be necessary. Nutritional suggestions include foods that are soft, moist, and nonspicy and liquids at room temperature or slightly chilled. Patients may also experience coughing, dry throat, and excessive mucus secretions.

A chronic side effect caused by irritation of the trachea and bronchi is a dry, nonproductive cough. Other chronic effects include fibrosis of the lung and subcutaneous fibrosis of the skin.

Complications are different from side effects because they are usually a result of doses that exceed organ tolerance. Complications are serious and, in the case of pneumonitis, may be life threatening. If spinal cord tolerance is exceeded, myelopathy may occur. With serious neurologic complications the resulting infections can lead to death.

Treatment Data Capture and Treatment Planning

Critical Structures. Three critical structures are of primary concern in treatment planning for lung cancer: the spinal cord, heart, and normal lung.[47] Frequently, with utilization of definitive dose levels, the radiation tolerances of these organs can be exceeded. Additional concerns and uncertainties may be faced with inclusion of various drug programs into the treatment regimen or with underlying intrinsic organ disease. Therefore, doses to these structures must be carefully documented during planning and throughout the treatment course. Fields are designed so that organ tolerance is not exceeded. Advance planning before organ tolerance is reached is critically important so that the optimal dose distributions can be achieved.[15] Prescriptions for definitive chest radiation should include specific normal tissue dose constraints, and care should be exercised that these constraints are not exceeded during treatment delivery without specific approval.

The first critical structure considered is the spinal cord. Doses of radiation required to control lung cancer exceed the spinal cord tolerance of 4500 to 5500 cGy[52] (Table 32-1). Although higher spinal cord tolerance doses are discussed in the literature,[39,52] radiation oncologists generally take a conservative approach to the spinal cord dose by prescribing treatments that do not exceed the 4500-cGy limit. Remaining under that dose tolerance limit is especially important when large treatment fields are used and multiple vertebral segments exposed.[27] Standard practice for radiation therapists is to require a written order for all cord doses greater than 4500 cGy. In charting daily treatments, radiation therapists should monitor a spinal cord dose column to ensure that tolerance is not exceeded. When cord doses become close to 4000 cGy, if not already carried out, planning should commence for technique changes that will spare the cord so that treatment can continue without disruption. Frequently, the cord receives a daily dose that is higher than the prescribed dose to the tumor. The quality of a patient's life will be diminished and even death may result if these standards are not followed.

Radiation therapists should always monitor the status of spinal cord doses throughout the course of therapy to ensure that tolerance is not exceeded without a written order by a radiation oncologist.

If cord tolerance is exceeded, neurologic signals that normally move along the spinal cord may be blocked. Demyelination of the oligodendrocytes that conduct nerve impulses is responsible for some of the neurologic complications. In addition, damages in the form of fibrosis and occlusion of capillaries and arterioles result in a reduced blood supply to the neurons and oligodendrocytes in the region treated. Because nervous system tissue has severely limited or no regenerative abilities, damage is irreparable.[51] Clinical manifestations of cord damage such as myelitis (inflammation of the spinal cord) can occur. Depending on the level of the cord affected, quadriplegia or paraplegia may follow. Necrosis and infarction of the cord can occur. When radiation-induced transection of the cord occurs, Brown-Séquard's syndrome results, with paralysis and loss of sensations such as pain and temperature. The extent and nature of loss will be dependent on the spinal cord level involved in the damage.[47]

The second critical structure in the treatment of lung cancer is the heart. When 60% or more of the heart is treated with 4500 to 5500 cGy, pericarditis (inflammation of the pericardium) and pancarditis (inflammation of all parts of the heart) may result[51] (see Table 32-1). Pericarditis caused by radiation is often constrictive rather than effusive, meaning that scar tissue formation can constrict cardiac motion, rather than a fluid buildup within the pericardium. Surgical intervention may be necessary to relieve the constriction, but this is typically hampered by the previous cardiopulmonary radiation. Long-term complications can follow because of damage of the interstitial components of cardiac tissue, and the resulting fibrosis may damage the valves.[47]

The third critical structure to be considered in the treatment of lung cancer is the adjacent normal lung. The major complication that occurs is radiation pneumonitis, followed by fibrosis. Pneumonitis occurs from 1 to 3 months after radiation. Fibrosis occurs from 2 to 4 months after treatment.[47] Pneumonitis is the clinical manifestation of vascular, epithelial, and interstitial injuries. Patients exhibit dyspnea, fevers, night sweats, and/or cyanosis.[11] The chronic phase consists of severe dyspnea and coughing, clubbing of the fingers, and an abscess that can be followed by infection and sepsis.

Other structures included in fields designed to treat lung cancers are important but not critical. The esophagus, bone marrow, skin, and sometimes the liver with right lower lobe lung tumors have dose tolerances identified in Table 32-1. Generally, however, tolerance of these organs is not exceeded.

Parallel-Opposed Fields. The simplest fields used in the treatment of lung cancer are anterior and posterior parallel-opposed mediastinal fields, which typically include the primary tumor volume and adjacent mediastinum (Figure 32-6). Typically, AP/PA (anteroposterior/posteroanterior) field arrangements are designed to include the primary tumor volume or clinical target volume (CTV) (defined by radiographic techniques) with a 2.0- to 2.5-cm margin of apparently normal tissue (planning target volume [PTV]). If induction chemotherapy is used, the definition of tumor volume should be that obtained before initiation of chemotherapy. If a primary tumor is located in an upper lobe, or involves the mainstem bronchus, ipsilateral supraclavicular lymph nodes may be included. Ipsilateral hilar and superior mediastinal lymph nodes should be included with a 2.0-cm margin along with subcarinal lymph nodes to at least 5.0 cm below the carina. If the primary lesion involves the lower lobe or inferior mediastinum, the field should extend to the bottom of T10 or to the diaphragm. Although contralateral hilar lymph nodes had been routinely included in AP/PA fields in the past, they are generally excluded at present, unless disease involves the contralateral mediastinum, subcarinal, or contralateral hilar region.

When possible, normal tissues should be shielded to provide only the appropriate margins as noted previously. Ideally, this shielding is accomplished with customized blocking, such as alloys, Cerrobend, or MLC (see Figure 32-6). Doses to the tumor and critical structures such as the heart and spinal cord should also be monitored (Figure 32-7).

Modern radiation therapy delivery techniques for intrathoracic tumors typically involve high doses of radiation to critical and noncritical normal structures. For this reason, and the increasing availability of CT-directed treatment planning, two-dimensional treatment techniques have been largely supplanted

Table 32-1	Organ Tolerances	
Organ	**TD 5/5 (cGy)**	**TD 50/5 (cGy)**
Spinal cord	5000	6000
Normal lung	2000	3000
Heart	4300	5000
Esophagus	5000	5500
Bone marrow	2500	3500
Skin	5500	7000
Liver	3500	4000
Bone	6500	7000

Modified from Rubin P, Williams J, editors: Clinical *oncology a multidisciplinary approach for physicians and students*, ed 8, Philadelphia, 2001, Saunders.

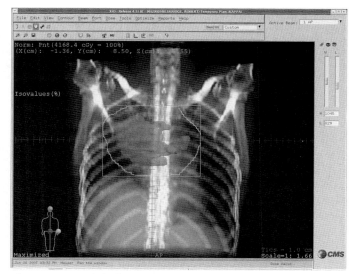

Figure 32-6 Digitally reconstructed radiograph for parallel-opposed fields for right lung tumor with extension across the midline. (Courtesy of Bayhealth Medical Center at Kent General Hospital, Dover, DE.)

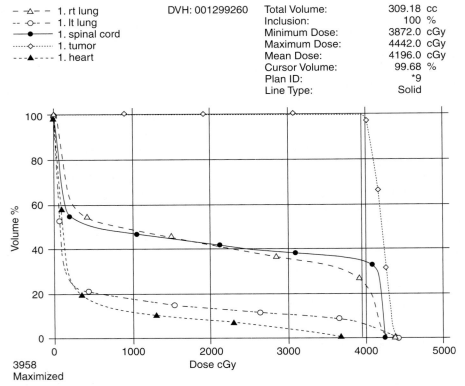

Figure 32-7. Dose-volume histogram measuring dose to the right and left lungs, spinal cord, tumor, and heart. Tumor received a maximum of 4442 cGy; spinal cord and heart received less than tolerance. See Figure 32-6 for DRR of fields. (Courtesy of Bayhealth Medical Center at Kent General Hospital, Dover, Del.)

by three-dimensional, volume-based techniques. Three-dimensional therapy (and the continuum of sophistication of three-dimensional methods such as IMRT and IGRT) currently represents the optimum standard level of care.

It is now apparent that the primary driver of lung motion is diaphragmatic excursion and that the variation in position of locally advanced lung tumors during a single treatment fraction can exceed 1 cm. The simplest intervention to reduce intratreatment motion is breath-holding, but this effect may be unpredictable, and the technique is frequently problematic for patients with underlying pulmonary disease. A number of studies have evaluated the impact and potential solutions for respiratory motion and a variety of technical solutions are entering the market place.[36]

Boosts Fields. **Boost fields** are used to deliver a high dose to a small volume. With boost fields the radiation dose is generally delivered to the gross tumor volume (GTV) only, excluding regional lymph nodes. Boost fields may be administered using AP/PA, or multiple-field combinations using three-dimensional or IMRT techniques, or employing customized beam shaping with MLC. Care must be taken to calculate doses to adjacent critical structures, such as the spinal cord, to ensure safe doses to those tissues. Investigators have reported studies utilizing concurrent (or field-within-a-field) boost techniques, in an attempt to optimize biological effectiveness of treatment and reduce duration.

Multiple-Field Combinations. Because patients with bronchogenic cancers typically have compromised pulmonary

function before initiation of radiation, the use of progressively reduced field sizes becomes even more essential.

Accurate positioning of the patient is essential, and immobilization devices and lasers should be used when possible. A sagittal laser and lasers aligned with marks on the sides of the patient increase the accuracy of the setup. Of critical importance is the arm position with off-cord boosts because the probability of the patient rolling to one side or the other increases if the arms are raised above the patient's head. Treatment planning should be carried out with the arms placed in the actual treatment position. In addition, the spinal cord can receive doses above tolerance if lasers are not aligned properly. Geographical misses can occur if the patient is not aligned accurately for every treatment. This goal of reproducibility is improved with the use of lasers and immobilization for alignment.[57]

During the planning process the depth of the spinal cord must be determined. If available, CT images are useful; the depth of the cord in the patient is determined from the images of the individual vertebral bodies in the field to be treated. In radiographic simulation, **orthogonal images**[57] are taken to determine the cord depth. Generally, anterior and lateral films of the thorax (orthogonal radiographs) are taken at right angles. The physical depth of the cord in the patient is measured from the image through the use of a demagnification calculation.

The depth of the spinal cord is important for two reasons. First, tumoricidal doses exceed the tolerance of the spinal cord. Second, because the depth of the spinal cord varies along the vertebral column, the dose calculated to one point in the spinal cord is not the same for the remainder of the cord. For example, the depth of the cord in the lower cervical area may be 5 cm, whereas the depth in the lower thorax may be 8 cm. If the tumor is close to the midplane (approximately 10 cm), overdoses to both areas of the spinal cord can occur. Even if cord tolerance is considered in the prescription, the dose the patient receives to the cord must be monitored closely because the dose along the length of the field varies as the depth of the cord changes. In situations with significant dose gradients along the spinal cord, additional running total columns in the treatment chart may be appropriate to monitor the dose differences for the various regions.

When the spinal column is not midplane the image of the anterior field is different from that of the posterior field. This is caused by divergence. The effect of divergence can be seen through a comparison of the disc spaces on the anterior and posterior images. When fields are exactly parallel-opposed the images may not be identical.[7]

In the planning of treatments for patients with lung cancer, magnification-measuring devices are particularly useful in finding the spinal cord depth. The cord depth can be determined from the lateral orthogonal film. The amount of the conventional simulation table on the film causes a distortion because of the width of the table and the distance the beam travels. Tables can be marked with a radiopaque wire in the center to reduce distortion.[7] Alternatively, the therapist can palpate the spinous processes and carefully tape on the patient's back a piece of solder wire that will relate the vertebral column to the skin surface. During simulation in the supine position the wire will be in contact with the table, thereby indicating the table on the radiographic image.

In the planning of fields for lung tumors near the heart, the volume of the heart treated should be considered. In particular, when parallel-opposed beams are weighted anteriorly to reduce the spinal cord dose, the dose to the heart should also be measured so that tolerance is not exceeded Use of chemotherapy should be monitored closely. Drugs such as doxorubicin (Adriamycin) have cardiac toxicity that has a synergistic effect when the drug is used in combination with radiation.[47]

The volume of lung treated and the total dose must be considered to avoid complications related to the lung. The dose tolerance to the lung generally ranges from 2000 to 3000 cGy[52] (see Table 32-1). Large volumes of lung are projected to have at least a 50% complication rate at 3000 cGy (TD 50/5, or 50% of the patients in 5 years). Fraction sizes range from 180 to 200 cGy. Care is taken throughout the planning process to minimize the amount of noncancerous lung in the fields. Customized beams such as reduced and boost fields, MLCs, and off-cord arrangements are used to limit the beam transmission through unaffected lung. The nature of lung tissue itself is notable. Lung density is less than the density of other tissue because of the presence of air (oxygen and carbon dioxide) in the organs. Therefore, the dose to the tumor and lung tissue is increased by 15% to 20%.[29,47] Heterogeneity corrections can be used to compensate for this phenomenon.[37]

Off-Axis Points. Typically, doses are calculated to the center of a field or to a normalized dose point (or volume) within a three-dimensional field. With lung tumors, however, knowledge about the structures not in the center is important. For example, a patient with a left upper lobe tumor will have off-axis points to include the tumor, supraclavicular nodes, and mediastinum.

Customized Beams. Optimal patient care frequently requires combinations of several types of field designs. For example, multiple fields with boosts, collimator rotations, and weighting may be needed to deliver the best dose distribution. Mixed beams of photons and electrons may be used to meet specific clinical challenges, such as a mass extending through the chest wall. Also, dual-energy accelerators have the capacity to customize the beam to an effective energy level that is not possible with a single-energy conventional accelerator. Beam arrangements are selected to cover the tumor and simultaneously limit the dose to the normal tissue. IMRT and IGRT represent newer steps on the continuum of beam customization.

Specific anatomic features, such as a **kyphosis** or **scoliosis** (excessive curvature of the spine), require special attention. With curvatures of the spine the collimator can be rotated to follow the vertebral column. Another approach is the use of MLCs to tailor the field to meet the individual patient's anatomy without rotating the collimator. Patients with barrel-shaped chests may benefit from the use of a compensating wedge (Figure 32-8).

There is increasing evidence that the use of IMRT may enable delivery of higher doses to irregularly shaped tumor volumes with reduced doses to normal tissue structures. Extensive studies in this regard have been carried out for tumor sites such as the prostate, but the normal movement of the lung and mediastinal structures during respiration presents added challenges in this regard. IMRT techniques have not as yet been adopted for routine use.

Doses. Total doses vary depending on the intent of therapy and precise tissue. Patients treated with a curative intent typically require higher doses and more complex field arrangements. Patients treated with palliative intent generally have the option of lower total doses, shorter courses of therapy, and more simple field arrangements. Definitive doses to control or cure localized SCLC generally range from 4500 to 5400 cGy at 180 to 200 cGy per fraction. Doses for definitive management of NSCLC generally range from 6000 to 7500 cGy at 180 to 200 cGy daily dose fractions. When used with systemic chemotherapy, especially concomitantly, total doses may be somewhat reduced.[14]

Definitive doses to control or cure localized bronchogenic carcinomas range from 6000 to 7500 cGy[13,15,45] (Table 32-2). Initial field arrangements are generally prescribed between 4000 and 4500 cGy. Boost fields follow in various combinations until tumoricidal doses are achieved. Various fraction patterns can be used, depending on whether conventional fractionation, hyperfractionation, accelerated fractionation, or accelerated hyperfractionation is prescribed.[35,55] **Conventional fractionation** uses a 180 to 200-cGy dose given once per day. The other fraction patterns change the conventional approach by altering the fraction size (either increased or decreased), daily dose (based on fraction size and number of fractions per day), number of treatment days, and/or total dose in an effort to improve patient tolerance and survival. Table 32-3 displays these different approaches to fractionation in a hypothetical patient.

Palliative treatment is given to relieve symptoms. For lung cancer, treatment can be given to relieve an airway obstruction. In these situations the total tumor dose ranges from 4000

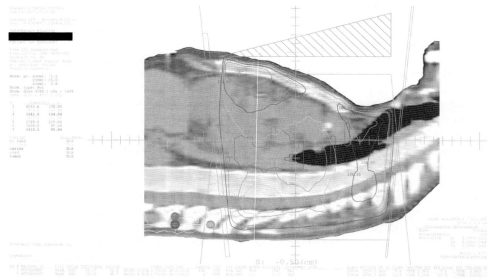

Figure 32-8. Use of compensating wedge to address dose distribution across a sloping chest. (Courtesy of Bayhealth Medical Center at Kent General Hospital, Dover, Del.)

to 5000 cGy.[47] Delivery of biological equivalent doses (BED) may permit shorter courses of therapy with altered fractionation patterns, depending on the patient's response.

For a patient with superior vena cava syndrome, initial doses are high for the first one to three treatments and range from 350 to 400 cGy.[13] Because of the large volume and high doses, the daily doses should be reduced after the initial treatments. Initial prescribed doses are generally 350 to 1200 cGy, followed by 200-cGy fractions to a total dose of 4500 to 5000 cGy.

Brachytherapy can be used in the treatment of lung cancer. High-dose-rate (HDR) remote afterloading is used in the treatment of endobronchial disease.[32] For example, during a course of external beam radiation a supplemental dose of radiation can be given with HDR, using 500 cGy for two to four treatments. In the event of recurrent disease, HDR may also be useful, particularly if spinal cord tolerance has been reached or the airway is compromised.

Role of Radiation Therapist

Education. Opportunities exist for the radiation therapist to evaluate the patient daily for needs related to education,

Table 32-2	External Beam Treatment Doses	
Treatment Approach	**Total Dose (cGy)**
Primary radiation	6000-7500
Surgery + radiation (postoperative)	5000-6500
Chemotherapy + radiation	3000-5000
Palliation and/or recurrence	4000-5000
Preoperative (superior sulcus)	3000-4500

Modified from Cox JD, editor: *Moss' radiation oncology: rationale, technique, results,* ed 7, St. Louis, 1994, Mosby; DeVita V, Hellman S, Rosenburg S: *Principles and practice of oncology,* ed 4, Philadelphia, 1993, JB Lippincott; and Pancoast HK: Superior pulmonary sulcus tumor, *JAMA* 99:17.

communication, and assessment. Frequently, patients need education regarding testing procedures such as x-ray examinations and blood tests. The information should include the reason that the tests are needed, the location and time to report, and special requirements such as fasting and other preparations. Procedures that seem uncomplicated to medical professionals may be overwhelming to patients and family members. Radiation therapists should take time to explain carefully and at the appropriate level the how, why, and when details of a particular study. Patient education is important from the time of consultation and continues to the last day of treatment. Education continues when patients return for follow-up visits. Patients have a right to this education as defined in the "Patient's Bill of Rights" supported by the American Hospital Association. At any point, a patient can refuse care (i.e., refuse further treatment). When possible the therapist must try to ensure patient understanding. Sometimes questions can be one-sided; the patient is not given the opportunity to indicate an understanding of the information received. The therapist should use a questioning style permitting the patient to reflect an answer that indicates an understanding of the explanation. Patient compliance is important to achieve the goal of therapy, whether definitive or palliative, and patient (and caregiver) education is a critical step in maximizing compliance.

Communication. Communication with patients and family members is essential. Details related to daily treatments, appointment times, and the length of treatment require initial education followed by frequent reinforcement. Communication is almost continuous throughout the day. As related to the patient, the scheduling of daily treatments and other planning times throughout the course of therapy requires reinforcement. Also of concern to patients is the management of the other commitments in their lives. Radiation therapists need to be sensitive and responsive to the demands placed on the patient by competing forces. For example, the scheduling of a simulation appointment for off-cord boosts and subsequent patient notification

Table 32-3	Fraction Patterns and Total Doses for Primary Radiation			
Type of Fractionation	**Fraction Size**	**Daily Dose**	**Treatment Days**	**Total Dose (cGy)**
Conventional fractionation	180-200	180-200	30-34	6000-6120
Hyperfractionation	120	240	30	7200
Accelerated fractionation	160	320	19	6080
Accelerated hyperfractionation	160	320	23	7360

should be done in advance. In this way the patient is given the opportunity to determine the best way to keep this appointment. If a problem arises, enough time should exist for the therapist and patient to collaborate in a positive manner on the way to work through the patient's special needs and concerns.

The Health Insurance Portability and Accountability Act of 1996 (HIPAA), Public Law 104-191, established sweeping new guidelines for patient privacy and access to patient information and records. Because of the complexity of this act and variations in interpretations under specific circumstances, it is incumbent on radiation therapists to acquaint themselves with policies of their specific facility or institution, especially related to contact with family members and others who play significant support roles in the treatment of lung cancer.

Assessment. Assessment is the process of evaluating a patient's condition. With lung cancer therapy, as with other types of treatment, the condition of a patient's skin should be assessed before daily treatment is given. Ongoing monitoring of dermatitis and erythema and appropriate skin care is necessary to prevent skin breakdown. If the skin is blistered, cracked or open, and oozing, treatment should be withheld until a physician's medical opinion is obtained.

A nutritional evaluation of the ability to swallow solid foods, liquids, and medications should be done to determine whether dietary counseling or medical intervention is required. Adequate fluid intake is particularly important to prevent dehydration because patients may reduce or stop their fluid intake as a result of the discomfort associated with esophagitis.

The status of blood counts should be reviewed. White blood cell counts of 2000/mm^3 or less and platelets of 50,000/mm^3 or less should not be treated without a written order. Patients receiving chemotherapy must be monitored closely.

Changes in a patient's condition can be observed during therapy. As described previously, lung cancer often metastasizes to the central nervous system and skeletal system. Clinically, evidence of brain metastasis may be observed with personality changes, headaches, and visual disturbances. With spinal metastases, patients may complain of severe neck and/or back pain and they may describe bowel and/or bladder dysfunctions such as incontinence. In addition, patients may experience leg and/or motor weakness that the therapist may observe as an unsteady gait or limp. Changes in gait or unusual difficulty getting on or off of the treatment couch should be questioned as they could be indications of early tumor spread. Symptoms related to pleural or pericardial effusion include dyspnea, increased respiratory effort,

chest pain, a change in a cough, or a fever.[25] Such observations, as well as apparent onset of difficulty with respiration when assuming a supine treatment position must be reported to the radiation oncologist for medical evaluation.

Radiation therapists should monitor a patient's condition throughout therapy especially:
- *Headaches, changes in personality and visual changes as these can be signs of brain metastases.*
- *Neck and/or back pain, incontinence, leg or motor weaknesses, changes in gait or unusually difficulty getting on and off the treatment table as these may be signs of tumor spread to the spinal column or cord.*
- *Dyspnea, chest pain, change in cough, or fever, as these may be related to pleural or pericardial effusion.*

CASE I

Disease Management in Practice

Non–Small Cell Lung Cancer

A 55-year-old man presented to the emergency department with a recent history of increasing swelling of the legs, face, and arms associated with increasing shortness of breath. CT of the chest showed a large anterior mediastinal mass with a clot in the pulmonary vein. The patient had a history of left upper lobectomy 13 years earlier without subsequent therapy. Emergent radiation therapy was planned for 25 Gy in 10 fractions, followed by a biopsy. Diagnosis: NSCLC with superior vena cava syndrome.

Radiation therapy was instituted using AP/PA fields with 18-MV beams with 250-cGy fractions totaling 2500 cGy (Figure 32-9). Reduced fields using AP/PA fields with 18-MV beams and 180 cGy for seven treatments totaling 1,260 cGy followed (Figure 32-10). A second boost was delivered using 6-MV and 18-MV beams, 180-cGy fractions for eight treatments totaling 1440 cGy. The total dose was 5400 cGy. Following completion of radiation therapy, the patient was referred for chemotherapy.

Lung Cancer

A 60-year-old man complained of pain down the medial aspect of his right arm and across his upper right anterior chest area. The initial diagnosis was arthritis. As the pain became more intense, he noticed weight loss and also required narcotics for pain control. He has smoked 1.5 packs of cigarettes daily since age 15.

PET-CT was done and showed thickening at the right apex with bony erosion of the first and second thoracic vertebrae and adjacent ribs highly suggestive of a Pancoast tumor (see Figure 32-11). The mass measured 2.6 cm and there

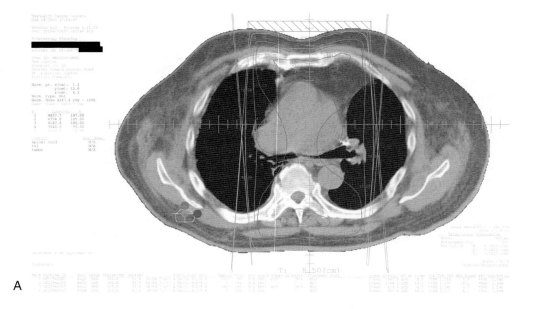

A

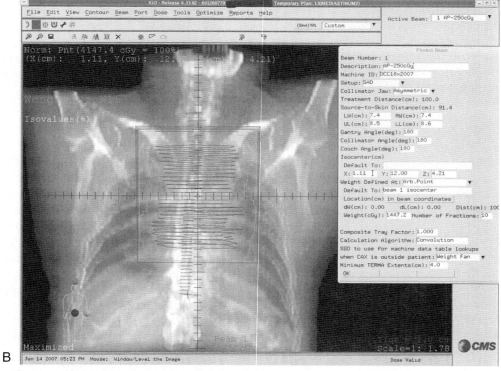

B

Figure 32-9. A, Anteroposterior (AP)/AP fields to right upper lobe and mediastinum. **B**, Beam's eye view of AP field.

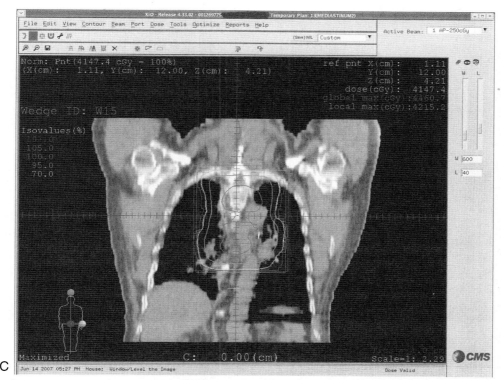

Figure 32-9, cont'd C, Beam's eye view of isodose values. (See Color Plate 20.) (Courtesy of Bayhealth Medical Center at Kent General Hospital, Dover, Del.)

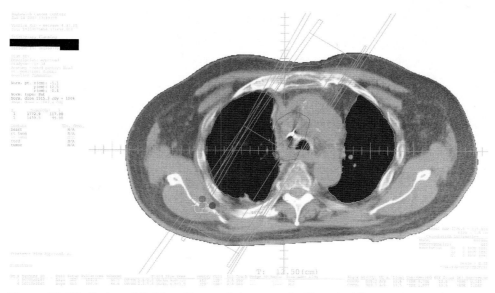

Figure 32-10. Reduced fields with parallel-opposed off-cord obliques. (See Color Plate 21.) (Courtesy of Bayhealth Medical Center at Kent General Hospital, Dover, Del.)

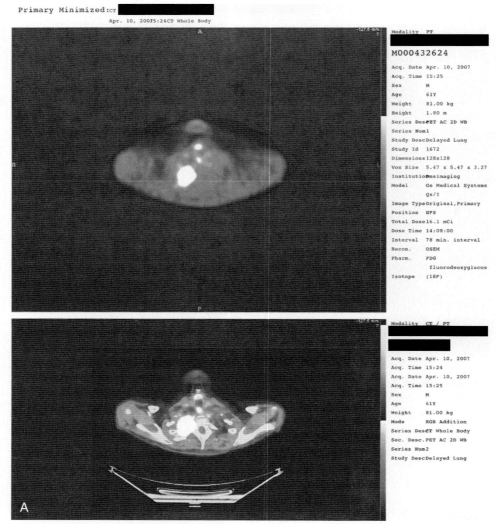

Figure 32-11. A, Positron emission tomography (PET)-computed tomography (CT) of the chest with right upper lobe mass preradiation therapy.

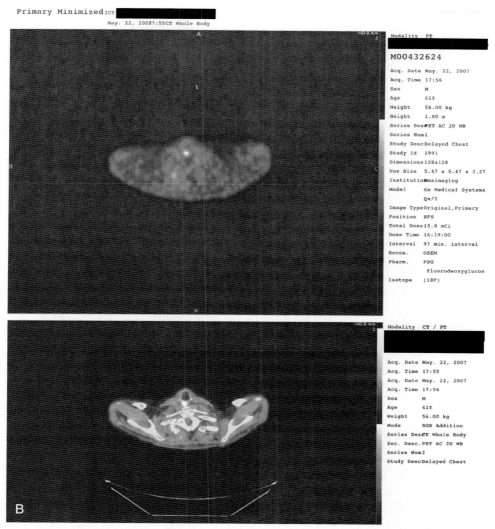

Figure 32-11, cont'd B, PET-CT of the chest with significantly reduced activity in the right upper lobe postradiation therapy. (**A** and **B**, Courtesy of Bayhealth Medical Center at Milford Memorial Hospital, Milford, DE.)

was no sign of region lymph node involvement. Subsequent PET imaging revealed an intense, hypermetabolic area measuring 4.5 × 1.8 × 3 cm at the right apex and superior sulcus with no other activity seen. In order to obtain a diagnosis, he underwent a limited thoracotomy. Pathology was confirmed for NSCLC. *Diagnosis:* Right apical lung cancer, non small-cell of the Pancoast type.

Triple modality therapy was planned starting with chemotherapy and radiation therapy.

Preoperative radiation therapy was completed to the right upper lobe primary and mediastinal lymph nodes with an off-cord boost. The technique used was AP/PA three-dimensional conformal therapy with 6-MV and 18-MV beams with the oblique boost fields using the same combination of energies. Then, 3789 cGy was administered to the AP/PA fields (Figure 32-12) plus 720 cGy to the parallel-opposed oblique fields (Figure 32-13). The patient received a total of 45 Gy (Figure 32-14, *A* and *B*).

The patient was pain free at his 1-month follow-up visit. Post radiation therapy PET-CT scan revealed complete regression of the tumor. Surgery followed with a right upper lobectomy with no tumor noted. Patient's follow-up plan is for monthly visits and PET-CT monitoring every 3 to 4 months.

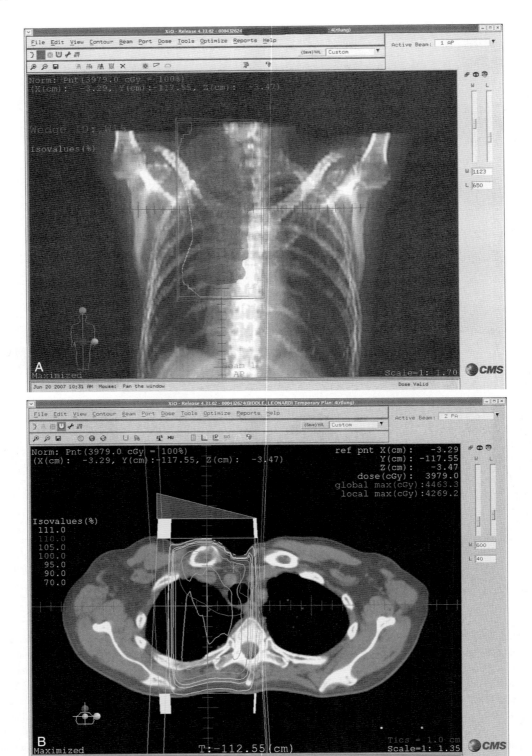

Figure 32-12. A, Digitally reconstructed radiograph of anterior field using multileaf collimation and a single wedge with tumor mass noted. **B,** Isodose distribution of anteroposterior (AP)/posteroanterior (PA) fields.

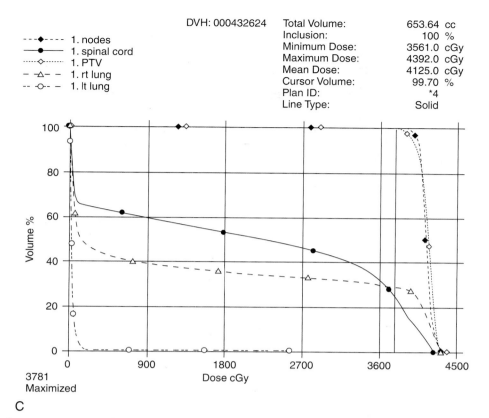

Total Volume: 653.64 cc
Inclusion: 100 %
Minimum Dose: 3561.0 cGy
Maximum Dose: 4392.0 cGy
Mean Dose: 4125.0 cGy
Cursor Volume: 99.70 %
Plan ID: *4
Line Type: Solid

C

Figure 32-12, cont'd C, Dose-volume histogram of AP/AP fields. (Dosimetry courtesy of Bayhealth Medical Center at Milford Memorial Hospital, Milford, DE.)

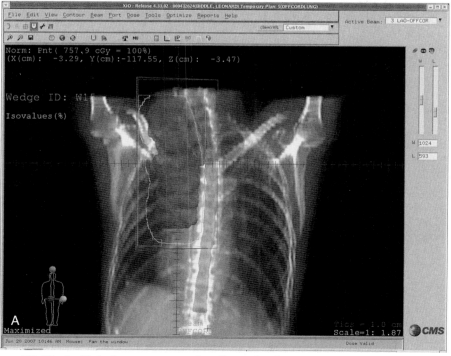

Figure 32-13. A, Digitally reconstructed radiograph of anterior oblique boost field with multileaf collimation and wedges. Note: tumor and spinal cord location.

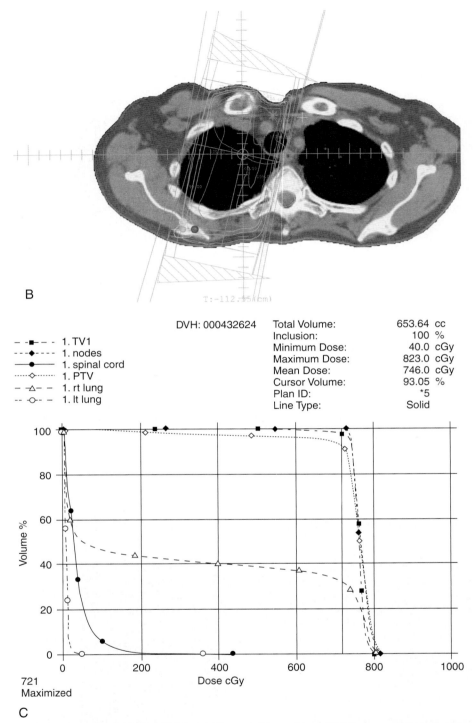

B

DVH: 000432624	Total Volume:	653.64	cc
	Inclusion:	100	%
	Minimum Dose:	40.0	cGy
— –■– – 1. TV1	Maximum Dose:	823.0	cGy
– – – ◆ – – – – 1. nodes	Mean Dose:	746.0	cGy
—●—— 1. spinal cord	Cursor Volume:	93.05	%
·····◇····· 1. PTV	Plan ID:	*5	
– –△– – 1. rt lung	Line Type:	Solid	
– –○– – 1. lt lung			

721
Maximized

C

Figure 32-13, cont'd B, Isodose distribution of oblique boost fields. **C**, Dose-volume histogram of off-cord boost fields. (Dosimetry courtesy of Bayhealth Medical Center at Milford Memorial Hospital, Milford, Del.)

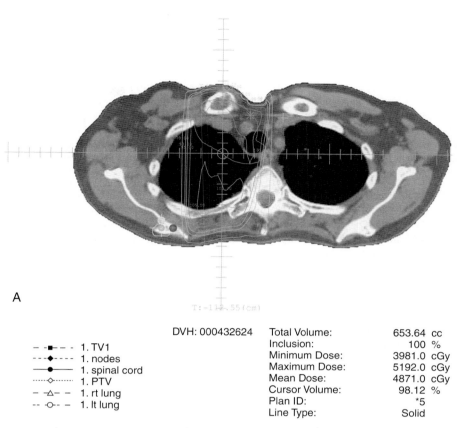

A

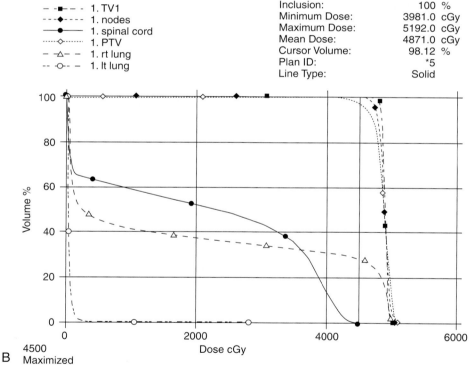

DVH: 000432624

- ---■--- 1. TV1
- ---◆--- 1. nodes
- ——●—— 1. spinal cord
- ········◇········ 1. PTV
- --△-- 1. rt lung
- --○-- 1. lt lung

Total Volume:	653.64	cc
Inclusion:	100	%
Minimum Dose:	3981.0	cGy
Maximum Dose:	5192.0	cGy
Mean Dose:	4871.0	cGy
Cursor Volume:	98.12	%
Plan ID:	*5	
Line Type:	Solid	

B   4500
Maximized

Figure 32-14. A, Composite isodose distribution of all fields. **B,** Dose-volume histogram composite of all fields. (Dosimetry courtesy of Bayhealth Medical Center at Milford Memorial Hospital, Milford, Del.)

SUMMARY

- Tobacco exposure is the leading cause of lung cancer, followed by occupational and radon exposure.
- Performance ability at the time of diagnosis is closely related to prognosis.
- A chest x-ray is the most common study used to detect lung cancer.
- The carina is important because malignant cells can break away from the tumor and travel from one hila of the lung to the other.
- Lung cancer spreads by direct extension to adjacent anatomy; via the lymphatics that drain the tumor site; and into the circulatory system via the thoracic duct and aorta, and the blood vessels that feed the local lymphatic structures.
- Common sites of lung cancer metastasis include liver, brain, bones, adrenal glands, contralateral lung, cervical lymph nodes, and kidneys.
- Common signs and symptoms of lung cancer include cough, hemoptysis, dyspnea, and chest pain.
- Surgery is performed for diagnosis of lung cancer as well as to remove the tumor mass. Surgery may be used pre and post radiation therapy and/or chemotherapy depending on stage.
- Chemotherapy using multiagent cycles may be used to treat lung cancer, especially in combination with surgery and/or radiation therapy.
- Radiation therapy either preoperatively or postoperatively typically consists of external beam plans to help control local and/or residual disease.

Review Questions

1. Microscopically, diffusion of oxygen and carbon dioxide takes place at the:
   a. bifurcation of the trachea
   b. right and left primary bronchi
   c. bronchiolar ducts
   d. alveolar-capillary membranes
2. Symptoms associated with local disease include:
   I. hemoptysis
   II. dyspnea
   III. orthopnea
   a. I only
   b. II only
   c. I and II only
   d. I, II, and III
3. Symptoms associated with regional disease include:
   I. dysphagia
   II. superior vena cava syndrome
   III. orthopnea
   a. I only
   b. II only
   c. I and II only
   d. I, II, and III
4. In what part of the lung are primary squamous cell carcinomas usually found?
   a. superiorly
   b. centrally

   c. laterally
   d. peripherally
5. Critical structures frequently located in the treatment fields for lung cancer include:
   a. normal lung and trachea
   b. esophagus and trachea
   c. spinal cord and heart
   d. heart and esophagus
6. Describe three criteria related to an individual's tobacco exposure that appear to increase the risk of developing lung cancer.
7. What are three variables that appear to affect significantly the prognosis of patients with lung cancer?
8. Name the two groups of lymphatics that are primarily responsible for the regional spread of bronchogenic carcinoma.
9. With conventional fractionation, what is the commonly accepted definitive dose range for localized bronchogenic carcinomas?
10. List at least three common acute side effects a patient may experience during the course of treatment.

The answers to the Review Questions can be found by logging on to our website at: *http://evolve.elsevier.com/Washington+Leaver/ principles*

Questions to Ponder

1. Discuss reasons that the incidence of lung cancer is rising.
2. Compare and contrast the various issues related to radiosensitivity and radiocurability of lung cancer.
3. What are common signs and symptoms of bronchogenic carcinomas? What are uncommon signs and symptoms?
4. Discuss the nonrespiratory signs and symptoms of lung cancer (i.e., neurologic findings).
5. Analyze the anatomic considerations in treatment field design.

REFERENCES

1. Agarawal JP, et al. The role of external beam radiotherapy in the management of bone metastases, *Clin Oncol (R Coll Radiol)* 18:747-760, 2006.
2. American Cancer Society. Cancer prevention and early detection, facts and figures 2008 (website): www.cancer.org. Accessed August 22, 2008.
3. American Joint Committee on Cancer: *The staging of cancer*, ed 6, New York, 2002, Springer-Verlag.
4. Antman KA, et al: Update on malignant mesothelioma, *Oncology* 19:1301-1316, 2005.
5. Bauer M, et al: Prognostic factors in cancer of the lung. In Cox JD, editor: *Syllabus: a categorical course in radiation therapy: lung cancer*, Oak Brook, IL, 1985, Radiological Society of North America.
6. Baum GL, Wolinski E: *Textbook of pulmonary diseases*, ed 5, New York, 1994, Little, Brown.
7. Bentel GC, Nelson CE, Noell KT: *Radiation therapy planning: including problems and solutions*, ed 2, New York, 1996, McGraw-Hill.
8. Brambilla WD, et al: The new World Health Organization classification of lung tumours, *Eur Respir J* 18:1059-1068, 2001.
9. Choy H, MacCrae RL: Irinotecan in combined modality therapy for locally advanced non-small cell lung cancer, *Oncology* 15:31-36, 2001.
10. Chung CK, et al: Evaluation of adjuvant postoperative radiotherapy for lung cancer, *Int J Radiat Oncol Biol Phys* 8:1877-1880, 1982.
11. Clark R, Idh DC: Small-cell lung cancer treatment progress and prospects, *Oncology* 12:647-658, 1998.

12. Cohen MH: Signs and symptoms of bronchogenic carcinoma. In Straus MJ, editor: *Lung cancer clinical diagnosis and treatment*, New York, 1977, Grune and Stratton.

13. Cox JD, Ang KK, editors: *Radiation oncology: rationale, technique, results*, ed 8, St. Louis, 2003, Mosby.

14. Curran WJ Jr: Combined modality therapy for limited stage small cell lung cancer, *Semin Oncol* 28:1422, 2001.

15. DeVita V, Hellman S, Rosenberg S, editors: *Principles and practice of oncology*, ed 6, Philadelphia, 2001, JB Lippincott.

16. Dillman RO, et al: A randomized trial of induction chemotherapy plus high dose radiation vs. radiation alone in stage III non-small cell lung cancer, *N Engl J Med* 323:940-945, 1999.

17. Eisert DR, Cox JD, Komaki R: Irradiation for bronchial carcinoma: reasons for failure. I. Analysis as a function of dose-time-fractionations, *Cancer* 37:2655-2670, 1976.

18. Emami B, et al: Phase I/II study of treatment of locally advanced (T3/T4) non-oat cell lung cancer with high dose radiotherapy (rapid fractionation): radiation therapy oncology group study, *Int J Radiat Oncol Biol Phys* 15:1021-1025, 1988.

19. Erozan YS, Frost JK: Cytopathological diagnosis of lung cancer, *Semin Oncol* 1:191-198, 1974.

20. Fishman AP: *Pulmonary diseases and disorders*, ed 2, New York, 1988, McGraw-Hill.

21. Gazdar AF: Pathology's impact on lung cancer management, *Contemp Oncol* 3:22-31, 1993.

22. Ginsberg RJ: Multi-modality treatment of resectable non-small lung cancer, *Clin Lung Cancer* 1:194-200, 2000.

23. Gordon GS, Vokes EEL: Chemoradiation for locally advanced unresectable non-small carcinoma of the lung, *Oncology* 13:1075-1084, 1999.

24. Green N, et al: Postresection irradiation for primary lung cancer, *Radiology* 116:405-407, 1975.

25. Groenwald SL, et al: *Manifestations of cancer and cancer treatment*, Boston, 1992, Jones and Bartlett.

26. Haagensen CD, et al: *The lymphatics in cancer*, Philadelphia, 1972, WB Saunders.

27. Hall TC, editor: Paraneoplastic syndromes, *Ann N Y Acad Sci* 230:367-377, 1974.

28. Henschke CI, et al: Survival of patients with stage I lung cancer detected on CT screening. *N Engl J Med* 355:1763-1771, 2006.

29. Kahn FM: *The physics of radiation therapy*, ed 3, Philadelphia, 2003, Lippincott Williams and Wilkins.

30. Karnofsky DA, Burchenal JH: The clinical evaluation of chemotherapeutic agents in cancer. In Macleod CM, editor: *Evaluation of chemotherapeutic agents*, New York, 1949, Columbia University Press.

31. Kelsey CR, Light KL, Marks LB: Patterns of failure after resection of non-small cell lung cancer: implications for postoperative radiation therapy volumes. *Int J Radiat Oncol Biol Phys* 65:1097-1105, 2006.

32. Komaki R: Preoperative radiation therapy for superior sulcus lesions, *Chest Surg Clin North Am* 1:13-35, 1991.

33. Komaki R, Garden AS, Cundiff JH: Endobronchial radiotherapy. In Roth HA, Cox JD, Hong WK, editors: *Advances in diagnosis and therapy of lung cancer*, Cambridge, MA, 1993, Blackwell.

34. Lally BE, et al. Postoperative radiotherapy for stage II and III non-small-cell lung cancer using the Surveillance, Epidemiology, and End Results database, *J Clin Oncol* 24:2998-3006, 2006.

35. Levitt SH, Kahn FM, Potish RA: *Levitt and Tapley's technological basis of radiation therapy practical clinical applications*, ed 2, Philadelphia, 1992, Lea and Febiger.

36. Liu HH, et al: Assessing respiration-induced tumor motion and internal target volume using four-dimensional computed tomography for radiotherapy of lung cancer. *Int J Radiat Oncol Biol Phys* 68:531-540, 2007.

37. Mah K, van Dyk J: On the impact of tissue inhomogeneity corrections in clinical thoracic radiation therapy, *Int J Radiat Oncol Biol Phys* 21:1257-1267, 1991.

38. Mantravadi RVP, et al: Unresectable non-oat cell carcinoma of the lung: definitive radiation therapy, *Radiology* 172:851-855, 1989.

39. Marcus RB, Million RR: The incidence of myelitis after irradiation of the cervical spinal cord, *Int J Radiat Oncol Biol Phys* 19:3-8, 1990.

40. Mew D, Pass H: Malignant mesotheliomas: a clinical challenge, *Contemp Oncol* 3:50-67, 1993.

41. Murray KJ, et al. A randomized phase III study of accelerated hyperfractionation versus standard in patients with unresected brain metastases: a report of the Radiation Therapy Oncology Group (RTOG), *Int J Radiat Oncol Biol Phys* 39:571-574, 1997.

42. Murray N: Small-cell lung cancer at the millennium: radiotherapy innovations improve survival while new chemotherapy treatments remain unproven, *Clin Lung Cancer* 1:181-190, 2000.

43. National Comprehensive Cancer Network: Non-small cell lung cancer (website): www.nccn.org. Accessed June 15, 2007.

44. National Comprehensive Cancer Network: Small-cell lung cancer (website): www.nccn.org. Accessed June 15, 2007.

45. Pancoast HK: Superior pulmonary sulcus tumor, *JAMA* 99:17, 1932.

46. Patz EF Jr, Erasmus J: Positron emission tomography imaging in lung cancer, *Clin Lung Cancer* 1:42-48, 1999.

47. Perez CA, Brady LW, editors: *Principles and practice of radiation oncology*, ed 3, Philadelphia, 1998, JB Lippincott.

48. Rapp E, et al: Chemotherapy can prolong survival in patients with advanced non-small-cell lung cancer: report of a Canadian multicenter randomized trial, *J Clin Oncol* 6:633-641, 1988.

49. Richardson RH, et al: The use of fiberoptic bronchoscopy and brush biopsy in the diagnosis of suspected pulmonary malignancy, *Am Rev Respir Dis* 109:63-66, 1974.

50. Rigler LG: The earliest roentgenographic signs of carcinoma of the lung, *JAMA* 195:655, 1966.

51. Rubin P, editor: *Radiation biology and radiation pathology syllabus*, Reston, VA, 1975, American College of Radiology.

52. Rubin P, Casarett GW: *Clinical radiation pathology*, Philadelphia, 1968, WB Saunders.

53. Rubin P, Williams J, editors: Clinical *oncology a multidisciplinary approach for physicians and students*, ed 8, Philadelphia, 2001, WB Saunders.

54. Saikh AY, et al: Chemotherapy and high dose radiotherapy followed by resection for locally advanced non-small-cell lung cancer, *Am J Clin Oncol* 30:258-263, 2007.

55. Seydel HG, et al: Hyperfractionation in the radiation therapy of unresectable non-oat cell carcinoma of the lung: preliminary report of a RTOG pilot study, *Int J Radiat Oncol Biol Phys* 11:1841-1847, 1985.

56. Siegfried JM: Lung cancer screening in high risk populations, *Clin Lung Cancer* 1:100-106, 1999.

57. Stanton R, Stinson D: *Applied physics for radiation oncology*, Madison, WI, 1996, Medical Physics Publishing.

58. Strauss GM: Potential treatment options for early stage non-small cell lung cancer patients, clinical decision-making in non-small cell lung cancer, *Cancer* 48:6-9, 1998.

59. Tazelaar HD: Screening, pathologic classification, prognostic factors and staging: clinical decision-making in non-small lung cancer, *Cancer* 48:3-6, 1998.

60. Tortora GJ, Derrickson BH: *Principles of anatomy and physiology*, ed 9, New York, 2006, Biological Sciences Textbooks, John Wiley & Sons.

61. U.S. Environmental Protection Agency: Radon (Rn) (website): www.epa.gov/radon. Accessed June 12, 2007.

62. Wagner H: Image-guided conformal radiation therapy planning and delivery for non-small-cell lung cancer, *Cancer Control* 10:277-288, 2003.

63. Wakelee HA, et al: Lung cancer incidence in never smokers, *J Clin Oncol* 25:472-478, 2007.

64. Wakelee H, Dubey S, Gandara D: Optimal adjuvant therapy for non-small cell lung cancer—how to handle stage I disease, *Oncologist* 12: 331-337, 2007.

65. Wozniak AJ, Gadgeel SM: Adjuvant treatment of non-small-cell lung cancer: how do we improve the cure rates further, *Oncology* 21:163-182, 2007.

BIBLIOGRAPHY

Nakhashi H, et al: Results of surgical treatment of patients with T3 non-small cell lung cancer, *Ann Thorac Surg* 46:178-181, 1988.

Schultheiss TE: Spinal cord radiation "tolerance": doctrine versus data, *Int J Radiat Oncol Biol Phys* 19:219-221, 1990.

U.S. Department of Health and Human Services: Summary of the HIPAA Privacy Rule (website): http://www.hhs.gov/ocr/privacysummary.pdf. Accessed June 12, 2007.

Valley JF, Mirimanoff RO: Comparison of treatment techniques for lung cancer, *Radiother Oncol* 28:168-173, 1993.

Head and Neck Cancers

Ronnie G. Lozano

Outline

Key Terms

Objectives

- Identify the medical professionals that would be involved in the multidisciplinary care and treatment of the head and neck patient.
- Name some of the advances having an impact on the localization and treatment of head and neck cancers.
- Identify the most common site of distant metastasis and other common sites of distant metastasis.
- Name the specific type of head and neck cancer with the greatest incidence of distant metastasis.
- Name the specific type of head and neck cancer known to involve the facial nerves, causing face paralysis.
- Describe a specific, primary objective of using intensity-modulated radiation therapy for the treatment of head and neck cancers.
- Name the specific head and neck cancer that consistently shows the greatest positive trend in the SEER reports and is noted as being the leading primary cancer among all ages, races, and genders.
- Identify four *general* etiologic risk factors for head and neck cancer.
- Name three occupations associated with greater risk of head and neck cancers.

- Name the virus associated with nasopharyngeal cancer in all races.
- Identify the histopathology that is present in 80% of the head and neck cancers.
- Describe the various distinctive functions of a mouth stent (tongue blade and cork or other similar device).
- Describe the general radiation therapy treatment techniques for the following head and neck sites:
  - Lip
  - Floor of the mouth
  - Tongue
  - Buccal mucosa
  - Hard palate
  - Retromolar trigone
  - Oropharynx region
  - Hypopharynx region
  - Nasopharynx region
  - Larynx region
  - Salivary glands
  - Maxillary sinus

The management of head and neck malignancies requires a multidisciplinary team approach, with an understanding that this disease can produce significant morbidity. Survival cannot be measured only in terms of mortality. Reducing deformity and restoring the function are essential to the management of head and neck cancer. The cure of cancer, with preservation of structure, function, and aesthetics, has become more evident with advances in modern radiation oncology, based on technologic gains in radiation physics and insights into radiation biology and pathophysiology.[32] From a structural standpoint, mutilation is no longer an acceptable condition of cure. Treatment that causes the permanent loss of vision, smell, taste, or hearing should be evaluated concerning its effect on quality of life and survival. Maintaining food paths and airways is vital, but the treatment decision should also preserve the patient's ability to interact as a human. The loss of the ability to speak results in significant changes in the patient's lifestyle, and it can significantly alter the patient's quality of life. With early detection techniques, head and neck cancers treated with radiation therapy allow for greater preservation of voice and swallowing. The effective management of patients with head and neck cancer involves the close cooperation of the radiation oncologists, medical oncologists, dentists, maxillofacial prosthodontists, nutritionists, head and neck surgeons, neurosurgeons, plastic surgeons, oral surgeons, pathologists, oncology nurses, radiologists, social workers, radiation therapists, speech therapists, pain service, and neurology service, without forgetting the patient's involvement. The patient may decide to select a treatment approach that offers a slightly lower probability of survival in return for a better functional or cosmetic result if the treatment is successful.[32] This is an important reason to bring the patient into the decision-making process regarding treatment. Despite many major advances, the treatment of locoregional recurrence remains a major challenge as indicated by low success rates for salvage therapy. Most patients with locoregional recurrence develop progressive disease resulting in a high degree of suffering.[25]

With the continued improvements in imaging, and the increasing accuracy of treatment techniques, tumors involving critical structures and selected parts of the brain can be eliminated with preservation of vision and minimal neurologic impairment.[32] Current inverse planning processes deliver nonuniform dose distributions based on detailed tissue metabolic information. This technology is something our predecessors could not even imagine before the advent of the computer. By systematically monitoring treatment variations, adaptive radiation therapy allows reoptimization of the treatment plan during the course of treatment. This process adjusts field margin and treatment dose, routinely customizing to each individual patient to achieve a safe dose escalation. Integrating image guidance technology with intensity-modulated radiation therapy (IMRT) and using functional image information with positron emission tomography (PET) fused with treatment planning have the potential to improve both tumor control and normal tissue sparing. The integration of robotics and new accelerator design coupled with image-guided tracking of bony landmarks or implanted fiducials has surpassed a degree of beam angle versatility and level of "exactitude" in treatment delivery ever desired. This effort has been further enhanced with the emergence of tomotherapy megavoltage units and the utilization of computed tomography (CT) images for analysis of interfractional variations in patient setup and anatomic changes.

NATURAL HISTORY

Head and neck cancer has been marked in American history by public accounts and newspaper articles describing the extensive suffering and death of Ulysses S. Grant in the late 1800s. This event significantly added to the public fears of cancers and the useless treatments of that era. Contemporary figures include the late Sammy Davis Jr., who reportedly said he would rather keep his voice than have a part of his throat removed when dealing with cancer of the larynx, and Roger Ebert, who had part of his mandible removed due to spread from cancer of the salivary gland. Today, only one third of affected patients present at an early disease stage. An estimated two thirds of oral cavity/pharynx patients present with locally advanced disease, either at the primary site or in the cervical lymph nodes, stages III and IV.[31] The lungs are the most common site of distant metastasis. Other sites of distant metastasis include the mediastinal lymph nodes, liver, brain, and bones. The incidence of distant metastasis is greatest with tumors of the nasopharynx and hypopharynx. A direct correlation appears to exist between the bulk of cervical nodal disease and the development of distant metastasis. Atypical metastatic spread may occur in patients who have had a radical neck dissection or previous radiation therapy. These patients are at high risk of developing atypical metastasis to the neck and to subcutaneous and cutaneous sites. Tumors may also spread along the nerves. Direct nerve invasion may occur from tumors in the affected area. Nerve routes are an important consideration in treatment planning. High-grade parotid tumors are known to involve the facial nerves and to cause paralysis.[25] The standard treatment for these patients is either surgery with preoperative or, more commonly, postoperative radiation therapy, or primary radiation therapy followed by surgery. A combination of chemotherapy and radiation therapy is used in patients with inoperable or unresectable (stages III and IV) disease in an attempt to increase cure rates over radiation therapy alone. The advantage of the treatment combinations is the preservation of cosmesis and function that result compared to radical surgeries. A challenge of another form involves cancerization, which refers to the higher risk for forming a second primary tumor in the same anatomic field of a previous treatment. It has been shown that patients cured for their first head and neck cancer have a greater than 20% lifetime risk of developing a second cancer. Second primary tumors (SPTs) are the leading cause of death among patients with early tumors of the head and neck. This has stimulated research on adjuvant chemoprevention regimens in preventing SPTs.[4]

Epidemiology

The Surveillance Epidemiology and End Results (SEER) data show that 4.48% of all cancer cases for 2007 are estimated to be that of the oral cavity and pharynx (34,360).[31] The 2008 estimates according to the American Cancer Society Surveillance Research report indicate that of the total 1,437,180 estimated cancer cases in the country, 25,310 cancer cases (3%) will be of the oral cavity and pharynx for males.[2] Females will present 10,000 oral cavity/pharynx cases (1.4%). Within the oral cavity/pharynx region, the estimated cases for both males and females are as follows, tongue (10,140), mouth (10,820), pharynx (12,410), and other (1,940).[2] Though the larynx is perceived as a head and neck site, SEER reports categorize the larynx under Respiratory Systems. If one includes the 12,250 expected larynx cases, the total estimated head and neck cases increases to 47,560 cases for 2008. Garden, Morrison, and Ang[15] write the following regarding larynx cancers: "Carcinomas of the hypopharynx are often considered together with carcinomas of the larynx as the anatomy of the hypopharynx is essentially created by the location of the voice box in the throat. Hypopharyngeal tumors frequently involve the larynx and vice versa. In these situations, it is one's best guess whether the epicenter of a large tumor is laryngeal or hypopharyngeal" (p. 727).

The SEER reports that head and neck cancer shows a significant decreasing trend over the period of 1995 to 2004. Larynx cancer is reported to have the greatest decreasing trend for that time period and oral/pharynx cancers are in sixth place (Figure 33-1).[3] Table 33-1 includes SEER estimates for 2006 and 2007.[2,31] While the SEER study over the 9-year period classifies the annual percent changes of head and neck (oral cavity/pharynx) and the larynx cases as significantly decreasing, the estimated data for 2006 and 2007 show an increasing trend for those 2 years. The longitudinal SEER report reflects the broader trend using more historical numbers and a greater data set versus 1-year differences in data.

It is worth noting that thyroid cancer consistently shows the greatest positive trend in the SEER reports. It leads among all ages, race, and gender in trending incidence of primary cancers and is second only to liver cancer and inflammatory bowel disease in trending U.S. cancer death rates for the time period reported. SEER 17 data (2000–2004) show the leading age group incurring cancer of the oral cavity/pharynx is 55 to 64 years old (24.7%). Larynx cancer most frequently involves people from the age of 65 to 74 (29.7%). Figure 33-2 provides

age distributions for the top five age groups. Although the age distribution chart may show the largest percentage of incidence to be cancer of the larynx, this represents breakdown by age groups only and may be misleading. A detailed study of the NCI: SEER Cancer Statistics Review indicates that the total

Table 33-1	**National Cancer Institute Surveillance Epidemiology and End Results**		
	Men	**Women**	**Total**
2007 ESTIMATES			
Oral cavity and pharynx			
New cases	24,180	10,180	34,360
Deaths	5,180	2,370	7,550
Larynx			
New cases	8,960	2,340	11,300
Deaths	2,900	760	3,660
2006 ESTIMATES			
Oral cavity and pharynx			
New cases	20,180	10,810	30,990
Deaths	5,050	2,380	7,430
Larynx			
New cases	7,700	1,810	9,510
Deaths	2,950	790	3,740

Trends in SEER Incidence and US Death Rates by Primary Cancer Site 1995-2004

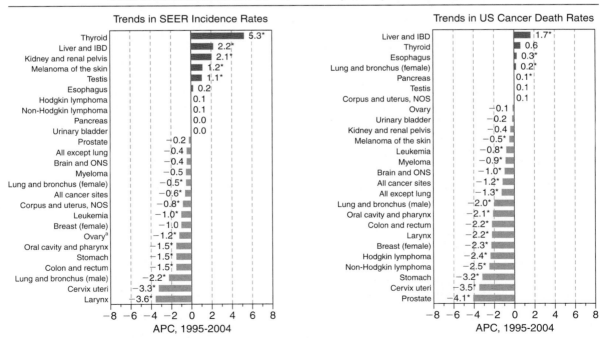

Source: SEER 13 areas (San Francisco, Connecticut, Detroit, Hawaii, Iowa, New Mexico, Seattle, Utah, Atlanta, San Jose-Monterey, Los Angeles, Alaska Native Registry and Rural Georgia) and NCHS public use file for the total US. For sex-specific cancer sites, the population was limited to the population of the appropriate sex. Underlying rates are per 100,000 and age-adjusted to the 2000 US Std Population (19 age groups - Census P25-1103).
The APC is the Annual Percent Change over the time interval.
*The APC is significantly different from zero (p <.05).
[a]Ovary excludes borderline cases or histologies 8442, 8451, 8462, 8472, and 8473.

Figure 33-1. Trends in SEER incidence and death rates by primary cancer site, 1995-2004. Note the decrease in incidence and death rates of oral cavity and pharynx tumors. (Used by permission, *SEER cancer statistics review, 1975-2004,* Bethesda, MD, 2005, National Cancer Institute.)

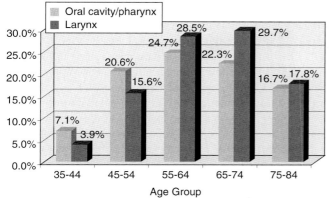

Oral Cavity/Pharynx and Larynx Cases 2000-2004
Age Distribution of Incidence (Top 5 Groups)

NCI: SEER Cancer Statistics Review 1975-2004 Table I-10

Figure 33-2. Comparitive statistics for 2006 and 2007 for head and neck cancers. (Used by permission, *SEER cancer statistics review, 1975-2004*, Bethesda, MD, 2005, National Cancer Institute.)

cases of larynx cancers were 13,225 and the total cases for oral cavity/pharynx cancers were 37,724 for that study period.[31]

The SEER advises that survival rates can be calculated by different methods for different purposes. The survival rates presented by the SEER Stat Fact Sheets are based on the relative survival rate, which measures the survival of the cancer patients in comparison to the general population to estimate the effect of cancer. It is reported that the overall 5-year relative survival rate for 1996–2003 for oral cavity and pharynx was 59.1% and 62.9%, respectively, for cancer of the larynx for the 17 SEER geographic areas. Table 33-2 presents the breakdown of the 5-year relative survival rates by race and by stage.

Table 33-2	National Cancer Institute Surveillance Epidemiology and End Results		
Overall 5-Year Relative Survival Rates By Race		**Men**	**Women**
Oral cavity and pharynx			
White		60.2%	62.8%
Black		35.5%	51.3%
Larynx			
White		65.4%	60.7%
Black		53.8%	45.2%
Overall 5-Year Relative Survival Rates By Stage		**Distribution**	**Survival**
Oral cavity and pharynx			
Localized		33.0%	81.8%
Regional		52.0%	52.1%
Distant		10.0%	26.5%
Unstaged		5.0%	46.2%
Larynx			
Localized		47.0%	81.1%
Regional		42.0%	50.0%
Distant		7.0%	23.9%
Unstaged		3.0%	45.7%

Cancers of the nasopharynx are uncommon in the United States in comparison to Hong Kong and southern China, areas of southeast Asia including Taiwan, Vietnam, and Thailand as well as the Philippines, Malaysia, some Mediterranean, north African populations, and Eskimos.[23,29] These areas are considered to be endemic for nasopharyngeal cancer (NPC). The incidence outside these areas is much lower and considered to be associated with tobacco.[29] A decreased incidence of NPC in successive generations of Chinese born in America suggests an etiologic role for environmental factors.[23,29] Tumors of the oral cavity and base of tongue are more common in India, which also indicates a strong environmental and cultural influence in the prevalence of this type of disease. In the Indian subcontinent, oral squamous cell carcinoma (SCC) may account for 50% of all cancers. The high incidence of buccal mucosal cancer in particular is due to betel nuts, the chewing of pan, a mixture of betel leaf, lime, catechu, and areca nut.[31,23] The alkaloids released when the nut is chewed provoke excessive and abnormal synthesis of collagen by cultured fibroblasts, causing submucous fibrosis. Environmental and genetic predisposition results in nasopharynx cancer being the most common tumor in the Kwantung province of southern China. Recurrences usually occur within the first 2 years and rarely after 4 years, establishing a 5-year follow-up for most sites.

Etiology and Predisposing Factors

The large number of disease processes that can affect the head and neck region can have a multitude of histologies. This is a reflection of the many specialized tissues present and at risk for specific diseases. This chapter refers to those tumors of an epithelial character arising from the mucosal lining of the aerodigestive tract. The most common sites of the aerodigestive tract affected are the oral cavity, pharynx, paranasal sinuses, larynx, thyroid gland, and salivary glands. General etiologic risk factors for head and neck cancer include (1) tobacco and alcohol use, (2) ultraviolet (UV) light exposure, (3) viral infection, and (4) environmental exposures.

Smoking. Tobacco was first introduced to Western civilization by the Spanish explorers of America in the early 16th century. At first, it was simply smoked in pipes but, as it became more popular, it was also chewed and snuffed. Cigarettes were first made in Spain in the mid 17th century and, in the 20th century, they became the most popular form of the tobacco habit. The incidence of head and neck cancers correlates most closely with the use of tobacco and alcohol.[4] Head and neck tumors occur six times more often among cigarette smokers than among nonsmokers. The mortality from laryngeal cancer appears to rise with increased cigarette consumption. For the heaviest smokers, death from laryngeal cancer is 20 times more likely than for nonsmokers.[30] Pipe and cigar smoking results in extensive intraoral keratosis. Unfiltered cigarettes cause lip carcinoma, especially when habitually held in the same place. The use of unfiltered cigarettes or dark, air-cured tobacco is associated with further increases in risk. Certain cancers like oropharynx cases, closer to the esophagus, are associated with the pooling of saliva carrying carcinogens related to tobacco.[30]

Alcohol. Alcohol consumption alone is a risk factor for the development of pharyngeal and laryngeal tumors.[30] Alcohol has been described to damage mucosa, making it more permeable to contaminants. Secondary etiologic factors of head and neck cancers that have been related to chronic drinking include factors that fit the usual characteristics of alcoholism like nutritional deficiencies and environmental carcinogens (due to smoking) that increase susceptibility to cancer in general.

Smoking, Tobacco, and Alcohol. This combination has been regarded as the most important risk factor for this disease.[4,29] Alcohol seems to have a synergistic effect on the carcinogenic potential of tobacco. This combination facilitates the pathogenic effects of the thousands of substances produced in the combustion process of smoking. These include "tars" (the basis for the tobacco taste) or aromatic hydrocarbons that contain the most potent carcinogens. Evidence suggests that ethanol suppresses the efficiency of DNA repair after exposure to nitrosamine compounds.[29] Nitrosamines (N-nitrosonornicotine) has been identified as the most potent noncombustible product in snuff and chewing tobacco that possesses carcinogenic activity.[35]

Smokeless Tobacco. There is a higher frequency of premalignant and malignant oral lesions in young Americans because of the increasing use of smokeless tobacco.[31] Smokeless tobacco users frequently develop premalignant lesions, such as oral leukoplakia, at the site where the tobacco quid rests against the mucosa (Figure 33-3). Over time, these lesions may progress to invasive carcinomas.[30] Tobacco may clearly induce a benign clinical condition involving the oral mucosa into malignant tumor. The most common conditions found with the use of smokeless tobacco are gingival recession, hyperkeratosis, and staining. The risk of oral epithelial dysplasia or carcinoma increases with long-term use.[35]

Ultraviolet Light. Exposure to UV is a risk factor for the development of lip cancer. At least 33% of lip cancer patients have outdoor occupations.

Occupational Exposures Occupations associated with greater risk include (1) nickel refining, (2) furniture and woodworking (cancers of the larynx, nasal cavity, and paranasal sinuses), and (3) steel and textile workers (oral cancer).[29]

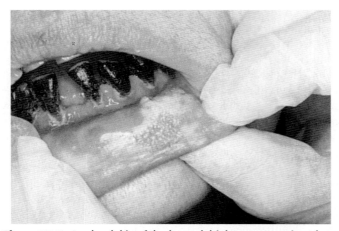

Figure 33-3. Leukoplakia of the lower labial mucosa at site where patient held tobacco during a 27-year habit. Microscopic epithelial dysplaia and intense dental staining occurred. (From Silverman S: *Oral cancer*, ed 5, Hamilton, 2003, BC Decker. Reprinted by the permission of the American Cancer Society, Inc.)

Exposure to dust, fumes, and formaldehyde has been associated with NPC.[9] Carpenters and sawmill workers who are exposed to dust of mainly hard and exotic woods develop adenocarcinoma of the nasal cavity and ethmoid sinus. Other carcinogens include synthetic wood, binding agents, and glues.

Radiation Exposure. Exposure, particularly in childhood, is implicated in the development of thyroid cancer and salivary gland tumors.[31] Salivary gland malignancies have been radiation induced in patients treated for benign conditions like acne, tinea capitis, infected tonsils, etc. Radiation-induced salivary gland tumors have also been reported among survivors of the atomic bomb in Hiroshima and Nagasaki.[10] Cancer of the maxillary sinus has been associated with the radioactive contrast medium, Thorotrast, used for imaging of the maxillary sinus during the 1960s.[33]

Viruses. Increasing evidence suggests a role for viruses in the development of head and neck cancer. Epstein-Barr virus (EBV) (one of eight herpes viruses that infect human tissue) and viral DNA have been identified in nasopharyngeal tissue in this type of cancer.[5,29] EBV has been associated with NPC in all races.[31]

Herpes simplex virus 1 (HSV-1) is the well-known cause of primary herpetic stomatitis and of recurrent herpes labialis (cold sores). The virus remains latent in the trigeminal or other sensory ganglion for an entire lifetime. Reactivation occurs to produce recurrent lesions or to be shed asymptomatically in the saliva. The virus has the ability to transform cells to a malignant phenotype under certain conditions. In an experimental situation, the infected cells can become immortal in cell culture and will invade and metastasize if they are injected into an experimental animal. Experiments with hamsters show that if tissue is exposed to low doses of the tobacco carcinogen benzo(a)pyrene and to HSV-1 simultaneously, tumors can be produced. This may have implications for a population of smokers, HSV-1, and oral cancer.

Human papillomavirus (HPV) has also been linked to head and neck carcinogenesis.[29] HPV has been found in oral papillomas, in leukoplakia lesions, and in oral carcinomas. Laryngeal papillomatosis and carcinoma of the larynx have been linked with HPV.[31] Cell studies show that high-risk HPVs can transform epithelial cells from cervix, foreskin, and the oral cavity to produce malignancy. Carcinomas of the tonsil, oral tongue, and the floor of mouth have been found to have a high prevalence of HPV DNA. Ang and Garden[5] describe a study suggesting that the HPV is found frequently in oropharyngeal carcinoma patients who have no history of smoking or alcohol use. It is noted that an increasing number of younger patients with SCCs of the upper aerodigestive track without the typical social history of smoking and alcohol has been observed. There is evidence to suggest that viruses such as the HPV may be linked to these cases.

Syphilis. Syphilis was implicated in tongue carcinoma in the preantibiotic era. Past reports of patients with oral cancer have indicated positive histories; however, little evidence currently supports an association between syphilis and oral cancer.[31,35]

Diet. Dietary factors leading to hypopharyngeal cancer include nutritional deficiency (vitamins A and E), especially in alcoholics and most prevalent in females.[31] Iron deficiency anemia has been associated with postcricoid cancers in (90%) women in Scandinavia and Great Britain who usually present with dysphagia from hypopharyngeal webs and atrophy of the oral mucosa.[44] The Plummer-Vinson syndrome (esophageal web, iron-deficiency anemia, dysphasia due to glossitis) is associated with a high incidence of postcricoid and tongue carcinoma, most prevalent in Europe. The web refers to an inflammation condition associated with a weblike formation on the wall of the esophagus or hypopharynx. It consists of a thin mucosal membrane covered by normal squamous epithelium. The term *Plummer-Vonson syndrome* originates from Scandinavia, and the condition is referred to as the *Paterson-Brown-Kelly syndrome* in Great Britain.[44] Fruits, vegetables, and carotenoids are suggested to have a preventive role by epidemiologic data.[29] Nasopharyngeal cases among southern Chinese and Hong Kong populations have been associated with ingestion of salted fish since childhood. Dimethylnitrosamine, a carcinogen in the nitrosamine group also found in snuff and chewing tobacco, has also been found in salted fish. This compound has induced carcinoma of the upper respiratory tract in rats.[15,24]

Marijuana. Chronic abuse of marijuana has been linked to head and neck cancer. While some literature report that the degree of risk is unknown,[29,30] other publications make the comparison of smokers using filtered cigarettes and the lack of such filter in smoking marijuana. An increased risk is established considering a higher concentration of tar and aromatic hydrocarbons.[44]

Dentures, Fillings, and Poor Oral Hygiene. While lacking studies with conclusive evidence, cases exist in which some carcinomas develop in areas covered by or adjacent to a prosthetic device. Even though the risk is low, chronic denture irritation in addition to other unidentified factors may possibly promote neoplastic activity. The same principle may apply to patients who have poor oral hygiene or jagged teeth or fillings that may act as irritants (Figures 33-4 and 33-5). Denture material per se has not been shown to be carcinogenic.[35]

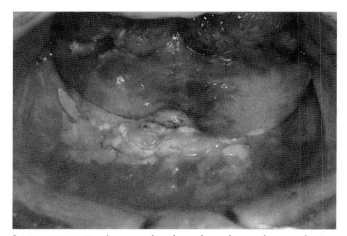

Figure 33-4. Carcinoma developed under a lower denture in anterior alveolar mucosa after 15-year history of leukoplakia. (From Silverman S: *Oral cancer*, ed 5, Hamilton, 2003, BC Decker. Reprinted by the permission of the American Cancer Society, Inc.)

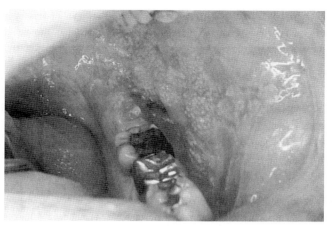

Figure 33-5. Atrophic lichen planus, an inflammatory disease. Buccal oral lesion transforming to carcinoma in posterior buccal after 13 years. (From Silverman S: *Oral cancer*, ed 5, Hamilton, 2003, BC Decker. Reprinted by the permission of the American Cancer Society, Inc.)

Genetics. Genetic predisposition to head and neck cancer has been suggested by its sporadic occurrence in unexpected populations like young adults and nonusers of tobacco and alcohol.[2] Increased susceptibility to environmental carcinogens has been attributed to genetic anomalies and/or other cofactors like viral infections. Current studies have identified at least 10 genetic alterations that generate an invasive tumor phenotype in cells. The research focuses on the inactivation of tumor suppressor genes and oncogene amplification. These types of studies continue to provide a greater understanding of the influence of genes and may be used in the future of screening. Chemoprevention of malignant transformation is a strategy that may be implemented upon identification of high risk based on key genetic changes and markers of carcinogenesis.[4]

An association with the Bloom syndrome and the Li-Fraumeni syndrome has been implicated in head and neck cancers.[35] Bloom syndrome is a rare autosomal recessive disorder characterized by telangiectases (erythema appears as macules or plaques in a butterfly distribution on the face and other areas exposed to the sun), photosensitivity, and growth abnormalities. Patients with Bloom syndrome have an overall 150 to 300 times increased risk of malignancy compared with the general population. Li-Fraumeni syndrome, an autosomal dominant disorder, has been linked to germline mutations of the tumor suppressor gene *p53*. Several types of cancers have been associated with these genetic disorders. It is estimated that SCC of the head and neck requires the accumulation of 8 to 11 mutations, and 4 to 7 genetic mutations may be sufficient for the development of salivary gland malignancies.[31]

Prognostic Indicators

In general, the morbidity of treatments increases and the prognosis decreases as the affected area progresses backward from the lips to the hypopharynx, excluding the larynx. Common characteristics of advanced stages and unfavorable prognosis include tumors that cross the midline, exhibit endophytic growth (invasion of the lamina propria and submucosa), are poorly differentiated, and are non-SCCs. Advanced stages also involve cases that have fixed lymph nodes, a fixed lesion, or have cranial nerve involvement. As with all cancer cases, the extent of lympadenopathy directly impacts prognosis. Vascular invasion may identify tumors with an aggressive biologic nature due to their ability to invade normal anatomic structures. An established association of vascular invasion in primary tumors and presence of cervical metastases as well as an increased risk for subsequent locoregional recurrence indicate a poor prognosis. Smith and Haffty report that "postoperative radiotherapy may mitigate the poor prognosis associated with vascular invasion" (p. 53).[37]

Anatomy and Physiology

The organs comprising the head and neck region serve dual purposes in that respiratory and digestive activities take place. For a better appreciation of this complex system, a brief anatomical review is necessary.

The staging and classification of head and neck tumors are based on involvement of subsites. Understanding the structure and physiological relationships of these adjacent structures is important. The opening of the nasal cavities into the nasopharynx (Figure 33-6) provides a natural pathway for tumor spread. During the act of swallowing, the soft palate elevates and prevents food from entering the nasopharynx. Tumors in this location do not allow this activity to occur. An enlargement of

the pharyngeal tonsil can obstruct the upper air passage and allow breathing only through the mouth, resulting in the passing of unfiltered, cool, dry air to the lungs. Collectively, the tonsils are bands of lymphoid tissue that provide protection against airway infections and form a barrier between the respiratory tubes (nasopharynx) and digestive tubes (oropharynx and hypopharynx). This anatomy may be referred to as the aerodigestive tract. In addition, knowing the location of a cervical vertebral body provides boundary locations of the soft tissue aspects of the head and neck region. The first cervical vertebra (C1) lies at the inferior margin of the nasopharynx, whereas the second and third cervical vertebrae (C2-3) contain the oropharynx. The epiglottis is in line with C3, whereas the true vocal cords lie along the fourth cervical vertebra (C4) (Figure 33-6).

Salivary gland tumors can involve facial nerves, major cranial nerves, arterial neck blood flow, and several lymph node groups (Figure 33-7). Tumors in this area can cause facial paralysis, nerve pain, and interruption of the neck muscles' blood supply (Figure 33-8).

Because tumors can damage the cranial nerves, which control our major senses, involvement of the cranial nerves leads to signs and symptoms that can point to a possible location of a tumor. Table 33-3 lists the 12 cranial nerves and their associated functions.

Lymphatics

Nearly one third of the body's lymph nodes are located in the head and neck area. Lymphatic drainage is mainly ipsilateral, but structures like the soft palate, the tonsils, the base of the tongue, the posterior pharyngeal wall, and especially the nasopharynx have bilateral drainage. However, sites like the true vocal cord, the paranasal sinuses, and the middle ear have few or no lymphatic vessels at all. Lymphatic drainage of the neck was described by Rouvière in 1938. Variations exist in lymph node group level classifications.[16,18] Variation is based on specific objectives of standardizing the terminology. The six-level classifications were developed to standardize terminology for neck dissection procedures, and only the node groups routinely removed during surgical neck dissection are considered (Robbins classification).[18] The six (surgical oncology) level classification and node groups have been identified and illustrated in Figure 33-9. Lymph node levels have also been defined according to anatomic landmarks and regarded as an imaging-based nodal classification. Figure 33-10, B, illustrates seven category levels, and Table 33-4 defines the category landmarks and depicts the major chains of the head and neck. Figure 33-11 provides correlation of the node group levels with axial cadaveric sections and axial CT images.

 For more CT-based lymph node delineation information, see http://www.rtog.org/pdf_file2.html?pdf_document= atlasneck_ctv.pdf.

Some nodes have two names. The **jugulodigastric lymph node** is called the *subdigastric node*, the **node of Rouvière** is also called the *lateral retropharyngeal node*, the *spinal accessory chain* is also referred to as the **posterior cervical lymph node chain**, and the *mastoid node* is also called the **retroauricular node**. The degree of lymph node involvement dictates the

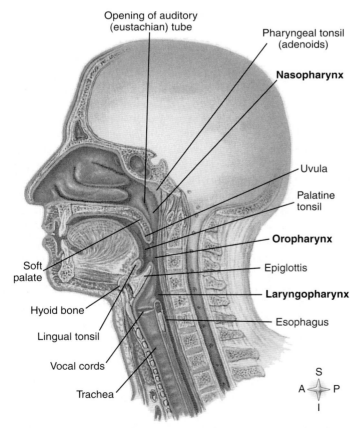

Figure 33-6 Pharynx. This midsagittal section shows the three divisions of the pharynx (nasopharynx, oropharynx, and laryngopharynx) and nearby structures. (From Thibodeau GA, Patton KT: *Anatomy and physiology*, ed 6, St. Louis, 2007, Mosby.)

Opening of auditory (eustachian) tube

Pharyngeal tonsil (adenoids)

Nasopharynx

Uvula

Palatine tonsil

Oropharynx

Epiglottis

Laryngopharynx

Esophagus

Soft palate

Hyoid bone

Lingual tonsil

Vocal cords

Trachea

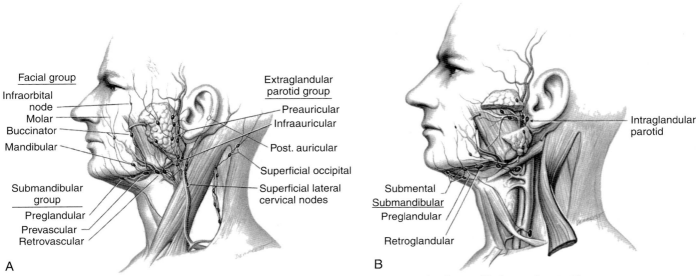

Figure 33-7. **A,** Extraglandular parotid, facial, and superficial submandibular nodes. **B,** The deep submandibular and parotid lymph nodes. (From Haagensen CD: *The lymphatics in cancer*, Philadelphia, 1972, Saunders.)

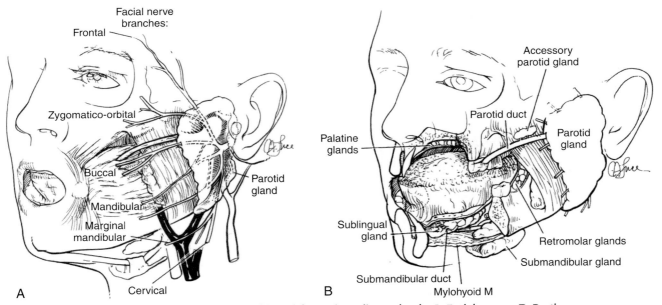

Figure 33-8. Anatomic relationships of the major salivary glands. **A,** Facial nerves. **B,** Portion of mandible removed to show minor salivary glands in the palate. (From McCarthy JG: *Plastic surgery: volume 5 Tumors of the head and neck and skin*, Philadelphia, 1990, Saunders.)

size of the radiation portal and the treatment plan. Figure 33-12 illustrates the major lymph node chains of the head and neck.

Figure 33-13 shows the jugulodigastric group (the group of neck nodes below the mastoid tip), which receives nearly all the lymph from the head area and is usually treated; the Rouvière node (the lateral retropharyngeal node) is included as the minimum target volume for NPC. This node is inaccessible to the surgeon and is a source of high risk for dissemination of disease if not treated due to its proximity to the carotid artery. The transverse slice shown as Figure 33-13, B, illustrates the proximity of the retropharyngeal node and the carotid artery.

Clinical Presentation

Most head and neck cancers are infiltrative lesions found in the epithelial lining. They can be raised or indurated (hard and firm). These growths are sometimes classified as **endophytic** tumors, which are more aggressive in spread and harder to control locally. **Exophytic** tumors are noninvasive neoplasms characterized by raised, elevated borders. Symptoms usually center on the anatomic area affected, with 60% of patients complaining of **otalgia** (ear pain).[41] Specific signs and symptoms correlate with anatomical sites. Box 33-1 provides a list of the

Table 33-3	Cranial Nerves and Their Functions		
Name	**Number**	**Function**	**Classification**
Olfactory	I	Smell	Sensory
Optic	II	Sight	Sensory
Oculomotor	III	Eye movement (up and down)	Motor
Trochlear	IV	Eye movement (rotation)	Motor
Trigeminal	V	Sensory (facial) and motor (jaw)	Mixed
Abducens	VI	Eye movement (lateral)	Motor
Facial (masticator)	VII	Expressions, muscle contractions, and mouthing	Mixed
Acoustic	VIII	Hearing	Sensory
Glossopharyngeal	IX	Tongue and throat movement	Mixed
Vagus	X	Talking and sounds	Mixed
Spinal accessory	XI	Movement of shoulders and head	Motor
Hypoglossal	XII	Movement of tongue and chewing	Motor

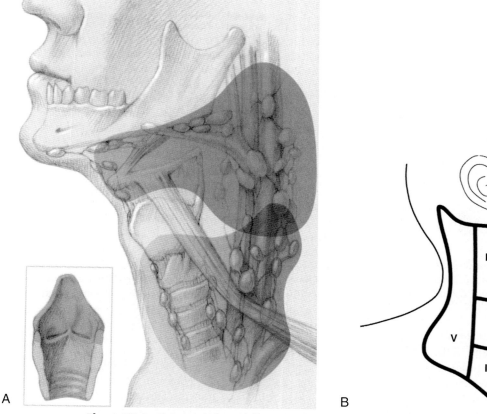
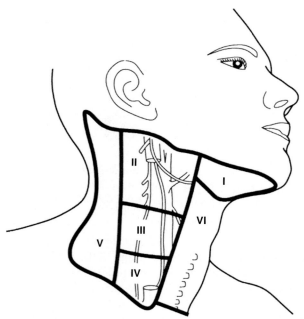

A

B

Figure 33-9. A, Lateral view of the superficial and deep node groups. Groups include the Ia, submental; Ib, submandibular; II, upper jugular; III, middle jugular; IV, lower jugular; V, posterior triangle; VI, anterior compartment. **B,** Nodal grouping by regions as generally used by the head and neck surgical oncologist. (**A,** From Werner JA, Davis KR: *Metastases in head and neck cancer*, Berlin, 2004, Springer; **B,** From Rubin P: *Clinical oncology: a multidisciplinary approach for physicians and students*, ed 8, Philadelphia, 2001, Saunders.)

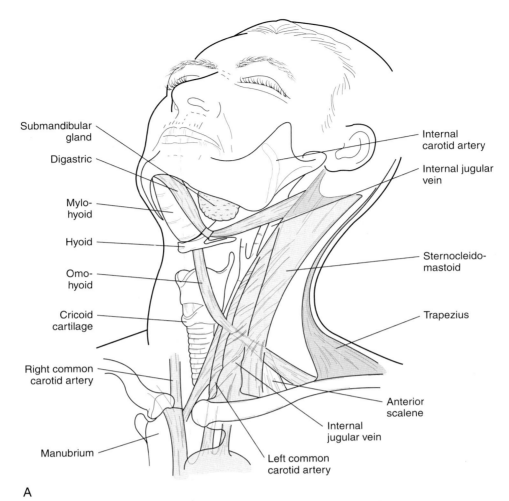

Submandibular
gland

Digastric

Mylo-
hyoid

Hyoid

Omo-
hyoid

Cricoid
cartilage

Right common
carotid artery

Manubrium

Internal
carotid artery

Internal jugular
vein

Sternocleido-
mastoid

Trapezius

Anterior
scalene

Internal
jugular vein

Left common
carotid artery

A

Figure 33-10. A, Line drawing of neck from left anterior view demonstrates anatomy relevant to nodal classification.

common symptoms by site. A cervical lymph node mass can be present clinically from any of these sites. In an adult, any enlarged cervical node that persists for 1 week or more should be regarded as suspicious and should be evaluated for a malignancy.

Detection and Diagnosis

Most of the structures of the aerodigestive track as well as the soft tissue within the facial/cervical regions can be directly examined by means of palpation, direct inspection, or biopsy. Frequently, findings correlate with presenting symptoms during the physical examination although accurate detection and staging requires radiographic evaluation.

Frank and Boyn[14] write "the combination of traditional laying on of the hands and contemporary technology leads to accurate assessment and appropriate therapy" (p. 3). A similar message is delivered by Beitler, Amdur, and Mendenhall,[7] who write "despite increasingly sophisticated imaging, the cancer-directed physical examination is essential. Tumor diagrams and photographs of the lesions are an important resource for the

patient record" (p. 357). Without dismissing the effectiveness of contemporary technology, it is clear that a well-executed basic physical examination along with good old-fashioned documentation using diagrams and photographs (perhaps now digital instead of the older Polaroid prints) still holds much value among practices of radiation therapy.

Careful examination and inspection of the head and neck via indirect laryngoscopy, palpation, and fiberoptic endoscopy are important. A systemic, step-by-step examination of all the anatomical compartments for any suspicious growths or nodes is needed. Nodes that are hard, greater than 1 cm, nontender, nonmobile, and raised suggest characteristics of metastasis. The number of nodes should also be assessed. The location of neck masses can often suggest the site of the primary tumor.

Box 33-2 lists common clinical presentations relative to the origin of the head and neck primary cancers. Biopsies are performed on all suspicious lesions to determine a precursor benign condition or to evaluate the predominant malignant growth pattern (grading). A fine-needle aspiration biopsy (FNAB) is performed for neck masses. Anti-EBV antibody titers —

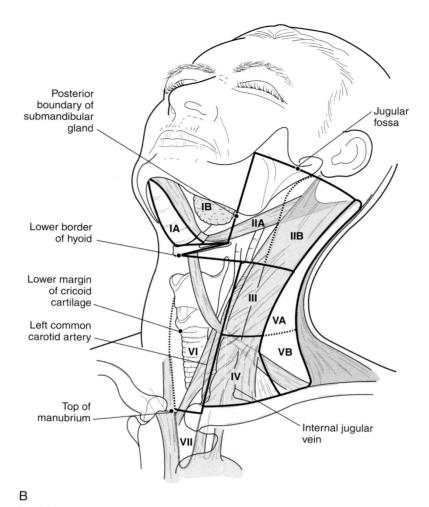

B

Figure 33-10 cont'd. B, Nodal classification levels are indicated with regard to anatomic landmarks. Posterior margin of the submanibular gland separates levels I and II, while the separation of levels II and III from level V is the posterior edge of the sternocleidomastoid muscle. The posterior edge of the internal jugular vein separates level IIA and IIB nodes. (From Leibel SA, Phillips TL: *Textbook of radiation oncology*, ed 2, Philadelphia, 2004, Saunders.)

immunoglobulin G and immunoglobulin A are fairly specific for NPC and may aid in the diagnosis of cervical node cancer with unknown primary cancer.

Image Acquisition

Radiographic studies performed routinely include CT, magnetic resonance imaging (MRI), and x-ray examinations of the skull, sinuses, and soft tissue. For symptomatic patients, barium swallow is recommended, along with chest films and bone scans to rule out metastases. PET may be useful in locating occult tumor in situations of an unknown primary setting and in ascertaining tumor recurrence after treatment. PET has been shown to have advantages over physical examination and CT imaging in follow-up of patients. Fluorodeoxyglucose (FDG) PET has been reported to accurately assess treatment response after IMRT; however, the same study reported a high false-positive rate. The study reported that "these lead to repeat biopsies that can result in non-healing tissues, especially after high dose radiation" (p. 1416).[42]

Staging entails a history and physical examination with CT or MRI of the head and neck, a chest radiograph, and routine blood cell counts and serum chemistries. Advanced nodal disease indicates a chest CT.[25] CT with intravenous contrast is the main imaging modality,[7,41] although MRI can provide important supplemental information. Some patients with advanced disease may benefit from PET/CT scanning to precisely define locoregional disease and detect distant metastases (Figure 33-14). However, Beitler, Amdur, and Mendenhall[7] report that PET may underestimate the extent of locoregional disease that is apparent in the CT (p. 357). CT is performed to determine extent of disease, especially deep invasion, to determine bone invasion, and for regional lymph nodes assessment.[26] MRI is useful to assess muscle invasion with retromolar trigone lesions. Hinerman, Foote, Sandow, and Mendenhall[17] write that regular chest radiography is used to detect pulmonary metastases. The authors also state that routine use of PET is not recommended in cancers of the oral cavity.

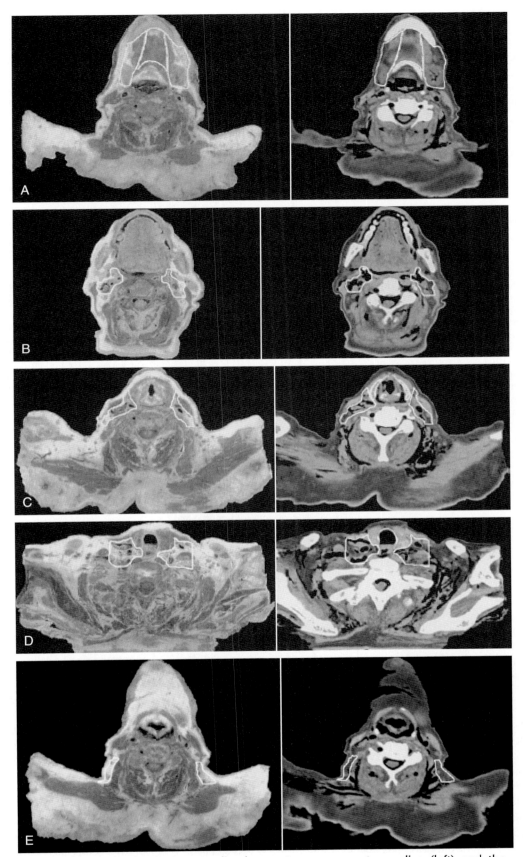

Figure 33-11. The borders are outlined on a transverse anatomy slice (left) and the matched CT slice (right). **A**, *Level 1:* This region is divided into subregions 1A (submental lymph nodes) and 1B (submandibular lymph nodes). The slices are at the upper region of 1A. **B**, *Level 2:* Illustration of high-jugular lymph nodes. **C**, *Level 3:* Mid-jugular lymph nodes. **D**, *Level 4:* Low-jugular lymph nodes. **E**, *Level 5:* Posterior triangle lymph nodes. (From Nowak P, et al: A 3D CT-based target definition for elective irradiation of the neck, *Int J Radiat Oncol Biol Phys* 45:33, 1999.)

Table 33-4	Imaging-Based Nodal Classification		
Nodes	**Anatomic Boundries**	**Subcategories**	**Anatomy and Lymphatic Drainage Patterns**
Level I	Above hyoid bone, below mylohyoid muscle, anterior to back of submandibular gland	IA: between medial margins of anterior bellies of digastric muscles IB: posterolateal to level IA	Includes the submental and submandibular triangles
Level II	From skull base to lower body of hyoid bone, posterior to back of submandibular gland and anterior to back of sternocleidomastoid muscle	IIA: anterior, lateral, medial,or posterior to internal jugular vein IIB: posterior to internal jugular vein with a fat plane separating nodes and vein	Includes the superior jugular chain nodes extending from the mandible down to the carotid bifurcation and posteriorly to the posterior border of the sternocleidomastoid muscle
Level III	From lower body of hyoid to lower cricoid cartilage arch, anterior to back of sternocleidomastoid muscle		Consists of the middle jugular nodes from the carotid bulb inferiorly to the omohyoid muscle
Level IV	From lower cricoid arch to level of clavicle, anterior to line connecting back of sternocleidomastoid and posterolateral margin of anterior scalene muscle, lateral to carotid arteries		Continues from the omohyoid muscle inferiorly to the clavicle including the lower jugular nodes. The posterior border of regions II, III, and IV is the posterior border of the sternocleidomastoid muscle, which is the anterior border of the level V group.
Level V	Posterior to back of sternocleidomastoid from skull base to clavicle. Below cricoid arch, posterior to line connecting back of sternocleidomastoid muscle and posterolateral margin of anterior scalene muscle	VA: from skull base to bottom of cricoid arch, posterior to sternocleodomastoid muscle VB: from cricoid arch to clavicle, posterior to line connecting back of sternocleidomastoid muscle and posterolateral margin of anterior scalene muscle	Includes the spinal accessory group and represents the posterior triangle bounded by the sternocleidomastoid anteriorly, the trapezius posteriorly, and the omohyoid inferiorly. Few lesions metastasize to level V without involvement of more central nodes.
Level VI	Between carotid arteries from level of lower body of hyoid bone to top of manubrium		Denotes the anterior nodal compartment consisting of the pretracheal and paratraacheal nodes, the Delphian node, and the perithyroid nodes
Level VII	Between carotid arteries below level of top of manubrium, caudal to level of innominate vein		Sometimes level VII is used to indicate the upper mediastinal nodes, although this designation is less common

Adapted from Som PM, Curtin HD, Mancuso AA: Imaging-based nodal classification for evaluation of neck metastatic adenopathy, *Am Jour of Roentgenology* 174: 837–844, 2000. http://www.ajronline.org

A PET scan is overall most helpful in patients with locally advanced disease. In initial staging, PET has a sensitivity and specificity of about 90% for nodal staging. This makes PET more sensitive and specific than CT or MRI. Although a high specificity has been reported, a limitation has been identified with early-stage tumors (clinically N0 stages) due to its lower sensitivity of nodal disease at this early stage.

CT and MRI can identify up to 50% of primary tumors that show no clinical evidence of tumor on physical examinaation. Tumors that are not identified using CT or MRI are detected with a stand-alone PET scan (without fusion with CT). Stand-alone PET has a detection rate of 25% for localizing undetected tumors with these other two imaging modalities and an endoscopy examination. Fusion studies with CT are expected to produce a higher detection rate and should be performed instead of MRI or CT and before endoscopy.[20] PET demonstrates high sensitivity for re-staging after radiation therapy; however, the optimal time for a PET study has been controversial. The recommended time is 3 months post treatment. A PET study prior to that will produce a higher chance of false-positive findings.[20]

Pathology

More than 80% of head and neck cancers arise from the surface epithelium of the mucosal linings of the upper digestive tract. These cancers are mostly SCCs. Adenocarcinomas are found to a lesser extent in the salivary glands. SCCs seen in the head and neck region include lymphoepithelioma, spindle cell carcinoma, verrucous carcinoma, and undifferentiated carcinoma.

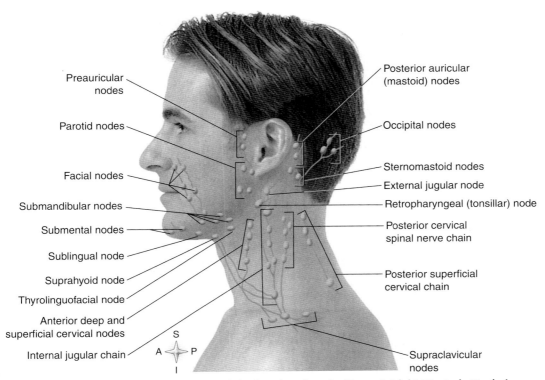

Figure 33-12. Lymphatic drainage of the head and neck. (From Seidel HM et al: *Mosby's guide to physical examination,* ed 5, St. Louis, 2002, Mosby.

Lymphoepithelioma occurs in places of abundant lymphoid tissue (i.e., the nasopharynx, tonsil, and base of the tongue). Patients with this histologic type have a better cure rate than do patients with SCC.[12]

Spindle cell carcinoma has a nonneoplastic background and responds to radiation therapy in much the same manner as SCC. Verrucous carcinoma is most often found in the gingiva and buccal mucosa. This type of carcinoma has an indolent pattern of growth and is associated with chewing tobacco or snuff. Verrucous carcinomas tend to be exophytic, have distinct margins, and look like warts. They are often hyperkeratotic, treated according to their appearance alone, and watched for further growth.

Undifferentiated lymphomas are similar histopathologically to undifferentiated carcinomas and should be treated as carcinomas if doubt exists after a microscopic evaluation. Box 33-3 lists some cell types found in the head and neck region. Tumor grading is classified as G-1 (well differentiated), G-2 (moderately well differentiated), or G-3 (poorly differentiated). Better differentiated tumors generally have a lower cell proliferation rate and are less likely to have aggressive behavior.[40] A variety of nonepithelial malignancies, melanomas, soft tissue sarcomas, and plasmacytomas can also occur in the head and neck region.

Staging

Current staging criteria are based on the 6th edition (2002) of the American Joint Committee on Cancer (AJCC) *Manual for Staging of Cancer*. This is a clinical staging system, not a pathologic staging system. The staging system for head and neck cancers is based mostly on clinical diagnostic information that determines the size, extent, and presence of positive nodes. CT, MRI, and sonography have added to the accuracy of tumor (T) and nodal (N) staging in advanced stages, especially in cases involving the nasopharynx, paranasal sinuses, and regional lymph nodes. Endoscopic evaluation also assures accuracy of the primary tumor staging. Any diagnostic information that contributes to the overall accuracy of the pretreatment assessment should be considered. Fine needle biopsy may confirm the presence of tumor and its histopathologic nature. This clinical staging system is based on the best possible estimate of the extent of disease before the first treatment. According to the AJCC handbook, when surgery is conducted, the cancer can be staged following pathologic staging (pTNM). This adds the pathologic findings of the resected specimen to the clinical staging but will not replace it.[3]

The three basic descriptors—tumor, node, metastasis (TNM)—are grouped into stage categories. Box 33-4 provides brief summaries of the sixth edition staging categories. Staging criteria for the primary lesion are site specific. However, except for tumors in the nasopharynx, there is more uniformity in the nodal staging criteria and stage grouping for the 6th edition system. NPCs are designated according to modified Uniform International Committee on Cancer (UICC) staging. The sixth edition system provides a uniform description of advanced tumors whereby T4 lesions are divided into T4a (resectable) and T4b (unresectable). This allows description of patients with

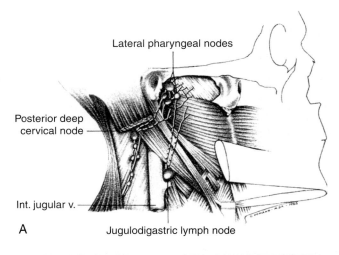

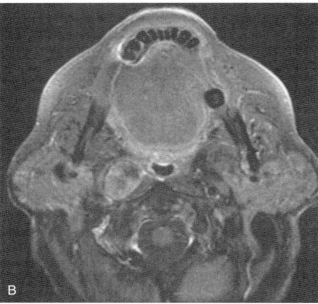

Figure 33-13. A, Major lymphatic drainage of the nasopharynx. **B**, shows a large, right retropharyngeal lymph node in a patient with tongue base cancer. (**A**, From Leibel SA, Phillips TL: *Textbook of radiation oncology*, ed 2, Philadelphia, 2004, Saunders; **B**, From Morrison WH, Garden AS, Ang KK: Oropharyngeal cancer. In Gunderson LL, Tepper JE: *Clinical radiation oncology*, ed 2, Philadelphia, 2007, Churchill Livingstone.)

advanced stage disease into three categories: stage IVA, advanced resectable disease; stage IVB, advanced unresectable disease; and stage IVC, advanced distant metastatic disease. Careful attention is given to the mobility of the nodes. Fixed nodes result in a poor prognosis. Contrast-enhanced CT and MRI scans can define the size and shape of the tumor better than a clinical evaluation. Three-dimensional multiplanar imaging has made staging much more precise and accurate for deeply invading disease or in the assessment of inaccessible neck nodes.

Spread Patterns

The port sizes of the irradiated fields in the head and neck area are large because of the risk of nodal spread. The inferior cervical

---

nodes are clinically positive in 6% to 23% of the cases for NPC. For this reason, the supraclavicular area requires treatment using an anterior port. Generally, hematogenous spread below the neck is rare, except in NPC or in the parotid gland. Over 75% of all head and neck cancers recur locally or regionally above the clavicle.

NPC with known bilateral cervical node involvement has shown a 25% chance of blood-borne distant spread first to the bone and then to the lung. The normal lymphatic drainage by site is listed in Box 33-5. Box 33-6 lists areas of the head and neck region and the expected direct spread of a tumor in each area.

TREATMENT CONSIDERATIONS

General Principles

Radiation and surgery are major curative modalities for head and neck cancers with adjuvant chemotherapy for advanced stages. The eradication of the disease, maintenance of physiologic function, and preservation of social cosmesis determine the best modality. The ability to cure and eradicate the disease

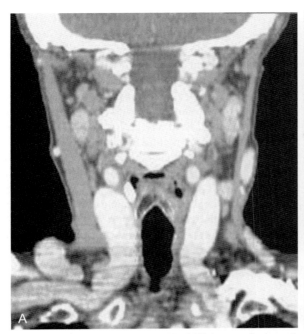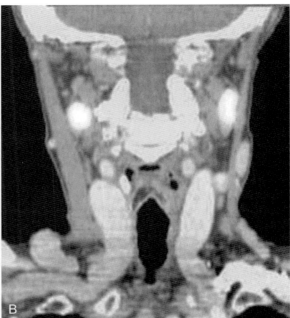

Figure 33-14. CT-MRI-PET image fusion. **A,** Post contrast, reformatted CT image in the coronal plane shows bilateral, mildly enlarged metastatic modes in the carotid-jugular chains. Tumoral involvement of the nodes remains speculative because of borderline short-axis diameter and absence of obvious necrotic changes. **B,** Superimposition of F-fluorode-oxyglucose positron emission tomography (FDG-PET) data on a CT image demonstrates increased glucose uptake within the nodes. (From Gregoire V, Duprez T, Lengele B, Hamoir M: Management of the neck. In Gunderson LL, Tepper JE: *Clinical radiation oncology*, ed 2, Philadelphia, 2007, Churchill Livingstone.)

without severe complications necessitates extremely selective treatment criteria. Radiation therapy is indicated in the majority of head and neck cancers because the tumors located in this region are often inaccessible for surgery. The goals of treatment, however, can only be achieved through a multidisciplinary approach involving many specialists as described in the first part of this chapter, but the patient plays an important role. Emphasis is given to age and general condition, comorbidity

factors (associated diseases; i.e., emphysema, cardiovascular disease), habits and lifestyle, occupation, and patient's desires. It is pleasing to see that new editions of mainstream textbooks have now included sections devoted to quality of life, placing a new emphasis of the post treatment aspect of care. Generally, small primary lesions with negative nodes are treated with one modality (surgery or radiotherapy). Small lesions with involved nodes may need both surgery and radiotherapy for control of neck disease. Large primary lesions (T3 and T4) or extensive cervical node disease, or both, usually need surgery and irradiation and chemotherapy. Follow-up at regular intervals to detect early recurrence, extension, or complications is important. Patients can often be salvaged if tumor recurrence is detected early.

Surgery

Surgical oncologists play a crucial role in staging. While clinical staging is based on the results of a noninvasive physical examination and radiology, pathologic staging is based on findings in resected tumor specimens and biopsies. These reveal microscopic disease that is undetectable with imaging and serves to enhance the accuracy of the evaluation. Sabel[34] writes that clinical and pathologic staging may have two dramatically different outcomes.

Surgical resection and reconstructive techniques produce good outcomes in most patients with early stage tumors.[5] The use

Box 33-3	Head and Neck Cancer Cell Types

- Squamous cell carcinoma
- Lymphoepithelioma
- Spindle cell carcinoma
- Verrucous carcinoma
- Undifferentiated carcinoma
- Transitional cell carcinoma
- Keratinized carcinoma
- Nonkeratinized carcinoma
- Adenocarcinoma
- Malignant mixed carcinoma
- Adenocystic carcinoma
- Mucoepidermoid carcinoma
- Acinic cell carcinoma

of surgery as a curative modality is correlated to the possibility of an en bloc resection. Partial resections involve a high risk of recurrence. Wide margins (>2 cm) are usually necessary. A biopsy of the cervical nodes and lesion is mandatory and should be performed by experienced oncologic surgeons. Surgery is the mode of treatment for early-stage lesions of the oral cavity and floor of the mouth if no clinically positive nodes are present or if the risk of deep cervical node involvement is low. Surgery reduces the risk of dental or salivary damage seen with radiation therapy. Laser therapy, cryotherapy, and electrocautery are conventional curative surgical modalities.

Surgery has a higher success rate for palliative salvage therapy in the event of failure after radiation therapy. This holds true for conventional treatment only, as accelerated treatments result in severe acute toxic effects often requiring a feeding tube and mucosal healing time that take several months. Salvage surgery in these cases is often challenging. Especially in cases of oropharyngeal cancers treated via accelerated fractionation, results include a high incidence of complications and poor survival rates.[38]

Surgery offers better local control of disease that has invaded bone because curative radiation therapy doses have shown a high risk of necrosis. Microsurgery has revolutionized the approach to reconstruction of head and neck defects. Reconstructive procedures involve microvascular free flaps (a unit of tissue transferred enbloc from a donor to another recipient site) consisting of skin, myocutaneous tissue, the jejunum for replacement of the cervical esophagus, and bone grafts (Figure 33-15). Reconstruction of the midface, the oral cavity including the mandible, the base of tongue, and the hypopharynx has made the plastic surgeon an essential member of the head and neck disease management team.

Box 33-4	**American Joint Committee on Cancer Head and Neck Staging**

PRIMARY TUMOR (T)

GENERAL—FOR ALL SITES
TX Primary tumor cannot be assessed
T0 No evidence of primary tumor
Tis Carcinoma in situ

ORAL CAVITY AND LIP
T1   2 cm or less
T2   >2 but <4 cm
T3   >4 cm
T4a   (oral cavity) Invades adjacent structures (e.g., through cortical bone, into deep [extrinsic] muscle of tongue [genioglossus, hypoglossus, palataglossus, and styloglossus], maxillary sinus, skin of face)
T4b   Tumor invades masticator space, pterygoid plates, or skull base and/or encases internal carotid artery. *Note:* Superficial erosion alone of bone/tooth socket by gingival primary is not sufficient to classify as T4.

OROPHARYNX
T1   2 cm or less
T2   >2 but <4 cm
T3   >4 cm
T4   Invades adjacent structures
T4a   Invades larynx, deep/extrinsic muscle of tongue, medial pterygoid, hard palate, or mandible
T4b   Invades lateral pterygoid muscle, pterygoid plates, lateral nasopharynx, or skull base or encases carotid artery

NASOPHARYNX
T1   Confined to nasopharynx
T2   Extends to soft tissue of oropharynx and/or nasal fossa
T2a   Without parapharyngeal extension
T2b   With parapharyngeal extension
T3   Invades bony structures and/or paranasal sinuses
T4   Intracranial extension, and/or involvement of cranial nerves, infratemporal fossa, hypopharynx, or orbit

HYPOPHARYNX
T1   Limited to one subsite of hypopharynx and 2 cm or less
T2   >2 but <4 cm without fixation or more than one subsite or adjacent site

T3   > 4 cm or with hemilarynx fixation
T4a   Invades thyroid/cricoid cartilage, hyoid bone, thyroid gland, esophagus, or central compartment soft tissue
T4b   Invades prevertebral fascia, encases carotid artery, or involves mediastinal structures

SUPRAGLOTTIS
T1   Limited to one subsite, with normal vocal cord mobility
T2   Invades mucosa of more than one adjacent subsite of supraglottis or glottis or region outside the supraglottis; without fixation of larynx
T3   Limited to larynx with vocal cord fixation and/or or invades postcricoid area, pre-epiglottic tissues, paraglottic space, and/or minor thyroid cartilage erosion
T4a   Invades through thyroid cartilage and/or tissues beyond larynx
T4b   Invades prevertebral space, encases carotid artery, or invades mediastinal structures

GLOTTIS
T1   Limited to vocal cord(s), with normal mobility
T1 a   Limited to one vocal cord
T1 b   Involves both vocal cords
T2   Extends to supraglottis, and/or subglottis, and/or with impaired cord mobility
T3   Limited to larynx with vocal cord fixation
T4   Invades thru thyroid cartilage and/or other tissues beyond larynx
T4a   Invades through thyroid cartilage and/or tissues beyond larynx
T4b   Invades prevertebral space, encases carotid artery, or invades mediastinal structures

SUBGLOTTIS
T1   Limited to subglottis
T2   Extends to vocal cord(s) with normal/impaired mobility
T3   Limited to larynx with vocal cord fixation
T4a   Invades cricoid or thyroid cartilage and/or tissues beyond larynx
T4b   Invades prevertebral space, encases carotid artery, or invades mediastinal structures

Box 33-4	American Joint Committee on Cancer Head and Neck Staging—Cont'd

MAXILLARY SINUS

T1 Limited to maxillary sinus mucosa with no erosion or destruction of bone

T2 Causing bone erosion or destruction including extension into hard palate and/or middle nasal meatus, except extension to posterior wall of maxillary sinus and pterygoid plates. Tumor invades any of the following: bone of the posterior wall of maxillary sinus, subcutaneous tissues, floor or medial wall of orbit, pterygoid fossa, ethmoid sinuses

T3 Tumor invades any of the following: bone of posterior all of maxillary sinus, subcutaneous tissues, skin of cheek, floor or medial all of orbit, infratemporal fossa, pterygoid plates, ethmoid sinuses

T4a Invades anterior orbital contents, skin of cheek, pterygoid plates, infratemporal fossa, cribiform plate, sphenoid or frontal sinuses invades any of the following: orbital apex, dura, brain, middle cranial fossa, cranial nerves other than maxillary division of trigeminal nerve (V2), nasopharynx, or clivus

T4b Tumor invades orbital contents beyond floor or medial all, including any of the following: orbital apex, cribriform plate, base of skull, nasopharynx, sphenoid, frontal sinuses

ETHMOID SINUS AND NASAL CAVITY

T1 Confined to ethmoid with or without bone erosion

T2 Invading two subsites in single region or extending to involve adjacent region within nasoethmoidal complex, with or without bony invasion

T3 Extends to invade medial wall or floor of orbit, maxillary sinus, palate, or cribiform plate

T4a Invades any of the following: anterior orbital contents, skin of nose or cheek, minimal extension to anterior cranial fossa, pterygoid plates, sphenoid or frontal sinuses

T4b Invades any of the following: orbital apex, dura, brain, middle cranial fossa, cranial nerves other than (V2), nasopharynx or clivus

NODE STAGING OF HEAD AND NECK TUMORS

Nasopharyngeal carcinomas are designated according to modified Uniform International Committee on Cancer (UICC) staging

NASOPHARYNGEAL CANCER (NPC)

NX Regional lymph nodes cannot be assessed

N0 No regional lymph node metastasis

N1 Unilateral metastasis in lymph node(s), <6 cm in greatest dimension, above the supraclavicular fossa

N2 Bilateral metastasis in lymph node(s), <6 cm in greatest dimension, above the supraclavicular fossa

N3 Metastasis in a lymph node(s)

N3a >6 cm in greatest dimension

N3b Extension to the supraclavicular fossa

ALL OTHER SITES EXCEPT THE THYROID GLAND

NX Regional lymph nodes cannot be assessed

N0 No regional lymph node metastasis

N1 Metastasis in a single ipsilateral lymph node, < 3 cm in greatest dimension

N2 Metastasis in a single ipsilateral lymph node, > 3 cm but < 6 cm in greatest dimension; or in multiple ipsilateral lymph nodes, none > 6 cm in greatest dimension; or in bilateral or contralateral lymph nodes, none > 6 cm in greatest dimension

N2a Metastasis in a single ipsilateral lymph node > 3 cm but < 6 cm in greatest dimension

N2b Metastasis in multiple ipsilateral lymph nodes, none >6 cm in greatest dimension

N2c Metastasis in bilateral or contralateral lymph nodes, none > 6 cm in greatest dimension

N3 Metastasis in a lymph node > 6 cm in greatest dimension

Mx Presence of distant metastasis cannot be assessed

M0 No distant metastasis

M1 Distant meetastasis

Notes: Histologic examination of a selective neck dissection specimen should include 6 or more lymph nodes. A radical or modified radical neck dissection specimen should include 10 or more lymph nodes.

AJCC STAGE GROUPING FOR HEAD AND NECK TUMORS EXCEPT NPC

Stage 0	Tis N0 M0
Stage 1	T1 N0 M0
Stage 2	T2 N0 M0
Stage 3	T3 N0 M0
	T1 N1 M0
	T2 N1 M0
	T3 N1 M0
Stage 4	T4 Any N M0
	Any T N2,3 M0
	Any T Any N

AJCC STAGE GROUPING FOR HEAD AND NECK TUMORS FOR NPC

Stage I	T1 N0 M0
Stage IIA	T2a N0 M0
Stage IIB	T1 N1 M0 or T2a N1 M0 or T2b N0-1 M0
Stage III	T1-2 N2 M0 or T3 N0-2 M0
Stage IVA	T4 N0-2 M0
Stage IVB	Any T N3 M0
Stage IVC	Any T Any N M11

Greene FL, et al: *AJCC cancer staging manual,* ed 6, New York, 2002, Springer-Verlag.

A common surgical treatment that students may see in their clinical experience is the total or partial laryngectomy along with a tracheostomy. Figure 33-16 provides a general illustration.

Neck Dissection

Crile described the first removal of the regional neck nodes in 1906 for treating metastatic spread. Some form of a neck dissection has been included in the majority of treatment plans since then. The radical neck dissection (RND) is regarded as the gold standard for the treatment of neck disease.[41] RND removes the lymph nodes from levels I through V, the sternocleidomastoid muscle (SCM), the internal jugular vein (IJ), and the spinal accessory/eleventh cranial nerve. The modified radical neck dissection (MRND) attempts to decrease morbidity by sparing the SCM, the IJ and 11th cranial nerve depending on the location of the metastatic nodes. Various selective neck

Box 33-5 Lymphatic Drainage by Site

ORAL CAVITY
- Lips into the submandibular, preauricular, and facial nodes
- Buccal mucosa into the submaxillary and submental nodes
- Gingiva into the submaxillary and jugulodigastric nodes
- Retromolar trigone into the submaxillary and jugulodigastric nodes
- Hard palate into the submaxillary and upper jugular nodes
- Floor of mouth into the submaxillary and jugular (middle and upper) nodes
- Anterior two thirds of the tongue into the submaxillary and upper jugular nodes

OROPHARYNX
- Base of the tongue into the jugulodigastric, low cervical, and retropharyngeal nodes
- Tonsillar fossa into the jugulodigastric and submaxillary nodes

- Soft palate into the jugulodigastric, submaxillary, and spinal accessory nodes
- Pharyngeal walls into the retropharyngeal nodes, pharyngeal nodes, and jugulo-digastric nodes

NASOPHARYNX
- Retropharyngeal nodes into the superior jugular and posterior cervical nodes

SINUSES
- Retropharyngeal and superior cervical nodes

LARYNX
- Glottis—extremely rare nodal involvement
- Subglottis into the peritracheal and low cervical nodes
- Supraglottis into the peritracheal, cervical submental, and submaxillary nodes

Box 33-6 Expected Direct Spread of a Tumor

1. Lips
   a. Skin
   b. Commissure
   c. Mucosa
   d. Muscle
2. Gingiva
   a. Soft tissue and buccal mucosa
   b. Periosteum
   c. Bone and maxillary antrum
   d. Dental nerves
3. Buccal mucosa
   a. Side walls of the oral cavity
   b. Lips
   c. Retromolar trigone
   d. Muscles
4. Hard palate
   a. Soft palate
   b. Bone and maxillary antrum
   c. Nasal cavity
5. Trigone
   a. Buccal mucosa
   b. Anterior pillar
   c. Gingiva
   d. Pterygoid muscle
6. Floor of mouth
   a. Soft tissue, tonsils, and salivary glands
   b. Root of tongue
   c. Base of tongue
   d. Geniohyoid-mylohyoid muscles
7. Tongue
   a. Anterior two thirds of tongue
   b. Lateral borders

   c. Base and underside of tongue
   d. Floor of mouth
8. Soft palate
   a. Tonsillar pillars
   b. Pharyngeal walls
   c. Hard palate
   d. Nasopharynx
9. Larynx
   a. True cords
   b. False cords
   c. Arytenoid muscles
   d. Epiglottis
   e. Hypopharynx
   f. Aryepiglottic folds
   g. Ventricles
10. Pharynx
   a. Anterior walls
   b. Posterior tongue
   c. Base of tongue
   d. Lateral walls
   e. Tonsillar pillars
   f. Uvula
   g. Soft palate
   h. Posterior walls
   i. Muscles and epiglottis
11. Tonsils
   a. Palatine-linguinal tonsil
   b. Tonsillar pillars
   c. Base of tongue
   d. Soft palate
   e. Pharyngeal wall

dissections (SNDs) preserve whole nodal levels reducing morbidity further.[41] Figure 33-17 illustrates steps of an RND.

The relation between wound healing and radiation therapy is not favorable after high doses. Both acute inflammatory changes in tissues and late radiation changes that include fibrosis and decreased vascularity require careful consideration. Wound healing is impaired by factors that include diminished blood supply, impaired collagen formation, and increased risk of infection in part due to decreased leukocyte function. Healing complications are common in cases of myocutaneous flaps involving tissue that is considered to be "severely injured" by high doses of radiation. An interesting note involves an irradiated hollow organ such as the trachea that requires resection and anastomosis. It is suggested that sparing one side from radiation exposure maintains a path of vascularity for better blood supply to the healing anastomosis and reduces fistula formation and leakage.[6]

Chemotherapy

Induction or neoadjuvant chemotherapy is useful in cases such as treatment of advanced NPCs before radiation therapy, as a radiosensitizer during treatment, or as an adjuvant after treatment.

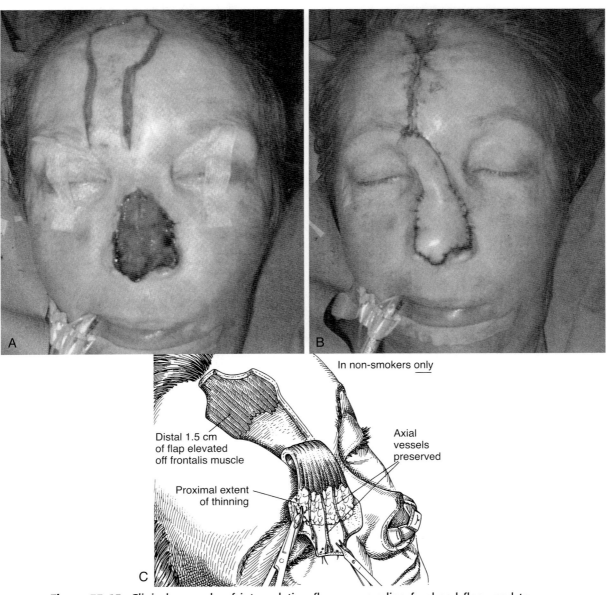

Figure 33-15. Clinical example of interpolation flap; paramedian forehead flap used to resurface a large nasal defect. **A**, Nasal defect, **B**, Intraoperative transfer of flap, **C**, Forehead flap in full thickness with all its vascular layers. (**A** and **B**, From Spector JA, Levine JP: Cutaneous defects: Flaps, grafts, and expansion; **C**, From Spicer GJ, Lisman RD: Upper and lower eyelid reconstruction. In McCarthy JG, Galiano RD, Boutros SG, editors: *Current therapy in plastic surgery*, Philadelphia, 2006, Saunders.)

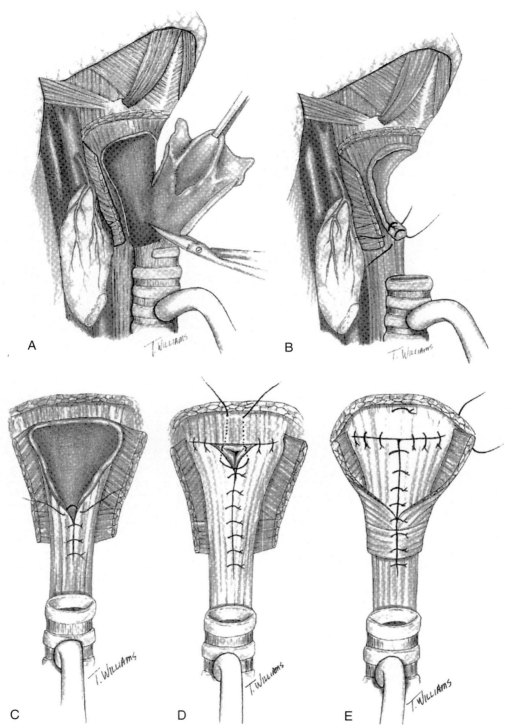

Figure 33-16. A, Excision of the larynx from the pharynx. Note scissors transecting the airway, well above the tracheotomy site. Thyroid gland has been transected. **B**, Right lateral view of the neopharynx following removal of the larynx. The pharyngeal mucosa is ready for closure. **C**, Frontal view of the neopharynx, partially closed. **D** and **E**, Postlaryngectomy pharyngeal reconstruction. Note that at this stage the airway is completely separate from the digestive system. (From Clayman GL, et al: Advanced stage cancer of the larynx. In Harrison LB, Sessions RB, Hong WK: *Head and neck cancer: a multidisciplinary approach*, ed 2, Philadelphia, 2004, Lippincott Williams & Wilkins.)

Combination chemotherapy for palliation of recurrence or metastases of NPC produces complete response rates up to 44%.[21]

The role of chemotherapy in head and neck cancer is standard for metastatic disease, locally recurrent disease, or salvage therapy, for which surgery and radiation therapy can no longer be used. Chemotherapy's role is limited, but it is evolving. Single-agent therapy with methotrexate, cisplatin, carboplatin, bleomycin, 5-fluorouracil (5-FU), hydroxyurea, ifosfamide, and the taxanes paclitaxel and docetaxel produces responses lasting from 2 to 6 months. Combination drug therapy has produced higher

response rates, but the prognosis has not improved, and the toxicity to the patient is higher. Cisplatin-containing combinations have produced the highest overall and complete remission rates. The average duration of response has been 11.3 months for patients with complete remission. Cisplatin and 5-FU continue to be the most frequently used combination regimen. Among the newer multiagent chemotherapeutic regimens are those that combine cisplatin with agents such as the taxanes or ifosfamide. Overall survival rates for combination chemotherapy has been similar to that of single-agent therapy.[31] Neoadjuvant (induction)

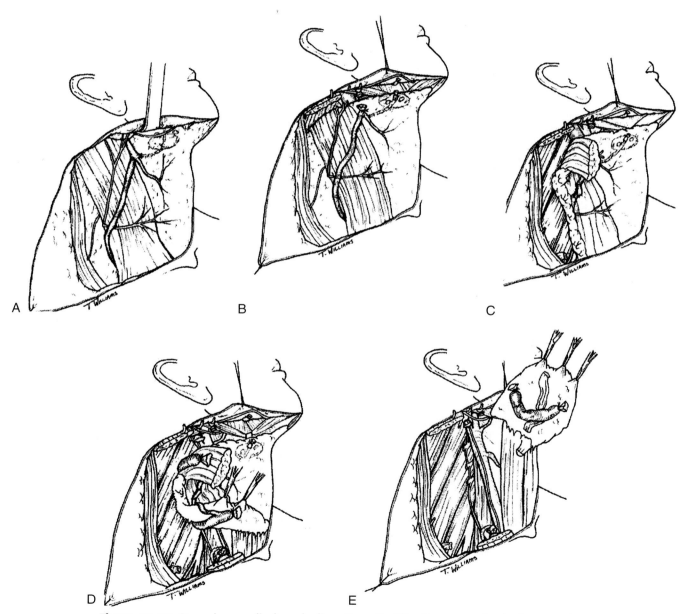

Figure 33-17. Steps in a radical neck dissection. **A,** Skin flaps are raised. The SCM is exposed, along with cranial nerves. **B,** A flap is raised to protect the marginal mandibular nerve. **C,** The SCM is detached from the mastoid and the posterior border is delineated. **D,** The IJ is ligated, and the neck-dissection specimen is raised from posterior to anterior. **E,** The specimen is removed from the carotid sheath and medial attachment. (From Wolfe MJ, Wilson K: Head and neck cancer. In Sabel MS, Sondak VK, Sussman JJ: *Essentials of surgical oncology; surgical foundations,* Philadelphia, 2007, Mosby.)

chemotherapy is the initial utilization of chemotherapy before local therapy, as a first-line modality. Neither induction chemotherapy nor adjuvant chemotherapy has improved survival when added to locoregional therapy; this includes multiagent regimens. Concurrent irradiation and chemotherapy yields a small increase in survival rate relative to irradiation alone, but complication rates also increased.[4] Because of the poor health and nutritional status of head and neck cancer patients, the use of chemotherapy as a front-line modality has not been favorable.

Radiation Therapy

The use of radiation is considered the mainstay of cancer management for the treatment of cancer in the head and neck region. The choice of external beam radiation therapy (EBRT) and/or brachytherapy depends on the individual and location of the tumor. Customization of the treatment technique is essential. Although Khan reports in 2007 that the simple electron beam provides a useful ancillary technique for boosting doses to superficial regions in the head and neck area still in use today,[19] the complexity of more modern radical radiation therapy requires that therapy be administered only by specially trained and experienced radiation oncologists who have full dosimetric and physics support facilities.[31]

Contemporary treatment planning allows three-dimensional (3D) planning with patient data obtained from CT, MRI, and PET. Advances in software provide complex treatments such as 3D conformal radiation therapy (3D-CRT), IMRT, image-guided radiation therapy (IGRT), and high-dose-rate brachytherapy (HDR). Sophisticated computer and imaging technology make inverse treatment planning the basis for IMRT. Standard fractionation schedules use daily treatments, 5 days per week, for approximately 6.5 to 7.5 weeks. Altered fraction schedules show improvement in tumor control; however, accelerated treatments also show a higher incidence of morbidity. SCCs with long doubling times are treated effectively with standard fractionation (200 cGy per day, 5 days a week). SCCs vary in doubling times, those with shorter doubling times demonstrate poorer control and may be treated more effectively with accelerated hyperfractionation (120 cGy, twice daily).[36]

Adherence to the TD 5/5 is required for irradiation of the total volume to a tumoricidal dose. Table 33-5 gives the tolerance doses for special organs found in the head and neck area.

Patient Positioning and Immobilization

Accurate and reproducible treatment has always been an important aspect of high-quality radiation therapy. The importance of precise reproducibility has grown with increased interest in 3D conformal therapy and dose escalation. The objective of tumor control with these new techniques involves higher doses while using tighter target margins to limit the dose to adjacent normal tissues. Precision calls for the use of numerous noninvasive immobilization techniques based on thermoplastic mask immobilization, customized polyurethane cradles and extended head to shoulder/upper thorax immobilization, and longer head boards extending from the head to the upper thorax for additional support of the head and shoulders. IGRT systems have been useful as an effective tool for confirming reproducibility, once the patient has been immobilized.

The treatment of head and neck cancers involves the following general patient positioning for many cases. Patient positioning for the treatment of head and neck cancers, however, may be dependent on the specific type of cancer being treated and the radiation oncologist's objectives regarding tumor volume and the sparing of normal tissue. For instance, the treatment of a parotid gland may require the patient to lie on the side with the affected side, while the treatment of a maxillary antrum usually requires that the patient's head be positioned with the chin extended to include the cephalad extent of the maxillary antrum in an anterior field without also including the eye.[8] For most cases, the patient is in the supine position with the neck extended and the head resting on an appropriate headrest. Clinically palpable nodes may be outlined with metallic wires during the simulation process. Surgical scars, orbital canthi, lacrimal glands, oral commissures may be identified in the same manner. It is generally believed that tumor cells trapped in the surgical scars are less well oxygenated and therefore more radioresistant, and that higher radiation doses are required to eradicate them.[17] This may be achieved with an additional electron boost field or by maximizing the dose to the skin in the area using tissue equivalent bolus material. A tongue blade with a cork attached to one end, or another similar device may be inserted between the incisor teeth to depress the tongue, displace the tongue from the treatment volume, or displace the palate (Figure 33-18). The head is immobilized with a customized thermoplastic face mask that is fixed to a base plate under the patient's head, which in turn may or may not be attached to the treatment couch. A small hole may be made in the mask when a bite block, positional stent, or nasogastric tube is used (Figure 33-19).

The lateral photon portals of the typical head and neck treatment should encompass as much of the clinical target volume as possible without having the entrance beam (as determined by the light field on the skin) go through the shoulder. The shoulders may be displaced inferiorly as much as possible to maximize the utility of the lateral portals. Inferior displacement of the shoulders can be accomplished by the patient's pulling on two ends of a strap wrapped around a footboard.[24] In a similar fashion, a shoulder strap that uses Velcro to secure the strap

Table 33-5	Doses Allowed for Special Organs in the Head and Neck Region		
Organ	**TD 5/5 (cGy)**	**TD 50/5 (cGy)**	**Whole/Partial Organ**
Muscles (adult)	6000	8000	Whole
Oral cavity	6000	8000	50 cm²
Spinal cord	4500	5500	Whole or partial
Lens of eye	500	1200	Whole
Brain	6000	7000	Whole
Retina	5500	7000	Whole
Cornea	5000	>6000	Whole
Ear	5000	7000	Whole
Thyroid gland	4500	15000	Whole
Pituitary gland	4500	20000	Whole

Modified from Bentel GC: *Treatment planning and dose calculation*, ed 4, New York, 1989, Pergamon Press.

around the patient's wrists and feet while the knees are bent, can be used to straighten their knees in order to pull the shoulders down. Patients with short necks or those unable to displace their shoulders inferiorly pose a treatment planning problem. One solution involves the use of lateral fields that are angled inferiorly to obtain better inferior coverage. This is done by rotating the foot of the treatment table 10 to 20 degrees away from the gantry.

 A mouth stent or tongue blade may serve more than one purpose. Mouth stents may separate/displace the palate, thereby sparing it from treatment. A tongue blade may serve to either depress and fix the tongue within a field or displace it from the field.

Treatment Data Capture and Treatment Planning

Imaging and modern treatment planning are inseparable. The most useful modalities are CT and MRI. Meticulous communication and a supervising form of continuity of care must exist from aspects of proper patient positioning as the process goes from initial image acquisition and localization to actual treatment delivery. Factors of error typically include imaging without a flat table and inconsistency in shape, form, and thickness

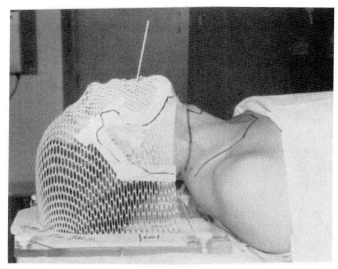

Figure 33-19. Treatment position of a patient with nasopharyngeal carcinoma.(From Leibel SA: Textbook of radiation oncology, Philadelphia, 1998, Saunders.)

or placement of positioning aids as the patient moves from the planning to the treatment stage. Improvement has been shown with more sophisticated and patient dedicated devices and with dedicated imaging staff within the radiation therapy department. Dedicated staff and imaging capabilities integrated within the radiation therapy department has become the standard for progressive treatment planning. Conventional simulators, equipped with fluoroscopy, are quickly disappearing from the forefront. Once useful for final verification of a CT simulation, the development of digitally reproduced radiographs (DRRs), special CT simulation software, the portal imaging system, and especially IGRT have made the conventional simulator obsolete. A dedicated CT scanner with wide apertures and flat tabletops and accessories to accurately reproduce treatment conditions has placed more demand on the CT simulator. Imaging has progressed from using the conventional simulation film, to viewing slice–by-slice transverse cuts of anatomy and gross tumor on a monitor. These data can be processed using computer software to view images in any plane. Added information for treatment planning heterogeneity corrections is provided by Hounsfield (CT) numbers for tissue density (see Chapter 23).

With the use of sophisticated imaging in radiation therapy, new terminology has emerged from other sciences. For example, conventional simulation has evolved to CT simulation. In addition, new terms such as virtual simulation, pixel (picture element), voxel, (volume element), window leveling, and contouring expand the medical terms used by the practicing radiation therapist. Other new terms are emerging. Beam arrangements can be either coplanar or noncoplanar. A highly conformal plan typically includes multiple beams facilitated by computer-driven multileaf collimation (MLC). Although custom-made cerrobend blocks are still being used, the demands of conformal radiation therapy call for facilitated beam shaping. Dynamic multileaf collimation (DMLC) allows changing the beam shape during the "beam-on" of treatment delivery to affect beam shape as well as dose distribution. Field-in-field techniques may

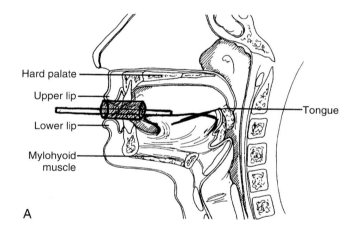

A

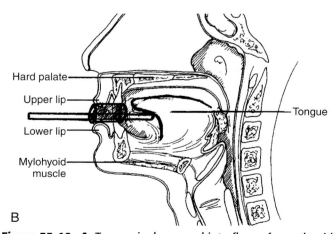

B

Figure 33-18. A, Tongue is depressed into floor of mouth with tongue blade and cork or bite-block if tumor invasion includes the tongue. **B,** Tip of tongue is displaced from treatment field when a lesion is limited to the anterior floor-of-mouth. Tongue blade is positioned under the tongue.

be facilitated using MLC to deliver additional dose to a subset of a larger treatment field. The manual beam patching technique referred to as the *field-in field technique* is a forward planning technique to achieve a more desirable dose distribution.[15]

Treatment planning by means of prescribing a target dose and letting the computer generate the optimal plan is how most advanced conformal radiation therapy is designed. Inverse treatment planning systems work with the defined target dose and programmed normal tissue tolerance doses to optimize the number of beam portals and the beam intensity pattern within each portal to generate the best dose distribution to fit the prescription. IMRT is based on this "inverse scheme of treatment planning. Methods of delivery vary from the step-and-shoot method to dynamic treatment. The Peacock multileaf intensity modulating collimator (MIMiC), also referred to as serial tomotherapy due to continuous fan beams delivered through an arc treatment, was the first treatment system on the market. Treatment planning systems today include ADAC Pinnacle, Eclipse, and CMS (Computerized Medical Systems).[19]

SITE-SPECIFIC STUDY OF CANCERS OF THE HEAD AND NECK

The Oral Cavity Region

Anatomy. The oral cavity extends from the skin-vermilion junction of the lip to the posterior border of the hard palate superiorly and to the circumvallate papillae inferiorly. Subdivisions within the oral cavity include the anterior two-thirds of the tongue (anterior to the circumvallate papillae), lip, buccal mucosa, lower alveolar ridge, upper alveolar ridge, retromolar trigone, floor of mouth, and hard palate (Figures 33-20 and 33-21).

Clinical Presentation. Patients who have oral cavity cancer often demonstrate poor oral and dental hygiene. In females, Plummer-Vinson syndrome (iron deficiency anemia) is considered an important etiologic factor. Because premalignant conditions are usually asymptomatic, the general practitioner or dentist is responsible for clinical detection. Early diagnosis is essential for a good prognosis. The areas cited to be least commonly examined are the paralingual gutters.

As previously stated, leukoplakia and erythroplasia represent severe dysplastic changes and should be regarded as serious pathologic problems. Most often, oral cavity cancers appear as nonhealing ulcers with little pain. Localized pain is considered a symptom of advanced disease.

Diagnostic Procedures and Staging. Inspection and palpation are important first steps. The malignant ulcer is typically raised, centrally ulcerated, with indurated edges and an infiltrated base. Biopsy is mandatory. Imaging modalities include both CT and MRI for staging of advanced tumors. The use of PET is not mentioned for staging and diagnosis in some literature; its routine use was specifically not recommended in others.

Histopathology. SCC accounts for 90% to 95% of the histopathologic types, either well or moderately well differentiated. Unusual variants of SCC include verrucous carcinoma and spindle cell SCC. Adenocarcinomas of the salivary gland may be identified.

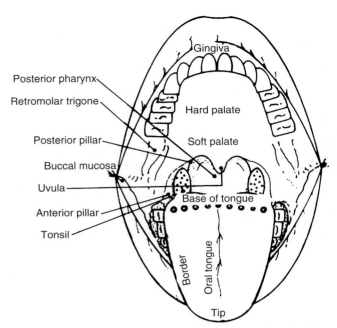

Figure 33-20. A front open-mouth view of the oral cavity. (From Cox JD: *Moss' radiation oncology: rationale, technique, results,* ed 7, St. Louis, 1994, Mosby.)

Staging. The staging system is listed in Box 33-4.

Metastatic Behavior. Cervical lymph node involvement at the time of presentation is uncommon, and oral cavity cancer demonstrates the lowest incidence (except glottic cancer) of nodal metastasis in the head and neck region. Blood-borne spread occurs in fewer than 20% of patients. Of those patients, most have cervical node involvement at the time of presentation and advanced-stage disease.

General Treatment Techniques. Early-stage (<1 to 1.5 cm) and premalignant lesions are candidates for surgery alone. If inadequate surgical margins and neck node involvement are present, combination radiation therapy and surgery is indicated. The sequence of the therapy is usually dictated by the first treatment's design. If radical surgery is planned, the radiation therapy should not be given before surgery. Elective irradiation of the lymph nodes is included if a lesion demonstrates a high rate of spread or has a history of bilateral movement (anatomically) via the lymphatics. A 5-year follow-up plan is recommended because lesions in most sites recur within 2 years and rarely after 4 years.

The Oral Cavity: The Lip. The lymphatics of the upper lip drain into the submandibular and preauricular nodal beds (Figure 33-22). Lymphatics from the mid-lower lip and anterior floor of the mouth rain into the submental nodal group (Figure 33-23). Lymphatics from the oral tongue drain into the anterior cervical chain; more anteriorly placed lesions drain lower in the neck than lesions placed more posteriorly (Figure 33-24).

Lip cancer is treated with radiation therapy in the same manner as skin cancer; however, the majority of cases can be surgically removed. Tumors that should be treated with radiation therapy are those involving a commissure in order to obtain better cosmesis and local control in cases of more advanced disease.

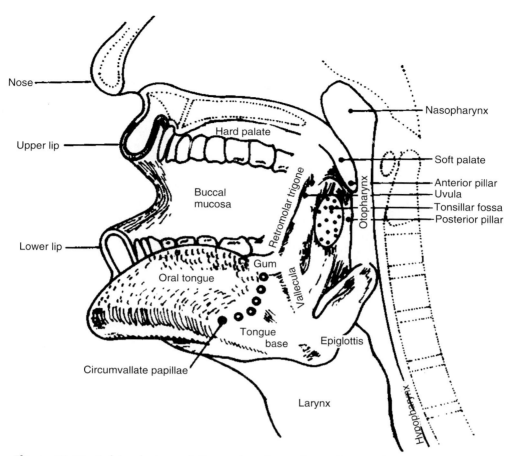

Figure 33-21. A lateral view of the oral cavity and oropharynx depicting anatomical subdivisions. (From Cox JD: *Moss' radiation oncology: rationale, technique, results,* ed 7, St. Louis, 1994, Mosby.)

Successful control is achievable, though, by EBRT, interstitial implants, or both. Single, anterior source-skin distance (SSD) ports, 100- to 200-kVp x-rays or 3- to 7-MeV electrons at the 100% isodose line is a common regimen. Protracted treatment schedules (4 to 6 weeks) with deliveries of 200 to 300 cGy per day can be given for lesions less than 2 cm. Larger, bulkier lesions require doses of 5000 to 6000 cGy. Regional (submental) lymphatics are rarely treated, whereas patients with advanced-stage or recurrent disease should have neck irradiation. Face shielding must be constructed to delineate the target volume and thus only expose 1 to 2 cm of normal tissue. A lead shield is designed and positioned in place to expose the lip lesion. The lesion may be treated with 100-kVp x-rays through a cone. To reduce complications to teeth and gums, a stent coated with wax or a low-atomic-number compound (tissue equivalent) can be made to fit over the teeth. A stent is a lead shield that may consist of two sheets of lead (each ⅛ inch thick) overlaid with one sheet of aluminum and is coated with wax or vinyl. The face-mask shielding should also be coated with wax to reduce the electron scatter to the adjacent tissues. Exit radiation to the bone and gums needs to be controlled at safe levels to prevent progressive, long-term physiological changes. With megavoltage electron energies, a tissue

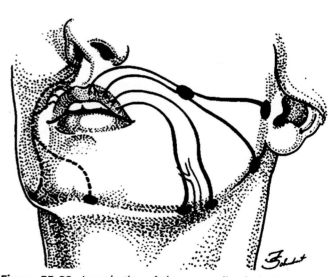

Figure 33-22. Lymphatics of the upper lip drain into buccal, parotid, upper cervical, and submandibular nodes. Lymphatics of the skin of the upper lip (dotted line) may cross midline to terminate in submental and submandibular nodes of the contralateral side. (From Cox JD: *Moss' radiation oncology: rationale, technique, results,* ed 7, St. Louis, 1994, Mosby.)

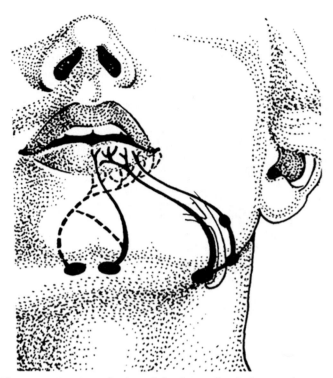

Figure 33-23. Lymphatics of the lower lip drain to submental and submandibular nodes. Sometimes disease involves facial nodes. Lymphatics of the skin of the lower lip (dotted line) may cross midline to end in submental or submandibular nodes on the contralateral side. (From Cox JD: *Moss' radiation oncology: rationale, technique, results*, ed 7, St. Louis, 1994, Mosby.)

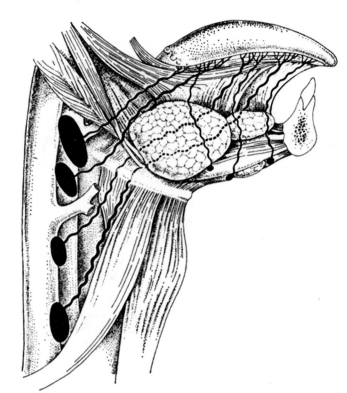

Figure 33-24. Lymphatics of the tongue, illustrating that the more anteriorly they originate in the tongue, the lower in the neck their draining nodes may lie. (From Cox JD: *Moss' radiation oncology: rationale, technique, results*, ed 7, St. Louis, 1994, Mosby.)

compensator is sometimes used to make the dose more uniform. Local control by interstitial implant is comparable to that achieved with EBRT. For larger lesions, better cosmetic results are obtained with EBRT. Death due to lip carcinoma is uncommon.

The Oral Cavity: The Floor of the Mouth. The medical literature suggests that most cancers of the floor of the mouth are treated with resection at some institutions (Figure 33-25). Megavoltage external beam alone gives inferior control results, even for T1 lesions. However, reports of several studies show that good local control may be achieved with a combination of external irradiation interstitial implants or intraoral cone.[24]

Cancers in this area arise on the anterior surface on either side of the midline. They can spread to the bone and tongue. About 30% of these cancers have positive submaxillary and subdigastric nodes. Therefore, opposed lateral ports are used. If the lesion is small and confined to the floor of the mouth, the tip of the tongue is elevated out of the portal with a cork. If the lesion has grown into the tongue, the tongue is flattened to reduce the superior border of the portal (see Figure 33-18, *A*, *B*). A small stainless steel pin may be inserted into the posterior border of the tumor and serves as a marker for treatment planning (simulation) and brachytherapy. The entire width of the mandibular arch is included in the port. The superior border is designed to spare the maxillary antrum. An off-cord boost via opposed laterals occurs at 4500 cGy. If the neck nodes are clinically positive, the lateral ports are enlarged to include all the

upper cervical nodes, and an anterior, bilateral, supraclavicular neck field is added.

The lateral borders of the anterior supraclavicular field extend to the coracoid process. The inferior borders extend horizontally 1 to 2 cm below the suprasternal notch, and the superior borders abut via (megavoltage x-ray) the lateral borders at the thyroid notch. The supraclavicular field is taken to 5000 cGy. The bilateral neck fields receive a minimum of 5000 cGy, with boost fields added to bring the dose between 6000 and 7000 cGy. The reduced boost fields can be treated with an intraoral cone, needle implants, or small external photon beams using 3D conformal radiotherapy. This is followed by radical neck dissection or limited nodal resection depending on the extent of disease.[8] The literature cites a recent report using HDR with good results delivering a dose of 6000 cGy. The advantage described of HDR versus LDR was the elimination of exposure to staff. Despite good local control, actuarial survival of these patients is poor, owing to a significant number of deaths from intercurrent disease or a second primary cancer.[24]

Bone and soft tissue necrosis is reported in up to 21% of patients within 2 years after treatment. Some patients require hemimandibulectomy. An overall 5-year disease-specific survival rate of 56% has been reported.[23]

The Oral Cavity: The Tongue. Both the anterior tongue and the base of tongue will be discussed in this section. The reader is advised that only the anterior two thirds is included in

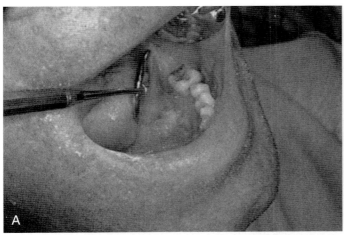
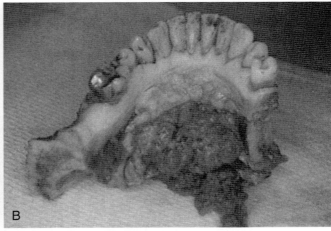

Figure 33-25. A, A deeply infiltrating squamous cell carcinoma involving the entire anterior floor of mouth and mandible. **B,** Treatment involved composite resection followed by radiation. Reconstruction was critical to function, appearance, and quality of life. (From Silverman S: *Oral cancer*, ed 5, Hamilton, 2003, BC Decker. Reprinted by the permission of the American Cancer Society, Inc.)

the oral cavity. The base of tongue is considered to be in the oropharynx. The oral tongue is the freely mobile portion of the tongue that extends anteriorly from the line of circumvallate papillae to the undersurface of the tongue at the junction of the floor of the mouth. It is composed of four areas: the tip, the lateral borders, the dorsum, and the undersurface (nonvillous surface of the tongue).

Small tumors arising in the anterior two thirds of the tongue also known as the oral tongue are usually resected. Radiation therapy is used in patients who are medically inoperable. Postoperative radiation therapy to the primary site and the cervical lymph nodes is used to cover positive margins, extensive primary tumor with bone or skin invasion, and multiple positive nodes. The anterior tongue drains into the submandibular lymph nodes, while the posterior portion of the tongue drains more to the jugulodigastric, posterior pharyngeal, and upper cervical lymph nodes.

Lesions of the tongue usually appear on the lateral borders near the middle and posterior third section. The lesions can be quite large and still confined to the tongue (Figure 33-26). Only a limited number of tongue cancers can be excised. Therefore, EBRT can achieve the best control with interstitial boost fields.

Lesions on the tip of the tongue are seen first and are commonly in an early stage, whereas lesions at the base and posterior one third of the tongue that invade the floor of the mouth, the tonsils, or the muscles are advanced and have a higher incidence of nodal metastasis. Base of tongue cancer is highly infiltrative and clinical understaging is common.[7] An early-stage lesion of the tongue can be cured with a local excision or hemiglossectomy (surgical removal of half the tongue). For the preservation of speech and swallowing functions, EBRT is the best choice for large T3-4 lesions. Iridium 192 implants follow the external beam. Brachytherapy requires a preprocedure tracheotomy because the tongue wells massively after

the implant. Figure 33-27 depicts radiation ports for the base of a tongue. A depressor, a tongue blade and cork, or some other type of mouth stent is sometimes inserted to push the tongue back and keep as much of the mandible out of the field as possible. The subdigastric and submaxillary nodes must always be included in the port. A three-field technique that uses isocentric lateral-opposed are used, with the posterior borders encompassing the upper cervical nodes and the superior border aligned to miss the maxillary antrum matched to a lower anterior neck field.[17] External beam is delivered to a dose of 5400 cGy in 30 fractions with 180 cGy/fraction. The fields are reduced off the spinal cord at 4500 cGy. At that point, the tongue and upper anterior neck is boosted with photons and the posterior neck is treated with electrons for a total dose of 5400 cGy.

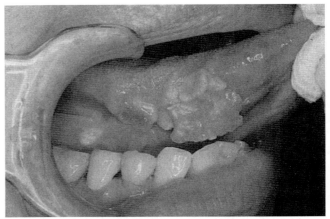

Figure 33-26. Advanced exophytic carcinoma that had been noticed for more than 6 months. (From Silverman S: *Oral cancer*, ed 5, Hamilton, 2003, BC Decker. Reprinted by the permission of the American Cancer Society, Inc.)

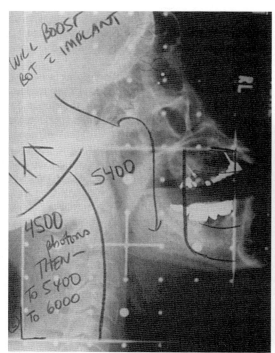
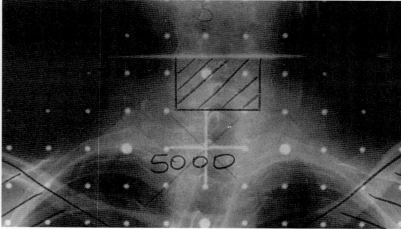

Figure 33-27. Simulation film, base of tongue, external beam radiation therapy. Patients are immobilized using custom designed Aquaplast masks and placement of a bite block. The superior border includes the retropharyngeal and upper jugular lymph nodes (levels I, II). The inferior border is at the hyoid bone; clinically this is just above the thyroid notch and can be palpated. The posterior border is placed at the posterior aspect of the spinal process. The anterior border is approx. 2 cm from the primary tumor. Even in the situation of a small primary, both the lateral and anterior neck are treated. The treatment field should include lymph node levels I, II, III, and V. There should be generous coverage of the retropharyngeal nodes. (From Leibel SA: *Textbook of radiation oncology*, Philadelphia, 1998, Saunders.)

Palpable nodes are treated with electrons at an additional 600 cGy, to a total dose to 6000 cGy. The patient then undergoes an iridium implant and a neck dissection.[42] The patient may be treated with IMRT as an alternative. The low neck is treated with an anterior field with a tapered midline block.[7] Survival after radiation therapy for carcinoma of the oral tongue is directly related to staging. The overall 5-year survival rates reported are 84% (T1), 78% (T2a), and 72% (T2b). Overall 5-year actuarial survival and determinate survival rates of 32% and 47%, respectively, have been reported.[23]

The Oral Cavity: The Buccal Mucosa. The buccal mucosa is the mucous membrane lining the inner surface of the cheeks and lips. Most lesions originate on the lateral walls, have a history of leukoplakia, and appear as a raised, exophytic growth. As it grows, the lesion invades the skin and bone. Usually, the patient notices a bump with the tip of the tongue. Pain is not associated with this lesion unless the nerves to the tongue or ear become involved. Advanced lesions bleed. Early lesions often appear as an inflammatory process, so care should be taken during a biopsy to obtain a differential diagnosis.

Stensen's duct can become obstructed. This enlarges the parotid gland, thereby necessitating surgical intervention. Small (1-cm) lesions can be excised, whereas larger lesions are treatable with combination surgery/radiation therapy, radical surgery, or aggressive radiation therapy alone. If radiation therapy is chosen as a treatment modality, a single-plane photon or electron beam that spares contralateral tissues, especially the contralateral parotid, can be used. The submaxillary and subdigastric nodes are at risk. If positive, these nodes require a controlling dose. Radiation therapy usually consists of 5500 to 6000 cGy in 6 weeks, followed by a boost of 2000 cGy sparing the mandible.[8] A total additional dose of up to 3000 cGy has been documented through an interstitial implant.[24] In advanced tumors, radiation therapy is followed by surgical resection of the lesion and regional lymph nodes. Fibrosis of the cheek and trismus are not infrequent complications following radical radiotherapy. T1 lesions can be treated with oral cone alone, 6000 cGy in 15 fractions or an implant to deliver 6000 cGy in 6 to 7 days. Three-dimensional conformal therapy has been exclusively recommended to spare the contralateral parotid.[23]

Large buccal mucosal tumors may be treated with 3D conformal therapy, delivering 7500 cGy with sparing of normal structures using right anterior and left anterior oblique beams (Figure 33-28). A 5-year actuarial disease-free survival after surgical salvage of 59.7% has been reported.[23]

The Oral Cavity: The Hard Palate. The hard palate is the semilunar area between the upper alveolar ridge and the mucous membrane covering the palatine process of the maxillary palatine bones. It extends from the inner surface of the superior alveolar ridge to the posterior edge of the palatine bone. Hard palate carcinomas are quite rare and are mostly adenocarcinomas, adenoid cystic carcinomas known for its perineural (around nerves) pattern of spread. The majority of malignant tumors of the hard palate are of minor salivary gland origin. SCC is rare. They tend to spread to the bone and invade the maxillary antrum. Adenoid cystic types spread hematogenously to lungs and bone and along the second branch of the fifth cranial nerve to the middle fossa. These types of tumors seldom metastasize to lymph nodes. Surgical resection is the usual treatment, with postoperative radiation therapy given as needed in high-risk patients. Irradiation with surface molds can treat very superficial lesions.[23] Cancers in this area have been noted to be the result of secondary spread from the upper gum. A history of ill-fitting dentures or trauma is common. Postoperative radiation therapy is added in high-risk patients. The typical treatment technique involves opposed lateral fields or wedge pairs to 6500 or 7000 cGy in 6.5 to 7.5 weeks. Postoperative cases doses of 6200 to 6500 cGy are delivered in 6.5 to 7.0 weeks. A balloon filled with water can be used to compensate for postsurgical tissue defects.[24] In addition, neutron therapy may be considered for advanced unresectable tumors, and/or mixed beam therapy using photon/proton combination, or proton therapy alone may also be considered as an alternative.[7] The following 5-year disease-free survival rates have been reported, 75% (stage I) (surgery alone), 46% (stage II) (all surgery except one postoperative irradiation), 40% (stage III) (all surgery except one postoperative irradiation), and 8% (stage IV).[23]

The Oral Cavity: The Retromolar Trigone. The retromolar trigone is the triangular space behind the last molar tooth. Carcinomas of this area are rare. Lesions can cause tongue pain, ear canal pain, or, if the muscles become involved, trismus. Indirect extension begins with early invasion of the anterior tonsillar pillar or the buccal mucosa. The retromolar trigone is included in the minimum target volume for the treatment of early tonsillar cancers.[7] Lee and Phillips[23] write, "Frequently, they are indistinguishable from carcinomas arising from the anterior tonsillar pillar" (p. 649). Most are moderately differentiated SCCs. CT scan and MRI in selected cases can demonstrated deep extension like bone invasion and positive neck nodes. Invasion of the pterygoid muscles that produce trismus is better imaged on MRI than by CT.[17] Lymphatic spread occurs to the submaxillary and subdigastric nodes. Hinerman, Foote, Sandow, and Mendenhall[17] report that local control rates for T1 and T2 lesions are similar using surgery or radiation therapy. Small lesions without bone invasion can be resected, but superficial T3 lesions can be treated by radiation therapy alone.[17] Lee and Phillips[23] report that lesions of the retromolar trigone are

treated in a "highly selected manner." T1 and T2 tumors are treated with radiation therapy, but surgical resection is the preferred modality. More advanced tumors require surgery and postoperative radiation therapy.

Early lesions may be treated with external radiation therapy alone using mixed electrons and photons with single lateral fields or parallel opposing fields with 2:1 loading favoring the diseased side. The typical treatment consists of 6600 to 7400 cGy, 200 cGy/fraction. Treatment techniques may also involve anterior and lateral wedged pair fields or anterior and posterior oblique fields using wedges. Small, well-defined lesions may be boosted via an intraoral cone using an electron beam. Large lesions that involve the base of tongue, invading bone, may be treated using parallel-opposed lateral fields to the primary lesion and cervical nodes. It is emphasized that lesions in this area have a high tendency for metastases to the neck; therefore, prophylactic neck treatment is critical.[23] An anterior field is included to treat the lower cervical nodes and bilateral supraclavicular fossa.[8] Surgery has been noted to be reserved for salvage of radiation therapy failures, but a recent report indicated that better locoregional control and disease-free survival was obtained with surgery and postoperative radiation therapy.[23] Moderately advanced lesions are usually managed with resection and postoperative radiation therapy. A 5-year determinate survival rate of 83% has been reported.

The subdivisions of the oral cavity include (1) the anterior two thirds of the tongue, (2) the lip, (3) the buccal mucosa, (4) the retromolar trigone, (5) the floor of the mouth, and (6) the hard palate.

The Pharynx Region

Anatomy. The pharynx is subdivided into three anatomical divisions: the oropharynx, nasopharynx, and hypopharynx, also referred to as the laryngopharynx (see Figure 33-6). Attention should be provided to the distinct anatomic structures that define each subdivision—the nasopharynx, located behind the nose and extending from the posterior nares to the level of the soft palate; the oropharynx, located behind the mouth from the soft palate above to the level of the hyoid bone below; and the laryngopharynx or hypopharynx, extending from the hyoid bone to its termination in the esophagus.[39]

Clinical Presentation. The most common symptoms include persistent sore throat, painful swallowing, and referred otalgia. Enlargement of cervical nodes is present. Fetor oris, dyspnea, dysphasia, hoarseness, dysarthria, and hypersalivation may indicate advanced disease.[31]

Diagnostic Procedures and Staging. The patient history is part of a comprehensive evaluation. If the history includes strong tobacco and alcohol use, determining habitual use is important and intervention may be required to guide the patient toward cessation programs. Cessation is important for the patient to tolerate the treatment better and for better results. Inspection includes indirect mirror examination (essential), palpation, biopsy (essential), fiberoptic endoscopy, and CT and MRI imaging to detect occult primaries and defining anatomic

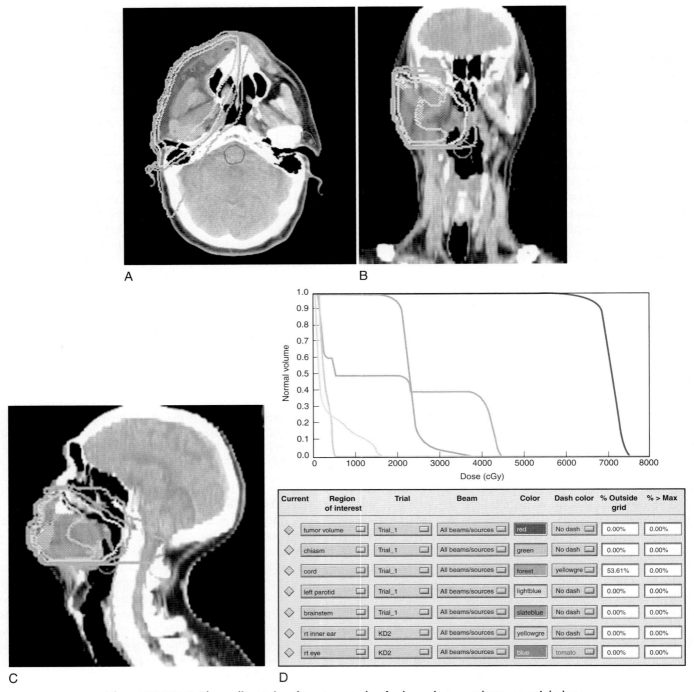

Figure 33-28. A, Three-dimensional treatment plan for buccal mucosal cancer, axial plane. **B**, Three-dimensional plan, coronal plane. **C**, Three-dimensional plan, sagittal view. **D**, Dose-volume histogram. (From Leibel SA, Phillips TL: *Textbook of radiation oncology*, ed 2, Philadelphia, 2004, Saunders.)

extensions. In addition to the history, physical examination, CT or MRI of the head and neck, a chest radiograph, and routine blood cell counts and serum chemistries are part of the staging evaluation. Other pretreatment diagnostic evaluations, especially for nasopharyngeal tumors, include EBV-specific serologic tests and liver function tests. CT of the chest and a

bone scan may be required for advanced nodal disease.[21,28] Pretreatment dental evaluation and initiation of dental prophylaxis are also recommended.

Histopathology. These tumors are predominantly SCCs (90%). Well-differentiated tumors are less common than in the oral cavity. Lymphoepithelioma may occur in the tonsil and base of tongue. Minor salivary gland carcinomas have been identified in this region. Non-Hodgkin's lymphoma is seen in approximately 5% of tonsillar malignancies.

Staging. The staging system is listed in Box 33-4.

Metastatic Behavior. Cervical lymph node involvement is common with oropharyngeal carcinoma. Base of tongue tumors may have palpable nodes upon presentation. The incidence of bilateral neck disease is up to 40%. Tonsillar lesions have palpable metastatic nodes at diagnosis in 60% to 70% of cases, pharyngeal wall lesions have involved nodes in 50% to 60% of cases, and soft palate carcinoma metastasizes about 40% to 50% of cases to the jugulodiagstric nodes. Bilateral nodal disease is frequent and retropharyngeal node involvement is common. Hematogenous metastasis is related with tonsillar and base of tongue primaries. Lung is the most common site.

GENERAL TREATMENT TECHNIQUES

The Oropharynx Region. The oropharynx consists of the base of the tongue, the tonsils (fossa and pillars), the soft palate, and the oropharyngeal walls. The oropharynx is situated between the axis and C3 vertebral bodies. The soft tissue regions include the anterior tonsillary pillars, the soft palate, the uvula, the base of the tongue, and the lateral-posterior pharyngeal walls (Figures 33-29 and 33-30; see Figure 33-6).

Tumors in this region and treatment can have a profound effect on all of the basic aerodigestive functions. The tonsils are the most common site of disease. Clinically, a sore throat and pain during swallowing are the most common presenting symptoms. Upper spinal accessory nodes are involved bilaterally in 50% to 70% of the patients. Early T1-2 lesions are treatable with EBRT alone. Large ports are required for T3-4 lesions that encompass the cervical and supraclavicular neck nodes. Debate exists for the treatment of small and intermediate cancers, T$_{1-3}$ tumors of the tonsillar fossa and/or soft palate. The issues are in regard to "the choice between conventional fractionated EBRT and accelerated fractionation, the optimal boost technique (external vs. interstitial radiation therapy), planned neck dissection after previous EBRT, and/or the use of adjuvant, neoadjuvant, or concomitant chemotherapy." A general trend is to aim for organ function preservation.[26]

 The oropharynx is located posterior to the oral cavity from the soft palate above to the level of the hyoid bone below.

Figure 33-31 shows a typical field for treatment of early stage cancer of the soft palate. The anterior border is 2 cm from known tumor; the superior border should be 1.5 to 2.0 cm superior to the soft palate. If there is extension into the tonsillar fossa, the field should encompass the medial pterygoid muscle at its insertion into the pterygoid plate. The posterior border is at the posterior spinous processes, and the inferior border at the level of the hyoid. This is matched to a low anterior neck field, with the spinal cord blocked on the lateral portals. With more advanced-stage lesions, the field may have to include portions of the base of tongue, tonsillar fossa, tonsillar pillar, soft palate, and medial pterygoid muscle. For more advanced tumor, the pterygoid plates up to the base of skull should be covered and, if there is extension into the nasopharynx or hypopharynx, this area too must be incorporated into the treatment field. Doses up to 6600 cGy to 7000 cGy in 6½ to

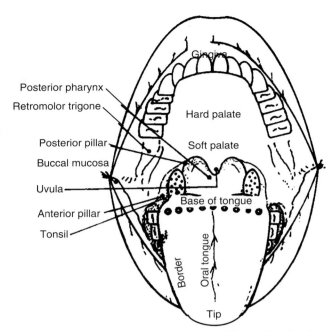

Figure 33-29. A front open-mouth view of the oral cavity. (From Cox JD: *Moss' radiation oncology: rationale, technique, results,* ed 7, St. Louis, 1994, Mosby.)

7 weeks with conventional fractionation are delivered for definitive treatment of T1 and T2 lesions that include the soft palate, tonsil, pharyngeal wall, and T1 lesions of the tongue.[18] Better locoregional control has been reported using accelerated or hyperfractionated regimens for T3-4 oropharyngeal and T2 base of tongue cancers with doses of 7000 to 8160 cGy. A delayed, accelerated, hyperfractionated schedule in which a concomitant boost is delivered as a second daily dose to the final cone-down field during the fifth and sixth weeks of treatment is described as a favored treatment regimen by Hu and colleagues.[18] A total of 7000 cGy in 6 weeks is delivered by delivering 180 cGy to the first (morning treatment) and 160 cGy after 6 hours. The total dose to the first field is 5400 cGy and 1600cGy is delivered as the concomitant boost, for a total of 7000cGy in 6 weeks.

For treatment of the neck, clinically negative neck nodes, all patients receive 5000 to 5400 cGy in 5 to 6 weeks. An additional boost to therapeutic doses to the neck or neck dissection follows for clinically positive neck nodes. The preference is neck dissection for palpable nodes after boosting to 6000 cGy.[18]

Beitler, Amdur, and Mendenhall[7] report that patients treated conventionally usually receive 7440 to 7680 cGy with 120 cGy/fraction administered twice daily. Those treated with IMRT receive 7200 cGy in 42 fractions using the concomitant boost technique. Unless the larynx is involved, it is excluded from the primary tumor portal. Acute mucosa reactions are common, and complications from the radiation pose a significant medical problem. With the currently available CT-based neck level definitions, more conformal contours and tighter boundaries can be designed. Critical structures like the temporomandibular joint and part of the pterygoid muscles can be avoided more easily. When using conformal treatment techniques (IMRT), the major salivary glands and oral mucosa can be spared to a greater extent. These measures lead to less trismus and xerostomia.[39]

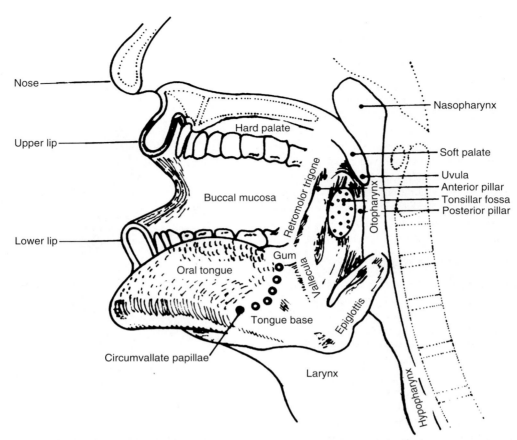

Figure 33-30. A lateral view of the oral cavity and oropharynx depicting anatomical subdivisions. (From Cox JD: *Moss' radiation oncology: rationale, technique, results*, ed 7, St. Louis, 1994, Mosby.)

The soft palate and tonsils have the best prognosis. Stage III and IV cancers are treated with definitive radiation therapy and concurrent chemotherapy.

The Hypopharynx Region. The hypopharynx (see Figures 33-6 and 33-30) is composed of the pyriform sinuses, postcricoid, and lower posterior pharyngeal walls below the base of the tongue. It is anatomically situated between the vertebral bodies C3-6. The cricoid cartilage represents the inferior border, and the epiglottis is the superior border. Most common presenting symptoms include sore throat, odynophagia (painful swallowing), and a neck mass. Up to 25% of cases present with a neck mass only, dysphagia and weight loss are common symptoms of locally advanced disease. More than 90% of cases present with dysphagia known as the hallmark of postcricoid carcinoma.[44]

Typically, disease of the hypopharynx is advanced. The pyriform sinus is the site of highest incidence of hypopharyngeal cancer. The male-to-female ratio ranges from 5:1 to 7:1 for pyriform sinus cancer and 3:1 to 4:1 for pharyngeal wall cancer. Postcricoid cancers occur predominantly in women.[44] There is a high rate (70% to 75%) of nodal metastasis in pyriform sinus cancers and the tumor is highly infiltrative. Treatment can also be debilitating. The rare T1-2 lesions are controllable through radiation or surgery, but most cases present as advanced, T2-4 lesions and are not candidates for laryngeal preservation.[7] Most patients receive combined radical surgery and radiation therapy for curative purposes. Large radiation ports are common. The most commonly used technique for the treatment of pyriform sinus, posterior pharyngeal wall, and postcricoid cancers remains the classically defined beam arrangements. This includes the opposed lateral photon fields, a low anterior neck photon field, and posterior cervical electron fields.[44]

Tumors of the posterior pharyngeal wall are considered unresectable. Radiation therapy consists of large fields, including the entire pharynx and upper cervical esophagus and extending superiorly to include the nasopharynx vault; superior deep, middle, and low jugular; and Rouviére's (lateral retropharyngeal) lymph nodes at the base of the skull. The large fields are typically treated to 4500 cGy and are then reduced off the spinal cord. The smaller fields are continued to 6500 to 7000 cGy or 7500 cGy with a twice-daily regimen. Attention is brought to a required sharp edge in order to treat the primary and Rouviére's lymph node while shielding the spinal cord.[8] Placement of the posterior border of the off-cord portal for tumors involving the posterior pharyngeal wall is challenged by adequately treating the tumor and limiting the dose to the spinal cord, even with a

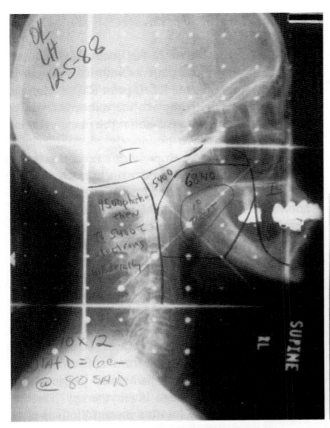

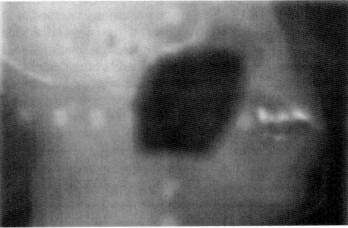

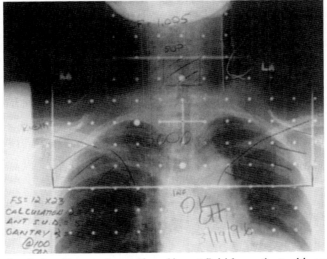

Figure 33-31. Simulation films and port film of boost field for patient with early stage cancer of the soft palate. (From Hu KS, et al: Cancer of the oropharynx. In Leibel SA, Phillips TL: *Textbook of radiation oncology*, ed 2, Philadelphia, 2004, Saunders.)

half-beam block to "sharpen" the beam edge. Placing the posterior beam edge anywhere within the vertebral body risks underdosage to the posterior pharyngeal wall.[7] Cases involving tumor or lymphadenopathy extending posterolaterally around the anterior aspect of the vertebral column to produce a horseshoe-shaped target volume have been reported. Zelefsky[44] reports that conformal radiation therapy using either an isocentric rotational technique with MLC or a static five-field technique may effectively

address the problem of a horseshoe-shaped target. Beitler, Amdur, and Mendenhall[7] describe this and any tumor that is wrapped around a vertebral body as a perfect case for IMRT.

The radiation ports for tonsillar, pharyngeal-wall, and posterior cricoid are quite similar stage for stage. Figure 33-32 depicts a typical field alignment for treatment of the region of the hypopharynx. Cumulative postoperative dose of 6300 cGy is delivered to the primary tumor bed after a field reduction off of the spinal cord at 4500 cGy and a second field reduction to exclude low-risk regions of the neck after 5400 cGy. The dose is divided in daily fractions of 180 cGy each. Posterior neck is boosted with appositional electron fields to 5400 cGy for negative nodes or 6300 if positive.[44] The inferior border of the lateral port is difficult to treat because of interference of the shoulders. Care must be taken to ensure that the shoulders are pulled down toward the feet and remain that way during treatment. Note that the lateral retropharyngeal and jugular chain nodes are treated, even if they are clinically negative. Anterior "**shine over**" (fall-off) is usually not necessary from the laterals unless the larynx is involved. Substantial soft tissue, cord damage, airway damage, or fibrosis is possible with these fields if the radiation dose to the critical organs is not carefully monitored. Full-course therapy can last 7 to 8 weeks.

Five-year survival rates above 70% have been reported for early lesions. However, the majority of cases are advanced and overall survival rarely exceeds 25%. Radical treatment measures achieve better locoregional control, but the 5-year survival outcomes are little improved compared to conservative measures. This result is related to the discovery of hematogenous metastases despite improved locoregional control.[31]

 The laryngopharynx or hypopharynx extends from the hyoid bone to its termination in the esophagus.

The Nasopharynx Region. The nasopharynx includes the posterosuperior pharyngeal wall and lateral pharyngeal wall, the Eustachian tube orifice, and the adenoids. The nasopharynx is a cuboidal structure lying on a line from the zygomatic arch to the external auditory meatus (EAM), extending inferiorly to the mastoid tip. The nasopharynx lies behind the nasal cavities and above the level of the soft palate (see Figure 33-6). The nasal cavity drains into the nasopharynx via the two posterior nares and also has on its lateral walls the two eustachian tubes, which connect to the middle ear. Disease in the nasopharynx can mimic an inflammatory process and cause considerable respiratory or auditory dysfunction.

Cranial nerve involvement occurs frequently. The ninth to the twelfth cranial nerves can be affected by enlargement of the retropharyngeal nodes (see Figure 33-12), as can the external carotid artery. Because of its proximity to the base of the brain, a lesion can directly invade the third and most commonly involves the sixth nerve. Any cranial nerve involvement signifies advanced, widespread disease. The involvement of the trigeminal (V), the oculomotor nerves (III), and the trochlear (IV) nerves has been referred to as petrosphenoidal syndrome with diplopia being the most common cranial nerve finding. The three branches of the trigeminal nerve, the ophthalmic, the maxillary, and the mandibular are most frequently involved. See Table 33-3 for the cranial nerves and their related functions; Figure 33-33 illustrates the ventral surface of the brain showing attachment of the cranial nerves.

 The nasopharynx is located behind the nose and extends from the posterior nares to the level of the soft palate.

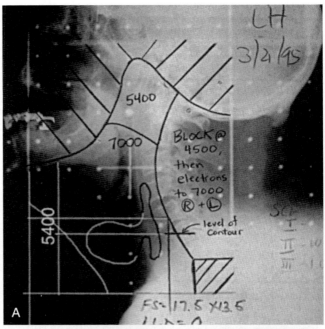

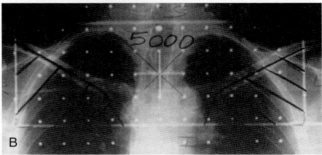

Figure 33-32. **A,** Typical lateral photon portals, cone-down fields, and doses for hypopharyngeal cancer. Level of contour is indicated. Horizontal white line above of contour and vertical dark line posterior to thyroid cartilage delineate the region encompassed by tissue compensators. Anterior curved white line delineates the skin surface at the anterior neck. A strip of the superior and anterior neck is blocked after 5400 cGy, as indicated by the vertical white line inside the anterior border of the treatment portal. **B,** Typical low anterior neck portal. (From Zelefsky MJ: Cancer of the hypopharynx. In Leibel SA, Phillips TL: *Textbook of radiation oncology,* ed 2, Philadelphia, 2004, Saunders.)

Staging for NPC differs from that for other head and neck cancers. The distribution and the prognostic impact of regional lymph node spread, particularly of the undifferentiated type, are different from those of other head and neck mucosal cancers and justify the use of a different N classification scheme. Lymphatic spread from a primary goes to the retropharyngeal, upper jugular, and spinal accessory nodes (level V). A solitary nodal mass in this level indicates examination of the nasopharynx.[41] Ninety percent of these lesions are SCC or its variants. NPC has a tendency toward poor differentiation and unusual growth patterns. Pathologic types have been grouped by The World Health Organization. The following is a breakdown of types within North America. The figures are approximations that vary according to source.

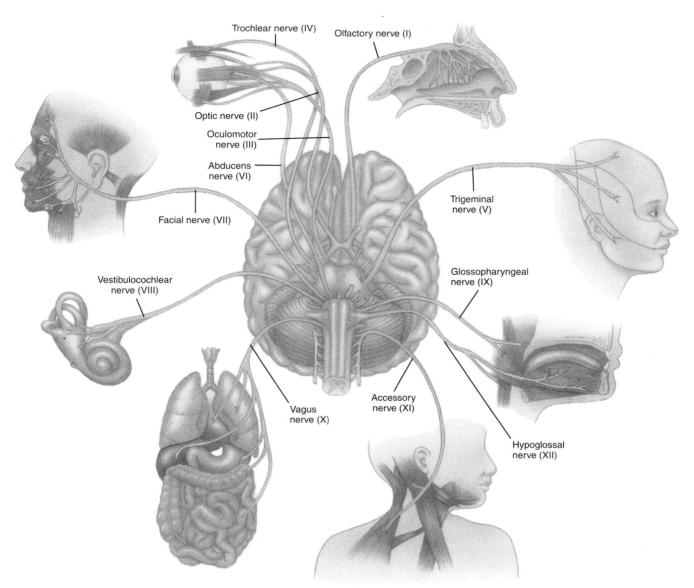

Figure 33-33. Cranial nerves and related functions. (From Thibodeau GA, Patton KT: *Anatomy and physiology*, ed 6, St. Louis, 2007, Mosby.)

Type 1: Keratinizing SCC (20% of cases)
Type 2: Nonkeratinizing carcinoma (10% of cases)
Type 3: Lymphoepithelioma (poorly differentiated carcinoma) (70% of cases)[8]

Nonkeratinizing carcinoma and lymphoepithelioma are variants of SCC. Surgical intervention in the nasopharynx is extremely difficult. This disease is not associated with tobacco consumption. EBV is associated with NPC. The age distribution is bimodal, with a small peak in adolescence and young adulthood and a major peak occurring between 50 and 70 years of age. The disease is uncommon in white populations, consisting of only 2% of all cases of head and neck cancer in the United States.[31] It has been noted to be rare among Japanese populations as well,[8] although the literature makes reference to a study of an early-staged population from Hong Kong in the United States.[44]

A high incidence in southern Chinese (57% of all head and neck cancers) and Middle Eastern countries may be attributed to nitrosamines in salted fish among southern China. Eskimos and the mixed populations of Southeast Asia are included among the higher cases.

From 75% to 85% of NPC patients have clinically positive cervical nodes, with about half of all cases having bilateral or contralateral disease. Radiation ports are quite large to encompass all the nodes and at-risk tissue. The lateral retropharyngeal (node of Rouviére), which usually cannot be surgically removed, and jugulodigastric are nearly always treated as tumor volume during any cone-down procedure.

NPC demonstrates an overall incidence of 25% of blood-borne metastasis. The nodal disease can be extensive, while the primary lesion is small. Patients with bilateral cervical nodes have up to a 40% to 70% likelihood of developing a distant metastasis, with bone, lung, and liver being the most common sites. NPC disease spreads to adjacent subsites rather quickly and demonstrates a 30% to 40% local recurrence rate. For these reasons, aggressive, large-volume radical radiation therapy is necessary.

Radiation treatment fields are arranged to cover the possible pathways of spread. The treatment portals are designed to deliver appropriate dose to gross disease (gross tumor volume [GTV]) and areas at risk of microscopic extension (clinical target volume [CTV]). This remains as the treatment objective regardless of treatment technique, in classically defined beam arrangements and in modern techniques using IMRT and inverse treatment planning. The following serve as general guidelines for the field arrangement according to the Intergroup study 0099.[44] The borders serve as general guidelines for patients with NPC and must be modified for each patient accounting for specific disease extension. There is debate regarding the treatment of the entire base of skull with margin and treatment to the pituitary to doses that eradicate disease but produce complications.[44] A general field arrangement includes:

- Superiorly—at least 2 cm beyond tumor that is visible on CT including the base of skull and sphenoid sinus.
- Posteriorly—allow 2 cm of margin beyond the mastoid process. The posterior margin may extend further to allow at least a 1.5-cm margin on enlarged modes.
- Anteriorly—include the posterior third of the maxillary sinus and nasal cavity. This anterior border can be modified to accommodate adequate margin (2 cm) for tumors with anterior extension.
- Inferiorly—border is at the thyroid notch to allow sparing of the larynx by a central block on the anterior lower neck field, which is matched to these lateral fields.
- The lower neck is generally treated with an anterior field with a central larynx block that extends inferiorly to the cricoid.

Figure 33-34 depicts a three-field setup. Opposing laterals with a matching anterior supraclavicular field are used to deliver a minimum of 5000 cGy to all areas. Subsequent cone down fields boost the dose to 6500 cGy, with careful consideration of the dose to the spinal cord, optic nerve, pituitary, and brainstem. An electron boost of 7000 cGy to bulky disease or positive nodes is warranted if lymphadenopathy is present.

Treatment of NPC has seen dramatic changes in the past several years. Much of the early work on IMRT has centered on NPC due to accurate immobilization, the extent of critical structures in proximity to tumor, and the high incidence of morbidity with conventional treatment techniques. Although treatments using modified fractionation such as hyperfractionation to 7440 cGy in 62 twice-daily fractions[7] are still being reported, IMRT is replacing conventional radiotherapy in an increasing number in the United States.[21] Several institutions have shown potential dosimetric improvement for IMRT over conventional techniques and 3D conformal techniques.[4] The preservation of

salivary function by sparing at least one parotid gland has been a primary objective of head and neck IMRT. Ove, Foote, and Bonner[29] report that "the ability to tailor dose to a desired distribution allows the simultaneous delivery of different fractionation schemes to different portions of the target. The primary target can be hypofractionated and conventional fractionation can be delivered to subclinical neck disease, or conventional fractionation can be applied to the target while delivering doses of less than 1.8 Gy to the secondary targets." Fusion of diagnostic MRI and treatment planning CT images provide accurate delineation of GTV and surrounding critical normal structures. The CTV is defined as the GTV and areas with potential microscopic disease. The CTV should also include lymph node groups of high risk—the upper deep jugular, submandibular, subdigastric, midjugular, posterior cervical, and retropharyngeal nodes. Also included as CTV are the lower neck and supraclavicular nodes considered as lower risk for microscopic spread, along with margin for movement and setup error.[21] One prescribed treatment includes 7000 cGy delivered to the GTV and positive neck nodes. The high-risk CTV receives 5940 cGy, and the low-risk CTV receives 5000 to 5400 cGy (negative neck nodes). And 180 cGy/fraction per day for 5 days per week is delivered to the CTV for a total dose of 5940 cGy to the high-risk CTV. The low-risk CTV receives 5040 cGy and the GTV receives a higher 212 cGy/fraction per day. Figure 33-35 shows an inverse IMRT plan using DMLC for a T4N1 NPC. Notice the varying doses to the right and left parotid glands.

Concomitant chemotherapy should be used along with radiation for stage III and IV (localized) tumors. Retreatment of local failures with a combination of external beam followed by an intracavitary brachytherapy boost is considered feasible.

This disease has an overall 45% survival rate. Survival decreases from 50% to 60% for T1 lesions to 10% to 20% for T4 lesions treated with radiation alone. Overall, lymphoepithelioma and undifferentiated carcinomas have been reported to be more radiosensitive and have a better prognosis that SCC. Local control has improved with improved radiotherapy.[21] Unlike other head and neck tumors, adjuvant chemotherapy seems to improve both local control and survival.[31]

The Larynx Region

The larynx is contiguous with the lower portion of the pharynx above and is connected with the trachea below. It extends from the tip of the epiglottis at the level of the lower border of the C3 vertebra to the lower border of the cricoid cartilage at the level of the C6 vertebra. The larynx is subdivided into three sites (Figure 33-36): the glottis, supraglottis, and subglottis region. Glottic cancer accounts for roughly 65% of larynx cancers, with a 30% site incidence in the supraglottic region. The remainder of the larynx cancers appear in the subglottic area.

Lee and Phillips[22] report that cancers of the larynx are the most common cancers of the upper aerodigestive tract. The propensity of cancer of the larynx has also been described as being "the most common head and neck cancer, if one excludes skin malignancies" (p. 352).[27] The ratio of glottic to supraglottic

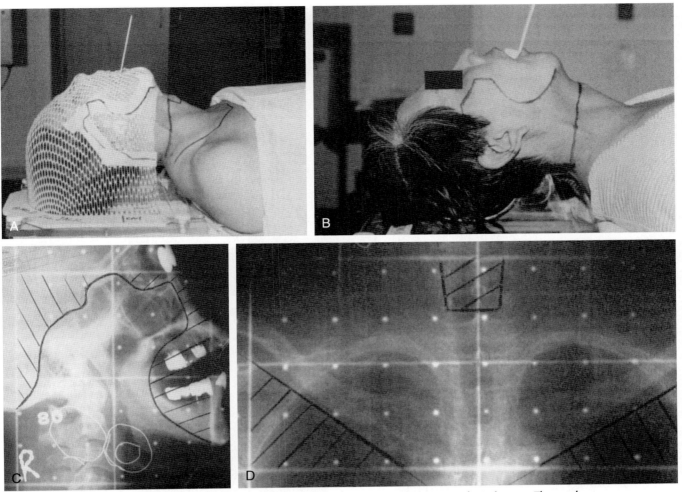

Figure 33-34. A, Treatment position of a patient with nasopharyngeal carcinoma. The neck is extended, a tongue blade with a cork attached to one end is inserted between the incisor teeth to depress the tongue. The head is immobilized. **B,** Outline of the primary treatment field on the face and neck **C,** Initial lateral photon portal of a patient with T1 N2 carcinoma of the nasopharynx. The neck nodes are outlined with metallic wires. **D,** Typical low anterior neck portal. A 2 × 2 block is placed at midline over the spinal cord at the junction of the lateral and anterior fields. (From Leibel SA, Phillips TL: *Textbook of radiation oncology,* ed 2, Philadelphia, 2004, Saunders.)

carcinomas is about 3:1. Carcinomas of the glottis (true vocal cord) are not considered life threatening, and the choice of therapy is based on the preservation of speech and maintenance of the airway. Historically, the treatment of larynx cancer focused on cure by aggressive surgery, leaving the survivor with a difficult and challenged life by the inability to communicate. The loss of vocalization has a profound psychological and socioeconomic impact on quality of life.

Incidence characteristics are consistent regardless of culture.[27] Larynx cancer is mostly (90%) a male-dominated disease, with a peak incidence in the 50- to 60-year age group.

Laryngeal carcinomas display an extremely high etiology toward smoking. The use of black tobacco is associated with a higher risk than the use of blond tobacco. People who use their voices extensively in their work also appear to be at higher risk. The role of alcohol has been associated with the incidence of supraglottic cancer; the role related to glottic cancer is not clear. A synergistic role of alcohol with tobacco is favored instead of alcohol being an independent factor. Studies have involved the relation to gastroesophageal reflux (GERD). It is believed that chronic irritation from acid may predispose patients to cancer.[15]

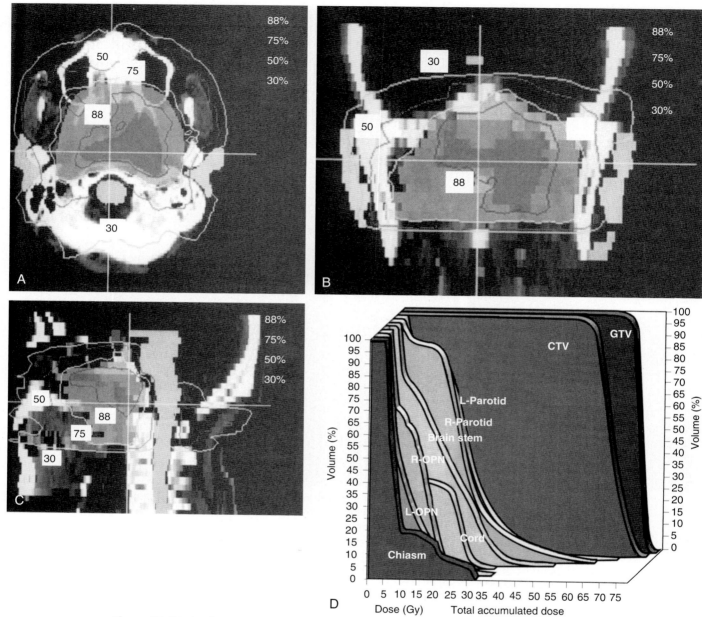

Figure 33-35. Isodose curves for an inverse IMRT plan delivered using multivane dynamic multi-leaf collimator (MIMiC) for a patient with T4 N1 NPC displayed on the axial (**A**), coronal (**B**), and sagittal (**C**) planes through the primary tumor and the dose-volume histogram for the relevant structures (**D**). (From Lee M, Fu KK: Cancer of the nasopharynx. In Leibel SA, Phillips TL: *Textbook of radiation oncology*, ed 2, Philadelphia, 2004, Saunders.)

Studies involve the molecular basis for laryngeal cancer. Mutation of the *p53* gene is common and is seen in 47% of the patients who are smokers but in only 14% of nonsmokers. This mutation has been identified in 55% of the tumors among drinkers and 20% among nondrinkers. The transformation of this gene and antigen proliferation are suspected to be associated with HPV infection that may play a role in laryngeal cancer.[22] Garden, Morrison, and Ang[15] refer to this as a causal link that also affects the tonsil.

A persistent sore throat and hoarseness are classic presenting symptoms. Cervical lymph node involvement, if present, is seen in supraglottic lesions but not in glottic lesions. Carcinoma in situ (Tis) is rather common on the vocal cords. Glottic lesions are well to moderately differentiated, with supraglottic lesions being less differentiated and more aggressive. About 65% to 75% of glottic lesions appear on the anterior two thirds of one cord. Cord mobility is a factor in the classification of the lesions. Early lesions are treated successfully with either surgery or radiation therapy; it has been reported that voice quality is better after radiation therapy alone.[22] Advanced lesions with fixed vocal cords due to extensive cartilage invasion are best treated with surgery and postoperative radiation therapy. Exophytic lesions are more responsive to radiation therapy than are infiltrative lesions. Radiation therapy alone or concurrent with

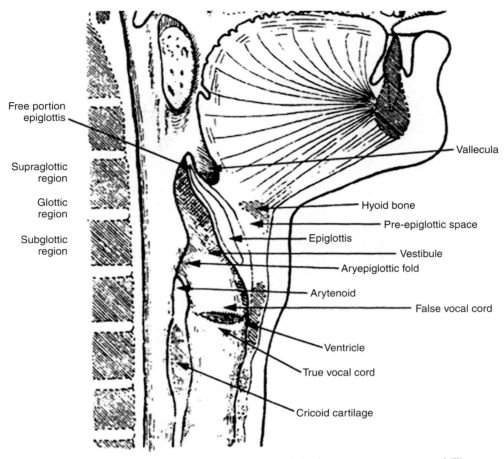

Figure 33-36. Anatomical regions and structures of the larynx. (From Lee NL, Phillips TL: Cancer of the larynx. In Leibel SA, Phillips TL: *Textbook of radiation oncology,* ed 2, Philadelphia, 2004, Saunders.)

chemotherapy may be the preferred treatment for poorly differentiated carcinoma. Conservation surgery may be the preferred treatment for early verrucous carcinoma of the vocal cord.[22] Verrucous carcinoma is generally a well-differentiated, slow-growing, wartlike lesion that is relatively radioresistant. It has a tendency to convert to a highly anaplastic neoplasm following radiation therapy.[15]

Proper selection in treating carcinoma in situ (Tis) with transoral laser excision requires an experienced team. Laser excision performed to a narrow margin treats microinvasive cancer and spares the anterior commissure, allowing mucosal waves to travel across the glottis unimpeded. Voice problems worsen as the extent of resection increases. Generally, radiation therapy for carcinoma in situ is based on anterior commissure involvement when the mucosal wave is impaired or when the patient is not in good medical condition. Limited risk of subclinical disease to the cervical lymphatics in the treatment of Tis and T1 lesions indicates a field encompassing the primary lesion only.[10]

The accurate definition of gross tumor volume using CT treatment planning is reportedly correlated with effective local control. Glottic cancer is treated with opposing lateral fields angled to be parallel to the trachea, 5 × 5 cm (for T1 and early T2) to 6 × 6 cm. Wedges are indicated if the tissue inhomogeneities produce unacceptable hot spots in the posterior margins. Daily doses can be 200 to 220 cGy, up to a total dose of 6000 to 7000 cGy, depending on the size of the lesion and mobility of the cord. Multiple studies suggest that 120 cGy fractions of twice-daily treatments to 7440 to 7900 cGy are appropriate. If hyperfractionation is not feasible, daily fractions of greater than 200 cGy per day result in superior outcomes to smaller daily doses.[6] The treatment of small fields for early glottic cancers rarely results in severe complications. Large, fixed lesions need more aggressive therapy; T3 and T4 lesions of the glottis and subglottis are treated as supraglottic lesions.[22]

The radiation port borders can be clinically determined before simulation, but CT scans and a contour of the neck are used for computerized treatment planning. Figure 33-37 depicts a typical lateral port, and Figure 33-38 illustrates the isodose distribution for a typical T1 N0 glottic lesion.

The typical radiation field borders are as follows:

Superior—upper thyroid notch
Inferior—cricoid cartilage (lower border of C6)
Anterior—1- to 1½-cm shine over (flash) over the skin
   surface at the level of the vocal cords
Posterior—just anterior to the vertebral body, including the
   anterior portion of the posterior pharyngeal wall

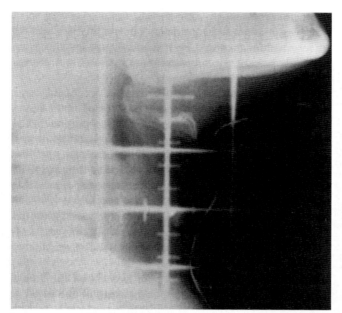

Figure 33-37. Simulation film of a lateral port, T1 N0 glottic cancer. (From Cox JD: *Moss' radiation oncology: rationale, technique, results*, ed 7, St. Louis, 1994, Mosby.)

Large T3-4, transglottic lesions are treated with radiation alone. In the event of a recurrence, salvage surgery is an option. However, the voice is usually sacrificed. Radiation therapy offers the best method of voice preservation.

Supraglottic lesions are frequently large and bulky but (despite appearances) do not usually invade the inferior false cord or the ventricles. These lesions tend to spread superiorly to the epiglottis.

Lymph node metastasis is expected in 40% to 50% of the patients. Therefore, the radiation ports are much larger than the glottic ports. Posteriorly, the spinal accessory chain is included in the lateral treatment fields, then boosted superficially. Superiorly, the field border extends along the mandible (Figure 33-39). If necessary, an anterior bilateral supraclavicular field is matched to the laterals. The midline block, placed below the cricoid, should only shield the trachea and cord. Because of the risk of blocking tumor, no midline block is used in some instances, thereby requiring that a safety block be placed in the lateral fields at the match line junction. Positioning and immobilizing the head are critical for this type of treatment port. Various treatment techniques have been described for supraglottic lesions. Recommendations include accelerated fractionated radiation therapy using a concomitant boost technique for a T3 N0 lesion. Lateral fields are treated to 5400 cGy reducing off the cord at 4500 cGy. A boost to the primary delivers 1800 cGy for a total dose of 7200 cGy. Twice-a-day hyperfractionation is also recommended for T2 and greater supraglottic lesions delivering 7440 to 7680 cGy at 120 cGy/fraction with two fractions per day at 6-hour interfraction intervals. The cord is blocked after 4560 cGy.[22]

Computer optimized or inversed-planned IMRT has been described as an ideal treatment technique for a T3 N1 supraglottic carcinoma. Though the expected benefits include voice preservation and less xerostomia than conventional treatment, the 50 minute treatment times are not tolerated well by all patients. Figure 33-40 illustrates an inverse-planned IMRT technique for T3 N1 SCC of the supraglottic larynx.

Surgery can control 80% of supraglottic T1-2 lesions, whereas radiation therapy offers 75% local control. Radiation therapy alone for T3-4 supraglottic lesions is contraindicated. Relapses are treated with surgery. The tumor dose needed to achieve control is 6600 to 7000 cGy. Electron beam boosts are needed for the cervical lymph nodes. Subglottic cancers are treated with a total laryngectomy, with postoperative radiation therapy given for any residual disease. Survival rates are good for glottic cancer: 80% to 90% without cord fixation, and 50% to 60% if fixation exists. Patients with supraglottic cancers have a 60% to 70% 5-year survival rate with negative nodes, but this rate drops to 30% to 50% if positive clinical nodes are present.[31] Garden and colleagues[15] note that because nearly all published series are retrospective single-institution studies, obtaining valid data on control rates remains a challenge. In comparing results of various treatment options, "it is thus difficult to ascertain if small differences in control rates between series are real" (p. 735). The management of early glottic carcinomas remains controversial and is often determined by the preference of the attending physician. Oncologists advocate either radiation therapy or voice-preserving partial laryngectomy. Equivalent control rates have been published with surgery (excision, cordectomy, or hemilaryngectomy) and radiation therapy.

Salivary Glands

The salivary glands consist of three large, paired major glands—the parotid, submandibular, and sublingual glands—and many smaller minor glands located throughout the upper aerodigestive tract. They play a role in digestion and tooth protection. The parotid gland is the largest of the three salivary glands, is located superficial to and partly behind the ramus of the mandible, and covers the masseter muscle. It fills the space between the ramus of the mandible and the anterior border of the sternocleidomastiod muscle. The parotid contains an extensive lymphatic capillary plexus, many aggregates of lymphocytic cells, and numerous intraglandular lymph nodes in the superficial lobe. Lymphatics drain from more laterally on the face, including parts of the eyelids, diagonally downward and posteriorly toward the parotid gland, as do the lymphatics from the frontal region of the scalp. Associated with the gland, both superficially and deeply, are parotid nodes that drain down along the retromandibular vein to empty into the superficial lymphatics and nodes along the outer surface of the sternocleidomastoid muscle and into upper nodes of the deep cervical chain. Lymphatics from the parietal region of the scalp drain partly to the parotid nodes in front of the ear and partly to the retroauricular nodes in back of the ear, which, in turn, drain into upper deep cervical nodes.

Chong and Armstrong[10] report that tumors of the salivary gland are rare, constituting from 3% to 4% of all cancers of the head and neck region. Foote and colleagues[13] write that malignant tumors of the salivary glands account for 7% of head and neck cancers diagnosed in North America each year. The parotid is the site of the highest incidence of salivary gland tumors

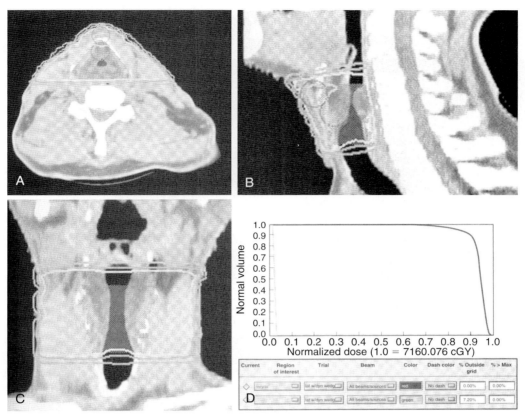

Figure 33-38. Isodose distribution on the axial plane (**A**), sagittal plane (**B**), and coronal plane (**C**). Dose-volume histogram for the tumor and spinal cord (**D**). (From Lee NL, Phillips TL: Cancer of the larynx. In Leibel SA, Phillips TL: *Textbook of radiation oncology*, ed 2, Philadelphia, 2004, Saunders.)

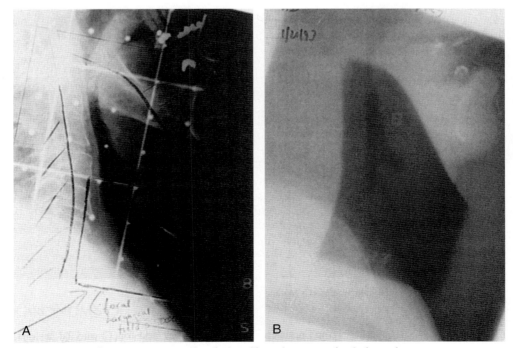

Figure 33-39. A, Simulation film of a supraglottis lateral port. **B**, Port film of a supraglottic lateral port. (From Leibel SA: *Textbook of radiation oncology*, Philadelphia, 1998, Saunders.)

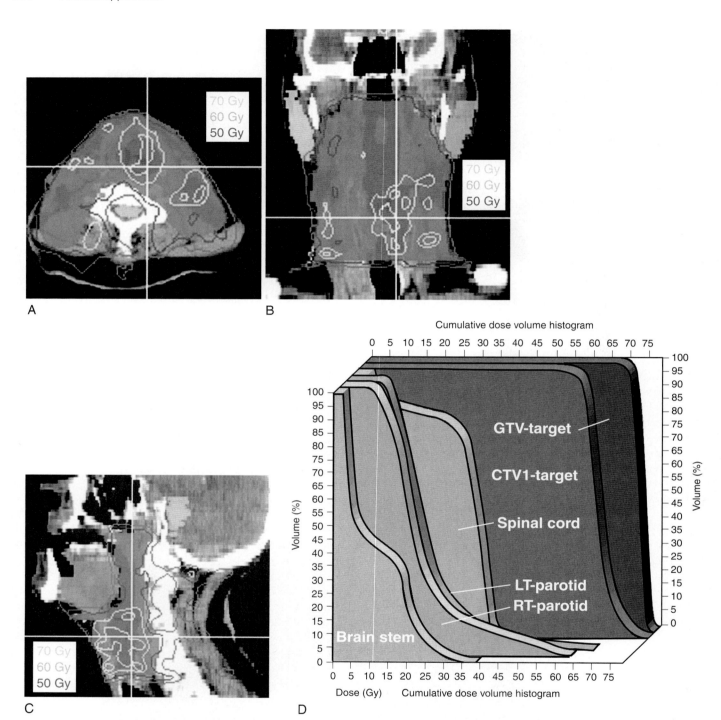

Figure 33-40. Isodose curves of an inverse IMRT plan using seven coplanar gantry angles delivered with MLC for treatment of T3N1 supraglottic laryngeal cancer. Axial (**A**), coronal (**B**), sagittal (**C**) planes through the centroid of the primary tumor, and the dose-volume histogram (**D**). (From Lee NL, Phillips TL: Cancer of the larynx. In Leibel SA, Phillips TL: *Textbook of radiation oncology,* ed 2, Philadelphia, 2004, Saunders.)

(80% to 90%). Of these tumors, more than two thirds are benign, and between 15% and 33% are malignant. Tumors of the minor salivary glands account for 2% to 3% of all head and neck cancers; about 65% and 85% of these are malignant.[13,31] The submandibular gland is involved in about 10% of all instances. Although the causes of these glandular tumors are stated to be unknown, low-dose ionizing radiation in childhood may account for some cases of malignant salivary tumors. Radiation-induced malignancies have been associated with early radiation treatments for benign conditions such as acne, tinea capitis, and infected tonsils. These malignancies have also been associated with the atomic bomb survivors.

Female patients with a history of carcinoma of the major salivary glands have an incidence of breast cancer 8 times higher than the normal population.[13] Chong and Armstrong[10] report that firm epidemiologic data of this association are lacking. The majority of major and minor salivary cancers are of unknown origin, and etiologic factors are poorly understood. However, risk factors such as dental radiographs have been implicated for both benign and malignant salivary gland tumors. Parotid gland tumors in children are more likely to be malignant compared with the same tumors in adults.[13] Exposure to hardwood dust has been linked to the development of nasal cavity and paranasal sinus minor salivary gland adenocarcinomas.[27] Malignant neoplasms occur in patients with an average age of 55; benign tumors occur in 40-year-olds. The incidences among genders are about equal with a slight male predominance.

Histologically, the more common cell types for malignant tumors are the adenoid cystic, mucoepidermoid, and adenocarcinoma. Most patients develop an asymptomatic parotid mass lasting on average from 4 to 8 months before presentation.[27] Presenting symptoms are localized swelling and pain, facial palsy, and rapid growth. Facial nerve involvement is highly suggestive of a malignancy. CT and MRI are not routinely used because they are ineffective in differentiating between benign and malignant salivary gland tumors. PET scans show an increased FDG uptake for both benign and malignant lesions as well. Although not useful in the evaluation of primary tumor, PET may play a role in the evaluation of distant metastasis.[10] FNAB is reported to be an accurate diagnostic technique with overall sensitivities of greater than 90% and specificities of greater than 95%.[13] Controversy exists regarding diagnostic procedures involving FNAB. A diagnosis via a lobectomy is done and submandibular lesions are excised for a frozen section.[31] Some institutions reserve FNAB for inoperable and recurrent lesions. Incisional or excisional biopsies are never performed to establish a tissue diagnosis, as such procedures increase the risk of recurrence, the risk of injury to the facial nerve, and subsequent surgical morbidity.[10]

The incidence of cervical node involvement varies according to the histologic subtype. High-grade mucoepidermoid tumors display a 44% metastatic behavior. The rate for this behavior is 5% in adenoid cystic tumors, 21% in malignant mixed tumors, 37% in SCC, and 13% in acinic cell carcinoma. Hematogenous metastases are common and range from about 13% for acinic cell carcinoma to 41% for adenoid cystic carcinoma. Lung metastases from adenoid cystic carcinomas may lie quiescent for years after presentation.[31]

Although tumors in this area are mostly benign, the risk of local recurrence is high. They are treated as low-grade cancer and are optimally treated via total resection, with generous margins for sparing facial nerves.

Radiation therapy is given postoperatively for residual, recurrent, or inoperable lesions. The field borders include the zygomatic arch or higher as indicated by tumor extension or scars superiorly. The anterior border includes the anterior edge of the masseter muscle, the inferior border is at the thyroid notch, and the posterior border is just behind the mastoid process.[13]

In the postoperative case, the primary resection bed is given 6000 to 6300 cGy if the margins are clear; 7000 to 7500 cGy is delivered if there is gross residual disease. The clinically negative neck is generally treated to 5000 cGy.[31] High-grade mucoepidermoid and undifferentiated cancers of the parotid often spread to ipsilateral lymph nodes but seldom involve contralateral lymph nodes. Consequently, the target volume is commonly designed to fit the local invasion and lymphatic spread. Because the opposite side is seldom at risk, most cancers of the parotid can be irradiated with a wedge pair or electron to spare the other parotid, the brainstem, and spinal cord. A strip of bolus should be placed over the scar to raise the surface dose and prevent recurrence in the scar. The patient may be positioned on his or her side with the lateral side of the head up when it is necessary to irradiate the parotid and cervical lymph nodes or supine when irradiating a local field.

Treatment is administered via one of several external beam techniques. Fields are best designed with the aid of 3D simulation and treatment planning. Treatment may be delivered using a wedge-pair technique, the ipsilateral photon/high-energy electron combination, or an opposed lateral field if the target volume extends beyond the midline. The usual wedge pair is a superior oblique and inferior oblique combination directed away from the opposite oral cavity and orbit. This involves rotating the table 90 degrees off the usual axis. An anterior and posterior oblique combination is possible if the exit is not through the contralateral orbit (requires maximum extension of the neck). This may involve matching the low-neck portal to the primary fields. It is important to use CT scan–based treatment planning to derive the maximum benefit from a wedge-pair technique.[8,10,13] An ipsilateral mixed-beam treatment using photons and high-energy electrons produces a homogeneous dose distribution and delivers 3000 cGy or less to the opposite salivary glands. Care should be taken to monitor the dose to the base of the brain and contralateral maxillary antrum with this technique. Local control with conventional fractioned radiation therapy is only about 25%.

IMRT is effective in cases of perineural involvement of the facial, trigeminal, hypoglossal, and lingual nerves requiring treatment of the proximal nerve to the brainstem while sparing the contralateral salivary gland, the eyes, temporal lobes, and brainstem itself. Subclinical intracranial disease in the cavernous sinus, adjacent to the brainstem, or within the petrous bone can be treated at 180 cGy/fraction, while higher-risk areas in the original tumor bed and high-risk neck can be treated at 200 cGy/fraction. Positive distal nerve margins may also be effectively treated with IMRT. The entire span of the nerve can be treated distally while sparing critical normal structures such as the lacrimal gland and eye.[13] Figure 33-41 illustrates IMRT to a postoperative right submandibular salivary gland with perineural invasion.

Improved results have been reported using accelerated fractionation.[31] Accelerated fractionation techniques provide similar dose levels of radiation therapy in a shorter amount of overall time. This counteracts quick cellular proliferation of aggressive tumors by giving more dose in a shorter time. Treatment complications should be monitored. Postoperative radiation therapy of major salivary gland tumors improves locoregional control in selected areas. Reported 5-year actuarial local control rates range from 100% (T1) to 83% (T2), 80% (T3), and 43% (T4).[10]

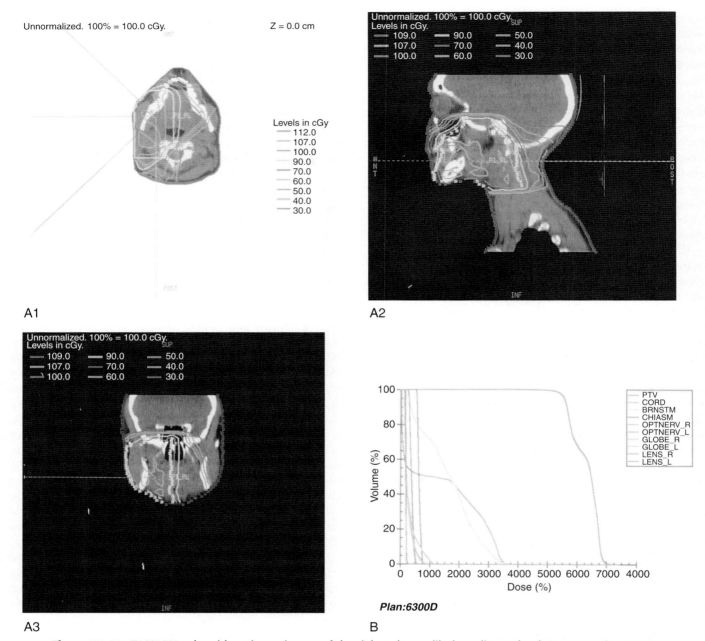

Figure 33-41. T1 N0 M0 adenoid cystic carcinoma of the right submandibular salivary gland. Postoperative IMRT to the right submandibular area and the pathways of the adjacent lingual nerve and the hypoglossal nerve to the base of skull to a dose of 5400 cGy, submandibular bed is boosted to 6300 cGy. **A**, Isodose distributions: *A1*, axial; *A2*, sagittal; *A3*, coronal. **B**, Dose volume histogram. (From Chong LM, Armstrong JG: Tumors of the salivary glands. In Leibel SA, Phillips TL: *Textbook of radiation oncology*, ed 2, Philadelphia, 2004, Saunders.)

Maxillary Sinus

The maxillary sinus is a pyramid-shaped cavity lined by ciliated epithelium and bound by thin bone or membranous partitions. Carcinomas arising from the ciliated epithelium or mucous glands perforate the bony walls almost from the start. The roof of the maxillary sinus is also the floor of the orbit. Tumors involving the superior portion of the sinus readily extend into the orbit. The more posterior wall or infratemporal surface separates the sinus from the pterygopalatine fossa and the postero-superior alveolar nerves. The nasal surface of the antrum is visible through the nostril, with the ostium of the sinus inferior to the middle turbinate. The alveolar process and hard palate separate the maxillary sinus from the oral cavity.

Maxillary sinus disease accounts for 80% of all sinus cancers with a 2:1 male prevalence. Most patients with carcinoma in the sinonasal region are older than 40. Adenocarcinoma of the nasal cavity and ethmoid sinus has been associated with wood dust exposure. SCCs of the maxillary sinus and nasal cavity are associated with chemical agents found in work related to nickel refinery and leather tanning. Thorotrast, an imaging contrast media used to image the maxillary sinus in the 1960s, includes radioactive thorium, which is now known to be a carcinogen. Ryu and colleagues[33] report that unlike other respiratory tract carcinomas, cancers of the nasal cavity and paranasal sinus have no association with smoking (p. 731). This is in contrast to Ahamad and colleagues,[1] who write that "cigarette smoking is reported to increase the risk of nasal cancer, with a doubling of risk among heavy or long-term smokers and a reduction in risk after long-term cessation" (p. 756). Patients with this type of cancer have a history of long-standing sinusitis, nasal obstructions, and bloody discharge. Although chronic sinusitis is frequently a symptom with the malignant tumor, sinusitis is not a causative agent.[33] These cancers are mostly SCCs and tend to invade the floor of the orbit, ethmoid sinuses, hard palate, and zygomatic arch. Displacement of the eye is common. Physical examination should include inspection and bimanual palpation of the orbit, oral and nasal cavities, and nasopharynx and direct fiberoptic endoscopy. Neurologic examination should emphasize cranial nerve function, because nasal cavity and paranasal sinus tumors are frequently associated with cranial nerve palsies, especially of the trigeminal branches. Cervical lymph nodes are palpated for adenopathy. Imaging has essentially replaced surgical exploration for staging and tumor mapping in this region. The most useful studies are CT and MRI. CT defines early cortical bone erosion more clearly, whereas MRI better delineates soft tissue and can differentiate among opacification of the sinuses due to fluid, inflammation, or tumor. MRI may demonstrate subtle perineural spread and involvement of the cranial nerve foramen and canals. In addition, visualization of sagittal and coronal images using MRI advances visualization compared with CT in evaluating intracranial or leptomeningeal spread.[33] Fusion of MRI with planning CT is useful in defining tumor not visible on CT alone. MRI or PET fusion with planning CT is also useful when induction chemotherapy is given where prechemotherapy images facilitate accurate mapping of the initial volume of gross tumor for precise target delineation.[1]

GENERAL TREATMENT TECHNIQUES

Cervical nodal spread is uncommon, but if it is present, the submandibular node is the first station involved and will be treated. Surgery and radiotherapy are complicated because these tumors are often located close to multiple critical structures including the eye, brain, optic nerves, brainstem, and cranial nerves. Adjuvant radiation therapy is favored based on aesthetic considerations as opposed to radical resections. But surgery is the principal treatment for control of small lesions of the nasal septum or those limited to the infrastructure of the maxillary sinus. Although primary radiation therapy for small lesions has a high cure rate, this approach has a significant chance of optic nerve injury from the high dose required to achieve good tumor control.[33]

Maxillary cancers are usually diagnosed at advanced stages. Most cases warrant treatment with combined surgery and postoperative radiation therapy. This is considered standard treatment. The results of radical surgical excisions such as craniofacial resection, total maxillectomy, or orbital exenteration have improved, especially with aggressive plastic reconstruction. However, these operations still produce significant morbidity.

Massive tumors with extensive involvement of the nasopharynx, base of skull, sphenoidal sinuses, brain, or optic chiasm are considered unresectable. Primary radiation therapy has been used with differing success depending on stage and extent of tumor. Treatment rational for radiation therapy has incurred a change over the past decade from preoperative to postoperative treatment. Preoperative radiation therapy may obscure the initial extent of disease and erroneously lead to a more conservative resection, leaving microscopic disease behind. Preoperative radiation therapy also has been shown to increase infection rate and the risk of postoperative wound-healing complications. Radiation therapy after surgery has the advantage of accurate pathologic review of all structures at risk. Radiation therapy target volumes for the nasal cavity, ethmoid sinuses, and maxillary sinuses include both halves of the nasal cavity and the ipsilateral maxillary sinus in the typical postoperative setting. If tumor extends superiorly into the ethmoid air cells, the ethmoid sinuses and the ipsilateral medial orbital wall are included. A tongue depressor is used to displace the tongue from the field.

In the postoperative radiation therapy setting, doses of 6000 to 6300 cGy are delivered via an external beam, wedged-pair technique. From 180 to 200 cGy per fraction and a cone-down boost may be delivered to gross residual tumor. Doses over 7000 cGy are recommended for unresectable tumors.[33] Lateral and anterior ports are custom designed to follow the expected route of spread. If the orbit is involved, eye blocking should not be used. Most of the cases would have had orbital exenteration during surgery, and the entire orbital defect is then included in the tumor volume (Figure 33-42). Care should be taken to miss the cord and contralateral lens. Angling the anterior beam a few degrees off the vertical spares brain tissue. If the nasal cavity is at risk, bolus material should be inserted to improve dose homogeneity. Angling the lateral port a few degrees off the horizontal plane spares the contralateral optic nerve and lens. Extensive disease may require the use of bilateral wedged fields. Attempts to shield the lacrimal gland and to retract the upper lid superior to the beam edge should be emphasized in order to reduce eye injury. Four fields using an anterior and two lateral wedged portal, plus an intraorbital electron portal, is reported to be more commonly used than the three-field technique (without using the anterior electron portal).[33]

It is most advantageous to base the treatment volume on treatment planning CT, with MRI correlation. The complex anatomy of this region and the presence of numerous critical, dose-limiting structures (optic nerves, chiasm, eyes, lacrimal gland, pituitary, brainstem, etc.) render these tumors ideal candidates for a sophisticated treatment-planning system.[33] A 3D system allows careful definition and comprehensive visualization of the tumor and normal anatomy through "beam's eye view." The use of nonaxial and noncoplanar fields allows greater flexibility in treatment planning so that dose distribution conforms to tumor volume in 3D space, sparing the surrounding normal tissue to a greater extent. This type of treatment planning has great potential for improving tumor control by allowing dose escalation. Compared to a classic treatment plan, which routinely includes one half to one third of the ipsilateral eye, greater sparing of the ipsilateral eye is possible without sacrificing tumor control by using a 3D conformal plan. The presentation of inhomogeneity

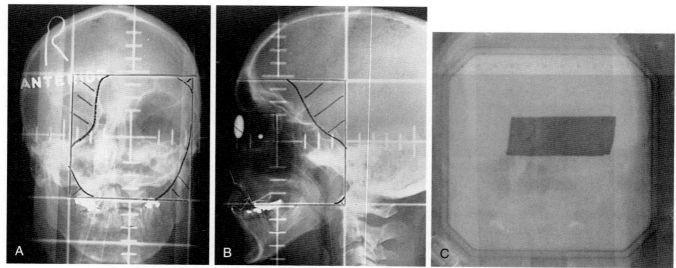

Figure 33-42. Postoperative radiation therapy for a locally advanced paranasal sinus tumor requiring left orbital exenteration. The treatment volume encompasses all the ipsilateral nasal cavity and sinuses including the frontal sinus and orbital bed, contralateral ethmoidal sinus and nasal cavity, and medial maxillary sinus. The patient was treated using a four-field technique that included left and right lateral photon portals, an anterior photon portal, and an electron portal to make up the dose to the left orbital bed, which was blocked from the lateral portals to protect the contralateral eye. **A,** Anterior photon portal including the entire orbital bed. **B,** Lateral photon portal blocking the eye (a dime is placed over the intact eyelid and a canthal marker is placed over the bony canthus). **C,** Anterior electron portal film. (From Ryu JK: Cancer of the nasal cavity and paranasal sinuses. In Leibel SA, Phillips TL: *Textbook of radiation oncology,* ed 2, Philadelphia, 2004, Saunders.)

corrections for air cavities and dense bone is a significant advantage of this type of conformal planning system. Inverse-planned IMRT may render a great therapeutic ratio for tumor of the paranasal sinuses compared with the more standard forward planning 3D conformal therapy (Figure 33-43). IMRT improves sparing of the optic critical structures, especially in unresectable, definitive cases where high doses are required for eradication of gross tumor. The SEER database shows an improving trend of overall survival rate for maxillary sinus. The overall survival for the 1970s was 31%; for the 1980s, 39%; and for the 1990s, 45%. The overall treatment outcome is still poor, though, with less that 55% of patients surviving longer than 5 years. The most common patterns of treatment failure are local recurrence and distant metastasis.[1]

MANAGEMENT OF SYMPTOMS AND MORBIDITY

The incidence of morbidity is related to the treatment technique used, the size of the irradiated volume, the time/dose fractionation scheme use, the location and the extent of the disease, and the patient's age and nutritional status. The early and late responding tissues are affected differently by these factors. The interaction of radiation in cells is random and has no selectivity for any structure or site. This forms the basis of the great challenge in radiation therapy.

The amount of dose prescribed to eradicate a cancer ultimately is dependent on normal tissue tolerance of that dose. Radiosensitivity is the innate sensitivity of cells, tissues, or tumors to radiation. Both normal and cancer cells are affected by radiation. Cells vary in their expressed sensitivity to radiation. Generally, rapidly dividing cells are most sensitive (e.g., mucosa); nondividing or slowly dividing cells generally are less radiosensitive, or radioresistant (e.g., muscle cells, neurons). Exceptions include small lymphocytes and salivary gland cells, which are nondividing but are radiosensitive. The incidence of morbidity is also higher when radiation therapy and surgery are combined. The difficulties consist of delayed wound healing due to impaired blood supply and infection.[31] Specific curative doses for head and neck cancers are listed in Table 33-6. The tissue tolerance doses (TD 5/5 and TD 50/5), the radiation doses to which a normal tissue can be irradiated and continue to function, are listed in Table 33-5. The radiation therapist should know the dose limitations to the specific tissues included in the typical head and neck port. Table 33-7 provides an approximate dose-tissue response schedule for a conventional fractionation scheme. The student may also refer to Chapter 4 on radiobiology.

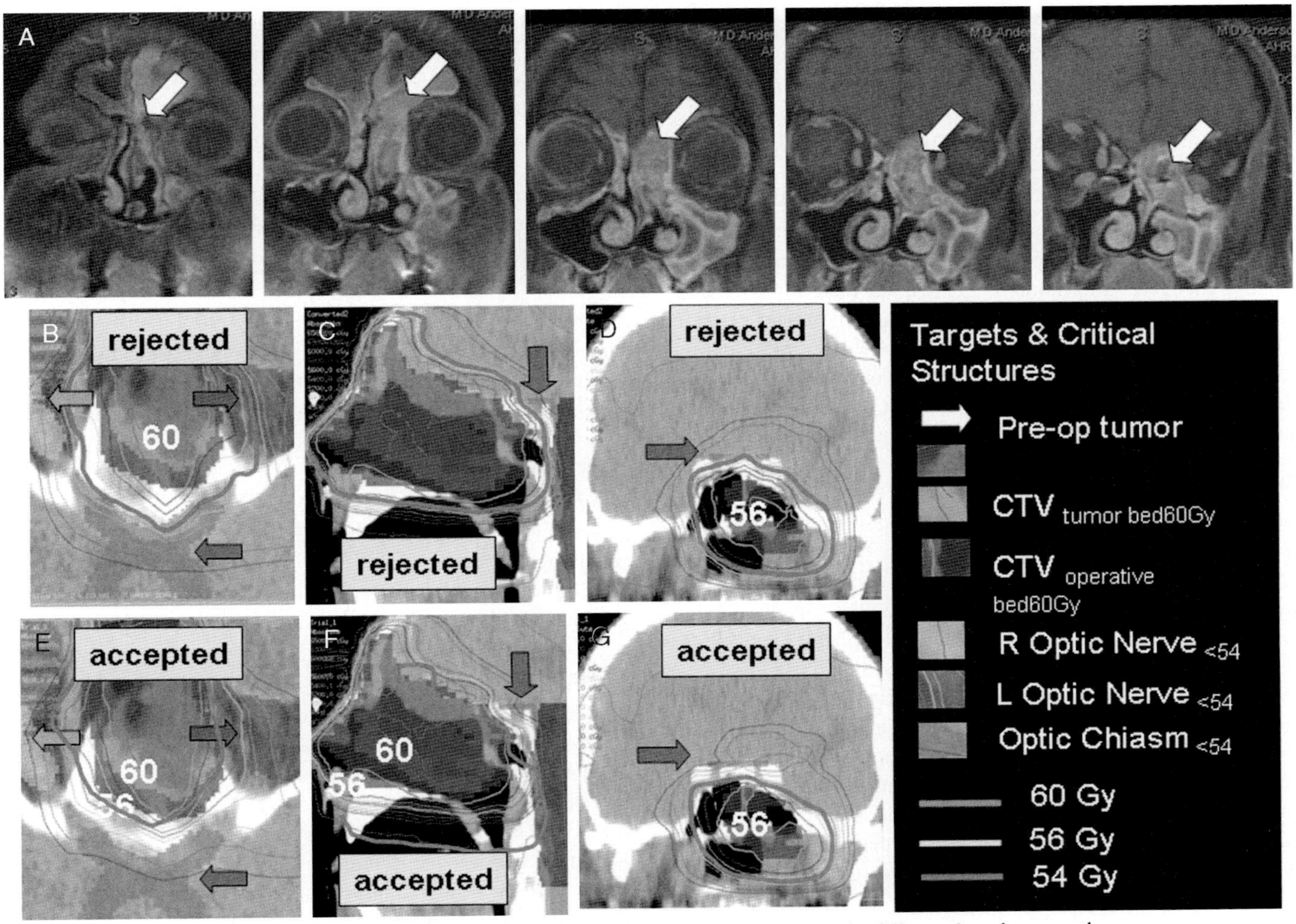

Figure 33-43. Diagnostic MRI shows a left-sided, invasive, poorly differentiated, nasoethmoid carcinoma invading the bone. After resection, the goal was to deliver a dose of 60 Gy in 30 fractions to the tumor bed and 54 Gy to the operative bed using IMRT (**A**). The plan was rejected because the 54-Gy isodose line (*light color*) was very close to the optic nerves and chiasm (*arrow*) (**B-D**). The optimized plan was accepted (**E-G**).(From Ahamad A, et al: Sinonasal cancer. In Gunderson LL, Tepper JE: *Clinical radiation oncology*, ed 2, Philadelphia, 2007, Churchill Livingstone.

Table 33-6	Typical Curative Radiation Doses for Head and Neck Lesions
5000 cGy	Nodes
5000 cGy	Any subclinical disease
6000-6500 cGy	T1 lesions
6500-7000 cGy	T2 lesions
7000-7500 cGy	T3-4 lesions

Table 33-7	Approximate Dose-Tissue Response Schedule for a Conventional Fractionation Scheme
Response	**Dose (cGy)**
Dry mouth	2000
Erythema	2000
Brachial plexus	5500
Spinal cord	4500
Lhermitte's sign	2000-3000
Mandible, teeth and gums	5000-6000
Mucositis	3000
Ears	4000
Cataracts	500-1000
Dry eye	4000
Optic nerve	5000
Retina	5000
Trismus	6000
Laryngitis	5000

Periodontal Disease and Caries

Because healing is poor after treatment, extractions of carious teeth after radiation therapy are not recommended. Aggressive extractions after high doses can lead to osteoradionecrosis. The teeth should be extracted prior to radiation therapy if the patient has carious teeth.

Nutrition

At the time of diagnosis, many patients will have lost a significant amount of weight. Maintaining adequate nutrition is a major problem for these patients, as both the tumor and treatment side effects, such as mucositis from both chemotherapy and radiation therapy (after 2000 to 3000 cGy), may contribute to this problem. Placement of a gastrostomy tube or nasogastric feeding may be required in order to maintain adequate nutrition.

Mucositis/Stomatitis

The epithelial cells of the mucous membrane lining the oral cavity are extremely radiosensitive. Inflammation of the oral mucous membranes with edema and tenderness can occur. A pseudomembrane may form along the mucosal surface. This membrane can slough off, leaving a friable, painful ulcerated surface. Areas that are adjacent to metallic tooth fillings within the treatment field may develop an increased reaction because of scatter radiation from the filling. Dental accessories may be available to eliminate scatter during treatment. Mouth care should involve avoiding drying agents, such as alcohol or glycerin-based products, and brushing/rinsing the oral cavity frequently. An oral-care regimen and the need for routine follow-up with a dentist should be part of the patient and family education (Box 33-7).

Xerostomia

Xerostomia occurs after 1000 to 2000 cGy and may be permanent after 4000 cGy, posing a significant long-term side effect. The patient then becomes at risk for dental caries and

---

Box 33-7	Recommended Oral-Hygiene Program

- Clean teeth and brush gums after meals.
- Use fluoride toothpaste or fluoride rinses daily.
- Floss daily.
- Rinse the mouth with salt and a baking-soda solution (1 qt water, ½ Tsp salt, ½ Tsp baking soda).
- See a dentist regularly during treatment for a teeth and gum examination.
- To reduce the severity of any head and neck complication, the patient should be encouraged to avoid the following:
  - Spicy hot foods, coarse or raw vegetables, dry crackers, chips, and nuts
  - Smoking, chewing tobacco, and alcohol
  - Sugary snacks
  - Commercial mouthwash that contains alcohol because it dries the mouth
- Cold foods and drinks

---

oral infections. When the salivary glands are within the treatment field, the saliva may become scant and is thick and ropy. In some patients, pilocarpine hydrochloride (Salagen) has been useful in stimulating the production of saliva. The use of saliva substitutes is required along with other oral lubricants—XeroLube or vegetable oils help decrease the sensation of mouth dryness. The use of reinforced daily fluoride application to the teeth may strengthen the tooth enamel and minimize dental caries.

Cataract Formation

One of the most radiosensitive tissues in the head and neck area is the lens, and formation of cataracts, which can be removed surgically, may develop following doses lower than 1000 cGy.[8]

Lacrimal Glands

Irradiation of the lacrimal gland may cause a dry, painful eye. Severe dry eye syndrome has been reported in 100% of patients receiving more that 5700 cGy. Obstruction to the tear duct, which is rare and usually associated with tumor involvement of the lacrimal duct, causes a constantly wet eye.[8]

Taste Changes

Treatment may affect the taste buds, which line the tongue and other parts of the oral cavity. While the sensation affected (sweet, sour, salty, or bitter) varies, reports indicate that the sweet sensation is affected more than the salty sensation.[9] The incidence is dose dependent. The taste buds are radiosensitive, and atrophy and degeneration are noted at 1000 cGy. Although some recovery may occur within a few months after treatment, many patients continue to report persistent taste changes for several months following irradiation. The therapist should educate the patient and family regarding temporary or permanent affects and maintenance of nutritional status. One should encourage the patient to identify and consume foods that have or retain some taste (sweet and sour foods retain some taste). Patients should be encouraged to chew foods longer to allow more contact of the food with the taste buds. The sense of taste and smell are closely linked. Because the olfactory senses are not affected, having the patient smell the food before eating it can give the sense of some taste.[9]

Skin Reactions

Most patients will experience some degree of acute skin effects. Affects vary depending on total dose, dose of daily fraction, type and energy of radiation used, the use of radiosensitizing/chemotherapy agents (methotrexate, 5-fluorouracil), the use of beam modifiers (bolus material), and individual differences among patients (complexity and nutrition). Reactions range from erythema or dryness to dry or moist desquamation. Adhering to principles of good wound care and maintaining a clean environment is recommended. Moisturizing lotions and gels can be applied to areas of dry desquamation; hydrocortisone cream can be applied to irritated, inflamed skin but should not be used on areas of moist skin reactions because it may enhance infection.[9] Box 33-8 lists elements of a recommended skin care program.

Box 33-8	Recommended Skin-Care Program

- Wash the skin with lukewarm water, pat dry, and do not wash off marks.
- Use mild soaps (e.g., Basis, Neutrogena).
- Use water-based lotions or creams (e.g., Aquaphor, Eucerin).
- Avoid lotions with perfume and deodorants.
- Avoid direct sunlight.
- Do not use straight razors.
- Avoid tight-fitting collars and hat brims.
- Do not use aftershave lotions or perfumes.
- Apply only nonadherent, hydrophilic dressings to wounds.

ROLE OF RADIATION THERAPIST

The extent of radiation therapy side effects varies from patient to patient. During the initial consultation, the radiation oncologist should inform the patient of all possible complications that can arise from the treatment or disease process; this is usually accomplished while completing an informed consent. The entire oncology team is responsible for assessing the efficiency of the treatment in terms of the health and well-being of the patient. The importance of adequate knowledge regarding treatment complications is to be emphasized to the radiation therapy student. The radiation therapist's role in patient assessment and as a gatekeeper to direct care or to avoid significant patient reactions (perhaps by interrupting treatment) is dependent on this knowledge.

Head and neck cancer patients need to know that the side effects encountered are site specific and related to dose dependency. Patients also need to understand that communicating any discomfort they are experiencing to the radiation therapists or other team members is vital to good cancer treatment management of the head and neck region. Radiation therapists should encourage patients to express any fears they have about the side effects, disease outcomes, or procedures that can alter speech, food intake, or breathing. Patients should also be informed that follow-up after treatment is an important aspect of the management of head and neck cancer because they are at risk for a recurrence. Radiation therapists should give patients explicit instructions regarding physical changes to look for in tissue color, texture, new growths, or unexplained pain. Patients should be instructed to seek medical advice as soon as possible.

Soreness of the throat and mouth is expected to appear in the second or third week of standard fractionated EBRT. Minor irritations often remain for about a month after treatments end. Xylocain viscus or dyclonine are good liquid pain relievers. Over-the-counter medication (approved by a physician) such as Ora-gel for babies and Ambersol can provide temporary relief.

Denture wearers may notice that the dentures no longer fit as a result of swelling of the gums. Loss of saliva is a common side effect of radiation to the oral cavity. Sipping cool carbonated drinks during the day may alleviate some of this. Lemon drops (sugar free) help promote saliva production and taste. The radiation therapist should instruct the patient to choose foods that are easy to eat. As chewing and swallowing become more difficult, the therapist should recommend more liquid, semisolid meals moistened with sauces, and gravies to make eating easier. Artificial saliva is a possible remedy; a physician should be consulted.

The cancer care team including the therapist should instruct the patient about wound care, cleaning of tracheostomies, and speech-rehabilitation options. The therapist should be mindful of any weeping surgical sites or a change in the healing process that can indicate an infection. Proper skin care during treatment is an important aspect of patient care management. To better facilitate communication with a speech-impaired patient, the therapist should provide a pad and pencil. Hand signals should be arranged with the patient in the event something goes wrong in the treatment room during beam-on conditions. The radiation therapist must understand that the head and neck cancer patient will undergo some structural and functional losses; the therapist should be ready to answer any questions or provide for the specific needs of the patient.

FUTURE DIRECTIONS

Greater results in radiation therapy may be achieved by the use of techniques such as 3D conformal therapy, proton-beam therapy, or intracavitary boost delivery for limited tumors. A report on proton-beam therapy for nasopharyngeal tumors has shown promising results. It suggests that the use of proton beams result in a significant increase in dose with increased sparing to normal tissue. The high cost and time-consuming planning is noted to be a disadvantage. Examples of the advantages of 3D conformal therapy and IMRT have been cited in several sections of this chapter. Computer-assisted multileaf collimators with a real-time portal imaging device allow the delivery of multiple beams with minimal human interventions. This development adds to available quality assurance which is growing in importance as treatment volumes become more specific with escalating doses. Local control has been reported to be enhanced. Sparing of structures such as the unaffected parotid gland is achieved using IMRT and tumor failure within the clinical tumor volume has led to studies of radioresistant tumor subvolumes. These studies bring a new awareness for the selection of more aggressive treatment techniques where hypoxic regions are identified.[11]

Fast neutrons has been investigated clinically, potential advantages over photons include less dependence on tumor oxygenation, less absorption of bone, and shorter overall treatment time. Results of treatment for primary or recurrent unresectable (T4) tumors of the paranasal sinus include complete regression in 86% of cases with local control to 68%. The disadvantages included adverse skin reactions, blindness or pain although overall local control rates are as high as 88%. Clinical trials of neutron treatment to salivary gland tumors show great advantages as well.

Recent studies involving the treatment of head and neck cancer patients using a helical tomotherapy unit focus on the elimination of systematic errors and random setup errors. Consideration of error includes the progressive deformation of the patient's soft tissue structures during the course of treatment. Protocols that use megavolt CT image guidance are under study. Variables under consideration include increased patient imaging dose and machine time in addition to precision.[43]

SUMMARY

- The effective management of patients with head and neck cancer involves the close cooperation of the radiation oncologists, medical oncologists, dentists, maxillofacial prosthodontists, nutritionists, head and neck surgeons, neurosurgeons, plastic surgeons, oral surgeons, pathologists, oncology nurses, radiologists, social workers, radiation therapists, speech therapists, pain service, and neurology service, without forgetting the patient's involvement.
- Integrating image guidance technology with intensity-modulated radiation therapy (IMRT), and using functional image information with positron emission tomography (PET) fused with treatment planning have the potential to improve both tumor control and normal tissue sparing.
- The lungs are the most common site of distant metastasis.
- The incidence of distant metastasis is greatest with tumors of the nasopharynx and hypopharynx.
- High-grade parotid tumors are known to involve the facial nerve and to cause paralysis.
- The preservation of salivary function by sparing at least one parotid gland has been a primary objective of head and neck IMRT. A general benefit involves producing minimal side effects and morbidity due to minimizing exposure to healthy tissue.
- Thyroid cancer consistently shows the greatest positive trend in the SEER reports. It leads among all ages, race, and gender in trending incidence of primary cancers and is second only to liver cancer and inflammatory bowel disease in trending U.S. cancer death rates for the time period reported.
- General etiologic risk factors for head and neck cancer include (1) tobacco and alcohol use, (2) ultraviolet light exposure, (3) viral infection, and (4) environmental exposures.
- Occupations associated with greater risk include (1) nickel refining, (2) furniture and woodworking (cancers of the larynx, nasal cavity, and paranasal sinuses), and (3) steel and textile workers (oral cancer).
- Epstein-Barr virus has been associated with nasopharyngeal carcinoma in all races.
- More than 80% of head and neck cancers arise from the surface epithelium of the mucosal linings of the upper digestive tract. These cancers are mostly squamous cell carcinomas.
- For the treatment of the floor of the mouth, if the lesion is small and confined to the floor of the mouth, the tip of the tongue is elevated out of the portal with a cork. If the lesion has grown into the tongue, the tongue is flattened with the tongue blade and cork to reduce the superior border of the portal. For the treatment of the tongue, a depressor, a tongue blade, and cork are sometimes inserted to push the tongue back and keep as much of the mandible out of the field as possible. A tongue blade with a cork attached to one end or a similar device may be inserted between the incisor teeth to depress the tongue, displace the tongue from the treatment volume, or displace the palate.

Review Questions

Multiple Choice

1. Multiple tumor types are included in the head and neck region. Which type of primary tumor is most common?
   a. adenocarcinoma
   b. squamous cell carcinoma
   c. basal cell carcinoma
   d. fibrosarcoma
2. The primary lymphatic drainage of the lower lip would be to:
   a. submental nodes
   b. submaxillary nodes
   c. subdigastric node
   d. the posterior cervical chain
3. What normal tissue would be at most risk of radiation damage when treating the maxillary antrum?
   a. brain
   b. eye
   c. skin
   d. pituitary
4. The most common sign/symptom of oral cancer is:
   a. ulceration
   b. hoarseness
   c. odynophagia
   d. xerostomia
5. The most commonly involved group of nodes in oropharyngeal cancer is the:
   a. submandibular nodes
   b. retropharyngeal nodes
   c. jugulodigastric nodes
   d. supraclavicular nodes
6. A tumor confined to the larynx with cord fixation in glottic cancer is staged as a:
   a. T1
   b. T2
   c. T3
   d. T4
7. Palpation of the cricoid cartilage indicates the inferior border of the:
   a. oral cavity
   b. oropharynx
   c. larynx
   d. hypopharynx
8. For patients with carious teeth, when is dental work recommended when anticipating oral cavity irradiation?
   a. following treatment
   b. preceding treatment
   c. both a and b
   d. neither a nor b
9. Postcricoid cancers occur predominantly in women.
   a. true
   b. false

10. Tumors of the head and neck may involve the cranial nerves that control our major senses. This may lead to signs and symptoms that can point to a possible location of a tumor. The cranial nerve that may be involved in facial paralysis is the cranial nerve.
    a. XII
    b. I
    c. VIII
    d. VII

The answers to the Review Questions can be found by logging on to our website at: *http://evolve.elsevier.com/Washington+Leaver/principles*

Questions to Ponder

1. A majority of head and neck cancers are grouped together by anatomical site. Why then is there such diverse difference in biological and clinical behavior between the same cell type and structures that are only a few millimeters apart?
2. What is the reason for the high incidence of a second primary for patients with early-stage squamous cell disease that was cured?
3. Are there biological markers that can be identified early and will decrease the toxicity and morbidity from treatments?
4. Will nonstandard radiation therapy fractionation schemes improve survivability at the expense of second malignancies?
5. Does chemotherapy have a role in the elective treatment of premalignant conditions seen in head and neck disease?

REFERENCES

1. Ahamad A, et al: Sinonasal cancer. In Gunderson LL, Tepper JE, editors: *Clinical radiation oncology*, ed 2, Philadelphia, 2007, Churchill Livingstone.
2. American Cancer Society: *Cancer facts & figures 2008*, Atlanta, 2008, American Cancer Society.
3. American Joint Committee on Cancer: *Manual for staging of cancer*, ed 6, New York, 2002, Springer-Verlag.
4. Ang KK: Head and neck tumors. In Gunderson LL, Tepper JE, editors: *Clinical radiation oncology*, ed 2. Philadelphia, 2007, Churchill Livingstone.
5. Ang KK, Garden AS: *Radiotherapy for head and neck cancers: Indications and techniques*, ed 3, Philadelphia, 2006, Lippincott Williams & Wilkins.
6. Barry MK, Donohue JH: Surgical principles. In Gunderson LL, Tepper JE, editors: *Clinical radiation oncology*, ed 2, Philadelphia, 2007, Churchill Livingstone.
7. Beitler JJ, Amdur RJ, Mendenhall WM: Cancers of the head and neck. In Khan FM, editor: *Treatment planning in radiation oncology*, ed 2, Philadelphia, 2007, Lippincott Williams & Wilkins.
8. Bentel GC: *Radiation therapy planning*, ed 2, New York, 1996, McGraw-Hill.
9. Bruner DW: *Manual for radiation oncology nursing practice and education*, ed 3, Pittsburgh, 2004, Oncology Nursing Press.
10. Chong LM, Armstrong JG: Tumors of the salivary glands. In Leibel SA, Phillips TL, editors: *Textbook of radiation oncology*, ed 2, Philadelphia, 2004, WB Saunders.
11. Clifford KS, et al: Patterns of failure in patients receiving definitive and postoperative IMRT for head and neck cancer, *Int J Radiat Oncol Biol Phys* 55:312-321, 2003.
12. Fajardo LF: *Radiation pathology*, New York, 2001, Oxford.
13. Foote RL, et al: Salivary gland cancer. In Gunderson LL, Tepper JE, editors: *Clinical radiation oncology*, ed 2, Philadelphia, 2007, Churchill Livingstone.
14. Frank DK, Sessions RB: Physical examination of the head and neck. In Harrison LB, Sessions RB, Hong WK, editors: *Head and neck cancer: a multidisciplinary approach*, ed 2, Philadelphia, 2004, Lippincott Williams & Wilkins.
15. Garden AS, Morrison WH, Ang KK: Larynx and hypopharynx cancer. In Gunderson LL, Tepper JE, editors: *Clinical radiation oncology*, ed 2, Philadelphia, 2007, Churchill Livingstone.
16. Gregoire V, et al: Management of the neck. In Gunderson LL, Tepper JE, editors: *Clinical radiation oncology*, ed 2, Philadelphia, 2007, Churchill Livingstone.
17. Hinerman RW, et al: Oral cavity cancer. In Gunderson LL, Tepper JE, editors: *Clinical radiation oncology*, ed 2, Philadelphia, 2007, Churchill Livingstone.
18. Hu KS, Harrison LB, Culliney B, Dicker A, Sessions RB: Cancer of the oropharynx. In Leibel SA, Phillips TL, editors: *Textbook of radiation oncology*, ed 2, Philadelphia, 2004, Saunders.
19. Khan FM: Introduction: Process, equipment, and personnel. In Khan FM, editor: *Treatment planning in radiation oncology*, ed 2, Philadelphia, 2007, Lippincott Williams & Wilkins.
20. Khandani AH, Sheikh A: Nuclear medicine. In Gunderson LL, Tepper JE, editors: *Clinical radiation oncology*, ed 2, Philadelphia, 2007, Churchill Livingstone.
21. Lee M, Fu KK: Cancer of the nasopharynx. In Leibel SA, Phillips TL, editors: *Textbook of radiation oncology*, ed 2, Philadelphia, 2004, WB Saunders.
22. Lee NL, Phillips TL: Cancer of the larynx. In Leibel SA, Phillips TL, editors: *Textbook of radiation oncology*, ed 2, Philadelphia, 2004, WB Saunders.
23. Lee NL, Phillips TL: Cancer of the oral cavity. In Leibel SA, Phillips TL, editors: *Textbook of radiation oncology*, ed 2, Philadelphia, 2004, WB Saunders.
24. Leibel S: *Textbook of radiation*, ed 2, Philadelphia, 2004, WB Saunders.
25. Lenhard E, Osteen R, Gansler T: *American Cancer Society's clinical oncology*, Atlanta, 2001, The Society.
26. Levendag P, et al: Brachytherapy versus surgery in carcinoma of tonsillar fossa and/or soft palate: Late adverse sequelae and performance status: can we be more selective and obtain better tissue sparing? *Int J Radiat Oncol Biol Phys* 59:713-724, 2004.
27. Mendenhall WM, Sulica L, Sessions RB: Early stage cancer of the larynx. In Harrison LB, Sessions RB, Hong WK, editors: *Head and neck cancer: a multidisciplinary approach*, ed 2, Philadelphia, 2004, Lippincott Williams & Wilkins.
28. Morrison WH, Garden AS, Ang KA: Oropharyngeal cancer. In Gunderson LL, Tepper JE, editors: *Clinical radiation oncology*, ed 2, Philadelphia, 2007, Churchill Livingstone.
29. Ove R, Foote RL, Bonner JA: Nasopharyngeal carcinoma. In Gunderson LL, Tepper JE, editors: *Clinical radiation oncology*, ed 2. Philadelphia, 2007, Churchill Livingstone.
30. Pazdur R: *Cancer management: a multidisciplinary approach*, ed 5, New York, 2001, PRR.
31. Ries LAG, et al, editors: *SEER cancer statistics review, 1975-2004*, Bethesda, MD, 2005, National Cancer Institute (website): http://seer.cancer.gov/csr/1975_2004. Accessed 2007.
32. Rubin P: *Clinical oncology: a multidisciplinary approach for physicians and students*, ed 8, Philadelphia, 2001, WB Saunders.
33. Ryu JK: Cancer of the nasal cavity and paranasal sinuses. In Leibel SA, Phillips TL, editors: *Textbook of radiation oncology*, ed 2, Philadelphia, 2004, WB Saunders.
34. Sabel M: Principles of surgical therapy. In Sabel MS, Sondak VK, Sussman JJ, editors: *Surgical foundations: essentials of surgical oncology*, Philadelphia, 2007, Mosby.
35. Silverman S, Miller C, Thompson J: Etiology and predisposing factors. In Silverman S, editor: *Oral cancer*, ed 5, Hamilton, 2003, BC Decker and American Cancer Society.

36. Singer MI, et al: Treatment. In Silverman S, editor: *Oral cancer*, ed 5, Hamilton, 2003, BC Decker.

37. Smith BD, Haffty BG: Prognostic factors in patients with head and neck cancer. In Harrison LB, Sessions RB, Hong WK, editors: *Head and neck cancer: a multidisciplinary approach*, ed 2, Philadelphia, 2004, Lippincott Williams & Wilkins.

38. Temam S, et al: Salvage surgery after failure of very accelerated radiotherapy in advanced head-and-neck squamous cell carcinoma, *Int J Radiat Oncol Biol Phys* 62:1078-1083, 2005.

39. Thibodeau GA, Patton KT: *Anatomy and physiology*, ed 6, St. Louis, 2007, Mosby.

40. Weng BM, Cohen JM: General principles of head and neck pathology. In Harrison LB, Sessions RB, Hong WK, editors: *Head and neck cancer: a multidisciplinary approach*, ed 2, Philadelphia, 2004, Lippincott Williams & Wilkins.

41. Wolfe MJ, Wilson K: Head and neck cancer. In Sabel MS, Sondak VK, Sussman JJ, editors: *Surgical foundations: essentials of surgical oncology*, Philadelphia, 2007, Mosby.

42. Yao M, et al: Value of EDG PET in assessment of treatment response and surveillance in head and neck cancer patients after intensity modulated radiation treatment: a preliminary report, *Int J Radiat Oncol Biol Phys* 60:1014-1418, 2004.

43. Zeidan OA, et al: Evaluation of image-guidance protocols in the treatment of head and neck cancers, *Int J Radiat Oncol Biol Phys* 67:670-677, 2007.

44. Zelefsky MJ: Cancer of the hypopharynx. In Leibel SA, Phillips TL, editors: *Textbook of radiation oncology,* ed 2, Philadelphia, 2004, WB Saunders.

BIBLIOGRAPHY

DeVita V, Hellman S, Rosenberg S: *Cancer: principles and practice of oncology*, ed 6, Philadelphia, 2001, Lippincott.

Mills SE, Gaffey MJ, Frierson HF: *Atlas of tumor pathology: tumors of the upper aerodigestive tract and ear*, Washington, DC, 2000, Armed Forces Institute of Pathology.

Myers E, Suen J: *Cancer of the head and neck*, ed 2, Philadelphia, 1996, WB Saunders.

Rice DH, Batsakis JG: *Surgical pathology of the head and neck*, Philadelphia, 2000, Lippincott.

Central Nervous System Tumors

Robert D. Adams, Dennis Leaver

Outline

Cancer of the central nervous
   system
Epidemiology
Etiology
Prognostic indicators

Anatomy and lymphatics
Natural history of disease and
   patterns of spread
Clinical presentation
Detection and diagnosis

Pathology
Staging
Treatment techniques
Role of radiation therapist
Summary

Objectives

- Discuss epidemiologic factors of this tumor site.
- Identify, list, and discuss etiologic factors that may be responsible for inducing tumors in this anatomic site.
- Describe the symptoms produced by a malignant tumor in this region.
- Discuss the methods of detection and diagnosis for tumors in this anatomic region.
- List the varying histologic types of tumors generic to this region.
- Describe the diagnostic procedures used in the workup and staging for this site.
- Differentiate between histologic grading and staging.
- Describe in detail the anatomy and physiology of this anatomic region/organ.
- Identify the treatment(s) of choice for this malignancy.
- Discuss the rationale for treatment with regard to treatment choice, histologic type, and stage of the disease.

- Describe in detail the treatment methods available for this diagnosis.
- Describe the differing types of radiation treatments that can be used for treating this tumor site.
- Identify the appropriate tumor lethal dose for various stages of this malignancy.
- Discuss the expected radiation reactions for the area based on time-dose-fractionation schemes.
- Discuss tolerance levels of the vital structures and organs at risk.
- Describe the instructions that should be given to a patient with regard to skin care, expected reactions, and dietary advice.
- Identify the psychological problems associated with a malignancy in this site.
- Describe the various treatment planning techniques for this anatomic site.
- Discuss survival statistics and prognosis for various stages for this tumor site.

Key Terms

Blood-brain barrier
  (BBB)
Cerebellum
Cerebrospinal fluid
  (CSF)
Cerebrum
Debulking
Edema
Gamma knife
Intracranial pressure
  (ICP)
Karnofsky Performance
  Scale (KPS)
Necrosis
Papilledema
Positron emission
  tomography (PET)
Radiation necrosis
Radiosensitizers
Regeneration
Tentorium
Ventricles

Central nervous system (CNS) tumors include brain and spinal cord tumors. The tumors can be primary or secondary (metastatic) and benign or malignant. Some are regarded as benign because of slow growth rates and their response to therapy.[4] In recent years, radiation therapy has played a significant role in the treatment of CNS tumors, provided a means of increased survival time, resulted in a regression of the effects of neurologic deficit, and enhanced the quality of life of many patients with brain tumors.[6]

Although CNS tumors rarely metastasize, they are often locally invasive and create significant problems. Structures that become involved with these neoplasms are not capable of **regeneration** (repair or regrowth). Tumors of the CNS, even if benign histologically, are considered malignant in part because of their inaccessible location.[16] As shown in Table 34-1, many different cell types are believed to produce CNS and spinal axis tumors. Because CNS tumors arise in different areas of the cranium and spinal axis, the belief is that different molecular and genetic mechanisms are at work during various times of life.

CANCER OF THE CENTRAL NERVOUS SYSTEM

Epidemiology

Approximately 21,810 cases of primary brain tumors and other nervous system tumors are diagnosed annually in the United States. Brain tumors account for 1.5% of all malignancies. About 80% of CNS tumors involve the brain, whereas 20% involve the spinal cord. Primary CNS neoplasms results in 13,070 deaths annually.[1] The incidence rate is 5 per 100,000 people and varies according to race,

Table 34-1	Classification of Tumors of the Central Nervous System	
Tumor Type	**Normal Tissue Origin**	**General Function of Tissue**
Glioma (includes glioblastoma, astrocytoma, glioblastoma multiforme, brainstem and thalamus tumors)	Astrocytes	These are star-shaped cells that are commonly found between neurons and blood vessels that provide support and help regulate ions. They are an important part of the blood-brain barrier.
Medulloblastoma	Primitive neuroectodermal cell or Primitive nerve tumors (PNET)	These cells comprise a family of the small blue round cell mass and are the most common malignant nervous system tumors of childhood. These cells do not usually remain in the body after birth.
Oligodendroglioma	Oligodendrocyte	Smaller cell that resembles an astrocyte. They produce a fatty insulating substance called myelin, which may be provided to many nearby axons.
Ependymoma	Ependyma	Lines the ventricles and spinal cord. These cuboidal-shaped cells aid in the production and circulation of cerebrospinal fluid.
Meningioma	Meninges	Comprised of three distinct coverings that protect the brain and spinal cord. CSF circulates within the meninges.
Lymphoma	Lymphocyte and microglia	Part of the immune system, the cells body's primary defense against infection and foreign substances. Microglial cells help support neurons and phagocytize bacteria and cellular debris.
Schwannoma	Schwann cell	They produce a fatty insulating substance called myelin, which insulates and protects nerves outside the CNS.

gender, and age. Brain tumors are the second leading cause of death in children (behind leukemia).[1]

Age is a dominant variable, with the incidence of CNS tumors in older patients appearing to rise. Nelson et al.[15] attribute this increase to three possible factors: (1) an increase in life expectancy, (2) the increasing availability and use of computer tomography (CT) and magnetic resonance imaging (MRI), and (3) an increased interest in geriatrics and an overall improvement in health care of the elderly. Most CNS tumors occur in persons between the ages of 50 and 80. The incidence is higher than 20 per 100,000 for older men and fewer than 2 per 100,000 for children younger than 15. Most brain tumors occur in two age peaks: childhood (3 to 12 years) and later in life.[4] Many different tumor types are included in the CNS category. In the United States in 2008, it is estimated that 21,810 CNS tumors will be diagnosed.[1] Of these, approximately 16,400 will occur in the cerebrum. Half of them will be gliomas—75% will be high-grade gliomas and 25% will be low-grade gliomas.[19]

 Recent statistics regarding brain cancer incidence can be found at the American Cancer Society's website: www.cancer.org.

The function of the **cerebrum** includes interpretation of sensory impulses and voluntary muscular activities; it is the center for memory, learning, reasoning, judgment, intelligence, and emotions. Gliomas commonly occur in persons between the ages of 40 and 75 years old.[19] Approximately 45% of childhood tumors are gliomas, with most involving the cerebellum and, to a lesser degree, the brainstem.[20] The **cerebellum** is the part of the brain that plays a role in the coordination of voluntary muscular movement.

Primary brain tumors are relatively uncommon. However, cerebral metastases occur in approximately 30% of patients with cancer and are the most common brain lesions.[17] The most common primary site of disease responsible for producing brain metastases is the lung. Most metastatic lesions occur in the cerebral hemispheres. Single metastases occur 40% to 45% of the time.[17] Brain metastases may be the only indication of malignant disease. These metastases can occur early in the disease process or may not appear until years later. Long-term survival for patients with CNS tumors is uncommon.[6] Factors such as the patient's age, Karnofsky Performance Scale (KPS) score, and neurologic signs and symptoms at the time of diagnosis are important in the changes of survival. Most spinal-axis tumors are extradural (on the outside of or unconnected to the dura mater). They are predominately metastatic carcinomas, lymphomas, or sarcomas. Most primary spinal-axis tumors are intradural (within or enclosed by the dural mater).

 The **Karnofsky Performance Scale (KPS)** scores, which range from 0 to 100, are a clinical method of measuring the ability of cancer patients to perform ordinary tasks. A higher score means the patient is better able to carry out daily activities. KPS may be used to determine a patient's prognosis, measure changes in a patient's ability to function, or decide if a patient is available for inclusion in a clinical trial.

Etiology

The origin of primary CNS tumors is largely unknown. Brain tumor associations include occupational and environmental exposures, lifestyle and dietary factors, medical conditions, and genetic factors. Occupational and environmental factors include chemicals, synthetic rubber, pesticides, herbicides, ionizing radiation, and electromagnetic fields. The association between chemical exposure and brain tumors is limited to a few occupations. Workers in agriculture and health care delivery have demonstrated higher incidence rates than normal. Lifestyle and dietary factors include cells phones, nitrates, hair dyes, and smoking.

Medical conditions include drugs, viral infections, and AIDS. Genetic factors, which include less than 5% of the etiology of brain tumors, include von Recklinghausen's disease, and autosomal dominant disorder (*NF1* and *NF2* genes).[3] Most recently, the origin and stimulus for the progression of brain tumors have been attributed to stem cells.[8]

Prognostic Indicators

The 5-year survival rates for patients with primary CNS tumors during the past four decades has ranged from 19% from 1960 to 1985, and has risen to an overall survival of 35% during the past two decades.[6] Several factors have been identified as prognostic indicators for CNS disorders. The three most important factors are age, the performance status, and tumor type. In numerous clinical trials involving malignant gliomas, these prognostic factors have had a greater influence on survival than has the type or extent of the therapy being evaluated. Unfortunately, one of the most common adult brain tumors, glioblastoma multiforme (GBM), is one of the most lethal and, despite years of clinical research, progress has been slow and disappointing.[14] The prognosis tends to be better in younger patients, with one exception. Children younger than 4 present a particular problem with respect to treatment regimen. Therapy must be modified because of the developing brain, which is more sensitive to radiation; therefore, radiation treatment in children younger than 4 years old must be avoided if possible.

Late effects after CNS treatment in children are an area of concern. A study by Avizonis et al.[2] focused on several areas of interest. Mean intelligent quotient (IQ) scores after treatment indicated slightly decreased scores as whole-brain dose radiation increased. However, learning disabilities can be overcome so that the children can go on to lead productive lives. Another area monitored in the study, the regrowth of hair, appeared to be dose related with diminished regrowth as the dose increased. The measured late effects after radiation did not seem to vary with regard to age at the time of treatment, gender, tumor type, or tumor location.

The location of the tumor is of great importance, serving as a natural prognostic indicator for survival time and neurologic defects. In addition, the KPS measures the neurologic and functional status, allowing for measurements of the quantity and quality of neurologic defects. The KPS ranges from 0 to 100 and is measured in decades. Patients who are able to work have scores in the 80, 90, 100 range. Patients who are unable to work but can still care for themselves have scores in the 50 to 70 range (Box 34-1). Patients who are chronically ill from the disease process have scores of 40 or below.

Tumor grade rather than size is the primary factor involved with prognosis. The tumors are normally grouped into benign, or low-grade, and malignant, or high-grade, categories. The presence or absence of **necrosis** has prognostic significance. Necrosis is the death of a cell or cell group resulting from disease or injury. The process is caused by the action of enzymes and can also affect part of a structure or an organ.

A pathologist examining a biopsy specimen under the microscope will grade the specimen to describe its growth rate and prognosis. With astrocytoma, there are several grading systems used by pathologists to describe the growth rate of the tumor.

Box 34-1 | Karnofsky Performance Scale

PERFORMANCE CRITERIA

Able to carry on normal activity; no special care needed	100	Normal; no complaints; no evidence of disease
	90	Ability to carry on normal activity; minor signs or symptoms of disease
	80	Normal activity with effort; some signs or symptoms of disease
Unable to work; able to live at home and care for most personal needs; a varying amount of assistance needed	70	Self-care; inability to carry on normal activity or do active work
	60	Occasional care for most needs required
	50	Considerable assistance and frequent medical care required
	40	Disabled; special care and assistance required
Unable to care for self; required equivalent of institutional or hospital care; disease may be progressing rapidly	30	Severely disabled; hospitalization indicated, although death not imminent
	20	Extremely sick; hospitalization necessary; active support treatment necessary
	10	Moribund; fatal processes progressing rapidly
	0	Dead

PERFORMANCE SCALE (EASTERN COOPERATIVE ONCOLOGY GROUP)

Grade

0 Fully active; able to carry on all predisease activities without restriction (Karnofsky score of 90 to 100)

1 Restricted in physically strenuous activity, but ambulatory and able to carry out work of a light or sedentary nature, such as light housework or office work (Karnofsky score of 70 to 80)

3 Capable of only limited self-care; confined to bed or chair 50% or more of waking hours (Karnofsky score of 30 to 40)

4 Completely disabled; Unable to carry on any self-care; totally confined to bed or chair (Karnofsky score of 10 to 20)

Modified from Carter S, et al: *Principles of cancer treatment*, New York, 1982, McGraw-Hill.

Some have a three-grade designation, some have four-grade designations, and others use *names* instead of a number. Most pathology reports will indicate how many grades have been used to describe the tumor. For example, grade II/IV represents grade 2 in the 4-grade system; grade II/III represents grade 2 using a 3-grade system. Other reports may indicate the tumor's growth rate by using descriptive words such as "well-differentiated astrocytoma," which would indicate the lowest grade of both the 3- and 4-grade systems, In addition, using descriptive terms such as glioblastoma multiforme represents the highest grade of both the 3- and 4-grade system.

Low-grade tumors have cellularity patterns that look similar to those found in reactive hyperplasia, whereas marked cellularity has been recognized in high-grade tumors, with necrosis seen in the most aggressive tumors, Typically, the higher the grade, the shorter is the survival time. Almost all patients experience a recurrence (with high-grade tumors) postoperatively, and 80% of all recurrences are within a 2-cm margin.[15]

Anatomy and Lymphatics

The brain is one of the most complex organs in the body (Figure 34-1). It is composed of two cerebral hemispheres and two cerebellar hemispheres. The cranial bones, meninges, and **cerebrospinal fluid (CSF)** provide an outer covering of protection for the brain.

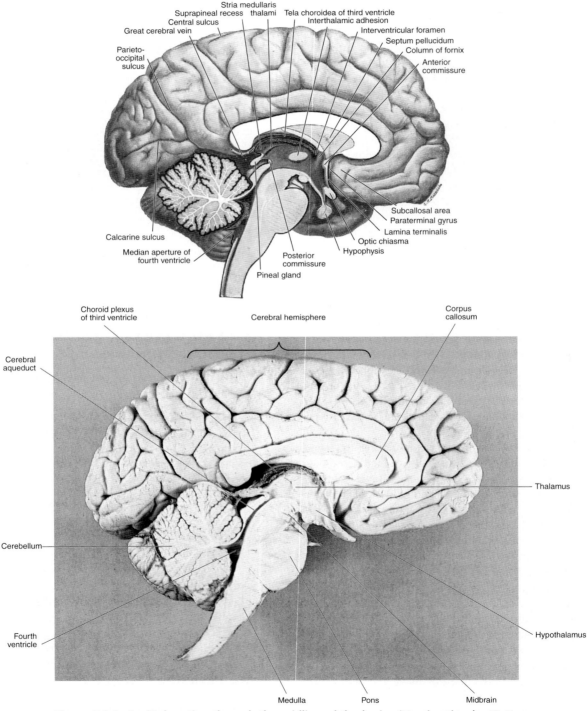

Figure 34-1. Sagittal section through the midline of the brain. (Hemisection by EL Rees; photograph by Kevin Fitzpatrick on behalf of GKT School of Medicine, London.) (From Strandring S, et al: Neuroanatomy. In Standring S, editor: *Gray's anatomy: the anatomical basis of clinical practice,* ed 39. Philadelphia, 2005, Churchill Livingstone.)

The **ventricles** are cavities that form a communication network with each other, the center canal of the spinal cord, and the subarachnoid space. They are filled with CSF. These cavities are the right and left lateral ventricles and the third and fourth ventricles. The lateral ventricles are located below the corpus callosum and extend from front to back. Each opens into the third ventricle. The lateral ventricles are able to communicate with the third ventricle via the interventricular foramen, which is a small oval opening. The third ventricle is connected to the fourth ventricle. The fourth ventricle lies between the cerebellum and inferior brainstem. Three small openings also allow the CSF to pass into the subarachnoid space. The openings also allow communication with the cord and subarachnoid space (see Figure 34-1).

The supratentorial and infratentorial regions comprise the two major intracranial compartments, the cerebral and cerebellar hemispheres. The **tentorium** (a fold of dura mater, or the outer covering of the brain) separates these compartments. It passes transversely across the posterior cranial fossa in the transverse fissure and acts as a line of separation between the occipital lobe of the cerebrum and the upper cerebellum. The cerebral hemispheres and the sella, pineal, and upper brainstem regions are located in the supratentorial region. The infratentorial region, which leads to the upper spinal cord, houses the brainstem, pons, medulla, and cerebellum.

The CNS is composed of 40% gray matter and 60% white matter. The gray matter contains the supportive nerve cells and related processes. It forms the cortex, or outer part of the cerebrum, and surrounds the white matter. The white matter is composed of bundles of nerve fibers, axons carrying impulses away from the cell body, and dendrites carrying impulses toward the cell body. The nerve cells process and integrate nerve impulses from other neurons. The spinal cord is also composed of a gray substance that forms the inner core, which contains the nerve cells. The outer layer, or white substance, is the location of the nerve fibers. The gray matter varies at different levels of the spinal cord.

The blood supply for the brain comes from the internal carotid arteries and vertebral arteries via the circle of Willis. The blood that enters the brain contains oxygen, nutrients, and energy-rich glucose, which is the primary source of energy for the brain cells. If the blood supply to the brain is interrupted, dizziness, convulsions, or mental confusion may result.

The spinal cord is the continuation of the medulla oblongata and forms the inferior portion of the brainstem. The anterior and lateral portions contain motor neurons and tracts, whereas the posterior portions contain the sensory tracts. The motor neurons are nerve cells that convey impulses from the brain to the cord. This system allows communication between the spinal cord and various parts of the brain. The cord continues down to the level of the first and second lumbar vertebrae. This is an important anatomic reference point for the radiation therapy student. Many times doses to the spinal cord must be calculated, and it is important to have an understanding of where the spinal cord ends. From the spinal cord come 31 pairs of nerves. The spinal cord is surrounded by the same material that surrounds the brain. The CSF flows between the arachnoid and pia arachnoid. Blood is supplied to the cord from the vertebral

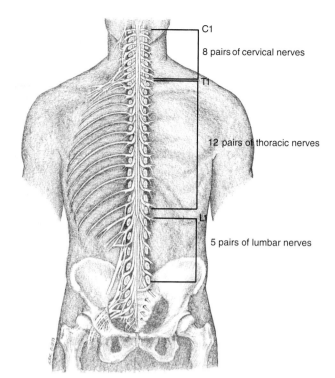

Figure 34-2. Spinal cord and nerves.

arteries and radicular branches of the cervical, intercostal, lumbar, and sacral arteries (Figure 34-2). No lymphatic channels exist in the brain substance.

The **blood-brain barrier (BBB)**, which hinders the penetration of some substances into the brain and CSF, exists between the vascular system and brain. Its purpose is to protect the brain from potentially toxic compounds. Substances that can pass through the BBB must be lipid soluble. Water-soluble substances require a carrier molecule to cross the barrier by active transport. Lipid-soluble substances include alcohol, nicotine, and heroin. Examples of water-soluble substances are glucose, some amino acids, and sodium. Various drugs pass the barrier with varying degrees of difficulty but never easily. Tumor cells infiltrating normal brain tissue cannot be reached by drugs that do not cross the BBB (Figure 34-3).

The CSF is a clear, colorless fluid resembling water. The entire CNS contains 3 to 5 oz of this fluid, which is composed of proteins, glucose, urea (a compound formed in the liver and excreted by the kidney), and salts. The CSF performs several functional roles, including buoyancy to protect the brain, a link in the control of the chemical environment of the CNS, a means of exchanging nutrients and waste products with the CNS, and a channel for intracerebral transport. Blockage of CSF, because of tumor growth, may have disastrous effects on the patient. If the flow of CSF is interrupted it may contribute to increased **intracranial pressure (ICP)**, which is pressure that occurs within the cranium.

Natural History of Disease and Patterns of Spread

With few exceptions, most gliomas tend to spread invasively because they do not form a natural capsule that inhibits growth.

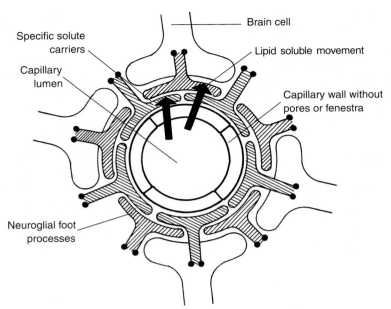

Specific solute carriers

Capillary lumen

Brain cell

Lipid soluble movement

Capillary wall without pores or fenestra

Neuroglial foot processes

Figure 34-3. Blood-brain barrier. (Redrawn from Maisey M, Britton KE, Gilday DL: *Clinical nuclear medicine,* ed 2, New York, 1992, Chapman and Hall.)

These neoplasms are unique because they do not metastasize through a lymphatic drainage system and rarely metastasize outside the CNS unlike many epithelial tumors and tumors of connective tissue origin that commonly metastasize to lymph nodes and other distant anatomic locations. The common route of spread for medulloblastomas and primitive neuroectodermal tumors (PNETs) is via CSF to points in the CNS.

Local invasion and CSF seeding provide the major patterns of spread for CNS tumors. These tumors tend to have cells that can invade normal brain. Drop metastases occur via the CSF and can form secondary tumors. The confines of the brain itself limit the spread of disease, but local recurrence is a major concern. Secondary seeding may grow along nerve roots, causing pain or cord compression. Although the lumbosacral area is the most frequent site of CSF seeding, any area along the spinal axis can become involved. Hematogenous spread is rare.

CNS tumors are characterized by their heterogeneity, which makes understanding their biology difficult. With an improved understanding of the reason and way that CNS tumors develop, grow, and progress, new treatment approaches can be developed and implemented.

Clinical Presentation

As stated, the location of the tumor correlates with the presenting symptoms. Table 34-2 provides an excellent correlation between common symptoms and tumor location. The initial symptom may be a headache, which is usually worse in the morning. This is due to the differences in the CSF drainage from the recumbent to upright positions. Seizures and difficulties with balance, gait, and ambulation are also common presenting signs. Focal signs are usually unilateral. Other neurologic symptoms can include aphasia, hemiplegia, and paresis. Ocular symptoms may result in decreased vision, oculomotor defects, proptosis, and ophthalmic defects. Other presenting signs may be expressive aphasia, sensory aphasia, mental and personality

changes, short-term memory loss, hallucinations, and changes in intellectual functions. Increased ICP can result from the obstruction of CSF flow. The symptoms can result from direct invasion of the tissue by the tumor, destruction of brain tissue and bone, and increased pressure.

Patients with spinal cord tumors have pain, weakness, loss of sensation, and bowel- and bladder-control problems. Although pain may be an early symptom, additional symptoms may signal a cord compression or vascular problems. Weakness usually occurs in the distal part of the extremity first and progresses proximally. Rapid deterioration of motor and sensory functions soon follows. Immediate treatment is required for patients who have a sudden onset of symptoms so that permanent paralysis may be prevented (Table 34-3). In contrast to brain lesions, the symptoms are more frequently bilateral.

Detection and Diagnosis

The initial workup is critical to a definitive diagnosis, and a complete history and physical examination are necessary. Because some CNS tumors are genetic, associated with exposure to chemicals, or related to infection, previous medical, family, and social histories are extremely important.

Information gathered from people other than the patient may also be beneficial in making a diagnosis. Mental changes, personality changes, and changes in behavior are not often noticed by the patient but are noticed by other individuals. Symptoms of long duration may indicate a slow-growing tumor, whereas the sudden onset of symptoms may point toward a tumor of higher grade and size.

A neurologic workup includes an evaluation in several key areas. The patient's mental status at the time of the diagnosis often reflects changes in behavior, mood, thought and speech patterns, and intelligence. Intellectual function is crucial, and the level of consciousness must be evaluated quickly. One test for intellectual function includes orientation to person, place,

| Table 34-2 | Symptoms, Signs, and Diagnostic Characteristics of Various Intracranial Tumors | | |

Tumor	Common Symptoms	Common Signs	Diagnostic Characteristics*
PRIMARY			
Malignant astrocytoma	Headache, seizure, unilateral weakness, mental changes	Focal presentation related to tumor location	Enhancing CT lesion, tumor blush on angiography
Glioblastoma multiforme (GM)			CT lesion
Astrocytoma with anaplastic foci (AAF)			No hypodense interior enhanced MR or CT lesion
Brainstem or thalamus	Nausea, vomiting, ataxia	Increased intracranial pressure (papilledema) abducens and oculomotor nerve defects	May not enhance CT; biopsy may not be appropriate
Meningioma (B, M)	Localized headache, seizure	Focal presentation related to tumor location	Enhancing MR or CT lesion associated with dura
Astrocytoma (B, M)	Headache, seizure, unilateral weakness, mental changes	Focal presentation related to tumor location	May not enhance on CT or MR
Cerebral	Headache, seizure, unilateral weakness, mental changes	Focal presentation related to tumor location	
Cerebellar	Occipital headache	Increased intracranial pressure (papilledema), abducens and oculomotor nerve defects, coordination	
Brain stem or thalamus	Nausea, vomiting, ataxia	Increased intracranial pressure (papilledema), abducens and oculomotor nerve defects, coordination	May be seen only on MR image biopsy may not be appropriate
Optic nerve	Ocular changes	Ocular changes	Detailed MR or CT scan
Pituitary (B, M)	Vertex headache, ocular changes	Ocular and endocrine abnormalities	Hormone analysis, resection histopathology
Medulloblastoma (M)	Morning headaches, nausea vomiting	Coordination, increased intracranial pressure (papilledema), abducens and oculomotor nerve defects	MR or CT scan, lumbar puncture recommended
Ependymoma (B, M)	Morning headaches, nausea vomiting	Coordination, increased intracranial pressure (papilledema), aducens and oculomotor nerve defects	MR or CT scan, lumbar puncture recommended
Hemangioma, arteriovenous malformation (B, M)	"Migrainous" headache	Focal presentation related to tumor location	Angiography, biopsy may not be appropriate
Oligodendroglioma (B, M)	Insidious headache, mental changes	Focal presentation related to tumor location	Radiographic calcification
Sarcoma (M), neurofibroma (B)	Focal presentation related to tumor location	Focal presentation related to tumor location	
Pinealoma (B, M) germinoma	Various (ocular, vestibular endocrine)	Parinaud's syndrome, endocrine changes, ocular changes, increased intracranial (papilledema), abducens and oculomotor nerve defects	Biopsy or resection may not be obtained, markers in CSF may be informative
Lymphoma (M), reticulum cell sarcoma, microglioma	Focal presentation related to tumor location	Focal presentation related to tumor location	"soft" CT enhancement
Unspecified (B, M)	Focal presentation related to tumor location	Focal presentation related to tumor location	
OTHER			
Craniopharyngioma	Headache, mental changes hemiplegia, seizure, vomiting (and ocular changes)	Cranial nerve defects (II-VII)	Cystic/calcified lesion on MR, bone erosion, mass effect from base of skull

Modified from Scally LT, Lin C, Beriwal S, et al: Brain, brain stem and cerebellum. In Perez C, Brady, editors: *Principles and practice of radiation oncology*, ed 4, Philadelphia, 2004, Lippincott Williams & Wilkins.
*Unless noted, a biopsy is assumed.
B, Benign; *CSF*, cerebrospinal fluid; *CT*, computed tomography; *M*, malignant; *MRI*, magnetic resonance.

Table 34-3	Clinical Manifestations of Spinal Cord Tumors
Location	**Findings**
Foramen magnum	Eleventh and twelfth cranial nerve palsies; ipsilateral arm weakness early; cerebellar ataxia; neck pain
Cervical spine	Ipsilateral arm weakness with leg and opposite arm in time; wasting and fibrillation of ipsilateral neck, shoulder girdle, and arm; decreased pain and temperature sensation in upper cervical regions early; pain in cervical distribution
Thoracic spine	Weakness of abdominal muscles; sparing of arms; unilateral root pains; sensory level with ipsilateral changes early and bilateral with time
Lumbosacral spine	Root pain in groin region and sciatic distribution; weakened proximal pelvic muscles; impotence; bladder paralysis; decreased knee jerk and brisk ankle jerks
Cauda equina	Unilateral pain in back and leg, becoming bilateral when the tumor is large; bladder and bowel paralysis

Modified from Levins V, Guten P, Leibel S: Neoplasms of CNS. In DeVita VT, Hellman S, Rosenberg SA, editors: *Cancer: principles and practice of oncology,* ed 4, Philadelphia, 1993, JB Lippincott.

and time and the quickness of the responses to these questions. Further intellectual functions are determined by studying speech, memory, and logical thought processes.

Coordination skills (including walking, balance, and gait), sensations, reflexes, and motor skills are also examined. Lesions that inhibit motor function tend to affect fine motor skills first and produce a spastic paralysis. Sensory functions can be tested with a pin, temperature, and vibrations. These functions can be affected before motor skills. Reflexes may be hyperactive with intracranial tumors early but may become hypoactive in later stages.

If spinal cord tumors are suspected, the evaluation of motor, sensory, and reflex functions is also important. Sensory testing is helpful in determining the level of the lesion. Motor testing may reveal weakness.

Ophthalmoscopy is a test designed to check for **papilledema** (edema of the optic disc), which results from increased ICP. Visual fields may decrease and blind spots increase as the disease progresses. An increase in ICP is usually the result of the flow of CSF becoming obstructed. This can indicate an increase in the tumor mass. If CSF flow is obstructed or production of the fluid is changed, hydrocephalus may appear on CT scans. Infection, **edema** (swelling caused by the abnormal accumulation of fluid in interstitial spaces), or hemorrhage may also cause rising pressure.

Invasion, irritation, and compression of the brain by the tumor cause symptoms. Benign tumors generally cause symptoms produced by pressure, whereas malignant tumors can cause pressure and destruction of CNS tissue. The initial presentation of symptoms depends on different anatomic locations. The involvement of specific regions of the brain generally produces symptoms specific to the areas controlled by those regions, thereby making tumor localization possible (Table 34-4).

Therefore, patients typically have symptoms that reflect the site of involvement. For example, if a tumor occurs in the frontal portion of the brain, symptoms likely to be identified include personality changes, memory defects, gait disorders, and speech difficulties. Lesions occurring in the parietal regions of the brain can produce symptoms such as loss of vision, spatial disorientation, and seizures.

Radiographs of the skull may show several changes that have occurred as a result of an ongoing tumor process. The pineal body may be calcified and deviated, increasing pressure may

show erosion of the posterior clinoid process of the sphenoid bone, or calcification of certain tumors may be seen. Radiographs may show a hammered-metal appearance, which results from chronic pressure on the inner table of the skull. This condition is seen more often in radiographs of children. Erosive changes also may occur if the tumor invades the skull by eroding through the dura or outermost, toughest, and most fibrous membranes covering the brain and spinal cord.

The CT scan can distinguish the CSF, blood, edema, and tumor from normal brain tissue. The risks to the patient are minimal with CT. The use of iodine-based contrast to enhance the study increases the risk of an allergic reaction. Localization of the tumor is achievable through the use of a contrast-enhanced study. This also provides information regarding tumor extension, grade, and growth patterns. An area of higher or lower x-ray scattering power differentiates between necrosis or edema and calcification. Contrast-enhanced volume is indicative of a tumor. If used in conjunction with MRI, CT can confirm calcification or verify hemorrhage (Figure 34-4).

CT scanning for brain tumors can distinguish between soft issue structures using CT numbers or Hounsfield units (HU). Each pixel used to reconstruct a CT image is assigned a CT number from +1000 (bone) to −1000 (air) that corresponds to the density of the tissue within the pixel.

MRI is useful for showing the normal anatomic structure and changes in the parenchyma. Having several advantages over CT scanning, MRI is the best noninvasive procedure. After radiation therapy or surgery, MRI provides a method of evaluating tumor response or recurrence. Iodine contrast is not necessary to perform the procedure, reducing the risk for a patient's reaction. Tumors smaller than 1 cm can be detected. With MRI, three-dimensional imaging is possible and bone artifacts are absent. MRI and some CT scans may be displayed in transverse, sagittal, and coronal sections. Contrast-enhanced studies can be performed through the use of gadolinium, which is a non–iodine-based intravenous (IV) contrast agent. Gadolinium helps differentiate between edema and the tumor and can detect surface seeding. MRI may not be able to detect treatment-related changes from recurrent disease. CT is more cost effective, allowing for more economical use in follow-up posttreatment (Figure 34-5).

Table 34-4	**Brain Tumor Localization Chart**			
	Frontal	**Parietal**	**Temporal**	**Occipital**
SYMPTOMS	Often asymptomatic until late Symptoms of increased ICP Bradyphrenia Personality changes Libido changes Impetuous behavior Excessive jocularity Defective memory Urinary incontinence Seizures (generalized, becoming focal) Gait disorders Weakness Loss of smell Speech disorder Tonic spasms of fingers and toes	Symptomatic earlier than frontal lobes Symptoms of increased ICP Loss of vision Spatial disorientation Tingling sensation Dressing apraxia Loss of memory Seizures (focal sensory epilepsy) Weakness (anterior extension)	Speech disorders (left hemisphere dominant; not only for right-handed, but for most left-handed persons) Loss of smell (superior lesion) Disturbance in hearing, tinnitus, etc. Speech disturbance Uncinate fits Seizures with vocal phenomena in aura, including speech arrest Hallucinations, dreams, déja vu Space-perception disturbances Dysarthria Dysnomia Disturbance of comprehension	Seizures (relatively less common, but with auras including flashing lights and unformed hallucinations) Loss of vision Tingling (early) Weakness (late)
SPECIAL CEREBRAL FUNCTIONS	Behavioral problems (anterior location) Labile personality Mental lethargy Defective memory Motor aphasia	Anosognosia Autotopagnosis Visual agnosia Graphesthesia (X) Loss of memory Proprioceptive agnosia	Dysarthria Sensory asphasia Defective hearing	Visual agnosia Visual impulses
CRANIAL NERVE FUNCTIONS	Anosima (inferior lesion) Nerve VI palsy with increased ICP Papilledema with increased ICP Foster Kennedy's syndrome Proptosis	Hemianopsia Papilledema (with increased ICP)	Superior quadrantanopsia (X) (could be homonymous hemianopsia with tumor extension) Central weakness of the cranial nerve VI Papilledema with increased ICP	Macular-sparing hemianspsia Horizontal nystagmus
MOTOR SYSTEM	Contralateral weakness (late) Paresis (flaccid spastic) Disturbed gait (midline lesion) Automatism Persistence of induced movement (Kral's phenomenon) Diagonal rigidity [arm (X): leg (−)] Loss of skilled movement (X) Urinary incontinence (super lesion)	Weakness Atrophy Clumsiness Dysdiadochokinesia Independent movements (unrecognized by patient)	Dysdiadochokinesia (early) Drift (secondary in later stages, involving arm more than leg)	Late appearance of motor signs, manifested by drift or dysdiadochokinesia
SENSORY FUNCTIONS	Rare involvement initially, unless invasion of sensory area (posterior lesion)	Dysesthesias (tingling) (X) Pallesthesia (loss of vibratory sense) (X) Loss of touch, press and position sense (X), but pain and temperature usually unaffected	Initially minimal	Somatosensory disturbances earlier than motor changes as adjacent structures are involved Visual phenomena, such as persisting images, unformed hallucinations, and aura
REFLEX CHANGES	Tonic plantar reflex Hoffmann's sign Grasp reflex Babinski's sign	Babinski's sign Hoffmann's sign	May occur contralateral to tumor	No effect in early stages

Modified from Wara WM, et al: In Perez C, Brady L, editors: *Principles and practice of radiation oncology*, ed 3. Philadelphia, 1993, JB Lippincott.
ICP, Intracranial pressure; *(X)*, contralateral; *(−)*, ipsilateral.

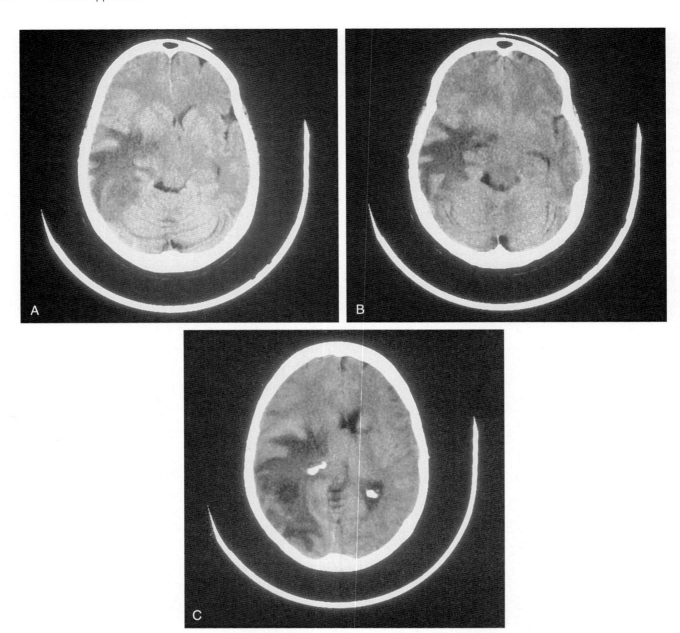

Figure 34-4. A and **B**, Noncontrast computed tomography (CT) scans of the head. Extensive edema can be seen through the white matter of the right temporal, parietal, and occipital lobes. A relatively well-circumscribed central area of low density appears to represent necrotic debris in the nidus (nucleus) of a tumor. This is strongly suggestive of a glioblastoma. **B** and **C**, Edema results in a midline shift approaching 1 cm to the left. **C**, Calcifications in the choroid plexus.

Positron Emission Tomography. Positron emission tomography (PET) is a beneficial diagnostic tool that may be useful in determining differences between necrosis and malignancy, which are associated with areas of high metabolism. PET uses the radionuclide FDG to help detect lesions. PET incorporates the localizing ability of CT scanning with the ability of the FDG agent to concentrate lesions and help differentiate between various types of CNS lesions, infections, and degenerative processes.[19]

A stereotactic biopsy (a procedure commonly performed during neurosurgery to guide the insertion of a needle into a specific area of the brain) allows all areas of the tumor and its borders to be studied before surgery causes changes in the appearance of the tumor. A biopsy is indicated if a lesion is deep seated, is probably malignant, and occurs in older or debilitated patients who cannot tolerate a surgical procedure. The risks of a biopsy include approximately a 30% rate of inadequate diagnosis. Other risks include hemorrhage in the area of the biopsy and postoperative swelling.[13]

Debulking procedures are performed if the tumor location is accessible and the tumor volume is large. **Debulking** accomplishes a reduction in tumor size and the opportunity to

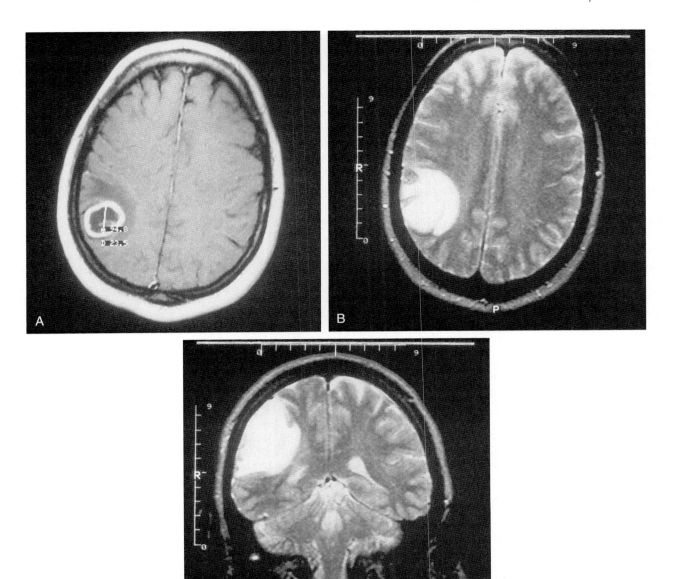

Figure 34-5. A 3-cm mass located in the right posterior parietal lobe with surrounding edema. The peripheral aspect of the lesion exhibits gadolinium enhancement. **A**, Axial magnetic resonance imaging (MRI) cut showing a lesion with a necrotic center. **B**, The mass is enhanced by gadolinium and shows surrounding edema. **C**, Coronal image.

obtain a pathologic diagnosis. A reduction in tumor size may sometimes make it easier to treat with postoperative radiation therapy.

Cerebral angiography has value for planning surgical intervention as a means for surgeons to study the intrinsic vasculature (blood supply) of the tumor and surrounding blood vessels. However, this tool is of little value in establishing a definitive diagnosis.

Because electroencephalography is imprecise and not specific for brain tumors, it is of little diagnostic value. Pneumoencephalography and ventriculography are now obsolete.

Pathology

The most important prognostic factor for CNS tumors is the histopathologic diagnosis. Benign lesions are indicative of a better prognosis, and the potential for a cure with the use of surgery and/or radiation therapy exists. Intracranial tumors are considered locally malignant based on the limited space for expansion in the cranium. Treatment of the neuralaxis is indicated for some histopathologically malignant lesions such as medulloblastoma because of the risk of metastatic seeding.

Tumor growth is not hindered in most gliomas because CNS tumors do not form a natural capsule to contain them. Cellularity patterns differ according to the tumor grade. Low-grade tumors exhibit reactive hyperplasia with low cellularity, whereas marked cellularity is common in high-grade tumors. Necrosis is an important feature in high-grade tumors. Survival rates, with or without treatment, are clearly associated with tumor grade. Histopathology is more important than anatomic staging in determining the clinical outcome and behavior of the tumor. In other words, the cell type associated with brain tumors is more important than the size of the tumor. Tissue diagnosis should be obtained in all patients with a brain tumor. The few exceptions include patients with diffuse intrinsic brainstem gliomas and optic nerve gliomas.[15]

Staging

No universal staging system is currently in use, and problems result because of the lack of a standardized method of staging. The American Joint Committee on Cancer uses a system based on the grade, tumor, metastasis (GTM) classification. Grade (G) has prognostic significance, ranging from well differentiated to poorly differentiated (G1 to G3).

The Kernohan grading system has also been used. It is also a 4-grade system, but it is difficult to use. The Kernohan system considers cellularity, anaplasia, mitotic figures, giant cells, necrosis, blood vessels, and proliferation.

Treatment Techniques

A multidisciplinary approach is necessary for the treatment of CNS tumors (Table 34-5). A biopsy is extremely important for diagnostic purposes and essential for therapeutic decision making.

Surgery. With the development of new surgical techniques, preoperative evaluation is even more important to further aid the surgeon. The tumor size and extent should be determined before surgery. The introduction of microsurgery, the ultrasonic aspirator, the laser, and perioperative sonography have made the surgeon's job easier. Computer-assisted stereotactic neuronavigation provides a new tool with the potential for great medical value.

When possible, surgery should be performed on tumors that are symptomatic and offer a chance for complete resection. Debulking is indicated with a large tumor volume and if a complete resection is not possible. Surgery can range from a debulking procedure to complete microsurgical removal. The primary goal for surgery is to remove the tumor and to obtain a histologic diagnosis. Surgery can be limited by the tumor location and extent, patient status, and risk of causing debilitating neurologic deficits. The patient's chances for survival are not enhanced by partial removal of the tumor. Tumor recurrence occurs from residual tumor that invades healthy brain tissue. Decreases in morbidity and mortality rates result from an earlier diagnosis, the use of steroid therapy, improvements in anesthetic techniques, and improved surgical methods. Surgical approaches to tumors depend on anatomic pathways, the tumor size, and the tumor location. According to Fransen and de Tribolet,[10] general opinion in the surgical world is that early and radical excision provide the best chance for a good outcome because of an accurate histologic diagnosis, control of a mass effect, and cytoreduction, which allow or enhance adjuvant therapy.

Surgery also plays a crucial role in the management of some spinal cord tumors. Surgery can establish a diagnosis and make

Table 34-5	Multidisciplinary Treatment Decisions for Various Brain Tumors			
Tumor Type	**Surgery**	**Radiation Therapy**	**Chemotherapy**
Astrocytoma (low grade)	Gross total resection* followed by observation	At tumor progression, postop RT 50-55 Gy	NR
	Gross total resection*	Postop RT 50-55 Gy	NR
Astrocytoma, mixed astrocytoma (high grade)	Gross total resection*	Postop RT 60-70 Gy + 50-60 Gy BT/RS	BCNU (patients <60 years)
Oligodendroglioma	Gross total resection*	Postop RT 60-70 Gy + 50-60 Gy BT/RS	NR
Anaplastic oligodendroglioma	Gross total resection*	Postop RT 60-70 Gy	PCV
Meningioma	Subtotal resection	Postop RT 50-55 Gy	NR
	Gross total resection	NR	
Malignant meningioma	Gross total resection*	Postop RT 60 Gy	
Ependymoma	Subtotal resection	Postop RT 54-59 Gy	
	Gross total resection	Postop RT 54 Gy + RS boost	
Medulloblastoma, anaplastic ependymoma	Gross total resection*	Postop RT 30-36 Gy to entire brain and spine; 20-25 Gy tumor boost	
Spinal cord tumors	Biopsy vs. resection	Postop RT 50 Gy	BCNU
CNS lymphoma	Biopsy	WBI 40-45 Gy	MTX or MAC

From Nelson D, et al: Central nervous system tumors. In Rubin P, editor: *Clinical oncology: multidisciplinary approach for physicians and students*, ed 8, Philadelphia, 2001, Saunders.
BCNU, Carmustine; *BT*, brachytherapy; *CNS*, central nervous system; *MAC*, multiagent chemotherapy; *MTX*, methotrexate; *NR*, not recommended; *PCV*, procarbazine, lomustine (CCNU), and vincristine; *Postop RT*, immediate postoperative radiation therapy (unless otherwise stated); *RS*, radiosurgery; *WBI*, whole brain irradiation.
*Gross total resection where possible; also includes subtotal resection or biopsy.

possible the removal of the tumor. Because of the location of the cord, a surgical resection is difficult at best to perform and impossible in some instances. Serious neurologic deficits are always a risk.

Radiation Therapy. Radiation therapy is indicated for malignant tumors that are incompletely excised, inaccessible from a surgical approach, and associated with metastatic lesions.

Several factors are considered in determining the doses for treatment. Tumor type, tumor grade, and patterns of recurrence are particularly important. The radioresponsiveness of the tumor must also be considered.[11] The total dose must be limited by normal tissue tolerance because **radiation necrosis** (tissue destruction) develops if tissue tolerance is exceeded. The risk of tumor progression must be balanced against the potential risk of necrosis when the dose is determined. In addition, consideration should be given to the side effects that may be induced. These side effects include acute reactions (or those encountered during the course of treatment), early-delayed reactions occurring from a few weeks until up to 3 months after treatment, and late-delayed reactions occurring months to years later. Threshold doses and the therapeutic ratio also must be considered.

Several approaches are available for treating tumors of the brain, depending on the type of disease, tumor location and extent, and whether the spinal axis requires treatment. Because brain malignancies can result from primary brain tumors, metastases from another site, or meningeal involvement, each type of malignancy must be handled appropriately.

The total surgical resection of a brain tumor for cure is an extremely difficult task to accomplish, partly because of the difficulty in obtaining generous enough resection margins in brain tissue. Radiation therapy usually follows surgery in an attempt to prevent tumor regrowth or recurrence. In the past, whole-brain irradiation has been used via lateral portals with a boost to the tumor bed after initial treatment. With the advent of CT and MRI, more accurate tumor localization allows smaller fields to be simulated and treated. Smaller field designs and unique configurations through the use of specialized blocking make simulation and daily reproducibility of the setup an even more important part of the treatment process.

If brain metastases are present from another primary site of involvement, whole-brain irradiation is the preferred treatment. Even with a solitary mass, occult disease is often present, although undetected. Therefore, the whole brain should be treated.

Simulation provides the foundation for all radiation treatment (see Chapters 22 and 23). The simulation procedure should be carefully explained to the patient before it begins. The patient's understanding of the complexity of the procedure and the necessity for daily reproducibility of the treatment setup should be stressed. Patients should be aware of the importance of their compliance and cooperation in relation to the outcome of the treatment. Accurate reproducibility is a must. Head rotation and tilting create the potential for difficulties in reproducibility. Immobilization is extremely important and can be achieved through the use of head-holding devices. The use of an immobilization system is beneficial for treating patients via lateral ports to a limited brain field with the patient in the supine position. The use of a thermoplastic mask greatly reduces errors in the reproducibility of the setup.

Lateral portal fields are used for treating the whole brain for palliative reasons. The inferior margin of the field intersects the superior orbital ridge and external auditory meatus (EAM). In selecting the field size, 1 cm of flash or shine over should be seen at the anterior, posterior, and superior borders of the field (Figure 34-6). The flash reduces the chances of clipping any of the anatomy as a result of the field size being too small. The fields may be treated isocentrically or with a fixed source-skin distance (SSD). Isocentric setups are quicker to set up and carry out because the patient and table are not moved between lateral fields. This approach also reduces error rates.

For complex treatment to the craniospinal axis (the brain and spinal cord), the patient is simulated and treated most frequently in the prone position, Lateral fields are used for treatment of the whole brain, whereas a gapped posterior field is used for treatment of the spinal cord. Care must be taken to match the beam divergence, allowing no overlap. Hot or cold spots can be avoided by feathering the gap. This can be accomplished by shifting the gap by 1 cm every 1000 cGy. Other methods of feathering the gap can be used. This approach allows a 1-cm gap between fields daily. With this technique the length of the brain and spine fields change daily. The central axis of the spine fields is shifted superiorly to accommodate the gap. The central axis of the brain field remains constant, whereas the field size changes. (Chapter 24 provides more details on the treatment of adjacent fields.)

International Commission on Radiation Units 50 and 62. The International Commission on Radiation Units (ICRU) report Numbers 50 and 62 are the international standard that determines the radiation tumor volumes. The Gross tumor volume (GTV) is the gross tumor seen on the MRI, CT, or other imaging studies. The Clinical target volume (CTV) is the central nervous

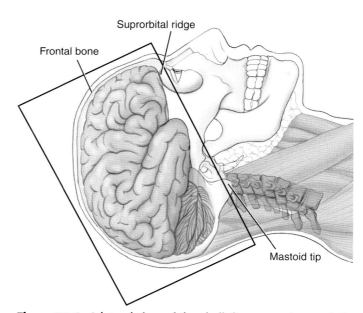

Figure 34-6. A lateral view of the skull demonstrating a whole brain radiation therapy field set up using the supraorbital ridge and mastoid tip as topographical bony reference marks. Note an equal amount of fall-off or "flash" surrounding the cranium on the anterior, superior, and posterior margins.

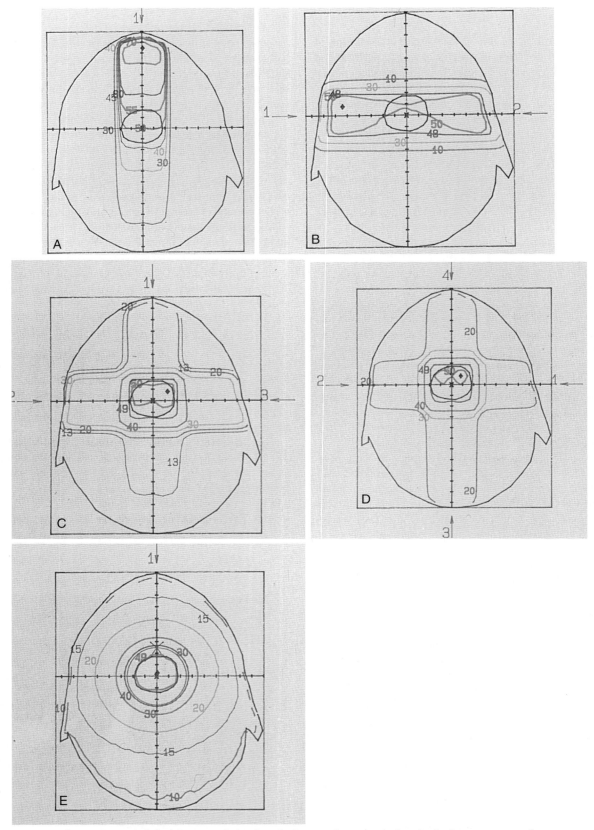

Figure 34-7. Axial contours of the head show a hypothetical spherical target centrally located. Dose distributions shown are for various two-dimensional treatment plans, all of which deliver 50 Gy to the isocenter. **A**, Single anteriorposterior (AP) field. **B**, Opposed lateral fields. **C**, Three fields (AP plus opposed lateral fields). **D**, Four fields (AP-postero anterior plus opposed lateral fields). **E**, 360-Degree arc rotation. (From Shaw EG, Debinski W, Robbins ME: Central nervous system tumors, overview. In Gunderson LL, Tepper JE, editors: *Clinical radiation oncology*, ed 2. Philadelphia, 2007, Churchill Livingstone.)

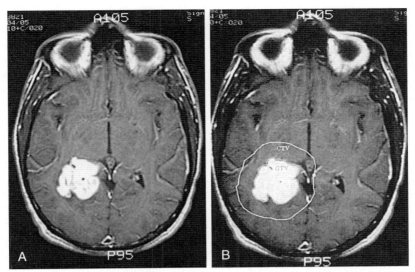

Figure 34-8. A, Magnetic resonance image with contrast of a patient with a right temporo-parietal pilocytic astrocytoma. **B,** The clinical target volume (CTV) is the gross tumor volume (GTV) plus a 1-cm margin. (From Shaw EG, Debinski W, Robbins ME: Central nervous system tumors, overview. In Gunderson LL, Tepper JE, editors: *Clinical radiation oncology,* ed 2, Philadelphia, 2007, Churchill Livingstone.)

system tissue with suspected microscopic tumor: this usually extends 1 to 3 cm beyond the GTV. The planning target volume (PTV) is the margin beyond the GTV and CTV and accounts for factors such as internal organ motion, setup variation, and patient movement. This usually contains and extends 0.5 to 1 cm beyond the GTV and CTV. The treated volume (TV) is the volume enclosed by the desired prescription isodose line (usually greater than 95%), and this contains the GTV, CTV, and PTV. The irradiated volume (IR) is the tissue volume that receives a significant dose of radiation and contains the GTV, CTV, PTV, and TV.[12]

Organs at risk (OAR) and planning organ at risk volume (PRV) should be delineated and the dose recorded based on the recommendations of ICRU Reports. Depending on the tumor site, the OAR that may receive a radiation dose may include the lens of the eye, the optic nerve and chiasm, the brainstem, the parotid glands, and the spinal cord.

The treatment volume for gliomas is determined by the tumor's extent, which (as shown by CT and MRI) includes the gross tumor volume (GTV) and related tumor edema. Figure 34-7 shows various dose distributions for two-dimensional treatment plans. Because tumor cells have been found in edema, this area should be included in the treatment field with a 1- to 3-cm margin for malignant tumors.[9] Figure 34-8 outlines the GTV on an MRI scan of a patient with an astrocytoma.

Conventional therapy has been enhanced through the use of three-dimensional treatment planning, intensity-modulated radiation therapy (IMRT), portal imaging, and multileaf collimators. Irregularly shaped fields can be created in seconds through the use of these collimators, eliminating the need to construct custom blocks. Three-dimensional treatment planning allows the use of multiple non-coplanar fields to a well-defined target volume (Figure 34-9). Checking the accuracy of the patient's

setup before treatment is possible through the use of portal imaging and image-guided radiation therapy (IGRT).

As a result of radiation treatments to the cranium, temporary hair loss occurs with doses ranging from 2000 to 4000 cGy. With doses of greater than 4000 cGy, hair loss may be permanent. Erythema, tanning, dry and moist desquamation, and edema are also side effects of the treatments. Early-delayed reactions include drowsiness, lethargy, a decreased mental status, and a worsening of symptoms. These reactions can occur up to 3 months after treatment, are usually temporary, and disappear without therapy. The occurrence of apparently new symptoms at this time is not necessarily indicative of treatment failure or the need for any change in therapy. Radiation necrosis is a complication that rarely occurs from 6 months to many years after irradiation. Late reactions are usually irreversible and progressive. Radiation cataracts can be avoided by shielding or keeping the eyes out of the field.

 Radiation tolerance for normal tissues within the CNS include 5000 cGy for whole brain, 6000 cGy for partial brain, and 4500-5000 cGy for the spinal cord. These tolerances are based on TD 5/5, which assumes a 5% incidence of complications at a 5-year period.

Chemicals that enhance the lethal effects of radiation are known as **radiosensitizers**. Hypoxic cell sensitizers and halogenated pyrimidines are under investigation. Hypoxic cells are more radioresistant than are well-oxygenated cells. The use of sensitizers makes the cells more susceptible to the radiation without increasing the radiation effects to the normal tissue, which is well oxygenated. Mitotically active tumor cells use these compounds more than replicating normal glial cells and vascular cells.

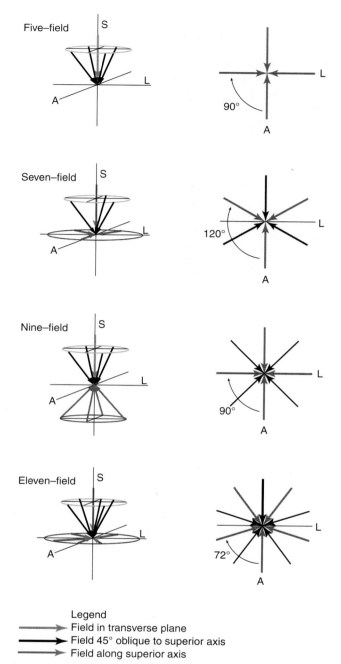

Legend
→ Field in transverse plane
→ Field 45° oblique to superior axis
→ Field along superior axis

Figure 34-9. Comparison of various non-coplanar, three-dimensional treatment approaches using 5, 7, 9, and 11 static, non-coplanar treatment beams. Beam orientations are shown from a lateral prospective (*left*) and as viewed from above (*right*). (From Shaw EG, Debinski W, Robbins ME: Central nervous system tumors, overview. In Gunderson LL, Tepper JE, editors: *Clinical radiation oncology*, ed 2. Philadelphia, 2007, Churchill Livingstone.)

Interstitial implants (brachytherapy) are done with the use of radioactive seeds that are temporarily placed in tumors. Adjacent normal tissue is spared from excessively high doses because of the rapid decrease of dose outside the high-dose volume. Conceptually normal tissue can better tolerate the low-dose rate (given over a longer period as compared with external beam radiation therapy), so a higher dose can be delivered. Interstitial implants provide a less invasive treatment modality than surgery if recurrence occurs.

Interstitial irradiation may provide an alternative in the treatment of infants and children. Brachytherapy may be beneficial to patients suffering from recurrent disease, but it does not play a major role in the management of the disease.

Stereotactic radiosurgery is an important treatment option for patients with CNS tumors. The process combines stereotactic localization techniques with a sharply collimated beam to direct the dose of radiation to a specific, well-defined lesion. The patient is positioned in a halo device that is used as an immobilization device to ensure the accuracy and reproducibility of the treatment setup. The target volume should be spherical and only up to 3 cm at its maximum dimension. Accuracy approaches 1 mm. A necrosing dose of radiation can be given in a single-fraction treatment or in multiple fraction. A local dose to the tumor can be increased while sparing surrounding tissue. The process can be accomplished with the use of different sources of radiation. Heavy charged particles, a **gamma knife** using multiple cobalt-60 sources (a type of radiosurgery with a sharply defined field, considered by some to be equivalent to resecting the irradiated region) and linear-accelerator–based systems can be used with comparable results. The role of radiosurgery in the management of primary, metastatic, and recurrent disease is still under investigation. (Chapter 16 provides more detailed information on stereotactic radiosurgery.)

 Radiosurgery using external beam treatment modalities includes linear accelerator–based and cobolt-60 accelerator–based treatments. More information is available at www.accuray.com, www.irsa.org/linac, and www.gammaknife.org.

Chemotherapy. Progress has been slow in the area of chemotherapeutic drugs. Several reasons account for this. According to Chatel, Lebrun, and Freny,[5] the number of effective drugs is limited, adjuvant therapy has not changed the time to progression, adjuvant chemotherapy only slightly increases the percentage of survival at 18 and 24 months, a 20% to 25% response rate exists when drugs are given at recurrence, and multidrug therapy does not seem to be more efficient than single-agent chemotherapy. Other reasons for the difficulty in finding useful drugs include the small number of patients with CNS tumors for use in clinical trials compared with more prevalent diseases, difficulties measuring the tumor response, and the fact that one measurement of response is survival time. Effective chemotherapy for CNS tumors is further hindered by the BBB, which impedes the penetration of the drugs into the brain. "High concentration in cerebral tumors can nevertheless be reached because of the frequent extensive disruption of the BBB, but tumor cells infiltrating normal tissue are theoretically inaccessible to drugs that do not cross the BBB."[7]

Chemotherapeutic drugs can be administered orally, intravenously, directly into the tumor bed, and via direct carotid perfusion. Most chemotherapeutic drugs cause cytotoxic effects by disrupting DNA synthesis in rapidly dividing cells.

The designing of new drugs that allow better penetration of the BBB and can exhibit better distribution and lower toxicity has become extremely important. Limited studies suggest that the drug concentrations in the area around the tumor or in normal brain may be lower than those in the tumor itself, where the BBB is inefficient. The concentrations of drugs in the normal brain tissue decrease as the distance from the tumor increases. Therefore, drug concentrations in the brain surrounding the tumor may be too low to eliminate infiltrating tumor cells. This can be a reason for therapeutic failures.[7] The nitrosourea drugs are lipid soluble, allowing them to cross the BBB. Because of this ability, these drugs can work against brain tumors.

Drugs of choice for CNS neoplasms include carmustine, procarbazine, vincristine, and Lomostine. Temozolomide, also a lipid-soluble alkalating agent developed especially for the treatment of malignant gliomas, has been studied and shows some positive results, especially in patients with recurrent disease.[9] Multiagent chemotherapy plays a major role in the treatment of recurrent gliomas

Role of Radiation Therapist

Patient education is a primary goal of the physician, radiation therapist, and oncology nurse. Although the physician and nurse initially discuss treatment procedures, side effects, skin care, nutrition, and psychosocial issues with the patient and family members, the emotional state of those persons at that time is generally not conducive to remembering and complying with all the information they are given. It becomes the responsibility of the therapist, who sees the patient daily, to reiterate and reinforce all these educational issues with the patient.

Daily contact allows the therapist to build a professional bond of trust, understanding, and communication with the patient. The therapist must be ready to step in and provide patients with emotional support, answers to their questions and concerns, and referrals to persons they may need to see (e.g., social worker, pastor, nutritionist, business office personnel, and support groups).

In addition, the therapist's daily contact also allows monitoring of the patient's mental and physical well-being. Some patients still feel overwhelmed, angry, and vulnerable and are in denial at the beginning of treatments.

A separate patient waiting area allows patients to talk and share their thoughts with other persons who have the same concerns. This area allows discussions regarding issues the patient may not be able to discuss with family members.

Patients undergoing treatment for CNS neoplasms can expect specific side effects. Most commonly, patients complain of fatigue. Reassuring patients that this is not unusual helps them a great deal to cope with the situation. Explaining to patients that the body requires plenty of rest while it tries to heal itself from the disease and effects of daily treatment eliminates some concern. Suggesting that patients pamper themselves and take a nap when they feel tired, rather than fight the fatigue, is an option.

A proper diet is a must for the healing process and well-being of the patient. If food becomes unappealing in looks, taste, and smell, the patient will not want to eat. The patient can try eating smaller portions several times a day rather than sitting down to a large meal. Large portions are sometimes discouraging to someone with no appetite. A change in the location of eating can sometimes help, as well as having someone else cook. Nutritional supplements should be available to patients, including different kinds of supplements so patients can then purchase the brand that appeals to them most.

Frequent blood tests are not required, with the exception of patients receiving craniospinal irradiation. The white cell count and platelet counts may decrease in patients treated with

craniospinal irradiation. These counts require close monitoring in the event the patient requires a break in treatment until the situation corrects itself.

Permanent hair loss for persons being treated for primary brain tumors occurs. A loan closet with wigs, turbans, and kerchiefs ranging in a wide variety of colors and styles should be available to patients. Shops specializing in these items should also be suggested. Therapists should caution patients to use a mild shampoo to prevent skin irritation. Moisturizing creams can be prescribed for dry desquamation and other products for moist desquamation. Therapists can also recommend skin conditioners if erythema tanning occurs.

The patient should be cautioned against exposing to direct sunlight areas of the body being treated. The radiation from the sun in combination with the radiation from treatment enhances the adverse side effects.

Most patients begin to feel a sense of security that develops over the course of treatment from the daily contact with the therapy team. When treatment ends, patients feel a sense of loss and abandonment after weeks of daily attention being focused on them and their needs. In some facilities, patients can be called 1 week to 10 days after the completion of treatment (before the first follow-up visit) just to check on them and evaluate their physical and mental condition. This may provide the patient with a sense of ongoing care.

The therapist must also be watchful for signs of medical complications that may arise as a result of the treatment. Early intervention of potential problems can prevent unnecessary suffering later in the course of treatment. Attention to detail regarding treatment setups and parameters is a must, and providing professional, competent, efficient, and accurate treatment in a relaxed and friendly atmosphere completes the role of the therapist.

CASE I

Germinoma

A 31-year-old white man noted a change in vision and headaches. An initial workup included an MRI scan about 4 months later that revealed gadolinium enhancement in the region of the hypothalamus. Separate disease was noted in the corpus callosum. The pineal gland was enlarged but not enhanced.

A spinal MRI showed no evidence of spinal tumors. An additional workup included serum alpha-fetoprotein (AFP) and human chorionic gonadotropin (hCG), which were within normal limits. A lumbar puncture for cytology was performed. CSF was negative for malignant cells. The patient's history revealed that, at the age of 15, the patient was treated for failure to grow and diabetes insipidus. Diabetes insipidus sometimes occurs for years before other symptoms develop. A CT scan performed at that time revealed a questionable suggestion of abnormality in the hypothalamic region but apparently was not pursued. The patient was treated at the time with growth hormones, thyroid supplements, and vasopressin with response.

A biopsy was performed via a right frontotemporal craniotomy 5 months after the onset of symptoms. A preoperative diagnosis considering the patient's long history indicated a glioma. A postoperative diagnosis was probable hypothalamic glioma. A pathology report was positive for hypothalamic germinoma with metastasis to the corpus callosum. Several special stains of the biopsy specimen were used to confirm this diagnosis, and several pathologists reviewed the slides because the patient's history was unusual for a diagnosis of germinoma.

The patient's visual-field deficits were unchanged postoperatively. The craniotomy incision healed well.

The patient presented himself for radiation therapy consultation shortly after surgery. His history revealed panhypopituitarism manifested by hypothyroidism, high prolactin levels, adrenal insufficiency, diabetes insipidus, and abnormal testosterone levels. The family history was unremarkable. The patient's mental status was intact. A neurologic review was within normal limits. Vision testing revealed greater deficits on the right. The patient had blurred vision on the right and denied having a headache.

Because the patient had spread to the corpus callosum, he was a candidate for curative radiation therapy to the cranial spinal axis. Risks and benefits of the treatment were explained to the patient. Side effects during treatment can include skin irritation, hair loss, and fatigue. The white cell count and platelet counts tend to become lower in adults who are treated with craniospinal irradiation. The patient's blood counts were monitored weekly. Long-term risks included radiation damage to the brain, lens with cataract formation, and spinal cord.

Because there was no seeding to the spinal cord, the plan was to administer 2550 cGy in 17 fractions to the craniospinal axis. After this a cone-down boost of 2500 cGy was given to the gross disease, as seen on an MRI scan. The craniospinal axis was treated with 6-MV photons. The boost to the cone-down used 10-MV photons. If seeding to the spinal column had been present, those areas would also have been boosted.

The patient was simulated in the prone position with an alpha cradle to ensure reproducibility. Lateral fields to the whole brain and a posteroanterior (PA) spinal field were planned. Multileaf collimation was used to shape the portals.

The patient experienced minimal nausea after his first treatment. Prochlorperazine (Compazine) spansules given before further treatments helped relieve this problem. The patient's blood counts dropped after receiving 750 cGy. Because the white count was below 1000/mm³, the patient was given time off with orders for a stat complete blood count to be done before resuming treatment. A 1-week break resolved this problem. He was cautioned not to use a toothbrush because of his decreased platelet count. He was told to sponge his teeth or gargle. The patient's visual deficits remained unchanged since the beginning of treatment.

Shifting of the fields to incorporate a gap began at 2100 cGy. A cone-down began after 2500 cGy. At 3090 cGy, the patient experienced less nausea but had complaints of altered taste with salty taste buds. At 3990 cGy, he was doing well but had flulike symptoms. He continued to have poor visual acuity but had improved visual-field changes with a decrease in bilateral hemianopsia. The patient finished treatment at a total dose of 5070 cGy. He had only a 1-week break because of falling blood counts. The patient was suffering from severe fatigue and had complaints of indigestion and gastric reflux. He lost a total of 10 lb during treatment.

The patient was feeling well and eating better at the time of his 1-month follow-up visit. He continued to have some fatigue, which the oncologist thought would resolve itself after a little more time. The patient was able to regain some of the weight he had lost. Vision testing revealed no papilledema. The patient's vision was still poor, and he was unable to read a page in a book. Visual fields revealed marked improvement in the inferior aspect fields. Cranial nerves III to XII were intact. No motor or sensory abnormalities were present, and cerebellar findings were intact. There was epilation over his skull consistent with the treatment portal. No evidence existed of skin changes along his spine or cranium. A recent MRI scan showed no evidence of remaining germinoma.

At a follow-up 3 months later, the patient had a good appetite with his energy level improving, although he was still having problems gaining weight. An ophthalmologist examined the patient for his poor vision. Other than

magnifying glasses, nothing could be done to help him. Optic nerve deficits were again noted with greater difficulty on the right than on the left. The patient had moderate alopecia with patchy regrowth. His blood counts had improved and were expected to continue to do so. The long-term survival prognosis for patients who have germinomas is 85% at 5 years. The patient is doing well 6 years after completion of treatment.

SUMMARY

- Approximately 21,810 cases of primary brain tumors and other nervous system tumors are diagnosed annually in the United States. The tumors account for 1.5% of all malignancies. About 80% of central nervous system (CNS) tumors involve the brain, whereas 20% involve the spinal cord.
- CNS tumors can be primary or secondary (metastatic) and benign or malignant.
- In recent years, radiation therapy has played a significant role in the treatment of CNS tumors, providing a means of increased survival time and enhancing the quality of life of many patients with brain tumors.
- The three most important as prognostic indicators for CNS tumors are age, the performance status, and tumor type.
- Tumors are normally grouped into benign, or low-grade, and malignant, or high-grade, categories with grade rather than size as the primary prognostic factor.
- The blood-brain barrier, which hinders the penetration of some substances into the brain and cerebrospinal fluid, exists between the vascular system and brain. Its purpose is to protect the brain from potentially toxic compounds.
- Positron emission tomography is a beneficial diagnostic tool that may be useful in determining differences between necrosis and malignancy, which are associated with areas of high metabolism.
- A multidisciplinary approach is necessary for the treatment of CNS tumors, as a biopsy is extremely important for diagnostic purposes and essential for therapeutic decision making.
- Radiation therapy is indicated for malignant tumors that are incompletely excised, inaccessible from a surgical approach, and associated with metastatic lesions.
- Daily contact allows the therapist to build a professional bond of trust, understanding, and communication with the patient. The therapist must be ready to step in and provide patients with emotional support, answers to their questions and concerns, and referrals.

Review Questions

Multiple Choice

1. Karnofsky Performance Status (KPS) is:
   a. a measure of the biologic grade of the tumor
   b. a measure of the neurologic and functional status of the patient
   c. measured in cGy
   d. directly measures the chance of 5-year survival
2. The purpose of the blood-brain barrier is to:
   I. hinder the penetration of some substances into the brain and CSF
   II. protect the brain from potentially toxic substances

III. protect the brain from radiation
IV. prevent the passage of lipid- or water-soluble substances into the brain
   a. I and III
   b. II and III
   c. I and II
   d. II and IV

3. Which of the following are important factors to consider in the initial workup for a definitive diagnosis of CNS neoplasms?
   a. family and social histories
   b. changes in behavior or personality
   c. difficulties with speech, memory, or logical thought processes
   d. all of the above

4. What does *not* belong in this group?
   a. high dose fractionation
   b. increased intracranial pressure
   c. edema
   d. papilledema

5. Surgery for CNS neoplasms can be limited by:
   a. tumor location and extent
   b. patient status
   c. risk of causing neurologic deficits
   d. all of the above

6. The most common brain lesion Is:
   a. astrocytoma
   b. glioma
   c. metastatic
   d. medulloblastoma

7. Little is known concerning the _____, development, and growth mechanisms of CNS tumors.
   a. etiology
   b. dose response
   c. effects of alcohol
   d. BBB

8. Which of the following does *not* provide protection for the brain?
   a. cerebellum
   b. cranial bones
   c. meninges
   d. cerebrospinal fluid (CSF)

9. Weakened proximal pelvic muscles, impotence, bladder paralysis, and decreased knee jerk may be signs of a spinal tumor in the _____ region.
   a cervical
   b. upper thoracic
   c. lower thoracic
   d. lumbosacral

10. Side effects from radiation treatment of primary brain tumors include:
   a. dry and moist desquamation
   b. edema
   c. hair loss
   d. spinal cord damage

The answers to the Review Questions can be found by logging on to our website at: *http://evolve.elsevier.com/Washington+Leaver/ principles*

Questions to Ponder

1. Explain the benefits and risks involved in treating patients who have CNS neoplasms with surgery, radiation therapy, and chemotherapy.
2. What are the presenting signs and symptoms you would anticipate with patients who have CNS tumors?
3. Explain the purpose of the feathered-gap technique for treating patients to the craniospinal axis.
4. Analyze the expected side effects from radiation therapy to the CNS.
5. Explain the use and effect of steroids when treating patients with CNS neoplasms.
6. Discuss the clinical application of two-dimensional and three-dimensional treatment approaches used to treat CNS tumors.

REFERENCES

1. American Cancer Society. *Cancer Facts & Figures 2008*. Atlanta, American Cancer Society, 2008.
2. Avizonis VN, et al: Late effects following central nervous system radiation in pediatric population, *Neuropediatrics* 23:228-234, 1992.
3. Bohner NI, et al: Descriptive and analytic epidemiology of brain tumors. In Black PM, Loeffler JS, editors: *Cancer of the nervous system*. Oxford, 1997, Blackwell Scientific Publications.
4. Central Brain Tumor Registry United States (CBTRUS): *Statistical Report: Primary brain tumors in the United States*. Chicago, 2003, CBTRUS.
5. Chatel M, Lebrun C, Freny M: Chemotherapy and immunotherapy in adult malignant gliomas, *Curr Opin Oncol* 5:464-473, 1993.
6. Deorah S, et al: Trends in brain cancer incidence and survival in the United States: Surveillance, Epidemiology, and End Results program, 1973 to 2001, *Neurosurg Focus* 20:E1, 2006.
7. Donnelli MG, Zucchetti M, D'Incali M: Do anticancer agents reach the tumor target in the human brain? *Cancer Chemother Pharmacol* 30:251-260, 1992.
8. Fomchenko EI, Holland EC: Stem cells and brain cancer, *Exp Cell Res* 306:323-329, 2005.
9. Fiveash JB, et al: High grade gliomas. In Gunderson LL, Tepper JE, editors: *Clinical radiation oncology*, ed 2, Philadelphia, 2007, Churchill Livingstone.
10. Fransen P, de Tribolet N: Surgery for supratentorial tumors, *Curr Opin Oncol* 5:450-457, 1993.
11. Hall EJ: *Radiobiology for the radiologist*, ed 6, New York, 2005, Lippincott Williams & Wilkins.
12. International Commission on Radiation Units and Measurements (ICRU): *Prescribing, recording, and reporting, photon beam therapy: report 50*, Washington, DC, 1993, ICRU.
13. Kreiger MD, et al: Role of stereotactic biopsy in the diagnosis and management of brain tumors, *Semin Surg Oncol* 14:13-25, 1998.
14. McLendon RE, Halperin, EC: Is the long term survival of patients with intracranial glioblastoma multiforme overstated? *Cancer* 98:1745-1748, 2003.
15. Nelson D, et al: Central nervous system tumors. In Rubin P, editor: *Clinical oncology: a multidisciplinary approach for physicians and students*, ed 8. Philadelphia, 2001, Saunders.
16. Ohgahi H, Kleinhues P: Epidemiology and etiology gliomas, *Acta Neuropathol* 109:93-108, 2005.
17. Patchell RA: The management of brain metastases, *Cancer Treat Rev* 29:533-540, 2003.
18. Rohen EM, et al: Screening for cerebral metastasis with FDG PET in patients undergoing whole body of central nervous system malignancy, *Radiology* 226:181-187, 2003.
19. Shaw EG, et al: Ethnic differences in survival of glioblastoma (GBM): a secondary analysis of the RTOG recursive partitioning analysis database, *Neurooncology* 5:296, 2003.
20. Smith M, Hare ML: An overview of progress in childhood cancer survival, *J Pediatr Oncol Nurs* 10:160-164, 2004.

Digestive System Tumors

Leila Bussman-Yeakel

Outline

Key Terms

Abdominoperineal
  resection
Achalasia
Anterior resection
Barrett's esophagus
Chronic ulcerative
  colitis
Endocavitary radiation
  therapy
Familial adenomatous
  polyposis
Gardner's syndrome
Hematochezia
Hereditary nonpolyposis
  colorectal syndrome
Intraoperative radiation
  therapy (IORT)
Leukopenia
Low anterior resection
Neoadjuvant
Odynophagia
Orthogonal radiographs
Peritoneal seeding
Plummer-Vinson
  syndrome
Tenesmus
Three-point setup
Thrombocytopenia
Tylosis

Objectives

- Identify, list and discuss epidemiologic and etiologic factors that may be responsible for inducing tumors in the colon, rectum, anus, esophagus, and pancreas.
- Describe the symptoms produced by a malignant tumor arising in the colon, rectum, anus, esophagus, and pancreas.
- Discuss the methods of detection and diagnosis for tumors in the colon, rectum, anus, esophagus, and pancreas.
- List the varying histologic types of tumors that occur in the colon, rectum, anus, esophagus, and pancreas.
- Describe the diagnostic procedures used in the work-up and staging for these sites.
- Describe in detail the most common routes of tumor spread for these digestive system sites.
- Describe and diagram the lymphatic routes of spread for tumors of the colon, rectum, anus, esophagus, and pancreas.
- Differentiate between histologic grading and staging.
- Describe in detail the anatomy and physiology of the colon, rectum, anus, esophagus, and pancreas.
- Identify the treatment(s) of choice for cancers of the colon, rectum, anus, esophagus, and pancreas.

- Discuss the rationale for treatment with regard to treatment choice, histologic type and stage of the disease.
- Describe in detail the treatment methods available for cancers of the gastrointestinal tract.
- Describe the differing types of radiation treatment techniques that can be used for treating tumors of the rectum, anus, esophagus, and pancreas.
- Identify the appropriate tumor lethal dose or prescribe dose for each site.
- Discuss the expected radiation reactions for the area based on time-dose-fractionation schemes.
- Discuss tolerance levels of the vital structures and organs at risk.
- Describe the instructions that should be given to a patient with regard to skin care, expected reactions, and dietary advice.
- Identify the psychological problems associated with a malignancy in each site.
- Discuss the rationale for using multi-modality treatments for each diagnosis.
- Describe the various treatment planning techniques.
- Discuss survival statistics and prognosis for various stages of each cancer listed: rectum, anus, esophagus, and pancreas.

This chapter discusses the three major malignancies of the gastrointestinal system that are managed with radiation therapy (i.e., cancers of the rectum, esophagus, and pancreas). Colorectal cancer is the most common gastrointestinal malignancy and is associated with the best prognosis. Cancers of the esophagus and pancreas are usually diagnosed with advanced-staged disease and do not have many long-term survivors.

COLORECTAL CANCER

Epidemiology and Etiology

The incidence of colorectal cancer has been steadily declining since 1980. However, about 108,070 colon cancer and 40,740 cases of rectal cancer are projected to occur in 2008.[5] The disease affects men and women equally. Cancer of the colon is ranked third in incidence when comparing men and women separately. The risk of developing cancer of the large bowel increases with age with more than 90% occurring in people over 50 years of age.[5,94] Cancer of the large bowel more commonly affects the rectum or distal colon. However, an increase has occurred in right (proximal) colon lesions, especially in older women. The reason for this is unclear, but the increase may be the result of earlier detection of precancerous lesions in the distal colon. Colorectal cancer is the second leading cause of cancer death in the United States, accounting for approximately 51,000 deaths annually.[5,11,24,33,81,99]

The cause of colorectal cancer has largely been attributed to a diet high in animal fat and low in fiber. The excess fat in a person's diet may act as a promoter of the development of colon cancer. A diet high in processed and red meats and low in fruit and vegetables has been associated with an increase risk of colorectal cancer. The intake of fiber into diets may act as an inhibitor, diluting fecal contents and increasing fecal bulk, resulting in quicker elimination, and therefore minimizing the exposure of the bowel epithelial lining to the carcinogens.[5, 33,81, 94,103] Other risk factors for the development of colorectal cancer include: obesity, smoking, excessive alcohol consumption (more than two drinks/day in men or 1/day in women), and minimal physical activity.[5,33,72,94]

Recent studies have shown that the risk of colorectal cancer may be decreased by the regular use of nonsteroidal anti-inflammatory drugs and postmenopausal hormone therapy. However, the use of these drugs as a preventative measure is not recommended.[5,33,72,94]

Other principal factors in the development of colon cancer include **chronic ulcerative colitis**, carcinomas arising in preexisting adenomatous polyps, and the hereditary cancer syndromes. These syndromes are **familial adenomatous polyposis** (FAP) and hereditary nonpolyposis colorectal syndrome (HNPCC).[33,81,88,103]

Individuals also at an increased risk for the development of colorectal cancer are those persons whose first-degree relative developed colorectal cancer or adenomatous polyps before age 60. An increased risk also exists if two or more first-degree relatives at any age developed colorectal cancer or adenomatous polyps in the absence of a hereditary syndrome.[99]

Chronic ulcerative colitis usually occurs in the rectum and sigmoid area of the bowel but may spread to the rest of the colon. This condition is characterized by extensive inflammation of the bowel wall and ulceration. A patient experiences attacks of bloody mucoid diarrhea up to 20 times a day. These attacks persist for days or weeks and then subside, only to recur.[96] The risk of developing colon cancer depends on the extent of bowel involvement, age of onset, and severity and duration of the active disease.[24,33,93] The earlier the age at onset and the longer the duration of the active disease, the higher the risk of developing cancer. Studies have shown the risk to be 3% at 15 years' duration, increasing to 5% at 20 years.[24,33,93] Only 1% of patients with a diagnosis of colorectal cancer have a history of chronic ulcerative colitis.

Adenomatous polyps are growths that arise from the mucosal lining and protrude into the lumen of the bowel. They are classified as tubular or villous, based on their growth pattern and microscopic characteristics. Polyps are considered a precursor to the development of a malignancy.[24,33,88,93,103] The larger the polyp, the greater is the risk of malignant transformation.[24,33,88] Villous adenomas are 8 to 10 times more likely than tubular adenomas to be malignant.[24,88,93]

Virtually all patients with the hereditary condition FAP, if left untreated, develop colon cancer.[24,33,81,93] FAP is characterized by the studding of the entire large bowel wall by thousands of polyps. Persons affected with this disease do not have polyps at birth. Progression to extensive involvement of the colon usually occurs by late adolescence. The cause of FAP is associated with a mutation on the adenomatous polyposis coli gene on chromosome 5.[79,99] FAP is treated by the complete removal of the colon and rectum. **Gardner's syndrome** is another inherited disorder similar to FAP. Patients with Gardner's syndrome have adenomatous polyposis of the large bowel and other abnormal growths, such as upper gastrointestinal polyps, periampullary tumors, lipomas, and fibromas.[24,33,93]

The frequent occurrence of colorectal cancer in families without polyposis has been termed **hereditary nonpolyposis colorectal syndrome** (HNPCC) also called Lynch syndrome.[11,24,33] The cause of HNPCC has been attributed to mutations in repair genes located on chromosome 2, 3, or 7. HNPCC has classically been defined as colorectal cancer that develops in three or more family members. At least two must be first-degree relatives and involve people in at least two generations with one family member being diagnosed before the age of 50.[99] Patients with this family history of colon cancer usually develop right-sided colon cancers at a much younger age than the general population. These patients are also at an increased risk for the development of a second cancer of the colon and adenocarcinomas of the breast, ovary, endometrium, and pancreas.[24,33] Individuals with this family history should undergo physical examinations regularly and consider genetic testing.

Anatomy and Lymphatics

Cancer of the large bowel is usually divided into cancer of the colon or rectum because the symptoms, diagnosis, and treatment are different based on the anatomic area involved. A major factor determining the treatment and prognosis is whether a lesion occurs in a segment of bowel that is located retroperitoneally or intraperitoneally. This is discussed further in the section on the anatomy and lymphatic drainage of these areas.

The colon is divided into eight regions: the cecum, ascending colon, descending colon, splenic flexure, hepatic flexure, transverse colon, sigmoid, and rectum. Located intraperitoneally, the cecum, transverse colon, and sigmoid have a complete mesentery and serosa and are freely mobile[24,54,81,87] (Figure 35-1). Lesions occurring in these regions can usually be surgically removed with an adequate margin unless the tumor is adherent

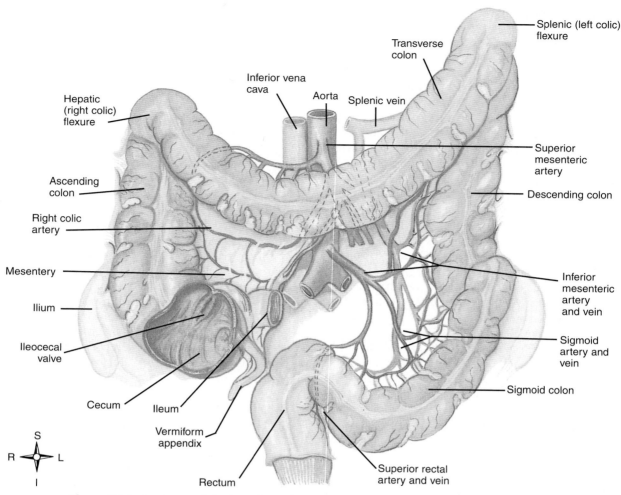

Figure 35-1. Anatomy of the large bowel. (From Thibodeau GA, Patton KT: *Anatomy and physiology*, ed 3, St. Louis, 1996, Mosby. Courtesy Ernest W. Beck.)

or invades adjacent structures.[24,52,80] Treatment failure or recurrence is most likely attributed to peritoneal seeding.

Located retroperitoneally, the ascending and descending colon and the hepatic and splenic flexures are considered immobile. They lack a true mesentery and a serosal covering on the posterior and lateral aspect. Because of the retroperitoneal location and lack of a mesentery for these regions, early spread outside the bowel wall and invasion of the adjacent soft tissues, kidney, and pancreas are common. Thus, adequate surgical margins are more difficult to achieve and may result in a local recurrence.[24,54, 81]

The rectum is continuous with the sigmoid and begins at the level of the third sacral vertebra. Like the sigmoid, the upper rectum is covered by the peritoneum but only on its lateral and anterior surfaces. The peritoneum is then reflected over the anterior wall of the rectum onto the seminal vesicles and bladder in males or the vagina and uterus in females, forming a cul-de-sac termed the rectovesical pouch or rectouterine pouch, respectively. The lower half to two thirds of the rectum is located retroperitoneally. Three transverse folds divide the rectum into areas known as the upper valve, middle valve, and lower valve, or ampulla (Figure 35-2). The middle valve is located 11 cm

superior from the anal verge and represents the approximate location of the peritoneal reflection.[81,87] Because of the retroperitoneal location, tumors of the rectum can invade adjacent structures of the pelvis, such as the prostate, bladder, vagina, and sacrum. Treatment options depend on the location of the lesion. As mentioned earlier, retroperitoneally located lesions are more apt to fail locally because of close surgical margins and may require adjuvant treatment subsequent to a complete surgical resection.[54,77]

A cross section through a segment of large bowel reveals four main layers: the mucosa, submucosa, muscularis propria, and serosa[41,81] (Figure 35-3). These layers are used in the staging system to define the amount of involvement through the bowel wall. The mucosa, or innermost layer, forms the lumen of the bowel and consists of two supporting layers: the lamina propria and muscularis mucosa. The next layer, the submucosa, is rich in blood vessels and lymphatics. The muscularis propria contains two muscle layers, one circular and one longitudinal, which are responsible for peristalsis. Beneath the muscularis layer is a lining of fat termed the subserosal layer. The outermost layer is the serosa. Not all segments of the colon have a serosal layer. This layer is provided by the visceral peritoneum.[24]

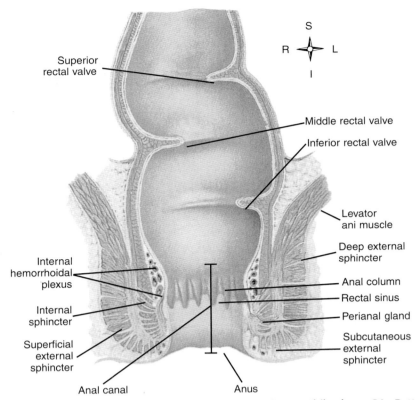

Figure 35-2. A coronal section through the rectum. (From Thibodeau GA, Patton KT: *Anatomy and physiology*, ed 6, St. Louis, 2007, Mosby.)

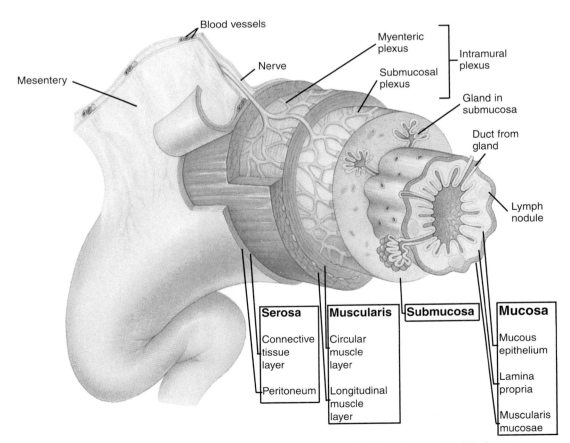

Figure 35-3. A cross section of the bowel wall. (From Thibodeau GA, Patton KT: *Anatomy and physiology*, ed 3, St. Louis, 1996, Mosby. Courtesy Barbara Cousins.)

The lymphatic drainage of the colon follows the mesenteric vessels. The right colon follows the superior mesenteric vessels and includes the ileocolic and right colic nodes (see Figure 35-3). The left colon follows the inferior mesenteric vessels and includes the regional nodes termed the midcolic, inferior mesenteric, and left colic. The sigmoid region drains into the inferior mesenteric system but also includes the nodes along the superior rectal, sigmoidal, and sigmoidal mesenteric vessels.[41] Lymphatic drainage of the upper rectum follows the superior rectal vessels into the inferior mesenteric system. Middle and lower rectum lymphatic drainage is along the middle rectal vessels, with the principal nodal group comprising the internal iliac nodes.[34,54,81] Other nodal groups at risk for involvement with rectal cancer are the perirectal, lateral sacral, and presacral nodes.[34,41] Low rectal lesions that extend into the anal canal can drain to the inguinal nodes (Figure 35-4).

With any of these regions, other nodal groups may be involved or at risk for involvement if the tumor has invaded an adjacent structure. For example, if a rectal cancer has invaded the vagina or prostate, the external iliac nodes may be involved with disease. For a lesion in the ascending colon that has invaded the posterior abdominal wall, the paraaortic nodes may be positive for disease.[54,81]

Clinical Presentation

Patients with rectal cancer usually have rectal bleeding. This may be bright red blood on the toilet paper or mixed in or on the stool.[23,81] This is termed **hematochezia**. Other symptoms include a change in bowel habits, diarrhea versus constipation, or a change in the stool caliber.[23,51,81] Pencil-thin stools, constipation, or diarrhea may be indicative of a tumor filling the rectal valve area and causing an obstructive-type process. **Tenesmus** (spasms of

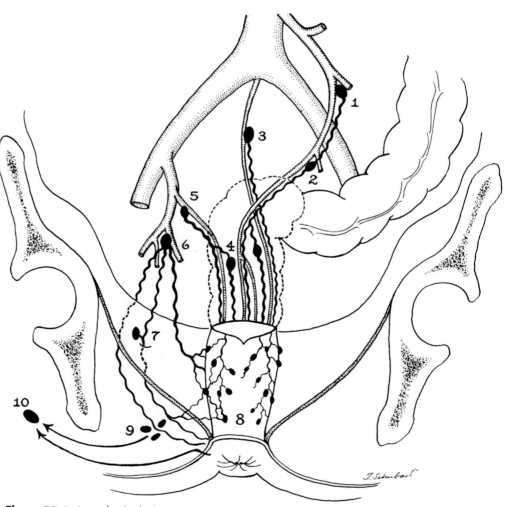

Figure 35-4. Lymphatic drainage of the rectum: 1 and 2, nodes at the origin of the inferior mesenteric artery and origin of the sigmoid vessels; 3, nodes of the sacral promontory; 4, sacral nodes; 5 and 6, internal iliac nodes, hypogastric; 7, external iliac nodes may be involved in low rectal lesions; 8, nodes located at the rectal wall; 9, ischiorectal nodes; and 10, inguinal nodes. (From Del Regato JA, Spjut HJ, Cox JD: *Ackerman and del Regato's cancer: diagnosis, treatment, and prognosis,* ed 6, St. Louis, 1985, Mosby.)

the rectum accompanied by a desire to empty the bowel) may be a patient's complaint with locally advanced rectal cancer. Pain in the buttock or perineal area may occur from tumor extension posteriorly.[23]

Presenting symptoms of patients with lesions in the left colon are similar to those of rectal cancer. Blood in the stool, a change in stool caliber, obstructive symptoms, and abdominal pain are the most common complaints.[24,91] In contrast, patients with right-sided colon lesions usually have abdominal pain, which is often accompanied by an abdominal mass. Nausea and vomiting are other possible symptoms. Occult blood in the stool and microcytic anemia are two other symptoms of colon cancer.[24,81]

Detection and Diagnosis

In general, a cancer in the large bowel is diagnosed via findings of the physical examination and radiographic and endoscopic studies. Together, these findings provide crucial information in the detection and extent of the disease process. According to the American Cancer Society screening guidelines for the early detection of colorectal cancer, beginning at age 50, it is recommended that an average-risk person undergo an annual fecal occult blood test or fecal immunochemical test, a flexible sigmoidoscopy and double contrast barium enema every 5 years, and a colonoscopy every 10 years. A colonoscopy should follow any positive test results. High-risk individuals, those with a family history of FAP or HNPCC, should undergo colonoscopies before age 50 and should determine a plan for screening with their health care provider.[5,94] These persons would also benefit from counseling to consider genetic testing.[99]

The initial procedure for any patient with a malignancy is a thorough history and physical examination. For all colorectal cancer patients, a digital rectal examination should be performed and attention should be given to the approximate size of the lesion, the mobility, the location from the anal verge, and the rectal wall involved.[81] Enlarged perirectal nodes may also be detected during the digital examination.

A proctosigmoidoscopy is performed as a complementary procedure and allows a more accurate depiction of the size and location of the lesion. This procedure also determines whether the mass is exophytic or ulcerative. A tissue diagnosis is obtained from a biopsy during the endoscopic procedure. A pelvic examination should be performed for colon or rectal cancer to rule out any other pelvic masses. An anterior extrarectal mass (a lesion in the cul-de-sac) may be indicative of peritoneal seeding. In women an anterior rectal mass may invade the vaginal wall, putting the external iliac nodes at risk for involvement. The left supraclavicular and inguinal lymph nodes should also be palpated, especially in patients with low rectal lesions nearing the dentate line.[81] Supraclavicular lymph node involvement indicates extensive incurable disease and generally occurs as a result of spread from metastatically involved paraaortic nodes via the thoracic duct. The physical examination should also assess potential sites of distant spread. Palpation of the abdomen should be performed to check for masses in the abdomen, liver, and ascites.

Endoscopic procedures, colonoscopies, and proctosigmoidoscopies can assess the size, location of lesion, and circumferential extent and provide the distance of the lesion from the anal verge. They are also used for obtaining biopsies of lesions or removing polyps for histologic confirmation of malignancy. Endorectal ultrasound (ERUS) is another useful tool. It can demonstrate the depth of invasion through the bowel wall into adjacent tissues and is useful in determining the T stage of the tumor.[6,94] It also can detect enlarged perirectal lymph nodes.[41,81]

After a diagnosis is established, a patient undergoes a staging workup to determine the extent or amount of spread of the disease. A chest radiograph is usually obtained to detect metastasis to the lungs. Computed tomography (CT) or magnetic resonance imaging (MRI) of the pelvis is done to evaluate whether the tumor has extended into other pelvic organs or structures and to determine pelvic lymph node involvement. An abdominal CT scan may also be obtained to detect metastasis to the liver or other abdominal structures.[94]

Laboratory studies used in the diagnosis and workup of colon cancer include a complete blood count (CBC) and blood chemistry profile. Elevated liver function tests indicate the need for imaging of the liver by CT or by sonography.

Positron emission tomography (PET) has been used as part of the staging workup to locate areas of uptake in the primary tumor, lymph nodes, or distant metastasis. PET scans have demonstrated uptake in lymph nodes that was not seen on initial CT scan. A combined PET-CT examination provides better anatomic correlation of areas of involvement than PET alone. PET-CT is becoming a commonly used examination for cancer staging and radiation treatment planning.[10,42]

Pathology and Staging

Adenocarcinoma is the most common malignancy of the large bowel, accounting for 90% to 95% of all tumors.[23,91] Other histologic types include mucinous adenocarcinoma, signet-ring cell carcinoma, and squamous cell carcinoma.[91]

Three principal staging systems exist. Two of the systems, Dukes classification and the modified Astler-Coller (MAC) system, are postoperative, whereas the American Joint Committee on Cancer (AJCC) tumor, node, metastases (TNM) system may be used clinically (preoperatively) or postoperatively (Box 35-1) The TNM system is the more commonly used system.

The staging system devised by Cuthbert Dukes in the 1930s was the first useful system. Tumors of the rectum are classified according to the level of invasion into the bowel wall and the absence or presence of nodes positive for tumor. The tumors are given a letter designation from A to C. Dukes A designation indicates a lesion that has not penetrated through the bowel wall. The B designation indicates a lesion that has penetrated the bowel wall with nodes negative for tumor, and the C designation indicates a lesion with nodes positive for tumor.

Astler-Coller expanded Dukes' system, making it more specific regarding the level of penetration through the bowel wall and nodal status. These modifications in the staging system were based on studies showing that penetration through the bowel wall, the number of nodes positive for tumor, and tumor adherence to adjacent structures were important predictors of survival.[24,81] In the MAC system, Gunderson and Sosin created separate categories for tumors that microscopically or grossly (B2m or B2g) involved surrounding organs or structures.[24]

Box 35-1	American Joint Committee on Cancer Staging Classification for Colorectal Cancer

PRIMARY TUMOR (T)

TX	Primary tumor cannot be assessed
T0	No evidence of primary tumor
Tis	Carcinoma in situ: intraepithelial or invasion of lamina propria
T1	Tumor invades submucosa
T2	Tumor invades muscularis propria
T3	Tumor invades through the muscularis propria into the subserosa, or into nonperitonealized pericolic or perirectal tissues
T4	Tumor directly invades other organs or structures, and/or perforates visceral peritoneum

REGIONAL LYMPH NODES (N)

NX	Regional lymph nodes cannot be assessed
N0	No regional lymph node metastasis
N1	Metastasis in 1 to 3 regional lymph nodes
N2	Metastasis in 4 or more regional lymph nodes

DISTANT METASTASIS (M)

MX	Distant metastasis cannot be assessed
M0	No distant metastasis
M1	Distant metastasis

STAGE GROUPING

Stage	T	N	M	Dukes	MAC
0	Tis	N0	M0	—	—
I	T1	N0	M0	A	A
	T2	N0	M0	A	B1
IIA	T3	N0	M0	B	B2
IIB	T4	N0	M0	B	B3
IIIA	T1-T2	N1	M0	C	C1
IIIB	T3-T4	N1	M0	C	C2/C3
IIIC	Any T	N2	M0	C	C1/C2/C3
IV	Any T	Any N	M1	—	D

HISTOLOGIC GRADE (G)

GX	Grade cannot be assessed
G1	Well differentiated
G2	Moderately differentiated
G3	Poorly differentiated
G4	Undifferentiated

With permission from American Joint Committee on Cancer (AJCC), Chicago, IL: *AJCC Cancer Staging Manual*, ed 6, New York, 2002, Springer-Verlag.

The TNM system incorporated these changes into the current system (Table 35-1), which is similar to the MAC system.[24,41] The revisions in the staging systems reflect that the two most important prognostic indicators of survival are the number of nodes positive for tumor and depth of penetration through the bowel wall.[24,54]

Over 95% of colon and rectal cancers are adenocarcinomas. These are cancers of the cells that line the inside of the colon and rectum. There are some other, more rare, types of tumors of the colon and rectum.[7]

Routes of Spread

As implied in the staging system, malignancies of the large bowel usually spread via direct extension, lymphatics, and hematogenous spread. Direct extension of the tumor is typically in a radial fashion, penetrating into the bowel wall rather than longitudinally.[24]

Lymphatic spread occurs if the tumor has invaded the submucosal layer of the bowel. The initial lymphatic and venous channels of the bowel wall are found in the submucosal layer. Lymphatic spread is orderly. The initial nodes involved for rectal cancer are the perirectal nodes.[24,54] Approximately 50% of patients have nodes positive for tumor at the time of diagnosis.[54]

Blood-borne spread to the liver is the most common type of distant metastasis. The mechanism of spread involves the venous drainage of the gastrointestinal system (the portal circulation). The second most common site of distant spread is the lung. This spread results from tumor embolus into the inferior vena cava (IVC).[24]

Table 35-1	TNM Colorectal Staging Systems

T1	Tumor invades submucosa
T2	Tumor invades muscularis propria
T3	Tumor invades through the muscularis propria into subserosa or into pericolic or perirectal tissues
T4	Direct extension into other organs or structures and/or perforation of visceral peritoneum
N0	Nodes negative
N1	1–3 regional nodes positive
N2	4 or more positive regional nodes
M0	No distant metastasis
M1	Distant metastasis

Modified from Fleming ID, et al, editors: *AJCC manual for staging of cancer*, ed 5, Philadelphia, 1997, Lippincott-Raven.

Lesions may also spread within the peritoneal cavity. The growth of a tumor through the bowel wall onto the peritoneal surface of the colon can result in tumor cells shedding into the abdominal cavity. These shed cells then take up residence on another surface (i.e., peritoneal lining, cul-de-sac) and begin to grow. This process is called **peritoneal seeding**. The implantation of tumor cells onto a surface at the time of surgery is another mechanism of spread.[24,56]

Treatment Techniques

Surgery is considered the treatment of choice. The tumor, an adequate margin, and draining lymphatics are removed. The type of procedure depends on the location of the tumor.

For colon tumors the removal of a large segment of bowel, adjacent lymph nodes, and the immediate vascular supply by procedures such as a right hemicolectomy or left hemicolectomy is common. Some colon surgeries are being done laparoscopically instead of the traditional open procedure. Patients who underwent laparoscopic colectomy recovered from the procedure sooner, had a shorter hospital stay than patients who underwent an open procedure. For rectal cancer the two most common procedures are the low anterior resection (LAR) and abdominoperineal resection (APR). The use of a laparoscopic surgical procedure for rectal cancer is more difficult to perform. Additional research studies are being done to evaluate treatment outcomes of this technique.[42,48]

The **low anterior resection** involves the removal of the tumor plus a margin (an en bloc excision) and immediately adjacent lymph nodes.[38] The bowel is then reanastomosed. Therefore, a colostomy is not required. This procedure is used in the treatment of colon cancers and select rectal cancers.[23,24] Patients with disease in the upper third or middle third of the rectum (6 to 12 cm above the verge) are usually candidates for this sphincter-preserving surgery.[23,38,49,76]

An APR is used in patients with rectal cancer in the lower third (distal 5 cm) of the rectum. An anterior incision is made into the abdominal wall to construct a colostomy. Then, a perineal incision is made to resect the rectum, anus, and draining lymphatics, pulling the entire en bloc specimen out through the perineal opening. Because of the narrow, bony configuration of the pelvis and closeness of adjacent structures (i.e., prostate and vagina), adequate margins laterally, anteriorly, and posteriorly are difficult to achieve.[76,81] Surgical clips placed to outline the tumor area assist the radiation oncologist in the design of treatment portals.[23,81] The final phase of the procedure involves the reconstruction or reperitonealization of the pelvic floor through the use of an absorbable mesh, omentum, or peritoneum. This is extremely important for the patient who needs postoperative radiation therapy. Reperitonealization allows the small bowel to be displaced superiorly, reducing the amount of small bowel in the treatment field and minimizing the treatment toxicity from radiation therapy.[23,38,81]

Radiation Therapy. Radiation therapy is most commonly used as an adjuvant treatment for rectal cancer. This is either done preoperatively or postoperatively and in conjunction with chemotherapy.

Postoperative adjuvant radiation therapy with concurrent chemotherapy is advocated based on the high local failure rate of surgery alone in rectal cancer patients who have nodes positive for tumor or tumor extension beyond the wall. Postoperative radiation therapy and chemotherapy have consistently been shown to improve local control and survival rates in rectal cancer patients. A major advantage of postoperative adjuvant treatment is that the physician has pathologic confirmation of the extent of the tumor spread through the wall to nodes or distant sites. This information is critical in determining whether adjuvant treatment is necessary.[82] Studies have shown that patients with nodes positive for tumor (N1) but with a tumor confined to the bowel wall (T2) have a 20% to 40% recurrence rate.[24,54,81] A similar local recurrence rate (20% to 35%) is found with T3 or T4 lesions, tumors that extend through the bowel

wall with or without adherence and nodes for tumor. A patient with both poor prognostic factors (extension through the wall and nodes positive for tumor (T3 N1, N2) has almost twice the risk for local recurrence. Various studies have reported recurrence rates in these patients of 40% to 65% in a clinical series and up to 70% in a reoperative series.[56,57]

Preoperative radiation therapy is another commonly used technique for patients with large rectal cancers that have invaded through the muscle layer (T3) or on imaging studies (ERUS or MRI) have enlarged lymph nodes indicating N1 or N2 disease. The goal of this treatment is sphincter preservation. Radiation therapy combined with chemotherapy is done prior to surgery (**neoadjuvant**) to shrink the tumor so that a low anterior resection can be done rather than an APR sparing the patient a colostomy. Preoperative radiation therapy has the potential advantages of downstaging the primary tumor, decreasing the chance of tumor spillage or seeding at the time of surgery, increased radiosensitivity due to well oxygenated cells in the nonoperative pelvis, and less acute side effects.[17,81,105] A disadvantage to preoperative radiation therapy is not having pathologic tumor (T) staging that results in the irradiation of a patient with a T1 or T2 tumor.[17,81,105] Preoperative chemoradiation followed by LAR has demonstrated good local control in patients whose T3 tumors responded to the preoperative chemoradiation.[17,81,105] Preoperative chemoradiation is also recommended when the tumor is locally advanced (T4) and has invaded through the bowel wall into pelvic tissues or organs.[6]

Endocavitary radiation therapy is a sphincter-preserving procedure done for curative intent in a select group of patients with low- to middle-third rectal cancers that are confined to the bowel wall. Papillon established the following characteristics for patients eligible for this procedure: no extension of the tumor beyond the bowel wall, a maximum tumor size of 3 × 5 cm, a mobile lesion with no significant extension into the anal canal, a well to moderately well-differentiated exophytic tumor that is accessible by the treatment proctoscope (≤10 cm from the anal verge).[51,89,94] Patients receive four doses of 3000 cGy each, separated by a 2-week interval. This is done on an outpatient basis through the use of a 50-kVp contact unit (4-cm source-skin distance [SSD]), with 0.5- to 1.0-mm aluminum filtration at a dose rate of 1000 cGy per minute. Treatments are delivered directly to the rectal tumor through an applicator inserted into the rectum and held in place by the radiation oncologist (Figure 35-5). If the size of the lesion exceeds the diameter of the applicator (3 cm), overlapping fields are necessary. Treatment results have been excellent with this technique. Papillon reported only a 11% locoregional failure rate with a 5-year follow-up out of 207 patients treated.[81,89]

Radiation alone has also been used in patients who are medically inoperable or who have locally advanced rectal cancer and are deemed unresectable.[23,81] In this setting, radiation provides palliation and is rarely curative. Radiation combined with chemotherapy (5-fluorouracil [5-FU]) has proved more effective than radiation alone in relieving symptoms, decreasing tumor progression, and increasing overall survival.

Chemotherapy. The addition of adjuvant chemotherapy combined with radiation therapy in the pre-operative or postoperative setting in high-risk rectal and colon cancer patients

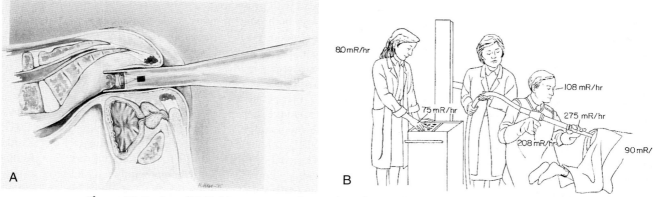

Figure 35-5. A and **B**, Sphincter-preserving endocavitary radiation therapy of the low rectal tumor. (Courtesy Dr. Alan J. Stark.)

(T3 or N1, N2) has demonstrated an increase in overall survival rates[31,55,56,81,82] (Figure 35-6). Many studies have demonstrated a decreased disease recurrence and improved survival rates with a combination of 5-FU and pelvic radiation therapy. The National Comprehensive Cancer Network (NCCN) has established treatment guidelines for patients with colon and rectal cancer. The current recommendations for T3 rectal cancer employ continuous venous infusion 5-FU during radiation therapy in the preoperative or postoperative setting. In the preoperative setting, the chemoradiation is followed by curative resection and then additional 5-FU with or without leucovorin or the FOLFOX (5-FU, leucovorin, oxaplatin) regimen. In the postoperative setting, 5-FU with or without leucovorin or FOLFOX is done first followed by radiation therapy with continuous 5-FU. Once the radiation therapy is completed, additional chemotherapy with 5-FU with or without leucovorin or FOLFOX is done. In the case of recurrent or metastatic rectal cancer the same drugs can be used or a regimen called FOLFIRI may be used. FOLFIRI consists of 5-FU, leucovorin, and irinotecan.[6,94] Two new monoclonal antibodies, Bevacizumab and cetuximab, are being studied in the use of advanced or metastatic colon or rectal cancer. Bevacizumab (avastin) is a drug that blocks the growth of new blood vessels to the tumor hindering the supply of oxygen and nutrients necessary for continued growth of the tumor. This drug is used in combination with FOLFOX or FOLFIRI. Cetuximab (erbitux) blocks the effects of hormone like factors on the cell surface that promote cancer cell growth causing cell death. Cetuximab may be used alone or in combination with other chemotherapy drugs in patients that are not responding to the chemotherapy agent irinotecan.[5,6,94]

Field Design and Critical Structures. Patients receiving preoperative or postoperative adjuvant radiation therapy for rectal cancer are at a high risk for local recurrence. These patients include those with extension beyond the bowel wall, tumor adherence (T3, T4), or lymph nodes positive for tumor (N1, N2). The treatment fields are typically designed to encompass the primary tumor volume and pelvic lymph nodes, shrinking the field to treat the primary target volume to a higher dose. Anatomic boundaries of the portals depend on whether the

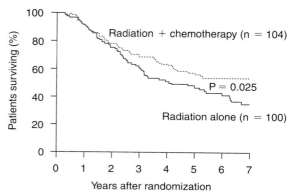

Figure 35-6. Improved survival rates with postoperative radiation and chemotherapy versus radiation alone. (Modified from Krook JE, et al: Effective surgical adjuvant therapy for high-risk rectal carcinoma, *N Engl J Med* 324:713, 1991.)

patient underwent an anterior resection or AP resection directly relating to the areas at risk for recurrence. For patients with rectal cancer, most recurrences occur in the posterior aspect of the pelvis, including metastasis to the internal iliac and presacral lymph nodes.[54,81] These two nodal groups are not included in a standard surgical resection for rectal cancer and need to be encompassed in radiation portals.[81] For irradiation of the pelvis, the dose-limiting structure or organ at risk (OAR) is the small bowel. The small bowel dose should be less than 45 Gy. Radiation treatment techniques and the field design must take into consideration the amount of small bowel in the field to minimize treatment-related toxicities. The reduction of the small-bowel dose is achieved through patient positioning and positioning devices, bladder distention, multiple-shaped fields, and dosimetric weighting.[24,54,81] The dose to the small bowel is more easily reduced during preoperative radiation therapy than postoperative radiation. This is because with postoperative radiation the rectum and peritoneum have been removed allowing the small bowel to fall lower in the pelvis which results in having more small bowel within the radiation field. The dose delivered to the large volume (tumor plus regional nodes) is 4500 cGy, with the coned-down volume (primary tumor bed) receiving 5000 cGy to 5500 cGy in 6 to 6½ weeks. Doses in excess of 5000 cGy are not achievable unless the small bowel can be excluded from the field.[23,54,81]

Traditionally, a three-field technique (PA and opposed laterals wedged) is used, allowing a homogenous dose to the tumor bed while sparing anterior structures, such as the small bowel. A four-field posteroanterior/anteroposterior (PA/AP) and opposed laterals may be used when the anterior structures such as the prostate or vagina are at risk for involvement or are involved. For patients who have undergone an anterior resection the superior extent of the field is placed 1.5 cm superior to the sacral promontory, which correlates to L5-S1 innerspace.[23,54,81] Depending on the superior extent of the lesion and clinical indications, the field may need to be placed at the L4-5 interspace or extend superiorly to include the paraaortic lymph node chain.[54] The more superiorly the field extends, the more precautions are necessary to avoid small-bowel injury and complications. The width of the PA/AP fields is designed to provide adequate coverage of the iliac lymph nodes. This border is placed 2 cm lateral to the pelvic brim and inlet. The inferior border generally includes the entire obturator foramina, although this may vary depending on the location of the lesion. The recommended inferior margin is 3 to 5 cm on the gross tumor preoperatively or below the most distal extent of dissection postoperatively[54] (Figure 35-7). A rectal tube is inserted at the time of simulation. Barium or Gastrografin contrast (30 to 40 cm²) is injected into the rectum to facilitate the

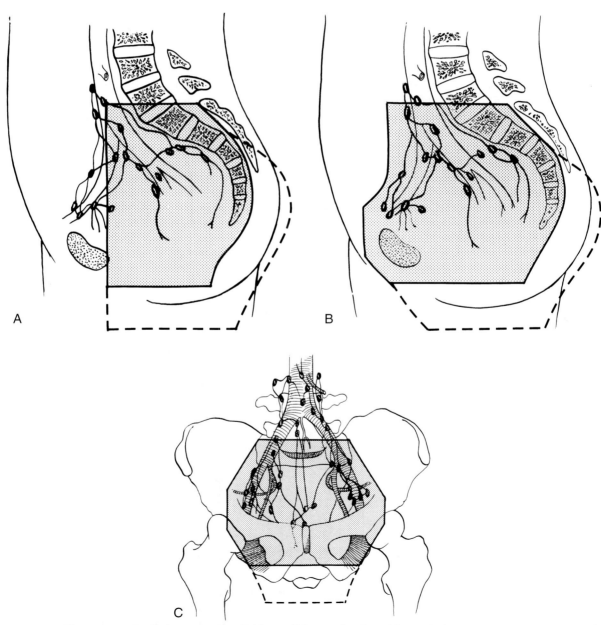

Figure 35-7. Radiation treatment fields. In all figures the dotted line indicates the field extension to be used after an abdominal-perineal resection. **A**, A standard lateral field. **B**, A lateral field to include external iliacs in patients who have involvement of structures with external iliac lymph node drainage. **C**, A standard anteroposterior/posteroanterior (AP/PA) field.

localization of critical structures and design of treatment fields. Lead shot or a BB is placed on the anal verge to reference the perineal surface on simulation films.

Lateral treatment portals and prone positioning with full bladder distention allows the small bowel to be excluded from the treatment volume. This position also assists in the localization of critical posterior structures. Anatomically, the rectum and perirectal tissues are extremely close to the sacrum and coccyx. In locally advanced disease the tumor may spread along the sacral nerve roots, resulting in tumor recurrence in the sacrum. Therefore the posterior field edge is placed 1.5 to 2.0 cm behind the anterior bony sacral margin. In advanced situations the entire sacral canal plus a 1.5-cm margin is recommended.[54,81] This margin allows day-to-day variances in the patient setup caused by movement. Anteriorly, the field border is placed at the anterior edge of the femoral heads to ensure coverage of the internal iliac nodes. The lower third of the rectum lies immediately posterior to the vaginal wall and prostate, placing these organs and their draining lymphatics at risk for involvement. If the rectal lesion has invaded anterior structures (prostate or vagina), the anterior border is placed on pubic symphysis for inclusion of the external iliac nodes[23,54,81] (Figure 35-7, B). In female patients, a tampon soaked with iodinated contrast is inserted into the vagina to ensure adequate coverage of the vagina in the radiation portals.

The use of a CT simulator rather than a fluoroscopic simulator allows the physician to more accurately localize and outline the pertinent anatomic structures described previously. With conventional simulation, these structures are transferred onto the simulation radiograph from measurements taken off a previous CT scan. Errors in measurements or the shift of anatomic structures because of change in patient position from the original scan may result in inadequate margins. The CT simulator

software enables physicians to digitize in different colors the target volume and critical normal structures, such as the rectum, bladder, and lymph nodes on each CT slice. The intimate relationships of target versus normal tissues are available at the time of simulation and with the patient in treatment position. This assists the physician and the dosimetrist in the accurate placement of the isocenter and in the design of the fields. A digitally reconstructed radiograph (DRR) is produced, which shows the radiation field outline, the treatment isocenter, and pertinent anatomic structures (see Figure 35-8). The CT images can be sent electronically directly to dosimetry for treatment planning.

The CT simulation procedure requires the radiation therapist to position the patient prone on a positioning device ensuring elbows are "in" so that they will not hit the sides of the CT gantry during the scan. It is extremely important to get the patient as straight as possible before the scan because they cannot be repositioned once the scan is complete. The patient is given oral contrast to drink 45 minutes prior to the CT simulation. This will allow the small bowel to be localized on the CT scans. Contrast is typically placed in the rectum at the time of simulation and the tubes removed before scanning. Unlike fluoroscopic simulation, a more dilute mixture of contrast (12-ml water and 3-ml Gastrografin) is used to prevent artifacts on the CT images. A tampon soaked with a more dilute iodinated contrast may be used in female patients. A reference isocenter or three points are placed on the patient's pelvis and marked with small BBs. The reference isocenter is used to ensure that the patient did not move during the scan. The reference isocenter is also used as the zero coordinates from which the treatment isocenter will be marked. After the reference isocenter is placed, couch parameters, scanning limits, and length of pilot or scout are recorded. A typical scan may extend from the level of the

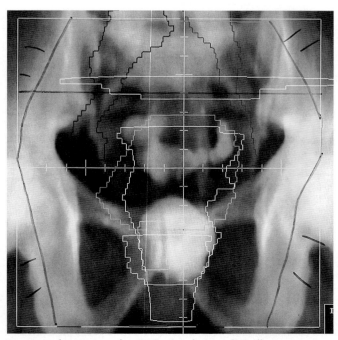

Figure 35-8. Computed tomography (CT) simulation digitally reconstructed radiograph (DRR) of standard posteroanterior (PA) field.

second lumbar vertebrae to below the lesser trochanters. Following the scan, the physician will determine the treatment isocenter and give the therapist the measurements to shift anterior or posterior and so forth to the appropriate location. The therapist then places marks or tattoos on the treatment isocenter or three points. Most CT simulators are not equipped with a patient marking system like a conventional simulator is. Only the treatment isocenter or three points can be marked. It is helpful if the radiation therapist uses the sagittal laser to place additional straightening lines superior and inferior to the isocenter. The patient may proceed to treatment following the completion of the treatment plan.

In patients having an AP resection the field design is similar, except the posterior and inferior borders are extended to include the entire perineal incision. The perineal region is included in the treatment volume to decrease the risk of tumor recurrence in the scar from implantation of tumor cells at the time of surgery. The entire perineal scar is outlined at the time of simulation with solder wire or lead BBs. The posterior and inferior margins are established by placing the field edge 1.5 to 2.0 cm beyond the radiopaque perineal markers. This corresponds to flashing the posterior and inferior perineal skin surfaces[54,81] (see Figure 35-7). The perineal scar is then bolused (thickness/energy dependent) during the PA treatment. The buttocks are taped apart, and bolus is placed on the entire perineal scar to have a controlled measurable bolusing effect. Because of the tangential radiation beam, the perineal tissue and thinner upper thigh tissue may exhibit acute skin reactions, requiring interruption of the planned treatment course. In male patients the penis and scrotum are shifted superiorly under the pubic region to lessen this reaction. Alternatively, the reaction to male genitalia can be reduced by the use of a three-field technique (PA and laterals).

Intensity-modulated radiation therapy (IMRT) is another technique that is used in the treatment of rectal cancer. This technique uses multiple oblique fields instead of the traditional three fields At Mayo Clinic the field arrangement used consists of P20R, P60R, A80R, A40R, ANT, A40L, P80L, P60L, and P20L. IMRT uses inverse forward planning to place dose limits on organs at risk such as the small bowel and femoral heads. IMRT allows more dose conformity to the planning target volume and spares the small bowel more than conventional methods. IMRT is more costly than traditional methods and although more tissues are exposed to low doses of irradiation with IMRT, the benefits of sparing more normal tissues is considered a greater advantage.

An extrapelvic colon cancer field design should include an initial margin of 3 to 5 cm beyond the tumor plus high-risk nodal groups and adjacent structures. If the tumor invaded or was adherent to an organ such as the ovary or stomach, the majority of the organ and its draining lymphatics should be encompassed in the treatment portal unless the organ was completely resected. Adherent structures should be included with a 3- to 5-cm margin. Usually, an AP/PA technique is used. However, CT treatment planning and clip placement may determine that a multifield approach more optimally spares normal tissue. The initial large volume is treated to 4500 cGy with a shrinking-field technique used to boost the tumor bed (with a 2- to 3-cm margin) an additional 540 to 900 cGy.[54,81]

Dose-limiting structures for treating an ascending or descending colon cancer include the kidney and small bowel. Contrast studies for assessing renal function and kidney localization films should be performed before treatment or at the time of simulation to ensure the adequate sparing of at least one kidney. For example, when treating a right-sided colon lesion, 50% or more of the right kidney may be in the field; therefore the left kidney must be spared.[54,81] Three-dimensional conformal radiation therapy techniques and IMRT may be used. IMRT allows more sparing of the kidneys, liver, and small bowel and is more commonly used.

In patients with locally advanced colorectal cancer or recurrent disease, local control is difficult to achieve. This is due to the limited surgical options because of fixation of the tumor to pelvic organs (prostate, uterus) or unresectable structures such as the presacrum or pelvic sidewall. If microscopic residual disease exists, an external beam dose of 6000 cGy or greater is necessary to provide a reasonable chance for control. This dose is even higher (≥7000 cGy) if gross residual disease exists.[53,59] These doses exceed the normal tissue-tolerance dose of abdominal or pelvic structures and cannot be safely delivered with conventional external beam irradiation.[52,53]

 Recall the dose limits of radiation for the kidneys, liver, and small bowel. What is the TD 5/5 for each of these organs at risk (OARs)? Which of the three organs is most sensitive to radiation damage? Intensity-modulated radiation therapy (IMRT) may help reduce the dose to organs at risk.

Intraoperative Radiation Therapy. Intraoperative radiation therapy (IORT) is a mechanism for supplementing the external beam dose to assist in obtaining local control of the tumor while sparing dose-limiting normal structures.[46] IORT is a specialized boost technique similar to brachytherapy. IORT is also used when cancer recurs in the pelvis. As the name implies, IORT involves an operative procedure requiring general anesthesia. The radiation oncologist and surgeon must work closely with one another to determine whether IORT is appropriate and which diagnostic tests would be helpful in planning the IORT and external beam radiation treatments. A contraindication for IORT is the presence of distant metastasis. The surgeon and radiation oncologist also determine the optimal sequence of surgery and external radiation by discussing the benefits and side effects of each.[52,59]

Patients undergoing an IORT procedure receive a dose of 1000 to 2000 cGy of electrons in a single fraction directly to the tumor bed. Critical dose-limiting structures (i.e., kidney, bowel) are shielded or surgically displaced out of the radiation portal so that these normal tissues receive little or no radiation. This dose, delivered in a single fraction, is two to three times the dose if delivered at conventional fractionation of 180 to 200 cGy/fraction. For example, an IORT single dose of 1500 cGy equals 3000- to 4500-cGy fractionated external radiation. When adding the effective IORT dose to the 4500 to 5000 cGy, delivered with conventional external beam radiation, the total effective dose equals 7500 to 9500 cGy.[52,59] A dose this high cannot be safely given with standard external irradiation.

The IORT dose is calculated at the 90% isodose line, with the energy and dose delivered depending on the depth or amount of residual disease. Electron energies of 9 to 12 MeV are used after a gross total resection or minimal residual and high energies of 15 to 18 MeV are used for patients who have recurrent disease with gross residual or unresectable disease.[52,54] The target volume is encompassed in a Lucite cylinder that projects from the patient and is docked to the treatment head of the linear accelerator. The beam of electrons travel through the Lucite cylinder directly onto the tumor bed (Figure 35-9).

The precise role of IORT in the treatment of large bowel cancer is still being studied. IORT continues to be used in locally advanced and recurrent colorectal cancer. This treatment in addition to combined modality therapy is associated with better local control and survival rates.[66,94] Moreover, toxicity can be significant. Further study is needed before IORT becomes a widely accepted tool in the treatment of colorectal cancer.

Side Effects. The acute and chronic side effects of irradiation to the pelvis or abdomen are directly related to the dose, volume, and type of tissue irradiated. The larger the area treated, the greater is the associated toxicities. The toxicities of treatment increase with escalating doses and depend on the normal tissue tolerances of the structures in the irradiated volume. For patients with colorectal cancer the main dose-limiting structure for acute and chronic side effects is the small bowel. Acute toxicities of treatment include diarrhea, abdominal cramps and bloating, proctitis, bloody or mucus discharge, and dysuria. Patients may also experience **leukopenia** (an abnormal decrease in the white blood cell count) and **thrombocytopenia** (an abnormal decrease in the platelet count). Gastrointestinal and hematologic toxicities are increased when chemotherapy is used with radiation therapy.[23,58,71,81] In patients who have their perineum treated, a brisk skin reaction (moist desquamation) may result, sometimes requiring a treatment break.[54]

Chronic effects occur less often than acute side effects but are more serious. Persistent diarrhea, increased bowel frequency, proctitis, urinary incontinence, and bladder atrophy have occurred in patients after radiation therapy. The most common long-term complication is damage to the small bowel, resulting in enteritis, adhesions, and obstruction.[23] The incidence of small-bowel obstruction requiring surgery may be decreased by radiation oncologists and surgeons working together to determine methods for minimizing the amount of small bowel in the radiation field.

As mentioned earlier, treatment techniques and fields are designed to limit the dose to the small bowel. These include surgical and radiation therapy interventions. For example, the surgeon can reconstruct the pelvis to minimize the amount of small bowel in the pelvis after an AP resection. The surgeon can help limit the volume of tissue irradiated by placing clips to demarcate the tumor bed, allowing the radiation oncologist to more precisely outline the area at risk instead of requiring a more generous treatment volume.[23]

Radiation therapy techniques for limiting the small-bowel dose are numerous and involve the efforts of the radiation oncologist, radiation therapists, and dosimetrists. Prior to CT simulation the patient is given oral contrast to drink to highlight the small bowel on the CT simulation scan. Since the patient is scanned in treatment position, the physician can use this information along with previous imaging studies, such as CT and barium studies, to determine the tumor–small bowel relationship and design the radiation field. Treating the patient in a prone position with a full bladder, shifts the small-bowel superiorly out of the treatment field further reducing the dose to the small bowel (Figure 35-10). Other devices used to minimize the small-bowel dosage are a false tabletop (FTT), or belly board, and an external compression device. The FTT fits over the treatment couch and has an opening to allow the bowel to shift

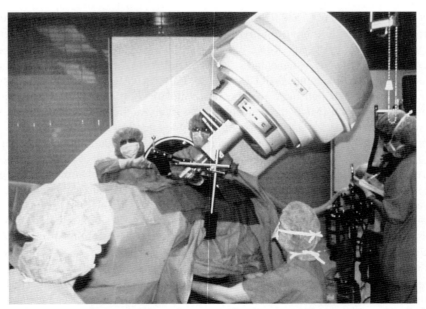

Figure 35-9. Intraoperative radiation therapy with a linear accelerator. Direct irradiation of the tumor bed with a single dose of megavoltage electrons.

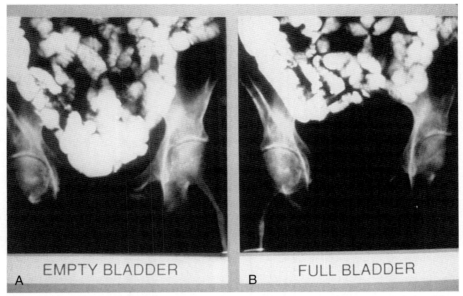

Figure 35-10. Radiographs of the small bowel demonstrating a superior shift of bowel with bladder distention. **A**, Empty bladder. **B**, Full bladder.

anteriorly as a result of gravity when the patient is in the prone position. An FTT is used with bladder distention or an external compression device to shift the small bowel superiorly.[13,23,81 94] Care must be taken to ensure reproducibility of the setup if using any positioning device.

The radiation oncologist and dosimetrist work together to further reduce the small-bowel dose by carefully planning the initial and boost-field volumes through the use of three-dimensional (3D) conformal treatment planning using multileaf collimation (MLC). High-energy beams (≥6 MV) are preferable with 3D conformal because of the depth-dose characteristics that deliver a homogeneous dose to the target volume while allowing the more anterior normal structures to be spared. A multiple-field approach (three or four fields) coupled with weighting of the fields to the posterior in rectal cancer patients further reduces the dose to the anteriorly located small bowel[23,51,53] (Figure 35-11). The use of IMRT is another method reducing dose to small bowel and other normal tissues.[21,83,94]

Role of Radiation Therapist

The radiation therapist plays a major role in the education of patients and their families. Communication is the key factor in making a patient's experience with a cancer diagnosis and treatment less traumatic and anxiety ridden. The therapist's first major role with the patient is in simulation. The therapist should inform the patient that the simulation is not a treatment but a planning session to locate and outline the area requiring treatment. The therapist should describe the procedure to the patient, indicating the length of time it will take and pointing out that the treatments do not require the same amount of time. The patient's position during the treatment should also be discussed. The therapist should inform the patient about the contrast materials that will be used during the procedure, the skin marks to be used to outline radiation portals, and the importance of

maintaining those marks. If using tattoos to indicate treatment isocenter or positioning marks, the patient should be told about the process of a needle stick and the permanency of these marks prior to the simulation to obtain consent. Most patients are treated in the prone position; therefore the therapist should explain the procedure before the patient is positioned. After the simulation begins, the therapist should continually update the patient on what is happening throughout the procedure. Keeping patients informed reduces the anxiety that they may be experiencing. Playing instrumental music during the simulation or treatment can calm and further reduce a patient's anxieties and fears.

At the time of the first treatment, therapists should familiarize patients with the treatment room and the location of the camera and audio equipment and explain what to do if they need something (e.g., raising their right hand). A common fear of patients is being alone in the room. Therapists should discuss the actual length of time that the machine is on per treatment. Therapists should also inform the patients about the types of noises that will be heard as the machine is programmed and treatment is initiated. If the patient's family members are also present, the therapist may offer to show them the treatment room and control area so that they may see the videocamera; however, the family should not be in the control area during the initiation of treatment so that the therapist's performance is not hindered.

The therapist should assess the information given to the patient regarding treatment instructions (e.g., full bladder) and potential side effects. Written materials regarding bladder distention, a low-residue diet, and available support services should be distributed during the first week of treatment.

As treatments progress, the therapist is responsible for inquiring about how the patient is feeling, monitoring any treatment-related side effects, and checking on the patient's

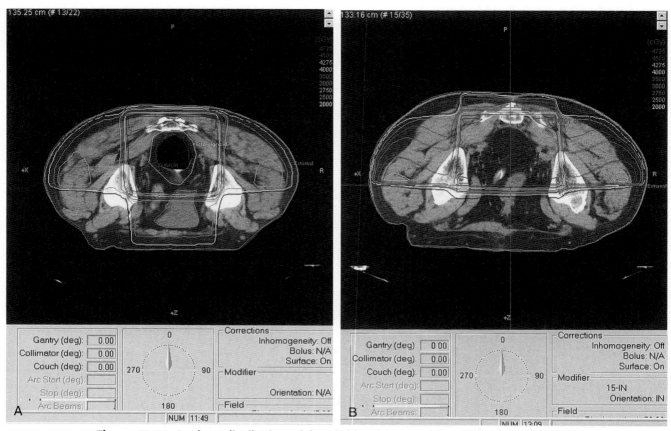

Figure 35-11. Isodose distribution of four-field pelvis technique (**A**) versus three-field technique (**B**). Note the sparing of the anteriorly located small bowel with the three-field technique.

emotional well-being. If the patient complains of abdominal cramping and diarrhea, the therapist should determine whether the patient is following a low-residue diet or has a prescription for an antidiarrheal agent, such as diphenoxylate (Lomotil) or loperamide (Imodium). The therapist should ask the patient about the physician's instructions regarding the prescription. In some instances the patient may not be taking the medication correctly. Dietary suggestions regarding which foods to avoid or recommendations for a low-residue diet are the therapist's responsibility. If the patient is experiencing diarrhea, instructions to avoid whole-grain breads or cereals, fresh fruits, raw vegetables, fried or fatty foods, milk, and milk products may be helpful. Recommended foods include white bread; meats that are baked, broiled, or roasted until tender; peeled apples; bananas; macaroni and noodles; and cooked vegetables[106] (Table 35-2). If the patient still complains of diarrhea after a diet and medications have been discussed, the patient may need to be referred back to the physician or dietitian for further evaluation.

Skin reactions on the perineum are common, especially in patients who have had a combined AP resection in which the entire perineal surface is treated with bolus. Skin reactions range from brisk erythema (treated with topical steroid creams) to moist desquamation (requiring sitz baths, Domeboro's solution, and possibly a treatment break). Therapists play an

important role in monitoring the perineal area, which the patient cannot easily see. The therapist meets with the patient daily and can assess whether the reaction has intensified. The therapist can question patients to determine the way that they are caring for their skin. If the patient has a moist desquamation, recommendations include taking sitz baths in tepid water, wearing loose undergarments or none at all, and allowing the area to be exposed to air and kept dry after the bath. These suggestions keep the area clean, dry and less irritated.

The physical side effects of treatment are often the most visible and easiest to address; however, the therapist must be alert to the emotional needs of the patient and family.

Table 35-2	Dietary Guidelines for Patients Receiving Pelvic Irradiation
Recommended Foods	**Foods to Avoid**
White bread	Whole-grain breads or cereals
Meat baked, broiled, or roasted until tender	Fried or fatty foods
Macaroni	Milk and milk products
Cooked vegetables	Raw vegetables
Peeled apples and bananas	Fresh fruit

The psychosocial aspect of a cancer diagnosis and treatment can be just as painful as the treatment or cancer itself. Therapists are not expected to diagnose but should listen to what the patient is saying and be available to offer suggestions and support. Sometimes, all the patient needs is for someone to listen and know someone cares. The therapist should provide the patient with information about community or hospital services, such as the American Cancer Society (ACS) "I Can Cope" series, the hospital oncology social worker or chaplain, and other support groups in the area. Patients with a colostomy may be having difficulty adjusting to their appliance, so the therapist can refer them to an endostomal therapist for assistance. The therapist should listen to patients and determine the way their diagnosis and treatment has affected their self-image and self-esteem. The ACS has a program called "Look Good, Feel Better" to assist patients in dealing with cosmetic side effects of cancer (primarily hair loss), but the program can also place a more positive outlook on a person's everyday life by stressing the message, "looking good and feeling better."

The ACS's written materials about specific types of cancer or other publications for cancer patients should be handed out or made available to the patient. These are documents that patients can use as references and share with families and friends because the physician gives much of this information verbally to the patient, who may have trouble remembering it. Many patients today access much of the information about their cancer and its treatment on the Internet (for instance, much useful information is posted on the ACS website, www.cancer.org).

The radiation therapist is also responsible for the ensuring the accurate delivery of the radiation treatments. Today, image-guidance radiation therapy (IGRT) is used to ensure radiation fields are correctly aligned before initiating treatment. There are many different types of image guidance technologies. One type is the linear accelerator equipped with a kV imager along with electronic portal imaging device (EPID). The kV imager produces an image of greater contrast and detail than the equivalent EPID image taken with 6 MV photons. Radiation therapists have the responsibility of taking the pretreatment port of the treatment field or orthogonal pair and then matching the bony anatomy on the kV image with the DRR from simulation and applying any shifts (i.e., anterior, posterior, superior) in treatment position prior to turning the beam on. Another IGRT system is cone-beam CT. The Varian Trilogy linear accelerator has the ability to do a one-revolution CT scan. The resultant scan is used to compare cone-beam scan with the simulation CT scan. The simulation CT scan is registered allowing the cone-beam CT to be compared with it. Bony anatomy is matched to determine if any shifts in isocenter are necessary. A physician may be present to confirm or approve shifts in isocenter prior to treatment.

CASE I

Postoperative Rectal

A 70-year-old woman noticed hematochezia (blood in stool) beginning in September 2006. This was not associated with any pain or change in her bowel movements. She was seen by her primary care provider who suggested this was due to hemorrhoids, and she added some fiber to her diet. Over the next several months, the hematochezia persisted and worsened. The patient did not have any weight loss. She did notice some loose stools, and she had some urgency with some bleeding. She then sought medical attention in August 2007. She underwent a sigmoidoscopy that showed a high rectal or sigmoid mass lesion at approximately 20 cm. Biopsy demonstrated grade 3 (of 4) invasive adenocarcinoma. She then underwent a full colonoscopy. This was an incomplete examination due to poor bowel preparation, but the same mass lesion was seen. The patient then had a CT scan of the abdomen and pelvis. The CT showed some thickening of the rectal wall near the area of the sigmoid but no lymphadenopathy. The patient underwent surgery to remove the rectum. The initial plan was to do this laparoscopically, but the patient had difficulty with ventilation during the procedure. There were no other complications and no evidence of any metastatic disease intraoperatively. Pathology demonstrated a 6.6 × 5.2 × 1.1 cm ulcerating mass. The tumor infiltrated through the muscularis propria to involve the perirectal fat and the serosa. Surgical margins were negative. Forty lymph nodes were removed and were negative for tumor. The patient has a stage IIA (T3 N0, M0) rectal adenocarcinoma. Postoperative adjuvant chemoradiation is being recommended due to the risk for local recurrence with a T3 tumor. The patient was treated with a three-field technique, PA, and opposed laterals to a dose of 5040 cGy and received concomitant chemotherapy.

ANAL CANCER

Epidemiology and Etiology

Cancers of the anus occur more often in women than in men and constitute approximately 1% to 2% of all large-bowel malignancies.[98] In 2008, the American Cancer Society predicts 5070 new cases of anal cancer will occur—3050 will occur in women, while 2020 will occur in men.[4] The median age at the time of diagnosis is 60. A general age distribution of 30 to 90 years is reported. There has been an increased incidence of cancers in men younger than 45 years. This trend has been attributed to male homosexuality and anal intercourse. The etiologic factors for the development of anal cancer are associated with genital warts, genital infections, human papillomaviruses (HPVs), anal intercourse in men or women before age 30, and immunosuppression.[4] HPV-16 is the type of HPV found in squamous cell cancers of the anus. It is also found in some genital and anal warts. HPV has been found to make two proteins, E6 and E7, that are able to shut down two tumor suppressor proteins, p53 and Rb, in normal cells. When these tumor suppressors are rendered inactive, cells can become cancerous.[4,64] Cigarette smoking has also been associated with the development of anal cancer.[31,49,98,100]

Anatomy and Lymphatics

The anal canal is 3 to 4 cm long and extends from the anal verge to the anorectal ring at the junction of the anus and rectum. The anal canal is lined with a hairless, stratified squamous epithelium up to the dentate or pectinate line. At this line the mucosa becomes cuboidal in transition to the columnar epithelium found in the rectum.[31,98]

Lymphatic spread occurs initially to the perirectal and anorectal lymph nodes. If the tumor extends above the dentate line, the nodal groups at risk are the internal iliac and lateral sacral nodes; this is similar to rectal cancer. With involvement below the dentate line, inguinal lymph nodes may be involved. Inguinal lymph node involvement is found in approximately 10% to 30% of patients.[64,98]

Clinical Presentation

The most common presenting symptoms is rectal bleeding. Other symptoms are pain, change in bowel habits, and the sensation of a mass.[4,64] Pruritus or itching has been reported less often and is associated with a perianal lesion.[4,31,98]

Detection and Diagnosis

A thorough physical examination should be performed. This includes a digital anorectal examination (noting anal sphincter tone and direct extension to other organs) and palpation of the inguinal lymph nodes. Anoscopy and/or proctoscopic examination and biopsy should be obtained. A further workup includes a CT scan of the abdomen and pelvis to evaluate the liver and perirectal, inguinal, pelvic, and paraaortic nodes. A PET scan to further assess spread of tumor to lymph nodes or liver or MRI has been advocated. Transrectal sonography may also be done to determine depth of invasion into the bowel wall.[4,64] A chest radiograph, a CBC, and liver function tests will also be performed.

Pathology, Staging, and Routes of Spread

Squamous cell carcinoma is the most common histology of anal cancer, comprising approximately 80% of the cases. The next most frequent type is basaloid, or cloacogenic, cancer. These tumors occur in the region of the dentate line where the epithelium is in transition. Also found in this region are adenocarcinoma (arising from the anal glands), mucoepidermoid tumors, and melanoma. Cancers occurring in the perianal region are typically squamous or basal cell carcinomas consistent with skin cancers.

The most commonly used staging system is the AJCC system. This is a clinical system in which tumors are staged according to their size and extent (Box 35-2).

Tumors of the anal canal spread most frequently by direct extension into the adjacent soft tissues. Lymphatic spread occurs relatively early, whereas hematogenous spread to the liver or lungs is less common.

Treatment Techniques

Combination radiation therapy and chemotherapy (5-FU and mitomycin C) is advocated as the preferred method of treatment and considered the standard of care for most patients.[64] Radiation alone is advocated for patients who cannot tolerate chemoradiation.[100] Studies have shown that the multimodality (radiation and chemotherapy) approach provides good local control and colostomy-free survival.[80,98,100] Most series report survival rates from 65% to 80% at 5 years, with a local control rate of 60% to 89%.[64,98] An AP resection with a wide perineal dissection is the most common surgical procedure for anal cancer. This procedure is no longer done as the initial treatment but is done in the case of local recurrence following conventional chemoradiation.[4,64]

A variety of radiation techniques exist for the treatment of anal cancer. Traditionally, a four-field or AP/PA pelvic-field with electron fields to the inguinal nodes including a boost to the tumor bed with a perineal electron field or another multifield technique has been used. The pelvic field extends from the

---

Box 35-2	American Joint Committee on Cancer Staging System for Anal Cancer

DEFINITION OF TNM
The following is the TNM classification for the staging of cancers that arise in the anal canal only. Cancers that arise at the anal margin are staged according to the classification for cancers of the skin.

PRIMARY TUMOR (T)
TX   Primary tumor cannot be assessed
T0   No evidence of primary tumor
Tis Carcinoma in situ
T1   Tumor 2 cm or less in greatest dimension
T2   Tumor more than 2 cm but not more than 5 cm in greatest dimension
T3   Tumor more than 5 cm in greatest dimension
T4   Tumor of any size invades adjacent organ(s), e.g., vagina, urethra, bladder (involvement of the sphincter muscle[s] alone is not classified as T4)

REGIONAL LYMPH NODES (N)
NX   Regional lymph nodes cannot be assessed
N0   No regional lymph node metastasis
N1   Metastasis in perirectal lymph node(s)
N2   Metastasis in unilateral internal iliac and/or inguinal lymph node(s)

N3   Metastasis in perirectal and inguinal lymph nodes and/or bilateral internal iliac and/or inguinal lymph nodes

DISTANT METASTASIS (M)
MX   Distant metastasis cannot be assessed
M0   No distant metastasis
M1   Distant metastasis

STAGE GROUPING

Stage	T	N	M
Stage 0	Tis	N0	M0
Stage I	T1	N0	M0
Stage II	T2	N0	M0
	T3	N0	M0
Stage IIIA	T1	N1	M0
	T2	N1	M0
	T3	N1	M0
	T4	N0	M0
Stage IIIB	T4	N1	M0
	Any T	N2	M0
	Any T	N3	M0
Stage IV	Any T	Any N	M1

With permission from American Joint Committee on Cancer (AJCC), Chicago, IL: *AJCC Cancer Staging Manual*, ed 6, New York, 2002, Springer-Verlag.

lumbosacral-sacroiliac region to 3 cm distal to the lowest extent of the tumor (noted by a radiopaque marker at the time of simulation). The inferior border typically flashes the perineum, resulting in brisk erythema and moist desquamation of the perineal tissues. The lateral border may extend to include treatment of the inguinal lymph nodes on the AP field only, placing that field edge at the midlateral aspect of the femoral heads. The PA field is kept narrower because the anteriorly located inguinal nodes do not receive much contribution from the posterior field. This also avoids an excessive dose to the femoral heads, yet encompasses the tumor bed and deep pelvic nodes. Anterior electron fields centered over each inguinal region and abutting the PA lateral border are used to further supplement the dose to the inguinal lymph nodes.[100]

The dose regimen used with radiation alone is 6000 to 6500 cGy delivered to the region of the primary tumor with a field reduction after 4500 cGy to reduce small bowel toxicity. With combined modality treatment, a dose of 3060 to 4500 cGy to the pelvis and inguinal nodes is used followed by a shrinking field boost with an additional 1440 to 2440 cGy delivered to the primary tumor. A higher total dose is advocated for T3 or T4 disease.[64]

Chemoradiation, although a very effective treatment, is associated with much acute toxicity. Almost all patients experience a perineal skin reaction, with about half of the patients encountering a moist desquamation. Nausea, vomiting and mild to moderate diarrhea is also reported. The most severe and life-threatening complication is bone marrow suppression from the irradiation to the pelvis and the 5-FU and mitomycin regimen.[64] Radiation therapists are responsible for monitoring a patient's blood counts and reporting any low counts, including the absolute neutrophil count, to the radiation oncologist. The radiation therapist sees the patient daily and should keep a watchful eye on the perineal skin and advise patient on proper skin care. The radiation therapist should also refer patient to the oncology nurse or radiation oncologist for further advisement on skin care in case a break in treatment is warranted.

There are many structures identified as OARs when treating anal cancer such as the femoral head and necks, genitalia/perineum, small bowel, and bladder. For this reason, IMRT is being used and studied in the treatment of anal cancer. The structures to avoid and respective dose limits are entered into the planning system as are the prescribed dose to the primary target volume and lymph nodes. IMRT's inverse planning allows doses to be conformed to the primary tumor and has shown improved dosimetric coverage of inguinal lymph nodes. The use of IMRT greatly reduces the doses to normal tissues (OARs) compared with the conventional 3D conformal AP/PA technique.[43,84]

In conclusion, radiation therapy in combination with chemotherapy or radiation therapy alone is considered the standard of care for the treatment of anal cancer providing sphincter preservation and satisfactory cure rates.

CASE II

Inguinal Lymph Node

A 66-year-old woman has noticed some blood on the toilet paper over the past couple of years. She recently has also had some fullness in her anal canal.

Her last colonoscopy was about 4 years ago and she was told it was normal. She was seen by a gastroenterologist who noted there was a 1.5-cm nodule in the posterior aspect of her anal canal. Several biopsies were taken and were not found conclusive for invasive squamous cell carcinoma but were positive for squamous cell carcinoma in situ. The patient was then seen by colorectal surgery consultants. At this consult, it was thought that the lesion was extending from the anal verge above the dentate line and the tissue above it. This was again biopsied. While biopsy results were pending, the patient underwent a CT scan of the abdomen and pelvis. The scan showed evidence of a large inguinal lymph node on the left hand side measuring approximately 2.5 cm in greatest dimension. The patient underwent an sonography-guided biopsy of the left inguinal lymph node with an 18-gauge core biopsy device. The lymph node at the time was barely palpable, but it was seen on a CT scan. Unfortunately, the pathology from that biopsy was positive for metastatic squamous cell carcinoma. She was referred to radiation and medical oncology.

The radiation oncologist recommended a course of radiation therapy in conjunction with chemotherapy. A dose of 5400 cGy with 180-cGy daily fraction size for 30 treatments was prescribed. The radiation oncologist did discuss with the patient the short- and long-term side effects of radiation with concurrent chemotherapy for invasive anal carcinoma. The patient was informed that this can be quite a morbid treatment with irritation of the perineum and anal canal, particularly toward the end of an approximately 6-week course of radiation therapy. The long-term side effects can also include anal stricture, vaginal dryness, thinning of the bone, and change in bowel habits from her prechemoradiation habits. The patient was treated using IMRT technique with nine fields. The fields consisted of eight obliques (P20R, P60R, A80R, A40R, P20L, P60L, A80L, A40L) and one anterior field. The patient also received 5-FU and mitomycin C during her radiation therapy.

ESOPHAGEAL CANCER

Epidemiology and Etiology

Cancer of the esophagus accounts for 1% of all cancers in the United States, with approximately 16470 cases estimated in 2008.[8] Men are 3 to 4 times more commonly affected than are women (12,970 versus 3500, respectively). African Americans have a 50% higher incidence than do whites.[5,8] Most cancers of the esophagus are diagnosed in patients between 55 and 85 years of age.[8] Esophageal cancer is usually diagnosed at an advance stage and is nearly a uniformly fatal disease. In 2008, the American Cancer Society estimated 14280 esophageal cancer–related deaths will occur in the United States. Esophageal cancer is the seventh leading cause of cancer-related deaths in men in the United States.[5,8] Survival rates have been improving, with 17% of whites and 12% of African Americans surviving 5 years after diagnosis.[8]

Cancer of the esophagus occurs with the greatest frequency in northern China, northern Iran, and South Africa.[8] This has been attributed to environmental and nutritional factors.[37,40,96]

There are many risk factors or etiologic factors that contribute to the development of esophageal cancer. Certain risk factors increase one's chance of developing a squamous cell carcinoma or adenonocarcinoma of the esophagus.[8] For example, the most common and important etiologic factors in the development of squamous cell cancer of the esophagus in Western countries are excessive alcohol and tobacco use. Alcohol and tobacco abuse are associated with 80% to 90% of all cases diagnosed in North America and Western Europe. The combination of these two factors has a synergistic effect on the mucosal surfaces, increasing the risk of esophageal cancer and other aerodigestive malignancies.[37,40,96] Excessive alcohol use has been an implicated risk factor for the development of squamous cell carcinomas. The use of tobacco products has shown to cause about 50% of squamous cell carcinomas. Tobacco use has also been shown to increase an individual's chance of developing adenocarinoma of the esophagus.[8]

Barrett's esophagus is a condition in which the distal esophagus is lined with a columnar epithelium rather than a stratified squamous epithelium. This mucosal change usually occurs with gastroesophageal (GE) reflux. One theory to explain this phenomenon is that chronic chemical trauma resulting from reflux causes the mucosa to undergo metaplasia leading to various degrees of dysplasia that are precancerous.[8,93,96] Adenocarcinoma of the esophagus occurs in patients with a history of Barrett's esophagus.

Longstanding gastroesophageal reflux disease (GERD) is associated with the development of adenocarcinomas of the distal esophagus. Approximately 30% of esophageal cancers are associated with GERD.[8] Patient's with GERD may or may not develop Barrett's esophagus.[8]

Dietary factors have also been implicated in the development of cancer of the esophagus. Diets low in fresh fruits and vegetables and high in nitrates (i.e., cured meats and fish, pickled vegetables) have been cited as risk factors for persons from Iran, China, and South Africa. A diet high in fruits and vegetables is considered a preventive measure against the development of esophageal and other cancers. Overweight and obesity have been linked to the development of adenocarcinomas in men.[8]

Other conditions predispose individuals to the development of esophageal cancer. They include achalasia, Plummer-Vinson syndrome, caustic injury, and tylosis.

Achalasia is a disorder in which the lower two thirds of the esophagus loses its normal peristaltic activity. The esophagus becomes dilated (termed megaesophagus), and the esophagogastric junction sphincter also fails to relax, prohibiting the passage of food into the stomach. Clinical symptoms include progressive dysphagia and regurgitation of ingested food. Patients with achalasia have a 5% to 20% risk of developing squamous cell cancer of the esophagus.[8,93,96]

Plummer-Vinson syndrome (also known as Paterson-Kelly syndrome) is an iron-deficient anemia characterized by esophageal webs, atrophic glossitis, and spoon-shaped, brittle fingernails. This syndrome occurs mostly in women. This condition is a risk factor for the development of squamous cell carcinoma.[8]

Caustic injuries and burns caused by the ingestion of lye are responsible for 1% to 4% of esophageal squamous cell cancers. Malignancies develop in the scarred, or stricture, area years after an injury.[93,96]

Tylosis is a rare inherited disorder that causes excessive skin growth on the palms of the hands and soles of the feet. Individuals with this condition are at significant risk of about 40% of developing a squamous cell carcinoma. A mutation on chromosome 17 is thought to cause tylosis and the associated squamous cell carcinoma.[8]

Many believe that some risk factors, such as use of tobacco or alcohol abuse, cause esophageal cancer by damaging the DNA of cells that line the inside of the esophagus. The DNA of esophageal cancer cells microscopically often shows many abnormalities; however, there have been no special changes described that are typical of this cancer. Long-term irritation of the lining of the esophagus—as with GERD, Barrett esophagus, achalasia, esophageal webs, or scarring from swallowing lye—can promote the formation of cancers.[8]

Prognostic Indicators

Tumor size is an important prognostic tool. According to a series by Hussey et al.,[40] patients with tumors less than 5 cm in length had a better 2-year survival rate (19.2%) than did patients with lesions larger than 9 cm (1.9%). Tumors 5 cm or less in length were more often localized (40% to 60%), whereas tumors larger than 5 cm had distant metastasis 75% of the time.[40,96] Other factors indicating a poor prognosis are weight loss of 10%, a poor performance status, and age greater than 65.

Anatomy and Lymphatics

The esophagus is a thin-walled 25-cm-long tube lined with stratified squamous epithelium. The esophagus begins at the level of C6 and traverses through the thoracic cage to terminate in the abdomen at the esophageal gastric (E-G) junction (T10-11).

For accurate classification, staging, and recording of tumors in the esophagus, the AJCC has divided the esophagus into four regions: cervical, upper thoracic, middle thoracic, and lower thoracic. Because lesions are localized by an endoscopy, reference is made to the distance of the lesion from the upper incisors (front teeth). This distance is also used in defining each region[41,96] (Figure 35-12).

The cervical esophagus extends from the cricoid cartilage to the thoracic inlet (suprasternal notch [SSN]), corresponding to vertebral levels C6 to T2-3 and measuring about 18 cm from the upper incisors. The thoracic inlet (SSN) to the level of the tracheal bifurcation (carina)—24 cm from the incisors—defines the upper thoracic portion. The middle thoracic esophagus begins at the carina and extends proximally to the E-G junction, or 32 cm from the incisors. The lower thoracic portion includes the abdominal esophagus and is approximately 8 cm long at a level of 40 cm from the incisors.[41,96]

The esophagus lies directly posterior to the trachea and is anterior to the vertebral column. Located laterally and to the left of the esophagus is the aortic arch. The descending aorta is situated lateral and posterior to the esophagus (see Figure 35-12). During an endoscopy an indentation is visible where the aorta and left mainstem bronchus are in contact with the esophagus. Because of the esophagus' intimate relationship with these structures, tumors are often locally advanced, fistulas may occur, and surgery is often not feasible.[34,87,96]

Histologically, the esophagus consists of the usual layers of the bowel common to the gastrointestinal tract (i.e., the mucosa, submucosa, and muscular layers). However, the esophagus lacks a serosal layer. The outermost layer, the adventitia, consists of a thin, loose connective tissue. This is another factor

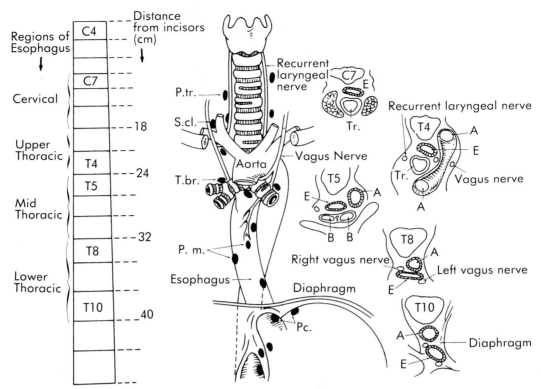

Figure 35-12. The relationship of the esophagus with surrounding anatomic structures, including divisions of the esophagus and their location from the upper central incisors. (From Cox JD: *Moss' radiation oncology: rationale, techniques, results*, ed 7, St. Louis, 1994, Mosby.)

contributing to the early spread of these tumors to adjacent structures.[40,87]

The esophagus has numerous small lymphatic vessels in the mucosa and submucosal layers. These vessels drain outward into larger vessels located in the muscular layers (Figure 35-13). Lymph fluid can travel the entire length of the esophagus and drain into any adjacent draining nodal bed, placing the entire esophagus at risk for skip metastasis and nodal involvement.[39,40,87,96]

Although the entire length of the esophagus is at risk for lymphatic metastasis, each region still has primary or regional nodes that specifically drain the area. For example, the upper third (cervical area) of the esophagus drains into the internal jugular, cervical, paraesophageal, and supraclavicular lymph nodes. The upper and middle thoracic portion has drainage to the paratracheal, hilar, subcarinal, paraesophageal, and paracardial lymph nodes. Finally, the principal draining lymphatics for

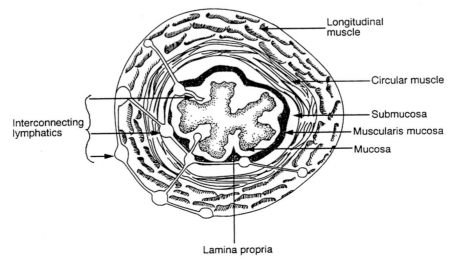

Figure 35-13. Lymphatic vessels located in the wall of the esophagus. (From Cox JD: *Moss' radiation oncology: rationale, techniques, results*, ed 7, St. Louis, 1994, Mosby.)

the distal or lower third of the esophagus include the celiac axis, left gastric nodes, and nodes of the lesser curvature of the stomach (Figure 35-14). Lymphatic spread is unpredictable and may occur at a significant distance from the tumor. Nodes positive for tumor outside a defined region represent distant metastasis rather than regional spread. For example, supraclavicular nodal involvement in a primary tumor located in the cervical esophagus is considered regional lymph node involvement, but this would be a distant metastasis for tumors arising in the thoracic esophagus.[34,41]

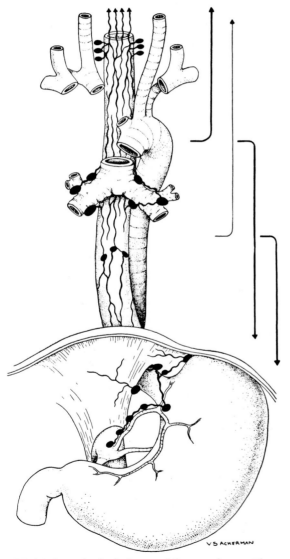

Figure 35-14. Lymphatic drainage of the esophagus. The *arrows* represent potential spread to cervical, mediastinal, and subdiaphragmatic lymph nodes, based on the location of the esophageal lesion. Subdiaphragmatic involvement is unusual in the upper-third tumors. (From del Regato JA, Spjut HJ, Cox JD: *Ackerman and del Regato's cancer: diagnosis, treatment, and prognosis,* ed 6, St. Louis, 1985, Mosby.)

Clinical Presentation

The most common presenting symptoms are dysphagia and weight loss, which occur in 90% of patients. Patients complain of food sticking in their throat or chest and may point to the location of this sensation. Initially, patients have difficulty with bulky foods, then with soft foods, and finally even with liquids. Patients may recall having this difficulty in swallowing for 3 to 6 months before the diagnosis. Regurgitation of undigested food and aspiration pneumonia may also occur. **Odynophagia** (painful swallowing) is reported in approximately 50% of patients. Symptoms of a locally advanced tumor include the following: hematemesis (vomiting blood), coughing (caused by a tracheoesophageal fistula), hemoptysis, Horner's syndrome, or hoarseness as a result of nerve involvement.[15,37,40,96]

Detection and Diagnosis

A thorough history and physical examination should be performed. Information should be obtained regarding weight loss and the use of alcohol and tobacco. The physical examination should include palpation of the cervical and supraclavicular lymph nodes and abdomen to assess potential spread to the nodes or liver. A chest radiograph and barium swallow are necessary for localizing the lesions causing the dysphagia. A barium swallow will depict characteristic features of esophageal cancers. The reported incidence of tumors located in each third of the esophagus varies in the literature. Lesions in the upper third of the esophagus occur with the least frequency, accounting for 10% to 25% of tumors. Approximately 40% to 50% of tumors are located in the middle third of the esophagus, and 25% to 50% are located in the lower third.[37,40,96]

A CT scan of the chest and upper abdomen should be obtained. This scan may demonstrate extramucosal spread and invasion of adjacent structures such as the trachea or aorta. Spread to lymph nodes in the thorax and abdomen can be also assessed. Bloodborne metastases to the liver and adrenals may be imaged via CT, although small lesions may not be detectable.[8,15]

A sonogram of suspicious liver nodules is performed to differentiate metastasis from a cystic mass.[15,37,40,96] Laboratory studies include a CBC and blood chemistry group to assess the liver and kidney function.

A histologic confirmation is obtained during an esophagoscopy. A rigid or flexible endoscope can be used to examine the entire esophagus, obtaining brushings and biopsies of all suspicious lesions. EUS is also helpful for visualizing the tumor, its depth of invasion, and lymph node status.[2,25,41,96] A bronchoscopy should also be performed for all upper- or middle-third lesions to detect any possible communication or fistula of the tumor with the tracheobronchial tree.[37,40,96]

PET has become a more routine test for the staging work-up of patients with esophageal cancer. Fluorodeoxyglucose (FDG), a sugar, is taken up by cancer cells because of their high mitotic activity. The PET scan has detected smaller, microscopic metastasis to lymph nodes and distant organs such as the liver that did not show up on a CT scan.[8,15]

DEFINITION OF TNM

PRIMARY TUMOR (T)

TX	Primary tumor cannot be assessed
T0	No evidence of primary tumor
Tis	Carcinoma in situ
T1	Tumor invades lamina propria or submucosa
T2	Tumor invades muscularis propria
T3	Tumor invades adventitia
T4	Tumor invades adjacent structures

REGIONAL LYMPH NODES (N)

NX	Regional lymph nodes cannot be assessed
N0	No regional lymph node metastasis
N1	Regional lymph node metastasis

DISTANT METASTASIS (M)

MX	Distant metastasis cannot be assessed
M0	No distant metastasis
M1	Distant metastasis

TUMORS OF THE LOWER THORACIC ESOPHAGUS

M1a	Metastasis in celiac lymph nodes
M1b	Other distant metastasis

TUMORS OF THE MIDTHORACIC ESOPHAGUS

M1a	Not applicable
M1b	Nonregional lymph nodes and/or other distant metastasis

TUMORS OF THE UPPER THORACIC ESOPHAGUS

M1a	Metastasis in cervical nodes
M1b	Other distant metastasis

STAGE GROUPING

Stage 0	Tis	N0	M0
Stage I	T1	N0	M0
Stage IIA	T2	N0	M0
	T3	N0	M0
Stage IIB	T1	N1	M0
	T2	N1	M0
Stage III	T3	N1	M0
	T4	Any N	M0
Stage IV	Any T	Any N	M1
Stage IVA	Any T	Any N	M1a
Stage IVB	Any T	Any N	M1b

With permission from American Joint Committee on Cancer (AJCC), Chicago, IL: *AJCC Cancer Staging Manual*, ed 6, New York, 2002, Springer-Verlag.

Pathology and Staging

The most common pathologic types of esophageal cancer are squamous cell carcinoma and adenocarcinoma. Squamous cell carcinomas are found most frequently in the upper and middle thoracic esophagus.[15] Adenocarcinoma typically occurs in the distal esophagus and GE junction, however, it can occur in other regions of the esophagus. In the United States, the incidence of squamous cell carcinoma has been declining while adenocarcinoma has been increasing in frequency.[8,15] Squamous cell carcinoma is the most common type of cancer that occurs in African Americans. Adenocarcinoma is more common in whites.[8,15] A variety of other epithelial tumors arise in the esophagus but are rare. These include adenoid cystic carcinoma, mucoepidermoid carcinoma, adenosquamous carcinoma, and undifferentiated carcinoma.[40,96]

Nonepithelial tumors also arise in the esophagus, although this is rare. Leiomyosarcoma (a tumor of the smooth muscle) is the most common nonepithelial tumor. Leiomyosarcomas yield a more favorable prognosis than squamous cell carcinomas. Malignant melanoma, lymphoma, and rhabdomyosarcoma are other nonepithelial tumors that can occur in the esophagus.[40,96]

The AJCC staging system for esophageal cancer is shown in Box 35-3.

Routes of Spread

Because the esophagus is distensible, lesions are large before causing obstructive symptoms. Spread is usually longitudinal. Occasionally, skip lesions may be present at a significant distance from the primary lesion. This is principally due to submucosal spread of the tumor through interconnecting lymph channels. Locally advanced disease, invasion into adjacent structures, and early spread to draining lymphatics are common in esophageal cancer. Because the esophagus lacks a serosa layer, tracheoesophageal fistula or bronchoesophageal fistulas may easily occur.[15] Distant metastasis can occur in many different organs, with the liver and lung being the most common.

Treatment Techniques

The treatment of esophageal cancer is highly complex and technically difficult. Most patients have locally advanced or metastatic disease at the time of diagnosis and require multimodality treatment. Treatment is usually categorized as curative or palliative and may be given with surgery or radiation for the locoregional problem and chemotherapy for distant spread of disease. Patients who receive either modality (surgery or radiation) alone have a significant risk of local recurrence and distant metastasis. The primary goal of either treatment is to provide relief of the dysphagia and a chance for cure. Many different combined modality treatment regimens are being studied to determine if one approach provides a better local control and survival outcome than others. The two most commonly used combined modality techniques are definitive chemoradiation therapy and neoadjuvant preoperative chemoradiotherapy.[3,15,45,70,78,95,102] Definitive chemoradiation therapy has been the current nonsurgical standard for the treatment of esophageal cancer.[53,67] Current studies are evaluating preoperative chemoradiotherapy with different chemotherapeutic agents and definitive chemoradiotherapy for locoregional cancers of the esophagus.

A variety of surgical techniques exist for the resection of esophageal cancer. In many centers, surgical resection is limited to the middle and lower thirds of the esophagus. The cervical esophagus is not considered a surgically accessible site in many institutions and is often managed with radiation therapy and chemotherapy. Curative surgery usually involves a subtotal or total esophagectomy. The type of procedure chosen depends on the location of the lesion and extent of involvement. Typically, the entire esophagus is removed. The continuity of the gastrointestinal system is maintained by placing either the stomach or left colon in the thoracic cavity. The Ivor Lewis procedure, also called transthoracic resection, consists of a laparotomy and right thoracotomy to remove the esophagus and mobilize the stomach into the thoracic cavity (Figure 35-15). The transhiatal approach esophagectomy also requires multiple surgical incisions. A laparotomy is performed to mobilize the stomach and remove the esophagus. A second incision is made at the neck to assist in the anastomosis of the stomach to the remaining cervical esophagus* (Figure 35-16).

Both of these procedures are technically difficult and associated with a high morbidity and mortality rate. Operative mortality rates from either procedure have ranged from 8% to 31%, although recent studies have demonstrated a decrease in these rates. Complications from surgery include anastomotic leaks (which can be life threatening), respiratory failure, pulmonary embolus, and myocardial infarctions. Strictures, difficulty in gastric emptying, and GE reflux are mechanical side effects resulting from surgery.

Even after a curative resection, most patients fail distantly with blood-borne spread to the lungs, liver, or bone.

Radiation Therapy. Radiation and concomitant chemotherapy remain the treatment standard.[2,25,26,97] Preoperative chemoradiation followed by curative surgery is also routinely being done with ongoing studies to evaluate the outcome of the treatment. Preliminary results show a slight improvement in survival.[3,15,45,78,95,102] Radiation therapy with chemotherapy is considered the current nonsurgical treatment of choice for esophageal cancer. Recent studies demonstrated a clear advantage for radiation therapy and chemotherapy compared with radiation therapy alone.[2,25,26,97] Radiation therapy alone might be used in patients who are medically unable to undergo combined modality treatment.

Chemotherapy. The poor survival rates resulting from esophageal cancer are associated with the high percentage of patients who fail locally and with distant metastases after curative treatment. The addition of combination chemotherapy has resulted in a decrease in local and distant failures and an increase in the overall survival rate compared with radiation alone[67] (Figures 35-17 and 35-18).

Continuous-infusion 5-FU and cisplatin are the standard drugs used in the treatment of esophageal cancer administered during weeks 1, 5, 8, and 11 of the radiation therapy treatments. Combined modality therapy has definite local control and survival benefits. However, the side effects from this regimen are worse.[26] New drugs and different combinations of chemotherapy and radiation are being researched. Paclitaxel, taxotere, CPT-11, and carboplatin are being evaluated.[†] Induction chemotherapy prior to preoperative chemoradiotherapy and surgery is a regimen currently being studied. This has also been called the three-step approach. The first step is induction

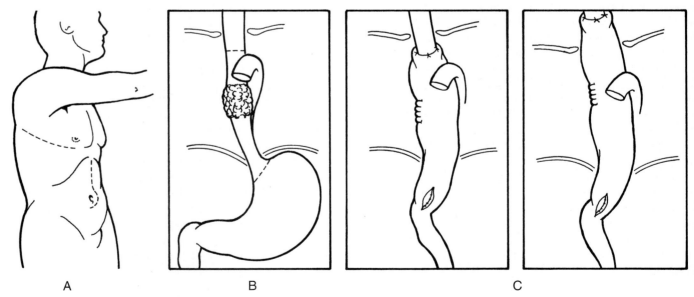

A   B   C

Figure 35-15. The Ivor Lewis procedure. **A,** Laparotomy and right thoracotomy. **B,** Tumor and margin of resection. **C,** Mobilization of the stomach into the chest cavity with anastomosis to the remaining esophagus (esophagogastrostomy). (Redrawn from Ellis FH Jr: Esophagogastrectomy for carcinoma: technical considerations based on anatomic location of lesion, *Surg Clin North Am* 60:273, 1980.)

*References 2, 15, 25, 26, 37, 47, 68, 96, 97.
†References 1, 3, 45, 59, 78, 95, 102.

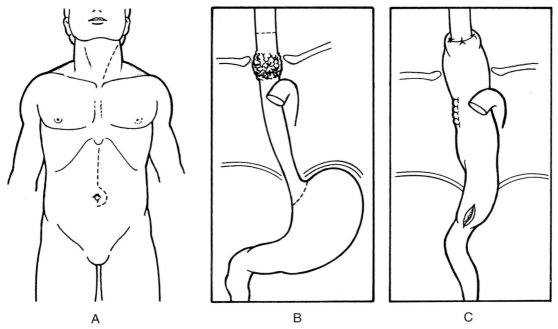

Figure 35-16. A, Laparotomy and left cervical incision. **B**, Tumor and margin of the resection. **C**, Mobilization of the stomach into the chest cavity with anastomosis to the cervical esophagus via a neck incision. (Redrawn from Ellis FH Jr: Esophagogastrectomy for carcinoma: technical considerations based on anatomic location of lesion, *Surg Clin North Am* 60:275, 1980.)

chemotherapy. CPT-11 (camptothecin-11) and cisplatin was given in one study as induction therapy, while another study used 5-FU, cisplatin, and paclitaxel. This was followed by chemoradiotherapy, with continuous-infusion 5-FU and paclitaxel. The third step was surgery.[3,78] Administering chemotherapy prior to the chemoradiotherapy is thought to shrink the primary tumor and make the chemoradiotherapy more effective.[3,78] Preliminary results showed an increase in tumor response in the induction chemotherapy group versus conventional chemoradiotherapy that may translate into longer disease free and overall survival.[78]

Field Design and Critical Structures. Esophageal cancer spreads longitudinally with skip lesions up to 5 cm from the primary. Regional spread to draining lymphatics is a common early presentation and must be taken into consideration in the design of the radiation field. The cervical, supraclavicular, mediastinal, and subdiaphragmatic (celiac axis) lymph node regions are at risk. The degree to which these nodal groups are

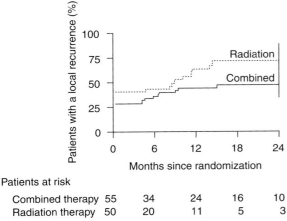

Patients at risk

Combined therapy	55	34	24	16	10
Radiation therapy	50	20	11	5	3

Figure 35-17. A comparison of radiation alone with combined radiation and chemotherapy regarding the time to a local recurrence in patients with esophageal cancer. (From Herskovic A, et al: Combined chemotherapy and radiotherapy compared with radiotherapy alone in patients with cancer of the esophagus, *N Engl J Med* 326:1596, 1992.)

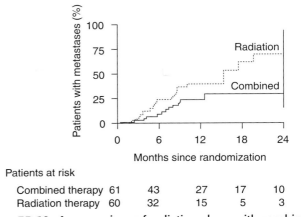

Patients at risk

Combined therapy	61	43	27	17	10
Radiation therapy	60	32	15	5	3

Figure 35-18. A comparison of radiation alone with combined radiation and chemotherapy regarding the time to a distant metastasis in patients with esophageal cancer. (Modified from Herskovic A, et al: Combined chemotherapy and radiotherapy compared with radiotherapy alone in patients with cancer of the esophagus, *N Engl J Med* 326:1595, 1992)

at risk depends on the location of the primary tumor. Supraclavicular nodes are involved more often with a proximal lesion than a distal lesion. However, neck or abdominal nodal-disease involvement can occur with any esophageal primary site.[2,26,44,97]

Because of the potential for longitudinal spread of these cancers, radiation portals encompassing the areas at risk are typically large. This volume is necessary for including the regional lymphatics and encompassing the primary tumor with a 5-cm margin above and below the gross tumor volume (GTV). The planning target volume (PTV) is also expanded to 2 to 2.5 cm for radial or lateral margins.[3,15,70,78,95,102] Lesions of the upper third of the esophagus are treated with a field that begins at the level of the thyroid cartilage and ends at the level of the carina to include supraclavicular, low anterior cervical, and mediastinal lymph nodes.[15] In patients with tumors of the distal third of the esophagus the inferior margin must include the celiac-axis lymph nodes, which are located at the T12-L1 vertebral level. The superior extent of the treatment field should include the mediastinal nodes and may not include the supraclavicular nodes because they are at a low risk of being involved.[2,3,15,40,60,70,96,97] For tumors of the mid-thoracic esophagus the anatomic borders included in the treatment field include the periesophageal lymph nodes and mediastinal nodes but may not include the supraclavicular fossa or the esophagogastric junction.[15]

The standard technique for treating the initial large fields is an AP/PA field, followed by shrinking fields of various arrangements. For treatment with radiation alone the prescribed dose is 65 Gy. With combined radiation and chemotherapy the total dose is 50.4 Gy to minimize normal tissue toxicity. Both of these doses exceed the radiation-tolerance dose of the spinal cord, which is 45 to 50 Gy. Careful dosimetry planning is necessary to avoid overdosing the spinal cord. AP/PA fields are used initially; as cord tolerance is approached, an off-cord technique is implemented. With CT simulation and 3D conformal planning capabilities, the AP/PA fields and oblique off-cord fields are frequently treated simultaneously. The AP/PA fields are discontinued as cord tolerance is reached. In recent years, the off cord technique at some institutions is initiated when the spinal cord has reached a dose of 30 to 36 Gy instead of 45 Gy.[70,102] A variety of off-cord field arrangements can be used, depending on the location of the tumor. The most common field arrangements are oblique and lateral radiation portals. Many institutions use a three-field approach: an anterior field and two posterior-wedged obliques, especially for lesions of the thoracic esophagus. Two anterior-wedged obliques or parallel-opposed oblique fields have also been used for lesions of the upper or middle third of the esophagus[40,60,70,96] (Figure 35-19). Another common off-cord technique in distal esophageal or GE junction lesions is opposed laterals with AP/PA fields.[2,3,15,25,26,70,97,102]

For the simulation of a patient with esophageal cancer, a variety of patient positions have been advocated. Some authors advise placing the patient in the prone position, using gravity to help place the esophagus at a greater distance from the spinal cord. This facilitates lower cord doses without compromising the tumor dose.[27,40] More universal is the standard supine position for patient simulation and treatment. Older patients and those who are more ill can tolerate this position easier and for a longer time than the prone position.

Other patient-positioning issues deal with the placement of the patient's arms. Because lateral treatment-field arrangements may be used, the patient's arms are often positioned above the head, with the patient clasping the elbows or wrists. This position can be difficult for the patient to hold and maintain, causing reproducibility problems later during treatment. Custom-made immobilization devices such as body casts, foaming cradles, and vacuum-bag devices greatly assist the daily reproducibility of the setup. With or without a custom-made device, measurements of the elbow-to-elbow separation and a photograph of the patient arm position will assist in the consistency of the daily setup.

For the simulation of patients with their arms along their sides for isocentric fields, the elbows should be bent slightly out from the body so that a set of marks can be placed on the thoracic cage for a **three-point setup**. This is extremely important if the lateral positioning marks are on the arms and shoulders, because they are in an upper-third esophageal lesion. The arms are mobile and are not reliable for positioning and maintaining the established isocenter daily. Therefore a second set of three reference points are placed lower on the thoracic cage and are used to establish the isocenter. The upper three points are used to maintain the shoulder position. The anteroposterior SSD, or setup distance, is double-checked and maintained, especially with oblique treatment fields.

Orthogonal radiographs are taken 90 degrees apart if there is an initial conventional simulation. This includes an anterior film (defining the actual treatment volume) and a lateral film (establishing the isocenter or depth). Both films should be taken with barium contrast in the esophagus to delineate the esophagus and its relationship to normal structures. These radiographs, along with multiple-level contours or a CT scan with the patient in treatment position, assist the dosimetrist in planning the necessary off-cord field arrangements (Figure 35-20). After the treatment plan is complete a second simulation is often needed to film the oblique treatment fields.

CT simulation more accurately defines the location of the target volume, lymph node regions, and spinal cord interface than a conventional simulation. CT simulation also allows pertinent information to be obtained in one procedure instead of having a postsimulation treatment-planning CT scan. A second simulation to film the obliques or boost fields is not required with CT simulation. All fields can be designed from the original CT scan and treatment isocenter.

The patient will typically be positioned supine with arms above the head in an immobilization device as described previously. The device is measured to ensure that it fits inside the scanner and a photograph of patient setup is taken. Oral contrast used for CT imaging may be given to the patient 30 minutes to 1 hour before the scan. A pudding-type contrast may also be given at the time of the CT simulation to visualize the esophagus. Patients with severe dysphagia may not tolerate this, especially in the supine position.

The radiation therapist will ensure that the patient is straight and place reference marks on the thoracic cage and place radiopaque markers on these marks for visualization on the scan. The coordinates of these reference marks, superior and inferior scanning limits, pilot or scout length will all be recorded.

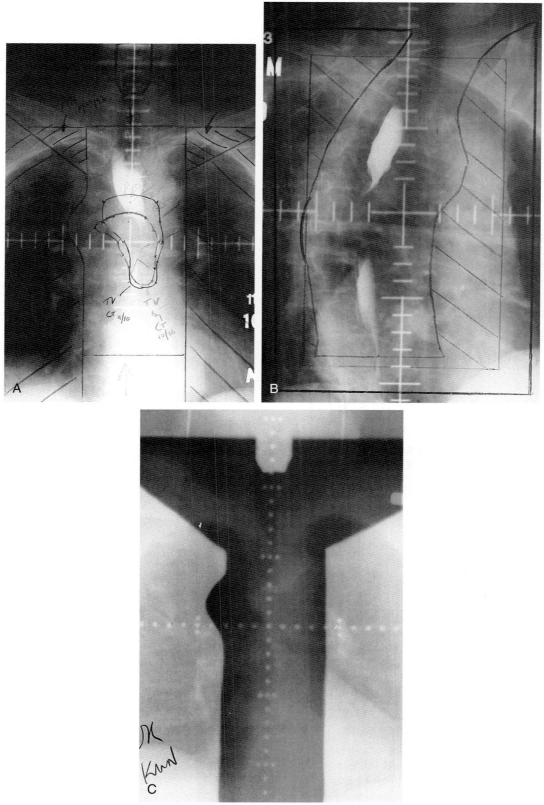

Figure 35-19. Radiation treatment fields for cancer of the esophagus. **A**, An anteroposterior/posteroanterior (AP/PA) field with barium to localize the esophageal lesion. **B**, Off-cord oblique fields. **C**, Port film of the initial anteroposterior field.

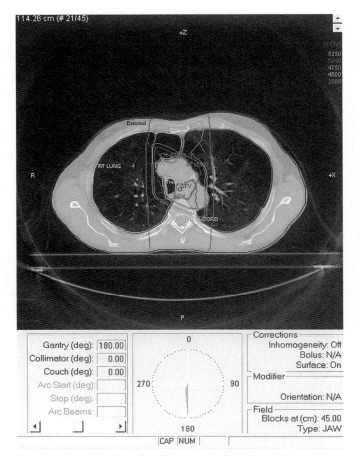

114.26 cm (# 21/45)

Gantry (deg): 180.00
Collimator (deg): 0.00
Couch (deg): 0.00
Arc Start (deg):
Stop (deg):
Arc Beams:

Corrections
Inhomogeneity: Off
Bolus: N/A
Surface: On
Modifier
Orientation: N/A
Field
Blocks at (cm): 45.00
Type: JAW

CAP NUM

Figure 35-20. Isodose distribution resulting from anteroposterior/ posteroanterior (AP/PA) and parallel-opposed obliques. AP/PA fields are discontinued as cord tolerance is reached. Note the sparing of the spinal cord with oblique fields.

A scan from above the mandible to iliac crest to include the entire esophagus and stomach may be obtained. Following the scan, the physician will digitize in different colors the target volume and critical anatomy as listed previously. The treatment isocenter will also be identified. The therapist is given the measurements to shift anterior or posterior and so forth from the reference marks to the appropriate location. The therapist then places marks or tattoos on the treatment isocenter or three points. Because the CT Simulator is not equipped with a field localization graticule like a conventional simulator, only the three points can be marked on the patient's skin. Additional straightening lines drawn superiorly and inferiorly on the anterior chest using the sagittal laser are beneficial. Patient setup information, such as positioning and immobilization devices, is recorded at the time of simulation. Field size parameters and gantry and/or couch angles will be recorded once planning is complete. The patient will proceed to treatment following the completion of the treatment plan. 3D conformal treatment planning may be done to spare vital organs such as heart, lungs, and spinal cord.[59] A DRR of a treatment field with pertinent anatomy identified and a transverse CT simulator image of the treatment isocenter is seen in Figure 35-21. A block check with

contrast may be done on a conventional simulator to verify field design and patient setup before treatment.

Side Effects

After 2 weeks of radiation treatment, patients begin to experience esophagitis. They complain of substernal pain during swallowing and the sensation of food sticking in their esophagus. Patients may be unable to eat solid foods and require a diet of bland, soft, or pureed foods. In addition, patients should eat small, frequent meals that are high in calories and protein (Table 35-3). High-calorie liquid supplements such as Carnation Instant Breakfast and Ensure are good alternatives for a high-calorie snack during the day or at bedtime.[36,67,106]

To ease the pain of swallowing, the physician may suggest that the patient take liquid analgesics or viscous lidocaine before meals. These drugs provide local and systemic pain relief. Esophagitis can become severe by the end of the treatment and may even require the placement of a nasogastric tube.

Concomitant chemotherapy increases the sensitivity of the esophageal mucosa to radiation. Therefore, more severe esophagitis and possibly ulceration may occur. The radiation tolerance of the esophagus is 65 Gy delivered with 1.8- to 2.0-Gy fractions. When concurrent chemotherapy is administered, the total radiation dose safely delivered is 50 Gy, based on the increased treatment-related toxicities associated with combined-modality treatment. Decreased blood counts, nausea, and vomiting also occur with chemotherapy. A break in a patient's treatment may be necessary if the leukocyte or platelet count becomes too low.

Radiation pneumonitis or pericarditis may occur if a large volume of lung or heart is in the radiation field. Proper field shaping, multiple fields per day, and careful treatment planning greatly reduce the likelihood of severe complications. Perforation and fistula formation can result from rapid shrinkage of a tumor that was adherent to the esophageal-tracheal wall.

Long-term side effects from irradiating the esophagus include stenosis or stricture as a result of scar formation. Dilatations of the esophagus can be performed, relieving the obstructive symptoms and restoring the patient's ability to swallow.[1,9,10,22,30,44,59] Transverse myelitis is a late complication that should not occur if the radiation treatments are delivered and planned precisely and accurately.

 Recall the dose limits of radiation for the lung, heart and spinal cord. What is the TD 5/5 for each of these organs at risk (OARs)? Which of the three organs is most sensitive to radiation damage? Careful planning using intensity-modulated radiation therapy (IMRT) may help reduce the dose to organs at risk.

Role of Radiation Therapist

Patients receiving radiation therapy for esophageal cancer require a lot of supportive care. They usually experience substantial weight loss as a result of the tumor's obstructive process and are nutritionally compromised. Esophagitis, as a result of the treatment, can cause more weight loss and further debilitate the health of the patient. The therapist should question patients about the way they are feeling, their appetite, and their food intake.

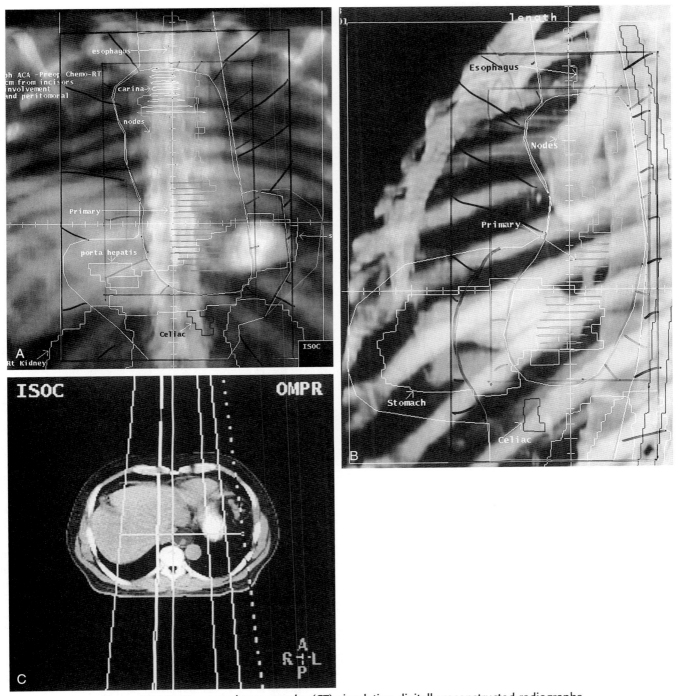

Figure 35-21. Computed tomography (CT) simulation digitally reconstructed radiographs (DRRs) of radiation treatment fields for cancer of the esophagus. **A**, Anteroposterior/posteroanterior (AP/PA) field with pertinent anatomy identified. **B**, Off-cord oblique field. **C**, CT simulation image at treatment isocenter. Note divergent beam outline.

Dietary suggestions regarding recommended foods or those to avoid should be made available to the patient. Some radiation therapy centers have printed sheets for the therapist or nurse to give to the patient. Many centers also have a dietitian to whom the patient may be referred for meal planning and dietary supplements.

Esophagitis can be emotionally and physically draining for these patients. The therapist should try to monitor the patient's emotional well-being as much as the physical aspects. The therapist should inform the patient about local cancer support groups that assist in coping with side effects of radiation treatments and disease.

Table 35-3	Dietary Guidelines for Patients Receiving Thoracic Irradiation
Recommended Foods	**Foods to Avoid**
Cottage cheese, yogurt, and milkshakes	Hot and spicy foods
Puddings	Dry to coarse foods
Casseroles	Crackers, nuts, and potato chips
Scrambled eggs	Raw vegetables, citrus fruits, and juices
Meats and vegetables in sauces or gravies	Alcoholic beverages

CASE III

Mid-Esophagus

A 54-year-old gentleman presented to his local physician with complaints of occasional intermittent chest discomfort. His local physician ordered a thorough cardiac evaluation that was negative. A few months later he began to notice some discomfort in his mid-chest with swallowing solids or even water. He mentioned this to his local physician and subsequently underwent evaluation by a gastroenterologist. An esophogastroduedenoscopy (EGD) was done that revealed a mass approximately 34 cm from the incisors that measured about 2 cm. The mass was noted to be firm and not polypoid. The surface was ulcerated, and the mass was firmly adherent to the esophageal wall. Biopsies of the mass were obtained. There was no stricture or narrowing at the gastroesophageal junction, but there was some slight irregularity consistent with esophagitis. This area was also biopsied. The gastroesophageal junction was noted at 45 cm from the incisors. The esophagus biopsy specimen was reviewed. The GE junction had hyperplastic squamous esophageal mucosa consistent with reflux. Fragments of cardia-type gastric mucosa had mild active gastritis. There was no evidence of *Helicobacter pylori*. The mid-esophagus mass biopsy was positive for invasive grade 2 (of 4) squamous cell carcinoma.

The patient underwent a CT scan of the abdomen and chest. This examination revealed a soft tissue mass measuring approximately 2 cm in the mid-thoracic esophagus. A PET/CT scan was also obtained. This examination revealed an FDG uptake in the mid-esophagus consistent with the patient's known esophageal carcinoma. There was no evidence for metastatic disease. The focal intense area of FDG uptake was noted just below the carina into the right side consistent with the patient's cancer. A second EGD was done this time with endoscopic sonography and biopsies. This examination revealed a long linear polypoid tumor extending from 32 to 36 cm from the incisors. There was some erythematous tissue around this area suggestive of high-grade dysplasia. Biopsies of the tumor and from the reddish tissues surrounding the tumor were obtained. A small lymph node was noted in the perigastric area, measuring approximately 4 mm. Closer to the tumor, there were multiple lymph nodes noted. The tumor had some peritumoral adenopathy suggestive of local, regional metastasis. At 26 cm from the incisors, above the tumor, a group of periesophageal lymph nodes were biopsied. The tumor was staged as a T2 lesion. The external wall of the esophagus was intact, but tumor was seen breaching into the muscularis propria. The fairly hypoechoic lymph nodes at 26 cm from the incisors were biopsied. Pathology from the lymph node biopsy was negative for malignancy. Because there are many lymph nodes suspicious for involvement, the patient was staged a T2 N1 M0 or stage IIB. It was recommended that the patient undergo preoperative chemoradiation consisting of 5040 cGy in 28 fractions with concomitant continuous infusion 5-FU and cisplatin followed by a 4-week interval and surgery as indicated. The patient was treated with AP, PA, and right and left Lateral fields.

PANCREATIC CANCER

Epidemiology and Etiology

Cancers of the pancreas account for approximately 2% of all cancers diagnosed annually in the United States. In 2008, the American Cancer Society estimates that 37,680 new cases of pancreatic cancer will occur. Pancreatic cancer is the fourth leading cause of cancer-related deaths in the United States, with an estimated 34,290 deaths expected to occur in 2008.[5,9] Pancreatic cancer has a high mortality rate and is considered one of the deadliest malignancies. It occurs slightly more commonly in men than in women, with incidence and mortality rates greater in African Americans than in whites. The disease rarely occurs in persons younger than 40 years with most patients in the 50- to 80-year-old age group.[49,75,101] Seventy percent of patients are older than 70 with a median age at diagnosis of 72.[9]

No known cause exists for the development of pancreatic cancer, although smokers have a 2 to 3 times higher risk of developing pancreatic cancer. Cigarette smoking is thought to cause about 20% to 30% of pancreatic cancers.[9] Hereditary nonpolyposis colorectal cancer, familial breast cancer associated with the *BRCA2* mutation, Peutz-Jeghers syndrome linked to polyps and other cancers, *p16* gene mutations in familial pancreatic cancer, and hereditary pancreatitis have been implicated as risk factors for the development of pancreatic cancer.[1,9] Exposure to industrial chemicals such as benzidine and beta napthylamine over an extended period is related to an increased incidence of pancreatic cancer. However, definitive evidence establishing a causal relationship is lacking.[1,9,19,57,75,101] Obesity, lack of physical activity, and diets high in fats, red meat, and processed meat (bacon, sausage) are thought to increase one's risk of developing pancreatic cancer. Conversely, diets high in vegetables and fruits will lower one's risk of developing pancreas cancer. More studies are being conducted to determine if high-fat diet does indeed cause pancreatic cancer. Pancreatic cancer is also more common in people with type 2 (adult-onset) diabetes.[1,9]

Anatomy and Lymphatics

The pancreas is located retroperitoneally at the L1-2 level and lies transversely in the upper abdomen. The pancreas is divided into three anatomic regions: the head, body, and tail. The head of the pancreas is located in the C-loop of the duodenum. The body lies just posterior to the stomach near the midline and is anterior to the IVC. Extending laterally to the left, the tail terminates in the splenic hilum. The pancreas is in direct contact with the duodenum, jejunum, stomach, major vessels (IVC), spleen, and kidney. Tumors of the pancreas commonly invade these structures and are therefore usually unresectable at the time of diagnosis.[19,57]

Numerous lymph node channels drain the pancreas and its surrounding structures. The main lymph node groups include the superior and inferior pancreaticoduodenal nodes, porta hepatis, suprapancreatic nodes, and paraaortic nodes. Tumors arising in the tail of the pancreas drain to the splenic hilar nodes

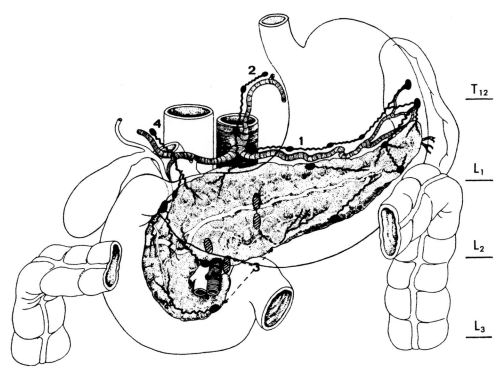

Figure 35-22. Anatomy and lymphatic drainage of the pancreas. Note the intimate relationship of the pancreas with the duodenum, stomach, transverse colon, spleen, and common bile duct. The four main trunks of lymphatic drainage. 1, The left side drains along the tail into splenic hilar nodes; 2, superior pancreatic lymph nodes and the celiac axis; 3, inferior pancreatic, mesenteric, and left paraaortic nodes; 4, right-side drainage to anterior and posterior pancreaticoduodenal nodes and right paraaortic nodes. (From del Regato JA, Spjut HJ, Cox JD: *Ackerman and del Regato's cancer: diagnosis, treatment, and prognosis,* ed 6, St. Louis, 1985, Mosby.)

(Figure 35-22). Most patients have advanced local and/or metastatic disease at the time of diagnosis.[19,34,57]

Clinical Presentation

The four most common presenting symptoms of pancreatic cancer are jaundice, abdominal pain, anorexia, and weight loss. Tumors arising in the head of the pancreas may obstruct the biliary system, resulting in jaundice. An obstruction of the biliary system results in excess bilirubin to be excreted in urine and less bilirubin to enter the bowel. This results in patients having dark urine and light-colored stools. Patients who are jaundiced also complain of pruritis or itching.[1,9] Tumors that occur in the body or tail of the pancreas are not associated with obstruction of the biliary system and commonly involve severe back pain and weight loss. Pancreatic cancers occur most frequently in the head and neck of the pancreas.[1,9,19,60,75]

Detection and Diagnosis

A thorough history and physical examination are extremely important. The abdomen should be assessed for palpable masses. The tumor's obstruction of the biliary system can result in an enlarged pancreas, gallbladder, or liver. Palpable supraclavicular nodes or rectal masses discovered during a digital rectal examination indicate peritoneal spread. All these signs suggest an advanced-stage disease. The presence or absence of jaundice

is assessed by paying particular attention to the sclera, skin, and oral-cavity mucosa.[1,9,19,57]

The most valuable and important diagnostic test is a spiral CT scan of the abdomen. This scan provides a complete view of the abdominal structures most likely involved with the tumor. This image localizes the mass in the pancreas and depicts whether it is a head, body, or tail primary. The scan also demonstrates whether the tumor has invaded surrounding structures such as the duodenum, superior mesenteric vessels, or celiac-axis vessels. Spread to the regional lymph nodes, peritoneal implants, and distant metastasis to the liver can also be assessed.[1,9,16,75,90]

The resectability of the tumor can be determined by the information found on the CT scan. Liver metastasis and the involvement of the superior mesenteric artery or other major vessels are two contraindications to surgery. A CT-guided fine-needle biopsy of the primary tumor or metastatic lesions may be performed to establish the diagnosis.[19,57,75]

Endoscopic retrograde cholangiopancreatography (ERCP) is used in evaluating the obstruction and potential involvement of the biliary system. A biopsy of the ampulla or duodenum may be obtained at the time of the ERCP. This procedure is even more beneficial for the diagnosis of a primary tumor of the biliary system. Ultrasonography has also been used to assess ductal obstruction, blood vessel invasion, and liver metastasis.

EUS is a relatively new procedure used to image the pancreas. A transducer is passed down the esophagus to the duodenum adjacent to the pancreas. This examination is more useful than CT for visualizing small lesions in the head of the pancreas and to evaluate the potential involvement of lymph nodes and vasculature.[9] EUS along with fine-needle aspiration is being used as a tool to obtain tissue for diagnosis with less chance of tumor seeding as compared with a percutaneous approach.

A laparoscopy to obtain a biopsy is commonly performed before any surgical intervention and may rule out small liver metastases (1 to 2 mm) that were undetectable on a CT scan.[9,57] A laparoscopic procedure does not require a big incision and is much easier on the patient.[9] According to a study done by Warshaw and colleagues,[65] laparotomy results indicated that 40% of patients had small metastases in the liver or on parietal peritoneal surfaces. These patients were spared the morbidity of unnecessary abdominal surgery. If the patient's tumor appears to be resectable, based on the diagnostic workup, exploratory surgery and a biopsy are performed to determine the histology of the pancreatic mass.

Pathology and Staging

Adenocarcinomas comprise 80% of pancreatic cancers. Other histologic types include islet cell tumors, acinar cell carcinomas, and cystadenocarcinomas.[1,9,19,57,75]

A formal TNM staging system for pancreatic cancer is available and is found in Table 35-4. Patients with disease confined to the pancreas, T1-3, are generally considered resectable.[1] More than 50% of patients that are diagnosed with pancreatic cancer have distant metastasis at the time of diagnosis.[9]

Routes of Spread

Cancers of the pancreas are locally invasive. Lymph node involvement or direct extension into the duodenum, stomach, and colon is not uncommon at the time of diagnosis. The tumor often encases or invades the superior mesenteric artery, portal vein, and celiac axis artery, rendering the tumor unresectable. Hematogenous spread to the liver via the portal vein is another common pathway of spread. Because of the propensity of these tumors to invade other abdominal structures, peritoneal seeding of tumor cells can also occur.[1,9,19,44,57,69,75]

Treatment Techniques

Surgery is the treatment of choice. Most tumors, however, are unresectable. Contraindications for undergoing a curative surgical procedure are liver metastasis, extra pancreatic serosal implantation, and invasion or adherence to major vessels.[1,9,19,74]

The most common potentially curative surgical procedure is a pancreaticoduodenectomy (Whipple procedure), which involves a resection of the head of the pancreas, entire duodenum, distal stomach, gallbladder, and common bile duct (Figure 35-23). Reconstruction is done to maintain the continuity of the biliary-gastrointestinal system. The remaining pancreas, bile ducts, and stomach are anastomosed onto various sites of the jejunum (Figure 35-24). The operative mortality rate from this procedure has greatly improved in recent years; it has been as high as 30%, but it is now less than 5%. The surgeon should place clips outlining the extent of the tumor to assist the radiation oncologist in planning adjuvant radiation therapy fields.[1,9,19,57,75,90,92]

Palliative biliary bypass procedures are often performed for unresectable tumors to redirect the flow of bile from obstructed ducts back into the gastrointestinal system. Typically, this is done by anastomosing the uninvolved bile ducts into the jejunum. Resolving the obstruction provides patients with relief of jaundice.

Even with a potentially curative resection, the 5-year survival rate is usually less than 10%, with a median survival time of approximately 11 to 14 months.[44,63,69,92] This is due to a high locoregional recurrence rate and a high risk of distant metastases.[44,60,69]

Table 35-4	American Joint Committee on Cancer Staging of Pancreas Cancer			

PRIMARY TUMOR

Tx	Primary tumor cannot be assessed
T0	No evidence of primary tumor
Tis	Carcinoma in situ
T1	Tumor limited to the pancreas ≤2cm or less in greatest dimension
T2	Tumor limited to the pancreas 2.1cm or greater in greatest dimension
T3	Tumor extends beyond the pancreas but without involvement of celiac axis or the superior mesenteric artery
T4	Tumor involves the celiac axis or the superior mesenteric artery (unresectable)

REGIONAL LYMPH NODES

Nx	Regional lymph nodes cannot be assessed
N0	No regional lymph nodes
N1	Regional lymph nodes

DISTANT METASTASIS

Mx	Distant metastasis cannot be assessed
M0	No distant metastasis
M1	Distant Metastasis

STAGE GROUPING

Stage 0	Tis	N0	M0
Stage IA	T1	N0	M0
Stage IB	T2	N0	M0
Stage IIA	T3	N0	M0
Stage IIB	T1	N1	M0
	T2	N1	M0
	T3	N1	M0
Stage III	T4	Any N	M0
Stage IV	Any T	Any N	M1

With permission from American Joint Committee on Cancer (AJCC), Chicago, IL: *AJCC Cancer Staging Manual*, ed 6, New York, 2002, Springer-Verlag.

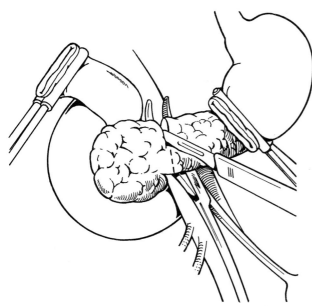

Figure 35-23. Pancreaticoduodenectomy (Whipple procedure); resection of the head of the pancreas, duodenum, distal stomach, gallbladder, and common bile duct. (From Beazley RM, Cohn I Jr: Tumors of the pancreas, gallbladder, and extrahepatic ducts. In Murphy G, Lawrence W, Lenhard R: *American Cancer Society textbook of clinical oncology*, 1995, American Cancer Society.)

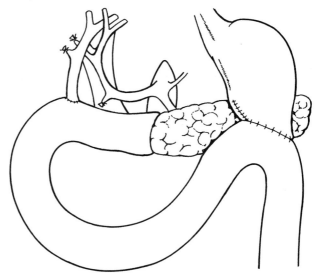

Figure 35-24. Reconstruction of the biliary and gastrointestinal system. The remaining pancreas, stomach, and bile ducts are anastomosed to the jejunum. (From Beazley RM, Cohn I Jr: Tumors of the pancreas, gallbladder, and extrahepatic ducts. In Murphy G, Lawrence W, Lenhard R: *American Cancer Society textbook of clinical oncology*, 1995, American Cancer Society.)

There are two general types of surgery used to treat cancer of the pancreas[9]:
- Potentially curative surgery *is used when imaging tests suggest that it is possible to remove all the cancer.*
- Palliative surgery *may be done if imaging tests show that the tumor is too widespread to be completely removed. This is done to relieve symptoms or to prevent certain complications such as blockage of the bile ducts or the intestine by the cancer.*

Several studies have shown that removing only part of the cancer does not help patients to live longer. Pancreatic cancer surgery is one of the most difficult operations a surgeon can do. It is also one of hardest for patients to undergo. There may be multiple complications and it may take several weeks for patients to recover.

Radiation Therapy. Because of the high rate of distant metastasis and locoregional failure rate after surgery alone, combined-modality therapy versus observation was investigated in a randomized trial of patients with resected tumors. Adjuvant combined-modality treatment after surgery resulted in a significant improvement in the overall survival rate of 18 to 29 months compared with no further treatment. Chemoradiation, the delivery of radiation and chemotherapy simultaneously, has become the main method for the adjuvant treatment of pancreatic cancer.[1,9,14]

Radiation therapy and chemotherapy are considered the preferred treatments for locally advanced, unresectable pancreatic cancers. Studies comparing radiation alone with radiation and chemotherapy alone have demonstrated that the combined-modality treatment provides modestly improved survival rates.[1,9,14,16,75,86,90,92]

Specialized radiation therapy techniques have been investigated to determine whether higher doses to the tumor bed would translate into an increase in local control and better survival rates. One method of delivering a higher dose to the primary tumor is IORT. A single dose of 10 to 20 Gy intraoperative electrons is delivered as a boost dose, following 50.4 Gy delivered by external beam radiation therapy. The main theoretical advantage of IORT is that it allows a higher dose to be delivered to the primary site than conventional external beam therapy because of the many dose-limiting structures located in the upper abdomen. Critical structures such as the kidney, liver, stomach, and small bowel can be moved out of the way or shielded during IORT. Studies evaluating the efficacy of this specialized boost technique have demonstrated an increase in local control when this method is added to the standard external beam therapy and chemotherapy treatment regimen. However, overall survival rates were not improved because of systemic failures in the liver or peritoneal seeding. Accordingly, IORT should not be used for pancreatic cancer in routine clinical practice. Different chemotherapy regimens are being investigated that may improve the systemic failures and increase survival rates.[1,16,29,43,44,75,90]

Chemotherapy. As mentioned, chemotherapy is used with radiation therapy as an adjuvant treatment in resected pancreatic tumors and as the primary treatment with radiation for unresectable disease. Gemcitabine is the most common drug used in the treatment of pancreatic cancer and was found to result in better survival rates than with 5-FU.[1,9] Different drug combinations and sequences are being investigated for improving survival rates. Gemcitabine has been paired with cisplatin and 5-FU to see if this combination results in better survival. Continuous infusion 5-FU is still being used as part of some chemoradiotherapy regimens. Other drugs that are being explored are irinotecan, capecitabine, oxaliplatin, and paclitaxel.[9,12,35,65] Neoadjuvant preoperative chemoradiotherapy has also been studied.[1] The preliminary results have not shown a survival benefit to preoperative chemoradiotherapy versus adjuvant chemoradiation therapy.[1] More research is needed to determine what drugs and in what combinations provide the best outcome for patients with pancreatic cancer.[1] Even with combined-modality treatment, the overall survival rate of patients with pancreatic cancer is extremely poor.[16,44,63,75]

Field Design and Critical Structures. Traditionally, a four-field technique is used for encompassing the primary tumor bed and draining lymphatics as defined by surgical clips or CT. A dose of 45 to 50 Gy is delivered in 1.8-Gy fractions with high-energy photons and a reduction in the field volume after 45 Gy. The upper abdomen contains many dose-limiting structures that must be considered for the designing and planning of radiation treatments. These structures include the kidneys, liver, stomach, small bowel, and spinal cord. Table 35-5 contains the TD 5/5 of these structures. The dose through the lateral fields is limited to 18 to 20 Gy because of the large volume of liver and kidneys in these fields.

Conformal 3D treatment planning and IMRT systems may allow higher doses of radiation to be delivered while keeping the dose-limiting structures within tolerance. Three-dimensional treatment planning permits the design of coplanar and non-coplanar beams that use a couch rotation to enter at unique angles to avoid critical structures allowing a higher dose to be achieved. Intensity-modulated systems use unique beam directions; however, they also vary the beam intensity and shape of the field with the use of MLCs.[16,62] Studies comparing IMRT with 3D conformal have shown that IMRT further reduces the dose to the liver, kidneys, stomach, and small bowel than 3D conformal.[1,12,20,35,73,85] Ongoing research studies are being conducted to see if dose escalation is possible with IMRT techniques due to the improved dose conformality to the tumor volume and sparing of critical structures.[12,20,73]

Typical AP/PA field volumes for the head of a pancreatic lesion extend approximately from T10-11 for inclusion of the tumor bed, draining lymphatics, and celiac axis (T12-L1). The width of the field should encompass the entire duodenal loop and the margin extending across the midline on the left. The lateral fields are designed to provide a 1.5- to 2-cm margin anteriorly beyond the known disease. Posteriorly, the field extends 1.5 cm behind the anterior vertebral body for adequate coverage of the paraaortic nodes (Figure 35-25). For body or tail lesions, the volume treated does not need to include the duodenal loop but must extend farther to the left to provide an adequate margin on the primary tumor and to include the splenic hilar nodes.[1,44,57]

For CT simulation, the patient is placed in the supine position with the arms above the head for easier placement of the lateral isocenter marks. A vacuum device or foaming cradle immobilization device is made before the simulation. The therapist should make sure the patient is straight on the table prior to making the immobilization device. This can be accomplished by using the sagittal laser and lining up midline structures such as suprasternal notch, xiphoid, and pubic bone. The device is measured to ensure that it fits inside the scanner, and a photograph of patient setup is taken. The CT simulation also requires that contrast be administered. With this simulation, the patient is instructed to drink contrast 30 minutes to 1 hour before the scan. Some centers may inject contrast for kidney localization, although the kidneys can be visualized on the scan without contrast.

The radiation therapist will place reference marks on the patient's abdomen before scanning. A scan from above the diaphragm to below the iliac crest will be obtained. The physician can digitize in the location of the target volume, lymph nodes, porta hepatis, and superior mesenteric artery to ensure coverage of these structures in the treatment field. The dose-limiting structures, kidneys, liver, stomach, small bowel, and spinal cord, may be outlined on the DRRs as well (Figure 35-26). Once the treatment isocenter has been identified, the radiation therapist will make the appropriate shifts from the reference isocenter and mark the final three points to be used for treatment. The CT images are then sent to the dosimetrist for 3D conformal planning or IMRT planning (Figure 35-27). For treating a head of pancreas lesion, approximately 50% of the right kidney is in the treated volume; therefore, at least two thirds of the left kidney should be shielded to preserve normal kidney function. MLC or shielding blocks are designed to block as much as possible of the kidneys, liver, and stomach on the AP/PA fields, and the lateral field is used to shield the spinal cord and small bowel.[1,57]

For fluoroscopic simulation, the patient is placed in the supine position and positioned with the arms above the head in an immobilization device as mentioned earlier. The device is measured to ensure it will fit in a CT scanner following the simulation procedure. A photograph of the patient in the device is taken to ensure reproducibility of the setup later. Preliminary borders and an isocenter are established and marked on the patient's skin. At many centers, renal contrast is injected, and a reference anteroposterior and/or lateral film is taken to determine the kidney location relative to other structures. This film assists in the design of custom shielding used to avoid unnecessary irradiation to the kidneys. The location of the kidneys may also be transferred from measurements of a CT scan onto the simulation film.

After the films for kidney localization are completed, the patient is instructed to drink barium for localization of the duodenum and stomach. This is done to ensure adequate margins on the duodenum, especially for unresectable head of pancreas lesions. Another set of anteroposterior and lateral radiographs are then taken. This final set of films is representative of the actual volume to be treated.

Table 35-5	Tolerance Doses (TD 5/5)
Kidneys	1800-2300 cGy
Liver	3000-3500 cGy
Small bowel	4000-4500 cGy
Spinal cord	4500-4700 cGy
Stomach	5000 cGy

Modified from Emami B, et al: Tolerance of normal tissue to therapeutic irradiation, *Int J Radiat Oncol Biol Phys* 21:109-122, 1991.

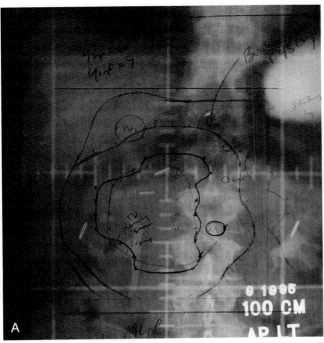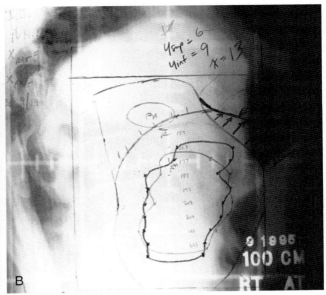

Figure 35-25. Radiation therapy treatment fields for pancreatic cancer. **A**, Anteroposterior/posteroanterior (AP/PA). **B**, Opposed laterals.

Side Effects. The most common complaints of patients receiving radiation for pancreatic cancer are nausea and vomiting. Antiemetics may be given to mitigate these adverse effects. Other potential acute side effects include leukopenia, thrombocytopenia, diarrhea, and stomatitis. Long-term side effects, such as renal failure, are rare and suggest the possibility of improper shielding of the kidney.[13,86]

CASE IV

Obstructive Jaundice

A 57-year-old woman presented with a 2-week history of nausea and dyspepsia with abdominal bloating, obstructive jaundice, dark urine and pale stools, elevated liver function tests, and a 24-pound weight loss over the preceding 6 months. The patient had also complained of postprandial discomfort and decreased appetite. A CT scan noted a distended gallbladder and common hepatic bile duct. No pancreatic mass was noted. An ERCP was performed to place a stent to relieve the obstructed ducts. At this time brushings from the common bile duct were obtained that were found positive for adenocarcinoma. An endoscopic sonogram was subsequently performed and noted a 1.5 × 1.5 cm pancreatic mass. A couple of lymph nodes were biopsied and found to be negative for malignancy. A repeat CT scan performed per pancreatic protocol noted a faint low-density lesion medial to the distal common bile duct in the head of the pancreas.

The patient underwent surgery and a Whipple procedure was performed. There was no evidence of peritoneal or hepatic metastasis. The tumor was noted at the junction of the head and neck of the pancreas and was attached to the lateral aspect of the portal vein. Pathology revealed invasive adenocarcinoma grade 3 (of 4) forming a 2.2 × 1.5 × 1.2 cm ill-defined mass in the head of the pancreas constricting the common bile duct with invasion through the wall of the common bile duct to erode the mucosal surface. Three of five

peripancreatic lymph nodes were positive for metastatic adenocarcinoma. The patient was referred to radiation and medical oncology for adjuvant treatment of her T3 N1 M0 pancreatic cancer.

It was recommend that the patient receive two cycles of gemcitabine followed by radiation with 5-FU. The gemcitabine will be given weekly for 3 (of 4) weeks for 2 months followed by combined chemoradiation with continuous infusion 5-FU. This would then be followed by 2 additional months of gemcitabine-based chemotherapy.

The patient was treated to 4500 cGy at 180 cGy per treatment using a 3D conformal technique with six oblique fields. Two of the obliques are angled cephalad and caudally with a couch rotation to further reduce kidney and liver doses. A shrinking field boost to an additional 540 cGy was done using five of the same obliques bringing the total cumulative dose to 5040 cGy.

CASE V

Pancreatic Duodenectomy

A 55-year-old man presented with episodes of fever and dark urine. He was found on endoscopy to have a polypoid lesion in the periampullary region of the pancreas that was biopsied and found to be a grade 3 adenocarcinoma. His CT scan demonstrated no evidence of metastatic disease in the liver or upper abdomen. The patient underwent a pylorus-sparing pancreatic duodenectomy. At the time of surgery the tumor had invaded minimally into the pancreas, and 1 of 16 nodes was found to be positive for tumor. Because of the high risk of local and distant failure with surgery alone, he was referred to radiation oncology for adjuvant chemoradiation. The patient underwent a CT simulation, and a 3D treatment plan was performed to provide adequate dose to the tumor bed and regional nodes while minimizing dose to sensitive organs such as the kidneys, liver, and spinal cord. The patient was treated with a four-field with a shrinking field cone-down boost to 5040 cGy.

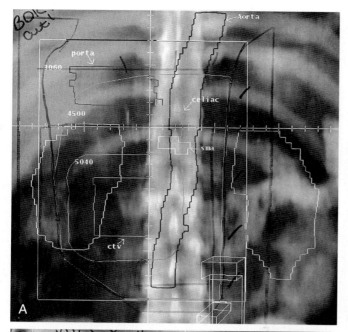

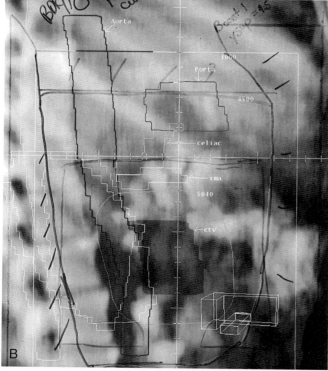

Figure 35-26. Computed tomography (CT) simulation digitally reconstructed radiographs (DRRs) of radiation treatment fields for cancer of the pancreas. **A**, Anteroposterior/posteroanterior (AP/PA). **B**, Opposed laterals.

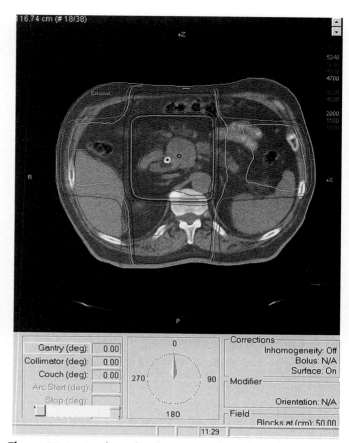

Figure 35-27. Isodose distribution resulting from anteroposterior/posteroanterior (AP/PA) and opposed lateral fields. Note dose to kidneys.

SUMMARY

COLORECTAL CANCER

- The risk of developing cancer of the large bowel increases with age with more than 90% occurring in people over 50 years of age. Cancer of the large bowel more commonly affects the rectum or distal colon. Colorectal cancer is the second leading cause of cancer death in the United States, accounting for approximately 51,000 deaths annually.
- The colon is divided into eight regions: cecum, ascending colon, descending colon, splenic flexure, hepatic flexure, transverse colon, sigmoid, and rectum.
- Patients with rectal cancer usually have rectal bleeding. Other symptoms include a change in bowel habits, diarrhea versus constipation, or a change in the stool caliber.
- Cancers in the large bowel is diagnosed via findings of the physical examination and radiographic and endoscopic studies.
- Adenocarcinoma is the most common malignancy of the large bowel, accounting for 90% to 95% of all tumors. Other histologic types include mucinous adenocarcinoma, signet-ring cell carcinoma, and squamous cell carcinoma.
- Surgery is considered the treatment of choice. Radiation therapy is most commonly used as an adjuvant treatment for rectal cancer, either done preoperatively or postoperatively and in conjunction with chemotherapy.

ANAL CANCER

- The etiologic factors for the development of anal cancer are associated with genital warts, genital infections, human papillomaviruses, anal intercourse in men or women before age 30, and immunosuppression.

- The most common presenting symptoms is rectal bleeding. Other symptoms are pain, change in bowel habits, and the sensation of a mass.
- Squamous cell carcinoma is the most common histology of anal cancer, comprising approximately 80% of the cases.
- Combination radiation therapy and chemotherapy is advocated as the preferred method of treatment and considered the standard of care for most patients. A variety of radiation techniques exist for the treatment of anal cancer, including a four-field or AP/PA pelvic-field with electron fields to the inguinal nodes.

ESOPHAGEAL CANCER

- Risk factors, such as use of tobacco or alcohol abuse, cause esophageal cancer. Long-term irritation of the lining of the esophagus, as with GERD, Barrett esophagus, achalasia, esophageal webs, or scarring from swallowing lye, can cause esophageal cancers.
- The esophagus is a 25-cm-long tube lined with stratified squamous epithelium. The esophagus begins at the level of C6 and traverses through the thoracic cage to terminate in the abdomen at the esophageal gastric junction (T10-11).
- The most common presenting symptoms are dysphagia and weight loss, which occur in 90% of patients.
- The most common pathologic types of esophageal cancer are squamous cell carcinoma and adenocarcinoma. Squamous cell carcinomas are found most frequently in the upper and middle thoracic esophagus. Adenocarcinoma typically occurs in the distal esophagus and GE junction.
- Because the esophagus is distensible, lesions are large before causing obstructive symptoms. Spread is usually longitudinal. Occasionally, skip lesions may be present at a significant distance from the primary lesion.
- The treatment of esophageal cancer is highly complex and technically difficult. Radiation therapy with chemotherapy is considered the current nonsurgical treatment of choice for esophageal cancer.

PANCREATIC CANCER

- Cancers of the pancreas account for approximately 2% of all cancers diagnosed annually in the United States, with a high mortality rate. No known cause exists for the development of pancreatic cancer, although smokers have a 2 to 3 times higher risk of developing pancreatic cancer.
- The pancreas is located retroperitoneally at the L1-2 level, lies transversely in the upper abdomen, and is divided into three anatomic regions: the head, body, and tail.
- The four most common presenting symptoms of pancreatic cancer are jaundice. abdominal pain, anorexia, and weight loss.
- The most valuable and important diagnostic test is a spiral CT scan of the abdomen, which provides a complete view of the abdominal structures most likely involved with the pancreatic tumor.
- Adenocarcinomas comprise 80% of pancreatic cancers.
- Surgery is the treatment of choice. Most tumors, however, are unresectable.

- Radiation therapy and chemotherapy are considered the preferred treatments for locally advanced, unresectable pancreatic cancers.

Review Questions

Multiple Choice

1. Which of the following methods may reduce dose to the small bowel during pelvic radiation therapy?
   a. supine position
   b. prone position
   c. treatment with a full bladder
   d. both b and c
2. The principal advantage(s) of intensity-modulated radiation therapy over conventional 3D conformal in the treatment of rectal, anal, or pancreatic cancer is:
   a. fewer long-term radiation side effects
   b. better dose conformity to target volumes
   c. more sparing of normal structures (OARs)
   d. all of the above
3. The principal lymph node group involved in patients with rectal cancer is the:
   a. common iliac nodes
   b. inguinal nodes
   c. paraaortic nodes
   d. internal iliac nodes
4. The principal etiologic factor(s) in the development of squamous cell carcinoma of the esophagus cancer in North America is(are):
   a. a diet high in fat and high in nitrate content
   b. a diet low in fat and high in vegetables and fruits
   c. excessive alcohol and tobacco use
   d. achalasia and Plummer-Vinson syndrome
5. A common site of blood-borne metastasis from rectal, pancreatic, or esophageal malignancies is the:
   a. brain
   b. bone
   c. adrenal gland
   d. liver
6. For radiation treatment to the thorax for esophageal cancer, the dose-limiting structure of most concern is the:
   a. spinal cord
   b. heart
   c. esophagus
   d. trachea
7. The radiation-field design most commonly used to avoid the critical structure in question 6 is:
   a. lateral-opposed fields
   b. AP/PA fields
   c. oblique fields
   d. wedge pair
8. Which of the following are common presenting symptoms of pancreatic cancer?
   I. jaundice
   II. nausea and vomiting
   III. 10% weight loss
   IV. anorexia

a. I and II
b. II and III
c. I, II, and IV
d. I, III, and IV
e. I, II, III, and IV

9. Which of the following statements regarding pancreatic cancer is *not* correct?
   a. It is locally invasive into surrounding structures.
   b. Hematogenous spread to the liver at the time of diagnosis is common.
   c. The 5-year survival rate is 80%.
   d. Most tumors are unresectable.

10. For irradiation of the upper abdomen for pancreatic cancer, the most radiosensitive dose-limiting structure is the:
    a. kidneys
    b. liver
    c. small bowel
    d. spinal cord

The answers to the Review Questions can be found by logging on to our website at: *http://evolve.elsevier.com/Washington+Leaver/principles*

Questions to Ponder

1. Describe the rationale for the use of neoadjuvant preoperative radiation therapy and adjuvant postoperative radiation therapy for rectal cancer.
2. Compare and contrast the postoperative radiation treatment field design used for a rectal cancer patient who has undergone an anterior resection versus an abdominoperineal resection.
3. What are the theoretical advantages of using IORT as a boost technique for the treatment of colorectal or pancreatic cancer?
4. What techniques are used to decrease or limit the radiation dose to the small bowel? Why are these important?
5. In treating the thorax for esophageal cancer, the arms and shoulders can create problems with the reproducibility of the setup. What can be done to ensure consistency in the daily setup of the treatment fields?
6. What is the main advantage of CT simulation and 3D conformal irradiation techniques?
7. What is the purpose of chemoradiation?
8. Barrett's esophagus and GERD are factors that are associated with the development of what histologic type of esophageal cancer?

REFERENCES

1. Abrams RA, Choo J: Pancreatic cancer. In Gunderson LL, Tepper JE, editors: *Clinical radiation oncology,* ed 2, Philadelphia, 2007, Churchill Livingstone.
2. Adlestein DJ, et al: Does paclitaxel improve the chemoradiotherapy of locoregionally advanced esophageal cancer? A nonrandomized comparison with fluorouracil based therapy, *J Clin Oncol* 18:2032-2039, 2000.
3. Ajani JA, et al: Preoperative induction of CPT-11 and cisplatin chemotherapy followed by chemoradiation therapy in patients with locoregional carcinoma of the esophagus or gastroesophageal junction, *Cancer* 100:11: 2347-2354, 2004.
4. American Cancer Society: *Anal cancer: detailed guide* (website): http://www.cancer.org/docroot/home/index.asp. Accessed August 23, 2008.
5. American Cancer Society: *Cancer facts and figures 2008.* Atlanta, 2008, American Cancer Society.
6. American Cancer Society and National Comprehensive Cancer Network: *Colon and rectal cancer treatment guidelines for patients, Version IV 2005.* Atlanta, 2005, American Cancer Society.
7. American Cancer Society: *Colorectal cancer facts and figures, special edition 2005* (website): http://www.cancer.org/downloads/STT/CAFF2005 CR4PWSecured.pdf. Accessed August 20, 2007.
8. American Cancer Society: *A detailed guide: esophageal cancer* (website): http://www.cancer.org/docroot/home/index.asp. Accessed August 22, 2008.
9. American Cancer Society: *Pancreatic cancer* (website): http://www.cancer.org/docroot/home/index.asp. Accessed August 22, 2008.
10. Anderson C, et al: PET-CT fusion in radiation management of patients with anorectal tumors, *Int J Radiat Oncol Biol Phys* 69:155-162, 2007.
11. Beart RW: Colorectal cancer. In Holleb AI, Fink DJ, Murphy GP, editors: *American Cancer Society clinical oncology,* Atlanta, 1991, American Cancer Society.
12. Ben-Josef E, et al: Intensity-modulated radiotherapy (IMRT) and concurrent capecitabine for pancreatic cancer, *Int J Radiat Oncol Biol Phys* 59 (2):454-459, 2004.
13. Bentel GC: *Radiation therapy planning,* New York, 1992, Macmillan.
14. Bilimoria KY, et al: Multimodality therapy for pancreatic cancer in the U.S., *Cancer* 110(6):1227-1234, 2007.
15. Blackstock AW: Cancer of the Esophagus, In Gunderson LL, Tepper JE, editors: *Clinical radiation oncology,* ed 2, Philadelphia, 2007, Churchill Livingstone.
16. Bodner WR, Hilaris BS, Mastoras DA: Radiation therapy in pancreatic cancer: current practices and future trends, *J Clin Gastroenterol* 30:230-233, 2000.
17. Bonnen M, et al: Long-term results using local excision after preoperative chemoradiation among selected T3 rectal cancer patients, *Int J Radiat Oncol Biol Phys* 60:1098-1105, 2004.
18. Boring CC, et al: Cancer statistics, 1994, *CA Cancer J Clin* 44:7-26, 1994.
19. Brennan MF, Kinsella TJ, Casper ES: Cancer of the pancreas. In Devita VT, Hellman S, Rosenburg SA, editors: *Cancer principles and practice of oncology,* Philadelphia, 1993, JB Lippincott.
20. Brown MW, et al: A dosimetric analysis of dose escalation using two intensity-modulated radiation therapy techniques in locally advanced pancreatic carcinoma, *Int J Radiat Oncol Biol Phys* 65(1):274-283, 2006.
21. Callister MD, Ezzell, GA, Gunderson LL: IMRT reduces dose to the small bowel and other pelvic organs in the preoperative treatment of rectal cancer, *Int J Radiat Oncol Biol Phys* 66:A290, 2006.
22. Chen YJ, et al: Organ sparing by conformal avoidance intensity-modulated radiation therapy for anal cancer: dosimetric evaluation of coverage of pelvis and inguinal/femoral nodes, *Int J Radiat Oncol Biol Phys* 63(1): 274-281, 2005.
23. Cohen AM, Minsky BD, Friedman MA: Rectal cancer. In Devita VT, Hellman S, Rosenburg SA, editors: *Cancer principles and practice of oncology,* Philadelphia, 1993, JB Lippincott.
24. Cohen AM, Minsky BD, Schilsky RL: Colon cancer. In Devita VT, Hellman S, Rosenburg SA, editors: *Cancer principles and practice of oncology,* Philadelphia, 1993, JB Lippincott.
25. Coia LR, et al: Outcome of patients receiving radiation for cancer of the esophagus: results of the 1992-1994 patterns of care study, *J Clin Oncol* 18:455-462, 2000.
26. Cooper JS, et al: Chemoradiotherapy of locally advanced esophageal cancer: long term follow up of a prospective randomized trial, *JAMA* 281:1623-1627, 1999.
27. Corn BW, et al: Significance of prone positioning in planning treatment for esophageal cancer, *Int J Radiat Oncol Biol Phys* 21:1303-1309, 1991.
28. Cotter SH, et al: FDG-PET-CT in the evaluation of anal carcinomas, *Int J Radiat Oncol Biol Phys* 65:720-725, 2006.
29. Crane CH, Beddar AS, Evans DB: The role of intraoperative radiotherapy in pancreatic cancer, *Surg Oncol Clin North Am* 12:965-977, 2003.
30. Cummings BJ: Adjuvant radiation therapy for colorectal cancer, *Cancer Suppl* 70:1372-1381, 1992.
31. Cummings BJ: Anal canal. In Perez CA, Brady LW, editors: *Principles and practices of radiation oncology,* Philadelphia, 1998, Lippincott-Raven.
32. Czito C, Willet CG: Colon Cancer. In Gunderson LL, Tepper JE, editors: *Clinical Radiation Oncology,* ed 2, St. Louis, 2007, Churchill Livingstone.
33. DeCosse JJ, Tsioulias GJ, Jacobson JS: Colorectal cancer: detection, treatment, and rehabilitation, *CA Cancer J Clin* 44:27-42, 1994.

34. Del Regato JA, Spjut HJ, Cox JD: Cancer of the digestive tract. In Ackerman LV, Del Regato JA, editors: *Cancer: diagnosis, treatment and prognosis*, ed 6, St. Louis, 1985, Mosby.

35. Dickler A, Abrams RA: Radiochemotherapy in the management of pancreatic cancer—part II: use in adjuvant and locally unresectable settings, *Semin Radiat Oncol* 15:235-244, 2005.

36. National Institutes of Health: *Eating hints* (pp 10-11), Washington, DC, 1983, U.S. Department of Health and Human Services, National Institutes of Health.

37. Ellis FH Jr, Levitan N, Lo TCM: Cancer of the esophagus. In Holleb AI, Fink DJ, Murphy GP, editors: *American Cancer Society clinical oncology*, Atlanta, 1991, American Cancer Society.

38. Enker WE: Adenocarcinomas of the appendix and colon: surgical management. In Copeland EM, editor: *Surgical oncology*, New York, 1983, John Wiley & Sons.

39. Fisher SA, Brady LW: Esophagus. In Perez CA, Brady LW, editors: *Principles and practices of radiation oncology*, Philadelphia, 1992, JB Lippincott.

40. Fisher SA, Brady LW: Esophagus. In Perez CA, Brady LW, editors: *Principles and practices of radiation oncology*, Philadelphia, 1998, JB Lippincott-Raven.

41. Fleming ID, et al, editors: *AJCC manual for staging of cancer*, ed 5, Philadelphia, 1997, Lippincott-Raven.

42. Fleshmann J, et al: Laparoscopic colectomy for cancer is not inferior to open surgery based on 5-year data from the COST Study Group Trial, *Ann Surg*, 246:4:655-664, 2007.

43. Foo ML, Gunderson LL: Adjuvant post-operative *radiation* therapy +/- 5-FU in resected carcinoma of the pancreas, *Hepato-gastroenterology* 45:613-623, 1998.

44. Foo ML, et al: Patterns of failure in grossly resected pancreatic ductal adenocarcinoma treated with adjuvant irradiation 5 fluorouracil, *Int J Radiat Oncol Biol Phys* 26:483-489, 1993.

45. Gamliel Z, Krasna MJ: Multimodality treatment of esophageal cancer, *Surg Clin North Am* 85:621-630, 2005.

46. Garton GR, et al: High-dose preoperative external beam and intraoperative irradiation for locally advanced pancreatic cancer, *Int J Radiat Oncol Biol Phys* 27:1153-1157, 1993.

47. Gockel I, et al: Transhiatal and transthoracic resection in adenocarcinoma of the esophagus: Does the operative approach have an influence on the long-term prognosis? *World J Surg Oncol* 3:40, 2005 (serial online): http://www.wjso.com/content/3/1/40.

48. Greene FL: Minimal access cancer management, *CA Cancer J Clin* 57:130-146, 2007.

49. Greenlee RT, et al: Cancer statistics 2001, *CA Cancer J Clin* 51:15-36, 2001.

50. Guillem JG, Paty PB, Cohen AM: Surgical treatment of colorectal cancer, *CA Cancer J Clin* 47:113-128, 1997.

51. Gunderson LL: Colorectal cancer. In Perez CA, Brady LW, editors: *Principles and practice of radiation oncology*, Philadelphia, 1987, Lippincott.

52. Gunderson LL, Dozois RR: Intraoperative irradiation for locally advanced colorectal carcinomas, *Perspect Colon Rectal Surg* 5:1-23, 1992.

53. Gunderson LL, Martenson JA: Gastrointestinal tract radiation tolerance, *Front Radiat Ther Oncol* 23:277-298, 1989.

54. Gunderson LL, Martenson JA: Cancers of the colon and rectum. In Levitt S, Khan F, Potish R, editors: *Technological basis of radiation therapy*, ed 2, Philadelphia, 1991, Lea and Febiger.

55. Gunderson LL, Martenson JA: Colorectal cancer: radiation therapy. In *Current therapy in hematology-oncology*, ed 4, Philadelphia, 1992, BC Decker.

56. Gunderson LL, Martenson JA: Postoperative adjuvant irradiation with or without chemotherapy for rectal carcinoma, *Semin Radiat Oncol* 4:55-63, 1993.

57. Gunderson LL, Willett CG: Pancreas and hepatobiliary tract. In Perez CA, Brady LW, editors: *Principles and practices of radiation oncology*, Philadelphia, 1992, JB Lippincott.

58. Gunderson LL, Martenson JA, Smalley SR: Gastrointestinal toxicity. In John MJ, et al, editors: *Chemoradiation: an integrated approach to cancer treatment*, Philadelphia, 1993, Lea and Febiger.

59. Gunderson LL, et al: Indications for and results of intraoperative irradiation for locally advanced colorectal cancer, *Front Radiat Ther Oncol* 25:284-306, 1991.

60. Gunderson LL, et al: Upper gastrointestinal cancers: rationale, results, and techniques of treatment, *Front Radiat Ther Oncol* 28:121-139, 1994.

61. Gunderson LL, et al: Locally advanced primary colorectal cancer: intraoperative electron and external beam irradiation +/– 5 FU, *Int J Radiat Oncol Biol Phys* 37:601-614, 1997.

62. Gunderson LL, et al: Conformal irradiation for hepatobiliary malignancies, *Ann Oncol* 10 (suppl 4):2221-225, 1999.

63. Gunderson LL, et al: Future role of radiotherapy as a component of treatment in biliopancreatic cancers, *Ann Oncol* 10 (suppl 4):291-295, 1999.

64. Haddock MG, Martenson JA: Anal Carcinoma. In Gunderson LL, Tepper JE, editors: *Clinical radiation oncology*, ed 2, St. Louis, 2007, Churchill Livingstone.

65. Haddock MG, et al: Gemcitabine, cisplatin and radiotherapy for patients with locally advanced pancreatic adenocarcinoma: results of the North Central Cancer Treatment Group phase II study N9942, *J Clin Oncol* 25:2567-2572, 2007.

66. Hahnloser D, Haddock MG, Nelson H: Intraopreative radiotherapy in the multimodality approach to colorectal cancer, *Surg Oncol Clin North Am* 4:993-1013, 2003.

67. Herskovic A, et al: Combined chemotherapy and radiotherapy compared with radiotherapy alone in patients with cancer of the esophagus, *N Engl J Med* 326:1593-1631, 1992.

68. Hulscher JBF, et al: Extended transthoracic resection compared with limited transhiatal resection for adenocarcinoma of the esophagus, *N Engl J Med* 347:1662-1669, 2002.

69. Kalser MH, Ellenberg SS: Pancreatic cancer: adjuvant combined radiation and chemotherapy following curative resection, *Arch Surg* 120:899-903, 1985.

70. Kelsey CR, et al: Paclitaxel based chemoradiotherapy in the treatment of patients with operable esophageal cancer, *Int J Radiat Oncol Biol Phys* 69:770-776, 2007.

71. Krook JE, et al: Effective surgical adjuvant therapy for high-risk rectal carcinoma, *N Engl J Med* 324:709-715, 1991.

72. Kushi LH: American Cancer Society guidelines on nutrition and physical activity for cancer prevention, *CA Cancer J Clin* 56:254-281, 2006.

73. Landry JC, et al: Treatment of pancreatic cancer tumors with intensity-modulatedradiation therapy (IMRT) using the volume at risk approach (VARA): employing dose-volume histogram (DVH) and normal tissue complication probability (NTCP) to evaluate small bowel toxicity, *Med Dosim* 27:121-129, 2002.

74. Lee P, et al: Image Guided radiation therapy (RT) for rectal cancer using cone beam CT (CBCT), *Int J Radiat Oncol Biol Phys* 66:S276, 2006.

75. Lilliemoe KD, Yeo CJ, Cameron JL: Pancreatic cancer: state-of the-art care, *CA Cancer J Clin* 50:241-268, 2000.

76. Lynch HT, et al: Familial colon cancer: delineation of clinical subsets with etiologic and treatment considerations. In Levin B, editor: *Gastrointestinal cancer: current approaches to diagnosis and treatment*, Austin, 1988, University of Texas Press.

77. Macdonald JS: Adjuvant therapy of colon cancer, *CA Cancer J Clin* 49:202-219, 1999.

78. Malaisrie SC, et al: The addition of induction chemotherapy to preoperative, concurrent chemoradiotherapy improves tumor response in patients with esophageal adenocarcinoma, *Cancer* 107:967-974, 2006.

79. Markowitz AJ, Winawer SJ: Management of colorectal polyps, *CA Cancer J Clin* 47:93-112, 1997.

80. Martenson JA, Gunderson LL: External radiation therapy without chemotherapy in the management of anal cancer, *Cancer* 71:1736-1740, 1993.

81. Martenson JA, Gunderson LL: Colon and rectum. In Perez CA, Brady LW, editors: *Principles and practices of radiation oncology*, Philadelphia, 1998, JB Lippincott-Raven.

82. Martenson JA, et al: Prospective phase I evaluation of radiation therapy, 5-fluorouracil, and levamisole in locally advanced gastrointestinal cancer, *Int J Radiat Oncol Biol Phys* 28:439-443, 1994.

83. Meyer J, et al: Advanced radiation therapy technologies in the treatment of rectal and anal cancer: intensity-modulated photon therapy and proton therapy, *Clin Colorectal Cancer* 6:348-356, 2007.

84. Milan MT, et al: Intensity-modulated radiation therapy (IMRT) in the treatment of anal cancer: toxicity and clinical outcome, *Int J Radiat Oncol Biol Phys* 63:354-361, 2005.

85. Milano MT, et al: Intensity-modulated radiotherapy in treatment of pancreatic and bile duct malignancies: toxicity and clinical outcome, *Int J Radiat Oncol Biol Phys* 59:445-453, 2004.

86. Moertel CG, et al: Therapy of locally unresectable pancreatic carcinoma: a randomized comparison of high dose (6000 rads) radiation alone, moderate dose radiation (4000 rads + 5-fluorouracil), and high dose radiation + 5-fluorouracil, *Cancer* 48:1705-1710, 1981.

87. Netter FH: Digestive system, vol 3 parts I and II. In Oppenheimer E, editor: *CIBA collection of medical illustrations*, West Caldwell, NJ, 1987, Donnelly & Sons.

88. O'Brien MJ, et al: Precursors of colorectal carcinoma, *Cancer Suppl* 70:1317-1325, 1992.

89. Papillon J: *Rectal and anal cancers: conservative treatment by irradiation: an alternative approach to radical surgery*, New York, 1982, Springer-Verlag.

90. Paulino AC: Resected pancreatic cancer treated with adjuvant radiotherapy with or without 5-fluorouracil: treatment results and patterns of failure, *Am J Clin Oncol* 22:489, 1999.

91. Peacock JL, Keller JW, Asbury RF: Alimentary tract cancers. In Rubin P, editor: *Clinical oncology: a multidisciplinary approach for physicians and students*, ed 7, Philadelphia, 1993, WB Saunders.

92. Pisters PW, et al: Preoperative chemoradiation for patients with pancreatic cancer: toxicity of endobiliary stents, *J Clin Oncol* 18:860-867, 2000.

93. Robbin SL, Cottran RS: *Pathologic basis of disease*, ed 2, Philadelphia, 1979, WB Saunders.

94. Rodel C, Valentini V, Minsky BD: Rectal Cancer. In Gunderson LL, Tepper JE, editors: *Clinical Radiation Oncology*, ed 2, St. Louis, 2007, Churchill Livingstone.

95. Rohatgi P, et al: Characterization of pathologic complete response after preoperative chemoradiotherapy in carcinoma of the esophagus and outcome after pathologic complete response, *Cancer* 104(11):2365-2372, 2004.

96. Roth JA, et al: Cancer of the esophagus. In Devita VT, Hellman S, Rosenburg SA, editors: *Cancer principles and practice of oncology*, Philadelphia, 1993, JB Lippincott.

97. Schnirer II, et al: Pilot study of concurrent 5 fluorouracil/paclitaxel plus radiotherapy in patients with carcinoma of the esophagus and GE junction, *Am J Clin Oncol* 24:91-95, 2001.

98. Shank B, Cohen AM, Kelsen D: Cancer of the anal region. In Devita VT, Hellman S, Rosenburg SA, editors: *Cancer principles and practice of oncology*, Philadelphia, 1993, JB Lippincott.

99. Smith RA, et al: American Cancer Society guidelines for the early detection guidelines for prostate, colorectal, and endometrial cancers, *CA Cancer J Clin* 51:38-75, 2001.

100. Stafford SL, Martenson JA: Combined radiation and chemotherapy for carcinoma of the anal canal, *Oncology* 12:373-377 1998.

101. Steele GD Jr, et al: Clinical highlights from the National Cancer Data Base: 1994, *CA Cancer J Clin* 44:71-80, 1994.

102. Urba SG, et al: Concurrent cisplatin, paclitaxel, and radiotherapy as preoperative treatment for patients with locoregional esophageal carcinoma, *Cancer* 98:2177-2183, 2003.

103. Vargas PA, Alberts DS: Primary prevention of colorectal cancer through dietary modification, *Cancer Suppl* 70:1229-1233, 1992.

104. Warshaw AL, Swanson RS: What's new in general surgery: pancreatic cancer in 1988, possibilities and probabilities, *Ann Surg* 208:541, 1988.

105. Wiltshire KL, et al: Preoperative radiation with xoncurrent chemotherapy for resectable rectal cancer: effect of dose escalation on pathologic complete response, local recurrence-free survival, and overall survival, *Int J Radiat Oncol Biol Phys* 64:709-716, 2005.

106. Yasko JM: *Care of the client receiving external radiation therapy*, Reston, VA, 1982, Reston Publishing.

Gynecological Tumors

George M. Uschold, Joy E. Anderson

Outline

Key Terms

Objectives

- Discuss epidemiologic factors of this tumor site.
- Identify, list, and discuss etiologic factors that may be responsible for inducing tumors in this anatomic site.
- Describe the symptoms produced by a malignant tumor in this region.
- Discuss the methods of detection and diagnosis for tumors in this anatomic region.
- List the varying histologic types of tumors characteristic to this region.
- Describe the diagnostic procedures used in the workup and staging for this site.
- Describe the clinical classification used for this area.
- Describe in detail the most common routes of tumor spread for this site.
- Describe and diagram the lymphatic routes of spread for tumors in this region.
- Differentiate between histologic grading and staging.
- Describe in detail the anatomy and physiology of this anatomic region/organ.
- Identify the treatment(s) of choice for this malignancy.
- Discuss the rationale for treatment with regard to treatment choice, histologic type, and stage of the disease.

- Describe in detail the treatment methods available for this diagnosis.
- Describe the differing types of radiation treatments that can be used for treating this tumor site.
- Identify the appropriate tumor lethal dose for various stages of this malignancy.
- Discuss the expected radiation reactions for the area based on time-dose-fractionation schemes.
- Discuss tolerance levels of the vital structures and organs at risk.
- Describe the instructions that should be given to a patient with regard to skin care, expected reactions. and dietary advice.
- Identify the psychological problems associated with a malignancy in this site.
- Discuss the rationale for using multimodality treatments for this diagnosis.
- Describe the various treatment planning techniques for this anatomic site including external beam and brachytherapy options.
- Discuss survival statistics and prognosis for various stages for this tumor site.

This chapter provides radiation therapists with basic knowledge of gynecologic malignancies. An initial section on epidemiology and etiology discusses the relative number of cancers and deaths resulting from the various sites. This section is followed by a site-specific discussion regarding the populations at risk and various risk factors. The anatomy of the pelvic gynecologic structures is then reviewed. Knowledge of radiation tolerances and lymphatic drainage is of critical importance in radiation therapy treatment planning. These issues are discussed in depth.

Following this general review, the organ areas (vulva, vagina, cervix, endometrium, and ovaries) are discussed in individual sections. Each section begins with a clinical presentation that includes symptoms, data regarding lymphatic spread, and prognostic features. This is followed by a brief description of the clinical workup, expected pathology, and staging. To minimize confusion, the staging is limited to the system provided by the International Federation of Gynecology and Obstetrics (FIGO).[21] Treatment considerations specific to each organ are then presented. This is done to orient the radiation therapist to required modifications in the treatment design beyond the basic pelvic treatment plan and to provide the rationale for these modifications. Each section closes with a case study that synthesizes the principles presented.

After the sections concerning specific organs, general principles of external beam radiation therapy and brachytherapy are discussed in detail. The goal is to promote a clear knowledge of the basic design of treatment fields and enable the radiation therapist to understand the rationale underlying the various simulations. Dose schedules are presented generally and with the specific sites. In general, the radiation therapist should be able to use data in this section to understand and critique most gynecologic treatment plans.

The chapter closes with a discussion of expected side effects from radiation therapy and the radiation therapist's role in evaluating and managing these sequelae. The radiation therapist has three main functions during the course of therapy: treatment delivery, ongoing patient assessment, and patient reassurance.

EPIDEMIOLOGY AND ETIOLOGY

An estimated 78,490 patients develop gynecologic cancer in the United States each year. This type of malignancy is divided into endometrial (50%), ovarian (29%), cervical (14%), and other gynecologic cancers (7%). An estimated 28,490 deaths occur each year, with ovarian being the most prevalent (56%), followed by endometrial (27%), cervical (14%), and other gynecologic cancers (3%).[1]

Ovarian cancer has the highest death rate due to non-specific early symptoms that result in a late-stage disease diagnosis.

Alternatively, considering the ratio of deaths to new cases, ovarian cancer has the highest death rate at 68%, followed by cervical cancer (excluding carcinoma in situ) at 33%, and endometrial cancer at 19%. Although there are 24% more endometrial than ovarian cancers, ovarian cancer deaths have 250% more incidence than endometrial-related deaths. The high death rate for ovarian cancer is primarily due to the relatively nonspecific early symptoms with a consequent diagnosis of later-stage disease. A secondary reason is less effective treatment. Endometrial cancer has a relatively higher cure rate because the early symptom of postmenopausal bleeding usually results in a physical evaluation at an earlier stage, during which effective local therapy can be initiated.

Overall, cervical carcinoma is more prevalent than other gynecologic cancers among younger women. Although cervical intraepithelial neoplasia affects mainly younger women, invasive cervical cancer rates reach their peak in women aged 50 to 60.[24] Women of lower socioeconomic status have a greater than average risk of developing cervical cancer and a less than average participation rate in cancer screening programs.[42]

Early sexual activity, multiple partners, and multiple pelvic infections (especially with genital warts and human papillomaviruses [HPVs] and herpes simplex type 2 [HSII]) have been associated with an increase in the risk of this disease and an earlier onset. Incidence is also higher among wives of men with penile cancer.[19] As with vaginal cancers, there is an increased risk of clear cell adenocarcinoma and abnormalities of the stratified epithelium in women whose mothers used diethylstilbestrol (DES) during the early months of pregnancy.[44] However, all women are at some risk and need effective and safe screenings. The widespread use of Papanicolaou (Pap) smears has resulted in early detection; two thirds of cervical cancers are now detected in the noninvasive stage and are therefore highly curable with local therapy.

Thanks to Papanicolaou smears, two thirds of cervical cancers are detected in the noninvasive stage and are highly curable with local therapy.

The prevalence of endometrial cancer has increased as a result of the aging population, high-calorie and high-fat diets, and the use of unopposed estrogen in the 1960s and 1970s. The incidence peaks at about 58 years, and more than 75% of patients are women older than 50. Diabetes and hypertension are both linked with an increase in prevalence of endometrial cancer.[45] Women who are 50 pounds overweight have a ninefold increase in risk.[38] A higher risk also results from an increase in estrogen or the estrogen-to-progesterone ratio, as occurs with nulliparity, infertility secondary to anovulation (with a deficit in progesterone), dysfunctional bleeding during menopause (secondary to estrogen overstimulation), or prolonged hormone replacement therapy (HRT). In the case of HRT, the increased risk seems to be treatment duration dependent.[6]

Vaginal and vulvar cancers are rare and usually occur in older women. Vulvar carcinoma, which is three times as common as vaginal cancer, has been associated with diabetes and sexually transmitted diseases.[1] Atrophic and dysplastic changes in the normal vaginal lining, a loss of hormone stimulation, and poor hygiene may also be associated with vulvar cancers. An unusual clear-cell type of vaginal cancer seen in young women (median age of 19) has been associated with DES use by their pregnant mothers while they were in utero.[44] Melanoma is also seen more frequently in the vulva than in the vagina. If the cervix is involved with a vaginally located cancer, the tumor is classified as a cervical cancer with vulvovaginal spread and is treated in the same way as other advanced cervical cancers.

Ovarian carcinoma occurs primarily in women between the ages of 50 and 70. At approximately 15,280 estimated deaths annually, it is the fifth leading cause of cancer deaths in women, following lung (70,880), breast (40,460), colon (26,180), and pancreatic (16,530) cancer.[1] Risk factors include an older age, late or few pregnancies, late menopause, a lack of oral contraceptive use, a family history of ovarian cancer, and a personal history of breast, colon, or endometrial cancer.[37] Diets high in meat and/or animal fat and living in industrialized nations (except Japan) are risk factors. Screening tools are inadequate because the disease is only intermittently detectable during physical examinations, radiographic studies, and serologic tests and usually is found at an advanced stage. With the low prevalence of this disease, even a 100% **sensitive test** (0% false negative) for detecting tumors and a 99% **specific test** (1% false positive) for patients with disease result in over 100 laparotomies for every early ovarian cancer detected with an iatrogenic death rate equal to or higher than the disease. For patients with hereditary ovarian cancer syndrome the lifetime risk increases from 1% to 40%, and a screening with an annual rectovaginal pelvic examination, CA-125 serum determinations, and **transvaginal sonography*** is recommended to reduce this significant risk.

ANATOMY AND LYMPHATICS

The vulva is the outermost portion of the gynecologic tract. The major parts include the labia majora and labia minora, the clitoris, and the area bound by these three called the vestibule. The vestibule is triangular, is located anterior to the vaginal opening, and usually contains the urethral meatus, unless the meatus exits within the outer third of the vaginal canal. The **perineum** refers to the area between the vulvovaginal complex and anal verge. The vagina is a muscular tube that extends 6 to 8 inches superiorly from the vulva and is located anterior to the rectum and posterior to the bladder. The cervix (the part of the uterus that extends into the apex of the vagina) is a firm, rounded structure from 1.5 to 3 cm in diameter. The cervix often protrudes into the vagina, producing lateral spaces in the vaginal apex called the fornices. A canal called the cervical os extends from the vagina, through the central cervix, and into the uterine cavity, or pelvic portion of the uterus. The uterus is a hollow, muscular structure that extends at a right angle from the vagina to overlie the bladder. Extending laterally from the superior uterus are the twin fallopian tubes. These are hollow structures designed to transfer the ova from the ovaries located adjacent to them to the uterus. The **parametrium** refers to the connective tissue immediately lateral to the uterine cervix (Figure 36-1).

Radiation therapy treatment requires an understanding of the radiosensitivity of the various gynecologic structures and their lymphatic drainage. The vulva and perineum usually show the most acute short-term side effects, partly because of their radiation sensitivity and the often parallel and tangential nature of the treatment beams applied to them. Doses above 40 Gy at standard fractions (1.8 to 2 Gy) often cause significant acute erythema and desquamation, and doses above 50 Gy cause late telangiectasis. Significant fibrosis can result from doses approaching 70 Gy. The vagina is more tolerant, with the upper vaginal mucosa tolerating up to 140 Gy and the lower up to 100 Gy before extensive fibrosis.[17] Early mucositis and later telangiectasis occur with much lower treatment-range doses (60 to 85 Gy). The uterus and cervix tolerate extremely high doses of radiation and allow the effectiveness of brachytherapy to these structures. Low-dose-rate brachytherapy, in combination with fractionated external radiation therapy, can be delivered locally to the cervical canal without necrosis when the total dose does not exceed 200 Gy.[15] The ovary is the most radiosensitive gynecologic structure. The dose response is age dependent. For example, a dose of 4 to 5 Gy produces the permanent cessation of menses in about 65% of women younger than 40, 90% of those aged 40 to 44, and 100% of those 50 years or older.[35]

Many other organs surrounding the gynecologic structures have dose tolerances that must be respected. The bladder, which is located anterior to the vagina and cervix and somewhat under the uterus, expands forward and away from these structures when it is filled. The point tolerance is about 75 to 80 Gy, but whole-bladder treatment results in acute cystitis at doses as low as 30 Gy. This results in acute bladder irritation with dysuria, frequency, and urgency but usually resolves in a couple of weeks. Chronic cystitis occasionally occurs 6 months after radiation with doses above 50 to 60 Gy, and contracture and/or hemorrhagic cystitis occurs with doses above 65 Gy. The rectum, which is immediately posterior to the vagina and cervix, also has a point tolerance of about 70 Gy. The rectum continues superiorly with the sigmoid colon, with a whole-organ tolerance of about 50 Gy. Diarrhea, bleeding, urgency, and pain can occur acutely at 30 to 40 Gy. Stricture, bleeding, and perforation are late complications that occur with doses above the tolerance level. The small bowel is variably looped down in the pelvis and may overlie the uterus and bladder. This bowel has a lower tolerance at 45 Gy, can yield the same acute toxicity as the large bowel (but at lower doses), and is more likely to obstruct as a chronic complication.

The treatment design must consider the extent of the primary lesion and the probability of metastases to the draining lymph nodes. Lymphatic drainage includes the inguinal lymph nodes (superficial and deep), pelvic nodes (the internal iliac chain, which originates approximately with the obturator node, and external iliac chain), and periaortic nodes (Figure 36-2). The deep inguinals drain into the external iliac chain, and the internal and external iliac chains join and then drain into the periaortics. Drainage is approximately contiguous. Therefore, if involvement of the nodes occurs at one level, including the next higher nodal group in the treatment field may be appropriate.

Ovarian and upper endometrial lymphatics follow the ovarian blood supply to terminate in periaortic lymph nodes at the level of the kidneys and then they follow the round ligament to involve the inguinal lymphatics. The primary drainage pattern of the cervix and additional drainage patterns of the ovary and uterus are to the external iliac, obturator, and hypogastric (internal iliac) chains. Upper vaginal lymphatic drainage follows the cervical pathways. Lower vaginal drainage may follow the vulvar drainage into the inguinal nodes.

VULVA

Clinical Presentation

Vulvar cancer patients usually have a subcutaneous lump or mass. Patients with more advanced disease have an ulcerative exophytic mass. The disease is usually unifocal, with the labia majora as the most common location. Often, the patient has a

---

*A test used to detect abnormalities in the reproductive system and possible complications with pregnancy by way of a vaginally inserted sonographic transducer that emits high-frequency sound waves that are electronically converted to diagnostic images.

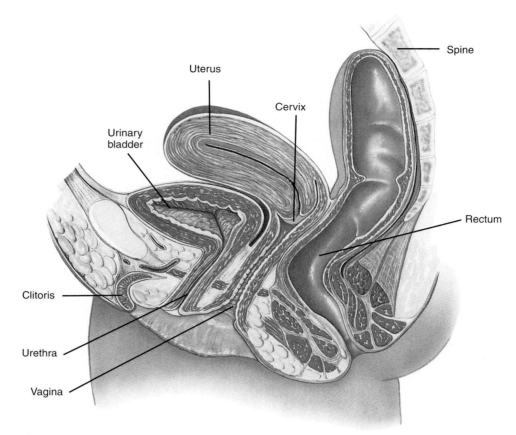

Figure 36-1. A sagittal view of the female pelvis. (From Seely R: *Essentials of anatomy and physiology*, St. Louis, 1991, Mosby.)

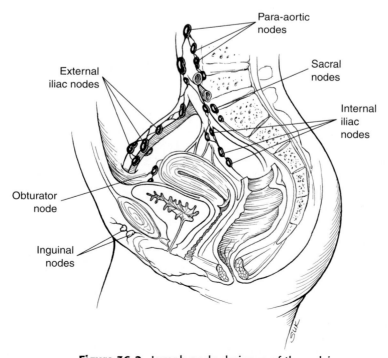

Figure 36-2. Lymph node drainage of the pelvis.

long history of local irritation. Lymphatic spread is predictable, involving the superficial inguinal nodes first, then the deep femoral nodes, and eventually the pelvic nodes. However, lymph nodes are falsely enlarged in about 40% of patients due to reactive hyperplasia. The incidence of lymph node involvement is related to the depth of invasion (less than 10% at 1 to 3 mm and about 25% at 3 to 4 mm) and tumor size (38% for tumors greater than 5 mm and 46% for those greater than 20 mm).[28] Occult disease is common, as is inflammation, so that a high level of false negatives and false positives may result from the physical examination and clinical suspicion alone. Prognostic factors include the size of the lesion, depth of invasion, and histologic subtype. The presence and extent of lymph node involvement are the strongest predictor of overall survival rates.

Detection and Diagnosis

A diagnostic workup should include a biopsy, with histologic examination, a history, a physical examination, blood counts and chemistries, a urinalysis, chest radiographs, an intravenous pyelogram (IVP) and/or a computed tomography (CT) scan, and a cystourethroscopy. Liver scans, a bone scan, a sigmoidoscopy, and a pelvic CT scan are usually performed if the tumor is locally advanced or if clinically suggested by other staging studies.

Pathology and Staging

Squamous cell carcinomas account for more than 90% of vulvar cancers, and adenocarcinomas represent most of the remaining cases.[37]

Staging is as follows:

Stage I: Tumor confined to the vulva or vulva and perineum with a maximum diameter of 2 cm or less in greatest dimension

Stage II: Tumor confined to the vulva or vulva and perineum with a maximum diameter greater than 2 cm in greatest dimension

Stage III: Tumor of any size with contiguous spread to the lower urethra and/or vagina or anus

Stage IVA: Tumor invades any of the following: upper urethra, bladder mucosa, rectal mucosa, or is fixed to the pelvic bone

Treatment Considerations

Historically, treatment has involved a radical vulvectomy with a groin node dissection. For stage III disease with inguinal nodes positive for tumor, deep pelvic nodes must be addressed, either with a pelvic node dissection or pelvic irradiation. Recent studies have indicated that a more conservative approach using wide local excision with external irradiation of the primary and inguinal nodes produces similar tumor control, 5-year disease-free survival and overall survival rates, while causing less morbidity.[3,16,29]

Radiation therapy may be administered preoperatively, but it is increasingly used as the sole local treatment, with or without chemotherapy (simulation techniques are discussed at the end of the chapter). For stage I and II disease, radiation therapy is usually given after wide local excision (50 Gy) and after a simple vulvectomy (60 Gy plus a 5- to 10-Gy boost if margins are close or positive for tumor). For stage III disease, radiation therapy is given postoperatively if the primary is larger than 4 cm, margins are positive for tumor or less than 8 mm, or two or more lymph nodes are positive for tumor. A dose of 50 Gy is delivered to control microscopic disease, with a 15 Gy boost if margins are microscopically positive for tumor and 20 Gy for grossly involved margins. Boosts may be delivered using photons, en face perineal electrons, and via brachytherapy. The inguinal region (nodes) is treated to 45 to 50 Gy for control of microscopic disease and to 65 to 70 Gy for clinically involved lymph nodes that were not dissected. If the pelvic nodes are included, 45 to 50 Gy is delivered for microscopic disease and 60 Gy for macroscopic disease. Treatment interruptions are usually needed at 40 Gy or less if chemotherapy is given concomitantly. The vulva and perineum usually develop significant moist desquamation as a result of the smaller thickness of tissue in the region relative to the pelvic separation, the tangential delivery of the external beam, and the need for use of bolus.

The overall 5-year survival rate is about 70%,[22,25] and the disease-free survival rates in surgically treated patients with stages I through IV disease are 100%, 86%, 59%, and 25%, respectively.[32] Hacker et al.[16] have shown the influence of regional lymph node involvement, with actuarial 5-year survival rates of 96% if nodes are negative for tumor, 94% with one node positive for tumor, 80% with two nodes positive for tumor, and 12% with three or more nodes positive for tumor.

Simulation and Treatment

Vulvar fields include the primary site and inguinal region. A pelvic field is added to the top or bottom of L5 if the primary is greater than 2 cm or if deep femoral nodes are positive for tumor. Pelvic fields should include the **pelvic inlet**, which is the opening in the pelvis into which a baby's head enters. The pelvic inlet is defined by the sacral promontory, the inner sidewalls, and the pubic bones. The pelvic field includes a 2 cm lateral margin to cover pelvic lymph nodes. The field is often wider in the region of the inguinal lymph nodes so as to encompass these nodes if they are considered to be at risk for involvement or if they are involved with disease. The patient is usually simulated in the "frog-leg" position, with wires over surgical scars and palpable nodes so that they may be included within the field. Bolus is placed over the vulva and perineum. The fraction size is limited to 1.7 to 1.8 Gy, and treatment breaks are often necessary by 40 Gy because of severe vulvar skin reactions (Figure 36-3). Inguinal nodes are best treated mainly from the anterior field in order to minimize dose to the femoral head and neck. Techniques to minimize femoral head and neck dose include partial transmission blocks, weighting of the anterior field more heavily, anterior bolus, use of lower energies anteriorly and higher energies posteriorly, and anterior electron fields for boosts. Use of a CT scan of the pelvis is important for determining the location of the inguinal and femoral lymph nodes, and also the other pelvic lymph nodes. Intensity modulated radiotherapy will increasingly be utilized to achieve these goals.

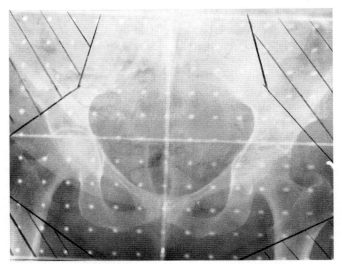

Figure 36-3. A simulation radiograph demonstrating a treatment field used to treat the vulva, pelvic, and inguinofemoral lymph nodes.

CASE I

Vulvectomy

An 83-year-old white woman with underlying peripheral vascular disease from her hypertension, diabetes, and hypercholesterolemia consulted with her gynecologist, and a pelvic examination exhibited a 5-cm right labial mass. A wide local excision and bilateral lymph node dissections revealed no nodes positive for tumor. The disease was therefore stage II and no additional treatment was given. The mass recurred 6 months later on the right side, and the patient underwent a simple vulvectomy and rhomboid skin flap grafts. Because of the recurrence, deep invasion, and close margins, she was referred for postoperative radiation therapy.

The treatment design included anteroposterior/posteroanterior (AP/PA) lower pelvic fields and anteriorly treated inguinal fields. Initially, 6-MV photons were used with anterior bolus. The initial dose was 50.4 Gy at 1.8 Gy/fraction. The perineum and operative sites received a boost of 10 Gy with en face 9-MeV electrons at 2 Gy/fraction. The patient required several treatment breaks for moist desquamation and urethral irritation. Diarrhea was not a major problem.

The patient remained free of disease for 18 months, until a recurrence was detected in the periurethral area. A low-dose rate iridium **interstitial implant** was performed to a small volume surrounding the area of recurrence at a dose of 40 Gy over 4 days. This treatment controlled the local disease, but she experienced recurrence again in the perineal body and anal canal. She is considering a type of exenterative procedure.

VAGINA

Clinical Presentation

Vaginal cancer is a malignancy that arises in the vagina and has not extended to the vulva or cervix at initial presentation. This definition helps make vaginal cancer a rare disease that accounts for approximately 2% of all gynecologic cancers. No etiologic associations are definite, except for the rarer clear cell carcinoma seen in 1 per 1000 women who had been exposed to DES while they were in utero. The usual squamous cell

carcinomas occur in older women (median age of 65), whereas clear cell carcinomas occur in young women between the ages of 15 and 27 (median age of 19 at diagnosis).[26] Abnormal vaginal bleeding and/or painful intercourse are the usual presenting symptoms. The most common location is the posterior upper third of the vagina. The risk of lymphatic involvement increases with the depth of invasion. Pelvic lymphatic involvement is similar to cervical cancer, with lesions of the lower third of the vagina also potentially involving the inguinal nodes.

Detection and Diagnosis

The workup should include a biopsy, a cytologic examination, a careful history, a physical examination, blood counts and chemistries, a urinalysis, chest radiographs, an IVP or abdomino-pelvic CT scan, and a cystourethroscopy. If the disease is advanced, liver and bone scans, a proctosigmoidoscopy, and a pelvic CT scan are recommended.

Pathology and Staging

Squamous cell carcinomas total 80% to 90% of vaginal cancers. Malignant melanomas account for about 5% of vaginal cancers. Other vaginal cancers include sarcomas, malignant lymphomas, and clear cell adenocarcinomas. Staging is as follows:

Stage I: Tumor confined to the vagina
Stage II: Tumor invades the paravaginal tissue but not to the pelvic wall
Stage III: Tumor extends to the pelvic wall (muscle, fascia, neurovascular structures, or skeletal portions of the bony pelvis)
Stage IVA: Tumor invades the mucosa of the bladder or rectum and/or extends beyond the true pelvis

Treatment Considerations

Radiation therapy is the treatment of choice for most vaginal cancers. Surgery is used for recurrent or persistent squamous cell cancers and in young women who have early clear cell adenocarcinoma. For small, superficial lesions, only the vaginal tissues are treated (via local excision or brachytherapy), but for invasive lesions the entire pelvis must be treated. Doses of 45 to 50 Gy are given to the pelvis, and the entire vagina is included in the external beam field. If the tumor involves the middle or lower third of the vagina and is stage II or higher, the inguinal nodes are also treated as in vulvar cancer. Microscopic disease is treated to 50 Gy and macroscopic to 65 to 80 Gy. Brachytherapy implants are used to bring the primary and adjacent macroscopic disease to curative doses. Problems with early acute dermatitis are similar to those seen in vulvar cancer patients.

Simulation and Treatment

Vaginal carcinomas are usually treated with radiation therapy. Surgery is most often reserved for recurrences, early-stage clear cell adenocarcinoma especially in a young patient, and persistent masses after radiotherapy. Brachytherapy alone or as a boost is dependent on the size of the primary and nodal disease. For carcinoma in situ and stage I well-differentiated cancer, the entire vagina may be treated via brachytherapy alone to a dose to 60 Gy using a **vaginal cylinder**, which is a canal-filling cylinder into which an isotope, usually cesium-137, is placed. This is the low-dose rate brachytherapy procedure, and the high-dose rate technique uses an equivalent dose and treatment is administered in a fractionated manner. Further brachytherapy can be done as a boost of 20 Gy to minimal disease, with the cylinder and/or another brachytherapy device consisting of needles placed directly into the at-risk tissues (an interstitial implant) for more deeply invasive tumors. For lesions larger than early stage I, doses of 45 to 50 Gy are given to a pelvic field and the entire vagina. A four-field technique is customarily used to cover the at-risk tissues, but the AP/PA technique or intensity-modulated radiation therapy (IMRT) may provide an advantage if the inguinal lymph nodes are to be treated and with modifications to allow a lower dose to the femoral head and neck. The inguinal nodes are included for tumors involving the lower two thirds of the vagina. Low-dose rate or high-dose rate brachytherapy interstitial implants are used to bring macroscopic primary doses up to 65 to 85 Gy (Figure 36-4, *A* and *B*). For superficial residual disease, intracavitary techniques are used. Deeply invasive disease requires boosting with combination implants that include an interstitial component (Figure 36-5, *A-F*).

CASE II

Vaginal Cylinder

A 61-year-old white woman with underlying chronic obstructive pulmonary disease (COPD) and hypertension complained to the gynecologist of 2 months of vaginal bleeding, especially after intercourse. A pelvic examination revealed a mass at the right lateral aspect of the vagina near to, but discontinuous from the cervix. A biopsy confirmed poorly differentiated, invasive squamous cell carcinoma. The results of other staging studies were negative for tumor. Her disease was classified as stage II (T2 N0).

Radiation therapy consisted of AP/PA (or four-field box) pelvic and vaginal treatment, with 18-MV photons at 2 Gy/fraction to 20 Gy. A **midline block** (shielding block used to eliminate dose to centrally located anatomy) was then added, and she was treated to an additional 20 Gy. A reduced parametrial boost with midline blocking of the small bowel was given an additional 10 Gy (or 45 to 50 Gy pelvis + vagina and one internal brachytherapy treatment insertion of 25 to 30 Gy).

Brachytherapy consisted of a vaginal cylinder implant, giving the mucosa 20 Gy over 2 days at the beginning of the midline-blocked pelvic treatment, and a second complex implant with a vaginal cylinder and right-sided interstitial needles given at the end of the initial pelvic treatment. The second implant yielded an additional 40 Gy to the vaginal mucosa and 25 Gy to the right-sided vaginal extension of the tumor.

The patient experienced some diarrhea, cystitis, and vaginal dryness but is still sexually active and free of disease 2 years later.

CERVIX

Clinical Presentation

Cervical cancer is a slowly progressive disease, with the earliest phase (noninvasive or carcinoma in situ) occurring approximately 10 years earlier than invasive cancer. The earlier cervical cancer is detected, the better is the local and overall control. Routine Papanicolaou smears have played a crucial role in the early detection of cervical cancer and in the improved overall

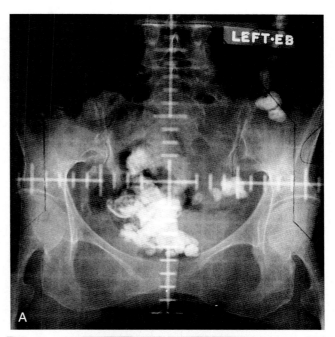

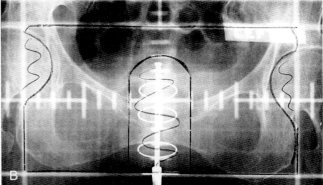

Figure 36-4. Radiographs of vaginal simulation and brachytherapy implant procedures. **A,** Typical anteroposterior/posteroanterior (AP/PA) simulation portal for a vaginal cancer treatment. **B,** Brachytherapy implant using a domed-cylinder technique. Note that the midline is blocked. The parametrial boost field with midline block is also shown.

survival rate. Screening should begin at age 18 or earlier in sexually active women.

Common presenting signs of invasive cancer are postcoital bleeding, increased menstrual bleeding, and discomfort with intercourse. A malodorous discharge, pelvic pain, and urinary or even rectal symptoms may accompany more advanced disease. Invasive cancer appears as a friable, ulcerative, or exophytic mass originating from or involving the cervix. It may be barrel-shaped and concentrically involve the cervix. The mass may extend into the vaginal canal and onto the vaginal sidewalls, or it may invade adjacent tissues such as the parametrium, bladder, or rectum. Lymphatic involvement is usually orderly, involving parametrial nodes, followed by pelvic, common iliac, periaortic, and even supraclavicular nodes. With periaortic nodal involvement, a 35% risk exists for supraclavicular spread.[8]

Survival rates and local control decrease as the stage and bulk of the disease increase. Ureter invasion has been associated

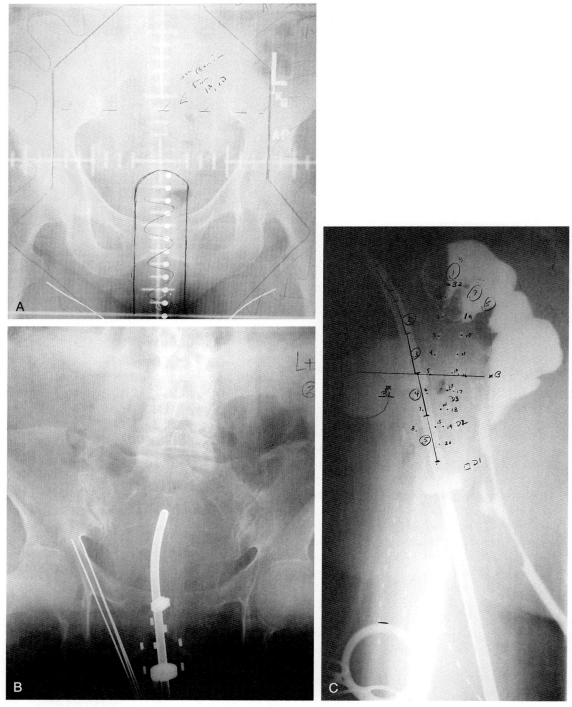

Figure 36-5. Treatment of vaginal cancer. **A**, Pelvic anteroposterior/posteroanterior (AP/PA) ports with a midline block. This particular arrangement used a 6-MV anterior field and an 18-MV posterior field. **B**, AP view of an intrauterine tandem, vaginal cylinder, and interstitial needles used during a brachytherapy boost. **C**, Lateral view of an intrauterine tandem, vaginal cylinder, and interstitial needles used during a brachytherapy boost.

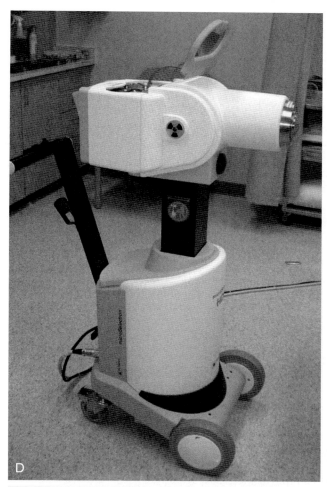

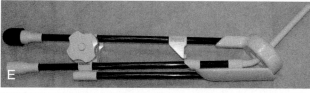

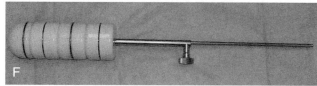

Figure 36-5. cont'd D, Microselectron HDR transportable unit. **E**, Tandem and ring HDR brachytherapy applicator set. **F**, Vaginal applicator set. (**D–F**, Courtesy Nucletron Corporation.)

with a reduction in 5-year survival rates from 92% to 54%.[30] Bulky or barrel-shaped cervical cancer is associated with a 22% chance of developing distant metastases within 5 years.[20] For stages IB and IIA, the involvement of lymph nodes results in approximately a 50% reduction in survival rates.[10-12] Anemia is an extremely common side effect of treatment, and restoring optimal hemoglobin levels is priority in improving the physical and quality of life status in patients,[4] and iron-based treatments are also being studied to ameliorate symptoms.[21] In addition, a recent study by Milosevic et al.[27] found that patients with an interstitial fluid pressure (IFP) greater than 19 mm Hg had a significantly lower disease-free survival rate compared with those whose IFP was less than 19 mm Hg (34% versus 68%, respectively).

Detection and Diagnosis

The workup should initially include a pelvic examination, Papanicolaou smear, and biopsy of any suspicious lesions. Further staging studies include a complete history, a physical examination under anesthesia, dilatation and curettage to assess uterine involvement, complete blood counts, chemistries, and a urinalysis. Chest radiographs, barium enema, and an IVP are used for FIGO staging. However, abdominal and pelvic CT scanning has essentially replaced the use of IVP. For more advanced disease, abdominopelvic CT or magnetic resonance imaging (MRI) scans, a cystoscopy, and a proctoscopy are recommended. A lymphangiogram may help with the radiotherapy treatment design but it is infrequently used today. Surgical evaluation with lymph node dissection is associated with a significant increase in pelvic side effects, but a laparoscopic or CT-directed biopsy of suspicious lymph nodes may be useful in designing treatment portals. PET scanning is becoming increasingly important for clinical staging and it further reduces the need for laparotomy. However, not all insurance companies are willing to allow or cover PET scanning.

Pathology and Staging

Squamous cell carcinoma is the most common pathologic type, as with vaginal and vulvar cancers. Adenocarcinomas of the cervix arise from the mucous-secreting endocervical glands and account for about 10% of these tumors. Small cell and clear cell types account for about 2% of the remaining tumors and have a higher metastatic potential.[37] Staging is as follows:

Stage 0: Carcinoma in situ

Stage I: Cervical cancer confined to the uterus

Stage IA: Invasive carcinoma diagnosed only by microscopy. Stromal invasion with a maximum depth of 5.0 mm measured from the base of the epithelium and a horizontal spread of 7.0 mm or less. Vascular space involvement, venous or lymphatic, does not affect classification.

Stage IA1: Measured stromal invasion 3.0 mm or less in depth and 7.0 mm or less in horizontal spread

Stage IA2: Measured stromal invasion more than 3.0 mm and not more than 5.0 mm in depth and 7.0 mm or less in horizontal spread or horizontal spread greater than 7.0 mm

Stage IB: Clinically visible lesion confined to the cervix or microscopic lesion greater than IA2

Stage IB1: Clinically visible lesion 4.0 cm or less in greatest dimension

Stage IB2: Clinically visible lesion more than 4.0 cm in greatest dimension

Stage II: Cervical cancer invades beyond the uterus but not to the pelvic sidewalls or lower third of the vagina

Stage IIA: Tumor without parametrial invasion

Stage IIB: Tumor with parametrial invasion

Stage III: Tumor extends to the pelvic wall and/or to the lower third of the vagina, and/or causes hydronephrosis or nonfunctioning kidney

Stage IIIA: Tumor involves lower third of the vagina, no extension to pelvic wall

Stage IIIB: Tumor extends to the pelvic wall and/or causes hydronephrosis or nonfunctioning kidney

Stage IVA: Tumor invades mucosa of the bladder or rectum and/or extends beyond the true pelvis

Staging is based on a clinical examination before the initiation of therapy and may be supplemented by a blood analysis, chest radiographs, an IVP, a cystoscopy, a barium enema, and bone scans. A CT scan, laparotomy findings, MRI scan, and lymphangiograms may modify treatment but do not change the FIGO staging. For statistical purposes, the cancer is staged at the earlier level if disagreement or doubt exists.

The incidence of pelvic and periaortic nodal involvement is local-stage dependent, with less than 5% and less than 1% for stage I, 15% and 5% for stage Ib, 30% and 15% for stage II, and 50% and 30% for stage III, respectively).[23] For stages IB and IIA, the involvement of lymph nodes results in approximately a 50% reduction in survival rates.[10-12]

Treatment Considerations

For early stage 0 (carcinoma in situ) and for stage Ia1 invasive cancer, the usual treatment is a total abdominal hysterectomy (TAH) with a small amount of vaginal tissue, known as the **vaginal cuff**. Alternately, a conization limited to the cervix may be performed in women who desire additional children. A tandem and ovoid implant, delivering 45 to 55 Gy to point A, is occasionally used for medically inoperable patients. For stage Ia2, TAH or a more aggressive modified radical hysterectomy is usually performed. In the medically inoperable patient, 70 to 80 Gy to the cervix and parametrial tissues may be delivered with the tandem and ovoids implant in 2 to 3 low-dose rate brachytherapy insertions, or 25 to 30 Gy in 5 to 6 treatments with high-dose rate brachytherapy insertions. Stages Ib1 and small IIa are somewhat controversial because surgery and radiation therapy yield similar control and survival data. Because of the preservation of vaginal pliability and ovarian function, surgery is often used for younger women, whereas radiation is used for women who have a higher risk for surgical complications. Radiation treatments consist of a combination of external beam therapy and implants. For bulky stage Ib2 cervical disease, radiation therapy doses of 80 to 85 Gy are given using the combined treatments. Postoperative irradiation is given to patients with pelvic nodes positive for tumor, surgical margins positive for tumor, and if disease is an incidental finding in a less-than-definitive surgical procedure as for benign disease. Patients with stages IIb, III, and IVa carcinoma are treated with irradiation combined with chemotherapy, unless chemotherapy is contraindicated. Total tumor doses are increased to 80 to 85 Gy for advanced or bulky disease, with the pelvic sidewall dose being taken to 60 to 65 Gy. Brachytherapy is a very important aspect of the treatment, and local control and survival are decreased if brachytherapy is not a part of the treatment (external beam treatment, implant doses and techniques, and side effects are further discussed later in this chapter).

Approximate 5-year survival rates are 95% for stage Ia cervical cancer, 85% for stage Ib, 70% for stage II, 50% for stage III, and less than 10% for stage IV. Local control rates are 92% for stage Ib, 85% for stage IIa, 75% for stage IIb, and 60% for stage IIIb.

Simulation and Treatment

Radiation therapy may be used to treat all stages of cervical cancer. Surgery is reserved for medically operable patients in early stages (in situ, Ia, Ib1, and IIa) for whom cure rates are similar and morbidity may be less. For bulky cervical disease, radiation may be followed by an extrafascial hysterectomy, but it is preferable to treat with only one local modality. Conversely, surgery may be followed by radiation therapy if pelvic nodes are positive for tumor, surgical margins are positive for tumor, and if simple hysterectomy was performed and more radical surgery was indicated because the disease was more advanced. Patients with stages Ib2, IIb, III, and IVa are usually treated with irradiation alone or in combination with chemotherapy.

The whole pelvis is initially treated using a four-field or high-energy (minimum 16-MV photons) AP/PA technique. The lower border generally falls at the inferior aspect of the obturator foramen, unless the vagina is involved, in which case the lower extent of the border is at least 4 cm below the most inferior extent of the disease (and may include the entire vaginal length). The upper border is usually at the top or bottom of L5 or may be extended upward to L4 for a portion of the treatment depending on the suspected level of potential nodal involvement. The lateral borders are 1.5 to 2.0 cm lateral to the pelvic sidewall in the AP/PA plane. Laterally, the anterior border is at or anterior to the pubic symphysis, with a block designed to include the external iliac nodes; the posterior border includes S3. In patients with anterior or posterior extension, AP/PA fields alone or widening of the laterals is necessary to extend anterior to the pubis or posterior to include S4 and S5. The actual field borders are best finalized by incorporating a CT or MRI in the treatment planning and localizing the lymph nodal areas of involvement (or those at risk) and the cervical disease. AP/PA fields allow midline blocking early if a greater percentage of the dose is to be administered with brachytherapy, and so possibly decrease the dose given to the entire rectum and bladder. The four-field technique allows exclusion of the anterior bladder and posterior rectum in patients for whom the external beam dose is to be taken to 45 to 50 Gy (Figure 36-6, *A-E*). In patients with a high risk for periaortic nodes to be treated, extended AP lateral fields are delineated (Figure 36-7).

Anal markers, rectal barium, vaginal markers, and bladder contrast may be helpful for delineating critical structures during the simulation process. Prone positioning with a belly board or full bladder may allow the exclusion of the small bowel without jeopardizing the tumor coverage. Small bowel contrast can allow minor field reductions that prevent complications, while allowing higher tumor or nodal doses.

Doses are escalated with increasing stage and volume of the disease. The higher the volume of the tumor, the later implants are done in the course of treatment. Also, the greater the bulk and stage, the smaller the percentage of the dose contribution from implants. Shrinkage of bulky tumor during the

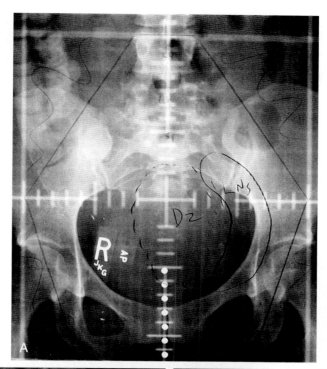

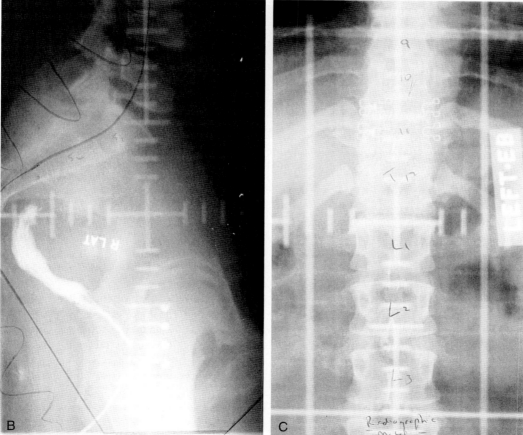

Figure 36-6. Radiographs of cervical simulation and implant procedures. **A**, Anteroposterior/posteroanterior (AP/PA) radiographs of a four-field technique for a bulky cervical cancer. Note the vaginal marker in place. **B**, Lateral view of a four-field technique for a bulky cervical cancer with rectal contrast and a vaginal marker. **C**, Matched AP/PA paraaortic fields used in the treatment of lymphatic drainage involved in regionally advanced cervical cancer.

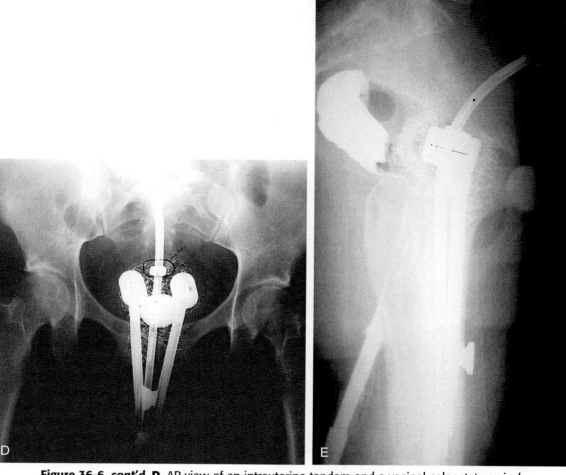

Figure 36-6. cont'd D, AP view of an intrauterine tandem and a vaginal colpostat cervical implant. **E**, Lateral view of an intrauterine tandem and a vaginal colpostat cervical implant.

external beam portion of the treatment will result in achieving better geometry for the brachytherapy implant. A standard **intrauterine tandem** (a small, hollow, curved cylinder that fits through the cervical os and into the uterus) and **vaginal colpostats** (two golf-club–shaped, hollow tubes placed laterally to the tandem into the vaginal fornices) may require supplementation with interstitial implant and with use of a vaginal cylinder as the disease bulk increases. Numerous dose, field, and sequencing arrangements are possible for external beam radiation therapy and brachytherapy. The actual protocol used is based on the radiation oncologist's clinical experience. Examples of doses and configurations include the following: a 70-Gy tumor dose via an implant alone for stage Ia disease, 75-Gy via 40-Gy pelvic radiation therapy plus 10 Gy with midline blocking plus a 35-Gy tumor dose from brachytherapy for stages Ib and IIa disease, 80-Gy via 40-Gy pelvic radiation therapy plus 20 Gy with midline blocking plus 40 Gy from brachytherapy for stages IIb and IIIa disease, and 85-Gy via 45-Gy pelvic radiation therapy plus 20 Gy with midline blocking plus 45 Gy from brachytherapy for stages IIIb and IVa disease. Some centers give a greater percentage of the dose with midline blocking to allow

higher implant doses, and some give higher pelvic radiation therapy doses without midline blocking to cover the volume more evenly and sacrifice the amount of the brachytherapy dose. Low-dose rate implants are usually paired (i.e., two are given approximately 2 weeks apart to achieve higher tolerated doses and allow further tumor regression). This also allows some correction for imperfections in the first implant dose distribution and in the patient's geometry. High-dose-rate implants are further fractionated for biologic reasons. The goal is to deliver 50 to 60 Gy to microscopic disease, 60 to 70 Gy to small macroscopic disease, and 70 to 90 Gy to large macroscopic disease (or its high-dose-rate equivalent) while limiting the volume and dose to the bladder, colorectal tissues, and small intestine. Central doses are traditionally prescribed to the **Point A** prescription point, usually defined as 2 cm superior to the cervical os and 2 cm lateral to the endocervical canal. **Point B** is 3 cm lateral to point A. Increasingly, with image-guided brachytherapy, the doses to tumor and tissues at risk for disease involvement are described by the isodose line that adequately covers the volume to be treated once the plan is generated.

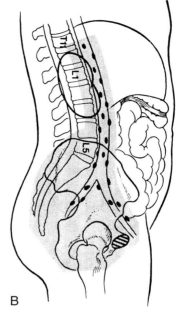

Figure 36-7. Extended field irradiation. **A,** Anterior and posterior portals. **B,** Lateral portals. (From Russel A, et al: High dose para-aortic lymph node irradiation for gynecological cancer: technique, toxicity and results, *Int J Radiat Oncol Biol Phys* 13:267-271, 1987.)

CASE III

Tandem and Ovoid

A 42-year-old woman presented with a 6-month history of progressively increased vaginal bleeding after intercourse. Her periods were otherwise normal, and she did not have any pelvic or vaginal pain. She had Papanicolaou smears performed in her 20s and early 30s but none recently.

During an examination, the cervix was enlarged to about 5 cm, and an ulcerative lesion was seen extending from the posterior aspect of the cervix into the posterior fornix. The Papanicolaou smear was positive for squamous cell carcinoma, and biopsies from the lesion, endocervix, and endometrium demonstrated invasive, poorly differentiated squamous cell carcinoma. A pelvic examination confirmed the bulky lesion, and the extension onto the vaginal wall was palpable; no parametrial extension was present (stage IIa). A chest radiograph and abdominopelvic CT scan were negative for metastatic disease. Within the pelvis was the enlarged cervical mass, but no discernible pelvic adenopathy or other masses were present.

Because of the lesion's bulk, the patient was not considered a surgical candidate and definitive radiation therapy was initiated. She received 4500 cGy via a four-field technique, with the treatment of customized 16 × 18.5 cm AP/PA and 14 × 18.5 cm right and left parallel-opposed fields. Photons of 15 MV were used to deliver 180-cGy daily fractions. Pelvic evaluation during the fifth week revealed marked shrinkage of the tumor. The first tandem and ovoid implant procedure was performed 3 days after the completion of the 4500 cGy dose. The tandem was loaded with 15-, 10-, and 10-mg radium-equivalent cesium-137 (Cs-137) sources, and the small ovoids were each loaded with 15 mg sources. The point-A dose rate was 50 cGy per hour, and the implant was left in place for 48 hours. The dose rate at the pelvic sidewall was 12 cGy per hour, whereas the bladder and rectum maximum dose rates were 30 cGy per hour. The week after the first implant, 540 cGy was delivered in three fractions as a pelvic-sidewall boost via 16 × 16 cm AP/PA fields, with a midline (rectal and bladder sparing)

rectangular block designed using the isodose distribution of the implant as a guide. A second, nearly identical implant was performed the week after the boost field, with a total implant time of 30 hours. The cumulative dose to point A was 8400 cGy, whereas the pelvic sidewall received 5980 cGy. The doses for the bladder and rectal points were each 6000 cGy.

Beginning the fourth week of treatment, the patient experienced diarrhea that was initially managed with a low-fiber diet, and she eventually required antidiarrheal agents. The diarrhea gradually improved throughout the implants, and the patient was without a complaint within 4 days after the second implant. She otherwise tolerated the treatment well.

At a follow-up visit 1 week after the second implant, the cervix size was normal. Considerable necrotic debris was present at the vaginal apex, and no bleeding occurred during the examination. The following month she described a brown vaginal discharge with sparse matter that resembled coffee grounds. At her next examination, there were patchy, hypopigmented areas alternating with **telangiectasis** (fine, superficial blood vessels) in the vaginal apex, and the cervix was nearly healed.

She continued to have control of the local disease and no pelvic side effects. About 1 to $1\frac{1}{2}$ years after therapy, she exhibited multiple lung nodules. A chemotherapeutic regimen was begun, but the patient expired 5 months later.

ENDOMETRIUM

Clinical Presentation

Recent studies have highlighted the increased risk of endometrial cancer in women who take the drug tamoxifen, which has led some to suggest that surveillance of this subset of patients is warranted.[7,39] About 75% of women with endometrial cancer experience vaginal bleeding and about 30% have a putrid vaginal discharge. Approximately one third of postmenopausal bleeding cases are cancer related, usually cervical or endometrial.

Most endometrial cancers are early stage, with about 70% in stage I and 10% each in stages II, III, and IV. Poor prognostic factors include higher grade, increased depth of invasion into the myometrial muscle, lymph node involvement, and cancer cells in the peritoneal fluid (peritoneal cytology positive for tumor) or on serosal surfaces.

Lymphatic spread occurs initially to the internal and external iliac pelvic nodes. For stage I disease, about 10% of patients have nodes positive for tumor. This increases to between 25% and 35% for stage II disease, a poorly differentiated histology, or a deep myometrial invasion. If pelvic nodes are involved, about a 60% chance exists for periaortic node involvement.

Detection and Diagnosis

Aspiration curettage has long been the gold standard for endometrial cancer screening, mostly because it improved on the sensitivity and accuracy of the **Papanicolaou smear**, a detection modality with only a 50% or less diagnostic accuracy in endometrial cancer.[9] However, it is increasingly the case that women with abnormal uterine bleeding are evaluated in the office setting using endometrial sampling or aspiration,[9] the latter of which has a reported sensitivity rate of 94% in some studies.[34] A thorough history is taken, and a physical examination is performed. Additional studies include chest radiographs, blood counts and chemistries, and a urinalysis. Surgery is now the standard initial definitive management. Before proceeding, pelvic sonographic evaluation is often performed, and a pelvic CT or an MRI scan is often performed if disease is suspected beyond the uterus. Standard surgery includes an exploratory laparotomy with staging biopsies, washings, and a radical hysterectomy.

Pathology and Staging

Adenocarcinoma of the endometrial lining is the most common type of endometrial cancer. Adenocarcinoma with squamous differentiation is a variant seen about 20% of the time and is usually more advanced in stage. Papillary serous adenocarcinoma is an extremely malignant form of endometrial carcinoma that tends to spread rapidly and widely throughout the abdominal cavity and usually has a poor outcome. Clear cell adenocarcinoma behaves similarly. Sarcomas rarely have a good outcome and deserve aggressive combined-modality therapy (usually surgery and radiation therapy). Staging is as follows:

Stage IA: Tumor limited to the endometrium
Stage IB: Tumor invading less than one half of the myometrium
Stage IC: Tumor invading one half or more of the myometrium
Stage IIA: Tumor limited to the glandular epithelium of the endocervix. No evidence of connective tissue stromal invasion
Stage IIB: Invasion of the stromal connective tissues of the cervix
Stage IIIA: Tumor involves serosa and/or adnexa and/or cancer cells in ascites or peritoneal washings
Stage IIIB: Vaginal involvement
Stage IIIC: Pelvic and or periaortic lymph node involvement
Stage IVA: Tumor invades bladder mucosa and/or bowel mucosa

Treatment Considerations

Treatment can involve surgery and/or radiation therapy, depending on the stage, grade, medical condition of the patient, and experience of the institution administering the therapy. Preoperative therapy is given in some institutions for high grade and high clinical stages to downstage the patient before surgery. Usually, patients who have already undergone operations are referred for postoperative therapy, and nonoperative candidates are referred for definitive therapy. After a TAH, patients with stage Ia, grade 1 disease are not treated further. At many institutions, patients with stage Ib, grades 1 and 2 and sometimes stage Ia, grade 2 disease are treated postoperatively with brachytherapy alone. Low surface doses of 60 to 70 Gy are typically used in one application, or high doses of 5 to 7 Gy to a 0.5-cm depth are used for three applications. Patients with stage Ic (or higher) or grade 3 disease have an increased risk of pelvic node involvement, so external beam radiation therapy is a component of postoperative treatment. Minimal nodal doses of 45 to 50 Gy are supplemented with implants to bring the vaginal mucosa dose up to 80 Gy or more. Residual pelvic nodes or masses can be boosted up to 60 to 65 Gy with shaped, small-volume external fields.

Irradiation alone may be used for medically inoperable patients and for stages III and IV. Usually, at least a 50-Gy external beam pelvic dose is recommended with an implant sufficient to bring the tumor dose above 75 Gy. Bulky disease can be brought to 100 Gy with careful implant techniques and midline shielding (see the section on simulation techniques at the end of the chapter).

For stage I disease, the local recurrence rate can be reduced from 12% with surgery alone to 3% with preoperative radiation therapy, and to 0% with postoperative radiation therapy.[14] The 5-year survival rates are 64%, 76%, and 81%, respectively. Overall, there is a 90% 5-year survival rate for all stage I patients, including the most common and nonirradiated stage I, grade 1 patients. For stage II, 5-year disease-free survival rates are about 80% with surgery and radiation therapy versus 50% for radiation therapy alone. The 5-year survival rate for stage III disease treated with radiation therapy alone is only 25%. Overall, patients treated with surgery and radiation therapy have an overall survival rate of 81.6%, a 5-year disease-free survival rate of 80.7%, and a 5-year recurrence-free survival rate of 94.6%.[46]

Simulation and Treatment

Most endometrial cancers are seen postoperatively. For stage Ib, grades 1 and 2 and sometimes stage Ia, grade 2, a vaginal cylinder or colpostats alone are used to treat the vaginal cuff. Orthogonal simulation films may be taken for treatment planning purposes. Typical low-dose-rate brachytherapy doses, a 60- to 70-Gy surface dose in two sessions, or high-dose rate brachytherapy dose fractions of 5 to 7 Gy to a 0.5-cm depth are prescribed for three to five fractions. For stage Ic or higher or for grade 3 disease, an increased risk of pelvic nodal involvement exists and pelvic radiation therapy is given. Fields are similar to cervical fields, and midline blocking may be used if brachytherapy is included as part of the preoperative, postoperative, or definitive treatment. Heyman capsule techniques or an intrauterine tandem is used if the uterus is still present for implantation. For postoperative treatment, a domed cylinder or vaginal colpostats are used if brachytherapy is necessary. Pelvic nodal doses of 40-50 Gy are recommended, with boosting up to 65 Gy for gross involvement. The endometrial cavity can be taken to 75 to 90 Gy with combined external beam therapy and low-dose rate brachytherapy, but the bladder and rectum must be kept to about 65 to 75 Gy or less, and the small bowel must be kept at or below 45 to 50 Gy (Figure 36-8). High-dose-rate brachytherapy may also be used to equivalent doses. Simulation with CT guidance is needed for the pelvic external beam treatment, and possibly also for the brachytherapy portion, but image-guided treatment planning is increasingly utilized.

CASE IV

HDR For Endometrial Cancer Post Hysterectomy

A 62-year-old postmenopausal woman had been having annual Papanicolaou smears, all of which were normal. She developed intermittent vaginal bleeding and consulted her gynecologist the same week. Another Papanicolaou smear was normal, but an endometrial biopsy showed a moderately differentiated endometrial carcinoma. A chest radiograph, blood work, and a pelvic sonogram showed thickened endometrial stripel. She underwent a total abdominal hysterectomy and the removal of both ovaries. No lymph nodes were palpable during the surgery and none were sampled. A pathology report confirmed a moderately differentiated adenocarcinoma on the posterior wall and that nearly invaded through the entire thickness of the myometrium. The cervix and parametrial tissues were not involved, and her disease was classified as FIGO stage IC.

Her postoperative course was unremarkable, and she was referred for adjuvant radiation therapy. She was treated with 18-MV photons to 4500 cGy as 180-cGy daily fractions via a four-field technique with customized 16 × 16 cm AP/PA and 16 × 14 cm right and left parallel-opposed fields. After completing the external beam radiation therapy, she underwent three high-dose-rate vaginal cylinder insertions. Then 5 Gy was prescribed at 0.5-cm vaginal mucosal depth for 3 fractions to be administered 1 week apart. A 3-cm-diameter domed cylinder was placed and the Ir-192 source was used to deliver the treatments to the vaginal mucosa. The patient tolerated the treatments well, experiencing mild diarrhea and fatigue at the completion of the external irradiation. The implant was well tolerated. Six years after treatment, she was without evidence of disease. She complained of having to urinate more frequently, but this was not problematic, and she was without dysuria. She had experienced periodic rectal irritation during the first 2 years after treatment, and each episode responded to steroid suppositories after several days.

OVARIES

Clinical Presentation

Ovarian cancer is the most deadly of the gynecologic carcinomas because it has few symptoms until it is widely disseminated. The most common presenting symptoms are abdominal and/or pelvic pain, abdominal distention, or nonspecific gastrointestinal symptoms (e.g., nausea, constipation, and heartburn). These are due to the presence of the tumor or fluid in the abdominal cavity. Occasionally, ovarian cancer may be diagnosed in the early stages at pelvic examination as a palpable mass adjacent to the uterus.

The disease is most common in women aged 50 to 70 years old. It is considered early if it is confined to the ovaries. Progression occurs within the pelvis, to the abdominal cavity, and to lymph nodes. Serum CA-125 is often elevated in the serum of epithelial ovarian cancer and has also been found to be a useful prognostic indicator of successful chemotherapy treatment.[5] In apparently early ovarian cancer, subclinical metastases are noted during surgery in the peritoneal fluid, periaortic nodes, and diaphragm in 33%, 10%, and 10% of the cases, respectively.[40,41] About 80% of ovarian cancer patients have abdominal cavity involvement at the time of presentation. Spread occurs through the lymphatic channel of the peritoneal lining and the diaphragm and lymph nodes as the peritoneal fluid circulates.

Detection and Diagnosis

Diagnosis and staging are surgical. The preoperative workup usually includes a history, a physical examination, liver and renal function blood work, chest radiographs, pelvic sonograms (including transvaginal views), abdominopelvic CT or MRI scans, and serum CA-125. Additional workups may include a barium enema (BE), an upper or lower endoscopy, and upper gastrointestinal (UGI) series depending on the presenting symptoms. The surgical evaluation includes a cytologic evaluation of the peritoneal fluid; an intraoperative evaluation for ovarian, fallopian tube, or other masses; and an examination and biopsy of the peritoneal surfaces. Removal of as much of the tumor as possible produces the best outcomes.

Pathology and Staging

About 90% of ovarian cancers are epithelial (from ovary surfaces), 7% are stromal, and 3% are from the ovarian germ cell. These include dysgerminomas, which are treated like seminomas. Staging is as follows:

Stage I: Tumor limited to the ovaries (one or both).
Stage IA: Tumor limited to one ovary, capsule intact, no tumor on ovarian surface. No malignant cells in ascites or peritoneal washings.
Stage IB: Tumor limited to both ovaries, capsules intact, no tumor on ovarian surface. No malignant cells in ascites or peritoneal washings.
Stage IC: Tumor limited to one or both ovaries with any of the following: capsule ruptured, tumor on ovarian surface. Malignant cells in ascites or peritoneal washings.
Stage II: Tumor involves one or both ovaries with pelvic extension and/or implants.
Stage IIA: Extension and/or implants on the fallopian tubes and/or uterus. No malignant cells in ascites or peritoneal washings.
Stage IIB: Extension to and/or implants on other pelvic tissues. No malignant cells in ascites or peritoneal washings.
Stage IIC: Pelvic extension and/or implants, with malignant cells in ascites or peritoneal washings.
Stage III: Tumor involves one or both ovaries with microscopically confirmed peritoneal metastases outside the pelvis.

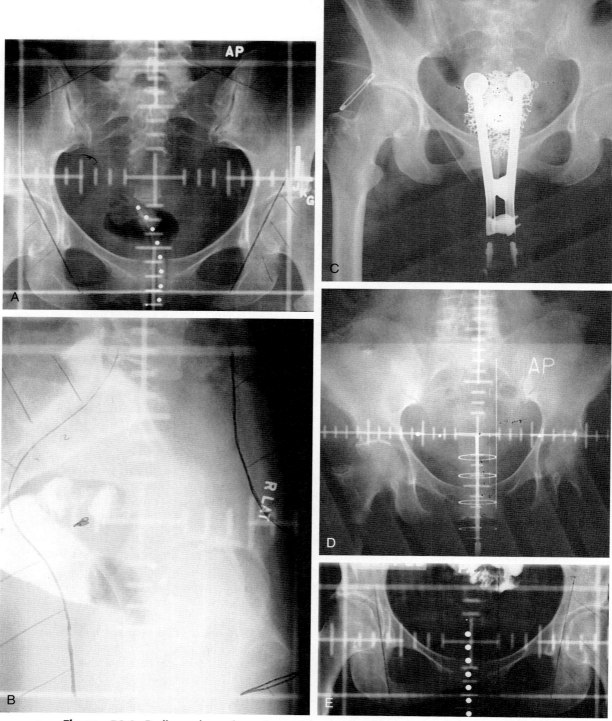

Figure 36-8. Radiographs of endometrial simulation and implant procedures. **A**, Anteroposterior/posteroanterior (AP/PA) simulation radiographs of a four-field treatment for postoperative endometrial cancer. Note the placement of the vaginal marker. **B**, Right and left lateral radiograph of a four-field treatment for postoperative endometrial cancer. Note the placement of the vaginal marker along with rectal contrast. **C**, Brachytherapy implant for postoperative endometrial cancer using colpostats. **D**, Brachytherapy implant using a high-dose-rate domed cylinder. **E**, Midline-blocked parametrial boost (small bowel excluded).

Stage IIIA: Microscopic peritoneal metastases beyond the pelvis (no macroscopic tumor).

Stage IIIB: Macroscopic peritoneal metastases beyond the pelvis 2 cm or less in greatest dimension.

Stage IIIC: Peritoneal metastasis beyond the pelvis more than 2 cm in greatest dimension and/or regional lymph node metastasis.

Treatment Considerations

For epithelial tumors, the initial treatment involves surgical evaluation and debulking. Postoperative therapy is standardly single agent or combination chemotherapy and whole abdominal and pelvic radiation therapy is now rarely used. Use of the radioisotope P-32 as a colloidal solution placed into the peritoneal cavity is an accepted alternative to single agent chemotherapy for treating high-risk stages I and II cases. For most epithelial tumors, postoperative therapy consists of platinum-based chemotherapy, although abdominopelvic radiation therapy yields similar results, but with increased rates of complications.[10-13,33,37] The two approaches are not additive, but toxicities are. Peritoneal radioisotope treatment is best not used in addition to external beam therapy for similar reasons.

Survival rates are 90% at 5 years for stage I, 20% for stage III, and 5% for stage IV disease. About 22 months of increased survival time occurs with optimal (with <1- to 2-cm sites of residual disease after surgery) versus suboptimal surgical reduction of intra-abdominal disease.[33]

For well-differentiated stage IA and IB disease, the 5-year survival rates are between 90% and 100%.[43] The 5-year survival rate for radiation therapy–treated stage II is 74% for microscopic residual disease, 58% for residual disease less than 2 cm, and 39% for residual disease greater than 2 cm. Comparable results for stage III are 48%, 43%, and 18%.[10-12]

Simulation and Treatment

Ovarian fields are also treated postoperatively after staging and optimal debulking by the gynecologic oncologist. The entire peritoneal cavity must be covered with an open-field technique that extends from the diaphragm to the pelvic floor. When no liver shielding is used, the upper abdominal dose is limited to 25 to 28 Gy in 1.0- to 1.2-Gy fractions. Partial renal blocking is used to limit the dose to a total of 18 to 20 Gy. The pelvis is then boosted up to a total dose of 50 Gy at 1.8 Gy/fraction. Higher energy photons are recommended with AP/PA fields to limit the dosage variation to less than or equal to 5% (Figure 36-9, *A* and *B*).

SIDE EFFECTS OF TREATMENT

Acute side effects of pelvic radiation therapy include fatigue, diarrhea, dermatitis, and dysuria. Fatigue may develop as early as the first week of treatment, and it could be exacerbated or complicated by anemia and depression as the patient continues to come to terms with the disease. Rest, reassurance, adequate nutrition, and antidepressants may make the course of treatment more tolerable. Anemia, secondary to blood loss or due to treatment of disease, should be corrected, especially if the patient is symptomatic, to a hemoglobin level above 10 g/dl and ideally above 11 g/dl. Diarrhea usually occurs the second or third week of treatment and is related to large and small bowel treatment. The addition of chemotherapy can significantly worsen this problem. Low-fiber diets, sucralfate (Carafate) as a small bowel–coating agent, diphenoxylate (Lomotil), and loperamide are useful in alleviating this problem. Excluding as much bowel as possible from the radiation therapy fields also helps. This is done with the use of belly boards, the prone position with a full bladder on smaller fields, custom shielding, serial field-size reduction, and, increasingly, IMRT. Other acute effects of treating abdominal fields include nausea and

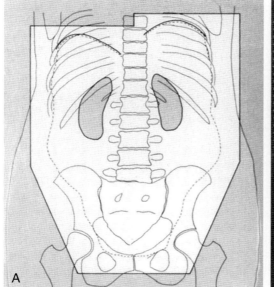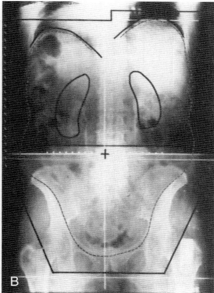

Figure 36-9. A line drawing **(A)** and prone simulator radiograph **(B)** showing the field margin for abdominopelvic irradiation (*nonshaded area*), peritoneal outline (*dotted line*), and renal shields. The pelvic boost field is not shown. (From Cox JD: *Moss' radiation oncology: rationale, techniques, results,* ed 7, St. Louis, 1994, Mosby.)

upper gastrointestinal bleeding. Nausea can be treated prophylactically with agents such as prochlorperazine (Compazine) or granisetron (Kytril), and gastritis can be treated with H_2 blockers (e.g., Tagamet, Zantac, Pepcid, and Axid), sucralfate, or other acid inhibitors. Dermatitis is more common with treatment using low-energy beams, with AP/PA only fields, with perineal flash or with use of bolus when indicated, and with concomitant chemotherapy. Domboro soaks, Aquaphor ointment, and natural care gels can lessen the severity and speed healing. The prevention and early treatment of local infection, and correction of anemia and nutritional problems may also speed skin healing. Dysuria usually occurs during the third or fourth week of treatment and can be lessened by treatment with a full bladder, partial bladder exclusion on lateral fields, and maintenance of a partially full bladder during brachytherapy. Medications such as phenazopyridine (Pyridium) and Urised can be used to anesthetize the bladder, or oxybutynin (Ditropan), hyoscyamine (Levsin), and terazosin (Hytrin) can be used to relax the bladder and relieve urinary frequency. Infections should be treated early and completely. Bleeding may also complicate the treatment as a result of anal irritation, bladder irritation, and a hemorrhagic tumor. Superficial **en face** radiation therapy using orthovoltage energy, high-energy photons, or electrons can be applied directly to vaginal and cervical tumors with a large fraction size and not count against the total prescribed dose (this can rapidly correct tumor bleeding). Rectal irritation can be treated with hemorrhoidal preparations, steroids, topical anesthetic agents, and sitz baths.

Late side effects can include menopause, vaginal dryness/narrowing/shortening, chronic cystitis, proctosigmoiditis, enteritis, and bowel obstruction. Use of replacement hormonal therapy may be considered, vaginal dryness can be treated with moisturizing agents such as Replens or hormonal creams, and shrinkage can be prevented with vaginal dilators or regular sexual activity. Chronic tissue inflammation or ulceration is treated with local medications, pentoxifylline (Trental), nutritional support, anti-inflammatory agents, and pain medications. Bowel obstruction is treated surgically.

ROLE OF RADIATION THERAPIST

Treatment Delivery

The primary role of the radiation therapist in the control of disease is simulation and treatment delivery. Patient positioning is an important component. Radiation therapists must often rely on their own experience regarding the way to position a particular patient for optimal comfort and stability. The pelvis can present considerable difficulty for simulation and reproducibility, especially when body habitus requires placement of setup markings on loose skin overlying fat folds. The meticulous assessment of the patient's rotation is critical to prevent the shifting of the marks. Reminding the patient to maintain a full bladder when it is used to exclude the small bowel, encouraging the patient to remain on a low-residue diet when diarrhea is a problem, and remaining open and responsive to patient concerns helps to get the patient through treatment in the shortest possible time (optimal cure) and with minimal discomfort.

Patient Assessment

The radiation therapist is a critical link in patient assessment. The radiation therapist is in daily contact with the patient, allowing monitoring of early changes in the patient's physical status. In addition, there is often better, closer communication between the patient and radiation therapist compared with the physician. Concerns and observations should be communicated to the medical staff members initially for more in-depth assessment. In some institutions, standing orders are written with specific expectations for suggestions to the patient and communications with medical staff members. Knowledge of institutional policy is important.

The skin should be carefully assessed beginning the third week of radiation therapy. The infraabdominal, gluteal, and inguinal folds are the earliest to show a skin reaction. The vulvar folds will also exhibit skin reaction early. Pelvic irradiation may cause diarrhea, with consequent weight loss and electrolyte imbalance. Loose or soft stools are common, but the primary concern is watery diarrhea, which should be communicated immediately to medical staff members.

 Skin irritation and bowel irregularities are common outcomes of pelvic irradiation. Close monitoring of symptoms is required, and specific medical attention may need to be initiated in the event of increasing severity.

Reassurance

The radiation therapist has a responsibility to maintain a caring, professional atmosphere. Questions should be answered as much as knowledge permits, and medical staff members should be kept aware of patient concerns and questions. Chart rounds are an excellent forum for this communication, but otherwise the radiation therapist should communicate with the nurse or physician.

SUMMARY

Gynecologic malignancies are common and may account for a significant proportion of the routine workload at a radiation oncology facility. For no other group of malignancies are the treatment options so diverse. The basic knowledge presented here should enhance the radiation therapist's role in managing these patients while enabling a deeper understanding of the treatment rationale and potential outcome.

- The most prevalent gynecologic cancer is endometrial, followed by ovarian, cervical, and other gynecologic cancers.
- Treatment options for gynecologic malignancies are the most diverse in the field of radiation therapy.
- The radiation therapist has three main functions during the course of therapy: treatment delivery, ongoing patient assessment, and patient reassurance.
- The radiation therapist is often more involved in the physical assessment of the patient than the physician. Concerns and observations should be reported to the appropriate medical staff. Knowledge of institutional policy is a must.
- Positioning a patient for treatment with regard for comfort and stability is dependent on the radiation therapist's own experience with that patient.

- Gynecologic radiation therapy treatment requires an understanding of the radiosensitivity of the various gynecologic structures. For instance, the most radiotolerant structure is the uteral canal, whereas the most radiosensitive is the ovary.
- Gynecologic radiation therapy planning requires consideration of lymphatic drainage patterns to ensure appropriate field coverage. Treatment design must also consider the extent of the primary lesion and probability of metastases to draining lymph nodes.
- The dose response for radiation side effects is dependent on age.
- Anemia is among the most common side effects of treatment, especially for cervical cancer. Hemoglobin restoration to optimal levels greatly increases treatment tolerability for the patient.
- Rest, reassurance, adequate nutrition, and antidepressants may help make treatment more tolerable for patients.

Review Questions

Multiple Choice

1. The most radiotolerant gynecologic structure is the:
   a. vulva
   b. uteral canal
   c. endocervix
   d. ovary
2. The most radiosensitive gynecologic structure is the:
   a. vulva
   b. uteral canal
   c. endocervix
   d. ovary
3. The dose response for radiation side effects in gynecologic structures is dependent on:
   a. age
   b. race
   c. both a and b
   d. neither a nor b
4. Gynecologic radiation therapy planning requires consideration of which drainage pattern(s) to ensure appropriate field coverage?
   a. arterial and venous
   b. lymphatic
   c. both a and b
   d. neither a nor b
5. Bladder and rectal doses are more important to gynecologic radiation therapy planning than kidney or ovarian doses.
   a. true
   b. false

Matching

Match the average age of onset with the disease.
6. ovarian cancer
7. cervical cancer
8. uterine cancer
9. clear cell vaginal cancer

10. vulvar cancer
    a. 48 years
    b. 60 years
    c. 19 years
    d. 58 years
    e. 65+ years

The answers to the Review Questions can be found by logging on to our website at: *http://evolve.elsevier.com/Washington+Leaver/principles*

Questions to Ponder

1. Why is the Point A dose more important in the treatment design for cervical cancer than in that for uterine cancer?
2. What important structures in and around the pelvis may MLCs help to reduce the dose while allowing full doses to at-risk tissues?
3. What are the tolerated (expected to have minimal long-term toxic effects) radiation therapy doses to the various pelvic structures?
4. Why is surgery less important for moderately advanced cervical cancer than for endometrial cancer?
5. In the United States, is preoperative or postoperative radiation therapy more commonly used for endometrial cancer? Explain the potential rationale for the most common approach.

REFERENCES

1. American Cancer Society: *Cancer facts and figures: 2008*, Atlanta, 2008, American Cancer Society.
2. Ansink AC, et al: Human papillomavirus, lichen sclerosis, and squamous cell carcinoma of the vulva: detection and prognostic significance, *Gynecol Oncol* 52:180-184, 1994.
3. Balat O, Edwards C, Delclos L: Complications following combined surgery (radical vulvectomy versus wide local excision) and radiotherapy for the treatment of carcinoma of the vulva: report of 73 patients, *Eur J Gynecol Oncol* 21:501-503, 2000.
4. Barrett-Lee P, et al: Management of cancer-related anemia in patients with breast or gynecologic cancer: new insights based on results from the European Cancer Anemia Survey, *Oncologist* 10:743-757, 2005.
5. Bast RC Jr, et al: CA-125: the past and the future, *Int J Biol Mark* 13:179-187, 1998.
6. Beral V, et al: Use of HRT and the subsequent risk of cancer, *J Epidemiol Biostat* 4:191-210, 1999.
7. Bergman L, et al: Risk and prognosis of endometrial cancer after tamoxifen for breast cancer. Comprehensive Cancer Centres' ALERT group. Assessment of liver and endometrial cancer risk following Tamoxifen, *Lancet* 356:881-887, 2000.
8. Buchsbaum HJ: Extrapelvic lymph node metastases in cervical carcinoma, *Am J Obstet Gynecol* 133:814-824, 1979.
9. Chambers JT, Chambers SK: Endometrial sampling: when? where? why? with what? *Clin Obstet Gynecol* 35:28-39, 1992.
10. Dembo AJ: Abdominopelvic radiotherapy in ovarian cancer: a 10 year experience, *Cancer* 55:2285-2290, 1985.
11. Dembo AJ, Bush RD: Choice of postoperative therapy based on prognostic factors, *Int J Radiat Oncol Biol Phys* 8:893-897, 1982.
12. Dembo AJ, Thomas GM, Friedlander ML: Prognostic indices in gynecologic cancer, *Dev Oncol* 48:239-250, 1987.
13. Fyles AW, et al: A randomized study of two doses of abdominopelvic radiation therapy for patients with optimally debulked Stage I, II, and III ovarian cancer, *Int J Radiat Oncol Biol Phys* 41:543-549, 1998.
14. Graham J: The value of preoperative or postoperative treatment by radium for carcinoma of the uterine body, *Surg Gynecol Obstet* 132:855, 1971.

15. Grigsby PW: Late injury of cancer therapy on the female reproductive tract, *Int J Radiat Oncol Biol Phys* 31:1281-1299, 1995.

16. Hacker NF, et al: Management of regional lymph nodes and their prognostic influence in vulvar cancer, *Obstet Gynecol* 61:408-412, 1983.

17. Hintz BL, et al: Radiation tolerance of the vaginal mucosa, *Int J Radiat Oncol Biol Phys* 6:711-716, 1980.

18. International Federation of Gynecology and Obstetrics (FIGO) classification, *FIGO* 18:190, 1989.

19. Iverson T, et al: Squamous cell carcinoma of the penis and of the cervix, vulva and vagina in spouses: is there any relationship? An epidemiological study from Norway, 1960-1992, *Br J Cancer* 76:658-660, 1997.

20. Kim HK, et al: Bulky, barrel-shaped cervical carcinoma (stages IB, IIA, IIB): the prognostic factors for pelvic control and treatment outcome, *Am J Clin Oncol* 22:232-236, 1999.

21. Kim YT, et al: Effect of intravenously administered iron sucrose on the prevention of anemia in cervical cancer patients treated with concurrent chemoradiotherapy, *Gynecol Oncol* 105:199-204, 2007.

22. Kohler U, Schone M, Pawlowitsch T: Results of an individualized surgical therapy of vulvar carcinoma from 1973-1993. *Zentralblatt fur Gynakologie* 119(S1):8-16, 1997.

23. Lanciano RM, Corn BW: Gynecologic cancer. In Coia LR, Moylan DJ, editors: *Introduction to clinical radiation oncology*, ed 2, Madison, WI, 1994, Medical Physics Publishing.

24. Lawson HW, et al: Cervical cancer screening among low-income women: results of a national screening program, *Obstet Gynecol* 92:745-752, 1998.

25. Magrina JF, et al: Primary squamous cell cancer of the vulva: radical versus modified radical vulvar surgery, *Gynecol Oncol* 71:116-121, 1998.

26. Melnick S, et al: Rates and risks of diethylstilbestrol-related clear-cell adenocarcinoma of the vagina and cervix. An update, *N Engl J Med* 316:514-516, 1987.

27. Milosevic M, et al: Interstitial fluid pressure predicts survival in patients with cervix cancer independent of clinical prognostic factors and tumor oxygen measurements, *Cancer Res* 61:6400-6405, 2001.

28. Montana GS, et al: Carcinoma of the vulva. In Perez CA, Brady LW, editors: *Principles and practices of radiation oncology*, ed 4, Philadelphia, 2004, JB Lippincott.

29. Moore DH, et al: Vulva. In Hoskine WJ, Perez CA, Young RC, editors: *Principles and practices of gynecologic oncology*, ed 4, Philadelphia, 2004, JB Lippincott.

30. Noguchi H, et al: Uterine body invasion of carcinoma of the uterine cervix as seen from surgical specimens, *Gynecol Oncol* 30:173-182, 1988.

31. Orbalic N, Bilenjki D, Bilbija Z: Prognostic importance of anemia related parameters in patients with carcinoma of the cervix uteri, *Acta Oncol* 29:199-201, 1990.

32. Origoni M, et al: Surgical staging of invasive squamous cell carcinoma of the vulva. Analysis of treatment and survival, *Int Surg* 81:67-70, 1996.

33. Ozols RF, et al: Epithelial ovarian cancer. In Hoskins WJ, Perez CA, Young RC, editors: *Principles and practice of gynecologic oncology*, ed 4, Philadelphia, 2004, JB Lippincott.

34. Paley P: Screening for the major malignancies affecting women: current guidelines, *Am J Obstet Gynecol* 184:1021-1030, 2001.

35. Peck WS, et al: Castration of the female by irradiation, *Radiology* 34:176-186, 1940.

36. Perez CA, Garipagaoglu M: Vagina. In Perez CA, Brady LW, editors: *Principles and practices of radiation oncology*, ed 4, Philadelphia, 2004, JB Lippincott.

37. Perez CA, et al: Gynecologic tumors. In Rubin P, Williams JP, editors: *Clinical oncology: a multidisciplinary approach for physicians and students*, ed 8, Philadelphia, 2001, WB Saunders.

38. Pettigrew R, Hamilton-Fairley D: Obesity and female reproductive function, *Br Med Bull* 53:341-358, 1997.

39. Physicians desk query 2002. *Endometrial cancer: screening*, Bethesda, MD, 2002, National Cancer Institute.

40. Piver MS, Chung WS: Prognostic significance of cervical lesion size and pelvic node metastasis in cervical carcinoma, *Obstet Gynecol* 46:507-510, 1975.

41. Piver MS, Barlow JJ, Lele SB: Incidence of subclinical metastasis in stage I and II ovarian carcinoma, *Obstet Gynecol* 52:100, 1978.

42. Segnan N: Socioeconomic status and cancer screening, *IARC Sci Pub* 138:369-376, 1997.

43. Thigpen JT: Limited-stage ovarian carcinoma, *Semin Oncol* 26(6 S18):29-33, 1999.

44. Treffers PE, et al: Consequences of diethylstilbestrol during pregnancy: 50 years later still a significant problem, *Netherlands Tijdschrift voor Geneeskunde* 145:675-680, 2001.

45. Weiderpass E, et al: Body size in different periods of life, diabetes mellitus, hypertension, and risk of postmenopausal endometrial cancer, *Cancer Caus Contr* 11(2):185-192, 2000.

46. Yalman D, et al: Postoperative radiotherapy in endometrial carcinoma: analysis of prognostic factors in 440 cases, *Eur J Gynecol Oncol* 21:3311-3315, 2000.

BIBLIOGRAPHY

Greene FL, et al, editors: *AJCC cancer staging manual*, ed 6, New York, 2002, Springer-Verlag.

Male Reproductive and Genitourinary Tumors

Deborah A. Kuban, Megan L. Trad

Outline

Key Terms

Bowen's disease
Bulbous urethra
Corpora cavernosa
Corpus spongiosum
Cryptorchidism
Fossa navicularis
Impotence
Morphology
Penile urethra
Prostate gland
Prostatic hypertrophy
Proton therapy
Smegma
Superior surface
Trigone

Objectives

- Understand the route of lymphatic spread from the prostate.
- Compare and contrast the treatment techniques and modalities for prostate carcinoma along with associated pros and cons.
- Describe how computed tomography and improvements in treatment planning have enabled physicians to increase the dose delivered to the prostate.

- Recognize the importance of rectal and bladder filling in the treatment of prostate cancer and the need for daily prostate targeting.
- Understand the treatment methods and techniques for seminoma patients.
- List the routes of spread for renal cell carcinoma.
- Understand the principles of bladder sparing radiation for bladder carcinoma.

PROSTATE

Epidemiology

Carcinoma of the prostate is the most common malignancy in males in the United States. Approximately 1:6 men will develop prostate cancer in their lifetime. It is estimated that 186,320 new cases will be diagnosed in the United States in 2008, and approximately 28,660 men will die of the disease that year.[3] The incidence increases with each decade of life; more than 65% of prostate carcinomas occur in men 65 years and older. African American men in the United States have one of the highest incidences, of prostate cancer in the world, significantly higher than that of white men of comparable age.[3]

Prognostic Indicators

Tumor Stage and Histologic Differentiation. Strong prognostic indicators in prostate carcinoma are the clinical stage and pathologic grade of tumor differentiation. Larger and less-differentiated tumors are more aggressive and have a greater incidence of lymphatic and distant metastases.

Age. Conflicting reports on age as a prognostic factor have been published. A Radiation Therapy Oncology Group (RTOG) study found a higher locoregional failure rate in patients younger than 60 years; however, survival was not significantly correlated with age.[71] Men younger than 65 years had an equivalent outcome at 5 years, as measured by post treatment prostate-specific antigen (PSA), compared with men older than 65.[33,38] The two groups had similar stages and prognostic factors.

Race. Although higher incidence and mortality rates have been reported for African American males, they have also been shown to present with more advanced disease.[3] Zagars et al.[109] compared outcome in white versus black patients after radiation and found no difference when stratified by pretreatment prognostic factors.

Prostate-Specific Antigen Level. Several reports strongly suggest a close correlation between pretreatment and also post treatment PSA levels and the incidence of failure-free survival.[49] Although a rising PSA level after radiation is more predictive than a single value, the higher the post treatment nadir, the greater is the risk of failure. For example, patients with a nadir of 0.5 ng/ml or higher had a 17% risk of subsequent failure, and those with a nadir of 1.0 ng/ml or higher had a 32% risk as shown by a large, multiinstitutional study.[92]

Lymph Node Status. The presence and location of lymph node metastases have great prognostic significance. Bagshaw et al.[6] reported 10-year disease-free survival rates of 75% in patients with localized disease and lymph nodes negative for tumor, versus 20% with pelvic nodes positive for tumor. The outcome with paraaortic nodal metastasis is worse still. Reporting on a group of more than 1000 patients treated by pelvic node dissection and iodine-125 (I-125) prostate implant, Leibel et al.[56] found lymph node involvement to be the most significant covariate affecting distant metastasis–free survival. At 10 years post treatment, 90% of patients with nodes positive for tumor had developed distant disease.

Anatomy

The **prostate gland** surrounds the male urethra between the base of the bladder and the urogenital diaphragm. The prostate is a walnut-shaped, solid organ that consists of fibrous, glandular, and muscular elements. It is attached anteriorly to the pubic symphysis by the puboprostatic ligament and separated posteriorly from the rectum by Denonvilliers' fascia (retrovesical septum), which attaches above to the peritoneum and below to the urogenital diaphragm. The seminal vesicles and vas deferens pierce the posterosuperior aspect of the gland and enter the urethra at the verumontanum (Figure 37-1).

Natural History of Disease

Local Growth Patterns. Most prostate carcinomas are multifocal and develop in the peripheral glands of the prostate,

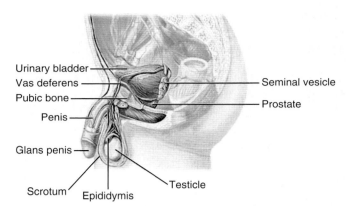

Figure 37-1. Anatomy of the prostate in relationship to the bladder, rectum and other surrounding structures. (Retrieved from http://www.prostatehealth.org.au/v1/html/sheet_3.htm.)

whereas benign prostatic hyperplasia arises from the central (periurethral) portion. As the tumor grows, it may extend into and through the capsule of the gland, invade periprostatic tissues and seminal vesicles and, if untreated, involve the bladder neck or rectum. The incidence of microscopic tumor extension beyond the capsule of the gland, at the time of radical prostatectomy, in patients with clinical stages T1b/c or T2 disease ranges from 10% to 50% and is also very much dependent on tumor grade and PSA. Seminal vesicle involvement has been observed in 1% to 30% of patients with stage T1 tumors and in 1% to 38% of patients with stage T2 lesions depending on the grade and PSA covariates.[68] The tumor may invade the perineural spaces, lymphatics, and blood vessels, producing lymphatic or distant metastases as well.

Regional Lymph Node Involvement and Distant Metastases. The tumor size and degree of differentiation affect the tendency of prostatic carcinoma to metastasize to regional lymphatics.

As smaller, nonpalpable tumors are diagnosed with the use of PSA screening, the incidence of metastatic pelvic lymph nodes decreases (Table 37-1). Periprostatic and obturator nodes are involved first, followed by external iliac, hypogastric, common iliac, and periaortic nodes (Figure 37-2). Approximately 7% of patients have involvement of the presacral lymph nodes, including the promontorial and middle hemorrhoidal group, without evidence of metastases in the external iliac or hypogastric lymph nodes. Metastases to the paraaortic nodes occur in 5% to 25% of patients. Patients with pelvic lymph node metastases are more likely to develop distant metastases than those with nodes negative for tumor. The incidence of distant metastases ranges from 20% in stage T1b to 90% in stage N1-3.

Clinical Presentation

Patients with prostate carcinoma may complain of decreased urinary stream, frequency, difficulty in starting urination, dysuria, and infrequently even hematuria. These symptoms may also be caused by conditions other than cancer, such as benign **prostatic hypertrophy** (enlargement of the prostate gland, leading to narrowing of the urethra) and infection. Some tumors are diagnosed

	Incidence of Metastatic Pelvic Lymph Nodes in Carcinoma of the Prostate	
Clinical Stage	**Nerve-Sparing Radical Prostatectomy***	**Radiation Therapy Series: Lymph Node Dissection†**
A2 (T1b)	2/61 (3.3%)	1/21 (5%)
B (T2)	33/425 (7.8%)	38/135 (28%)
C (T3, T4)	—	48/95 (51%)

Table 37-1

*Data from Petros J, Catalona WJ: Lower incidence of unsuspected lymph node metastases in 521 consecutive patients with clinically localized prostate cancer, *J Urol* 147:1574, 1992.
†Data from Hanks G, et al: Comparison of pathologic and clinical evaluation of lymph nodes in prostate cancer: implications of RTOG data for patient management and trial design and stratification, *Int J Radiat Oncol Biol Phys* 23:293, 1992.
T, tumor.

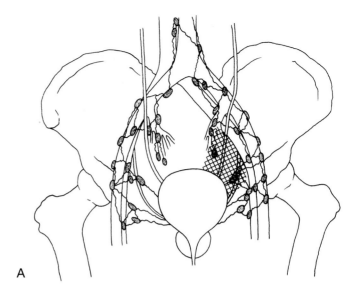

A

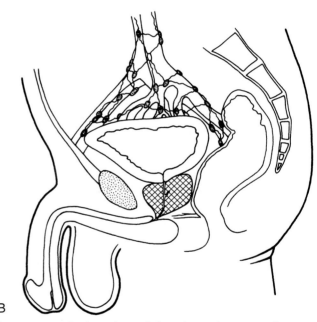

B

Figure 37-2. A, Location of lymph nodes most frequently involved in carcinoma of the prostate. The hatched area outlines the zone usually dissected in a limited staging lymphadenectomy. **B**, Sagittal view. (**A** from Perez CA: Prostate. In Perez CA, Brady LW, editors: *Principles and practice of radiation oncology,* ed 3, Philadelphia, 1998, Lippincott-Raven.)

at the time of a transurethral resection (a surgical procedure of the prostate performed for lower urinary tract obstructive symptoms), although this procedure is being performed much less often due to the efficiency of current medications. Bone pain or other symptoms associated with distant metastasis are seen less frequently at the time of the initial diagnosis.

Almost 40% of patients diagnosed with carcinoma of the prostate 20 years ago had M1 disease (distant metastasis). Increasing awareness by the public and physicians and the growing use of PSA have reduced this percentage to less than 5%. The American Cancer Society suggests that men without a family history of prostate cancer begin screening at age 50. Earlier screening is suggested for men with a higher propensity for developing the disease.[3]

Detection and Diagnosis

Complete physical and rectal examinations are mandatory. In most patients the seminal vesicles cannot be palpated, but a firm area extending above the prostate suggests that the seminal vesicles are involved by malignancy. Approximately 50% of prostatic nodules found during rectal examination are confirmed to be malignant at the time of a biopsy.

The diagnosis of prostatic carcinoma can be obtained only through histologic confirmation. A transrectal sonography-guided needle biopsy is the standard method of diagnosis in the United States. In Europe, especially Scandinavia, an aspiration biopsy has been used for many years with impressive results.[7] False-negative diagnoses range from less than 5% to 30%.

The standard tests required in the evaluation of patients with prostatic carcinoma are listed in Box 37-1.

Some have concluded that in many cases there are no specific characteristics on transrectal sonograms that differentiate benign prostatic disease from malignancy. Therefore, a biopsy is always required.[81] A sensitivity rate of 86% and a specificity rate of only 41% have been reported for sonography. Tumors less than 1 cm are the most difficult to detect.[13] Transrectal magnetic resonance imaging (MRI) is increasingly used in the evaluation of these patients.[87]

Screening. Carcinoma of the prostate can be asymptomatic until reaching a significant size. An annual digital rectal examination of the prostate should be performed in all men older than 50 years. A digital rectal examination has a 70% sensitivity rate and 50% specificity rate in detecting prostate cancer. Radioimmunoassays for prostatic acid phosphatase, which have a sensitivity rate of only 10% and a specificity rate of 90% for malignant tumors, have been largely replaced by PSA testing.

PSA Testing. PSA blood levels are routinely obtained in men older than 50 years. PSA is detected in normal prostatic tissue,

- Clinical
  - History and clinical examination
  - Rectal examination
- Laboratory
  - CBC and blood chemistry
  - Serum PSA
- Radiographic imaging
  - CT or MRI scan of the pelvis and abdomen
  - Chest x-ray examination
  - Radioisotope bone scan
  - Transrectal ultrasonography
- Biopsy
  - Needle biopsy of prostate (transrectal, sonography guided)

CBC, Complete blood count; *PSA,* prostate-specific antigen.

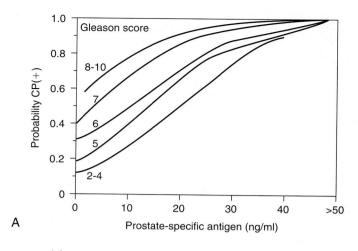

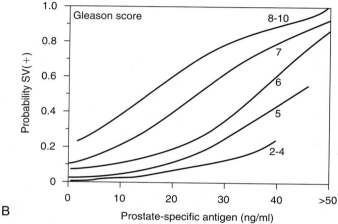

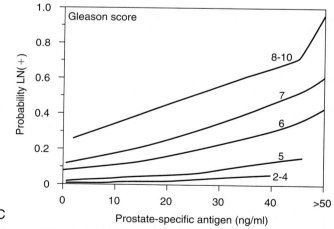

benign hyperplasia, malignant tumors, and seminal fluid and is measured by serum analysis. Although a normal PSA value, in general, is said to be 4 ng/ml or less, PSA level must be adjusted for age. For a 49-year-old man, a normal PSA would be 2.5 ng/ml or less, whereas a 70-year-old man would have a low risk of prostate cancer with a PSA of 6.5 ng/ml. As men age, prostate size increases, with higher PSA levels secondary to benign hypertrophy. An elevated PSA with no palpable disease of the prostate (stage T1c) is now the most common presentation for this disease because of increased screening and awareness.

PSA in the Selection of Patients for Therapy and Post Treatment Evaluation. Several have shown a close correlation between PSA levels and clinical and pathologic tumor stage and lymph node status, especially in conjunction with Gleason score, the histologic tumor grade. A group of patients with a PSA level below 2.8 ng/ml and a Gleason score below 4 had an incidence of nodal disease or seminal vesicle involvement of approximately 1% at the time of prostatectomy, but 60% of patients with a PSA level above 40 ng/ml and a Gleason score above 8 had these findings[68] (Figure 37-3). PSA is also of great value in the follow-up of patients treated with radical prostatectomy or radiation therapy.[19]

Pathology and Staging

Most malignant tumors of the prostate are adenocarcinomas. Gleason devised a quantitative histologic grading system based on the morphologic tumor characteristics.[34] The pathologist evaluates the predominant degree of differentiation of the tumor (primary pattern) and the less-frequent component (secondary pattern) based on the **morphology** of the lesion (e.g., glandular pattern, distribution of glands, stromal invasion) (Figure 37-4, A). The primary and secondary tumor grades are each labeled from 1 to 5. The two grades are added for a Gleason score of 2 to 10. The Gleason score correlates closely with prognosis, with lower scores representing more slowly growing, nonaggressive tumors and higher scores their more invasive, metastatic counterparts (Figure 37-4, B). Perez et al.[70] found that the histologic differentiation of the tumor was strongly correlated with the

Figure 37-3. A, Probability of capsular penetration *(CP+)* as a function of the serum prostate-specific antigen (PSA) and preoperative Gleason score. **B,** Probability of seminal vesicle involvement *(SV+)* as a function of the serum PSA and preoperative Gleason score. **C,** Probability of lymph node involvement *(LN+)* as a function of the serum PSA and preoperative Gleason score. (From Partin AW, et al: The use of prostate specific antigen, clinical stage and Gleason score to predict pathological stage in men with localized prostate cancer, *J Urol* 150:110-114, 1993.)

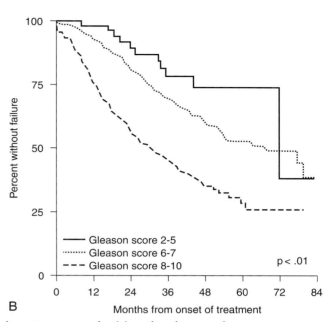

Figure 37-4. A, Simplified drawing of histologic patterns, emphasizing the degree of glandular differentiation and relation to stroma. The all-black area in the drawing represents the tumor tissue and glands with all cytologic detail obscured, except in the right side of pattern 4, where tiny open structures are intended to suggest the hypernephroid pattern. **B,** Survival correlated with the Gleason score (*N* = 566). (**A** from Gleason DF, et al: Histologic grading and clinical staging of prostatic carcinoma. In Tannenbaum M, editor: *Urologic pathology: the prostate*, Philadelphia, 1977, Lea and Febiger; **B** from Pilepich MV, et al: Prognostic factors in carcinoma of the prostate: analysis of RTOG Study 75-06, *Int J Radiat Oncol Biol Phys* 13:339-349, 1987.)

incidence of distant metastases and survival but not as closely with locoregional failure.

Findings from the digital examination of the prostate and imaging studies determine the stage of the disease, which is classified according to the American Joint Committee on Cancer (AJCC)[37] (Box 37-2).

Stage T1 lesions are not detectable on digital rectal examination. T1a lesions are well-differentiated adenocarcinomas that are incidentally found during a transurethral resection of the prostate. They involve 5% or less of resected tissue. Stage T1b tumors are also subclinical, but they are more diffuse or have a larger volume, frequently with multifocal involvement of the prostate (>5% of tissue resected). T1c tumors are identified by a needle biopsy (e.g., because of elevated PSA levels).

Stage T2 tumors are palpable and confined within the capsule of the prostate gland. T2a tumors involve one lobe; T2b involve both lobes.

Stage T3 lesions are more locally extensive, beyond the edges of the prostate or into the seminal vesicles. T3a denotes extracapsular extension, either unilateral or bilateral. T3b indicates seminal vesicle invasion.

Stage T4 tumors are fixed to the pelvic sidewall or invade adjacent structures such as rectum or bladder. Regional nodal status is described as negative (N0) or positive (N1).

Distant disease is designated M1a: nonregional nodes, M1b: bone, and M1c: other sites.

Whether prostate cancer is localized (T1 and T2), is more extensive (T3 and T4), or has metastasized to lymph nodes (N1) or distantly (M1) has great bearing on subsegment survival (Figure 37-5).

Treatment Techniques

Several areas of controversy surround the management of patients with prostatic carcinoma. The natural history of this tumor is variable and influenced by multiple prognostic factors. The different forms of therapy can affect the quality of life and sexual function to varying degrees.

In general, localized carcinoma of the prostate has a fairly slow clinical course. The National Cancer Institute Consensus Development Conference on Management of Localized Prostate Cancer concluded that radical prostatectomy and radiation therapy are clearly effective treatments in appropriately selected patients for tumors limited to the prostate.

Observation. Several have reported on patients who, after a histologic diagnosis of prostatic carcinoma, were managed conservatively and monitored without specific anticancer treatment until symptoms developed.[1,2,14] The literature indicates that the tumors that are not poorly differentiated can have a protracted course associated with significant competing mortality and

PRIMARY TUMOR (T)[1]

pT2	Organ confined
pT2a	Unilateral, one-half of one lobe or less
pT2b	Unilateral, involving more than one-half of lobe but not both lobes
pT2c	Bilateral disease
pT3	Extraprostatic extension
pT3a	Extraprostatic extension[2]
pT3b	Seminal vesicle invasion
pT4	Invasion of bladder, rectum

REGIONAL LYMPH NODES (N)

pNX	Regional nodes not sampled
pN0	No positive regional nodes
pN1	Metastases in regional nodes(s)

DISTANT METASTASIS (M)[5]

MX	Distant metastasis cannot be assessed (not evaluated by any modality)
M0	No distant metastasis
M1	Distant metastasis
M1a	Nonregional lymph node(s)
M1b	Bone(s)
M1c	Other site(s) with or without bone disease

PRIMARY TUMOR (T)

TX	Primary tumor cannot be assessed
T0	No evidence of primary tumor
T1	Clinically inapparent tumor neither palpable nor visible by imaging
T1a	Tumor incidental histologic finding in 5% or less of tissue resected
T1b	Tumor incidental histologic finding in more than 5% of tissue resected
T1c	Tumor identified by needle biopsy (e.g., because of elevated PSA)
T2	Tumor confined within prostate[3]

T2a	Tumor involves one-half of one lobe or less
T2b	Tumor involves more than one-half of one lobe but not both lobes
T2c	Tumor involves both lobes
T3	Tumor extends through the prostate capsule[4]
T3a	Extracapsular extension (unilateral or bilateral)
T3b	Tumor invades seminal vesicle(s)
T4	Tumor is fixed or invades adjacent structures other than seminal vesicles: bladder neck, external sphincter, rectum, levator muscles, and/or pelvic wall

REGIONAL LYMPH NODES (N)

NX	Regional lymph nodes were not assessed
N0	No regional lymph node metastasis
N1	Metastases in regional nodes(s)

STAGE GROUPING

I	T1a	N0	M0	G1
II	T1a	N0	M0	G2, 3-4
	T1b	N0	M0	Any G
	T1c	N0	M0	Any G
	T1	N0	M0	Any G
	T2	N0	M0	Any G
III	T3	N0	M0	Any G
IV	T4	N0	M0	Any G
	Any T	N1	M0	Any G
	Any T	Any N	M1	Any G

HISTOLOGIC GRADE (G)

GX	Grade cannot be assessed
G1	Well differentiated (slight anaplasia) (Gleason 2-4)
G2	Moderately differentiated (moderate anaplasia) (Gleason 5-6)
G3-4	Poorly differentiated/undifferentiated (marked anaplasia) (Gleason 7-10)

With permission from American Joint Committee on Cancer (AJCC), Chicago, IL: *AJCC cancer staging manual*, ed 6, New York, 2002, Springer-Verlag.
Notes:
1. There is no pathologic T1 classification.
2. Positive surgical margin should be indicated by an R1 descriptor (residual microscopic disease).
3. Tumor found in one or both lobes by needle biopsy, but not palpable or reliably visible by imaging, is classified as T1c.
4. Invasion into the prostatic apex or into (but not beyond) the prostatic capsule is classified not as T3, but as T2.
5. When more than one site of metastasis is present, the most advanced category is used. pM1c is most advanced.

marginal benefit from therapy at 10 years.[1,2,11] Observation is reasonable management for patients older than 75 years. It can also be offered to younger patients, 65 to 75 years old, with small, well-differentiated tumors. However, in today's health environment in the United States, most patients do not readily accept delaying definitive therapy unless they are very elderly with indolent-behaving disease or in very poor general health from other medical illness.

According to many urologists, stage T1a disease, which is found incidentally, requires no treatment; many years of natural evolution may pass before the disease becomes a clinical problem. According to one study, only 6.8% of 148 patients with this stage disease progressed.[11] A literature review showed a death rate of only 1.9% in 262 patients with stage T1a carcinoma. Some authors have noted decreased survival rates

with poorly differentiated tumors, however.[14,45] In 313 patients treated with external irradiation, the 5-year survival rate was comparable to that of a matched-age normal male group but the 10-year survival rate was below the normal life expectancy, 51% versus 62%.[38] Both stage T1a and T1b (diagnosis by transurethral resection) prostate cancer have been more infrequently diagnosed since the introduction of PSA as a tool for screening in the mid-1980s. Patients with an elevated PSA, who are subsequently found to have prostate cancer on biopsy, are staged as T1c. Furthermore, benign prostate hypertrophy is now largely treated with medication, reserving transurethral resection for only the most severe cases.

Prostatectomy. Patients with resectable stage T1 or T2 prostate cancer who are in good general medical condition and have a life expectancy of at least 10 years are candidates for

Overall survival for patients with prostate carcinoma by stage

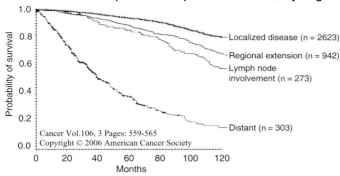

Figure 37-5. Overall survival for patients with prostate cancer by stage. (From Taylor SH, et al: Inadequacies of the current American joint committee on cancer staging system for prostate cancer. Retrieved February 4, 2008, from http://www3.inter-science.wiley.com/cgi-bin/abstract/112221260/ABSTRACT.)

radical prostatectomy. Impetus has been given to the use of nerve-sparing surgery because an increasing number of tumors are being diagnosed at earlier stages, and a lower incidence of sexual **impotence** (the inability to obtain an erection) has been reported with this surgery (40% to 60%, depending on the patient's age and tumor extent) compared with classic radical prostatectomy (close to 100%).[12] Radiation therapy has been shown to provide a very similar outcome for these patients. A recent report from the Cleveland Clinic compared stage T1 and T2 patients treated by surgery versus radiation.[51] For good prognosis patients (initial PSA 10 ng/ml or less, Gleason 6 or less), 78% of irradiated patients and 80% of prostatectomy patients were disease free 5 years after treatment by PSA criteria, which is the strictest and most objective measure. In those patients at higher risk for recurrence based on prognostic factors, 25% and 38% of those treated by radiation versus surgery, respectively, were PSA disease free. This difference was not statistically significant. Of note is that these results were reported for patients treated by conventional radiation doses and techniques. Reported outcome for patients treated to higher doses using three-dimensional (3D) conformal or intensity-modulated radiation therapy (IMRT) techniques seems to indicate that even better results are attainable.[111]

For stage T3 disease, most urologists and radiation oncologists agree that external beam radiation is the treatment of choice, usually with hormonal therapy. Because of the significant tumor bulk and high metastatic potential in this category, results with radiation alone have been less than satisfactory, with 10% to 35% PSA disease-free survival at 10 years.[55] The addition of hormone therapy to radiation has markedly improved disease control. Zagars et al.[110] report PSA disease-free survival of 78% versus 33% at 6 years dependent on hormonal therapy. A randomized European Cooperative Group Trial (European Organization for Research and Treatment of Cancer [EORTC]) showed significant improvement not only in PSA progression–free survival but overall survival as well for patients treated with 3 years of hormonal therapy (androgen deprivation) in addition to radiation. PSA progression–free survival was 76% and overall survival was 78% at 5 years after treatment for patients treated with the combination therapy versus 45% and

60%, respectively, for patients treated with radiation alone.[10] Dose escalation studies have not shown nearly as marked a benefit to date for this group.

Radioisotopic implant is also an option for patients with early stage (T1c, T2a-b), low-grade (Gleason ≤6), low-PSA (≤10 ng/ml) prostate cancer. I-125 and palladium-103 (Pd-103) are the permanent sources used. The current technique is a transperineal template sonography-guided approach. PSA disease-free survival appears to be equivalent to external beam therapy, in the 80% to 90% range, if candidates are carefully selected.[8,9]

Hormonal Therapy. In 1941, Huggins et al.[42] demonstrated prostate tumor regression and diminished serum acid phosphatase levels after orchiectomy or estrogen administration. Many types of hormonal therapy, all seeking to reduce the androgenic stimulation of prostatic carcinoma, have been used since then. Orchiectomy removes 95% of circulating testosterone and is followed by a prompt, long-lasting decline in serum testosterone levels. Estrogen appears to suppress pituitary gonadotropin, causing reduced stimulus for testicular testosterone synthesis, direct interference with hormonal synthesis, or a direct effect on the prostatic cell competing with hormonal receptors. Gonadotropin-releasing hormone agonists such as goserelin (Zoladex) and leuprolide acetate (Lupron) cause an initial rise in gonadotropin levels, followed by a sharp decline within 2 to 3 weeks. Parallel changes occur in levels of circulating testosterone. Results with these compounds are similar to those obtained with bilateral orchiectomy.

Aminoglutethimide, which is administered with a glucocorticoid, inhibits the synthesis of all adrenal steroids and can further reduce serum testosterone levels in castrated patients.[105]

Flutamide (Eulexin) and bicalutamide (Casodex) are both nonsteroidal antiandrogens. Flutamide inhibits androgen uptake and nuclear binding in the prostate cancer cell, and bicalutamide competitively inhibits the action of androgens by binding to cytosol androgen receptors. Hormonal therapy has long been used to reduce metastatic tumor burden and palliate symptoms; however, more recently hormonal therapy has been added to radiation in locally advanced and high-grade tumors. The RTOG 86-10 and 92-02 studies have shown an advantage in disease control and survival with short-term hormonal administration (2 months before and during radiation) in bulky Gleason score 2 to 6 tumors and with long-term hormonal therapy (2 years) in Gleason score 8 to 10 tumors. It appears that testosterone ablation helps by reducing tumor bulk locally and also by controlling microscopic, clinically undetected metastatic disease.[39,72]

Chemotherapy. Several drugs have been evaluated in patients for whom hormonal therapy has failed. Response rates with single-agent doxorubicin (Adriamycin) are 25% to 35%. With cyclophosphamide, the rate of partial response plus stable disease ranges from 26% to 41%. In about 10% of patients, 5-fluorouracil (5-FU) has induced partial responses. A partial response rate of only 8% was observed with hydroxyurea. Yagoda and Petrylak[106] reviewed multiple chemotherapy trails and found an overall 9% clinical response rate. Multiple drug combinations were also tested and the combination of paclitaxel (Taxol), etoposide, and estramustine appeared promising. Because patients with locally advanced, high-grade, high-PSA tumors typically have a poor outcome even with a combination of radiation and hormonal therapy, the RTOG initiated a protocol (RTOG 99-02) randomizing one arm to chemotherapy (Taxol, etoposide, etramustine) in addition to radiation and hormonal therapy. Although this study closed early because of deep venous thrombosis on the chemotherapy arm attributed to estramustine, a second study is now in progress with different drugs, docetaxel and prednisone. In randomized trials, docetaxel plus prednisone has shown a response in PSA and pain relief as well as a small survival advantage in patients with metastatic disease.[25] Therefore, this regimen is now considered standard for test metastatic patients when hormone therapy is no longer effective. The hypothesis of the RTOG randomized trial described here is that earlier application of chemotherapy may prevent the development of disseminated disease. It is thought that effective cytotoxic systemic treatment will be necessary to truly eradicate the occult metastatic disease, which is so prevalent in patients with locally advanced, poorly differentiated tumors.

External Radiation. A decision must first be made regarding treatment volume and whether seminal vesicles and/or pelvic lymph nodes will be irradiated. Seminal vesicles are usually included in the treatment volume when the risk of involvement is at least in the 10% to 15% range. The risk of involvement can be calculated from an equation[82,83] or estimated from a table wherein surgically dissected patients are categorized by prognostic factors.[68] In general, these are usually patients with PSA greater than 10 ng/ml and with tumors with Gleason score greater than 6. Treating the seminal vesicles usually results in a larger volume of rectum irradiated. Although it would seem prudent to include the seminal vesicles under the conditions noted previously on the basis of general radiation therapy principles, there are no study results to date that document improved outcome.

Pelvic lymph node irradiation is controversial as well. Studies disagree as to the ultimate benefit in terms of disease progression and survival. An RTOG study addressing lymph node irradiation recently reported negative results overall but improved outcome in patients who received hormonal therapy specifically given before and during nodal radiation compared to afterward.[54,84] Thus, the benefit of irradiated pelvic lymph nodes remains debatable. Currently, decisions on lymph node therapy are left to the discretion of the treating physician and institutional policy. In general, a risk of involvement in the 20% range would prompt therapy by those who believe it may be beneficial. When the pelvic lymph nodes are treated, the field size is usually 15 × 15 cm at the patient surface (16.5 cm at the isocenter) (Figure 37-6, A). The reduced field for treatment of the prostate and seminal vesicles is determined by computed tomography (CT) scan, and therefore size will vary according to prostate and seminal vesicle size, usually in the range of 8 to 10 cm including margins. A final cone-down may be done to encompass only the prostate. Location varies as well but is generally related to the pubic symphysis. The inferior margin may be determined by retrograde urethrogram, implanted marker, or CT scan. When CT scan is used, margins should be more generous because the inferiormost extent of the gland may be difficult to determine exactly. Blocking devices or multileaf collimation (MLC) is, of course, used to shape the fields.

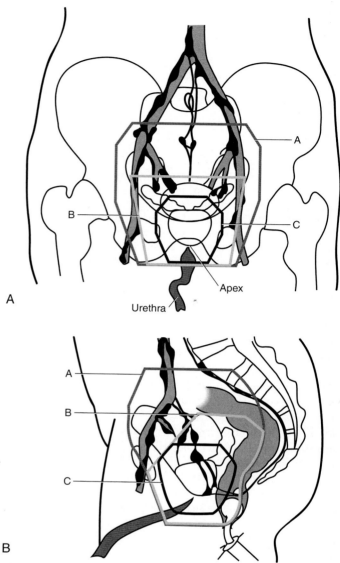

Figure 37-6. A, Anteroposterior (AP) fields for *(A)* prostate, seminal vesicles, and pelvic nodes, *(B)* prostate and seminal vesicles, *(C)* prostate only. **B**, Lateral fields for same regions. (From Kuban DA, El-Mahdi AM: Cancers of the genitourinary tract. In Khan FM, Potish RA, editors: *Treatment planning in radiation oncology*, Baltimore, 1998, Lippincott Williams & Wilkins.)

A four-field box technique with lateral portals has typically been used to treat pelvic lymph nodes, although intensity-modulated radiation therapy (IMRT) techniques have been applied more recently. Nodes can be mapped on CT scan and planning done individually, or a more standard field can be applied. With the latter technique, the upper border is at the midsacral level and the lower border determined by the inferiormost aspect of the prostate. The lateral margins of the anterior field are 1.5 to 2 cm from the lateral pelvic brim (see Figure 37-6, A). For the lateral field, the anterior margin is 1 cm posterior to the projection of the anterior cortex of the pubic symphysis (Figure 37-6, B). Small bowel is spared anteriorly at the upper aspect of the field, being mindful of the location of the external iliac nodes. The posterior border is generally at the posterior ischium with shielding of the posterior rectal wall as appropriate. Barium or a plastic catheter with radiopaque markers can be used to define the rectum if CT planning is not used. The position of the seminal vesicles must be verified by CT scan, and the posterior field margin must allow for coverage of these structures with adequate margin. Typical simulation films for a pelvic nodal field are shown in Figure 37-7, A and B. Field dimensions and blocking are then defined by CT scan contours and planning.

Simulation. Patients are most often simulated in the supine position. Immobilization by a foaming cradle, vacuum bag, or other leg/pelvis immobilization device is first carried out. If a conventional simulator is used, a standard isocenter can be marked (usually tattooed) on the patient. For a typical field to encompass the prostate or prostate and seminal vesicles, the isocenter is placed 1.5 to 2 cm below the top of the symphysis pubis, at midline on the anterior projection and 5.5 to 6.5 cm posterior to the tip of the pubic symphysis on the lateral projection. If a CT simulator is available, a preliminary scan is done by obtaining slices every 5 mm from the inferior aspect of the sacroiliac joints through the inferior ischia. An isocenter is set within the prostate using the CT images. It is marked anteriorly and laterally, both right and left, with BBs. The patient is then scanned every 3 mm using the same superior and inferior margins with care to scan through the plane of the BBs. The isocenter is tattooed on the patient at the three points (see Figure 37-7, A and B). Scans are transferred to the treatment-planning computer.

CT scanning does not allow for very accurate visualization of the inferiormost extent of the prostatic apex because it appears to blend with the urogenital diaphragm, so the field length is often overestimated to ensure that the entire prostate is well within the radiation portal. This can cause undue radiation of the penile bulb and perhaps a higher risk of impotence. In addition to CT, two other methods may be used to determine the inferior field margin. A retrograde urethrogram performed at the time of treatment simulation defines the apex of the urethra or the point where the urethra passes through the urogenital diaphragm, by a narrow point, or beak, in the column of contrast media (see Figure 37-7, C). The inferiormost aspect of the prostate is typically located approximately 1 cm above the urethral apex; therefore, by using the urethrogram, an appropriate margin can be applied. A more recent technique uses MRI to define the inferior border of the prostate because this imaging modality can better distinguish the prostate from the soft tissues of the urogenital diaphragm.[87]

Conformal Three-Dimensional Treatment Planning and Delivery. The development of sophisticated radiation treatment–planning computers has allowed the planning CT to be reconstructed in three dimensions. The target (prostate or prostate and seminal vesicles) and the surrounding normal structures can be anatomically defined. These organs are outlined on each CT slice. Margins are generally dependent on intended dose, setup error, and internal organ motion. The latter two may vary depending on external immobilization and techniques for correcting for internal prostate movement such as fiducial markers, rectal balloon, or transabdominal sonography (B-mode acquisition technology [BAT]). In general, required margins on the clinical target volume (CTV) to achieve the planning target volume (PTV), are usually in the range of 0.55 to 1.0 cm

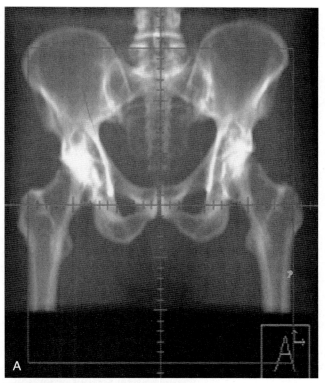

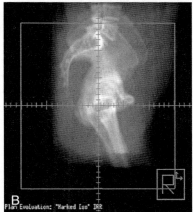

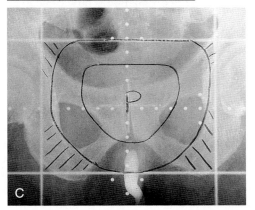

Figure 37-7. A, Anteroposterior (AP) projection and isocenter placement simulation films for CT scan planning. **B**, Lateral simulation field. **C**, AP urethrogram showing inferior field margin. (**C**, From Kuban DA, El-Mahdi AM: Cancers of the genitourinary tract. In Khan FM, Potish RA, editors: *Treatment planning in radiation oncology*, Baltimore, 1998, Lippincott Williams & Wilkins.)

for conformal and IMRT techniques when daily pre-prostate localization is carried out. When techniques with less accuracy are used, margins must be larger to prevent marginal misses.

Sonography is commonly associated with visualizing a fetus in the mother's womb; however, in the field of radiation therapy, it is a common way of ensuring accurate delivery of dose to the prostate on a daily basis. The prostate is located inferior to the bladder, posterior to the pubic symphysis, and just anterior to the rectum. Bladder and rectal filling and slight differences in patient positioning on the treatment table can change the prostate position from day to day. Sonography (BAT) can be done just before treatment each day to ensure proper radiation field alignment. The prostate, bladder, and rectum can all be seen on sonograms. Patients are treated with a full bladder, which helps in visualizing the bladder-prostate interface and in moving the bladder out of the field. By properly aligning the prostate within the radiation field, not only is the proper dose delivered, avoiding marginal misses, but also the bladder and rectum are maximally spared.

Beam design may vary. A common technique is six fields consisting of a right and left lateral pair and two parallel-opposed oblique pairs 45 degrees off lateral. If an anterior beam is used, mainly for the purpose of portal imaging, this may be referred to as a seven-field arrangement. A four-field, typical "box" approach, followed by six fields as just described, is another technique frequently used, especially if lymph nodes are treated initially. To shape or conform each field, Cerrobend blocks or MLC settings on the treatment machine are applied as specified by the computer plan (Figure 37-8). The dose to pelvic nodes is typically 45 to 50 Gy with 54 to 56 Gy to seminal vesicles at high risk but not proved to be involved by tumor. Prostate doses typically range from 72 to 80 Gy at 1.8 to 2.0 Gy/day.

A word should be said about dose prescription. Care should be taken to define the prescription point. There can be up to a 5% difference with standard conformal techniques and more for IMRT depending on whether the total dose is prescribed to isocenter, the CTV, or PTV. Although doses prescribed to isocenter may appear higher on paper, the dose to the CTV and PTV is actually considerably lower. For definitions of tumor and planning volumes, see Table 37-2.

IMRT is a more advanced technique that specifies the chosen dose to the tumor volume as well as acceptable dose levels for surrounding normal structures such as bladder, rectum, and femoral heads. Although five to eight different beam angles are typically used, MLC settings change while each field is being treated, shielding the critical structures a portion of the time and thus treating the tumor volume to a higher dose than the organs of lesser tolerance. Although this technique tends to produce extremely conformal fields with tight margins, inhomogeneity of dose tends to be greater with differentials in the 5% to 15% range. Care must be taken that the highest doses are within the tumor volume and not in normal structures where tolerance will be exceeded. It is with this technique that doses of 80 Gy or more can be delivered to the prostate (Figure 37-9). Dose-volume histograms (DVHs) must be constructed to determine the volume of the critical organs (rectum, bladder, and femur) receiving high doses (Figure 37-9, E). These parameters have been proved to be related to late radiation-induced complications.

Proton Therapy. Proton therapy offers another way to deliver high radiation doses to a tumor. Protons are positively charged particles and deposit their radiation differently than do x-rays. Compared with an x-ray beam, a proton beam has a low "entrance dose" (the dose delivered between the surface and the tumor), a high dose designed to cover the entire tumor, and no "exit dose" beyond the tumor[103] (Figure 37-10, A and B). This unique characteristic gives proton therapy the ability to deposit a radiation dose in a precise manner and thus minimize damage to the surrounding normal tissue. This may lead to better cancer control with fewer side effects and long-term complications.

For this type of treatment, patients are treated from right and left lateral fields up to a dose of 76 to 82 Gy. Brass apertures are placed in the beams path in order to shape the beam to the desired field size. Because proton beams are very sensitive to the amount and density of tissue traversed, lateral beams provide the most accurate, reproducible arrangement for prostate cancer therapy. Lateral beams are not always well suited to treating seminal vesicles, however. This beam arrangement treats far too much rectum when seminal vesicles wrap around the rectum posteriorly. Therefore, some patients with more extensive tumors, which require seminal vesicle irradiation, may not be good candidates for proton therapy.

Interstitial Brachytherapy. Although a prostate implant was done through an open retropubic technique similar to prostatectomy in the mid-1970s to mid-1980s, the advent of transrectal sonography permitted a less invasive transperineal template technique that was pioneered in the late 1980s. This procedure is done with either spinal or general anesthesia and uses a grid or template against the perineum with the patient in the dorsal lithotomy position. Transrectal sonography is used to direct the needles, which are either preloaded or attached to the Mick applicator that deposits the radioactive seeds. Dosimetry planning may be done in advance by taking sonographic images every 5 mm from the base of the prostate through the apex and then loading these into the treatment-planning computer. Seeds are then distributed throughout the prostate 1 cm apart. Isodoses are computed (Figure 37-11, A and B). Alternatively, this planning can be done in the operating room just before the procedure. In general, for the average gland, approximately 25 needles and 100 or so seeds are used. The commonly used permanent isotopes are I-125 (half-life = 60 days) and Pd-103 (half-life = 17 days). The usual dose for implant alone with iodine is 145 Gy, and with palladium, 115 Gy. Postimplant dosimetry is done postoperatively by obtaining a CT scan, usually at approximately 30 days after the procedure to allow for edema to subside, and entering the seeds and prostate as seen on the scan into the treatment-planning computer. The prostate volume that receives 100% of the prescribed dose (V_{100}) and the dose to 90% of the prostate volume (D_{90}) are the parameters typically recorded. Outcome data suggest that recurrence rates increase with D_{90} values less than 140 Gy.[98] Implants with V_{100} values of 80% or greater are considered good quality. Doses to the rectum and urethra are also evaluated.

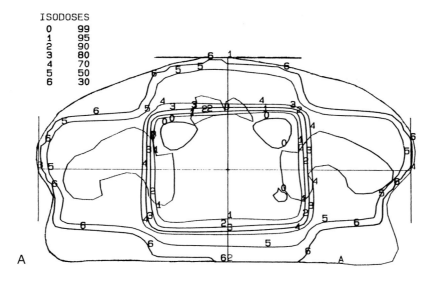

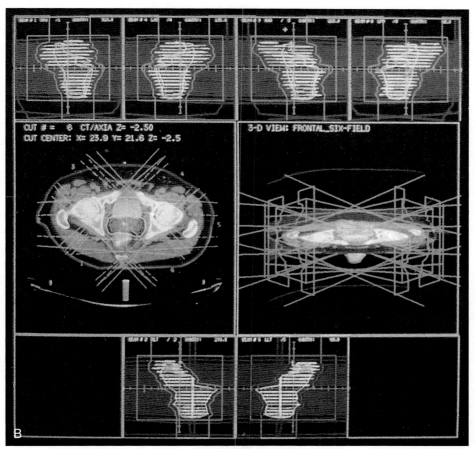

Figure 37-8. A, Isodose distribution for four-field box pelvic treatment technique. **B**, Three-dimensional beam's eye view treatment plan and fields. (**A**, From Kuban DA, El-Mahdi AM: Cancers of the genitourinary tract. In Khan FM, Potish RA, editors: *Treatment planning in radiation oncology*, Baltimore, 1998, Lippincott Williams & Wilkins. **B**, Reprinted with permission from Ten Haken RK, et al: Boost treatment of the prostate using shaped, fixed fields, *Int J Radiat Oncol Biol Phys* 16:193-200, 1989.)

Table 37-2	Volume Definitions for Treatment Planning	
Volume	**Definition**	
GTV Gross tumor volume	Palpable or visible extent of tumor	
CTV Clinical target volume	GTV plus margin for subclinical disease extension	
PTV Planning target volume	CTV plus margin for treatment reproducibility (patient/organ movement, daily setup error)	
Treatment volume	Volume enclosed by appropriate isodose in achieving the treatment purpose	

Interstitial implant can also be used as a boost after moderate-dose external beam radiation. Patients chosen for this procedure are those with significant risk of tumor extension outside the prostate capsule. Typically, a dose of 45 Gy to the prostate, seminal vesicles, and possibly pelvic nodes is delivered with external beam. This is then followed 2 to 4 weeks later by an implant, as a boost, to the prostate. The implant dose is decreased to 110 Gy with I-125 and 90 Gy with Pd-103.

High-dose-rate (HDR) iridium is another way to deliver a boost following moderate dose external beam. Compared with I-125 and Pd-103, which are permanent implants, this is a temporary implant technique. Similar to permanent isotopes, a perineal template is used to introduce needles and catheters into

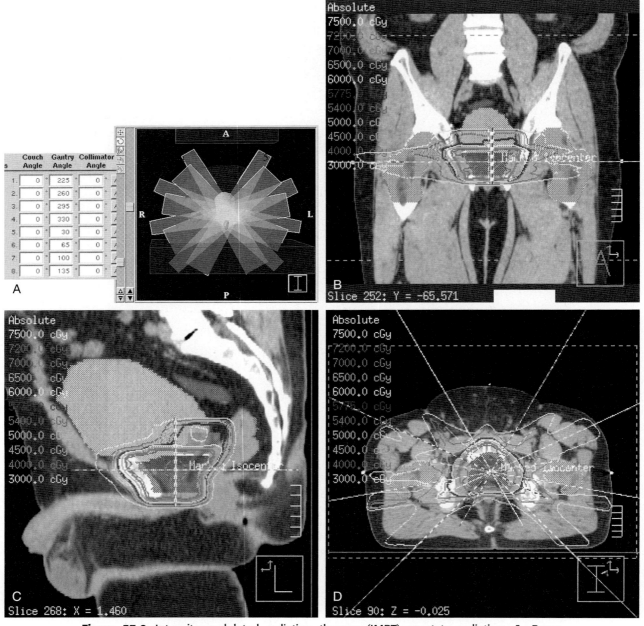

Figure 37-9. Intensity-modulated radiation therapy (IMRT) prostate radiation. **A**, Beam angles (8). **B**, Coronal dose distribution. **C**, Sagittal dose distribution. **D**, Axial dose distribution. (See Color Plate 22.)

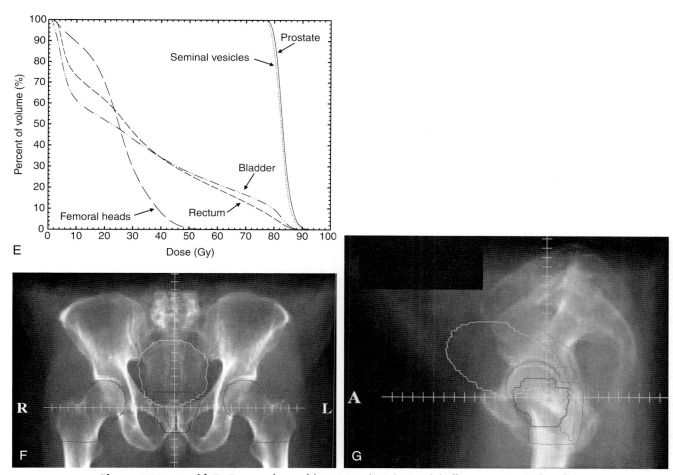

Figure 37.9. cont'd E, Dose-volume histogram (DVH) **F**, Digitally reconstructed radiograph (DRR) for treatment setup, anterior view. **G**, DRR for treatment setup.

the prostate. The catheters are left in place and the patient is hospitalized. Doses have ranged from 500 cGy in each of three fractions to 900 cGy for two fractions. This is generally delivered over 2 days. Total doses and fraction sizes have varied as radiobiologic dose equivalents of these large fraction sizes are being established.

Postprostatectomy Radiation. Three situations arise in the postprostatectomy setting: (1) PSA does not decrease to the undetectable range immediately after prostatectomy, signaling that all tumor has not been removed; (2) PSA is undetectable postoperatively but tumor margins contain tumor or seminal vesicles are involved; and (3) PSA is undetectable immediately after surgery but after a period begins to rise. In the latter two circumstances, radiation to the prostate fossa is commonly applied. In the first situation, the PSA may still be detectable because of metastatic disease, and therefore local radiation would not be beneficial. Care must be taken to prove that the only disease remaining is in the surgical bed before local therapy is applied.

CT scan planning can be used similar to the procedure for an intact prostate. The surgical bed, or area where the prostate and seminal vesicles are normally found, is contoured as the target volume. Care is taken to include any site found worrisome by the surgeon or noted as being involved by the pathology report. Four-field or six-field conformal techniques have been typically used, although IMRT is now applied at some centers. Field sizes tend to be in the 10 × 8 cm range. Doses for microscopic disease immediately postoperatively with undetectable PSA are generally at the 64 to 66 Gy level with higher doses, in the 70 Gy range, for rising PSA. Care must be taken to evaluate rectal and bladder DVHs. Following surgical removal of the prostate, the bladder and rectum tend to move into the prostatic space, necessitating inclusion of a significant portion of these organs if the area at risk is to be adequately treated. It is not unusual that desired dose levels are compromised by critical organ (rectum and bladder) tolerance.

Results of Treatment

Surgery. Overall, survival is a poor measure of treatment outcome for prostate cancer therapy because this is a slowly progressive disease that many men die *with* but not because *of*. There are many other medical conditions in elderly men that affect

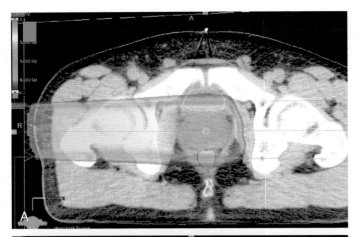

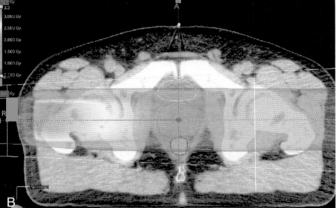

Figure 37-10. A, Lateral proton beam. **B,** Lateral photon beams. Both images are a single right lateral beam. Notice the lack of exit dose on the proton beam. (See Color Plate 23.)

the death rate. Therefore, cause-specific survival based on death from cancer per se is a better measure. To evaluate a particular therapy and its efficacy in eradicating the disease, PSA disease-free survival is generally used in the case of prostate cancer. Because a rising PSA post treatment signals disease recurrence, it is an objective and early measure of disease status. Outcome is also very much dependent on prognostic factors such as tumor stage, histologic grade (Gleason score), and pretreatment PSA. Patients who have had prostatectomy can be additionally classified according to pathologic features: extracapsular tumor extension, seminal vesicle involvement, and lymph node status.

For prostatectomy, overall PSA progression-free survival rates range from 70% to 85% at 5 years and 45% to 75% at 10 years. For those patients with the best prognosis, T1 to T2, PSA of 10 ng/ml or less, Gleason of 6 or less, the PSA progression–free rate is 80% to 85% at 10 years.[23,67] On the contrary, however, the PSA progression–free rate at 10 years is only 50% for pretreatment PSA greater than 10 ng/ml, 70% with extracapsular extension, 40% with seminal vesicle involvement, and 10% with lymph nodes positive for tumor.[23,67] Clinical disease usually becomes detectable long after the PSA rise. In the Johns Hopkins surgical series, only 4% of men had local recurrence and 8% had distant disease 10 years after prostatectomy.[67]

Radiation. Results with both external beam radiation and radaoisotopic implant are much the same as for surgery if like groups are compared. When treating patients with radiation, we do not, of course, have the pathologic factors such as extracapsular extension, seminal vesicle involvement, and lymph node status by which to group patients into prognostic categories. Tumor stage, grade, and PSA, however, provide substantial information for comparison. With external beam therapy, the best prognostic group—T1 to T2, PSA of 10 ng/ml or less, Gleason of 6 or less—has a PSA disease-free survival of 80% at 10 years just as for surgery,[51] and newer techniques (IMRT) with higher doses provide even better results.[111] Similar patients show PSA disease-free survival of 80% to 90% of the time with implant.[8,9] The implant patients tend to be a more highly select group with smaller amounts of disease, which may account for slightly better outcome statistics. Patients with more advanced disease, T3 or PSA greater than 10 ng/ml or Gleason 7 to 10, tend to have more guarded prognosis—again, similar to those surgically treated.[10,55]

As radiation techniques become more highly conformal and doses are increased, early reports on outcome appear promising. The randomized study from the University of Texas M. D. Anderson Cancer Center comparing 70 Gy with 78 Gy reported a 39% absolute gain in PSA disease-free survival at 8 years for patients with pretreatment PSA greater than 10 ng/ml treated to 78 Gy[48,73] (Figure 37-12). There was no advantage for higher dose in patients with pretreatment PSA of 10 ng/ml or less. Other investigators have seen improved outcome results with higher doses as well (Table 37-3). A randomized study has shown improvement in 5-year PSA progression–free survival for both low- and intermediate-/high-risk patients treated with 79.2 Gy compared with 70 Gy.[113] Because serum PSA is a good marker for recurrent disease and has been shown to highly correlate with prostate biopsy results, routine postradiation biopsies are no longer done except in randomized trials. Biopsies become important, however, when local treatment for prostate recurrence is planned. Because these therapies, such as prostatectomy, cryotherapy, and repeat irradiation, usually carry significant complication rates, it is essential to ensure that there is, in fact, local disease present because a PSA rise could also be caused by nodal or distant disease.

Palliative Radiation. Irradiation doses of 50 to 60 Gy may be effective in the treatment of massive, locally extensive prostatic carcinoma or significant-size pelvic lymph node disease, which may produce pain, hematuria, urethral obstruction, or leg edema.

Radiation is frequently used in the treatment of distant metastases secondary to carcinoma of the prostate. Marked symptomatic relief is noted in more than 80% of patients treated with doses of 30 Gy in 2 weeks. Most commonly, osseous sites are treated with localized fields. Although unusual, brain metastases may be successfully treated with doses of 30 Gy in 10 fractions to the entire cranial contents just as for other primary sites. For palliation of pain, larger doses per day are also effective and may be especially prudent in patients in poor general condition and very limited life span.

If multiple skeletal sites are involved by the tumor and produce symptoms, radioactive strontium-89 can be administered intravenously, with some degree of pain relief occurring in 80% of patients.[74] Samarium-153 is a newer isotope that is also used for this purpose.[4]

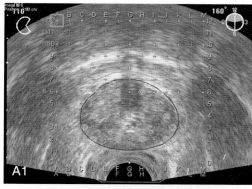

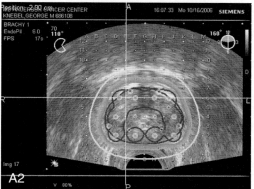

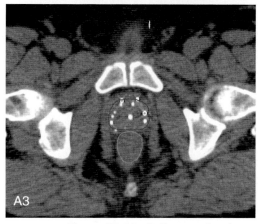

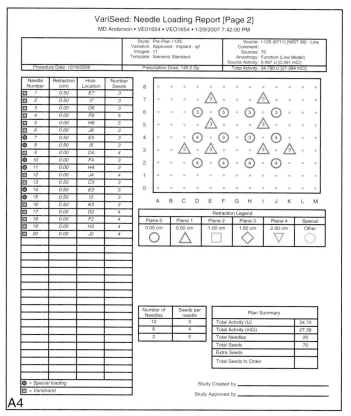

Figure 37-11. A, Prostate implant treatment planning. (See Color Plate 24.)

Side Effects and Complications

Surgery. With improved anesthesia and surgical techniques and the availability of antibiotics and other supportive care, operative mortality has been reduced to 1% or less. Wound infection, hematoma, or pelvic abscess occurs in less than 5% of patients. If a lymphadenectomy is done, patients may develop lymphocele (5%) or penile, scrotal, or lower extremity edema (less than 5%). Thrombophlebitis and pulmonary emboli rarely occur (less than 5%).[12] The most significant morbidity is incontinence and sexual impotence, which is related to the type of radical prostatectomy. Moderate stress incontinence requiring pads is reported to be 5% to 8% by major university centers.[23]

Surveys of patients, however, show this rate to be considerably higher at 25% to 30%.[58] The preservation of potency is related to the tumor stage, unilateral or bilateral resection of the neurovascular bundle, and patient age. With a bilateral nerve sparing procedure, potency rates range from 76% in men younger than 60 years to 49% for those older than 65. Potency rates are less, of course, if nerves can only be spared unilaterally because of close proximity to tumor or if the patient did not have full erectile function preoperatively.[23]

Radiation Therapy. Acute gastrointestinal (GI) side effects of radiation include diarrhea, abdominal cramping, rectal discomfort, and occasionally rectal bleeding, which may

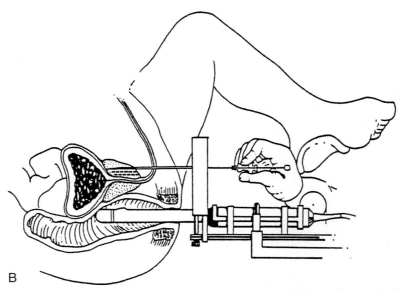

Figure 37-11. cont'd B, Sonography-guided transperineal template implant technique. (From Kuban DA, El-Mahdi AM: Cancers of the genitourinary tract. In Khan FM, Potish RA, editors: *Treatment planning in radiation oncology,* Baltimore, 1998, Lippincott Williams & Wilkins.)

be caused by transient proctitis. Patients with hemorrhoids may develop discomfort earlier than other patients, and aggressive symptomatic treatment should be instituted promptly. A higher incidence of both acute and late GI effects occurs when larger volumes of the pelvis are irradiated.

Severe late sequelae of treatment include persistent proctitis, rectal bleeding, and ulceration. Although the incidence of grade 2 (moderate) GI complications is low, 5%, with doses in the 64 to 70 Gy range, this rate can more than double (14%) when higher doses of 75 to 81 Gy are used.[112] Storey et al.[99] have shown that the rectal complication rate is related to the amount of rectum treated to doses of 70 Gy or higher. Therefore, attention to DVHs is imperative when dose escalating. When the amount of treated rectum is kept to a minimum, grade 2 complication rates can be reduced to 5% or less.[111,112] Fortunately, severe grade 3 and 4 GI complications occur infrequently, in less than 2% of patients. To date no strong relationship to irradiated bladder volume has been shown for urinary complications. It is thought that urinary toxicity may be related to a great extent to the urethra, which is contained within the prostate and cannot be spared. Moderate (grade 2) urinary complication occur in 10% to 15% of patients and mainly require medication for urgency or frequency. More severe (grade 3) urinary complications such as urethral strictures occur in only 1% to 3% of patients.[99,111,112] Late gastrointestinal and urinary complication rates for implant patients are similar to those for patients treated with external beam.[5,8]

Sexual impotence (erectile dysfunction) has been observed in 30% to 60% of formerly potent patients treated with external irradiation and in 20% to 30% of those treated with interstitial

Months	0	10	20	30	40	50	60
70 Gy	53	43	33	20	13	9	5
78 Gy	53	50	40	29	18	12	8

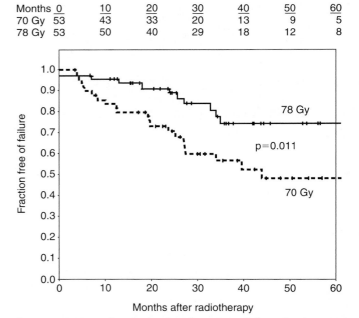

Figure 37-12. Kaplan-Meier freedom from failure (FFF) curves for patients with PSA levels of more than 10 ng/mL by dose randomization (70 Gy versus 78 Gy). The numbers of patients at risk at 10-month intervals are shown above the graphs. (From Kuban DA, et al: Long term results of the MD Anderson randomized dose-escalation trial for prostate cancer, *Int J Radiat Oncol Biol Phys* 70:67-74, 2008.)

Table 37-3	5-Year PSA Disease-Free Survival With Higher Versus Lower Dose Irradiation				
			% 5-Year PSA-DFS PSA (ng/ml)		
Study	**Total No. of Patients**	**Dose (Gy)**	**≤10**	**10-20**	**>20**
Hanks	232	<71.5	ND	29	8
		71.5-75.7	ND	57	28
		≥75.7	ND	73	30
			≤10	>10	
Kuban	301	70	85	61	
		78	87	81	
			Favorable	Unfavorable	
Lyons	738	<72	81	41	
		≥72	98	75	
			Favorable	Intermediate	High
Zelefsky	1100	64.8-70.2	79	49	21
		75.6-86.4	90	67	50

Data from Hanks G, et al: *Int J Radiat Oncol Biol Phys* 41:501, 1998; Kuban D, et al: *Int J Radiat Oncol Biol Phys* 70:67,2008; Lyons JA, et al: Urology 55:85, 2000; Zelefsky MJ, et al: *J Urol* 166:876, 2001.
Favorable, PSA ≤10 ng/ml, Gleason ≤6, T1-T2; *intermediate,* one factor worse; *ND,* no difference based on dose; *PSA-DFS PSA,* prostate-specific antigen disease-free survival; *unfavorable or high,* ≥2 factors worse.

implant.[5,58] These percentages are, of course, dependent on patient age, definition of potency, and degree of potency pretreatment. Data are also greatly influenced by physician versus patient reporting via survey. The latter tends to produce higher rates of dysfunction and complications.

PENIS AND MALE URETHRA

Epidemiology

Carcinoma of the penis is relatively rare in the United States; the estimated incidence is 1 per 100,000 each year, accounting for less than 1% of cancers in men. This tumor is extremely rare in circumcised Jewish men; circumcision performed early in life protects against carcinoma of the penis, but this is not true if the operation is done in adult life. The higher incidence in some areas of South America, Africa, and Asia and in African Americans seems to be related to the absence of the practice of neonatal circumcision. Phimosis (narrowing of the opening of the prepuce) is common in men suffering from penile carcinoma. **Smegma** (a white secretion that collects under the prepuce of the foreskin) is carcinogenic in animals, although the component of smegma responsible for its carcinogenic effect has not been identified.[16]

Carcinoma of the male urethra is also rare. There are no recognized racial or geographic predisposing factors. Although the cause remains unknown, some correlation exists between the incidence of carcinoma of the urethra and chronic irritation and infections, venereal diseases, and strictures. The average age at the time of presentation is 58 to 60 years, although 10% of these tumors occur in men younger than 40 years.[16]

Prognostic Indicators

The principal prognostic factors in carcinoma of the penis are the extent of the primary lesion and status of the lymph nodes. The incidence of nodal involvement is related to the extent and location of the primary lesion. Tumor-free regional nodes imply an excellent long-term disease-free survival rate, 85% to 90%.[17,96]

Patients with involvement of the inguinal nodes do considerably worse, and only 40% to 50% experience long-term survival. Pelvic lymph node involvement implies an even worse prognosis; less than 20% of these patients survive. Tumor differentiation is another important prognostic factor.[32]

The overall prognosis for carcinoma of the urethra in males varies considerably with the location of the primary lesion. The prognosis for distal lesions is generally similar to that for carcinoma of the penis. Lesions of the bulbomembranous urethra are usually extensive and associated with a dismal prognosis. Tumors of the prostatic urethra have prognostic features similar to those of bladder carcinoma. Superficial lesions have a good prognosis and may be managed with a transurethral resection, whereas deeply invasive tumors have a greater tendency to develop inguinal or pelvic lymph node and distant metastases.

Anatomy and Lymphatics

The basic structural components of the penis include two **corpora cavernosa** and the **corpus spongiosum** (Figure 37-13, A). These are encased in a dense fascia (Buck's fascia), which is separated from the skin by a layer of loose connective tissue. Distally, the corpus spongiosum expands into the glans penis, which is covered by a skin fold known as the *prepuce.*

Composed of a mucous membrane and the submucosa, the male urethra extends from the bladder neck to the external urethral meatus (Figure 37-13, B). The posterior urethra is subdivided into the membranous urethra, the portion passing through the urogenital diaphragm, and the prostatic urethra, which passes through the prostate. The anterior urethra passes through the corpus spongiosum and is subdivided into *fossa navicularis* (a widening within the glans), the **penile urethra** (which passes through the pendulous part of the penis), and the **bulbous urethra** (the dilated proximal portion of the anterior urethra).

The lymphatic channels of the prepuce and the skin of the shaft drain into the superficial inguinal nodes located above the fascia lata. For practical purposes lymphatic drainage may be

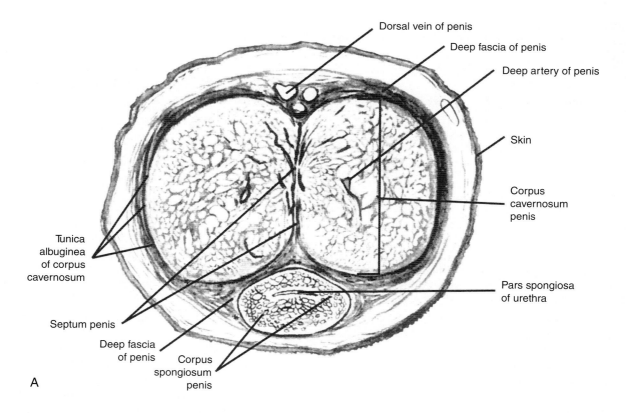

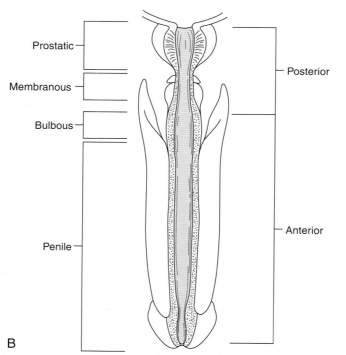

Figure 37-13. A, Cross section of the penis shaft. **B**, Anatomic subdivisions of the male urethra. (**A**, From Sobotta J: *Atlas der Anatomie des Menschen*, 17, Aufl., Urban and Schwarzenberg, 1972; **B**, From Perez CA, Pilepich MV: Penis and male urethra. In Perez CA, Brady LW, editors: *Principles and practice of radiation oncology*, ed 2, Philadelphia, 1992, JB Lippincott.)

considered bilateral. Some disagreement exists regarding whether the glands and deep penile structures drain into the superficial or deep inguinal lymph nodes. The lymphatics of the fossa navicularis and penile urethra follow the lymphatics of the penis to the superficial and deep inguinal lymph nodes. The lymphatics of the bulbomembranous and prostatic urethra may follow three routes: external iliac, obturator and internal iliac, and presacral lymph nodes. The pelvic (iliac) lymph nodes are rarely involved in the absence of inguinal lymph node involvement.

Clinical Presentation

The presence of phimosis may obscure the primary lesion. Secondary infection and an associated foul smell are common, whereas urethral obstruction is unusual. Inguinal lymph nodes are palpable at the time of presentation in 30% to 45% of patients.[17] However, the lymph nodes contain tumor in only half the patients; enlargement of the lymph nodes is often related to inflammatory (infectious) processes. Conversely, 20% of patients with clinically normal inguinal lymph nodes have occult metastases.

Patients with urethral carcinoma may exhibit obstructive symptoms, tenderness, dysuria, urethral discharge, and occasionally initial hematuria (blood in the urine). Lesions of the distal urethra are often associated with palpable inguinal lymph nodes at the time of presentation.

Detection and Diagnosis

Penile lesions can be seen on examination and documented by biopsy. Urethral lesions are evaluated by urethroscopy and cystoscopy. Inguinal lymph nodes should be thoroughly evaluated. Radiographic assessment of the regional lymphatics is of questionable value because of the extensive inflammatory changes often present in the lymph nodes. CT is useful in the identification of enlarged pelvic and paraaortic lymph nodes in patients with involved inguinal lymph nodes. Nodal involvement can be confirmed by biopsy or dissection.

Pathology and Staging

Most malignant penile tumors are well-differentiated squamous cell carcinomas. No significant correlation between the histologic grade and survival time has been found. Bowen's disease is squamous cell carcinoma in situ that may involve the shaft of the penis and hairy skin of the inguinal and suprapubic areas. Erythroplasia of Queyrat is an epidermoid carcinoma in situ that involves the mucosal or mucocutaneous areas of the prepuce or glans. This carcinoma appears as a red, elevated, or ulcerated lesion. Some patients with erythroplasia of Queyrat have invasive squamous cell carcinoma at the time of the diagnosis. Extramammary Paget's disease is a rare as intraepithelial apocrine carcinoma. The most common sites are the scrotum, inguinal folds, and perineal region. Primary lymphoma of the penis is extremely rare as well.

Cancers metastatic to the penis are also rare. The most common neoplasms metastasizing to the penis are carcinomas from the genitourinary organs, followed by carcinomas from the GI and respiratory systems. Priapism as an initial presenting feature or later development occurs in 40% of these patients.[75] Approximately 80% of urethral carcinomas in males are well-differentiated or moderately differentiated squamous cell

carcinomas.[69] Others include transitional cell carcinomas (15%), adenocarcinomas (5%), and undifferentiated or mixed carcinomas (1%). More than 90% of carcinomas of the prostatic urethra are of the transitional cell type. Adenocarcinomas occur only in the bulbomembranous urethra. The AJCC staging systems for carcinoma of the penis and male urethra are shown in Boxes 37-3 and 37-4.[37]

Routes of Spread

Most carcinomas of the penis start in the preputial area, arising in the glands, the coronal sulcus, or the prepuce. Extensive primary lesions may involve the corpora cavernosa or even the abdominal wall. The inguinal lymph nodes are the most common site of metastatic spread. About 20% of patients with clinically nonpalpable inguinal nodes have micrometastases. Pathologic evidence of nodal metastases is reported in about 35% of all patients and in approximately 50% of those with palpable lymph nodes.[17,26,96] Distant metastases are uncommon, about 10%, even in patients with advanced locoregional disease. They usually occur in patients who have inguinal lymph node involvement.

The natural history of carcinoma of the male anterior urethra is similar to that of carcinoma of the penis. Most tumors are low grade and progress slowly at primary and regional sites rather than spread to distant areas. Tumors of the penile urethra spread to the inguinal lymph nodes, and tumors of the bulbomembranous and prostatic urethra metastasize first to the pelvic lymph nodes.[69]

Treatment Techniques

Carcinoma of the Penis. Therapy is usually performed in two phases: initial management of the primary tumor and later treatment of the regional lymphatics. Surgery for the primary tumor ranges from local excision or chemosurgery in a small group of highly selected patients, particularly those with small lesions of the prepuce, to a partial or total penectomy. Although surgical resection is usually a highly effective and expedient treatment modality, it may not be acceptable to sexually active patients.

Bowen's disease and erythroplasia of Queyrat can be treated with topical 5-FU (5% cream), a local excision, or superficial x-rays (4500 to 5000 cGy in 4 to 5 weeks). The principal advantage of radiotherapeutic management of the primary lesion in penile carcinoma is organ preservation. Many different techniques, doses, and fractionation schemes have been used.[26,69] Interstitial implants, molds, and contact orthovoltage and megavoltage irradiation have improved tumor control in some modern series and decreased the incidence of treatment-related sequelae. Most patients who experience local failure after radiation therapy can be salvaged surgically.

Nodal management by observation with delayed intervention when signs of nodal involvement appear has replaced elective nodal dissection for the following reasons: (1) the 1% to 3% surgical mortality rate, (2) the morbidity associated with lymphadenectomy, and (3) the relatively low incidence of nodal metastasis (10% to 20%) in patients with clinically normal lymph nodes. Survival rates are high with this treatment.[86,96] Patients with lymph nodes clinically negative for tumor who are at risk for microscopic nodal metastases because of a primary tumor more advanced than stage I or a moderately to poorly

---

Box 37-3	American Joint Committee on Cancer Staging System for Carcinoma of the Penis

PRIMARY TUMOR (T)

TX   Primary tumor cannot be assessed
T0   No evidence of tumor
Tis   Carcinoma in situ
Ta   Non-invasive verrucous carcinoma
T1   Tumor invades subepithelial connective tissue
T2   Tumor invades corpus spongiosum or cavernosum
T3   Tumor invades urethra or prostate
T4   Tumor invades other adjacent structures

REGIONAL LYMPH NODES (N)

NX   Regional lymph nodes cannot be assessed
N0   No regional lymph node metastasis
N1   Metastasis in a single superficial inguinal lymph node
N2   Metastasis in a multiple or bilateral superficial inguinal lymph node
N3   Metastasis in deep inguinal or pelvic lymph node(s), unilateral or bilateral

DISTANT METASTASIS (M)

MX   Distant metastasis cannot be assessed
M0   No distant metastasis
M1   Distant metastasis

STAGE GROUPING

0	Tis	N0	M0
	Ta	N0	M0
I	T1	N0	M0
II	T1	N1	M0
	T2	N0	M0
	T2	N1	M0
III	T1	N2	M0
	T2	N2	M0
	T3	N0	M0
	T3	N1	M0
	T3	N2	M0
IV	T4	Any N	M0
	Any T	N3	M0
	Any T	Any N	M1

HISTOLOGIC GRADE (G)

GX   Grade cannot be assessed
G1   Well differentiated
G2   Moderately well differentiated
G3-4   Poorly differentiated or undifferentiated

With permission from American Joint Committee on Cancer (AJCC), Chicago, IL: *AJCC cancer staging manual*, ed 6, New York, 2002, Springer-Verlag.

Box 37-4	American Joint Committee on Cancer Staging System for Carcinoma of the Urethra

PRIMARY TUMOR (T) (MALE AND FEMALE)

TX   Primary tumor cannot be assessed
T0   No evidence of primary tumor
Ta   Noninvasive papillary, polypoid, or verrucous carcinoma
Tis   Carcinoma in situ
T1   Tumor invades subepithelial connective tissue
T2   Tumor invades any of the following: corpus spongiosum, prostate, periurethral muscle
T3   Tumor invades any of the following: corpus cavernosum, beyond prostatic capsule, anterior vagina, bladder neck
T4   Tumor invades other adjacent organs

UROTHELIAL (TRANSITIONAL CELL) CARCINOMA OF THE PROSTATE

Tis pu   Carcinoma in situ, involvement of the prostatic urethra
Tis pd   Carcinoma in situ, involvement of the prostatic ducts
T1   Tumor invades subepithelial connective tissue
T2   Tumor invades any of the following: prostatic stroma, corpus spongiosum, periurethral muscle
T3   Tumor invades any of the following: corpus cavernosum, beyond prostatic capsule, bladder neck (extraprostatic extension)
T4   Tumor invades other adjacent organs (invasion of the bladder)

REGIONAL LYMPH NODES (N)

NX   Regional lymph nodes cannot be assessed
N0   No regional lymph node metastasis
N1   Metastasis in a single lymph node 2 cm or less in greatest dimension
N2   Metastasis in a single node more than 2 cm in greatest dimension, or in multiple nodes
N3   Metastasis in deep inguinal or pelvic lymph node(s), unilateral or bilateral

DISTANT METASTASIS (M)

MX   Distant metastasis cannot be assessed
M0   No distant metastasis
M1   Distant metastasis

STAGE GROUPING

0a	Ta	N0	M0
0ais	Tis	N0	M0
	Tis pu	N0	M0
	Tis pd	N0	M0
I	T1	N0	M0
II	T2	N0	M0
III	T1	N1	M0
	T2	N1	M0
	T3	N0	M0
	T3	N1	M0
IV	T4	N0	M0
	T4	N1	M0
	Any T	N2	M0
	Any T	Any N	M1

HISTOLOGIC GRADE (G)

GX   Grade cannot be assessed
G1   Well differentiated
G2   Moderately well differentiated
G3-4   Poorly differentiated or undifferentiated

With permission from American Joint Committee on Cancer (AJCC), Chicago, IL: *AJCC cancer staging manual*, ed 6, New York, 2002, Springer-Verlag.

differentiated histology can receive elective radiation to the inguinal lymph nodes (5000 cGy in 5 weeks) with a high probability of tumor control and low morbidity. Generally, clinically involved and resectable regional lymph nodes are managed by radical lymphadenectomy. Some patients can be treated with combined radiation and lymphadenectomy and, if necessary, pelvic lymph node dissection.

Chemotherapy. The use of chemotherapy for carcinoma of the penis is limited. Some degree of tumor regression has been described with systemic agents, such as bleomycin, 5-FU, and methotrexate. A response to cisplatin has also been reported.[25] Systemic therapy is usually reserved for metastatic and recurrent disease or those lesions so advanced as to be incurable by surgery and radiation.

Carcinoma of the Male Urethra. Noninvasive carcinoma of the proximal urethra can be treated with a transurethral resection. For lesions of the distal urethra, results with penectomy or radiation therapy are similar to those for carcinoma of the penis, and the 5-year survival rates of 50% to 60% are comparable.[78] Involved regional lymph nodes are treated with

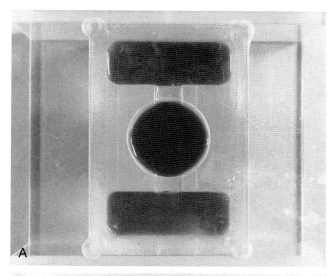

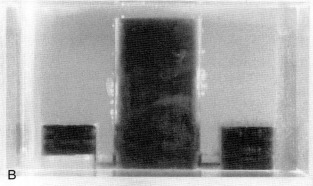

Figure 37-14. A, View from above of a plastic box with a central cylinder for external irradiation of the penis. The patient is treated in the prone position. The penis is placed in the central cylinder, and water is used to fill the surrounding volume in the box. The depth dose is calculated at the central point of the box. **B**, Lateral view. (From Perez CA, Pilepich MV: Penis and male urethra. In Perez CA, Brady LW, editors: *Principles and practice of radiation oncology*, ed 3, Philadelphia, 1998, Lippincott-Raven.)

lymphadenectomy. Most patients, however, exhibit advanced invasive lesions, which are difficult to manage with radical surgery or radiation therapy.

Radiation Therapy Techniques. If indicated, circumcision must be performed before the start of radiation therapy to minimize radiation therapy-associated morbidity.

External Irradiation. External beam therapy requires specially designed accessories, including bolus, to achieve homogeneous dose distribution to the entire organ involved. One device consists of a plastic box with a central circular opening that can be fitted over the penis. The space between the skin and box must be filled with tissue-equivalent material (Figure 37-14). This box can be treated with parallel-opposed megavoltage beams. An ingenious alternative to the box technique is the use of a water-filled container to envelop the penis while the patient is in a prone position.

A more complex device consists of a Perspex tube attached to a baseplate resting on the skin. This device is placed as close as possible to the base of the penis, and a flexible tube is connected to a vacuum pump. The suction effect keeps the penis in a fixed position during treatment. Appropriate bolus is placed outside the tube. The patient can also be treated in the prone position, with the penis hanging through a small hole placed in the Perspex's cylinder.

A well-established association exists between large fraction size and late tissue damage. The daily fraction in most reported series is 250 to 350 cGy for a total dose of 5000 to 5500 cGy, although a smaller daily fraction size, 180 to 200 cGy, and a higher total dose are preferable. A total dose of 6500 to 7000 cGy, with the last 500 to 1000 cGy delivered to a reduced portal, should result in reduced incidence of late fibrosis.

Regional lymphatics can be treated with external beam megavoltage radiation. The fields should include bilateral inguinal and pelvic (external iliac and hypogastric) lymph nodes (Figure 37-15). The posterior pelvis may be partially spared by anterior loading of the beams. Depending on the extent of nodal

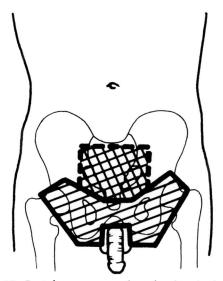

Figure 37-15. Portals encompassing the inguinal and pelvic lymph nodes. (From Perez CA, Pilepich MV: Penis and male urethra. In Perez CA, Brady LW, editors: *Principles and practice of radiation oncology*, ed 2, Philadelphia, 1992, JB Lippincott.)

disease and proximity of the detectable tumor to the skin surface or presence of skin invasion, the application of a bolus to the inguinal area should be considered. If clinical and radiographic evaluations show no gross enlargement of the pelvic lymph nodes, the dose to these nodes may be limited to 5000 cGy. In patients with palpable lymph nodes, doses of 6500 to 7000 cGy in 7 to 8 weeks, 180 to 200 cGy per day, with reduced fields after 5000 cGy are required. If grossly involved nodes are respectable, this is typically the preferred treatment. Radiation can be applied postoperatively for extracapsular extension or microscopic residual disease.

Brachytherapy. A mold is usually built in the form of a box or cylinder with a central opening and channels for the placement of radioactive sources (needles or wires) in the periphery of the device. The cylinder and sources should be long enough to prevent under dosage at the tip of the penis. A dose of 6000 to 6500 cGy at the surface and approximately 5000 cGy at the center of the organ is delivered in 6 to 7 days. The mold can be applied continuously, in which case an indwelling catheter or intermittent catheterization is used. Single- or double-plane implants can also be used to deliver 6000 to 7000 cGy in 5 to 7 days.[26] In extensive lesions involving the shaft of the penis (stage III), obtaining an adequate margin with brachytherapy procedures is difficult, similar to the situation seen in attempting a partial penectomy.

Results of Treatment

Carcinoma of the Penis. Reports of treatment results are scarce because cancer of the penis is uncommon in the Western world. A significant proportion of patients have been treated surgically, with 5-year survival rates ranging from 25% to 80%, depending on the stage of the primary tumor and inguinal lymph node involvement.[65,69]

A summary of tumor control rates achieved with irradiation is presented in Table 37-4. In patients 41 to 57 years old treated with various radiation techniques (mold, interstitial, and external beam), 5-year survival rates range from 45% to 68%. A 5-year survival rate of 66% and tumor control rate of 86% have been reported in patients with stage I carcinoma of the penis treated with radiation, compared with a 5-year survival rate of 70% and tumor control rate of 81% in surgically treated patients.[69] Survival and local control rates were only slightly affected by the treatment modality in stage II but were lower in stage III patients treated surgically. If radiation did not control the primary lesion after 6 months, the penis was amputated and a significant number of patients were salvaged. Of patients initially treated surgically or with radiation, 8% and 20%, respectively, developed inguinal lymph node metastases. Overall, 8% of patients treated surgically and 10% of those irradiated died of inguinal lymph node metastases and tumor spread.

In one study, 80% of patients treated with radiation therapy had tumor control and conservation of the penis.[86] Although irradiation alone or combined with lymph node dissection controlled lymph node metastases smaller than 2 cm in four patients, radiation therapy was successful in controlling lymph node metastases in only one of seven patients who had N2 or N3 disease.

Table 37-4	**Overall Control of Primary Carcinoma of the Penis with Radiation Therapy**			
Author	**No. of Patients**	**Treatment Method**	**Dose**	**Local Control (%)**
Almgard and Edsmyr	16	Radium implant and external beam therapy		
Engelstad	72	Mold therapy and teleradium	3500-3700 R (500-700 R/day)	50
Jackson	39	Mold (most patients) and external beam therapy (some patients)	Doses not noted	49
Marcial, et al.	25	External beam, interstitial, and mold therapy	4000 R in 2 weeks	
			5000 R in 4 weeks	
		Mold	5000-6000 R in 5-6 days	64
Murrell and Williams	108	External beam therapy	3000-6700 cGy (200 cGy/day)	52
Kelley, et al.	10	External beam therapy (electrons)	5100-5400 cGy (300 cGy/day)	100
Knudson and Brennhovd	145	Mold therapy	3500-3700 cGy in 3-5 days	32
Haile and Delclos	20	Mold therapy, implant, and External beam therapy	Doses not noted 6000 cGy	90
Mazeron, et al.	23	Iridium-192 implant	6000-7000 cGy	78
Pointon	32	External beam therapy	5250-5500 cGy (16 Fractions in 22 days)	84.4
Sagerman, et al.	15	External beam therapy	4500 cGy (15 Fractions in 3 weeks) to 6400 cGy (32 Fractions in 6.5 weeks)	60
Salaverria, et al.	41	Iridium mold therapy	6000 cGy over several days	84.3

Modified from Perez CA, Pilepich MV: Penis and male urethra. In Perez CA, Brady LW, editors: *Principles and practice of radiation oncology*, ed 2, Philadelphia, 1992, JB Lippincott.
R, Roentgen.

Table 37-5	Results of Radiation Therapy for Carcinoma of the Penis Tumor Control				
Author	**Modality**	**Stages I–II**	**Stages III–IV**	**Complications**	**Penis Preservation**
Duncan and Jackson	Teletherapy	16/20 (80%)		2/20 (10%)	16/20 (80%)
Jackson	Mold therapy	20/45 (44%)		2/45 (4%)	20/45 (44%)
Haile and Delclos	External beam therapy	6/6 (100%)	2/2 (100%)	16/20 (80%)	
	Brachytherapy	7/7 (100%)			
Kaushal and Harma	Cobalt-60	14/16 (88%)		2/16 (12%)	13/14 (93%)
Kelley et al.	Electron beam	10/10 (100%)			10/10 (100%)
Pierquin et al.	Iridium implant	14/14 (100%)	12/31 (39%)	3/45 (6.7%)	
Sagerman et al.	External beam therapy	9/12 (75%)	1/3 (33%)		2/15 (13%)
Salaverria et al.	Mold brachytherapy	12/13 (92%)			10/13 (77%)

From Perez CA, Pilepich MV: Penis and male urethra. In Perez CA, Brady LW, editors: *Principles and practice of radiation oncology*, ed 2, Philadelphia, 1992, JB Lippincott.

Duncan and Jackson[20] observed 3-year tumor-control rates of 90% with external beam irradiation and only 47% with mold therapy. Other authors have reported a 5-year survival rate of 92% in patients with stages I and II tumors treated with radium-226 or iridium-192 molds, compared with 77% in patients treated with partial penectomy.[86]

Table 37-5 shows a summary of treatment results correlated with the tumor stage, preservation of the organ, and morbidity.

Carcinoma of the Male Urethra. Most patients with male urethral carcinoma are treated surgically. Partial or total penectomy is performed for distal urethral lesions, depending on the tumor location and extent. Associated 5-year disease control is in the 50% range in the absence of lymph node involvement. Tumors of the proximal urethra require total penectomy and those located even more proximally at the prostatic urethra require prostatectomy and often cystectomy as well. The prognosis for these patients is not nearly as good.[100]

Side Effects and Complications

Irradiation of the penis produces brisk erythema, dry or moist desquamation, and swelling of the subcutaneous tissue of the shaft in almost all patients. Although they are uncomfortable, these reversible reactions subside within a few weeks with conservative treatment. Telangiectasia and fibrosis are usually asymptomatic, common, late consequences of radiation therapy.

Most strictures after radiation therapy are at the meatus. Meatal-urethral strictures occur with a frequency of up to 40%.[26,62] This incidence compares with that of urethral strictures after penectomy.

Ulceration, necrosis of the glans, and necrosis of the skin of the shaft are rare complications. Lymphedema of the legs has occurred after inguinal and pelvic radiation therapy and is related to field size, dose, and whether lymph node dissection proceeded radiation.

URINARY BLADDER

Epidemiology

Approximately 68,810 new cases and 14,100 deaths from bladder cancer will be reported in the United States annually.[3] The incidence peaks in the seventh decade, and in men this cancer is the fourth most prevalent malignant disease. It occurs about four times more often in men than in women.

Prognostic Indicators

The tumor extent and depth of muscle invasion are important factors affecting the tumor's behavior and outcome of therapy. Tumor morphology is also important because papillary tumors are usually low grade and superficial with a favorable prognosis. Infiltrating lesions tend to be higher grade, sessile, and nodular; they invade muscle, vascular, and lymphatic spaces and generally have a worse prognosis. The degree of histologic differentiation must also be considered because well-differentiated tumors are less aggressive and have a better prognosis than poorly differentiated tumors, which are usually more invasive.[90]

Anatomy and Lymphatics

The urinary bladder, when empty, lies entirely within the true pelvis. The empty bladder is roughly tetrahedral; each of its four surfaces is shaped like an equilateral triangle. The base of the **superior surface** (the only surface covered with peritoneum) is behind, and the apex is in front. The apex of the bladder is directed toward the upper part of the pubic symphysis and is joined to the umbilicus by the middle umbilical ligament, the urachal remnant. The sigmoid colon and the small intestine rest on the superior surface.

In the male, the rectovesical pouch separates the upper part of the bladder base from the rectum. The seminal vesicles and deferent duct separate the lower part of the base from the rectum.

The parietal peritoneum of the suprapubic region of the abdominal wall is displaced so that the bladder lies directly against the anterior abdominal wall without any intervening peritoneum.

The ureters pierce the wall of the bladder base obliquely. During the contraction of the muscular bladder wall the ureters are compressed, preventing reflux. The orifices of the ureters are posterolateral to the internal urethral orifice, and, with the urethral orifice, they define the **trigone** (the triangular portion of the bladder formed by the openings of the ureters and urethra orifice). The sides of the trigone are approximately 2.5 cm in length in the contracted state and up to 5 cm in the distended state (Figure 37-16). In the male, the bladder neck rests on the prostate.

The epithelium, or urothelium, is transitional. The mucous membrane is only loosely attached to the subjacent muscle layer by a delicate vascular submucosa (lamina propria), except over the trigone, where the mucosa is firmly attached.

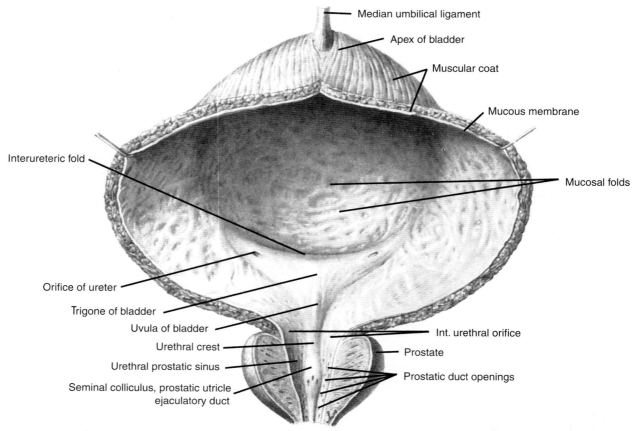

Figure 37-16. A ventral view of the urinary bladder and prostate, illustrating the location of the trigone of the bladder. (From Sobotta/Becher: *Atlas der Anatomie des Menschen*, 17, Aufl., Urban and Schwarzenberg, 1972.)

The lymphatics of the bladder form two plexuses, one in the submucosa and one in the muscular layer. They accompany the blood vessels into the perivesical space and ultimately terminate in the internal iliac lymph nodes. Some lymphatics may find their way into the external iliac nodes. From these nodes, the lymphatics progress to the common iliac and paraaortic lymph nodes.

Clinical Presentation

Most patients with bladder cancer, 75% to 80%, present with gross painless hematuria. Clotting and urinary retention may occur. Approximately 25% of patients have symptoms of vesical irritability, although almost all patients with carcinoma in situ experience frequency, urgency, dysuria, and hematuria.

Detection and Diagnosis

In addition to a complete history and physical examination, including rectal and pelvic examination, each patient should have a chest x-ray examination, urinalysis, complete blood cell count, liver function tests, cystoscopic evaluation, and bimanual examination performed under anesthesia. Biopsy is done for diagnosis. An abdominal CT scan with contrast should be obtained before cystoscopy so that the upper tracts can be evaluated. Retrograde pyelogram, ureteroscopy, brush biopsy, and cytology can then be done, if necessary. CT or MRI is used to evaluate bladder-wall thickening and detect extravesical extension and lymph node metastases. Bone scans are

obtained for patients with T3 and T4 disease and those with bone pain.

Pathology and Staging

Most bladder cancers (98%) are epithelial in origin. In the Western Hemisphere, approximately 92% of epithelial tumors are transitional cell carcinomas, 6% to 7% are squamous cell carcinomas, and 1% to 2% are adenocarcinomas. Squamous or glandular differentiation can be seen in 20% to 30% of transitional cell carcinomas. Patients whose bladders are chronically irritated by long-term catheter drainage (e.g., paraplegics) or bladder calculi are at risk of developing squamous cell carcinoma.

Morphologically, bladder cancers can be separated into the following four categories: (1) papillary, (2) papillary infiltrating, (3) solid infiltrating, and (4) nonpapillary, noninfiltrating, or carcinoma in situ. At the time of diagnosis, 70% of these cancers are papillary, 25% show papillary or solid infiltration, and 3% to 5% indicate carcinoma in situ.

The TNM, AJCC V staging system is given in Box 37-5.[37] This system combines histologic findings from transurethral resection specimens and clinical findings from bimanual examination under anesthesia. Pathologic staging is based on histologic examination of cystectomy specimens. In the AJCC system these stages are preceded by the prefix p (e.g., pT3).

The presence of muscle invasion categorizes the lesion as T2 to T4b. Although a bimanual examination with the patient under

Box 37-5	American Joint Committee on Cancer Staging System for Carcinoma of the Urinary Bladder

PRIMARY TUMOR (T)

TX	Primary tumor cannot be assessed
T0	No evidence of primary tumor
Ta	Non-invasive papillary carcinoma
Tis	Carcinoma in situ: "flat tumor"
T1	Tumor invades subepithelial connective tissue
T2	Tumor invades muscle
pT2a	Tumor invades superficial muscle (inner half)
pT2b	Tumor invades deep muscle (outer half)
T3	Tumor invades perivesical tissue
pT3a	microscopically
pT3b	macroscopically (extravesical mass)
T4	Tumor invades any of the following: prostate, uterus, vagina, pelvic wall, abdominal wall
T4a	Tumor invades prostate, uterus, vagina
T4b	Tumor invades pelvic wall, abdominal wall

REGIONAL LYMPH NODES (N)

NX	Regional lymph nodes cannot be assessed
N0	No regional lymph node metastasis
N1	Metastasis in a single lymph node 2 cm or less in greatest dimension
N2	Metastasis in a single lymph node, more than 2 cm but not more than 5 cm in greatest dimension; or multiple lymph nodes, none more than 5 cm in greatest dimension
N3	Metastasis in a lymph node, more than 5 cm in greatest dimension

DISTANT METASTASIS (M)

MX	Distant metastasis cannot be assessed
M0	No distant metastasis
M1	Distant metastasis

STAGE GROUPING

0a	Ta	N0	M0
0is	Tis	N0	M0
I	T1	N0	M0
II	T2a	N0	M0
	T2b	N0	M0
III	T3a	N0	M0
	T3b	N0	M0
	T4a	N0	M0
IV	T4b	N0	M0
	Any T	N1	M0
	Any T	N2	M0
	Any T	N3	M0
	Any T	Any N	M1

HISTOLOGIC GRADE (G)

GX	Grade cannot be assessed
G1	Well differentiated
G2	Moderately differentiated
G3-4	Poorly differentiated or undifferentiated

With permission from American Joint Committee on Cancer (AJCC), Chicago, IL: *AJCC cancer staging manual*, ed 6, New York, 2002, Springer-Verlag.

anesthesia and radiographic studies are helpful in further separating the various stages, understaging is common.

Routes of Spread

Bladder cancer spreads via direct extension into or through the wall of the bladder. In a small proportion of cases, the tumor spreads submucosally under intact, normal-appearing mucosa. Intraepithelial involvement of the distal ureters, prostatic urethra, and periurethral prostatic ducts is frequently found with multifocal or diffuse carcinoma in situ. Approximately 75% to 85% of new bladder cancers are superficial (Tis, Ta, or T1), and about 15% to 25% of patients have evidence of muscle invasion

at the time of the diagnosis. Those with superficial disease can develop muscle invasion when tumors recur after conservative therapy. Of all patients with muscle-invasive bladder cancer, approximately 50% have evidence of muscle invasion at the time of the initial diagnosis, and the remaining 40% initially exhibit more superficial disease that later progresses. Perineural invasion and lymphatic or blood vessel invasion are common after the tumor has invaded muscle.

Lymphatic drainage occurs via the external iliac, internal iliac, and presacral lymph nodes. Published data correlate the incidence of pelvic lymph node metastases with the depth of tumor invasion in the bladder wall[94] (Table 37-6). The most common sites of distant metastasis are the lung, bone, and liver.

Treatment Techniques

For carcinoma in situ, a radical cystectomy is usually curative. However, most patients and urologists prefer more conservative initial management. For lesions that are smaller than 5 cm, reasonably well delineated, and without involvement of the bladder neck, prostatic urethra, or ureters, treatment consists of electrofulguration followed by intravesical chemotherapy or bacillus Calmette-Guérin (bCG).

Ta and T1 disease is usually treated with a transurethral resection and fulguration. Patients with diffuse grade 3, T1 disease, or involvement of the prostatic urethra or ducts are difficult to treat locally and may be initially treated with a cystectomy.

Intravesical immunotherapy chemotherapy is often administered after a transurethral resection for T1, grade 2 or 3 lesions.

Table 37-6	Incidence of Histologically Positive Lymph Nodes Correlated With Pathologic Stage in Bladder Cancer

Pathologic Stage	No. of Patients	Positive Lymph Nodes (%)
pT1	41	5
pT2	20	30
pT3a	13	31
pT3b	28	64
pT4	8	50

Modified from Skinner DG, Tift JP, Kaufman JJ: High dose, short course preoperative radiation therapy and immediate single stage radical cystectomy with pelvic node dissection in the management of bladder cancer, *J Urol* 127:671-674, 1982.

Most physicians withhold intravesical treatment for patients with T1, grade 1 tumors. The most commonly used agents are BCG, mitomycin-C and interferon. Patients require close follow-up with cystoscopy, cytology, and resection as indicated.

Definitive treatment with transurethral resection is not applicable to most patients with muscle-invasive disease. Failure to completely eradicate high-grade disease, progression to muscle invasion, or involvement of the prostatic urethra or prostatic periurethral ducts usually signals the need for radical cystectomy.

Partial Cystectomy. Carefully chosen patients with relatively small, solitary, well-defined lesions with muscle invasion or superficial disease not suitable for transurethral resection may be treated by segmental resection. However, recurrence rates can be as high as 50% to 70%, and the primary lesion must be located at the bladder dome, right or left bladder wall, and well removed from the ureteral orifices and trigone area such that partial cystectomy is technically feasible. Many patients who are disease free 5 years after partial cystectomy owe their survival to salvage treatment with total cystectomy or radiation. In the Stanford series, radical cystectomy was the most successful salvage treatment.[28]

Radical Cystectomy With or Without Preoperative Radiation Radical cystectomy is recommended for superficial disease (Tis, Ta, T1) in which all attempts at conservative management have proved unsuccessful. Patients are included whose recurrences after each successive transurethral resection and/or intravesical chemotherapy treatment increase in frequency or grade or progress to muscle invasion. Cystectomy is also indicated for patients with recurrent tumors in whom bladder capacity has been so reduced by repeated transurethral resections and intravesical chemotherapy treatments that the successful eradication of the tumor by these conservative means would produce an unsatisfactory functional result.

For clinical stage T2, T3, and resectable T4a disease, radical cystectomy is commonly used. Preoperative radiation was recommended in years past for large tumors with deep muscle invasion because the risk of understaging was high and local recurrence rates were substantial. More recently, however, staging evaluation and surgical technique has improved such that local recurrence rates are in the 7% to 15% range.[63,93] Furthermore, neither the Southwest Oncology Group trial nor a meta-analysis of six randomized radiation trials showed a benefit associated with preoperative radiation.[43,95] Because most patients with bladder cancer fail therapy because of distant disease, attention was instead turned toward chemotherapy.[97] For T3 and T4a disease, preoperative radiation may be used if resectability is questionable.[66] Although lower doses and shorter fractionation schedules have been used, 45 Gy in 25 fractions has the greatest potential for downstaging with the least complications.

Full-Dose External Beam Radiation With Surgery Reserved for Salvage. Patients treated with radical radiation ideally should have adequate bladder capacity without substantial voiding symptoms or incontinence. The completeness of transurethral resection before radiation may influence local control. Studies show that approximately 40% of patients will have a bladder free of tumor after radiation alone.[36,44] Doses are in the 65 to 70 Gy range.

After radiation, patients undergo cystoscopy every 3 months for 2 years and every 6 months thereafter. Some persistent or recurrent lesions, particularly low-grade tumors, that were downstaged with radiation therapy have been successfully managed with endoscopic resection. If a local tumor persists 3 months after resection, a cystectomy is indicated.[77]

Bladder Sparing With Chemotherapy Plus Irradiation. Because of the high rate of local recurrence after radiation alone and the high incidence of distant metastasis, several investigators began to administer chemotherapy concurrently with radiation in an attempt to sensitize the local tumor and address the metastatic component.[22,46,89,91] A trimodality approach was found to be effective: maximal transurethral resection, chemotherapy and radiation. Patients with T2 to T3 muscle-invasive tumors are candidates for this procedure. Those with poor renal function will not tolerate the necessary chemotherapy, and those with an irritable bladder may have severe symptoms secondary to radiation such that these factors must be considered before embarking on this treatment regimen.

A recent RTOG trial compared the classic regimen of methotrexate, cisplatin, and vinblastine (MCV) given for two cycles before concurrent radiation and cisplatin with radiation and cisplatin alone.[91] There was no benefit in overall survival, survival with an intact bladder, or reduction of distant metastases secondary to the MCV. This regimen, as a neoadjuvant approach, has now been largely discontinued because it was also more difficult for patients to tolerate.

Doses with the previous regimen are typically 40 to 45 Gy to the larger pelvic field to include lymph nodes, followed by a boost to the involved area of the bladder for a total of 65 Gy. Cystoscopy with biopsy and cytology is done after the first 40 to 45 Gy, and, if residual tumor is documented and the patient is a surgical candidate, cystectomy is performed. Cystectomy can also be used for salvage should patients fail after completing the entire regimen.

Interstitial Implants. Interstitial radiation therapy for bladder cancer is used more commonly in Europe than in the United States. This technique may be used alone, with external beam radiation, or following partial cystectomy. Suitable patients are those with solitary T1 high-grade to T3a lesions measuring less than 5 cm whose general medical condition permits a surgical procedure. In experienced hands, selected patients can achieve excellent local control and survival. Overall, however, results appear similar to external beam approaches and no comparative trials have been attempted.

Radiation Therapy

Initial Target Volume. Portals should include the total bladder and tumor volume, prostate and prostatic urethra, and pelvic lymph nodes. Typically, a four-field (anteroposterior/posteroanterior [AP/PA], laterals) pelvic technique is used. Fields extend 1 cm inferiorly to the caudal border of the obturator foramen and superiorly to just below the sacral promontory or just below the S1-L5 disc interspace on the AP projection. These fields include the perivesical, obturator, external iliac, and internal iliac lymph nodes but clearly not the common iliac nodes. The field widths should extend 1.5 cm laterally to the bony margin of the pelvis at its widest point. The irradiation portals are usually at least 12 × 12 cm to include the empty bladder.[27] The anterior boundary of the lateral fields should be at least 1 cm anterior to the most anterior portion of the bladder mucosa seen on an air contrast cystogram or CT scan or 1 cm

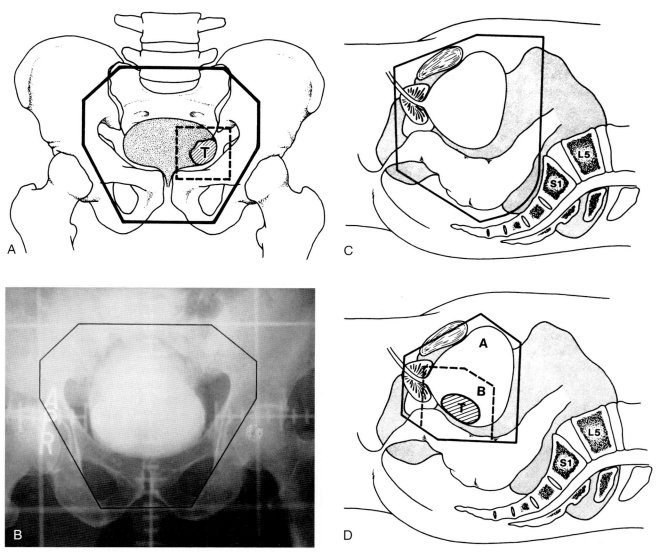

Figure 37-17. A, Diagram of the anteroposterior (AP) pelvic field used for carcinoma of the bladder. The boost volume is outlined with dashed lines. *T*, Residual primary tumor. **B**, Simulation film of the AP portal. **C**, Diagram of the lateral pelvic field encompassing the bladder and pelvic lymph nodes. **D**, Reduced portals after 4500 to 5000 cGy *(A)* and 6500 or 7000 cGy *(B)*.

anterior to the anterior tip of the symphysis, whichever is more anterior. Posteriorly, the fields should extend at least 2 cm posterior to the most posterior portion of the bladder or 2 cm posterior to the tumor mass if it present on a pelvic CT scan. The lateral fields should be shaped with MLCs inferiorly to shield the tissues outside the symphysis anteriorly and to block the entire anal canal and as much of the posterior rectal wall as possible (Figure 37-17). Planning is now largely done by CT scan. High-energy photons (10 to 20 MV) are most suitable.

Boost Target Volume. The contour of the primary bladder tumor volume is obtained from findings gathered via a bimanual examination, cystoscopy, and CT scan. If the radiation oncologist is satisfied that all initial sites of the tumor are limited to one section of the bladder, the high-dose volume should exclude the uninvolved areas of the bladder (see Figure 37-17). Treating the bladder while full can help in this regard. Lateral or oblique beams, arcs, or other field combinations can be used.

Simulation is performed with the patient in the supine position. A Foley catheter is inserted into the bladder through the use of sterile technique, and 150 to 250 ml of iodinated contrast material (20% concentration) is injected to outline the posterior portion of the bladder. For visualization of the anterior wall of the bladder on lateral (cross-table) radiographs, 100 to 150 ml of air is injected. Currently, CT scan planning is preferred and is helpful for large tumor masses with extravesical extension.

Doses. The larger pelvic field to include the bladder and pelvic lymph nodes is generally treated to a dose of 45 to 50 Gy at 180 cGy/day, which requires 5 to 5½ weeks of treatment. With chemotherapy, the nodal dose is usually kept at 45 Gy. A smaller boost volume, as previously described is taken to 65 Gy, or possibly 70 Gy, if radiation alone is being used.

Results of Treatment

The rate of complete response for radical radiation alone for muscle-invasive bladder cancer is in the 45% range for all

T stages.[21,61,77] Approximately 40% to 50% of patients who achieved complete response developed local recurrence later, yielding 5-year local control rates of approximately 25% to 30% for T2 and T3 lesions. The 5- and 10-year local control rates for T4 cancers are lower at 16%. A complete response is associated with significantly improved survival rates. Within each T stage, 5-year survival rates for patients with papillary, solid, or mixed tumors do not differ significantly after external beam irradiation alone.[77]

Using the trimodality bladder-sparing approach as described previously, maximal transurethral resection of the prostate (TURP), radiation, and concomitant chemotherapy, 5-year overall survival is 50% to 60% and with an intact bladder is approximately 40%.[22,46,89,91] Unfortunately, the distant metastatic rate remains high at 40%. Contrary to concern expressed by some urologists regarding a dysfunctional bladder and severe urinary symptoms following this regimen, quality of life remains good and bladder damage requiring cystectomy is very infrequent, with a reported 1.5% rate.[46,89,91]

TESTIS

Epidemiology

The American Cancer Society estimates that 8,090 new cases of testicular cancer and 380 deaths from the disease will occur each year in the United States.[3] The incidence of this tumor has been reported to be 3.8 per 100,000 in the United States. Although testicular tumors are relatively rare, they are the most common malignancy in men between 20 and 34 years of age. The incidence is lowest in Asians, Africans, Puerto Ricans, and North American blacks. Higher rates are reported among whites in the United States, United Kingdom, and Denmark. The origin of testicular tumors may be related to gonadal dysgenesis, as strongly suggested by a higher incidence in men with undescended testes. **Cryptorchidism** (undescended testes) also increases the risk of intraabdominal testicular tumors. Patients with one testicular tumor are at increased risk for developing a contralateral malignancy; 5% may develop a contralateral lesion within 5 years.

The greatest incidences of testicular carcinomas are found in men ranging in age of 20 to 34 years. Many individuals in this age range have not even begun or are not finished having children. Because treatment techniques for these types of cancers include chemotherapy and often radiation therapy, the option of sperm banking must be presented to the patient. Chemotherapy commonly causes infertility during treatment and for an undetermined amount of time afterwards. It is thought that radiation therapy does not affect the patient's fertility, but a small dose does reach the opposite testicle. For this reason, it is often necessary to deposit sperm in a sperm bank before any treatment has started, in order to plan for the future.

Prognostic Indicators

In seminoma, the tumor stage is a significant prognostic factor. The histologic subtype and mild elevation of serum beta human chorionic gonadotropin (hCG) likely have no prognostic implications. In stages II and III, the outcome is related to the bulk of the retroperitoneal disease, which is associated with an increased propensity for distant metastasis. Patients with stage III or IV disease have a worse prognosis because of the possibility of mediastinal and supraclavicular lymph node involvement or distant metastasis.

The prognosis of nonseminomatous tumors is related to the stage of the disease as well. Most patients with stage I or II disease survive with modern multiagent chemotherapy. In these patients, the levels of tumor markers and the volume of metastasis do have prognostic value. Patients with choriocarcinoma have a poor prognosis.

Anatomy and Lymphatics

The testes are contained in the scrotum and suspended by the spermatic cords. The left testis is usually longer than the right. The testis is invested by the tunica vaginalis, tunica albuginea, and tunica vasculosa. The functioning testis houses the spermatozoa in different stages of development and is responsible for testosterone production.

A close network of anastomosing tubes in a fibrous stroma at the upper end of the testis constitutes the rete testis and vasa efferentia. These small tubes converge in the vas deferens, a continuation of the epididymis, which is a hard, cordlike structure about 2 feet in length and 5 mm in diameter. The vas deferens enters the pelvis along the spermatic cord and empties into the seminal vesicles (two lobulated membranous pouches located on top of the prostate). The ejaculatory ducts, one on each side, begin at the base of the prostate, run forward and downward between its middle and lateral lobes, and end in the verumontanum after entering the prostate.

The lymphatics from the hilum of the testes accompany the spermatic cord up to the internal inguinal ring along the cords of the testicular-spermatic veins. These lymphatics drain into the retroperitoneal lymph nodes between the level of T11 and L4 but are concentrated at the level of the L1 through L3 vertebrae. They drain to the left renal hilum on the left side and to the pericaval lymph nodes on the right. Crossover from the right to the left side is common, but crossover in the opposite direction is rare. From the retroperitoneal lumbar nodes, drainage occurs through the thoracic duct to lymph nodes in the mediastinum and supraclavicular fossa and occasionally to the axillary nodes.

Clinical Presentation

Usually, a testicular tumor appears as a painless swelling or nodular mass in the scrotum and is sometimes noted incidentally by the patient or a sexual partner. Occasionally, patients complain of a dull ache, heaviness, or pulling sensation in the scrotum or an aching sensation in the lower abdomen. Approximately 10% of patients have acute and severe pain, which may be related to torsion of the spermatic cord. Frequently, patients relate the appearance of the mass to a previous trauma, although this is coincidental rather than etiologic. Rarely, patients exhibit symptoms of metastatic disease, such as a neck mass, respiratory symptoms, or low back pain. Gynecomastia occurs in approximately 5% of patients with testicular germ cell tumors.[24]

Detection and Diagnosis

A complete history and physical examination are mandatory. If a testicular tumor is suspected, a testicular sonogram should be performed. The appropriate surgical procedure to make the diagnosis and remove the primary tumor is radical orchiectomy through an inguinal incision. Although beta hCG levels are slightly elevated in 17% of patients with pure seminoma, any elevation of alpha-fetoprotein (AFP) signals nonseminomatous disease. Beta HCG and/or AFP levels are elevated in more than 80% of patients with disseminated nonseminomatous disease. Serum markers (beta hCG, AFP) are assayed before and after orchiectomy because they can be used to document persistent or recurrent cancer and may predict the responsiveness of nonseminomas to surgery or chemotherapy.

A CT scan of the chest, abdomen, and pelvis forms the basis of the staging process to evaluate pelvic, abdominal, mediastinal, and supraclavicular lymph nodes as well as the pulmonary parenchyma. A semen analysis and sperm banking should be considered for patients in whom treatment is likely to compromise fertility and who intend to have children in the future.

Pathology and Staging

A representation of the dual origin of testicular tumors is shown in Figure 37-18. About 95% of testicular neoplasms originate in germinal elements. The most common type of testicular tumor is seminoma, which has three histologic subtypes: classic, anaplastic, and spermatocytic. The prognosis is not significantly different for the various subtypes. The nonseminomatous tumors include embryonal carcinoma, teratoma, choriocarcinoma, and yolk sac tumor (embryonal adenocarcinoma in the prepubertal testis). The most common single-cell type is embryonal carcinoma. Yolk sac tumors are the most common in children. Choriocarcinoma accounts for about 1% of these tumors. It is not uncommon that more than one cell type can be found in the same patient.

The EORTC/International Union Against Cancer (UICC) and the AJCC staging systems are contained in Box 37-6. The EORTC/UICC or some modification is perhaps the most widely used.

Routes of Spread

Although the routes of dissemination are similar for seminoma and nonseminoma, the propensity for involvement of various sites differs. Pure seminoma has a much greater tendency to remain localized or involve only lymph nodes, whereas nonseminomatous germ cell tumors of the testes may spread by lymphatic or hematogenous routes.

Seminoma spreads orderly, initially to the lymph nodes in the retroperitoneum. From the retroperitoneal nodes, the seminoma spreads to the next echelon of draining lymphatics in the mediastinum and supraclavicular fossa (stage III disease). Only rarely and late does pure seminoma spread hematogenously to involve the lung parenchyma, bone, liver, or brain (stage IV disease). Less than 5% of patients have stage III or IV disease at the time of presentation. The orderly route of spread for pure seminoma has been confirmed by surveillance studies. In one study of 255 patients, of 33 patients with relapses, 29 had disease in the retroperitoneal lymph nodes. The site of the second relapse when infradiaphragmatic irradiation was used for the first relapse was the supradiaphragmatic nodes.[18]

Nonseminomatous tumors that metastasize outside the lymph nodes usually involve the lungs and liver.

Treatment Techniques

The initial management goal for a suspected malignant germ cell tumor of the testis is to obtain serum AFP and beta hCG measurements and, after staging procedures, to perform a radical inguinal orchiectomy with high ligation of the spermatic cord. Further management depends on the pathologic diagnosis of the stage and extent of the disease.

Seminoma. The most commonly applied treatment for patients with stage I seminoma is radical orchiectomy and postoperative irradiation of the paraaortic or paraaortic and ipsilateral pelvic nodes. Because of the low incidence of pelvic nodal involvement, 0.5% to 3% as shown by the Leeds Conference and surveillance studies, it has been suggested that paraaortic radiation alone may be adequate.[59,101,104] Additionally, a randomized trial has shown equally good results with paraaortic radiation alone.[29] While for years the standard radiation dose for seminoma has been 2500 cGy/fraction, a randomized trial showed that

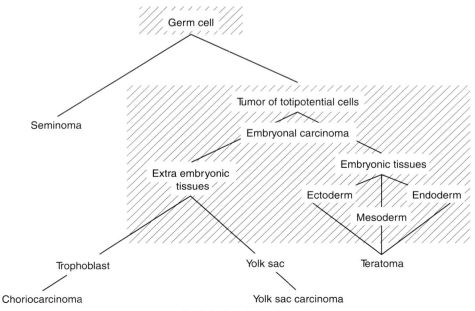

Figure 37-18. Dual origin for derivation of testes tumors.

Box 37-6	Testis Staging Systems

EORTC   UICC/AJCC

PRIMARY TUMOR (T) (PATHOLOGIC CLASSIFICATION)

Stage I

	pT_1	Tumor limited to testis (including rete)
	pT_2	Tumor invasion beyond tunica albuginea or into epididymis
	pT_3	Tumor invasion of spermatic cord
	pT_4	Tumor invasion of scrotum

LYMPH NODES (N)

Stage II

IIA	N_1	Metastasis in single node (<2 cm maximum diameter)
IIB	N_2	Metastasis in a single node (2 to 5cm in maximum diameter)
IIC, D	N_3	Metastasis in a lymph node (>5 cm in maximum diameter)

Stage III   Supradiaphragmatic and infra- diaphragmatic nodes: abdominal sites A, B, C, and D

DISTANT METASTASIS (M)

	M0	No distant metastasis
Stage IV	M1	Distant metastases (specific site)

STAGE GROUPINGS

I	T1, T2, N0, M0
II	T3, T4, N0, M0
III	Any T, N1, M0
IV	Any T, N2 or N3, M0
	Any T, any N, M1

AJCC, American Joint Committee on Cancer; *EORTC*, European Organization for Research on Treatment of Cancer; *UICC*, International Union Against Cancer.

2000 cGy in 10 fractions produced the same low relapse rate as 3000 cGy in 15 fractions.[45] Therefore, some are moving to the shorter fractionation scheme. Surveillance studies performed in Canada and the United Kingdom with patients receiving no further treatment after orchiectomy have indicated recurrence rates of approximately 20%.[18,104] Of patients in whom the tumor recurred, 99.5% were salvaged by subsequent radiation or chemotherapy. If surveillance is chosen over radiation, consistent follow-up is mandatory. Studies have been done using one or two cycles of cisplatin chemotherapy for stage I seminoma. Although the outcome is similar to nodal radiation, radiation remains the mainstay of therapy in the United States for stage I disease.

For patients with stage IIA disease (<2 cm diameter mass), the radiation dose and portals for the paraaortic and ipsilateral pelvic lymph nodes are similar to those used for stage I disease including adequate margin to cover the enlarged nodes. For stage IIB disease (<5 cm diameter mass), the paraaortic and ipsilateral pelvic lymph nodes should be irradiated with appropriate modification of the treatment field to encompass the larger mass. The dose to the entire nodal volume is 2500 cGy in 160- to 180-cGy fractions or 2000 cGy in 10 fractions, with an additional boost of 500 to 1000 cGy in 180- to 200-cGy fractions with reduced fields to cover the gross tumor.[53] At some institutions, the preferred primary treatment modality for stage IIB disease is chemotherapy.

The optimal therapy for patients with stage IIC retroperitoneal disease (5 to 10 cm in transverse diameter) must be individualized. If the mass is centrally located and does not overlap most of one kidney or significantly overlap the liver, primary radiation therapy can be applied, with chemotherapy reserved for relapse. However, if the location of the mass is such that the radiation volume covers most of one kidney or a significant volume of the liver, the potential morbidity of radiation therapy can be avoided by the use of primary cisplatin-containing combination chemotherapy.

Stage IID is rare. Patients in this stage should be treated with primary cisplatin-containing combination chemotherapy.

The current standard therapy for stages III and IV disease is four courses of cisplatin-containing combination chemotherapy. Often, residual masses may exist in the abdominal or mediastinal area after four cycles of chemotherapy. The 1989 Germ Cell Consensus Conference in Leeds, England, concluded from the available data that patients should be observed after appropriate chemotherapy and that further exploratory surgery or consolidative irradiation should be given only for overt disease progression.[101] This, however, is a controversial issue.

Nonseminoma. The initial treatment for nonseminoma is radical inguinal orchiectomy, followed by cisplatin-based chemotherapy. The most commonly accepted standard regimens include four courses of (a) cisplatin, vinblastine, and bleomycin (PVB) or (b) bleomycin, VP-16, cisplatin (BEP). Several investigators are exploring the use of fewer courses of cisplatin-containing combination chemotherapy and the use of single-agent cisplatin, carboplatin, or ifosfamide. One third of chemotherapy-treated patients have a radiographically apparent residual mass or masses after chemotherapy. In general, these masses should be excised because approximately 40% are teratomas and another 10% to 15% are carcinomas. Presumptive evidence exists indicating that unresected teratomas may give rise to later relapse and that patients have a lower risk of recurrence after surgical excision. Patients with persistent carcinoma require additional chemotherapy but generally do well following treatment.

Irradiation has little role in the management of patients with disseminated nonseminoma, except in the palliation of brain and other metastatic sites. Chemotherapy is the mainstay of treatment in this advanced state.

Radiation Therapy. Patients with stage I testicular seminoma should receive megavoltage irradiation to the paraaortic or paraaortic and ipsilateral pelvic lymph nodes. The top of the portal should be at the T10 to T12 level to ensure treatment of nodes at the level of the renal hilum. The inferior border should be at the bottom of L5 or at the top of the obturator foramen, depending on whether pelvic nodes will be treated. The lateral border must include the paraaortic lymph nodes and ipsilateral renal hilum (usually 10 to 12 cm wide). A shaped field with 2-cm margins is designed to encompass the ipsilateral pelvic lymph nodes (Figure 37-19). CT planning, to be sure that nodal areas are included and the kidneys are avoided, is now commonly done. Previously, renal contrast was given so that the kidneys could be seen on plain x-rays. Testicular shielding for decreasing primary and, to a lesser degree, scattered irradiation should be applied if the patient wants to preserve fertility.[30,51]

The recommended dose to retroperitoneal and pelvic lymphatics for stages I and IIA disease is 2500 cGy in fractions of 160 to 180 cGy or 2000 cGy in 10 fractions with AP/PA fields given 5 days per week and both fields treated daily. For IIA disease, a boost of 500 to 600 cGy to the known nodal involvement is often delivered. For stages IIB and IIC tumors, the portals are the same as those in stages I and IIA, except that

the fields should be modified to cover the palpable or radiographic mass with an adequate margin. The first 2000 to 2500 cGy is delivered to the entire nodal volume followed by a boost of 500 to 1000 cGy in 180- to 200-cGy fractions to a reduced field to encompass the mass with an adequate margin of at least 2 cm.

If the primary radiation therapy field encompasses most of one kidney, care must be taken to protect at least two thirds of the kidney from receiving doses higher than 1800 cGy. Care should also be taken to limit the radiation dose to a significant volume of the liver to less than 3000 cGy. If these parameters cannot be met, chemotherapy typically becomes the treatment of choice.

Controversial Issues

Scrotal or Inguinal Irradiation. A standard recommendation has been to modify the treatment volume to include both inguinal regions if there has been previous inguinal surgery and to include the scrotum if it has been violated. Reports from the Princess Margaret and Royal Marsden Hospitals demonstrated that previous inguinal or scrotal violation without irradiation of these sites results in little increased risk of relapse. The 1989 Consensus Conference in Leeds, England, recommended that inguinal or scrotal irradiation be omitted even if scrotal interference has occurred.[101]

Mediastinal irradiation

In the 1960s and early 1970s, the use of prophylactic mediastinal irradiation to treat patients who had stage I or II testicular seminoma was common. Compiled data from six series suggest that supradiaphragmatic relapse is extremely rare, even for relatively poorly staged patients with stage IIA or IIB disease, if prophylactic mediastinal irradiation is withheld. Mediastinal relapse occurred in only 8 of 250 patients, and 7 of 8 patients were salvaged with radiation. Because the possible survival benefit of elective mediastinal irradiation is only 0.4%, most radiation oncologists have abandoned its use for stages IIA and IIB disease.[85]

Paraaortic Versus Ipsilateral Iliac and Paraaortic Irradiation. There is growing interest in Europe and the United Kingdom in reducing the radiation volumes for the treatment of stage I disease by omitting irradiation of the pelvic lymph nodes.[29] Less than 3% of patients have involved pelvic nodes, and it is unlikely that the reduction of the irradiated volume will cause a significant increase in relapse rate. Furthermore, salvage chemotherapy is very effective. The most commonly used field in the United States, however, still encompasses both paraaortic and ipsilateral pelvic nodes (see Figure 37-19).

Results of Treatment

Rates of disease-free survival for stage I testicular seminoma are in the 95% to 97% range at 5 years according to multiple studies.[29,30,45,104,107] Corresponding cause-specific survival is 100%.

For patients with stage IIA and IIB disease, rates of disease-free and cause-specific survival are 90% and 95%, respectively.[53,85,108]

Survival for patients with stage IIC, IID, and III disease depends on the initial bulk of the tumor and the therapeutic approach.

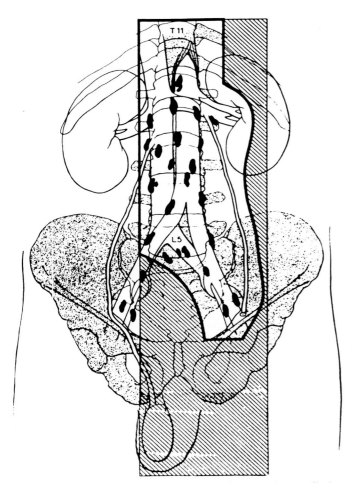

Figure 37-19. Contoured anterior and posterior radiation treatment fields for clinical stage I or IIA left testicular cancer. (From Kubo H, Shipley WU: Reduction of the scatter dose to the testicle outside the radiation treatment fields, *Int J Radiat Oncol Biol Phys* 8:1741-1745, 1982.)

With radiation alone, tumor-free survival rates range from 30% to 50%, and primary chemotherapy yields a progression-free survival rate of 91%.[108] Chemotherapy is highly effective as salvage treatment for failure after radiation as well.

Side Effects and Complications. In general, paraaortic and pelvic radiation is well tolerated. Patients often develop nausea and occasionally diarrhea during the treatment course, which is usually controlled with appropriate medication. Severe dyspepsia or a peptic ulcer occurs in only 3% to 5% of irradiated patients.[30]

Patterns of case studies have shown that a significant increase in late complications occurred with wide-field irradiation for seminoma and Hodgkin's disease with doses greater than 2500 cGy. However, no late complications were reported with lower doses.[15] The complication rate increased to 2% with 3500 cGy and to 6% with 4000 to 4500 cGy. Reports have also suggested an increased risk of cardiovascular disease following mediastinal radiation, which is no longer routinely prescribed.[15]

Approximately 50% of patients with seminoma have a decreased sperm count at the time of diagnosis. Further decreases are noted after pelvic and paraaortic irradiation, even if gonadal shielding is used. Typically, the uninvolved testicle receives 1% to 2% of the prescription dose because of scattered radiation through the body tissues.[31] Spermatogenesis may be affected by doses as low as 50 cGy, and cumulative doses above 200 cGy will likely induce permanent sterility.[88]

Second Primary Malignancy. A 5% to 10% incidence of second malignancy has been reported in patients treated with radiation therapy for testicular seminoma. These second malignancies arise from inside and outside the radiation treatment portal. Whether they result from radiation treatment, the predisposition of patients with testicular seminoma to develop a second primary, or a combination of both is not clear. Among 10-year survivors diagnosed with testicular cancer, the overall risk of developing a second solid tumor is approximately twice that of the general population. The risk of developing tumors of the bladder, pancreas, and stomach, organs typically at least partially within the treatment portal, is as high as 3 to 4 times that of the general population according to a large study in which patients had long-term follow-up.[102] Risk appears to be similar with either radiation or chemotherapy but is highest when the two are combined—3 times that of the normal population.

KIDNEY

Epidemiology

Renal Cell Carcinoma. The estimated number of new cases of kidney and renal pelvis cancers reported each year in the United States is 54,390, which will result in approximately 13,010 deaths, representing 2% of all new cancers and cancer deaths annually.[3] The average age at the time of diagnosis is 55 to 60 years, with a male-to-female ratio of 2:1.

Several environmental, occupational, hormonal, cellular, and genetic factors are associated with the development of renal cell carcinoma.[57] Cigarette and tobacco use, obesity, and analgesic abuse (i.e., phenacetin-containing analgesics) have been correlated with an increased risk and incidence of kidney cancer. A higher incidence of renal cell carcinoma has also been reported among leather tanners, shoe workers, and asbestos workers. Exposure to cadmium, petroleum products, and thorium dioxide (a radioactive contrast agent used in the 1920s) may cause renal cell carcinoma in humans.

The association of renal cell cancer and von Hippel-Lindau disease has long been established. Various tumor-produced growth factors have been described in the initiation or progression of renal cell carcinoma.[57]

Renal Pelvic and Ureteral Carcinoma. About 7% of all renal neoplasms and less than 1% of all genitourinary tumors are transitional cell carcinomas of the upper urinary tract.[79] For renal pelvic tumors, the incidence in men versus in women is 3:1, and the peak incidence is in the fifth and sixth decades of life. About one third of patients with upper urinary tract tumors develop bladder carcinoma. Etiologic factors for renal pelvic and ureteral cancer are similar to those for tumors of the urinary bladder. Urban residency, cigarette and tobacco use, aminophenol exposure (e.g., benzidine, β-naphthylamine), renal stones, and analgesics (e.g., chronic phenacetin abuse) have been associated with an increased risk of developing upper urinary tract tumors.

Prognostic Indicators

Renal Cell Carcinoma. The major prognostic factors for survival in patients with renal cell carcinoma are the stage and histologic grade of the tumor. Reported 5-year survival rates are 88% for stage I, 67% for stage II, 40% for stage III, and 2% for stage IV disease.[35] Renal vein or vena cava involvement, without corresponding regional lymph node metastasis, is not a poor prognostic sign if the entire tumor thrombus is removed. The mean survival time for patients with metastasis at the time of diagnosis is approximately 4 months, and only about 10% of patients survive 1 year.[76]

Renal Pelvic and Ureteral Carcinoma. Stage and grade are important prognostic factors in carcinoma of the renal pelvis and ureter. One report noted that 54 patients with transitional cell carcinoma of the renal pelvis and ureter had a median survival time of 91.1 months for early-stage tumors and 12.9 months for more advanced tumors.[41] When patients were stratified according to low or high tumor grade, the median survival time was 66.8 months versus 14.1 months, respectively.

Anatomy and Lymphatics

The kidneys and ureters and their vascular supply and lymphatics are located in the retroperitoneal space between the parietal peritoneum and the posterior abdominal wall. The kidneys are located at a level between the eleventh rib and the transverse process of the third lumbar vertebra. The renal axis is parallel to the lateral margin of the psoas muscle. Each kidney is about 11 to 12 cm in length, with the right kidney usually 1 to 2 cm lower than the left. Gerota's fascia envelops the kidney in its fibrous capsule and the perinephric fat.

The collecting system lies on the anteromedial surface of the kidney and forms a funnel-shaped apparatus that is continuous with the ureter. The ureters course posteriorly, parallel to the lateral border of the psoas muscle, until they curve anteriorly in the pelvis to join the base of the bladder.

The lymphatic drainage of the kidney and renal pelvis occurs along the vessels in the renal hilum to the paraaortic and paracaval nodes. The lymphatic drainage of the ureter is segmented and diffuse, involving any of the following: renal hilar, abdominal paraaortic, paracaval, common iliac, internal iliac, or external iliac nodes.

The topographical relationship of the kidneys, renal pelvis, and ureters to other abdominal organs is illustrated in Figure 37-20.

Clinical Presentation

Renal Cell Carcinoma. Renal cell carcinoma may appear as an occult primary tumor or with signs and symptoms. In one report, the classic triad of gross hematuria, a palpable abdominal mass, and pain occurred in only 9% of patients. Two of three components of the triad occurred in 36% of patients, whereas hematuria, gross or microscopic, was noted in 59% of patients.[76] Several paraneoplastic syndromes or systemic symptoms of renal cell carcinoma have been described, and the tumor may masquerade behind a variety of symptom patterns.

Renal Pelvic and Ureteral Carcinoma. Gross or microscopic hematuria is the most common sign in patients who have a renal pelvic or ureteral tumor, occurring in 70% to 95%

of cases.[79] The other less common symptoms include pain (8% to 40%), bladder irritation (5% to 10%), and other constitutional symptoms (5%). Approximately 10% to 20% of patients have a flank mass secondary to the tumor or associated hydronephrosis. Otherwise, physical findings are unremarkable.

Detection and Diagnosis

Renal Cell Carcinoma. The diagnosis of renal cell carcinoma is established clinically and radiographically in most patients. After a radiographic diagnosis is made, a thorough staging workup is performed to determine resectability. A metastatic workup that includes a bone scan, chest radiograph, and CT or MRI scan of the abdomen and pelvis should be performed before surgery. If metastatic lesions are detected, a histologic confirmation of the most easily accessible lesion should be obtained.

An intravenous pyelogram (IVP) can identify the tumor, determine its location, and show the function of the contralateral kidney when surgery is contemplated. However, an IVP is not sensitive or specific for small to medium-sized tumors. Ultrasonography provides accurate anatomic detail of extrarenal extension of the tumor. In addition, it differentiates solid

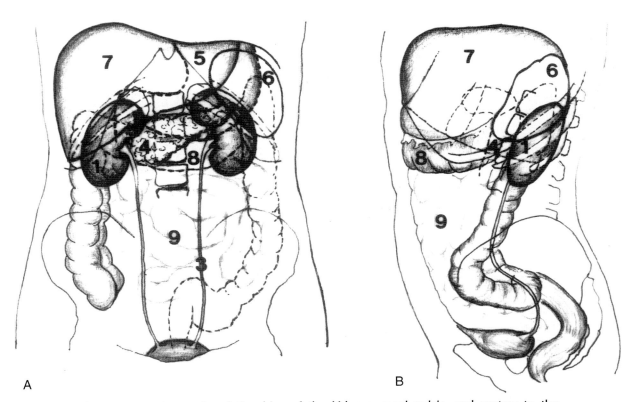

A   B

Figure 37-20. Anatomic relationships of the kidneys, renal pelvis, and ureters to the abdominal viscera. The surrounding structures as numbered (*1*, right kidney; *2*, left renal pelvis; *3*, left ureter; *4*, pancreas; *5*, stomach; *6*, spleen; *7*, liver; *8*, transverse colon; *9*, small bowel) become dose-limiting factors in the planning of abdominal or retroperitoneal irradiation. **A,** Anteroposterior view. **B,** Lateral view. (Courtesy Peter P. Lai, MD.)

from cystic renal lesions. Renal arteriography detects neovascularity, arteriovenous fistula, and pooling of contrast medium, and it accentuates capsular vessels. Contrast-enhanced or dynamic CT provides extremely accurate information about the location and size of the tumor and lymph node enlargement. CT plus digital subtraction angiography provides adequate diagnostic and anatomic details with much less morbidity than arteriography. Inferior venacavography is sometimes used to detect the extent of the tumor thrombus involvement within the vena cava.

Renal Pelvic and Ureteral Carcinoma. Excretory urography is frequently used to evaluate patients with renal pelvic carcinoma. The most common finding is a filling defect in the renal pelvis or collecting system. Retrograde pyelography accurately delineates upper-tract filling defects and defines the lower margin of the ureteral lesion. CT or MRI of the abdomen and pelvis before and after contrast gives useful information regarding tumor extension. Angiography is not often used. Endoscopic ureteroscopy with percutaneous nephroscopy is a recently developed technique. A brush cytology or biopsy from such an endoscopic retrograde procedure has a diagnostic accuracy of 80% to 90%.[57]

Pathology and Staging

The proximal tubular epithelium is the tissue of origin for renal cell carcinoma. Clear cell carcinoma is the predominant subtype. Some reports indicate that spindle cell (sarcomatoid variant) carcinoma is associated with a poor prognosis. A tumor's high nuclear grade is associated with an increased incidence of lymph node involvement and a short survival time.[76]

Transitional cell carcinoma accounts for more than 90% of malignant tumors of the renal pelvis and ureter, and squamous cell carcinoma accounts for 7% to 8%.[57] Adenocarcinoma of the upper urothelial tract is rare. Squamous cell carcinoma of the renal pelvis is often deeply invasive and is associated with a worse prognosis than transitional cell carcinoma. High-grade renal pelvic or ureteral tumors are associated with poor survival rates.[41]

The AJCC system for the classification of renal cell carcinoma of the kidney is shown in Box 37-7. T1 and T2 refer to cancers that are intrarenal and have not invaded through the capsule. T3 and T4 cancers are based on the local extension of the primary tumor. The N classification depends on the size and number of involved lymph nodes and not on laterality.

The AJCC staging classification for renal pelvic and ureteral carcinoma is shown in Box 37-8. The grouping of the T categories depends on the tumor's extent with regard to depth of penetration of the lesion.

Routes of Spread

Renal Cell Carcinoma. A tumor may spread in the following ways: (1) by local infiltration through the renal capsule to involve the perinephric fat and Gerota's fascia; (2) by direct extension in the venous channels to the renal vein or inferior vena cava; (3) by retrograde venous drainage to the testis; (4) by lymphatic drainage to the renal hilar, paraaortic, and paracaval nodes; and 5) by hematogenous route to any part of the body, including the lung, liver, central nervous system, skeleton, and other organs. The incidence of lymph node metastasis is 12% to 23%.[57]

Box 37-7	American Joint Committee on Cancer Staging Classification for Cancer of the Kidney

PRIMARY TUMOR (T)

TX	Primary tumor cannot be assessed
T0	No evidence of tumor
Tis	Carcinoma in situ
Ta	Papillary noninvasive carcinoma
T1	Tumor invasion of subepithelial connective tissue
T2	Tumor invasion of muscularis
T3	Tumor invasion beyond muscularis into periureteric-peripelvic fat or renal parenchyma
T4	Tumor invasion of adjacent organs or through the kidney into perinephric fat

REGIONAL LYMPH NODES (N)

NX	Regional lymph nodes cannot be assessed
N0	No regional lymph node metastasis
N1	Metastasis in a single lymph node (2 cm or less in greatest dimension)
N2	Metastasis in a single lymph node (more than 2 cm but not more than 5 cm in greatest dimension) or multiple lymph nodes (none more than 5 cm in greatest dimension)
N3	Metastasis in a lymph node (more than 5 cm in greatest dimension)

DISTANT METASTASIS (M)

MX	Distant metastasis cannot be assessed
M0	No distant metastasis
M1	Distant metastasis

STAGE GROUPING

Stage 0	Tis	N0	M0
	Ta	N0	M0
Stage I	T1	N0	M0
Stage II	T2	N0	M0
Stage III	T3	N0	M0
Stage IV	T4	N0	M0
	Any T	N1, N2, N3	M0
	Any T	Any N	M1

HISTOPATHOLOGIC GRADE

GX	Grade cannot be assessed
G1	Well differentiated
G2	Moderately well differentiated
G3-4	Poorly differentiated or undifferentiated

Box 37-8	American Joint Committee on Cancer Staging Classification for Renal Pelvic and Ureteral Cancer

PRIMARY TUMOR (T)

TX   Primary tumor cannot be assessed
T0   No evidence of tumor
Tis   Carcinoma in situ
Ta   Papillary noninvasive carcinoma
T1   Tumor invasion of subepithelial connective tissue
T2   Tumor invasion of muscularis
T3   Tumor invasion beyond muscularis into periureteric-peripelvic fat or renal parenchyma
T4   Tumor invasion of adjacent organs or through the kidney into perinephric fat

REGIONAL LYMPH NODES (N)

NX   Regional lymph nodes cannot be assessed
N0   No regional lymph node metastasis
N1   Metastasis in a single lymph node (2 cm or less in greatest dimension)
N2   Metastasis in a single lymph node (more than 2 cm but not more than 5 cm in greatest dimension) or multiple lymph nodes (none more than 5 cm in greatest dimension)
N3   Metastasis in a lymph node (more than 5 cm in greatest dimension)

DISTANT METASTASIS (M)

MX   Distant metastasis cannot be assessed
M0   No distant metastasis
M1   Distant metastasis

STAGE GROUPING

Stage 0	Tis	N0	M0
	Ta	N0	M0
Stage I	T1	N0	M0
Stage II	T2	N0	M0
Stage III	T3	N0	M0
Stage IV	T4	N0	M0
	Any T	N1, N2, N3	M0
	Any T	Any N	M1

HISTOPATHOLOGIC GRADE

GX   Grade cannot be assessed
G1   Well differentiated
G2   Moderately well differentiated
G3-4   Poorly differentiated or undifferentiated

With permission from American Joint Committee on Cancer (AJCC), Chicago, IL, *AJCC cancer staging manual*, ed 6, New York, 2002, Springer-Verlag.

Approximately 45% of patients with renal cell carcinoma have localized disease, 25% have advanced disease, and 30% have radiographic evidence of metastasis at the time of the diagnosis.[57] Approximately 50% of patients with renal cell carcinoma eventually develop metastasis. Common metastatic sites include the lung (75%), soft tissue (36%), bone (20%), liver (18%), cutaneous areas (8%), and central nervous system (8%).[60]

Spontaneous regression of metastatic renal cell carcinoma after nephrectomy has been reported but is extremely rare.

Renal Pelvic and Ureteral Carcinoma. Upper urinary tract carcinoma is a multifocal process; patients with cancer at one site in the upper urinary tract are at greater risk of developing tumors elsewhere in the urinary tract.

Transitional cell carcinoma of the upper urothelial tract may spread via direct extension, blood, or lymphatics. The implantation of tumor cells in the bladder has been demonstrated, especially in previously traumatized areas.[80]

Treatment Techniques

Renal Cell Carcinoma. Standard treatment for patients with localized renal cell carcinoma T1 and T2 is radical nephrectomy, which consists of the complete removal of the intact Gerota's fascia and its contents, including the kidney, adrenal gland, and perinephric fat. Regional lymphadenectomy is often performed at the time of radical nephrectomy.

The role of preoperative radiation therapy before nephrectomy has not been defined. Tumor shrinkage and increased resectability have been reported in patients who received preoperative irradiation, but no survival benefit has been noted.[52]

Definitive radiation treatment may be indicated if the patient is not a candidate for surgical resection. It is limited, of course, by the inability to deliver high doses of radiation to the upper abdomen, where most surrounding structures have low tolerance. Therefore, the intent typically becomes palliative.

Chemotherapy and immunotherapy, such as interferon and interleukin, are used, although survival gains are marginal. The newer antiangiogenic targeting agents are showing promise.

Patients with a solitary bony metastasis are at risk of developing multiple metastases, but these patients also have a 30% to 40% chance of surviving for 5 years.[47] Thus, these lesions are often treated surgically or with high-dose palliative radiation therapy in an attempt to ensure a long symptom-free survival time.

Renal Pelvic and Ureteral Carcinoma. Management of renal pelvic and ureteral carcinoma consists of nephroureterectomy with the excision of a cuff of bladder and bladder mucosa. Less aggressive surgery, such as nephrectomy and partial ureterectomy, is accompanied by a ureteral stump recurrence rate of 30%. More conservative surgical excision has been advocated for patients with low-stage, low-grade, and solitary lesions. The survival rate for patients with solitary, well-differentiated tumors after surgical resection is greater than 90%.[64]

Combination chemotherapy consisting of methotrexate, vinblastine, doxorubicin [Adriamycin], and cisplatin (MVAC) produces an objective response of more than 70% in limited groups of patients who have metastatic transitional cell carcinoma of the bladder, ureter, or renal pelvis.[97] For patients who have high-stage and high-grade tumors with local extension or patients with regional lymph node metastases, combination chemotherapy and radiation offer the best chance of disease control.

Radiation Therapy Techniques

Renal Cell Carcinoma. Radiation is most commonly delivered in the postoperative setting when tumor is left behind or for recurrence following surgery. The treatment volume includes the renal fossa and site of gross recurrence, if present, along with the paraaortic nodal drainage sites in the adjuvant setting.

Postoperative radiation doses range from 4500 to 5500 cGy; the usual recommended dose that can be safely given to the upper abdomen with an acceptable complication rate is 5040 cGy at 180 cGy/fraction over 5 to 6 weeks. A boost of 540 cGy in three fractions to a smaller volume may be added, with special care, to bring the total tumor dose to 5580 cGy. The remaining kidney should not receive doses above 1800 cGy. For a right-sided tumor, a field reduction may be needed at 3600 to 4000 cGy to ensure that no more than 30% of the liver parenchyma is irradiated to a higher dose. The nominal dose for the spinal cord should be limited to 4500 cGy with 180-cGy fractions. No attempt is made to include the entire surgical incision in the treatment field for patients who receive postnephrectomy irradiation, unless specific knowledge exists of significant wound contamination by tumor spillage.[52]

The patient is usually treated via isocentric, parallel-opposed AP/PA-shaped fields. CT planning is used to define the area at risk and normal structures. Treatment plans include (1) equal weighting of parallel-opposed AP/PA fields, (2) bias loading (i.e., 3:1 or 2:1 posterior loading), and (3) other wedge pair techniques. A shrinking-field technique should be used to reduce exposure to dose-limiting adjacent structures. High-energy photons, 10 MV or higher, should be used. An example of a typical postoperative treatment field and technique is shown in Figure 37-21. Although the kidney is shown, this would, of course, represent the renal bed after surgical removal.

Radiation can also be used to palliate a symptomatic renal mass that is unresectable or in the patient who is inoperable. Depending on the patient's symptoms and longevity, a shorter treatment scheme can be used. Similar treatment plans encompassing the kidney are applied.

Renal Pelvic and Ureteral Carcinoma. Postoperative radiation has been applied to patients with renal pelvic and ureteral carcinoma. The treatment portal usually includes the entire renal fossa, ureteral bed, and ipsilateral bladder trigone. The extent is dictated by clinical information obtained at the time of surgery and a pathologic analysis of the resected specimen (Figure 37-22). Because of the high incidence of lymph node involvement, the treatment portal should also include the

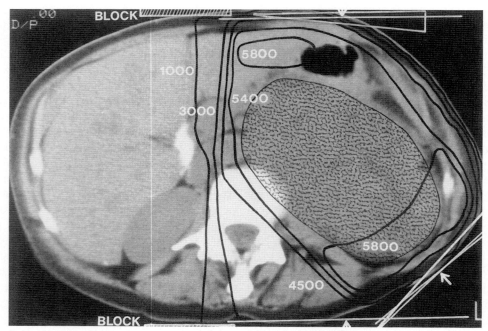

Figure 37-21. Radiation dose distribution corresponding to the treatment portal in Figure 37-21. Notice that a combination of anteroposterior/posteroanterior (AP/PA) plus oblique portals with wedges is used to encompass the entire lesion with an isodose curve of 5400 cGy. The spinal cord dose is less than 4150 cGy. (From Lai PP: Kidney, renal pelvis, and ureter. In Perez CA, Brady LW, editors: *Principles and practice of radiation oncology,* ed 2, Philadelphia, 1992, JB Lippincott.)

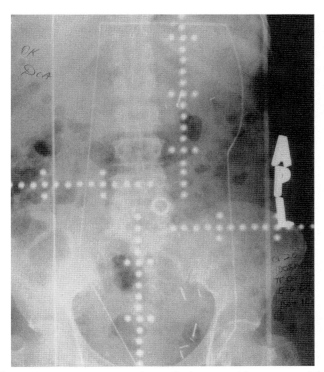

Figure 37-22. A postoperative radiation portal for cancer of the renal pelvis and ureter. Usually, the entire renal fossa, urethral bed, and ipsilateral trigone are included; the exact extent is determined by pathologic information. (From Lai PP: Kidney, renal pelvis, and ureter. In Perez CA, Brady LW, editors: *Principles and practice of radiation oncology,* ed 2, Philadelphia, 1992, JB Lippincott.)

paraaortic and paracaval areas. As in renal cell carcinoma of the kidney, the postoperative radiation dose is limited by the tolerance of normal tissues in the treatment field. The usual dose is 5040 cGy in 180-cGy fractions, with a possible boost of an additional 540 cGy in three fractions to a reduced volume. The technique is generally AP/PA parallel opposed for the large field with the same technique or oblique beams for the boost.

Results of Treatment

Results of studies of postoperative radiation therapy for renal cell carcinoma have varied, making it difficult to draw conclusions regarding efficacy (Table 37-7). Survival benefit remains questionable. Of note is that locoregional failure is rarely reported and compared. Older treatment techniques without CT planning were used, often, with severe or even fatal complications. Therefore, postoperative radiation is not widely applied for renal, renal pelvis, and ureteral malignancies. Sufficient evidence of residual disease from evaluation of surgical findings and specimens must be present to warrant postoperative radiation. Similarly, preoperative radiation has shown questionable benefit in past studies and is generally no longer applied.

Side Effects. The side effects and complications from radiation treatment of cancer of the kidney, renal pelvis, and ureters are similar to those expected from irradiation of the abdomen and pelvis. Acute side effects include nausea, vomiting, diarrhea, and abdominal cramping, which usually respond to conservative medical management.[52] The complication rate is related to the total dose and fraction size. With careful attention given to the treatment technique and dose-volume distribution, many complications can be eliminated.

ROLE OF RADIATION THERAPIST

Treatment Plan Implementation

Accurate dose delivery, daily observation of the patient's tolerance to therapy, and the psychological needs of the patient are important aspects of the radiation therapist's role. Reproducibility of the daily treatment is of prime importance because the patient's outcome depends on accurate dose delivery to the target volume and the sparing of critical structures. A positive outcome, however, can be overshadowed if the patient is unhappy because of a lack of appropriate psychological support and understanding of potential side effects during the course of therapy.

Treatment Information and Psychological Support

Accurate dose delivery is important for the control of disease. However, patients are just as concerned with potential side effects of radiation treatments and the way that the side effects affect their daily routine and interaction with family and friends. The potential side effects of treatment to the abdomen and pelvis are similar to those of other sites treated with radiation, including skin reaction, fatigue, weight loss, nausea and vomiting, diarrhea, and hair loss in the area being irradiated.

Skin changes caused by radiation exposure depend on the beam energy and dose. Because most tumors in the abdomen and pelvis (>85%) are treated with a beam energy greater than 6 MV or with multiple beams such as with IMRT, skin reactions are usually not more severe than dry desquamation or slight tanning. Single or parallel-opposed treatment fields given with lower beam energies may produce more severe skin reactions because of higher surface doses and the thick body parts involved. Patients should be instructed to avoid the use of harsh creams or soaps in the irradiated area. Topical preparations usually provide some comfort.

Many patients are more easily fatigued during radiation treatments because much of the body's energy is being used to fight the disease process or repair the effects of radiation on normal tissues. The therapist should counsel patients not to be alarmed if they are more easily tired during the course of treatment; patients should be told to maintain good nutrition and get plenty of rest to minimize weight loss and fatigue. If the patient encounters problems with nausea, vomiting, or diarrhea, the physician can prescribe medications to alleviate these symptoms. Fatigue may also be caused by treatment induced anemia. Blood counts should be checked.

Hair loss can occur in the irradiated field because of the sensitivity of the follicles to radiation. This hair loss may be permanent, depending on the dose of radiation.

The therapist should encourage the patient and family to discuss with the physician any problems concerning treatment. Problems dealing with transportation, work, or financial concerns should be referred to social service personnel to minimize

Table 37-7	Renal Cell Carcinoma: 5-Year Survival Rates After Nephrectomy or Postoperative Irradiation and Nephrectomy					
Author	Stage	No. of Patients	Radiation Dose/ Fraction Size (cGy)	Treatment	5-year Survival Rate	Local Recurrence (%)
Peeling, et al. (1969)*		96		N	52% (50/96)	
		68		N + RT	25% (17/68)	
Rafla (1970)†	All	96		N	37% (35/94)	
		94		N + RT	57% (46/81)	
	Renal vein	36		N	30% (11/36)	
	± others	40		N + RT	40% (14/35)	
	Renal pelvis	50		N	32% (16/49)	
	± others	60		N + RT	60% (30/50)	
	Renal capsule	52		N	28% (15.52)	
	± others	69		N + RT	57% (34/59)	
Rafla and Parikh (1984)‡		135		N	18% (24/135)	
		105	4500	N + RT	38% (40/105)	
Finney (1973)§		48		N	47% (17/35)	7
		52	5500/204	N + RT	36% (14/39)	7
Kjaer et al. (1987)¶		33		N	63%§	1
		32	5000/250	N + RT	38%¶	0

Modified from Lai PP: Kidney, renal pelvis, and ureter. In Perez CA, Brady LW, editors: *Principles and practice of radiation oncology*, 1992, JB Lippincott.

N, Nephrectomy; *RT*, postoperative radiation therapy.

*This is a retrospective study with incomplete staging information and no description of the radiation dose or technique. The endpoint was 5-year survival, with no mention of local recurrence.

†This is the only report that described the benefits of irradiation with survival *and* local recurrence as endpoints. Unfortunately, there was no description of the radiation dose or technique. The study was performed in the pre-CT era; therefore local recurrence is an underestimate. Subgroup analysis (involvement of renal vein, renal pelvis, renal capsule + others) indicated an effect of radiation therapy on survival.

‡The authors also showed some data attesting to the benefits of radiation therapy in patients with renal capsular, renal vein, and regional lymphatic involvement.

§This is a randomized study, but no staging information is available. The incidences of local recurrence and distant metastasis are similar. However, there are four fatal liver complications among the patients who received radiation therapy.

¶ In this randomized study 27 or 32 patients assigned to the irradiation arm completed treatment; 12 of 27 (44%) reported significant complications, with five fatal complications related to irradiation.

the patient's emotional stress. A pleasant, friendly, and helpful attitude can also provide good emotional support.

Treatment Planning and Delivery

The basic steps in the planning and delivery of the physician's treatment plan generally apply to all sites. However, some issues that improve the daily reproducibility of the treatment apply specifically to abdominal and pelvic sites. For example, rectal and bladder filling can have a significant effect on prostate position. Procedures should be developed and followed to improve consistency in the setup between simulation and treatment units.

Simulation

Immobilization. The construction of immobilization devices, an important part of the treatment-planning process, should be accomplished during the initial simulation. The patient's treatment position must be established, and appropriate immobilization and repositioning devices should be constructed before any simulation images are taken or treatment-planning CT data are obtained. This helps ensure agreement in the transfer of information between the simulator and treatment unit.

Reproducibility of the patient setup can be improved with a treatment position that the patient can maintain through proper immobilization and repositioning devices. The methods most commonly used for immobilization during treatment of abdominal and pelvic sites are polyurethane foam molds or vacuum devices with the patient in the supine position. However, thermal plastic molds are also being used at some facilities with the patient in the prone position. These immobilization devices may extend from the chest through the thighs for abdominal fields or the hips to the feet for pelvic fields. The length tends to vary between institutions. Of greatest importance is that the therapists are experienced and comfortable with a device which consistently provides a reproducible setup.

Simulation and Treatment Variations. Daily isocenter variation in the AP/PA direction can be reduced by setting the isocenter based on the digital couch height or lateral lasers rather than using the optical distance indicator projected on the patient's skin surface. The depth of the isocenter should be checked daily for consistency and verification that the depth of calculation is not changing as a result of weight loss or bloating. Daily fluctuations of 1 to 2 cm in the skin's isocenter depth for an anterior abdominal or pelvic field are not uncommon. If the depth of calculation is consistently off in one direction, the physicist and physician should be notified so that the resulting change in dose may be evaluated for a new monitor unit calculation. Differences in the skin's isocenter depth on lateral or posterior fields are generally less than 1 cm when patients are carefully aligned with the sagittal lasers and the vertical height is set with a digital readout or lateral lasers.

Systematic errors can also occur from differences in the alignment of lasers and optical distance indicators from the simulator and the treatment unit. A tolerance of 2 mm on the laser alignment or optical distance indicator can result in a 4-mm discrepancy in the setup from the simulator to the treatment unit. Similar discrepancies can occur from differences in the alignment of blocking trays from machine to machine caused by worn or damaged parts.

Studies of variation in the daily setup of portals relative to bony landmarks in treatment of the prostate show greater maximum and average variation without immobilization devices versus with foam-mold or other immobilization devices.

Treatment Verification

Portal images of the treatment fields should be taken before treatment on the first day and compared with the simulation images for correct field placement. The first-day images serve as a guide for subsequent images taken during the course of therapy. Both portals for parallel-opposed beams should be taken on the same day with a fiducial grid in place to distinguish block-mounting errors from patient-positioning or patient-movement errors. The fiducial grid provides a means for determining the magnification factor on the portal image so that required adjustments can be made easily. Interpreting anatomic changes resulting in a magnification change of corresponding anatomy on each of the images is also much easier with a fiducial grid in place.

Most conformal treatment techniques use multiple oblique beam arrangements, which are difficult to interpret for anatomical coverage and positional accuracy of the isocenter. For these reasons conformal beam arrangements are best evaluated from a set of orthogonal films that allow vertical and horizontal shifts in the isocenter position to be viewed separately. A set of portal images taken with the exact treatment angles may still be useful for documentation and comparison with the simulation images for anatomic coverage.

Dose-verification measurements can be taken on all photon portals through the use of a diode detector or thermoluminescent dosimeter. The dose measurements are meant to discover errors resulting from incorrect or missing wedges, compensating filters, or incorrect monitor unit calculations.

Record-and-verify systems are also highly recommended to ensure that daily setups are consistent and correct.

Site-Specific Instructions

Some type of immobilization or repositioning device is always used for patients treated definitively with conformal techniques. Lasers aid in setup accuracy as well. Typical simulation procedures are listed in the simulation section, and these must be reproduced on the treatment machine.

Prostate. Patients should be treated with a full bladder to minimize the amount of bladder in the treatment portals. The rectum is often simulated empty to ensure that a full rectum does not move the prostate anteriorly during simulation. An empty rectum during treatment would then allow the prostate to move posteriorly, outside the treatment field. Since the prostate can be in a slightly different position each day due to rectal and bladder filling, accurate prostate targeting must be assured. Transabdominal sonographic (BAT) implanted fiducial markers or CT scan can be used to align a daily image with the planning CT. Field changes can then be made to follow the internal movement of the gland.

Bladder. Patients should be treated with an empty bladder when the entire bladder is being treated to maintain an adequate margin. During a boost field, a full bladder will reduce the amount of bladder treated to the boost dose.

Kidney. Considerations relative to abdominal treatments should be applied to treatment of the kidney. Tolerance of abdominal organs is relatively low.

Penis. The treatment approach depends on the need to treat only the penis or the penis and regional lymphatics. External beam therapy requires specially designed accessories, including bolus, to achieve homogeneous dose distribution to the entire organ involved.

SUMMARY

- Male reproductive and genitourinary tumors range from the most common form of cancers found in men such as prostate cancer, to the relatively rare such as penile and urethral carcinomas.
- Testicular cancer, although relatively, rare is the most common malignancy found in men between the ages of 20 and 34.
- As with all other types of cancers, early detection is the most important factor in gaining control over the disease.
- A clear understanding of lymphatic drainage and surrounding anatomy is vital to gaining a better understanding of the treatment rational and dose limitations.
- Several areas of controversy surround the many treatment options available to patients with prostate cancer. Different forms of treatment can affect quality of life and sexual function to varying degrees.
- Ever evolving technology such as CT simulation and IMRT, with associated increases in radiation dose, have improved disease control rates and decreased the side effects related to radiation therapy.
- The potential side effects of treatment to the abdomen and pelvis are similar to those of other sites treated with radiation, including skin reaction, fatigue, weight loss, nausea and vomiting, diarrhea, and hair loss in the area being irradiated.
- Genitourinary cancer management has proven to be a fruitful proving ground in the development of dose escalation treatment regimens and conformal treatment delivery. The treatment of these cancers with today's technology has led to the refinement of intensity

modulated radiation therapy treatment delivery, image guided radiation therapy, and to a degree particulate therapies.

Review Questions

Multiple Choice

1. The most common pathology of malignant tumors of the prostate is:
   a. squamous cell carcinoma
   b. adenocarcinoma
   c. transitional cell carcinoma
   d. Burkitt's cell carcinoma
2. The most common type of kidney tumor is:
   a. transitional cell lymphoma
   b. choriocarcinoma
   c. adenocarcinoma
   d. seminoma
3. The cancer with the highest incidence rate for males is:
   a. prostate cancer
   b. penile cancer
   c. kidney and ureteral cancer
   d. lung cancer
4. Which of the following are common immobilization-repositioning devices used in the treatment of prostate cancer?
   I. polyurethane foam molds
   II. vacuum devices
   III. belly board
   IV. rubber bands or other devices to position the feet.
   a. I and III only
   b. I and IV only
   c. II and III only
   d. I, II, and IV only
5. For patients with bladder cancer, the bladder should be _____ during whole-bladder radiation.
   a. empty
   b. partially full
   c. full
   d. localized with contrast material
6. A side effect associated with the treatment of prostate cancer, in which the adult male is unable to obtain an erection, is:
   a. benign prostatic hypertrophy
   b. transurethral resection of the prostate
   c. impotence
   d. none of the above
7. The prostate gland is located _____ to the rectum.
   a. posterior
   b. anterior
   c. superior
   d. both a and c
8. The tumor of the male reproductive and genitourinary system that requires the lowest dose to control the disease is:
   a. prostate
   b. kidney
   c. seminoma
   d. bladder
9. The tumor of the male reproductive and genitourinary system for which a brachytherapy implant would be most likely used to control the disease is:
   a. prostate
   b. kidney
   c. testis
   d. bladder
10. The most common testicular tumor pathology is:
    a. seminoma
    b. choriocarcinoma
    c. teratoma
    d. embryonal carcinoma

The answers to the Review Questions can be found by logging on to our website at: *http://evolve.elsevier.com/Washington+Leaver/principles*

Questions to Ponder

1. Discuss the role of a digital rectal examination and prostate-specific antigen (PSA) in the screening of the prostate cancer.
2. Compare and contrast the following prognostic indicators related to carcinoma of the prostate: tumor stage, grade, PSA level, and race.
3. Examine the following specific treatment options for carcinoma of the prostate: surgery, external beam radiation therapy, brachytherapy, hormonal therapy, and chemotherapy.
4. Discuss the general management of cancer of the urinary bladder, surgery versus radiation.
5. Compare the treatments for testicular seminoma and nonseminoma.
6. Discuss the role of the radiation therapist in the treatment of patients with genitourinary tumors.

REFERENCES

1. Adolfsson J, Steineck G, Whitmore WF Jr: Recent results of management of palpable clinical localized prostate cancer, *Cancer* 72:310-322, 1993.
2. Albertsen PC, Hanley JA, Fine J: 20-year outcomes following conservative management of clinically localized prostate cancer, *JAMA* 293: 2095-2101, 2005.
3. American Cancer Society: *Cancer facts and figures: 2008*, Atlanta, 2008, American Cancer Society.
4. Anderson PM, et al: High-dose samarium-153 ethylene diamine tetramethylene phosphonate: low toxicity of skeletal irradiation in patients with osteosarcoma and bone metastases, *J Clin Oncol* 20:189-196, 2002.
5. Arterbery VE, et al: Quality of life after permanent prostate implant, *Semin Surg Oncol* 13:461-464, 1997.
6. Bagshaw MA, Ray GR, Cox RS: Radiotherapy of prostatic carcinoma: long-or short-term efficacy (Stanford University experience), *Urology* 25: 17-23, 1985.
7. Benson MC: Fine-needle aspiration of the prostate, *NCI Monogr* 7:19-24, 1988.
8. Blasko JC, et al: Prostate specific antigen based disease control following ultrasound guided 125 iodine implantation for stage T1/T2 prostatic carcinoma, *J Urol* 154:1096-1099, 1995.
9. Blasko JC, et al: Palladium-103 brachytherapy for prostate carcinoma, *Int J Radiat Oncol Biol Phys* 46:839-850, 2000.
10. Bolla, M, et al: Long-term results with immediate androgen suppression and external irradiation in patients with locally advanced prostate cancer (an EORTC study): a phase III randomized trail, *Lancet* 360:103-106, 2002.

11. Byar DP, Veterans Administration Cooperative Urological Research Group: Survival of patients with incidentally found microscopic cancer of the prostate: results of a clinical trial of conservative treatment, *J Urol* 108:908-913, 1972.

12. Catalona WJ, Bigg SW: Nerve-sparing radical prostatectomy: evaluation of results after 250 patients, *J Urol* 143:538-544, 1990.

13. Chodak GW, et al: Comparison of digital examination and transrectal ultrasonography for the diagnosis of prostate cancer, *J Urol* 135-951-954, 1986.

14. Chodak GW, et al: Results of conservative management of clinically localized cancer, *N Engl J Med* 330:242-248, 1994.

15. Coia LR, Hanks GE: Complications from large field intermediate dose infradiaphragmatic radiation: an analysis of the Patterns of Care Outcome Studies for Hodgkin's disease and seminoma, *Int J Radiat Oncol Biol Phys* 15:29-35, 1988.

16. Crawford ED, Dawkins CA: Cancer of the penis. In Skinner DG, Lieskovsky G, editors: *Diagnosis and management of genitourinary cancer*, Philadelphia, 1988, WB Saunders.

17. DeKernion JB, et al: Carcinoma of the penis, *Cancer* 32:1256-1262, 1973.

18. Duchesne GM, et al: Orchidectomy alone for stage I seminoma of the testis, *Cancer* 65:1115-1118, 1990.

19. Dugan TC, et al: Biopsy after external beam radiation therapy for adenocarcinoma of the prostate: correlation with original histological grade and current prostate specific antigen levels, *J Urol* 148:1565-1566, 1992.

20. Duncan W, Jackson SM: The treatment of early cancer of the penis with megavoltage X-rays, *Clin Radiol* 23:246-248, 1972.

21. Duncan W, Quilty PM: The results of a series of 963 patients with transitional cell carcinoma of the urinary bladder primarily treated by radical megavoltage x-ray therapy, *Radiother Oncol* 7:299-310, 1986.

22. Dunst J, et al: Organ-sparing treatment of advanced bladder cancer: a 10-year experience, *Int J Radiat Oncol Biol Phys* 30:261-266, 1994.

23. Eastham JA, Scardino PT: Radical prostatectomy for clinical stage and T2 prostate cancer. In Volgelzang NJ, et al, editors: *Comprehensive textbook of genitourinary oncology*, ed 2, Philadelphia, 2000, Lippincott Williams & Wilkins.

24. Einhorn LH, Richie JP, Shipley WU: Cancer of the testis. In DeVita VJ Jr, Hellman S, Rosenberg SA, editors: *Cancer: principles and practice of oncology*, ed 4, Philadelphia, 1993, JB Lippincott.

25. Eisenberger MA, De Witt R, Berry W, et al: A multicenter phase III comparison of docetaxel (D) + prednisone (P) and mioxantone (MTZ) + P in patients with hormone-refractory prostate cancer (HRPC). *J Clin Oncol* 22(Suppl):4, 2004.

26. Elwell CM, Jones, WG: *Comprehensive textbook of genioturinary oncology*, ed 2, Philadelphia, 2000, Lippincott Williams & Wilkins.

27. Emami BE, Pilepich MV: Anatomic considerations in radiotherapeutic management of bladder cancer, *Am J Clin Oncol* (CCT) 6:593-597, 1983.

28. Faysal MH, Freiha FS: Evaluation of partial cystectomy for carcinoma of bladder, *Urology* 14:352-356, 1979.

29. Fossa SD, et al: Optimal planning target volume for stage I testicular seminoma: A Medical Research Council randomized trail. Medical Research Council Testicular Tumor Working Group, *J Clin Oncol* 17(4):1146, 1999.

30. Fossa SD, Aass N, Kaalhus O: Radiotherapy for testicular seminoma stage I: treatment results and long-term post-irradiation morbidity in 365 patients, *Int J Radiat Oncol Biol Phys* 16:383-388, 1989.

31. Fraas BA, et al: Peripheral dose to the testes: the design and clinical use of a practical and effective gonadal shield, *Int J Radiat Oncol Biol Phys* 11:609-615, 1985.

32. Fraley EE, et al: Cancer of the penis: prognosis and treatment plans, *Cancer* 55:1618-1624, 1985.

33. Freeman GM, et al: Young patients with prostate cancer have an outcome justifying their treatment with external beam radiation, *Int J Radiat Oncol Biol Phys* 35:243-250, 1996.

34. Gleason DF, Veterans Administration Cooperative Urological Research Group: Histologic grading and clinical staging of prostatic carcinoma. In Tannenbaum M, editor: *Urologic pathology: the prostate*, Philadelphia, 1977, Lea and Febiger.

35. Golimbu M, et al: Renal cell carcinoma: survival and prognostic factors, *Urology* 27:291-301, 1986.

36. Gospodarowicz MK, et al: Radical radiotherapy for muscle invasive transitional cell carcinoma of the bladder: failure analysis, *J Urol* 142: 1448-1454, 1989.

37. Greene FL, et al: *AJCC Cancer Staging Handbook*, ed 6, New York, 2002, Springer-Verlag.

38. Hanks GE, et al: The outcome of treatment of 313 patients with T-1 (UICC) prostate cancer treated with external beam irradiation, *Int J Radiat Oncol Biol Phys* 14:243-248, 1988.

39. Hanks GE, et al: RTOG Protocol 92-02: A phase III trial of the use of long term total androgen suppression following neoadjuvant hormonal cytoreduction and radiotherapy in locally advanced carcinoma of the prostate, *Int J Radiat Oncol Biol Phys Suppl* 48(3):112, 2000.

40. Heaney JA, et al: Prognosis of clinically undiagnosed prostatic carcinoma and the influence of endocrine therapy, *J Urol* 118:283-287, 1977.

41. Huben RP, Mounzer AM, Murphy GP: Tumor grade and stage as prognostic variables in upper tract urothelial tumors, *Cancer* 62:2016-2020, 1988.

42. Huggins C, Stevens RE, Hodges CV: Studies on prostatic cancer II. The effects of castration on advanced carcinoma of the prostate gland, *Arch Surg* 43:209-223, 1941.

43. Huncharek M, Muscat J, Gesehwind JF: Planned preoperative radiation therapy in muscle invasive bladder cancer: results of a meta-analysis, *Anticancer Res* 18:1931-1934, 1998.

44. Jenkins BJ, et al: Reappraisal of the role of radical radiotherapy and salvage cystectomy in the treatment of invasive bladder cancer, *Br J Urol* 62:343-346, 1988.

45. Jones WG, et al: Randomized trail of 30 versus 20 Gy in the adjuvant treatment of stage I Testicular Seminoma: a report on medical research council trial TE188, European Organization for research and treatment of cancer trial 30942, *J Clin Oncol* 23(6): 1200-1208, 2005.

46. Kachnic LA, et al: Bladder preservation by combined modality therapy for invasive bladder cancer, *J Clin Oncol* 15:1022-1029, 1997.

47. Kjaer M: The treatment and prognosis of patients with renal adenocarcinoma with solitary metastasis 10 year survival results, *Int J Radiat Oncol Phys* 13:619-621, 1987.

48. Kuban DA, et al: Long term results of the MD Anderson randomized dose-escalation trial for prostate cancer, *Int J Radiat Oncol Biol Phys* 70:67-74, 2008.

49. Kuban DA, El-Mahdi AM, Schellhammer PF: PSA for outcome prediction and post-treatment evaluation following radiation for prostate cancer: do we know how to use it? *Semin Radiat Oncol* 8:72-78, 1998.

50. Kubo H, Shipley WU: Reduction of the scatter dose to the testicle outside the radiation treatment fields, *Int J Radiat Oncol Biol Phys* 8:1741-1745, 1982.

51. Kupelian P, et al: External beam radiotherapy versus radical prostatectomy for clinical stage T1-2 prostate cancer: therapeutic implications of stratification by pretreatment PSA levels and biopsy Gleason scores, *Cancer J Sci Am* 3:78-87, 1997.

52. Lai PP: Kidney, renal pelvis, and ureter. In Perez CA, Brady LW, editors: *Principles and practice of radiation oncology*, ed 2, Philadelphia, 1992, JB Lippincott.

53. Lai PP, et al: Radiation therapy for stage I and IIA testicular seminoma, *Int J Radiat Oncol Biol Phys* 28:373-379, 1993.

54. Lawton CA, et al: An update of the phase III trail comparing whole pelvic to prostate only radiotherapy and neoadjuvant to adjuvant total androgen suppression: updated analysis of RTOG 94-13, with emphasis on unexpected hormone/radiation interactions, *Int J Radiat Oncol Biol Phys* 69:646-655, 2007.

55. Lee RW, Hanks GE, Schultheiss TE: Role of radiation therapy in the management of stage T3 and T4 prostate cancer: rationale, technique, and results. In Volgelzang NJ, et al., editors: *Comprehensive textbook of genitourinary oncology*, ed 2, Philadelphia, 2000, Lippincott Williams & Wilkins.

56. Leibel SA, et al: The effects of local and regional treatment on the metastatic outcome in prostatic carcinoma with pelvic lymph node involvement, *Int J Radiat Oncol Biol Phys* 28:7-16, 1993.

57. Linehan WM, Shipley WU, Longo DL: Cancer of the kidney and ureter. In DeVita VT, Hellman S, Rosenberg SA, editors: *Cancer: principles and practice of oncology*, ed 3, Philadelphia, 1989, JB Lippincott.

58. Litwin MS, et al: Quality of life outcomes in men treated for localized prostate cancer, *JAMA* 273:129-135, 1995.

59. Logue JP, et al: Para-aortic radiation for stage I seminoma of the testis. *Int J Radiat Oncol Biol Phys* 48(suppl):208 (abstract no 192), 2000.

60. Maldazys JD, deKernion JB: Prognostic factors in metastatic renal carcinoma, *J Urol* 136:376-379, 1986.

61. Mameghan H, et al: Analysis of failure following definitive radiotherapy for invasive transitional cell carcinoma of the bladder, *Int J Radiat Oncol Biol Phys* 31:247-254, 1995.

62. Mandler JI, Pool T: Primary carcinoma of the male urethra, *J Urol* 96:67-72, 1966.

63. Montie JE, Straffon RA, Stewart RH: Radical cystectomy in men treated for localized prostate cancer, *JAMA* 273:129-135, 1995.

64. Mufti GR, et al: Transitional cell carcinoma of the renal pelvis and ureter, *Br J Urol* 63:135-140, 1989.

65. Narayana AS, et al: Carcinoma of the penis: analysis of 219 cases, *Cancer* 49:2185-2191, 1982.

66. Parsons JT, Million RR: Planned preoperative irradiation in the management of clinical stage B2-C (T3) bladder carcinoma, *Int J Radiat Oncol Biol Phys* 14:797-810, 1988.

67. Partin AW, Walsh PC: Management of stage B (T1c-T2) prostate cancer. Surgical management of localized prostate cancer. In Radhavan D, et al., editors: *Principles and practice of genitourinary oncology*, Philadelphia, 1997, Lippincott-Raven.

68. Partin AW, et al: Combination of prostate specific antigen, clinical stage and Gleason score to predict pathological stage in men with localized prostate cancer, *JAMA* 277:1445-1451, 1997.

69. Perez CA, Pilepich MV: Penis and male urethra. In Perez CA, Brady LW, editors: *Principles and practice of radiation oncology*, ed 2, Philadelphia, 1992, JB Lippincott.

70. Perez CA, et al: Factors influencing outcome of definitive radio-therapy for localized carcinoma of the prostate, *Radiother Oncol* 16:1-21, 1989.

71. Pilepich MV, et al: Prognostic factors in carcinoma of the prostate: analysis of RTOG Study 75-06, *Int J Radiat Oncol Biol Phys* 13:339-349, 1987.

72. Pilepich MV, et al: Androgen deprivation with radiation therapy compared with radiation therapy alone for locally advanced prostatic carcinoma: a randomized comparative trial of the Radiation Therapy Oncology Group, *Urology* 45:616-623, 1995.

73. Pollack A, et al: Prostate cancer radiation dose response: results of the M.D. Anderson phase III randomized trail. *Int. J Radiat Oncol Biol Phys*, 53:1097-1105, 2002.

74. Porter AT, et al: Results of randomized phase III trial to evaluate the efficacy of strontium-89 adjuvant to local external beam irradiation in the management of endocrine metastatic prostate cancer, *Int J Radiat Oncol Biol Phys* 25:805-813, 1993.

75. Powell BL, Craig JB, Muss HB: Secondary malignancies of the penis and epididymis: a case report and review of the literature, *J Clin Oncol* 3:110-116, 1985.

76. Pritchett TR, Lieskovsky G, Skinner DG: Clinical manifestations and treatment of renal parenchymal tumors. In Skinner DG, Lieskovsky G, editors: *Diagnosis and management of genitourinary tumors*, Philadelphia, 1988, WB Saunders.

77. Quilty PM, et al: Results of surgery following radical radiotherapy for invasive bladder cancer, *Br J Urol* 58:396-405, 1986.

78. Radhavaiah NV: Radiotherapy in the treatment of carcinoma of the male urethra, *Cancer* 41:1313-1316, 1978.

79. Reitelman C, et al: Prognostic variables in patients with transitional cell carcinoma of the renal pelvis and proximal ureter, *J Urol* 138:1144-1145, 1987.

80. Richie JP: Carcinoma of the renal pelvis and ureter. In Skinner DG, Lieskovsky G, editors: *Diagnosis and management of genitourinary tumors*, Philadelphia, 1988, WB Saunders.

81. Rifkin MD, et al: Comparison of magnetic resonance imaging and ultrasonography in staging early prostate cancer: results of a multi-institutional cooperative trial, *N Engl J Med* 323:621-626, 1990.

82. Roach M: The use of prostate specific antigen, clinical stage and Gleason score to predict pathological stage in men with localized prostate cancer, *J Urol* 150:1923-1924, 1993.

83. Roach M, et al: Predicting the risk of lymph node involvement using the pre-treatment prostate specific antigen and Gleason score in men with clinically localized prostate cancer, *Int J Radiat Oncol Biol Phys* 28:33-37, 1994.

84. Roach M III, et al: Phase III trial comparing whole-pelvic versus prostate-only radiotherapy and neoadjuvant versus adjuvant combined androgen suppression: Radiation Therapy Oncology Group 9413, *J Cln Oncol* 21(10):1904-1011, 2003.

85. Sagerman RH, et al: Stage II seminoma: results of postorchiectomy irradiation, *Radiology* 172:565-568, 1989.

86. Salaverria JE, et al: Conservative treatment of carcinoma of the penis, *Br J Urol* 51:32-37, 1979.

87. Schnall MD, et al: Prostate cancer: local staging with endorectal surface coil MR imaging, *Radiology* 178:797-802, 1991.

88. Shapiro E, et al: Effects of fractionated irradiation on endocrine aspects to testicular function, *J Clin Oncol* 3:1232-1239, 1985.

89. Shipley WU, et al: Selective bladder preservation by trimodality therapy for patients with muscularis propria-invasive bladder cancer and who are cystectomy candidates- The Massachusetts General hospital and Radiation Therapy Oncology Group Experiences, *Semin Radiat Oncol* 15:36-41, 2004.

90. Shipley WU, et al: Full-dose irradiation for patints with invasive bladder carcinoma: clinical and histological factors prognostic of improved survival, *J Urol* 134:679-683, 1985.

91. Shipley WU, et al: Phase III trial of neoadjuvant chemotherapy in patients with invasive bladder cancer treated with selective bladder preservation by combined radiation therapy and chemotherapy: Initial results of RTOG 89-03, *J Clin Oncol* 16:3576-3583, 1998.

92. Shipley WU, et al: Radiation therapy for clinically localized prostate cancer—a multi-institutional pooled analysis, *JAMA* 281:1598-1604, 1999.

93. Skinner DG, Liekovsky G: Management of invasive and high grade bladder cancer. In Skinner DG, Liekovsky G, editors: *Diagnosis and management of genitourinary cancer*, Philadelphia, 1988, WB Saunders.

94. Skinner DG, Tift JP, Kaufman JJ: High dose, short course preoperative radiation therapy and immediate single stage radical cystectomy with pelvic node dissection in the management of bladder cancer, *J Urol* 127:671-674, 1982.

95. Smith JA, et al: Treatment of advanced bladder cancer with combined preoperative irradiation and radical cystectomy versus radical cystectomy alone: a phase III intergroup study, *J Urol* 157:805-808, 1997.

96. Stadler WM, et al: *Comprehensive textbook of genitourinary oncology*, ed 2, Philidelphia, 2000, Lippincott, Williams and Wilkins.

97. Sternberg CN, et al: Chemotherapy for bladder cancer: treatment guidelines for neoadjuvant chemotherapy, bladder preservation, adjuvant chemotherapy, and metastatic cancer, *Urology* 69:62-79, 2007.

98. Stock RG, et al: A dose-response study for I-125 prostate implants, *Int J Radiat Oncol Biol Phys* 41:101-108, 1998.

99. Storey MR, et al: Complications from dose escalation in prostate cancer: preliminary results of a randomized trial, *Int J Radiat Oncol Biol Phys* 48:635-642, 2000.

100. Terry PJ, Cookson MS, Sarosdy MF: Carcinoma of the urethra and scrotum. Om Ragajavon D, et al, editors: *Principles and practice of genitourinary oncology*, Philadelphia, 1997, Lippincott-Raven.

101. Thomas G, et al: Consensus statement on the investigation and management of testicular seminoma 1989, *EORTC Genitourinary Group Monogr* 7:285-294, 1990.

102. Travis LB et al: Second cancers among 40,576 testicula cancer patients: focus on long-term survivors. *J Natl Cancer Inst* 97(18): 1354-1365, 2005.

103. University of Texas MD Anderson Cancer Center: *Proton Therapy Centre* (website): http://www.mdanderson.org/care_centers/radiationonco/ptc/. Accessed November 28, 2007.

104. Warde P, et al: Stage I testicular seminoma: results of adjuvant irradiation and surveillance, *J Clin Oncol* 13:2255-2262, 1995.

105. Worgul TJ, et al: Clinical and biochemical effect of aminoglutethimide in the treatment of advanced prostatic carcinoma, *J Urol* 129:51-55, 1983.

106. Yagoda A, Petrylak D: Cytotoxic chemotherapy for advanced hormone-resistant prostate cancer. *Cancer* 71:1098, 1993.

107. Zagars GK: Stage I testicular seminoma following orchidectomy: to treat or not to treat, *Eur J Cancer* 14:1923-1924, 1993.

108. Zagars GK, Babaian RJ: The role of radiation in stage II testicular seminoma, *Int J Radiat Oncol Biol Phys* 13:163-170, 1987.

109. Zagars GK, Pollack A, Pettaway CA: Prostate cancer in African-American men: outcome following radiation therapy or without adjuvant androgen ablation, *Int J Radiat Oncol Biol Phys* 42:517-523, 1998.

110. Zagars GK, Pollack A, Smith LG: Conventional external-beam radiation therapy alone or with androgen ablation for clinical stage III (T3, NX/N0, M0) adenocarcinoma of the prostate, *Int J Radiat Oncol Biol Phys* 44:809-819, 1999.

111. Zelefsky MJ, et al: High dose radiation delivered by intensity modulated conformal radiotherapy improves the outcome of localized prostate cancer, *J Urol* 176:1415-1419, 2006.

112. Zelefsky MJ, et al: High dose radiation delivered by intensity modulated conformal radiotherapy improves the outcome of localized prostate cancer, *J Urol* 166:876-881, 2001.

113. Zietman Al, et al: *JAMA* 294:1233-1239, 2005.

Breast Cancer

George M. Uschold, Hong Zhang

Outline

Key Terms

Objectives

- Discuss epidemiologic factors of this tumor site.
- Identify, list, and discuss etiologic factors that may be responsible for inducing tumors in this anatomic site.
- Describe the symptoms produced by a malignant tumor in this region.
- Discuss the methods of detection and diagnosis for tumors in this anatomic region.
- List the varying histologic types of tumors generic to this region.
- Describe the diagnostic procedures used in the work-up and staging for this site.
- Describe the clinical classification used for this area.
- Describe in detail the most common routes of tumor spread for this site.
- Describe and diagram the lymphatic routes of spread for tumors in this region.
- Differentiate between histologic grading and staging.
- Describe in detail the anatomy and physiology of this anatomic region/organ.
- Identify the treatment(s) of choice for this malignancy.
- Discuss the rationale for treatment with regard to treatment choice, histologic type, and stage of the disease.

- Describe in detail the treatment methods available for this diagnosis.
- Describe the differing types of radiation treatments that can be used for treating this tumor site.
- Identify the appropriate tumor lethal dose for various stages of this malignancy.
- Discuss the expected radiation reactions for the area based on time-dose-fractionation schemes.
- Discuss tolerance levels of the vital structures and organs at risk.
- Describe the instructions that should be given to a patient with regard to skin care, expected reactions, and dietary advice.
- Identify the psychological problems associated with a malignancy in this site.
- Discuss the rationale for using multimodality treatments for this diagnosis.
- Describe the various treatment planning techniques for this anatomic site including external beam and brachytherapy options.
- Discuss survival statistics and prognosis for various stages for this tumor site.

HISTORICAL PERSPECTIVE

The recorded history of the treatment of breast cancer dates back 5000 years to a document known as the "Edwin Smith Papyrus." Written between 3000 and 2500 BC, the papyrus discusses surgical and other treatments for illnesses afflicting the ancient Egyptians. A translation of the document, first published in 1930, reveals that at the time there was thought to be no treatment for what were most likely malignant tumors of the breast.

Several millennia later, Hippocrates (460 to 370 BC), the revered Greek physician who gave the name *carcinoma* to malignant disease, referred only twice to breast cancer. Both references describe advanced disease that resulted in the patient's death. He thought that it was better not to treat deep-seated cancer, because in his experience, treatment only hastened death. Hippocrates taught that cancer was caused by an excess or imbalance of "black bile" in the body.[46] Therefore, medical belief of the day was that cancer is a systemic disease and essentially incurable.

During the time of the Roman Empire, physicians performed surgery for breast cancer, sometimes using an extremely aggressive approach that included removal of the pectoralis muscles. This approach was later discouraged by Aulus Celsus, an important scholar of the early first century AD. Celsus argued that cancer of the breast was "irritated" by the surgeon's intervention, which hastened the patient's death; therefore, he recommended treatment with "mild medicines."

Leonidus, a Greek physician from the first century AD, described the surgical procedure he used for breast cancer. He removed the breast with a margin of normal-appearing tissue and was careful to stop the bleeding during surgery through the use of cautery (heat).

Claudius Galen (138 to 201 AD), a physician who was educated in Greece and practiced in Rome, became the authority on medicine for the next 1000 years. Galen subscribed to Hippocrates' black bile theory of the systemic nature of cancer, and he recommended no intervention in the course of the disease.

During the 1000 years that comprised the Medieval period, or Dark Ages, which followed the fall of the Roman Empire, essentially no advances were made in the scientific understanding of cancer or any human illnesses. This was a period of political and religious activity, to the exclusion of scientific endeavor. Restrictions placed on the study and practice of medicine by religious authorities, and adherence to the teachings of Galen as all encompassing left the world of medicine basically unchanged for a millennium. Despite the lack of advancement between 500 and 1500 AD, knowledge of medicine and an appreciation for learning were kept alive in monasteries. Eventually, the foundations for future progress were laid in the eleventh century, when several medical schools came into existence in cities such as Paris and Oxford.

In the middle of the sixteenth century, Andreas Vesalius published *De Humani Corporis Fabrica*, the work that established the science of human anatomy. Humans were no longer bound by religious dictum and centuries of tradition. Increasingly, extensive surgical techniques were developed. The seventeenth century saw the treatment of breast cancer evolve to include the excision of enlarged axillary lymph nodes at the time of mastectomy. However, in the days before anesthesia and asepsis, surgery of any kind was fraught with danger for patients, many of whom died from overwhelming infection.

A revolution in thinking relative to the nature of breast cancer occurred in the mid-eighteenth century, when French surgeons Henri Le Dran and Jean Louis Petit theorized that the disease originated locally in the breast and was not initially systemic. They believed the malignancy spread from its primary site in the breast to involve regional lymph nodes and ultimately to disseminate widely via the circulatory system. As a result, physicians of the day realized an opportunity to cure patients if the cancer could be removed early in its course and if local control could be established. Therefore, wide surgical excision with axillary dissection and removal of the pectoralis muscle was advised.

With the advent of anesthesia, antisepsis, and the ability to examine tissue microscopically in the mid-nineteenth century, radical breast surgery evolved rapidly. William Stewart Halsted perfected the technique of radical mastectomy at the end of the nineteenth century (Figure 38-1). For the first time, a dramatic improvement in local recurrence and overall survival rates could be demonstrated. The Halstedian approach remained preeminent until the mid-twentieth century.

Current concepts in the treatment of breast cancer include a much less radical role for surgery and the emergence of radiation therapy and systemic drug treatment, all of which have permitted a conservative, breast-preserving approach for women with relatively early disease. Although great strides have been made in the detection and treatment of breast cancer, it remains a disease that defies complete control. Approximately 21% of women who have breast cancer die of the disease.[55] Therefore, the need exists for continued research into improved treatment modalities, earlier diagnoses, and, ultimately, the prevention of breast cancer.

EPIDEMIOLOGY

Incidence

According to American Cancer Society (ACS) statistics, breast cancer is the most common malignant disease in American women. It affects an estimated 182,460 new patients each year in the United States, making it the second major cause of cancer death preceded only by lung cancer.[1] Current data indicate that every woman has approximately a one-in-eight chance of developing breast cancer over her lifetime. The incidence rate rose in the 1980s, correlating with diagnostic advances and the increased use of mammography. However, incidence rates dropped significantly in 2003, when many postmenopausal women began discontinuing the long-term use of hormone replacement therapy after it was found to be associated with an increased risk of having breast cancer.[39] In addition, breast cancer is diagnosed in about 1990 men each year.[1]

Risk Factors

Gender. The most significant risk factor for breast cancer is gender. The female-to-male incidence ratio is approximately 100:1. In men, breast cancer represents less than 1% of all malignancies.[1] Major risk factors for women are listed in Box 38-1.

Age. Older women have the highest probability of developing breast cancer. Women 65 to 79 years old have an incidence rate of 423 per 100,000. This is double the rate for women 40 to 59 years old, whose incidence rate is 215 per 100,000.[41] Although incidence rates are higher for older persons, these patients represent only a small number of the total cases.

Incidence rises steadily during the reproductive years after age 30. The median age of onset is approximately 55 years, with the predominant age group between 40 and 70 years.[15]

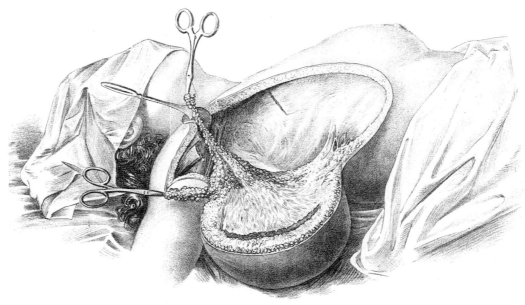

Figure 38-1. A technique of radical mastectomy at the end of the nineteenth century at Johns Hopkins. This is where Dr. William Halsted perfected the technique of radical mastectomy. (Courtesy of The Alan Mason Chesney Medical Archives of the John Hopkins Medical Institution, Baltimore, MD.)

A slight decrease in incidence occurs in the perimenopausal years, followed by a gradual rise during postmenopausal years. The decrease in incidence is attributed to hormonal changes that occur during menopause.

Family History. Genetic associations and racial differences in breast cancer rates suggest inherited tendencies toward development of the disease. Although hereditary patterns may be partially attributed to shared risk factors such as dietary and environmental factors, a genetic association is strongly suggested. Family history appears to be significant because female relatives of women with breast cancer have a higher incidence than the general population. Indeed, a recent population-based, case-control study concluded that 33% of breast cancer cases in patients aged 20 to 29 are genetically attributable. This rate, however, markedly decreases in older patients, down to nearly 2% in patients aged 70 to 79.[10]

The probability of developing breast cancer is double or triple for women whose mothers and/or sisters (first-degree relatives) have the disease, especially if the family members were diagnosed at a young age.[37] Women with a strong family history of breast cancer must follow a good breast health program.

The genes *BRCA1* and *BRCA2* are associated with up to an 85% likelihood of breast cancer development. This particular type of heritable breast cancer accounts for less than 10% of all cases. Currently, women of families with multiple cases of breast cancer may be tested for this gene so that the risk will be known.

Hormonal Factors. Risk factors for breast cancer are influenced by hormonal variables, as listed in Box 38-2. These risk factors appear to reflect menstrual and childbearing history. Early **menarche** (the beginning of menstruation) and late **menopause** (the ending of menstruation) increase breast cancer risk. **Oophorectomy** (removal of one or both ovaries) before age 50 appears to reduce risk.[55] These facts lead to a general assumption that the overall length of ovarian function is related to breast cancer risk.

Women who have given birth to a child (parous women) have less risk than women who have never been pregnant

Box 38-1	Major Risk Factors for Breast Cancer

- Gender
- Age
- Family history
- Hormonal factors
- Personal history of breast cancer
- History of benign breast disease
  - Atypical hyperplasia
  - Lobular carcinoma in situ

Box 38-2	Hormonal Influences on Breast Cancer Risk

- Ovarian function
  - Age at menarche
  - Age at menopause
  - Oophorectomy
- Parity
- Hormonal manipulation

(nulliparous women). Pregnancy later in life increases the risk more than nulliparity. Women who give birth to their first child after age 35 are twice as likely to develop breast cancer as are women who give birth to their first child before age 20.[55]

Hormonal manipulation, relative to progesterone and estrogen, has also been associated with an increased incidence of breast cancer. Women who are taking hormone replacement therapy (used to alleviate menopausal symptoms) are at an increased risk of being diagnosed with breast cancer, and this risk further increases with prolonged use.[11,12] However, any increased risk disappears approximately 5 years after cessation of therapy. Women taking oral contraceptives (used to prevent ovulation) are at a slightly increased risk of being diagnosed with breast cancer during use and within 10 years of cessation of oral contraceptive use, but there is no increased risk noted after 10 years.[11,12]

History of Malignancy. A history of breast cancer, either invasive or **ductal carcinoma in situ (DCIS)** (cancer confined to the breast), in one breast increases the risk for development of cancer in the opposite breast. This risk increases for women treated curatively for breast cancer at a relatively young age. Breast cancer patients must be closely monitored for the development of a contralateral breast malignancy.

History of Benign Breast Disease. Benign breast disease encompasses a variety of histologic subcategories associated with varying degrees of cancer risk. Women with **atypical hyperplasia** or lobular carcinoma in situ have an increased risk of developing breast cancer. These abnormal findings, in association with a family history of breast cancer, may have increased the risk by 11-fold.[17,36]

Dietary and Environmental Factors. International differences in breast cancer rates have been well documented. Incidence rates are higher in Europe, Canada, and the United States and lower in Asia and developing countries such as Mexico. Dietary fat intake, long suspected as a risk factor for breast cancer, has been found to have no association.[27] However, a positive association of alcohol consumption and breast cancer risk has been documented, correlating with the amount of intake.[47]

Radiation Exposure. Radiation exposure causes breast cancer. However, the issue is complicated by numerous variables, including the type and quality of radiation, frequency of exposure, and magnitude of dose. Retrospective studies of women exposed to low levels of radiation for the monitoring of tuberculosis or treatment of benign conditions such as postpartum mastitis or fibroadenomas of the breast indicate increased breast cancer incidence. Subsequently, the treatment of nonmalignant conditions with radiation has been almost completely abandoned.

Much information on cancer induction by radiation exposure has been gained from the study of Hiroshima and Nagasaki atomic bomb survivors. A series of reports have been prepared by the National Research Council's committees on the biological effects of ionizing radiations (BEIR). The BEIR V report indicates that radiation-induced cancer is dose and time dependent and that the latent period appears to be relatively long (between 20 and 30 years).[13] The risk of breast cancer resulting from radiation appears to be greatest for women exposed at a relatively young age.

A threshold dose for breast cancer induction by radiation has not been determined. It is possible that exposure at levels similar to that of natural background radiation carries no risk. Based on current knowledge, the risk of radiation-induced breast cancer rarely contraindicates medically necessary radiation exposure.

PROGNOSTIC INDICATORS

Box 38-3 lists prognostic indicators for breast cancer; however, the list continues to expand through clinical and laboratory research. The pathologic staging system incorporates the most important factors, including the lymph node status, extent of the tumor, and presence of distant metastasis.

Lymph Node Status

The number of axillary lymph nodes involved by a tumor is the most important prognostic indicator and is a significant aspect of staging. A higher number of involved nodes correlates with an increased recurrence rate and a decreased survival rate. At least 10 axillary nodes must be evaluated to separate low risk (fewer than three nodes positive for tumor) from high risk (four or more nodes positive for tumor). The prognosis for patients with more than 10 axillary lymph nodes positive for tumor is extremely poor. The involvement of internal mammary (IM) lymph nodes by cancer, with or without axillary lymph node involvement, further reduces disease-free survival rates. Similarly, supraclavicular lymph node involvement implies a poor prognosis.

Tumor Extent

The size of the primary tumor is another aspect of the staging system that serves as a prognostic indicator. Larger tumors increase the likelihood of involvement of the skin, muscle, chest wall, and regional lymph nodes, resulting in a worse overall prognosis. The 5-year survival rate for patients with lesions less than 0.5 cm is 99%, whereas the rate associated with lesions larger than 0.5 cm is 82%. With regional lymph node metastasis, 4.5-cm tumors have a 70% incidence rate of nodal involvement, whereas 1.5-cm tumors have a 38% incidence rate.[7]

Although tumor location by quadrant influences the pattern of lymph node metastasis, no evidence indicates that the location of the primary tumor directly affects the prognosis. The fixation of a mass to the chest wall involves significant negative staging and prognostic implications.

Histology

Infiltrating ductal carcinoma is the most common histologic type of breast malignancy, accounting for 70% to 80% of all

Box 38-3	Prognostic Indicators for Breast Cancer

- Lymph node status
- Tumor extent
- Histology grade
- Estrogen and progesterone receptor, *HER-2/neu* status
- Other laboratory studies

breast cancers. Infiltrating lobular carcinoma is the next most common type, comprising about 5% to 10% of breast cancers.

There are several other relatively rare types of infiltrating breast cancer, such as mucinous or colloid, tubular, and papillary carcinoma. These lesions have distinct histologic characteristics and tend to yield a more favorable prognosis.

Inflammatory Carcinoma

Tumors classified as inflammatory carcinoma yield an extremely poor prognosis. The diagnosis of inflammatory cancer is based on pathologic evidence of malignancy and clinical findings of breast tenderness and enlargement, peau d'orange appearance, erythema, warmth, and diffuse induration of the skin.

Estrogen and Progesterone Receptor, HER-2/neu Status

Samples of tumor tissue should be analyzed to determine the level of expression of estrogen, progesterone, and *HER-2/neu* receptors on the cells. This information and other factors indicate the potential response to hormonal therapy. Patients who are receptor positive are more likely to respond to hormonal therapy. In general, patients with estrogen/progesterone receptor (ER/PR) receptor–positive tumors have a better outcome than those with receptor-negative tumors.[55] *HER-2/neu* expression has been associated with poor outcome.[56]

Other Laboratory Studies

Tumor proliferation rate, extent of angiogenesis, expression of *p53* gene, and other gene profiling studies may provide important prognostic information and guide treatment decision making in this era of molecular targeting.

Survival

Advancements in methods of detection and treatment of breast cancer have resulted in improved survival rates at all stages. The overall 5-year survival rate, as indicated by women who survive 5 years after the initial diagnosis (regardless of disease status), is 89%. The 5-year survival rate decreases to 83% if evidence exists of regional spread and to 20% if distant metastasis is present at the time of the diagnosis.[1] Survival rates correlate with early detection, tumor characteristics, the treatment approach, and the patient's general condition.

However, 5-year survival is not the best indicator of survival for breast cancer patients. Because of breast cancer's systemic nature, patients may relapse up to 20 years or more after treatment, and few options are available for cure after relapse.

ANATOMY

Embryology

The breast evolves from sudoriferous (sweat) gland tissue. Early in human fetal development, the galactic band or milk streak develops, extending bilaterally from the axilla to the inguinal region. The portion of the band located on the thoracic trunk continues to develop, with the appearance of cells that form the nipple, areola, and ultimately all tissues of the breast. The remainder of the band regresses and disappears.

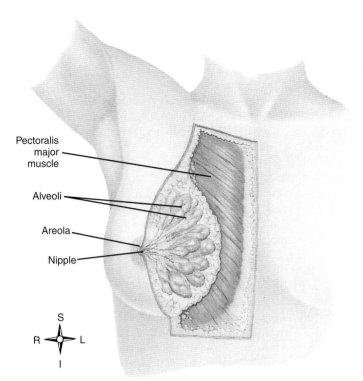

Figure 38-2. Dissected view of the breast. (From Thibodeau GA, Patton KT: *Anatomy and physiology*, ed 6, St. Louis, 2007, Mosby.)

Location and Extent

The protuberant portion of the adult breast is located between the second and sixth ribs in the sagittal plane and extends from the sternochondral junctions to the midaxillary line in the axial plane. Additional breast tissue is often present beyond these margins, particularly medially and superiorly. Breast tissue is also in the axilla, which is referred to as the axillary tail of Spence. The average diameter of the gland at its base is 10 to 12 cm, and the average central thickness is 5 to 6 cm.

Structure

The breast parenchyma consists of 15 to 20 sections or lobes that are embedded in adipose (fat) tissue. Each lobe is drained by a system of ducts that open at the nipple. In each lobe are numerous lobules that contain the milk-producing alveoli. The subcutaneous tissues of the breast also include fat, connective tissue, circulatory and lymphatic vessels, and nerve supply (Figures 38-2 and 38-3).

The skin overlying the breast is thin and contains sweat glands, hair follicles, and sebaceous (oil) glands. The circular, pigmented area surrounding the nipple is the areola. The nipple and areola are largely composed of smooth muscle tissue and contain sweat and sebaceous glands.

Musculature

The breast is contiguous with or in close proximity to several functionally important muscles: the pectoralis major and minor, serratus anterior, and latissimus dorsi. The breast lies over the pectoralis major and serratus anterior muscles and is attached to them by a layer of connective tissue, the deep pectoral fascia.

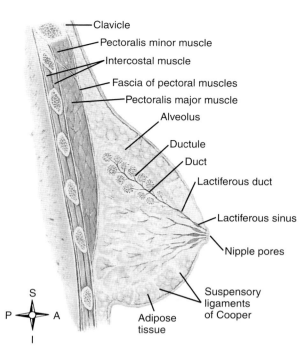

Figure 38-3. Sagittal section of the breast. (From Thibodeau GA, Patton KT: *Anatomy and physiology*, ed 6, St. Louis, 2007, Mosby.)

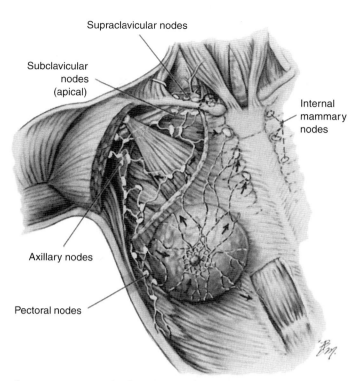

Figure 38-4. Lymph drainage and lymph node groups of the breast. (From Cox JD, editor: *Moss' radiation oncology: rationale, technique, results*, ed 7, St. Louis, 1994, Mosby.)

The superficial pectoral fascia encompasses the breast tissue and is attached to the deep fascia by bands of connective tissue called Cooper's suspensory ligaments, which support the breast. Surgical approaches to breast cancer have historically involved the removal of several of these muscles, at times producing significant disfigurement and functional deficit.

Blood Supply

Arteries. The major arterial supply to the breast is via the branches of the IM artery. Several branches of the axillary artery provide blood to the lateral aspect of the breast, most notably the lateral thoracic artery.

Veins. The deep venous drainage of the breast lies along three major routes that play significant roles in the development of blood-borne metastasis from breast cancer. The IM vein, axillary vein, and intercostal veins empty into the pulmonary capillaries via the superior vena cava, allowing metastatic spread into the lung.

In addition, the intercostal veins communicate with the vertebral plexus of Batson, a system of small veins running vertically through and around the vertebral column. This system drains the proximal humeri, shoulders, skull, vertebral bodies, bony pelvis, and proximal femurs. Venous blood can flow in both directions in this system because of the absence of valves and low pressure in the channels. Malignant cells in the blood draining through the intercostal veins from the breast can therefore enter the axial skeleton, resulting in metastatic disease.

Lymphatic Drainage

Lymph Vessels. Two sets of lymphatic channels are associated with the breast. These were first delineated in the late eighteenth century by Cruikshank and Mascagni, who used injections of mercury on cadavers to visualize the lymphatics of this area.[14,35] The first group of lymphatics is superficial and drains the skin covering the breast. The second is a deep group that drains the internal breast tissues. The superficial and deep groups of lymphatics communicate with each other extensively, a fact that has implications for the management of breast cancer.[23] Figure 38-4 illustrates lymphatic channels of the breast.

Axillary Lymph Nodes. Primary deep lymphatic drainage of the breast occurs to the ipsilateral axilla. Between 10 and 38 lymph nodes are in each axilla. These can be divided into three major sections (levels I, II, and III) based on location and sequential drainage patterns. Nodes in level I are located lowest, or most superficially, in the axilla and represent the first station of drainage from the breast. These are followed by nodes in levels II and III, which are positioned at increasing height in the axilla.[24] Studies in the 1800s first demonstrated that 70% of the lymphatic drainage of the breast occurs to the axilla, with 30% going to the IM nodes.

Internal Mammary Lymph Nodes. The IM lymph nodes are located near the edge of the sternum, embedded in fat in the intercostal spaces. Most IM nodes are in the first, second, and third intercostal spaces, with the average person having approximately eight small nodes (four per side).[24]

Supraclavicular Lymph Nodes. In addition to direct drainage to the previously mentioned nodal groups, lymphatic drainage occurs from the breast to the supraclavicular nodes, liver, and contralateral IM nodes.

NATURAL HISTORY

Sites of Origin

The location of a primary breast tumor is best described by dividing the breast into quadrants. As shown in Figure 38-5, approximately 48% of breast cancers arise in the upper-outer quadrant, 15% in the upper-inner quadrant, 11% in the lower-outer quadrant, 6% in the lower-inner quadrant, and 17% in the subareolar area (around the nipple, where the ducts converge); an additional 3% are multicentric.[55] The higher frequency of cancers in the upper-outer quadrant is explained by the fact that more breast tissue is contained in this area. Breast cancer rarely appears in both breasts (bilaterally).

The term *multicentric* describes tumors that appear in several areas of the breast. Multifocal breast cancer denotes a situation in which elements of a tumor are contained in tissue near the primary lesion in the same quadrant. Multifocal breast cancer is more common than multicentric cancer and is prognostically more favorable.[55]

Tumor Progression

Breast cancer tends to grow locally, involving the ducts and adjacent tissues, and may spread to local and regional lymphatics. Left untreated, the cancer can become fixed in position, and the overlying skin may become infiltrated by the tumor, eventually causing ulceration. Disease involving the dermal lymphatics is a sign of inflammatory cancer.

The involvement of axillary lymph nodes occurs in an orderly and progressive manner. Large tumor size and multicentricity are highly associated with axillary lymph node involvement. Lesions of the upper-outer quadrant more frequently metastasize to the axillary lymph nodes, whereas lesions of the medial quadrants and central area have a tendency to metastasize to the IM lymph nodes. Progressive involvement of supraclavicular lymph nodes may also occur.

Recurrence

Breast cancer can recur in the breast (local recurrence), in the lymphatics (regional recurrence), or at distant metastatic sites. Patients with local recurrence after conservative treatment can be treated with additional surgery. Patients who experience regional recurrence are usually treated with systemic therapy and, if possible, surgical resection.

Distant Metastasis

Breast cancer can spread to distant sites via invasion of the blood vessels, followed by hematogenous spread to other sites. Distant metastatic sites include bone, lung, brain, liver, eyes, ovaries, and the adrenal and pituitary glands.

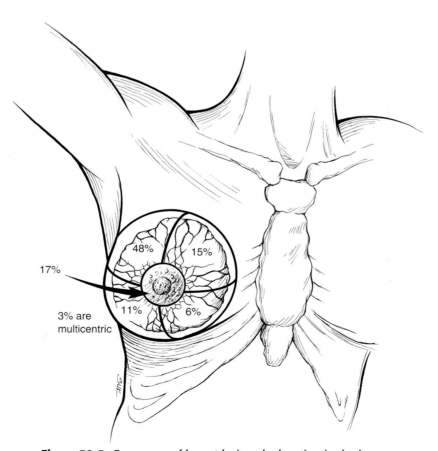

Figure 38-5. Frequency of breast lesions by location in the breast.

CLINICAL PRESENTATION

With early detection, breast cancer is one of the most curable malignant diseases. A three-step breast health program is recommended for all women. This program includes a monthly self-examination, an annual clinical examination by a qualified medical professional, and a routine mammographic examination as defined by established guidelines. Women must pay careful attention to breast cancer warning signs. Presenting symptoms of breast cancer are listed in Box 38-4.

Although most changes of the breast are benign, 20% of all masses are malignant. The potential for a diagnosis of malignancy, combined with the shortness of breast tumor doubling time, warrants immediate attention and close follow-up of women with breast complaints. Women who follow a good breast health program and seek medical attention promptly after the detection of breast changes may benefit from an early diagnosis and treatment, ultimately leading to a better outcome.

Breast Mass

The most common presentation of breast cancer is a painless lump. Unfortunately, by the time a breast lesion is palpable, it has already grown to about 0.5 cm. Small lesions can be difficult to detect, especially if they are deep within breast tissues. The assessment of a breast mass must address the size, shape, consistency, mobility, pain or tenderness, location in the breast, and relation to skin and surrounding tissues. The opposite breast should be compared for asymmetry. A clinical history relative to known risk factors, a physical assessment of the mass, and a biopsy of a suspicious lesion are critical to the proper management of a patient who has a breast mass.

In premenopausal women, glandular breast tissues tend to change throughout the menstrual cycle. For this reason the evaluation of a breast mass over one or two menstrual cycles may be necessary. An aspiration, biopsy, or both may be recommended for a persistent mass.

 Because benign breast conditions (including cysts) are more rare postmenopausally, palpable breast masses in postmenopausal women tend to be highly suspicious and warrant a biopsy.

Nipple Discharge or Retraction

The sudden onset of nonlactational serous discharge from one breast is the second most common symptom of breast cancer. Nipple retraction and tenderness or pain in the nipple may also

suggest cancer. Nipple changes must also be investigated for benign diagnoses, including cystic mastopathy, intraductal papilloma, and Paget's disease.

Skin Changes and Alterations in Breast Contour

Changes in skin texture, dimpling, irritation, increased warmth, scaling, pain, and ulceration of the skin are breast cancer symptoms requiring careful evaluation. Other types of symptomatic changes include distortion of the normal breast contour, swelling, and thickening of subcutaneous tissues. Peau d'orange, a condition in which the skin develops an orange peel appearance, is a clinical sign of inflammatory breast cancer.

Lymphadenopathy

Occasionally, the first sign of breast cancer is the enlargement of an axillary lymph node. Cervical, supraclavicular, and axillary lymph nodes drain breast tissues and require careful assessment. Arm edema may also be a sign of lymph node involvement.

Mammographic Abnormality

A mammogram and a clinical examination of the breast can detect small, discrete lesions and chest wall involvement. On a mammogram, breast cancer typically appears as an ill-defined, opacified lesion with or without spiculated margins, as demonstrated in Figure 38-6.

Mammographic breast cancer screening is recommended for improving survival rates through early detection. Patients with

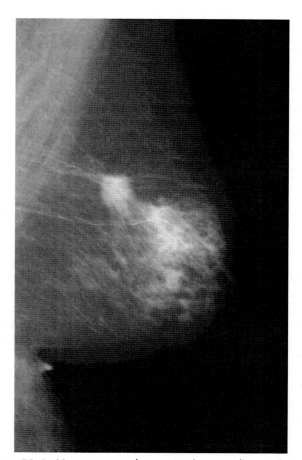

Figure 38-6. Mammogram demonstrating a malignant lesion.

Box 38-4	Clinical Presentation of Breast Cancer

- Breast mass
- Nipple discharge or retraction
- Skin changes
- Alteration in breast contour
- Lymphadenopathy
- Mammographic abnormality
- Distant metastasis

an incidental finding of breast cancer through a mammography tend to have the best prognosis.

Distant Metastasis

Distant metastasis (most commonly in the form of bone, lung, brain, or liver involvement) may be present at the time of the diagnosis. Patients with distant metastasis (stage IV disease) have an extremely poor prognosis. Discomfort from the metastatic site is usually not the patient's only symptom; however, it provides the patient with the impetus for seeking medical attention. As a result of improvements in health education, awareness, detection, and diagnosis, fewer patients exhibit distant metastasis at the time of the diagnosis.

DETECTION AND DIAGNOSIS

As the most common malignancy in women, cancer of the breast affects one in every eight women in the United States.[1] Such a widespread disease merits the continued development of screening and detection methods that provide the earliest possible diagnosis because early lesions can be highly curable.[45,49] Important features of breast cancer screening and detection methods include cost effectiveness, accuracy, **specificity** (the probability that a test will be negative for an instance when no disease if present), safety, and availability.

The medical community has made great progress in this regard. As recently as several decades ago, most breast cancer patients were first treated in an advanced stage of disease. Fear and ignorance played a large role in preventing earlier diagnoses. Women were not cognizant of the need to examine their own breasts and thus were often not aware of any change until it became obtrusive. In addition, women were not anxious to hear that they needed a radical mastectomy, and they often delayed seeking medical attention. Surgical treatment for breast cancer was perceived as disfiguring and defeminizing and was often psychologically traumatic for the patient.

Detection

As a result of public education campaigns by the ACS and other groups, many breast cancers are diagnosed early (i.e., at a smaller size and before involvement of the lymph nodes). Such tumors can often be successfully treated without removal of the breast.

The ACS periodically publishes updated recommendations for the detection of breast cancer. The current cornerstones of breast cancer detection are breast self-examination (BSE), clinical breast examination, and mammographic screening.

Breast Self-Examination. BSE is widely regarded as a simple and effective means of familiarizing women with the consistency and feel of their breasts, thereby allowing them to detect changes. The ACS recommends that women examine their breasts monthly, particularly at the same point each month relative to their menstrual cycle.

Varying reports describe the effectiveness of BSE in terms of its influence on the stage of disease at the time of the diagnosis and on survival rates. Some retrospective studies found a lower mortality rate among women who had breast cancer and practiced BSE. One reported that women who had been given a brochure on BSE had somewhat smaller tumors at the time of diagnosis.

BSE can be effective only if performed correctly. Educational materials are available that describe the technique, the frequency of examinations, the position of the body during an examination, and the way to palpate the breast and axillary tissue.

Clinical Breast Examination. A clinical breast examination is an important aspect of breast cancer detection. Physicians and other health professionals perform this procedure, which can detect tumors as small as 0.5 cm in diameter. The skin over the breast is evaluated for color and textural changes. With the patient in the sitting and supine positions, the breast is examined visually and by palpation for mobility and the presence of a mass. The presence of chest wall fixation is assessed through a series of muscle-tensing maneuvers by the patient. Dimpling of the skin, nipple discharge, and axillary lymph node enlargement are evaluated during the clinical examination.

Mammographic Screening. Mammography is a powerful tool in the quest for early detection of breast cancer. However, aspects of mammographic screening remain controversial. One of the major sources of contention is disagreement concerning the ideal interval for mammographic screening. The ACS and American College of Obstetrics and Gynecology recommend that asymptomatic women between the ages 35 and 39 who are at an average risk for developing breast cancer should obtain a baseline mammogram.

 Starting at age 40, all women should have a mammogram done every year.

Numerous prospective, randomized trials have demonstrated the efficacy of mammography in the screening of asymptomatic women for breast cancer. In addition, mammography remains the only modality that routinely detects breast cancer if the lesion is too small to feel during a clinical examination.

Mammography is not without limitations. Mammograms miss 10% to 15% of small and moderate-size breast cancers. This is often due to radiographic overlap between glandular and tumor tissue, rendering the tumor difficult to discern. Because of the relative radiographic similarity of glandular and tumor tissue, mammographic findings are often not specific for malignancy, resulting in numerous invasive diagnostic procedures (biopsies) that are negative for malignancy. Several studies have shown as few as one biopsy positive for tumor for every seven performed. Other series show that approximately one of three and one-half biopsies are positive for cancer. Most centers today have similar results.

Another problem affecting the efficacy of mammography as a screening tool is the lack of its access for many women. Not all insurance policies cover mammographic screening, and uninsured women in lower socioeconomic strata are often unable to pay the cost of screenings. Through the efforts of many individuals and organizations, low-cost screening programs have been made available, but a pressing need for services remains for millions of economically disadvantaged women.

Many factors are involved in the production of an optimal mammographic study. These include the age, upkeep, and type of equipment and the competency of the radiographer, mammographer, and radiologist. Proper positioning of the breast is essential to produce a useful mammogram. Even the film processor must be appropriately maintained to avoid the appearance of artifacts and to optimize the quality of the mammogram. For many years, the American College of Radiology (ACR) conducted a voluntary program that granted accreditation to mammographic facilities meeting their quality standards. Since October 1994, the U.S. Food and Drug Administration (FDA) has required the certification of all mammographic facilities. The major agency approved by the FDA to grant mammography accreditation is the ACR.

The two primary modalities of mammography are low-dose film and screen mammography and xerography. The standard low-dose film mammogram involves exposures in two views, a craniocaudad and a medial-lateral view. Although the current maximum acceptable radiation dose from a two-view mammogram is 0.01 Gy, the average optimally performed procedure delivers only 0.002 Gy. With radiation doses at this level, mammography presents a favorable risk-benefit ratio to patients.

Xerography is a technique of mammography that provides greater visualization of the area close to the chest wall but lacks the detail of good quality film mammography. As a result, xerography is reserved for obtaining additional detail in the patient whose lesion is adjacent to the chest wall.

Digital mammography and computer-aided detection (CAD) are two recent developments. Digital mammography may help improve the accuracy of detection.[38] However, a more recent study has challenged the efficacy of CAD.[16]

Sonography. Sonography has been used fairly extensively in breast cancer detection. Sonography is currently used as an adjunct to mammography for its ability to distinguish between cystic and solid masses and to guide biopsy procedures. Ultrasonography is not a suitable screening modality for breast cancer for several reasons. It cannot detect microcalcifications, it is not sensitive enough to detect small breast cancers, and it can miss subtle structural irregularities indicative of breast malignancy.

Magnetic Resonance Imaging. Magnetic resonance imaging (MRI) of the breast has been used for approximately a decade. It has been of some value in women with silicone breast implants, extremely dense breast tissue, or changes in the breast secondary to radiation treatment. MRI of the breast has several significant limitations, including its inability to detect microcalcifications and its high cost. Advances in the development of surface coils have resulted in several studies on the efficacy of MRI for breast cancer. The ACS has recommended involving high-risk women in routine screenings.[44]

Computed Tomography. The expense of computed tomography (CT) is sufficiently high to rule out its use as a screening method. However, it is an important tool for the evaluation of local and regional disease in selected patients who have an established diagnosis of breast cancer.

Diagnosis

A definitive diagnosis of breast cancer can only be made through a microscopic examination of tissue removed from the breast. This tissue is obtained from a biopsy through one of several techniques.

Fine-Needle Biopsy. Fine-needle biopsy involves the careful placement of a relatively small-gauge needle into the suspicious tissue in the breast. The needle is attached to a syringe in which the evacuated blood and/or tissue is collected. This material is prepared on slides for cytologic evaluation.

Core-Needle Biopsy. Core-needle biopsy is similar to fine-needle biopsy in that a syringe and a larger-gauge needle are used to aspirate a core of tissue from the breast mass. The pathologist then examines this tissue histologically.

Incisional Biopsy. An incisional biopsy involves the partial removal of a breast mass to make a histologic diagnosis. This procedure is usually performed if the mass is too large to be completely removed without compromising subsequent surgical treatment.

Excisional Biopsy. Excisional biopsy, sometimes referred to as lumpectomy, removes the mass in its entirety with or without a portion of surrounding normal tissue. This has become the method of choice for removing small breast masses. The placement of the surgical incision is extremely important. Cosmetic effect and treatment considerations (radiation therapy and surgical) are directly related to the type and placement of the incision. Curvilinear rather than radial incisions must be used.[23] The incision should be placed directly over the mass to avoid tunneling through breast tissue (a situation with implications for the placement of the boost field during radiation treatment).

PATHOLOGY

Two basic methods are used for obtaining pathologic information. Gross examination is performed to record the dimensions of the specimen, the size of the tumor, and the tumor's relationship to the excisional margin. Microscopic examination is performed through an analysis of the specimen under a microscope whereby tumor margins are assessed to evaluate the adequacy of the excision. In addition, the pathologist determines the tumor histology and presence of associated DCIS and lymphatic invasion, if any.

Histopathologic types of breast cancer are listed in Box 38-5. Most breast cancers arise in the terminal ductal lobular units of the breast and are classified as ductal or lobular, depending on the specific site of origin. The specific type is defined based on cytologic features and growth patterns. Carcinoma in situ (CIS) is also classified as ductal or lobular and is characterized by a proliferation of malignant epithelial cells that do not invade the basement membrane.

More than 70% of invasive breast cancers are infiltrating ductal carcinoma. These tumors usually contain some component of DCIS and tend to spread to the axillary lymph nodes. Infiltrating lobular carcinoma comprises about 5% to 10% of breast cancers.[55] The prognosis and likelihood of lymph node involvement is similar to that of ductal carcinoma.

Inflammatory breast cancer can be composed of any histologic cell type. However, its clinical features are distinct. Accounting for less than 1% of all breast cancer, it is characterized by obvious skin changes such as peau d'orange, erythema, thickening, increased warmth, and diffuse induration caused by dermal lymphatic involvement. The entire breast may be tender and enlarged. Inflammatory cancer involves a grave prognosis of a survival time of less than 2 years because it tends to be fast growing and aggressive. Therefore, combined-modality treatment (including surgery, chemotherapy, and radiation therapy) is used for these patients.

In addition to defining the histologic type of breast cancer, the pathologist can assess the tumor grade. The degree of

<table>
<tr><td>

Box 38-5   **Histopathologic Types of Breast Cancer**

- Cancer, NOS
  - Ductal
  - Intraductal (in situ)
  - Invasive with predominant intraductal component
  - Invasive, NOS
  - Comedo
  - Inflammatory
  - Medullary with lymphocytic infiltrate
  - Mucinous (colloid)
  - Papillary
  - Scirrhous
  - Tubular
  - Other
- Lobular
  - In situ
  - Invasive with predominant in situ component
  - Invasive
- Nipple
  - Paget's disease, NOS
  - Paget's disease with intraductal carcinoma
  - Paget's disease with invasive ductal carcinoma
- Other
  - Undifferentiated carcinoma

</td></tr>
</table>

NOS, Not otherwise specified.

differentiation assesses the morphologic features of tubule formation, nuclear pleomorphism, and mitotic count of the tissue being reviewed. In the assessment of these components, a value of 1 (favorable) to 3 (unfavorable) is assigned for each feature and is then added together. A combined score of 3 to 5 points is a grade 1, a combined score of 6 to 7 is grade 2, and a combined score of 8 to 9 is grade 3. The higher the grade, the more undifferentiated is the disease, which equates to a more aggressive disease (Box 38-6).

STAGING

Patients with breast cancer are staged for a variety of reasons. Staging aids in the selection of the treatment technique, allows the evaluation of treatment methods, and indicates the prognosis. The two methods of staging breast cancer are clinical and pathologic. Clinical staging involves all physical examinations, imaging, and pathologic examination of the primary tumor or other related tissue to establish the diagnosis. Pathologic staging includes all these factors plus data from surgical procedures

<table>
<tr><td>

Box 38-6   **Histopathologic Grade (G)**

GX   Grade cannot be assessed
G1   Well differentiated
G2   Moderately differentiated
G3   Poorly differentiated
G4   Undifferentiated

</td></tr>
</table>

as well as pathologic evaluation of primary tumor, lymph node, and metastases (if applicable). If gross involvement of the tumor margin is present, then the true extent of the primary tumor cannot be assessed and is therefore coded as TX. Sentinel lymph nodes should also be pathologically assessed for staging purposes.

The currently accepted staging system is that of the American Joint Committee on Cancer (AJCC), which is based on tumor, node, metastasis (TNM) definitions, and stage groupings (Box 38-7). The primary tumor, regional lymph node status, pathologic classification status, and distant metastasis are parameters used to place patients into four main groups. With simultaneous bilateral breast cancers, the tumors are staged independently.

ROUTES OF SPREAD

Cancer of the breast is a relatively slow disease process, with distant metastases sometimes occurring decades after definitive treatment of the primary tumor.[24] Some researchers believe that cancer of the breast is a systemic disease, even in the earliest clinical stages, based on the following facts: (1) little change has occurred in long-term survival rates since the radical mastectomy was developed and (2) late distant metastases continue to appear, even with the use of advanced treatment techniques.[26]

Extension in the Breast

A basic therapeutic tenet of this disease is that all ipsilateral breast tissue is at risk and requires treatment. This is due to the fact that extension throughout the breast is possible as a result of the following mechanisms:

1. Direct invasion into surrounding breast tissue
2. Extension via the duct system
3. Spread along the lymphatic channels in the breast

Direct extension of a primary breast lesion can be demonstrated mammographically. The tumor has fingerlike projections that extend into the parenchyma of the breast (Figure 38-7). Without treatment, such lesions ultimately involve the skin of the breast and/or the chest wall.

Cancer also spreads in the breast by progressive involvement of the ducts. Whether this process represents actual direct extension along the ducts or a more generalized development of cancer in multiple ducts simultaneously is not fully understood.

The extensive lymphatic system of the breast provides an avenue for the primary spread of tumor cells in breast tissue. Cells can migrate via lymphatic channels deep into the chest wall or central portion of the breast beneath the nipple-areola complex.

Regional Lymph Node Involvement

Lymph nodes in the axillary and IM areas are the most likely sites of regional involvement of breast cancer. The supraclavicular nodes are only occasionally involved. The presence or absence of disease in these nodal groups is an important factor in treatment decisions and as an indicator of the prognosis.

Axillary Lymph Node Involvement. Lymph nodes located in the axilla represent the primary lymphatic drainage

Box 38-7 | **American Joint Committee on Cancer Staging System for Breast Cancer**

PRIMARY TUMOR (T)

TX	Primary tumor cannot be assessed
T0	No evidence of primary tumor
Tis	Carcinoma in situ
Tis	(DCIS) Ductal carcinoma in situ
Tis	(LCIS) Lobular carcinoma in situ
Tis	(Paget's) Paget's disease of the nipple with no tumor

Note: Paget's disease associated with a tumor is classified according to the size of the tumor

T1	Tumor 2 cm or less in greatest dimension
T1mic	Microinvasion 0.1 cm or less in greatest dimension
T1a	Tumor more than 0.1 cm but not more than 0.5 cm in greatest dimension
T1b	Tumor more than 0.5 cm but not more than 1 cm in greatest dimension
T1c	Tumor more than 1 cm but not more than 2 cm in greatest dimension
T2	Tumor more than 2 cm but not more than 5 cm in greatest dimension
T3	Tumor more than 5 cm in greatest dimension
T4	Tumor of any size with direct extension to (a) chest wall or (b) skin, only as described below
T4a	Extension to chest wall, not including pectoralis muscle
T4b	Edema (including peau d'orange) or ulceration of the skin of the breast, or satellite skin nodules confined to the same breast
T4c	Both T4a and T4b
T4d	Inflammatory carcinoma

REGIONAL LYMPH NODES (N)

NX	Regional lymph nodes cannot be assessed (e.g., previously removed)
N0	No regional lymph node metastasis
N1	Metastasis in a movable ipsilateral axillary lymph node(s)
N2	Metastasis in ipsilateral axillary lymph node(s) fixed or matted, or in clinically apparent[1] ipsilateral internal mammary nodes in the *absence* of clinically evident axillary lymph node metastasis
N2a	Metastases in ipsilateral axillary lymph node fixed to one another (matted) or to other structures
N2b	Metastasis only in clinically apparent[1] ipsilateral internal mammary nodes in the *absence* of clinically evident axillary lymph node metastasis
N3	Metastasis in ipsilateral infraclavicular lymph node(s) with or without axillary lymph node involvement, or in clinically apparent[1] ipsilateral internal mammary node(s) and in the *presence* of clinically evident axillary lymph node metastasis; or metastasis in ipsilateral supraclavicular lymph node(s) with or without axillary or internal mammary lymph node involvement
N3a	Metastasis in ipsilateral infraclavicular lymph node(s) and axillary lymph node(s)
N3b	Metastasis in ipsilateral internal mammary lymph node(s) and axillary lymph node(s)
N3c	Metastasis in ipsilateral supraclavicular lymph node(s)

REGIONAL LYMPH NODES (PN)[2]

pNX	Regional lymph nodes cannot be assessed (e.g., previously removed, or not removed for pathologic study)
pN0	No regional lymph node metastasis histologically, no additional examination for isolated tumor cells (ITC)[3]
pN0(i–)	No regional lymph node metastasis histologically, negative IHC
pN0(i+)	No regional lymph node metastasis histologically, positive IHC, no IHC cluster greater than 0.2 mm
pN0(mol–)	No regional lymph node metastasis histologically, negative molecular findings (RT-PCR)[4]
pN0(mol+)	No regional lymph node metastasis histologically, positive molecular findings (RT-PCR)[4]
pN1	Metastasis in 1 to 3 axillary lymph nodes, and/or in internal mammary nodes with microscopic disease detected by sentinel lymph node dissection but not clinically apparent[5]
pN1mi	Micrometastasis (greater than 0.2 mm, none greater than 2.0 mm)
pN1a	Metastasis in 1 to 3 axillary lymph nodes
pN1b	Metastasis in internal mammary nodes with microscopic disease detected by sentinel lymph node dissection but not clinically apparent[5]
pN1c	Metastasis in 1 to 3 axillary lymph nodes and in internal mammary lymph nodes with microscopic disease detected by sentinel lymph node dissection but not clinically apparent[5,6]
pN2	Metastasis in 4 to 9 axillary lymph nodes, or in clinically apparent[1] internal mammary lymph nodes in the absence of axillary lymph node metastasis
pN2a	Metastasis in 4 to 9 axillary lymph nodes (at least one tumor deposit greater than 2.0 mm)
pN2b	Metastasis in clinically apparent[1] internal mammary lymph nodes in the *absence* of axillary lymph node metastasis
pN3	Metastasis in 10 or more axillary lymph nodes, or in infraclavicular lymph nodes, or in clinically apparent[1] ipsilateral internal mammary lymph nodes in the *presence* of 1 or more positive axillary lymph nodes; or in more than 3 axillary lymph nodes with clinically negative microscopic metastasis in internal mammary lymph nodes; or in ipsilateral supraclavicular lymph nodes
pN3a	Metastasis in 10 or more axillary lymph nodes (at least one tumor deposit greater than 2.0 mm), or metastasis to the infraclavicular lymph nodes
pN3b	Metastasis in clinically apparent[1] ipsilateral internal mammary lymph nodes in the *presence* of 1 or more positive axillary lymph nodes; or in more than 3 axillary lymph nodes in internal mammary lymph nodes with microscopic disease detected by sentinel lymph node dissection but not clinically apparent[5]
pN3c	Metastasis in ipsilateral supraclavicular lymph node

Continued

DISTANT METASTASIS (M)

MX Distant metastasis cannot be assessed
M0 No distant metastasis
M1 Distant metastasis

STAGE GROUPING

0	Tis	N0	M0
I	T1[7]	N0	M0
IIA	T0	N1	M0
	T1[7]	N1	M0
	T2	N0	M0
IIB	T2	N1	M0
	T3	N0	M0
IIIA	T0	N2	M0
	T1[7]	N2	M0
	T2	N2	M0
	T3	N1	M0
	T3	N2	M0
IIIB	T4	N0	M0
	T4	N1	M0
	T4	N2	M0
IIIC	Any T	N3	M0
IV	Any T	Any N	M1

Note: Stage designation may be changed if post-surgical imaging studies reveal the presence of distant metastases, provided that the studies are carried out within 4 months of diagnosis in the absence of disease progression and provided that the patient has not received neoadjuvant therapy.

HISTOLOGIC GRADE (G)

All invasive breast carcinomas with the exception of medullary carcinoma should be graded. The Nottingham combined histologic grade (Elston-Ellis modification of Scarff-Bloom-Richardson grading system) is recommended. The grade for a tumor is determined by assessing morphologic features (tubule formation, nuclear pleomorphism, and mitotic count), assigning a value of 1 (favorable) to 3 (unfavorable) for each feature, and adding together the scores for all three categories. A combined score of 3-5 points is designated as grade 1; a combined score of 6-7 points is grade 2; a combined score of 8-9 points is grade 3.

HISTOLOGIC GRADE (NOTTINGHAM COMBINED HISTOLOGIC GRADE IS RECOMMENDED)

GX   Grade cannot be assessed
G1   Low combined histologic grade (favorable)
G2   Intermediate combined histologic grade (moderately favorable)
G3   High combined histologic grade (unfavorable)

Notes:
1. Clinically apparent is defined as detected by imaging studies (excluding lymphoscintigraphy) or by clinical examination.
2. Classification is based on axillary lymph node dissection with or without sentinel lymph node dissection. Classification based solely on sentinel lymph node dissection without subsequent axillary lymph node dissection is designated (sn) for "sentinel node," e.g., pN0(i+)(sn).
3. Isolated tumor cells (ITC) are defined as single tumor cells or small cell clusters not greater than 0.2 mm, usually detected only by immunohistochemical (IHC) or molecular methods but which may be verified on HandE stains. ITCs do not usually show evidence of metastatic activity (e.g., proliferation or stromal reaction.)
4. RT-PCR, reverse transcription–polymerase chain reaction.
5. Not clinically apparent is defined as not detected by imaging studies (excluding lymphoscintigraphy) or by clinical examination.
6. If associated with greater than three positive axillary lymph nodes, the internal mammary nodes are classified as pN3b to reflect increased tumor burden.
7. T1 includes T1mic.

of the breast. About one third of patients with clinical negative study have microscopic involvement of the axillary nodes.[54] The incidence of axillary lymph node involvement is a function of several factors, including the following:

1. Size of the primary tumor—as tumor size increases, so does the likelihood of axillary node involvement.[9]
2. Quadrant location of the primary tumor—lesions located in the upper-outer or lower-outer quadrants have a greater chance of axillary node involvement.[21]

Lymph nodes in the axilla can be divided into three subsections. Because of the sequential drainage pattern, the lowest (level I) nodes are the first and most likely to be involved, followed by levels II and III. Occasionally, lymph nodes in a higher level may be involved while the nodes in the lower level(s) are negative for tumor, a situation referred to as **skip metastasis**. The two largest series studying this process demonstrated a 3.5% rate of skip metastasis in patients with axillary lymph node involvement.[42,51]

Internal Mammary (IM) Lymph Node Involvement.

IM lymph nodes are the second most common nodal site of involvement from breast cancer. Of all breast cancer patients, 20% have IM nodes positive for tumor.[23] The incidence of IM involvement is directly related to axillary node involvement and the size of the primary tumor. The age of the patient also influences IM node involvement, with younger patients demonstrating a higher incidence.[50] Most studies also show that the primary tumor location in the medial quadrants or center of the breast increases the incidence of IM involvement.

Assessing the status of IM nodes as a result of their intrathoracic location, which is relatively inaccessible for a biopsy, can be difficult. CT and lymphoscintigraphy are used to image the IM nodes.

Supraclavicular Lymph Node Involvement

Supraclavicular lymph node involvement from breast cancer is correlated with extensive axillary metastasis and medial quadrant location.[24] The involvement of IM and supraclavicular nodes is considered a grave prognostic indicator in breast cancer.

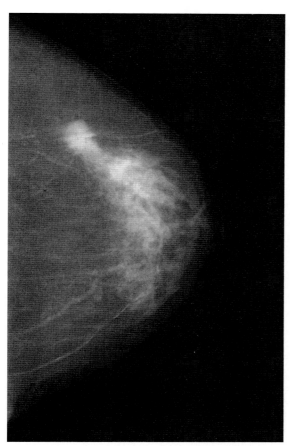

Figure 38-7. Mammographic demonstration of a primary breast lesion.

Distant Metastasis

Breast cancer has a propensity to metastasize via embolization (i.e., spread via tumor cells entering the circulatory system and traveling to a distant organ). The length of time between the initial diagnosis and discovery of distant metastasis varies widely in this disease but can be extremely long, measured sometimes in decades. The development of distant metastasis is linked to the size and histology of the primary tumor and extent of lymph node involvement.

TREATMENT MANAGEMENT

A multidisciplinary approach that includes surgery, radiation therapy, and chemotherapy is required for breast cancer treatment. Historically, breast cancer was treated aggressively via radical mastectomy with or without radiation therapy. In addition to single-institution studies, large national cooperative groups, such as the National Surgical Adjuvant Breast and Bowel Project (NSABP) and the Radiation Therapy Oncology Group (RTOG), contribute to continuing breast cancer research and the development of treatments. The research of these and other groups carried out over the past 30 years indicates that breast cancer appears to be systemic in its progression. Aggressive local treatment via radical mastectomy has not improved survival rates; therefore, current surgical and radiation treatment techniques are more conservative. Chemotherapy has been used increasingly to address microscopic, lymphatic,

and systemic disease. When indicated, radiation therapy is usually delivered postoperatively.

Decisions regarding treatment are influenced by the extent of the primary tumor, the patient's general medical condition, and the patient's personal preference. Although limited surgery (breast conservation) with or without radiation treatment is popular, it is not appropriate for all patients. If the breast is small relative to the tumor or multicentric tumor involvement is present, then a mastectomy may be the best treatment choice. In addition, limited surgery is not an option for patients with advanced breast cancer, although it may become feasible following preoperative chemotherapy to reduce the amount of disease.

Surgery

Radical Mastectomy. Introduced by William S. Halsted in the late 1800s, the Halsted radical mastectomy was the treatment of choice for breast cancer through the 1970s. Before this, patients were more likely to have large, bulky tumors, and early, limited surgical techniques were ineffective in reducing the incidence of chest wall recurrence. To address the high incidence of chest wall recurrence and lymph node involvement, Halsted devised the radical mastectomy, which involves the removal of the breast with its overlying skin, all the axillary lymph nodes, and the pectoral muscles (Figure 38-8).

Although the Halsted radical mastectomy did not lead to improved long-term survival rates, chest wall recurrences were

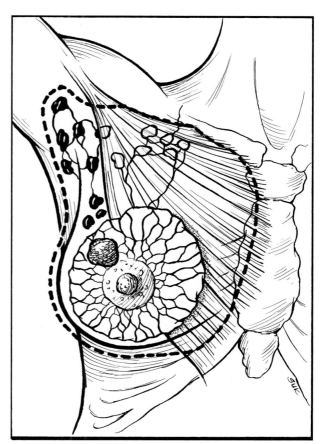

Figure 38-8. Radical mastectomy: removal of the breast with its overlying skin, the axillary lymph nodes, and the pectoralis major and minor muscles.

reduced, which accounted for the procedure's initial popularity. Unfortunately, the complication rate from radical mastectomy is high and complications can be severe, often leaving the patient with a concave chest wall, arm weakness, shoulder stiffness, and lymphedema (arm swelling). Eventually, the extent of surgery was reduced because radical mastectomy did not reduce the incidence of metastatic disease and because of the high risk of complications. Currently, radical mastectomy is rarely performed, comprising less than 2% of all breast surgeries in the United States.

Modified Radical Mastectomy. Radical mastectomy was subsequently modified to preserve muscle, some skin, lymphatics, and blood vessels, thereby improving cosmetic results, reducing arm edema, and improving arm strength. Modified radical mastectomy involves removal of the breast and some or all of the axillary lymph nodes. It may also include removal of the pectoralis minor muscle, while preserving the pectoralis major (Figure 38-9). Sometimes the lymph nodes are sampled through a separate axillary incision. The use of modified radical mastectomy resulted in survival rates similar to those for radical mastectomy; therefore, this modified procedure eventually replaced the more extensive operation.

Lumpectomy. The excisional biopsy of a breast mass is sometimes referred to as lumpectomy, tylectomy, or tumorectomy. This procedure involves removal of the tumor with a

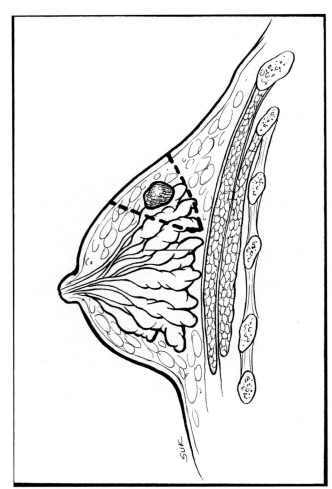

Figure 38-10. Lumpectomy: removal of the tumor with a margin of normal-appearing tissue.

margin of normal-appearing tissue (Figure 38-10). Overlying skin and underlying tissue are left intact. Lymph nodes are sampled through a separate axillary incision.

Axillary Dissection. Removal of a sample of axillary lymph nodes in the axilla on the side of the involved breast (ipsilateral) is necessary for staging the patient's disease. The pathologic status of axillary lymph nodes influences the selection of the treatment technique and helps indicate the prognosis.

Sentinel Node Biopsy. This procedure has been used extensively in staging the patients with clinically negative axillae. The sentinel nodes are the first group of lymph nodes to which the primary tumor will spread. After visualizing these nodes by ^{99m}Tc colloid or/and isosulfan blue dye, these nodes will be removed by limited dissection of axilla. Randomized control trials have shown that sentinel mapping has resulted in less shoulder and arm morbidity compared with full axillary dissection. There are no significant differences in effectiveness of accurately staging the axillae. [33,34,52]

Breast Reconstruction. Breast reconstruction may be an option for women who have undergone a mastectomy. Expander/implant breast reconstruction is achieved through the gradual expansion of existing skin and muscle and the subsequent placement of an artificial breast implant. If remaining tissues are

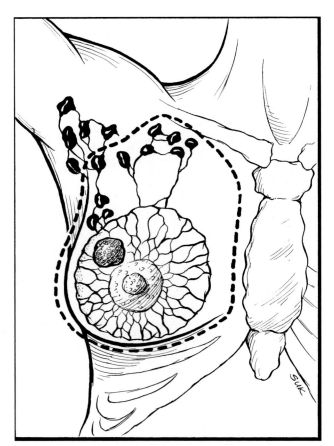

Figure 38-9. Modified radical mastectomy: removal of the breast with its overlying skin, some or all of the axillary lymph nodes. The pectoralis minor muscle may be removed, leaving the pectoralis major muscle intact.

inadequate for expansion after a mastectomy, then skin and muscle may be transferred to the chest area from other parts of the body. A normal breast contour may be obtained by matching the size and shape of the implant with that of the opposite breast. It is possible to reconstruct just the contour of the breast or, in some patients, the entire breast, including the nipple and areola. A plastic surgeon performs the procedure, which may require several operations over 6 to 12 months. Autologous tissue flap reconstruction, on the other hand, using either latissimus dossi or transverse rectus abdominis offers more predictable results in terms of cosmesis. It requires transposition of muscle, subcutaneous tissue, and skin into the mastectomy defect. This type of reconstruction is more technically demanding than prosthetic reconstruction.

Systemic Therapy

Systemic therapy may be combined with surgery and/or radiation therapy and consists of chemotherapy or endocrine therapy (hormonal manipulation). The goal of systemic treatment is the destruction, prevention, or delay of tumor spread to distant sites in the body. When systemic therapy is used before surgery, it is referred to as primary or neoadjuvant therapy. When systemic therapy is used after the surgery, it is referred to as **adjuvant therapy**.

Chemotherapy. Chemotherapy consists of the following cancer-killing agents (used alone or in combination): cyclophosphamide (C), doxorubicin (Adriamycin) (A), and paclitaxel. Combination chemotherapy is the use of several agents together. For example, combination chemotherapy consisting of AC means that doxorubicin and cyclophosphamide are used together.

A treatment regimen is defined according to the order of administration, specific agent(s), dosages, routes of administration, and exact administration schedule. Drugs can be administered through the patient's mouth or via an injection into a vein or muscle. A schedule of administration indicates whether the drugs are given daily, weekly, or monthly. The duration of treatment is expressed in terms of months or years. Chemotherapy may be administered before or after surgery, before or after radiation therapy, or with radiation treatment. The sequence of chemotherapy, surgery, and radiation therapy continues to be studied for its effect on local control and survival. In addition, a variety of adjuvant treatment regimens are under investigation.

Endocrine Therapy. Current endocrine therapy consists of a variety of drugs used to deprive cancer cells of the hormones needed for growth. The most commonly used agents are tamoxifen and aromitase inhibitors. Tamoxifen and aromitase inhibitors are frequently a component of adjuvant therapy for postmenopausal women. They are used alone or with other chemotherapeutic agents. The estrogen receptor status also plays a role in the selection of hormonal therapy as an element of treatment.[28]

Treatment Approach, Each patient is considered unique, and management depends on the patient's stage of disease, lymph node status, estrogen receptor and progesterone receptor (ER/PR) status, and menopausal status. Although no single treatment exists that is best for any group of patients, some general comments can be made. In general, stage I breast cancer

patients have a low incidence of relapse; therefore chemotherapy is reserved for high-risk patients in this group. For stages II and III breast cancer patients, systemic therapy is useful in reducing relapse rates and increasing overall survival rates. Multiagent chemotherapy is the present treatment of choice for premenopausal women with ipsilateral lymph node involvement, whereas tamoxifen and aromitase inhibitors alone or with chemotherapy are beneficial for postmenopausal women.[22,26,28] A combination of systemic and local treatment is usually required for patients with advanced disease (stage IV).[28] For patients with unresectable tumors, chemotherapy is frequently sequenced first to achieve a systemic effect and to potentially downstage the tumor. Although data suggest that delaying irradiation during chemotherapy increases the risk of local failure, this risk may be acceptable for patients with locally advanced disease because distant metastasis is a predictor of overall survival. Optimal sequencing of chemotherapy, surgery, and radiation therapy has not yet been determined.

Treatment of Advanced Breast Cancer. For metastatic breast cancer, current chemotherapy can often prolong the survival time or inhibit progression of the disease. For some patients, chemotherapy is used as a palliative measure.

Side Effects. Endocrine and chemotherapeutic agents can also affect healthy tissues, causing side effects such as nausea and vomiting, loss of appetite, fatigue, change in menstruation, mouth ulcers, and hair loss. The type of side effects that the patient experiences depends on the agent(s) used and the patient's response to the drugs. For example, some patients may experience hot flashes (a short-term side effect of tamoxifen) as a result of lowered levels of estrogen. Most side effects are acute, resolving after the completion of treatment. A few side effects are permanent. For example, doxorubicin may cause cardiac damage. In addition, a small chance exists that the chemotherapy will cause a second cancer.

Radiation Therapy

Mastectomy Management of Breast Cancer. Current methods for conservative breast cancer management have been well established. The ACR adopted "Standards for Breast Conservation Treatment" in 1992. The American College of Surgeons, the College of American Pathologists, and the Society of Surgical Oncology have endorsed this document. A variety of research efforts have provided the evidence necessary to conclude that mastectomy and breast conservation treatment (lumpectomy, ipsilateral axillary lymph node dissection, and radiation therapy) are equally effective for selected patients with early-stage breast cancer (stages I and II).

Mastectomy and breast conservation treatment (surgery and radiation) are equally effective for selected patients with early-stage breast cancer (stage I and II).

As defined by ACR standards, the four critical elements used to select patients for breast conservation are as follows:
1. The patient's history and a physical examination are used to establish familial patterns and assess physical findings.
2. A mammographic evaluation is used to define the extent of the tumor, investigate the potential presence of multicentric or multifocal disease, and evaluate the contralateral breast.

3. A pathologic evaluation of the tumor including a gross and microscopic examination and additional data such as ER/PR analysis, extent of CIS, DNA ploidy, S phase fraction, and mitotic grade are obtained.

4. An assessment of the patient's needs and expectations is a difficult but essential consideration. Long-term survival, possibility and consequences of local recurrence, treatment options for potential local recurrence, follow-up procedures, physical and cosmetic outcomes, psychological adjustment, and quality of life are factors requiring careful consideration.

Although properly staged and selected patients may be eligible for conservative treatment, some contraindications have been identified. Pregnancy, multicentric disease, and scleroderma are contraindications of breast conservation treatment. A history of vascular disease, a large tumor in a small breast, an extremely large or pendulous breast, and the specific location of the tumor in the breast are factors requiring special consideration and potentially contraindicating the use of a conservative approach to treatment.

Total gross removal of the tumor and a margin of surrounding tissue with maintenance of good cosmesis is the main goal of conservative breast surgery. A separate sentinel node or axillary dissection is performed. After a 2- to 4-week surgical recovery, if chemotherapy is not given, radiation therapy may begin. Proper simulation and treatment planning are critical factors in establishing an appropriate treatment technique. Special attention to physical and technical considerations substantially reduces the risk of complications. Specific techniques are addressed in the following section. Generally, however, lower megavoltage beam energies (4 to 8 MV) and tissue compensators are used to improve dose homogeneity. Tangential fields are used to encompass the entire breast and chest wall. The amount of lung projected at the center of the tangential fields should be limited to between 1.0 and 3.4 cm, thereby reducing the risk of radiation pneumonitis. If peripheral lymphatic irradiation is required, then overlapping or excessive gapping between fields must be avoided. If the axillary dissection includes level III, then axillary irradiation should be avoided so that lymphedema does not result.

Fields are treated daily with standard fractionation (180 to 200 cGy/fraction) to a total dose of 4500 to 5000 cGy. A boost dose may be delivered with a reduced photon field electron beam or interstitial technique, increasing the total dose to the primary tumor site to 6000 to 6600 cGy. Although precise indications for performing the boost remain controversial, patients with margins positive for tumor or close margins of surgical resection usually receive boost irradiation.

Follow-up assessment of patients receiving conservative breast treatment is carefully scheduled to evaluate new or recurrent disease status, treatment sequelae, and cosmetic outcome. The patient's medical history, physical examination, and follow-up mammograms contribute to the evaluation process. The acute and late radiation morbidity scoring schemes of the RTOG and European Organization for Research on Treatment of Cancer are provided in Tables 38-1 and 38-2. An assessment of the cosmetic result is based on the physician's evaluation (using a four-point scoring index) and the patient's perception.

Mastectomy Management of Breast Cancer. Currently, the role of radiation therapy in postoperative breast cancer treatment is not well defined. Radiation therapy was initially used in breast cancer management as an adjuvant to radical mastectomy for the purpose of prophylaxis. The main goal was to reduce the local recurrence rate, thereby improving survival. The risk of radiation-induced cardiac damage and the evolution of the role of chemotherapy have reduced the use of radiation therapy in postoperative patients. The tumor size, number of axillary lymph nodes positive for tumor, and margin status may be indications for adjuvant radiation therapy.

If radiation therapy is indicated, then the chest wall is treated via tangential fields with lower megavoltage beam energies, using tissue compensators as necessary. In some cases, a single electron field may provide good coverage. Peripheral (supraclavicular and/or axillary) lymphatic irradiation may also be required. Fields are treated daily with standard fractionation (180 to 200 cGy/fraction) to a total dose of 4500 to 5000 cGy. Wider tangential ports that extend across the midline may be used to treat IM nodes. Another technique for treating the IM nodes combines photon and electron treatment, helping to limit the cardiac dose. Adjoining fields must be carefully planned to avoid overdosage or underdosage of tissues in these areas, leading to potential match-line **fibrosis** (abnormal formation of fiberlike scarring) or local recurrence, respectively.

Radiation Treatment Techniques

Radiation treatment for primary breast malignancy is one of the more technically challenging and relatively high-volume procedures performed in a radiation oncology department. Therefore, straightforward, reproducible techniques are advantageous, affording optimal target-volume-dose homogeneity and acceptable dose limits for normal structures.

There are almost as many techniques for breast irradiation as there are radiation oncology centers. Many techniques are only slight variations on a theme. Current standard of practice incorporates several essential elements in the treatment of breast cancer. This section presents these elements and details one specific technique.

Positioning and Immobilization. Radiation treatment of breast cancer is demanding, requiring stringent positioning and immobilization techniques. One of the key elements involves the mobility of the patient's arm. Many postoperative patients (whether the surgery involved a mastectomy or an axillary dissection) experience initial difficulty in raising the arm to an acceptable position for radiation treatment. Most patients who encounter this problem can correct it with exercise in several days. Therefore, the simulation and start of therapy should be delayed until the patient's arm moves appropriately. If the patient is simulated before mobility is restored, then the shoulder girdle will assume a different position for treatment than for simulation, leading to poor reproducibility of the treatment fields. At the time of consultation, before the simulation appointment, the radiation oncologist can give the patient a handout detailing exercises and explaining their necessity.

Many commercially available devices are available to assist in patient positioning for treatment of breast cancer.

Table 38-1	RTOG Acute Radiation Morbidity Scoring Criteria

Organ Tissue	Grade 0	Grade 1	Grade 2	Grade 3	Grade 4
Skin	No Change over baseline	Follicular, faint or dull erythema; epilation; dry desquamation; decreased sweating	Tender or bright erythema and patchy, moist desquamation; moderate edema	Confluent, moist desquamation other than skin folds and pitting edema	Ulceration; hemorrhage; necrosis
Mucous membrane	No Change over baseline	Injections; possible expeience of mild pain not requiring analgesic	Patchy mucositis that may produce an imflammatory serosanguineous discharge; possible experience of moderate pain requiring analgesia	Confluent fibrinous mucositis; possibility of severe pain requiring narcotic	Ulceration; hemorrhage; necrosis
Eye	No Change over baseline	Mild conjunctivitis with or without scleral injection; increased tearing	Moderate conjunctivitis with or without keratitis requiring steroids and/or antibiotics; dry eye requiring artificial tears; iritis with photophobia	Severe keratitis with corneal ulceration; objective decrease in visual acuity or in visual fields; acute glaucoma; panophthalmitis	Loss of vision (unilateral or bilateral)
Ear	No Change over baseline	Mild external otitis with erythema and pruritis secondary to dry desquamation not requiring medication; audiogram unchanged from baseline	Moderate external otitis requiring topical medication; serous ototis medius; hypoacusis on testing only	Severe external otitis with discharge or moist desquamation; symptomatic hypoacusis; tinnitus, not drug related	Deafness
Salivary gland	No Change over baseline	Mild mouth dryness; slightly thickened saliva; possibility of slightly altered taste, such as metallic taste (these changes not reflected in alteration in baseline feeding behavior, such as increased use of liquids with meals)	Moderate to complete dryness; thick, sticky saliva; markedly altered test	—	Acute salivary gland necrosis
Pharynx and esophagus	No Change over baseline	Mild dysphagia or odynophagia; possible requirement of topical anesthetic or nonnarcotic analgesics and soft diet	Moderate dysphagia or odynophagis; possible requirement of narcotic analgesics and puree or liquid diet	Severe dysphagia or odynophagia with dehydration or weight loss (>15% from pretreatment baseline) requiring NG feeding tube, intravenous fluids, or hyperalimentation	Complete obstruction; ulceration; perforation; fistula
Larynx	No Change over baseline	Mild or intermittent hoarseness; cough not requiring antitussive; erythema of mucosa	Persistent hoarseness but ability to vocalize; referred ear pain, sore throat, patchy fibrinous exudates or mild arytenoids edema not requiring narcotic; cough requiring antitussive	Whispered speech and throat pain or referred ear pain requiring narcotic; confluent fibrinous exudates and marked arytenoid edema	Marked dyspnea; stridor or hemoptysis with tracheostomy or intubation necessary
Upper gastrointestinal system	No change	Anorexia with ≤5% weight loss from pretreatment baseline; nausea not requiring antiemetics; abdominal discomfort not requiring parasympatholytic drugs or analgesics	Anorexia with ≤15% weight loss from pretreatment baseline; nausea and/or vomiting requiring antiemetics; abdominal pain requiring analgesics	Anorexia with >15% weight loss from pretreatment baseline or requiring NG tube or parenteral support. Nausea and/or vomiting requiring tube or parenteral support; abdominal pain (severe despite medication; hematemesis or melana; abdominal distention (flat plate radiograph demonstrates distended bowel loops)	Ileus, subacute or acute obstruction, perforation, and bleeding requiring transfusion; abdominal pain requiring tube decompression or bowel diversion

NG, Nasogastric.

Table 38-2	RTOG and EORTC Late Radiation Morbidity Scoring Scheme

Organ Tissue	Grade 0	Grade 1	Grade 2	Grade 3	Grade 4
Skin	None	Slight atrophy; pigmentation change, some hair loss	Patch atrophy; moderate telangiectasia; total hair loss	Market atrophy; gross telangiectasia	Ulceration
Subcutaneous tissue	None	Slight induration (fibrosis) and loss of subcutaneous fat	Moderate fibrosis but asymptomatic; slight field contracture; <10% linear reduction	Severe induration and loss of subcutaneous tissue; field contracture >10% linear measurement	Necrosis
Mucous membrane	None	Slight atrophy and dryness	Moderate atrophy and telangiectasia; little mucus	Marked atrophy with complete dryness; severe telangiectasia	Ulceration
Salivary glands	None	Slight dryness of mouth; good response on stimulation	Moderate dryness of mouth; poor response on stimulation	Complete dryness of mouth; no response on stimulation	Fibrosis
Spinal cord	None	Mild L'hermitte's sign	Severe L'hermitte's sign	Objective neurologic findings at or below cord level treated	Mono; paraquadraplegia
Brain	None	Mild headache; slight lethargy	Moderate headache; great lethargy	Severe headaches; severe central nervous system dysfunction (partial loss of power or dyskinesia)	Seizures or paralysis; coma
Eye	None	Asymptomatic cataract; minor corneal ulceration or keratitis	Symptomatic cataract; moderate corneal ulceration; minor retinopathy or glaucoma	Severe keratitis; severe retinopathy or detachment; severe glaucoma	Panopthalmitis; blindness
Larynx	None	Hoarseness; slight arytenoid edema	Moderate arytenoid edema; chondritis	Severe edema; severe chondritis	Necrosis
Lung	None	Asymptomatic or mild symptoms (dry cough); slight radiographic appearances	Moderate symptomatic fibrosis or pneumonitis (severe cough); low-grade fever; patchy radiographic appearances	Severe symptomatic fibrosis or pneumonitis; dense radiographic changes	Severe respiratory insufficiency; continuous O_2; assisted ventilation
Heart	None	Asymptomatic or mild symptoms; transient T wave inversion and ST changes; sinus tachychardia >110 (at rest)	Moderate angina on effort; mild pericarditis; normal heart size; persistent abnormal T wave and ST changes; low QRS	Severe angina; pericardial effusion; constrictive pericarditis; moderate heart failure; cardiac enlargement; electrocardiogram abnormalities	Tamponade; severe heart failure; severe constrictive pericarditis
Esophagus	None	Mild fibrosis; slight difficulty in swallowing solids; no pain on swallowing	Inability to take solid food normally; swallowing semisolid food; possible indication for dilatation	Severe fibrosis; ability to swallow only liquids; possibility of pain on swallowing; dilation required	Necrosis; perforation; fistula
Small and large intestine	None	Mild diarrhea; mild cramping; bowel movement five times daily; slight rectal discharge or bleeding	Moderate diarrhea and colic; bowel movement >5 times daily; excessive rectal mucus or intermittent bleeding	Obstruction of bleeding requiring surgery	Necrosis; perforation; fistula
Liver	None	Mild lassitude; nausea, dyspepsia; slightly abnormal liver function	Moderate symptoms; some abnormal liver function tests; serum albumin normal	Disabling hepatic insufficiency; liver function tests grossly abnormal; low albumin; edema or ascites	Necrosis; hepatic coma or encephalopathy
Kidney	None	Transient albuminuria; mild impairment of renal function; urea 25–35 mg%; creatinine 1.5-2.0 mg% creatinine clearance >75%	Persistent moderate albuminuria (2+); mild hypertension; no related anemia; moderate impairment of renal function; urea >36-60 mg%; creatinine clearance (50–74%)	Severe albuminuria; severe hypertension; persistent anemia (<10%); severe renal failure; urea >60 mg%; creatinine >4.0 mg%; creatinine clearance<50%	Malignant hypertension; uremic coma; urea >100%
Bladder	None	Slight epithelial atrophy; minor telangiectasia (microscopic hematuria)	Moderate frequency; generalized telangiectasia; intermittent macroscopic hematuria	Severe frequency and dysuria; severe generalized telangiectasia (often with petechiae); frequent hematuria; reduction in bladder capacity (<150 ml)	Necrosis; contracted bladder (capacity >100 ml); severe hemorrhagic cystitis

Table 38-2 **RTOG and EORTC Late Radiation Morbidity Scoring Scheme–Cont'd**

Organ Tissue	Grade 0	Grade 1	Grade 2	Grade 3	Grade 4
Bone	None	Asymptomatic; no growth retardation; reduced bone density	Moderate pain or tenderness; growth retardation; irregular bone sclerosis	Severe pain or tenderness; complete arrest of bone growth; dense bone sclerosis	Necrosis; spontaneous fracture
Join	None	Mild joint stiffness; slight limitation of movement	Moderate stiffness; intermittent or moderate joint pain; moderate limitation of movement	Severe joint stiffness; pain with severe limitation of movement	Necrosis; complete fixation

These range from custom-molded foam casts to boards with adjustable head and arm supports. One such device is illustrated in Figure 38-11. An important element of reproducibility in immobilization is the ability to index the patient to the immobilization device exactly the same way daily.

For this type of treatment the patient should, at minimum, disrobe from the waist up. The patient lies supine in the selected positioning device on the simulator-treatment table. The patient's body must be straight (in the sagittal plane) and level from side to side. Laser triangulation points are marked on the patient's anterior and side surfaces in the area between the waist and inframammary fold to assist in the daily positioning process.

The arm on the uninvolved (contralateral) side may rest on the tabletop with the hand palm down. Patients must not place the contralateral hand on the abdomen or grasp the belt or waistband of their clothing. Such a position of the contralateral hand and arm (particularly in large-breasted women) can result in distortion of the thoracic anatomy, including rotation and/or displacement of the uninvolved breast into the treatment field. Preferably, the contralateral arm should be positioned the same as the ipsilateral arm.

The ipsilateral arm is raised and supported far enough in a cephalad direction to allow the tangential radiation beam to treat the breast or chest wall while avoiding the patient's upper arm. Adjustment of the patient's arm position can help reduce or eliminate skin folds in the axilla and supraclavicular areas.

The patient's head should be straight if treatment is limited to the breast or chest wall. If the peripheral lymphatics also require irradiation, then the head should be turned slightly to the contralateral side. Identical daily positioning of the patient's arm and head is extremely important for the accuracy of the treatment process.

The feet should be held together with a band or masking tape around the toes. This helps eliminate rotation of the patient's lower abdomen, thereby enhancing setup reproducibility. A triangular sponge or bolster may be placed under the patient's knees to relieve pressure on the lumbar region. The same immobilization devices must be used each time the patient is treated.

When lying supine, patients with large and/or pendulous breasts often have breast tissue displaced up into the infraclavicular area. These patients can be positioned on an incline board so that their head and thorax are elevated relative to their pelvis and lower extremities. This position can be useful in keeping the breast tissue in a more normal location, which is necessary to adequately irradiate the breast and avoid treating the upper arm. This position can also help alleviate the problem of deep skin folds in the supraclavicular area. Care must be taken, however, to avoid overtilting the patient and causing redundancy of the skin in the inframammary area.

The patient position should be well documented and explained in the setup instructions. For patients with unusual conditions or situations in which the setup needs further clarification, Polaroid photographs or digital images of the patient in the treatment position are essential.

Intact Breast or Chest Wall Treatment Technique. Women who require only breast or chest wall irradiation are treated with tangential (glancing) fields. The purpose of this field arrangement is to maximize coverage of the tissues at risk and minimize the radiation dose to underlying structures, primarily the lung and heart. Radiation beams produced by lower energy linear accelerators (4 to 6 MV) and cobalt units are ideally suited to this type of treatment. Considerations for field margins for tangential fields are as follows:

- Superior, at the most cephalad of the following points:
  - First intercostal space
  - As far cephalad as possible without including the arm

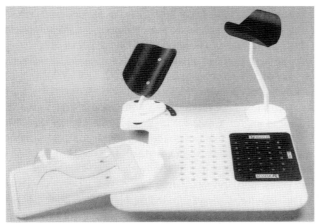

Figure 38-11. Diacor immobilization device used to assist in patient positioning for radiation treatment. (Courtesy Diacor, Salt Lake City, UT.)

- Superior extent of the palpable breast tissue
- Cephalad (>2 cm) to original location of the mass
- Inferior
  - Caudad (1 to 2 cm) to the inframammary fold
  - In a postmastectomy patient, this can be extrapolated from inframammary fold of contralateral breast
- Medial
  - At midline of patient, as determined by palpation of suprasternal notch and xiphoid process
  - Exceptions include patient whose mass or incision extends to or beyond midline and patient who will receive IM lymphatic irradiation
- Lateral
  - Corresponding to midaxillary line (a line drawn from the center of the patient's axilla in a caudad direction)
  - Including drain sites or incisions considered at risk, original tumor bed, and appropriate amount of lung margin

Most current techniques use an isocentric method of tangential field irradiation. In these techniques the isocenter is placed at some depth in the patient's breast or chest wall. At many institutions the isocenter is placed approximately halfway between the ribs and skin, at a point approximately midway between the medial and lateral entrance points of the beam. Other techniques place the isocenter at the deep edge of the tangential field and split the radiation beam in half, blocking the deep half of the beam.

An important feature of the tangential field arrangement is the **coplanar** nature of the deep (or posterior) margin of the ports (Figure 38-12). In coplanar fields, the deep border of the medial tangent and the deep border of the lateral tangent form a single plane. This is important in ensuring a dose as homogeneous as possible throughout the treatment volume. Coplanar tangential fields may be achieved with a split-beam technique, as just mentioned, or an unblocked technique.

Asynchronous jaws or multileaf collimator (MLC) provides the best result with a split-beam technique. Suspended blocks are least desirable because of transmission through the block and scatter that reaches the contralateral breast. Unintended irradiation of the contralateral breast is of concern, especially in

younger patients. Several investigators have demonstrated a small but finite incidence of radiation-induced cancer in the contralateral breast of women who received radiation treatment for breast cancer.[5,14]

Perhaps the most desirable method of treating coplanar tangential fields (from the standpoint of limiting dose to the contralateral breast) is the unblocked isocentric technique. Coplanar tangential fields are not parallel opposed. The number of degrees from parallel opposition is a function of field size and may be calculated.

Planning tangential fields can be a relatively complex process. Several techniques described in the literature over the past 20 years have become well-established methods for planning comprehensive radiation treatment of the breast or chest wall and peripheral lymphatic areas.[35,43,48,50] Techniques used at many institutions today are exact replicas or variations of these themes. Several commercial vendors market systems that include immobilization devices and programmable calculators capable of performing the necessary mathematical calculations. Other techniques use factors that are derived empirically.

The following method is reproducible, satisfies all essential criteria, and incorporates the advantage of a stable setup point. The patient will be placed on the breast board. It is available through several commercial vendors. The breast bridge, also available commercially, can easily make all the necessary measurements for conventional simulation techniques.

1. Set the patient up on the breast board. Make sure the patient is centered and leveled.
2. Mark superior, inferior, medial, and lateral borders on the patient. The medial and lateral borders are marked by radiopaque makers. The central axis is placed midpoint between superior and inferior borders.
3. Use the breast bridge to get chest wall angle, chest wall separation, sternal angle, and field width.
4. A formula can be generated by physicists at each institution to calculate the shift and depth of central axis, the gantry angles, and collimator angles of medial and lateral tangents. The formula can be programmed into an Excel file to be readily available to the therapist doing the simulation.
5. Make the shift and depth to set up the isocenter.
6. Set up the medial tangent field first. Rotate the gantry to the desired angle. Adjust the angle as needed under the fluoroscopy to make sure the markers from the medial and lateral margins are aligned (coplanar). Adjust the collimator angle as needed such that the medial field edge is parallel to the chest wall (Figure 38-13). Make sure the skin flash is adequate.
7. Set up the lateral tangent by rotating the gantry to the desired angle. Adjust the angle as needed under the fluoroscopy to make sure the markers from the medial and lateral margins are aligned. Make sure the skin flash is adequate. Rotate the collimator the same number of degrees in the opposite direction of that used in step 6.
8. The amount of lung included in the tangential fields should be carefully considered. If insufficient lung is in the field, adjust the lateral border in a posterior direction (if clinically allowable). If there is too much lung, move the lateral border anteriorly (if clinically allowable).

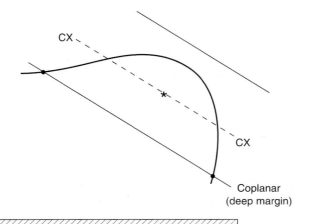

Figure 38-12. Tangential breast irradiation field arrangement features a coplanar deep margin.

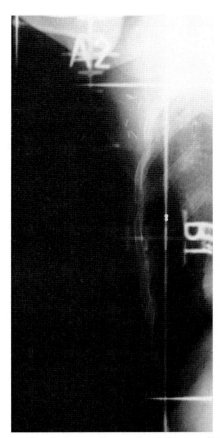

Figure 38-13. Simulation radiograph of the medial tangential field.

It may also be possible to adjust the medial border, depending on the location of the lesion. If adjustments are necessary, return to step 6 and continue.

9. Mark the setup points and field borders on the patient for accurate realignment of the fields for treatment.
10. Complete the setup documentation form.

Computerized treatment planning of the tangential field pair is necessary to visualize the dose distribution throughout the treatment volume and surrounding normal tissues (i.e., lung and heart). Wedges or a compensator may be needed to improve dose homogeneity. Skin doses are often adequate because of tangentially configured radiation beams; therefore, bolus is not usually required.

Comprehensive Breast or Chest Wall and Peripheral Lymphatics Treatment Technique. One critical aspect of comprehensive irradiation for breast cancer is the avoidance of junctional inconsistency between the peripheral lymphatic fields (i.e., supraclavicular-axillary and tangential fields). If overlap occurs, hot or overdosed areas result from a combination of divergence and geometrical distortion of the radiation beams. Such excess dose can lead to match-line fibrosis and a poor cosmetic result. Conversely, a cold or underdosed area provides the potential for tumor recurrence. Avoidance of junctional irregularities can be achieved through the establishment of a vertical straight edge in the axial plane, perpendicular to the floor where the fields meet.

Supraclavicular Field. When used, the supraclavicular field is planned before the tangential fields. Considerations for field margins for the supraclavicular field are as follows:

- Superior
  - Approximately 5 cm above the suprasternal notch (SSN)
  - Avoidance of flash over the skin of the supraclavicular area
- Medial
  - Midpoint of the SSN
- Lateral
  - Approximately 2 to 3 cm of the humeral head
- Inferior, at one of the following:
  - Approximately at the angle of Louis
  - Just above the superior extent of the palpable breast tissue
  - A point >2 cm cephalad to the original location of the mass

The central ray of the supraclavicular field is placed at the inferior margin of the volume to be treated. The inferior half of the beam is blocked by multileaf collimation and an asymmetrical jaw, creating a vertical straight edge at the inferior border of the supraclavicular field. The gantry is angled 10 to 15 degrees mediolaterally to avoid exiting through the spinal cord. A simulation film of the supraclavicular field is provided in Figure 38-14.

Posterior Axillary Boost Field. A posterior axillary boost (PAB) field is sometimes used to increase the midaxillary dose to the prescribed level in a subset of patients whose axillary fossa requires radiation. This is done because at midplane the radiation dose from an anterior supraclavicular field alone may be insufficient. A simulation film of the PAB field is provided in Figure 38-15.

The PAB field should be parallel opposed to the supraclavicular field and uses the identical inferior margin, preserving the vertical straight edge. Considerations for field margins of the PAB field are as follows:

- Superior
  - Mid to upper clavicle

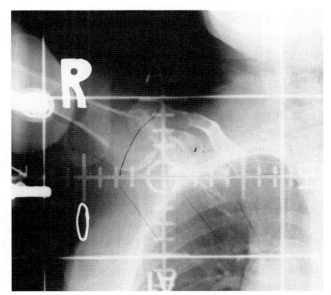

Figure 38-14. Simulation radiograph of the supraclavicular field.

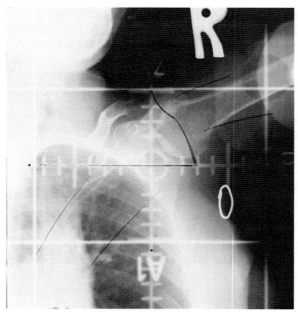

Figure 38-15. Simulation radiograph of the posterior axillary boost field.

- Medial
  - A strip of lung approximately 1 cm wide
- Lateral
  - Approximately 1 to 2 cm of the humeral head, which is subsequently blocked
- Inferior
  - Corresponding to the inferior border of the supraclavicular field

Its relatively small total dose notwithstanding, the PAB should be treated with the same fractionation scheme as the supraclavicular field. Considering larger boost fractions (about 1.8 or 2.0 Gy delivered over a few days) may be tempting; however, this dose must be considered as additive to that being delivered via the supraclavicular field, and a large boost fraction would result in an extremely large daily dose to the PAB site.

Tangential Breast or Chest Wall Fields. The tangential photon fields in comprehensive irradiation for breast cancer are planned in the same way as those described in the section on tangential breast or chest wall irradiation, with several notable additions necessary for an appropriate junction with the supraclavicular-axillary fields. To establish a vertical straight edge at the superior border of the tangential fields, correction must be made for the divergence of the tangential fields into the supraclavicular-axillary field and for geometrical distortion of the radiation beam. The couch assembly is rotated in such a way that the patient's feet are directed away from the collimator and a block is placed at the superior edges of the tangential fields. This is done to force correspondence to the vertical straight edge created by the inferior border of the supraclavicular-axillary field pair. The exact location of the block can be determined by placing a rod with a dependent chain on the patient's skin at the level of the supraclavicular field's inferior border. Steps in comprehensive breast irradiation are as follows:

1. After imaging the supraclavicular-axillary fields, follow steps 1 through 10 of the previously described tangential

technique with some modification. A device composed of a metal rod with an attached chain is used to help define the inferior border of the supraclavicular-axillary field. The metal rod is taped to the patient's skin at the level of the inferior border of the supraclavicular-axillary field, allowing the dependent chain to hang freely over the patient's side.
2. Rotate the collimator so that the medial field edge is parallel to the chest wall.
3. Rotate the couch until fluoroscopic images of the rod and chain are superimposed. Film this field (Figure 38-16).
4. To align the lateral tangent field, rotate the gantry approximately 180 degrees, and confirm via fluoroscopy that the two lead markers are superimposed (coplanar). Adjustment of the gantry angle may be necessary to obtain superimposition. There should be 1 to 3 cm of lung in the field (Figure 38-17). Rotate the collimator the same number of degrees in the opposite direction of that used in step 2.
5. Mark the edge of the lateral tangential light field on the patient's skin.
6. Rotate the couch in the opposite direction from that in step 3 until fluoroscopic images of the rod and chain are superimposed.
7. Readjust the gantry and collimator angles to match the line marked on the patient in step 5.
8. Verify superimposition of the medial field edge markers and the rod and chain via fluoroscopy. Image this field.

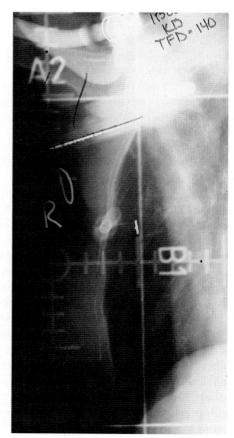

Figure 38-16. Simulation radiograph of the medial tangential field, illustrating the use of the rod and chain.

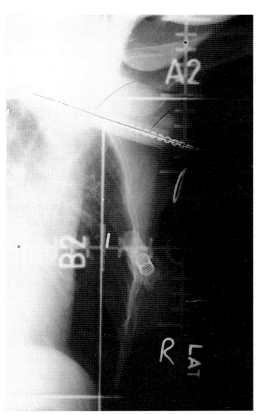

Figure 38-17. Simulation film of the lateral tangential field, illustrating the use of the rod and chain.

9. Mark the setup points and field borders on the patient for accurate realignment of the fields for treatment.

10. Complete a setup documentation form.

Single isocenter setup is another way to treat both supraclavicular field and breast if the field length is less than 20 cm, half of the field length of treatment machine limit. This method has its advantage of simple setup during daily treatment, with no need of blocking and coach rotation.

Internal Mammary Lymph Nodes. A relatively small proportion of patients with breast cancer may be at risk for involvement of the IM lymph nodes. Whether to irradiate the IM nodes remains controversial, partly because current techniques are potentially damaging to normal tissues. One method of irradiating the IM nodes is the extended or deep tangential field configuration. Rather than placing the edge of the medial tangential field at the patient's midline, the field is extended beyond the midline to the contralateral side by approximately 3 cm. Although this arrangement is usually successful in encompassing the ipsilateral IM nodes, it results in a significant increase in the volume of lung irradiated. The extended tangential field also encroaches on the contralateral breast tissue, causing an increase in scattered dose to the breast. Furthermore, in the treatment of left-sided lesions, a fairly large portion of the heart is often included in the extended tangential field.

An alternative method of irradiating the IM nodes involves the use of an en face (perpendicular to the skin surface with a slight angle towards the patient) IM field with a combination of electrons and photons. This field arrangement is subject to the difficulties of matching en face and tangential fields, as well as the problems of joining photon and electron ports, and may result in a hot or cold spot at the junctional area. In addition, an increased volume of cardiac tissue is included in the en face configuration. The photon portion of the IM node treatment contributes less exit dose to the vertebral bodies and spinal cord once is angled. Conversely, if electrons are used for most or all of the IM treatment, the skin dose may be unacceptably high, contributing to acute and chronic sequelae and a potentially less acceptable cosmetic result.

Breast Boost. Patients with conservatively managed breast cancer usually receive additional radiation treatment to the tumor bed immediately after the completion of tangential irradiation. This boost may be delivered with electron teletherapy or radioactive implantation. Electrons are the technique of choice at most institutions because of patient convenience, cost, and cosmetic considerations. In planning the electron boost, care must be taken to ensure that the treatment volume adequately encompasses the tumor bed. The assumption that the location and length of the scar accurately reflect the position and size of the tumor bed may be inaccurate.[3,40,48] If the surgeon places clips on the tumor bed at the time of resection, then the position and size of the electron field can be optimized via fluoroscopy and/or radiographs obtained in the simulator room.

Occasionally, the tumor bed boost is delivered via radioactive implantation. Potential indications for this method include the presence of a gross residual tumor at the time of resection, a deep-seated lesion in an extremely large breast, and, rarely, patient preference. Because implantation is invasive, relatively expensive, and labor intensive and because it requires anesthesia and sometimes inpatient admission, current practice does not routinely include boosting the tumor bed with a radioactive implant.

Virtual Computed Tomography Simulation. Many institutions now use CT for breast setup. The patient is placed with an immobilization device. The treatment borders and scars are outlined with radiopaque catheters. The patient is taken to the CT scanner where slices are taken to include all the borders. The 3-mm slices provide digitally reconstructed high-resolution radiographs. The scan information can be transferred to the treatment planning computer and used for field design. The treatment volume can then be verified using a digitally reconstructed radiograph.

Evolving Technology. Breast geometry poses a significant challenge for delivering homogeneous doses of radiation. Intensity-modulated radiation therapy (IMRT) has the potential to reduce these discrepancies in breast irradiation. The most common IMRT technique for breast cancer treatment is multiple static MLC segments.[6,19,30,32,53] The treatment is delivered through sequential open fields and MLC fields with fixed gantry angles. As a result, improved dose distribution can be achieved with reduced dose exposure to the lung and heart. By strategic use of dose homogeneity, concomitant boost is also being explored to treat the whole breast and boost the tumor bed at the same time. At this time, there are only limited clinical data that have demonstrated decreased morbidity by improving dose homogeneity using IMRT.[16]

Accelerated partial breast irradiation (APBI) has been investigated as a possible alternative treatment option for women undergoing breast-conserving therapy. Instead of treating the whole breast, partial breast irradiation targets the tumor bed with a margin. The treatment can be completed in 5 days with twice-a-day treatment. There are various techniques to deliver partial breast irradiation. Multicatheter interstitial brachytherapy has been used longest but is technically challenging. Balloon catheter brachtherapy has been used widely in the United States since Food and Drug Administration (FDA) clearance in 2002. Three-dimensional conformal external beam radiotherapy is a noninvasive alternative. Outside of the United States, intraoperative radiotherapy has been the main method to deliver the treatment. A paper by D. Arthur and F. Vicini provides an excellent review of all these treatment techniques and supporting clinical data.[2] The efficacy of APBI is currently being investigated by an ongoing phase III randomized control study sponsored by NSABP and RTOG.

Special Problems. Occasionally, patients requiring radiation therapy for breast malignancy have special circumstances that render planning and treatment difficult. These include a lack of arm mobility, extreme breast size, and very pendulous breasts.

Lack of Arm Mobility. When planned appropriately in terms of energy selection, field placement, and junction considerations, electron beams offer a viable method of treating postmastectomy patients who have severely compromised arm mobility, as in instances of brachial plexopathy. Because electron fields are treated en face as opposed to tangentially, the problem of avoiding the patient's arm is circumvented. The ideal candidate for this technique has a relatively flat chest wall of uniform thickness. The patient's arm can rest on the treatment table, at her side, and in as abducted a position as the patient can manage. Typically, a minimum of two electron fields are used to encompass the chest wall margins listed previously. One field treats the anterior-medial chest wall, and the other covers the lateral chest wall. The precise matching of adjacent electron field edges can be difficult, so care must be taken to shift the match-line or use junctional wedges or some other means of enhancing dose uniformity where the fields meet.

Some postoperative patients are completely unable to abduct the arm, usually as a result of advanced disease. These individuals can be treated with their arm in an abducted position through the use of an anterior photon field that encompasses the supraclavicular, axillary, and lateral chest wall regions in a single field. The anterior chest wall can be treated with an en face electron field.

Extreme Breast Size and Pendulous Breasts. Patients with extremely large and/or pendulous breasts are particularly challenging to treat. Numerous devices and techniques have been developed to stabilize the breast and position it on the chest, permitting a reasonably accurate setup and treatment. Elastic netting can be placed over the breasts; however, this works best on smaller breasts because the material is not strong enough to support an extremely large breast on the chest wall. Systems that use thermoplastic materials to mold the breast into an appropriate position are available commercially. Thermoplastic sheets may also be molded to the patient and fastened around the patient's back with bandage material. A simple ring can be placed around the breast to immobilize and retain the breast in position on the anterior chest.[4] A Styrofoam crutch can also be

fashioned and positioned to support pendulous breast tissue located far to the patient's lateral chest. Prone position using a commercially available board may also be advantageous to give homogeneous dose to the breast. Care must be taken not to underdose the chest wall.

Side Effects. The aim of radiation therapy to the breast is the complete eradication of tumor cells with minimal structural and functional damage to normal tissue. A compromise of accepting a certain degree of acute and chronic tissue damage in return for a potential cure is necessary. In every situation, careful planning and treatment delivery are essential to minimize side effects.

Combining radiation treatment and chemotherapy may intensify toxicity. In breast cancer patients, the use of doxorubicin is of particular concern. When used concomitantly, radiation and doxorubicin may be hazardous. If doxorubicin is given after radiation therapy, then a recall phenomenon may occur in previously treated areas, displayed by exacerbation of reactions of the esophagus, skin, lungs, and heart.

Skin Changes. Skin and subcutaneous tissue changes are expected in the irradiated treatment volume. The skin dose depends on the exact treatment technique used for each patient. Variables in the treatment plan that affect the skin dose include the type of radiation (photons or electrons), beam energy, boost technique (external beam or brachytherapy), wedge, bolus, fraction size, total dose, and physical conformation of the patient.

Special consideration must be given to the physical conformation of the patient. Skin folds tend to intensify skin reactions as a result of bolus effect and are therefore the most sensitive areas. Proper positioning is necessary to help minimize folds in potential problem areas. Axillary folds may be minimized by adjusting arm abduction. Skin folds in the inframammary, supraclavicular, and neck areas may be altered or eliminated by increasing or decreasing the cephalocaudad incline of the patient. Obese patients or those with large, pendulous breasts may require netting or thermoplastic material for the immobilization and reduction of skin folds.

During a standard radiation treatment schedule, skin reaction intensifies according to the escalating dose. The RTOG categorizes acute and chronic skin reactions, as shown in Tables 38-1 and 38-2. Dryness and redness (erythema) of the skin are common after a skin dose of about 3000 cGy (3 to 4 weeks into treatment). Dry desquamation, which involves flaking of superficial layers of the epidermis, may appear after the delivery of about 4000 cGy to the skin. Moist desquamation, involving the loss of superficial and deep epidermal layers, occurs when doses to the skin exceed 5000 cGy. Moist desquamation may arise earlier in treatment in areas where skin folds or bolus intensify the prescribed dose. Treatment of the large breast is more difficult secondary to such acute effects and can result in a less acceptable cosmetic outcome.

Care of irradiated skin varies according to the type and severity of the reaction. Patients should be advised regarding measures that protect the skin from further irritation and damage. The treatment area must be kept clean through normal, gentle cleansing, and sun exposure should be avoided. Cornstarch is often recommended as a soothing agent for early skin reactions and as a substitute for commercial deodorant. The use of lotions, creams, deodorants, or powders in the treatment area should be discouraged because they may contain irritating agents such as perfumes, alcohol, or metals. Shaving under the arm is not recommended, and clothing should be soft and loose fitting. Extreme temperatures from hot water bottles, heating pads, and ice packs should also be avoided over the skin of the treated area.

Patients experiencing moist desquamation may require daily skin care to help prevent infection and minimize fluid loss. Gentle cleansing may be performed with a solution of hydrogen peroxide diluted by sterile water and dabbed carefully onto the affected area. Proper wound dressing using nonstick bandaging techniques is essential, as care must be taken to avoid placing adhesives or tape in the treatment area. Cornstarch should never be used in areas of moist desquamation because it may promote fungal growth and increase the risk of wound infection.[25] Instead, Silvadene Cream is often prescribed to promote proper healing.

Severe acute reactions may result in a longer healing time and higher incidence of chronic skin changes. Such skin changes progress slowly and can persist for months or years after irradiation. Most chronic skin changes are cosmetic and rarely problematic, and they include hyperpigmentation (excessive coloration), hair loss, epidermal thinning, **telangiectasia** (permanent dilation of vessels, producing small, red lesions), and subcutaneous fibrosis. Rare cases of delayed wound healing, ulceration, and necrosis (death of skin cells) may occur after skin doses of over 70 Gy.[18]

Fatigue. Most patients receiving radiation therapy complain of generalized fatigue. The incidence appears to be related to the radiation dose, treatment volume, and site of involvement. Breast cancer patients may experience a comparatively minor degree of fatigue. Other factors (such as a history of recent surgery or chemotherapy, the patient's general medical and psychologic condition, current medications, pain, or anemia) may contribute to fatigue.

Cardiac Effects. Portions of the heart are sometimes necessarily included in the radiation fields used in breast cancer treatment. Tangential fields used to treat the left chest wall may include a small to moderate volume of the heart, depending on the patient's anatomy and physical configuration. A larger volume of the heart may be included during irradiation of the IM lymph nodes. Although the myocardia (heart muscle) is relatively radioresistant, the risk of promoting arteriosclerosis, leading to pericarditis, is of concern. The incidence of pericarditis is less than 5% for small heart volumes treated to 60 Gy with standard fractionation or for large heart volumes treated to 40 Gy.[8,18] In addition, larger fraction sizes may intensify cardiac damage.

Pulmonary Effects. Tangential fields used to irradiate the breast and/or chest wall always include a small volume of lung tissue. Peripheral lymphatic fields may also irradiate lung tissue. Some degree of **radiation pneumonitis** (inflammation of the lung tissue) and fibrosis can be expected after the administration of more than 2500 cGy to any portion of lung via standard fractionation.[31] These effects are directly related to the total dose, fraction size, and irradiated lung volume. The incidence of pulmonary damage grows as the volume, dose, and fraction size increase. The time of onset and degree of severity also vary depending on the volume, dose, and fraction size of lung irradiated.

Although initial morphologic changes are not clinically manifested, symptoms may appear after a latent period of 1 to 3 months.[31] These symptoms may include coughing, dyspnea, sputum production, fever, and night sweats and may subside after several months. Scarring or fibrosis may begin 3 to 7 months after irradiation, and depending on its severity, chronic respiratory distress may develop. The degree of severity can be monitored via a chest radiograph, CT scan, and pulmonary function tests. Fortunately, the incidence of chronic pulmonary effects is rare in breast cancer patients because of the small volume of lung irradiated.

Lymphedema. Lymphedema of the arm may occur as a result of axillary lymphatic obstruction. Some acute lymphedema usually occurs immediately after breast surgery and axillary dissection. The severity and risk of lymphedema are directly related to the extent of the axillary dissection and may be further complicated by radiation and chemotherapy. Approximately 25% to 30% of patients receiving radiation therapy after level III axillary lymph node dissection experience arm edema. Tumor infiltration, infection, inflammation, scarring of the lymph nodes, and radiation-induced fibrosis (alone or in combination) may cause lymphatic obstruction. If a collateral circulatory pathway develops in response to the obstruction, allowing for lymphatic drainage, then the edema will resolve. Where the obstruction is severe or the damage is irreparable, lymphatic circulation may be permanently compromised, resulting in chronic edema of the arm.

Radiation-induced lymphedema is relatively rare and similar to other chronic effects in that the incidence and severity are directly related to the radiation dose and treatment volume. Depending on the degree of edema, this condition may be disfiguring and uncomfortable and may impair mobility and function of the arm.

Brachial Plexopathy. The brachial plexus (a network of nerves supplying the upper extremities) originates between C5 and T1 and extends downward over the first rib, behind the middle of the clavicle, and into the axilla. Damage to these nerves in the form of fibrosis is termed brachial plexopathy. High doses of radiation (5500 to 6000 cGy) may lead to this condition.[4,25] Fortunately, standard dose levels prescribed for breast cancer treatment do not exceed 4500 to 5400 cGy and rarely result in this complication. The incidence of brachial plexopathy may also be related to surgery and chemotherapy. Symptoms include a loss of motor function (paresthesia of the arm and hand), weakness, and pain, for which the only treatment is symptomatic pain relief.

Myelopathy. Although the spine is usually avoided entirely during breast irradiation, portions of the cervical and thoracic spine may need to be included in the IM and supraclavicular fields. Care must be taken not to exceed the spinal cord's tolerance dose to avoid delayed complications of chronic progressive myelopathy (ranging from severe to fatal). The TD 5/5 (minimal tolerance dose) is 4500 to 5000 cGy for instances in which portions of the spinal cord are irradiated with standard fractionation.[4,18]

The supraclavicular field may be angled 10 to 15 degrees mediolaterally to avoid the spinal cord completely. The IM chain field may be treated via expanded tangential fields that entirely avoid the spinal cord or with a combination of en face photons and electrons to reduce the spinal cord dosage. Any adjoining of fields over the spinal cord must be planned carefully to avoid overlap, which can result in an overdose of radiation to the spinal cord.

Osteoradionecrosis. Tangential treatment fields of the chest wall may incidentally deliver a relatively high dose of radiation to the ribs. The incidence of a resulting rib fracture is relatively low (less than 1%), and the ribs appear to heal on their own.

SUMMARY

Breast cancer represents an enigmatic yet fascinating challenge in cancer management. The incidence of breast cancer is widespread, and it is sometimes fatal, recurring sometimes two or three decades after the initial diagnosis and treatment. Breast cancer is especially important because it affects a part of the female anatomy that is functionally and culturally associated with beauty, femininity, sexuality, and nurturing. With recorded history dating back several millennia, the pendulum of breast cancer treatment has swung between extremes of belief that breast cancer is an incurable systemic disease and the notion that it is a local, therefore curable, problem. This debate continues today, with many researchers occupying a rational middle ground in which each patient is evaluated against the backdrop of multiple prospective and retrospective analyses to maximize survival potential.

- Approximately one in eight women are diagnosed with breast cancer in the United States.
- The most common presenting symptom of early-stage breast cancer is a palpable mass.
- Microscopic examination of tissue removed from the breast via biopsy is the best insurance of a definitive diagnosis.
- The pathologic staging system incorporates lymph node status, tumor extent, and distant metastasis. Staging aids in the selection of treatment and indicates the prognosis.
- Involvement of supraclavicular lymph nodes implies a poor prognosis.
- A multidisciplinary approach that includes surgery, radiation therapy, and chemotherapy is required for breast cancer treatment.
- Occasionally, patients requiring radiation therapy for breast malignancy have special circumstances that render planning and treatment difficult. These include a lack of arm mobility, extreme breast size, and very pendulous breasts.
- Many postoperative patients (whether the surgery involved a mastectomy or an axillary dissection) experience initial difficulty in raising the arm to an acceptable position for radiation treatment. Therefore, the simulation and start of therapy should be delayed until the patient's arm moves appropriately via an exercise regimen.
- Patients undergoing radiation treatment to the breast should be advised to wear nonrestrictive clothing, avoid using commercial deodorant, and avoid sun exposure to the affected area.
- Common side effects include skin erythema, dry or wet skin desquamation, fatigue, and breast discomfort. Most side effects resolve after completion of treatment.

Review Questions

Multiple Choice

1. The pathologic staging system for breast cancer incorporates:
   - I. lymph node status
   - II. tumor extent
   - III. distant metastasis
   - a. I and II
   - b. II and III
   - c. I and III
   - d. I, II, and III

2. The most common presenting symptom of early-stage breast cancer is:
   - a. nipple discharge
   - b. pain
   - c. palpable mass
   - d. ulceration

3. Which of the following is proper advice for a patient receiving radiation treatment to the breast?
   - I. Do not wear restrictive clothing.
   - II. Avoid using commercial deodorant.
   - III. Avoid sun exposure to the skin of the treated area.
   - a. I and II
   - b. II and III
   - c. I and III
   - d. I, II, and III

4. TD 5/5 refers to:
   - a. minimal tolerance dose
   - b. maximum tolerance dose
   - c. tumor dose of 5 Gy in 5 days
   - d. tumor dose of 5 cGy in 5 days

5. The TD 5/5 for the spinal cord delivered through standard fractionation is:
   - a. 1500 cGy
   - b. 3000 cGy
   - c. 4500 cGy
   - d. 6000 cGy

6. Which of the following is *not* currently a standard technique for breast surgery?
   - a. radical mastectomy
   - b. modified radical mastectomy
   - c. lumpectomy
   - d. tylectomy

7. Chemotherapy for breast cancer may consist of:
   - I. drug therapy
   - II. endocrine therapy
   - III. immunotherapy
   - a. I and II
   - b. II and III
   - c. I and III
   - d. I, II, and III

8. In treating a breast cancer patient via tangential fields plus an electron field boost, the usual total dose to the tumor bed delivered through a standard fractionation schedule is:
   - a. 4000 to 4600 cGy
   - b. 5000 to 5600 cGy

c. 6000 to 6600 cGy

d. 7000 to 7600 cGy

9. The technique that may be used to adequately irradiate the internal mammary lymph nodes on a patient with left breast cancer and simultaneously deliver the least cardiac dose is:

a. anterior photon field, 50 Gy in 5 weeks

b. anterior photon-electron fields, equally weighted, 50 Gy in 5 weeks

c. wide tangential fields, extending 5 cm across the midline, 50 Gy in 5 weeks

d. anterior electron field, 50 Gy in 5 weeks

10. The skin usually reacts in a pattern that is dose dependent. Which of the following would you expect to see first for radiation administered using a standard fractionation schedule?

a. dry desquamation

b. erythema

c. moist desquamation

d. radiation pneumonitis

The answers to the Review Questions can be found by logging on to our website at: *http://evolve.elsevier.com/Washington+Leaver/principles*

Questions to Ponder

1. Discuss the significant prognostic indicators for breast cancer.
2. Describe the signs of inflammatory breast cancer.
3. Describe the acute effects experienced by patients undergoing radiation treatment to the breast.
4. Define the three elements of treatment in conservative management of early-stage breast cancer.
5. Describe the field arrangements most commonly used for patients receiving conservative management of breast cancer.
6. Discuss important considerations for positioning the conservatively managed patient for breast irradiation.
7. Describe the methods for detection and diagnosis of breast cancer.
8. Identify the common presenting symptoms of breast cancer.
9. Discuss the importance of staging breast cancer.
10. Describe the primary lymphatic drainage of breast tissue.

REFERENCES

1. American Cancer Society: *Cancer facts and figures: 2008*, Atlanta, 2008, American Cancer Society.
2. Arthur DW, Vicini FA: Accelerated partial breast irradiation as a part of breast conservation therapy, *J Clin Oncol* 23:1726-1735, 2005.
3. Bedwinek J: Breast conserving surgery and irradiation: the importance of demarcating the excision cavity with surgical clips, *Int J Radiat Oncol Biol Phys* 26:675-679, 1993.
4. Bentel GC, Nelson CE, Noell KT: *Treatment planning and dose calculation in radiation oncology,* ed 4, Elmsford, NY, 1989, Pergamon Press.
5. Boice JD, et al: Risk of breast cancer following low dose radiation exposure, *Radiology* 131:589-597, 1979.
6. Buchholz TA: Breast. In Chao KSC, editor: *Practice Essentials of Intensity Modulated Radiation Therapy*, ed 2, Philadelphia, 2005, Lippincott Williams & Wilkins.
7. Buchholz TA, et al: The breast. In Cox JD, editor: *Moss' radiation oncology: rationale, technique, results*, ed 8, St. Louis, 2003, Mosby.
8. Byhardt RW, Moss WT: The heart and blood vessels. In Cox JD, editor: *Moss' radiation oncology rationale, technique, results*, ed 8, St. Louis, 2003, Mosby.
9. Carter C, Allen C, Henson D: Relation of tumor size, lymph node status, and survival in 24,740 breast cancer cases, *Cancer* 63:181-187, 1989.
10. Claus EB, et al: The genetic attributable risk of breast and ovarian cancer, *Cancer* 77:2318-2324, 1996.
11. Collaborative Group on Hormonal Factors in Breast Cancer: Breast cancer and hormonal contraceptives: collaborative reanalysis of individual data on 53,297 women with breast cancer and 100,239 women without breast cancer from 54 epidemiological studies, *Lancet* 347:1713-1727, 1996.
12. Collaborative Group on Hormonal Factors in Breast Cancer: Breast cancer and hormonal replacement therapy: collaborative reanalysis of individual data on 53,297 women with breast cancer and 100,239 women without breast cancer from 54 epidemiological studies, *Lancet* 350:1047-59, 1997.
13. Committee on the Biological Effects of Ionizing Radiations, Board on Radiation Effects Research, Commission on Life Sciences, National Research Council: *Health effects of exposure to low levels of ionizing radiation BEIR V*, Washington, DC, 1990, National Academy Press.
14. Cruikshank WC: *The anatomy of the absorbing vessels of the human body*, London, 1786, G. Nicol.
15. Donegan WL, Spratt JS: *Cancer of the breast*, ed 5, Philadelphia, 2002, WB Saunders.
16. Donovan E, et al: Randomised trial of standard 2D radiotherapy (RT) versus intensity modulated radiotherapy (IMRT) in patients prescribed breast radiotherapy. *Radiother Oncol* 82:254-264, 2007.
17. Dupont WD, et al: Breast cancer risk associated with proliferative breast disease and atypical hyperplasia, *Cancer* 71:1258-1265, 1993.
18. Emami B, et al: Tolerance of normal tissue to therapeutic radiation, *Int J Radiat Oncol Biol Phys* 22:109-122, 1991.
19. Evans PM, et al: The delivery of intensity modulated radiotherapy to the breast using multiple static fields. *Radiother Oncol* 57:79-89, 2000.
20. Fenton JJ, et al: Influence of computer-aided detection on performance of screening mammography, *N Engl J Med* 356:1399-1409, 2007.
21. Fisher B, et al: Location of breast carcinoma and prognosis, *Surg Gynecol Obstet* 129:705-716, 1969.
22. Goldhirsch A, Gelber RD: Understanding adjuvant chemotherapy for breast cancer, *N Engl J Med* 330:1308-1309, 1994.
23. Haagensen CD: *Diseases of the breast*, ed 3, Philadelphia, 1986, WB Saunders.
24. Harris JR, et al: *Diseases of the breast*, ed 3, Philadelphia, 2004, Lippincott Williams & Wilkins.
25. Hassey Dow K, Hilderley L: *Nursing care in radiation oncology*, ed 2, Philadelphia, 1997, WB Saunders.
26. Henderson IC: Adjuvant systemic therapy for early breast cancer, *Cancer Suppl* 74(1):401-408, 1994.
27. Hunter DJ, et al: Cohort studies in fat intake and the risk of breast cancer: a pooled analysis, *N Engl J Med* 334:356-361, 1996.
28. John MJ, et al: *Chemoradiation: an integrated approach to cancer treatment*, Malvern, PP, 1993, Lea and Febiger.
29. Kelsey JL: A review of the epidemiology of human breast cancer, *Epidemiol Rev* 1:74-109, 1979.
30. Kestin LL, et al: Intensity modulation to improve dose uniformity with tangential breast radiotherapy: initial clinical experience. *Int J Radiat Oncol Biol Phys* 48:1559-1568, 2000.
31. Komaki R, Cox JD: The lung and thymus. In Cox JD, editor: *Moss' radiation oncology: rationale, technique, results*, ed 8, St. Louis, 2003, Mosby.
32. Krueger EA, et al: Potential gains for irradiation of chest wall and regional nodes with intensity modulated radiotherapy. *Int J Radiat Oncol Biol Phys* 56:1023-1027, 2003.
33. Kuehn T, et al: Sentinel-node biopsy for axillary staging in breast cancer: results from a large prospective German multi-institutional trial, *Eur J Surg Oncol* 30:252-259, 2004.
34. Mansel RE, et al: Randomized multicenter trial of sentinel node biopsy versus standard axillary treatment in operable breast cancer: The ALMANAC trial, *J Natl Cancer Inst* 98:599-609, 2006.

35. Mascagni P: *Vasorum lymphaticorum corporis humani historia et ichnographia*, Siena, Italy, 1787, P. Carli.

36. Page DL, et al: Subsequent breast carcinoma risk after biopsy with atypia in a breast papilloma. *Cancer* 78:258-266, 1996.

37. Pharoah PDP, et al: Family history and the risk of breast cancer: A systemic review and meta-analysis, *Int J Cancer* 71:800-809, 1997.

38. Pisano ED, et al: Diagnostic performance of digital versus film mammography for breast cancer screening, *N Engl J Med* 353:1773-1783, 2005.

39. Ravdin PM, et al: The decrease in breast cancer incidence in 2003 in the United States, *N Engl J Med* 356:1670-1674, 2007.

40. Regine WF, et al: Computer-CT planning of the electron boost in definitive breast irradiation, *Int J Radiat Oncol Biol Phys* 20:121-125, 1991.

41. Ries, LAG et al (eds): SEER cancer statistics review, 1975-2003, National Cancer Institute, Bethesda, MD, http://seer.cancer.gov/csrr/1975_2003/ based on November 2005 SEER data submission, posted to the SEER website, 2006.

42. Rosen PP, et al: Discontinuous or "skip" metastases in breast carcinoma: analysis of 1228 axillary dissections, *Ann Surg* 276-283, 1983.

43. Saphillo O, Parker MI: Metastases of primary carcinoma of the breast with special reference to spleen, adrenal glands and ovaries, *Arch Surg* 42:1003, 1941.

44. Saslow D, et al: American Cancer Society guidelines for breast screening with MRI as an adjunct to mammography, *CA Cancer J Clin* 57:75-89, 2007.

45. Shapiro S, et al: Ten- to fourteen- year effect of screening on breast cancer mortality, *J Natl Cancer Inst* 69:349-355, 1982.

46. Shinkin MB: *Contrary to nature*, Washington, DC, 1977, United States Printing Office.

47. Singletary KW, Gapstur SM: Alcohol and breast cancer: review of epidemiologic and experimental evidence and potential mechanisms, *JAMA* 286:2143-2151, 2001.

48. Solin LJ, et al: A practical technique for the localization of the tumor volume in definitive irradiation of the breast, *Int J Radiat Oncol Biol Phys* 11:1215-1220, 1985.

49. Tabár L, et al: Update of the Swedish two-county program of mammographic screening for breast cancer, *Radiol Clin North Am* 30:187-210, 1992.

50. Veronesi U, et al: Prognosis of breast cancer patients after mastectomy and dissection of internal mammary nodes, *Ann Surg* 202:702-707, 1985.

51. Veronesi U, et al: Distribution of axillary node metastases by level of invasion: an analysis of 539 cases, *Cancer* 59:682-687, 1987.

52. Veronesi U, et al: A randomized comparison of sentinel-node biopsy with routine axillary dissection in breast cancer, *N Engl J Med* 349:546-553, 2003.

53. Vicini FA, et al: Optimizing breast cancer treatment efficacy with intensity-modulated radiotherapy. *Int J Radiat Oncol Biol Phys* 54:1336-1344, 2002.

54. Voogd AC, et al: The risk of nodal metastases in breast cancer patients with clinically negative lymph nodes: a population-based analysis, *Breast Cancer Res Treat* 62:63-69, 2000.

55. Wood WC, et al: Cancer of the breast. In DeVita VT, Hellman S, Rosenberg SA, editors: *Cancer principles and practice of oncology*, ed 7, Philadelphia, 2005, Lippincott Williams & Wilkins.

56. Yamauchi H, et al: The role of c-erbB-2 as a predictive factor in breast cancer, *Breast Cancer* 8:171-183, 2001.

Pediatric Solid Tumors

Jeffrey Young

Outline

Key Terms

Objectives

- Discuss epidemiologic factors related to pediatric cancers.
- Identify, list, and discuss etiologic factors that may be responsible for inducing pediatric tumors.
- Describe how pediatric cancers are different than adult cancers in the same organ system.
- Discuss the methods of detection and diagnosis for pediatric tumors.
- Describe the diagnostic procedures used in the workup and staging for various pediatric malignancies.
- Differentiate between histologic grading and staging.
- Discuss the rationale for treatment with regard to treatment choice, histologic type, and stage of the disease.
- Describe in detail the treatment methods available for pediatric malignancies.

- Discuss the expected radiation reactions for pediatric malignancies based on time-dose-fractionation schemes, and discuss how three-dimensional planning can reduce late effects.
- Discuss tolerance levels of the vital structures and organs at risk.
- Describe the instructions that should be given to a patient with regard to skin care, expected reactions, and dietary advice.
- Identify the psychological problems associated with a pediatric malignancy.
- Discuss the rationale for using multimodality treatments.
- Discuss survival statistics and prognosis for various tumors related to pediatric cancers.

A lthough older groups dominate the patient population of radiation oncology centers, childhood cancer (age 20 years or younger) is a significant problem. An estimated 10,500 new cases are expected to occur each year among children aged 0 to 14 years along with up to another 5000 in those aged 15 to 20 years. This yields a rate of 16 cancer cases per 100,000 population under 20 years old. An estimated 1500 deaths are expected annually, about one third of them from leukemia.[4] The types of cancers that develop, their treatments, and cure rates are distinctly different than those of the adult population (Table 39-1).

Predisposing genetic conditions include xeroderma pigmentosa; ataxia telangiectasia; Bloom, Fanconi's, and Down syndromes; neurofibromatosis; and others. Genetic abnormalities and oncogenes such as *p53*, retinoblastoma tumor suppressor gene, and chromosome translocations lead to loss of growth control in cancer cells.[45] Cytogenetic and molecular markers that correlate to prognosis are being increasingly identified, which allows treatment intensity stratification. Acute leukemias and

Table 39-1	Cancer in Children	
Cancer Type	**Percentage Occurring in Children**	**Predominant Age at Occurrence**
Acute leukemia	31.0	2-8 years
Acute lymphoblastic leukemia	21.0	2 years, then stable
Other	10.0	2-18 years
Central nervous system	19.0	Varies with histology
Malignant lymphoma	8.0	Varies with type
Hodgkin's disease	6.0	Increases with age
Neuroblastoma	8.0	0-3 years
Wilms' tumor	6.0	<5 years
Soft tissue sarcomas	5.0	<5 years >10-12 years
Bone sarcomas	5.0	Increases with age >10 years
Retinoblastoma	2.5	0-2 years
Germ cell tumors	2.5	<1 year; >8-10 years
Liver tumors	2.5	4 years

From Cox JD, Ang KK: *Radiation oncology, rationale, technique, result*, St. Louis, 2003, Mosby.

Table 39-2	Relative Incidence of Brain Tumors
Type of Tumor	**Percentage of Total**
SUPRATENTORIAL (45%-50%)	
Low-grade astrocytoma	25
Anaplastic astrocytoma, glioblastoma, and PNET	10
Ependymoma	3
Pineal and germ cell tumors	4
Pituitary and craniopharyngioma	5
INFRATENTORIAL (50%-55%)	
Medulloblastoma	25
Low-grade astrocytoma	15
Ependymoma	5
Brainstem glioma	10

Data from Duffner PK, et al: Survival of children with brain tumors: SEER program, 1973-1980, *Neurology* 36:597-601, 1986.
PNET, Primitive neuroectodermal tumor.

lymphomas account for about 40% of pediatric cancers. Central nervous system (CNS) tumors are the most frequent solid tumors, and radiation has a critical role in their treatment. Although a shift toward other effective therapies has taken place, radiation is still used in patients who have soft tissue sarcoma, Ewing's sarcoma of bone, Wilms' tumor, neuroblastoma, Hodgkin's lymphoma, and other benign and malignant conditions.

The treatment of childhood malignancies is always multidisciplinary and requires close attention to the physical and emotional needs of the child and family. Care is coordinated with medical, surgical, and nursing oncology colleagues and supported from social services, physical therapists, nutritionists, educators, and others. This team approach usually requires referral to a specialized children's cancer program. More than 50% of patients are involved in clinical trial investigations led by the Children's Oncology Group (COG) in the United States and similar international groups. Therapists have special demands for such protocol patients including strict treatment and data guidelines, concurrent chemotherapy, immobilization and anesthesia. Because many radiation therapists do not see pediatric patients, the remainder of this chapter highlights selected childhood cancers and their unique treatments.

BRAIN TUMORS

Epidemiology

CNS cancer cases annually involve a wide spectrum of lesions histologically and anatomically. In children (compared with adults), low-grade and infratentorial (posterior fossa) tumors are more frequent and metastatic lesions from non-CNS primaries are rare. For long-term survivors, late effects of treatment are a major concern. Table 39-2 illustrates relative incidences

from a combination of patient series. Infratentorial and primitive neuroectodermal tumors (PNETs) lesions tend toward younger ages. Neurofibromatosis is linked to risk of low-grade glioma, and retinoblastoma suppressor gene defects on chromosome 13 can be inherited, leading to a high risk of bilateral disease. However, most benign and high-grade tumors occur sporadically. Because the disease and its treatment can have major long-term side effects for children, individualized multidisciplinary care involving neurosurgery, endocrinology, pediatric and radiation oncology, neuro-psychology, rehabilitation, social work, and other services is a must.

Low-Grade Astrocytoma

Astrocytomas are tumors originating from the supporting cells of the brain. These tumors can be histologically similar to normal glial cells but have continued slow, relentless growth. They occur about equally in the cerebrum and posterior fossa. A long history of mild symptoms dependent on the area of brain involved is the usual course. Headaches, degenerating coordination, visual impairment, or poor school performance can worsen subtly for months or years, and seizures can eventually develop. Radiologically, a cystic component may be present, and there is less surrounding edema than with high-grade lesions (Figure 39-1, *A*).

If discovered in an extremely young child without major neurologic deficits, a low-grade brain tumor can be followed with serial physical and radiologic examinations. After the child reaches an age at which the brain is more mature (usually 3 to 5 years old), neurosurgery is the primary treatment. If the lesion can be completely removed, the long-term prognosis is excellent. A recurrence-free survival rate of 90% to 100% has been achieved in juvenile astrocytomas.[60] Although historically thought to be resistant, modern chemotherapy has induced responses in some low-grade gliomas, allowing delay and occasionally avoidance of radiation.

Radiation therapy has been reserved for surgically inaccessible or recurrent lesions and those with postsurgical residual

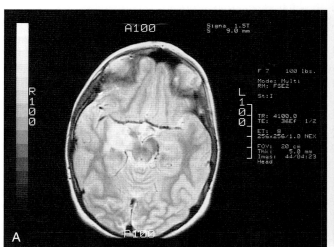

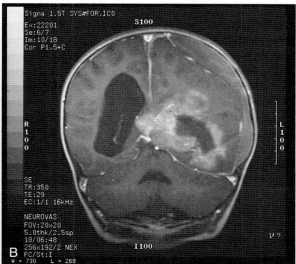

Figure 39-1. A, Low-grade astrocytoma. Note the regular border and minimal edema. **B**, Glioblastoma multiforme. Invasive borders, edema, and shift of normal structures.

tumor in locations where further growth could lead to significant neurological problems. A dose of 5000 to 5400 cGy at 180 cGy/day is routinely used. Because infiltration of surrounding brain tissue is usually limited with low-grade gliomas, only a 1.0-cm clinical target volume (CTV) beyond the lesion plus an additional 0.5 cm for the planning target volume (PTV) is generally an adequate margin with three-dimensional treatment planning. Computed tomography (CT) and magnetic resonance imaging (MRI) image fusion helps to design precise three-dimensional and IMRT fields to better spare critical normal tissues. Radiation has enhanced the long-term control of residual tumors in most series, [6] but progression may occur years later. Long-term follow-up with imaging and neurologic evaluation is required.

High-Grade Astrocytoma

In contrast to their low-grade counterparts, high-grade astrocytomas definitely behave malignantly. They grow rapidly, invade and destroy adjacent brain tissues, and can occasionally spread through the CNS or distantly. Neuropathologists commonly classify high-grade gliomas in order of escalating malignancy as anaplastic astrocytoma and glioblastoma multiforme. High-grade gliomas are usually supratentorial, with neurologic symptoms progressing quickly. Headaches and lethargy are followed by motor or sensory loss, seizures, and occasionally intracranial hemorrhage. Radiologically, these lesions have indistinct borders, areas of necrosis, and surrounding edema (see Figure 39-1, *B*). Steroids are used to reduce edema before surgery.

Neurosurgery is the important first step of multidisciplinary treatment for high-grade brain tumors. Surgery yields the histologic diagnosis, removes the gross tumor, and decompresses adjacent structures, but residual tumor invariably remains. The extent of resection is important to prognosis even requiring repeat surgery by a skilled pediatric neurosurgeon in some instances. Radiation is routinely used postoperatively. The benefit and

optimal sequencing of chemotherapy are still uncertain. CNS tumor research groups have demonstrated improvements in survival rates with some combinations.[24] Chemotherapy is especially vital in infants to delay the need for radiation while the brain matures, to hopefully reduce late sequelae of radiation.

The radiation technique requires large fields. Anaplastic astrocytomas and glioblastomas may be treated with a margin of 2.5 cm or more. The overall prognosis is poor, even with aggressive treatment. Neither hyperfractionated radiation to over 7000 cGy nor high-dose chemotherapy with stem cell transplant has made a major impact on cure. Local recurrence is still a major problem. The survival rate at 5 years is 20% to 35% in many series.[28]

Optic Glioma

Optic tract and hypothalamic gliomas are usually pilocytic or low-grade astrocytomas. Children with neurofibromatosis are at a higher risk to develop these tumors. Observation may be employed for asymptomatic patients, but because visual and hormonal functions can be impaired they frequently require treatment. Those who progress radiologically or develop symptoms receive carboplatin-based chemotherapy or radiation[34] depending on age. Potential bilateral, chiasmatic, and distal optic tract involvement must be considered during radiation field design. In such instances, larger tailored fields with about 1.5-cm margins are required, and the prognosis is worse. Long-term follow-up is required before any conclusions can be made about the treatment of this indolent disease.

Ependymoma

Ependymomas arise from the ventricular linings and can be cerebral or posterior fossa in location. The presenting symptoms and preoperative imaging results often mimic medulloblasroma. Cerebrospinal fluid (CSF) metastatic seeding is unusual but far more likely in infratentorial and anaplastic ependymomas. Although neuropathologists debate the grading of ependymomas, a definite relationship exists with higher rates of CSF seeding and primary tumor relapse in highly malignant histology lesions.[47] Staging of the entire brain and spinal cord is necessary. Surgery should have the goal of gross total resection. Radiation is used for residual tumor or recurrence. If CSF seeding is noted, then cranial spinal irradiation (CSI) with techniques similar to those for medulloblastoma are needed. Supratentorial and low-grade tumors can be treated with a 2-cm margin using three-dimensional techniques. Doses of 5400 to 5940 cGy to the primary mass are recommended. Chemotherapy is being used in some investigational trials, especially for the youngest patients or to improve resectability, but the value has yet to be established.

Medulloblastoma

Epidemiology. Medulloblastoma is the prototype posterior fossa malignancy and constitutes about 25% of all childhood brain tumors. It usually occurs in children 2 to 12 years old with a peak at 5 years, but can rarely occur in adults.[14] Medulloblastoma is believed to arise from primitive neuroepithelial cells and histologically appears as small, round blue cells forming pseudorosettes.[65] The tumor usually arises in the midline of the cerebellum, can invade the fourth ventricle and brainstem, and has a high propensity to spread throughout the CSF.

Diagnosis and Staging. The presenting symptoms of medulloblastoma usually occur over a period of weeks to a few months. Several symptoms develop as a result of the invasion and compression of the fourth ventricle, thus stopping the inferior flow of CSF with resultant hydrocephalus. Headaches and early-morning vomiting occur intermittently at first and then steadily. Later findings are ataxia and cranial nerve abnormalities from invasion of the brainstem. CT and MRI scans usually show a round, central cerebellar, enhancing mass (Figure 39-2), and hydrocephalus is often noted. Steroids and a ventriculostomy can be used to reduce pressure in the acute situation. Because of the propensity for CSF seeding, imaging the entire CNS via MRI is critical. Supratentorial and spinal cord drop metastases can be present in up to 25% of patients at diagnosis.[20]

Chang et al.[12] initially developed a staging system at Columbia University that related to tumor size, invasion of the fourth ventricle and brainstem, and amount of CSF spread. With the known importance of surgical debulking, therapy is now based on residual tumor of greater than 1.5 cm^2 and the extent of CSF or gross neuroaxis metastases. Medulloblastoma is one CNS tumor that can develop distant metastases, usually in bone. The intense, technical multidisciplinary therapy necessary for medulloblastomas must be performed in a center with pediatric cancer expertise.

Treatment Techniques. After the patient is stabilized neurologically, every attempt should be made for neurosurgical removal of the gross tumor. A posterior occipital craniotomy is used. The purple, friable, bulging tumor is usually quickly evident. Although the central mass is removed easily, it is the anterior extent into the brainstem or laterally into the cerebellar peduncle that often leads to residua. Most studies have demonstrated a survival benefit with gross total removal, but surgery is not considered curative. The routine use of ventriculoperitoneal (VP) shunts is discouraged because of the risk of tumor seeding into the peritoneal cavity. Draining CSF can potentially contain tumors cells that may seed in the peritoneal cavity.

The benefit of postoperative radiation therapy was documented by Patterson and Farr[61] as early as 1953. Craniospinal irradiation (CSI) is a technical challenge, and several methods have been used. The most common technique uses lateral-opposed fields for the brain and CSF spaces from the retroorbital space down through the midcervical cord. Careful shielding must be done for the anterior globe, oropharynx, and neck. The treatment couch is angulated a few degrees to compensate for divergence over the spinal cord. The divergence of the spinal radiation field determines the collimator angle for the brain field. Depending on the height of the child, one or two posterior fields are used to encompass the spine down to the level of the second or third sacral segment where the CSF space ends on MRI. This technique is illustrated in Figure 39-3.[75] Some centers have used electrons or protons to treat the spinal CSF space avoiding radiation exposure to normal tissues anterior to the spine. However, this requires precise physics and extensive tissue compensators and is not available in most centers. Usually 6-MV x-rays are used for each field. Present physics recommendations are for a 0- to 0.5-cm gap between the spinal field and lateral brain fields. Usually, this junction and the one between the two spine fields in taller children are moved superiorly and inferiorly 1 cm daily or weekly. This prevents excessive dose gradients at the field junctions eliminating the potential for a spinal cord overdose or a low dose area that can allow tumor cells to survive. Optimally these children should be immobilized in a prone position unless doing so is deemed unsafe. Some centers have perfected a similar CSI technique with the patient in the supine position. Custom head holders or body cradles are helpful. Because of the critical importance of field junctions reproducible positioning of the head and careful marking of treatment portal edges are paramount. If sedation is needed, the anesthesia staff members may require some modifications of the previous technique for airway safety and monitoring equipment.

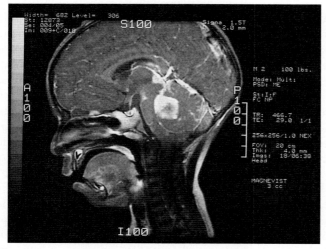

Figure 39-2. Magnetic resonance imaging (MRI) scan of medulloblastoma. Pressure on the brainstem and cerebrospinal fluid (CSF) obstruction are evident. Diffuse CFS seeding can be present.

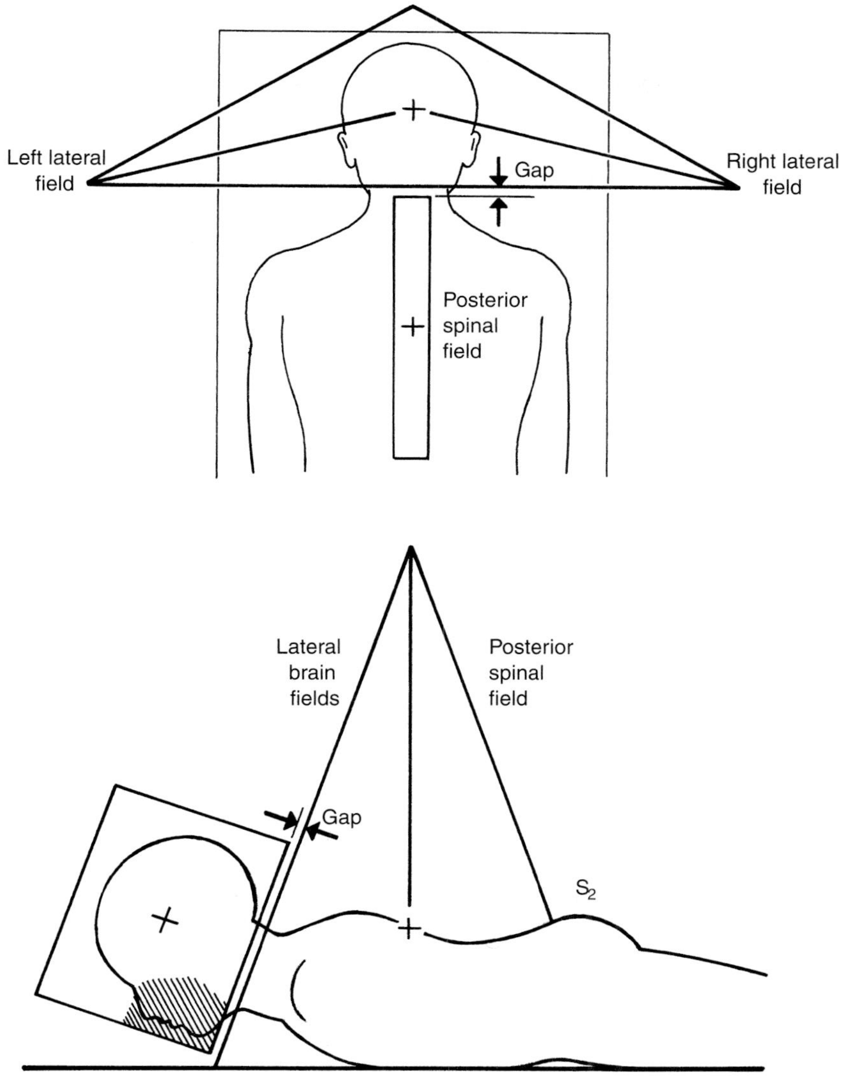

Figure 39-3. Radiation portal alignment for medulloblastoma. The brain portal collimator angle is adjusted for spinal field divergence. The junction gap is moved 1 cm daily or weekly.

CSI can usually proceed at 150 to 180 cGy/day. Premedication for nausea is often needed because of the exit beam of the spinal field interacting with the gastrointestinal tract. Because of late sequelae, an attempt has been made to reduce the CSI dose or use chemotherapy as a substitute. Some now prescribe 2340 cGy CSI with higher doses if CSF metastases are seen.[77] Chemotherapy is used during and after radiation. Because the most frequent site of recurrence is still the posterior fossa, that region is boosted with three-dimensional fields after CSI. This boost field should extend from the posterior clinoids to the back of the skull and from beyond the superior aspect of the tentorium (usually over halfway from the skull's base to its top) down to the level of C2. Studies are underway to treat only the decompressed tumor bed with 1.5 cm margin rather than the entire posterior fossa. Three-dimensional treatment planning can avoid excessive doses to the cochlea and ear canals improving long

term hearing. The daily fraction is usually 180 cGy/day up to a total of 5580 cGy because dose response in earlier studies noted lower control rates with doses under 5000 cGy.[73]

Chemotherapy was initially used in relapsed patients, and some lasting responses were seen. Over the past few years, cooperative research groups in Europe and the United States have added chemotherapy in a randomized fashion to standard surgery and radiation. In most studies, a 10% to 20% benefit has been noted with chemotherapy, with most of the improvement in T3, T4, or M1 situations.[33] The sequencing of chemotherapy before or after radiation is still under evaluation. High-dose chemotherapy with stem cell transplant has salvaged some relapsed patients.[51]

The entire radiation treatment course for medulloblastoma is 6 to 7 weeks, excluding any potential treatment breaks that are possible due to surgical complications, low blood counts and infection, or gastrointestinal toxicity. In addition to weekly blood counts, nutrition must be carefully monitored in these children. The psychological trauma of alopecia (hair loss) and a daily hospital trip is significant. Despite the rigors of the treatment, the addition of radiation and chemotherapy has increased survival rates to more than 70%.[59] However, recurrences 5 or more years later can occur, necessitating long-term follow-up by imaging as well as for neuropsychological late effects.

> *Brain tumors are the most common solid tumor in children and adolescents. They are often treated with radiation after surgery. Each type and location of brain tumor requires individualized multidisciplinary treatment. Three-dimensional dosimetry is utilized to spare normal tissues and reduce late effects which are more severe the younger the patient age when irradiated. Medulloblastoma craniospinal radiation is the most technically challenging treatment regimen for therapists. More information is available via Children's Oncology Group and Childhood Brain Tumor Foundation (www.cbtf.org).*

Central Nervous System Germ Cell Tumors

CNS germ cell tumors develop from embryologic nests of tissue in the midline brain usually in the suprasellar or pineal region. Before neurosurgical biopsy became safe, empirical treatment of the tumor mass with radiation was common. In most instances, a biopsy can now be performed to guide the treatment. Germinoma is the most common histology and is quite radiosensitive. It can be treated with low dose CSI followed by primary tumor boost to 5000 cGy, or with cisplatin-based chemotherapy followed by local field irradiation.[3,5] In non-CSI cases, usually the primary mass and the supratentorial CSF ventricle spaces are treated to 3000 to 4500 cGy depending on the response to chemotherapy.[70] Nongerminomatous germ cell tumors often require chemotherapy, CSI, and primary tumor boost.

Brainstem Glioma

Brainstem gliomas typically cause cranial nerve deficits that can affect vision, facial motosensory function, and swallowing. Most of these lesions are diffuse in the pons and thus are entirely unresectable. If biopsied, most of these diffuse tumors are found to be high-grade astrocytomas. If the MRI images are typical of the diffuse glioma, biopsy is not routinely performed.

The mainstay of treatment is radiation therapy. The fields should cover the entire MRI abnormality with an additional 1.5- cm margin. Doses of 180 cGy/day were historically delivered with lateral-opposed fields, but now this truly central lesion can best be treated with three-dimensional or IMRT conformal therapy. Doses of 5400 cGy in the past resulted in poor cure rates. The use of hyperfractionation with doses escalated to 7800 cGy delivered at 100 to 117 cGy twice daily and concomitant chemotherapy have not yielded much improvement. Local progression and worsening neurologic function typically occurs within a few months requiring prolonged supportive care. Unfortunately, the survival rate in diffuse lesions remains only 10%.[31]

Rarely, the brainstem glioma is an exophytic lesion extending from the posterior aspect of the brainstem. These lesions tend to have a low-grade histology and are amenable to surgical resection by select pediatric neurosurgeons. The survival rate for patients with these lesions can be more than 50%.[44]

Benign Tumors of the Central Nervous System

Pituitary adenomas usually occur in adolescents and adults but can also be seen in young children. These patients can have excessive hormone production, visual disturbance from pressure on the optic chiasm, or diabetes insipidus (DI). Transphenoidal hypophysectomy or medical management to counteract hormone production usually supplants radiation in the treatment of children. Localized radiation therapy with multiple fields or stereotactic radiation therapy with a dose of 4500 cGy can be given if other methods fail and can control more than 70% of tumors.[13]

Craniopharyngiomas arise from embryologic remnants of pharyngeal pouch tissues. These tumors eventually enlarge (usually with a prominent cystic component) and disrupt the hypothalamic pituitary axis (DI or precocious puberty), impair vision, or induce seizures. Surgery and radiation therapy can be effective with the goal of reducing visual or late side effects. Today these tumors are usually treated with three-dimensional conformal fields with narrow margins to 5000 to 5400 cGy. Because panhypopituitarism almost always develops, a pediatric endocrinologist must be included on the management team for these patients. Some physicians have injected radionuclides into the cysts, with good results in selected patients.[78]

Meningiomas and acoustic neuromas are histologically benign lesions that occur far more often in patients who have neurofibromatosis. These lessons are treated by observation or surgery if they progress and cause neurologic symptoms. Radiation may be required for unresectable lesions. Arteriovenous malformations (AVMs) in surgically difficult regions can be treated with stereotactic radiosurgery. Usually 1500 to 2000 cGy is delivered in a single fraction, with control of potentially deadly rebleeding in 80% of patients.[29] Doses and control rates depend on the size of the AVM.

Late Effects of Treatment

The treatment of large areas of the brain and spinal cord can have a variety of devastating late sequelae. These effects are definitely worse the younger the child's age at the time of treatment. Because survival rates were so poor for many decades, only now are these late effects being adequately assessed.[55] Postsurgical deficits of motor sensory loss, poor coordination, or cranial nerve dysfunction can last a lifetime. The acute hair loss can be psychologically traumatic, and high doses of radiation can lead to permanent hair loss for some children. Parents are always extremely concerned about the child's subsequent intellectual abilities. Changes of cortical atrophy and basal ganglia calcifications can occur, even with lower radiation doses used in leukemic CNS prophylaxis, but do not correlate with neurologic impairment. Whole-brain radiation with high doses for high-grade gliomas and CSF seeding tumors has decreased the median intelligence quotient of survivors 10% to 20%.[43] Cisplatin and radiation doses over 3000 cGy to the cochlea can decrease hearing. Doses over 2000 cGy to the pituitary and hypothalamus can cause delayed decreases in pituitary hormones. Thyroid and growth hormone deficits are most likely and with early detection can be reversed via supplemental hormones.[58]

CSI can decrease the height of vertebral bodies, leading to a short-waisted adult. Second malignancies may develop many years later in the CNS, bones and soft tissues, or bone marrow from the damage that earlier radiation and chemotherapy induced.[35] Careful follow-up and early intervention, both medically and educationally, can lessen many of the late effects just mentioned. Although doing so may frighten parents, mentioning the risks for late effects when obtaining informed consent for a child's radiation treatment is necessary. Despite these risks, parents are almost always ecstatic that even an impaired child has survived a life-threatening brain tumor.

RETINOBLASTOMA

Epidemiology

Although **retinoblastoma** (the primitive neuroectodermal tumor of the retina) is the most common intraocular tumor in young children, it only occurs about 300 times annually in the United States. Most retinoblastomas occur in children 6 months to 4 years of age.[1] A well-documented hereditary pattern is present in 25% to 35% of patients. The retinoblastoma gene is located on chromosome 13 (13q-14 deletion) and is a tumor-suppressor gene.[81] Therefore, both halves of the chromosome must suffer a deletion of the gene for retinoblastoma to occur. These patients account for most cases of bilateral retinoblastoma and have a significant risk of development of later second malignancies. However, at least 65% of retinoblastomas are unilateral and without evidence of inheritance.[1]

Diagnosis and Staging

Retinoblastoma is usually discovered as a result of an abnormal retinal light reflex (white rather than red). This tumor may be noted from a flash photograph or during the pediatrician's routine examination. An ophthalmologist should examine both eyes with the child under anesthesia to document multifocality or bilaterality. A biopsy is not done because of the risk of vitreous seeding. CT of the brain and orbit can detect unusual cases with extraocular extension or simultaneous supratentorial-pineal lesions (trilateral retinoblastoma). The CSF is assessed by lumbar puncture cytology, and a bone marrow biopsy may be indicated. Clinical staging systems have developed to suggest preferred treatments and predict success rates. The initial system was developed by Reese[64] and correlated tumor size and location with visual preservation. A newer system from St. Jude's investigators stages disease both inside and beyond the distant metastases that can occur in bone or bone marrow[68] (Box 39-1).

Treatment Techniques

As mentioned, the pediatric ophthalmologist must detail the extent of local disease. With small focal tumors away from the optic disc and macula, photocoagulation or cryosurgery may yield control. With more extensive but unilateral retinoblastoma not involving the optic nerve, enucleation leads to almost certain cure while sacrificing the globe.

External beam radiation has classically been used in cases of bilateral or inoperable unilateral disease. If both eyes are involved, both can be treated with organ-sparing intent because visual preservation may occur on the side with more advanced initial disease. It is a technical challenge with external beam

Box 39-1	St. Jude Children's Research Hospital Staging System for Retinoblastoma

Intraocular disease
    Ia. Retinal tumor, single or multiple
    Ib. Extension to lamina cribrosa
Orbital disease
    IIa. Orbital tumor
    IIb. Optic nerve invasion
Intracranial metastases
    IIIa. Positive cerebrospinal fluid
    IIIb. Central nervous system mass lesion
Hematogenous metastases

From Schwartzman E, et al: Results of a stage based protocol for the treatment of retinoblastoma, *J Clin Oncol* 14: 1532-1536, 1996.

therapy to treat the entire retina, which extends anterior to the lateral bony canthus, and still spare the cornea and lens. Methods include (1) combined lateral and anterior fields with a divergent hanging lens block, (2) a suction cup to displace the anterior globe (pioneered in Europe), (3) three-dimensional/IMRT conformal volumes, especially when tumor is beyond the globe, or (4) conformal proton therapy. Daily general anesthesia is required, with specialized dosimetry verifying doses in such small-shaped radiation portals. The usual dose is 180 to 200 cGy daily to 4000 to 5000 cGy. Several series report local control and visual preservation ranging from 50% to 100%, depending on the stage.[1,64,67]

If the tumor masses are less extensive, radiation implant plaques can be used. Cobalt-60 and iodine-125 are the most widely used radionuclides. Doses of 4000 to 6000 cGy over 1 week are delivered, with a cure rate of more than 80% and visual preservation in most patients.[41,71] Implants reduce radiation exposure to bones, contralateral globe, and anterior structures, with a resultant decrease in long-term effects.

Because retinoblastoma is a small blue cell tumor of neuroectodermal origin, a good response to chemotherapeutic agents is expected. Vincristine, cyclophosphamide, and the platinols have shown good response rates when extraocular or disseminated disease is present. Subsequent trials have involved neoadjuvant chemotherapy in hope of avoiding external radiation therapy or enucleation. This has been successful in 40% to 90% of lower-stage patients.[32]

Late Effects of Treatment

Long-term sequelae of retinoblastoma therapies include the cosmetics of the face, effects on vision, and a high risk of a **second malignant neoplasm (SMN)**, a new cancer developing years after treatment of the initial tumor. If enucleation is chosen, the child will require several prosthetic eyes as growth occurs. Because external radiation uses doses of 4000 cGy or more and occurs in children who are young, facial growth will definitely be impaired. As adults, these patients have small orbits and are narrow between the temples. Cured tumors can leave blind spots. Radiation retinitis, dry eyes from decreased tear gland function, and cataracts can limit useful vision. However, overall survival rates and visual acuity are often high.

As noted earlier, the retinoblastoma gene is a tumor-suppressor gene. If this gene is absent, then other cancers, especially sarcomas, develop later in life with alarming frequency. Sarcomas can be induced in the radiation therapy portal but occur as a new primary outside the radiation therapy field more often. Eng et al.[25] reported a 25% incidence at 30 years.

NEUROBLASTOMA

Epidemiology

Neuroblastoma is a small, round blue cell tumor derived from cells of neural crest origin. These cells migrate embryologically to form paravertebral sympathetic ganglia, the adrenal medulla, and peripheral nerves. Neuroblastoma-like cells occur in fetal adrenals and in 1% of infant autopsies. Because only about 600 clinically apparent tumors develop in the United States annually, most of these precursor lesions must spontaneously regress. However, neuroblastoma is the second most common solid tumor (after brain tumors). Patients range from newborns to children several years old, with a median age of younger than 24 months.[46]

Like the normal adrenal tissues, neuroblastoma cells can manufacture epinephrine-like compounds such as vanilmandelic acid (VMA) and homovanillic acid (HVA), which can be detected in the urine. Molecular genetic studies have demonstrated a deletion on the short arm of chromosome 1 in up to 80% of patients.[9] Surprisingly, neuroblastomas with an excessive or aneuploid number of chromosomes yield a better prognosis. The **oncogene** (a gene regulating the development and growth of cancerous tissues) primarily associated with neuroblastoma is n-*myc*. This gene occurs on the short arm of chromosome 2 and is a promoter of growth. Thus when excessive copies of this gene are present (called n-*myc* amplified tumors), aggressive growth and poor survival are typical.[10] Other chromosomal abnormalities on 1, 11, and 17 can be found and may relate to prognosis as well.[62]

Diagnosis and Staging

Most neuroblastomas occur in the abdomen, with the origin in the adrenal gland or paraspinal ganglia. A lethargic, ill-appearing child younger than 2 years with an abdominal mass is common. Invasion of the spinal canal in a dumbbell fashion from a paravertebral neuroblastoma can cause symptoms of neurologic compromise or even spinal cord compression. Flushing and diarrhea may occur in response to the vasoactive peptides. In the newborn, a large abdominal mass or liver metastases can cause respiratory compromise necessitating emergency intervention.

Unfortunately, many children present with symptoms of metastatic disease. Patients older than 18 months have a 70% chance of developing metastatic disease.[46] Weakness and anemia from bone marrow invasion, painful bony metastases, blue skin lesions, or massive liver involvement may occur, even with a small primary tumor. In general, these patients are younger and sicker than those with a corresponding-sized **Wilms' tumor** (the childhood embryonal kidney cancer). The radiologic evaluation depends on the presentation in the abdomen or chest. Abdominal sonography or CT and chest CT are appropriate. Sometimes calcifications are visible in the mass on a plain film

---

Box 39-2	International Staging System for Neuroblastoma

Stage 1—Localized tumor confined to area of origin; complete gross excision, with or without microscopic residual disease; identifiable ipsilateral and contralateral lymph nodes negative microscopically

Stage 2A—Unilateral tumor with incomplete gross excision; identifiable ipsilateral and contralateral lymph nodes negative microscopically

Stage 2B—Unilateral tumor with complete or incomplete gross excision; with positive ipsilateral regional lymph nodes; identifiable contralateral lymph nodes negative microscopically

Stage 3—Tumor infiltrating across the midline with or without regional lymph node involvement; unilateral tumor with contralateral regional lymph node involvement; or midline tumor with bilateral regional lymph node involvement

Stage 4—Dissemination of tumor to distant lymph nodes, bone, bone marrow, liver, and/or other organs (except as defined in stage 4S)

Stage 4S—Localized primary tumor as defined for stage 1 or 2, with dissemination limited to liver and skin

Adapted from Brodeur GM, et al: International criteria for diagnosis, staging and response to treatment with neuroblastoma, *J Clin Oncol* 6:1874-1881, 1988.

---

or CT scan. The lungs and liver must be assessed for metastases. MRI of the spine is used for paravertebral masses to delineate spinal canal invasion. A bone marrow biopsy is required and a bone scan is done to look for bone cortex metastases. More recently, radioiodinated catecholamine precursors (MIBG) have been used to detect occult metastatic involvement.

Staging systems have historically evolved based on radiographic and surgical findings. Initially, Evans[26] developed the first prognostic staging system. An international staging committee expanded their concept to include more surgical findings. This system is commonly used now and is summarized in Box 39-2. This system relates to prognosis and directs the treatment.

The age at the time of presentation is extremely important regarding the prognosis. The special category 4S predominantly occurs in infants younger than 1 year. Many of these patients spontaneously regress, and the cancerous elements turn benign if acute situations can be managed.[18] Increasingly, histologic subtypes and molecular genetic markers (especially n-*myc* amplification) are being used to predict clinical behavior and direct the aggressiveness of therapy in most clinical research groups. Variations in molecular genetics may explain the differential age prognosis observed clinically.

Treatment Techniques

The therapy for neuroblastoma remains an enigma to most pediatric oncologists. Although it may spontaneously regress in the newborn, neuroblastoma often has a progressive metastatic course in older children. Individual masses may regress well with low doses of chemotherapy or radiation, but cure of the usual advanced disease presentation is infrequent. Completely resected localized disease without nodal metastases is often

Table 39-3	Five-Year Survival Rates in 550 Neuroblastoma Patients on POG protocols, 1981–1989	
Stage	**Children <1 Year Old**	**Children >1 Year Old**
I and II	95%	85%
III	80%	60%
IV	50%	15%

Modified from Ries LAG et al, editors: *SEER Cancer Statistics Review, 1973-1991: tables and graphs*, NIH publication No. 94-2789, Bethesda, MD, 1994, National Cancer Institute.
POG, Pediatric Oncology Group.

cured with surgery alone. In 1967, Lingley et al.[50] showed 100% local control and long-term survival in 8 of 13 patients after they underwent incomplete surgery followed by radiation. The use of multiagent chemotherapy has supplanted radiation in most resected patients, even those with nodal metastases or microscopic residua. More extensive stage 3 and 4 tumors definitely benefit from tumor bed irradiation, usually to doses of 2100 cGy in recent protocols.[11,52] Radiation commonly is directed to residua after surgery and chemotherapy, rather than to all areas of initial disease.

The likelihood of children older than 2 years developing metastatic disease demands the use of multiagent chemotherapy. In Europe and the United States, aggressive regimens involving platinum compounds, vincristine, doxorubicin (Adriamycin), etoposide, and cyclophosphamide have been used. Although such treatment has improved the previously almost uniformly fatal stage 4 results, overall survival rates had been disheartening (Table 39-3). Newer efforts involving the use of high-dose chemotherapy stem cell transplant up to three consecutive times are increasing cure rates to 30%.[53]

Radiation therapists can also be called on to palliatively treat patients who have progressive metastatic disease. Low doses of 1000 cGy may achieve pain relief or regression of soft tissue masses, which are important for short-term quality of life to terminally ill patients and their families.

Late Effects of Treatment

Because neuroblastoma patients are often infants, the late effects of radiation can be significant. In the acute situation with a newborn, doses of only 500 cGy may be effective with almost no long-term side effect. In older patients receiving over 2000 cGy, the bones and soft tissues of the treated region may have decreased or asymmetric growth. Kidney and liver tissues must be shielded from high doses of radiation to prevent impaired function. Lung fibrosis can occur with thoracic radiation. The intense doses of multiagent chemotherapy and stem cell transplants used for neuroblastoma can adversely affect many organ systems. Although late second malignancies are always a risk after radiation and chemotherapy, the oncogenes associated with neuroblastoma do not intensify the risk to retinoblastoma survivors.

WILMS' TUMOR

Epidemiology

Wilms' tumor is a malignant embryonal cancer of the kidney. It was first described in the German medical literature in 1899. Nearly 500 cases occur annually in the United States, and about 5% are bilateral. The average age at the time of presentation is 3 or 4 years, and almost all such tumors occur before the age of 8. A higher risk of Wilms' tumor occurs in patients with multiple genitourinary (GU) abnormalities, hemihypertrophy and aniridia, and Beckwith-Wiedemann syndrome. Wilms' tumor genetic abnormalities have recently been discovered and include a deletion on chromosome 11p13, 1p, and 16q.[22,39] Benign embryonal rests called nephroblastomatoses can be associated with malignant Wilms' tumor, especially in bilateral cases. Wilms' tumors can contain renal tubular, glomerular, and connective tissue elements. Unfavorable histologic appearances occur in up to 15% of patients and include highly anaplastic pathology, clear cell sarcomas, and rhabdoid tumors. These unfavorable tumors have a cure rate only half that of their usual histologic Wilms' tumor counterpart and clear cell and rhabdoid tumors tend to metastasize to bone or brain, respectively.[8]

Diagnosis and Staging

Wilms' tumor most often appears as a painless abdominal mass noted at the pediatrician's examination or when parents bathe the child. As the cancers enlarge, they can cause pain and pressure on the gastrointestinal tract. They may even hemorrhage and rupture. Despite large tumors, children do not often appear severely ill. A differential diagnosis includes neuroblastomas, lymphomas, sarcomas, and liver tumors.

After the physical examination, an abdominal sonogram is usually the first step in making a diagnosis. In the United States, this is followed by a CT scan of the chest and abdomen because of the tendency for lymph node and pulmonary metastases. Because Wilms' tumor can be bilateral, the contralateral kidney must be carefully examined (Figure 39-4, *A*). With right-sided tumors, direct liver invasion can mimic liver metastases. The unfavorable histologies of clear cell sarcomas and rhabdoid tumors can metastasize to bone and brain. The initial staging system focused on tumor size, tumor spill or postoperative residua, and metastases. The National Wilms' Tumor Study Group (NWTS) was formed in the United States to investigate treatment options. Members have now conducted Protocol Study No. 5. The staging system of the NWTS is based on operative findings and is listed in Box 39-3. These stages relate to prognosis and direct the aggressiveness of treatment options. Because surgery alone led to cure rates of less than 30% many years ago, radiation therapy by the 1940s and chemotherapy by the 1960s have greatly increased survival rates.

Treatment Techniques

In the United States, the removal of the malignant kidney via nephrectomy is nearly always the first step. Careful examination of the other kidney for bilateral tumors is done intraoperatively. A biopsy is performed on the lymph nodes, and tumor

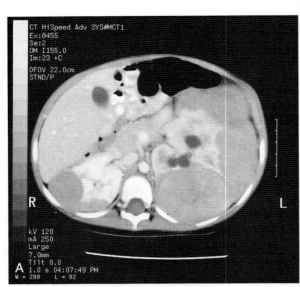
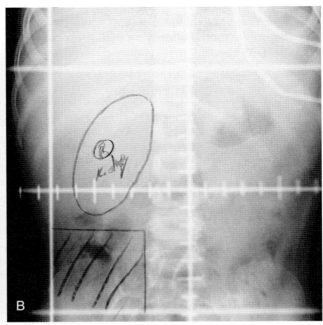

Figure 39-4. Wilms' tumor. **A,** Preoperative computed tomography (CT) scan of a bilateral Wilms' tumor in a 3-year-old girl. **B,** Postoperative radiation portal received 1200 cGy to the left tumor bed and remaining involved right kidney. Note the shielding for the bowel and pelvic structures inferiorly on the right side.

thrombi in the renal vein or inferior vena cava can be removed during surgery. Because large Wilms' tumors are often soft and necrotic, rupture of the mass and tumor spill into the abdominal cavity are risks. Because widespread tumor spill adversely affects the prognosis and demands more subsequent treatment, SIOP studies usually use chemotherapy or radiation preoperatively. In the first SIOP cooperative study, this method reduced intraoperative tumor spill from 32% to 4%.[48] This was verified in SIOP 93-01 when over 400 patients had an average 60% reduction in tumor size after preoperative chemotherapy.[38] In patients with bilateral disease, a partial resection can be done on the minimally affected side.

Radiation was initially used to cover the entire tumor bed and abdomen. If tumor spill occurred, the whole abdomen was treated. Doses higher than 3000 cGy were successful but led to

significant late effects.[19] The first four NWTS studies have resulted in conclusions for reduced radiation indications. With the addition of effective chemotherapy, routine radiation for completely removed stages I and II tumors is not necessary. Data from NWTS 3 indicated no significant difference in local control between 1080 and 2000 cGy.[77] This lower dose is still indicated for microscopic residual disease, lymph node metastases, bilateral disease, and pulmonary metastases. All cases of unfavorable histology are treated as high-stage lesions and uniformly irradiated. Known areas of gross residual disease are usually boosted to at least 2000 cGy.

In designing the radiation portals, it is important to use the preoperative imaging and surgeon's intraoperative findings to delineate the radiation portal. If treating only unilateral disease, it is still important to cover the entire width of the vertebral body plus 1 cm contralaterally. This allows para-aortic nodal coverage and homogeneous irradiation of the vertebral bodies to reduce the risk of scoliosis. At the low dose of 1080 cGy, which is often used now, the risk of bony or visceral toxicity (including the remaining kidney) is minimal. Still, it is wise to shield the growth plates of long bones. Figure 39-4, B, represents a postoperative radiation portal for a bilateral Wilms' tumor patient whose large left-sided cancer was removed before postoperative radiation. This patient is without recurrent disease many years later. Because recurrence is still a major problem in histologically unfavorable Wilms' tumor, the fields are similar but doses are usually higher.

Farber[27] first reported the encouraging survival improvement associated with Wilms' tumor by using actinomycin-D in 1966. The addition of vincristine and doxorubicin for advanced stages

Box 39-3	The National Wilms Tumor Study Staging System

I Tumor limited to kidney and completely excised

II Tumor beyond kidney but completely excised
    Local tumor spillage or vessel invasion permitted but resected

III Residual nonhematogenous tumor confined to abdomen
    Involved lymph nodes, diffuse tumor spillage, or grossly unresected tumor

IV Hematogenous metastases
    Usually lung, liver, bone, or brain

V Bilateral kidney involvement at time of diagnosis

Table 39-4	4-year survival rates of NWTS-3 patients	
Stage	**Relapse-Free Rate (%)**	**Overall Rate (%)**
I FH	90	96
II FH	88	92
III FH	79	86
IV FH	75	82
I-III UH	65	68
IV UH	55	55

Modified from Green DM, et al: Wilms tumor. In Pizzo PG, Poplack DG, editors: *Principles and practice of pediatric oncology,* ed 2, Philadelphia, 1993, JB Lippincott.
FH, Favorable histology; *NWTS-3,* National Wilms Tumor Study Group protocol study No. 3; *UH,* unfavorable histology.

led to cure rates of 80% to 100% in later NWTS studies. Even patients with metastatic disease can be cured more than 70% of the time (Table 39-4). Patients with late pulmonary metastases can often be salvaged with chemotherapy, lung irradiation, and lung resections. With the high overall cure rates, the present aim of studies is to reduce late effects and find more successful multidisciplinary combinations for patients who have advanced disease and unfavorable histology.

Late Effects of Treatment

Historically, when doses of 3000 to 4000 cGy of orthovoltage radiation were used, atrophy of soft tissues on the treated side and scoliosis were common. With modification of the technique to include the entire vertebral body and the use of doses less than 2000 cGy, such late effects should rarely occur now. For the treatment of pulmonary metastases, doses must be kept below 1500 cGy to prevent diffuse lung fibrosis. If thoracic radiation is needed for a prepubertal female, breast development can be impaired. High doses of actinomycin-D have resulted in liver damage. Because these children go through life with only one kidney, any urinary tract symptoms must be addressed quickly to prevent infections, stones, or other diseases from damaging the remaining kidney.

Neuroblastoma, Wilms' tumor of the kidney, sarcomas, and lymphomas can all present as abdominal masses in children. Their staging, treatments, and prognosis are different, so accurate diagnosis must occur initially. While radiation is now used less often than in decades past, it can still play a pivotal role with residual disease after surgery and chemotherapy. Cure is still possible even with metastatic disease.

SOFT TISSUE SARCOMAS
Epidemiology

Soft tissue sarcomas arise from mesenchymal tissues and can occur anywhere in the body. A wide variety of histologic appearances can be seen, but **rhabdomyosarcomas (RMS)** constitute about 40% of cases.[40] The embryonal histologic subtype is associated with loss of heterozygosity on chromosome 11p[69] and familial soft tissue sarcoma cases may be related to the *p53* oncogene mutation, as noted by Li and Fraumeni.[49] About 75% of soft tissue sarcomas occur before the age of 10. The rhabdomyosarcoma sites are nearly evenly divided between the head and neck area (including the orbit), GU region, and extremities and trunk.[63]

Rhabdomyosarcoma has distinct histologic variants. The more favorable prognosis embryonal subtype tends to occur in the orbit and GU regions. The alveolar subtype has a worse prognosis and a predilection for extremities and the trunk.[56] Other undifferentiated sarcomas are usually treated along guidelines established by the Intergroup Rhabdomyosarcoma Study Group (IRS), which is now merged into the Children's Oncology Group (COG).

Diagnosis and Staging

The presenting symptoms of soft tissue sarcomas depend on the area of involvement. A painless mass can enlarge relatively asymptomatically in an extremity, whereas a small mass in the orbit can cause pain, tearing, and outward displacement of the globe, known as proptosis. The GU occurrences in the prostate and bladder in males cause urinary difficulties. A fleshy, exophytic mass extruding from the vagina in young girls has been called sarcoma botryoides because of its resemblance to clusters of grapes.

The staging of rhabdomyosarcomas and other soft tissue sarcomas has historically included size and resectability, nodal involvement, and metastases. The latter are most likely to occur in the lung and bone marrow. The IRS first developed a clinical grouping system based on surgical findings, but some now favor the TGNM system (Table 39-5), which also includes histology, a known prognostic factor. After the histologic diagnosis is obtained from an incisional biopsy, staging includes a physical examination and sonographic, CT, or MRI scans to determine the tumor's size and involvement of adjacent structures. A bone marrow biopsy and chest CT scan are done to detect metastases. The stage and histology dictate the treatment regimen in IRS and other international studies. Metastatic disease is extremely rare with orbital presentations but may be present in about 25% of patients who have tumors in the extremities and trunk.[53]

Treatment Techniques

After the biopsy and staging, the surgical possibilities must be assessed. The first choice, if possible, is the complete removal of the mass with appropriate margins without the destruction of precious anatomy. The initial IRS study proved that small, fully resected lesions have good curability without additional treatment. In more advanced cases, the local relapse rate was extremely high with surgery alone. The original approach of removing the entire organ or extremity is no longer necessary because of multidisciplinary treatment including chemotherapy and radiation. The removal of a child's eye or GU structures is generally not preferred and has led to organ-sparing treatments with chemotherapy and radiation.

Table 39-5	Intergroup Rhabdomyosarcoma Study Staging Systems	
Clinical System	**TGNM System**	
I. Localized, completely resected	**TUMOR**	
II. Grossly resected with microscopic residue or involved lymph nodes	T_1 — Confined to site origin T_2 — Extension to surrounding tissues	
III. Gross residual tumor	a. <5cm	
IV. Distant metastases	b. ≥5cm	
	HISTOLOGY	
	G_1 — Favorable: embryonal, undifferentiated, mixed	
	G_2 — Unfavorable; alveolar	
	NODES	
	N_0 — Not clinically involved	
	N_1 — Clinically involved by tumor	
	METASTASES	
	M_0 — No distant metastases	
	M_1 — Metastatic disease at time of diagnosis	

Modified from Raney RB et al: Rhabdomyosarcoma and other undifferentiated sarcomas. In Pizzo PA, Poplack DG, editors: *Principles and practice of pediatric oncology*, Philadelphia, 1989, JB Lippincott. *TGNM,* Tumor, grade, node, metastases.

Radiation improves local control and organ preservation in all rhabdomyosarcoma groups, except small and fully excised lesions. Fortunately, the frequently unresectable tumors of the orbit and pelvis are usually the more favorable embryonal histology, and local control rates of 90% or more have been obtained with combinations of chemotherapy and radiation.[76] Originally the margins of radiation fields included the entire muscular compartment. More recently, the IRS has decreased margins to as low as 2 cm if critical normal tissues can be spared. Around the orbit three-dimensional planning can spare the contralateral eye, facial bones, optic chiasm, and most brain tissues. In the pelvis or along extremities, the growth plates of the long bones must be shielded. With the routine use of chemotherapy, the bone marrow in the pelvic wings should be spared if possible. For locally positive intraoperative margins and some surface gynecologic presentations, brachytherapy implants have been used with success.[36] In general, the external beam radiation portals include the prechemotherapy tumor volume with at least a 2-cm margin. IRS-IV included hyperfractionated radiation without advantageous results.[21] Using three-dimensional dosimetry, standard doses of 180 cGy/day to a total of 3600 to 5040 cGy are directed to the area of postsurgical residual disease.

Chemotherapy was initially used only for metastatic disease, but its subsequent use postoperatively led to higher survival rates because of the elimination of occult metastatic disease.[42] In serial IRS studies, vincristine and actinomycin-D have been effective. New regimens have combined these agents with etoposide and ifosfamide. With good tumor reduction, some inoperable cancers can be resected or radiation fields greatly reduced. Surgery or radiation therapy is now performed for local control within the first 3 months of the treatment regimen

because resistant clones of cells can lead to tumor growth and lost opportunities. The tumor's histology, stage, and location affect survival rates (Table 39-6). Although the survival rate for patients with orbital lesions is more than 90%, patients with metastatic disease still fare poorly with survival rates of 10% to 35%.[4] Overall, in IRS-IV, the 3-year failure-free survival rate was 77%.[16]

Late Effects of Treatment

The long-term sequelae of rhabdomyosarcoma and other soft tissue sarcoma treatment depend on the tumor's location and treatment modality. Amputations and pelvic exenterations are generally reserved for the salvaging of organ-sparing treatment failures. However, some patients' families may prefer bladder removal rather than the long-term effects of chemoirradiation on their young child's reproductive structures. With the high radiation doses, bone and soft tissue growth is affected unless the growth points of bones can be excluded. In the head and neck region, cosmetic changes may require reconstructive surgery. If invasion of the cranial contents occurs necessitating CNS radiation to 3000 cGy or more, the survivor may develop some of the side effects noted in the brain tumor section. Dryness of the treated eye or retinal damage from chemotherapy and radiation sometimes necessitates enucleation, even if the sarcoma is cured. The appropriate use of brachytherapy implants in select cases can spare many of the surrounding normal tissues from damage. Chemotherapeutic agents can cause acute and chronic neurologic, kidney, heart, and liver damage. The risk of treatment-induced second malignancies is present for many years. As survivors grow to adulthood, fertility is questionable after chemotherapy and highly unlikely for those receiving pelvic radiation.

MISCELLANEOUS CHILDHOOD TUMORS

Germ Cell Tumors

According to embryologic development, benign and malignant germ cell tumors can occur anywhere in the midline— from the CNS through the mediastinum, retroperitoneum, and down to the ovaries and testicles. CNS germ cell tumors are discussed in the brain tumor section of this chapter. Sacrococcygeal teratomas often occur in newborns. The majority of these tumors are histologically benign and are almost always cured by surgery.

Ovarian and testicular tumors that occur in adolescents differentiate along seminoma-dysgerminoma or nonseminomatous lines. The latter group includes embryonal carcinoma, choriocarcinoma, and yolk sac tumors. The nonseminomatous tumors often produce alpha-fetoprotein (AFP) or human chorionic gonadotropin (hCG), which can be used as chemical markers for response to therapy. Surgical removal of the testicles or ovaries is done first and is often curative in stage I disease. For nonseminomatous cancers, chemotherapy with regimens containing cisplatin, bleomycin, etoposide, and vinblastine has led to a high rate of success.[82]

For testicular seminoma seen mostly in older adolescents and young adults, radical orchiectomy and CT staging of the draining pelvic and para-aortic nodes are performed. Historically moderate doses of radiation in the 2000- to 2500-cGy range have been used to prevent pelvic and para-aortic nodal relapse.

Table 39-6	Actuarial Survival Rates at 3 Years: Results of the Intergroup Rhabdomyosarcoma Studies I and II	
Prognostic Factors	**IRS I (%)**	**IRS II (%)**
CLINICAL GROUP		
I	79	88
II	68	77
III	42	68
IV	18	32
HISTOLOGIC TYPE		
Embryonal	—	69
Alveolar	—	56
Other	—	66
PRIMARY SITE		
Orbit	91	93
GU (mainly group III)	—	64
Trunk and extremity	53	57
Retroperitoneum and pelvis	39	46

Modified from Pizzo PA, et al: Solid tumors of children. In DeVita T, Hellman S, Rosenberg SA, editors: *Cancer: principles and practice of oncology*, ed 4, Philadelphia, 1993, JB Lippincott.
GU, Genitourinary; *IRS*, Intergroup Rhabdomyosarcoma Study Group.

Now close surveillance can be used with radiation or chemotherapy in the 20% who experience relapse.[80] Cure rates overall are close to 100%.

Liver Tumors

Liver tumors appear as right upper quadrant abdominal masses, much like Wilms' tumor or neuroblastoma. Sonographic or CT scanning can usually determine the organ of origin. Benign vascular or fetal remnant tumors can be observed if they are small, or if necessary because of their large size, they can be resected with excellent results. Hepatoblastoma is a malignancy usually occurring in patients younger than 2 years. Hepatocellular carcinoma occurs in the second decade of life and can be multifocal. AFP can be elevated in both hepatic malignancies.[30]

Primary surgical resection is the goal. If this is not possible or postoperative residua are present, chemotherapy with doxorubicin and cisplatin is often used. Radiation has demonstrated some good response but is rarely used except for palliation. Unfortunately, overall survival rates for unresectable lesions are usually less than 50%.[37]

Hematologic Diseases

Leukemia. Acute lymphoblastic leukemia is the most common childhood cancer. Patients require extensive chemotherapy regimens for 2 years. Radiation can be used for CNS or testicular involvement because those sites have diminished chemotherapy penetration. Doses of 1200 to 1800 cGy along with systemic and intrathecal chemotherapy dramatically reduce CNS relapse rates in high-risk patients.[79] Total body radiation (TBI) is often given as part of the bone marrow transplant preparatory regimen in relapse patients. This requires very specialized facilities, techniques, and dosimetry.

Langerhans' Cell Histiocytosis. This is a spectrum of diseases that involves abnormal proliferation of the immune system's histiocytic Langerhans' cells. Infants can have multifocal visceral disease involving the lung, skin, liver, and bone marrow, creating a life-threatening condition known as Letterer-Siwe syndrome. More commonly, bones can be involved with a lytic lesion referred to as an eosinophilic granuloma. Individual histiocytosis lesions may vary over time and occasionally spontaneously regress. Focal bony lesions can be treated via surgical curettage with success. If an impending fracture is a concern or the lesion is in a surgically unresectable region such as the base of skull or spinal column, low doses of radiation are usually effective. Although no direct dose-response curve has been substantiated, doses from 400 to 1200 cGy can be effective. Steroids, vinblastine, or cyclophosphamide can be used as well.

Hodgkin's Lymphoma. In children, Hodgkin's is almost always treated with chemotherapy initially. Increasingly, risk and response adapted doses are being used. Sites of original bulk disease are now treated with low dose involved field radiation (1500 to 2500 cGy) after chemotherapy to reduce recurrence. High cure rates are being achieved with fewer long-term effects.[72] Second malignancy risks are significant in long-term survivors.[57] Refer to the Hodgkin's disease section earlier in this text for more detailed information.

Nasopharynx

Male adolescents may develop nasopharyngeal angiofibromas. They are highly vascular and can erode bone. Usually, vascular embolization and surgical resection are used. Moderate doses of radiation (such as 3000 cGy) can control relapses or unresectable lesions.[17]

Undifferentiated nasopharyngeal carcinomas can occur in children and require high-dose radiation, as they do in adults. Recently, chemotherapy has been used to reduce radiation fields and doses. High cure rates can be achieved, but long-term dry mouth and dental problems are of concern.[83]

Benign and malignant thyroid tumors can arise in adolescents (more often in girls). These tumors are surgically approached, and even lymph node metastases do not imply a bad prognosis. External radiation is rarely used, but iodine-131 can be helpful for thyroid ablation or treatment of metastatic lesions.

Keloids and Kaposi's Sarcoma

Keloids (excess scar formation) can be bothersome and cosmetically disfiguring for young people. If repeated resections and steroid injections are not successful, the best control is obtained via resection, followed immediately by low-dose radiation (900 to 1200 cGy in three fractions).[74] Unfortunately, the human immunodeficiency virus (HIV) infection epidemic has led to the occurrence of Kaposi's sarcoma of the skin in children. Focal painful or disfiguring lesions can be palliated with single doses of 700 cGy, although more lasting results are obtained by a short course to 2000 cGy.[15]

PALLIATIVE RADIATION

Despite the obvious goal of cure for pediatric malignancies, **palliation** or symptom-relieving treatments are sometimes necessary. Mediastinal malignancies may cause airway or vascular compromise. Spinal cord compression at the time of presentation or late in the course of the illness demands immediate treatment to reduce pain and avoid paralysis. Painful bone metastases can be treated to reduce analgesic needs.

The palliative needs of children in the final stages of cancer must be addressed carefully and compassionately. The goal of such treatments is much different than the usual curative protocols. The attempt must be made to relieve symptoms quickly with a minimum number of treatments to limit the invasion of the family's remaining time together. The successful treatment of painful or disfiguring masses can reduce the need for narcotics or hospitalization and improve cosmetics and quality of life during precious final days or weeks. In these instances immobilization and simulation techniques are altered in deference to the comfort of the child. Frequently, high daily doses are used for rapid palliation when long-term effects are not of concern.[84] Although this is a difficult time for radiation staff members, such palliative efforts in times of great need are of immeasurable importance to the children and their families. End-of-life care is increasingly being addressed by trained pediatric specialists.

ROLE OF RADIATION THERAPIST

Almost all patients in radiation oncology centers are adults. In addition to the diseases and their treatment, the personal needs of pediatric patients pose a challenge. Immobilization, small treatment fields, and techniques such as CSI are technically demanding. For general anesthesia, treatment techniques may need to be altered for anesthetic safety. Close cooperation among radiation therapists, nurses, and anesthesia staff members is necessary for patient positioning and visibility of monitors. These complex procedures are often lengthy, sometimes up to an hour. Allowing adequate time in the schedule is important. Usually this is done early in the morning to reduce disruption of the child's feeding patterns and avoid other treatment day conflicts. Therapists often must juggle an already crowded schedule of adults, but most patients are willing to change in deference to children and their families.

Many pediatric patients are on an investigational protocol, requiring careful documentation of treatment setups, daily doses, and quality assurance. Clear instructions between the radiation therapist on the simulator and treatment machine are essential. Digital images of patient positioning, verification of initial portal films, and dose calculations are usually sent for immediate review by national clinical research groups. Careful adherence to protocol guidelines reflects positively on the quality of a radiation oncology department.

The psychosocial elements of pediatric oncology can be immense. Families who are constantly at the hospital have an extremely difficult time maintaining jobs and homes. In addition, children evoke sympathy and compassion from everyone involved. However, behavioral limits may need to be placed on patients or families to ensure quality treatments. Rewards such as stickers or toys should not be used daily, but therapists may be the best judges of when a difficult or sick child needs an uplifting gift. When children with terminal cancer come for palliation, it is an especially difficult time. However, the value of the radiation therapist's technical expertise and heartfelt compassion cannot be overstated.

Table 39-7	5-year survival trends for cancers in children ages 0 to 14 years		
Diagnosis	**Survival Rate (%) for 1960-1963**	**Survival Rate (%) for 1974-1976**	**Survival Rate (%) for 1996-2003**
Acute lymphocytic leukemia	4	52	85
Brain tumor	35	53	70
Neuroblastoma	25	52	66
Wilms' tumor	33	74	92
Hodgkin's disease	52	79	95
All sites	28	55	80

Modified from Parker SL, et al: Cancer statistics, 1996, *CA Cancer J Clin* 46:5-27, 1996; and U.S government SEER cancer incidence data (website): seer.cancer.gov/. Accessed 2007.

Table 39-8	Childhood Cancer Radiation Treatment Summary
Type of Childhood Cancer	**Role for Radiation**
Acute leukemia	CNS relapse prevention
	Bone marrow transplantation regimen
Brain tumors	Three-dimensional localized RT for gliomas, ependymomas
	Craniospinal RT plus tumor boost for medulloblastomas
Hodgkin's lymphoma	Involved fields for initial bulky masses after chemotherapy
Neuroblastoma	Local boost for advanced disease
	Bone marrow transplantation regimen
Wilms' tumor	Tumor bed RT for stage III, IV and
	Unfavorable histology
	Metastatic lesions—especially lung
Sarcomas	Locoregional RT for all but small resected
	Soft tissue tumors
	Unresected Ewing's bone sarcoma
Palliative radiation	Noncurative comfort and compassion

Modified from Kun L: Childhood cancers: part I, 1569-1573. In Gunderson L, Tepper J, editors: *Clinical radiation oncology,* Philadelphia, 2007, Churchill Livingstone.

SUMMARY

• The multidisciplinary protocol approach to pediatric oncology is always a learning experience. This strategy has led to dramatic increases in cure rates for childhood cancers over the past 40 years to reach an overall survival rate of over 70% (see Table 39-7).

• Numerous late side effects must be considered in pediatric cases.

• In addition to organ toxicities and risk of second malignancies, childhood cancer survivors have psychological scars. Social, employment, and insurance discrimination may exist throughout adulthood.

• The Children's Oncology Group not only directs clinical trials and research but also acts as an advocate for survivors of childhood cancer.

• A summary of radiation treatment for childhood cancers can be found in Table 39-8.

• For the radiation therapist, the treatment of children is demanding and often heart wrenching. However, great joy occurs when a cured child and grateful parent return years later.

Review Questions

Multiple Choice

1. A tumor that does *not* spread through the entire central nervous system is:
   a. medulloblastoma
   b. craniopharyngioma
   c. ependymoma
   d. CNS germ cell tumor

2. The approximate survival rate for patients with stage IV Wilms' tumor is:
   a. 10%
   b. 30%
   c. 50%
   d. 70%

3. The factor *not* related to survival in neuroblastoma cases is:
   a. age
   b. stage
   c. n-*myc* amplification
   d. male gender

4. The retinoblastoma gene is a(n):
   a. tumor promoter
   b. tumor suppressor
   c. active haploid
   d. inactive haploid

5. The present protocol dose for occult Wilms' tumor is approximately:
   a. 1000 cGy
   b. 2000 cGy
   c. 4000 cGy
   d. 6000 cGy

6. The tolerance of the kidney is about:
   a. 100 cGy
   b. 1000 cGy
   c. 1500 cGy
   d. 3000 cGy

7. The most likely second malignant neoplasm after radiation for retinoblastoma is:
   a. leukemia
   b. lung cancer
   c. lymphoma
   d. osteosarcoma

8. Which of the following has the highest incidence in children?
   a. retinoblastoma
   b. neuroblastoma
   c. ALL
   d. Wilms' tumor

9. Craniospinal irradiation is usually administered for treatment of:
   a. retinoblastoma
   b. neuroblastoma
   c. leukemia
   d. medulloblastoma

The answers to the Review Questions can be found by logging on to our website at: *http://evolve.elsevier.com/Washington+Leaver/ principles*

Questions to Ponder

1. List examples of chromosome and gene abnormalities associated with pediatric cancer.
2. Why is shifting the junction between the brain and spinal fields important during craniospinal irradiation?
3. Detail some technical considerations for the simulation and treatment of craniospinal irradiation cases.
4. Note possible long-term effects of high-dose brain radiation and discuss methods to reduce such late effects.
5. What organ-sparing techniques are possible by combining chemotherapy, radiation, and surgery for solid tumors?
6. Discuss the unique characteristics and prognosis of stage IV-S neuroblastoma.
7. What types of counseling and advice are needed for long-term survivors of childhood cancer?
8. How much have childhood cancer cure rates improved over the past four decades?

REFERENCES

1. Abramson DH: Retinoblastoma: diagnosis and management, *CA Cancer J Clin* 32:130-140, 1982.
2. Abramson DH, et al: Outcome following initial external beam radiotherapy in patients with Reese-Ellsworth group IV retinoblastoma, *Arch Ophthal* 122:1316-1333, 2004.
3. Allen JC, Kim JH, and Packer RJ: Neoadjuvant chemotherapy for newly diagnosed germ cell tumors of the central nervous system, *J Neurosurg* 67:65-70, 1987.
4. American Cancer Society: *Cancer facts and figure: 2008*, Atlanta, 2008, American Cancer Society.
5. Baranzelli MC, et al: Nonmetastatic intracranial germinoma: the experience of the French Society of Pediatric Oncology, *Int J Radiat Biol Oncol Phys* 43:783-788, 1999.
6. Bouchard J: *Radiation therapy of tumors and diseases of the nervous system*, Philadelphia, 1988, Lea and Febiger.
7. Breneman JC, et al: Prognostic factors and clinical outcomes in children with metastatic rhabdomyosarcoma: a report from the IRS IV, *J Clin Oncol* 21:78-84, 2003.
8. Breslow N, et al: Prognosis for Wilms tumor patients with nonmetastatic disease at diagnosis: results of the Second National Wilms Tumor Study, *J Clin Oncol* 3:521-531, 1985.
9. Brodeur GM, Sekhon GS, Goldstein MN: Chromosomal aberrations in human neuroblastomas, *Cancer* 40:2256-2263, 1977.
10. Brodeur GM, et al: Gene amplification in human neuroblastomas: basic mechanisms and clinical implications, *Cancer Genet Cytogenet* 19:101-111, 1986.
11. Castleberry RP, et al. Radiotherapy improves the outlook for patients older than one year with Pediatric Oncology Group Stage C neuroblastoma, *J Clin Oncol* 9:789-795, 1991.
12. Chang CH, Housepian EM, Herbert C: An operative staging system and a megavoltage radiotherapeutic technique for cerebellar medulloblastoma, *Radiology* 93:1351-1359, 1969.
13. Chun MS, Masko GD, Hetelekidis S: Radiation therapy in the treatment of pituitary adenomas, *Int J Radiat Oncol Biol Phys* 15:305-309, 1988.
14. Cohen ME, Duffner PK: *Brain tumors in children: principles of diagnosis and treatment*, New York, 1984, Raven Press.
15. Cooper JS, Fried PR: Defining the role of radiotherapy for epidemic Kaposi's sarcoma, *Int J Radiat Oncol Biol Phys* 13:35-39, 1987.
16. Crist WM, et al: Intergroup Rhabdomyosarcoma Group IV: Results for patients with nonmetastatic disease, *J Clin Oncol* 19: 3091-3102, 2001.
17. Cummings BJ, Blend R: Primary radiation therapy for juvenile nasopharyngeal angiofibroma, *Laryngoscope* 94:1599-1605, 1984.
18. D'Angio GJ, Evans A, Koop CE: Special pattern of widespread neuroblastoma with a favorable prognosis, *Lancet* 1:1046, 1971.
19. D'Angio GJ, et al: Radiation therapy of Wilms tumor:results according to dose, field, post-operative timing, and histology, *Int J Radiat Biol Oncol Phys* 4:769-780, 1978.
20. Deutsch M: The impact of myelography on the treatment results of medulloblastoma, *Int J Radiat Oncol Biol Phys* 10:999-1003, 1989.
21. Donaldson SS, et al: Results from the IRS-IV trial of hyperfractionated radiotherapy in children with rhabdomyosarcoma: a report from the IRSG, *Int J Radiat Oncol Biol Phys* 51:718-728, 2001.
22. Douglas EC, et al: Abnormalities of chromosome 1 and 11 in Wilms tumor, *Cancer Genet Cytogenet* 14:331-338, 1985.
23. Druja TP, et al: Homozygosity of chromosome 13 in retinoblastoma, *N Engl J Med* 310:550-553, 1984.
24. Duffner PK, et al: Postoperative chemotherapy and delayed radiation in children less than 3 years of age with malignant brain tumors, *N Engl J Med* 328:1725-1731, 1993.
25. Eng C, et al: Mortality from second tumors among long term survivors of retinoblastoma, *J Natl Cancer Inst* 85:1121-1128, 1993.
26. Evans AE: Staging and treatment of neuroblastoma, *Cancer* 45:1799-1802, 1980.
27. Farber S: Chemotherapy in the treatment of leukemia and Wilms tumor, *JAMA* 138:826, 1966.
28. Finley JL, Uteg R, Giese WL: Brain tumors in children. II. Advances in neurosurgery and radiation oncology, *Am J Pediatr Hematol Oncol* 9:256-263, 1987.
29. Flickinger JC, Kondziolka D, Lunsford LD: Radiosurgery of benign lesions, *Semin Radiat* Oncol 5:220-224, 1995.
30. Fraumeni JF, Miller RW, Hill JA: Primary carcinoma of the liver in childhood: an epidemiologic study, *J Natl Cancer Inst* 40:1087-1099, 1968.
31. Freeman CR, et al: Hyperfractionated radiation therapy of brainstem tumors, *Cancer* 68:474-481, 1991.
32. Friedman DL, et al: Chemoreduction and local ophthalmologic therapy for intraocular retinoblastoma, *J Clin Oncol* 18:12-17, 2000.
33. Friedman HS, Schold SC: Rational approaches to the chemotherapy of medulloblastoma, *Neurol Clin* 3:843-854, 1985.
34. Garvey M and Packer RJ: An integrated approach to the treatment of chiasmatic-hypothalamic gliomas, *J Neurooncol* 28:167-183, 1996.
35. Garwicz S, et al: Second malignant neoplasms after cancer in childhood and adolescence: a population-based case control study in the 5 Nordic countries, *Int J Cancer* 88:672-678, 2000.
36. Gerbaulet A, et al: Iridium afterloading curietherapy in the treatment of pediatric malignancies, *Cancer* 56:1274-1279, 1985.
37. Giacomantonio M, et al: 30 years of experience with pediatric primary malignant liver tumors, J Pediatr Surg 19:523-526, 1984.
38. Graf N, Tournade MF, de Kraker J: The role of preoperative chemotherapy in the management of Wilms' tumor. The SIOP studies, *Urol Clin North Am* 27:443-454, 2000.
39. Grund PE, et al: Loss of heterozygosity for chromosomes 1p and 16q is an adverse prognostic factor in favorable histology Wilms' tumor: a report from the National Wilms Tumor Study Group, *J Clin Oncol* 23:7312-7321, 2005.
40. Gurney JG, et al: Incidence of cancer in children in the United States, *Cancer* 75:2186, 1995.
41. Hernandez JC, et al: Conservative treatment of retinoblastoma: the use of plaque brachytherapy, *Am J Clin Oncol* 16:397-401, 1993.
42. Heyn RM, et al: The role of combined chemotherapy in the treatment of rhabdomyosarcoma, *Cancer* 34:2128-2142, 1974.
43. Hirsch JE, et al: Medulloblastoma in childhood: survival and functional results, *Acta Neurochir* 48:1-15, 1979.
44. Hoffman HJ, Becker I, Craven MA: A clinically and pathologically distinct group of benign brainstem gliomas, *Neurosurgery* 7:243-248, 1980.
45. Israel MA: Molecular and cellular biology of pediatric malignancies. In Pizzo PA, Poplack DG, editors: *Principles and practice of pediatric oncology*, Philadelphia, 1989, JB Lippincott.
46. Kissane JM, Smith MG: *Pathology of infancy and childhood*, St. Louis, 1967, Mosby.
47. Kun LE: Patterns of failure in tumors of the central nervous system, *Cancer Treat Symp* 2:285-294, 1983.
48. Lemere J, et al: Effectiveness of preoperative chemotherapy in Wilms tumor: results of SIOP clinical trials, *J Clin Oncol* 1:604-610, 1983.

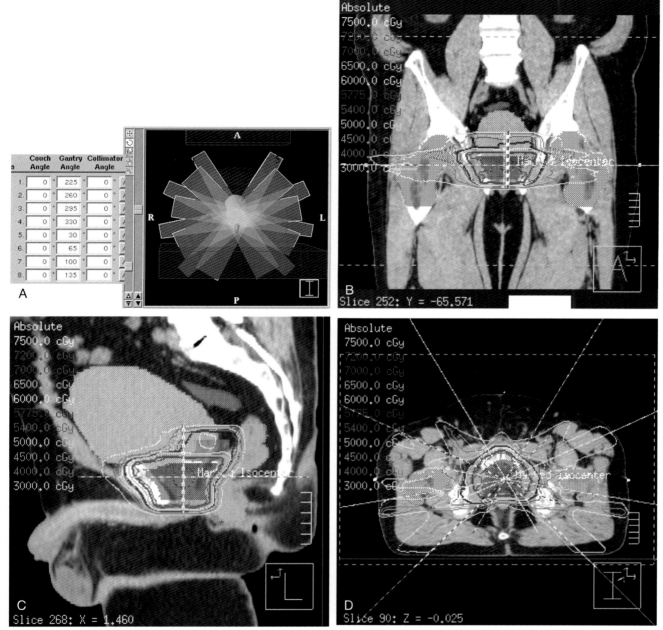

Color Plate 22. Intensity-modulated radiation therapy (IMRT) prostate radiation. **A,** Beam angles (8). **B,** Coronal dose distribution. **C,** Sagittal dose distribution. **D,** Axial dose distrubution. (See Figure 37-9.)

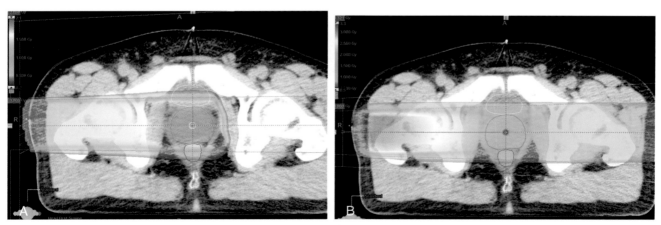

Color Plate 23. A, Lateral proton beam. **B,** Lateral photon beams. Both images are a single right lateral beam. Notice the lack of exit dose on the proton beam. (See Figure 37-10.)

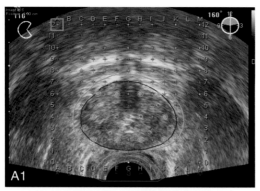

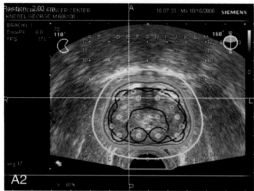

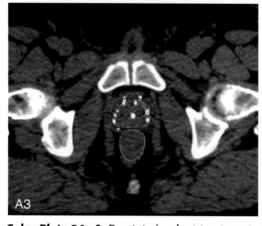

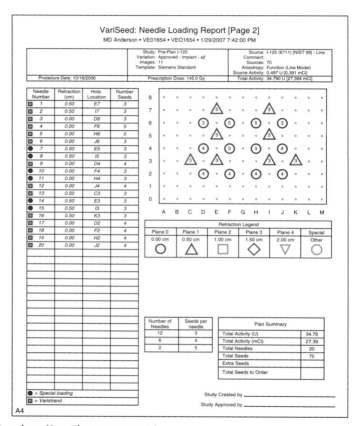

VariSeed: Needle Loading Report [Page 2]

MD Anderson • VE01654 • VEO1654 • 1/29/2007 7:42:00 PM

	Study: Pre-Plan I-125		Source: I-125 (6711) [NIST 99] - Line
	Variation: Approved - Implant - sjf		Comment:
	Images: 11		Sources: 70
	Template: Siemens Standard		Anisotropy: Function (Line Model)
			Source Activity: 0.497 U [0.391 mCi]
Procedure Date: 10/16/2006		Prescription Dose: 145.0 Gy	Total Activity: 34.790 U [27.394 mCi]

Needle Number	Retraction (cm)	Hole Location	Number Seeds
▣ 1	0.50	E7	3
▣ 2	0.50	I7	3
▣ 3	0.00	D6	3
▣ 4	0.00	F6	5
▣ 5	0.00	H6	5
▣ 6	0.00	J6	3
● 7	0.50	E5	3
● 8	0.50	I5	3
▣ 9	0.00	D4	4
● 10	0.00	F4	3
● 11	0.00	H4	3
▣ 12	0.00	J4	4
▣ 13	0.50	C3	3
▣ 14	0.50	E3	3
● 15	0.50	I3	3
▣ 16	0.50	K3	3
▣ 17	0.00	D2	4
▣ 18	0.00	F2	4
▣ 19	0.00	H2	4
▣ 20	0.00	J2	4

Retraction Legend

Plane 0	Plane 1	Plane 2	Plane 3	Plane 4	Special
0.00 cm	0.50 cm	1.00 cm	1.50 cm	2.00 cm	Other
○	△	□	◇	▽	○

Number of Needles	Seeds per needle
12	3
6	4
2	5

Plan Summary	
Total Activity (U)	34.79
Total Activity (mCi)	27.39
Total Needles	20
Total Seeds	70
Extra Seeds	
Total Seeds to Order	

● = Special loading
▣ = Varistrand

Study Created by _____

Study Approved by _____

Color Plate 24. A, Prostate implant treatment planning. (See Figure 37-11, A.)

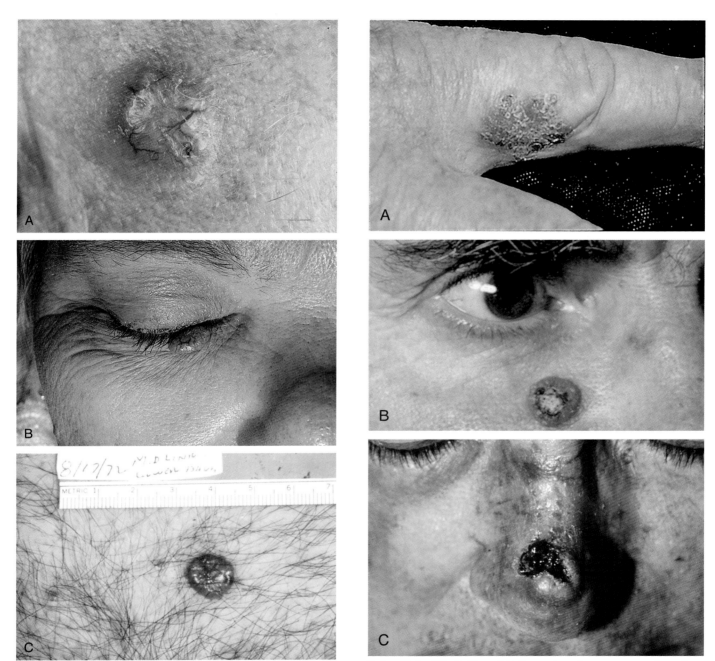

Color Plate 25. A, B, and **C,** Examples of basal cell carcinomas. (See Figure 40-10.) (**A,** From Habif: *Clinical dermatology: a color guide to diagnosis and therapy,* ed 4, Philadelphia, 2004, Mosby. **B,** From Callen, et al: *Color atlas of dermatology,* ed 2, Philadelphia, 2000, Saunders. **C,** Courtesy the National Cancer Institute.)

Color Plate 26. A, B, and **C,** Examples of squamous cell carcinomas. (See Figure 40-11.) (**A,** From Goldstein BG, Goldstein AO: *Practical dermatology,* ed 2, St. Louis, 1997, Mosby. Courtesy Department of Dermatology, Medical College of Georgia. **B,** From Bomford CK, Kunkler IH: *Walter and Miller's textbook of radiotherapy: radiation physics, therapy and oncology,* ed 6, Edinburgh, 2003, Churchill Livingstone. **C,** Courtesy the National Cancer Institute.)

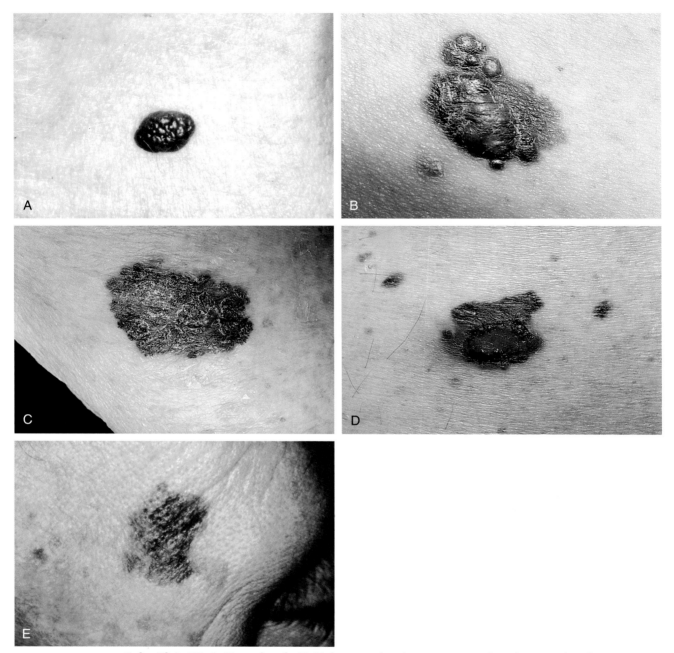

Color Plate 27. A, Normal mole. **B**, Melanoma showing asymmetry. **C**, Melanoma showing irregular borders. **D**, Melanoma showing uneven color. **E**, Melanoma showing a large diameter. (See Figure 40-12.) (**A** an d **E**, Courtesy the National Cancer Institute. **B**, **C**, and **D**, From Callen, et al: *Color atlas of dermatology*, ed 2, Philadelphia, 2000, Saunders.)

49. Li FP, Fraumeni JF. Rhabdomyosarcoma in children: epidemiologic study and identification of a familial cancer syndrome, *J Natl Cancer Inst* 43:1365, 1999.

50. Lingley JF, et al: Neuroblastoma: management and survival, *N Engl J Med* 277:1227-1230, 1967.

51. Mahoney DH, et al: High dose melphalan and cyclophosphamide with autologous bone marrow rescue for recurrent/progressive malignant brain tumors in children: a pilot Pediatric Oncology Group study, *J Clin Oncol* 14:382-388, 1996.

52. Matthay KK, et al: Patterns of relapse after ABMT for neuroblastoma, *Proc ASCO* 10:312, 1991.

53. Matthay KK, et al: Treatment of high risk neurobladtoma with intensive chemotherapy, radiotherapy, autologous bone marrow transplantation, and 13-cis-retinoic acid, *N Engl J Med* 341:1165-1173, 1999.

54. Maurer HM, et al: The Intergroup Rhabdomyosarcoma Study—I: a final report, *Cancer* 61:209-220, 1988.

55. Mulhern RK, Hancock J, Fairclough D, et al: Neuropsychologic status of children treated for brain tumors: critical review and integrative analysis, *Med Pediatr Oncol* 20:181-191, 1992.

56. Newton WA Jr, et al: Histopathology of childhood sarcomas, IRS I and II: clinicopathologic correlation, *J Clin Oncol* 6:67-75, 1988.

57. Ng AK, et al: Second malignancy after Hodgkin's disease treated with radiation therapy with or without chemotherapy: long term risks and risk factors, *Blood* 100:1989-1996, 2002.

58. Oberfield SE, et al: Thyroid and gonadal function and growth of long term survivors of medulloblastoma/PNET. In Green DM, D'Angio GJ, editors: *Late effects of treatment for childhood cancer*, New York, 1992, Wiley-Liss.

59. Packer RJ, et al: Treatment of children with medulloblastoma with reduced craniospinal radiation and adjuvant chemotherapy: a Children's Cancer Group study, *J Clin Oncol* 17:2127-2136, 1999.

60. Palma L, Guidetti B: Cystic pilocytic astrocytomas of the cerebral hemispheres: surgical experience with 51 cases and long term results, *J Neurosurg* 62:811-815, 1985.

61. Patterson E, Farr RF: Cerebellar medulloblastoma: treatment by irradiation of the whole central nervous system, *Acta Radiol* 39:323-336, 1953.

62. Plantaz D, et al: Gain of chromosome 17 is the most frequent abnormality detected in neuroblastoma by comparative genomic hybridization, *Am J Pathol* 150:81-89, 1997.

63. Raney B: Soft tissue sarcoma in adolescents. In Tebbi CK, editor: *Adolescent oncology*, Mt. Kisco, NY, 1987, Futura Publishing.

64. Reese A: *Tumors of the eye*, Hagerstown, MD, 1976, Harper and Row.

65. Rorke L: The cerebellar medulloblastoma and its relationship to primitive neuroectodermal tumors, *J Neuropathol Exp Neurol* 42:2-15, 1983.

66. Rudoler S, et al: Patterns of presentation, treatment, and outcome of children referred for emergent/urgent therapeutic irradiation. Presented at the Evolving Role of Radiation in Pediatric Oncology Conference, Philadelphia, 1995.

67. Schipper JJ, Tan KE, Von Peperzel HA: Treatment of retinoblastoma by precision megavoltage radiation therapy, *Radiother Oncol* 3:117-132, 1985.

68. Schwartzman E, et al: Results of a stage based protocol for the treatment of retinoblastoma, *J Clin Oncol* 14:1532-1536, 1996.

69. Scrable H, et al: Molecular differential pathology of rhabdomyosarcoma, *Genes Chromosomes Cancer* 23, 1989.

70. Shibamoto Y, et al: Intracranial germonoma: radiation therapy with tumor volume based dose selection, *Radiology* 218:452-456, 2001.

71. Shields CL, et al: Plaque radiotherapy for retinoblastoma: long term control and treatment complications in 208 tumors, *Ophthalmology* 108:2116-2121, 2001.

72. Sieber M, et al. Two cycles ABVD plus extended field radiotherapy is superior to radiotherapy alone in early stage Hodgkin's disease: Results of the German Hodgkin's Lymphoma Study Group Trial HD7, *Blood* 100:A341, 2002.

73. Silverman CL, Simpson JR: Cerebellar medulloblastoma: the importance of posterior fossa dose to survival and patterns of failure, *Int J Radiat Oncol Biol Phys* 8:1869-1876, 1982.

74. Stevens KR Jr: The soft tissue. In Moss WT, Cox JD, editors: *Radiation oncology: rationale, techniques, results*, ed 6, St. Louis, 1989, Mosby.

75. Tarbell NJ, Buck BA: *Postgraduate advances in radiation oncology: the treatment of medulloblastoma*, Berryville, VV, 1990, Forum Medicum.

76. Tefft M, Wharam M, Gehan E: Local and regional control of rhabdomyosarcoma by radiation in IRS II, *Int J Radiat Oncol Biol Phys* 15(suppl 1):159, 1988.

77. Thomas PRM, et al: Validation of radiation dose reductions used in the Third National Wilms Tumor Study, *Proc ASCO* 29:227, 1988.

78. Van den Berge JH, et al: Intracavitary brachytherapy of cystic craniopharyngiomas, *J Neurosurg* 77:545-550, 1992.

79. Waber DP, et al: Excellent therapeutic efficacy and minimal late neurotoxoicity in children treated with 18 Gray of cranial radiation therapy for high risk acute lymphoblastic leukemia: a 7 year follow-up study of the Dana Farber Cancer Institute Consortium protocol 87-01, *Cancer* 92: 15-22, 2001.

80. Warde P, et al: Results of adjuvant radiation and surveillance in stage I seminoma, *Br J Urol* 80:291, 1997.

81. Weinberg RA: The retinoblastoma gene and gene product, *Cancer Surv* 12:43-57, 1992.

82. Williams S, et al: Treatment of disseminated germ cell tumors with cisplatin, bleomycin and either vinblastine or etoposide, *N Engl J Med* 316: 1435-1440, 1987.

83. Wolden SL, et al: Improved long term survival with combined modality therapy for pediatric nasopharynx cancer, *Int J Radiat Biol Oncol Phys* 46:859-864, 2000.

84. Young JA, Eslinger P, Galloway M: Radiation treatment for the child with cancer, *Issues Comp Pediatr Nurs* 12:159-169, 1989.

BIBLIOGRAPHY

D'Angio GJ, et al: *Practical pediatric oncology*, New York, 1989, Raven.

Green DM, D'Angio GJ, editors: *Late effects of treatment for childhood cancer*, New York, 1992, Wiley-Liss.

Halperin EC, et al: *Pediatric radiation oncology*, Philadelphia, 2005, Lippincott Williams & Wilkins.

Kun LE, et al: Childhood cancers: Chapters 64-72, p 1569-1680. In Gunderson L, Tepper J, editors: *Clinical radiation oncology*, Philadelphia, 2007, Churchill Livingstone.

Pizzo PA, et al: *Principles and practice of pediatric oncology*, Philadelphia, 1993, JB Lippincott.

Schwartz CL, et al: *Survivors of childhood cancer*, St. Louis, 1994, Mosby.

Skin Cancers and Melanoma

Charles M. Washington

Outline

Skin and melanoma
  Epidemiology
  Etiology
  Anatomy and physiology

Clinical presentation
Detection and diagnosis
Pathology and staging
Treatment techniques

Radiation therapy
Prevention
Role of radiation therapist
Summary

Objectives

- Discuss epidemiologic factors of skin and melanoma tumors.
- Identify, list, and discuss etiologic factors that may be responsible for inducing skin and melanoma tumors.
- Describe the common symptoms produced by skin and melanoma malignancies.
- Discuss the methods of detection and diagnosis.
- List the varying histological types for tumors generic to this region.
- Describe the diagnostic procedures used in workup and staging for skin and melanoma tumors.
- Describe the clinical classification used for this area.
- Describe in detail the most common routes of tumor spread.
- Differentiate between histologic grading and staging.
- Describe the anatomy and physiology of the skin.
- Identify the options of treatment(s) for these tumors.

- Discuss the rationale for treatment with regard to treatment choice, histologic type, and stage of the disease.
- Describe the treatment methods available for this diagnosis.
- Describe the differing types of radiation treatments that can be used for treating skin and melanoma tumors.
- Discuss the expected radiation reactions for the area based on time-dose-fractionation schemes.
- Describe the instructions that should be given to a patient with regard to skin care, expected reactions and dietary advice.
- Discuss the rationale for using multimodality treatments for this diagnosis.
- Discuss survival statistics and prognosis for various stages for this tumor site.

Key Terms

Actinic (solar) keratoses
Basal cell carcinoma (BCC)
Dermits
Desquamation
Epidermis
Erythema
Keratin
Keratinocytes
Keratoacanthoma
Melanin
Melanocytes
Mohs' surgery
Mycosis fungoides
Nevus
Squamous cell carcinoma
Subcutaneous layer
Telangiectases
Xeroderma pigmentosum

D uring a lifetime, the skin, one of the most visible and vulnerable organs of the body, is subjected to macny external influences, including cold, heat, friction, ultraviolet (UV) light, pressure, and chemicals. As a result, the skin is especially susceptible to trauma, infection, and disease.

This chapter focuses on the three main types of skin cancer: basal cell carcinoma (BCC), squamous cell carcinoma, and malignant melanoma. Basal cell and squamous cell carcinomas are commonly referred to as *nonmelanoma cancers of the skin*.

SKIN CANCERS AND MELANOMA

Epidemiology

Cancer of the skin is the most common type of malignancy. Approximately 50% of all people who live to age 65 will develop at least one skin cancer during their lifetime.[4,7] In 2008 the incidence of basal cell and squamous cell skin cancer was estimated to be more than 1 million new cases (BCCs outnumber squamous cell cancers of the skin approximately 5:1), whereas malignant melanoma of the skin was expected to account for 62,480 new cases, an increase seen over the past few years.[2,3] Figure 40-1 shows the estimated new melanoma cases per year for a 10-year period. The reason that such a large range for nonmelanoma skin cancer estimates exists is that many early skin cancer lesions are easily treated by primary physicians and dermatologists and are not reported to the various cancer-tracking agencies.

Unfortunately, the incidence of skin cancers and melanomas is rising and continues to grow throughout the world. BCCs are more abundant than squamous cell carcinomas in the skin by approximately

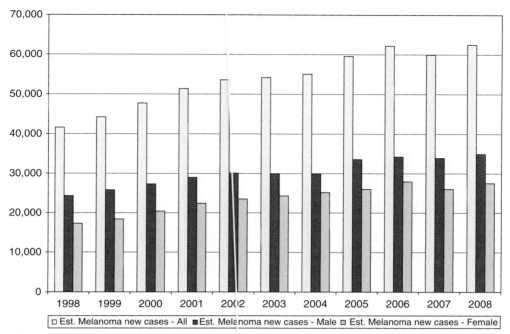

Figure 40-1. Estimated new melanoma cases per year in the United States. (Compiled from "1998-2008 Cancer facts and figures" on the American Cancer Society's website: http://www.cancer.org/docroot/STT/stt_0 asp. Accessed September 16, 2008.)

5:1 in males and 10:1 in females, accounting for about one-third of all cancer diagnoses. The annual incidence of malignant melanoma of the skin also is trending upward.[39] More young people are being affected; a few theories that might account for this trend are as follows:

1. The "healthy tan" has become fashionable in recent years. Crowded beaches and the proliferation of tanning salons seem to indicate people are interested in that look.
2. Clothing trends have changed in recent years. Everyday fashions and swimwear have become more liberal, allowing for more skin to be exposed to the sun's rays.
3. The depletion of the ozone layer has diminished the atmosphere's ability to protect the earth and its inhabitants from the sun's harmful UV rays. Rays that were formerly filtered by the ozone layer now reach the earth's surface and its inhabitants.

In contrast to increasing rates of incidence, death rates as a result of skin cancer have stayed virtually the same over the past 11 years (Figure 40-2). Melanoma mortality for the most recent period is increasing slightly in white men, and it has stabilized in white women.[3] Nonmelanomas, however, have experienced a decreasing death rate. The fact that death rates are so low and declining for nonmelanoma skin cancer is good news, but the comparatively higher death rates for melanomas are concerning.

Melanomas are much more lethal than their nonmelanoma counterparts. About 8,420 people (5,400 males and 3,020 females) will die from melanoma in 2008. Although nonmelanomas outnumber melanomas approximately 30:1, more people die each year from melanoma than from nonmelanoma skin cancers.

Some individuals are more prone to skin cancer than others. Tendencies for people to develop skin cancers and melanomas can be grouped into four main categories: geographic location, skin type, multiplicity, and gender.

Geographic Location. People who live near the equator have a high chance of developing skin cancer because the sun's rays are intense and direct. At latitudes away from the equator, the sun's rays are angled and are not as intense. This angulation causes the rays to travel through more of the atmosphere, allowing it to absorb more harmful rays in areas away from the equator than those at the equator itself (Figure 40-3). Table 40-1 shows annual UV levels in selected cities, with Anchorage's level as an arbitrary baseline. On average, the closer a city is to the equator, the higher is the UV exposure. The greater the UV exposure, the higher are the rates for skin cancer. For example, melanoma rates in Honolulu are twice those in Detroit. This difference corresponds roughly with that in the UV index. Similarly, people living at high altitudes are more prone to develop skin cancer because high levels have fewer atmospheres to filter the sun's rays. As elevation increases, there is an increase in UV radiation exposure.

Skin Type. Individuals with fair complexions are 10 times more likely to develop skin cancer than those with dark skin. Especially susceptible are albinos, people with freckles or light-colored eyes, and people who suffer from **xeroderma pigmentosum** (a genetic condition caused by a defect in mechanisms that repair deoxyribonucleic acid [DNA] damage caused by UV light, characterized by the development of pigment abnormalities and multiple skin cancers in body areas exposed to the sun). These people tend to tan poorly and burn easily.

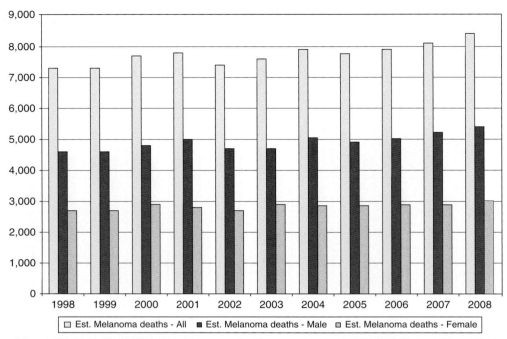

Figure 40-2. Estimated new melanoma deaths per year in the United States. (Compiled from "1998-2008 Cancer facts and figures" on the American Cancer Society's website: http://www.cancer.org/docroot/STT/stt_0.asp. Accessed September 16, 2008.)

People with dark skin have greater quantities of **melanin** (a natural protective substance that gives color to the skin, hair, and iris of the eye) in their skin, giving them more protection from the UV rays of the sun. This does not mean that dark-skinned individuals are free of skin cancers, but they get them less often and in more unusual places, such as on the palm of the hand, on the sole of the foot, or in the mucous membranes.

Among African Americans, squamous cell carcinoma is more common than BCC. Squamous cell carcinoma tends to occur in sites not exposed to the sun and is often aggressive.[44]

Multiplicity. Prior skin cancer occurrence increases the odds that a second primary skin cancer will develop. Reasons for this may include the following: (1) other areas of the skin may have been exposed to the same carcinogens that caused the

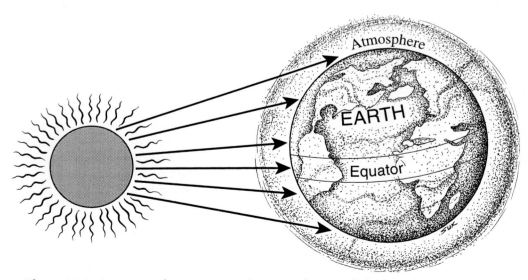

Figure 40-3. Areas near the equator receive more direct sunlight than areas closer to the poles. Notice the way the angled rays near the poles are filtered through larger amounts of the atmosphere before they reach the earth.

Table 40-1	Comparison of Latitude on Ultraviolet Exposure		
City	Degrees of Latitude	Elevation (ft)	Ultraviolet Index
Anchorage	61	118	100
Seattle	47	10	477
Detroit	42	585	630
Philadelphia	40	100	656
Boise*	43	2704	715
Phoenix	33	1090	889
Denver*	39	5280	951
Houston	29	40	999
Miami	25	10	1028
Honolulu	21	21	1147

Modified from Roach M, Hastings J, Finch S: Sun struck: here's the hole story about the ozone and your chances of getting skin cancer, *Health* 11:40, May-June, 1992.

*UV readings for Boise and Denver seem to be out of place, but in comparing the elevations of those two cities, a significant difference is evident. High elevations also contribute to higher UV exposures.

initial skin cancer and (2) the individual may have a weakness in the immune system that hinders the ability to naturally fight off skin cancers.

A previous melanoma of the skin increases the risk of another primary melanoma by 5 to 9 times. The rate of second primary melanomas is higher in persons younger than 40 years at the original time of diagnosis compared with persons diagnosed at age 40 or older. The risk is highest in the first year after the original diagnosis but remains highly elevated long afterward.[44]

For individuals with at least one nonmelanoma cancer occurrence, the chances of developing a second malignancy are 17% within 1 year and 50% within 5 years.[44] Because of these elevated risks, any patient diagnosed with skin cancer should be closely monitored for signs of recurrence or new primaries.

Gender. Rates for melanoma skin cancers are slightly higher for men than women, but men are 3 times more likely than women to develop nonmelanomas, except on the legs, where women have higher rates of nonmelanoma skin cancers.[47] This trend seems to be related to skin care habit differences between the genders rather than genetics. Men tend to work outside more often and do not wear sunscreens as often (50% less) as women. Also, men have a more nonchalant attitude about sun exposure and its effects. In general, women seem to pay more attention to their skin than do men.

Etiology

Many factors are directly and indirectly responsible for the development of the various forms of skin cancer, but the major cause is exposure to UV light.

UV Light. The American Cancer Society estimates that approximately 90% of all skin cancers would be prevented if people protected their skin from the sun's rays.[4,7] The risk of developing melanoma increases 4 to 5 times after three or more blistering sunburns during adolescence.[1] The time between the initial stimulus (sunburn) and the appearance of a melanoma is believed to be between 10 and 20 years.[48] At greatest risk for developing a malignant melanoma is the person who primarily stays indoors and receives occasional sun exposure. In contrast, people who spend a majority of the time in the sun (e.g., farmers, construction workers) are most apt to develop BCCs or squamous cell carcinomas.

Sunlight contains two types of UV rays that are harmful to the skin: ultraviolet A (UVA) and ultraviolet B (UVB). UVB is thought to cause cancer by damaging DNA and its repair systems, resulting in mutations that may lead to cancer. It is also thought to play a role in cellular immunity by impairing T-cell function and increasing suppressor T-cell numbers.[42]

 Tanning salons have marketed their product as safe for everyone by stating that their machines only put out UVA rays and they filter out UVB radiation, which is the most damaging to the skin. However, a 2002 study in the JNCI found that tanning-bed enthusiasts have up to 2½ times the risk of squamous cell carcinoma and 1½ times the risk of basal cell carcinoma compared with nonusers. The amount of UVA radiation emitted from tanning beds is actually 2 to 5 times stronger than natural sunlight.[32] According to recent studies, a person who goes to a tanning salon more than 10 times a year increases their odds of getting melanoma by 8. A safer choice would be tanning lotions and the spray-on tan.[32]

UVA rays have long been considered relatively harmless compared with UVB rays. In fact, "most tanning equipment emits ultraviolet A light."[42]

Studies have shown that the stratum corneum absorbs UVB (see anatomy and physiology section in this chapter), whereas 50% of UVA radiation is able to penetrate to the highly mitotic basal layer of the skin, where the potential for malignant changes and premature aging of the skin exists. Evidence also suggests that UVA acts to promote tumors initiated by UVB.[48]

Like many other cancers, skin cancer is a disease of aging. Most skin cancers appear after age 50, but the damaging effects of the sun's rays are accumulated over a lifetime. However, skin cancers can develop in infants, children, and young adults, especially those with high-risk factors (e.g., xeroderma pigmentosum, giant hairy nevi).

Other Factors Associated With Nonmelanoma Skin Cancers. Other factors that contribute to nonmelanoma skin cancers include exposure to arsenic (an element used in medicines and poisons) and therapeutic or occupational exposure to radiation. After irradiation, the risk to the exposed individual is up to 20%, and latent periods may extend up to 50 years beyond the initial exposure. Squamous cell carcinomas account for two thirds of these radiation-induced lesions, which tend to be aggressive and result in a 10% mortality rate.[17]

Besides xeroderma pigmentosum, another genetic condition associated with the formation of BCCs is called basal cell nevus syndrome (a genetically linked condition that appears during the late teen years). Symptoms include multiple BCCs of the skin, cysts of the jaw bones, pitting of the palms and soles, and skeletal anomalies (particularly of the ribs).[2]

Squamous cell carcinomas of the skin have also been associated with the following[5]:

- Human papillomavirus infection
- Immunosuppression as a result of organ transplant, lymphoma, or leukemia
- Thermal or electrical burns and chronic heat exposure
- Scars or chronic inflammatory conditions
- Hydrocarbons derived from coal and petroleum
- Areas of chronic drainage (e.g., fistulas, sinuses)

Smoking is a proven cause of squamous cell carcinoma of the lip. It has also been linked to the development of squamous cell skin cancer in other anatomic areas. However, it is not known whether cigarette smoke acts directly as a skin carcinogen or has an adverse effect on the immune system, inhibiting the body's ability to defend itself from cancer.[5]

Other Factors Associated With Melanoma Skin Cancers. Melanomas tend to develop from melanocytes (the skin cells that produce melanin), which grow in clusters to form a mole, or **nevus**. Moles can be broadly classified according to when they are acquired: congenital melanocytic nevi (those present at birth) and common acquired nevi (those that develop later in life).

Congenital melanocytic nevi can be classified into three sizes: small (less than 1.5 cm in diameter), medium (1.5 cm to

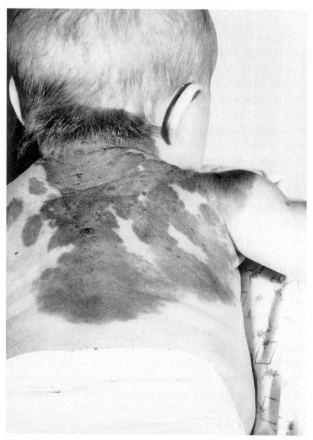

Figure 40-4. This child with a giant hairy nevus has approximately an 8% chance of developing a melanoma within the first 15 years of life. Because of the high risk, this lesion will be removed in a series of prophylactic surgical procedures. (Photograph and information courtesy R. Dean Glassman, MD.)

19.9 cm in diameter), and large (20 cm or more in diameter). Large nevi (Figure 40-4) are accompanied by an approximate 6% to 8% risk of developing melanoma compared with a 1% risk in the general population. Accordingly, some surgeons believe that these moles should be removed prophylactically before malignant changes can occur. Prophylactic removal of small and medium lesions should be made individually because the chance of malignant change in them is small.[50]

Melanocytic nevi can be grouped into three main categories: junctional, compound, and intradermal. Junctional nevi tend to be small (usually less than 6 mm), well-circumscribed, flat lesions with smooth surfaces that are uniformly brown or black and circular. The melanocyte clusters in junctional nevi are found above the basement layer. Compound nevi contain melanocyte clusters in the dermis and epidermis. They appear as small, well-circumscribed, slightly raised papules that often contain excess hair. The surface is rough and color ranges from tan to brown throughout. Over time, these lesions may take on a nodular appearance. Intradermal nevi are small, well-circumscribed, dome-shaped lesions that range from flesh to brown. They too may contain excess hair. Melanocytic clusters are found only in the dermal layer in these moles.[23]

The propensity of a mole to develop into a melanoma is related to the location of the melanocytic clusters found in the moles. Intradermal nevi rarely transform into melanomas; the likelihood of junctional and compound nevi transforming into melanomas is far greater. One theory for this pattern is that melanocytes located in the dermis do not receive as much UV exposure because they are located deep in the skin. **Melanocytes** in junctional and compound nevi are closer to the skin's surface and receive higher amounts of melanoma-inducing UV radiation.

Dysplastic nevi, also known as B-K or atypical moles, are acquired pigmented lesions of the skin that have one or more of the clinical features of melanoma—asymmetry, border irregularity, color variation, or a diameter greater than 6 mm.[23] "The presence of dysplastic moles marks an individual as having an increased risk of melanoma. Even a single dysplastic mole appears to be a significant risk factor for melanoma."[5,6]

The number of moles a person has also influences the chances of acquiring melanoma. One study showed that "persons who have twelve moles at least 5 mm in diameter have an estimated 41-fold increased risk of melanoma while those who have fifty or more moles at least 2 mm in diameter have a 64-fold increased risk of melanoma."[45]

People with a family history of melanoma have an eightfold increase in their chances of acquiring the disease.[44] Several studies have pinpointed a region on the short arm of chromosome 9 (9p) as one involved in the early-stage development of melanoma tumors.[29] Genetic material from this area is thought to play a vital role in the suppression of tumor formation. Without this material a person may be more susceptible to tumor formation because one of the normal defense mechanisms may be missing. Other chromosomal abnormalities associated with melanomas can be found on chromosomes 1, 6, 7, 11, and 19.[29]

"Some families are affected with an inherited familial atypical mole and melanoma (FAM-M) syndrome, also known as B-K mole syndrome or dysplastic nevus syndrome (DNS).

The syndrome is defined by (1) occurrence of melanoma in one or more first- or second-degree relatives; (2) large number of moles (often 50+), some of which are atypical and often variable in size; and (3) moles that demonstrate certain distinct histologic features. Persons with this syndrome have a markedly increased risk of developing melanoma. Their lifetime risk may be as much as 100%."[11] These patients require close monitoring because of the high risks involved. This syndrome has also been described in the nonfamilial setting.[23]

"Hormones, pregnancy, birth control pills, and certain environmental exposures have also been linked to the development of malignant melanoma, but these factors need further study."[3]

Anatomy and Physiology

The skin is the largest organ of the body, covering about 17 to 20 sq ft on the average person. The skin provides many functions, including the following:

- Regulates body temperature through perspiration (as perspiration evaporates, it carries heat away from the body) and blood flow through vessels located in the skin (the skin allows heat carried by the blood to radiate off its surface)
- Acts as a barrier between the external environment and the body, offering protection against factors such as trauma, UV light, and bacterial invasion
- Participates in the production of vitamin D, which is vital to the process enabling the body to absorb and use calcium in the gastrointestinal tract
- Provides receptors for external stimuli such as heat, cold, pressure, and touch, allowing the body to be aware of its environment

Vitamin D is often referred to as the "sunshine vitamin" because the body manufactures vitamin D after being exposed to the sun.[36] Vitamin D is very important in the body's absorption of calcium, and it also helps the body keep the right amount of calcium and phosphorus in the blood. Tanning salon marketers have recently advertised the use of tanning beds to make up for vitamin D deficiency, however, 10 to 15 minutes of natural sunlight three times a week is more than enough to keep up with the body's requirements. Vitamin D can also be found in most dairy products such as milk and cheese and in fish, oysters, and many fortified cereals.[36]

The skin is an example of an epithelial membrane, a connective tissue covered by a layer of epithelial tissue. The connective tissue layer in the skin is called the **dermis**; the epithelial layer is called the **epidermis** (Figure 40-5). These layers are held together by an intermediate layer called the basement membrane.[52]

The dermis is the deeper layer of the skin composed of connective tissue that contains blood and lymphatic vessels, nerves and nerve endings, sweat glands, and hair follicles. It contains mainly elastic and collagen fibers that allow for the flexibility and strength of the skin. The upper 20% of the dermis is referred to as the papillary region and contains dermal papillae, ridges that are responsible for the formation of fingerprints. The lower 80% of the dermis is the reticular region and contains many accessory structures of the skin, such as the following: hair follicles, sebaceous (oil) and sudoriferous (sweat) glands and their ducts, nerve endings, and blood vessels.[52]

A **subcutaneous layer** containing nerves, blood vessels, adipose (fat) tissue, and areolar connective tissue lies beneath the dermis. Because the epidermis is avascular, the blood vessels of the dermis and subcutaneous layer are responsible for the nutritional status of the epidermis.

The epidermis is the extremely thin outer layer of the skin, composed of four to five layers (depending on its location). These layers are as follows, from deepest to most superficial[52]:

1. **Stratum basale (stratum germinativum)**—This is the basal layer containing stem cells capable of producing **keratinocytes** (stratified epithelial cells, which comprise 90% of the epidermal cells of the skin and provide a barrier between the host and the environment, prevent the entry of toxic substances from the environment and the loss of important constituents from the host) and cells that give rise to glands and hair follicles. This layer also contains melanocytes (which comprise 8% of the epidermal cells of the skin), cells with branching processes that produce the pigment melanin. In hairless skin a third type of cell, Merkel's cells, can also be found. Together with a flattened portion of a neuron called a tactile (Merkel's disc), Merkel's cells function in the sensation of touch.
2. **Stratum spinosum**—This layer contains 8 to 10 rows of keratinocytes, which have a spiny appearance microscopically. Branches from the melanocytes reach into this layer, allowing the keratinocytes to absorb the protective pigment melanin via exocytosis.
3. **Stratum granulosum**—This layer contains three to five rows of somewhat flattened cells. The keratinocytes begin to produce a substance called keratohyalin, which is a precursor to a waterproof protein called **keratin**.
4. **Stratum lucidum**—This layer is normally found only in areas in which thick skin is present (soles and palms) and contains three to five rows of clear, flat cells that contain eleidin, another keratin precursor.
5. **Stratum corneum**—This layer forms the skin surface and contains 25 to 30 rows of flat, dead, scaly (squamous) cells that are completely filled with keratin and have lost all their internal organelles, including nuclei. The lower layers of cells are closely packed and adhere to each other, whereas the upper layers of cells are loosely packed and continually flake away from the surface.

Basically, the outer, protective layer of the skin is composed of dead cells filled with keratin. Each day, millions of these cells are sloughed off and continually replaced by cells from the lower layers of the epidermis. Germ cells in the stratum basale give rise to keratinocytes, which go through a process called keratinization as they are pushed toward the surface by new cells. As the cells are relocated, they accumulate keratin to the point that the cells can no longer function and dies. The mature keratinocytes serve their protective function and are eventually shed from the surface of the skin. The time necessary for the cell to travel from the germ layer to the surface is approximately 2 to 4 weeks. This cycle continually repeats itself.

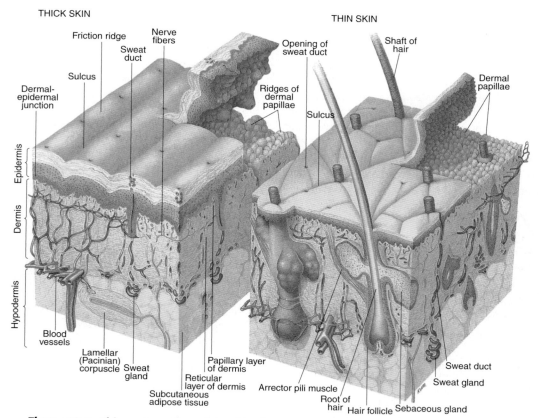

THICK SKIN

Friction ridge
Nerve fibers
Sweat duct
Sulcus
Dermal-epidermal junction
Epidermis
Dermis
Hypodermis
Blood vessels
Lamellar (Pacinian) corpuscle
Sweat gland
Subcutaneous adipose tissue
Reticular layer of dermis
Papillary layer of dermis

THIN SKIN

Opening of sweat duct
Shaft of hair
Ridges of dermal papillae
Dermal papillae
Sulcus
Arrector pili muscle
Root of hair
Hair follicle
Sebaceous gland
Sweat duct
Sweat gland

Figure 40-5. This cross section of the skin shows the relationship between the epidermis, dermis, and subcutaneous layers. Notice how thick the dermis is compared with the epidermis. Also shown are the various accessory structures of the skin and their location. (From Thibodeau GA, Patton KT: *Anatomy and physiology*, ed 6, St. Louis, 2007, Mosby.)

Melanin is a pigment that serves a protective function of the skin. It is produced by the melanocytes and absorbed by the keratinocytes in the stratum spinosum layer of the epidermis. UV light damages the keratinocytes by inhibiting synthesis of DNA and ribonucleic acid (RNA) (genetic material in the cell), leading to cell dysfunction or death. The melanin absorbed by the keratinocytes is placed in the cell so that it lies between the skin surface and nucleus of the cell, thus protecting it from the sun's rays like an umbrella (Figure 40-6).

Melanin is one of the pigments responsible for differences in skin color among individuals. The more melanin a person's skin contains, the darker the skin. The number of melanocytes is about the same in all races. Differences in skin darkness are attributed to the amount of melanin that the melanocytes produce. The systemic release of melanocyte-stimulating hormone (MSH) from the anterior pituitary gland controls overall skin darkness. The more MSH released by the pituitary, the more melanin the melanocytes produce and the darker the person's skin. Variations in skin darkness can occur in localized areas of the body as a result of exposure to UV light. Brief exposure to UV light causes melanin already present in the epidermis to darken considerably, whereas long-term exposure causes melanocytes to increase melanin production.

Both processes result in darker or tanned skin. A tan is actually a response by the body to damage caused by UV light.[52] In the absence of UV stimulation, melanocytes decrease melanin production to normal levels and the skin returns to normal color.[47]

Skin cancers can be classified according to the cell of the skin from which they originate. Malignant melanoma, the most lethal form of skin cancer, arises from the melanocytes located in the stratum basale. The most common sites for melanoma are the legs of women and the trunk and face of men. Melanomas can also arise in other areas of the body, such as the choroid or ciliary body of the eye, the eyelids, the mucosa of the oral cavity, the genitalia, and the anus.

Basal cell carcinoma (BCC), a slow-growing form of skin cancer that does not tend to metastasize, arises from the stem cells of the stratum basale. It is the most prevalent cancer in humans and, if left untreated, can cause extensive damage.

Squamous cell carcinoma, a faster-growing cancer than the basal cell type with a higher propensity for metastasis, arises from the more mature keratinocytes of the upper layers of the epidermis. This type of nonmelanoma skin cancer can arise anywhere on the body but is especially common on sun-exposed areas such as the head, neck, face, arms, and hands.

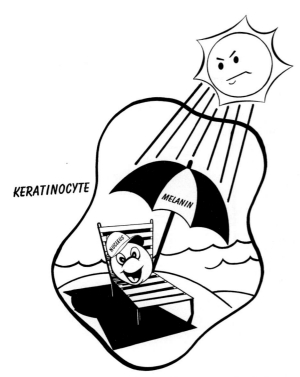

Figure 40-6. This cartoon depicts the way melanin is strategically placed inside the keratinocyte between the nucleus and sun's rays, protecting it from ultraviolet radiation.

Other types of cancers can arise in the skin but are not covered in detail in this chapter. These include, but are not limited to, the following[31]:

1. **Adenocarcinoma** of the sebaceous and sudoriferous glands—This type of cancer arises in the dermal layer of the skin and is a slow-growing lesion capable of metastasis. It tends to be radioresistant; therefore, surgery is the treatment of choice.

2. **Cutaneous T-cell lymphoma**, including mycosis fungoides—This is a disease of the T lymphocytes. It resembles eczema or other inflammatory conditions and tends to remain localized to the skin for long periods. Total-body irradiation with electrons and topical nitrogen mustard has been used to control early stages of the disease.

3. **Kaposi's sarcoma**—This is a slow-growing, temperate tumor thought to arise from vascular tissue. The associated nodular purple lesions are often multifocal and common in individuals affected with acquired immunodeficiency syndrome (AIDS) and those living in the Mediterranean region. Surgical excision is indicated for individual lesions and radiation therapy for multiple lesions.
The AIDS epidemic has introduced an aggressive variant of this disease. Although associated lesions are radiosensitive, AIDS patients who acquire this disease have a poor prognosis and are best treated systemically with chemotherapy. Radiation therapy is used to palliate local areas.

4. **Merkel's cell carcinoma**—This is a rare tumor thought to arise from Merkel's (tactile) cells. It is known for high rates of recurrence after surgical excision, frequent involvement of regional lymph nodes, and distant metastatic failure.

These tumors are structurally similar to small cell carcinomas and appear as firm, nontender, pink-red nodular lesions with an intact epidermis.[26] These types of cancers are often treated with a combination of chemotherapy and radiation therapy or surgery.

Clinical Presentation

Although skin cancers and melanomas occur in a wide variety of shapes, sizes, and appearances, similarities exist that facilitate lesion classification. Following is a discussion concerning the tumors seen most often and premalignant growths that may precede them.

Nonmelanoma Precursors and Characteristics. Premalignant lesions are those that, if left untreated or not closely monitored, can develop into cancer. Squamous cell carcinomas tend to arise more often from precursor lesions compared with BCCs.[54] The American Cancer Society classifies some of the precancerous lesions for nonmelanomas as follows[2]:

1. **Actinic (solar) keratoses**—These are warty lesions or areas of red, scaly patches occurring on the sun-exposed skin of the face or hands of older, light-skinned individuals (Figure 40-7). Because actinic keratoses have a 5% to 10% chance[17] of degrading into squamous cell carcinoma, some physicians remove them surgically or treat them with 5-fluorouracil (5-FU), liquid nitrogen, or electrodesiccation to destroy them and eliminate the possibility of cancerous change.[17]

2. **Arsenical keratoses**—These are multiple, hard, cornlike masses on the palms of hands or soles of feet resulting from long-term arsenic ingestion.

3. **Bowen's disease**—This is a precancerous dermatosis or carcinoma in situ characterized by the development of pink or brown papules covered with a thickened, horny layer (Figure 40-8).

4. **Keratoacanthoma**—This is a rapid-growing lesion that can appear suddenly as a dome-shaped mass on a sun-exposed area (Figure 40-9). Microscopically, the nodules are composed of well-differentiated squamous epithelia with a necrotic center or central keratin mass. They can be difficult to distinguish from squamous cell cancer and usually resolve themselves if left untreated.

Nonmelanoma skin cancers have a multitude of appearances (Figures 40-10 and 40-11). BCCs tend to arise as smooth, red,

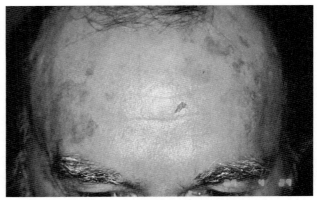

Figure 40-7. Actinic keratosis. (Courtesy Mark McLaughlin, MD.)

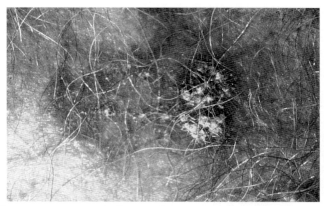

Figure 40-8. Bowen's disease. (Courtesy Mark McLaughlin, MD.)

or milky lumps and have a pearly border and multiple **telangiectases** (tiny blood vessels visible on the skin's surface). BCCs can be shiny or pale. About 80% of BCCs occur on the head and neck. Squamous cell carcinomas tend to have a scaly, crusty, slightly elevated lesion that may have a cutaneous horn. Approximately 80% of UV-induced squamous cell carcinomas develop on the arms, head, and neck.[49] Other symptoms possibly indicating a BCC or squamous cell carcinoma include a sore that takes longer than 3 weeks to heal, a recurrent red patch that may itch or be tender, and a wart that bleeds or scabs. Some BCCs may contain melanin, causing the lesion to appear black and resemble a melanoma. In general, any new growths that persist or change in appearance should be reported to a physician.

Melanoma Precursors and Characteristics. Approximately 70% of melanomas occur as the result of a change in a preexisting nevus. The other 30% arise from de novo melanomas, growths not associated with previously observed nevi.[17] The American Cancer Society[6] has released the ABCD rules for early detection of melanoma (Figure 40-12). These are as follows:

A, *Asymmetry*—Melanomas tend to be asymmetrical; most benign moles tend to be symmetrical.

B, *Border*—Melanomas tend to have notched, uneven borders; most benign moles tend to possess clearly defined, smooth borders.

C, *Color*—Melanomas can contain different shades of black, brown, or tan; benign moles tend to be uniformly tan or brown.

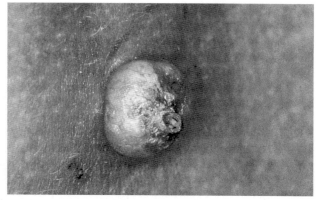

Figure 40-9. Keratoacanthoma. (Courtesy Mark McLaughlin, MD.)

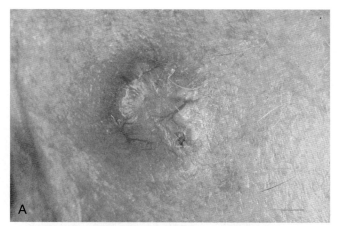

A

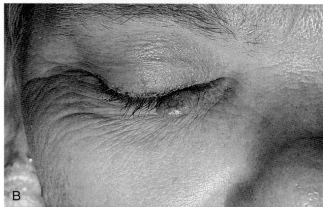

B

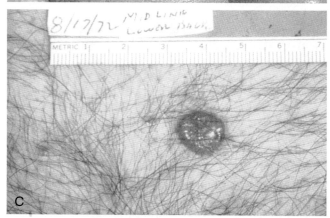

C

Figure 40-10. A, **B**, and **C**, Examples of basal cell carcinomas. (See Color Plate 25.) (**A**, From Habif: *Clinical dermatology: a color guide to diagnosis and therapy*, ed 4, Philadelphia, 2004, Mosby. **B**, From Callen, et al: *Color atlas of dermatology*, ed 2, Philadelphia, 2000, Saunders. **C**, Courtesy the National Cancer Institute.)

D, *Diameter*—Most melanomas have a diameter greater than 6 mm; most benign moles tend to be less than 6 mm in diameter.

In addition to the ABCD rules, the following changes in the appearance of a mole should be monitored as possible signs of melanoma[5]:

1. Change in *color*—red, white, and/or blue areas in addition to black and tan

2. Change in *surface*—scaly, flaky, bleeding, or oozing moles or a sore that does not heal

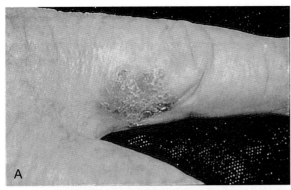

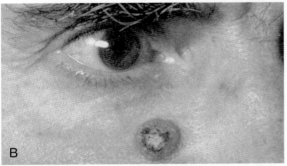

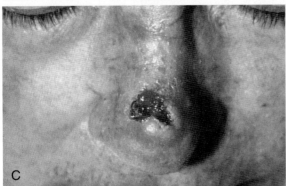

Figure 40-11. A, B, and **C,** Examples of squamous cell carcinomas. (See Color Plate 26.) (**A,** From Goldstein BG, Goldstein AO: *Practical dermatology,* ed 2, St. Louis, 1997, Mosby. Courtesy Department of Dermatology, Medical College of Georgia. **B,** From Bomford CK, Kunkler IH: *Walter and Miller's textbook of radiotherapy: radiation physics, therapy and oncology,* ed 6, Edinburgh, 2003, Churchill Livingstone. **C,** Courtesy the National Cancer Institute.)

3. Change in *texture*—hard, lumpy, or elevated moles
4. Change in *surrounding skin*—spread of pigmentation, swelling, or redness to surrounding skin
5. Change in *sensation*—unusual pain or tenderness in a mole
6. Change in *previously normal skin*—pigmented areas that arise in previously normal skin

A few pigmented lesions of the skin are benign, but these can be difficult to distinguish from melanoma.[23] They are as follows:

1. **Simple lentigo**—This is a small (1 to 5 mm), brown to black macule. It is round with sharply defined edges, and the surface is flat, similar to a freckle. Thought to be the precursor to the common mole, some simple lentigines are clinically indistinguishable from junctional nevi.

2. **Solar lentigo**—This is a small to medium, flat, lightly pigmented macule better known as a liver spot. It is especially common in older white people on areas of the skin chronically exposed to the sun.

3. **Seborrheic keratoses**—These are round or ovoid, wartlike papules ranging from a few to several millimeters. These growths tend to be raised (often with a warty, "stuck-on" appearance) and composed of proliferating epidermal cells, especially of the basal type.

4. **Others**—Some common moles may be difficult to distinguish from melanoma. For a description of common moles, see the section on etiology.

Although all these lesions tend to be benign, they should be watched for signs of malignant change. Questionable lesions should be biopsied and analyzed to rule out malignancy.

Detection and Diagnosis

Theoretically, no one should die from skin cancer because the skin lends itself easily to self-inspection and cancer detection. If people were educated on the way to detect skin cancer and actually took the time to inspect themselves, cancer should be found at an early stage and therefore be easily treatable. Following are some of the methods used to detect and diagnose skin cancer.

Everyone should inspect the total surface area of the skin monthly for signs of cancer (Box 40-1). High-risk individuals should have photographs of the skin taken to document existing moles to which they can refer when questions arise concerning factors such as the size, color, and shape of moles. Body charts indicating the location and size of moles may also be useful.

Inspections should take place in well-lighted areas. Familiarity with existing moles, freckles, and blemishes is important so that newly pigmented areas or blemishes can be distinguished from older ones. When surveying the skin, individuals should remember the ABCD rules. In addition, people should watch for sores that do not heal or other areas of unexplained changes in the skin.

Any unusual changes should be brought to the attention of a physician. The earlier skin cancer is detected, the better is the chance it will be cured. People who find unusual lesions must not let their fears of pain, cost, and disfigurement get in the way of seeking a proper diagnosis and treatment. Skin cancer is obviously not something that will go away by itself.

A routine physical examination should include a thorough inspection of the skin's surface by the physician. Physicians must be knowledgeable in distinguishing between benign and malignant conditions. Also, regional lymph nodes should be inspected for signs or symptoms of metastasis.

A family history should be taken to determine whether a person is at a higher risk for developing melanoma because a family member previously had the disease. Patients with a family history of melanoma should be monitored closely.

Individuals should have a biopsy performed for unusual or suspicious lesions. Depending on the size and location of the lesion, the biopsy may be incisional (only a portion of the lesion is removed for tissue diagnosis—usually reserved for large lesions) or excisional (entire lesion is removed). Excisional biopsies (including punch, saucerization, or elliptical incision)

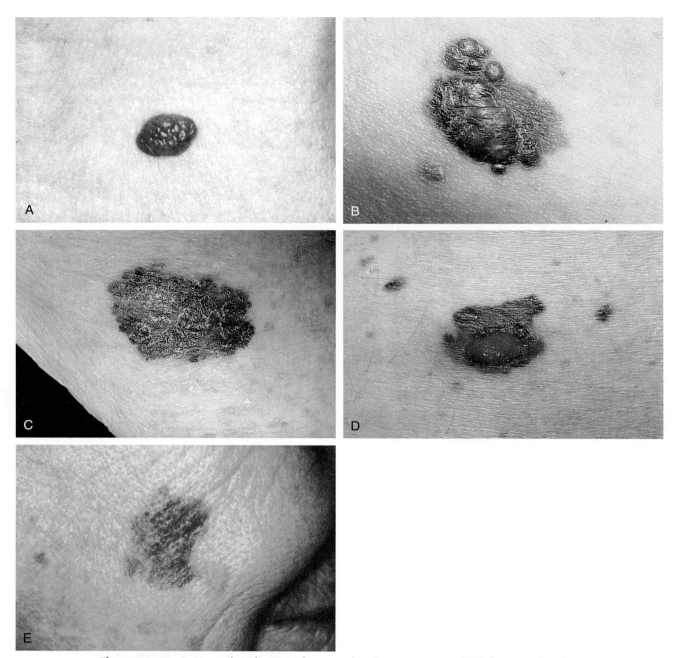

Figure 40-12. A, Normal mole. **B**, Melanoma showing asymmetry. **C**, Melanoma showing irregular borders. **D**, Melanoma showing uneven color. **E**, Melanoma showing a large diameter. (See Color Plate 27.) (**A** and **E**, Courtesy the National Cancer Institute. **B**, **C**, and **D**, From Callen, et al: *Color atlas of dermatology*, ed 2, Philadelphia, 2000, Saunders.)

may be indicated for suspected squamous cell carcinomas or melanomas to ascertain the depth of the tumor's penetration and should include a portion of the underlying subcutaneous fat for accurate microstaging. A shave or curettage may be adequate to diagnose BCC but is not recommended for lesions suspected to be melanoma.[38]

To the naked eye, some lesions are difficult to define as malignant or nonmalignant without a biopsy. A relatively new technique in diagnosing melanomas is in vivo (in tissue) *epiluminescence microscopy (ELM)*, or *dermatoscopy*. ELM is a noninvasive procedure that allows physicians to differentiate between benign and malignant lesions while they are in the early phases of development and have not yet begun to exhibit the features displayed by later melanomatous lesions. The procedure uses a *dermatoscope*, which looks similar to an ophthalmoscope. Mineral oil is placed on the surface of the lesion, causing the stratum corneum to become almost invisible and facilitating the examination of the epidermis, particularly the dermal-epidermal junction. ELM images can be digitized by primary care physicians and sent to ELM experts via telephone for quick analysis.[13] Digitized ELM images can also be fed into computers run by specially designed software. These programs

<table>
<tr><td>

Box 40-1   **Performing a Skin Self-Examination**

- A simple skin self-examination performed regularly can aid in the early detection of cancer. The best time to do this self-examination is after a shower or bath. Check the skin in a well-lighted room using a full-length mirror and a handheld mirror. It is best to begin by noting the location of birthmarks, moles, and blemishes and what they usually look like. Check for anything new—a change in the size, texture, or color of a mole, or a sore that does not heal.
- Check **all** areas, including the back, the scalp, between the buttocks, and the genital area.
- Look at the front and back of your body in the mirror, then raise your arms and look at the left and right sides.
- Bend your elbows and look carefully at your palms; forearms, including the undersides; and the upper arms.
- Examine the back and front of your legs. Also look between your buttocks and around your genital area.
- Sit and closely examine your feet, including the soles and the spaces between the toes.
- Look at the face, neck, and scalp. Use a comb or a blow dryer to move hair to see better.

</td></tr>
</table>

Modified from the National Cancer Institute: *What you need to know about skin cancer,* (website): http://www.cancer.gov/cancerinfo/wyntk/skin#25. Accessed on April 15, 2003.

evaluate lesions based on factors such as shape, size, color, and border and attempt to make an objective analysis on a previously subjective science.[23]

A dermatologist should be able to identify a type of lesion just by its appearance. Based on this information, the dermatologist should also have a good idea concerning the metastatic potential of the lesion. Again, BCCs have an extremely small chance of metastasis, squamous cell carcinomas have a slightly higher chance, and malignant melanomas have the highest chance of all the major skin cancers.

If the physician suspects that a patient may have an advanced squamous cell carcinoma or melanoma, an evaluation for metastasis should be conducted. This evaluation should include the following:

- Physical examination of the patient to find evidence of lymphadenopathy, secondary lesions of the skin, or second primaries
- Evaluation of motor skills to detect possible brain involvement
- Chest x-ray examination to rule out lung metastasis
- Liver function tests to rule out liver involvement
- Evaluation of alkaline phosphatase levels and bone scan if patient complains of bone pain
- Complete blood counts (CBCs) to detect anemias that may be the result of gastrointestinal bleeding caused by metastasis
- Biopsy of regional lymph nodes to compare the number of lymph nodes positive for tumor with the total number of nodes in the biopsy

Computed tomography (CT) and magnetic resonance imaging (MRI) examinations, because of their cost, are often done only when signs and symptoms point to metastatic disease. Because melanoma can spread to virtually any part of the body, CT scans of the head, chest, abdomen, and pelvis may be ordered to rule out involvement of the brain, lung, liver, bowel, adrenals, and subcutaneous skin. MRI is often used as an adjuvant to CT.

Pathology and Staging

Melanoma. After it has been removed, the biopsy specimen is sent to a pathologist, who examines it microscopically and provides much useful information that is used to diagnose, stage, and develop a prognosis for the patient. Essential to a pathology report for melanoma are the diagnosis (whether the biopsy specimen indicates cancer), thickness of the tumor, and status of the margins (whether tumor cells are present on the edges of the biopsy specimen). If cancer is diagnosed, additional information may include the following:

- Specific cancer subtype
- Depth of tumor penetration
- Degree of mitotic activity (reproductive rate of cells)
- Growth pattern (radial versus lateral)
- Level of host response (number of lymphocytes present in and/or around the tumor)
- Presence, if any, of tumor ulceration, tumor regression, or satellitosis (lymphatic extensions of the tumor that result in small lesions adjacent to the primary)

Melanomas can be classified according to their growth patterns, and histologic appearances can be grouped into the following four major categories[17]:

1. *Superficial spreading melanomas (SSMs)*, also called radial spreading melanomas, are the most common melanoma subtype, accounting for approximately 70% of all lesions. They generally arise on any anatomic site as preexisting lesions that evolve over several years and have a radial (horizontal) growth pattern. The periphery of these deeply pigmented lesions is often notched or irregular and colors in the tumors can vary from brown, black, red, pink, or white. Partial regression of the tumor is common. As time passes, the tumor tends to grow more vertically, resulting in a more elevated, irregular surface.

2. *Nodular melanomas (NMs)* account for approximately 15% of all lesions and can also occur on any anatomic site. They are twice as common in men than in women. Lesions tend to be raised throughout and vary in color from dark brown, blue, or blue-black. Some lesions may not contain any pigment at all (amelanotic). These tumors are particularly lethal because they lack a radial growth phase, making an early diagnosis difficult. They tend to invade early and frequently show ulceration when advanced.

3. *Lentigo maligna melanomas (LMMs)*, also called Hutchinson's freckles, account for approximately 5% of all lesions and tend to occur in chronically sun-exposed skin of older white people, especially females. LMM begins with a relatively benign radial growth phase that may last for decades before it enters its vertical growth phase. The appearance of an LMM is similar to that of an SMM but lacks the red hues and has minimal elevation during its vertical growth phase.

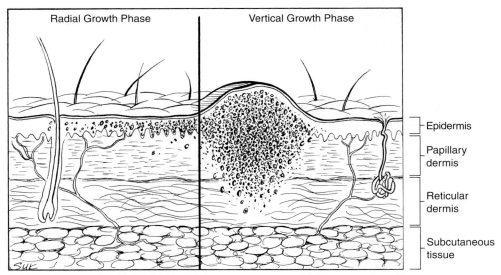

| Radial Growth Phase | Vertical Growth Phase |

Epidermis
Papillary dermis
Reticular dermis
Subcutaneous tissue

Figure 40-13. A cross section of a superficial spreading melanoma showing the radial growth phases indicative of most early melanomas (*left*), and the vertical phase indicative of most late melanomas (*right*).

4. *Acral lentiginous melanomas (ALMs)* account for approximately 10% of all lesions and are found mainly on the palms, soles, nail beds, or mucous membranes. The ALM is the most common form of melanoma in blacks and Asians and has a tan or brown flat stain on the palms or soles. An ALM can also appear as a brown to black discoloration under the nail bed and is often mistaken for a fungal infection.

Because melanocytes are found in the basal layer of the epidermis, melanoma formation takes place in this area. Most melanomas begin their development with a radial (horizontal) growth phase (Figure 40-13), during which abnormal melanocytes form nests along the basal layer. Later, some of the melanocytes begin to migrate into and form nests in the upper layers of the epidermis. The horizontal phase can last as long as 15 years in instances of SSM, 5 years in instances of LMM, or an extremely short (or nonexistent) period in instances of NM.

The second phase of development is the vertical growth phase. During this phase, melanocytes descend across the basal lamina and into the dermis. Also during this phase, nodules can become raised on the skin's surface. After invasion into the dermis has taken place, inflammatory cells arrive to defend the body from foreign invaders. If these cells are successful, a spontaneous regression takes place. If they are not successful, the melanoma grows deeper into the dermis and may involve the blood and lymphatic vessels, thus possibly helping the melanoma spread to regional lymph nodes and/or virtually any organ of the body.[28]

Dr. Wallace Clark and Dr. Alexander Breslow developed the main microstaging systems for melanomas. Both systems are basically indirect measures of tumor volume. Clark's system categorizes melanomas based on their level of invasion through the epidermis and layers of the dermis. Clark's levels (Figure 40-14) may indicate the potential for metastasis because the access of tumor cells to lymphatic and vascular structures are assessable. Also, the extent of invasion may indicate the tumor's progression from relatively harmless radial growth to more aggressive vertical growth.[37] Clark's levels are as follows:

- Level 1—confinement to the epidermis above the basement membrane
- Level 2—invasion through the basement membrane to the papillary dermis
- Level 3—presence of tumor cells at the papillary-reticular junction of the dermis
- Level 4—invasion into the reticular dermis
- Level 5—invasion into subcutaneous fat

Breslow's system categorizes melanomas based on tumor thickness from the top of the granular layer of the epidermis or, if the primary tumor is ulcerated, from the ulcer surface to the deepest identifiable melanoma cell as measured by an ocular micrometer.[16] Figure 40-15 demonstrates how melanoma thickness should be measured using Breslow microstaging. Breslow's microstaging levels are as follows:

- Level 1—melanoma in situ, limited to the epidermis
- Level 2—less than 0.75 mm
- Level 3—0.76 mm to 1.5 mm
- Level 4—1.51 mm to 4 mm
- Level 5—greater than 4 mm

Because Breslow's system has more to do with tumor bulk than penetration, the current thought is that this system is more reproducible and correlates more accurately with the risk of metastatic disease and prognosis than Clark's system. One problem that Clark's system does not address is the variation in skin thickness throughout the body. In contrasting the extremely thin skin of the eyelids with the extremely thick skin of the soles of the feet, a 0.75-mm lesion would be far more penetrating in the eyelid than on the sole of the foot, yet the size of the tumor is the same in both instances. Other problems that

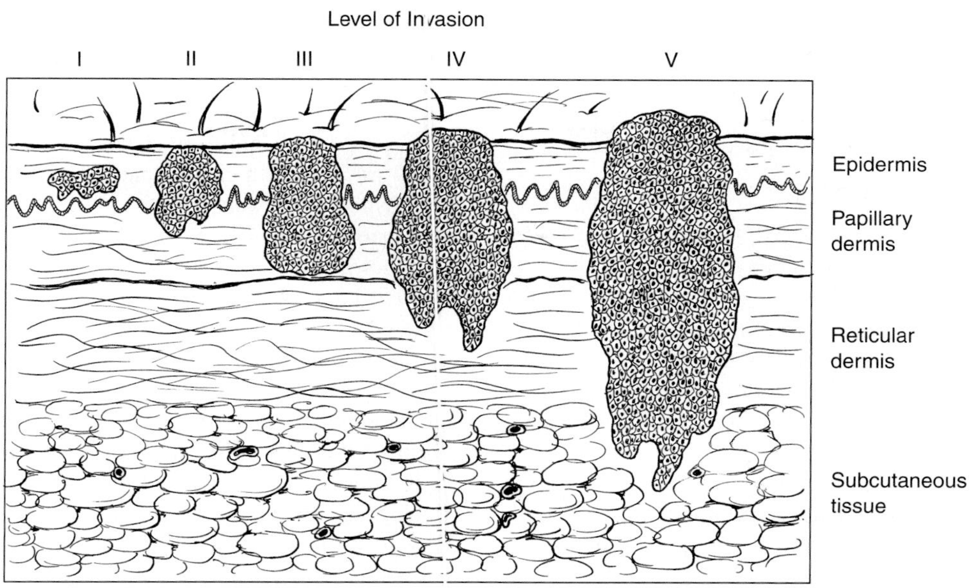

Level of Invasion

I II III IV V

Epidermis

Papillary dermis

Reticular dermis

Subcutaneous tissue

Figure 40-14. A schematic relating Clark's levels to the layer of the skin through which the tumor has penetrated.

pathologists may encounter with Clark's system occur when specimens are taken from areas of the body where the papillary-reticular junction of the dermis (an important demarcation point) is not well defined or when the integrity of the tissue layers in the surgical specimen is compromised.

The American Joint Committee on Cancer (AJCC) has recently revised its assessment system for malignant melanoma of the skin to reflect the following changes:

- Melanoma thickness and ulceration, but not level of invasion, are used in all T categories except T1.
- The number of metastatic lymph nodes, rather than their gross dimensions and the delineation of clinical occult (microscopic) versus clinically apparent (macroscopic) nodal metastases, are used in the N category.

- The site of distant metastases and the presence of elevated serum lactic dehydrogenase (LDH) are used in the M category.
- All patients with stage I, II, or III disease are upstaged when a primary melanoma is ulcerated.
- Satellite metastases around a primary melanoma and in- transit metastases have been merged into a single staging entity that is grouped into stage IIIc disease.
- A new convention for defining clinical and pathologic staging has been developed that takes into account the new staging information gained from intraoperative lymphatic mapping and sentinel node excision.[8]

With these changes, the TNM system has been modified to take into account these changes. Familiar to most radiation oncology professionals, this system for melanoma assesses primary tumor thickness, regional node status, and distant metastatic sites as follows:

Primary Tumor (T)

TX	Primary tumor cannot be assessed
T0	No evidence of primary tumor
Tis	Melanoma in situ
T1	Melanoma <1.0 mm in thickness with or without ulceration
T1a	Melanoma <1.0 mm in thickness and level II or III, no ulceration
T1b	Melanoma <1.0 mm in thickness and level IV or V or with ulceration
T2	Melanoma 1.01-2.0 mm in thickness with or without ulceration
T2a	Melanoma 1.01-2.0 mm in thickness, no ulceration
T2b	Melanoma 1.01-2.0 mm in thickness, with ulceration
T3	Melanoma 2.01-4.0 mm in thickness with or without ulceration
T3a	Melanoma 2.01-4.0 mm in thickness, no ulceration

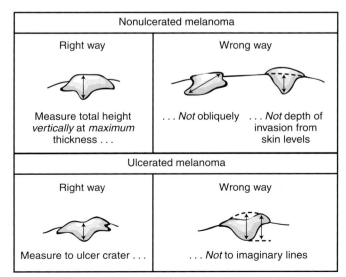

Figure 40-15. Measuring melanoma thickness correctly and incorrectly for Breslow microstaging.

T3b   Melanoma 2.01-4.0 mm in thickness, with ulceration
T4   Melanoma greater than 4.0 mm in thickness with or without ulceration
T4a   Melanoma >4.0 mm in thickness, no ulceration
T4b   Melanoma >4.0 mm in thickness, with ulceration

Regional Lymph Nodes (N)

NX   Regional lymph nodes cannot be assessed
N0   No regional lymph node metastasis
N1   Metastasis in one lymph node
N1a   Clinically occult (microscopic) metastasis
N1b   Clinically apparent (macroscopic) metastasis
N2   Metastasis in two or three regional nodes or intralymphatic regional metastasis without nodal metastasis
N2a   Clinically occult (microscopic) metastasis
N2b   Clinically apparent (macroscopic) metastasis
N2c   Satellite or in-transit metastasis without nodal metastasis
N3   Metastasis in four or more regional nodes, or matted metastatic nodes, or in-transit metastasis, or satellite(s) with metastasis in regional node(s)

Distant Metastasis (M)

MX   Distant metastasis cannot be assessed
M0   No distant metastasis
M1   Distant metastasis
M1a   Metastasis to skin, subcutaneous tissues or distant lymph nodes
M1b   Metastasis to lung
M1c   Metastasis to all other visceral sites or distant metastasis at any site associated with an elevated serum LDH

After a tumor has been classified according to the TNM system, it is typically organized into specific stages. Stage groupings allow health care workers to assemble patients with similar disease patterns to aid physicians in treatment planning, facilitate information exchange, indicate disease spread risk and prognosis, and help evaluate treatment results. In assessing metastatic spread potential, stage I tumors demonstrate a low risk, stages II through IIIA have an intermediate risk, stage IIIB has a high risk, and stages IIIC and IV are at a very high risk.[8] The presence of melanoma ulceration upstages the prognosis of stages I to III patients compared with patients with melanoma of the same thickness without ulceration or those with nodal metastases arising from a nonulcerating melanoma. The clinical groupings that relate TNM and stage are as follows:

Stage 0	Tis	N0	M0
Stage IA	T1a	N0	M0
Stage IB	T1b	N0	M0
	T2a	N0	M0
Stage IIA	T2a	N0	M0
	T3a	N0	M0
Stage IIB	T3b	N0	M0
	T4a	N0	M0
Stage IIC	T4b	N0	M0
Stage III	Any T	N1	M0
	Any T	N2	M0
	Any T	N3	M0
Stage IV	Any T	Any N	M1

Survival rates for patients with an ulcerated melanoma are proportionately lower than those with a nonulcerated melanoma of the same T category, but similar to those for patients with a nonulcerated melanoma of the next higher T category.[8]

The two most significant characteristics of the primary melanoma are tumor thickness and ulceration. Other significant prognostic factors were age, site of the primary melanoma, level of invasion and gender, as noted in the following list:

1. *Tumor thickness*—Thicker tumors yield a poorer prognosis.
2. *Ulceration*—Ulcerated tumors have a worse prognosis than nonulcerated.
3. *Age*—The prognosis for older patients is worse than that for younger patients.
4. *Location of primary tumor*—Tumors located on the extremities, excluding the feet, have a better prognosis than do tumors on the head and neck, which have a better prognosis than a tumor found on the trunk.[20]
5. *Depth of invasion*—The deeper the level of penetration, the poorer is the prognosis.
6. *Gender*—All things being equal, women have a 22% survival advantage over men when the disease is found before it has metastasized.[46]

Because the epidermis does not contain any blood vessels or lymphatics, skin cancers confined to that area have virtually no chance of spreading other than via direct extension. After a tumor invades the superficial lymphatic plexus of the dermis (which is devoid of valves characteristic of deeper lymphatic vessels), it can spread in any direction from the tumor. Because melanomas can occur on a multitude of different locations throughout the body, physicians must be aware of the lymphatic drainage patterns of the specific area where the melanoma is found. Obviously, a melanoma found on the shoulder will affect different regional nodes than a melanoma found on the leg. The following are areas of the body and the regional nodes that may be affected if a melanoma has developed there[8]:

- Ipsilateral preauricular, submandibular, cervical, and head and neck—supraclavicular nodes
- Thorax—ipsilateral axillary lymph nodes
- Arm—ipsilateral epitrochlear and axillary lymph nodes
- Abdomen, loins, and buttocks—ipsilateral inguinal lymph nodes
- Leg—ipsilateral popliteal and inguinal lymph nodes
- Anal margin and perianal skin—ipsilateral inguinal lymph nodes

Some melanomas do not fit into specific drainage categories but rather between drainage areas. In those cases, regions on both sides of the area containing the tumor must be considered potential drainage sites. Procedures have been developed to aid physicians in determining the actual lymphatic flow patterns from the primary melanoma site. A study called *lymphoscintigraphy* uses a radioactive isotope that is injected into the primary melanoma site. The isotope then filters through the lymphatic channels that drain the tumor, and the patient is scanned to determine which lymph node stations could potentially harbor malignant cells. Another procedure, called *intraoperative lymphatic mapping*, uses special dyes that are injected into the primary tumor. As these dyes are transported through the lymphatic channels, they stain the tissues that they contact.

During surgery, the physician can identify the draining lymphatics and follow them to the lymph node closest to the tumor, or the sentinel node.

Sentinal lymph node mapping has evolved from the knowledge that tumors drain in a logical pattern through the lymphatic system. A sentinel lymph node is defined as the first lymph node to receive lymphatic drainage from a tumor. During a sentinel lymph node mapping procedure, blue dye is injected into the tumor site, and this indicates the most likely route of lymphatic drainage from the tumor. This allows the surgeons to then go in and remove and biopsy only the first lymph nodes that would be affected from the tumor, saving the patient from a nodal basin dissection, which often causes lymphedema.

The most likely site of early metastases, the sentinel node is removed and analyzed to determine whether it contains malignant cells.[38]

Melanomas can spread to virtually any organ of the body and tend to spread in the following order: (1) direct extension of the primary, including invasion into the subcutaneous tissues; (2) regional lymphatics; (3) distant skin and subcutaneous tissues; (4) lung; and (5) liver, bone, and brain.

Nonmelanoma. After a biopsy sample is taken (incisional or excisional), the cell type of the carcinoma must be determined.

The four main subtypes of BCC are as follows[20]:

1. *Nodular-ulcerated* BCC is the most common type and is found mainly on the head and neck. Lesions are generally smooth, shiny, and translucent and accompanied by telangiectasis, an abnormal dilation of capillaries and arterioles that may be visible on the skin's surface. Ulceration is common and lesions may be pigmented. Pigmented lesions may sometimes be mistaken for melanoma.
2. *Superficial* BCC is found mainly on the trunk and appears as a red plaque, which may develop areas of translucent papules as it spreads over the skin's surface. These lesions may also develop areas of pigmentation.
3. *Morphea-form*, or *sclerosing*, BCC often appears as a scar-like lesion, often with indistinct margins. This type of lesion is uncommon, is found mainly on the head and neck, and has a rather high propensity for invasion and recurrence after treatment.
4. *Cystic* BCC is an uncommon cancer that "undergoes central degeneration to form a cystic lesion."[17]

Although BCCs do not tend to metastasize, they are capable of extensive local invasion and destruction. They commonly follow the path of least resistance, although they have been known to destroy bone and cartilage if left untreated.

However, rare cases of metastatic BCC have been reported. The rate of metastasis is less than 1 per 4000 cases, and the condition is often detected 10 or more years after treatment of the primary. Tumors most likely to metastasize are large, ulcerated, resistant tumors found on the head or neck of middle-aged men.[33] Regional lymph nodes are usually involved, but the involvement of liver, lung, and bone has been reported.

Squamous cell carcinomas can take on a variety of appearances. As mentioned earlier, they can be scaly, slightly ulcerated, or nodular. Occasionally, tumors contain characteristics of BCC and squamous cell cancer.

A verrucous variety of squamous cell carcinoma has been described as a low-grade, warty neoplasm with a greasy, foul discharge. These lesions are most commonly found on the sole of the foot.[24]

Squamous cell carcinomas have a higher propensity to metastasize than BCCs. This tendency is based on a variety of factors, including the following[40]:

1. *Differentiation*—Poorly differentiated lesions have a higher propensity to metastasize than well-differentiated lesions.
2. *Etiology*—Tumors developing in immunosuppressed patients or in areas of chronic inflammation, scar tissue, and radiation dermatitis have higher rates of metastasis compared with tumors that develop in sun-exposed areas.
3. *Size and invasion*—Tumors greater than 1 cm in size and more than 4 mm deep have a higher propensity for metastasis, even in sun-exposed areas.

Most studies report a 3% to 10% rate of metastasis from squamous cell skin cancer, but patients with high-risk factors can have up to a 30% chance of developing metastasis. Regional lymph nodes are affected 85% of the time in metastatic patients, with possible involvement of liver, bone, brain, and especially lung.[41]

Because nonmelanoma skin cancers can occur anywhere on the skin's surface, multiple lymphatic regions may be affected. Lymphatic drainage patterns for nonmelanomas are the same as those for melanomas. The following describes the TNM categories for nonmelanomas:

Primary Tumor (T)

TX	Primary tumor cannot be assessed
T0	No evidence of primary tumor
Tis	Melanoma in situ
T1	Tumor <2 cm in greatest dimension
T2	Tumor >2 cm but <5 cm, in greatest dimension
T3	Tumor >5 cm in greatest dimension
T4	Tumor invades deep extradermal structures (bone, cartilage, etc.)

Regional Lymph Nodes (N)

NX	Regional lymph nodes cannot be assessed
N0	No regional lymph node metastasis
N1	Regional lymph node metastasis

Distant Metastasis (M)

MX	Distant metastasis cannot be assessed
M0	No distant metastasis
M1	Distant metastasis

BCC and squamous cell cancer of the skin are not reportable diseases. In other words, physicians are not responsible for keeping accurate records concerning factors such as incidence and survival. Therefore, a strong database does not exist for calculating survival rates stage by stage. Although the overall survival rate is not known, early nonmelanoma lesions are almost 100% curable.[14]

Treatment Techniques

Melanoma. Surgical excision has been the mainstay in the treatment of primary melanoma and typically consists of en bloc removal of the intact tumor or biopsy site with a margin of normal-appearing skin and underlying subcutaneous tissue.[7,33] Chemotherapy, immunotherapy, and biochemotherapy are often used as a treatment for melanomas that have metastasized. The role of radiation therapy is limited primarily to the palliative treatment of metastatic disease sites. Melanoma has a reputation for being a radioresistant tumor, but radiation therapy has been a successful adjuvant to surgery and as the primary treatment modality in selected tumors and tumor sites.

Although surgery is currently the only form of curative therapy for malignant melanoma, controversy exists concerning surgical margins and the use of prophylactic lymph node removal to help prevent the occurrence of metastasis. Although early retrospective data suggested less sensitivity to radiation delivered at a conventional dose rate per fraction, it is now well documented that regardless of fractionation schedule, melanoma cells are radioresponsive if adequate total doses are delivered.[12]

Until the late 1970s, wide local excisions with 5-cm margins of normal skin surrounding the tumor were routine, sometimes creating large defects requiring skin grafts to close the wound. There are two reasons for use of these wide margins: a field effect surrounding tumors with a radial growth phase and the possibility for small groups of melanoma cells arising near the main tumor mass. Recent studies, however, indicate that wide margins are not always required. The thickness of the tumor, site of the tumor, and potential morbidity of the operation should determine the margin size around the primary. The decision to use wider margins should be based on the chance of local recurrence because no clear evidence exists to prove that creating larger margins increases the likelihood of survival.[33] In all excisions, surgical margins should include subcutaneous tissue down to the fascia and should show no involvement of the tumor.

Biopsies of questionable lesions often encompass a 0.5-cm margin around the tumor. If at the time of the pathologic examination the lesion is found to be a malignant melanoma beyond the in situ stage, the surgeon must go back and create the proper margins. In the case of sublingual lesions (found beneath the nail beds), all but the earliest lesions are treated by the amputation of the complete digit.

The key to melanoma treatment is the eradication of the tumor before it has a chance to metastasize. Although a tumor may be removed with clear margins, a few stray cells that can lead to recurrence or metastasis may be left behind. This is the area in which chemotherapy and immunotherapy play a role. These agents will hopefully cause the destruction of stray cells before they can reseed. (Specifics concerning chemotherapy and immunotherapy are discussed in the section concerning metastatic disease.)

Patients with proven lymph node metastasis should undergo a complete excision of regional lymph nodes, removing as much of the soft tissue and its associated lymphatics as possible between the tumor site and the regional lymph nodes. Even with such treatment the risk of distant metastasis is typically high.[25]

Patients who have melanomas on an extremity have been treated with isolated limb perfusion, which combines chemotherapy with hyperthermia. With this technique the extremity is isolated with a tourniquet while the blood in the limb circulates through a machine that pumps, oxygenates, and heats it. Because this blood is cut off from the rest of the body, large doses of chemotherapy can be introduced and circulated through the limb. Melphalan (L-PAM) is the agent of choice in most instances, although cisplatin (DDP) has been used successfully.[19] Because melanoma cells cannot survive above 105.8° F, the heating action provides an extra mode of cell killing to the process. After about 1 hour of treatment, the treated blood is completely drained and the tourniquet is removed, allowing the normal blood supply to return to the limb.[46]

For patients who have developed distant metastasis, no successful curative treatment options are available. The options available are for symptomatic relief and the prolongation of life.

Surgery can be used to remove local recurrences and localized metastatic areas such as nonregional lymph nodes, distant skin lesions, and subcutaneous metastases. Because surgery of this type is palliative, it is normally performed on patients whose quality of life would be enhanced with few side effects. Radiation therapy can also be used for palliation. It can be used to relieve symptoms caused by skin, soft tissue, bone, brain, and spinal cord metastases.

Chemotherapy has been successful in producing remissions in some patients, but its use in the treatment of malignant melanoma is largely palliative. Dacarbazine (DTIC) as a single agent is the drug of choice, although nitrosoureas and vinca alkaloids have also been used. Tumors of the skin, lymph nodes, and soft tissues respond better to drugs than do visceral metastases.[24] Unfortunately, the response rate is low and lasts an average of 4 to 6 months.[24] The problem with cytotoxic regimens is their lack of tumor specificity. They affect the surrounding tissue as much as they do the tumor, causing serious complications when administered in large doses. Through the study of the biochemical properties and behavior of melanomas, the addition of cytokines (immune system mediators) to a chemotherapeutic regimen improves the outcome of metastatic melanoma by increasing the time to progression of the disease.[15]

Studies have shown that some melanomas contain estrogen (hormones affecting the secondary sex characteristics as well as systematic effects such as the growth and maturity of long bones) receptors, allowing for responses to antiestrogen therapy. Antiestrogens block receptor sites for estrogen, denying the cell the effect that estrogen would have had on the cell. Research has shown that dacarbazine plus tamoxifen (TAM), an antiestrogen, is more effective than dacarbazine alone in terms of response rate and median survival. The effects of tamoxifen-aided treatment are more pronounced in women and in men and postmenopausal women with higher than normal body mass indexes (weight divided by height). Tamoxifen also has a synergistic effect with cisplatin.[35]

A bone marrow transplant using high-dose chemotherapy and autologous, or self-donated, marrow can also improve the response to chemotherapy treatment. Although improvements in short-term survival have been seen, long-term survival has not been affected.[34]

Immunotherapy also plays a role in metastatic melanoma treatments. Melanomas have a history of spontaneous regression in which the body is somehow able to fend off the disease using its own natural defenses. Basically, immunotherapy attempts to take advantage of this phenomenon and bolster the body's immune system so that it is able to fight off the melanoma on its own.

Immunotherapy can be divided into the following five major types[9]:

1. Active—stimulation of the body's natural defenses
   - Nonspecific—use of microbial or chemical adjuvants to activate macrophages, natural killer cells, and other nonspecific defenses; stimulation of the immune system in general
   - Specific—use of tumor cells or tumor-associated antigens sometimes mixed with haptens, viruses, or enzymes to activate T cells, macrophages, or other cells the body uses to fight specific tumor cells; stimulation of particular areas of the immune system
2. Adoptive—transfer of cells with antitumor properties into the tumor-bearing host to directly or indirectly cause tumor regression
3. Restorative—replacement of depleted immunologic subpopulations, such as T cells, or inhibition of the body's natural suppressor mechanisms (suppressor T cells or suppressor macrophages) to allow the body to replace the depleted subpopulations on its own
4. Passive—transfer of antibodies or other short-lived antitumor factors into the tumor-bearing host to control tumor growth
5. Cytomodularitive—enhancement of tumor-associated antigens and histocompatibility (HLA) antigens on the surface of tumor cells to make them more recognizable as foreign invaders by the body's immune system

Other agents used to promote a general immune response are interferons and interleukins. Interferons are special proteins that activate and enhance the tumor-killing ability of monocytes and produce chemicals toxic to cells. Interferons tend to be toxic to the patient and are not often used in single-agent therapy. Interleukins are substances that act as costimulators and intensifiers of immune responses.

Although the results of immunotherapy are not curative, the fact that the body is able to cause tumor regression at all gives researchers hope that someday immunology will play a bigger role in the fight against melanoma and other cancers.

Nonmelanoma. Patients with basal cell or squamous cell carcinomas of the skin have several treatment options. The technique selected depends on factors such as previous methods of treatment (if any), the location on the body, the risk of recurrence and metastasis, and the volume of tissue invasion. The number one goal of treatment is eradication of the tumor, followed by good cosmetic results. In instances in which cure rates are similar but the cosmetic results will differ, the modality offering better cosmetic results should be used. If control rates are similar and cosmetic results are similar or unimportant, the most cost-effective and/or quickest treatment method is preferred.[35]

Surgery can be performed to remove nonmelanoma skin cancers from areas where scarring is acceptable and patients want expedient results. Often, the original excisional biopsy contains all the tumor with acceptable margins, and no further treatment is needed. Otherwise, the surgeon may have to operate on the site a second time to ensure that safe margins around the tumor have been created. Although a uniform recommendation does not exist concerning the size of margins, many surgeons use 3- to 5-mm margins for small, well-defined lesions and at least 1-cm margins for larger or more aggressive tumors.[42]

For large, salvageable, eroding tumors, extensive surgery may be needed to remove not only the tumor but also additional tissue that may have been invaded, such as bone or muscle tissue. Such intervention may include the use of skin grafts and/or prosthetic devices.[17]

A more precise type of surgery, referred to as **Mohs' surgery** (developed by Dr. Fredric Mohs at the University of Wisconsin), is used in areas where normal tissue sparing is important; in areas of known or high risk of cancer recurrence; in areas where the extent of the cancer is unknown; or in instances of aggressive, rapidly growing tumors.[21]

Mohs', or microscopic, surgery is different from conventional surgery in that the tumor is completely mapped out through the examination of each piece of removed tissue to determine the presence and extent of any tumor. Through the removal of only tissue containing a tumor a major amount of tissue is preserved versus conventional surgery. Mohs' surgery is indicated for recurrent basal and squamous cell carcinomas, those in known high-risk sites for recurrence, and those with aggressive histologic subtypes.[20,21]

This surgery is performed on an outpatient basis with a local anesthetic. The tumor is removed one layer at a time and examined under a microscope. From the microscopic sample the surgeon knows where to obtain the next sample. This process repeats itself until the tumor is excised completely. The wound is then stitched or allowed to heal on its own. Of all therapeutic modalities, Mohs' surgery has the greatest success rate.[17]

One reason that Mohs' surgery has not replaced conventional surgery in the treatment of nonmelanoma skin cancers is that it is a time-consuming and expensive process. Cancers that are not viewed as problematic are treated almost as effectively and more inexpensively with conventional surgery.

Curettage and electrodesiccation are often used to treat BCC and early squamous cell carcinoma. With the patient under local anesthesia, the cancer is scooped out with a curette, an instrument in the form of a loop, ring, or scoop with sharpened edges. The destruction of any remaining tumor cells and stoppage of bleeding is carried out through a process called electrodesiccation, which uses a probe emitting a high-frequency electric current to destroy tissue and cauterize blood vessels. The advantage of this method, also known as electrosurgery, is that it often leaves a white scar, which is less noticeable on people with fair skin.[39]

Another method of treating early nonmelanoma skin lesions is cryosurgery, in which liquid nitrogen or carbon dioxide is applied to a lesion, lowering its temperature to around $-50°$ C and thereby freezing and killing the abnormal cells. This procedure may have to be repeated once or twice to completely eliminate the tumor. Again, a white scar is generally formed as a result. Cryosurgery is not recommended for lesions of the scalp or lower legs because of poor healing in those areas.[24]

Lasers (light amplification by stimulated emission of radiation) can also be used to treat early BCCs and in situ squamous cell carcinomas. Lasers use highly focused beams of light that are able to destroy areas of a tumor with pinpoint accuracy while preserving the surrounding normal tissue. Advantages of laser surgery include little blood loss or pain because the blood vessels and nerves are instantly sealed. In addition, laser surgery provides faster healing than conventional surgery.

Radiation therapy is used on BCC and squamous cell carcinoma located in places of cosmetic significance, such as the eyelids, lips, nose, face, and ears. It is also used on tumors in which surgical removal is difficult or in areas of recurrence. The major advantage of radiation therapy is normal tissue sparing. Disadvantages include its considerable cost, multiple treatments, and late skin changes in the treatment area. Doses and fractionation schedules should be carefully planned to avoid these late changes, which could include scarring, necrosis, and chronic radiation dermatitis.[24]

Finally, early nonmelanoma skin cancers can be treated with 5-FU in the form of a solution or cream. Applying 5-FU to the affected area daily for several weeks causes the area to become inflamed and irritated during treatment, but scarring does not usually result.[40]

A few investigational therapies are being researched that may someday be used to treat nonmelanoma skin cancers. In photodynamic therapy (PDT), a photosensitizing agent is injected into the body and absorbed by all cells. The agent is quickly discharged from normal cells but is retained longer by cancer cells. Light from a laser is directed on the tumor area, causing a reaction within the cells containing the photosensitizing agent that destroys the cell.[40]

As with melanomas, immunotherapy is also being researched for use against nonmelanoma cancers. Intralesional interferon alpha has been used, but because of side effects such as local pain, skin necrosis, and an influenza-type syndrome, it is not expected to be a major player in the treatment of skin cancer.[42]

Radiation Therapy

Nonmelanoma. Radiation therapy is effective in the treatment of nonmelanoma skin cancers, especially in the treatment of small tumors in which cosmetic results are important or in areas of extensive disease where the primary tumor and affected lymph nodes can be included in the radiation field. Because most skin lesions tend to be superficially located, electrons and kilovoltage x-rays are often used in their treatment. Megavoltage x-rays are rarely used in the treatment of skin cancers but may be used with or without electrons for special circumstances such as scalp lesions or tumors that are deeply infiltrating.[24]

Brachytherapy, including temporary implants or superficial molds using iridium-192 or cesium-137 sources and permanent implants using gold seeds, has produced good curative and cosmetic results. However, brachytherapy does not possess any significant advantages over external beam radiation therapy. There are disadvantages in the use of brachytherapy for skin cancer: cost, trauma, and length of stay required for the procedure;

radiation exposure to personnel; uncertain dose distribution; and risk associated with anesthesia.[18]

Radiation therapy is often used to treat lesions on the lips, nose, eyelids, face, and ears because they are highly visible and cosmetic results are important. The choice between treatment with kilovoltage x-rays and electrons comes down to the size of the treatment volume, depth of the lesion, underlying anatomic structures, physician preference, and equipment availability. Modern radiation therapy departments have linear accelerators capable of producing a wide range of electrons with energies from 3 to 4 MeV to more than 20 MeV; kilovoltage machines dedicated to therapy are becoming scarce.

Each modality has advantages and disadvantages that can be compared by using the following four main categories[18]:

1. **Field size**—For the treatment of next-to-critical structures such as the eye, kilovoltage x-rays allow the target volume to be covered with a smaller field size compared with that of a field producing similar effects near the skin surface through the use of electrons. Because of its physical properties, the electron field must be opened considerably to cover the same as the kilovoltage machines. One solution to help minimize this problem with electrons is to increase the field size and use tertiary collimation on the skin's surface.

2. **Depth of maximum dose (D_{max})**—A surface dose less than 90% to 95% is generally unacceptable in the treatment of skin cancer.[17] The characteristics of the beam to be used must be known for each specific setup to ensure that the skin surface is receiving the correct dose. This is relatively easy with low-energy x-rays because D_{max} is always at the surface regardless of field size or collimation technique. The D_{max} of electrons, in contrast, is a function of field size, location of secondary collimation, and surface contour. Because the D_{max} of electron beams is a function of energy and is usually found at a depth beneath the skin's surface, bolus material of appropriate thickness is often used to bring the dose toward the surface.

3. **Deep-tissue dose**—A characteristic of electrons is their rapid falloff; they penetrate the tissue to a certain point and dissipate, allowing for the sparing of some of the underlying tissues. Kilovoltage x-rays penetrate much deeper, however, and affect a greater volume of underlying tissue.

4. **Differential bone absorption**—Gram for gram, the absorbed dose is higher in bone and cartilage than in soft tissue with the use of kilovoltage x-rays. This can result in underlying bone and cartilage receiving higher doses than the dose at D_{max}. No significant difference exists between bone and soft tissue doses for electrons used in clinical practice.

5. **Cosmesis and control rates**—A study by Perez, Lovett, and Gerber[47] indicated excellent or good cosmesis in 95% of patients treated with kilovoltage x-rays, compared with 80% of patients treated with electrons. Also, cosmetic results were superior for patients in whom less than 50% of the dose was delivered with bolus.

Both electron and orthovoltage treatment use various cones to collimate the treatment field, although the shielding cutouts for each type of beam are manufactured by different processes.

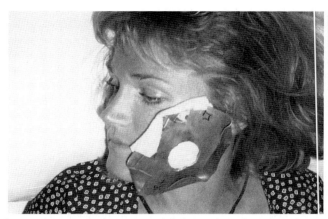

Figure 40-16. Blocking material for orthovoltage equipment often consists of a thin strip of lead shielding that rests directly on the patient's skin.

In electron therapy most departments manufacture custom cutouts by using low melting point alloys like Cerrobend. These cutouts outline the field and protect normal tissues as the radiation oncologist outlines. Custom cutouts may be substituted with a series of lead strips layered to produce the desired outline. These strips rest on the lower part of the cone and are commonly taped into position. Orthovoltage treatment requires a different type of blocking scheme. Instead of being attached to the machine, the blocking material typically rests on the patient's skin (Figure 40-16). Because lead is a soft metal, it can be formed into thin sheets that are somewhat pliable. These sheets can be contoured to the patient's anatomy, and holes can be cut into the sheets, creating the field through which the radiation passes. This type of blocking scheme can also be used as tertiary shielding in electron beam therapy. Regardless of the type of radiation used, the transmission factor for the blocking material should not exceed 5%.[30]

Radiation fields as a general rule should include a 2-cm margin completely surrounding the tumor to cover possible microscopic extension. A 1-cm margin may be adequate for small, superficial BCCs. Tumors and their full margins should receive a majority of the dose, with a boost field encompassing the clinical tumor to deliver the full dose to the tumor. In doing so the amount of normal tissue treated is reduced, and the cosmetic effect is improved. Although surgery accounts for the major means of management for most nonmelanomas, radiation therapy still plays a role with doses varying according to the size and penetration of the tumor and will differ from institution to institution.

Rapid fractionation schemes may be used in areas where late cosmetic results are not important or in instances in which transportation to and from the treatment site is difficult for the patient. Fraction size is the dominant factor in producing adverse reactions in late-responding normal tissue (the higher the daily dose, the greater the likelihood of adverse late effects).[54]

Depending on the area to be treated and type of radiation used, special considerations exist, including the following:
- Carcinomas of the skin overlying the *pinna of the ear or nasal cartilages* require special care in dose fractionation. Poorly designed treatment regimens can result in painful chondritis, which may require excision.[18]

- *Bolus* may be used with electron therapy to fill in gaps on uneven surfaces, maximize the surface dose, or reduce the underlying tissue dose.
- *Lip*—Cancers that cross the vermilion border of the lip have a higher risk of nodal metastasis, possibly indicating the need for prophylactic neck irradiation.[24] In the designing of a radiation field for the lip, a lead shield should be created to protect the teeth and gums. Paraffin wax on the outside of the shield helps prevent electron backscatter, reducing the dose to the buccal mucosa.
- *Nose*—Radiation treatments for skin cancers involving the nose should also include a wax-coated lead strip in the nostril to help protect the nasal septum. For more invasive lesions, tissue-equivalent material should be inserted into the nostril to remove the air gap and create a more uniform dose to the deeper tissues.
- *Eye*—For the treatment of carcinomas of the eyelid with radiation, the lens of the eye should be protected with an appropriately sized eye shield. Small-to-medium shields can be placed between the eyelid and eye, whereas larger shields can be used to cover the eyelid. A thin film of antibacterial ointment can be applied to the inside of the shield before insertion to aid in the prevention of infection and help protect against scratching of the lens. Concern about the increase in lid dose from backscatter is avoidable by coating the outer surface of the shield with a low-atomic-number material such as wax or dental acrylic.[30] The lens of the eye is one of the most radiosensitive structures. A single dose of 200 cGy may cause the development of cataracts (a loss of transparency in the lens of the eye).[49] Larger doses are required for cataractogenesis in fractionated regimens. The latent period between irradiation and the appearance of cataracts is also dose related. The latency is about 8 years after exposure to a dose in the range of 250 to 650 cGy.[27]
- *Ear*—In the treatment of skin cancers of the ear with radiation, treatment planning should be done so that doses to the inner ear do not exceed 1000 cGy.[18] Because of the unique and varied shape of the external ear and depending on the location and extent of the tumor, bolus material may be necessary to "flatten" the surface of the ear or get rid of the air gap behind the external ear in tumors involving the base of the auricle.

Malignant Melanoma. Traditionally, malignant melanoma has been considered a radioresistant tumor when treated with conventional dose fraction sizes; radiation therapy was reserved mainly for the treatment of metastases. Recently, however, the role of radiation therapy has expanded to that of an adjuvant and, in some instances, the primary treatment modality.

Researchers have discovered that treatment results improve with the use of larger fractions. Because of the initial shoulder of the cell survival curve of melanoma cells exposed to radiation, standard fraction sizes of 180 to 200 cGy are not effective. Larger doses per fraction are needed to overcome the apparent repair processes that melanoma cells seem to possess.[10]

Radiation therapy as the primary treatment modality is limited to large facial lentigo maligna melanomas for which wide surgical resection requires extensive reconstruction.

Most of these lesions are controllable with proper fractionation, but up to 24 months may be necessary for the lesion to regress completely.[10]

One of the problems physicians face in the treatment of melanoma patients with bad prognostic features (i.e., ulcerative lesions or positive nodes) is local recurrence or regional relapse after wide local excision with or without limited neck dissection. Physicians at the M. D. Anderson Cancer Center in Houston, Texas, continue to use radiation therapy as an adjuvant to surgery. Their aim is to reduce the morbidity associated with local-regional recurrences such as ulceration, disfigurement, and pressure symptoms and possibly improve the survival rate of a small subgroup of patients by helping to contain the disease before it has a chance to spread to distant sites. Patients were treated with five fractions of 600 cGy delivered twice per week via electron beams of appropriate energies when possible.[18]

The role of radiation therapy is greatest in the treatment of metastatic or recurrent disease. The role of megavoltage x-rays is also increased as deeper levels of tissue become involved or major organs become affected. Fractions of at least 500 cGy should be used to treat cutaneous, subcutaneous, lymph node, or visceral metastases in small treatment volumes or in areas in which late effects are irrelevant. When affected lymphatics or organs require large treatment volumes or if late effects may be detrimental, lower daily doses of 200 to 400 cGy may be used up to normal tissue tolerance or hyperfractionation may be used (115 cGy × 2 per day to a total dose of 3500 to 4000 cGy). The therapeutic outcome is based on the tumor size and dose per fraction.[20]

Side Effects. A major difference between megavoltage x-ray treatment of internal structures and kilovoltage x-ray or megavoltage-electron treatment of skin lesions is the location of the D_{max}. For the treatment of internal structures, having the D_{max} at least 0.5 cm beneath the skin surface is preferable for maintaining the skin-sparing effect (i.e., if the maximum dosage of radiation is absorbed beneath the skin, the epidermal layer receives a much smaller percentage of radiation and produces fewer side effects as a result). For the treatment of skin cancers, just the opposite should occur. Maximum doses should be applied at or near the skin surface where tumors are located, whereas underlying tissues are spared. As a result, skin reactions can be expected to be worse during the treatment of primary skin cancers than during the properly planned treatment of internal structures.

Radiation reactions can be divided into acute (early) or chronic (late) changes. The severity of the reaction depends on the volume, dose, and protraction of the treatment. High doses to large volumes in short amounts of time result in more severe reactions than low doses to small volumes over long periods.

Early reactions that can be expected during the course of radiation treatment for skin cancers include the following:

- **Erythema** (inflammatory redness of the skin) is usually the first sign of the effects of irradiation. This condition is caused by the swelling of the capillaries of the dermal layer, increasing the blood flow to the skin.[18]
- Pigmentation is caused by the increased production of melanin by the melanocytes, causing the skin to become darker. The melanocytes respond to x-rays and electrons the

same way that they do to UV rays and try to protect the young epithelial cells in the same fashion.
- Dry **desquamation**, or shedding of the epidermis, appears at intermediate doses of radiation. The radiation affects the sensitive basal cells, and, although not all are killed, enough are compromised that the basal layer has a hard time replacing the cells naturally sloughed off. The result is an abnormal thinning of the epithelial layer.[18]
- Moist desquamation* appears at the high-dose levels necessary to control skin cancer. As a result of these high doses, nearly all the cells of the basal layer are destroyed. After the cells of the epidermis have gone through their normal cycle, no cells from the germinal layer exist to replace them. The dermis then becomes exposed and begins producing a serous oozing from its surface. The epidermis is thought to be ultimately repopulated from more radioresistant cells surrounding hair follicles or sweat glands.[40]
- Temporary hair loss (alopecia) appears after moderate doses of radiation. Higher doses may result in permanent hair loss.
- Sebaceous (oil) and sudoriferous (sweat) glands may show decreased or absent function when subjected to curative doses for skin cancer.[40]
- Late reactions that can be expected after a curative course of radiation therapy include the following[22]:
  - The skin seldom returns to its previous state. Damage to the dermal layer results in fibrosis, giving the skin a firmer, rougher appearance. Capillaries are dilated and fewer, resulting in telangiectasia. Also, the epithelial layer is thin and more susceptible to injury. Damage to melanocytes results in hypopigmentation and increased sensitivity to the sun.
  - Necrosis is a common effect in patients who receive large doses in short amounts of time. The incidence of necrosis in carefully planned treatment regimens should not exceed 3%.

Prevention

Skin cancer is one of the few malignancies in which the causes are readily identifiable and preventable. About 90% of skin cancers can be avoided if people take proper precautions against the sun's rays.[2] If people take the time to educate themselves concerning skin cancer prevention and detection and follow through on that knowledge, the trend of rising skin cancer incidence could be reversed.

Exposure to UV light is the main triggering mechanism for skin cancer, so any type of preventive measures will stress ways to avoid UV exposure. Sun exposure also causes photoaging of the skin, including processes such as premature freckling, fine wrinkling, and dilation of the capillaries. Irregular pigmentation, commonly referred to as liver spots, often develops during later years in photodamaged skin.

---

*Moist desquamation is a skin reaction that can occur with exposure to radiation that is characterized by breakdown of the epidermis and presence of a white or yellow color. Raw skin may be apparent, and bleeding may occur.

The ozone layer is the portion of the atmosphere that protects the earth from harmful UV rays. In recent years this natural defense mechanism has been under attack by manmade substances such as chlorofluorocarbons, automobile exhaust, and other agents. The National Aeronautics and Space Administration (NASA) estimates a 2% increase in UV radiation for every 1% loss of the ozone layer.[51] Efforts are under way by many governments throughout the world to limit the release of these destructive agents into the atmosphere. Through the preservation of the ozone layer the amount of UV light that reaches the earth's surface can be limited.

With or without a healthy ozone layer, plenty of UV light reaches the planet's surface and is a potential cause of skin cancer. Not all sun exposure is bad, however. The human body needs sunlight to aid in the production of vitamin D, which is essential for calcium absorption in the intestines and may help protect against certain types of cancer. Not much sun exposure is needed; only about 5 minutes a day is required to produce sufficient amounts of vitamin D. Also, a little time in the sun after an extended period of cloudy days can often give a person a psychological boost.[43]

The following are some potential UV light sources about which people should be aware[45]:

- *Strong sun*—Avoid exposure to the sun between 10 AM and 2 PM because the rays are directly overhead and considered strongest during this time. In the continental United States, the UV intensity is reduced by half at 3 hours before and 3 hours after peak exposure time. The peak exposure time is 12:00 noon during standard time and 1:00 PM during daylight saving time. One way to judge the amount of UV exposure is by looking at a person's shadow. The longer the shadow, the lower is the intensity of the UV rays. The shorter the shadow, the greater is the intensity.
- *Reflected light*—Snow, sand, water, and cement are capable of reflecting UV light. Added to the direct rays of the sun, the reflective rays can increase overall exposure rates. Even people who wear hats or sit under umbrellas must be aware of the exposure risks of reflected light.
- *Cloudy skies*—UV rays can penetrate through clouds. Depending on cloud conditions, between 20% and 80% of UV rays still reach the ground. Proper precautions are needed even on cloudy days.
- *Fluorescent lights*—Fluorescent lights emit small amounts of UVA radiation, potentially boosting a desk worker's annual exposure by approximately 6%.
- *Tanning lamps*—Although most tanning salons and tanning equipment manufacturers would like the public to believe that tanning beds are safe, most emit UVA rays capable of skin injury, including skin cancer, premature skin aging, blood vessel damage, and immune system effects. A tan is the body's natural response to damage caused by UV light, whether that light is made by humans or nature.

If avoiding sources of UV light is impossible, certain protective measures must be undertaken. Slacks, long-sleeved shirts, hats, and visors offer excellent protection from UV light. Care must be taken to protect areas of the skin not directly covered by the various articles. These areas include the ears, tops of the feet, and backs of the knees.

Sunscreens are effective in protecting against UV exposure. The blocking ability of sunscreens is indicated by its sun-protection factor (SPF), which tells how long a person can stay in the sun with protection versus without protection before a sunburn develops. For example, a sunscreen with an SPF of 15 enables a person wearing it to stay in the sun 15 times longer than if the person was wearing no sunscreen.

Sunscreens contain different ingredients to protect against UVA and UVB rays. Agents that can block both types of rays are referred to as broad-spectrum sunscreens. The use of sunscreens and their role in the prevention of skin cancers is controversial. Some think that although the protective capacity of sunscreens against UVB is good, the protective capacity against UVA is lacking.

Some people think that the use of sunscreens may be counterproductive. They theorize that people using sunscreens are able to stay out in the sun for longer periods than without sunscreen because the UVB rays are being effectively blocked. With a minimum number of UVB rays available to cause the skin to feel burned, people are able to stay in the sun for longer periods. Because sunscreens are not as effective in blocking UVA, people are being exposed to higher levels of UVA than before sunscreens were developed. Increased UVA exposure can promote previous UVB damage or cause other types of damage on its own.

The American Academy of Dermatology, the Australian College of Dermatology, and the Canadian Dermatology Association strongly disagree with these views, stating, "One of the most powerful weapons in our fight against (skin cancers) is sun avoidance through the combination of protective clothing and sunscreens."[47] In fact, the Australians have initiated the "Slip, Slap, Slop" program, encouraging individuals to slip on protective clothing, slap on a hat, and slop on some sunscreen. Babies are very susceptible to sunburn and should be kept out of the direct sun. Therefore, they require extra sun protection.[49]

A sunscreen with an SPF of at least 15 is the best choice. Sunscreen should be applied at least 15 minutes before going outside to allow the skin to absorb it. Also, sunscreen should be reapplied every 2 hours and after swimming or heavy physical activity. Because the lips do not contain melanin and are a prime site for skin cancer, they should be protected with a lip balm or block having an SPF of 15.

Certain types of medications, such as antibiotics and diuretics, can increase a person's sensitivity to the sun. Before taking any medications, people should always consult drug labels, the physician, or the pharmacist regarding possible side effects, including those caused by UV exposure.

In 1994, the National Weather Service (NWS), the U.S. Environmental Protection Agency (EPA), and the Centers for Disease Control and Prevention (CDC) introduced the UV index to inform the public about the type of UV conditions to expect so that proper precautions can be taken. The index is a next-day forecast of the likely exposure to UV radiation for a specific location during the peak hour of sunlight around noon. The UV index ranges from 0 to 15; the higher the number, the more intense is the sun intensity. Although there is no direct link between SPF and UV index, the UV index can inform us what level of protection we should consider.[50] The index uses a

Table 40-2	The Four Skin Phototypes	
Skin Phototypes	**Skin Color in Unexposed Area**	**Tanning History**
Never tans, always burns	Pale or milky white; alabaster	Develops red sunburn; painful swelling occurs; skin peels
Sometimes tans, usually burns	Very light brown; sometimes freckles	Usually burns; pink or red coloring appears; can gradually develop light brown tan
Usually tans, sometimes burns	Light tan; brown, or olive; distinctively pigmented	Infrequently burns; shows moderately rapid tanning response
Always tans, rarely burns	Brown, dark brown, or black	Rarely burns; shows very rapid tanning response

set of four skin-type categories into which the public is divided based on the normal color of the person's skin and its propensity for sunburn. These are shown in Table 40-2.

In addition to analyzing primary protection against UV rays, the National Cancer Institute is researching chemoprevention of nonmelanoma skin cancer. Chemoprevention is the use of natural and manmade substances to prevent cancer. High doses of vitamin A, beta carotene, and isotretinoin (a synthetic form of vitamin A) may help individuals who lack natural defenses (persons with albinism and xeroderma pigmentosum) to fight skin cancer.

Helping people to realize the dangers of overexposure to the sun and the importance of early detection remains a major hurdle in skin cancer prevention. Young people especially feel invulnerable to the damaging and aging effects of the sun. To many, the short-term gratification a tan provides outweighs the seemingly small risks of the sun exposure that provides it. They think that skin cancer is for old people. In a way they are correct, because skin cancer usually shows up as people grow older. However, they do not realize that the cause of skin cancer is overexposure to the sun during a person's younger years.

Currently, mass media campaigns, educational posters, and brochures are aimed at educating the public concerning the dangers of sun exposure and the importance of early screening and detection. Health care institutions are trying to help by providing skin cancer screenings as a part of public health care fairs. Again, rising skin cancer rates can be reversed if people become educated on the prevention and detection of skin cancers and follow through on the recommendations.

Role of Radiation Therapist

The radiation therapist plays a prominent role in the management of skin cancer patients being treated with ionizing radiation. Patient education, technical expertise, assessment, and therapeutic communication are as important for the therapist to pay attention to as in treating any other cancer patient. The therapist typically blends their technical and psychosocial skills to achieve the best possible patient outcome.

The radiation therapist reiterates the physician instructions for the patient undergoing treatment, particularly the management of sensitive and injured skin during treatment. As they note changes in the integrity of skin being treated, that information can be relayed to the appropriate member of the patient care team so that any issues or problems are addressed.

It is not uncommon for patients to need to be reminded about cleaning treatment areas and keeping any treatment lines placed on their skin. This being the case, the daily interactions that the therapist has with the patient serves as a unique opportunity to remind them about such things as line management and skin care and to assess how the patient is coping with treatment, mentally and physically.

Technical skills and treatment delivery competencies in skin cancer treatment are paramount in the radiation therapist's role. Seeing the patient each day and delivering potentially dangerous doses of radiation require great attention to detail and careful consideration of each step of treatment. This end provider of care is the link to successful delivery of a planned course of therapy; the best plan delivered incorrectly does not serve the patient well.

CASE I

Pigmented Lesion

A 79-year-old white man with a past medical history significant for four prior nonmelanomatous skin cancers presented with a pigmented preauricular lesion and a lymph node at the angle of his left jaw. He was seen by his dermatologist, who performed a shave biopsy of the pigmented lesion and referred the patient for needle biopsy of the lymph node. The shave biopsy confirmed an invasive melanoma measuring 1.01 mm thick with Clark level IV invasion and positive resection margins. The lymph node biopsy revealed metastatic melanoma.

The patient was referred to a head and neck surgeon, radiation oncologist, and dental oncologist for further evaluation. A wide local excision of the primary tumor, superficial parotidectomy, and levels I through IV neck dissection were performed along with extraction of three teeth. The pathologic specimen revealed two of five involved intraparotid lymph nodes with associated extracapsular extension (growth outside the capsule of the lymph node into the surrounding adipose tissue). There were no involved lymph nodes in the cervical chain. The patient recovered well and was referred for radiation.

The patient was simulated in an open neck position (Figure 40-17) with a customized VacLoc immobilization device for his upper torso and a customized aquaplast immobilization device for his head and neck. The aquaplast mask was rolled up above the treatment field. A pillow between the patient's legs increases comfort during the simulation and radiation treatments.

The physician marked the borders of the treatment field, the borders of the temporal lobe (demarcated by a line drawn between the lateral canthus

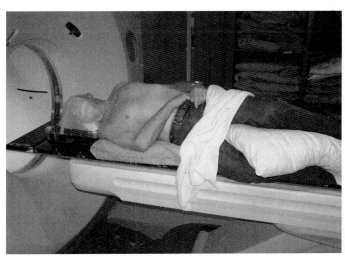

Figure 40-17. The patient is in an open neck position, which stretches the neck to the slide, eliminating skin folds and flattening out the area to be treated. This facilitates more even dose distribution.

of the eye and the mastoid process), and the larynx (by palpation) (Figure 40- 18). The ear is taped down, Domborro solution is instilled into the external ear canal, and TX-151 is placed within the folds of the ear. Tissue equivalent bolus measuring 1 cm thick is then placed over the temporal lobe and larynx to limit the radiation dose to these structures. The bolus must be beveled to avoid dose buildup below and just outside the tissue covered by the bolus.

A radiation dose of 30 Gy is delivered in five equal fractions of 6 Gy over a period of 2½ weeks. The radiation is delivered on Monday-Thursday-Monday-Thursday-Monday or on Tuesday-Friday-Tuesday-Friday-Tuesday. The radiation is delivered using a single appositional electron field with the dose specified to D_{max}

The evening after the first radiation treatment, the patient experienced parotiditis, but he had been warned by the therapist that this was a common side effect of radiation to the parotid gland and the patient took a non-narcotic analgesic with symptomatic relief. After the fourth radiation

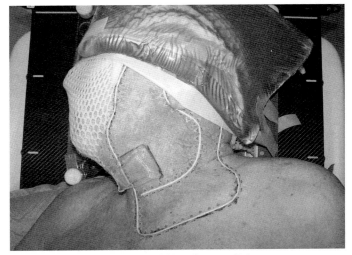

Figure 40-18. Treatment field borders outlining treatment area for patient with preauricular lesion.

treatment, the patient began to experience sore throat and moist desquamation behind his left ear, leading to some discomfort. Two weeks after the completion of the radiation, these symptoms had completely resolved.

SUMMARY

- Skin cancer represents the most commonly diagnosed malignancy, surpassing lung, breast, colorectal, and prostate cancer.
- More than 1 million Americans are diagnosed with skin cancer each year, yet many of these malignancies could have been prevented through the avoidance of prolonged exposure to the sun.
- Two types of skin cancer, basal cell and squamous cell skin cancer, are usually easily treated with surgery or cryotherapy and are unlikely to metastasize.
- Malignant melanoma is the most lethal of the skin cancers and must be taken very seriously.
- The only way to change this upward trend in the incidence of skin cancer is through education of the dangers of sun exposure and stressing the importance of skin cancer screening.

Review Questions

Multiple Choice

1. The main triggering mechanism for skin cancer is
   a. Exposure to ultraviolet light
   b. Therapeutic radiation exposure
   c. Chronic heat exposure
   d. Traumatic exposure
2. The layer of the epidermis that contains cells that is most sensitive to radiation is the:
   a. stratum basale
   b. stratum granulosum
   c. stratum lucidum
   d. stratum corneum
3. The disease that is occasionally treated by total skin irradiation with electrons is:
   a. Kaposi's sarcoma
   b. malignant melanoma
   c. mycosis fungoides
   d. glandular adenocarcinoma
4. The layers of the skin, starting with the most superficial to the deepest, are:
   - I. subcutaneous layer
   - II. epidermis
   - III. dermis
   - IV. basement layer

   a. I, III, IV, II
   b. II, IV, III, I
   c. II, III, I, IV
   d. IV, I, III, II
5. Melanocytes are found in the _____ layer of the skin stratum.
   a. basale
   b. granulosum
   c. spinosum
   d. corneum

6. The treatment of choice for most melanoma skin cancers is:
   a. surgery
   b. isolated limb perfusion
   c. chemotherapy
   d. radiation therapy

7. The technique in which the tumor is removed and examined one layer at a time is:
   a. curettage and electrodesiccation
   b. Mohs' surgery
   c. cryosurgery
   d. laser surgery

8. Tanning of the skin in the treated area after a course of radiation therapy is caused by:
   a. damage to the basal layer
   b. increased vascularity of the epidermis
   c. stimulation of the melanocytes
   d. inflammation of the dermis

9. With the use of shielding to protect the eye during irradiation, backscatter can be minimized by:
   a. using a shield composed of Cerrobend
   b. using a shield at least 1.7 mm in thickness
   c. using a larger diameter shield
   d. coating the outer surface of the shield with a low-atomic-number material such as wax

10. The use of kilovoltage x-rays allows the target volume to be covered with a smaller field size compared with a field that would produce similar effects near the skin through the use of electrons.
    a. true
    b. false

The answers to the Review Questions can be found by logging on to our website at: *http://evolve.elsevier.com/Washington+Leaver/principles*

Questions to Ponder

1. Describe the latest trends in the rates of incidence and rates of death in nonmelanoma and melanoma skin cancers.
2. Analyze circumstances that would render individuals more susceptible to developing skin cancer.
3. Contrast the microstaging systems for melanoma developed by Drs. Wallace Clark and Alexander Breslow.
4. Describe and outline the prognostic factors for malignant melanomas.
5. Compare the advantages and disadvantages of electron beam therapy versus kilovoltage x-rays in the treatment of nonmelanoma skin cancer.

REFERENCES

1. American Cancer Society: *Cancer facts and figures: 2008*, Atlanta, 2008, American Cancer Society.
2. American Cancer Society: *Cancer prevention and early detection facts and figures 2008*, Atlanta, 2008, American Cancer Society.
3. American Cancer Society: *Cancer response system: malignant melanoma*, No. 448257, Atlanta, American Cancer Society.
4. American Cancer Society: *Cancer response system: skin cancer*, No. 473157, Atlanta, American Cancer Society.
5. American Cancer Society: Overview skin cancer—basal and squamous cell (website): www.cancer.org/docroot/CRI/content/CRI_2_2_2X_What_causes_nonmelanoma_skin_cancer_51.asp?sitearea=. Accessed August 19, 2007.
6. American Cancer Society: *Prevention and early detection of malignant melanoma*, No. 3029-PE, Atlanta, 1990, American Cancer Society.
7. American Cancer Society: *Surgery* (website): www.cancer.org/docroot/ETO_1_2X_surgery.asp. Accessed August 19, 2007.
8. American Joint Committee on Cancer: *Manual for staging of cancer*, ed 6, Philadelphia, 2002, JB Lippincott.
9. American Cancer Society: *Immunotherapy* (website): www.cancer.org/docroot/ETU/eto_1_3_immunotherapy.asp. Accessed August 19, 2007.
10. Ang KK, et al: Postoperative radiotherapy for cutaneous melanoma of the head and neck region, *Int J Radiat Oncol Biol Phys* 30:795-798, 1994.
11. Atlas of genetics and cytogenetics in oncology and hemotology: dysplastic nevus syndrome (website): www.atlasgeneticsoncology.org/kprones/Dysp/NevusID10013.html. Accessed August 18, 2007.
12. Ballo MT, et al: Adjuvant irradiation for axillary metastatic metastases from malignant melanoma, *Int J Radiat Oncol Biol Phys* 52:964-972, 2002.
13. Barzegari M, et al: Computer-aided dermoscopy for diagnosis of melanoma, *BMC Dermotology* 5(8), 2005.
14. Bath-Hextal F, et al: *Interventions for basal cell carcinoma of the skin: systemic review*, *BMJ* 329(7468), 2004.
15. Boggs W: *Biochemotherapy extends survival in metastatic melanoma* (website): http://www.oncolink.com/custom_tags/print_article.cfm?Page=2&id=8354&Section=Reuters_Articles. Accessed August 20, 2007.
16. Breslow A: Cross-sectional areas and depth of invasion in the prognosis of cutaneous melanoma, *Ann Surg* 172:902, 1970.
17. Casciato DA, Lowitz BB: *Manual of clinical oncology*, ed 5, Philadelphia, 2004, Lippincott Williams & Wilkins.
18. Cox JD, Ang KK: *Radiation oncology rationale, techniques, results,* ed 8, St. Louis, 2002, Mosby.
19. Curnis F, Sacchi A, Corti A: Improving chemotherapeutic drug penetration in tumors by vascular targeting and barrier alteration, *J Clin Invest* 110:475-482, 2002.
20. De Vita VT, et al., editors: *Cancer: principles and practice of oncology*, ed 7, Philadelphia, 2004, Lippincott Williams & Wilkins.
21. Eide MJ, et al: Relationship of treatment delay with surgical defect size from keratinocyte carcinoma, *NIHPA Author Manuscripts* 124:308-314, 2005.
22. Escarlata L, et al: Early and late skin reactions to radiotherapy for breast cancer and their correlation with radiation induced DNA damage in lymphocytes, *Breast Cancer Res* 7, 2005.
23. Friedman RJ, et al: Malignant melanoma in the 1990's: the continued importance of early detection and the role of physician examination and self-examination of the skin, *CA Cancer J Clin* 41:201, 1991.
24. Fink DJ, Holleb AI, Murphy GP: *American Cancer Society textbook of clinical oncology*, Atlanta, GA, 1991, American Cancer Society.
25. Gietema HA, et al: Sentinal lymph node investigation in melanoma: detailed analysis of the yield from step sectioning and immunohisto-chemestry, *J Clin Pathol* 57:618-620, 2004.
26. Goessling W, Phillip MH, Mayer RJ: Merkel cell carcinoma, *J Clin Oncol* 20:588-598, 2002.
27. Hall EJ, Giaccia AJ: *Radiobiology for the radiologist*, ed 6, Philadelphia, 2005, JB Lippincott.
28. Harrell MI, Iritani BM, Ruddell A: Tumor-induced sentinel lymph node lymphagiogenesis and increased lymph flow precede melanoma metastasis, *Am J Pathol* 170(2), 2007.
29. Hussein MR, Wood GS: Molecular aspects of melanocytic dysplastic nevi, *J Mol Diagn* 4:71-80, 2002.
30. Kahn F: *The physics of radiation therapy*, Philadelphia, 2003, Lippincott Williams & Wilkins.
31. Kim EJ, et al: Immunopathogenesis and therapy of cutaneous T cell lymphoma, *J Clin Invest* 115:798-812, 2005.
32. Levine H: The killer tan, *Prevention Magazine* (website): http://www.msnbc.msn.com/id/4741472/. Accessed August 27, 2007.
33. Mackie RM: Observational study of type of surgical training and outcome of definitive surgery for primary malignant melanoma, *BMJ* 325: 1276- 1277, 2002.
34. Malignant melanoma: Report of a meeting of physicians and scientists, University College London Medical School, *Lancet* 340:948-951, 1992.

35. Mathews AB: Development of the facial skin index: a health related outcomes index for skin cancer patients, *NIHPA Author Manuscripts* 32:924-934, 2006.

36. McGee W: Vitamin D, MEDLINE PLUS (website): http://www.nlm.nih.gov/medlineplus/ency/article/002405.htm. Accessed August 27, 2007.

37. Morton DL, et al: Multivariate analysis of the relationship between survival and the microstage of primary melanoma by Clark level and Breslow thickness, *Cancer* 71:3737, 1993.

38. Murray CA, et al: Histopathologic patterns of melanoma metastases in sentinel lymph nodes, *J Clin Pathol* 57:64-67, 2004.

39. National Cancer Institute: *Research report: skin cancers: basal cell and squamous cell carcinomas*, National Institutes of Health publication No. 91-2977, Bethesda, MD, 1990, National Cancer Institute.

40. Preston DS, Stern RS: Nonmelanoma cancers of the skin, *N Engl J Med* 327:1649, 1992.

41. Perez CA, et al: *Principles and Practice of Radiation Oncology,* ed 4, Philadelphia, 2003, Lippencott Williams & Wilkins.

42. Reid K, Vikhanski L: The sun's ominous side: skin cancer, *Med World News* 33:18, 1992.

43. Rhee JS, et al: Creation of a quality of life instrument for nonmelanoma skin cancer patients, *NIH Public Access* 115:1178-1185, 2005.

44. Rhodes AR, et al: Risk factors for cutaneous melanoma: a practical method of recognizing predisposed individuals, *JAMA*, 258:3146, 1987.

45. Roach M, Hastings J, Finch S: Sun struck: here's the hole story about the ozone and your chances of getting skin cancer, *Health* May-June:40, 1992.

46. Scoggins CR, et al: Gender related differences in outcome for melanoma patients, *Ann Surg* 243:693-700, 2006.

47. Skolnick AA: Sunscreen protection controversy heats up, *JAMA* 265:3218, 1991.

48. Skin Cancer Foundation: Preventing and treating sunburn (website): www.skincancer.org/preventing-&-treating-sunburn/. Accessed August 19, 2007.

49. Stava C, et al: Health profiles of 996 melanoma survivors: the M. D. Anderson experience, *BMC Cancer* 6(95), 2006.

50. The ultraviolet index (website): http://www.cpc.ncep.noaa.gov/ products/stratosphere/uv_index/uv_what.html. Accessed August 25, 2007.

51. Thomas JM: Cure of cutaneous melanoma (website): www.bmj.com/cgi/content/full/332/7548/987. Accessed August 18, 2007.

52. Tortora CJ, Derrickson GH: *Principles of anatomy and physiology revised edition*, New York, 2005, Harper Collins.

53. Travis EL: *Primer of medical radiobiology*, ed 2, St. Louis, 1989, Year Book Medical Publishers.

54. Walter J, et al: *Walter and Millers textbook of radiotherapy,* ed 6, New York, 2002, Churchill Livingstone.

BIBLIOGRAPHY

Marx JL: Cancer vaccines show promise at last, *Science* 245:813, 1989.

Mitchell MS, et al: Effectiveness and tolerability of low-dose cyclophosphamide and low-dose intravenous interleukin-2 disseminated melanoma, *J Clin Oncol* 6:409, 1988.

Showers V: *World facts and figures*, ed 3, New York, 1989, John Wiley & Sons.

Sober AJ, Haluska FG: *American Cancer Society atlas of clinical oncology: skin cancer*, Hamilton, Ontario, 2001, BC Decker.

Wandycz W: Safe sun, *Forbes* 152:212, July 19, 1993.

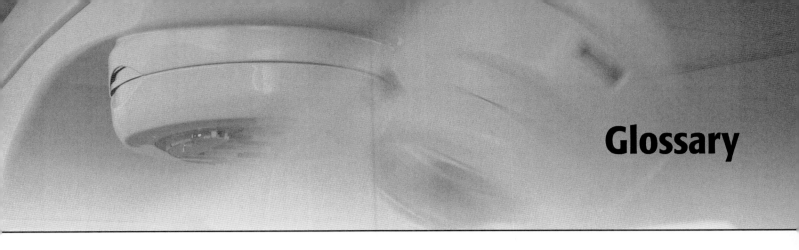

Glossary

abdominoperineal resection Anterior incision into the abdominal wall, with the construction of a colostomy followed by a perineal incision to remove the rectum and anus and draining lymphatics.

ablation Surgical excision or amputation of any part of the body.

absorbed dose Energy absorbed per unit mass of any material; units are the centigray or rad (older term).

abstracting Gathering data for measuring and evaluating patterns of care and outcomes among the general population. In oncology centers, this is done on an ongoing basis with a tumor registry system.

accelerated fractionation Technique in which the overall treatment time is shortened through the use of doses per fraction less than conventional doses two to three times per day.

accelerated hyperfractionation Technique in which there are more treatment days than accelerated fractionation. Total dose (cGy) of primary radiation is more than conventional fractionation, hyperfractionation, or accelerated fractionation.

accelerator structure Structure resembles a length of pipe and is the basic element of the linear accelerator. Accelerator structure allows electrons produced from a hot cathode to gain energy until they exit the far end of the pipe.

accreditation Process of voluntary external peer review in which a nongovernmental agency grants public recognition to an institution or specialized program of study that meets specific qualifications.

achalasia Loss of the normal peristaltic activity of the lower two thirds of the esophagus, resulting in dilation of the esophagus. This is a risk factor for the development of esophageal cancer.

actinic keratosis Warty lesion with areas of red, scaly patches occurring on the sun-exposed skin of the face or hands of older, light-skinned individuals.

active length In brachytherapy, the length of the area in which the radioactivity lies in the source.

activity Rate at which a radioactive isotope undergoes nuclear decay; units are the Curie (Ci) or Becquerel. (Bq = 1 disintegration per second). $1 \text{ Ci} = 3.7 \times 10^{10}$ Bq.

ADCZ Combination of the following drugs: doxorubicin, dacarbazine, cisplatin, and vincristine commonly used in chemotherapy.

ADDIE model Model is a step-by-step approach in which the Analysis, Design, Development, Implementation, and Evaluation can be used in creating an educational tool for patients or students.

adenocarcinoma Epithelial cells that are glandular. An example is the tissue lining the stomach. Tumor originating in the cells of this lining is called *adenocarcinoma of the stomach.*

adenohypophysis Anterior lobe of the pituitary.

adenomas Nonfunctioning pituitary tumors.

adjacent Refers to the length of the side of the right triangle that is close, or adjacent, to the specified angle.

adjuvant therapy Use of one form of treatment in addition to another.

advance directives Both the living will and the durable power of attorney for health care are considered advance directives, because they clearly describe the wishes of the patient when he or she was considered competent.

advisory agency Organization that collects and analyzes data and information and makes recommendations.

advocate Supporter who can act as a professor and friend. Advocate assists patients by ensuring that their needs are fulfilled and their rights enforced.

affective Content that may be verbal or nonverbal and comprises feelings, attitudes, and behaviors.

afferent lymphatic vessel Lymphatic vessels that flow into a lymph node. There are more afferent vessels than efferent vessels associated with each lymph node.

afterloading System that was developed to allow devices known as *applicators* to be inserted into the treatment area first, then loaded with radioactivity quickly and safely. In this way, dose to personnel is kept to a minimum.

agreement state State that enters into an agreement with the Nuclear Regulatory Commission to assume the responsibility of enforcing regulations for ionizing radiation.

akimbo Position in which the arms are bent by the side.

ALARA Abbreviation for As Low As Reasonably Achievable.

algebraic equation Mathematical formula that describes a physical phenomenon based on the interaction of several factors or variables

algorithms These are a finite set of instructions used by computers to compute a desired result.

allergic reaction Reaction resulting from an immunologic reaction to a drug to which the patient has already been sensitized.

alopecia Hair loss. Partial or complete lack of hair.

Alpha Cradle Trade name for an immobilization device created from a Styrofoam shell and foaming agents.

alpha particle Particulate radiation, positively charged, which consists of two protons and two neutrons; emitted during nuclear decay.

American Joint Committee on Cancer (AJCC) Classification and anatomic staging system.

American National Standards Institute (ANSI) Institute seeks to provide standardization of interfaces and data sources by outlining industry-specific requirements.

American Registry of Radiologic Technologists (ARRT) World's largest credentialing body tests and certifies radiologic technologists and the radiation therapist for practice in the United States.

American Society of Radiologic Technologists (ASRT) Mission of the ASRT is to foster the professional growth of radiologic technologists by expanding knowledge through education, research and analysis.

analytical model Also referred to as an *engineering model.* Identifies the caregiver as a scientist dealing only in facts and does not consider the human aspect of the patient.

anaphylactic shock Severe reaction (marked by respiratory arrest and vascular shock) to a sensitizing substance such as insect stings, contrast media, and other drugs.

anaplastic Pathologic description of cells, describing a loss of differentiation and more primitive appearance.

anatomic position Position in which the subject stands upright, arms straight down by the sides of the body with palms facing forward.

anemia Decrease in the peripheral red cell count.

anesthetic Agent that produces complete or partial loss of sensation with or without loss of consciousness.

aneuploid Condition in which the cells have an abnormal number of chromosomes.

Ann Arbor staging system Classification system used for non-Hodgkin's lymphomas and Hodgkin's disease.

anode Positive part of the x-ray tube that becomes a target for the source of electrons (the cathode).

anorexia Loss of appetite resulting in weight loss.

ANSI *See* American National Standards Institute (ANSI).

anterior Relates to anatomy nearer to the front of the body.

anterior resection Abdominal incision to remove an affected portion of the bowel with the margin plus the adjacent lymphatics.

antibody Protein substance manufactured by the immune system's plasma cells in a defensive response to the presence of a specific antigen.

antigen Substance or pathogen that is viewed as foreign by a person's immune system and induces the formation of antibodies.

anxiety Response to a perceived threat at an emotional level with an increased level of arousal associated with vague, unpleasant, and uneasy feelings.

application service providers (ASP) Provider who maintains computer servers. Web-based electronic medical records (EMR) use the Internet to gain controlled access to servers maintained by application service providers. Applications and data are stored off-site and maintained by the EMR provider.

applied dose *See* Given Dose (GD). *See also* Dose Maximum (D_{max}).

Aquaplast Trade name for a thermoplastic that is frequently used as an immobilization device.

articular cartilage Thin layer of hyaline cartilage covering the joint surface of the epiphyses.

artifact Unwanted image abnormalities, such as star and beam hardening artifacts that can be caused by patient motion, anatomy, design of the scanner or system failure.

asepsis Condition free from germs.

ASP *See* Application Service Providers (ASP).

aspect of care Those activities considered to be of the most importance in providing health care services.

assault Threat of touching in an injurious way.

assessment Information obtained through a continuous, systematic assessment allows the health care provider to (1) determine the nature of a problem, (2) select an intervention for that problem, and (3) evaluate the effectiveness of the intervention.

astrocytoma Central nervous system tumor originating from the nonneuronal supporting cells. It can be low grade or anaplastic.

asymmetric collimation Process using collimators in which the blade pairs are capable of independent movement.

asymptomatic Absence of symptoms. Patient who does not have or experience symptoms is asymptomatic.

atlas First cervical vertebral body with the specialized function of supporting the skull and allowing it to turn.

atom Smallest unit of an element that retains the properties of that element.

atomic mass unit (amu) Quantity that describes the very small masses of subatomic particles. Mass of an atom of carbon 12 is exactly 12.000 amu.

attenuation Removal of photons and electrons from a radiation beam by scatter or absorption as it travels through a medium, typically tissue or tissue equivalent materials.

attributable risk Risk that can be linked to a specific disease.

atypical hyperplasia Proliferation of unusual-appearing cells in a normal tissue arrangement.

auer rods Structures in the cytoplasm of myeloblasts, myelocytes, and monoblasts.

autoclave Device used for sterilization by steam under pressure.

autologous bone marrow transplant (ABMT) Technique of using a patient's own previously removed bone marrow to rescue the patient from the potentially fatal hematologic toxicity of extremely high-dose chemotherapy and radiation.

autonomy Quality or state of being self-governing; self-directing freedom, especially moral independence.

autoradiograph Signature exposure of a radioactive source obtained by placing the source on an unexposed x-ray film for a period of time.

axial Anatomical term used to describe the body in the transverse plane

axillary lymphatic pathway (principal pathway) Comes from trunks of the upper and lower half of the breast and moves toward the underarm.

B symptoms Group of symptoms (fevers, night sweats, weight loss) associated with lymphomas.

backscatter factor Ratio of the dose rate with a scattering medium (water or phantom) to the dose rate at the same point without a scattering medium (air).

backup timer setting Backup timer device refers to a safety device that will stop the treatment if the primary timer device fails.

barium sulfate Heavy metal salt; the most commonly used contrast agent for examinations of the gastrointestinal tract.

Barrett's esophagus Condition in which the distal esophagus is lined with a columnar epithelium rather than a stratified squamous epithelium. It usually occurs as a result of gastroesophageal reflux.

basal cell carcinoma Slow-growing, locally invasive, but rarely metastasizing neoplasm derived from basal cells of the epidermis or hair follicles.

base Special number (e = 2.718272…) discovered by Euler, a mathematician.

baseline study Initial study performed so that future studies can be compared with the original values.

battery Touching of a person without permission.

beam-flattening filter Located on the carousel with the scattering foil shapes the x-ray beam in its cross-sectional dimension.

beamlet Small photon intensity element, also referred to as a bixel, used to subdivide an IMRT beam for calculation purposes.

beam modifiers Devices that change the shape of the treatment field or distribution of the radiation at depth.

beam-restricting diaphragms Devices made of 2 mm to 3 mm of lead, the diaphragms (also called *x-ray shutters, blades,* or *collimators*) define both the size and the axis of the x-ray beam on a conventional simulator.

beam sculpting Producing a beam shape consistent with the three-dimensional volume of the tumor. Usually used with IMRT.

beam's eye views (BEVs) Visualization perspective that is "end-on" or positioned as if looking at a volume from the source or radiation. Made possible from collected CT data, this perspective is essential in three-dimensional planning.

becquerel (Bq) A Standard International (SI) unit of radioactivity that equals 1 disintegration per second.

bending magnet Used in high-energy linear accelerators to bend the electron stream within the head of the gantry, sometimes at right angles.

beneficence Doing or producing of good; acts of kindness and charity.

benign Tumors that are generally well differentiated and do not metastasize or invade surrounding normal tissue. Benign tumors are often encapsulated and slow growing.

benign prostatic hypertrophy (BPH) Enlargement of the prostate gland common in men older than 50 years. It generally causes a narrowing of the urethra.

beta particle Electrons (B−, negatively charged) or positrons (B+, positively charged) emitted during nuclear decay.

betatron Older megavoltage unit that can provide x-ray and electron therapy beams from less than 6 to more than 40 MeV.

bimodal Occurring with two peaks of incidence. With Hodgkin's disease, the disease occurs with greater frequency during the young adult years and then again in the fifth or sixth decade of life.

binding energy The amount of energy required to remove that electron from the atom. The electron binding energy has a negative value and is usually measured in kilo electron Volts (keV).

biometric technology Form of password security, such as fingerprint or retinal scanning.

biopsy Surgical removal of a small tissue sample from a solid tumor to determine the pathology for the diagnosis of disease.

bite block Object placed between the patient's teeth to assist in immobilization and to position the tongue. Positioning device made of cork, Aquaplast pellets, or dental wax that may also be used with a mask to position the chin and move the tongue out of the treatment area.

bitemporal hemianopsia Loss of peripheral vision.

blocked field size Squivalent rectangular field dimensions of the open treated area within the collimator field dimensions.

blood-brain barrier (BBB) Barrier system that hinders the penetration of some substances into the brain and cerebrospinal fluid. The BBB exists between the vascular system and brain.

body cavities Spaces within the body that contain internal organs.

body habitus Physique of the human body. Internal anatomy of a person varies with the physique. Four standard body habiti are hypersthenic, sthenic, hyposthenic, and asthenic.

Bohr atom Bohr atom model states that the electrons surrounding the nucleus exists only in certain energy states or orbits, and when an electron moves from one orbit to another it must gain or lose energy. This model has been replaced with complex quantum mechanical models of the atom, but it is still an excellent way to derive a mental picture of the atom's structure.

bolus Tissue equivalent material that is usually placed on the patient to increase the skin dose and/or even out irregular contours in the patient

boost fields Fields that are used to deliver a high dose to a small volume. With boost fields the radiation dose is generally delivered to the gross tumor volume only, excluding regional lymph nodes.

Bowen's disease Precancerous dermatosis or form of intraepidermal carcinoma characterized by the development of pink or brown papules covered with a thickened, horny layer.

brachytherapy Radiation treatment of disease accomplished by inserting radioactive sources directly into the tumor site.

Bragg peak Sharp increase in the dose distribution curve of a charged particle at a particular depth.

bremsstrahlung German term for "braking" radiation.

bronchogenic carcinoma Cancer of the lung that arises in the anatomy of the bronchial tree.

bronchoscope Long flexible tube used in the diagnosis and management of lung cancer, and is used to examine the bronchial tree, to obtain a specimen for biopsy, or in some cases to remove a foreign body.

build-up region Region between the skin surface and the depth of D_{max}. Build-up region is a characteristic of megavoltage irradiation. In this region, the dose increases with depth until it reaches a maximum at the depth of D_{max}.

bulbous urethra Dilated proximal portion of the anterior urethra.

cachexia State of general ill health and malnutrition with early satiety; electrolyte and water imbalances; and progressive loss of body weight, fat, and muscle.

caliper Graduated ruled instrument with one sliding leg and one that is stationary is used to figure out the thickness of the patient's tissue.

calvaria Part of the skull that protects the brain.

carcinoma in situ Malignant changes at the cellular level in epithelial tissues without extension beyond the basement membrane.

carfusion Dyelike liquid usually containing silver nitrate and phenol in a fuchsin base; magenta liquid that can be painted onto patients by using thin sticks or swabs.

carina Area in which the trachea divides into two branches.

carrier Person who carries a specific pathogen but is free of signs or symptoms of the disease and yet is capable of spreading the disease.

case manager Member of the health care team who is assigned to manage the continuum of care for the patient.

cassette Cassette provides the light-tight conditions necessary for x-ray film, photostimulable plates, and intensifying screens to work properly.

cathode One of the electrodes found in the x-ray tube that represents the negative side of the tube.

cell cycle Sequence of recurring biochemical and morphologic events observed in a population of reproducing cells.

cellular differentiation Degree to which a cell resembles its cell of origin in morphology and function.

centigray Unit of energy absorbed per unit mass of any material. 1 cGy = 1 rad.

central axis It is the central portion of the beam emanating from the target; the only part of the beam that is not divergent.

cerebellum Part of the brain that plays a role in the coordination of voluntary muscular movements located in the occipital region.

cerebrospinal fluid (CSF) Fluid that flows through and protects the brain and spinal canal.

cerebrum Largest part of the brain, consisting of two hemispheres.

Cerrobend A form of Lipowitz metal used for designing custom shielding blocks and consists of 50.0% bismuth, 26.7% lead, 13.3% tin, and 10.0% cadmium.

certification Process by which a government or nongovernment agency or association grants authority to an individual who has met predetermined qualifications to use a specific title.

cervical cancer Slowly progressive disease, with the earliest phase (noninvasive carcinoma in situ) occurring approximately 10 years earlier than invasive cancer.

cervix Part of the uterus that protrudes into the cavity of the vagina.

cesium Radioactive isotope with a half-life of 30 years that is commonly used as a low-dose brachytherapy source.

characteristic radiation Radiation that is created by the direct interaction of cathode electrons with inner-shell electrons of the target material.

chemotherapeutic agents Classified by their action on the cell or their source and include alkylating agents, antimetabolites, antibiotics,

hormonal agents, nitrosoureas, vinca alkaloids, and miscellaneous agents.

chemotherapy Use of chemical agents to induce specific effects on disease.

chief complaint Patient's reason for visiting with the clinician. Chief complaint is recorded by the clinician.

childhood cancer Incidence of malignancies in people less than 18 years old.

chin to suprasternal notch (SSN) measurement Measurement taken between the anatomic landmarks of the tip of chin and the suprasternal notch (SSN).

chromophobe Refers to histological structures of tissue that do not take up colored dye and, thus, appear more pale under the microscope.

chromosomes Gene-bearing protein structures in the nucleus of animal cells.

chronic ulcerative colitis Extensive inflammation and ulceration of the bowel wall resulting in bloody mucoid diarrhea several times a day, associated with an increased risk of colorectal cancer.

circulator One of four major components housed in the drive stand, which prevents backflow of microwave power.

civil law Law that governs relationships between individuals.

Clarkson integration or Clarkson technique Method used to calculate the dose in an irregularly shaped field.

clinical target volume (CTV) Visible (imaged) or palpable tumor plus any margin of subclinical disease that needs to be eliminated through the treatment planning and delivery process.

cobalt-60 Radioactive isotope with a half-life of 5.26 years that is used as a source for external-beam radiation therapy.

Code of Ethics Serves as a guide by which radiation therapist may evaluate their professional conduct as it relates to patients, health care consumers, employers, colleagues, and other members of the health-care team.

cognitive Pertaining to an individual's basic reasoning processes.

cold thyroid nodule Nodule having no uptake.

collegial model Cooperative method of pursuing health care for the provider and patient. It involves sharing, trust, and consideration of common goals.

collimation Edge definition of radiation beam size and dimensions.

collimator Arrangement of shielding material designed to define the "x" and "y" dimensions of the beam of radiation.

collimator assembly Collimator assembly in the conventional simulator provides support for essential equipment within the head of the gantry.

collimator field size Unblocked or open field size as defined by the collimator setting and projected at the reference distance, usually the isocenter of the machine.

colonization Presence of an agent that is infectious but does not initiate an immune response.

colostomy Surgical construction of an artificial excretory opening from the colon on the surface of the abdominal wall.

combination chemotherapy Selection of drugs that act on the cell during different phases of the cell cycle, increasing the cell killing potential. In addition, drugs with known toxicities are used for maximum effectiveness, resulting in fewer side effects.

common iliac nodes Nodes that lie at the bifurcation of the abdominal aorta at the level of L4. These nodes directly drain the urinary bladder, prostate, cervix, and vagina.

communication Ability to transfer concrete and abstract information from one person to another person or a group of people while keeping the same meaning. Communication can be verbal, nonverbal, or a combination of the two techniques.

compensator Beam modifier that changes radiation output relative to loss of attenuation over a changing patient contour.

compensatory vertebral curves Specific sections of the curvature of the vertebral column that form after birth because of the development of muscles as an infant grows. Cervical and lumbar curves are compensatory curves.

complex immobilization devices Individualized devices that restrict patient movement and ensure reproducibility in positioning.

Compton scattering Produced when an x-ray photon interacts with an outer-shell orbital electron with sufficient energy to eject it from orbit and alter its own path.

computer-based patient record (CPR) Electronic patient record stored digitally.

computerized physician online order entry (CPOE) Method of online management of medical orders, such as laboratory orders, radiology exams and medications for the computerized tracking and documentation process related to the electronic medical record.

concomitant Situation in which two types of treatment take place at the same time.

cone-beam CT It differs from fan beam CT in that the CT detector is an area detector. At certain degree intervals during the rotation of the gantry, single projection images are acquired. Net result is a three-dimensional reconstruction data set, which can project images in three orthogonal planes (axial, sagittal, and coronal).

confidentiality Principle that relates to the knowledge that information revealed by a patient to a health care provider, or information that is learned in the course of a health care provider performing her/his duties, is private and should be held in confidence.

conformal radiation therapy (CRT) Therapy that, with the use of three-dimensional treatment planning, allows the delivery of higher tumor doses to selected target volumes without increasing treatment morbidity.

consequentialism (the theory of utility) Evaluates an activity by weighing the good against the bad or the way a person can provide the greatest good for the greatest number.

Consumer Assurance of Radiologic Excellence (CARE) Bill The Consumer Assurance of Radiologic Excellence bill would require those who perform medical imaging and radiation therapy procedures to meet minimum federal education and credentialing standards.

contact therapy unit Machine that operates at potentials of 40 to 50 kV and uses an extremely short source-skin distance.

content specifications Document outlines the specific topics with corresponding number of questions that may appear on the ARRT certification examination.

contiguous Systematic and predictable, as in the spread of Hodgkin's disease.

continuous quality improvement (CQI) Same as for quality improvement; it is an ongoing improvement of health care services through the systematic evaluation of processes.

contour Reproduction of an external body shape, usually taken through the transverse plane of the treatment beam.

contour corrections Corrections for beam incidence onto surfaces other than flat surfaces and for angles of incidence other than 90 degrees ("normal" incidence). Also called *obliquity corrections*.

contractual model Model that maintains a business relationship between the provider and patient; a sharing of information and responsibility.

contralateral Opposite side of the body.

contrast Image contrast has been described as the tonal range of densities from black to white or the number of shades of gray in the image.

contrast media High-density substances used radiographically to visualize internal anatomy for imaging.

convalescence Period of recovery after an illness.

conventional fractionation Fractionation in which the total dose of radiation is typically divided into 180- or 200-cGy increments and delivered once a day, 5 days a week.

coping strategies Every patient brings a history of coping strategies to the cancer experience. Patients use whatever has worked for them in the past in managing their anxiety.

coplanar Geometrical principle describing two radiation fields configured in such a way that the beam edges lie in the same plane. (Central ray is not parallel opposed.)

coronal plane Perpendicular (at right angles) to the sagittal plane and vertically divides the body into anterior and posterior sections.

corpora cavernosa One of the basic structural components of the penis that is encased in a dense fascia (Buck's fascia), which is separated from the skin by a layer of loose connective tissue.

corpus spongiosum One of two basic structural components of the penis.

cortex Outer portion of a structure as in the adrenal gland. Inner portion of the adrenal gland is the medulla.

cosine One of three of the most common functions associated with the right triangle. Other two functions are the sine and tangent.

covenant model Model that deals with an understanding between the patient and health care provider and is based on traditional values and goals.

craniospinal irradiation (CSI) Complex irradiation of all central nervous system and cerebrospinal fluid regions from behind the eye down to the midsacrum for treatment of medulloblastoma and other cerebrospinal fluid seeding tumors.

critical structures Normal tissue whose radiation tolerance limits the deliverable dose.

critical thinking Cognitive process that allows mastery of theory and uses practical experiences. Critical thinking incorporates the use of cognitive, affective, and psychomotor domains.

cryotherapy Use of cold temperatures to treat a disease.

cryptorchidism Undescended testes.

CT imaging Cross-sectional information provided by CT scanning contributes considerable information to the radiation oncologist in four major areas: diagnosis, tumor and normal tissue localization, tissue density data for dose calculations, and follow-up treatment monitoring.

CT simulator Computed tomography scanner equipped with software that can provide information needed to design the patient's treatment parameters.

CT simulator/virtual simulation Type of simulation that operates along with a three-dimensional geometric planning computer.

cultural sensitivity Accepting and respecting patients for who they are is an important attribute of oncology caregivers.

cumulative effect Effect that develops if the body is unable to detoxify and excrete a drug quickly enough or if too large a dose is taken.

Curie (Ci) Historical unit of radioactivity that equals 3.7×10^{10} Bq.

curriculum Body of courses and formally established learning experiences presenting the knowledge, principles, values, and skills that are the intended consequences of a program's formal education.

customer Person who is not employed by the particular institution or hospital with whom employees come in contact.

cyclotron Charged particle accelerator used mainly for nuclear research and more recently for generating proton and neutron beams.

cystectomy Surgical removal of the bladder.

cytoplasm All the cellular protoplasm except the nucleus and its contents. It consists of a watery fluid (cytosol) in which numerous organelles are suspended.

cytotoxic Ability to kill cancer cells. Cytotoxic drugs are used to destroy cells of the primary tumor and those that may be circulating through the body.

CYVADIC Chemotherapy program that consists of the combination of the following drugs: cyclophosphamide (Cytoxan), vincristine, doxorubicin (Adriamycin), and dacarbazine. CYVADIC is one of the most used drug programs in chemotherapy.

daily treatment record Document recording the actual treatment delivery.

debulking surgery Surgical procedure used to reduce tumor size, reduce tumor burden, and increase the opportunity to obtain a pathologic diagnosis.

decay constant Total number of atoms that decay per unit time.

definitive Course of radiation therapy in which the objective is to cure by eradication of the disease.

de novo Latin term that means "anew."

densitometer Special device that measures the degree of blackening on the film.

density Degree of darkening on the image.

deontology One of three ethical theories. Deontology uses formal rules of right and wrong for reasoning and problem solving.

deoxyribonucleic acid (DNA) Large, double-stranded nucleic acid molecule that carries the genetic material of the cell on the chromosomes. This genetic information is composed of a sequence of nitrogen bases and molecular subunits.

depression Perceived loss of self-esteem resulting in a cluster of affective behavioral (e.g., change in appetite, sleep disturbances, lack of energy, withdrawal, and dependency) and cognitive (e.g., decreased ability to concentrate, indecisiveness, and suicidal ideas) responses.

depth Distance beneath the patient's skin to the point of calculation.

dermis Deeper layer of the skin composed of connective tissue that contains blood and lymphatic vessels, nerves and nerve endings, sweat glands, and hair follicles.

desquamation Acute effect of irradiation characterized by shedding of the epidermis.

detectors Solid state detectors in a CT scanner are designed to convert radiation to light.

diaphysis Shaft or long axis of the bone.

Digital Imaging and Communications in Medicine (DICOM) Standards produced by a joint committee of the National Electrical Manufacturers Association (NEMA) and the American College of Radiology (ACR) and affiliated with several international agencies. This committee was formed to provide communication standards for sharing image information regardless of manufacturer and has included radiation therapy treatment information. This facilitates the use of picture archival and communications systems (PACS) and allows diagnostic images to be widely distributed.

digitally reconstructed radiograph (DRR) Based on acquired CT information, these are images that render a beam's eye view display of the treatment field anatomy and areas of treatment interest. These images resemble conventional radiographs.

dimensional analysis Process that involves assessment of units of measure used in calculating some scientific quantity. This practice involves canceling of common units in an effort to leave the specified unit.

diplopia Double vision.

direct proportionality Relationship between measurable quantities and factors; as one increases, the other increases and vice versa.

divergence Divergence is the spreading out of the beam of radiation. Farther from the source, the more the beam has spread.

D_{max} See Dose Maximum (D_{max}).

D_0 Graphic representation of the cell's radiosensitivity.

doctrine of foreseeability Principle of law that holds a person liable for all consequences of any negligent acts to another individual to whom a duty is owed and should have been reasonably foreseen under the circumstances.

doctrine of personal liability Doctrine stating that all persons are liable for their own negligent conduct.

doctrine of *res ipsa loquitur* ("the thing speaks for itself") Doctrine, which is an accepted substitute for the medical expert, requiring the defendant to explain an incident and convince the court that no negligence was involved.

doctrine of respondent superior Legal doctrine that holds an employer liable for negligent acts of employees occurring while he or she is carrying out his or her orders or otherwise serving his or her interests.

domain Group of job activities related on the basis of required skills and knowledge.

dose calculation matrix Grid of points at which dose is computed and subsequently displayed.

dose distributions Spatial representations of the magnitude of the dose produced by a source of radiation. They describe the variation of dose with position within an irradiated volume.

dose equivalent Product of the absorbed dose and a quality factor (QF), which takes into account the biologic effects of different types of radiation on humans; units are the rem (1 rem = 1 rad × QF) or sievert (1 Sv = 1 Gy × QF). 1 Sv = 100 rem.

dose escalation Refers to the delivery of higher than traditional doses to a treatment volume.

dose maximum (D_{max}) The depth of maximum buildup, in which 100% of the dose is deposited beneath the skin. Depth at which electronic equilibrium occurs for photon beams. This is also the depth of maximum absorbed dose and ionization, for photons, from a single treatment field. Depth of maximum ionization and maximum absorbed dose are usually not the same depth for electrons. *See also* Given Dose (GD).

dose rate Also known as *output*, the dose rate of a treatment machine is the amount of radiation exposure produced by a treatment machine or source as specified at a reference field size and at a specified reference distance.

dose-volume histogram (DVH) Plot of target or normal structure volume as a function of dose.

dosimetrist Radiation therapy practitioner responsible for production of the patient's treatment plan and any associated quality assurance components.

D_q The quasi threshold dose. Measure of cell response at low doses. This parameter represents the dose at which survival becomes exponential. It is also a measure of the cell's ability to accumulate and repair sublethal damage.

drop metastases Secondary tumors that occur via the cerebrospinal fluid.

droplet nuclei Residual remains of airborne pathogens after the evaporation of moisture.

DRR See Digitally Reconstructed Radiograph (DRR).

drug Any substance that alters physiologic function, with the potential for affecting health.

drug interactions Mutual or reciprocal action or influence between drugs and/or food that can create positive or negative effects in the body.

durability power of attorney Legal document that allows an individual to designate anyone willing, eighteen years of age or older, to be their surrogate and make decisions in matters of health care.

dynamic wedge Use of a moving collimator jaw to produce a wedged isodose distribution.

dysphagia Difficulty in swallowing. Sensation of food sticking in the throat.

dysplopia Double vision.

dyspnea Difficult, labored, or uncomfortable breathing.

ecchymoses Escape of blood into the tissues, causing large, blotchy areas of discoloration.

edema Excessive accumulation of fluid in a tissue, producing swelling.

effective dose equivalent Dose equivalent weighted by the proportionate risk for various tissues. That is, it is the sum over specified tissues of the products of the dose equivalent in a tissue and the weighting factor for that tissue.

effective field size (EFS) Another term for blocked field size (BFS). Effective field size is the equivalent rectangular field dimensions of the open or treated area within the collimator field dimensions. Effective field size is the actual area treated.

efferent lymphatic vessels Lymphatic vessels that flow out of the hilum of a lymph node.

elapsed days Total time over which radiation treatment is delivered (protracted).

electrical charge Measure of how strongly the particle is attracted to an electrical field and can be either positive or negative.

electrocautery Instrument for directing a high-frequency current through a local tissue area.

electron binding energy Amount of energy required to remove an electron from its orbit in an atom.

electron density Number of electrons per unit mass.

electron gun Responsible for producing electrons and injecting them into the accelerator structure. This essential part of the linear accelerator is responsible for producing electrons and injecting them into the accelerator structure.

electron shields "Cutouts" that collimate and shape the electron treatment field.

electronic medical record (EMR) Patient's medical record stored on and accessed from a computer.

electronic portal imaging device (EPID) System producing near real-time portal images on a computer screen for evaluation. Most electronic portal-imaging systems are lightweight and come with a retracted arm along the gantry's axis. Arm may be equipped with Amorphous Silicon (aSi) imaging technology, which provides a quick and accurate comparison of its images with reference images.

electrons Negatively charged subatomic particles that can be accelerated by a variety of machines or are emitted from decaying isotopes and used for external beam treatment and brachytherapy.

empathy Identifying with the feelings, thoughts, or experiences of another person.

en bloc French term meaning "in one block." In surgical cancer care, it means "in one specimen."

endocavitary radiation therapy Sphincter-sparing procedure in which the radiation treatment is delivered by a 50-kVp contact unit inserted into the rectum.

endometrial cancer Cancer of the endometrium or uterus.

endophytic pattern Growth pattern that invades within the lamina propria and submucosa.

endoplasmic reticulum Continuous membrane in the cellular cytoplasm containing the ribosomes.

engineering model Model that identifies the caregiver as a scientist dealing only in facts and does not consider the human aspect of the patient.

ependymoma Tumors arising from the ependymal cells lining the brain ventricles and central spinal canal. They may be low or high grade.

epidemiology Study of defining the distribution and determinants causing disease and injury in human populations.

epidermis Extremely thin outer layer of the skin composed of four or five distinct layers of cells.

epiphyseal line Cartilage at the junction of the diaphysis and epiphysis in young bones that serves as a growth area for long-bone lengthening.

epiphyses Knoblike portions of a long bone made up of spongy bone. It is located at either end of a long bone.

epistaxis Nosebleed.

equivalent square Square field that has the same percentage depth dose and output of a rectangular field. This method takes different rectangular field sizes and compares them to square fields that demonstrate the same measurable scattering and attenuation characteristics.

erythema Acute radiation effect, manifested by redness and inflammation of the skin or mucous membranes, is effected by capillary congestion, caused by dilation of the superficial capillaries.

erythroplasia Reddened, velvetlike patches on the mucous membranes.

esophagitis Inflammation of the esophagus. Patients complain of substernal pain and food sticking. Esophagitis may begin after 2 weeks of radiation therapy and continues for 2 to 4 weeks after treatment with conventional fractionation.

ethics Discipline dealing with what is good and bad, with a concern for moral duty and obligations; a set of moral principles or values; a theory or system of moral values; the principles of conduct governing an individual or professional group.

etiology Study of the causes of disease.

evidence-based care Practitioners commonly base clinical decision making on their knowledge and experience, patient preference, and clinical circumstances. Evidence-based care combines this information with scientific evidence.

excisional biopsy Removal of the entire tumor by cutting it out so that a diagnosis can be made.

exenteration (pelvic) Radical removal of most or all pelvic organs.

exit dose Term exit dose is used for the dose at the exit surface of the patient or to a depth that is the equivalent of the depth of D_{max}.

exophytic Noninvasive neoplasm that projects out from an epithelial surface.

exponent Exponent, or "power," is a shorthand notation that represents the multiplication of a number by itself a given number of times.

exposure Amount of ionization produced by photons in air per unit mass of air; units are the roentgen (R) or Coulomb per kilogram (C/kg). $1 R = 2.58 \times 10^{-4}$ C/kg.

extended-field irradiation Extended distance setup occurs when the setup source-skin distance (SSD) is greater than the reference SSD. Reference SSD is normally 80 cm for cobalt-60 treatment machines and 100 cm for linear accelerators.

external auditory meatus (EAM) The ear canal that connects the outer and middle ear.

extrapolation number (n) Part of a graphic representation of a cell-survival curve, determined by extrapolating the linear portion of the curve back until it intersects the y-axis.

extravasation Accidental leakage into the surrounding tissues; a discharge or escape (e.g., of blood) from a vessel into the tissues.

false imprisonment Intentional confinement without authorization by a person who physically constricts another with force, threat of force, or confining clothing or structures.

false positive/false negative Screening tests may yield false-positive or false-negative readings. False-positive reading indicates disease when in reality none is present. False-negative reading is the reverse; the test indicates no disease when in fact the disease is present.

familial adenomatous polyps (FAP) Hereditary disease in which the entire large bowel is studded with polyps. If left untreated, the patient develops a cancer of the large bowel.

feathering Migration of a gap between treatment fields through the treatment course.

fibrosarcoma Soft tissue sarcoma (STS) derived from collagen-producing fibroblasts. *See also* Soft Tissue Sarcoma (STS).

fibrosis Abnormal formation of fibrous tissue caused by alterations in the structure and function of blood vessels.

fiducial marker Fiducial markers may include natural anatomy or be artificial markers placed internally or at the skin surface or fixed external to the patient to document location through various imaging modalities.

fiducial plate Plastic trays imbedded with lead markers at regular intervals. These trays, sometimes referred to as a reticule or beaded trays, are positioned in the head of the gantry between the field-defining wires and accessory holder.

field-defining wires They are small tungsten wires (also called *delineators*) located in the collimator assembly that represent the edge of the treatment field.

field size Dimensions of a treatment field at the isocenter (usually represented by width ¥ length).

filament Small coil of wire made of thoriated tungsten, which has an extremely high melting point (3380° C).

file server Central computer where the database and program executables reside.

film badge Device for measuring dose.

film speed Reciprocal of the exposure in roentgens needed to produce a density of 1.0.

filtered back projection Commonly used method of reconstructing CT data. It is also called the *summation method*.

flat panel detectors Imaging device that uses amorphous silicon and solid state integrated circuit technology to produce images with quality far superior to conventional film-screen combinations.

flatness Difference between the maximum and minimum intensity of the central 80% of the profile and specifying this difference as a percentage of the central axis intensity. Degree of evenness of dose across a beam profile.

flow chart Pictorial representation of the steps necessary in a process.

fluence pattern Refers to an intensity pattern of the IMRT beam. This may be described as the sequence and progression of dose delivered per beam, as a product of several segments.

fluoroscopy-based simulation Conventional simulation, also referred to as fluoroscopy-based simulation, implies the use of a piece of x-ray equipment capable of the same mechanical movements of a treatment unit.

focal spot Section of the target at which radiation is produced.

focusing cup Small oval depression in the cathode assembly.

fomite Any inanimate object (vehicle) involved in the transmission of disease.

forward planning Process of entering dose-altering parameters and beam modifiers into the treatment plan by the planner.

fosa navicularis Anterior urethra passes through the corpus spongiosum and is subdivided into *fossa navicularis* (a widening within the glans), the penile urethra (which passes through the pendulous part of the penis), and the bulbous urethra (the dilated proximal portion of the anterior urethra).

four-dimensional (4D) Uses three-dimensional treatment planning + Time = 4D

fractionation Radiation therapy treatments given in daily fractions (segments) over an extended period of time, sometimes up to 6 to 8 weeks.

free radical Atom or atom group in a highly reactive transient state that is carrying an unpaired electron with no charge.

free space Term used for dosimetry measurements using a build-up cap or miniphantom.

frequency of the wave Represented by the Greek letter ν (read as nu), the number of times that the wave oscillates or cycles per second and is measured in units of cycles per second.

friable tumors Tumors that are easily broken or pulverized.

gadolinium Non–iodine-based intravenous contrast agent used for computed tomography and magnetic resonance imaging scans. Gadolinium helps differentiate between edema and a tumor.

gamma rays Electromagnetic radiation emitted from decaying isotopes and used for external-beam treatment and brachytherapy. High-energy electromagnetic radiation of no mass and no charge emitted during nuclear decay.

gantry On a conventional simulator, it is a mechanical C-shaped device that supports the x-ray tube and collimator device at one end. On a CT scanner, it is the circular ring housing the x-ray tube and solid state detectors. On a linear accelerator, it is responsible primarily for directing the photon (x-ray) or electron beam at a patient's tumor.

gap Distance between the borders of two adjacent fields. Gap is usually measured on the patient's skin. Skin gap is usually calculated to verify the depth at which the two adjacent fields abut.

Gardner's syndrome Inherited disorder (similar to familial adenomatous polyps) consisting of adenomatous polyposis of the large bowel, upper gastrointestinal polyps, periampullary tumors, lipomas, fibromas, and other tumors. This condition is associated with an increased risk in the development of colorectal cancer.

gated treatments Radiation treatment where the beam is turned "on" when the target is within the treatment volume and turned "off" when the target is outside the target volume. Length of time required deliver the treatment will increase significantly.

generic name Drug name coined by the original manufacturer.

genetically significant dose Dose equivalent to the gonads weighted for the age and sex distribution in those members of the irradiated population expected to have offspring; units are the rem or sievert.

genome Complete complement of hereditary factors as found on a haploid distribution of chromosomes.

germ cell tumors Tumors developing from embryologic nests of tissue located throughout the body, from the brain down to the ovaries and testes.

germ theory Hypothesis that microorganisms cause disease.

given dose (GD) The dose delivered at the depth of maximum equilibrium (D_{max}) through a single treatment field. Also known as *applied dose* or D_{max} *dose*.

golgi apparatus Cytoplasmic organelle consisting of flattened membranes that modify, store, and route products of the endoplasmic reticulum.

grade Grade of a tumor provides information about its biological aggressiveness and is based on the degree of cell differentiation. For some tumors, such as a high-grade astrocytoma, grade is the most important prognostic indicator.

gradient Change in position with the rate of change of a value (dose).

grenz ray Low-energy x-ray in the range of 10 to 15 kV.

grid Device constructed with thin lead foil strips and plastic spacers. It should be employed during simulation both to absorb the scattered radiation emitted from the thicker body parts and to allow the use of beam energies needed to maximize differential absorption between similar tissues.

gross tumor volume (GTV) Gross palpable or visible tumor.

ground state Minimum amount of energy needed to keep the atom together.

half-life Time period in which the activity decays to one half of the original value. It is the essential value to employ the decay formula for a particular isotope.

half-value layer Thickness of absorbing material necessary to reduce the x-ray intensity to half its original value.

health care organization Generic term used to describe all types of groups that provide health care services.

Health Insurance Portability and Accountability Act (HIPAA) Congress passed HIPAA in 1996. HIPAA guidelines and regulations require security precautions not only to restrict access but also to keep records of who is accessing information.

Health Level 7, Inc. (HL7) ANSI-accredited organization that develops standards for exchanging clinical and administrative data. Specifically, HL7 defines standards for "the exchange, management and integration of data that supports clinical patient care and the management, delivery and evaluation of healthcare services." HL7 interfaces allow sharing of information available used across the entire health care facility.

heat units Capacity of the anode and x-ray tube housing to store thermal energy.

heavy charged particle Particles like carbon-12 ion lose their energy by Coulomb interaction with atomic electrons and nuclei. Additionally, they also undergo nuclear reactions with the nuclei.

helical CT Also referred to as spiral CT. Patient is positioned at a fixed point, and, while the x-ray tube is rotating, the patient moves into the aperture to create a scan pattern that resembles a "slinky" or coiled spring.

hematochezia Patients with rectal cancer usually have rectal bleeding. This may be bright red blood on the toilet paper or mixed in or on the stool.

hematuria Common symptom of bladder and kidney tumors with an abnormal presence of blood in the urine.

hemiglossectomy Surgical removal of half the tongue.

hereditary nonpolyposis colorectal syndrome Frequent occurrence of colorectal cancer in families without adenomatous polyposis. This syndrome is associated with an increased risk of developing a second malignancy of the colon and adenocarcinomas of the breast, ovary, endometrium, and pancreas.

heterogeneity corrections Corrections that account for the presence of irradiated media other than water are called *heterogeneity corrections*.

high-dose-rate (HDR) brachytherapy Delivery of brachytherapy on an outpatient basis using HDR brachytherapy equipment. Actual treatment delivery lasts about 5 to 10 minutes in contrast to a hospital stay that might take several days for low-dose-rate brachytherapy.

high osmolality High number of particles in solution.

hilum Area of an organ where blood, lymphatic vessels, and nerves enter and exit.

hinge angle Measure of the angle between central rays of two intersecting treatment beams. If a lateral and anteroposterior beam intersect at the isocenter, the hinge angle would be 90 degrees.

HIPAA *See* Health Insurance Portability and Accountability Act (HIPAA).

histiocyte Phagocytic cell found in loose connective tissue.

histiocytosis X Spectrum of diseases caused by abnormal proliferation of a variety of immune cells affecting single or multiple organs.

history and physical Initial presentation and plan for assessment and treatment that becomes part of the patient's medical record.

history of present illness Clinician records, through conversation with the patient, a history of the present illness, and this becomes part of the patient's medical record.

HL7 *See* Health Level 7, Inc. (HL7).

homogeneous radiation beam Producing a homogeneous beam attempts to deliver the same dose throughout a defined volume of tissue through multiple treatment angles and beam intensities.

Horner's syndrome Condition caused by paralysis of the cervical sympathetic nerves. It may cause sinking in of the eyeball, ptosis of the upper eyelid, slight elevation of the lower lid, constriction of the pupil, and flushing of the affected side of the face.

hospice Program that provides care for patients who have limited life expectancy. Care is provided in the patient's home or a hospital setting.

hospital information system Electronic medical record's functions and technical infrastructure requires special expertise in information systems (IS) to create and maintain. Hospital information system departments may employ several specialists in areas ranging from system analysts to hardware and network specialists.

hot thyroid nodule Nodule having a radionuclide uptake much higher than the rest of the thyroid gland.

Hounsfield units Also called *CT numbers*, which range from +1000 to −1000. Hounsfield units represent various tissue densities and linear attenuation coefficients.

hyperfractionation Fractional doses smaller than conventional, delivered two or three times daily to achieve an increase in the total dose in the same overall time.

hyperparathyroidism Condition, caused by a tumor in the parathyroid, in which calcium is leaked from the bones, resulting in softening and deformity as the mineral salts are replaced by fibrous connective tissue.

hyperpigmentation Excessive coloration to the skin.

hyperthyroidism Hyperactivity of the thyroid gland.

hypertrophic pulmonary osteoarthropathy Frequently seen phenomenon associated with lung cancer, which is manifested by clubbing of the distal phalanges of the fingers.

hypophysis Pituitary gland.

hypotenuse Length of the longest side of the triangle.

hypothesis Prediction of the relationship between certain variables.

hypothyroidism Underactivity of the thyroid gland.

iatrogenic Disease or illness created as a result of the treatment or diagnosis of another condition.

idiosyncratic response (effects) Inexplicable and unpredictable symptoms caused by a genetic defect in the patient.

image fusion Process of combining images from different modalities with a CT image. Properly fused images combine the enhanced imaging capabilities of MRI and/or PET with the spatial accuracy of CT. Anatomy can be defined on any of the image data sets and can then be displayed on the CT image.

image-guided radiation therapy (IGRT) It may be used in a variety of forms, including EPID, an in-room CT scanner, KV cone beam computed tomography, MV cone beam computed tomography, ultrasound and others.

Rational for IGRT is to image the patient just prior to treatment, compare the position of external set-up marks and internal anatomy to the treatment plan.

image intensifier It is a useful tool during fluoroscopy, because it converts an x-ray image into a light image.

image matrix Images seen on the monitor are a display of cells in rows and columns, called the *image matrix*. Matrix size can be selected. However, 512 × 512 is commonly used in CT.

image registration Process where the images of the patient are with respect to the isocenter of the accelerator.

immobilization Process of ensuring that a patient does not move out of treatment position, thus allowing for reproducibility and accuracy in treatment.

immobilization device Device that assists in reproducing the treatment position while restricting movement (i.e., casts, masks, or bite blocks).

immune serum globulin Serum-containing antibody; a form of artificial immunity.

immunity Ability of the body to defend itself against infectious organisms, foreign bodies, and cancer cells.

immunoglobulin System of closely related, although not identical, proteins capable of acting as antibodies. Humans have five main types.

immunotherapy Therapy producing or increasing immunity.

impotence Significant side effect associated with the treatment of prostate cancer in which the adult male is unable to obtain an erection or ejaculate after achieving an erection.

incidence Occurrence of a particular disease over a period of time in relationship to the entire population.

incident Any happening not consistent with the routine operation of the hospital or routine care of a particular patient.

incisional biopsy Act of cutting into tissue to remove part of the tumor so that a diagnosis can be made.

incubation Time interval between exposure to infection and the appearance of the first sign or symptom characteristic of the disease.

indexing Allows for increased accuracy in treatment set-up reproducibility from simulation to treatment delivery and through multiple treatments over the course of daily radiation therapy delivery.

induration Process of becoming hard and firm in soft tissues.

inferior Toward the feet.

infiltration Swelling around the injection site accompanied by cool, pale skin and possibly hard patches or localized pain.

information flow Process between multiple databases and primary information generating systems networking an essential part of accurate treatment delivery in radiation oncology.

information system department Department that may employ several computer specialists in areas ranging from hardware to network

to application support for managing the array of requirements, from running the computer system to ensuring that it is employed efficiently by clinicians and staff.

informed consent Assurance that the purpose, benefit, risk, and any alternative options have been explained and understood and a disclaimer (which will not always hold up in court) releasing the caregiver and facility from liability if complications develop or the treatment fail.

infundibulum Stalklike structure that attaches the pituitary to the hypothalamus.

intensifying screens Used to convert the invisible energy of an x-ray beam into visible light energy.

intensity-modulated radiation therapy (IMRT) Therapy that delivers nonuniform exposure across the beam's eye view (BEV) using a variety of techniques and equipment.

interdisciplinary All the disciplines cooperating in the management of the disease process, as in the cancer-management team.

interfraction Changes occurring between treatment sessions

interlocks Safety switches blocking or terminating radiation production.

internal mammary lymphatic pathway Lymphatic chain that runs toward the midline and passes through the pectoralis major and intercostal muscles close to the body of the sternum (T4 to T9).

International Standards Organization (ISO) Organization that accredits various specialty organizations that produce standards for industry specific requirements.

interpolation To estimate values between two measured, known values. Mathematical process used in radiation therapy in which unlisted values in tables can be derived.

interstitial brachytherapy Treatment technique that is characterized by the placement of radioactive sources directly into a tumor or tumor bed. Interstitial implants can be either permanent or temporary.

interstitial implant Application of a brachytherapy implant directly into the tissues via devices such as needles, ribbons, or seeds placed in the at-risk tissues.

interstitial radiation therapy Insertion of radioactive sources into the tissue to treat the disease.

intracavitary brachytherapy Radioactive sources are placed within a body cavity for treatment. This type of brachytherapy has been the mainstay in treatment of cervical cancer for more than 50 years.

intradermal Shallow injection between the layers of the skin.

intrafraction Changes or motion during the treatment administration.

intrahypophyseal tumors Pituitary tumor that stays in the pituitary gland.

intraluminal brachytherapy Places sources of radiation within body tubes such as the esophagus, uterus, trachea, bronchus, and rectum. Many high dose rate applications are performed for intraluminal applications.

intramuscular (IM) Administrative route for chemotherapy agents. It is used for large amounts or quick effects.

intraoperative radiation therapy (IORT) Boost technique in which a single dose of 10 to 20 Gy is delivered directly to the tumor bed with electrons or photons. Tumor bed has been surgically exposed, allowing critical normal structures to be shielded or displaced out of the radiation beam.

intrasellar lesions Pituitary tumors that grow within the confines of the sella.

intrathecal Injection that requires drugs to be instilled into the space containing cerebrospinal fluid.

intrauterine tandem Brachytherapy device placed through the cervical os into the uterus and subsequently afterloaded to give the dose application directly to the cervix, uterus, and upper vagina.

intravascular brachytherapy Rapidly emerging treatment modality that introduces radioactive source(s) through vascular routes.

intravenous (IV) Injection directly into the bloodstream providing an immediate effect.

intravenous pyelogram (IVP) Radiographic procedure using contrast media to outline the kidneys, ureters, and bladder.

invasion of privacy Revealing confidential information or improperly and unnecessarily exposing a patient's body.

inverse planning Treatment planning in which the clinical objectives are specified mathematically and computer software is used to determine the best beam parameters (mainly beamlet weighting) that will lead to the desired dose distribution.

inverse proportionality Relationship between measurable quantities and factors, in that as one increases, the other decreases, and vice versa.

inverse square law Mathematical relationship that describes the change in beam intensity as the distance from the source changes, where intensity is inversely proportional to the distance squared.

involved field radiation Radiation that includes only the affected lymph node region such as the supraclavicular, ipsilateral cervical, or the inguinal nodes.

ionic contrast media Media having high osmolality or a high number of particles in isolation. Large amount of iodine provides greater contrast but also increases toxicity and viscosity.

ionizing radiation Radiation with sufficient energy to separate an electron from its atom.

ipsilateral Refers to a body component on the same side of the body.

iridium Radioactive isotope with a half-life of 74 days. It is used in wire form for interstitial brachytherapy.

irradiated volume Volume of tissue receiving a significant dose (e.g., >50%) of the specified target dose.

ISO *See* International Standards Organization (ISO).

isocenter Point of intersection of the three axes of rotation (gantry, collimator, and base of couch) of the treatment unit.

isocentric technique Approach to three-dimensional treatment using multiple imaging modalities, including fluoroscopy, CT, MRI, PET, SPECT, and ultrasound, planning where the isocenter is placed in or near the target volume

isodose curve Plotted percentage depth dose at various points in the beam along the central axis and elsewhere.

isodose distributions Two-dimensional spatial representations of dose.

isodose lines Lines connecting points of equivalent relative radiation dose.

isthmus Connects the lobes of the thyroid gland.

iteration Refers to a repetitious process, which follows a sequence of instructions in a computer program, making slight adjustments in each treatment plan until the best result is achieved. It is usually used with IMRT.

Joint Commission on the Accreditation of Healthcare Organizations *See* The Joint Commission (TJC).

Joint Review Committee on Education in Radiologic Technology (JRCERT) Purpose of the JRCERT is to promote excellence in education and enhances quality and safety of patient care through the accreditation of educational programs.

jugulodigastric Group of high neck nodes below the mastoid tip and near the angle of the mandible.

justice Quality of being just, impartial, or fair; treatment that is fair or adequate.

Karnofsky performance scale (KPS) Scale that measures the neurologic and functional status. KPS allows measuring of the quantity and quality of neurologic defects. Scale ranges from 1 to 100.

keratin Extremely tough, waterproof, protein substance in hair, nails, and horny tissue.

keratinocyte Any one of the cells in the skin that synthesizes keratin.

keratoacanthoma Papular lesion filled with a keratin plug that can resemble squamous cell carcinoma. It is benign and usually subsides spontaneously within 6 months.

keratosis Lesion on the epidermis marked by the presence of a circumcised overgrowth of the horny layer.

kilovoltage units Equipment carrying out external-beam treatment by using x-rays generated at voltages up to 500 kVp.

kilovolts peak (kVp) Unit of measurement for x-ray voltages. (1 kV = 1000 V of electrical potential.)

klystron Equipment that converts kinetic energy to microwave energy in the linear accelerator.

kwashiorkor Protein malnutrition that includes an adequate intake of carbohydrates and fats but an inadequate intake of protein.

kyphosis Excessive curvature of the vertebral column that is convex posteriorly.

LAN *See* Local Area Network (LAN).

lasers Each positional laser projects a small red or green beam of light toward the patient during the simulation or treatment process. This provides the therapist several external reference points in relationship to the position of the isocenter.

latent image Image on the recording medium that is not visible until the image is processed or digitized.

latent period Time between the exposure and incidence of an abnormality.

lateral Toward one side or the other.

law Primarily concerned with the good of a society as a functioning unit.

law of Bergonié and Tribondeau Law stating that ionizing radiation is more effective against cells that (1) are actively mitotic, (2) are undifferentiated, and (3) have a long mitotic future.

LD$_{50/30}$ Lethal effect of acute whole-body exposure in which 50% of the total population exposed is affected in 30 days.

lean Systemwide set of methods and tools for improving a process by emphasizing speed and efficiency. It was first used in the early days of mass production of the automobiles (1910). It focuses on time and waste in a process.

legal concepts Sum of artificial rules and regulations by which society is governed in any formal and legally binding manner.

legal ethics Study of the law mandating certain acts and forbidding others under penalty of criminal sanction.

leiomyosarcoma Soft tissue sarcoma (STS) arising from smooth muscle. *See also* Soft Tissue Sarcoma (STS).

LET *See* Linear Energy Transfer (LET).

leukoencephalopathy Widespread demyelinating lesions of the brain, brainstem, and cerebellum.

leukopenia Abnormal decrease in the white blood cell count, usually below 5000 cells per mm^3.

leukoplakia Small, white, raised patches on the mucous membrane.

L'hermitte's syndrome Pain resembling sudden electric shock throughout the body. It is produced by flexing of the neck or some cervical trauma.

libel Written defamation of character.

licensure Process by which an agency or government grants permission to an individual to work in a specific occupation after finding that the individual has attained the minimal degree of competency to ensure the health and safety of the public.

life experiences Life experiences can be described as information gathered through a normal day's activity that is useful to enhance an existing cognitive knowledge base.

light cast Fiberglass tape that contains resin, which can be molded around a patient. When exposed to ultraviolet light, it hardens, creating a rigid immobilization device.

limb-sparing surgery (LSS) Radical or wide en bloc resection for soft tissue masses that requires a 1- to 3-cm normal tissue margin that allows the limb and extremity to remain intact (avoids amputation). Also called *limb salvage surgery*.

linear accelerator Radiation therapy treatment unit that accelerates electrons and produces x-rays or electrons for treatment.

linear energy transfer (LET) Average energy deposited per unit path length to a medium by ionizing radiation as it passes through that medium. An average value calculated by dividing the energy deposited in kiloelectron volts (keV) by the distance traveled in micrometers (μm or 10^{-6} meters).

linear interpolation Process of calculating unknown values from known values.

liposarcoma Soft tissue sarcoma (STS) arising from fat. *See also* Soft Tissue Sarcoma (STS).

living will Purpose of the living will is to allow the competent adult to provide direction to health care providers concerning their choice of treatment under certain conditions, should the individual no longer be competent by reason of illness or other infirmity, to make those decisions.

local area network (LAN) Geographically confined to an area in which a common communication service may be used. For larger geographic areas or when multiple LANs are to be connected, a wide area network is used.

localization Geometrical definition of the tumor and anatomic structures using surface or fiducial marks for reference.

logarithm Inverse or exponential notation. Exponent that indicated the power to which a number is raised to produce a given number.

low-dose rate (LDR) brachytherapy Brachytherapy that is delivered in a conventional low dose rate regimen that lasts several days and requires a hospital stay.

low osmolality Refers to contrast agents in which the iodides remain intact instead of splitting, and therefore they agitate the cells less.

lymph Excessive tissue fluid consisting mostly of water and plasma proteins from capillaries.

lymphangiography Radiographic study that uses special injected dyes that aid in visualizing the lymphatic system on x-ray.

lymphatic system Consists of lymphatic vessels, lymphatic organs, and the fluid that circulates through it, called *lymph*.

lysosome Membranous sac containing hydrolytic enzymes and found in the cellular cytoplasm. It functions in intracellular digestion.

lytic Pertaining to the destruction of cells.

magnetic resonance imaging (MRI) Diagnostic, nonionizing means of visualizing internal anatomy through noninvasive means. Imaging is based on the magnetic properties of the hydrogen nuclei.

magnetron A special type of electron tubes that are used to provide microwave power to accelerate electrons.

MAID One of the most often used chemotherapy drug programs consisting of the following drugs: methotrexate, doxorubicin, ifosfamide, and dacarbazine.

malignant Tumors that are malignant often invade and destroy normal surrounding tissue and, if left untreated, can cause the death of the host.

malignant fibrous histiocytoma (MFH) Deep STS tumor showing partial fibroblastic and histiocytic differentiation with a variable pattern and giant cells

malignant melanoma Most lethal form of skin cancer, which arises from the melanocytes found in the stratum basale of the epidermis.

mantle field Radiation field that treats the lymph nodes superior to the diaphragm.

mantoux tuberculin skin test Purified protein derivative (PPD) of tuberculin used in skin tests to show if a person has ever been "infected" by tuberculosis (TB) germs.

marasmus Calorie malnutrition that is observed in patients who are slender or slightly underweight and characterized by weight loss of 7% to 10% and fat and muscle depletion.

mass equivalence Measure of the mass of photons used to help explain related physical characteristics.

mass stopping power Sum of all energy losses. This includes both losses caused by collisions of electrons with atomic electrons and radiation losses or bremsstrahlung production.

mastoid process Extension of the mastoid temporal bone at the level of the ear lobe.

Mayneord's factor Used to convert the percentage depth dose at the reference distance to the percentage depth dose at a nonreference distance. This would occur, for example, at extended distance setups.

mean life Average lifetime for the decay of radioactive atoms.

medial Toward the midline of the body.

median sagittal plane Also called the *midsagittal plane*, divides the body into two symmetric right and left sides. There is only one median sagittal plane.

mediastinoscopy Small flexible tube frequently used for the evaluation of the superior mediastinal extent of disease.

mediastinum Tissue and organs separating the lungs. Mediastinum contains the heart and its large vessels, trachea, esophagus, thymus, lymph nodes, and other structures.

medical informatics Organization, analysis, management and use of information in healthcare and the electronic medical record.

medical information systems Medical information system departments may employ several specialists in areas ranging from system analysts to hardware and network specialists.

medical record All components used to document chronologically the care and treatment rendered to a patient.

medication Drug administered for its therapeutic effects.

medulla Inner portion of the adrenal gland.

medullary Cavity within the bone that contains fats or yellow bone marrow.

medulloblastoma Highly malignant cerebellar tumor usually arising in the midline with the propensity to spread via the cerebrospinal fluid.

megavoltage equipment Units using x-ray beams of energy 1 MeV or greater.

melanin Pigment that gives color to the skin and hair and serves as protection from ultraviolet light.

melanocyte Melanin-forming cell found in the stratum basale of the epidermis.

melanoma Dark pigmented malignant tumor arising from the skin.

menarche Beginning of a woman's first menstrual period.

menopause End of a woman's menstrual activity.

menorrhagia Pain during menstruation.

mesothelioma Malignant tumors that develop in the mesothelial lining, the pleura, and possibly the pericardium.

metastases Spread of cancer beyond the primary site.

metastasize Process of tumors spreading to a site in the body distant from the primary site.

meter setting Used for the monitor unit setting for linear accelerators and the minute setting for cobalt-60 treatment machines.

microadenomas Neoplasms that are less than 1.0 cm midline block shielding device used to spare the midline structures like the spinal cord from the effects of radiation.

microwaves Similar to ordinary radiowaves but have frequencies thousands of times higher. Microwave frequencies needed for linear accelerator operation are about 3 billion cycles per second (3000 MHz).

midline block Shielding block used to eliminate dose to centrally located anatomy.

milliamperes (mA) Units of measurement for x-ray currents in which the ampere (Å) is a measure of electrical current.

misadministration Incorrect application or delivery of a prescribed dose of radiation therapy, which can be minor or major and may cause death or serious injury to the patient depending on the extent of the dose.

mitochondria Cytoplasmic organelle serving as the site of cellular respirations and energy production.

mitosis Cell division involving the nucleus and cell body.

Mohs' surgery Surgical method in which the tumor is removed one layer at a time and examined microscopically.

monitor unit (MU) Unit of output measure used for linear accelerators. Accelerators are calibrated so that 1 MU delivers 1 cGy for a standard, reference field size at a standard reference depth at a standard source-to-calibration point.

monoclonal antibody Antibody derived from hybridoma cells that can be used to identify tumor antigens.

moral ethics Study of right and wrong as it relates to conscience, God, a higher being, or a person's logical rationalization.

morphology Glandular pattern, distribution of glands, and stromal invasion of the tumor.

multicentric Arising from many foci and having multiple origination.

multidisciplinary Use of several disciplines at the same time. Having two or more modalities in a combined effort to treat a disease process.

multileaf collimator (MLC) Distinct part of the linear accelerator that allows treatment field shaping and blocking through the use of motorized leaves in the head of the machine.

Musculoskeletal Tumor Society (MTS) Surgical staging system—classification and anatomic staging system used for soft tissue sarcomas.

mutation Change; transformation.

mycosis fungoides Chronic, progressive lymphoma arising in the skin. Initially, the disease stimulates eczema or other inflammatory dermatoses. In advanced cases, ulcerated tumors and infiltrations of lymph nodes may occur.

myelosuppression Reduction in bone marrow function.

nadir Lowest point and the time of greatest depression of blood values.

nasion Center depression at the base of the nose.

natural background radiation Ionizing radiation from natural sources including cosmic rays from outer space and the sun, terrestrial radiation from radioactive materials in the earth, and internal radiation from radioactive materials normally present in the body.

natural history Normal progression of a tumor without treatment.

necrosis Death or disintegration of a cell or tissue caused by disease or injury.

NED (no evidence of disease) At the time of patient follow-up examination, there is no residual cancer noted.

negligence Neglect or omission of reasonable care or caution.

network System of independent, interconnected computers or terminals communicating with one another over a shared medium, consisting of hardware and communication protocols.

neuroblastoma Cancer of neural crest tissues, usually adrenal medulla or spinal ganglia, with frequent metastases.

neurofibromatosis (von Recklinghausen's disease) Small, discrete, pigmented skin lesions (cafe au lait spots and/or pigmented nevi) that develop into multiple neurofibromas along the course of peripheral nerves; may undergo malignant transformation.

neurohypophysis Posterior lobe of the pituitary.

neutrons Neutral subatomic particles found in the nucleus of an atom.

nevus Benign, localized cluster of melanocytes arising in the skin, usually early in life.

node of Rouvière One of the lateral retropharyngeal lymph nodes located between the pharynx and the prevertebral fascia. They receive lymph from the nasopharynx and the auditory mode tube. Also called the *lateral retropharyngeal node*.

nonionic contrast media Media having low osmolality. Iodides remain intact instead of splitting; therefore they agitate the cells less. These agents are equally effective but cost much more than ionic agents.

nonmaleficence Not doing wrong or harm to an individual.

nosocomial Infection acquired in a hospital.

nuclear binding energy Total amount of energy that it takes to hold a nucleus together and is measured in MeV (10^6 electron volts).

nuclear energy level High energy states of the atom.

nuclear force Major force that holds the nucleus of an atom together.

nuclear medicine Branch of medicine that uses radioisotopes in the diagnosis and treatment of disease.

nuclear membrane Membranous envelope enclosing the nucleus and separating it from the cytoplasm.

nucleoli Rounded internuclear organelle serving as the site of construction of the ribosomes.

nucleoside Compound composed of a nitrogenous base and a five-carbon sugar. With the addition of a phosphate group, a nucleoside becomes a nucleotide.

nucleotide Compound composed of a nitrogenous base, five-carbon sugar, and phosphate group.

nucleotides Basic building blocks of the nucleic acids RNA and DNA.

nucleus Conspicuous cytoplasmic organelle containing most of the genetic material (a small amount is located in the mitochondria) and nucleolus.

objectives Define the required behaviors needed to achieve the desired results, including the knowledge, skills, and attitudes the student or patient will learn.

obliquity corrections *See* Contour Corrections.

occupancy factor (T) Fraction of time that an area adjacent to a source of radiation is occupied.

Occupational Safety and Health Administration (OSHA) Administrative regulatory agency requiring employers to ensure the safety of workers.

odontalgia Toothache.

odynophagia Painful swelling.

Ohngren's line Line that connects the medial canthus of the eye with the angle of the mandible. It divides the maxillary antrum into anterior-inferior and superior-posterior halves.

oncogene Gene that regulates the development and growth of cancerous tissues.

oophorectomy Surgical removal of the ovaries.

oophoropexy Fixation of the ovaries behind the uterus.

opposite Length of the side of the right triangle that is opposite the specified angle in equations.

optical distance indicator (ODI) Sometimes called a *rangefinder*, it projects a scale onto the patients' skin, which corresponds to the source-skin distance (SSD) used during the simulation or treatment process.

optimal contrast When technical factors (primarily kVp) are selected that maximize the rate of differential absorption between body parts of varying tissue density and effective atomic number.

optimization Procedure to make a system as effective as possible.

organ segmentation Process of identifying structures, target volumes or normal tissues, by creating contours around them.

organelle One of many membrane-bound particles suspended in the cytoplasm of cells and having specialized functional characteristics.

orthogonal Two images taken 90 degrees apart. They are required for treatment-planning purposes to define the location and relationship of various anatomic structures relative to the field's isocenter.

orthopnea Difficulty breathing, except in an upright position.

orthovoltage therapy Treatments using x-rays produced at potentials ranging from 150 to 500 kV.

osmolality Property of a solution that depends on the concentration of the solute per unit of solvent.

osseous Composed of bone or resembling bone; bony.

osteoblastic Bone-forming cells.

osteomyelitis Infection of bone and marrow caused by the growth of germs in the bone. Infection may reach the bone through the bloodstream or by direct injury.

otalgia Earache.

outcomes Result of the performance, or lack of performance, of a process.

output Referred to as the *dose rate of the machine*. Dose rate should be specified for field size, distance, and medium.

output factor Ratio of the dose rate of a given field size to the dose rate of the reference field size.

ovarian cancer Cancer of the ovaries.

ovoid Also called *colpostats*, these applicators are oval-shaped and insert into the lateral fornices of the vagina. They can accommodate radioactive sources and shielding material and are used in the treatment of gynecologic tumors.

oxygen-enhancement ratio (OER) Magnitude of the oxygen effect on cell death is termed the OER, which compares the response of cells with radiation in the presence and absence of oxygen.

Paget's disease Disease characterized by excessive and abnormal bone reabsorption and formation. It may affect any part of the skeletal system but primarily strikes the spine, pelvis, femur, and skull.

palliation Noncurative treatment to relieve pain and suffering when the disease has reached the stage at which a cure is no longer possible.

palpation Use of touch to acquire information about the patient. Physician palpates the patient by using the tips of the fingers.

pancoast tumor Malignant superior sulcus tumor in the apex of the lung with clinical symptoms that includes (1) pain around the shoulder and down the arm, (2) atrophy of the muscles of the hand, (3) Homer's syndrome caused by involvement of the brachial plexus, and (4) bone erosion of the ribs and sometimes vertebrae.

pantograph Most widely used and most accurate mechanical contouring device.

papilledema Swelling of the optic disc, usually associated with increased intracranial pressure.

paraaortic field Radiation field that treats the subdiaphragmatic nodes.

paraaortic nodes Efferent to the cisterna chyli, which is the beginning of the thoracic duct. These nodes run adjacent to the abdominal aorta from T12 to L4.

parallel-opposed field set Most common combined-field geometry in which two treatment fields share common central axes, 180 degrees apart.

parallel response tissues High-dose region of a serial-tissue DVH is of particular importance. Overall function of organs consisting of parallel response tissues is affected by the injury of a number of elements of that organ above a certain minimum "reserve."

parametrium Tissues lateral to and around the uterus.

paranasal sinuses Air spaces in the skull, lined by mucous membranes, that reduce the weight of the skull and give the voice resonance. Four paranasal sinuses are the ethmoid, maxillary, sphenoid, and frontal.

paraneoplastic syndrome Collective term for disorders arising from metabolic effects of cancer on tissues remote from the tumor. Such disorders may appear as endocrine, hematologic, or neuromuscular disorders.

parenteral Medication bypassing the gastrointestinal tract. Taken literally, this would include the topical and some mucous membrane routes, but the word has come colloquially to mean "by injection."

parity Viable pregnancy (500-g birth weight or 20-week gestation), regardless of the outcome.

pathogenicity Ability of an infectious agent to cause disease.

patient couch One of the mechanical components of the conventional simulator. Treatment couch, sometimes mounted on a turntable, allows rotation about a fixed axis that passes through the isocenter.

patient positioning aids Devices that place the patient in a particular position for treatment but do not ensure that the patient does not move.

patient support assembly (PSA) Also called a *couch* or *table*, it allows the tabletop its mobility, permitting the precise and exact positioning of the isocenter during simulation or treatment.

peak scatter factor Peak scatter factor is a backscatter factor sometimes normalized to a reference field size, usually 10×10 cm, for energies of 4 MV and above.

peer review Evaluation by health care professionals with the same credentials in which standards of practice are applied to evaluate professional performance and processes.

pelvic inlet Upper entrance into the pelvis, bordered by the sacral promontory, medial pelvic sidewalls, and pubic bones.

pendant Set of handheld local controls suspended from the ceiling or attached to the treatment couch that mimic those of the treatment unit.

penile urethra Urethra that passes through the pendulous part of the penis.

penumbra Area or region at the beam's edge where the radiation intensity falls to 0.

percentage depth dose (PDD) Ratio, expressed as a percentage, of the absorbed dose at a given depth to the absorbed dose at a fixed reference depth, usually D_{max}.

perineum Part of the body dorsal to the pubic arch; ventral to the tip of the coccyx; and lateral to the inferior rami of the pubis, ischium, and sacrotuberous ligaments. These are the tissues surrounding the genitals and anal opening.

periosteum Glistening-white, double-layered membrane covering the outer surface of the diaphysis.

peritoneal cytology Pathologic examination of cells obtained from the fluid surrounding the abdominal wall and its contained viscera.

peritoneal seeding Shedding or sloughing of tumor cells into the abdominal (peritoneal) cavity.

peroxisome Intracellular enzyme-containing body that participates in the metabolic oxidation of various substrates.

petechiae Minute red spots caused by the escape of small amounts of blood.

Peyer's patches Extra lymphatic tissue located within the submucosal layer in the distal ileum.

pharmacodynamics Way drugs affect the body.

pharmacokinetics Way drugs travel through the body to their receptor sites.

pharmocology Science of drugs and their sources, chemistry, and actions.

pharynx Membranous tube that extends from the base of skull to the esophagus and connects the oral and nasal cavities with the larynx and esophagus.

phase I, II, III studies Series of studies performed to assess the risk, benefits, and effects of proposed treatment options. Phase I study is the first step in testing a new treatment in humans, assessing the best way to give a new treatment and the best dose. Dose is usually increased a little at a time to find the highest dose that does not cause harmful side effects. Phase II study tests whether a new treatment has an appropriate tumoricidal effect against certain cancers. Phase III study compares the results of people taking a new treatment with the results of people taking the standard treatment to prove the safety and efficacy of a new treatment.

phlebitis Inflammation of a vein.

photoelectric effect Interaction, sometimes described as true absorption, occurs when the incident photon penetrates deep into the atom and ejects an inner-shell electron from orbit.

photon Small packet of electromagnetic energy (e.g., radiowaves, visible light, and x-rays and gamma rays).

photostimulable plate Method using x-ray detectors that convert x-rays to a digital image. Flat plate contains a layer of phosphor material, which when exposed to x-rays, stores the latent image as a distribution of electron charges

phototiming Form of automatic exposure control (AEC) in which one or more ionization cells automatically stop the exposure during the creation of a simulation image.

pigmentation Coloration of the skin caused by the presence or absence of melanin.

pitch Used in spiral CT, it is determined by the couch movement in the longitudinal direction during one rotation of the gantry, divided by the slice thickness.

pixels Small, discrete elements that make up an image.

planning target volume (PTV) Volume that indicates the clinical target volume (CTV) plus margins for geometric uncertainties, such as patient motion, beam penumbra, and treatment setup differences.

ploidy Number of chromosome sets in a cell. (Haploid cells have one set, and diploid cells have two sets.)

Plummer-Vinson syndrome Iron-deficiency anemia characterized by esophageal webs and atrophic glossitis. It predisposes an individual to the development of esophageal cancer.

pluripotent Pertaining to an embryonic cell that can form different kinds of cells.

pocket ionization chamber (pocket dosimeter) Device for measuring exposure. It uses the phenomenon that, when air is irradiated, the ions formed partially discharge the static electricity on a fine filament, allowing it to move across a scale. Filament and scale can be visualized by holding the cylindrical device up to a light and looking through one end.

polypeptide Chain of many amino acids linked by peptide bonds. Polypeptides are the subunits of proteins.

polyurethane mold Immobilization-repositioning device in which polyurethane (a synthetic rubber polymer) foam hardens and shapes to the patient's body build.

portal verification Documentation of treatment portals through radiographic images or electronic portal imaging devices.

positioning devices Common or customized devices that assist in ensuring patient treatment location during treatment.

positioning lasers Lasers that project a small red or green beam of light toward the patient during the simulation process. These lasers provide the therapist several external reference points in relationship to the position of the isocenter.

positron emission tomography (PET) Nuclear medicine procedure that has become useful in oncology to examine the biochemical or physiological (functional) aspects of a tumor. This diagnostic tool is useful in determining the physiology of the organ in question. Beneficial diagnostic tool that may be useful in determining differences between necrosis and malignancy, which are associated with areas of high metabolism.

positrons Positively charged electrons.

practice standards Authoritative statements established by the profession for judging the quality of practice, service, and education.

premalignant Physiologic characteristics of predisposing factors that may lead to malignancy.

prevention Effective strategy for saving lives lost from cancer and diminishing suffering. Prevention includes measures that stop cancer from developing.

priestly model Model that provides the caregiver with a godlike, paternalist attitude by making decisions for the patient and not with the patient.

primary site compartment Natural anatomic boundaries surrounding the soft tissue sarcoma primary. It is composed of common fascia plane(s) of muscles, bone, joint, skin, subcutaneous tissues, and major neurovascular structures.

primary tumor Main, or initial, source of malignant or benign tumor location, without reference to secondary sites of spread.

primary vertebral curves Vertebral curves that are developed *in utero* as the fetus develops in the C-shaped fetal position, and they are present at birth.

profile Description of radiation intensity as a function of position across the beam at a given depth.

progenitor Originator or precursor.

prognosis Estimation of life expectancy.

projection That part of the CT beam that falls on one detector is called a *ray*. One complete translation of rays is called a *view*, which generates a profile or projection that are then created and stored in digital form.

proliferation Rapid and repeated reproduction of a new part (e.g., through cell division).

proportion Two ratios that are equal. Proportion can also be an equation relating two ratios.

prospective study Study in which the theory of the cause of a condition or disease is tested by examining those who have a particular characteristic or trait. Population to be examined is selected in the beginning of the study.

prostate Walnut-shaped organ that surrounds the male urethra, located between the base of the bladder and urogenital diaphragm.

prostate gland Gland that surrounds the male urethra between the base of the bladder and the urogenital diaphragm.

prostate-specific antigen (PSA) Glycoprotein that is produced by epithelial cells in the prostate. Serum PSA level has been roughly correlated with prostate tumor volume

prostatic hypertrophy Enlargement of the prostate gland, leading to narrowing of the urethra.

protein Complex biologic compound composed of amino acids. Linked together in a determined, three-dimensional sequence, 20 different amino acids are commonly found in proteins.

protocols Specified treatment regimen. It describes the specifics of the type of treatment, the time schedule of the treatment, the total dose of the treatment, and specific areas to be included in the treatment.

proton Subatomic particle, located in the nucleus with a positive charge

protraction Time over which total dose is to be delivered.

protractor Gantry angle scale that is located at the central point of rotation of the gantry arm. It is an instrument in the shape of a graduated circular device. It is used to measure the gantry angle, which may range from 0 to 360 degrees.

programmatic accreditation Radiation therapy student's assurance the program meets the minimum professional curriculum developed by the ASRT.

pruritus Itching.

pseudocapsule Soft tissue sarcomas that are surrounded by compressed normal tissue, reactive inflammation, and fibrosis to give the gross anatomic appearance of a capsule.

psychosocial Psychological support of the patient during the course of disease, with the recognition that social aspects of the treatment and disease prognosis may require special care.

purpura Blotchyness and red spots caused by petechiae and ecchymoses.

quality assessment Systematic quality analysis and review of patient care data.

quality assurance (QA) Systematic monitoring of the quality and appropriateness of patient care with an emphasis on performance levels.

quality-assurance (QA) program Series of activities and documentation performed with the goal of optimizing patient care.

quality audit Review of the radiation therapy process that is routinely and continuously measured, the results analyzed, and corrective action taken as required to ensure quality patient care.

quality control (QC) Component of quality assurance used in reference to the mechanical and geometrical tests of the radiation therapy equipment.

quality improvement (QI) Continuous improvement of health care services through the systematic evaluation of processes.

quality indicator Measurement tool used to evaluate an organization's performance.

quality of life Person's subjective sense of well-being derived from current experience of life as a whole.

radiation necrosis Tissue death resulting from the effects of radiation.

radiation oncologist Physician who reviews the medical findings with the patient and discusses treatment options and the benefits of radiation therapy as well as the possible side effects.

radiation oncology team Group consisting of all staff employees in radiation oncology who come in contact with the patient and/or family members throughout the course of radiation treatments.

radiation pneumonitis Inflammation of the lung tissue.

radiation therapist Medical practitioner on the radiation oncology team who sees the patient daily and is responsible for treatment delivery and daily assessment of patient tolerance to treatment.

radiation therapy domain Confines of the radiation therapy department and the socialization that takes place inside.

radiation therapy prescription Legal document written by a radiation oncologist that provides the therapist with the information required to deliver the appropriate radiation treatment. It defines the treatment volume, intended tumor dose, number of treatments, dose per treatment, and frequency of treatment.

radical resection Surgical removal of structures.

radioactive decay Process of an unstable nuclei emitting radiation.

radioactivity Emission of energy in the form of electromagnetic radiation or energetic particles.

radiographic cassette Holder for radiographic film used in portal imaging or simulation.

radiographic contrast Element of imaging that provides visual evidence of the differential absorption rates of various body tissues. Radiographic contrast has been described as the tonal range of densities from black to white or the number of shades of gray in the radiograph.

radiographic density Degree of darkening on the film. Radiograph of high density is dark, and a radiograph of low density is light.

radiolysis Initial event in the radiolysis (splitting) of water involves the ionization of a water molecule, thus producing a water ion.

radiopaque marker Material with a high atomic number used to document structures radiographically.

radioprotectors Certain chemicals and drugs that diminish the response of cells to radiation.

radiosensitizers Chemicals and drugs that help enhance the lethal effects of radiation.

radium substitute Any isotope used for brachytherapy whose dosimetry is based on the original radium work.

random error Variation in individual treatment setup.

randomization Method by which patients are blindly assigned to participate in specific portions of a protocol called an *arm*. Use of randomization ensures an equitable distribution of patients in each arm without prejudices that can later be blamed for unfair patient selection and can be detrimental to the outcome of the trial.

randomize To make random for scientific experimentation.

ratio Mathematical comparison of two numbers, values, or terms that denotes a relationship between the two.

recombinant deoxyribonucleic acid (DNA) DNA molecule in which rearrangement of the genes has been artificially induced.

recombinant DNA technology (genetic engineering) Techniques that facilitate the manipulation and duplication of pieces of DNA.

reconstructed field of view Diameter or the area of a CT scan that is displayed on the computer. It should be large enough to display the entire contour of the patient.

reconstruction time Time it takes the CT computer to analyze and process the information received from the detectors and display it on a TV monitor.

Reed-Sternberg cell Giant multinucleated connective tissue cell that is characteristic of Hodgkin's disease.

reflective listening Health care workers can reflect the specific content or implied feelings of their nonverbal observations or communication they feel has been omitted or emphasized.

regeneration Repair, regrowth, or restoration of a part (as tissue).

regional accreditation Agencies that serve select regions of the United States.

regulatory Requirements for limits of exposure to radiation for various groups.

regulatory agency Organization that may promulgate rules and regulations that have the force of law, license users, and provide inspection and enforcement actions.

rehabilitation Dynamic process with the goal of enabling persons to function at their maximal level within the limitations of their disease or disability in terms of physical, mental, emotional, social, and economic potential.

relative biologic effectiveness (RBE) RBE equals dose from 250 keV x-ray divided by dose from test radiation to produce the same biologic effect.

reproductive failure Decrease in the reproductive integrity or the ability of a cell to undergo an infinite number of divisions after radiation.

respiratory cycle Healthy adult at rest breathes in and out, one respiratory cycle, about 12 to 16 times per minute or approximately 1 cycle every 4 seconds.

rest mass Mass (weight) of the particle when it is not moving.

restricted mass stopping power Refinement of the total mass stopping power. Restricted mass collisional stopping power better describes the absorbed dose by accounting for energy transferred by delta rays.

retinoblastoma Primitive neuroectodermal tumor of the retina that may be inherited. It usually occurs in children younger than 4 years.

retrospective studies Study of a group of individuals all having the same disease and common characteristics that might have caused the disease.

review of systems Includes the patient's description of the signs and symptoms that lead the patient to present to the doctor, including subjective report of overall feelings of wellness.

rhabdomyosarcoma (RMS) Malignancy of skeletal muscle origin that can occur in many areas of the body and disseminates early. Soft tissue sarcoma (STS) arising from striated muscle. *See also* Soft Tissue Sarcoma (STS).

ribosome Organelle constructed in the nucleolus and concerned with protein synthesis in the cytoplasm.

right angle Three-sided polygon on which one corner measures 90 degrees.

right lymphatic duct Serves only the right arm and right side of the head and neck and drains into the right subclavian vein. This duct is about 1 to 2 cm in length.

risk management Process of avoiding or controlling the risk of financial loss to the staff members and hospital or medical center.

role fidelity Principle that reminds health care professionals that they must be faithful to their role in the health care environment.

room's eye view Image rendering technique that demonstrates the geometric relationship of the treatment machine to the patient. This view may also help prevent possible orientations of the beam that could result in collisions with the patient.

Rouvier's node Node located just inferior to the base of the skull and medial to the internal carotid artery.

sarcoma Malignancy arising from other than epithelial tissues of the body.

scan field of view Area for which projection data is collected for a CT scan is determined by the scan field of view. It helps to position the patient in the center of the CT bore so the patient's contour is not cut off laterally and is centered in the scan field of view.

scanning beams Narrow "pencil beam" of electrons is scanned by magnetic fields across the treatment area. This constantly moving pencil beam distributes the dose evenly throughout the field.

scatter air ratio (SAR) Ratio of the scattered dose at a given point to the dose in free space at the same point.

scattering Produced when an x-ray photon interacts with an outer-shell orbital electron with sufficient energy to eject it from orbit and alter its own path

scattering foil Most common method of producing an electron beam wide enough for clinical use is to use a scattering foil. Scattering foil is a thin sheet of a material that has a high Z number placed in the path of the "pencil beam" of electrons. Second scattering foil may be added to create a "dual scattering foil" arrangement. First scattering foil is used to widen the beam; the second is used to improve the flatness of the beam.

scientific notation Special use of exponents that uses base 10 notation. It is used to represent either very large or very small numbers.

scientific revival Intellectual resurgence of the sixteenth century.

scope of practice Body of courses and formally established learning experiences presenting the knowledge, principles, values, and skills that are the intended consequences of formal education; the defining document to guide radiation therapists through the day-to-day responsibilities of the profession.

screening Selecting appropriate tests and studies to check for disease.

secondary vertebral curves (compensatory vertebral curves) Vertebral curves that develop after birth as the child learns to sit up and walk. Muscular development and coordination influence the rate of secondary curvature development.

second malignant neoplasm (SMN) Cancer developing years after the treatment of an initial tumor related to genetics and previous carcinogenic chemotherapy and radiation.

segment Refers to the shape that the mechanical aperture multileaf collimator (MLC) creates during part of the total IMRT dose delivered.

seminoma Most common malignant testicular tumor.

sensitive test A 100% sensitive test will give 0% false negative for detecting tumors.

sensitivity Ability of a test to give a true, positive result.

sensitometry Measurement of the film's response to exposure and processing.

sentinal node Primary drainage lymph node of a specific anatomic area. For example, the sentinel node for the breast is most commonly located near the axilla.

separation Measurement of the thickness of a patient along the central axis or at any other specified point within the irradiated volume.

serial response tissues Tissues in organs that can be affected by the incapacitation of only one element. Spinal cord is such an organ. High-dose region of a serial-tissue dose-volume histogram (DVH) is of particular importance.

shelling Surgical procedure that removes the primary tumor and its pseudocapsule, giving it the gross appearance of having removed all viable tumor.

shielding block Field-shaping material that reduces beam transmission to less than 5% of the original intensity.

shine over Fall off of the radiation beam over a surface that misses tissue and projects in the air; also known as *fall off*.

shrinking fields Technique that reduces the treated field area one or more times during the course of treatment in response to a tumor that reduces in size and/or the need to limit doses to normal structures.

significant figures Number of figures in a measurement or calculation that are known with some degree of reliability. For example, the number 10.2 is said to have 3 significant figures. Number 10.20 is said to have 4 significant figures.

simple immobilization devices Devices that restrict movement but require a patient's voluntary cooperation.

simulated CT Extension of a conventional simulator to allow the acquisition of axial "slices." They simulate CT slices. Usually these are limited to a small number of thick slices and are adequate for localization and two-dimensional treatment planning but generate poor quality digitally reconstructed radiograph (DRR) images.

simulation Process carried out by the radiation therapist under the supervision of the radiation oncologist. It is the mockup procedure of a patient treatment with radiographic documentation of the treatment portals.

simulators Radiographic x-ray units that mimic all the movements and parameters of the treatment units. They are used for imaging the target volume during treatment planning.

simulators with a CT mode Simulators that incorporate the conventional benefits with the added benefits of cross-sectional information obtained during the simulation process.

sine One of three most common functions associated with the right triangle. Other two are the cosine and tangent. Sine of the angle is the ratio opposite the hypotenuse.

Six Sigma Process improvement method Focuses on improving the process through precision and accuracy with the elimination of defects in the process. It was originally formulated by Bill Smith for the Motorola Corporation in 1986.

skin sparing Property of megavoltage irradiation where the maximum dose occurs at some depth beneath the skin surface.

skin squames Superficial skin cells that serve as vehicles for airborne pathogens.

skip metastasis Situation that may occur where lymph nodes in a higher level may be involved while the nodes in the lower level(s) are negative for tumor.

slander Oral defamation of character.

sliding window IMRT technique describing the movement of the MLC from one side of the field to the other within a narrow opening while the beam is on.

slip ring CT x-ray tube and detector can continue to rotate around the patient without concern of cables becoming tangled because of slip rings, which are metal strips carrying electronic signals and power that is swept up by special metal brushes.

smegma White secretion located under the prepuce of the foreskin in the adult male. It is carcinogenic in animals.

SOAP note Initial presentation and plan for assessment and treatment described in the history and physical (H&P) may be referred to as a "SOAP note." The acronym, SOAP, is described as follows: Subjective findings as reported by the patient; Objective or observations of the clinician, including vital signs and physical examination; Assessment of the disease or condition; and Plan for further examination and/or treatment. This information becomes part of the patient's medical record.

soft tissue sarcoma (STS) Malignant tumor arising primarily, but not exclusively, from mesenchymal connective tissues. *See also* Liposarcoma, Leiomyosarcoma, Rhabdomyosarcoma (RMS), and Fibrosarcoma, which are all types of sarcomas.

schwannoma Nonencapsulated tumor resulting from disorderly proliferation of Schwann cells that includes portions of nerve fibers; typically undergoes formation to malignant schwannomas

segmental MLC (SMLC) Refers to an IMRT technique describing the sequence of leaves moving for repositioning, then coming to rest while the beam is delivered in multiple segments at each gantry angle.

source-axis distance (SAD) Distance from the source of radiation to the axis of rotation of the treatment unit.

source head Housing for shielding that contains the device for positioning the cobalt-60 source.

source-skin distance (SSD) Distance from the source of radiation to the patient's skin.

spatial resolution Refers to the clarity or the measure of detail in a CT image.

specific activity Activity per unit mass of a radioactive material (Ci/g). Specific activity dictates the total activity that a small source can have.

specific test Test for detecting tumors, a 99% specific test gives 1% false positive results

specificity Ability of the test to obtain a true-negative result.

spiral CT Also referred to as *helical CT.* Patient is positioned at a fixed point, and, while the x-ray tube is rotating, the patient moves into the aperture to create a scan pattern that resembles a "slinky" or coiled spring.

squamous cell carcinoma As it relates to skin cancer, it is a faster growing cancer than the basal cell type with a higher propensity for metastasis, arises from the more mature keratinocytes of the upper layers of the epidermis. This type of nonmelanoma skin cancer can arise anywhere on the body but is especially common on sun-exposed areas such as the head, neck, face, arms, and hands.

staging Cancer is "staged" after a histologic diagnosis is made. Staging helps determine the anatomic extent of the disease. Treatment decisions are based on the histologic diagnosis and extent of the disease.

staging laparotomy Surgical procedure that includes a splenectomy, lymph node biopsy, and bone marrow biopsy; used in staging lymphomas

stand Drive stand appears as a large, rectangular cabinet, at least as large as the gantry. As its name indicates, the drive stand is a stand containing the apparatus that drives the linear accelerator.

standard precautions Precautions that should be followed because of potential contact with body fluids. These precautions include wearing gloves, a mask, and protective eyewear; properly handling needles; and disposing of used equipment into containers for biohazardous material.

step and shoot *See* segmental MLC (SMLC).

stereoscopic images Two images from different angles focused on the same point.

stereotactic radiosurgery Use of a high-energy photon beam with multiple ports of entry convergent on the target volume.

stomatitis Inflammation of the mouth.

stratified Segregate populations according to certain specific characteristics.

striae Lines or bands elevated above or depressed below surrounding tissue.

stridor Harsh, rasping breath.

subcutaneous Tissue just below the skin.

subcutaneous injection A 45- or 90-degree injection into the subcutaneous tissue just below the skin.

subcutaneous layer Layer of areolar connective tissue and adipose tissue that lies beneath the dermis that contains nerves and blood vessels.

superficial therapy Treatment with x-rays produced at potentials ranging from 50 to 150 kV.

superior vena cava syndrome Edema of the face, neck, or upper arms resulting from increased venous pressures caused by compression of the superior vena cava. It is most commonly caused by a metastatic, mediastinal lymph node tumor in lung cancer.

suprasternal notch (SSN) Depression in the manubrium, which occurs at the level of T2 and articulates with the medial ends of the clavicles.

Surveillance, Epidemiology, and End Results (SEER) program Program initiated in 1973 to collect data in an effort to determine the epidemiology and etiology of cancer.

symmetry Maximum point-to-point difference in the central 80% of the profile.

synergistic Body organ, medicine, or substance that cooperates with another or others to produce a total effect greater than the sum of the individual elements.

systemic error Variation in the translation of the treatment setup from the simulator to the treatment unit.

systemic treatment Cancer management treatment that encompasses the patient's entire system, generally through venous means. Chemotherapy affects not only cancerous cells but others also because of the systemic nature of its delivery.

tabletop Part of the patient support assembly (PSA) on which a patient is positioned during treatment or simulation; may be called a *treatment couch* or *patient tabletop*.

tandem Long narrow tube that inserts into the opening of the cervix (cervical os) into the uterus. They can hold radioactive sources and are used in the treatment of gynecologic tumors.

tangent Tangent of the angle is equal to the length of the opposite side divided by the length of the adjacent side.

target volume Area of a known and presumed tumor.

TD$_{5/5}$ Dose of radiation that is expected to produce a 5% complication rate within 5 years.

TD$_{50/5}$ Dose of radiation that is expected to produce a 50% complication rate within 5 years.

telangiectasia Dilation of the surface blood vessels caused by the loss of capillary tone, resulting in a fine spider-vein appearance on the skin surface.

teleology Also called *consequentialism*, an ethical theory where the consequences of an act or action should be the major focus when deciding how to solve an ethical problem.

teletherapy Treatment at a distance.

tenesmus Ineffective and painful straining during a bowel movement.

tennis racket May be a square or rectangular section of the tabletop, similar to a tennis or racquetball racquet woven tightly together.

tensile strength Resistance in lengthwise stress, measured in weight per unit area.

The Joint Commission (TJC) An independent, not-for-profit organization dedicated to improving quality of care in organized health care settings. It is the accrediting body for health care organizations.

therapeutic relationship Genuine collaborative effort between the patient and health care provider. This requires good reflective listening skills and paying careful attention to all the cues. In addition, these cues need to be interpreted in the context of the patient's values, beliefs, and culture to be truly meaningful and helpful in treating and respecting the uniqueness of each cancer patient.

thermionic emission In an oversimplification, x-rays are produced when a stream of electrons liberated from the cathode is directed across the tube vacuum at extremely high speeds to interact with the anode. These cathode electrons are freed from the tungsten filament atoms in a process called *thermionic emission*.

thermoluminescent dosimeter (TLD) Device for measuring dose. It uses the phenomenon that some solid materials, when irradiated, will subsequently give off light when heated. Amount of light emitted is proportional to the dose delivered to the crystal.

thoracic duct Located on the left side of the body, the thoracic duct is typically larger than the right lymphatic duct. It serves the lower extremities, abdomen, left arm, and left side of the head and neck and drains into the left subclavian vein. This duct is about 35 to 45 cm in length and begins in front of the second lumbar vertebra (L2) called the *cisterna chyli*.

three-dimensional (3D) conformal radiation therapy (3DCRT) Three-dimensional image visualization and treatment-planning tools are used to conform isodose distributions to only target volumes while excluding normal tissues as much as possible.

three-point setup Three marks placed on a patient to define the isocenter. It is used to position and level the patient daily to ensure reproducibility and consistency of the setup and treatment.

thrombocytopenia Abnormal decrease in the number of platelets.

tissue absorption factor Beam of radiation gives up energy as it travels through the body. The more tissue the beam traverses, the more it is attenuated. There are a number of different methods for measuring the attenuation of the beam as it travels through tissue; these are percentage depth dose, tissue-air ratio, tissue-phantom ratio, and tissue-maximum ratio. First method used was percentage depth dose.

tissue-air ratio Ratio of the absorbed dose at a given depth in phantom to the absorbed dose at the same point in free space.

tissue-maximum ratio Ratio of the absorbed dose at a given depth in phantom to the absorbed dose at the same point at the level of D_{max} in phantom.

tissue-phantom ratio Ratio of the absorbed dose at a given depth in phantom to the absorbed dose at the same point at a reference depth in phantom. If the reference depth is chosen to be the depth of D_{max}, then the tissue-phantom ratio is called the *tissue-maximum ratio*.

titers Measurement of the number of specific antibodies in a person's body or blood specimen.

tolerance Body's adaptation to a particular drug and requirement of ever greater doses to achieve the desired effect.

topical brachytherapy Radioactive sources are placed on top of the area to be treated. Molds of the body part to be treated may be taken and prepared to place the sources in definite arrangements to deliver the prescribed dose.

tort law Type of law that governs rights between individuals in noncriminal actions. This law deals with violations of civil as opposed to criminal law.

total nodal irradiation System of radiating all the major lymph nodes.

total quality management (TQM) Professional performance standards that define activities in the areas of education, interpersonal relationships, personal and professional self-assessment, and ethical behavior.

transcription Process resulting in the transfer of genetic information from a molecule of DNA to a molecule of RNA.

transfer Understanding of a subject matter to a depth that allows transfer of knowledge from one event to deal with another event. Ability to use knowledge in more than one setting. Use of preexisting knowledge to problem solve.

translation Process resulting in the construction of a polypeptide in accordance with genetic information contained in a molecule of RNA.

transmission factor Any device placed in the path of the radiation beam will attenuate the beam.

transmission filters Filters that allow the transmission of a predetermined percentage of the treatment beam.

transpectoral lymphatic pathway Lymphatic pathway that passes through the pectoralis major muscle and provides efferent drainage to the supraclavicular and infraclavicular fossa nodes.

transurethral resection (TURP) Surgical procedure of the prostate performed through the urethra.

travel time Length of time for a cobalt-60 source to advance and retract.

treatment console Operating center where timers and system-monitoring indicators are displayed.

treatment couch Part of the linear accelerator, the treatment couch is the area on which patients are positioned to receive their radiation treatment.

treatment field (portal) Volume exposed to radiation from a single radiation beam.

treatment number Number of treatments delivered.

treatment planning Process by which dose delivery is optimized for a given patient and clinical situation.

treatment record Documents the delivery of treatments, recording fractional and cumulative doses, machine settings, verification imaging; and the ordering and implementation of prescribed changes.

treatment technique Defined method by which a treatment is delivered to the patient.

treatment time Amount of time required to deliver a prescribed dose of radiation, taking all pertinent treatment factors such as field size, energy, depth, and so forth into account. Treatment time is used in treatment with cobalt-60.

treatment verification Process using diagnostic-quality radiographs of each treatment field from the initial simulation procedure to determine the accuracy of the treatment plan.

treatment volume Generally larger than the target volume, the treatment volume encompasses the additional margins around the target volume to allow for limitations of the treatment technique.

triangulation Treatment isocenter is located relative to three setup coordinates on the patient's surface or on the equipment fixed relative to their anatomy.

trigone Portion of the bladder (shaped like a triangle) formed by the openings of the two ureters and orifice of the urethra.

tuberculin skin test (Mantoux test) Intradermal injection of purified protein derivative (PPD) or tuberculin used to test for exposure to tuberculosis.

tumor localization May involve the use of a simulator in determining the extent of the tumor and location of critical structures.

tumor registry Tracking mechanism for cancer incidence, characteristics, management, and results in cancer-treatment facilities for patients diagnosed with cancer.

tumor staging Means of defining the tumor size and extension at the time of diagnosis. Tumor staging provides a means of communication about tumors, helps in determining the best treatment, aids in predicting prognosis, and provides a means for continuing research.

tumorcidal dose Dose high enough to eradicate the tumor.

tumor-suppressor gene Gene whose presence and proper function produces normal cellular growth and division. Absence or inactivation of such a gene leads to uncontrolled growth or neoplasia.

ulceration Rare, late radiation reaction exhibited by an open sore on the skin or mucous membrane. It is caused by the shedding of dead tissue.

ultrasound Imaging that involves high frequency sound waves sent into the body. Echo waves as the sound bounces back from various tissue interfaces is recorded.

universal precautions Method of infection control in which any human blood or body fluid is treated as if it were known to be infectious.

urticaria Hives.

use factor (U) Fraction of time that the radiation beam is directed at a barrier; the use factor for scatter and leakage radiation is always.

user interface (UI) Part of the electronic medical record that refers to the graphical, textual and auditory information the program presents to the user, and the input methods the user employs to control the program.

Vac-Lok Trade name for an immobilization device that consists of a cushion and a vacuum compression pump.

vacuole Membrane-bound cavity in the cytoplasm of a cell having a variety of storage, secretory, and metabolic functions.

vacuum-formed shell Immobilization device that is formed when a piece of plastic is molded over a plaster cast of a patient's anatomy.

vaginal cancer Malignancy that arises in the vagina and does not extend to the vulva or cervix. Vaginal cancer is a rare disease that accounts for approximately 2% of all gynecologic cancers.

vaginal colpostats Paired brachytherapy devices that allow insertion into the lateral vaginal fornices or apex of the vagina for intracavitary treatment. These are usually shielded anteriorly and posteriorly for greater lateral throw of the dose and often look like small golf clubs.

vaginal cuff Small rim of vaginal tissue at the apex of the vagina around the cervix. Some of this is removed during a hysterectomy,

and some remains as the new apex of the vagina with surgical scarring.

vaginal cylinder implant Domed-ended tubular brachytherapy device used to give even dose distribution to the apex or entire vaginal surface. This resembles a candle with a central hollow canal for later afterloading.

Van de Graaff generator Electrostatic accelerator designed to accelerate charged particles. In radiation therapy procedures the unit produces high-energy x-rays typically at 2 MeV.

vector Animal, usually an arthropod, that carries and transmits a pathogen capable of causing disease.

venipuncture Puncture of a vein.

ventricles Cavities that form a communication network with each other, the center canal of the spinal cord, and the subarachnoid space. They are filled with cerebrospinal fluid (CSF).

veracity Truthfulness within the realm of health care practice.

verification Final check that each of the planned treatment beams does cover the tumor or target volume and does not irradiate normal tissue structures.

verification simulation Final check that each of the planned treatment beams covers the tumor or target volume and does not irradiate normal tissue structures.

virtual simulation Target is defined first, and then the fields are shaped to conform to the target during three-dimensional CRT treatment planning. Patient need not be present to perform simulation or treatment planning.

virtue ethics Use of practical wisdom for emotional and intellectual problem solving.

virulence Relative power of a pathogen to cause disease. Severity expressed in terms of morbidity and mortality.

vital signs Information, such as blood pressure, pulse, and respiration, that may be gathered along with a chief complaint at the patient's initial encounter with a nurse or other clinical specialist.

voxel Volume elements.

vulva Female external genitalia composed of the mons veneris, labia majora, labia minora, vestibule of the vagina, and vestibular glands.

vulvar cancer Cancer of the outermost portion of the gynecologic tract. Vulvar cancer patients usually have a subcutaneous lump or mass. Patients with more advanced disease have an ulcerative exophytic mass.

Waldeyer's ring Ring of tonsillar tissue that encircles the nasopharynx and oropharynx: two palatine tonsils, lingual, and pharyngeal tonsils.

WAN *See* Wide Area Network (WAN).

warm thyroid nodule Nodule having a slightly higher concentration than the rest of the thyroid gland.

waveguide Hollow, tube-like structure within the linear accelerator that is used to accelerate injected electrons to near the speed of

light prior to striking a target to produce photons.

wavelength of the wave Physical distance between peaks of the wave.

wave particle duality Photons exhibit the characteristics of a particle at times and the characteristics of a wave at other times.

wedge Beam modifier that changes. Angle is defined relative to the horizontal plane at depth.

wedge angle Angle between the slanted isodose line and a line perpendicular to the central axis of the beam.

wedge filter Tool that modifies the isodose distribution of a beam to correct for oblique incidence or tissue inhomogeneities by progressively decreasing beam intensity across the field irradiated.

wide area network (WAN) For large geographic areas or when multiple LANs (local area networks) are to be connected, a WAN may be employed. WANs use a variety of communication services currently including telephone dial-up, T-1 or T-3 lines, or even the Internet to communicate over long or short distances.

wide resection Surgical procedure for soft tissue carcinoma. Procedure involves a wide en bloc excision for limb salvage and/or wide through-bone amputation.

Wilms' tumor Childhood embryonal kidney cancer.

window level Represents the central Hounsfield unit of all the CT numbers within the window width.

window width Range of numbers displayed or the contrast on a CT image.

windowing Technique allows the radiation therapist to change the appearance of the image after it has been acquired by the CT scanner. Two characteristics of the window are window level and window width.

wipe test Test done to evaluate the contamination or leakage of a sealed radioactive source.

workload (W) For superficial and orthovoltage units, the milliamperage (mA) used and beam on time per week; for high energy units, the Gy (rad) per week at isocenter.

xeroderma pigmentosum Rare disease of the skin starting in childhood and marked by disseminated pigment discolorations, ulcers, cutaneous and muscular atrophy, and death.

x-ray Electromagnetic radiation that is produced when a fast electron stream hits a target. Synergy of the resultant x-ray beam increases with the voltage that accelerates the electrons.

x-ray generator Generator that provides radiographic and fluoroscopic control of the simulator through the selection of various exposure factors, which include focal spot, mAs, kVp, and time.

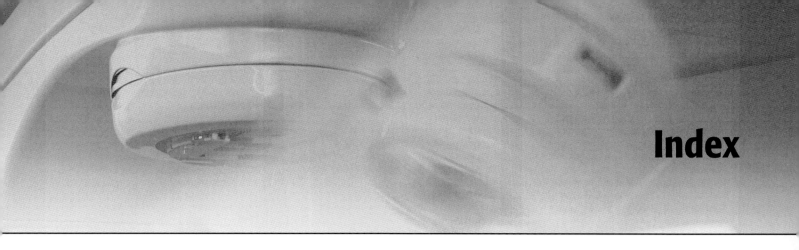

Index

Page numbers followed by *f* indicate figures; *t,* tables; *b,* boxes.